P9-DCR-467

**PDR NURSE'S HANDBOOK**

1 9 9 9   E D I T I O N

# PDR®

*Nurse's*
*Handbook*™

ISBN 0-7668-0913-7

90000

9 780766 809130

Announcing...

# www.nursespdr.com

With this book, you also get access to Live Internet Updates through our
World Wide Web site, **www.nursespdr.com**

Among the valuable features of the site:

► Searchable database of all drugs
► Monthly drug updates
► Daily pharmaceutical news headlines
► Additional drug listings not found in book
► Links to over 200 related sites

**www.nursespdr.com** represents our ongoing commitment to offering the most
dynamic and exciting products possible.

To register or visit, just point your browser to:

# http:// www.nursespdr.com

## PDR NURSE'S HANDBOOK

# 1999 EDITION

# PDR®

## *Nurse's Handbook*™

**THE INFORMATION STANDARD
FOR PRESCRIPTION DRUGS
AND NURSING CONSIDERATIONS**

**PUBLISHING STAFF**

*Vice President of Directory Services:* Stephen B. Greenberg
*Director of Product Management:* David P. Reiss
*Product Manager:* Mark A. Friedman
*Associate Product Manager:* Bill Shaughnessy
*Director, Professional Support Services:* Mukesh Mehta, RPh
*Senior Drug Information Specialist:* Thomas Fleming, RPh
*Drug Information Specialist:* Maria Deutsch, MS, RPh, CDE
*Manager of Production, Annuals:* Kimberly Hiller-Vivas
*Art Director:* Richard A. Weinstock
*Senior Digital Imaging Coordinator:* Shawn W. Cahill
*Digital Imaging Coordinator:* Frank J. McElroy, III

**DEVELOPMENT STAFF**

*Publisher:* William Brottmiller
*Developmental Editor:* Marjorie A. Bruce
*Production Coordinator:* Barbara A. Bullock
*Art and Design Coordinator:* Timothy J. Conners
*Technology Project Manager:* Lisa Santy
*On-Line Program Director:* Cliff Butler, PhD
*Editorial Assistant:* Diane Biondi

ISBN: 0-7668-0913-7

Manufactured in the United States of America

10 9 8 7 6 5 4 3 2

This book may be purchased in bulk at discounted rates for sales promotions, training or premiums by calling 800-347-7707 x4.

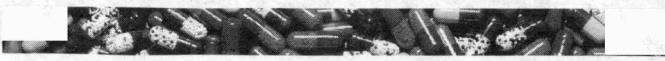

# Notice to the Reader

The monographs in this edition of the *PDR® Nurse's Handbook*™ are the work of two distinguished authors: George R. Spratto, PhD, Dean of the School of Pharmacy at West Virginia University, Morgantown, West Virginia, and Adrienne L. Woods, MSN, CRNP, FNP-C, Family Nurse Practitioner, Primary Care, at the Department of Veterans Affairs Medical and Regional Office Center, Wilmington, Delaware.

The publisher and the authors do not warrant or guarantee any of the products described herein or perform any independent analysis in connection with any of the product information contained herein. The publisher and the authors do not assume and expressly disclaim any obligation to obtain and include information other than that provided by the manufacturer.

The reader is expressly warned to consider and adopt all safety precautions that might be indicated by the activities described herein and to avoid all potential hazards. By following the instructions contained herein, the reader willingly assumes all risks in connection with such instructions.

The publisher and the authors make no representations or warranties of any kind, including but not limited to the warranties of fitness for a particular purpose or merchantability nor are any such representations implied with respect to the material set forth herein, and the publisher and the authors take no responsibility with respect to such material. The publisher and the authors shall not be liable for any special, consequential, or exemplary damages resulting, in whole or in part, from the reader's use of, or reliance upon, this material.

The authors and publisher have made a conscientious effort to ensure that the drug information and recommended dosages in this book are accurate and in accord with accepted standards at the time of publication. However, pharmacology and therapeutics are rapidly changing sciences, so readers are advised, before administering any drug, to check the package insert provided by the manufacturer for the recommended dose, for any contraindications for administration, and for any added warnings and precautions. This recommendation is especially important for new, infrequently used, or highly toxic drugs.

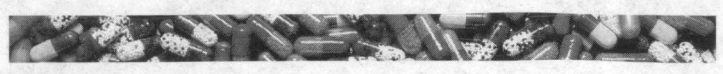

# Acknowledgments

We would like to extend our thanks to the Delmar team who work so diligently to ensure that the manuscript process flows smoothly and to try to keep us on track. Team members include Lisa Santy, Barbara Bullock, and Tim Conners. The other member of the team—Marge Bruce—deserves a special note of thanks and appreciation; her hard work and dedication to the project, as well as her understanding of the difficulty in meeting deadlines, is an inspiration for us to keep working. Thanks are also expressed to Bea Ruberto and to Datapage Technologies for their work in continuing to establish our database.

George Spratto extends appreciation to his colleagues at West Virginia University. Special thanks are extended to Marie Abate, Pharm.D. and Arthur Jacknowitz, Pharm.D. of the Drug Information Center, School of Pharmacy, West Virginia University, who assisted in researching information on new drugs. Greatest appreciation and love go to my wife, Lynne, sons, Chris and Gregg, and daughter-in-law Kim who continue to be supportive and maintain a high level of excitement for the project.

Adrienne Woods would like to extend her appreciation to Sally Marshall, MSN, CETN for her help on the wounds and dressings appendix. Also, to my husband, Howard, the best father, and friend, I have ever known, for his patience, love and understanding. To my children, Katy and Nate, for enduring hectic schedules, early mornings, and a few missed soccer and baseball games. Finally, to Peanut butter for his endless hours of companionship and contented purring as he lounged on the fax machine.

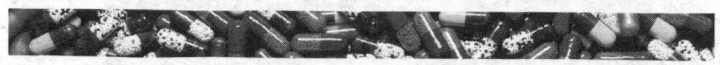

# Preface

Lately, major new drugs seem to be appearing at an ever faster pace, making the need for a truly up-to-date clinical reference guide an increasingly important concern for every nurse. To meet this challenge, we're proud to present the thoroughly revised and updated *PDR® Nurse's Handbook™* for 1999.

The first thing you'll notice about this brand new edition is a complete change in the way it's organized. To better fulfill your needs for quick, easy access to information on specific drugs, all entries in the handbook are now arranged alphabetically by generic name. In addition, you'll find a host of other handy features to aid you in finding the precise facts you need:

- Dosage forms and routes are clearly delineated and correlated, when appropriate, with the target disease state.
- Boldface italics highlight life-threatening side effects.
- For fast emergency reference, symptoms and treatment of overdose are summarized in the "Overdose Management" section of a drug.
- Nursing considerations are presented in nursing process format, with assessment, intervention, teaching, and evaluation guidelines all clearly labeled. Specific criteria for evaluating the outcomes of drug therapy are easily found in the "Outcome/Evaluate" section.
- Instant Internet updates are now available at the handbook's new website, **www.nursespdr.com.**

While the *PDR® Nurse's Handbook™* is specifically designed to serve as the core of every nurse's personal reference library, it's far from the only practice aid available from PDR. For instance, the new *PDR® Atlas of Anatomy™* now offers you a detailed exploration of the human body based on award-winning "peel-away" illustrations from A.D.A.M. Software. In addition, the new *PDR Companion Guide™* provides you with a unique, 1,800-page database of drug reactions and interactions, indications and off-label uses, contraindications, and U.S. equivalents of over 15,000 foreign medications.

Altogether, *PDR*'s continually expanding library of medical reference works now boasts a total of 10 titles. The complete list includes:

- *Physicians' Desk Reference®*
- *PDR For Nonprescription Drugs®*
- *PDR For Ophthalmology®*
- *PDR Companion Guide™*
- *PDR® Generics™*
- *PDR® Medical Dictionary™*
- *PDR® Nurse's Handbook™*
- *PDR® Nurse's Dictionary™*
- *PDR® Atlas of Anatomy™*
- *PDR Supplements*

*PDR*'s comprehensive drug information databases are available in a variety of electronic formats as well. For instance, the *PDR® Nurse's Handbook* is now available on a fast, easy-to-use CD-ROM. Equipped with powerful search tools, the new *PDR® Nurse's Handbook™ CD-ROM 1999 Edition* enables you to quickly zero in on the precise facts you need, instantly view full-color pictures of the products, even hear the correct pronunciation of each drug's name. Custom printing capabilities allow you to print patient handouts personalized with the individual's name. The Windows-ready disc runs on virtually all IBM-compatible PCs.

For busy nurses on the go, there's also *Pocket PDR®*, a unique handheld electronic database of drug information that literally fits in your pocket. The latest edition of this incredible device boasts a larger screen, easy-to-change batteries, a protective plastic lid, and key facts on dosage, administration, precautions, warnings, side effects, and contraindications for every fully described prescription drug in *PDR* and *PDR For Ophthalmology*.

*PDR* and its major companion volumes are also found in the *PDR® Electronic Library™* on CD-ROM, now used in over 40,000 medical practices. This Windows-compatible disc provides users with a complete database of *PDR* prescribing information, electronically searchable for instant retrieval. A standard subscription includes *PDR*'s sophisticated prescription-screening program and an extensive file of chemical structures, illustrations, and full-color product photographs. Optional enhancements include the complete contents of *The Merck Manual* and *Stedman's Medical Dictionary,* as well as a comprehensive database of billing codes. The disc is available for use on individual PCs and PC networks. For more information on this or any other members of the growing family of *PDR* professional references, please call, toll-free, 1-800-232-7379 or fax 201-573-4956.

For patient teaching purposes, you should also keep *PDR*'s library of consumer handbooks in mind. Available titles include:
- *The PDR® Family Guide to Prescription Drugs®*
- *The PDR® Pocket Guide to Prescription Drugs™*
- *The PDR® Family Guide to Over-The-Counter Drugs™*
- *The PDR® Family Guide Encyclopedia of Medical Care™*

In 1999, also be on the lookout for a major new *PDR* Family Guide to natural medicines and alternative therapies, boasting the most comprehensive encyclopedia of herbal remedies yet to be offered the public. This and other *PDR* Family Guides are presented in easy-to-read, plain-English style. They are available—in affordable soft-cover format—almost everywhere books are sold.

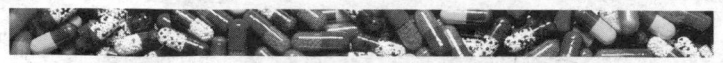

# USING THE HANDBOOK

An understanding of the format of *PDR® Nurse's Handbook*™ will help you reference information quickly.

- There are three chapters:
  1. Detailed information on "How to Use PDR-99"
  2. Alphabetical listing of therapeutic/chemical drug classes with general information for the class, plus a listing of drugs in the class covered in Chapter 3
  3. Alphabetical listing of drugs by generic name

The individual entries follow a similar format. All items listed below may not appear in each drug entry but are represented where appropriate and when information is available.

**General drug information** (similar in format to Chapter 2) includes the following categories:

— COMBINATION DRUG HEADING indicates when two or more drugs are combined in the same product

— GENERIC NAME OF DRUG

— PHONETIC PRONUNCIATION of generic name

— FDA PREGNANCY CATEGORY to which drug is assigned; see Appendix 3 for the definition of these categories

— TRADE NAME(S) by which the drug is marketed; a maple leaf (✤) indicates that the trade name is available only in Canada

— DRUG SCHEDULE If the drug is controlled by the U. S. Controlled Substances Act, the appropriate schedule is listed. See Appendix 1 for the definition of the five schedules as well as a listing of drugs with their schedules in both the United States and Canada

— Rx = prescription drug; OTC = nonprescription, over-the-counter drug

— See also reference to classification in Chapter 2, if applicable

— **Classification** is the chemical or pharmacologic class to which the drug has been assigned

— CONTENT (for combination drugs) is the generic name and amount of each drug in the combination product

— ACTION/KINETICS The action portion describes the mechanism(s) by which a drug achieves its therapeutic effect; not all mechanisms of action are known. The kinetics portion provides information about the rate of drug absorption, distribution, minimum effective serum or plasma level, biologic half-life, duration of action, metabolism and excretion.

The time it takes for half the drug to be excreted or removed from the blood, t½, is important in determining how often a drug is to be administered and how long to assess for side effects. Therapeutic serum or plasma levels indicate the desired concentration, in serum or plasma, for the drug to exert its beneficial effect and is helpful in predicting the possible onset of side effects, as well as achievement of the desired drug effects.

— USES are the approved therapeutic applications for the drug. Investigational uses, when available, are also listed for selected drugs.

——CONTRAINDICATIONS notes disease states or conditions for which the drug should not be used. The safe use of many of the newer pharmacologic agents during pregnancy, lactation, or childhood has not been established and therefore should generally not be used.

— SPECIAL CONCERNS cover considerations for use with pediatric, geriatric, pregnant, or lactating clients. Situations and disease states when the drug should be used with caution are also listed.

— SIDE EFFECTS include potential drug-related undesired or bothersome effects, organized by body system or organ affected. Nearly all potential side effects are listed. In any given clinical situation, a client may show no side effects, one or two side effects, or several side effects. Life-threatening side effects are identified by bold italic print.

— OVERDOSE MANAGEMENT lists the symptoms of drug overdose. The treatment portion of this category gives approaches and/or antidotes to treat the symptoms of the drug overdose. Designated by a special icon **OD**.

— DRUG INTERACTIONS lists the results of drugs interacting with one another, usually an increase or decrease in the effect. Drug interactions may result from a number of different mechanisms (e.g., additive or inhibitory effects, interference with degradation of drug, increased rate of elimination, decreased absorption from the GI tract, receptor site competition or displacement from plasma protein binding sites, and potential lethal/adverse drug interactions.).

Any side effects that accompany the administration of a specific drug may be increased as a result of a drug interaction.

Drug interactions are often listed for classes of drugs. Therefore drug interactions are likely to occur for all drugs in the class.

— LABORATORY TEST INTERFERENCES indicates the effect of the drug on laboratory test values for the client. Some of the interferences are caused by the therapeutic or toxic effects of the drugs; others result from interference with the testing method itself. Interferences are described as false positive (+), or increased ($\uparrow$), values and as false negative (-), or decreased ($\downarrow$), values. Many of the laboratory test interferences are addressed under *Nursing Considerations*.

— DOSAGE provides adult and pediatric doses as well as the dosage forms in which the drug is available. The dosage form or route of administration is clearly shown and is often followed by the disease state (in italics) for which the particular dosage is recommended. The listed dosage is to be considered as a general prescribing guideline; the exact amount of the drug to be given is determined by the provider. However, one should always question orders or prescriptions when dosages and routes of administration differ markedly from the accepted norm.

**Nursing Considerations** are guidelines to help the practitioner in applying the nursing process to pharmacotherapeutics to ensure safe practice.

- Administration/Storage: Guidelines to the practitioner in preparing medications for administration, administering the medication, and proper storage and disposal of the medication; specific IV Route delineated by a special icon **IV** .

- Assessment: Guidelines to assist the practitioner in what to obtain, identify, and assess before, during, and after drug therapy.

- Interventions: Guidelines for specific nursing actions related to the drug being administered.

- Client/Family Teaching: Guidelines to promote education, active participation, understanding, precautions, and compliance with drug therapy with desired outcome.

- Outcome/Evaluate: Identifies desired outcomes of drug therapy and client response.

— ADDITIONAL CONTRAINDICATIONS, ADDITIONAL SIDE EFFECTS, or ADDITIONAL NURSING CONSIDERATIONS provide information relevant to a specific drug but not necessarily to the class overall and serves to reinforce certain areas of importance. (Also refer to Chapter 2.)

— INDEX is extensively cross-referenced (multiple trade names and the generic name for each drug are paired); information is coded as follows:

- **boldface** = generic drug name

- *italics* = therapeutic drug class

- regular type = trade name

- CAPITALS = combination drugs

**VISUAL IDENTIFICATION GUIDE**

Products shown in this color insert are organized alphabetically by generic name. Included are more than 200 photographs of tablets, capsules, and other solid dosage forms, covering leading brands and the most frequently dispensed doses from generic manufacturers. All items are reproduced in actual size and in color. For products with distinguishing features on both sides, the front view is supplemented with a picture of the back. Each product is labeled with its brand name (unless it is labeled as generic) and the name of the supplier.

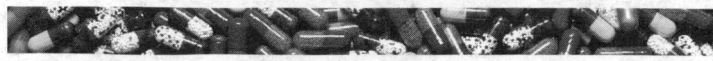

# Table of Contents

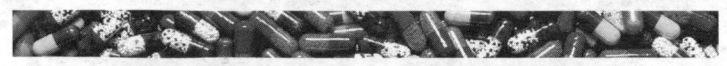

# Common Sound-Alike Drug Names

The following is a list of common sound-alike drug names; trade names are capitalized. In parentheses next to each drug name is the pharmacological classification/use for the drug.

Accupril (ACE inhibitor)

Accutane (antiacne drug)

acetazolamide (antiglaucoma drug)

acetohexamide (oral antidiabetic drug)

Adriamycin (antineoplastic)

Aredia (bone growth regulator)

albuterol (sympathomimetic)

atenolol (beta-blocker)

Aldomet (antihypertensive)

Aldoril (antihypertensive)

allopurinol (antigout drug)

Apresoline (antihypertensive)

alprazolam (anti-anxiety agent)

lorazepam (anti-anxiety agent)

Ambien (sedative-hypnotic)

Amen (progestin)

amiloride (diuretic)

amlodipine (calcium channel blocker)

amiodarone (antiarrhythmic)

amrinone (inotropic agent)

amitriptyline (antidepressant)

nortriptyline (antidepressant)

Apresazide (antihypertensive)

Apresoline (antihypertensive)

Arlidin (peripheral vasodilator)

Aralen (antimalarial)

Artane (cholinergic blocking agent)

Altace (ACE inhibitor)

asparaginase (antineoplastic agent)

pegaspargase (antineoplastic agent)

Atarax (antianxiety agent)

Ativan (antianxiety agent)

atenolol (beta-blocker)

timolol (beta-blocker)

Atrovent (cholinergic blocking agent)

Alupent (sympathomimetic)

bacitracin (antibacterial)

Bactroban (anti-infective, topical)

Benylin (expectorant)

Ventolin (sympathomimetic)

Brevital (barbiturate)

Brevibloc (beta-adrenergic blocker)

Bumex (diuretic)

Buprenex (narcotic analgesic)

Cafergot (analgesic)

Carafate (antiulcer drug)

calciferol (Vitamin D)

calcitriol (Vitamin D)

carboplatin (antineoplastic agent)

cisplatin (antineoplastic agent)

Cardene (calcium channel blocker)

Cardizem (calcium channel blocker)

Cataflam (NSAID)

Catapres (antihypertensive)

Catapres (antihypertensive)

Combipres (antihypertensive)

cefotaxime (cephalosporin)

cefoxitin (cephalosporin)

cefuroxime (cephalosporin)

deferoxamine (iron chelator)

chlorpromazine (antipsychotic)

chlorpropamide (oral antidiabetic)

chlorpromazine (antipsychotic)

prochlorperazine (antipsychotic)

chlorpromazine (antipsychotic)

promethazine (antihistamine)

Clinoril (NSAID) — Clozaril (antipsychotic)

clomipramine (antidepressant) — clomiphene (ovarian stimulant)

clonidine (antihypertensive) — Klonopin (anticonvulsant)

Cozaar (antihypertensive) — Zocor (antihyperlipidemic)

cyclobenzaprine (skeletal muscle relaxant) — cyproheptadine (antihistamine)

cyclophosphamide (antineoplastic) — cyclosporine (immunosuppressant)

cyclosporine (immunosuppressant) — cycloserine (antineoplastic)

Cytovene (antiviral drug) — Cytosar (antineoplastic)

Cytoxan (antineoplastic) — Cytotec (prostaglandin derivative)

Cytoxan (antineoplastic) — Cytosar (antineoplastic)

Dantrium (skeletal muscle relaxant) — danazol (gonadotropin inhibitor)

Darvocet-N (analgesic) — Darvon-N (analgesic)

daunorubicin (antineoplastic) — doxorubicin (antineoplastic)

desipramine (antidepressant) — diphenhydramine (antihistamine)

DiaBeta (oral hypoglycemic) — Zebeta (beta-adrenergic blocker)

digitoxin (cardiac glycoside) — digoxin (cardiac glycoside)

diphenhydramine (antihistamine) — dimenhydrinate (antihistamine)

dopamine (sympathomimetic) — dobutamine (sympathomimetic)

Edecrin (diuretic) — Eulexin (antineoplastic)

enalapril (ACE inhibitor) — Anafranil (antidepressant)

enalapril (ACE inhibitor) — Eldepryl (antiparkinson agent)

Eryc (erythromycin base) — Ery-Tab (erythromycin base)

etidronate (bone growth regulator) — etretinate (antipsoriatic)

etomidate (general anesthetic) — etidronate (bone growth regulator)

Fioricet (analgesic) — Fiorinal (analgesic)

flurbiprofen (NSAID) — fenoprofen (NSAID)

folinic acid (leucovorin calcium) — folic acid (vitamin B complex)

Gantrisin (sulfonamide) — Gantanol (sulfonamide)

glipizide (oral hypoglycemic) — glyburide (oral hypoglycemic)

glyburide (oral hypoglycemic) — Glucotrol (oral hypoglycemic)

Hycodan (cough preparation) — Hycomine (cough preparation)

hydralazine (antihypertensive) — hydroxyzine (antianxiety agent)

hydrocodone (narcotic analgesic) — hydrocortisone (corticosteroid)

hydromorphone (narcotic analgesic) — morphine (narcotic analgesic)

Hydropres (antihypertensive) — Diupres (antihypertensive)

Hytone (topical corticosteroid) — Vytone (topical corticosteroid)

imipramine (antidepressant) — Norpramin (antidepressant)

Inderal (beta-adrenergic blocker) — Inderide (antihypertensive)

Inderal (beta-adrenergic blocker) — Isordil (coronary vasodilator)

Indocin (NSAID) — Minocin (antibiotic)

Lanoxin (cardiac glycoside) — Lasix (diuretic)

Lioresal (muscle relaxant) — lisinopril (ACE inhibitor)

Lithostat (lithium carbonate) — Lithobid (lithium carbonate)

Lithotabs (lithium carbonate) — Lithobid (lithium carbonate)

Lodine (NSAID) — codeine (narcotic analgesic)

| | |
|---|---|
| Lopid (antihyperlipidemic) | Lorabid (beta-lactam antibiotic) |
| lovastatin (antihyperlipidemic) | Lotensin (ACE inhibitor) |
| metolazone (thiazide diuretic) | methotrexate (antineoplastic) |
| metolazone (thiazide diuretic) | metoclopramide (GI stimulant) |
| metoprolol (beta-adrenergic blocker) | misoprostol (prostaglandin derivative) |
| Monopril (ACE inhibitor) | minoxidil (antihypertensive) |
| Norlutate (progestin) | Norlutin (progestin) |
| Norvasc (calcium channel blocker) | Navane (antipsychotic) |
| Ocufen (NSAID) | Ocuflox (fluoroquinolone antibiotic) |
| Orinase (oral hypoglycemic) | Ornade (upper respiratory product) |
| Percocet (narcotic analgesic) | Percodan (narcotic analgesic) |
| paroxetine (antidepressant) | paclitaxel (antineoplastic) |
| Paxil (antidepressant) | paclitaxel (antineoplastic) |
| Paxil (antidepressant) | Taxol (antineoplastic) |
| penicillamine (heavy metal antagonist) | penicillin (antibiotic) |
| pindolol (beta-adrenergic blocker) | Parlodel (inhibitor of prolactin secretion) |
| Platinol (antineoplastic) | Paraplatin (antineoplastic) |
| Pravachol (antihyperlipidemic) | Prevacid (GI drug) |
| Pravachol (antihyperlipidemic) | propranolol (beta-adrenergic blocker) |
| prednisolone (corticosteroid) | prednisone (corticosteroid) |
| Prilosec (inhibitor of gastric acid secretion) | Prozac (antidepressant) |
| Prinivil (ACE inhibitor) | Prilosec (GE drug) |
| Prinivil (ACE inhibitor) | Proventil (sympathomimetic) |
| propranolol (beta-adrenergic blocker) | Propulsid (GI drug) |
| Provera (progestin) | Premarin (estrogen) |
| Prozac (antidepressant) | Proscar (androgen hormone inhibitor) |
| quinidine (antiarrhythmic) | clonidine (antihypertensive) |
| quinidine (antiarrhythmic) | Quinamm (antimalarial) |
| quinine (antimalarial) | quinidine (antiarrhythmic) |
| Regroton (antihypertensive) | Hygroton (diuretic) |
| Rifamate (antituberculous drug) | rifampin (antituberculous drug) |
| Seldane (antihistamine) | Feldene (NSAID) |
| Stadol (narcotic analgesic) | Haldol (antipsychotic) |
| terbinafine (antifungal agent) | terfenadine (antihistamine) |
| terbutaline (sympathomimetic) | tolbutamide (oral hypoglycemic) |
| tolazamide (oral hypoglycemic) | tolbutamide (oral hypoglycemic) |
| torsemide (loop diuretic) | furosemide (loop diuretic) |
| trifluoperazine (antipsychotic) | trihexyphenidyl (antiparkinson drug) |
| Trimox (amoxicillin product) | Diamox (carbonic anhydrase inhibitor) |

| | |
|---|---|
| Vancenase (corticosteroid) | Vanceril (corticosteroid) |
| Vasosulf (sulfonamide/decongestant) | Velosef (cephalosporin) |
| Versed (benzodiazepine sedative) | Vistaril (antianxiety agent) |
| Versed (benzodiazepine sedative) | VePesid (antineoplastic) |
| Xanax (antianxiety agent) | Zantac ($H_2$ histamine blocker) |
| Zebeta (beta-blocker) | DiaBeta (oral hypoglycemic) |
| Zinacef (cephalosporin) | Zithromax (macrolide antibiotic) |
| Zocor (antihyperlipidemic) | Zoloft (antidepressant) |
| Zofran (antiemetic) | Zantac ($H_2$ histamine blocker) |
| Zosyn (penicillin antibiotic) | Zofran (antiemetic) |

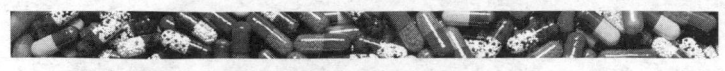

# Commonly Used Abbreviations and Symbols

| | |
|---|---|
| aa, A | of each |
| ABG | arterial blood gas |
| a.c. | before meals |
| ACE | angiotensin-converting enzyme |
| ACLS | advanced cardiac life support |
| ACTH | adrenocorticotropic hormone |
| ad | to, up to |
| a.d. | right ear |
| ad lib | as desired, at pleasure |
| ADP | adenosine diphosphate |
| ADA | adenosine deaminase |
| ADH | antidiuretic hormone |
| ADL | activities of daily living |
| AFB | acid fast bacillus |
| AHF | antihemophilic factor |
| AIDS | acquired immune deficiency syndrome |
| a.l. | left ear |
| ALT | alanine aminotransferase |
| a.m., A.M. | morning |
| AMI | acute myocardial infarction |
| AML | acute myeloid leukemia |
| AMP | adenosine monophosphate |
| ANA | antinuclear antibody |
| ANC | active neutrophil count |
| ANS | autonomic nervous system |
| APTT | activated partial thromboplastin time |
| aq | water |
| aq dist. | distilled water |
| ARC | AIDS-related complex |
| ARDS | adult respiratory distress syndrome |
| ASA | aspirin |
| ASAP | as soon as possible |
| ASHD | arteriosclerotic heart disease |
| AST | aspartate aminotransferase |
| ATC | around the clock |
| ATP | adenosine triphosphate |
| ATX | antibiotics |
| a.u. | each ear, both ears |
| AV | atrioventricular |
| b.i.d. | two times per day |
| b.i.n. | two times per night |
| BMR | basal metabolic rate |
| BP | blood pressure |
| BPH | benign prostatic hypertrophy |

| BS | blood sugar, bowel sounds |
| BSA | body surface area |
| BSE | breast self-exam |
| BSP | Bromsulphalein |
| BUN | blood urea nitrogen |
| C | Celsius/Centigrade |
| CABG | coronary artery bypass graft |
| C&DB | cough and deep breathe |
| CAD | coronary artery disease |
| caps, Caps | capsule(s) |
| CBC | complete blood count |
| CCB | calcium channel blocker |
| $C_{CR}$ | creatinine clearance |
| $CD_4$ | helper $T_4$ lymphocyte cells |
| CDC | Centers for Disease Control and Prevention |
| C&DB | cough and deep breathe |
| CF | cystic fibrosis |
| CHF | congestive heart failure |
| CLL | chronic lymphocytic leukemia |
| cm | centimeter |
| CML | chronic myelocytic leukemia |
| CMV | cytomegalovirus |
| CN | cranial nerve |
| CNS | central nervous system |
| CO | cardiac output |
| COPD | chronic obstructive pulmonary disease |
| CPAP | continuous positive airway pressure |
| CPB | cardiopulmonary bypass |
| CPK | creatine phosphokinase |
| CPR | cardiopulmonary resuscitation |
| C&S | culture and sensitivity |
| CSF | cerebrospinal fluid |
| CT | computerized tomography |
| CTS | carpal tunnel syndrome |
| CTZ | chemoreceptor trigger zone |
| CV | cardiovascular |
| CVA | cerebrovascular accident |
| CVP | central venous pressure |
| CXR | chest X ray |
| dATP | deoxy ATP |
| DBP | diastolic BP |
| dc | discontinue |
| DEA | Drug Enforcement Agency |
| DI | diabetes insipidus |
| DIC | disseminated intravascular coagulation |
| dil. | dilute |
| dL | deciliter (one-tenth of a liter) |
| DNA | deoxyribonucleic acid |
| DOE | dyspnea on exertion |
| dr. | dram (0.0625 ounce) |
| DTR | deep tendon reflex |
| DVT | deep vein thrombosis |
| EC | enteric-coated |
| ECB | extracorporeal cardiopulmonary bypass |
| ECG, EKG | electrocardiogram, electrocardiograph |
| EDTA | ethylenediaminetetraacetic acid |

| | |
|---|---|
| EEG | electroencephalogram |
| EENT | eye, ear, nose, and throat |
| e.g. | for example |
| elix | elixir |
| emuls. | emulsion |
| ENT | ear, nose, throat |
| EPS | electrophysiologic studies |
| ER | extended release |
| ESR | erythrocyte sedimentation rate |
| ET | endotracheal |
| ETOH | alcohol |
| ext. | extract |
| F | Fahrenheit, fluoride |
| FBS | fasting blood sugar |
| FDA | Food and Drug Administration |
| FEV | forced expiratory volume |
| FFP | fresh frozen plasma |
| FOB | fecal occult blood |
| FS | finger stick |
| FSH | follicle-stimulating hormone |
| F/U | follow-up |
| g, gm | gram (1,000 mg) |
| GABA | gamma-aminobutyric acid |
| GERD | gastroesophageal reflux disease |
| GFR | glomerular filtration rate |
| GGT | gamma-glutamyl transferase: *syn.* gamma-glutamyl transpeptidase |
| gi, GI | gastrointestinal |
| GnRH | gonadotropin-releasing hormone |
| G6PD | glucose-6-phosphate dehydrogenase |
| gr | grain |
| gtt | a drop, drops |
| GU | genitourinary |
| h, hr | hour |
| HA, HAL | hyperalimentation |
| HCG | human chorionic gonadotropin |
| HCP | health-care provider |
| HCV | hepatitis C virus |
| HDL | high density lipoprotein |
| HFN | high flow nebulizer |
| H&H | hematocrit and hemoglobin |
| HIV | human immunodeficiency virus |
| HMG-CoA | 3-hydroxy-3-methyl-glutaryl-coenzyme A |
| HOB | head of bed |
| HR | heart rate |
| h.s. | at bedtime |
| HSE | herpes simplex encephalitis |
| HSV | herpes simplex virus |
| 5-HT | 5-hydroxytryptamine |
| HTN | hypertension |
| IA | intra-arterial |
| IBD | inflammatory bowel disease |
| ICP | intracranial pressure |
| ICU | intensive care unit |
| Ig | immunoglobulin |
| im, IM | intramuscular |

| | |
|---|---|
| IMV | intermittent mandatory ventilation |
| INR | international normalized ratio |
| I&O | intake and output |
| IOP | intraocular pressure |
| IPPB | intermittent positive pressure breathing |
| ITP | idiopathic thrombocytopenia purpura |
| IU | international units |
| iv, IV | intravenous |
| IVPB | IV piggyback, a secondary IV line |
| JVD | jugular venous distention |
| kg | kilogram (2.2 lb) |
| KVO | keep vein open |
| l, L | liter (1,000 mL) |
| L | left |
| LDH | lactic dehydrogenase |
| LDL | low density lipoprotein |
| LFTs | liver function tests |
| LH | luteinizing hormone |
| LHRH | luteinizing hormone-releasing hormone |
| LOC | level of consciousness |
| LV | left ventricular |
| LVFP | left ventricular function pressure |
| M | mix |
| $m^2$, $M^2$ | square meter |
| m | meter |
| MAC | *Mycobacterium avium* complex |
| MAO | monoamine oxidase |
| MAP | mean arterial pressure |
| max | maximum |
| mcg | microgram |
| mCi | millicurie |
| MDI | metered-dose inhaler |
| mEq | milliequivalent |
| mg | milligram |
| MI | myocardial infarction |
| MIC | minimum inhibitory concentration |
| min | minute, minim |
| mist, mixt | mixture |
| mL | milliliter |
| MRI | magnetic resonance imaging |
| MS | multiple sclerosis |
| NaCl | sodium chloride |
| ng | nanogram |
| NG | nasogastric |
| NGT | nasogastric tube |
| NKA | no known allergies |
| NKDA | no known drug allergies |
| noct | at night, during the night |
| non rep | do not repeat |
| NPN | nonprotein nitrogen |
| NPO | nothing by mouth |
| NR | do not refill (e.g., a prescription) |
| NSAID | nonsteroidal anti-inflammatory drug |
| NSR | normal sinus rhythm |
| NSS | normal saline solution |
| N&V | nausea and vomiting |

| | |
|---|---|
| $O_2$ | oxygen |
| o.d. | once a day |
| O.D. | right eye |
| OH | orthostatic hypotension |
| OOB | out of bed |
| OR | operating room |
| os | mouth |
| O.S. | left eye |
| $O_2$ sat | oxygen saturation |
| OTC | over the counter |
| O.U. | each eye, both eyes |
| oz | ounce |
| PA | pulmonary artery |
| PABA | para-aminobenzoic acid |
| PAWP | pulmonary artery wedge pressure |
| PBI | protein-bound iodine |
| p.c. | after meals |
| PCA | patient-controlled analgesia |
| PCI | percutaneous coronary intervention |
| PCN | penicillin |
| PCP | *Pneumocystis carinii* pneumonia |
| PE | pulmonary embolus |
| PEEP | positive end expiratory pressure |
| per | by, through |
| PFTs | pulmonary function tests |
| pH | hydrogen ion concentration |
| PMH | past medical history |
| PMI | point of maximal intensity |
| PMS | premenstrual syndrome |
| PND | paroxysmal dyspnea |
| po, p.o., PO | by mouth |
| PPD | purified protein derivative |
| PR | by rectum |
| p.r.n., PRN | when needed or necessary |
| PSA | prostatic specific antigen |
| PT | prothrombin time |
| PTCA | percutaneous transluminal coronary angioplasty |
| PTSD | post traumatic stress disorder |
| PTT | partial thromboplastin time |
| PUD | peptic ulcer disease |
| PVC | premature ventricular contraction; polyvinyl chloride |
| PVD | peripheral vascular disease |
| q.d. | every day |
| q.h. | every hour |
| q2h | every two hours |
| q3h | every three hours |
| q4h | every four hours |
| q6h | every six hours |
| q8h | every eight hours |
| qhs | every night |
| q.i.d. | four times a day |
| q.o.d. | every other day |
| q.s. | as much as needed, quantity sufficient |
| RA | right atrium; rheumatoid arthritis |
| RBC | red blood cell |
| RDA | recommended daily allowance |

| | |
|---|---|
| REM | rapid eye movement |
| Rept. | let it be repeated |
| RNA | ribonucleic acid |
| ROM | range of motion |
| ROS | review of systems |
| RRMS | relapsing-remitting multiple sclerosis |
| R/T | related to |
| RV | right ventricular |
| RUQ | right upper quadrant |
| Rx | symbol for a prescription |
| SA | sinoatrial or sustained-action |
| SAH | subarachnoid hemorrhage |
| SBE | subacute bacterial endocarditis |
| SBP | systolic BP |
| sc, SC, SQ | subcutaneous |
| SCID | severe combined immunodeficiency disease |
| SGOT | serum glutamic-oxaloacetic transaminase |
| SGPT | serum glutamic-pyruvic transaminase |
| S., Sig. | mark on the label |
| SI | sacroiliac |
| SIMV | synchronized intermittent mandatory ventilation |
| SL | sublingual |
| SLE | systemic lupus erythematosus |
| SOB | shortness of breath |
| sol | solution |
| sp | spirits |
| SR | sustained-release |
| ss | one-half |
| S&S | signs and symptoms |
| stat | immediately, first dose |
| STD | sexually transmitted disease |
| SV | stroke volume |
| SVT | supraventricular tachycardia |
| syr | syrup |
| tab | tablet |
| TB | tuberculosis |
| TCA | tricyclic antidepressant |
| TENS | transcutaneous electric nerve stimulation |
| TIA | transient ischemic attack |
| t.i.d. | three times per day |
| t.i.n. | three times per night |
| TKR | total knee replacement |
| T.O. | telephone order |
| TPN | total parenteral nutrition |
| TSH | thyroid stimulating hormone |
| U | unit |
| µ | micron |
| µCi | microcurie |
| µg | microgram |
| µm | micrometer |
| UGI | upper gastrointestinal |
| ung | ointment |
| URI, URTI | upper respiratory infection |
| USP | U. S. Pharmacopeia |
| ut dict | as directed |
| UTI | urinary tract infection |

| | |
|---|---|
| UV | ultraviolet |
| VAD | venous access device |
| VF | ventricular fibrillation |
| vin | wine |
| VLDL | very low density lipoprotein |
| VMA | vanillylmandelic acid |
| V.O. | verbal order |
| VS | vital signs |
| VT | ventricular tachycardia |
| WBC | white blood cell |
| XRT | radiation therapy |
| & | and |
| > | greater than |
| < | less than |
| ↑ | increased, higher |
| ↓ | decreased, lower |
| - | negative |
| / | per |
| % | percent |
| + | positive |
| x | times, frequency |

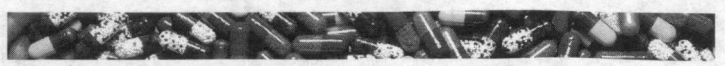

# Drugs Archived on the Web

The drugs listed here were removed from PDR® Nurse's Handbook - 1999 to make room for new drugs. The monograph for each of the drugs listed can be found in its entirety on the World Wide Web at **www.nursespdr.com**

Actifed

  Sinus Daytime/Nightime Caplets and Tablets
  Syrup
  Tablets

Advil Cold and Sinus Caplets and Tablets

Alka-Seltzer Plus

  Cold & Cough Medicine Liquigels and Tablets
  Night-Time Cold Medicine Liquigels and Tablets
  Sinus Medicine Tablets

Allerest

  12 Hour Caplets
  Children's Chewable Tablets
  Headache Strength Tablets
  Maximum Strength Tablets
  No Drowsiness Tablets
  Sinus Pain Formula Tablets

Aluminum hydroxide gel

Aluminum hydroxide gel, dried

Basic aluminum carbonate gel

Bisacodyl

Bisacodyl tannex

Buclizine hydrochloride

Calcium carbonate precipitated

Carprofen

Cascara sagrada

Castor oil

Castor oil, emulsified

Cefmetazole sodium

Cefonicid sodium

Chlorotrianisene

Excedrin

   Aspirin Free Analgesic Caplets
   Extra Strength Analgesic Caplets and Tablets
   P. M. Caplets, Liquigels, and Tablets

Fenfluramine

Gelusil

Glycerin

Insulin, zinc suspension, prompt

Insulin, human

Maalox

   Antacid Caplets
   Heartburn Relief Suspension and Tablets
   Magnesia and Alumina Oral Suspension
   Plus Tablets
   Extra Strength Plus Suspension
   Extra Strength Antacid Plus Anti-Gas Tablets

Magaldrate

Magnesium hydroxide

Magnesium oxide

Maprotiline hydrochloride

Methylcellulose

Microfibrillar Collagen Hemostat

Mineral Oil

Mylanta

   Gelcaps
   Liquid and Tablets
   Double Strength Liquid and Tablets

Naldecon Syrup and Tablets

Nitroglycerin transmucosal

Novahistine

   DMX
   Elixir

Ornade

Oxycodone and Aspirin

Oxymetazoline hydrochloride

Pantothenic acid

Pentaerythritol Tetranitrate Sustained-Release Capsules

Pentaerythritol Tetranitrate Sustained-Release Tablets

Pentaerythritol Tetranitrate Tablets

# CHAPTER 1
# How To Use PDR-99

PDR® Nurse's Handbook™ is intended to be a quick reference to obtain useful information on drugs. An important objective is also to provide information on the proper monitoring of drug therapy and to assist practitioners in teaching clients and family members about important aspects of drug therapy.

Chapter 2 includes general information on important therapeutic or chemical classes of drugs. The classes of drugs are listed alphabetically. Specific drugs in therapeutic or chemical classes are found in Chapter 3 (alphabetical listing of drugs). The information on each therapeutic or chemical class in Chapter 2 begins with a list of the drugs addressed in the drug class. Information on the specific drugs is provided under that drug in Chapter 3. Information on many other drugs also is provided in Chapter 3.

The format for information on individual drugs (and for drug classes when appropriate) is presented as follows:

**Drug Names:** The generic name for the drug is presented first; this is followed by the phonetic pronunciation of the generic name. The FDA pregnancy category A, B, C, D, or X (see Appendix 3 for definitions) to which the drug is assigned is also listed in this section. All trade names follow this; if the trade name is available only in Canada, the name is followed by a maple leaf ( ✦ ). Also, if the drug is controlled by the U.S. Federal Controlled Substances Act, the schedule in which the drug is placed follows the trade name (e.g., C-II, C-III, C-IV or I, II, III, IV, V). See Appendix 1 for a listing of controlled substances in both the United States

and Canada. A combination drug heading indicates that two or more drugs are combined in the same product.

**Classification:** This section defines the type of drug or the class under which the drug is listed. This information is most useful in learning to categorize drugs. To minimize the need to repeat general information, a cross reference to Chapter 2 is often made for drugs listed in Chapter 3. This information should also be consulted.

**General Statement:** Information about the drug class and/or what might be specific or unusual about a particular group of drugs is presented. In addition, brief information may be presented about the disease(s) for which the drugs are indicated.

**Action/Kinetics:** The action portion describes the proposed mechanism(s) by which a drug achieves its therapeutic effect. Not all mechanisms of action are known, and some are self-evident, as when a hormone is administered as a replacement. The kinetics portion lists pertinent pharmacologic properties, if known, about rate of drug absorption, distribution, minimum effective serum or plasma level, biologic half-life, duration of action, metabolism, and excretion. Metabolism and excretion routes may be important for clients with systemic liver disease, kidney disease, or both. Again, information is not available for all therapeutic agents.

The time it takes for half the drug to be excreted or removed from the blood, t½ (half-life), is important in determining how often a drug is to be administered and how long to assess for side effects. Therapeutic serum or plasma levels indicate the desired concentration, in serum or plasma, for the drug to exert its beneficial effect and is helpful in predicting the possible onset of side effects or the lack of effect. Drug therapy is often monitored in this fashion (e.g., antibiotics, theophylline, phenytoin, amiodarone). An additional feature is a listing of commonly accepted therapeutic drug levels (see Appendix 9).

**Uses:** Approved therapeutic use(s) for the particular drug are presented. Investigational uses are also listed for selected drugs.

**Contraindications:** Disease states or conditions in which the drug should not be used are noted. The safe use of many of the newer pharmacologic agents during pregnancy, lactation, or childhood has not been established. As a general rule, the use of drugs during pregnancy is contraindicated unless specified by the provider where the benefits of drug therapy far outweigh the potential risks.

**Special Concerns:** This section covers considerations for use with pediatric, geriatric, pregnant, or lactating clients. Situations and disease states when the drug should be used with caution are also listed.

**Side Effects:** Undesired or bothersome effects the client *may* experience while taking a particular agent are described. Side effects are listed by the body organ or system affected and are usually presented with the most common side effects for that organ system listed in descending order of incidence. This feature allows easy access to information on potential side effects of each drug. It is important to note that nearly all of the potential side effects are listed; in any given clinical situation, however, a client may show no side effects, or one or more side effects. If potentially life threatening, the side effect is indicated by boldface italic print.

**OD   Overdose Management:** When appropriate, this section provides a list of the symptoms observed following an overdose (*symptoms* ) of the drug as well as approaches for treatment of the overdose (*treatment*).

**Drug Interactions:** This is an alphabetical listing of drugs that may interact with one another. The study of drug interactions is an important area of pharmacology and is changing constantly as a result of the influx of new drugs, clinical feedback, and increased client usage. The compilation of such interactions is far from complete; therefore, listings in this handbook are to be considered *only* as general cautionary guidelines.

Drug interactions may result from a number of different mechanisms (e.g., additive or inhibitory effects, interference with degradation of drug, increased rate of elimination, decreased absorption from the GI tract, and competition or displacement from receptor sites or plasma protein binding sites). Such interactions may manifest themselves in a variety of ways; however, an attempt has been made throughout the text to describe these interactions whenever possible as an increase ($\uparrow$) or a decrease ($\downarrow$) in the effect of the drug, and a reason for the change.

It is important to realize that any side effects that accompany the administration of a particular agent also may be increased as a result of a drug interaction.

The reader should be aware that drug interactions are often listed for classes of drugs. Thus, the drug interaction is likely to occur for all drugs in a particular class. Consult this information in Chapter 2.

**Laboratory Test Interferences: (or Considerations):** The manner in which a drug may affect laboratory test values is presented. Some of these effects are caused by the therapeutic or toxic effects of the drugs; others result from interference with the testing method itself. The laboratory interferences or laboratory considerations are described as false positive (+), or increased ($\uparrow$), values and as false negative (–), or decreased ( ↓ ), values.

**Dosage:** The dosage form and route of administration is clearly shown and is followed by the disease state or condition (in italics) for which the dosage is recommended. This is followed by the adult and pediatric doses, when available. The listed dosage is to be considered as a general guideline; the exact amount of the drug to be given is determined by the provider. However, one should question orders when dosages differ markedly from the accepted norm. We have tried to give complete data for drugs that are frequently prescribed.

**Nursing Considerations:** These guidelines were developed to assist the nurse to apply the nursing process to pharmacotherapeutics. The Administration/Storage section assists the practitioner in preparing the medications for administration, administering the drug, and proper storage. All information relating to IV administration is listed under an IV icon to promote ready reference. Guidelines assessing the client before, during, and after prescribed drug therapy are identified, as are nursing interventions appropriate for the prescribed drug therapy. Important client/family teaching issues related to the particular drug therapy are addressed. Specific outcome criteria are listed to help evaluate the effectiveness of the prescribed drug therapy. Nursing considerations that include assessments and interventions may contain specifics such as:

1. Gathering of physical data and client history.

2. Assessment of specific physiologic functions that may be affected by the drug.

3. Specific laboratory tests to monitor during drug therapy.

4. Identification of sensitivities/interactions and conditions that may preclude a particular drug therapy.

5. Documenting specific indications for therapy and describing symptom characteristics related to this condition.

6. Physiologic, pharmacologic, and psychologic effects of the drug and how these may affect the client and impact on the nursing process.

7. Adverse reactions that can arise as a result of drug therapy and appropriate nursing interventions.

8. Ensuring client safety when receiving drug therapy.

The practitioner must also assess the client for the *Side Effects* listed for that drug. Side effects must be documented and reported to the provider. Severe side effects generally are cause for dosage modification or discontinuation of the drug.

Specific information for the client is provided for each drug. Client/family teaching emphasizes specifics to help the client/family recognize side effects, avoid potentially dangerous situations, and to alleviate anxiety that may result from taking a particular drug. Details on administration have been included to enhance client understanding and compliance. Side effects that require medical intervention are included as well as specifics on how to minimize side effects for certain medications (i.e., take medication with food to decrease GI upset or take at bedtime to minimize daytime sedative effects).

The proper education of clients is one of the most challenging aspects of nursing. The instructions must be tailored to the needs, awareness, and sophistication of each client. For example, clients who take medication to lower BP should assume responsibility for taking their own BP or having it taken and recorded. Clients should carry identification listing the drugs currently prescribed. They should know what they are taking and why, and develop a mechanism to remind themselves to take their medication as prescribed. Clients should carry this drug list with them whenever they go for a check-up or seek medical care. The drug list may also be shared with the pharmacist if there is a question concerning drugs prescribed, if the client is considering taking an over-the-counter medication, or if the client has to change pharmacies. The records, especially BP recordings, should be shared with the health care provider to ensure accurate evaluation of the response to the prescribed drug therapy. This may also alert the provider to any medication consumption by the client that they did not prescribe, were not aware of, or that may interfere with (i.e., potentiate, antagonize) the current pharmacologic regimen. The provider may also encourage the client to call with any questions or concerns about their therapy.

Finally, when taking the nursing history, emphasis should be placed on the client's ability to read and to follow directions. Clients with language barriers should be identified, and appropriate written translations should be provided. In addition, client life-style, cultural factors, and income as well as the availability of health insurance and transportation are important factors that may affect compliance with therapy and F/U care. The potential for a client being/becoming pregnant, and whether a mother is breast feeding her infant should be included in assessments. The age and orientation level, whether learned from personal observation or from discussion with close friends or family members, can be critical in determining potential relationships between drug therapy and/or drug interactions. Including these factors in the nursing assessment will assist all on the health care team to determine the type of therapy and drug delivery system best suited to a particular client and will promote the highest level of compliance.

An outcomes/evaluate section is included to assist in determining the effectiveness and positive therapeutic outcome of the prescribed drug therapy. Specific outcome criteria related to each drug are delineated.

*The previous points are covered for all drugs or drug classes. When drugs are presented as a group (as in*

*Chapter 2) rather than individually, the points may be covered only once for each group. In this case the practitioner should look for the appropriate entry in the drug class.* For example, the *Contraindications, Side Effects, Drug Interactions,* and *Nursing Considerations* for all the insulins are so similar that they generally are listed only once in Chapter 2, under Insulins, in order to prevent lengthy duplication. However, the individual drug entries are cross-referenced to this general information.

Information that requires emphasis or is relevant to a particular drug is listed under appropriate headings, such as *Additional Contraindications, Additional Side Effects,* or *Additional Nursing Considerations.* Such entries are *in addition to* and not *instead of* the regular entry, which is referenced and must also be consulted.

Additional information to assist the practitioner in administering drugs and monitoring drug therapy appropriately is also found in the text. For example, formulas for calculating IV flow rates and administration guidelines for some frequently administered IV antibiotics are included in Appendices 5 and 6, respectively. Dosage based on body surface area (BSA) is frequently used when calculating the dosage of potent drugs such as those used in chemotherapy (e.g., treatment of cancer) or for drug administration to children. Nomograms for computing the BSA (for children) are provided in Appendix 4. A list of sound-alike drug names is included in the front portion of the book to alert the practitioner to these similarities in an effort to prevent a potential lethal error. It is important to check drug names carefully to ensure that the prescribed drug is, indeed, the one that is being administered, as it is sometimes easy to confuse drugs that sound alike or are spelled similarly. Also helpful are the Table of Weights and Measures (Appendix 10), Commonly Used Abbreviations and Symbols (front portion of book), and the

Guide to Drug Compatibility (in the back of the handbook). Appendix 8, Drug Preview, contains information on the newest marketed drugs; however, due to time constraints, the information could not be incorporated into Chapter 3.

The wound/dressing classification section (Appendix 7) identifies the therapeutic class of wound care products as well as the types of wounds appropriate for this therapy. Additionally, vitamins and vaccines are addressed as a group in Chapter 2. Finally, due to the rapidly changing area of pharmacotherapy, a monthly Internet and e-mail update service has been developed to ensure that you have all the tools necessary to practice currently and safely.

You are now ready to use PDR® Nurse's Handbook™. We hope that the text will be useful and assist you in your education, profession, and practice. The safe administration of drugs, assessment of potential interactions and adverse effects, as well as outcome evaluation are crucial parts of the nursing process.

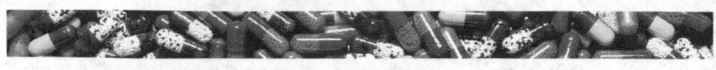

# CHAPTER 2
# Therapeutic Drug Classifications

## ALKYLATING AGENTS

*See also the following individual entries:*

- Busulfan
- Carboplatin for Injection
- Carmustine
- Chlorambucil
- Cisplatin
- Cyclophosphamide
- Dacarbazine
- Ifosfamide
- Lomustine
- Mechlorethamine hydrochloride
- Melphalan
- Mesna
- Streptozocin
- Thiotepa

**Action/Kinetics:** Under physiologic conditions alkylating agents donate an alkyl group (carbonium ion) to biologically important macromolecules, such as DNA. These reactions inactivate the molecule, bringing *cell division* to a halt. This cytotoxic activity affects replication of cancerous cells and other cells, especially in rapidly proliferating tissues, such as the bone marrow, intestinal epithelium, and hair follicles.

The toxic effects of the alkylating agents are usually cell-cycle nonspecific and become apparent when the cell enters the S phase and cell division is blocked at the $G_2$ phase (premitotic phase), resulting in cells having a double complement of DNA.

Resistance of cancer cells to alkylating agents usually develops slowly and gradually. The resistance seems to be the sum total of several minor adaptations, including decreased permeability of the cells, increased production of noncancer receptors (nucleophilic substances), and increased efficiency of the DNA repair system.

### NURSING CONSIDERATIONS

See *Nursing Considerations* for individual agents and *Nursing Considerations* for *Antineoplastic Agents*.
**Outcomes/Evaluate:** Clinical/radiographic evidence of tumor regression and disease stabilization

## ALPHA-1-ADRENERGIC BLOCKING AGENTS

*See also the following individual entries:*

- Doxazosin mesylate
- Prazosin hydrochloride
- Terazosin

See also *Beta-Adrenergic Blocking Agents*.
**Action/Kinetics:** Selectively block postsynaptic alpha-1-adrenergic receptors. Results in dilation of both arterioles and veins leading to a decrease in supine and standing BP. Diastolic BP is affected the most. Prazosin and terazosin do not produce reflex tachycardia. Terazosin also relaxes smooth muscle in the bladder neck and prostate, making it useful to treat BPH.

Adrenergic blocking agents have many undesirable effects which, although not toxic, limit their use. Always start treatment at low doses and increase gradually.
**Uses:** Alone or in combination with diuretics or beta-adrenergic blocking agents to treat hypertension. Doxa-

zocin and terazosin are used to treat BPH. *Investigational:* Prazosin is used for refractory CHF, management of Raynaud's vasospasm, and to treat BPH. Doxazosin, along with digoxin and diuretics, is used to treat CHF.

**Contraindications:** Hypersensitivity to these drugs (i.e., quinazolines).

**Special Concerns:** The first few doses may cause postural hypotension and syncope with sudden loss of consciousness. Use with caution in lactation, with impaired hepatic function, or if receiving drugs known to influence hepatic metabolism. Safety and efficacy have not been established in children.

**Side Effects:** The following side effects are common to alpha-1-adrenergic blockers. See individual drugs as well. *CV:* Palpitations, postural hypotension, hypotension, tachycardia, chest pain, arrhythmia. *GI:* N&V, dry mouth, diarrhea, constipation, abdominal discomfort or pain, flatulence. *CNS:* Dizziness, depression, decreased libido, sexual dysfunction, nervousness, paresthesia, somnolence, anxiety, insomnia, asthenia, drowsiness. *Musculoskeletal:* Pain in the shoulder, neck, or back; gout, arthritis, joint pain, arthralgia. *Respiratory:* Dyspnea, nasal congestion, sinusitis, bronchitis, **bronchospasm,** cold symptoms, epistaxis, increased cough, flu symptoms, pharyngitis, rhinitis. *Ophthalmic:* Blurred vision, abnormal vision, reddened sclera, conjunctivitis. *GU:* Impotence, urinary frequency, incontinence. *Miscellaneous:* Tinnitus, vertigo, pruritus, sweating, alopecia, lichen planus, headache, edema, weight gain, facial edema, fever.

**OD** **Overdose Management:** *Symptoms:* Extension of the side effects, especially on BP. *Treatment:* Keep supine to restore BP and normalize heart rate. Shock may be treated with volume expanders or vasopressors; support renal function.

**Drug Interactions:** Alpha-1 blockers ↓ the antihypertensive effect of clonidine.

**Laboratory Test Interferences:** ↑ Urinary VMA.

**Dosage** ───────────
See individual agents.

## NURSING CONSIDERATIONS
**Administration/Storage:** Take the first dose of prazosin and terazosin at bedtime.

**Assessment**
1. Note any history of PUD; drug should be used cautiously.
2. Document indications for therapy, type, onset, and characteristics of symptoms.
3. Monitor electrolytes, ECG, and VS.
4. Assess for heart or lung disease and note currently prescribed therapy. Some agents may cause vasospasm with Prinzmetal or vasospastic angina.

**Interventions**
1. Use cautiously in older clients due to possibility of orthostatic hypotension. They may tolerate a slower, more gradual increase in dosage (i.e., terazosin 1 mg/day for 7 days followed by 2 mg/day for 7 days, etc., until desired response).
2. Initiate with a low dose and at bedtime to prevent syncope and postural hypotensive effects.
3. Titration generally should be based on standing BP due to postural effects.
4. Drug does not affect glucose levels and may be useful with diabetes.

**Client/Family Teaching**
1. Take first dose at bedtime to minimize syncope and hypotensive effects. Use caution when performing activities that require mental alertness until drug effects realized.
2. Take with milk or meals to minimize GI upset.
3. Do not drive or undertake hazardous tasks for 12–24 hr after the first dose and after increasing dose or following an interruption of dosage.
4. Avoid symptoms of orthostatic hypotension by rising slowly from a sitting or lying position and waiting until symptoms subside.
5. Keep record of BP and weight. Report any weight gain or ankle

edema; without a diuretic, one may experience retention of salt and water due to vasodilation.

6. Dizziness, lassitude, headache, and palpitations may occur as well as transient apprehension, fear, anxiety, and/or palpitations. Report any persistent side effects so dosage may be evaluated and adjusted accordingly.

7. Review life-style changes and additional holistic interventions for BP control; i.e., dietary restrictions of fat, sodium, and cholesterol; weight reduction; regular physical activity and exercise; decreased use of alcohol; stress reduction; and smoking cessation.

8. Avoid excess caffeine and OTC agents (especially cold remedies) unless approved.

9. Do not interrupt therapy without approval.

**Outcomes/Evaluate**

• ↓ BP

• ↓ Nocturia, urgency, and frequency

# AMEBICIDES AND TRICHOMONACIDES

*See also the following individual entries:*

Atovaquone
Erythromycins
Metronidazole
Paromomycin sulfate
Tetracyclines

**General Statement:** Amebiasis is a widely distributed disease caused by the protozoan *Entamoeba histolytica*. *E. histolytica* has two forms: (1) an active motile form known as the trophozoite form and (2) a cystic form that is resistant to destruction and is responsible for the transmission of the disease. The overt manifestations of amebiasis vary. Some manifest violent acute dysentery (characterized by sudden development of severe diarrhea, cramps, and passage of bloody, mucoid stools); others have

few overt symptoms or are even completely asymptomatic.

Amoebae often migrate from the GI tract to other parts of the body (extraintestinal amebiasis). The spleen, lungs, or liver are frequently affected. The amoebae colonize in these organs and form abscesses that may rupture and thereby serve as infectious foci.

At present, no one drug can cure both intestinal and extraintestinal amebic infestations; thus, combination therapy is used. Often the more effective but toxic agents are used initially for a short period of time, while long-term eradication or prophylaxis is carried out with less toxic agents.

Infestation with the parasite *Trichomonas vaginalis* causes vaginitis. This is treated by various locally applied antitrichomonal agents—often effective amebicides—and also by the oral administration of metronidazole. This drug is usually prescribed for both sexual partners to prevent reinfection. Acid douches (vinegar or lactic acid) are a helpful adjunct to treatment.

The incidence of infections by another protozoan organism, *Giardia lamblia,* is transmitted in the feces. Infections are characterized by mucous diarrhea, abdominal pain, and weight loss. Drugs of choice are metronidazole and quinacrine.

## NURSING CONSIDERATIONS

See also *General Nursing Considerations for All Anti-Infectives.*

AMEBICIDES

**Assessment**

1. Document type and onset of symptoms; identify causative factors/conditions, any travel, and possible exposures.

2. Obtain CBC, electrolytes, nutrition profile, and cultures.

3. Assess for acute dysentery or extraintestinal amebiasis as agents of choice are highly toxic.

**Interventions**

1. Clients are frequently on combi-

nation-drug therapy for amebiasis; observe for toxic reactions.

2. Provide supportive nursing care to clients having acute dysentery; assist in the effort to control diarrhea, maintain fluid and electrolyte balance, skin integrity, comfort, and prevent complications caused by malnutrition. Activity may have to be curtailed during the acute disease phase.

3. Administer drugs only for the time ordered; allow for rest periods between courses of therapy.

**Client/Family Teaching**

1. Carriers must continue with drug therapy; review benefit to themselves, their families, and their coworkers.

2. Thorough hand washing is imperative, especially in factories, schools, and other institutions where disease is easily spread; disinfect toilets daily.

3. Food handlers must be particularly conscientious about washing hands after toileting; use soap, water, and clean towels.

4. Obtain regular periodic stool examinations to check for recurrence.

5. Client and carriers need to report for follow-up visits to ensure eradication of organisms. Do not self-medicate.

TRICHOMONACIDES

**Client/Family Teaching**

1. Review the prescribed method/frequency for administration.

2. Review methods for insufflation, suppositories, and douching; practice good feminine hygiene.

3. Wear a pad to prevent clothing or bed linen from becoming stained with vaginal suppositories, especially if they contain iodine (which does stain). Change pad frequently and immediately upon staining because it may serve as a growth medium for organisms.

4. Sexual partner may be an asymptomatic carrier and may also require therapy to prevent reinfection of female. Use condoms during sexual intercourse while undergoing treatment to prevent reinfections.

**Outcomes/Evaluate**

• Negative cultures; resolution of infection

• Clinical/microscopic confirmation of eradication/prophylaxis of amebiasis and trichomoniasis

# AMINOGLYCOSIDES

*See also the following individual entries:*

> Amikacin sulfate
> Gentamicin sulfate
> Kanamycin sulfate
> Neomycin sulfate
> Paromomycin sulfate
> Tobramycin sulfate

**Action/Kinetics:** Broad-spectrum antibiotics believed to inhibit protein synthesis by binding irreversibly to ribosomes (30S subunit), thereby interfering with an initiation complex between messenger RNA and the 30S subunit. This leads to production of nonfunctional proteins; polyribosomes are split apart and are unable to synthesize protein. Usually bactericidal as a result of disruption of the bacterial cytoplasmic membrane. Poorly absorbed from the GI tract; usually administered parenterally (exceptions: some enteric infections of the GI tract and prior to surgery). Also absorbed from the peritoneum, bronchial tree, wounds, denuded skin, and joints. Distributed in the extracellular fluid and cross the placental barrier, but not the blood-brain barrier. Penetration of the CSF is increased when the meninges are inflamed.

Rapidly absorbed after IM injection. **Peak plasma levels, after IM:** Usually ½–2 hr. Measurable levels persist for 8–12 hr after a single administration. **t½:** 2–3 hr (increases sharply in impaired kidney function). Ranges of t½ from 24 to 110 hr have been observed. Excreted mainly unchanged in urine. Resistance develops slowly.

**Uses:** Are powerful antibiotics that induce serious side effects—do not use for minor infections. Gram-negative bacteria causing bone and joint infections, septicemia (including neonatal sepsis), skin and soft tissue infections (including those from burns), respiratory tract infections, postoperative infections, intra-abdominal infections (including peritonitis), UTIs. In combination with clindamycin for mixed aerobic-anaerobic infections. Also, see individual drugs.

Used for gram-positive bacteria only when other less toxic drugs are either ineffective or contraindicated. Use in CNS *Pseudomonas* infections such as meningitis or ventriculitis is questionable.

**Contraindications:** Hypersensitivity to aminoglycosides, long-term therapy (except streptomycin for tuberculosis). Use with extreme caution with impaired renal function or preexisting hearing impairment. Safe use in pregnancy and during lactation not established.

**Special Concerns:** Assess premature infants, neonates, and older clients closely as they are particularly sensitive to toxic effects. Considerable cross-allergenicity occurs among the aminoglycosides.

**Side Effects:** *Ototoxicity:* Both auditory and vestibular damage have been noted. The risk of ototoxicity and vestibular impairment is increased with poor renal function and in the elderly. Auditory symptoms include tinnitus and hearing impairment, while vestibular symptoms include dizziness, nystagmus, vertigo, and ataxia.

*Renal Impairment:* This may be characterized by cylindruria, oliguria, proteinuria, azotemia, hematuria, increase or decrease in frequency of urination; increased BUN, NPN, or creatinine; and increased thirst. *Neurotoxicity:* Neuromuscular blockade, headache, tremor, lethargy, paresthesia, peripheral neuritis (numbness, tingling, or burning of face/mouth), arachnoiditis, encephalopathy, acute organic brain syndrome. CNS depression, characterized by stupor, flaccidity, and rarely, *coma, and respiratory depression in infants.* Optic neuritis with blurred vision or loss of vision. *GI:* N&V, diarrhea, increased salivation, anorexia, weight loss. *Allergic:* Rash, urticaria, pruritus, burning, fever, stomatitis, eosinophilia. Rarely, *agranulocytosis and anaphylaxis.* Cross-allergy among aminoglycosides has been observed. *Miscellaneous:* Joint pain, *laryngeal edema, pulmonary fibrosis,* superinfection.

**OD** **Overdose Management:** *Symptoms:* Extension of side effects. *Treatment:* Undertake hemodialysis (preferred) or peritoneal dialysis.

**Drug Interactions**
*Bumetanide* / ↑ Risk of ototoxicity
*Capreomycin* / ↑ Muscle relaxation
*Cephalosporins* / ↑ Risk of renal toxicity
*Ciprofloxacin HCl* / Additive antibacterial activity
*Cisplatin* / Additive renal toxicity
*Colistimethate* / ↑ Muscle relaxation
*Digoxin* / Possible ↑ or ↓ effect of digoxin
*Ethacrynic acid* / ↑ Risk of ototoxicity
*Furosemide* / ↑ Risk of ototoxicity
*Methoxyflurane* / ↑ Risk of renal toxicity
*Penicillins* / ↓ Effect of aminoglycosides
*Polymyxins* / ↑ Muscle relaxation
*Skeletal muscle relaxants (surgical)* / ↑ Muscle relaxation
*Vancomycin* / Additive ototoxicity and renal toxicity
*Vitamin A* / ↓ Effect of vitamin A due to ↓ absorption from GI tract
**Laboratory Test Interferences:** ↑ BUN, BSP retention, creatinine, AST, ALT, bilirubin. ↓ Cholesterol values.

## NURSING CONSIDERATIONS

See also *General Nursing Considerations for All Anti-Infectives.*
**Administration/Storage**
1. Check expiration date.

2. Warn if drug being administered stings or causes a burning sensation.

3. During IM administration
• Inject deep into muscle mass to minimize transient pain.
• Use a Z track method for thin, elderly clients.
• Rotate/document injection sites.

4. With IV administration
• Dilute with compatible solution.
• Infuse at the rate ordered to prevent excessive serum concentrations.

5. Administer for only 7–10 days and avoid repeating course of therapy unless a serious infection is present that does not respond to other antibiotics.

6. Administer around the clock to maintain therapeutic drug levels.

**Assessment**

1. Assess for allergic reactions; note adverse reactions and hypersensitivity to anti-infective medications.

2. Obtain weight to ensure correct dosage.

3. Determine baseline liver, renal, auditory, and vestibular function; assess for nephrotoxicity.

4. Assess for presence and source(s) of infection. Document fever, culture/lab reports, and wound characteristics (i.e., color, odor, drainage).

**Interventions**

1. Monitor VS and I&O; encourage fluids to prevent renal tubule irritation.

2. Monitor drug levels; withhold drug and report if elevated, (e.g., levels > 30 mcg/mL of amikacin are considered toxic.)

3. With vestibular dysfunction protect by supervising ambulation and providing side rails; note (potential for) fall hazard.

4. Assess for ototoxicity; pretreatment audiograms may be helpful, as hearing loss is a dose-related side effect of drug therapy most commonly associated with amikacin, kanamycin, neomycin, or paromomycin. Tinnitus, dizziness, and loss of balance are also signs of vestibular injury and more commonly seen with gentamicin and streptomycin. The onset of deafness may occur several weeks after drug has been discontinued.

5. Do not administer concurrently or sequentially with a topical or systemic nephrotoxic or ototoxic drug (e.g., potent diuretics such as ethacrynic acid or furosemide) unless provider designates benefits outweigh the risks.

6. Observe for neuromuscular blockade with muscular weakness leading to apnea, when administered with a muscle relaxant or after anesthesia. Have calcium gluconate or neostigmine available to reverse blockade.

7. Note cells or casts in the urine, oliguria, proteinuria, lowered specific gravity, or increasing BUN or creatinine, all of which indicate altered renal function.

**Client/Family Teaching**

1. Review goals of therapy and prescribed method of administration.

2. Take at the prescribed time intervals, ATC, until prescription is finished.

3. Follow a well-balanced diet and consume at least 2–3 L/day of fluids.

4. Report symptoms of superinfection (black, furry tongue; loose, foul-smelling stools; vaginal itching).

5. Alterations in hearing, vision, and/or ambulation should also be reported.

**Outcomes/Evaluate**

• Negative culture reports
• Resolution of infection with ↓ WBCs, ↓ fever, ↓ drainage; symptomatic improvement
• Therapeutic drug levels

# AMPHETAMINES AND DERIVATIVES

*See also the following individual entries:*

Amphetamine sulfate
Dextroamphetamine sulfate
Mazindol
Methamphetamine hydrochloride
Phendimetrazine tartrate
Phenylpropanolamine hydrochloride

**Action/Kinetics:** Thought to act on the cerebral cortex and reticular activating system (including the medullary, respiratory, and vasomotor centers) by releasing norepinephrine from central adrenergic neurons. High doses cause release of dopamine from the mesolimbic system. The stimulatory effect on the CNS causes an increase in motor activity and mental alertness, a mood-elevating effect, a slight euphoric effect, and an anorexigenic effect. The anorexigenic effect is thought to be produced by direct stimulation of the satiety center in the lateral hypothalamic feeding center of the brain. Peripheral effects are mediated by alpha- and beta-adrenergic receptors and include increases in both systolic and diastolic BP and respiratory stimulation. Readily absorbed from the GI tract and distributed throughout most tissues, with the highest concentrations in the brain and CSF. Duration of anorexia (PO): 3–6 hr. Metabolized in liver and excreted by kidneys. Excreted slowly (5–7 days); cumulative effects may occur with continued administration.

Psychic stimulation is often followed by a rebound effect manifested as fatigue. Tolerance will develop to all drugs of this class. There is a relatively wide margin of safety between the therapeutic and toxic doses of amphetamines. However, both acute and chronic toxicity can occur.

**Uses:** See individual drugs.

**Contraindications:** Hyperthyroidism, advanced arteriosclerosis, nephritis, diabetes mellitus, hypertension, narrow-angle glaucoma, angina pectoris, CV disease, and individuals with hypersensitivity to these drugs. Use in emotionally unstable persons susceptible to drug abuse and in agitated states. Psychotic children. Lactation. Appetite suppressants in children less than 12 years of age. Within 14 days of MAO inhibitors.

**Special Concerns:** Use with caution in clients suffering from hyperexcitability states; in elderly, debilitated, or asthenic clients; and in clients with psychopathic personality traits or a history of homicidal or suicidal tendencies.

**Side Effects:** *CNS:* Nervousness, dizziness, depression, headache, insomnia, euphoria, symptoms of excitation. Rarely, psychoses. In children, manifestation of vocal and motor tics and Tourette's syndrome. *GI:* N&V, cramps, diarrhea, dry mouth, constipation, metallic taste, anorexia. *CV:* Arrhythmias, palpitations, dyspnea, pulmonary hypertension, peripheral hyper- or hypotension, precordial pain, fainting. *Dermatologic:* Symptoms of allergy including rash, urticaria, erythema, burning. Pallor. *GU:* Urinary frequency, dysuria. *Ophthalmologic:* Blurred vision, mydriasis. *Hematologic:* **Agranulocytosis,** leukopenia. *Endocrine:* Menstrual irregularities, gynecomastia, impotence, and changes in libido. *Miscellaneous:* Alopecia, increased motor activity, fever, sweating, chills, muscle pain, chest pain.

Long-term use results in psychic dependence, as well as a high degree of tolerance.

**OD** **Overdose Management:** *Symptoms of Acute Overdose (Toxicity):* Restlessness, irritability, insomnia, tremor, hyperreflexia, rhabdomyolysis, rapid respiration, **hyperpyrexia,** assaultiveness, hallucinations, panic states, sweating, mydriasis, flushing, hyperactivity, confusion, hypertension or hypotension, extrasystoles, tachypnea, fever, delirium, self-injury, arrhythmias, **seizures, coma, circulatory collapse, death. Death usually results from CV collapse or convulsions.** *Symptoms of Chronic Toxicity:* Chronic use/abuse is characterized by emotional lability, loss of appetite, severe dermatoses, hyperactivity, insomnia, irritability, somnolence, mental impairment, occupational deterioration, a tendency to withdraw from social contact, teeth grinding, continuous chewing, and

---

ulcers of the tongue and lips. Prolonged use of high doses can elicit symptoms of paranoid schizophrenia, including auditory and visual hallucinations and paranoid ideation. *Treatment of Acute Toxicity (Overdosage):*

• Symptomatic treatment. After oral ingestion, induce emesis or perform gastric lavage, followed by use of activated charcoal. Acidification of the urine increases the rate of excretion. Give fluids until urine flow is 3–6 mL/kg/hr; furosemide or mannitol may be beneficial.

• Maintain adequate circulation and respiration.

• CNS stimulation can be treated with chlorpromazine and psychotic symptoms with haloperidol. Hyperactivity can be treated with diazepam or a barbiturate. Reduce stimuli and maintain in a quiet, dim environment. Treat clients who have ingested an overdose of long-acting products for toxicity until all symptoms of overdosage have disappeared.

• IV phentolamine may be used for hypertension, whereas hypotension may be reversed by IV fluids and possibly vasopressors (used with caution).

**Drug Interactions**

*Acetazolamide* / ↑ Effect of amphetamine by ↑ renal tubular reabsorption

*Ammonium chloride* / ↓ Effect of amphetamine by ↓ renal tubular reabsorption

*Anesthetics, general* / ↑ Risk of cardiac arrhythmias

*Antihypertensives* / Amphetamines ↓ effect of antihypertensives

*Ascorbic acid* / ↓ Effect of amphetamine by ↓ renal tubular reabsorption

*Furazolidone* / ↑ Toxicity of anorexiants due to MAO activity of furazolidone

*Guanethidine* / ↓ Effect of guanethidine by displacement from its site of action

*Haloperidol* / ↓ Effect of amphetamine by ↓ uptake of drug at its site of action

*Insulin* / Amphetamines alter insulin requirements

*MAO inhibitors* / All peripheral, metabolic, cardiac, and central effects of amphetamine are potentiated for up to 2 weeks after termination of MAO inhibitor therapy (symptoms include hypertensive crisis with possible intracranial hemorrhage, hyperthermia, convulsions, coma); death may occur. ↓ Effect of amphetamine by ↓ uptake of drug into its site of action

*Methyldopa* / ↓ Hypotensive effect of methyldopa by ↑ sympathomimetic activity

*Phenothiazines* / ↓ Effect of amphetamine by ↓ uptake of drug at its site of action

*Sodium bicarbonate* / ↑ Effect of amphetamine by ↑ renal tubular reabsorption

*Thiazide diuretics* / ↑ Effect of amphetamine by ↑ renal tubular reabsorption

*Tricyclic antidepressants* / ↓ Effect of amphetamines

**Laboratory Test Interferences:** ↑ Urinary catecholamines, ↑ plasma corticosteroid levels.

**Dosage**
See individual drugs. Many compounds are timed-release preparations.

## NURSING CONSIDERATIONS
### Administration/Storage
1. If prescribed to suppress appetite, administer 30 min before anticipated meal time.
2. Use a small initial dose; then increase gradually as necessary.
3. Unless otherwise ordered, give the last dose of the day at least 6 hr before bedtime.
### Assessment
1. Identify meds currently taking, indications, and effectiveness.
2. Note physical conditions that would contraindicate using drugs in this category.
3. Note age and whether debilitated.
4. Monitor electrolytes, ECG, weight, VS, and CBC.

5. These drugs are under the Controlled Substances Act; follow appropriate policy for dispensing/handling to restrict availability and discourage abuse.

**Interventions**

1. If agitated or complains of sleeplessness, reduce dosage of drug.

2. If receiving MAO inhibitors or received them 7–14 days before amphetamine therapy, assess for hypertensive crisis. Monitor and report fever, marked sweating, excitation, delirium, tremors, or twitching; pad side rails and have suction available.

3. Monitor VS. Assess for arrhythmias, tachycardia, or hypertension. CV changes accompanied by psychotic syndrome usually indicate acute toxicity.

4. If somnolent or appears mentally or physically impaired, stop the drug. Observe for signs of psychologic dependence and drug tolerance.

5. Measure height to assess for growth inhibition.

**Client/Family Teaching**

1. When anorexiants are used for weight reduction, their effect lasts only 4–6 weeks; use is short term. Follow an established dietary and exercise regimen to maintain weight loss and attend a behavioral modification weight control program.

2. Take only as prescribed, 1 hr before meals and last dose 6 hr before bedtime to ensure adequate rest. Abrupt withdrawal may cause symptoms.

3. Diets high in fiber, fruit, and fluids assist to reduce drugs' constipating effects. See dietitian to discuss weight control and/or reducing diets and to assist with food selections and meal planning when weight loss is the goal.

4. Record food intake and weight daily the first week and then at least once a week. May become anorexic; report any persistent, severe weight loss so therapy can be adjusted.

5. Report any changes in attention span and ability to concentrate.

6. Take only as directed; do not share meds. Report if drug tolerance occurs.

7. Amphetamines may cause a false sense of euphoria and well being and mask extreme fatigue. These may impair judgment and ability to perform potentially hazardous tasks, such as operating a machine or an automobile. Using amphetamines to treat fatigue is inappropriate because rebound effects may be severe.

8. Seek medical assistance if experiencing extreme fatigue and depression once drug is discontinued. Periodic "drug holidays" may be ordered to assess progress and prevent dependence.

9. Avoid OTC medications and ingesting large amounts of caffeine in any form. Read labels for the detection of caffeine since this contributes to CV side effects.

10. Dry mouth may be managed by frequent rinsing, chewing sugarless gum, or sucking sugarless hard candies.

11. May alter insulin and dietary requirements. With diabetes, monitor blood sugar closely; adjustments in insulin, oral hypoglycemic agent, and/or dietary requirements may be needed.

12. Store safely out of child's reach.

**Outcomes/Evaluate**

• Improved attention span; ability to concentrate

• Weight reduction

• ↓ Episodes of narcolepsy

---

# ANGIOTENSIN-CONVERTING ENZYME (ACE) INHIBITORS

*See also the following individual entries:*

Benazepril hydrochloride
Captopril
Enalapril maleate
Fosinopril sodium
Lisinopril
Moexipril hydrochloride

Quinapril hydrochloride
Ramipril
Trandolapril

**Action/Kinetics:** Believed to act by suppressing the renin-angiotensin-aldosterone system. Renin, which is synthesized by the kidneys, produces angiotensin I, an inactive decapeptide derived from plasma globulin substrate. Angiotensin I is converted to angiotensin II by ACE. Angiotensin II is a potent vasoconstrictor that also stimulates secretion of aldosterone from the adrenal cortex, resulting in sodium and fluid retention. The ACE inhibitors prevent the conversion of angiotensin I to angiotensin II. This results in a decrease in plasma angiotensin II and subsequently a decrease in peripheral resistance and decreased aldosterone secretion (leading to sodium and fluid loss) and therefore a decrease in BP. There may be either no change or an increase in CO. Several weeks of therapy may be required to achieve the maximum effect to reduce BP. Standing and supine BPs are lowered to about the same extent. Are also antihypertensive in low renin hypertensive clients. ACE inhibitors are additive with thiazide diuretics in lowering blood pressure; however, β-blockers and captopril have less than additive effects when used with ACE inhibitors.

**Uses:** Alone or in combination with other antihypertensive agents (especially thiazide diuretics) for the treatment of hypertension. See also individual drug entries.

**Contraindications:** History of angioedema due to previous treatment with an ACE inhibitor.

**Special Concerns:** Use during the second and third trimesters of pregnancy can result in injury and even death to the developing fetus. May cause a profound drop in BP following the first dose; initiate therapy under close medical supervision. Use with caution in renal disease (especially renal artery stenosis) as increases in BUN and serum creatinine have occurred. Use with caution in clients with aortic stenosis due to possible decreased coronary perfusion following vasodilator use. With the exception of fosinopril (contraindicated), use with caution during lactation. Geriatric clients may show a greater sensitivity to the hypotensive effects of ACE inhibitors although these drugs may preserve or improve renal function and reverse LV hypertrophy. For most ACE inhibitors, safety and effectiveness have not been determined in children.

**Side Effects:** See individual entries. Side effects common to most ACE inhibitors include the following. *GI:* Abdominal pain, N&V, diarrhea, constipation, dry mouth. *CNS:* Sleep disturbances, insomnia, headache, dizziness, fatigue, nervousness, paresthesias. *CV:* Hypotension (especially following the first dose), palpitations, angina pectoris, *MI,* orthostatic hypotension, chest pain. *Hepatic:* Rarely, cholestatic jaundice progressing to **hepatic necrosis and death.** *Miscellaneous:* Chronic cough, dyspnea, increased sweating, diaphoresis, pruritus, rash, impotence, syncope, asthenia, arthralgia, myalgia. *Angioedema* of the face, lips, tongue, glottis, larynx, extremities, and mucous membranes. **Anaphylaxis.**

**OD** **Overdose Management:** *Symptoms:* Hypotension is the most common. *Treatment:* Supportive measures. The treatment of choice to restore BP is volume expansion with an IV infusion of NSS. Certain of the ACE inhibitors (captopril, enalaprilat, lisinopril) may be removed by hemodialysis.

**Drug Interactions**
*Allopurinol* / ↑ Risk of hypersensitivity reactions
*Anesthetics* / ↑ Risk of hypotension if used with anesthetics that also cause hypotension
*Antacids* / Possible ↓ bioavailability of ACE inhibitors
*Capsaicin* / Capsaicin may cause or worsen cough associated with ACE inhibitor use
*Digoxin* / ↑ Plasma digoxin levels
*Indomethacin* / ↓ Hypotensive effects of ACE inhibitors, especially

in low renin or volume-dependent hypertensive clients

*Lithium* / ↑ Serum lithium levels → ↑ risk of toxicity

*Phenothiazines* / ↑ Effect of ACE inhibitors

*Potassium-sparing diuretics* / ↑ Serum potassium levels

*Potassium supplements* / ↑ Serum potassium levels

*Thiazide diuretics* / Additive effect to ↓ BP

**Laboratory Test Interferences:** ↑ BUN and creatinine (both are transient and reversible). ↑ Liver enzymes, serum bilirubin, uric acid, blood glucose. Small ↑ in serum potassium.

**Dosage**
See individual drugs.

## NURSING CONSIDERATIONS

**Administration/Storage:** Do not interrupt or discontinue ACE inhibitor therapy without consulting provider.

**Assessment**

1. Note any previous therapy with ACE inhibitors and antihypertensive agents and the results.

2. Monitor VS (BP—both arms while lying, standing, and sitting), electrolytes, CBC, and renal function studies; check urine for protein (microalbuminuria).

3. Document hereditary angioedema (especially if caused by a deficiency of C1 esterase inhibitor).

4. Assess understanding of hypertension (or CHF) and prescribed therapy.

5. Document weight, risk factors, and medical problems. Identify lifestyle changes needed to achieve and maintain lowered BP. Assess motivation and ensure a trial of "good behavior" with dietary modifications and regular exercise for 3–6 months has been done.

**Interventions**

1. Assess for neutropenia (esp. with captopril); precludes drug therapy.

2. Report any evidence of angioedema (swelling of face, lips, extremities, tongue, mucous membranes, glottis, or larynx) esp. after first dose

(but may also be delayed response). Relieve S&S with antihistamines. If involves laryngeal edema, observe for airway obstruction. *Stop* drug; use epinephrine (1:1000 SC).

3. Monitor VS, I&O, weight, serum potassium, and renal function studies. Those hypovolemic due to diuretics, GI fluid loss, or salt restriction may exhibit severe hypotension after initial doses; supervise ambulation until drug response evident.

4. If undergoing surgery or general anesthesia with drugs that cause hypotension, ACE inhibitors will block angiotensin II formation; correct hypotension by volume expansion.

**Client/Family Teaching**

1. Take 1 hr before meals and only as directed.

2. Review prescribed dietary guidelines; do not use salt substitutes containing potassium.

3. Medication controls but does not cure hypertension; take as prescribed despite feeling better and do not stop abruptly.

4. Take BP readings at various times during the day and record to prevent treating "white collar" readings.

5. Do not perform activities that require mental alertness until drug effects realized; initially may cause dizziness, fainting, or lightheadedness.

6. Rise slowly from a lying position and dangle feet before standing; avoid sudden position changes to minimize postural effects.

7. Practice birth control; report if pregnancy suspected.

8. Report adverse side effects:
• Nonproductive, persistent, chronic cough
• Sore throat, fever, swelling of hands or feet, irregular heartbeat, chest pains, difficulty breathing, or hoarseness
• Excessive perspiration, dehydration, vomiting, and diarrhea
• Itching, joint pain, fever, or skin rash

9. Report edema and weight gain of more than 3 lb/day or 5 lb/week.

---

10. With diabetes (with or without hypertension), ACE inhibitors have been shown to reduce proteinuria and to slow the progression of renal disease.

11. Avoid any OTC medications, especially cold remedies, without approval.

12. NSAIDs include aspirin and may impair the hypotensive effects of ACE inhibitors while antacids may decrease bioavailability.

13. Avoid excessive amounts of caffeine (e.g., tea, coffee, cola).

14. Regular exercise, proper diet, weight loss, stress management, and adequate rest in conjunction with medications are needed in the overall management of hypertension. Additional interventions such as reducing alcohol use, discontinuing tobacco products, and reducing salt intake may also assist in BP control.

**Outcomes/Evaluate**
- ↓ BP
- Improvement in S&S of CHF
- ↓ Proteinuria/renal damage
- ↓Morbidity post-AMI

# ANTACIDS

*See also the following individual entries:*

Sodium bicarbonate

**General Statement:** Hydrochloric acid maintains the stomach at a pH (1–2) necessary for optimum activity of the digestive enzyme pepsin and for stimulating the release of secretin when the acid contents of the stomach pass into the duodenum. Under certain circumstances, however, people suffer adverse reactions due to gastric acidity ranging from heartburn to life-threatening peptic or duodenal ulcers. Although production of acid has an important role in the development of gastric and duodenal ulcers, other factors are also involved. These include endogenous histamine (which can stimulate gastric acid secretion), antigen-antibody reactions, and the psychologic makeup of the client. Acute and chronic GI disturbances are among the most common medical conditions requiring treatment. Various drugs and dietary measures are used for the treatment of hyperacidity states and ulcers, and the use of antacids is an important part of such regimens.

**Action/Kinetics:** Antacids act by neutralizing or reducing gastric acidity, thus increasing the pH of the stomach and relieving hyperacidity. If the pH is increased to 4, the activity of pepsin is inhibited. The ability of a specific antacid to neutralize acid is termed *acid-neutralizing capacity,* and antacids are selected on this basis. Acid-neutralizing capacity (ANC) is expressed as milliequivalents per milliliter and is defined by the HCl required to maintain an antacid suspension at pH 3.5 for 10 min in vitro. An antacid should neutralize at least 5 mEq/dose; also, to be considered an antacid, the compound should contribute to at least 25% of the ANC of a product.

Ideally, antacids should not be absorbed systemically, although substances such as sodium bicarbonate or calcium carbonate may produce significant systemic effects. The most effective dosage form for antacids is suspensions. Antacids also promote healing of peptic ulcers.

Antacids containing magnesium have a laxative effect, whereas those containing aluminum or calcium have a constipating effect. This is why clients are often given alternating doses of laxative and constipating antacids. Antacids containing aluminum bind with phosphate ions in the intestine forming the insoluble aluminum phosphate, which is excreted in the feces. This is of value in treating hyperphosphatemia of chronic renal failure. **Onset:** Depends on ability of the antacid to solubilize in the stomach and react with hydrochloric acid. The poorly soluble antacids (e.g., magnesium trisilicate) react slower with hydrochloric acid than do the more soluble compounds. **Duration of antacids:**

30 min if fasting; up to 3 hr if taken after meals.

**Uses:** Treatment of hyperacidity (heartburn, acid indigestion, sour stomach), gastric ulcer, duodenal ulcer, gastroesophageal reflux. Adjunct (with histamine $H_2$-receptor antagonists) in the treatment of hypersecretory conditions (e.g., Zollinger-Ellison syndrome), systemic mastocytosis, and multiple endocrine adenoma. Treatment of hypocalcemia, hypophosphatemia. Prophylaxis of renal calculi.

**Contraindications:** Sodium-containing products are contraindicated in CHF, hypertension, or conditions requiring a low-sodium diet. Pregnant or lactating women should not use antacids without physician approval. Children less than 6 years of age.

**Special Concerns:** Chronic use of aluminum-containing antacids may aggravate metabolic bone disease seen in geriatric clients; also, chronic use of aluminum-containing antacids may contribute to development of Alzheimer's disease. Taking too much of an antacid may result in an increased secretion of stomach acid. Antacids may mask the warning signs associated with ulcers and GI bleeding caused by NSAIDs.

**Side Effects:** *Aluminum-containing antacids:* Constipation, intestinal obstruction, aluminum intoxication, hypophosphatemia, osteomalacia. *Calcium carbonate, aluminum-magnesium hydroxide, magnesium oxide, soluble bismuth salts, sodium bicarbonate:* Milk-alkali syndrome (acute: headache, nausea, irritability, weakness; chronic: alkalosis, hypercalcemia, renal impairment). Rebound hyperacidity. *Magnesium-containing antacids:* Diarrhea, hypermagnesemia in clients with renal failure.

**Drug Interactions**

1. *Aluminum-containing antacids:* ↑ Effect of benzodiazepines. ↓ Effect of allopurinol, chloroquine, corticosteroids, diflunisal, digoxin, ethambutol, histamine $H_2$ antagonists, iron products, isoniazid, penicillamine, phenothiazines, tetracyclines, thyroid hormones, and ticlopidine by ↓ absorption from GI tract.

2. *Aluminum- and magnesium-containing antacids:* ↑ Effect of levodopa, quinidine, sulfonylureas, and valproic acid probably by ↓ excretion. ↓ Effect of benzodiazepines, captopril, corticosteroids, fluoroquinolones, histamine $H_2$ antagonists, hydantoins, iron products, ketoconazole, penicillamine, phenothiazines, salicylates, tetracyclines, and ticlopidine either by ↓ absorption from GI tract or ↑ excretion.

3. *Calcium-containing antacids:* ↑ Effect of quinidine by ↓ excretion. ↓ Effect of fluoroquinolones, hydantoins, iron products, salicylates, and tetracyclines either by ↓ absorption from GI tract or ↑ excretion.

4. *Magnesium-containing antacids:* ↑ Effect of dicumarol, quinidine, and sulfonylureas probably by ↓ excretion. ↓ Effect of benzodiazepines, corticosteroids, digoxin, histamine $H_2$ antagonists, hydantoins, iron products, nitrofurantoin, penicillamine, phenothiazines, tetracyclines, and ticlopidine either by ↓ absorption from GI tract or ↑ excretion.

5. *Sodium bicarbonate:* ↑ Effect of amphetamines, flecainide, quinidine, and sympathomimetics probably by ↑ excretion. ↓ Effect of benzodiazepines, hydantoins, ketoconazole, lithium, methenamine, methotrexate, salicylates, sulfonylureas, and tetracyclines either by ↓ absorption from GI tract or ↑ excretion.

**Dosage** ————————
See individual drugs.

# NURSING CONSIDERATIONS
**Administration/Storage**

1. Clients who have an active peptic ulcer should take antacids every hour during waking hours for the first 2 weeks.
2. For PUD, it is recommended that most antacids be taken 1 hr and 3 hr after meals and at bedtime.
3. Tablets should be thoroughly

chewed before swallowing and followed by a glass of milk or water. Effervescent tablets should completely dissolve in water before ingestion.

4. Liquid preparations have a more rapid action time and greater activity than tablets. Refrigerate to improve palatability.

5. Shake liquid suspensions thoroughly before pouring the medication. After administering, follow with water to ensure passage to the stomach. When administering via feeding tube, flush tube with water.

6. The absorption rate of many drugs may be affected by antacids. Enteric-coated tablets may dissolve prematurely. Therefore, if other oral drugs are to be taken, it should be done at least 2 hr after ingestion of the antacid.

7. Administer laxative or cathartic dose at bedtime, as medication takes about 8 hr to be effective and the effect should not interfere with the client's rest.

**Assessment**

1. Document indications for therapy and type and onset of symptoms.

2. Note subjective reports of heartburn, indigestion, or epigastric pain. Document any precipitating factors such as foods as well as location, character, and duration of discomfort.

3. List other drugs taking to ensure none interact unfavorably.

4. Note if the client has problems with diarrhea. Antacids containing magnesium may have a laxative effect, worsening this problem; use aluminum-based product instead.

5. Determine if the client has a history of cardiac disease or hypertension. These clients often are on low-sodium diets, so prescribed antacids should also be low in sodium.

6. Note any radiologic studies or endoscopic findings; document H. pilorior urease or slant test results.

**Interventions**

1. Clients taking antacid preparations containing calcium or aluminum are prone to constipation. Encourage fluid intake of 2–3 L/day unless contraindicated and also increased consumption of foods high in bulk and fiber.

2. If the client has renal failure, increasing fluid intake to avoid constipation is not an option. Stool softeners may be necessary. Also, absorption of Na, Mg, Al, or Ca may precipitate alkalosis.

3. If constipation persists, determine if changing the antacid or using laxatives and/or enemas may be of some benefit.

4. Clients taking antacids that contain magnesium may report diarrhea. Document and report as a change in antacid or alternating a magnesium-based antacid with an aluminum- or calcium-based antacid may be indicated. Magnesium salts have a cathartic effect.

**Client/Family Teaching**

1. Take the tablets with water. The liquid acts as a vehicle, transporting the medication to the stomach, where the desired drug action occurs.

2. Take the drug at the prescribed times. Some may need to be taken on an empty stomach, whereas others, such as those used to bind phosphate, may need to be taken with meals.

3. Advise that refrigeration may improve taste.

4. Report any persistent constipation or diarrhea.

5. Advise that consumption of large amounts of TUMS can cause acid rebound.

6. Avoid taking OTC preparations unless specifically ordered.

7. Do not smoke or use alcoholic beverages as these alter drug effects.

8. Report any evidence of GI bleeding (dark black or tarry stools, coffee ground emesis).

9. Discuss the importance of following the specific dietary regime established as well as adhering to the medication protocol. Explain that antacids should be taken for 4–6 weeks after symptoms have disappeared as healing of the ulcer is not correlated with the disappearance of symptoms.

10. Instruct client to report if the

symptoms for which they are being treated show little or no improvement after 2 weeks of therapy.

**Outcomes/Evaluate**
- Improvement in or resolution of pretreatment symptoms
- ↓ gastric pain and irritation
- Evacuation of a soft, formed stool
- ↑ Gastric pH
- Duodenal ulcer healing
- Prophylaxis of renal calculi

---

# ANTHELMINTICS

*See also the following individual entries:*

> Albendazole
> Ivermectin
> Mebendazole
> Oxamniquine
> Praziquantel
> Pyrantel pamoate
> Thiabendazole

**General Statement:** Helminths (worms) may infect the intestinal lumen or the worm also may migrate to a particular tissue. Treatment of helminth infections is complicated by the fact that a worm may have one or more morphologic stages. Thus, it is important to ensure that therapy rids the body of eggs and larvae, as well as worms. Also, a client may be infected by more than one type of worm. Factors such as availability and cost of the drug, toxicity, ease of administration, and how long it takes to complete therapy also have a significant impact on successful treatment of helminths. Accurate diagnosis is extremely important before treatment is started because its success depends on selecting the drug best suited for the eradication of a specific infestation. Parasites that infest only the intestinal tract can be eradicated by locally acting drugs. Other parasites enter tissues and must be treated by drugs that are absorbed from the GI tract.

Since many parasitic infestations are transmitted by persons sharing bathroom facilities, the provider may wish to examine all members of the household for parasitic infestation. Treatment is often accompanied or followed by repeated laboratory examinations to determine whether the parasite has been eradicated.

Helminths can be divided into three groups: cestodes (flatworms, tapeworms), nematodes (roundworms), and trematodes (flukes). The following is a brief description of the more common helminths and the drug of choice to treat infections by that particular helminth.

**CESTODES (FLATWORMS, TAPEWORMS):** The more common tapeworms are the beef tapeworm (*Taenia saginata*), pork tapeworm (*T. solium*), dwarf tapeworm (*Hymenolepis nana*), and fish tapeworm (*Diphyllobothrium latum*). Tapeworm infestations are difficult to eradicate. **Drug treatment:** Praziquantel.

**NEMATODES: 1. Filaria (filariasis).** Infections due to *Wuchereria bancrofti, Brugia malayi,* and *B. timori* are transmitted by mosquitoes. Mosquito control is the best means of combating this infestation. Other filarial infections include *Loa loa,* transmitted by the bite of a horsefly, and *Onchocerca volvulus* (onchocerciasis, river blindness), which is transmitted by the bite of a blackfly. **Drug treatment:** Diethylcarbamazine. Suramin sodium (available from Centers for Disease Control) is used to treat onchocerciasis.

**2. Hookworm (uncinariasis).** Intestinal infection caused by *Ancylostoma duodenale* or *Necator americanus*. **Drug treatment:** Mebendazole or pyrantel pamoate.

**3. Pinworm (enterobiasis).** Caused by *Enterobius vermicularis*. **Drug treatment:** Mebendazole, pyrantel pamoate, thiabendazole.

**4. Roundworm (ascariasis).** Caused by *Ascaris lumbricoides.*

---

**Drug treatment:** Mebendazole, pyrantel pamoate.

**5. Trichinosis.** Caused by *Trichinella spiralis*, these parasites are transmitted by the consumption of raw or inadequately cooked pork. **Drug treatment:** Corticosteroids to control the inflammation caused by systemic infestation; mebendazole, thiabendazole.

**6. Threadworm (strongyloidiasis).** This parasite (*Strongyloides stercoralis*) infests the upper GI tract. **Drug treatment:** Thiabendazole.

**7. Whipworm (trichuriasis).** This threadlike parasite (*Trichuris trichiura*) lodges in the mucosa of the cecum. **Drug treatment:** Mebendazole.

**TREMATODES:** Schistosomiasis (blood flukes or bilharziasis) can be transmitted by *Schistosoma mansoni, S. japonicum, S. haematobium,* and *S. mekongi.* The infection is difficult to eradicate. **Drug treatment:** Praziquantel, oxamniquine (*S. mansoni* only).

**Side Effects:** N&V, cramps, and diarrhea are common to most.

## NURSING CONSIDERATIONS

See also *General Nursing Considerations for All Anti-Infectives.*

**Assessment**

1. Document type and onset of symptoms, causative factors, and exposure(s).

2. Obtain specimens for microscopic exam.

3. Determine if pregnant; note ulcer presence.

**Client/Family Teaching**

1. Review instructions regarding diet, cathartics, enemas, meds, and follow-up tests.

2. *Good hygienic practices reduce the incidence of helminthiasis.*

3. Notify school that child is undergoing therapy; identify close contacts that should also be treated.

4. Specific practices are as follows:

PINWORMS

1. Therapy consists of a single dose with meals and is repeated in 2 weeks.

2. Prevent infestation with pinworms by:

• Washing hands with soap and water before and after contact with infected person and when changing their clothes or bed linens

• Washing hands frequently during the day, always after toileting, and before meals

• Keeping nails short

• Washing ova from anal area in the a.m. to prevent itching

• Applying ointment to anal area to reduce scratching, which transfers pinworms. Scratching causes pinworms to attach to the fingers, which when placed in the mouth causes reinfection

• Changing clothes daily and checking for evidence of eggs or worms

• Wearing tight underpants

• Wearing gloves to prepare food

• Washing linens in hot water

• Not sharing washcloths and towels and changing/laundering regularly

• Disinfecting toilet daily

• For several days after therapy, wet mop or vacuum bedroom floor; do not sweep, as this spreads eggs

• Wash bed linens and night clothes after therapy and do not shake

3. Eggs are not visible but contaminate everything they come in contact with (i.e., food, hands, clothes, linens, rugs). Eggs floating in the air can be swallowed and cause infestation; is very contagious and easily transmissable and all family members need to be checked.

4. After treatment, swab the perianal area each morning with transparent tape and return to provider. A cure is considered when no further eggs are found on microscopic exam for 7 consecutive days.

ROUNDWORMS, HOOKWORMS, WHIPWORMS:

1. Two to 3 weeks after therapy, stools should be microscopically examined for fecal egg count.

2. Record stool color and consistency; examine for expulsed worm.

3. Examine results of the enema for the head of the worm.

4. Advise that:

• Stools must go to the lab warm and be examined daily until no further roundworm ova are found

• Wash hands with soap and water frequently during the day, always after toileting, and before eating

• Wash all fruits and vegetables before eating; cook meats and vegetables thoroughly

• Wear shoes, do not defecate outside, use a bathroom, and double flush to ensure proper excretion disposal

TREMATODES:

1. Dizziness, drowsiness, N&V, headache, diarrhea, and pruritis may occur 3 hr after dose of med and last for several hours.

2. Report any low-grade fever, discoloration of urine, or seizure activity.

3. With prior seizure disorder, should hospitalize for treatment due to change in seizure threshold.

**Outcomes/Evaluate**

• Knowledge of illness, prevention of transmission, and eradication/expulsion of organism

• Causes for repeated infestation; need for further treatment

# ANTIANEMIC DRUGS

*See also the following individual entries:*

Ferrous fumarate
Ferrous gluconate
Ferrous sulfate
Ferrous sulfate, dried

**General Statement:** Anemia refers to the many clinical conditions in which there is a deficiency in the number of RBCs or in the hemoglobin level within those cells. There are many types of anemia. However, the two main categories are (1) iron-deficiency anemias, resulting from greater than normal loss or destruction of blood cells, and (2) megaloblastic anemias, resulting from deficient production of blood cells. The cause of the iron deficiency must be determined before therapy is started.

**Action/Kinetics:** The RDA for iron is 90–300 mg/day. Iron is absorbed from the GI tract through the mucosal cells where it combines with the protein transferrin. This complex is transported in the body to bone marrow where iron is incorporated into hemoglobin. Absorption kinetics depend on the iron salt ingested and on the degree of deficiency. Under normal circumstances, iron is well conserved by the body although small amounts are lost through shedding of skin, hair, and nails and in feces, perspiration, urine, breast milk, and during menstruation. Iron is highly bound to protein.

**Uses:** Prophylaxis and treatment of iron-deficiency anemia. Iron preparations are particularly suitable for the treatment of anemias in infants and children, in blood donors, during pregnancy, and in clients with chronic blood loss. Optimum therapeutic responses are usually noted within 2–4 weeks. *Investigational:* Clients receiving epoetin therapy (failure to give iron supplements either IV or PO can impair the hematologic response to epoetin).

**Contraindications:** Hemosiderosis, hemochromatosis, peptic ulcer, regional enteritis, and ulcerative colitis. Hemolytic anemia, pyridoxine-responsive anemia, and cirrhosis of the liver.

**Special Concerns:** Allergic reactions may result due to certain products containing tartrazine and some products containing sulfites.

**Side Effects:** *GI:* Constipation, gastric irritation, nausea, abdominal cramps, anorexia, vomiting, and diarrhea. These effects may be minimized by administering preparations as a coated tablet. Soluble iron preparations may stain the teeth.

---

**OD** **Overdose Management:**
*Symptoms:* Symptoms occur in four stages—(1) Lethargy, N&V, abdominal pain, weak and rapid pulse, tarry stools, dehydration, acidosis, hypotension, and *coma* within 1–6 hr. (2) If client survives, symptoms subside for about 24 hr. (3) Within 24–48 hr symptoms return with *diffuse vascular congestion, shock, pulmonary edema, acidosis, seizures, anuria, hyperthermia, and death.* (4) If client survives, pyloric or antral stenosis, hepatic cirrhosis, and CNS damage are seen within 2–6 weeks. Toxic reactions are more likely to occur after parenteral administration.*Treatment (Iron Toxicity):*

- General supportive measures.
- Maintain a patent airway, respiration, and circulation.
- Induce vomiting with syrup of ipecac followed by gastric lavage using tepid water or 1%–5% sodium bicarbonate (to convert from ferrous sulfate to ferrous carbonate, which is poorly absorbed and less irritating). Saline cathartics can also be used.
- Deferoxamine is indicated for clients with serum iron levels greater than 300 mg/dL. Deferoxamine is usually given IM, but in severe cases of poisoning it may be given IV. Hydration should be maintained.
- It may be necessary to treat for shock, acidosis, renal failure, and seizures.

**Drug Interactions**
*Allopurinol* / May ↑ hepatic iron levels
*Antacids, oral* / ↓ Effect of iron preparations due to ↓ absorption from GI tract
*Chloramphenicol* / Chloramphenicol ↑ serum iron levels
*Cholestyramine* / ↓ Effect of iron preparations due to ↓ absorption from GI tract
*Cimetidine* / ↓ Effect of iron preparations due to ↓ absorption from GI tract
*Pancreatic extracts* / ↓ Effect of iron preparations due to ↓ absorption from GI tract

*Penicillamine* / ↓ Effect of penicillamine due to ↓ absorption from GI tract
*Fluoroquinolones* / ↓ Effect of fluoroquinolones due to ↓ absorption from GI tract due to formation of a ferric ion-quinolone complex
*Levodopa* / ↓ GI absorption and ↓ effect of levodopa due to formation of chelates with iron salts
*Methyldopa* / ↓ Effect of methyldopa due to ↓ absorption from GI tract
*Tetracyclines* / ↓ Effect of tetracyclines due to ↓ absorption from GI tract; also, ↓ absorption of iron salts
*Vitamin E* / Vitamin E ↓ response to iron therapy
**Laboratory Test Interferences:** Iron-containing drugs may affect electrolyte balance determinations.

**Dosage**
See individual drugs. Duration of therapy: 2–4 months longer than the time needed to reverse anemia, usually 6 or more months.

## NURSING CONSIDERATIONS
### Administration/Storage
1. For infants and young children, administer liquid preparation with a dropper. Deposit liquid well back against the cheek.
2. Eggs and milk or coffee and tea consumed with a meal or 1 hr after may significantly inhibit absorption of dietary iron.
3. Ingestion of calcium and iron supplements with food can decrease iron absorption by one-third; iron absorption is not decreased if calcium carbonate is used and taken between meals.
4. Do not crush or chew sustained-release products.

### Assessment
1. Take a drug history, including:
- Antacid use; any other drugs that may interact
- OTC drugs, i.e., iron compounds or vitamin E, being used
- Recent abdominal surgery; all currently prescribed drugs
- Allergy to sulfites or tartrazines (may be present in some products)

2. Ask about any GI bleeding; tarry stools or bright blood in stool or vomitus.

3. Assess for thalassemia; obtain hemoglobin electrophoresis, as iron administration could be lethal.

4. Note any complaints of fatigue, pallor, poor skin turgor, or change in mental status, especially among the elderly.

5. Assess nutritional status and diet history through questioning and intake if possible.

6. Pregnancy is an indication for iron prophylactically.

7. Review pregnancies and menstruation history; note frequency, amounts, and heavy or abnormal bleeding.

8. Monitor VS, CBC, chemistry profile, stool for occult blood, reticulocytes, serum transferrin, and iron panel results. Note cause (i.e., iron-deficient or megaloblastic anemia) or if further workup anemia is needed.

**Interventions**

1. Check stools for occult blood; drugs may alter color.

2. Discourage symptom-based self-medication with iron.

3. Coated tablets may diminish GI effects such as nausea, constipation or diarrhea, gastric irritation, and abdominal cramps.

4. Treatment for iron intoxication (see symptoms of iron toxicity):
- Stop parenteral administration; notify provider.
- Monitor VS for 48 hr; a second crisis may occur within 12–48 hr of the first.
- Follow guidelines for *Treatment of Iron Toxicity*.

5. Discontinue if 500 mg of iron daily does not cause a 1 g-rise of hemoglobin in 1 mo.

6. Will reduce tetracycline absorption. If to receive both, allow at least 2 hr to elapse between doses.

**Client/Family Teaching**

1. Adhere to prescribed regimen; report any problems immediately.

2. Review the form of iron prescribed (bi- or trivalent) and frequency of administration.

3. Take with meals to reduce gastric irritation. Milk products, eggs, and antacids inhibit absorption so avoid unless taking ferrous lactate. Coffee and tea consumed within 1 hr of meals may inhibit absorption of dietary iron.

4. Taking preparations with citrus juices enhances iron absorption.

5. May cause indigestion, change in stool color (black and tarry or dark green), abdominal cramps, diarrhea, or constipation; may be relieved by changing the med, dosage, or time of administration.

6. Increase intake of fruit, fiber, and fluids to minimize constipating effects. Eat a well-balanced diet, including foods high in iron (i.e., meat proteins, dried fruits). Poor families may consume foods they can afford (e.g., raisins, dark green leafy vegetables, and liver versus apricots or prunes).

7. Iron preparations are extremely dangerous for children; an overdosage can be fatal, so store out of reach.

8. Dilute liquid preparations well with water or fruit juice and use a straw to minimize teeth staining.

9. Pregnant women need an iron-rich diet. The American Academy of Pediatrics recommends an iron supplement for infants during their first year of life.

10. Follow administration guidelines for each product to minimize side effects. Do not self-medicate with vitamin, mineral, and iron supplements.

**Outcomes/Evaluate**

- Resolution of anemia; If hemoglobin has not increased 1 g in 4 weeks, then diagnosis should be reconfirmed.
- Improvement in exercise tolerance and level of fatigue
- Improvement in skin pallor, color of nail beds, hemoglobin and iron levels

# ANTIANGINAL DRUGS–NITRATES/ NITRITES

*See also the following individual entries:*

Amyl nitrite
Isosorbide dinitrate
Isosorbide mononitrate, oral
Nitroglycerin IV
Nitroglycerin sublingual
Nitroglycerin sustained release
Nitroglycerin topical ointment
Nitroglycerin transdermal system
Nitroglycerin translingual spray

**General Statement:** Three groups of drugs are currently used for the treatment of angina. These agents include the nitrates/nitrites, beta-adrenergic blocking agents, and calcium channel blocking drugs.

**Action/Kinetics:** Nitrates relax vascular smooth muscle by stimulating production of intracellular cyclic guanosine monophosphate. Dilation of postcapillary vessels decreases venous return to the heart due to pooling of blood; thus, LV end-diastolic pressure (preload) is reduced. Relaxation of arterioles results in a decreased systemic vascular resistance and arterial pressure (afterload). The oxygen requirements of the myocardium are reduced and there is more efficient redistribution of blood flow through collateral channels in myocardial tissue. Diastolic, systolic, and mean BP are decreased. Also, elevated central venous and pulmonary capillary wedge pressures, pulmonary vascular resistance, and systemic vascular resistance are reduced. Reflex tachycardia may occur due to the overall decrease in BP. Cardiac index may increase, decrease, or remain the same; those with elevated left ventricular filling pressure and systemic vascular resistance values with a depressed cardiac index are likely to see improvement of the cardiac index. The onset and duration depend on the product and route of administration (sublingual, topical, transder-

mal, parenteral, oral, and buccal).
**Onset:** Less than 1 min for amyl nitrite to 1 to 3 min for IV, sublingual, translingual, and transmucosal nitroglycerin or sublingual isosorbide dinitrate; 20 to 60 min for sustained-release, topical, and transdermal nitroglycerin or oral isosorbide dinitrate or mononitrate; and up to 4 hr for sustained-release isosorbide dinitrate. **Duration of action:** 3 to 5 min for amyl nitrite and IV nitroglycerin; 30 to 60 min for sublingual or translingual nitroglycerin; several hours for transmucosal, sustained-release, or topical nitroglycerin and all isosorbide dinitrate products; and up to 24 hr for transdermal nitroglycerin.

**Uses:** Treatment and prophylaxis of acute angina pectoris (use sublingual, transmucosal, or translingual nitroglycerin; amyl nitrite). Nitrates are first-line therapy for unstable angina. Prophylaxis of chronic angina pectoris (topical, transdermal, translingual, transmucosal, or oral sustained-release nitroglycerin; isosorbide dinitrate and mononitrate; erythrityl tetranitrate; pentaerythritol tetranitrate). IV nitroglycerin is used to decrease BP in surgical procedures resulting in hypertension, as well as an adjunct in treating hypertension or CHF associated with MI. *Investigational:* Nitroglycerin ointment has been used as an adjunct in treating Raynaud's disease. Also, isosorbide dinitrate with prostaglandin $E_1$ for peripheral vascular disease. Sublingual and topical nitroglycerin and oral nitrates have been used to decrease cardiac workload in clients with acute MI and in CHF.

**Contraindications:** Sensitivity to nitrites, which may result in severe hypotensive reactions, MI, or tolerance to nitrites. Severe anemia, cerebral hemorrhage, recent head trauma, postural hypotension, closed angle glaucoma, impaired hepatic function, hypertrophic cardiomyopathy, hypotension, recent MI. PO dosage forms should not be used in clients with GI hypermotility or with malabsorption syndrome. IV nitroglycerin should not be used in clients with hypotension, uncorrected hypovolemia, inadequate cerebral circulation, constrictive pericarditis, increased ICP, or pericardial tamponade.

**Special Concerns:** Use with caution during lactation and in glaucoma. Tolerance to the antianginal and vascular effects may occur. Safety and efficacy have not been determined during lactation and in children.

**Side Effects:** *CNS:* Headaches (most common) which may be severe and persistent, restlessness, dizziness, weakness, apprehension, vertigo, anxiety, insomnia, confusion, nightmares, hypoesthesia, hypokinesia, dyscoordination. *CV:* Postural hypotension (common) with or without paradoxical bradycardia and increased angina, tachycardia, palpitations, syncope, rebound hypertension, crescendo angina, retrosternal discomfort, *CV collapse,* atrial fibrillation, PVCs, *arrhythmias. GI:* N&V, dyspepsia, diarrhea, dry mouth, abdominal pain, involuntary passing of feces and urine, tenesmus, tooth disorder. *Dermatologic:* Crusty skin lesions, pruritus, rash, exfoliative dermatitis, cutaneous vasodilation with flushing. *GU:* Urinary frequency, impotence, dysuria. *Respiratory:* Upper respiratory tract infection, bronchitis, pneumonia. *Allergic:* Itching, wheezing, tracheobronchitis. *Miscellaneous:* Perspiration, muscle twitching, methemoglobinemia, cold sweating, blurred vision, diplopia, *hemolytic anemia,* arthralgia, edema, malaise, neck stiffness, increased appetite, rigors. **Topical use:** Peripheral edema, contact dermatitis.

Tolerance can occur following chronic use. Nitrites convert hemoglobin to methemoglobin, which impairs the oxygen-carrying capacity of the blood, resulting in *anemic hypoxia.* This interaction is dangerous in clients with preexisting anemia.

**OD** **Overdose Management:** *Symptoms (Toxicity):* Severe toxicity is rarely encountered with therapeutic use. Symptoms include hypotension, flushing, tachycardia, headache, palpitations, vertigo, perspiring skin followed by cold and cyanotic skin, visual disturbances, syncope, nausea, dizziness, diaphoresis, initial hyperpnea, dyspnea and slow breathing, slow pulse, *heart block,* vomiting with the possibility of bloody diarrhea and colic, anorexia, and increased ICP with symptoms of confusion, moderate fever, and paralysis. Tissue hypoxia (due to methemoglobinemia) may result in *cyanosis, metabolic acidosis, coma, seizures, and death due to CV collapse. Treatment (Toxicity):*
• Induction of emesis or gastric lavage followed by activated charcoal (nitrates are usually rapidly absorbed from the stomach). Gastric lavage may be used if the drug has been recently ingested.
• Maintain in a recumbent shock position and keep warm. Give oxygen and artificial respiration if required.
• Monitor methemoglobin levels.
• Elevate legs and administer IV fluids to treat severe hypotension and reflex tachycardia. Phenylephrine or methoxamine may also be helpful.
• Do not use epinephrine and similar drugs as they are ineffective in reversing severe hypotension.

**Drug Interactions**
*Acetylcholine* / Effects ↓ when used with nitrates
*Alcohol, ethyl* / Hypotension and CV collapse due to vasodilator effect of both agents
*Antihypertensive drugs* / Additive hypotension
*Aspirin* / ↑ Serum levels and effects of nitrates
*Beta-adrenergic blocking drugs* / Additive hypotension
*Calcium channel blocking drugs* / Additive hypotension, including significant orthostatic hypotension
*Dihydroergotamine* / ↑ Effect of dihydroergotamine due to increased bioavailability or antagonism resulting in ↓ antianginal effects

*Heparin* / Possible ↓ effect of heparin

*Narcotics* / Additive hypotensive effect

*Phenothiazines* / Additive hypotension

*Sympathomimetics* / ↓ Effect of nitrates; also, nitrates may ↓ effect of sympathomimetics resulting in hypotension

**Laboratory Test Interferences:** ↑ Urinary catecholamines. False negative ↓ in serum cholesterol.

**Dosage** —————————

See individual agents.

## NURSING CONSIDERATIONS

**Administration/Storage**

1. It is important to understand the appropriate use of each of the available dosage forms. Do not change from one brand to another without consulting the provider or pharmacist as products manufactured by different companies may not be equivalent.

2. Store tablets and capsules tightly closed in their original container. Avoid exposure to air, heat, and moisture.

3. Take oral nitrates on an empty stomach with a glass of water.

4. Use inhalation products either lying or sitting down.

5. Inhalation products are flammable; do not use under situations where they might ignite.

**Assessment**

1. Note any sensitivity to nitrites.

2. Document location, intensity, duration, extension, and any precipitating factors (i.e., activity, stress) surrounding anginal pain. Use a pain-rating scale to rank pain.

3. If history of anemia, administer with extreme caution.

4. Nitrates are contraindicated with elevated intracranial pressure.

5. Determine experience with self-administered medications; note if SL tablets ordered for the bedside.

6. Note any changes in ECG or elevated cardiac panel. Document results of echocardiogram, stress test, and/or catheterization.

**Interventions**

1. While hospitalized, note drug required to keep angina under control. Record:
- How frequently given
- Intensity of pain (use a pain-rating scale; rate pain initially and 5 min after administration)
- Duration of attacks
- Whether relief is partial or complete
- Time it takes for relief to occur
- Any side effects

2. Report when consumed so effectiveness can be determined and usage monitored.

3. Monitor VS. Assess for sensitivity to hypotensive effects of nitrites (N&V, pallor, restlessness, and CV collapse).

4. Monitor for hypotension when receiving additional drugs; adjustment may be necessary. Supervise activities/ ambulation until drug effects realized.

5. Assess for signs of tolerance, which occur following chronic use but may begin several days after starting treatment; manifested by absence of response to the usual dose. (Nitrites may be discontinued temporarily until tolerance is lost, and then reinstituted. During interim, other vasodilators may be used.)

6. Observe for nausea, vomiting, drowsiness, headache, or visual disturbances with long-term therapy (prolonged effects which require a change in drug).

7. Note change in activity and response to drug therapy. Determine if less discomfort experienced when performing regular activity.

**Client/Family Teaching**

1. Take PO medications on an empty stomach. The drug decreases myocardial oxygen demand and reduces workload of the heart.

2. To prevent postural hypotension, take SL tabs while sitting or lying down. Make position changes slowly and rise only after dangling feet for several minutes.

3. Elderly clients should sit or lie down when taking nitroglycerin;

prone to hypotensive effects and may become dizzy and fall.

4. Brand interchange is not recommended due to differences in effectiveness between products manufactured by different companies.

5. Always carry SL tablets for use in aborting an attack. Check expiration date; replace when needed or every 6 mo.

6. A burning sensation under the tongue attests to drug potency.

7. Carry SL tablets in a *glass* bottle, tightly capped. Keep in original container as heat, moisture, and air cause deterioration. Do not use plastic containers; drug deteriorates in plastic; avoid child-proof caps as client must get to the tablets quickly.

8. If pain is not relieved in 5 min by first SL tablet, take up to 2 more tablets at 5-min intervals. If pain has not subsided 5 min after third tablet, client should be taken to the emergency room; *do not* drive.

9. Take SL tabs 5–15 min prior to any situation likely to cause pain (e.g., climbing stairs, sexual intercourse, exposure to cold weather).

10. Record attacks; report any increase in the frequency/intensity of attacks and loss of effectiveness.

11. Schedule frequent rest periods, pace activities, and avoid stressful situations. Use Tylenol for drug-induced headaches.

12. Follow instructions on how to apply topical nitroglycerin. Some advise removing at bedtime and replacing upon arising; some studies support a nitrate-free period of at least 8 hr may reduce or prevent nitrate tolerance.

13. Avoid alcohol; nitrite syncope, a severe shock-like state, may occur.

14. Do not smoke. Review risks and life-style changes necessary to prevent further CAD (i.e., weight control, dietary changes, ↓ salt intake, modified regular exercise program, no alcohol/tobacco, and stress reduction).

15. Have family or significant other learn CPR; survival rate is greatly increased when CPR is initiated immediately.

16. Carry ID and list of prescribed drugs. Know what you are taking and why.

**Outcomes/Evaluate**
- ↓ Myocardial oxygen requirements; ↑ activity tolerance
- Improved myocardial perfusion
- Relief of coronary artery spasm

# ANTIARRHYTHMIC DRUGS

*See also the following individual entries:*

Adenosine
Amiodarone hydrochloride
Bretylium tosylate
Calcium Channel Blocking Drugs
Digitoxin
Digoxin
Diltiazem hydrochloride
Disopyramide phosphate
Flecainide acetate
Ibutilide fumarate
Lidocaine hydrochloride
Moricizine hydrochloride
Phenytoin
Phenytoin sodium
Procainamide hydrochloride
Propafenone hydrochloride
Propranolol hydrochloride
Quinidine bisulfate
Quinidine gluconate
Quinidine polygalacturonate
Quinidine sulfate
Tocainide hydrochloride
Verapamil

**General Statement:** Cardiac arrhythmias are altered patterns of contraction or marked increases or decreases in the rate of the heart which reduce the ability of the heart to pump blood. Some examples of cardiac arrhythmias are *premature ventricular beats, ventricular tachycardia, atrial flutter, atrial fibrillation, ventricular fibrillation,* and *atrioventricular heart block.*

**Action/Kinetics:** The various antiarrhythmic drugs are classified according to both their mechanism of action and their effects on the action potential of cardiac cells. Importantly, one drug in a particular class may be more effective and safer in an individual client. The antiarrhythmic drugs are classified as follows:

1. Group I. These drugs decrease the rate of entry of sodium during cardiac membrane depolarization, decrease the rate of rise of phase O of the cardiac membrane action potential, prolong the effective refractory period of fast-response fibers, and require that a more negative membrane potential be reached before the membrane becomes excitable (and thus can propagate to other membranes). Drugs classified as group I are further listed in subgroups (according to their effects on action potential duration) as follows:

• Group IA: Depress phase O and prolong the duration of the action potential. Examples: Disopyramide, procainamide, and quinidine.

• Group IB: Slightly depress phase O and are thought to shorten the action potential. Examples: Lidocaine, phenytoin, and tocainide.

• Group IC: Slight effect on repolarization but marked depression of phase O of the action potential. Significant slowing of conduction. Examples: Flecainide, indecainide, and propafenone.

*NOTE:* Moricizine is classified as a group I agent but it has characteristics of agents in groups IA, B, and C.

2. Group II. These drugs competitively block beta-adrenergic receptors and depress phase 4 depolarization. Examples: Acebutolol, esmolol, and propranolol.

3. Group III. These drugs prolong the duration of the membrane action potential (relative refractory period) without changing the phase of depolarization or the resting membrane potential. Examples: Amiodarone, bretylium, and sotalol.

4. Group IV. Verapamil, a calcium channel blocker that slows conduction velocity and increases the refractoriness of the AV node.

Two other drugs, adenosine and digoxin, are also used to treat arrhythmias. Adenosine slows conduction time through the AV node and can interrupt the reentry pathways through the AV node. Digoxin causes a decrease in maximal diastolic potential and duration of the action potential; it also increases the slope of phase 4 depolarization.

**Special Concerns:** Monitor serum levels of antiarrhythmic drugs since some drugs can cause toxic side effects which can be confused with the purpose for which the drug is used. For example, toxicity from quinidine can result in cardiac arrhythmias. Antiarrhythmic drugs may cause new or worsening of arrhythmias, ranging from an increase in frequency of PVCs to severe ventricular tachycardia, ventricular fibrillation, or tachycardia that is more sustained and rapid. Such situations (called proarrhythmic effect) may make it difficult to distinguish the proarrhythmic effect from the underlying rhythm disorder.

## NURSING CONSIDERATIONS

### Assessment

1. Note drug sensitivity and any previous experiences with these drugs.

2. Assess extent of palpitations, fluttering sensations, chest pains, fainting episodes, or missed beats; obtain ECG with arrhythmia documentation.

3. Assess heart sounds and VS.

4. Monitor BS, electrolytes, liver and renal function studies. Ensure that serum pH, electrolytes, $pO_2$ and/or $O_2$ saturations are WNL.

5. Assess life-style related to cigarettes and caffeine use, alcohol consumption, and lack of regular exercise. Certain foods, emotional stress, and other environmental factors may also trigger arrhythmias; identify and eliminate before instituting drugs.

### Interventions

1. Use a cardiac monitor if administering drugs by IV route. Monitor for

rhythm changes; report and document rhythm strips.

2. Monitor BP and pulse. A HR < 50 bpm or > 120 should be avoided. Review written parameters for BP and pulse ranges.

3. Monitor serum electrolyte and drug levels.

**Client/Family Teaching**

1. Drugs work by controlling the irregular heart beats so the heart can pump more efficiently.

2. Take drugs as ordered; If a dose is missed, do not double up on the next dose unless specifically ordered.

3. Record BP and pulse for review at next visit.

4. Avoid OTC products. Eliminate caffeine, cigarettes, and alcohol, as these alter drug absorption and may precipitate arrhythmias.

5. Keep follow-up visits so that therapy can be adjusted and evaluated.

6. Report concerns/fears or problems R/T sexual activity.

7. Always carry list of currently prescribed meds and condition being treated.

8. Family/significant other should learn CPR; survival rates are greatly increased when initiated immediately.

**Outcomes/Evaluate**

• ECG evidence of arrhythmia control; restoration of stable cardiac rhythm

• Laboratory confirmation that serum drug concentrations are within therapeutic range

# ANTICOAGULANTS

*See also the following:*

Antithrombin III (human)
Ardeparin sodium
Dalteparin sodium injection
Danaparoid sodium
Enoxaparin injection
Heparin sodium injection
Heparin sodium and Sodium chloride
Heparin sodium lock flush solution

Warfarin sodium

**Action/Kinetics:** Drugs that influence blood coagulation can be divided into three classes: (1) *anticoagulants,* or drugs that prevent or slow blood coagulation; (2) *thrombolytic agents,* which increase the rate at which an existing blood clot dissolves; and (3) *hemostatics,* which prevent or stop internal bleeding. The dosage of all agents must be carefully adjusted since overdosage can have serious consequences. The major anticoagulants are warfarin, heparin, and heparin derivatives. The following considerations are pertinent to all types. Anticoagulants do not dissolve previously formed clots, but they do forestall their enlargement and prevent new clots from forming.

**Uses:** Venous thrombosis, pulmonary embolism, acute coronary occlusions with MIs, and strokes caused by emboli or cerebral thrombi. Prophylactically for rheumatic heart disease, atrial fibrillation, traumatic injuries of blood vessels, vascular surgery, major abdominal, thoracic, and pelvic surgery, prevention of strokes in clients with transient attacks of cerebral ischemia, or other signs of impending stroke.

Heparin is often used concurrently during the therapeutic initiation period. *Investigational (Warfarin):* Reduce risk of postconversion emboli; prophylaxis of recurrent, cerebral thromboembolism; prophylaxis of myocardial reinfarction; treatment of transient ischemic attacks; reduce the risk of thromboembolic complications in clients with certain types of prosthetic heart valves; reduced risk of thrombosis and/or occlusion following coronary bypass surgery.

**Contraindications:** Hemorrhagic tendencies (including hemophilia), clients with frail or weakened blood vessels, blood dyscrasias, ulcerative lesions of the GI tract (including peptic ulcer), diverticulitis, colitis, SBE, threatened abortion, recent operations on the eye, brain, or spinal cord, regional anesthesia and lumbar block, vitamin K deficiency, leukemia with bleeding tendencies, thrombocytopenic purpura, open wounds or ulcerations, acute nephritis, impaired hepatic or renal function, or severe hypertension. Hepatic and renal dysfunction. In the presence of drainage tubes in any orifice. Alcoholism.

**Special Concerns:** Use with caution in menstruation, in pregnant women (because they may cause hypoprothrombinemia in the infant), during lactation, during the postpartum period, and following cerebrovascular accidents. Geriatric clients may be more susceptible to the effects of anticoagulants.

**Side Effects:** See individual drugs.

**Dosage**

See individual drugs.

## NURSING CONSIDERATIONS

See also *Nursing Considerations* for individual agents.

**Assessment**

1. Review history and drug profile to ensure none interact unfavorably.
2. Assess for defects in clotting mechanism or any capillary fragility.
3. Note indications for therapy, time frame (i.e., DVT 6 months; valve replacement—lifetime), and desired INR, PT, or PTT and record.
4. Review PMH for conditions that may preclude therapy: PUD, chronic GI tract ulcerations, severe renal or liver dysfunction, infections of the endocardium.
5. Assess for alcoholism as anticoagulants are contraindicated.
6. Monitor CBC, PT/INR or PTT.

**Interventions**

1. Post/advise that client receiving anticoagulant therapy.
2. Monitor PT/INR or PTT levels closely; adjust oral anticoagulant weekly, esp. if receiving one of the many drugs known to interact or compete.
3. Question about bleeding (gums, urine, stools, vomit, ecchymosis, and/or petechiae). If urine discolored, determine cause, i.e., from

drug therapy or hematuria. Indanedione-type anticoagulants turn alkaline urine a red-orange color; acidify urine or test for occult blood.

4. Sudden lumbar pain may indicate retroperitoneal hemorrhage.
5. GI dysfunction may indicate intestinal hemorrhage. Test for blood in urine and feces; check H&H to assess for abnormal bleeding.
6. Have vitamin K, FFP, or factor IX concentrate for warfarin overdoses and protamine sulfate for heparin overdose (generally for every 100 U of heparin administer 1 mg IV) available.
7. Apply pressure to all venipuncture and injection sites to prevent bleeding and hematoma formation.
8. With SC administration, do not aspirate or massage; administer in lower abdomen and rotate sites.

**Client/Family Teaching**

1. Take at the same time every day as prescribed; record to ensure that drug has been taken.
2. Report if dizziness, headaches, bleeding gums or wounds, or vomiting of coffee ground material are evident; esp. important with the elderly.
3. Report increased bleeding, black and blue areas on the skin, illness, heavy menstrual flow, or blood in the urine.
4. Avoid contact sports and any unsafe situations or activities that may result in injury, falls, bumps, or cuts.
5. To prevent cuts, use an electric razor for shaving instead of a razor blade.
6. To prevent bleeding gums, use a soft bristle toothbrush and brush gently; inform dentist of drug therapy.
7. If severe sight problems, teach family that furniture should not be moved from usual places. This creates confusion for someone without full vision and can cause accidents resulting in bleeding and/or bruising; wear shoes and use a night light to prevent falls and bumps in the dark.
8. Review dietary sources of vitamin K (asparagus, spinach, broccoli, brussels sprouts, cabbage, collards, turnips, mustard greens, milk, yo-

gurt, and cheese) that should be consumed in limited quantities; alters PT.

9. Avoid OTC drugs. Check prior to taking any nonprescription drugs that have anticoagulant-type effects such as salicylates, NSAIDs, steroids, or vitamin preparations with high levels of vitamin K, mineral preparations from health food stores, or alcohol.

10. Always carry ID, noting drug therapy, the name and number of the provider so they may be contacted if excessive bleeding or emergency surgery is required.

11. Identify social/economic situations that may alter compliance; identify available resources.

12. Must return for follow-up visits and lab studies to evaluate effectiveness and to ensure proper dosage.

**Outcomes/Evaluate**
• PT: 1.5–2 times control; INR: 2.0–3.0 (standard therapy); INR: 3–4 (valves)
• PTT: 2–2.5 times the control/normal
• Prevention of thrombus formation
• Resolution of DVT
• ↓Risk of thromboembolism with prosthetic heart valves

**Special Concerns**
1. The elderly are more prone to developing bleeding complications.
2. Unusual hair loss and itching are common with the elderly; report immediately.
3. Many elderly use multiple pharmacies and shop for value; make sure they carry the name and dosage of all drugs prescribed.

# ANTICONVULSANTS

*See also the following individual entries:*

Acetazolamide
Acetazolamide sodium
Carbamazepine
Clonazepam
Clorazepate dipotassium
Diazepam
Ethosuximide

Felbamate
Fosphenytoin sodium
Gabapentin
Lamotrigine
Magnesium sulfate
Methsuximide
Phenobarbital
Phenobarbital sodium
Phensuximide
Phenytoin
Phenytoin sodium extended
Phenytoin sodium parenteral
Phenytoin sodium prompt
Primidone
Tiagabine hydrochloride
Topiramate
Valproic acid

**General Statement:** Therapeutic agents cannot cure convulsive disorders, but do control seizures without impairing the normal functions of the CNS. This is often accomplished by selective depression of hyperactive areas of the brain responsible for the convulsions. Therefore, these drugs are taken at all times (prophylactically) to prevent the occurrence of the seizures. There are several different types of epileptic disorders; consult the International Classification of Epileptic Seizures. No single drug can control all types of epilepsy; thus, accurate diagnosis is important. Drugs effective against one type of epilepsy may not be effective against another. Therapy begins with a small dose of the drug, which is continuously increased until either the seizures disappear or drug toxicity occurs. If a certain drug decreases the frequency of seizures but does not completely prevent them, another drug can be added to the dosage regimen and administered concomitantly with the first. Failure of therapy most often results from the administration of doses too small to have a therapeutic effect or from failure to use two or more drugs together. With appropriate diagnosis and selection of drugs, four out of five cases of epilepsy can be controlled adequately, but it may take the provider some time to find the best drug or combination of drugs with which to treat the client.

## Dosage

Dosage is highly individualized. However, trauma or emotional stress may necessitate an increase in drug dosage requirements (e.g., if the client requires surgery and starts having seizures). For details, see individual agents.

## NURSING CONSIDERATIONS

### Administration/Storage

1. Shake oral suspensions thoroughly before pouring to ensure uniform mixing.

2. Drug therapy must be individualized according to client needs.

3. Do not discontinue abruptly unless provider approved. To avoid severe, prolonged convulsions, withdraw over a period of days or weeks.

4. If there is reason to substitute one anticonvulsant drug for another, withdraw the first drug at the same time the dosage of the second drug is being increased.

5. Be prepared, in case of acute oral toxicity, to assist with inducing emesis (provided the client is not comatose) and with gastric lavage, along with other supportive measures such as administration of fluids and oxygen.

### Assessment

1. Check medical history for hypersensitivity to anticonvulsant drugs. Note derivatives that should be avoided.

2. Assess orientation to time and place, affect, reflexes, and VS.

3. Document seizure classification (partial or generalized). Determine the frequency and severity of seizures, noting location, duration, consciousness, type, frequency and any precipitating factors, presence of an aura, and any other characteristics.

4. Assess skin, eyes, and mucous membranes.

5. Determine if pregnant; may cause fetal abnormalities.

6. Monitor CBC, glucose, uric acid, urinalysis, liver and renal function studies.

7. Determine why receiving therapy and when it was instituted. If no seizure experienced for over 1 year with prophylactic therapy, may try gradual drug discontinuation.

### Interventions

1. Monitor VS; observe for S&S of impending seizures.

2. With IV administration, monitor closely for respiratory depression and CV collapse.

3. Note any evidence of CNS side effects, such as blurred vision, dimmed vision, slurred speech, nystagmus, or confusion. Supervise ambulation until drug effects resolved.

4. Observe for muscle twitching, loss of muscle tone, episodes of bizarre behavior, and/or subsequent amnesia.

5. With phenytoin, check calcium levels; can contribute to bone demineralization which can result in osteomalacia in adults and rickets in children. The risk increases with inactivity.

6. Vitamin D supplementation may be used to prevent hypocalcemia (4,000 units of vitamin D weekly); folic acid may prevent megaloblastic anemia.

7. Administer vitamin K to pregnant women 1 month before delivery to prevent postpartum hemorrhage and bleeding in the newborn and the mother.

### Client/Family Teaching

1. Take the prescribed amount of drug ordered. Do not increase, decrease, or discontinue without approval; convulsions may result.

2. May initially cause a decrease in mental alertness, drowsiness, headache, vertigo, and ataxia. CNS symptoms are dose-related and should subside with continued therapy; avoid hazardous tasks until symptoms disappear.

3. Lessen GI distress by taking with large amounts of fluid or with food.

4. Dosage may require adjusting if undergoing physical trauma or emotional distress.

5. Avoid alcohol and any other CNS depressants.

6. Increase fluid intake and include fruit and other foods with roughage and bulk in the diet.
7. With gingival hyperplasia, intensify oral hygiene, use a soft tooth brush, massage the gums, use dental floss daily, and obtain routine dental checks.
8. If slurred speech develops, try to consciously slow speech patterns to avoid the problem.
9. Avoid situations/exposures that result in fever and low glucose and sodium levels; may lower seizure threshold.
10. Report if rash, fever, severe headaches, stomatitis, rhinitis, urethritis, or balanitis (inflammation of the glans penis) occur; symptoms of hypersensitivity which require med change.
11. Report sore throat, easy bruising, petechiae, or nosebleeds; signs of hematologic toxicity.
12. Jaundice, dark urine, anorexia, and abdominal pain may indicate hepatotoxicity; needs LFTs to detect for hepatitis, hepatocellular degeneration, and fatal hepatocellular necrosis.
13. Practice reliable birth control; may harm fetus.
14. If nursing, observe infant for signs of toxicity.
15. Carry ID with the form of epilepsy and prescribed therapy. Family should learn CPR and how to protect client during a seizure.
16. Identify support groups (Epilepsy Foundation; National Head Injury Group) that may assist to understand and cope with disorder.

**Outcomes/Evaluate**
• ↓ Frequency of seizures; improved seizure control
• Serum drug levels within desired range

# ANTIDEPRESSANTS, TRICYCLIC

*See also the following individual entries:*

Amitriptyline and Perphenazine
Amitriptyline hydrochloride
Amoxapine
Clomipramine hydrochloride
Desipramine hydrochloride
Doxepin hydrochloride
Imipramine hydrochloride
Imipramine pamoate
Nortriptyline hydrochloride
Trimipramine maleate

**General Statement:** The tricyclic antidepressants are chemically related to the phenothiazines and, as such, they exhibit many of the same pharmacologic effects (e.g., anticholinergic, antiserotonin, sedative, antihistaminic, and hypotensive). The tricyclic antidepressants are less effective for depressed clients in the presence of organic brain damage or schizophrenia. Also, they can induce mania; this possibility should be kept in mind when given to clients with manic-depressive psychoses.

**Action/Kinetics:** It is now believed that antidepressant drugs cause adaptive changes in the serotonin and norepinephrine receptor systems, resulting in changes in the sensitivities of both presynaptic and postsynaptic receptor sites. These effects may increase the sensitivity of postsynaptic -1 adrenergic and serotonin receptors and decrease the sensitivity of presynaptic receptor sites. The overall effect is a reregulation of the abnormal receptorneurotransmitter relationship. Well absorbed from the GI tract. All have a long serum half-life. Up to 46 days may be required to reach steady plasma levels and maximum therapeutic effects may not be noted for 24 weeks. Because of the long half-life, single daily dosage may suffice. More than 90% bound to plasma protein. Partially metabolized in the liver and excreted primarily in the urine.

**Uses:** Endogenous and reactive depressions. Preferred over MAO inhibitors because they are less toxic. See also individual drugs.

**Contraindications:** Severely impaired liver function. Use during acute recovery phase from MI. Concomitant use with MAO inhibitors.

**Special Concerns:** Use with caution during lactation and with epilepsy, CV diseases, glaucoma, BPH, suicidal tendencies, a history of urinary retention, and the elderly. Use during pregnancy only when benefits clearly outweigh risks. Generally not recommended for children less than 12 years of age. Geriatric clients may be more sensitive to the anticholinergic and sedative side effects.

**Side Effects:** Most frequent side effects are sedation and atropine-like reactions. *CNS:* Confusion, anxiety, restlessness, insomnia, nightmares, hallucinations, delusions, mania or hypomania, headache, dizziness, inability to concentrate, panic reaction, worsening of psychoses, fatigue, weakness. *Anticholinergic:* Dry mouth, blurred vision, mydriasis, constipation, paralytic ileus, urinary retention or difficulty in urination. *GI:* NV, anorexia, gastric distress, unpleasant taste, stomatitis, glossitis, cramps, increased salivation, black tongue. *CV:* Fainting, tachycardia, hypo- or hypertension, arrhythmias, *heart block,* possibility of palpitations, *MI, stroke. Neurologic:* Paresthesias, numbness, incoordination, neuropathies, extrapyramidal symptoms including tardive dyskinesia, dysarthria, seizures. *Dermatologic:* Skin rashes, urticaria, flushing, pruritus, petechiae, photosensitivity, edema. *Endocrine:* Testicular swelling and gynecomastia in males, increase or decrease in libido, impotence, menstrual irregularities and galactorrhea in females, hypo- or hyperglycemia, changes in secretion of ADH. *Miscellaneous:* Sweating, alopecia, nasal congestion, lacrimation, increase in body temperature, chills, urinary frequency including nocturia. Bone marrow depression including thrombocytopenia, leukopenia, *agranulocytosis,* eosinophilia.

High dosage increases the frequency of seizures in epileptic clients and may cause epileptiform attacks in normal subjects.

**OD** **Overdose Management:** *Symptoms:* CNS symptoms include agitation, confusion, hallucinations, hyperactive reflexes, choreoathetosis, *seizures, coma.* Anticholinergic symptoms include dilated pupils, dry mouth, flushing, and *hyperpyrexia.* CV toxicity includes depressed myocardial contractility, decreased HR, decreased coronary blood flow, tachycardia, intraventricular block, *complete AV block, re-entry ventricular arrhythmias, PVCs, ventricular tachycardia or fibrillation, sudden cardiac arrest, hypotension, pulmonary edema.Treatment:* Admit client to hospital and monitor ECG closely for 3 to 5 days.

• Empty stomach in alert clients by inducing vomiting followed by gastric lavage and charcoal administration **after insertion of cuffed ET tube.** Maintain respiration and avoid the use of respiratory stimulants.

• Normal or half-normal saline to prevent water intoxication.

• To reverse the CV effects (e.g., hypotension and cardiac dysrhythmias), hypertonic sodium bicarbonate, IM, is given by IV infusion. The usual dose is 0.52 mEq/kg by IV bolus followed by IV infusion to maintain the blood at pH 7.5. If hypotension is not reversed by bicarbonate, vasopressors (e.g., dopamine) and fluid expansion may be needed. If the cardiac dysrhythmias do not respond to bicarbonate, lidocaine or phenytoin may be used.

• Isoproterenol may be effective in controlling bradyarrhythmias and torsades de pointes ventricular tachycardia. Propranolol, 0.1 mg/kg IV (up to 0.25 mg by IV bolus) is used to treat life-threatening ventricular arrhythmias in children.

• Shock and metabolic acidosis are treated with IV fluids, oxygen, bicarbonate, and corticosteroids.

• Control hyperpyrexia by external means (ice pack, cool baths, spongings).

• To reduce possibility of convulsions, minimize external stimulation. If necessary, use diazepam or phenytoin to control convulsions. Avoid barbiturates if MAO inhibitors have been used recently.

**Drug Interactions**

*Acetazolamide* / Effect of tricyclics by renal tubular reabsorption of the drug

*Alcohol, ethyl* / Concomitant use may lead to GI complications and performance on motor skill tests-death has been reported

*Ammonium chloride* / Effect of tricyclics by renal tubular reabsorption of the drug

*Anticholinergic drugs* / Additive anticholinergic side effects

*Anticoagulants, oral* / Hypoprothrombinemia due to breakdown by liver

*Anticonvulsants* / Tricyclics may incidence of epileptic seizures

*Antihistamines* / Additive anticholinergic side effects

*Ascorbic acid* / Effect of tricyclics by renal tubular reabsorption of the drug

*Barbiturates* / Additive depressant effects; also, barbiturates may breakdown of antidepressants by liver

*Benzodiazepines* / Tricyclic antidepressants effect of benzodiazepines

*Beta-adrenergic blocking agents* / Tricyclic antidepressants effect of the blocking agents

*Charcoal* / Absorption of tricyclic antidepressants effectiveness (or toxicity)

*Chlordiazepoxide* / Concomitant use may cause additive sedative effects and/or additive atropine-like side effects

*Cimetidine* / Effect of tricyclics (especially serious anticholinergic symptoms) due to breakdown by liver

*Clonidine* / Dangerous BP and hypertensive crisis

*Diazepam* / Concomitant use may cause additive sedative effects and/or additive atropine-like side effects

*Dicumarol* / Tricyclic antidepressants may the t of dicumarol anticoagulation effects

*Disulfiram* / Levels of tricyclic antidepressant; also, possibility of acute organic brain syndrome

*Ephedrine* / Tricyclics effects of ephedrine by preventing uptake at its site of action

*Estrogens* / Depending on the dose, estrogens may or the effects of tricyclics

*Ethchlorvynol* / Combination may result in transient delirium

*Fluoxetine* / Fluoxetine pharmacologic and toxic effects of tricyclic antidepressants (effect may persist for several weeks after fluoxetine is discontinued)

*Furazolidone* / Toxic psychoses possible

*Glutethimide* / Additive anticholinergic side effects

*Guanethidine* / Tricyclics antihypertensive effect of guanethidine by preventing uptake at its site of action

*Haloperidol* / Effect of tricyclics due to breakdown by liver

*Levodopa* / Effect of levodopa due to absorption

*MAO inhibitors* / Concomitant use may result in excitation, increase in body temperature, delirium, tremors, and convulsions although combinations have been used successfully

*Meperidine* / Tricyclics enhance narcotic-induced respiratory depression; also, additive anticholinergic side effects

*Methyldopa* / Tricyclics may block hypotensive effects of methyldopa

*Methylphenidate* / Effect of tricyclics due to breakdown by liver

*Narcotic analgesics* / Tricyclics enhance narcotic-induced respiratory depression; also, additive anticholinergic effects

*Oral contraceptives* / Plasma levels of tricyclic antidepressants due to breakdown by liver

---

*Oxazepam* / Concomitant use may cause additive sedative effects and/or atropine-like side effects

*Phenothiazines* / Additive anticholinergic side effects; also, phenothiazines effects of tricyclics due to breakdown by liver

*Procainamide* / Additive cardiac effects

*Quinidine* / Additive cardiac effects

*Reserpine* / Tricyclics hypotensive effect of reserpine

*Sodium bicarbonate* / Effect of tricyclics by renal tubular reabsorption of the drug

*Sympathomimetics* / Potentiation of sympathomimetic effects hypertension or cardiac arrhythmias

*Tobacco (smoking)* / Serum levels of tricyclic antidepressants due to breakdown by liver

*Thyroid preparations* / Mutually potentiating effects observed

*Vasodilators* / Additive hypotensive effect

**Laboratory Test Interferences:** Alkaline phosphatase, bilirubin; or blood glucose. False or urinary catecholamines.

## Dosage

See individual drugs.

Dosage levels vary greatly in effectiveness from one client to another; therefore, dosage regimens must be carefully individualized.

## NURSING CONSIDERATIONS

### Administration/Storage

1. In adolescents and elderly clients, use a lower initial dosage than in adults; the dose may then be gradually increased as required.

2. Individualize the dose according to age, weight, physical and mental condition, and response to the therapy.

3. For maintenance therapy, a single daily dose may suffice.

4. Dose usually administered at bedtime, so any anticholinergic and/or sedative effects will not impact ADL.

5. To reduce incidence of sedation and anticholinergic effects, start with small doses and then gradually increase to desired dosage levels.

### Assessment

1. Document indications for therapy, behavioral manifestations, onset of symptoms, and any causative factors.

2. Assess for suicide ideations, extent of dysphoric mood, appetite, and excessive weight changes.

3. Note sleep disturbances, lethargy, apathy, impaired thought processes, or lack of responses.

4. List drugs currently prescribed; some that may intensify depressive reactions include antihypertensives (i.e., reserpine, methyldopa, beta blockers), antiparkinsonians, hormones, steroids, anticancers, and antituberculins (cycloserine) as well as barbiturates and alcohol.

5. Monitor CBC, liver and renal function studies.

6. Record ECG, assess heart sounds, note any CAD, and evaluate neurologic functioning. Assess for tachycardia and increase in anginal attacks; may precede MI or stroke.

7. Note eye exam; report visual changes, headaches, halos, eye pain, dilated pupils, or nausea. May require a med change, esp. with glaucoma.

8. Monitor I&O; Check for abdominal distention, urinary retention, and absence of bowel sounds (as in paralytic ileus).

9. Differentiate type of depression based on diagnostic features related to reactive, major depressive, or bipolar affective disorders. Review symptoms to determine if affective, somatic, psychomotor, or psychological.

### Interventions

1. Note signs of allergic response, i.e., skin rash, alopecia, and eosinophilia.

2. Sore throat, fever, easy bruising, unusual bleeding, presence of petechiae or purpura may be symptoms of blood dyscrasias. Check for evidence of agranulocytosis, esp. common among elderly women and during the second month of drug therapy.

3. With hyperthyroidism, assess for arrhythmias precipitated by tricyclic drugs.

4. Assess for adverse endocrine disturbances such as increased or decreased libido, gynecomastia, testicular swelling, and impotence.

5. Report symptoms of cholestatic jaundice and biliary tract obstruction such as high fever, yellowing of the skin, mucous membranes and sclera, pruritus, and upper abdominal pain.

6. TCAs may alter blood sugar levels and require adjustment of hypoglycemic agent.

7. If receiving electroshock therapy, report as combination may be hazardous.

8. Discontinue several days prior to surgery; may adversely affect BP.

9. Withdraw slowly to avoid any withdrawal symptoms.

10. Assess for epileptiform seizures precipitated by the drug.

**Client/Family Teaching**

1. GI complaints of anorexia, N&V, epigastric distress, diarrhea, blackened tongue, or a peculiar taste require a dosage adjustment. Take with or immediately following meals to reduce gastric irritation.

2. Take sedating meds at bedtime to minimize daytime sedation; take those that cause insomnia in the a.m. or upon arising.

3. Avoid other drugs and alcohol during and for 2 weeks following TCA therapy.

4. Use caution when performing tasks requiring mental alertness or physical coordination; may cause drowsiness or ataxia.

5. Rise slowly from a supine position; do not remain standing in one place for any length of time. If feeling faint, lie down to minimize orthostatic hypotension.

6. Increase oral hygiene, take frequent sips of water, suck on hard candy, or chew sugarless gum to maintain a moist mouth. A high-fiber diet, increased fluid intake, and a stool softener may prevent constipation.

7. May affect carbohydrate metabolism; an adjustment of hypoglycemic agent and diet may be indicated.

8. If photosensitive, stay out of the sun; wear protective clothing, sunglasses, and a sunscreen.

9. May alter libido or reproductive function.

10. Practice reliable birth control; report if pregnancy is suspected.

11. Report any alterations in perceptions, i.e., hallucinations, blurred vision, or excessive stimulations. Watch those recovering from depression for suicidal tendencies; remove firearms from the house.

12. May take 24 weeks to realize a maximum clinical response; stay on the treatment regimen.

13. Will see provider more often the first 23 weeks; scripts will be for only small amounts to ensure compliance and to prevent an overdose; excess consumption can be lethal. Provide a number to call for help.

14. Instruct family how help clients alter their behavior; encourage participation in psychotherapy programs.

**Outcomes/Evaluate**

• Understanding of illness and need for drug therapy and medical supervision

• ↓ Depression evidenced by improved appetite, renewed interest in outside activities, ↑ socialization, improved sleeping patterns, ↑ energy, and a general sense of well being

• ↓ Anxiety; improved coping skills

# ANTIDIABETIC AGENTS: HYPOGLYCEMIC AGENTS

See also *Antidiabetic Agents: Insulins.*

*See also the following individual entries:*

Acarbose
Acetohexamide
Chlorpropamide
Glimepiride

Glipizide
Glyburide
Metformin hydrochloride
Miglitol
Tolazamide
Tolbutamide
Tolbutamide sodium
Troglitazone

**General Statement:** The American Diabetes Association has developed new standards for treating clients with diabetes. If followed, the new standards will enable clients to decrease their blood glucose levels closer to normal; this will reduce the risk of complications, including blindness, kidney disease, heart disease, and amputations. The goals of the new standards include establishing specific targets for control of blood glucose (usually between 80 and 120 mg/dL before meals and between 100 and 140 mg/dL at bedtime) and increased emphasis on educating clients for self-management of their disease. Targets for BP and lipid levels are also provided. If the guidelines are followed, it is estimated that the risk of development or progression of retinopathy, nephropathy, and neuropathy can be reduced by 50%–75% in clients with insulin-dependent (type I) diabetes. The guidelines suggest the following treatment modalities:

• Frequent monitoring of blood glucose.

• Regular exercise.

• Close attention to meal planning; consult a registered dietitian.

• For type I diabetics, either continuous SC insulin infusion or multiple daily insulin injections; for type II diabetics, consider insulin administration in certain situations, although dietary modification, exercise, and weight reduction are the cornerstone of treatment.

• Instruction in the prevention and treatment of hypoglycemia and other complications (both acute and chronic) of diabetes.

• Development of a process for ongoing support and continuing education for the client.

• Routine assessment of treatment goals.

**Action/Kinetics:** Oral hypoglycemic drugs are classified as either first or second generation. *Generation* refers to structural changes in the basic molecule. Second-generation oral hypoglycemic drugs are more lipophilic and, as such, have greater hypoglycemic potency. Also, second-generation drugs are bound to plasma protein by covalent bonds, whereas first-generation drugs are bound to plasma protein by ionic bonds. The implication is that the second-generation drugs are potentially less susceptible to displacement from plasma protein by drugs such as salicylates and oral anticoagulants.

The oral hypoglycemics are believed to act by one or more of the following mechanisms: (1) stimulating insulin release from pancreatic beta cells, possibly due to increased intracellular cyclic AMP; (2) the peripheral tissues become more sensitive to insulin due to an increase in the number of insulin receptors or an increased ability of circulating insulin to combine with receptors; or (3) extrapancreatic effects, including decreased glucagon release and hepatic glucose production. To be effective, the client must have some ability for endogenous insulin production. Differences in oral hypoglycemic drugs are mainly in their pharmacokinetic properties and duration of action.

**Uses:** Non-insulin-dependent diabetes mellitus (type II) that does not respond to diet management alone. Concurrent use of insulin and an oral hypoglycemic for type II diabetics who are difficult to control with diet and sulfonylurea therapy alone. One method used is the BIDS system: bedtime insulin (usually NPH) with daytime (morning only or morning and evening) oral hypoglycemic.

Guidelines for oral hypoglycemic therapy include onset of diabetes in clients over 40 years of age, duration of diabetes less than 5 years, absence of ketoacidosis, client is obese or has normal body weight, fasting serum glucose of 200 mg/dL or less, has a daily insulin requirement of 40 units or less, and hepatic and renal function is normal.

**Contraindications:** Stress before and during surgery, ketosis, severe trauma, fever, infections, pregnancy, diabetes complicated by recurrent episodes of ketoacidosis or coma; juvenile, growth-onset, insulin-dependent, or brittle diabetes; impaired endocrine, renal, or liver function. Use in diabetics who can be controlled by diet alone. Relapse may occur with the sulfonylureas in undernourished clients. Long-acting products in geriatric clients.

**Special Concerns:** Use with caution in debilitated and malnourished clients and during lactation since hypoglycemia may occur in the infant. Safety and effectiveness in children have not been established. Geriatric clients may be more sensitive to oral hypoglycemics and hypoglycemia may be more difficult to recognize in these clients. Use of sulfonylureas has been associated with an increased risk of CV mortality compared to treatment with either diet alone or diet plus insulin. There may be loss of blood glucose control if the client experiences stress such as infection, fever, surgery, or trauma.

**Side Effects:** Hypoglycemia is the most common side effect. *GI:* Nausea, heartburn, full feeling. *CNS:* Fatigue, dizziness, fever, headache, weakness, malaise, vertigo. *Hepatic:* Cholestatic jaundice, aggravation of hepatic porphyria. *Dermatologic:* Skin rashes, urticaria, erythema, pruritus, eczema, photophobia, morbilliform or maculopapular eruptions, lichenoid reactions, porphyria cutanea tardia. *Hematologic:* Thrombocytopenia, leukopenia, **agranulocytosis, aplastic anemia,** pancytopenia, **hemolytic anemia.** *Endocrine:* Inappropriate secretion of ADH resulting in excessive water retention, hyponatremia, low serum osmolality, and high urine osmolality. *Miscellaneous:* Paresthesia, tinnitus,

resistance to drug action develops in a small percentage of clients.

**OD** **Overdose Management:** *Symptoms:* Hypoglycemia. The following symptoms of hypoglycemia are listed in their general order of appearance: tingling of lips and tongue, hunger, nausea, decreased cerebral function (lethargy, yawning, confusion, agitation, nervousness), increased sympathetic activity (tachycardia, sweating, tremor), seizures, stupor, coma. *Treatment:* Mild hypoglycemia is treated with PO glucose and adjusting the dose of the drug or meal patterns. Severe hypoglycemia requires hospitalization. Concentrated (50%) dextrose is given by rapid IV and is followed by continuous infusion of 10% dextrose at a rate that will maintain blood glucose above 100 mg/dL. Client should be monitored for at least 24–48 hr as hypoglycemia may recur (clients with chlorpropamide toxicity should be monitored for 3–5 days due to the long duration of action of this drug).

**Drug Interactions**
*Acetazolamide* / ↑ Blood sugar in prediabetics and diabetics on oral hypoglycemics
*Alcohol* / Possible Antabuse-like syndrome, especially flushing of face and SOB. Also, ↓ effect of oral hypoglycemic due to ↑ breakdown by liver
*Androgens/anabolic steroids* / ↑ Hypoglycemic effect
*Anticoagulants, oral* / ↑ Effect of oral hypoglycemics by ↓ breakdown by liver and ↓ plasma protein binding
*Beta-adrenergic blocking agents* / ↓ Hypoglycemic effect; also, symptoms of hypoglycemia may be masked
*Charcoal* / ↓ Hypoglycemic effect due to ↓ absorption from GI tract
*Chloramphenicol* / ↑ Effect due to ↓ breakdown by liver and ↓ renal excretion
*Cholestyramine* / ↓ Hypoglycemic effect

*Clofibrate* / ↑ Hypoglycemic effect due to ↓ plasma protein binding

*Diazoxide* / ↓ Effects of both drugs

*Digitoxin* / ↑ Digitoxin serum levels

*Fenfluramine* / ↑ Hypoglycemic effect

*Fluconazole* / ↑ Hypoglycemic effect

*Gemfibrozil* / ↑ Hypoglycemic effect

*Histamine H₂ antagonists* / ↑ Hypoglycemic effect to ↓ breakdown by liver

*Hydantoins* / ↓ Effect of sulfonylureas due to ↓ insulin release

*Isoniazid* / ↑ Requirements for sulfonylureas

*Magnesium salts* / ↑ Hypoglycemic effect

*MAO inhibitors* / ↑ Hypoglycemic effect due to ↓ breakdown by liver

*Methyldopa* / ↑ Hypoglycemic effect due to ↓ breakdown by liver

*Miconazole* / ↑ Effect of oral hypoglycemics

*Nicotinic acid* / ↓ Effect of oral hypoglycemics

*NSAIDs* / ↑ Hypoglycemic effect of oral antidiabetics

*Oral contraceptives* / ↓ Hypoglycemic effect of oral antidiabetics

*Phenobarbital* / ↓ Effect of oral hypoglycemics due to ↑ breakdown by liver

*Phenothiazines* / ↑ Requirements for sulfonylureas due to ↓ release of insulin

*Phenylbutazone* / ↑ Effect of oral hypoglycemics due to ↓ breakdown by liver, ↓ plasma protein binding, and ↓ renal excretion

*Probenecid* / ↑ Hypoglycemic effect

*Rifampin* / ↓ Effect of sulfonylureas due to ↑ breakdown by liver

*Salicylates* / ↑ Effect of oral hypoglycemics by ↓ plasma protein binding

*Sulfinpyrazone* / ↑ Hypoglycemic effect

*Sulfonamides* / ↑ Effect of oral hypoglycemics by ↓ plasma protein binding and ↓ breakdown by liver

*Sympathomimetics* / ↑ Requirements for sulfonylureas

*Thiazides* / ↑ Requirements for sulfonylureas

*Thyroid hormone* / ↑ Requirements for sulfonylureas

*Tricyclic antidepressants* / ↑ Hypoglycemic effect

*Urinary acidifiers* / ↑ Hypoglycemic effect due to ↓ renal excretion

*Urinary alkalinizers* / ↓ Hypoglycemic effect due to ↑ renal excretion

**Laboratory Test Interferences:** ↑ BUN and serum creatinine.

**Dosage** ———————————

**PO.** See individual preparations. Adjust dosage according to needs of client. Exercise and diet are of primary importance in the control of diabetes.

## NURSING CONSIDERATIONS

See also *Nursing Considerations* for *Insulins.*

**Administration/Storage**

1. To decrease the incidence of gastric upset, take PO drugs with food.

2. If ketonuria, acidosis, increased glycosuria, or serious side effects occur, withdraw the med.

3. Transfer from insulin:

• If the client has been receiving 20 units or less of insulin daily, initiate oral hypoglycemic therapy and discontinue insulin abruptly.

• For clients receiving 20–40 units of insulin daily, initiate oral hypoglycemic therapy and reduce insulin dose by 25%–50%. Discontinue insulin gradually, using the absence of glucose in the urine as a guide. With glyburide, insulin may be discontinued abruptly.

• For clients receiving more than 40 units of insulin daily, initiate PO therapy and reduce insulin by 20%. Discontinue insulin gradually, using glucose in the urine or finger sticks as a guide. It may be advisable to hospitalize clients on such high doses of insulin while they are being transferred to oral hypoglycemic agents.

4. Transfer from one oral hypoglycemic agent to another:

• Except for chlorpropamide, no transition period is necessary. When

transferring from chlorpropamide, caution should be exercised for 1–2 weeks due to the long drug half-life.
• Mild symptoms of hyperglycemia may appear during the transfer period. Clients should perform finger sticks and test their urine for ketones regularly (1–3 times daily) during the transfer period. Positive results must be reported.

5. Be prepared to treat if the client develops severe hypoglycemia.

6. Review the drugs with which oral hypoglycemic agents interact and determine if the client is taking any of them.

7. Type II diabetic clients who do not respond to the sulfonylureas are said to be *primary failures*. Responses to the sulfonylureas during the initial months of therapy followed by failure to respond are referred to as *secondary failures*. A glucophage or metformin trial may be useful in these clients.

**Assessment**

1. Obtain a thorough nursing history.

2. Document any stress. Clients about to undergo surgical procedures, who have suffered severe trauma, who have a fever and infection, or who are pregnant should generally not be placed on oral hypoglycemic agents.

3. Assess mental functions to determine if able to understand the complexities of the transfer process.

4. Note if taking oral contraceptives; effectiveness is lessened by oral hypoglycemic agents.

5. Note any previous experience with sulfonylureas and the outcome. Determine metformin trial and the outcome; elderly do better with a slower metformin titration (i.e., increase dose weekly or increase by ½ tablet instead of a whole tablet).

6. Identify clients that may benefit from ACE and vitamin E therapy.

7. Monitor electrolytes, CBC, HbA1c, and urine for microalbuminuria.

**Client/Family Teaching**

1. Use machine to test blood sugar (or urine for ketones) and record for provider review. (Urine testing is not an accurate reflection of true serum glucose levels and should not be used to modify treatment.)

2. With hypoglycemic episodes, check finger stick at the time of the reaction. Then drink 4 oz of juice (fast-acting CHO), followed by a longer acting CHO (approximately 10 g) such as half a meat sandwich or several peanut butter crackers, and recheck finger stick in 15 min. If glucose is less than 100, repeat the process, i.e., juice and a CHO and another finger stick. Report if this occurs often.

3. Medication helps to control hyperglycemia but does not cure diabetes; therapy is usually long term.

4. Must adhere to prescribed diet if drug is to be effective; most secondary failures are due to poor dietary compliance; see dietitian as needed.

5. Regular physical exercise, diet, and weight control are imperative.

6. Insulin may be necessary if complications occur. Review administration of insulin and how to rotate sites. Do not change brands of insulin or syringes. Review equipment, methods of storage and discarding used syringes.

7. Report illness or if unusual itching, skin rash, jaundice, dark urine, fever, sore throat, nausea/vomiting, or diarrhea occurs.

8. With thyroid scan advise lab as sulfonylureas interfere with the uptake of radioactive iodine.

9. Avoid alcohol; a disulfuram-like reaction may occur.

10. Do not take any OTC meds without approval.

11. Need close medical supervision for the first 6 weeks and periodic lab tests; oral agents may cause blood dyscrasias.

12. Carry ID, a list of prescribed drugs, juice, and hard candy (such as Lifesavers) or a fast-acting CHO (candy bar) at all times.

---

**Outcomes/Evaluate**
- Knowledge of diabetes; compliance with therapy and dietary regimen
- ↓ Hypo- or hyperglycemic episodes
- HbA1c within desired range

# ANTIDIABETIC AGENTS: INSULINS

See also *Antidiabetic Agents: Hypoglycemic Agents.*

*See also the following individual entries:*

Insulin injection
Insulin injection concentrated
Insulin lispro injection
Insulin zinc suspension (Lente)
Insulin zinc suspension, Extended
(Ultralente)

**General Statement:** Insulin preparations with different times of onset, peak activity, and duration of action have been developed. Such products are prepared by precipitating insulin in the presence of zinc chloride to form zinc insulin crystals and/or by combining insulin with a protein such as protamine. Based on these modifications, insulin products are classified as fast-acting, intermediate-acting, and long-acting. These preparations permit the provider to select the preparation best suited to the life-style of the client.

RAPID-ACTING INSULIN: Insulin injection (Regular Insulin, Crystalline Zinc Insulin, Unmodified Insulin)

INTERMEDIATE-ACTING INSULIN
1. Isophane insulin suspension (NPH)
2. Insulin zinc suspension (Lente)

LONG-ACTING INSULIN: Insulin zinc suspension extended (Ultralente)

*NOTE:* Insulin preparations with various times of onset and duration of action are often mixed to obtain optimum control in diabetic clients.

**Action/Kinetics:** Following combination with insulin receptors on cell plasma membranes, insulin facili-tates the transport of glucose into cardiac and skeletal muscle and adipose tissue. It also increases synthesis of glycogen in the liver. Insulin stimulates protein synthesis and lipogenesis and inhibits lipolysis and release of free fatty acids from fat cells. This latter effect prevents or reverses the ketoacidosis sometimes observed in the type I diabetic. Insulin also causes intracellular shifts in magnesium and potassium.

Since insulin is a protein, it is destroyed in the GI tract. Thus, it must be administered SC so that it is readily absorbed into the bloodstream and distributed throughout the extracellular fluid. Metabolized mainly by the liver.

**Uses:** Replacement therapy in type I diabetes. Diabetic ketoacidosis or diabetic coma (use regular insulin). Insulin is also indicated in type II diabetes when other measures have failed (e.g., diet, exercise, weight reduction) or with surgery, trauma, infection, fever, endocrine dysfunction, pregnancy, gangrene, Raynaud's disease, kidney or liver dysfunction.

Human insulins are used for local insulin allergy, lipodystrophy at the injection site, immunologic insulin resistance, temporary insulin use (e.g., surgery, acute stress, gestational diabetes), and newly diagnosed diabetes.

Regular insulin is used in IV HA solutions, in IV dextrose to treat severe hyperkalemia, and IV as a provocative test for growth hormone secretion.

Insulin and oral hypoglycemic drugs have been used in type II diabetics who are difficult to control with diet and PO therapy alone.

**Diet:** The dietary control of diabetes is as important as medication with appropriate drugs. The role of the nurse and dietitian in teaching the client how to eat properly cannot be underestimated. They must teach the client how to calculate exchange values of various foods. Food lists and food-exchange values published by the American Diabetes Association and the American Dietetic Association are valuable teaching aids.

Diabetic clients should adhere to a regular meal schedule. The frequency of meals and the overall caloric intake vary with the type of drug taken and individual client needs. Close attention to meal frequency and meal planning is imperative and a registered dietitian should be consulted. Diabetic children may be on a less restricted diet, adjusting the insulin dosage according to blood and urine glucose readings. Children with negative urine glucose tend to become hypoglycemic rapidly with exercise or decrease in appetite, and many providers allow for glucose spilling.

**Contraindications:** Hypersensitivity to insulin.

**Special Concerns:** Pregnant diabetic clients often manifest decreased insulin requirements during the first half of pregnancy and increased requirements during the latter half. Lactation may decrease insulin requirements.

**Side Effects:** *Hypoglycemia:* Due to insulin overdose, delayed or decreased food intake, too much exercise in relationship to insulin dose, or when transferring from one preparation to another. Even carefully controlled clients occasionally develop signs of insulin overdosage characterized by one or more of the following: hunger, weakness, fatigue, nervousness, pallor or flushing, profuse sweating, headache, palpitations, numbness of mouth, tingling in the fingers, tremors, blurred and double vision, hypothermia, excess yawning, mental confusion, incoordination, tachycardia, loss of sensitivity, and loss of consciousness. Level of awareness is markedly diminished after an attack.

Symptoms of hypoglycemia may mimic those of psychic disturbances. Severe prolonged hypoglycemia may cause brain damage, and in the elderly, may mimic stroke.

*Allergic:* Urticaria, angioedema, lymphadenopathy, bullae, anaphylaxis. Occurs mostly following intermittent insulin therapy or IV administration of large doses to insulin-resistant clients. Antihistamines or corticosteroids may be used to treat these symptoms. Clients who are highly allergic to insulin and cannot be treated with oral hypoglycemics may respond to human insulin products.

*At site of injection:* Swelling, stinging, redness, itching, warmth. These symptoms often disappear with continued use. Lipoatrophy or hypertrophy of subcutaneous fat tissue (minimize by rotating site of injection).

*Insulin resistance:* Usual cause is obesity. Acute resistance may occur following infections, trauma, surgery, emotional disturbances, or other endocrine disorders.

*Ophthalmologic:* Blurred vision, transient presbyopia. Occurs mainly during initiation of therapy or in clients who have been uncontrolled for a long period of time.

*Hyperglycemic rebound (Somogyi effect):* Usually in clients who receive chronic overdosage.

DIFFERENTIATION BETWEEN DIABETIC COMA AND HYPOGLYCEMIC REACTION (INSULIN SHOCK): Coma in diabetes may be caused by uncontrolled diabetes (high sugar content in blood or urine, ketoacidosis) or by too much insulin (insulin shock, hypoglycemia).

Diabetic coma and insulin shock can be differentiated in the following manner:

**Hyperglycemia (Diabetic Coma)**
*Onset* / Gradual (days)
*Medication* / Insufficient insulin
*Food intake* / Normal or excess
*Overall appearance* / Extremely ill
*Skin* / Dry and flushed
*Infection* / Frequent
*Fever* / Frequent
*Mouth* / Dry
*Thirst* / Intense

---

*Hunger* / Absent
*Vomiting* / Common
*Abdominal pain* / Frequent
*Respiration* / Increased, air hunger
*Breath* / Acetone odor
*BP* / Low
*Pulse* / Weak and rapid
*Vision* / Dim
*Tremor* / Absent
*Convulsions* / None
*Urine sugar* / High
*Ketone bodies* / High (type I only)
*Blood sugar* / High
**Hypoglycemia (Insulin Shock)**
*Onset* / Sudden (24–48 hr)
*Medication* / Excess insulin
*Food intake* / Probably too little
*Overall appearance* / Very weak
*Skin* / Moist and pale
*Infection* / Absent
*Fever* / Absent
*Mouth* / Drooling
*Thirst* / Absent
*Hunger* / Occasional
*Vomiting* / Absent
*Abdominal pain* / Rare
*Respiration* / Normal
*Breath* / Normal
*BP* / Normal
*Pulse* / Full and bounding
*Vision* / Diplopia
*Tremor* / Frequent
*Convulsions* / In late stages
*Urine sugar* / Absent in second specimen
*Ketone bodies* / Absent in second specimen
*Blood sugar* / Less than 60 mg/100 mL

Source: Adapted with permission from *The Merck Manual*, 11th ed.

Diabetic coma is usually precipitated by the client's failure to take insulin. Hypoglycemia is often precipitated by the client's unpredictable response, excess exertion, stress due to illness or surgery, errors in calculating dosage, or failure to eat.

TREATMENT OF DIABETIC COMA OR SEVERE ACIDOSIS: Administer 30–60 units regular insulin. This is followed by doses of 20 units or more q 30 min. To avoid a hypoglycemic state, 1 g dextrose is adminis-tered for each unit of insulin given. Treatment is often supplemented by electrolytes and fluids. Urine samples are collected for analysis, and VS are monitored as ordered.

TREATMENT OF HYPOGLYCEMIA (INSULIN SHOCK): Mild hypoglycemia can be relieved by PO administration of CHO such as orange juice, candy, or a lump of sugar. If comatose, adults may be given 10–30 mL of 50% dextrose solution IV; children should receive 0.5–1 mL/kg of 50% dextrose solution. Epinephrine, hydrocortisone, or glucagon may be used in severe cases to cause an increase in blood glucose.

**Drug Interactions**
*Alcohol, ethyl* / ↑ Hypoglycemia → low blood sugar and shock
*Anabolic steroids* / ↑ Hypoglycemic effect of insulin
*Beta-adrenergic blocking agents* / ↑ Hypoglycemic effect of insulin
*Chlorthalidone* / ↓ Hypoglycemic effect of antidiabetics
*Clofibrate* / ↑ Hypoglycemic effects of insulin
*Contraceptives, oral* / ↑ Dosage of antidiabetic due to impairment of glucose tolerance
*Corticosteroids* / ↓ Effect of insulin due to corticosteroid-induced hyperglycemia
*Dextrothyroxine* / ↓ Effect of insulin due to dextrothyroxine-induced hyperglycemia
*Diazoxide* / Diazoxide-induced hyperglycemia ↓ diabetic control
*Digitalis glycosides* / Use with caution, as insulin affects serum potassium levels
*Diltiazen* / ↓ Effect of insulin
*Dobutamine* / ↓ Effect of insulin
*Epinephrine* / ↓ Effect of insulin due to epinephrine-induced hyperglycemia
*Estrogens* / ↓ Effect of insulin due to impairment of glucose tolerance
*Ethacrynic acid* / ↓ Hypoglycemic effect of antidiabetics
*Fenfluramine* / Additive hypoglycemic effects
*Furosemide* / ↓ Hypoglycemic effect of antidiabetics

*Glucagon* / Glucagon-induced hyperglycemia ↓ effect of antidiabetics

*Guanethidine* / ↑ Hypoglycemic effect of insulin

*MAO inhibitors* / MAO inhibitors ↑ and prolong hypoglycemic effect of antidiabetics

*Oxytetracycline* / ↑ Effect of insulin

*Phenothiazines* / ↑ Dosage of antidiabetic due to phenothiazine-induced hyperglycemia

*Phenytoin* / Phenytoin-induced hyperglycemia ↓ diabetic control

*Propranolol* / Inhibits rebound of blood glucose after insulin-induced hypoglycemia

*Salicylates* / ↑ Effect of hypoglycemic effect of insulin

*Sulfinpyrazone* / ↑ Hypoglycemic effect of insulin

*Tetracyclines* / May ↑ hypoglycemic effect of insulin

*Thiazide diuretics* / ↓ Hypoglycemic effect of antidiabetics

*Thyroid preparations* / ↓ Effect of antidiabetic due to thyroid-induced hyperglycemia

*Triamterene* / ↓ Hypoglycemic effect of antidiabetic

**Laboratory Test Interferences:** Alters liver function tests and thyroid function tests. False + Coombs' test, ↑ serum protein, ↓ serum amino acids, calcium, cholesterol, potassium, and urine amino acids.

**Dosage**

Dosage highly individualized. Usually administered SC. Insulin injection (regular insulin) is the **only** preparation that may be administered IV. Give IV only for clients with severe ketoacidosis or diabetic coma. Dosage for insulin is always expressed in USP units.

Dosage is established and monitored by blood glucose (often using glucose monitoring machines in the home), urine glucose, and acetone tests. Furthermore, since requirements may change with time, dosage must be checked at regular intervals. It may be advisable to hospitalize some clients while their daily insulin and caloric requirements are being established. The main goal is to control the blood sugar and send the client home to fine tune as generally the home environment is more reliable for determining drug requirements.

In pregnancy, insulin requirements may increase suddenly during the last trimester. After delivery, requirements may suddenly drop to prepregnancy levels. To prevent the development of hypoglycemia, insulin is often discontinued on the day of delivery and glucose is administered IV.

The various insulin preparations can be mixed to obtain the combination best suited for the individual client. However, mixing must be done according to the directions received from the physician/provider and/or pharmacist.

---

## NURSING CONSIDERATIONS

*Also includes general applications for all clients with diabetes controlled by medication (whether it be insulin or an oral hypoglycemic agent).*

**Administration/Storage**

1. Read the product information and any important notes inserted into the insulin package.

2. Discard open vials not used for several weeks or any whose expiration date has passed.

3. Refrigerate stock supply of insulin but avoid freezing. Freezing destroys the manner in which insulin is suspended in the formulation.

4. Store vial in a cool place, avoiding extremes of temperature or exposure to sunlight.

5. Use the following guidelines with respect to mixing the various insulins:

• Regular insulin may be mixed with NPH or Lente insulins. However, to avoid transfer of the longer-acting insulin into the regular insulin vial, withdraw regular insulin into the syringe first.

---

• Give a mixture of regular insulin with NPH or Lente insulin within 15 min of mixing due to binding of regular insulin by excess protamine and/or zinc in the longer-acting preparations.

• Lente or Ultralente insulins may be mixed with each other in any proportion; however, do not mix these with NPH insulins.

• When used in an insulin infusion pump, insulin may be mixed in any proportion with either 0.9% NaCl injection or water for injection. Due to stability changes, use such mixtures within 24 hr of their preparation. Buffered insulin is usually the form prescribed and utilized with the insulin pump.

6. Store compatible insulin mixtures for no longer than 1 month at room temperature or 3 months at 2°C–8°C (36°F–46°F). However, bacterial contamination may occur.

7. To ensure a constant amount of precipitate in each dose, invert the vial several times to mix before the material is withdrawn. Avoid vigorous shaking and frothing of the material. (Regular and globin insulin are the only two insulins that do not have a precipitate.)

8. Discard any vial in which the precipitate is clumped or granular in appearance or which has formed a solid deposit of particles on the side of the vial.

9. To prevent dosage error, do not alter the order of mixing insulins or change the model or brand of syringe or needle.

10. Administer at a 90° angle with a 28- or 29-gauge needle. Syringes come in 0.3-cc (30-U), 0.5-cc (50-U) and 1-cc (100-U) sizes. Get the smallest syringe with the smallest needles to enhance dosage validity (e.g., if client is prescribed less than 30 U insulin, advise to obtain the 0.3- cc syringe).

11. Provide an automatic injector for clients fearful of injecting themselves.

12. Assist the visually impaired client with diabetes to obtain information and devices for self-administration by consulting their local diabetes association or by writing to the American Diabetes Association, 149 Madison Avenue, New York, NY 10016 (telephone: 212-725-4925), for their buyer's guide, which lists numerous available products for diabetics. Clients may also contact The Lighthouse, Inc., 800 Second Avenue, New York, NY 10017 (telephone: 212-808-0077) for additional information on visual impairments.

13. Lipoatrophy may occur. This may appear as mild dimpling of the skin or as deep pits in young girls and women and lipodystrophy, appearing as well-developed muscle on the anterior and lateral thighs of young boys and men. To prevent, rotate injection sites.

• Make a chart indicating the injection sites (see Figure 1).

• Allow 3–4 cm between injection sites.

• Do not inject in the same site for at least 1–2 weeks.

• Avoid injecting within 1 cm around the umbilicus because of the high vascularity in this area.

---

**Figure 1** Each injection area is divided into squares; each square is an injection site. Start in a corner of an injection area and move down or across the injection sites in order. Jumping from site to site will make it more difficult to remember where the last shot was administered. Keep track of the rotation pattern to assist in maintaining site rotation. A grid may be developed from this figure and numbered to keep track of injections. Systematically use all the sites in one area before moving to another (for example, use all the sites in both arms before moving to the legs). This will help keep the blood sugar more even from day to day. An important consideration when choosing injection sites is that insulin is absorbed into the bloodstream faster from some areas than from others; it enters the bloodstream most quickly from the abdomen (stomach), a little more slowly from the arms, even more slowly from the legs, and most slowly from the buttocks. (Courtesy Eli Lilly & Company.)

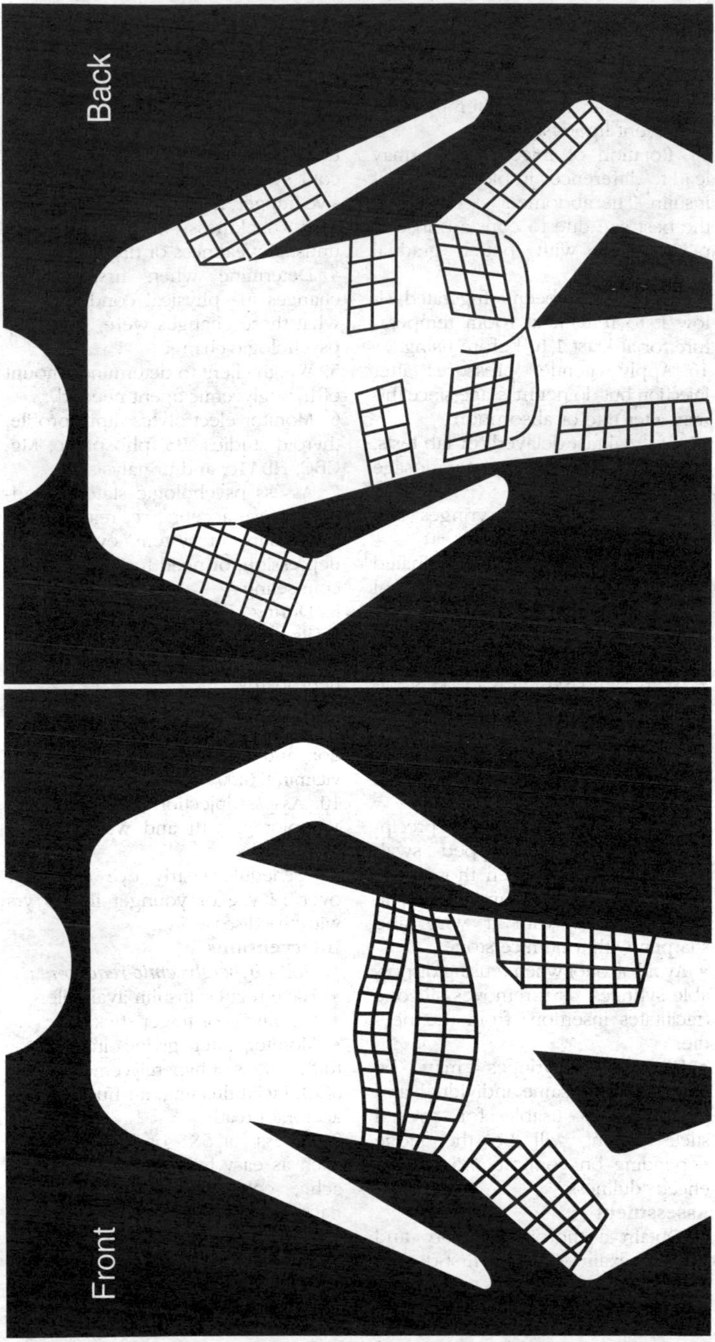

Back

Front

- Avoid injections around the waistline because of the sensitive nerve supply to this area and the potential for fabric irritation.
- Use insulin at room temperature to prevent lipodystrophy.

14. Rotation of injection sites may lead to differences in blood levels of insulin. The abdomen is considered the best site due to constant insulin peak times with better gradual absorption.

15. If insulin has been refrigerated, allow it to remain at room temperature for at least 1 hr before using.

16. Apply gentle pressure after injection but do not massage since this may alter rate of absorption.

17. If breakfast delayed for lab tests, check with the provider for dosage adjustment.

18. Care of reusable syringes and needles.

- Do not use heavily chlorinated water or water with a high chemical content for sterilizing syringes. To sterilize, boil the syringe and needle for 5 min.
- Needle and syringe can be sterilized by soaking in isopropyl alcohol for at least 5 min. The alcohol must evaporate from the equipment before use to prevent reduction in the strength (dilution) of the insulin.
- Clean syringes covered by a precipitate with a cotton-tipped swab soaked in vinegar; then thoroughly rinse syringe in water and sterilize it. Clean needles with a wire and sharpen with a pumice stone.
- Avoid alcohol when reusing disposable syringes, as it removes silicone (facilitates insertion) from the needle.
- Disposable syringes may be reused by the same individual and are generally usable for several sticks. Client will be the judge depending on comfort and experienced "dullness."

## Assessment

1. Obtain a thorough history and physical exam. Note any first-degree relatives with disease.

2. Assess for S&S of hyperglycemia: thirst, polydypsia, polyuria, drowsiness, blurred vision, loss of appetite, fruity odor to the breath, and flushed dry skin. Note state of consciousness.

3. Assess for S&S of hypoglycemia: drowsiness, chills, confusion, anxiety, cold sweats, cool pale skin, excessive hunger, nausea, headache, irritability, shakiness, rapid pulse, and unusual weakness or tiredness.

4. Determine when first noticed changes in physical condition and what these changes were. Note any psychologic changes.

5. Weigh client to determine amount of hypoglycemic agent needed.

6. Monitor electrolytes, lipid profile, thyroid studies, BS, phosphate, Mg, CBC, HbA1c, and urinalysis.

7. Assess psychologic state, including disease acceptance, readiness to learn, support system, evidence of depression, or need for client/family counseling.

8. During physical exam assess DTRs; check extremities (monofilament) to assess for sensation and neuropathy.

9. Identify candidates for ACE therapy to prevent/preserve renal function and inhibit organ damage and vitamin E (400 IU) for CAD protection.

10. Assess injection sites, monitor VS, plot growth and weight every 3–4 months.

11. Schedule yearly eye exams if over 12 yrs; or younger if > 5 yrs with the disease.

## Interventions

1. For a *hyperglycemic reaction:*
- Have regular insulin available.
- Obtain BS or finger stick.
- Monitor after giving insulin for further signs of hyperglycemia such as SOB, facial flushing, air hunger, and acetone breath.

2. Assess for S&S of *hypoglycemia,* such as easy fatigue, hunger, headache, cold, clammy, drowsiness, nausea, lassitude, and tremulousness. Most likely to occur before meals, during or after exercise, and at insulin peak action times (i.e., 3 a.m. with evening dosing).

• Weakness, sweating, tremors, and/or nervousness may occur later.

• Excessive restlessness and profuse sweating at night.

• Obtain BS or finger stick; promptly give 4 oz of juice and a CHO, if conscious.

• If conscious and taking long-acting insulin, also give a slowly digestible CHO, such as bread with corn syrup or honey. Give additional CHO such as crackers and milk for the next 2 hr.

• If unconscious, apply honey or Karo syrup to the buccal membrane or give glucagon.

• If hospitalized, minimally responsive or unconscious, give 10%–20% IV dextrose solution.

3. A Somogyi effect is often mistaken as client not following the prescribed therapy. This occurs when hypoglycemia triggers the release of epinephrine and glucocorticoids, which stimulates glycogenesis and results in a higher a.m. BS level. Reduction in bedtime insulin dosage is necessary to stabilize. If treated for hypoglycemia, check 3 a.m. BS; if normal and then BS rises between 3 a.m. and 7 a.m., this is related to growth hormone release—termed the Dawn Phenomenon. To control, give long-acting insulin at bedtime instead of at dinnertime.

4. Juveniles with diabetes demand closer attention and observation for infection or emotional disturbances andhypoglycemia. They are more susceptible to insulin shock and have a more limited response to glucagon. Determine if managed with intensive or conventional insulin therapy; adjust for hypoglycemia unawareness (when client passes out due to loss of catecholamine response).

5. For the newly diagnosed elderly client, the initial insulin doses should be low and gradually increased.

6. The usual dose of NPH insulin is 0.8–1.5 U/kg; give two-thirds of dose in a.m. and one-third of dose in p.m. If using regular insulin, try 1:2 in a.m. and 1:1 in p.m. with NPH.

7. Identify BS goals, i.e., young child 80–180 mg/dL premeal and 100–180 mg/dL at bedtime; adolescent 70–150 mg/dL premeal and 100–180 mg/dL at bedtime; adult 80–140 mg/dL premeal and 100–180 mg/dL at bedtime and adjust as symptoms and condition dictate.

**Client/Family Teaching**

1. Medications assist to control diabetes but do not cure it. Type I diabetes is usually early onset and the pancreas makes little or no insulin; individuals with type I diabetes must take insulin injections or they will die. Type II diabetes is usually later onset and the pancreas still makes insulin, but the body cannot use it (termed insulin resistance); individuals with type II diabetes can use either oral hypoglycemic agents or insulin to lower their blood sugar and to help them utilize their own insulin better.

2. Urine testing is not an accurate reflection of what the blood sugar is doing and is not generally used to adjust the treatment plan. If testing urine for sugar, review how to conduct this test. Follow instructions when testing for glycosuria with Clinitest Tablets, Tes-Tape, Diastix, or Clinistix.

• Test a fresh second-voided specimen.

• Empty bladder by voiding 1 hr before mealtime.

• As soon as able to void again, obtain and test specimen.

3. In type I diabetics, urine ketones indicate that there is not enough insulin present to get the body's sugar into the cells so it is burning body fat as an alternative and producing ketones as waste products; may lead to ketoacidosis, a life-threatening condition. Test urine for ketones with a "dip-and-read" product when:

• Finger sticks > 240 mg/dL

• Pregnant

• Experiencing severe stress

• Vomiting or sick to stomach

• Sick with flu/cold or virus infection

• Experiencing symptoms of hyperglycemia (unusual fatigue, vision difficulty, increased thirst and/or hunger, polydipsia, unusually tired or sleepy, stomach pain, increased nausea, fruity odor to breath, rapid respirations, weight loss without altering food intake or activity patterns)

4. If performing finger sticks to monitor glucose levels, review procedure. Review instructions for technique, calibration, operation, and device maintenance. Bring in periodically to double check machine accuracy and to review data bank to ensure values coincide with client log. Some general principles may be followed.

• Rotate sites.

• Cleanse area with soap and water or alcohol prior to stabbing.

• Stab finger outside, by nail, where the capillaries are abundant and let a bead of blood form.

• Wipe off with a cotton ball.

• Let blood bead re-form and apply to the test strip.

• Follow specific guidelines for the device in use.

5. Regimens are specific to the individual, based on age, severity of diabetes, weight, any other medical problems they have, as well as the philosophy of the health care team.

6. Take insulin 30 min before a meal (exception is Humalog, which can be taken at meal time). Administer at a 90° angle with a 28- or 29-gauge needle. Syringes come in 0.3-cc (30-U), 0.5-cc (50-U) and 1-cc (100-U) sizes. Purchase the smallest syringe with the smallest needles to enhance dosage validity (e.g., if prescribed less than 30 U insulin, obtain the 0.3-cc syringe). May reuse disposable insulin syringes; based on comfort and perceived dullness.

7. Use a chart to document and rotate injection sites to avoid lipohypertrophy of injection sites ( lumps from scar tissue after many injections). Avoid these areas due to unreliable absorption.

• For self-injection, brace the arm against a hard surface such as the wall or a chair.

• Cleanse the area thoroughly with alcohol, allow to dry, then, depending on the condition of the skin, either pinch between the thumb and forefingers of one hand, or spread the skin using the thumb and fingers of one hand.

• Insert into the subcutaneous tissue and aspirate to be sure needle is not in a blood vessel.

• Inject insulin and withdraw the needle.

8. Review use and care of equipment, proper disposal of needles and syringes, and provision and storage of drug.

9. *Always* check expiration dates; have an extra vial equipment on hand for traveling, away from home, or when hospitalized.

10. Have regular insulin for emergency use.

11. Must balance food, insulin, and exercise. Exercise increases the utilization of CHO and increases CHO needs. Have snacks available; 5–8 Lifesavers, juice, or hard candy helps counteract hypoglycemia.

12. Adhere to prescribed diet, weight control, and ingestion of food relative to the peak action of insulin being used. Record weekly weights; reduce intake of animal fats and salt; select a variety of foods to meet starch and sugar, protein, and fat requirements (usual recommendation; CHO 50%; protein 20%; fat 30%). Consume the kinds of fiber that help lower BS and fat levels (breads, cereals, and crackers made from whole grains, such as whole wheat and brown rice, fresh vegetables and fruits, dried beans, and peas), as well as low cholesterol and polyunsaturated and monosaturated fats.

13. Confer with dietitian for assistance in shopping, food selection/exchanges, diet, and meal planning. Consume premeal snacks in the a.m., in the afternoon, and at bedtime.

14. May experience allergic responses: itching, redness, swelling, stinging, or warmth may occur at the injection site and usually disappears

after a few weeks of therapy. Report as purified or human insulins are used for local allergy and lipohypertrophy at injection site.

15. Blurred vision may occur at beginning of insulin therapy; should subside in 6–8 weeks. The effect is caused by fluctuation of blood glucose levels, which produce osmotic changes in the lens of the eye and within the ocular fluids. If it does not clear up in 8 weeks, consult eye doctor.

16. If ill and omit a meal because of fever, nausea, or vomiting, replace solid foods that contain starch and sugar, such as bread and fruit, with liquids that contain sugar (fruit juice, regular sodas) and follow designated sliding scale for "sick days." Do not omit insulin or hypoglycemic agents unless instructed. Perform finger sticks q 4 hr, and with type I, also test urine for ketones; report if moderate or high.

17. Failure to take insulin will result in ketoacidosis. Adjust insulin based on BS and guidelines for insulin administration during sick days. Identify soft foods and liquids to consume for sick days (i.e., regular soda, apple juice, clear broth, cream soups, puddings, apple sauce, popsicle, ice cream ).

18. If ill, notify provider; to prevent coma, maintain adequate hydration by drinking 1 cup or more of noncaloric fluids such as coffee, tea, water, or broth every hour. Test finger sticks and urine more; identify when to go to the emergency room.

19. If there is no insulin/equipment to administer, decrease food intake by one-third and drink plenty of fluids. Obtain supplies as soon as possible and return to prescribed diet and insulin dosage.

20. Follow good hygienic practices to prevent infection. Bathe daily with mild soap and lukewarm water. Use lotion to prevent skin dryness. Avoid injury from punctures. Avoid scratches; wear gloves when working

with the hands. Always protect feet and wear shoes. Use sunscreen and protective clothing to avoid sunburn, and dress appropriately for the weather, taking care to prevent frostbite.

21. Establish a daily routine of checking and caring for the feet. Wear comfortable shoes (leather or canvas) and stockings (no garters or elastic tops) and do exercises. Clip toenails (straight across); do not undertake any self-treatment for ingrown toenails, corns, warts, or calluses. Do not use any heat treatments, hot water bottles, or heating pads, and do not smoke, as this decreases blood flow to the feet. Obtain annual foot screen.

22. Hyperglycemia compounds risk for tooth and gum problems; brush after meals, floss daily, and see dentist q 6 mo.

23. Diabetes can damage the small blood vessels to the eye; obtain yearly eye exams. Eye damage has no symptoms in the early, treatable stage. Report blurred or double vision, narrowed visual fields, increased difficulty seeing in dim light, pressure or pain in the eye, or seeing dark spots.

24. May experience decreased sensation in feet, legs, and hands; use care when handling hot or cold items, wear shoes to protect feet, and dress appropriately for the weather.

25. Carry ID and list of meds, who to notify and what to do if unable to respond.

26. Avoid alcohol; causes hypoglycemia. Excessive intake may require a reduction of insulin; also causes a disulfiram-type reaction with oral hypoglycemic agents.

27. Carry all medications, syringes, glucagon, and blood testing equipment in carry-on luggage when traveling. Always carry diabetes ID. Keep to the usual meal, exercise, and medication routines as closely as possible. Carry food and fast-acting sugar in the event meals are de-

layed. Request meds for vomiting/diarrhea and plan ahead for mealtimes when crossing two or more time zones. Protect insulin and test strips from extremes in heat or cold (keeping between 15°C and 30°C or 59°F and 86°F).

28. Use only the insulin prescribed; check for correct species (human, beef, pork, or mixed beef-pork), brand name (Humulin, Iletin I, Iletin II, etc.), and type (Regular, Lente, NPH, etc.).

29. Check vials before each dose is taken. Regular and Buffered Regular insulin (for pumps) should be clear and colorless, whereas other forms may be cloudy.

30. Two kinds of insulin can be mixed in the same syringe
• Regular insulin can be mixed with any other insulin.
• Lente forms can be mixed with other Lente insulins but cannot be mixed with other insulins except regular insulin.
• A single form of insulin in a syringe can be stable for weeks or a month.
• Except for the commercially prepared mixtures, mixtures of insulin are not stable and should be administered within 5 min of preparation.
• When mixed, regular (unmodified) insulin should always be drawn up in the syringe first.

31. Impotence may be caused by damaged nerves and reduced blood flow related to diabetes; should be evaluated to find cause and best treatment.

32. Silent heart attacks may occur. Identify risk factors and alter lifestyle to prevent CAD (i.e., regular exercise, low-fat, low-salt, low-cholesterol diet, no tobacco or alcohol, stress reduction).

33. Identify support groups to assist in understanding and coping with this disease. The American Diabetes Association, 1660 Duke Street, Alexandria, VA 22314 (telephone: 703-549-1500 or 1-800-ADA-DISC) and local diabetes support groups offer additional information and support.

**Outcomes/Evaluate**
• Understanding and management of diabetes
• Positive coping strategies
• Serum glucose, HbA1c, and renal function studies WNL
• Healthy intact skin at injection sites
• Prevention of target organ damage

# ANTIEMETICS

*See also the following individual entries:*

Dimenhydrinate
Diphenhydramine hydrochloride
Dronabinol
Granisetron hydrochloride
Hydroxyzine hydrochloride
Hydroxyzine pamoate
Meclizine hydrochloride
Ondansetron hydrochloride
Phosphorated carbohydrate solution
Prochlorperazine
Prochlorperazine edisylate
Prochlorperazine maleate
Scopolamine hydrobromide
Trimethobenzamide hydrochloride

**General Statement:** Nausea and vomiting can be caused by a variety of conditions, such as infections, drugs, radiation, motion, organic disease, or psychologic factors. The underlying cause of the symptoms must be elicited before emesis is corrected. Many drugs used for other conditions, such as the antihistamines, phenothiazines, barbiturates, and scopolamine, have antiemetic properties and can be used. However, CNS depression make their routine use undesirable.

**Drug Interactions:** Because of their antiemetic and antinauseant activity, the antiemetics may mask overdosage caused by other drugs.

**NURSING CONSIDERATIONS**
**Assessment**
1. Determine if nausea is an unusual occurrence or a recurring phe-

nomenon; establish onset, duration, and causative factors such as vertigo, chemotherapy, or illness.

2. Note any past use of antiemetics; under what conditions and the response.

3. Ensure no intestinal obstruction, drug overdose, or increased ICP.

4. Determine physiologic mechanism triggering N&V. Generally, if centrally mediated to the CTZ, would see nausea without vomiting, whereas if the vomiting center were triggered directly, then may see retching with vomiting.

5. Assess for other effects; antiemetics may mask signs of underlying pathology or overdosage of other drugs.

6. Monitor I&O; observe for dehydration. Offer liquids and then gradually advance to regular foods as tolerated.

**Client/Family Teaching**

1. Drug may cause drowsiness and dizziness. Avoid driving or performing other hazardous tasks until drug effects evaluated.

2. Review measures to decrease nausea such as ice chips, sips of water, nongreasy foods, removal of noxious stimuli (odors or materials), and frequent oral hygiene. Advance diet only as tolerated.

3. Dangle legs before standing, rise slowly to prevent symptoms of orthostatic hypotension.

4. Report any unresponsive N&V or abdominal pain.

5. Avoid alcohol and any other nonprescribed CNS depressants.

**Outcomes/Evaluate**

• Control of N&V; prevention of dehydration

• Improved nutritional status evidenced by weight gain and/or ↑ caloric intake

---

# ANTIHISTAMINES (H₁ BLOCKERS)

*See also the following individual entries:*

Astemizole
Brompheniramine maleate
Cetirizine hydrochloride
Chlorpheniramine maleate
Cyproheptadine hydrochloride
Dexchlorpheniramine maleate
Dimenhydrinate
Diphenhydramine hydrochloride
Fexofenadine hydrochloride
Levocabastine hydrochloride
Loratidine
Meclizine hydrochloride
Olopatadine hydrochloride
Promethazine hydrochloride
Terfenadine
Tripelennamine hydrochloride

**Action/Kinetics:** Compete with histamine at H₁ histamine receptors (competitive inhibition), thus preventing or reversing the effects of histamine. First-generation antihistamines bind to central and peripheral H₁ receptors and can cause CNS depression or stimulation. Second-generation antihistamines are selective for peripheral H₁ receptors and cause less sedation. Antihistamines do not prevent the release of histamine, antibody production, or antigen-antibody interactions. Antihistamines prevent or reduce increased capillary permeability (i.e., decrease edema, itching) and bronchospasms. Allergic reactions unrelated to histamine release are not affected by antihistamines. Certain of the first-generation antihistamines also have anticholinergic, antiemetic, antipruritic, or antiserotonin effects. Clients unresponsive to a certain antihistamine may regain sensitivity by switching to a different antihistamine.

From a chemical point of view, the antihistamines can be divided into the following classes.

**FIRST GENERATION:**

1. **Ethylenediamine Derivatives.** Moderate sedative effects; almost no anticholinergic or antiemetic activity. Frequently cause GI distress. Example: Tripelennamine.

2. **Ethanolamine Derivatives.** Moderate to high sedative effects.

---

Significant anticholinergic and antiemetic effects. Low incidence of GI side effects. Examples: Clemastine, diphenhydramine.

3. **Alkylamines.** Among the most potent antihistamines. Minimal sedation, moderate anticholinergic effects, and no antiemetic effects. Paradoxical excitation may also occur. Examples: Brompheniramine, chlorpheniramine, dexchlorpheniramine.

4. **Phenothiazines.** Significant antihistaminic action and sedation; high degree of both anticholinergic and antiemetic effects. Example: Promethazine.

5. **Piperidines.** Moderate antihistaminic activity, low to moderate sedation, moderate anticholinergic activity, and no antiemetic effects. Examples: Azatadine, cyproheptadine, phenindamine.

**SECOND GENERATION:**

1. **Piperazines.** Low to no sedation or anticholinergic effects and no antiemetic activity. Example: Cetirizine.

2. **Piperidines.** Moderate to high antihistamine activity, low to no sedation and anticholinergic activity, and no antiemetic action. Examples: Astemizole, fexofenadine, loratidine, terfenadine.

The kinetics of most first-generation antihistamines are similar. **Onset:** 15–30 min; **peak:** 1–2 hr; **duration:** 4–6 hr (piperidines have a longer duration). Many antihistamines are available as timed-release preparations. Most first-generation antihistamines are metabolized by the liver and excreted in the urine. The pharmacokinetics of the second-generation antihistamines vary; consult individual drugs.

**Uses: PO:** Treatment of vasomotor, perennial, or seasonal allergic rhinitis and allergic conjunctivitis. Treatment of angioedema, urticarial transfusion reactions, urticaria, pruritus. Atopic dermatitis, contact dermatitis, pruritus ani, pruritus vulvae, insect bites. Sneezing and rhinorrhea due to the common cold. Treatment of anaphylaxis, parkinsonism, drug-induced extrapyramidal reactions, vertigo. Prophylaxis and treatment of motion sickness, including N&V. Nighttime sleep aid.

*Parenteral:* Relief of allergic reactions due to blood or plasma. As an adjunct to epinephrine in treating anaphylaxis. Uncomplication allergic conditions when PO therapy is not possible.

See also the individual drugs.

**Contraindications:** *First-generation antihistamines.* Hypersensitivity to the drug, narrow-angle glaucoma, symptomatic prostatic hypertrophy, stenosing peptic ulcer, and pyloroduodenal or bladder neck obstruction. Use with MAO inhibitors. Pregnancy or possibility thereof (some agents), lactation, premature and newborn infants. The phenothiazine-type antihistamines are contraindicated in CNS depression from any cause, bone marrow depression, jaundice, dehydrated or acutely ill children, and in comatose clients. Use to treat lower respiratory tract symptoms such as asthma.

*Second-generation antihistamines.* Hypersensitivity. Astemizole and terfenadine use in significant hepatic dysfunction and concomitant use with clarithromycin, erythromycin, itraconazole, ketoconazole, quinine, and troleandomycin due to the possibility of serious CV effects (including torsades de pointes, prolongation of the QT interval, other ventricular arrhythmias, cardiac arrest, and death). Also terfenadine use with cisapride, HIV protease inhibitors, mibefradil, serotonin reuptake inhibitors, sparfloxacin, and zileuton.

**Special Concerns:** Administer with caution to clients with convulsive disorders and in respiratory disease. Excess dosage may cause hallucinations, convulsions, and death in infants and children. Use in geriatric clients may result in dizziness, excessive sedation, syncope, toxic confusional states, and hypotension.

**Side Effects:** *CNS:* Sedation ranging from mild drowsiness to deep sleep. Dizziness, incoordination, faintness, fatigue, confusion, lassitude, restlessness, excitation, nervousness, tremor, *tonic-clonic seizures,* headache, irritability, insomnia, euphoria, paresthesias, oculogyric crisis, torticollis, catatonic-like states, hallucinations, disorientation, tongue protrusion (usually with IV use or overdosage), disturbing dreams, nightmares, pseudoschizophrenia, weakness, diplopia, vertigo, hysteria, neuritis, paradoxical excitation, epileptiform seizures in clients with focal lesions. Extrapyramidal reactions include opisthotonus, dystonia, akathisia, dyskinesia, and parkinsonism. *CV:* Postural hypotension, palpitations, bradycardia, tachycardia, reflex tachycardia, extrasystoles, increased or decreased BP, ECG changes (including blunting of T waves and prolongation of the Q-T interval), *cardiac arrest.* *GI:* Epigastric distress, anorexia, increased appetite and weight gain, N&V, diarrhea, constipation, change in bowel habits, stomatitis. *GU:* Urinary frequency, dysuria, urinary retention, gynecomastia, inhibition of ejaculation, decreased libido, impotence, early menses, induction of lactation. *Hematologic:* Hypoplastic anemia, *aplastic anemia, hemolytic anemia,* thrombocytopenia, leukopenia, pancytopenia, *agranulocytosis,* thrombocytopenic purpura. *Respiratory:* Thickening of bronchial secretions, wheezing, nasal stuffiness, chest tightness, sore throat, *respiratory depression;* dry mouth, nose, and throat. *Ophthalmic:* Blurred vision, diplopia. *Miscellaneous:* Tinnitus, photosensitivity, acute labyrinthitis, obstructive jaundice, erythema, high or prolonged glucose tolerance curves, glycosuria, elevated spinal fluid proteins, increased plasma cholesterol, increased perspiration, chills; tingling, heaviness, and weakness of the hands.

*Topical use:* Prolonged use may result in local irritation and allergic contact dermatitis.

**OD** **Overdose Management:** *Symptoms (Acute Toxicity):* Although antihistamines have a wide therapeutic range, overdosage can nevertheless be fatal. Children are particularly susceptible. Early toxic effects may be seen within 30–120 min and include drowsiness, dizziness, blurred vision, tinnitus, ataxia, and hypotension. Symptoms range from CNS depression (sedation, *coma,* decreased mental alertness) to *CV collapse* and CNS stimulation (insomnia, hallucinations, tremors, or *seizures*). Also, *profound hypotension, respiratory depression, coma, and death* may occur. Anticholinergic effects include flushing, dry mouth, hypotension, fever, *hyperthermia* (especially in children), and fixed, dilated pupils. Body temperature may be as high as 107°F. In children, symptoms include hallucinations, toxic psychosis, delirum tremens, ataxia, incoordination, muscle twitching, excitement, athetosis, *hyperthermia, seizures,* and hyperreflexia followed by postictal depression and *cardiorespiratory arrest.* *Treatment:*

• Treat symptoms and provide supportive care.

• Vomiting is induced with syrup of ipecac (do not use for phenothiazine overdosage) followed by activated charcoal and a cathartic. If vomiting has not been induced within 3 hr of ingestion, gastric lavage can be undertaken.

• Hypotension can be treated with a vasopressor such as norepinephrine, dopamine, or phenylephrine (do not use epinephrine).

• For convulsions, use only short-acting depressants (e.g., diazepam). IV physostigmine can be used to treat centrally mediated convulsions.

• Ice packs and a cool sponge bath are effective in reducing fever in children.

---

*bold italic* = life threatening side effect

• Severe cases of overdose can be treated by hemoperfusion.

**Drug Interactions**

*Alcohol, ethyl* / See *CNS depressants*

*Anticoagulants* / Antihistamines may ↓ the anticoagulant effects

*Antidepressants, tricyclic* / Additive anticholinergic side effects

*CNS depressants, antianxiety agents, barbiturates, narcotics, phenothiazines, procarbazine, sedative-hypnotics* / Potentiation or addition of CNS depressant effects. Concomitant use may lead to drowsiness, lethargy, stupor, respiratory depression, coma, and possibly death

*Heparin* / Antihistamines may ↓ the anticoagulant effects

*MAO inhibitors* / Intensification and prolongation of anticholinergic side effects; use with phenothiazine antihistamine → hypotension and extrapyramidal reactions

NOTE: Also see *Drug Interactions* for *Phenothiazines*.

**Laboratory Test Interferences:** Discontinue antihistamines 4 days before skin testing to avoid false – result.

**Dosage**

**Usually PO.** Parenteral administration is seldom used because of irritating nature of drugs. Topical usage is also limited because antihistamines often cause hypersensitivity reactions. When given for motion sickness, antihistamines are usually given 30–60 min before anticipated travel. See individual drugs.

# NURSING CONSIDERATIONS

**Administration/Storage**

1. Inject IM preparations deep into the muscle; irritating to the tissues.

2. Swallow sustained-release preparations whole. Scored tablets may be broken before swallowing. If difficulty swallowing capsules, may open and put contents into soft food for ingestion.

3. Do not apply topical preparations to raw, blistered, or oozing areas of the skin.

4. Do not apply to the eyes, around the genitalia, or to mucous membranes.

5. PO preparations may cause gastric irritation; administer with meals, milk, or a snack.

**Assessment**

1. Note any drug sensitivity; document known allergens and all meds prescribed.

2. Avoid with any ulcers, glaucoma, or pregnancy.

3. Document type, onset, and duration of symptoms; note triggers.

4. Stop antihistamines 2–4 days prior to skin testing to avoid false negative results.

5. Document VS, CV status, and lung sounds; note characteristics of secretions.

6. Note extent and characteristics of any rash, if present.

**Client/Family Teaching**

1. Take med before or at the onset of symptoms; cannot reverse reactions but may prevent them.

2. Do not drive or operate equipment until drug effects realized or drowsiness worn off. Sedative effects may disappear after several days or may not occur at all.

3. Report sore throat, fever, unexplained bruising, bleeding, or petechiae; may cause blood dyscrasia.

4. May cause sensitivity to sun or ultraviolet light; avoid long exposures, use sunscreen, hat, sunglasses, and protective clothing when in the sun.

5. If used for motion sickness, take 30 min before travel time.

6. Reduce symptoms of dry mouth by frequent rinsing, good oral hygiene, and sugarless gum or candies.

7. Severe CNS depression is a symptom of overdosage. Report dizziness, weakness; avoid other CNS depressants.

8. Ensure adequate hydration. If bronchial secretions are thick, increase fluids to decrease secretion viscosity; avoid milk temporarily. If voiding problems, void prior to taking the drug.

9. Exercise regularly; consume 2 L fluids/day and more fruits, fruit juic-

es, and dietary fiber to prevent constipation. Stool softeners may be needed.

10. Recurrent reactions may be referred to an allergist. Protect self from undue exposure and create an allergen-free living area.

11. Raise BP, use with high BP only if medically supervised.

12. Avoid alcohol and OTC products.

13. Children may manifest excitation rather than sedation.

14. Clinical effectiveness may diminish with continued usage; switching to another class may restore drug effectiveness.

15. Family/significant other should learn CPR; survival is greatly increased when CPR is initiated immediately.

**Outcomes/Evaluate**

- ↓ Frequency/intensity of allergic manifestations; ↓ itching/swelling
- Prevention of motion sickness
- Effective nighttime sedation

# ANTIHYPERLIPIDEMIC AGENTS—HMG-COA REDUCTASE INHIBITORS

*See also the following individual entries:*

Atorvastatin calcium
Fluvastatin sodium
Lovastatin
Pravastatin sodium
Simvastatin

**General Statement:** The National Cholesterol Education Program Expert Panel on Detection, Evaluation, and Treatment of High Blood Cholesterol in Adults has developed guidelines for the treatment of high cholesterol and LDL in adults. Cholesterol levels less than 200 mg/dL are desirable. Cholesterol levels between 200 and 239 mg/dL are considered borderline-high while levels greater than 240 mg/dL are considered high. With respect to LDL, levels less than 130 mg/dL are considered desirable while levels between 130 and 159 md/dL are considered borderline-high and levels greater than 160 mg/dL are considered high. Depending on the levels of cholesterol and LDL and the number of risk factors present for CAD, the provider will develop a treatment regimen.

**Action/Kinetics:** The HMG-CoA reductase inhibitors competitively inhibit HMG-CoA reductase; this enzyme catalyzes the early rate-limiting step in the synthesis of cholesterol. HMG-CoA reductase inhibitors increase HDL cholesterol and decrease LDL cholesterol, VLDL cholesterol, and plasma triglycerides. The mechanism to lower LDL cholesterol may be due to both a decrease in VLDL cholesterol levels and induction of the LDL receptor, leading to reduced production or increased catabolism of LDL cholesterol. The maximum therapeutic response is seen in 4–6 weeks.

**Uses:** Adjunct to diet to decrease elevated total LDL and cholesterol in clients with primary hypercholesterolemia (types IIa and IIb) when the response to diet and other nondrug approaches has not been adequate. See also individual drugs.

**Contraindications:** Active liver disease or unexplained persistent elevated liver function tests. Pregnancy, lactation. Use in children.

**Special Concerns:** Use with caution in those who ingest large quantities of alcohol or who have a history of liver disease. Safety and efficacy have not been established in children less than 18 years of age.

**Side Effects:** The following side effects are common to most HMG-CoA reductase inhibitors. Also see individual drugs. *GI:* N&V, diarrhea, constipation, abdominal cramps or pain, flatulence, dyspepsia, heartburn. *CNS:* Headache, dizziness, dysfunction of certain cranial nerves (e.g., alteration of taste, facial paresis, impairment of extraocular movement), tremor, vertigo, memory loss, paresthesia, anxiety, insomnia, depression. *Musculoskeletal:* Localized pain, myalgia, muscle cramps or pain, myopathy, rhabdomyolysis, arthralgia. *Respiratory:* Upper respiratory infection, rhinitis, cough. *Ophthalmic:* Progression of cataracts (lens opacities), ophthalmoplegia. *Hypersensitivity:* **Anaphylaxis, angioedema,** vasculitis, purpura, thrombocytopenia, leukopenia, **hemolytic anemia,** lupus erythematosus-like syndrome, polymyalgia rheumatica, positive ANA, ESR increase, arthritis, arthralgia, eosinophilia, urticaria, photosensitivity, fever, chills, flushing, malaise, dyspnea, **toxic dermal necrolysis, Stevens-Johnson syndrome.** *Miscellaneous:* Rash, pruritus, cardiac chest pain, fatigue, influenza, alopecia, edema, dryness of skin and mucous membranes, changes to hair and nails, skin discoloration.

**Drug Interactions**
*Gemfibrozil* / Severe myopathy or rhabdomyolysis
*Warfarin* / ↑ Anticoagulant effect of warfarin.

**Laboratory Test Interferences:** ↑ AST, ALT, CPK, alkaline phosphatase, bilirubin. Abnormal thyroid function tests.

**Dosage**
See individual drugs.

## NURSING CONSIDERATIONS

**Administration/Storage:** Lovastatin should be taken with meals; fluvastatin, pravastatin, and simavastatin may be taken without regard to meals.

**Assessment**
1. Review life-style, duration of illness, and attempts made to control with diet, exercise, and weight reduction.
2. Note any alcohol abuse or liver disease.
3. Perform PMH, ROS, and physical exam; document risk factors.
4. Monitor LFTs as recommended. Transaminase levels 3 times normal may precipitate severe hepatic toxic-

ity. If CK elevated, assess renal function as rhabdomyolsis with myoglobinuria could cause renal shutdown. Stop drug therapy.
5. Note nutritional analysis by dietician; assess cholesterol profile (HDL, LDL, cholesterol, and triglycerides) after 3–6 months of exercise and diet therapy if risk factors do not require immediate drug therapy.

**Client/Family Teaching**
1. Take only as directed.
2. May cause photosensitivity; avoid prolonged exposure to the sun or UV light. Use sunscreens, sunglasses, and protective clothing when exposed.
3. Report any pain in skeletal muscles or unexplained muscle pain, tenderness, or weakness promptly, especially if accompanied by fever or malaise.
4. Continue life-style modifications that include low-fat, low-cholesterol, and low-sodium diets, weight reduction with obese clients, smoking cessation, reduction of alcohol consumption, and regular aerobic exercise in the overall goal of cholesterol reduction.
5. Do not take niacin; may cause hepatic failure.
6. Avoid any unprescribed or OTC agents.
7. Stop drug with any major trauma, surgery, or serious illness.
8. Report for labs to prevent liver toxicity and to assess results.

**Outcomes/Evaluate:** ↓ LDL, triglycerides, and total cholesterol levels; ↓ risk of CAD

# ANTIHYPERTENSIVE AGENTS

*See also the following drug classes and individual drugs:*

*Agents Acting Directly on Vascular Smooth Muscle*

    Diazoxide IV
    Hydralazine hydrochloride
    Nitroprusside sodium

*Alpha-1-Adrenergic Blocking Agents*

Doxazosin mesylate
Prazosin hydrochloride
Terazosin

*Angiotensin-II Antagonists*

Irbesartan
Losartan potassium

*Angiotensin-Converting Enzyme Inhibitors*

Benazepril hydrochloride
Captopril
Enalapril maleate
Fosinopril sodium
Lisinopril
Moexipril hydrochloride
Quinapril hydrochloride
Ramipril
Trandolopril

*Beta-Adrenergic Blocking Agents*

*Calcium Channel Blocking Agents*

Amlodipine
Bepridil hydrochloride
Diltiazem hydrochloride
Felodipine
Isradipine
Mibefradil dihydrochloride
Nicardipine hydrochloride
Nifedipine
Nimodipine
Nisoldipine
Verapamil

*Centrally-Acting Agents*

Clonidine hydrochloride
Guanabenz acetate
Guanfacine hydrochloride
Methyldopa
Methyldopate hydrochloride

*Combination Drugs Used for Hypertension*

Amiloride and
Hydrochlorothiazide
Amlodipine and Benazepril
hydrochloride
Bisoprolol fumarate and
Hydrochlorothiazide
Enalapril maleate and
Hydrochlorothiazide
Fosinopril sodium
Lisinopril and
Hydrochlorothiazide

Losartan potassium and
Hydrochlorothiazide
Methyldopa and
Hydrochlorothiazide
Propranolol and
Hydrochlorothiazide
Spironolactone and
Hydrochlorothiazide
Triamterene and
Hydrochlorothiazide

*Miscellaneous Agents*

Carvedilol
Epoprostenol sodium
Labetalol hydrochloride
Mecamylamine hydrochloride
Minoxidil, oral

*Peripherally-Acting Agents*

Guanadrel Sulfate
Guanethidine sulfate
Phentolamine mesylate

**General Statement:** The Sixth Report of the Joint National Committee on Prevention, Detection, Evaluation and Treatment of High Blood Pressure classifies BP for adults aged 18 and over as follows: Optimal as <120/<80 mm Hg, Normal as <130/<85 mm Hg, High Normal as 130–139/85–89 mm Hg, Stage 1 Hypertension as 140–159/90–99 mm Hg, Stage 2 Hypertension as 160–179/100–109 mm Hg, and Stage 3 Hypertension as 180 or greater/110 or greater mm Hg. Drug therapy is recommended depending on the BP and whether certain risk factors (e.g., smoking, dyslipidemia, diabetes, age, gender, target organ damage, clinical CV disease) are present. Life-style modification is an important component of treating hypertension, including weight reduction, reduction of sodium intake, regular exercise, cessation of smoking, and moderate alcohol intake.

The goal of antihypertensive therapy is a BP of <140/90 mm Hg, except in hypertensive diabetics where the goal is <135/85 mm Hg and those with renal insufficiency where the goal is <130/85 mm Hg. Generally speaking, the primary agents for initial monotherapy to treat uncomplicat-

---

♣ = Available in Canada                    ***bold italic*** = life threatening side effect

ed hypertension are diuretics and beta blockers. Alternative drugs include ACE inhibitors, alpha-1 blockers, alpha-beta blocker, and calcium antagonists.

**NURSING CONSIDERATIONS**
**Assessment**
1. Obtain history; note any family history of hypertension, stroke, CVD, CHD, dyslipidemia, and diabetes.
2. Determine baseline BP before starting any antihypertensive therapy. To ensure accuracy of baseline readings, take BP in both arms (lying, standing, and sitting) 2 min apart (30 min after last cigarette) at least three times during one visit and on two subsequent visits. Document weight and risk factors.
3. Ascertain life-style modifications (weight reduction, ↓ alcohol intake, regular exercise, reduced sodium/fat intake, and smoking cessation) needed to achieve lowered BP. Offer a trial following these modifications and reassess in 3–6 mo before starting therapy unless BP severe.
4. Monitor ECG, electrolytes, FBS, CBC, uric acid, urinalysis, and liver and renal function studies.
5. Note funduscopic and neurologic exam findings.
6. Assess for thyroid enlargement and presence of target organ damage. If difficult to control or complex, refer for 24-hr ambulatory BP monitoring.
**Client/Family Teaching**
1. Drugs control but do not cure hypertension. Take meds despite feeling fine and do not stop abruptly; may cause rebound hypertension.
2. Keep a record of BP readings for provider; helps identify "white collar syndrome."
3. Adhere to a low-sodium, low-fat diet; see dietitian as needed for education and meal planning, preparation, and food selections.
4. Weakness, dizziness, and fainting may occur with rapid changes of position from supine to standing. Rise slowly from a lying or sitting position and dangle legs for several minutes before standing to minimize orthostatic effects. Exercising in hot weather may enhance hypotensive effects.
5. If dose missed, do not double up or take two doses close together.
6. Have yearly eye exams to detect early retinal changes.
7. Avoid meds that may lower BP (e.g., alcohol, barbiturates, CNS depressants) or that could elevate BP (e.g., OTC cold remedies, oral contraceptives, steroids, NSAIDs, appetite suppressants, tricyclic antidepressants, MAO inhibitors). Sympathomimetic amines in products used to treat asthma, colds, and allergies must be used with extreme caution
8. Avoid excessive amounts of caffeine (tea, coffee, chocolate, or colas).
9. Notify provider if sexual dysfunction occurs as med can usually be changed to minimize symptoms or other options for sexual dysfunction explored.
10. Identify holistic interventions/life-style modifications necessary for BP control: dietary restrictions of fat and sodium (2–3 g/day), weight reduction, ↓ alcohol (i.e., less than 24 oz beer or less than 8 oz of wine or less than 2 oz of 100-proof whiskey per day), tobacco cessation, ↑ physical activity, regular exercise programs, proper rest, and methods to reduce and deal with stress.
**Outcomes/Evaluate**
• Understanding of illness/compliance with prescribed therapy
• ↓ BP (SBP < 140 and DBP < 90 mm Hg)
• Control/prevent target organ damage

# ANTI-INFECTIVE DRUGS

*See also the following individual drugs and drug classes:*

Amebicides and Trichomonacides
Aminoglycosides
4-Aminoquinolines
Anthelmintics
Antimalarials

Antiviral Drugs
Aztreonam for injection
Bacitracin
Butenafine hydrochloride
Cephalosporins
Chloramphenicol
Clindamycin
Erythromycins
Fluoroquinolones
Fosfomycin tromethamine
Imipenem-Cilastatin sodium
Lincomycin hydrochloride
Loracarbef
Macrolides
Meropenem
Mupirocin
Penicillins
Pentamidine isethionate
Spectinomycin hydrochloride
Sulfonamides
Tetracyclines
Trimetrexate glucuronate
Vancomycin hydrochloride

**General Statement**

The following general guidelines apply to the use of most anti-infective drugs:

1. Anti-infective drugs can be divided into those that are *bacteriostatic,* that is, arrest the multiplication and further development of the infectious agent, or *bactericidal,* that is, kill and thus eradicate all living microorganisms. Both time of administration and length of therapy may be affected by this difference.

2. Some anti-infectives halt the growth of or eradicate many different microorganisms and are termed *broad-spectrum antibiotics.* Others affect only certain specific organisms and are termed *narrow-spectrum antibiotics.*

3. Some of the anti-infectives elicit a hypersensitivity reaction in some persons. Penicillins cause more severe and more frequent hypersensitivity reactions than any other drug.

4. Because of differences in susceptibility of infectious agents to anti-infectives, the sensitivity of the microorganism to the drug ordered should

be determined before treatment is initiated. Several sensitivity tests are commonly used for this purpose.

5. Certain anti-infective agents have marked side effects, some of the more serious of which are neurotoxicity, including ototoxicity, and nephrotoxicity. Care must be taken not to administer two anti-infectives with similar side effects concomitantly, or to administer these drugs to clients in whom the side effects might be damaging (e.g., a nephrotoxic drug to a client suffering from kidney disease). The choice of anti-infective also depends on its distribution in the body (i.e., whether it passes the blood-brain barrier).

6. Anti-infective drugs can also eradicate the normal intestinal flora necessary for proper digestion, synthesis of vitamin K, and control of fungi that may gain access to the GI tract (superinfection).

**Action/Kinetics:** The mechanism of action of the anti-infectives varies. The following modes of action have been identified.* Note the considerable overlap among these mechanisms:

1. Inhibition of synthesis of or activation of enzymes that disrupt bacterial cell walls leading to loss of viability and possibly cell lysis (e.g., penicillins, cephalosporins, cycloserine, bacitracin, vancomycin, miconazole, ketoconazole, clotrimazole).

2. Direct effect on the microbial cell membrane to affect permeability and leading to leakage of intracellular components (e.g., polymyxin, colistimethate, nystatin, amphotericin).

3. Effect on the function of 30S and 50S bacterial ribosomes to cause a reversible inhibition of protein synthesis (e.g., chloramphenicol, tetracyclines, erythromycin, clindamycin).

4. Bind to the 30S ribosomal subunit that alters protein synthesis and leads to cell death (e.g., aminoglycosides).

---

*Chambers, H.F., Sande, M.A.: Antimicrobial agents. In *Goodman and Gilman's The Pharmacological Basis of Therapeutics,* 9th ed. Edited by Hardman, J.G., Limbud, L.E., New York, McGraw-Hill, 1996, p. 1029.

♣ = Available in Canada          **bold italic** = life threatening side effect

5. Effect on nucleic acid metabolism which inhibits DNA-dependent RNA polymerase (e.g., rifampin) or inhibition of gyrase (e.g., quinolones).

6. Antimetabolites that block specific metabolic steps essential to the life of the microorganism (e.g., trimethoprim, sulfonamides).

7. Bind to viral enzymes that are essential for DNA synthesis leading to a halt of viral replication (e.g., acyclovir, ganciclovir, vidarabine, zidovudine).

**Uses:** See individual drugs. The choice of the anti-infective depends on the nature of the illness to be treated, the sensitivity of the infecting agent, and the client's previous experience with the drug. Hypersensitivity and allergic reactions may preclude the use of the agent of choice.

**Contraindications:** Hypersensitivity or allergies to the drug.

**Side Effects:** The antibiotics and anti-infective agents have few direct toxic effects. Kidney and liver damage, deafness, and blood dyscrasias are occasionally observed.

The following undesirable manifestations, however, occur frequently:

1. Suppresion of the normal flora of the body, which in turn keeps certain pathogenic microorganisms, such as *Candida albicans, Proteus,* or *Pseudomonas,* from causing infections. If the flora is altered, *superinfections* (monilial vaginitis, enteritis, UTIs), which necessitate the discontinuation of therapy or the use of other antibiotics, can result.

2. Incomplete eradication of an infectious organism. Casual use of anti-infectives favors the emergence of *resistant* strains insensitive to a particular drug.

To minimize the chances for the development of resistant strains, anti-infectives are usually given at specified doses for a prescribed length of time after acute symptoms have subsided.

**OD** **Overdose Management:** *Treatment:* Discontinue the drug and treat symptomatically. Supportive measures should be instituted as needed. Hemodialysis may be used although its effectiveness is questionable, depending on the drug and the status of the client (i.e., more effective in impaired renal function).

**Laboratory Tests:** The bacteriologic sensitivity of the infectious organism to the anti-infective (especially the antibiotic) should be tested by the lab before initiation of therapy and during treatment.

## GENERAL NURSING CONSIDERATIONS FOR ALL ANTI-INFECTIVES

**Administration/Storage**

1. Check expiration date.

2. Store according to recommended method of drug storage.

3. Mark date and time of reconstitution, your initials, and the solution strength. Note and mark how long the drug may be stored after dilution; store under appropriate conditions.

4. Complete administration by IVPB (or as ordered) before the drug loses potency.

**Assessment**

1. Document type and onset of symptoms, location and source of infection (if known).

2. Note any unusual reaction or problems with any anti-infectives (usually penicillin).

3. Obtain cultures before administering empiric therapy. Use correct procedure for obtaining, storing, and transporting specimens.

4. Monitor CBC, liver and renal function studies.

**Interventions**

1. Conspicuously mark allergy in red on the chart, medication record, ID band, care plan, pharmacy record, and bed.

2. Assess for side effects such as hives, rashes, difficulty breathing, which may indicate a hypersensitivity or allergic response; stop drug and report.

3. Monitor VS, I&O; ensure adequate hydration.

4. If drug mainly excreted by the

kidneys, reduce dose with renal dysfunction. Nephrotoxic drugs are usually contraindicated with renal dysfunction because toxic levels of the drugs are rapidly attained when renal function is impaired.

5. Verify orders when two or more anti-infectives are ordered for the same client, especially if they have similar side effects, such as nephrotoxicity and/or neurotoxicity.

6. Assess for superinfections, particularly of fungal origin, characterized by black furred tongue, nausea, and/or diarrhea. *Prevent superinfections by:*

• Limiting exposure to persons suffering from an active infectious process
• Rotating IV site q 72 hr; changing IV tubing q 24–48 hr
• Providing/emphasizing good hygiene
• Washing hands carefully before and after contact with client

7. Schedule administration throughout 24-hr period to maintain therapeutic drug levels. Administration schedule is determined by the drug half-life (t½), severity of infection, evidence of organ dysfunction, and client's need for sleep. Assess drug levels (peak and trough) to ensure appropriate dosing.

**Client/Family Teaching**

1. Take meds at prescribed intervals; use only under medical supervision.

2. Do not share with friends or family members. Prevent recurrence by completing entire prescription, despite feeling well. This ensures that the organism is eradicated and diminishes the emergence of drug-resistant bacterial strains. Incomplete therapy may render client unresponsive to the antibiotic with the next infection.

3. Report any unusual bruising or bleeding, e.g., bleeding gums, blood in stool, urine, or other secretions; S&S of allergic reactions, including rash, fever, pruritis, and urticaria or superinfections such as pain, swelling, redness, drainage, perineal itching, diarrhea, rash, or a change in symptoms.

4. Discard any unused drug after therapy completed.

5. Take antipyretics as prescribed RTC (q 4 hr) for fever reduction when needed.

**Outcomes/Evaluate**

• Prevention/resolution of infection
• ↓ Fever, WBCs; ↑ appetite
• Negative culture reports
• Therapeutic serum drug levels

# ANTIMALARIAL DRUGS, 4-AMINOQUINOLINES

*See also the following individual entries:*

Chloroquine hydrochloride
Chloroquine phosphate
Hydroxychloroquine sulfate

**Action/Kinetics:** Several mechanisms have been proposed for the action of 4-aminoquinolines. These include (a) an active chloroquine-concentrating mechanism in the acid vesicles of the parasite causing inhibition of growth, (b) release of aggregates of ferriprotoporphyrin IX from erythrocytes in the parasite causing membrane damage and erythrocyte or parasite lysis, (c) interference with hemoglobin digestion by the parasite, and (d) interference with synthesis of nucleoprotein by the parasite. The drugs are active against the erythrocytic forms of *Plasmodium vivax* and *P. malariae* as well as most strains of *P. falciparum*. The aminoquinolines are rapidly and almost completely absorbed from the GI tract and are widely distributed throughout the body. **Peak serum levels:** 1–6 hr. Very slowly excreted; presence of drug has been demonstrated in the bloodstream weeks and even months after the drug has been discontinued. Up to 70% may be excreted unchanged. Urinary excretion is increased by acidifying the urine; excretion is slowed by alkalinization.

**Uses:** Treatment or prophylaxis of acute attacks of malaria caused by *Plasmodium falciparum, P. vivax, P. ovale,* and *P. malariae.* Will cause a radical cure of vivax and malariae malaria if combined with primaquine. Effective only against the erythrocytic stages and therefore will not prevent infections. However, complete cure of infections due to sensitive strains of falciparum malaria is possible.

Extraintestinal amebiasis caused by *Entamoeba histolytica.* Discoid or lupus erythematosus, scleroderma, pemphigus, lichen planus, polymyositis, sarcoidosis, porphyria cutanea tarda.

**Contraindications:** Hypersensitivity. Changes in retinal or visual field. Lactation. Use in psoriasis or porphyria only if benefits clearly outweigh risks. Concomitantly with gold or phenylbutazone or in clients receiving drugs that depress blood-forming elements of bone marrow.

**Special Concerns:** Use with extreme caution in the presence of hepatic, severe GI, neurologic, and blood disorders. Infants and children are sensitive to the effects of 4-aminoquinolines. Certain strains of *P. falciparum* are resistant to 4-aminoquinolines.

**Side Effects:** *GI:* N&V, diarrhea, cramps, anorexia, epigastric distress, stomatitis, dry mouth. *CNS:* Headache, fatigue, nervousness, anxiety, irritability, agitation, apathy, confusion, personality changes, depression, psychoses, **seizures.** *CV:* Hypotension, ECG changes (inversion or depression of T wave, widening of QRS complex). *Dermatologic:* Pruritus, changes in pigment of skin and mucous membranes, dermatoses, bleaching of hair. *Hematologic:* Neutropenia, **aplastic anemia,** thrombocytopenia, **agranulocytosis.** *Ocular:* Retinopathy that may be permanent and may lead to blindness. Blurred vision, difficulty in focusing or in accommodation; chronic use may lead to corneal deposits or keratopa-

thy. *Miscellaneous:* Peripheral neuritis, ototoxicity, neuromyopathy manifested by muscle weakness.

**OD** **Overdose Management:** *Symptoms:* Headache, drowsiness, visual disturbances, *CV collapse, seizures followed by sudden and early respiratory and cardiac arrest.* Infants and children have manifested respiratory depression, *CV collapse, shock, seizures, and death following overdoses of parenteral chloroquine.* ECG changes include nodal rhythm, atrial standstill, prolonged intraventricular conduction, and bradycardia, which lead to *ventricular fibrillation or arrest.* *Treatment:* Undertake gastric lavage or emesis followed by activated charcoal. Seizures should be controlled prior to gastric lavage. Seizures due to anoxia can be treated by oxygen, mechanical ventilation, or vasopressors (in shock with hypotension). Tracheostomy or tracheal intubation may be required. Forced fluids and acidification of the urine may hasten excretion. Peritoneal dialysis and exchange transfusions may also help.

**Drug Interactions**
*Acidifying agents, urinary (ammonium chloride, etc.)* / ↑ Urinary excretion of antimalarial and thus ↓ its effectiveness
*Alkalinizing agents, urinary (bicarbonate, etc.)* / ↓ Excretion of antimalarial and thus ↑ amount of drug in system
*Antipsoriatics* / 4-Aminoquinolines inhibit antipsoriatic drugs
*MAO inhibitors* / ↑ Toxicity of 4-Aminoquinolines due to ↓ breakdown in liver

**Laboratory Test Interferences:** Colors urine brown.

**Dosage** ———————————
See individual drug entries.

## NURSING CONSIDERATIONS

See also *General Nursing Considerations for All Anti-Infectives.*

**Administration/Storage:** Store in amber-colored containers.

**Assessment**
1. Identify if for prophylaxis or

acute drug therapy; identify source and exposure dates.

2. Obtain cultures. Note any hepatic, neurologic, or blood disorders; monitor lab parameters.

3. Assess for retinopathy manifested by visual disturbances. Retinal changes are not reversible. Mandate regular eye exams during prolonged therapy.

**Interventions**

1. Observe for overdosage and symptoms of acute toxicity (headache, drowsiness, visual disturbances, CV collapse, convulsions, and cardiac arrest) which develop within 30 min of ingestion. Death may occur within 2 hr; see *Overdose Management*.

2. Monitor VS, I&O, and state of consciousness.

3. With some therapies, fluids will have to be forced and ammonium chloride administered for weeks to months to acidify urine and promote renal excretion of the drug.

4. Check toxic effects of other drugs being used because the combination with chloroquine may intensify toxic effects.

5. When used for suppressive therapy, administer drug on the same day each week. Give immediately before or after meals to minimize gastric irritation (e.g., hydroxychloroquine).

6. Administer with the evening meal when managing discoid lupus erythematosus.

**Client/Family Teaching**

1. Take exactly as prescribed.

2. Report any persistent, new, or bothersome side effects.

3. Report as scheduled for F/U and labs to prevent relapse.

4. Ensure that adequate fluid intake as well as the meds to acidify urine are taken as prescribed. Some drugs may discolor urine brown.

5. Wear sunglasses to prevent photophobia.

6. Avoid alcohol during therapy.

7. Keep in child-proof containers and out of child's reach.

**Outcomes/Evaluate**

• Understanding of disease/compliance with prescribed therapy
• Malaria prophylaxis
• Elimination of causative organism
• Symptomatic improvement

# ANTINEOPLASTIC AGENTS

*See also the following individual entries:*

Aldesleukin
Altretamine
Amifostine
Anastrozole
Asparaginase
Bicalutamide
Bleomycin sulfate
Busulfan
Carboplatin for injection
Carmustine
Chlorambucil
Cisplatin
Cladribine injection
Cyclophosphamide
Cytarabine
Dacarbazine
Dactinomycin
Daunorubicin
Diethylstilbestrol diphosphate
Docetaxel
Doxorubicin hydrochloride
Doxorubicin hydrochloride liposomal
Estramustine phosphate sodium
Etoposide
Floxuridine
Fludarabine phosphate
Fluorouracil
Flutamide
Gemcitabine hydrochloride
Goserelin acetate
Hydroxyurea
Idrarubicin hydrochloride
Ifosfamide
Interferon Alfa-n3
Interferon Alfa-2a Recombinant
Interferon Alfa-2b Recombinant
Irinotecan hydrochloride
Letrozole
Leuprolide acetate

---

Levamisole hydrochloride
Lomustine
Mechlorethamine hydrochloride
Megestrol acetate
Melphalan
Mercaptopurine
Mesna
Methotrexate
Methotrexate sodium
Mitomycin
Mitotane
Mitoxantrone hydrochloride
Nilutamide
Octreotide acetate
Paclitaxel
Pegaspargase
Pentostatin
Plicamycin
Porfimer sodium
Procarbazine hydrochloride
Rituximab
Streptozocin
Strontium-89 chloride
Tamoxifen
Teniposide
Testolactone
Thioguanine
Thiotepa
Topotecan hydrochloride
Toremifene citrate
Vinblastine sulfate
Vincristine sulfate
Vinorelbine tartrate

**General Statement:** The choice of the chemotherapeutic agent(s) depends both on the cell type of the tumor and on its site of growth. All antineoplastic agents are cytotoxic (i.e., cell poisons) and therefore interfere with normal as well as neoplastic cells. However, neoplastic cells are more active and multiply more rapidly than normal cells and are thus more affected by the antineoplastic agents. Normal, rapidly growing tissue cells, such as those of the bone marrow, the GI mucosal epithelium, and hair follicles, are particularly susceptible to antineoplastic agents. The margin between the dose of antineoplastic drug needed to destroy the neoplastic cells and that needed to cause bone marrow damage, for example, is narrow. Since WBCs or platelets show the effect of an overdose more rapidly than do erythrocytes, the platelet and WBC counts are often used as a guide to dosage. If a blood or marrow test indicates a precipitous fall in the WBC or platelet count, the antineoplastic agent may have to be discontinued or the dosage modified significantly. Drugs are frequently withheld when the WBC count falls below $2,000/mm^3$ and the platelet count falls below $100,000/mm^3$. With the advent of granulocyte colony-stimulating factors, providers may now utilize this to support large dosing on an aggressive cancer, thus preventing postponement of therapy until recovery of the client's hematologic parameters. Sometimes the effect of the antineoplastic drugs on the bone marrow is cumulative, with the depression of WBCs and platelets occurring weeks or months after initiation of therapy.

GI tract toxicity is manifested by development of oral ulcers, intestinal bleeding, nausea, vomiting, loss of appetite, and diarrhea. Finally, alopecia often results from antineoplastic drug therapy.

**Action:** During division, cells go through a number of stages during which they may be susceptible to various chemotherapeutic agents (see *Action/Kinetics* of various agents). The various cell stages are described in Figure 2.

**Uses:** Most of the drugs discussed in this section are used exclusively for neoplastic disease. A few are used on an experimental basis for some of the rheumatic diseases.

**Contraindications:** Hypersensitivity to drug. Some antineoplastic agents may be contraindicated for a period of 4 weeks after radiation therapy or chemotherapy with similar drugs. During first trimester of pregnancy.

**Special Concerns:** Use with caution, and at reduced dosages, in clients with preexisting bone marrow depression, malignant infiltration of bone marrow or kidney, liver dysfunction, or previous recent chemotherapy usage. The safe use of these

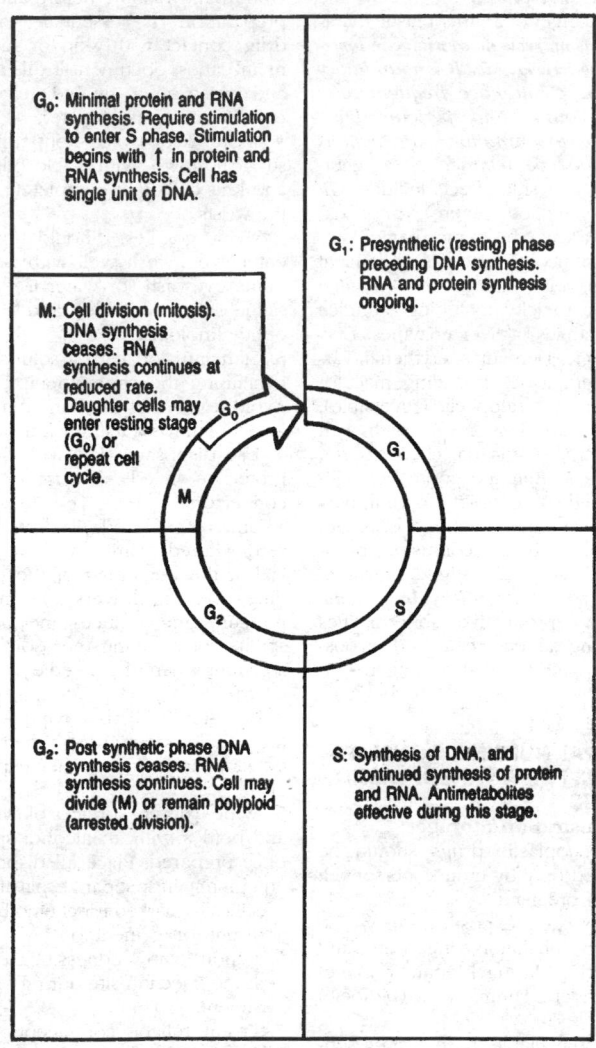

**Figure 2**   Cell stages.

drugs during pregnancy has not been established.

**Side Effects:** *Bone marrow depression* (leukopenia, thrombocytopenia, **agranulocytosis,** anemia) is the major danger of antineoplastic therapy. **Bone marrow depression can sometimes be irreversible.** *It is mandatory that the client have frequent total blood counts and periodic bone marrow examinations. Precipitous falls must be reported to a physician.* Other side effects include: *GI:* N&V (may be severe), anorexia, diarrhea (may be hemorrhagic), stomatitis, mucositis, enteritis, abdominal cramps, intestinal ulcers. *Hepatic:* Hepatic toxicity including jaundice and changes in liver enzymes. *Dermatologic:* Dermatitis, erythema, various dermatoses including maculopapular rash, alopecia (reversible), pruritus, staining of vein path with some drugs, urticaria, cheilosis. *Immunologic:* Immunosuppression with increased susceptibility to viral, bacterial, or fungal infections. *CNS:* Depression, lethargy, confusion, dizziness, headache, fatigue, malaise, fever, weakness. *GU:* **Acute renal failure,** reproductive abnormalities including amenorrhea and azoospermia. *NOTE:* Alkylating agents, in particular, may be both carcinogenic and mutagenic.

## GENERAL NURSING CONSIDERATIONS FOR ANTINEOPLASTIC AGENTS

### Administration/Storage

1. Antineoplastic drugs should be prepared only by trained personnel; avoid if pregnant.
2. Cytotoxic exposure may be through inhalation, ingestion, and absorption during preparation; prepare under a laminar flow (biologic) hood.
   • If not available, prepare in a separate room in a work area away from cooling or heating vents and away from other people. Cover work table area with a disposable plastic liner.

• Use latex gloves to protect the skin when reconstituting; do not use gloves made of PVC since these are permeable to some cytotoxic drugs. Good handwashing before and after preparation is essential. Prevent drug contact with skin or mucous membranes; document if this occurs and wash area immediately with copious amounts of water.
• Wear disposable, nonpermeable surgical gown with a closed front and knit cuffs that completely cover the wrists.
• Wear goggles. Should material enter eyes, wash well with isotonic saline eyewash (or water if isotonic saline is unavailable) and consult ophthalmologist.

3. Start infusion with a solution not containing the chemotherapy drug. Avoid dorsum of the hand, wrist, or antecubital fossa as infusion site.
4. Use disposable Luer-Lok fittings, protective needles, syringes, and connectors.
   • Under the hood, if drug to be reconstituted from a vial, vent the vial at the beginning of the procedure. Venting lowers the internal pressure and reduces the risk of spilling or spraying (aerosolization) solution when the needle is withdrawn.
   • Use sterile alcohol wipe around the needle and vial top when withdrawing the drug and when expelling air.
5. Wipe external surfaces of syringes and bottles with an alcohol sponge once prepared. Place all disposable equipment in a separate plastic bag specifically marked for chemotherapy and sent for incineration.
6. Report pain, redness, or edema near the injection site during or after treatment.
7. Ensure reliable contraception.
8. Wear latex gloves when disposing of vomitus, urine, or feces.
9. Record all exposure times during preparation, administration, cleanup, and spills. Follow appropriate institutional guidelines governing

exposures allowed, extravasation, and periodic lab evaluations.

# NURSING CONSIDERATIONS DURING INITIATION OF CHEMOTHERAPY

## Assessment

1. Identify condition requiring therapy and any previous radiation, surgery, or chemotherapy treatments.
2. Assess emotional status; note any hypersensitivity to drugs or foods.
3. Assess nutritional status; note height, weight, and VS; doses are based on BSA ($m^2$).
4. Examine oral mucosa for any abnormalities or problems.
5. Monitor bone marrow function (CBC with differential), platelets, liver and renal function.
6. Note prescribed route of administration: oral, IV, IM, or directly at the tumor site (intracavity, intrapleural, intrathecal, intravesical, intraperitoneal, intra-arterial, or topical).
7. Depending on the route, length of therapy, frequency of access, venous integrity, and client preference, determine if venous access device would be more comfortable.
8. Assess pain control regimen to ensure that meds are available in quantities sufficient to relieve pain.
9. Premedicate (antiemetic, antihistamine, and/or anti-inflammatory) 30–60 min before therapy and as needed.

## Interventions

1. Monitor VS, I&O.
2. Report any pain, redness, or edema near injection site during or after treatment. If extravasation occurs, stop infusion and follow institutional protocol for minimizing effects. General guidelines for managing an extravasation include
- Document and report.
- Aspirate drug through the cannula with a small syringe (tuberculin size).
- Administer antidote when indicated.
- Remove needle and apply ice (heat if vinca alkaloids).

- Assess and follow-up until site is healed.
3. Chart antineoplastic drugs on the medication administration record (MAR) and according to the established protocol.
- Record client's drug therapy on the MAR:
- Day 1: first day of the first dose.
- Number each day after that in sequence, even though may not receive drug daily.
- Indicate when nadir (the time of most severe physiologic depression) is likely to occur so that possible complications, such as infection and bleeding, can be anticipated, assessed for, and treated early; note recovery time.
- When repeating drug regimen, the first day of therapy is charted as day 1.
4. Establish interventions to promote client compliance. Keep informed and interpret complicated terminology/therapy; support client/family and help to understand unconventional emotions and anger.
5. Identify support groups to assist in coping with illness, complex therapy, and emotional turmoil within family unit.

## Client/Family Teaching

1. Comply with all aspects of the therapeutic regimen.
2. Review information/literature R/T condition requiring treatment. The American Cancer Society provides many free booklets on cancers, chemotherapy, and how to deal with the side effects of treatments. Go to the library, local cancer society, and provider with unanswered questions. May also call 1-800-4-CANCER, the Cancer Information Service at the National Cancer Institute, or access through the Internet for further information
3. Review drug side effects that may occur and a means for coping with these problems.
4. Identify community support groups that may assist in coping with illness.

---

★ = Available in Canada                    **bold italic** = life threatening side effect

5. Provide a number to reach provider to report adverse side effects or to request clarification of instructions.

6. When antineoplastic agents are prepared and administered in the home, advise families how to dispose of urine, feces, vomitus, and equipment and how to handle drug spills.

**Outcomes/Evaluate**

• Understanding of illness, drug side effects, and goals of therapy

• N&V, pain, anorexia, or diarrhea that may indicate inadequate levels of prescribed agents

• Evidence of acute renal failure, hepatic toxicity, or changes in liver enzymes

• Presence and extent of psychologic depression, lethargy, or other mental status changes

• Control of pain

• Control/regression of malignant cell proliferation

• Desired cure

## NURSING CONSIDERATIONS FOR BONE MARROW DEPRESSION (MYELOSUPPRESSION)

LEUKOPENIA

**Assessment**

1. Assess for granulocytopenia or decreased WBCs (normal values: 5,000–10,000/mm$^3$).

2. Review differential (normal values: neutrophils 60%–70%, lymphocytes 25%–30%, monocytes 2%–6%, eosinophils 1%–3%, basophils 0.25%–0.5%).

3. Note any sudden sharp drop in WBC count or a reduction below 2,000/mm$^3$; may require a reduction in dosage or withdrawal of drug.

4. Determine nadir (time the blood count reaches its lowest point after chemotherapy) for prescribed agent (generally 7–14 days). This assists to predict, monitor, and respond to effects of the bone marrow depression.

5. Report fever above 38°C (100°F); limited resistance to infection due to leukopenia and immunosuppression. Assess for early signs of infection: check oral cavity for sores/ulcerated areas and urine for odor or particulate matter. With reduced or absent granulocytes, local abscesses do not form with pus; infection becomes systemic.

6. Increased weakness or fatigue may indicate anemia or electrolyte imbalance. Fatigue is a significant side effect of therapy. With cytobines, e.g., interferon, fatigue may be overwhelming.

**Interventions**

1. *Prevent infection by* using strict medical asepsis and frequent handwashing.

2. Provide frequent, meticulous, physical hygiene; maintain clean environment.

3. Cleanse and dry rectal area after each bowel movement. Apply ointment if irritated; use Tucks and/or Nupercainal for discomfort.

4. Use a gentle antiseptic to wash with tendency for skin eruptions.

5. Provide mouth care q 4–6 hr; otherwise mucosal deterioration occurs. Avoid lemon or glycerin; these tend to reduce saliva production and change pH of the mouth.

6. If WBC falls below 1,500–2,000/mm$^3$, may protect with:

• Private room; explain reasons

• Universal precautions; use gloves, masks, and gowns

• Avoid indwelling urinary catheters

• Limit articles brought into room

• Provide private bathroom or bedside commode

• Minimize traffic in and out of room

• Screen visitors for infection before they enter room; limit visitations

• Avoid exposure to dust, sprays, contaminated medical equipment

• Avoid deodorants; blocks sebaceous gland secretion

• Keep fresh fruits, vegetables, cut flowers, and any source of stagnant water (water pitcher, humidifiers, flower vases) away from client

• Review/stress kitchen hygiene and food safety at home

• Dogs, cats, birds, and other animals may carry infection; avoid contact

• Assess orders for granulocyte colony-stimulating factors and ensure availability
7. Prevent nosocomial infections from invasive procedures by:
• Washing hands before and after any contact
• Cleansing skin with antiseptic before procedure
• Changing IV tubing q 24 hr
• Changing IV site q 48 hr, if no implanted device or other designated catheter for long-term use
• Practice strict asepsis with all treatments and dressing changes

THROMBOCYTOPENIA
**Assessment**
1. Obtain platelet count (normal values: 150,000–400,000/mm³). If platelet count below 50,000/mm³ monitor closely.
2. Check urine for blood cells; stool and gastric contents for occult blood.
3. Inspect skin for petechiae/bruising; assess all orifices for bleeding.
4. May hemorrhage spontaneously if platelets are below 20,000; transfuse platelets.
**Interventions**
1. Minimize SC or IM injections; apply pressure for 3–5 min to prevent leakage or hematoma.
2. Do not apply BP cuff or other tourniquet for excessive periods of time.
3. Avoid rectal temps and constipation; test all urine, GI secretions, and stool for occult blood.
4. Use safety precautions to avoid falls.
5. *Control bleeding*
• With epistaxis: pinch nose for 10 min and apply pressure to upper lip to stop; in severe cases, small sponges saturated with neosynephrine ¼% gently inserted into affected nare, or nasal packing, may be necessary.
• With transfusions, monitor VS before and q 15 min after transfusion started and for at least 2 hr after completed. Assess for histoincompatibility, indicated by chills, fever,

and urticaria. Stop transfusion, provide supportive care, and follow appropriate institutional protocol for transfusion reaction.
6. Advise client to *prevent bleeding* by:
• Not picking or forcefully blowing their nose
• Avoiding contact sports and any activities that may lead to injury
• Reporting any severe frontal headaches
• Using an electric razor for shaving rather than a blade
• Using a soft-bristled toothbrush or massaging gums with fingers or a cotton ball and avoiding dental floss to limit irritation
• Avoiding rectal irritation with enemas, suppositories, or thermometers
• Using a water-based lubricant before intercourse
• Consuming plenty of fluids, increasing activity, and taking stool softeners to prevent constipation
• Rearranging furniture so that area for ambulation is unimpeded and also to prevent bumping into furniture at night when getting out of bed to go to the bathroom
• Having a night light to permit visualization during the night
• Wearing shoes or slippers when ambulating

ANEMIA
**Assessment**
1. Monitor CBC, reticulocyte count, MCV and hemoglobin (normal values: men, 13.5–18.0 g/dL blood; women, 11.5–15.5 g/dL blood), and hematocrit (normal values: men, 40%–52%; women, 35%–46%), and iron panel.
2. Assess for pallor, lethargy, dizziness, increased SOB, or unusual fatigue.
**Interventions**
1. *Minimize anemia by:*
• Providing a nutritious tolerable diet
• Taking vitamins/iron supplements as ordered

---

2. *Assist with treatment of anemia by:*
- Administering diet high in iron
- Giving vitamins/iron supplements
- Administering blood transfusions
- Spacing/scheduling activities to permit frequent rest periods
- Positioning to facilitate ventilation; teaching breathing and relaxation techniques and administering oxygen
- Controlling room temperature for comfort and providing emotional support

## NURSING CONSIDERATIONS FOR GI TOXICITY

NAUSEA AND VOMITING; ANOREXIA

### Assessment

1. N&V may be due to either a CNS effect on the chemoreceptor trigger zone or direct irritation to the GI tract. With radiation therapy, N&V may be attributed to the accumulation of toxic waste products of cell destruction and localized damage to the lining of the throat, stomach, and intestine.
2. Anticipatory N&V is a conditioned response of unknown origin prior to chemotherapy which does respond to premedication.
3. Determine if refusing food or fluids or experiencing anorexia.
4. Monitor nutritional status and weights.
5. Examine the frequency, character, and amount of vomitus. List antiemetics prescribed and results.

### Interventions

1. *Prevent N&V by:*
- Premedicating with antiemetics. Usually given 30–60 min before or just after drug therapy.
- Administering therapy on an empty stomach, with meals, or at bedtime
- Using an antiemetic suppository
- Providing ice chips at onset of nausea
- Avoiding carbonated beverages
- Ingesting dry carbohydrates such as toast and dry crackers before any activity

- Waiting for N&V to pass before serving food
- Providing small, nutritious snacks and planning meal schedules to coincide with client's best tolerance time
- Encouraging cold foods and salads with little cooking aroma to minimize N&V
- Providing nourishing foods client likes
- Encouraging intake of a high-protein diet
- Freezing and serving dietary supplements like ice cream to make them more palatable
- Avoiding foods with overpowering aroma
- Chewing foods well
- Providing good oral hygiene both before and after meals (try 1 tsp baking soda in a glass of warm water)
- Eating favorite foods
- Eating meals with others, preferably at a table. Sharing encourages some clients to eat.
2. Antiemetics that have different actions/pharmacokinetics may be administered concurrently in an effort to control severe N&V.
3. *Treat N&V by:*
- Administering antiemetic(s). Report all vomiting; a change in therapy or electrolyte correction may be needed.
- Giving other medications after meals
- Offering simple foods: rice, toast, noodles, bananas, scrambled eggs, mashed potatoes, custards, ice cream
- Offering salty foods (pretzels, crackers)
- Avoiding solid and liquid foods at the same meal
- Eliminating any room odors; avoiding malodorous foods (e.g., cabbage, sauerkraut, etc.)
- Keeping as comfortable, clean, and free from odor as possible
- Trying another or concurrent antiemetic agents
- Correcting electrolytes; providing hyperalimentation
- Screening visitors and calls until client ready

4. *Approach anorexia by:*
• Providing small, frequent meals q 2 or 3 hr on schedule
• Maximizing caloric intake by offering nutrient-dense snacks and drinks (yogurt, cheese and crackers, peanut butter and jelly sandwiches, cereal, dried fruit, fruit nectars, and instant breakfast drink mixes)
• Making nutrient-dense supplements with whole milk
• Suggesting a walk or activity before eating to boost appetite
• Concentrating on and obtaining favorite foods
5. *Increase caloric intake and protein consumption by:*
• Adding high-calorie foods such as mayonnaise, butter, and gravy to foods
• Using whole milk in puddings, cream soups, custards
• Making double-strength milk by adding powdered milk to whole milk for gravies, hot cereals, mashed potatoes, eggs, casseroles, baked things, etc.
• Adding whipped cream to frosting and desserts
• Offering milkshakes, nectar, and eggnog when thirsty
• Offering peanut butter on crackers, bagels with cream cheese, trail mix, and nuts and seeds for snacks
• Cutting up meats and cheeses and adding to salads, soups, scrambled eggs, etc.

BOWEL DYSFUNCTION (DIAR-RHEA/ABDOMINAL CRAMPING)
**Assessment**
1. Note frequency and severity of cramping caused by hypermotility.
2. Document frequency, color, consistency, and amount of diarrhea; indicates tissue destruction. Check stool C&S.
3. Assess for dehydration and acidosis indicating electrolyte imbalance; monitor I&O.
**Interventions**
1. *Prevent diarrhea/abdominal cramping by:*
• Providing small, frequent meals on a schedule

• Identifying factors that aggravate/increase incidence
• Using constipating foods, i.e., hard cheeses
2. *Treat diarrhea by:*
• Administering antidiarrheal and narcotic agent (i.e., codeine, tincture of opium, imodium, or lomotil). Report diarrhea or abdominal cramping as a change in therapy or electrolyte correction may be needed.
• Increasing fluids to avoid dehydration
• Providing foods to correct sodium and potassium losses, e.g., bananas, potatoes, fish and meat, apricot nectar, tomato juice, and sports drinks with "electrolytes"
• Avoiding high-fiber foods that contain "insoluble fiber," such as wheat bran, brown rice, and popcorn
• Administering bulk-forming agents (i.e., metamucil)
• Offering "soluble-fiber" foods, i.e., white rice, oatmeal, applesauce, mashed potatoes, and pears
• Avoiding fried foods and greasy foods
• Avoiding excessive sweets; may aggravate diarrhea due to sorbitol, found in many gums and candies
• Using alumimum-containing antacids
• Avoiding gas-forming foods, such as broccoli, corn, onion, garlic, lentils, and kidney beans
• Considering lactose-free products or Lact-Aid, which facilitates digestion of lactose
• Restricting oral intake to rest the bowel if necessary
• Providing good skin care, especially to perianal area to prevent skin breakdown. Apply A&D ointment for perianal tenderness. Change gown and bed linens frequently; use special mattresses and room deodorizers as needed.
3. *Prevent constipation by:*
• Providing a high-fiber diet
• Administering stool softeners and bulk-forming agents
• Promoting increased fluid intake

---

✦ = Available in Canada                    *bold italic* = life threatening side effect

- Increasing activity levels
- Monitoring frequency, consistency, and amount of stool

4. *Prevent obstruction by:*
- Aggressive management of constipation
- Assessing for early S&S such as abdominal pain, N&V, and diminished or absent bowel sounds
- Keeping NPO, using NG suction to relieve before referring for surgical intervention

STOMATITIS (MUCOSAL ULCERATION)
**Assessment**
1. Assess for mouth dryness, erythema, soreness, painful swallowing, and white patchy areas of oral mucosa.
2. Symptom onset usually 5 days to 2 weeks after starting therapy; assess regularly.
**Interventions**
1. *Prevent stomatitis by:*
- Assessing oral cavity t.i.d. and reporting bleeding gums or burning sensation when acid liquids such as fruit juice are ingested
- Setting up a regular schedule for oral preventive care
- Providing good mouth care
- Applying lubricant (Vaseline) to lips t.i.d.
2. *Treat stomatitis by:*
- Providing good oral care
- Applying topical viscous anesthetic, such as benzocaine 20%, or a swish and gargle anesthetic dyclonine hydrochloride 0.5%, or a swish, swallow/discard agent such as lidocaine 2% (Xylocaine), before meals or as needed to anesthetize oral mucosa. May swallow lidocaine after swishing it around oral cavity but encouraged to expectorate it.
- Puncture a vitamin E capsule and apply to painful lesions to promote healing
- Offering "Magic Mouthwash," which consists of 4 g (approx. ⅛ teaspoon) baking soda, 30mL viscous xylocaine, 30mL benedryl elixir, and 30mL Maalox (optional) in 1 L NSS; swish and spit out q 1–2 hr as needed

- Providing allopurinol mouthwash for fluorouracil-related stomatitis; or try sucking ice chips ½ hr before and during treatment
- Offering small, frequent meals of bland foods at medium temperatures
- Administering nystatin solution or clotrimazole troches for fungal infections
3. Administer medications (antifungals, antivirals) to prevent general infections.

**NURSING CONSIDERATIONS FOR NEUROTOXICITY**
**Assessment**
1. Be aware of agents causing or having the potential to cause neurotoxic effects; further administration once symptoms have become prominent may be life threatening.
2. Report symptoms of minor neuropathies, i.e., tingling in hands and feet; loss of deep tendon reflexes. Use a monofilament to measure progressive loss of sensation.
3. Report serious neuropathies, i.e., weakness of hands, ataxia, loss of coordination, foot drop, wrist drop, or paralytic ileus.
**Interventions**
1. *Prevent functional loss due to neurotoxicity by:*
- Identifying neuropathies early so drug regimen can be adjusted
- Practicing/teaching seizure precautions
2. *Treat neuropathies by:*
- Using safety measures with functional losses
- Maintaining good body alignment by frequent and anatomically correct repositioning; ROM exercises.
- Providing stool softeners/laxatives as needed

**NURSING CONSIDERATIONS FOR OTOTOXICITY**
**Assessment:** Assess for hearing difficulties before initiating therapy.
**Interventions**
1. Report tinnitus or hearing impairment.
2. Perform audiometry testing p.r.n. during therapy.

## NURSING CONSIDERATIONS FOR HEPATOTOXICITY

**Assessment**

1. Obtain/assess the following LFTs:
- Total serum bilirubin (normal values: 0.1–1.0 mg/dL); elevations may indicate liver disease or increased rate of RBC hemolysis.
- AST (normal values: 8–33 units/L). Elevations indicative of changes in liver, skeletal muscles, lungs, pancreas, and heart. Hepatitis produces striking elevations in the AST.
- ALT (normal values: 8–20 units/L). Elevations may precede hepatic necrosis.
- LDH (normal values: 70–250 units/L). Elevations may indicate hepatitis, pulmonary infarction, and CHF.

2. Assess for liver involvement, i.e., abdominal pain, high fever, diarrhea, and yellowing of skin/sclera.

**Interventions**

1. Prevent further hepatotoxicity by reporting LFT elevations and signs of liver involvement so drug regimen can be changed.

2. Assist with the treatment for hepatotoxicity by providing supportive nursing care for pain, fever, diarrhea, and symptoms associated with jaundice.

## NURSING CONSIDERATIONS FOR RENAL TOXICITY

**Assessment**

1. Assess the following renal function tests:
- BUN (normal values: 5–20 mg/dL)
- Serum uric acid (normal values: men, 3.5–7.0 mg/dL; women, 2.4–6.0 mg/dL)
- Creatinine clearance (normal values: women, 0.8–1.7 g/24 hr; men, 1.0–1.9 g/24 hr)
- Quantitative uric acid (normal values: 250–750 mg/day)

2. Report stomach pain, swelling of feet or lower legs, shakiness, unusual body movement, or stomatitis.

**Interventions**

1. Monitor I&O.

2. Limit hyperuricemia with extra fluids to speed excretion of uric acid and to decrease hazard of crystal and urate stone formation. Administer uricosuric agents (i.e., probenecid) or antigout agents (i.e., allopurinol, colchicine) to lower uric acid levels.

3. Test pH and alkalinize urine.

## NURSING CONSIDERATIONS FOR IMMUNOSUPPRESSION

**Assessment**

1. Assess for the presence of fever, chills, or sore throat.

2. Note any changes in WBC and differential.

**Interventions**

1. Treat client with immunosuppression by:
- Preventing infection as noted under bone marrow depression for leukopenia
- Delaying active immunization for several months after therapy is completed; may experience a hypo- or hyperactive response
- Avoiding contact with children who have recently taken the oral polio vaccine
- Administering granulocyte colony-stimulating factor

2. Review food safety (e.g., storage, handling, washing, cooking meats thoroughly, avoiding raw eggs) and stress the importance of kitchen hygiene when preparing meals at home

## NURSING CONSIDERATIONS FOR GU ALTERATIONS

**Assessment**

1. Assess for altered GU function. Most symptoms, such as amenorrhea, cease after med is discontinued.

2. Review risks; sterility may be a permanent result of therapy.

**Client/Family Teaching**

1. Certain drugs may render individuals sterile. Advise that egg/sperm harvesting may be performed prior to therapy to accommodate future pregnancies.

2. To prevent teratogenesis, teach client and partner to use reliable contraceptive measures to avoid

---

pregnancy, both during and for several months after therapy.

## NURSING CONSIDERATIONS FOR ALOPECIA

### Client/Family Teaching

1. Hair loss is a normal occurrence with many during chemotherapy. Treatment disrupts the mitotic activity of the hair follicle which weakens the hair shaft which causes it to break off. This includes all hair, i.e., eyebrows, body, and pubic hair.
2. Alopecia may occur within 2–3 weeks after the initial treatment. Assist to understand, be prepared for, and expect this as normal with chemotherapy. People respond differently; some may lose hair with a certain agent, others may not.
3. Reinforce that hair will grow back but may be of a different texture or color. It should start to grow in again about 8 weeks after therapy is completed.
4. If receiving more than 4,500 rad to the cranium, hair loss may be permanent.
5. Alternatives for managing alopecia include
• Shopping for a wig before hair loss begins
• Wearing a bandana or hat to cover head, and taking special care to protect the bare head from sun exposure
• Shaving head, if hair starts to fall out in large clumps, and using a wig or scarf until scalp hair has grown in again
• Wearing a night cap at bedtime so hair that falls out during the night will be collected in one place and not all over the bed in the morning.
• Encouraging expression of feelings related to changes in self-image

## NURSING CONSIDERATIONS FOR ALTERATIONS IN SKIN

### Assessment

1. Document skin turgor and integrity.
2. Slight changes in skin color may occur during therapy.

### Interventions

1. Maintain cleanliness of skin through bathing and frequent linen changes.

2. Prevent dryness and replenish skin moisture with emollient lotions.
3. Prevent excessive exposure to sun or artificial ultraviolet light; use sunscreen and protective clothing when exposed.
4. Use a special mattress or bed to redistribute weight on bony prominences and to minimize pressure and friction on pressure points.
5. Establish and document a schedule for repositioning, massaging, and assessing skin condition.
6. Ensure adequate nutritional intake.
7. Refer for assistance with makeup application.
8. With pruritus, attempt to stop scratching as this may impair skin integrity. Administer antihistamines, corticosteroids, nonirritating moisturizers, and cool/ice compresses as needed.

# ANTIPARKINSON AGENTS

*See also the following individual entries:*

> Amantadine hydrochloride
> Benztropine mesylate
> Biperiden hydrochloride
> Bromocriptine mesylate
> Carbidopa
> Carbidopa/Levodopa
> Diphenhydramine hydrochloride
> Levodopa
> Pergolide mesylate
> Pramipexole
> Ropinirole hydrochloride
> Selegiline hydrochloride
> Trihexyphenidyl hydrochloride

**General Statement:** Parkinson's disease is a progressive disorder of the nervous system, affecting mostly people over the age of 50. Parkinsonism is a frequent side effect of certain antipsychotic drugs, including prochlorperazine, chlorpromazine, and reserpine. Drug-induced symptoms usually disappear when the responsible agent is discontinued. The cause of Parkinson's disease is unknown; however, it is associated with a depletion of the neurotransmitter dopamine in the nervous system. Administration of levodopa—the precursor of dopamine—relieves symptoms in 75%–80% of the clients. Anticholinergic agents also have a beneficial effect by reducing tremors and rigidity and improving mobility, muscular coordination, and motor performance. They are often administered together with levodopa. Certain antihistamines, notably diphenhydramine (Benadryl), are also useful in the treatment of parkinsonism. Clients suffering from Parkinson's disease need emotional support and encouragement because the debilitating nature of the disorder often causes depression. Comprehensive treatment also includes physical therapy.

**NURSING CONSIDERATIONS**

See *Nursing Considerations* for individual drugs.

**Assessment**

1. Document PMH, onset of symptoms, and their progression.
2. Determine if symptoms may be drug induced with agents such as haldol or phenothiazines.
3. Assess for depression, behavioral changes, and suicide ideations.

**Client/Family Teaching**

1. Parkinson's disease is a movement disorder of unknown origin; is usually progressive and leads to disability if untreated.
2. Drug therapy is aimed at restoring normal balances of cholinergic and dopaminergic influences in the brain (basal ganglia).
3. Take only as prescribed; some have many adverse side effects.
4. Close follow-up is imperative; some drugs may lose their effectiveness.

**Outcomes/Evaluate**

• Improved motor function and mood
• ↓ Drooling, ↓ rigidity, ↓ tremors
• Improvement in gait, posture, and muscle spasms

# ANTIPSYCHOTIC AGENTS, PHENOTHIAZINES

*See also the following individual entries:*

Chlorpromazine
Chlorpromazine hydrochloride
Fluphenazine decanoate
Fluphenazine enanthate
Fluphenazine hydrochloride
Mesoridazine besylate
Perphenazine
Prochlorperazine
Prochlorperazine edisylate
Prochlorperazine maleate
Promazine hydrochloride
Thioridazine hydrochloride
Trifluoperazine
Triflupromazine hydrochloride

**General Statement:** Antipsychotic drugs do not cure mental illness, but they calm the intractable client, relieve the despondency of the severely depressed, activate the immobile and withdrawn, and make some more accessible to psychotherapy.

Most phenothiazines induce some sedation, especially during the initial phase of the treatment. Medicated clients can, however, be easily roused. In this manner, the phenothiazines differ markedly from the narcotic analgesics and sedative hypnotics. However, phenothiazines potentiate the analgesic properties of opiates and prolong the action of CNS depressant drugs. These drugs also cause sedation, decrease spontaneous motor activity, and many lower BP.

According to their detailed chemical structure, the phenothiazines belong to three subgroups:
1. Dimethylaminopropyl compounds—includes chlorpromazine. Often the first choice for clients in acute excitatory states. Cause more sedation than other phenothiazines and are especially indicated for clients exhausted by lack of sleep.
2. Piperazine compounds—Act most selectively on the subcortical

sites. Minimal drowsiness and undesirable motor effects. Greatest antiemetic effects because they specifically depress the CTZ of the vomiting center.

3. Piperidine compounds—Less toxic in terms of extrapyramidal effects.

**Action/Kinetics:** It has been postulated that excess amounts of dopamine in certain areas of the CNS cause psychoses. Phenothiazines are thought to act by blocking postsynaptic mesolimbic dopamine receptors, leading to a reduction in psychotic symptoms. Phenothiazines block both $D_1$ and $D_2$ dopamine receptors. The antiemetic effects are thought to be due to inhibition or blockade of dopamine ($D_2$) receptors in the chemoreceptor trigger zone in the medulla as well as by peripheral blockade of the vagus nerve in the GI tract. Relief of anxiety is manifested as a result of an indirect decrease in arousal and increased filtering of internal stimuli to the brain stem reticular system. Alpha-adrenergic blockade produces sedation. Phenothiazines also raise pain threshold and produce amnesia due to suppression of sensory impulses. In addition, these drugs produce anticholinergic and antihistaminic effects and depress the release of hypothalamic and hypophyseal hormones. Peripheral effects include anticholinergic and alpha-adrenergic blocking properties.

**Peak plasma levels:** 2–4 hr after PO administration. Widely distributed throughout the body. **t½ (average):** 10–20 hr. Most metabolized in the liver and excreted by the kidney.

**Uses:** Psychoses, especially if excessive psychomotor activity manifested. Involutional, toxic, or senile psychoses. Used in combination with MAO inhibitors in depressed clients manifesting anxiety, agitation, or panic (use with caution). With lithium in acute manic phase of manic-depressive illness. As an adjunct in alcohol withdrawal to reduce anxiety, tension, depression, nausea, and/or vomiting. For severe behavioral problems in children, manifested by

hyperexcitable and/or combative behavior; also, for short-term use in hyperactive children who exhibit excess motor activity and conduct disorders.

Prophylaxis and control of severe N&V due to cancer chemotherapy, radiation therapy, postoperatively. Intractable hiccoughs, intermittent porphyria, tetanus (as adjunct). As preoperative and/or postoperative medications. Some phenothiazines are antipruritics. See also individual drugs.

**Contraindications:** Severe CNS depression, coma, clients with subcortical brain damage, bone marrow depression, lactation. In clients with a history of seizures and in those on anticonvulsant drugs. Geriatric or debilitated clients, hepatic or renal disease, CV disorders, glaucoma, prostatic hypertrophy. Contraindicated in children with chickenpox, CNS infections, measles, gastroenteritis, dehydration due to increased risk of extrapyramidal symptoms.

**Special Concerns:** Use with caution in clients exposed to extreme heat or cold and in those with asthma, emphysema, or acute respiratory tract infections. Use during pregnancy only when benefits outweigh risks. Children may be more sensitive to the neuromuscular or extrapyramidal effects (especially dystonias); those especially at risk include children with chickenpox, CNS infections, measles, dehydration, or gastroenteritis. Thus, generally, phenothiazines are not recommended for use in children less than 12 years of age. Geriatric clients often manifest higher plasma levels due to decreases in lean body mass, total body water, and albumin and an increase in total body fat. Also, geriatric clients may be more likely to manifest orthostatic hypotension, anticholinergic effects, sedative effects, and extrapyramidal side effects.

**Side Effects:** *CNS:* Depression, drowsiness, dizziness, lethargy, fatigue. Extrapyramidal effects, Parkinson-like symptoms including shuffling gait or tic-like movements of head and face, tardive dyskinesia (see what follows), akathisia, dystonia. **Seizures,** especially in clients with a history thereof. **Neuroleptic malignant syndrome (rare).** *CV:* Orthostatic hypotension, increase or decrease in BP, tachycardia, fainting. *GI:* Dry mouth, anorexia, constipation, paralytic ileus, diarrhea. *Endocrine:* Breast engorgement, galactorrhea, gynecomastia, increased appetite, weight gain, hyper- or hypoglycemia, glycosuria. Delayed ejaculation, increased or decreased libido. *GU:* Menstrual irregularities, loss of bladder control, urinary difficulty. *Dermatologic:* Photosensitivity, pruritus, erythema, eczema, exfoliative dermatitis, pigment changes in skin (long-term use of high doses). *Hematologic:* **Aplastic anemia,** leukopenia, **agranulocytosis,** eosinophilia, thrombocytopenia. *Ophthalmologic:* Deposition of fine particulate matter in lens and cornea leading to blurred vision, changes in vision. *Respiratory:* **Laryngospasm, bronchospasm, laryngeal edema,** breathing difficulties. *Miscellaneous:* Fever, muscle stiffness, decreased sweating, muscle spasm of face, neck, or back, obstructive jaundice, nasal congestion, pale skin, mydriasis, systemic lupus-like syndrome.

*Tardive dyskinesia* has been observed with all classes of antipsychotic drugs, although the precise cause is not known. The syndrome is most commonly seen in older clients, especially women, and in individuals with organic brain syndrome. It is often aggravated or precipitated by the sudden discontinuance of antipsychotic drugs and may persist indefinitely after the drug is discontinued. Early signs of tardive dyskinesia include fine vermicular movements of the tongue and grimacing or tic-like movements of the head and neck. Although there is no known cure for the syndrome, it may not progress if the dosage of the drug is slowly reduced. Also, a few drug-free days

may unmask the symptoms of tardive dyskinesia and help in early diagnosis.

**OD** **Overdose Management:** *Symptoms:* CNS depression including deep sleep and **coma,** hypotension, extrapyramidal symptoms, agitation, restlessness, seizures, hypothermia, **hyperthermia,** autonomic symptoms, **cardiac arrhythmias,** ECG changes. *Treatment:* Emetics are not to be used as they are of little value and may cause a dystonic reaction of the head or neck that may result in aspiration of vomitus.

• Hypotension: Volume replacement; norepinephrine or phenylephrine may be used (do not use epinephrine).

• Ventricular arrhythmias: phenytoin, 1 mg/kg IV, not to exceed 50 mg/min; may be repeated q 5 min up to 10 mg/kg.

• Seizures or hyperactivity: Diazepam or pentobarbital.

• Extrapyramidal symptoms: Antiparkinson drugs, diphenhydramine, barbiturates.

**Drug Interactions**
*Alcohol, ethyl* / Potentiation or addition of CNS depressant effects. Concomitant use may lead to drowsiness, lethargy, stupor, respiratory collapse, coma, or death
*Aluminum salts (antacids)* / ↓ Absorption from GI tract
*Amphetamine* / ↓ Effect of amphetamine by ↓ uptake of drug to the site of action
*Anesthetics, general* / See *Alcohol*
*Antacids, oral* / ↓ Effect of phenothiazines due to ↓ absorption from GI tract
*Antianxiety drugs* / See *Alcohol*
*Anticholinergic drugs* / Additive anticholinergic side effects and/or ↓ antipsychotic effect
*Antidepressants, tricyclic* / Additive anticholinergic side effects
*Antidiabetic agents* / ↓ Effect of antidiabetic agents, since phenothiazines ↑ blood sugar
*Bacitracin* / Additive respiratory depression

---

✽ = Available in Canada                    ***bold italic*** = life threatening side effect

*Barbiturate anesthetics* / ↑ Chance of tremor, involuntary muscle activity, and hypotension

*Barbiturates* / See *Alcohol;* also, barbiturates may ↓ effect due to ↑ breakdown by liver

*Bromocriptine* / Phenothiazines ↓ effect

*Capreomycin* / Additive respiratory depression

*Charcoal* / ↓ Effect of phenothiazines due to ↓ absorption from GI tract

*CNS depressants* / See *Alcohol;* also, ↓ effect of phenothiazines due to ↑ breakdown by liver

*Colistimethate* / Additive respiratory depression

*Diazoxide* / Additive hyperglycemic effect

*Guanethidine* / ↓ Effect of guanethidine by ↓ uptake of drug at the site of action

*Hydantoins* / ↑ Risk of hydantoin toxicity

*Lithium carbonate* / ↑ Risk of extrapyramidal symptoms, disorientation, or unconsciousness

*MAO inhibitors* / ↑ Effect of phenothiazines due to ↓ breakdown by liver

*Meperidine* / ↑ Risk of hypotension and sedation

*Metoprolol* / Additive hypotensive effects

*Narcotics* / See *Alcohol*

*Phenytoin* / ↑ Effect of phenytoin due to ↓ breakdown by liver

*Polymyxin B* / Additive respiratory depression

*Propranolol* / Additive hypotensive effects

*Quinidine* / Additive cardiac depressant effect

*Sedative-hypnotics, nonbarbiturate* / See *Alcohol*

*Succinylcholine* / ↑ Muscle relaxation

*Tricyclic antidepressants* / ↑ Serum levels of tricyclic antidepressant

**Laboratory Test Interferences:** False +: Bile (urine dipstick), ferric chloride, pregnancy tests, urinary porphobilinogen, urinary steroids, urobilinogen (urine dipstick). False –: Inorganic phosphorus, urinary steroids. *Caused by pharmacologic effects:* ↑ Alkaline phosphatase, bilirubin, serum transaminases, serum cholesterol, urinary catecholamines. ↓ Glucose tolerance, serum uric acid, 5-HIAA, FSH, growth hormone, LH, vanillylmandelic acid.

## Dosage

See individual drugs. Effective over a wide dosage range. Dosage is usually increased gradually to minimize side effects over 7 days until the minimal effective dose is attained. Dosage is increased more gradually in elderly or debilitated clients because they are more susceptible to the effects and side effects of drugs. After symptoms are controlled, dosage is gradually reduced to maintenance levels. It is usually desirable to keep chronically ill clients on maintenance levels indefinitely. Medication, especially in clients on high dosages, should not be discontinued abruptly.

## NURSING CONSIDERATIONS
### Administration/Storage

1. Do not interchange brands of PO form of drug or suppositories; may differ in bioavailability.
2. Do not use pink or markedly discolored solutions.
3. When preparing or administering parenteral solutions, nurse and client should avoid contact of drug with skin, eyes, and clothing to prevent contact dermatitis.
4. Do not mix antipsychotic drugs with other drugs in the same syringe.
5. Order a specific flow rate when administering parenteral solutions.
6. To lessen pain of injection, dilute commercially available injectable solutions in saline or local anesthetic.
7. When administering IM, inject drug deeply into the muscle.
8. Massage area of injection site after IM administration to reduce pain.
9. Prevent extravasation of the IV solution.
10. Store solutions in a cool dry place in amber-colored containers.

## Assessment

1. Take a complete medical and drug history; note any drug hypersensitivity or genetic predisposition. (These agents are referred to as neuroleptics in Europe.)
2. Determine any history of seizures; this class of drugs may lower seizure threshold.
3. Document indications for therapy. Assess baseline mental status, noting mood, behavior, and any depression.
4. If administering to children, note extent of hyperexcitability.
5. Assess child for chickenpox or measles.
6. Note any history of asthma or emphysema.
7. Monitor VS; assess BP in both arms in a reclining position, standing position, and sitting position, 2 min apart.
8. Monitor hematologic profile, liver and renal function studies, urinalysis, ECG, and ocular findings.

## Interventions

1. If administered IV, monitor flow rate and BP. Keep recumbent for at least 1 hr after IV completed, then slowly elevate HOB and observe for tachycardia, faintness, or dizziness; supervise ambulation.
2. If hospitalized, ensure that med has been swallowed. May give a liquid preparation to permit better control over drug taking and to improve compliance.
3. Measure I&O; report abdominal distention and urinary retention. May need to reduce dosage, add antispasmodics, or change therapy.
4. Note any changes in carbohydrate metabolism (e.g., glycosuria, weight loss, polyphagia, increased appetite, or excessive weight gain); may require a change in diet/drug therapy and can be significant with diabetes.
5. Some may develop a hypersensitivity reaction with fever, asthma, laryngeal edema, angioneurotic edema, and anaphylactic reaction. *Stop*

medication, notify provider, and treat symptomatically.
6. The antiemetic effects of phenothiazines may mask other pathology such as toxicity to other drugs, intestinal obstruction, or brain lesions.
7. If receiving barbiturates to relieve anxiety, reduce barbiturate dose. If administered as an anticonvulsant, do not reduce dosage.
8. Discontinue drug gradually to minimize severe GI disturbances or tardive dyskinesia.

## Client/Family Teaching

1. May take with food or milk to minimize GI upset. Take as directed, may be weeks or months before the full effects will be noticed
2. Do not stop taking abruptly. Abrupt cessation of high doses of phenothiazines can cause N&V, tremors, sensations of warmth and cold, sweating, tachycardia, headache, and insomnia.
3. Report distress when in a hot or cold room; may affect heat-regulating mechanism.
• Provide extra blankets if feeling cold.
• Bathe in tepid water if feeling too warm.
• Do *NOT* use heating pads or hot water bottles if feeling cold.
• Avoid hot tubs, hot baths, or hot showers; hypotension may occur.
4. Report if excessively active or depressed. Spasms of face, neck, back, or tongue may be treated with antihistamines, or provider may discontinue drug.
5. Report any elevation of body temperature, feeling of weakness, or sore throat (symptoms of blood dyscrasias).
6. Take slow, deep breaths if respiratory symptoms occur; may depress cough reflex.
7. May cause menstrual irregularity and false positive pregnancy tests; may develop engorged breasts and begin lactating. Keep accurate record of periods and report if pregnancy is suspected.
8. Males may experience decreased

libido and develop breast enlargement. Report so med can be adjusted.

9. May develop photosensitivity reactions; wear protective clothing, sunglasses, sunscreen and avoid sunbathing.

10. Drug may discolor the urine pink or reddish brown. With long-term therapy may develop a yellow-brown skin reaction that may turn grayish purple.

11. Avoid driving a car or operating heavy machinery or engaging in any activities that require mental alertness for at least 2 weeks after starting therapy. Consult provider before resuming these activities.

12. Long-term therapy may affect vision; schedule regular ophthalmic exams. Report blurred vision and avoid driving.

13. Report evidence of early cholestatic jaundice, such as high fever, upper abdominal pain, nausea, diarrhea, itching, and rash.

14. Withhold drug and report if yellowing of the sclera, skin, or mucous membranes occurs; may indicate biliary obstruction.

15. To prevent dry mouth, rinse mouth frequently, increase fluid intake, chew sugarless gum, and suck on sour hard candies.

16. Increase fluids and bulk in the diet to minimize constipation; may need laxatives. Report any urinary retention or persistent constipation.

17. Rise slowly from a lying or sitting position; dangle legs before standing to avoid orthostatic symptoms.

18. Avoid alcohol, OTC drugs, and any other CNS depressants without approval.

19. Report for periodic labs and follow-up care to evaluate and adjust drug dosage.

**Outcomes/Evaluate**

• ↓ Excitable, withdrawn, agitated, or paranoid behaviors

• Orientation to time and place, and an understanding of illness

• Adherence to prescribed drug regimen

• Relief of N&V

**Special Concerns**

1. When working with the elderly, be particularly observant for symptoms of tardive dyskinesia. May exhibit puffing of the cheeks or tongue; may develop chewing movements and involuntary movements of the extremities and trunk.

2. If administering to a child, note neuromuscular reactions, especially if dehydrated or has an acute infection making more susceptible to side effects.

# ANTITHYROID DRUGS

*See also the following individual entries:*

Methimazole
Propylthiouracil

**Action/Kinetics:** These drugs inhibit (partially or completely) the production of thyroid hormones by the thyroid gland by preventing the incorporation of iodide into tyrosine and coupling of iodotyrosines. They do not affect release or activity of preformed hormone; thus, it may take several weeks for the therapeutic effect to become established.

**Uses:** Hyperthyroidism; prior to surgery or radiotherapy. Adjunct in treatment of thyrotoxicosis or thyroid storm. Propylthiouracil is also used to reduce mortality due to alcoholic liver disease.

**Contraindications:** Lactation (may cause hypothyroidism in the infant).

**Special Concerns:** Use with caution in the presence of CV disease. PT should be monitored during therapy as propylthiouracil may cause hypoprothrombinemia and bleeding.

**Side Effects:** *Hematologic: Agranulocytosis,* thrombocytopenia, granulocytopenia, hypoprothrombinemia, *aplastic anemia,* leukopenia. *GI:* N&V, taste loss, epigastric pain, sialadenopathy. *CNS:* Headache, paresthesia, drowsiness, vertigo, depression, CNS stimulation. *Dermatologic:* Skin rash, urticaria, alopecia, skin pigmentation, pruritus, exfoliative dermatitis, erythema nodosum. *Miscellaneous:* Jaundice, arthralgia, myalgia, neuritis, edema, lymphadenopathy, vasculitis, lupus-like syndrome, drug fever, periarteritis, hepatitis, nephritis, interstitial pneumonitis, insulin autoimmune syndrome resulting in hypoglycemic coma.

**OD Overdose Management:** *Symptoms:* N&V, headache, fever, pruritus, epigastric distress, arthralgia, pancytopenia, *agranulocytosis* (most serious). Rarely, exfoliative dermatitis, hepatitis, neuropathies, CNS stimulation or depression. *Treatment:* Maintain a patent airway and support ventilation and perfusion. Very carefully monitor and maintain VS, blood gases, and serum electrolytes. Monitor bone marrow function.

**Dosage** ─────────────
See individual drugs.

---

## NURSING CONSIDERATIONS
### Assessment
1. Document onset of illness, symptoms experienced, physical presentation, and any underlying cause.
2. Determine if pregnant.
3. Monitor VS, I&O, and weights; PT, CBC, ECG, and thyroid function studies.
4. Assess thyroid gland noting any enlargement, pain, asymmetry, or nodules.

### Client/Family Teaching
1. It takes 6–12 weeks for the drug to produce full effect. Take regularly and exactly as directed q 8 hr around the clock. Hyperthyroidism may recur if not taken properly.
2. Report symptoms of hyperthyroidism or thyrotoxicosis (palpitations, increased HR, nervousness, sleeplessness, sweating, diarrhea, weight loss, fever).
3. Report symptoms of hypothyroidism (weak, listless, tired, headache, dry skin, cold intolerance, constipation) as dosage may require adjustment.
4. Report any sore throat, enlargement of the cervical lymph nodes, GI disturbances, fever, skin rashes, itching, or jaundice; may require either a dosage reduction or withdrawal of the drug.
5. May alter taste perception; increase use of herbs and nonsodium seasonings.
6. Report symptoms of iodism (cold symptoms, skin lesions, stomatitis, GI upset, metallic taste)
7. Identify dietary sources of iodine (iodized salt, shellfish, turnips, cabbage, kale) that may need to be omitted from the diet.
8. Report any unusual bleeding, alopecia, nausea, loss of taste, or epigastric pain.
9. When drug is taken for 1 year, more than half the clients achieve a permanent remission. Those who relapse are usually treated with radioiodine.
10. Carry ID listing medical problems and currently prescribed meds.

**Special Concerns:** Children must be checked every 6 months for appropriate growth and development; plot on a graph.

**Outcomes/Evaluate**
• Thyroid function studies within desired range (euthyroid)
• Control of symptoms associated with hyperthyroidism
• ↓ Vascularity and friability of the thyroid gland in preparation for surgery
• ↓ Mortality in clients with alcoholic liver disease

---

# ANTIVIRAL DRUGS

*See also the following individual entries:*

Acyclovir (Acycloguanosine)
Amantadine hydrochloride
Cidofovir
Delavirdine mesylate
Didanosine (ddI, Dideoxyinosine)
Famciclovir
Foscarnet sodium
Ganciclovir sodium
Idoxuridine (IDU)
Indinavir sulfate
Lamivudine
Lamivudine and Zidovudine

---

★ = Available in Canada    ***bold italic*** = life threatening side effect

Nelfinavir mesylate
Nevirapine
Penciclovir
Ribavirin
Rimantidine hydrochloride
Ritonavir
Saquinavir mesylate
Stavudine
Trifluridine
Valacyclovir hydrochloride
Vidarabine
Zalcitabine
Zidovudine (Azidothymidine, AZT)

**Action/Kinetics:** To maintain their growth and reproduce, viruses must enter living cells. Thus, it is difficult to find a drug that is specific for the virus and that does not interfere with the function of the host cell. However, there are enzymes and replicative mechanisms that are unique to viruses and an increasing number of drugs with specific antiviral activity have been developed. The antiviral drugs currently marketed act by one of the following mechanisms:

1. Inhibition of enzymes required for DNA synthesis. Example: Idoxuridine.

2. Inhibition of viral nucleic acid synthesis by interacting directly with herpes virus DNA polymerase or HIV reverse transcriptase. Example: Foscarnet.

3. Inhibition of viral DNA synthesis. Examples: Acyclovir, Cidofovir, Didanosine, Famciclovir, Ganciclovir, Penciclovir, Trifluridine, Valacyclovir, Vidarabine.

4. Prevent penetration of the virus into cells by inhibiting uncoating of the RNA virus. Examples: Amantadine, Rimantadine.

5. Protease inhibitors resulting in release of immature, noninfectious viral particles. Examples: Indinavir, Ritonavir, Nelfinavir, Saquinavir.

6. Inhibition of reverse transcriptase resulting in inhibition of replication of the virus. Examples: Lamivudine, Nevirapine, Stavudine, Zalcitabine, Zidovudine.It is becoming increasingly common to combine two antiviral drugs that have different mechanisms of action in order to treat HIV infections.

## NURSING CONSIDERATIONS

See *General Nursing Considerations For All Anti-Infectives.*

**Assessment**

1. Document indications for therapy, type and onset of symptoms, and exposure characteristics.

2. MonitorCBC, liver and renal function studies, and viral loads when indicated.

3. List other agents and route prescribed to ensure none interact unfavorably.

4. Note underlying medical conditions that may preclude drug therapy.

**Client/Family Teaching**

1. Review method and frequency for drug administration. Take exactly as directed; do not share meds.

2. Identify specific measures necessary to decrease or halt the spread of the disease.

3. Maintain adequate nutrition; consume 2–3 L/day of fluids during therapy to prevent crystalluria.

4. Report any rashes or unusual side effects of drug therapy.

5. If symptoms do not improve or worsen after specified time frame, report to provider.

6. Need close medical supervision and follow-up during drug therapy.

**Outcomes/Evaluate**

• Prophylaxis of viral infections
• Reduction in length and severity of symptoms of viral infections

# BARBITURATES

See also the following individual entries:

Pentobarbital
Pentobarbital sodium
Phenobarbital
Phenobarbital sodium
Secobarbital sodium

**Action/Kinetics:** Barbiturates produce all levels of CNS depression, ranging from mild depression (sedation) following low doses to hypnotic (sleep-inducing) effects, and even coma and death, as dosage is increased. Certain barbiturates are also effective anticonvulsants. The depressant and anticonvulsant effects may be related to their ability to increase and/or mimic the inhibitory activity of the neurotransmitter GABA on nerve synapses. Importantly, barbiturates are not analgesics and therefore should not be given to clients for the purpose of ameliorating pain. Sodium salts are readily absorbed after PO, rectal, or parenteral administration. They are distributed throughout all tissues, cross the placental barrier, and appear in breast milk. The main difference between the various barbiturates is in the onset of action, which ranges from 10 to 15 min for pentobarbital and secobarbital and 60 or more minutes for phenobarbital. Metabolized almost completely in the liver (except for phenobarbital) and are excreted in the urine.

**Uses:** Preanesthetic medication. Sedation, hypnotic, anticonvulsant (phenobarbital) and for the control of acute convulsive conditions (only phenobarbital, mephobarbital), as in epilepsy, tetanus, meningitis, eclampsia, and toxic reactions to local anesthetics or strychnine. The benzodiazepines have replaced barbiturates for the treatment of many conditions, especially daytime sedation. See also information on individual drugs.

**Contraindications:** Hypersensitivity to barbiturates, severe trauma, pulmonary disease when dyspnea or obstruction is present, edema, uncontrolled diabetes, history of porphyria, and impaired liver function and for clients in whom they produce an excitatory response. Also, clients who have been addicted previously to sedative-hypnotics.

**Special Concerns:** Use with caution during lactation and in clients with CNS depression, hypotension, marked asthenia (characteristic of Addison's disease, hypoadrenalism, and severe myxedema), porphyria,

fever, anemia, hemorrhagic shock, cardiac, hepatic or renal damage, and a history of alcoholism in suicidal clients. Geriatric clients usually manifest increased sensitivity to barbiturates, as evidenced by confusion, excitement, mental depression, and hypothermia. When given in the presence of pain, restlessness, excitement, and delirium may result. Intra-arterial use may cause symptoms from transient pain to gangrene; SC use produces tissue irritation, including tenderness and redness to necrosis.

**Side Effects:** *CNS:* Sleepiness, drowsiness, agitation, confusion, hyperkinesia, ataxia, CNS depression, nightmares, nervousness, psychiatric disturbances, hallucinations, insomnia, anxiety, dizziness, headache, abnormal thinking, vertigo, lethargy, hangover, excitement, appearance of being inebriated. Irritability and hyperactivity in children. *Musculoskeletal:* Localized or diffuse myalgic, neuralgic, or arthritic pain, especially in psychoneurotic clients. Pain is often most intense in the morning and is frequently located in the neck, shoulder girdle, and arms. *Respiratory:* Hypoventilation, ***apnea, respiratory depression.*** *CV:* Bradycardia, hypotension, syncope, ***circulatory collapse.*** *GI:* N&V, constipation, liver damage (especially with chronic use of phenobarbital). *Allergic:* Skin rashes, ***angioedema,*** exfoliative dermatitis (including ***Stevens-Johnson syndrome and toxic epidermal necrolysis***). Allergic reactions are most common in clients who have asthma, urticaria, angioedema, and similar conditions. Symptoms include localized swelling (especially of the lips, cheeks, or eyelids) and erythematous dermatitis).

*After SC use:* Tissue necrosis, pain, tenderness, redness, permanent neurologic damage if injected near peripheral nerves.

*After IV use. CV:* Circulatory depression, thrombophlebitis, ***peripheral vascular collapse, seizures*** *with cardiorespiratory arrest, myocardial depression, cardiac arrhythmias. Respiratory:* **Apnea, laryngospasm, bronchospasm,** dyspnea, rhinitis, sneezing, coughing. *CNS:* Emergence delirium, headache, anxiety, prolonged somnolence and recovery, restlessness, **seizures.** *GI:* N&V, abdominal pain, diarrhea, cramping. *Hypersensitivity:* **Acute allergic reactions, including erythema, pruritus, anaphylaxis.** *Miscellaneous:* Pain or nerve injury at injection site, salivation, hiccups, skin rashes, shivering, skeletal muscle hyperactivity, **immune hemolytic anemia with renal failure,** and radial nerve palsy.

*After IM use:* Pain at injection site.

Barbiturates can induce physical and psychologic dependence if high doses are used regularly for long periods of time. Withdrawal symptoms usually begin after 12–16 hr of abstinence. Manifestations of withdrawal include anxiety, weakness, N&V, muscle cramps, delirium, and even **tonic-clonic seizures.**

**OD** **Overdose Management:**
*Symptoms (Acute Toxicity):* Characterized by cortical and **respiratory depression; anoxia; peripheral vascular collapse;** feeble, rapid pulse; pulmonary edema; decreased body temperature; clammy, cyanotic skin; depressed reflexes; stupor; and **coma.** After initial constriction the pupils become dilated. **Death results from respiratory failure or arrest followed by cardiac arrest.** *Symptoms (Chronic Toxicity):* Prolonged use of barbiturates at high doses may lead to physical and psychologic dependence, as well as tolerance. Doses of 600–800 mg daily for 8 weeks may lead to physical dependence. The addict usually ingests 1.5 g/day. Addicts prefer short-acting barbiturates. Symptoms of dependence are similar to those associated with chronic alcoholism, and withdrawal symptoms are equally severe. Withdrawal symptoms usually last for 5–10 days and are terminated by a long sleep.

*Treatment (Acute Toxicity):*

• Maintenance of an adequate airway, oxygen intake, and carbon dioxide removal are essential.

• After PO ingestion, gastric lavage or gastric aspiration may delay absorption. Emesis should not be induced once the symptoms of overdosage are manifested, as the client may aspirate the vomitus into the lungs. Also, if the dose of barbiturate is high enough, the vomiting center in the brain may be depressed.

• Absorption following SC or IM administration of the drug may be delayed by the use of ice packs or tourniquets.

• Maintain renal function.

• Removal of the drug by peritoneal dialysis or an artificial kidney should be carried out.

• Supportive physiologic methods have proven superior to use of analeptics.

*Treatment (Chronic Toxicity):* Cautious withdrawal of the hospitalized addict over a 2–4-week period. A stabilizing dose of 200–300 mg of a short-acting barbiturate is administered q 6 hr. The dose is then reduced by 100 mg/day until the stabilizing dose is reduced by one-half. The client is then maintained on this dose for 2–3 days before further reduction. The same procedure is repeated when the initial stabilizing dose has been reduced by three-quarters. If a mixed spike and slow activity appear on the EEG, or if insomnia, anxiety, tremor, or weakness is observed, the dosage is maintained at a constant level or increased slightly until symptoms disappear.

**Drug Interactions**

GENERAL CONSIDERATIONS
1. Barbiturates stimulate the activity of enzymes responsible for the metabolism of a large number of other drugs by a process known as *enzyme induction.* As a result, when barbiturates are given to clients receiving such drugs, their therapeutic effectiveness is markedly reduced or even abolished.
2. The CNS depressant effect of the

barbiturates is potentiated by many drugs. Concomitant administration may result in coma or fatal CNS depression. Barbiturate dosage should either be reduced or eliminated when other CNS drugs are given.

3. Barbiturates also potentiate the toxic effects of many other agents.

*Acetaminophen* / ↑ Risk of hepatotoxicity when used with large or chronic doses of barbiturates

*Alcohol* / Potentiation or addition of CNS depressant effects. Concomitant use may lead to drowsiness, lethargy, stupor, respiratory collapse, coma, or death

*Anesthetics, general* / See *Alcohol*

*Anorexiants* / ↓ Effect of anorexiants due to opposite activities

*Antianxiety drugs* / See *Alcohol*

*Anticoagulants, oral* / ↓ Effect of anticoagulants due to ↓ absorption from GI tract and ↑ breakdown by liver

*Antidepressants, tricyclic* / ↓ Effect of antidepressants due to ↑ breakdown by liver

*Antidiabetic agents* / Prolong the effects of barbiturates

*Antihistamines* / See *Alcohol*

*Beta-adrenergic agents* / ↓ Beta blockade due to ↑ breakdown by the liver

*Carbamazepine* / ↓ Serum carbazepine levels may occur

*Charcoal* / ↓ Absorption of barbiturates from the GI tract

*Chloramphenicol* / ↑ Effect of barbiturates by ↓ breakdown by the liver and ↓ effect of chloramphenicol by ↑ breakdown by liver

*Clonazepam* / Barbiturates may ↑ excretion of clonazepam → loss of efficacy

*CNS depressants* / See *Alcohol*

*Corticosteroids* / ↓ Effect of corticosteroids due to ↑ breakdown by liver

*Digitoxin* / ↓ Effect of digitoxin due to ↑ breakdown by liver

*Doxorubicin* / ↓ Effect of doxorubicin due to ↑ excretion

*Doxycycline* / ↓ Effect of doxycycline due to ↑ breakdown by liver (effect may last up to 2 weeks after barbiturates are discontinued)

*Estrogens* / ↓ Effect of estrogen due to ↑ breakdown by liver

*Felodipine* / ↓ Plasma levels of felodipine → ↓ effect

*Fenoprofen* / ↓ Bioavailability of fenoprofen

*Furosemide* / ↑ Risk or intensity of orthostatic hypotension

*Griseofulvin* / ↓ Effect of griseofulvin due to ↓ absorption from GI tract

*Haloperidol* / ↓ Effect of haloperidol due to ↑ breakdown by liver

*MAO inhibitors* / ↑ Effect of barbiturates due to ↓ breakdown by liver

*Meperidine* / CNS depressant effects may be prolonged

*Methadone* / ↓ Effect of methadone

*Methoxyflurane* / ↑ Kidney toxicity due to ↑ breakdown of methoxyflurane by liver to toxic metabolites

*Metronidazole* / ↓ Effect of metronidazole

*Narcotic analgesics* / See *Alcohol*

*Oral contraceptives* / ↓ Effect of contraceptives due to ↑ breakdown by liver

*Phenothiazines* / ↓ Effect of phenothiazines due to ↑ breakdown by liver; also see *Alcohol*

*Phenylbutazone* / ↓ Elimination t½ of phenylbutazone

*Phenytoin* / Effect variable and unpredictable; monitor carefully

*Probenecid* / Anesthesia with thiobarbiturates may be ↑ or achieved at lower doses

*Procarbazine* / ↑ Effect of barbiturates

*Quinidine* / ↓ Effect of quinidine due to ↑ breakdown by liver

*Rifampin* / ↓ Effect of barbiturates due to ↑ breakdown by liver

*Sedative-hypnotics, nonbarbiturate* / See *Alcohol*

*Sulfisoxazole* / Sulfisoxazole may ↑ the anesthetic effects of thiobarbiturates

*Theophyllines* / ↓ Effect of theophyllines due to ↑ breakdown by liver

*Valproic acid* / ↑ Effect of barbiturates due to ↓ breakdown by liver

*Verapamil* / ↑ Excretion of verapamil → ↓ effect

*Vitamin D* / Barbiturates may ↑ requirements for vitamin D due to ↑ breakdown by the liver

**Laboratory Test Interferences**

1. **Interference with test method:** ↑ 17-Hydroxycorticosteroids.

2. **Caused by pharmacologic effects:** ↑ Creatinine phosphokinase, alkaline phosphatase, serum transaminase, serum testosterone (in certain women), urinary estriol, porphobilinogen, coproporphyrin, uroporphyrin. ↓ PT in clients on coumarin. ↑ or ↓ Bilirubin. False + lupus erythematosus test.

## Dosage

See individual drugs. Aim for minimum effective dosage. As hypnotics, barbiturates should be administered intermittently because tolerance develops. Elderly clients should receive one-half of the adult dose, and children should receive one-quarter to one-half the adult dose.

## NURSING CONSIDERATIONS

### Administration/Storage

1. Aqueous solutions of sodium salts are unstable and must be used within 30 min after preparation.

2. Discard parenteral solutions that contain precipitate.

3. During IV administration:

• Closely monitor for the correct rate of flow. A too rapid injection may produce respiratory depression, dyspnea, and shock.

• Monitor IV site closely for extravasation, which may cause pain, nerve damage, and necrosis.

• Note any redness or swelling along the site of the vein; evidence of thrombophlebitis.

4. Maintain an accurate record of the barbiturates on hand and the amounts dispensed following appropriate institutional and Drug Enforcement Agency guidelines.

### Assessment

1. Note any adverse reactions to any of the barbiturate family of drugs.

2. Note any trials with non-narcotic sedatives and the outcome.

3. Identify indications for therapy, associated symptoms, and anticipated time frame for administration.

4. When used for sleep disorders, review sleeping patterns with the client and family. This is important when considering the type of barbiturate to prescribe.

• Determine usual bedtime and usual wakening hours.

• Identify cause of insomnia. A person in pain who gains relief of the pain may not need sleeping medication. Note evidence of fear and anxiety that may interfere with sleep.

• Assess environmental preferences for sleep, such as room temperature, lights, and sounds.

• Note sensory alterations that could cause sleeplessness or disruptions in sleep time.

5. Determine if pregnant; identify other measures to encourage sleep if pregnancy is a probability.

6. Document any evidence or history of previous dependence on any sedative-hypnotics.

7. Assess for physical conditions that may preclude drug therapy.

8. Monitor CBC, liver and renal function studies. Many of the barbiturates are metabolized by the liver. Assess for hematologic disorders such as agranulocytosis, megaloblastic anemia, and/or thrombocytopenia.

### Interventions

1. Do not awaken to administer a sleeping medication.

2. Assist during ambulation and use side rails once in bed. Clients who receive hypnotic medications may become confused and unsteady; particular problem among elderly—"at risk for fall" should be prominently posted.

3. Use supportive measures such as a back rub, warm drinks, quiet atmosphere and a calm attitude to encourage relaxation.

4. When administered PO, remain with the client to determine that the drug has been swallowed. If disoriented or wearing dentures, check the buccal cavity, under the tongue, and under denture plates. Routinely check bedside area to ensure client not hoarding medication.

5. Some clients may experience a period of transitory elation, confusion, or euphoria before sedation; provide measures to calm and to prevent injury.

6. If confused after taking the barbiturate, do not apply cuffs or other restraints. Remain with client and try to soothe and orient them by turning on a light and talking quietly and calmly until they are relaxed.

7. If a second sleeping medication requested during the night, try to determine the cause of the sleeplessness. Institute comfort measures; relieve pain. Wait approximately 20–30 min and then give the second dose of sleeping medication if client has not yet fallen asleep.

8. Record length of time receiving barbiturates. Therapy that requires sedative doses of medication over an 8-week period will cause physical dependence. Review the need to alter the dose and explore other related factors, such as the environment, the existence of psychologic stress, or possibly drug dependence.

9. Assess for evidence of physical and/or psychologic dependence and tolerance. Document any changes in the VS and skin condition.

10. Be alert to S&S of porphyria, a metabolic disorder characterized by N&V, abdominal pain, and muscle spasms; stop drug and report.

11. With a child, supervise play activity, especially if riding a bicycle or engaging in other potentially dangerous forms of play.

12. When receiving barbiturates on an outpatient basis, be alert to the number of times they return for prescription refills. Increased frequency of refills may indicate dependency or that they may be selling the drug for profit.

**Client/Family Teaching**

1. Review goals of therapy and estimated time frame to accomplish.

2. Do not drive a car or operate other hazardous machinery after taking drug.

3. Take only as prescribed.

4. Avoid OTC drugs or any other agents unless prescribed.

5. Avoid the alcohol; potentiates effects of barbiturates.

6. If for insomnia, take 30 min before bedtime.

7. To avoid accidental overdose, keep in a medicine closet or drawer *away from* the bedside.

8. Keep out of the reach of children. Large doses may be fatal and the potential for abuse exists.

9. If taking for 8 or more weeks, do not stop suddenly without supervision; may result in withdrawal symptoms: weakness, anxiety, delirium, and tonic-clonic seizures.

10. Report any signs of hematologic toxicity such as infections (sore throat or fever) or increased bleeding tendencies (nosebleeds or easy bruising).

11. Identify factors contributing to insomnia. Try alternative methods to promote relaxation and sleep (such as progressive muscle relaxation, guided imagery, white noise simulator, or soft music). Consider sleep disorder center.

12. Daily exercise helps promote rest; identify a program and establish a daily routine such as with daily walks in the development or mall.

13. Limit caffeine intake and avoid after midafternoon.

14. Establish a regular bedtime routine; discourage dozing during the afternoon or early evening hours.

15. Take prescribed analgesics for adequate relief of pain. Allow sufficient time to unwind from a busy or overstimulating day, before attempting to sleep.

16. With continuous use of these drugs a decrease in responsiveness

---

(drug tolerance) may develop. Abuse and physical dependence limit the usefulness of these drugs in long-term therapy.

**Outcomes/Evaluate**
- ↓ Muscle spasms, ↓ tremulousness, and ↓ level of anxiety (in preparation for anesthesia)
- Effective sedation
- Improved sleeping patterns with less frequent awakenings
- Control of seizures

# BETA-ADRENERGIC BLOCKING AGENTS

*See also Alpha-1-Adrenergic Blocking Agents and the following individual agents:*

Acebutolol hydrochloride
Atenolol
Betaxolol hydrochloride
Bisoprolol fumarate
Carteolol hydrochloride
Esmolol hydrochloride
Levobunolol hydrochloride
Metipranolol hydrochloride
Metoprolol succinate
Metoprolol tartrate
Nadolol
Penbutolol sulfate
Pindolol
Propranolol hydrochloride
Sotalol hydrochloride
Timolol maleate

**Action/Kinetics:** Combine reversibly with beta-adrenergic receptors to block the response to sympathetic nerve impulses, circulating catecholamines, or adrenergic drugs. Beta-adrenergic receptors have been classified as beta-1 (predominantly in the cardiac muscle) and beta-2 (mainly in the bronchi and vascular musculature). Blockade of beta-1 receptors decreases HR, myocardial contractility, and CO; in addition, AV conduction is slowed. These effects lead to a decrease in BP, as well as a reversal of cardiac arrhythmias. Blockade of beta-2 receptors increases airway resistance in the bronchioles and inhibits the vasodilating effects of catecholamines on peripheral blood vessels. The various beta-blocking agents differ in their ability to block beta-1 and beta-2 receptors (see individual drugs); also, certain of these agents have intrinsic sympathomimetic action.

Certain of these drugs (betaxolol, carteolol, levobunolol, metipranolol, and timolol) are used for glaucoma. The drugs appear to act by reducing production of aqueous humor; metipranolol and timolol may also increase outflow of aqueous humor. These drugs have little or no effect on the pupil size or on accommodation.
**Uses:** See individual drugs.
**Contraindications:** Sinus bradycardia, second- and third-degree AV block, cardiogenic shock, CHF unless secondary to tachyarrhythmia treatable with beta blockers, overt cardiac failure. Most are contraindicated in chronic bronchitis, bronchial asthma or history thereof, bronchospasm, emphysema, severe COPD.
**Special Concerns:** Use with caution in diabetes, thyrotoxicosis, cerebrovascular insufficiency, and impaired hepatic and renal function. Withdrawing beta blockers before major surgery is controversial. Safe use during pregnancy and lactation and in children has not been established. May be absorbed systemically when used for glaucoma; thus, there is the potential for an additive effect with beta blockers used systemically. Certain of the products for use in glaucoma contain sulfites, which may result in an allergic reaction. Also, see individual agents.
**Side Effects:** *CV:* Bradycardia, hypotension (especially following IV use), CHF, cold extremities, claudication, worsening of angina, strokes, edema, syncope, arrhythmias, chest pain, peripheral ischemia, flushing, SOB, sinoatrial block, pulmonary edema, vasodilation, increased HR, palpitations, conduction disturbances, *first-, second-, and third-degree heart block,* worsening of AV block, thrombosis of renal or mesenteric arteries, precipitation or worsening of Raynaud's phenomenon. Sudden

withdrawal of large doses may cause angina, ventricular tachycardia, *fatal MI, sudden death,* or *circulatory collapse. GI:* N&V, diarrhea, flatulence, dry mouth, constipation, anorexia, cramps, bloating, gastric pain, dyspepsia, distortion of taste, weight gain or loss, retroperitoneal fibrosis, ischemic colitis. *Hepatic:* Hepatomegaly, acute pancreatitis, elevated liver enzymes, liver damage (especially with chronic use of phenobarbital). *Respiratory:* Asthma-like symptoms, *bronchospasms, bronchial obstruction, laryngospasm with respiratory distress,* wheeziness, worsening of chronic obstructive lung disease, dyspnea, cough, nasal stuffiness, rhinitis, pharyngitis, rales. *CNS:* Dizziness, fatigue, lethargy, vivid dreams, depression, hallucinations, delirium, psychoses, paresthesias, insomnia, nervousness, nightmares, headache, vertigo, disorientation of time and place, hypoesthesia or hyperesthesia, decreased concentration, short-term memory loss, change in behavior, emotional lability, slurred speech, lightheadedness. In the elderly, paranoia, disorientation, and combativeness have occurred. *Hematologic: Agranulocytosis,* thrombocytopenia. *Allergic:* Fever, sore throat, respiratory distress, rash, pharyngitis, *laryngospasm, anaphylaxis. Skin:* Pruritus, rashes, increased skin pigmentation, sweating, dry skin, alopecia, skin irritation, psoriasis (reversible). *Musculoskeletal:* Joint and muscle pain, arthritis, arthralgia, back pain, muscle cramps, muscle weakness when used in clients with myasthenic symptoms. *GU:* Impotence, decreased libido, dysuria, UTI, nocturia, urinary retention or frequency, pollakiuria. *Ophthalmic:* Visual disturbances, eye irritation, dry or burning eyes, blurred vision, conjunctivitis. When used ophthalmically: keratitis, blepharoptosis, diplopia, ptosis, and visual disturbances including refractive changes. *Other:* Hyperglycemia or hypoglycemia, lupus-like syndrome,

Peyronie's disease, tinnitus, increase in symptoms of myasthenia gravis, facial swelling, decreased exercise tolerance, rigors, speech disorders. *Systemic effects due to ophthalmic beta-1 and beta-2 blockers:* Headache, depression, arrhythmia, heart block, CVA, syncope, CHF, palpitation, cerebral ischemia, nausea, localized and generalized rash, bronchospasm (especially in those with preexisting bronchospastic disease), respiratory failure, masked symptoms of hypoglycemia in insulin-dependent diabetics, keratitis, visual disturbances (including refractive changes), blepharoptosis, ptosis, diplopia.

**OD** **Overdose Management:** *Symptoms:* CV symptoms include bradycardia, hypotension, CHF, *cardiogenic shock,* intraventricular conduction disturbances, *AV block, pulmonary edema, asystole,* and tachycardia. Also, overdosage of pindolol may cause hypertension and overdosage of propranolol may result in systemic vascular resistance. CNS symptoms include respiratory depression, decreased consciousness, *coma, and seizures.* Miscellaneous symptoms include *bronchospasm* (especially in clients with obstructive pulmonary disease), hyperkalemia, and hypoglycemia. *Treatment:*

• To improve blood supply to the brain, place client in a supine position and raise the legs.

• Measure blood glucose and serum potassium. Monitor BP and ECG continuously.

• Provide general supportive treatment such as inducing emesis or gastric lavage and artificial respiration.

• *Seizures:* Give IV diazepam or phenytoin.

• *Excessive bradycardia:* If hypotensive, give atropine, 0.6 mg; if no response, give q 3 min for a total of 2–3 mg. Cautious administration of isoproterenol may be tried. Also, glucagon, 5–10 mg rapidly over 30 sec, followed by continuous IV infusion of

5 mg/hr may reverse bradycardia. Transvenous cardiac pacing may be needed for refractory cases.

• *Cardiac failure:* Digitalis, diuretic, and oxygen; if failure is refractory, IV aminophylline or glucagon may be helpful.

• *Hypotension:* Place client in Trendelenburg position. IV fluids unless pulmonary edema is present; also vasopressors such as norepinephrine (may be drug of choice), dobutamine, dopamine with monitoring of BP. If refractory, glucagon may be helpful. In intractable cardiogenic shock, intra-aortic balloon insertion may be required.

• *Premature ventricular contractions:* Lidocaine or phenytoin. Disopyramide, quinidine, and procainamide should be avoided as they depress myocardial function further.

• *Bronchospasms:* Give a beta-2-adrenergic agonist, epinephrine, or theophylline.

• *Heart block, second or third degree:* Isoproterenol or transvenous cardiac pacing.

**Drug Interactions**

*Anesthetics, general* / Additive depression of myocardium

*Anticholinergic agents* / Counteract bradycardia produced by beta-adrenergic blockers

*Antihypertensives* / Additive hypotensive effect

*Ophthalmic beta blockers* / Additive systemic beta-blocking effects if used with oral beta blockers

*Chlorpromazine* / Additive beta-adrenergic blocking action

*Cimetidine* / ↑ Effect of beta blockers due to ↓ breakdown by liver

*Clonidine* / Paradoxical hypertension; also, ↑ severity of rebound hypertension

*Disopyramide* / ↑ Effect of both drugs

*Epinephrine* / Beta blockers prevent beta-adrenergic action of epinephrine but not alpha-adrenergic action → ↑ systolic and diastolic BP and ↓ HR

*Furosemide* / ↑ Beta-adrenergic blockade

*Hydralazine* / ↑ Beta-adrenergic blockade

*Indomethacin* / ↓ Effect of beta blockers possibly due to inhibition of prostaglandin synthesis

*Insulin* / Beta blockers ↑ hypoglycemic effect of insulin

*Lidocaine* / ↑ Effect of lidocaine due to ↓ breakdown by liver

*Methyldopa* / Possible ↑ BP to alpha-adrenergic effect

*NSAIDs* / ↓ Effect of beta blockers, possibly due to inhibition of prostaglandin synthesis

*Oral contraceptives* / ↑ Effect of beta blockers due to ↓ breakdown by liver

*Phenformin* / ↑ Hypoglycemia

*Phenobarbital* / ↓ Effect of beta blockers due to ↑ breakdown by liver

*Phenothiazines* / ↑ Effect of both drugs

*Phenytoin* / Additive depression of myocardium; also phenytoin ↓ effect of beta blockers due to ↑ breakdown by liver

*Prazosin* / ↑ First-dose effect of prazosin (acute postural hypotension)

*Reserpine* / Additive hypotensive effect

*Rifampin* / ↓ Effect of beta blockers due to ↑ breakdown by liver

*Ritodrine* / Beta blockers ↓ effect of ritodrine

*Salicylates* / ↓ Effect of beta blockers, possibly due to inhibition of prostaglandin synthesis

*Succinylcholine* / Beta blockers ↑ effects of succinylcholine

*Sympathomimetics* / Reverse effects of beta blockers

*Theophylline* / Beta blockers reverse the effect of theophylline; also, beta blockers ↓ renal clearance of theophylline

*Tubocurarine* / Beta blockers ↑ effects of tubocurarine

*Verapamil* / Possible side effects since both drugs ↓ myocardial contractility or AV conduction; bradycardia and asystole when beta blockers are used ophthalmically

**Laboratory Test Interferences:** ↓ Serum glucose.

**Dosage**
See individual drugs.

## NURSING CONSIDERATIONS
### Administration/Storage
1. Sudden cessation of beta blockers may precipitate or worsen angina.
2. The lowering of intraocular pressure (IOP) may take a few weeks to stabilize when using betaxolol or timolol.
3. Due to diurnal variations in IOP, the response to b.i.d. therapy is best assessed by measuring IOP at different times during the day.
4. If IOP is not controlled using beta blockers, add additional drugs to the regimen, including pilocarpine, dipivefrin, or systemic carbonic anhydrase inhibitors.

### Assessment
1. Note indications for therapy and any symptoms or history of depression; assess mental status.
2. Determine pulse and BP in both arms while lying, sitting, and standing.
3. Monitor EKG, glucose, CBC, electrolytes, liver and renal function studies.
4. Note any history of asthma, diabetes, or impaired renal function.
5. With asthma, avoid nonselective beta antagonists due to beta-2 receptor blockade which may lead to increased airway resistance.
6. Review drugs currently prescribed to ensure none interact unfavorably.

### Interventions
1. Monitor pulse rate and BP; obtain written parameters for medication administration (e.g., hold for SBP < 90 or HR < 50).
2. When assessing respirations note the rate and quality. Drugs in this category may cause dyspnea and bronchospasm.
3. Monitor I&O and daily weights. Observe for increasing dyspnea, coughing, difficulty breathing, fatigue, or edema—symptoms of CHF, may require digitalization, diuretics, and/or discontinuation of drug therapy.
4. Assess complaints of "having a cold, easy fatigue, or feeling of light-headedness."; may require a drug change.
5. With diabetics watch for symptoms of hypoglycemia, such as hypotension or tachycardia; most mask these signs.
6. During IV administration, monitor EKG (may slow AV conduction and increase PR interval) and activities closely until drug effects are realized.

### Client/Family Teaching
1. When prescribed for BP control, drug helps control hypertension but does not cure it. Must continue to take despite feeling better.
2. Record BP and take pulse immediately prior to first dose each day so medication can be adjusted as needed.
3. Review instructions when to call provider, i.e., if HR < 50 beats/min or SBP < 80 mm Hg.
4. Review life-style changes necessary for BP control: regular exercise, low-fat and reduced-calorie diet, decreased salt and alcohol intake, smoking cessation, and relaxation techniques.
5. Always consult provider before interrupting therapy because abrupt withdrawal of most beta-adrenergic blocking agents may precipitate angina, MI, or rebound hypertension. A 2-week taper is useful.
6. Some drugs may cause blurred vision, dizziness, or drowsiness; do not engage in activities that require mental alertness until drug effects become apparent.
7. Rise from a sitting or lying position slowly and dangle legs before standing to avoid symptoms of orthostatic hypotension. Elastic support hose may help decrease symptoms.
8. Dress warmly during cold weather because diminished blood supply to extremities may cause client to be more sensitive to the cold; check extremities for warmth.
9. Avoid excessive intake of alco-

---

✸ = Available in Canada        ***bold italic*** = life threatening side effect

hol, coffee, tea, or cola. Avoid OTC agents without approval.

10. If diabetic, perform finger sticks often and report symptoms of hypoglycemia.

11. Report any asthma-like symptoms, cough, or nasal stuffiness; may be symptoms of CHF and require further evaluation.

12. Report any bothersome side effects or changes, especially new-onset depression.

**Outcomes/Evaluate**

- ↓ BP
- ↓ IOP
- ↓ Frequency/severity of anginal attacks; improved exercise tolerance
- ↓ Anxiety levels; ↓ tremors
- Migraine prophylaxis
- Control of cardiac arrhythmias

# CALCIUM CHANNEL BLOCKING AGENTS

*See also the following individual entries:*

Amlodipine
Bepridil hydrochloride
Diltiazem hydrochloride
Felodipine
Isradipine
Mibefradil dihydrochloride
Nicardipine hydrochloride
Nifedipine
Nimodipine
Nisoldipine
Verapamil

**Action/Kinetics:** For contraction of cardiac and smooth muscle to occur, extracellular calcium must move into the cell through openings called *calcium channels.* The calcium channel blocking agents (also called *slow channel blockers* or *calcium antagonists*) inhibit the influx of calcium through the cell membrane, resulting in a depression of automaticity and conduction velocity in both smooth and cardiac muscle. This leads to a depression of contraction in these tissues. Drugs in this class have different degrees of selectivity on vascular smooth muscle, myocardium, and conduction and pacemaker

tissues. In the myocardium, these drugs dilate coronary vessels in both normal and ischemic tissues and inhibit spasms of coronary arteries. They also decrease total peripheral resistance, thus reducing energy and oxygen requirements of the heart. Also effective against certain cardiac arrhythmias by slowing AV conduction and prolonging repolarization. In addition, they depress the amplitude, rate of depolarization, and conduction in atria.

**Uses:** See individual drugs.

**Contraindications:** Sick sinus syndrome, second- or third-degree AV block (except with a functioning pacemaker). Use of bepridil, diltiazem, or verapamil for hypotension (<90 mm Hg systolic pressure). Lactation.

**Special Concerns:** Abrupt withdrawal may result in increased frequency and duration of chest pain. Hypertensive clients treated with calcium channel blockers have a higher risk of heart attack than clients treated with diuretics or beta-adrenergic blockers. Safety and effectiveness of bepridil, diltiazem, felodipine, and isradipine have not been established in children.

**Side Effects:** Side effects vary from one calcium channel blocker to another; refer to individual drugs.

**OD** **Overdose Management:** *Symptoms:* Nausea, weakness, drowsiness, dizziness, slurred speech, confusion, marked and prolonged hypotension, bradycardia, junctional rhythms, *second- or third-degree block.* *Treatment:*

- Treatment is supportive. Monitor cardiac and respiratory function.
- If client is seen soon after ingestion, emetics or gastric lavage should be considered followed by cathartics.
- *Hypotension:* IV calcium, dopamine, isoproterenol, metaraminol, norepinephrine. Also, provide IV fluids. Place client in Trendelenburg position.
- *Ventricular tachycardia:* IV procainamide or lidocaine; also, cardioversion may be necessary. Also, provide slow-drip IV fluids.

- *Bradycardia, asystole, AV block:* IV atropine sulfate (0.6–1 mg), calcium gluconate (10% solution), isoproterenol, norepinephrine; also, cardiac pacing may be indicated. Provide slow-drip IV fluids.

**Drug Interactions**
*Beta-adrenergic blocking agents /* Beta blockers may cause depression of myocardial contractility and AV conduction
*Cimetidine /* ↑ Effect of calcium channel blockers due to ↓ first-pass metabolism
*Fentanyl /* Severe hypotension or increased fluid volume requirements
*Ranitidine /* ↑ Effect of calcium channel blockers due to ↓ first-pass metabolism

**Dosage**
See individual drugs.

## NURSING CONSIDERATIONS
**Assessment**
1. Document indications for therapy, type and onset of symptoms. List other agents used and the outcome.
2. Note any experience with calcium channel blocking drugs and the response.
3. Assess and document CV and mental status. These drugs cause peripheral vasodilation. Any excessive hypotensive response and increased HR may precipitate angina.
4. Document VS, weight, ECG and BP in both arms while lying, sitting, and standing. Assess for symptoms of CHF (weight gain, peripheral edema, dyspnea, rales, jugular vein distention).
5. Monitor glucose, electrolytes, I&O, liver and renal function studies.

**Client/Family Teaching**
1. Take with meals to reduce GI irritation.
2. These agents work by decreasing myocardial contractile force, which in turn decreases the myocardial oxygen requirements.
3. Review goals of therapy (e.g., to decrease the DBP by 10 mm Hg, to

decrease the heart rate by 20 beats/min).
4. Take pulse and BP at the same time of day and at least twice a week as well as weights; review written instructions regarding when to withhold meds and when to contact the provider.
5. Do not perform activities that require mental alertness until drug effects are realized.
6. Report any side effects such as dizziness, vertigo, unusual flushing, facial warmth, edema, nausea, or persistent constipation, as they may be toxic drug effects
7. If postural hypotension occurs, advise to change positions slowly, especially when standing up from a reclining position. Sit down immediately if lightheadedness occurs. Move slowly from lying down to a sitting or standing position.
8. Long periods of standing, excessive heat, hot showers or baths, and ingestion of alcohol may exacerbate postural hypotension; take precautions to avoid these situations.
9. Any swelling of the hands or feet, pronounced dizziness, or chest pain accompanied by diaphoresis, SOB, or severe headaches should be reported immediately.
10. Review importance of life-style changes for BP control, i.e., regular exercise, low-fat, low-cholesterol, reduced-calorie diet, decreased salt and alcohol consumption, smoking cessation, and stress reduction.

**Outcomes/Evaluate**
- Control of hypertension
- ↓ HR
- ↓ frequency/intensity of anginal attacks
- Stable cardiac rhythm

# CALCIUM SALTS

*See also the following individual entries:*

Calcium carbonate
Calcium chloride
Calcium citrate

Calcium glubionate
Calcium gluceptate
Calcium gluconate
Calcium lactate

**Action/Kinetics:** Calcium is essential for maintaining normal function of nerves, muscles, the skeletal system, and permeability of cell membranes and capillaries. The normal serum calcium concentration is 9–10.4 mg/dL (4.5–5.2 mEq/L). Hypocalcemia is characterized by muscular fibrillation, twitching, skeletal muscle spasms, leg cramps, tetanic spasms, cardiac arrhythmias, smooth muscle hyperexcitability, mental depression, and anxiety states. Excessive, chronic hypocalcemia is characterized by brittle, defective nails, poor dentition, and brittle hair. Calcium is well absorbed from the upper GI tract. However, severe low-calcium tetany is best treated by IV administration of calcium gluconate. The presence of vitamin D is necessary for maximum calcium utilization. The hormone of the parathyroid gland is necessary for the regulation of the calcium level.

**Uses: IV:** Acute hypocalcemic tetany secondary to renal failure, hypoparathyroidism, premature delivery, maternal diabetes mellitus in infants, and poisoning due to magnesium, oxalic acid, radiophosphorus, carbon tetrachloride, fluoride, phosphate, strontium, and radium. To treat depletion of electrolytes. Also during cardiac resuscitation when epinephrine or isoproterenol has not improved myocardial contraction (may also be given into the ventricular cavity for this purpose). To reverse cardiotoxicity or hyperkalemia. **IM or IV:** Reduce spasms in renal, biliary, intestinal, or lead colic. To relieve muscle cramps due to insect bites and to decrease capillary permeability in various sensitivity reactions. **PO:** Osteoporosis, osteomalacia, chronic hypoparathyroidism, rickets, latent tetany, hypocalcemia secondary to use of anticonvulsant drugs. Myasthenia gravis, Eaton-Lambert syndrome, supplement for pregnant, postmenopausal, or nursing women. Also, prophylactically for primary osteoporosis. *Investigational:* As an infusion to diagnose Zollinger-Ellison syndrome and medullary thyroid carcinoma. To antagonize neuromuscular blockade due to aminoglycosides.

**Contraindications:** Digitalized clients, sarcoidosis, renal or cardiac disease, ventricular fibrillation. Cancer clients with bone metastases. Renal calculi, hypophosphatemia, hypercalcemia.

**Special Concerns:** Calcium requirements decrease in geriatric clients; thus, dose may have to be adjusted. Also, low levels of active vitamin D metabolites may impair calcium absorption in older clients. Use with caution in cor pulmonale, respiratory acidosis, renal disease or failure, ventricular fibrillation, hypercalcemia.

**Side Effects: Following PO use:** GI irritation, constipation. **Following IV use:** Venous irritation, tingling sensation, feeling of oppression or heat, chalky taste. Rapid IV administration may result in vasodilation, decreased BP and HR, *cardiac arrhythmias,* syncope, or *cardiac arrest.* **Following IM use:** Burning feeling, necrosis, tissue sloughing, cellulitis, soft tissue calcification. *NOTE:* If calcium is injected into the myocardium rather than into the ventricle, *laceration of coronary arteries, cardiac tamponade, pneumothorax, and ventricular fibrillation* may occur. *Symptoms due to excess calcium (hypercalcemia):* Lassitude, fatigue, GI symptoms (anorexia, N&V, abdominal pain, dry mouth, thirst), polyuria, depression of nervous and neuromuscular function (emotional disturbances, confusion, skeletal muscle weakness, and constipation), confusion, delirium, stupor, *coma,* impairment of renal function (polyuria, polydipsia, and azotemia), renal calculi, arrhythmias, and bradycardia.

**OD** **Overdose Management:** *Symptoms:* Systemic overloading from parenteral administration can result in an acute hypercalcemic syndrome with symptoms including markedly increased plasma calcium levels, lethargy, intractable N&V, weakness, **coma, and sudden death.** *Treatment:* Discontinue therapy and lower serum calcium levels by giving an IV infusion of sodium chloride plus a potent diuretic such as furosemide. Consider hemodialysis.

**Drug Interactions**

*Atenolol* / ↓ Effect of atenolol due to ↓ bioavailability and plasma levels

*Corticosteroids* / Interfere with absorption of calcium from GI tract

*Digitalis* / ↑ Digitalis arrhythmias and toxicity. Death has resulted from combination of digitalis and IV calcium salts

*Iron salts* / ↓ Absorption of iron from the GI tract

*Milk* / Excess of either may cause hypercalcemia, renal insufficiency with azotemia, alkalosis, and ocular lesions

*Norfloxacin* / ↓ Bioavailability of norfloxacin

*Sodium polystyrene sulfonate* / Metabolic alkalosis and ↓ binding of resin to potassium in clients with renal impairment

*Tetracyclines* / ↓ Effect of tetracyclines due to ↓ absorption from GI tract

*Thiazide diuretics* / Hypercalcemia due to thiazide-induced renal tubular reabsorption of calcium and bone release of calcium

*Verapamil* / Calcium antagonizes the effect of verapamil

*Vitamin D* / Enhances intestinal absorption of dietary calcium

**Dosage** ————————
See individual agents.

## NURSING CONSIDERATIONS
### Administration/Storage

ORAL

1. Administer 1–1.5 hr after meals. Alkalis and large amounts of fat decrease the absorption of calcium.
2. If difficulty swallowing large tablets, obtain a calcium in water suspension. Because calcium goes into suspension six times more readily in hot water than in cold water, the solution can be prepared by diluting the medication with *hot* water. Solution may then be cooled before administering.

IV

1. Warm solutions to body temperature and give slowly (0.5–2 mL/min), stop administration if client complains of discomfort.
2. Administer slowly, observing VS closely for evidence of bradycardia, hypotension, and cardiac arrhythmias.
3. Prevent leakage of medication into the tissues. These salts are extremely irritating.
4. Keep client recumbent for a short time following the injection.
5. Do not mix calcium salts with carbonates, phosphates, sulfates, or tartrates in parenteral admixtures.

IM

1. Rotate injection sites because calcium may cause tissue sloughing.
2. Do not administer IM calcium gluconate to children.

### Assessment

1. Perform a thorough nursing history, noting indications for therapy and any underlying causes.
2. Note if receiving digitalis products; drug may be contraindicated.
3. Monitor calcium levels and renal function; assess for renal disease. Administer vitamin D to facilitate absorption.
4. With hypocalcemic tetany, use safety precautions to protect from injury.
5. Assess for S&S of hypercalcemia, i.e., fatigue and CNS depression.

### Client/Family Teaching

1. Calcium requirements are best met by dietary sources (including milk in the diet). Supplements may need vitamin D to facilitate absorption.
2. Multivitamin and mineral preparations are expensive and do not con-

---

tain sufficient calcium to meet daily calcium requirements.

3. Consult a dietitian to assist with proper selection of foods and meal planning and preparation.

4. Review prescribed replacement regimen. Need close follow-up for dosage adjustments to prevent hypercalcemia and hypercalciuria.

**Outcomes/Evaluate**

- Resolution of hypocalcemia
- Relief of muscle cramps
- Osteoporosis prophylaxis
- Serum calcium levels within desired range (8.8–10.4 mg/dL)

# CARDIAC GLYCOSIDES

*See also the following individual entries:*

Digitoxin
Digoxin

**Action/Kinetics:** Cardiac glycosides increase the force and velocity of myocardial contraction (positive inotropic effect) by increasing the refractory period of the AV node and increasing total peripheral resistance. This effect is due to inhibition of sodium/potassium–ATPase in the sarcolemmal membrane, which alters excitation–contraction coupling. Inhibiting sodium, potassium–ATPase, results in an increase of calcium influx and an increased release of free calcium ions within the myocardial cells, which then potentiate the contractility of cardiac muscle fibers. The digitalis glycosides also decrease the rate of conduction and increase the refractory period of the AV node due to an increase in parasympathetic tone and a decrease in sympathetic tone. Clinical effects are not seen until steady-state plasma levels are reached. The initial dose of digitalis glycosides is larger (loading dose) and is traditionally referred to as the *digitalizing dose;* subsequent doses are referred to as *maintenance doses.*

**Uses:** All types of CHF, including that due to venous congestion, edema, dyspnea, orthopnea, and car-

diac arrhythmia. Control of rapid ventricular contraction rate in clients with atrial fibrillation or flutter. Slow HR in sinus tachycardia due to CHF. Supraventricular tachycardia. Prophylaxis and treatment of recurrent paroxysmal atrial tachycardia with paroxysmal AV junctional rhythm. Cardiogenic shock (value not established).

**Contraindications:** Ventricular fibrillation or tachycardia (unless congestive failure supervenes after protracted episode not due to digitalis), in presence of digitalis toxicity, hypersensitivity to cardiac glycosides, beriberi heart disease, certain cases of hypersensitive carotid sinus syndrome.

**Special Concerns:** Use with caution in clients with ischemic heart disease, acute myocarditis, hypertrophic subaortic stenosis, hypoxic or myxedemic states, Adams-Stokes or carotid sinus syndromes, cardiac amyloidosis, or cyanotic heart and lung disease, including emphysema and partial heart block. Those with carditis associated with rheumatic fever or viral myocarditis are especially sensitive to digoxin-induced disturbances in rhythm. Electric pacemakers may sensitize the myocardium to cardiac glycosides. Also use with caution and at reduced dosage in elderly, debilitated clients, pregnant women and nursing mothers, and newborn, term, or premature infants who have immature renal and hepatic function and in reduced renal and/or hepatic function.

**Side Effects:** Cardiac glycosides are extremely toxic and have caused death even in clients who have received the drugs for long periods of time. There is a narrow margin of safety between an effective therapeutic dose and a toxic dose. Overdosage caused by the cumulative effects of the drug is a constant danger in therapy with cardiac glycosides. Digitalis toxicity is characterized by a wide variety of symptoms, which are hard to differentiate from those of the cardiac disease itself.

*CV:* Changes in the rate, rhythm,

and irritability of the heart and the mechanism of the heartbeat. Extrasystoles, bigeminal pulse, coupled rhythm, ectopic beat, and other forms of arrhythmias have been noted. **Death most often results from ventricular fibrillation.** Cardiac glycosides should be discontinued in adults when pulse rate falls below 60 beats/min. All cardiac changes are best detected by the ECG, which is also most useful in clients suffering from intoxication. **Acute hemorrhage.** GI: Anorexia, N&V, excessive salivation, epigastric distress, abdominal pain, diarrhea, bowel necrosis. Clients on digitalis therapy may experience two vomiting stages. The first is an early sign of toxicity and is a direct effect of digitalis on the GI tract. Late vomiting indicates stimulation of the vomiting center of the brain, which occurs after the heart muscle has been saturated with digitalis. CNS: Headaches, fatigue, lassitude, irritability, malaise, muscle weakness, insomnia, stupor. Psychotomimetic effects (especially in elderly or arteriosclerotic clients or neonates) including disorientation, confusion, depression, aphasia, delirium, hallucinations, and, rarely, **convulsions.** Neuromuscular: Neurologic pain involving the lower third of the face and lumbar areas, paresthesia. Visual disturbances: Blurred vision, flickering dots, white halos, borders around dark objects, diplopia, amblyopia, color perception changes. Hypersensitivity (5–7 days after starting therapy): Skin reactions (urticaria, fever, pruritus, facial and **angioneurotic edema**). Other: Chest pain, coldness of extremities.

**OD** **Overdose Management:** The relationship of cardiac glycoside levels to symptoms of toxicity varies significantly from client to client; thus, it is not possible to identify glycoside levels that would define toxicity accurately. Symptoms (Toxicity): GI: Anorexia, N&V, diarrhea, abdominal discomfort, or pain. CNS: Blurred, yellow, or green vision and halo effect; headache, weakness, drowsiness, mental depression, apathy, restlessness, disorientation, confusion, **seizures,** EEG abnormalities, delirium, hallucinations, neuralgia, psychosis. CV: Ventricular tachycardia, unifocal or multiform PVCs (especially in bigeminal or trigeminal patterns), paroxysmal and nonparoxysmal nodal rhythms, AV dissociation, accelerated junctional rhythm, excessive slowing of the pulse, **AV block (may proceed to complete block),** atrial fibrillation, **ventricular fibrillation (most common cause of death).** Children: Visual disturbances, headache, weakness, apathy, and psychosis occur but may be difficult to recognize. CV: Conduction disturbances, supraventricular tachyarrhythmias (e.g., **AV block**), atrial tachycardia with or without block, nodal tachycardia, unifocal or multiform ventricular premature contractions, ventricular tachycardia, sinus bradycardia (especially in infants).Treatment in Adults:

• Discontinue drug and admit to the intensive care area for continuous monitoring of ECG.

• If serum potassium is below normal, potassium chloride should be administered in divided PO doses totaling 3–6 g (40–80 mEq). Potassium should not be used when severe or complete heart block is due to digitalis and not related to tachycardia.

• Atropine: A dose of 0.01 mg/kg IV to treat severe sinus bradycardia or slow ventricular rate due to secondary AV block.

• Cholestyramine, colestipol, activated charcoal: To bind digitalis in the intestine, thus preventing enterohepatic recirculation.

• Digoxin immune FAB: See drug entry. Given in approximate equimolar quantities as digoxin, it reverses S&S of toxicity, often with improvement seen within 30 min.

• Lidocaine: A dose of 1 mg/kg given over 5 min followed by an infusion of 15–50 mcg/kg/min to maintain normal cardiac rhythm.

• *Phenytoin:* For atrial or ventricular arrhythmias unresponsive to potassium, can give a dose of 0.5 mg/kg at a rate not exceeding 50 mg/min (given at 1–2 hr intervals). The maximum dose should not exceed 10 mg/kg/day.

• *Countershock:* A direct-current countershock can be used *only as a last resort*. If required, therapy should be initiated at low voltage levels.

   *Treatment in Children:* Give potassium in divided doses totaling 1–1.5 mEq/kg (if correction of arrhythmia is urgent, a dose of 0.5 mEq/kg/hr can be used) with careful monitoring of the ECG. The potassium IV solution should be dilute to avoid local irritation although IV fluid overload must be avoided. Digoxin immune FAB may also be used.

   Digoxin is not removed effectively by dialysis, by exchange transfusion, or during cardiopulmonary bypass as most of the drug is found in tissues rather than the circulating blood. Digitoxin is not effectively removed by either peritoneal or hemodialysis due to its high degree of plasma protein binding.

**Drug Interactions:** One of the most serious side effects of digitalis-type drugs is hypokalemia (lowering of serum potassium levels). This may lead to cardiac arrhythmias, muscle weakness, hypotension, and respiratory distress. Other agents causing hypokalemia reinforce this effect and increase the chance of digitalis toxicity. Such reactions may occur in clients who have been on digitalis maintenance for a long time.

*Albuterol* / ↑ Skeletal muscle binding of digoxin

*Amiloride* / ↓ Inotropic effects of digoxin

*Aminoglycosides* / ↓ Effect of digitalis glycosides due to ↓ absorption from GI tract

*Aminosalicylic acid* / ↓ Effect of digitalis glycosides due to ↓ absorption from GI tract

*Amphotericin B* / ↑ K depletion

caused by digitalis; ↑ risk of digitalis toxicity

*Antacids* / ↓ Effect of digitalis glycosides due to ↓ absorption from GI tract

*Beta blockers* / Complete heart block possible

*Calcium preparations* / Cardiac arrhythmias if parenteral calcium given with digitalis

*Chlorthalidone* / ↑ K and Mg loss with ↑ chance of digitalis toxicity

*Cholestyramine* / Binds digitoxin in the intestine and ↓ its absorption

*Colestipol* / Binds digitoxin in the intestine and ↓ its absorption

*Ephedrine* / ↑ Chance of cardiac arrhythmias

*Epinephrine* / ↑ Chance of cardiac arrhythmias

*Ethacrynic acid* / ↑ K and Mg loss with ↑ chance of digitalis toxicity

*Furosemide* / ↑ K and Mg loss with ↑ chance of digitalis toxicity

*Glucose infusions* / Large infusions of glucose may cause ↓ in serum potassium and ↑ chance of digitalis toxicity

*Hypoglycemic drugs* / ↓ Effect of digitalis glycosides due to ↑ breakdown by liver

*Methimazole* / ↑ Chance of toxic effects of digitalis

*Metoclopramide* / ↓ Effect of digitalis glycosides by ↓ absorption from GI tract

*Muscle relaxants, nondepolarizing* / ↑ Risk of cardiac arrhythmias

*Propranolol* / Potentiates digitalis-induced bradycardia

*Reserpine* / ↑ Chance of cardiac arrhythmias

*Spironolactone* / Either ↑ or ↓ toxic effects of digitalis glycosides

*Succinylcholine* / ↑ Chance of cardiac arrhythmias

*Sulfasalazine* / ↓ Effect of digitalis glycosides by ↓ absorption from GI tract

*Sympathomimetics* / ↑ Chance of cardiac arrhythmias

*Thiazides* / ↑ K and Mg loss with ↑ chance of digitalis toxicity

*Thioamines* / ↑ Effect and toxicity of cardiac glycosides

*Thyroid* / ↓Effectiveness of digitalis glycosides
*Triamterene* / ↑ Pharmacologic effects of digoxin
**Laboratory Test Interferences:** May ↓ PT. Alters tests for 17-ketosteroids and 17-hydroxycorticosteroids.

**Dosage**
**PO, IM, or IV.** *Highly individualized.* See individual drugs: digitoxin, digoxin. The rates at which clients become digitalized vary considerably. Clients with mild signs of congestion can often be digitalized gradually over a period of several days. Clients suffering from more serious congestion, for example, those showing signs of acute LV failure, dyspnea, or lung edema, can be digitalized more rapidly by parenteral administration of a fast-acting cardiac glycoside. Once digitalization has been attained (pulse 68–80 beats/min) and symptoms of CHF have subsided, the client is put on maintenance dosage. Depending on the drug and the age of the client, the daily maintenance dose is often approximately 10% of the digitalizing dose.

## NURSING CONSIDERATIONS
**Administration/Storage**
1. The names digoxin and digitoxin are similar. However, their dosage and duration of their effect differ markedly. Check client's name, the order, the medication administration record/card, and the drug bottle label to be administered.
2. Measure all oral liquid meds precisely, using a calibrated dropper or a syringe.
3. The half-life of cardiac glycosides is prolonged in the elderly. When working with elderly clients, anticipate smaller doses than for those in other age groups.
4. Obtain written parameters indicating the pulse rates, both high and low, at which cardiac glycosides are to be held; changes in rate or rhythm may indicate toxicity.

**FOR CLIENTS STARTING ON A DIGITALIZING DOSE**
**Assessment**
1. Document type, onset, and characteristics of symptoms. If administered for heart failure, note causes; ensure that failure not solely related to diastolic dysfunction as drug's positive inotropic effect may increase cardiac outflow obstruction with hypertrophic cardiomyopathy.
2. Note any drugs prescribed that would adversely interact with digitalis glycosides; diuretics may increase toxicity.
3. Monitor CBC, serum electrolytes, calcium, magnesium, liver and renal function tests.
4. Obtain ECG, noting rhythm and rate.
5. Document cardiopulmonary findings; note presence of S3, JVD, HJR, displaced PMI, HR above 100 bpm, rales, peripheral edema, DOE, PND, and echo, MUGA, and/or cardiac cath findings. Note New York Heart Association Classification based on client symptoms.

**FOR CLIENTS BEING DIGITALIZED AND FOR CLIENTS ON A MAINTENANCE DOSE OF A CARDIAC GLYCOSIDE**
**Interventions**
1. During digitalization, monitor closely.
2. Observe monitor for bradycardia and/or arrhythmias, or count apical pulse rate for at least 1 min before administering the drug. Obtain written parameters (e.g., HR > 50 or 60) for drug administration.
• Document adult HR below 50 bpm or if an arrhythmia (irregular pulse) occurs.
• If child's HR is 90–110 bpm or if an arrhythmia is present, withhold drug and report.
3. Anticipate more than once daily dosing in most children (up to age 10) due to higher metabolic activity.
4. With co-worker simultaneously take the apical and radial pulse for 1 min, and report pulse deficit (e.g., the wrist rate is less than the apical

rate); may indicate an adverse drug reaction.

5. Monitor weights and I&O. Weight gain may indicate edema. Adequate intake will help prevent cumulative toxic drug effects.

6. If taking non-potassium-sparing diuretics as well as a cardiac glycoside, will need potassium supplements. Provide the most palatable preparation available. (Liquid potassium preparations are usually bitter.)

7. If gastric distress experienced, use an antacid. Antacids containing aluminum or magnesium and kaolin/pectin mixtures should be given 6 hr before or 6 hr after dose of cardiac glycoside to prevent decreased therapeutic effects.

8. When given to newborns, use a cardiac monitor to identify early evidence of toxicity: excessive slowing of sinus rate, sinoatrial arrest, or prolonged PR interval.

9. Monitor digoxin levels periodically (therapeutic range 0.5–2.0 ng/mL) and assess for symptoms of toxicity; draw specimen more than 6 hr after last dose. Have digoxin antidote available (digoxin immune FAB) for severe toxicity.

10. Use caution; digoxin withdrawal may worsen heart failure.

**Client/Family Teaching**

1. Take after meals to lessen gastric irritation.

2. Initially, maintain a written record of pulse rates and weights; review guidelines for withholding medication and reporting abnormal pulse rates.

3. Do not change brands; different preparations have variations in bioavailability and could cause toxicity or loss of effect.

4. Follow directions carefully for taking the medication. If one dose of drug is accidentally missed, do not double up on the next dose.

5. Report toxic drug symptoms: anorexia, N&V, and diarrhea are often early symptoms and are due to the toxic effects on the GI tract and CTZ stimulation. Disorientation, agitation, visual disturbances, changes in color perception, and hallucinations may also occur.

6. Maintain a sodium-restricted diet. Read labels and review foods low in sodium; consult dietitian for assistance in shopping, meal planning, food selection, and preparation.

7. Consult provider before taking any other medications, whether prescribed or OTC, because drug interactions occur frequently with cardiac glycosides.

8. Report any persistent cough, difficulty breathing, or edema (S&S of CHF).

9. Identify community health agencies available to assist clients in maintaining health.

10. Return for scheduled follow-up visits and lab tests.

**Outcomes/Evaluate**

• Stable cardiac rate and rhythm, improved breathing patterns, ↓ severity of S&S of CHF, improved CO, improved activity tolerance, ↓ weight, and improved diuresis

• Serum drug levels within therapeutic range (e.g., digoxin 0.5–2.0 ng/mL)

**Special Concerns**

1. Elderly clients must be observed for early S&S of toxicity (N&V, anorexia, confusion, and visual disturbances) because their rate of drug elimination is slower.

2. The half-life of cardiac glycosides is prolonged in the elderly; anticipate smaller drug doses.

3. Be especially alert to cardiac arrhythmias in children. This sign of toxicity occurs more frequently in children than in adults.

# CEPHALOSPORINS

*See also the following individual entries:*

Cefaclor
Cefadroxil monohydrate
Cefamandole nafate
Cefazolin sodium
Cefepime hydrochloride
Cefixime oral

Cefoperazone sodium
Cefotaxime sodium
Cefotetan disodium
Cefoxitin sodium
Cefpodoxime proxetil
Cefprozil
Ceftazidime
Ceftibuten
Ceftizoxime sodium
Ceftriaxone sodium
Cefuroxime axetil
Cefuroxime sodium
Cephalexin hydrochloride monohydrate
Cephalexin monohydrate
Cephalothin sodium
Cephapirin sodium
Cephradine
Loracarbef

**General Statement:** Cephalosporins are broad-spectrum antibiotics classified as first-, second-, and third-generation drugs. The difference among generations is based on pharmacokinetics and antibacterial spectra. Generally, third-generation cephalosporins have more activity against gram-negative organisms and resistant organisms and less activity against gram-positive organisms than first-generation drugs. Third-generation cephalosporins are also stable against beta-lactamases. Cephalosporins can be destroyed by cephalosporinase. Also, the cost increases from first- to third-generation cephalosporins.

**Action/Kinetics:** The cephalosporins interfere with a final step in the formation of the bacterial cell wall (inhibition of mucopeptide biosynthesis), resulting in unstable cell membranes that undergo lysis (same mechanism of actions as penicillins). Also, cell division and growth are inhibited. The cephalosporins are most effective against young, rapidly dividing organisms and are considered bactericidal. Cephalosporins are widely distributed to most tissues and fluids. First- and second-generation drugs do not enter the CSF well but third-generation drugs

enter inflamed meninges readily. Rapidly excreted by the kidneys.

**Uses:** See individual drugs. Cephalosporins are effective against infections of the biliary tract, GI tract, GU system, bones, joints, upper and lower respiratory tract, skin, and skin structures. Also, gynecologic infections, meningitis, osteomyelitis, endocarditis, intra-abdominal infections, peritonitis, otitis media, gonorrhea, septicemia, and prophylaxis prior to surgery. A listing of the drugs in each generation follows:

First-Generation Cephalosporins: Cefadroxil, cefazolin, cephalexin, cephalothin, cephapirin, cephradine.

Second-Generation Cephalosporins: Cefaclor, cefamandole, cefmetazole, cefonicid, cefotetan, cefoxitin, cefprozil, cefuroxime, and loracarbef.

Third-Generation Cephalosporins: Cefepime, cefixime, cefoperazone, cefotaxime, cefpodoxime, ceftazidime, ceftibuten, ceftizoxime, ceftriaxone.

**Contraindications:** Hypersensitivity to cephalosporins or related antibiotics.

**Special Concerns:** Safe use in pregnancy and lactation has not been established. Use with caution in the presence of impaired renal or hepatic function, together with other nephrotoxic drugs, and in clients over 50 years of age. Perform $C_{cr}$ on all clients with impaired renal function who receive cephalosporins. If hypersensitive to penicillin, may occasionally cross-react to cephalosporins.

**Side Effects:** *GI:* N&V, diarrhea, abdominal cramps or pain, dyspepsia, glossitis, heartburn, sore mouth or tongue, dysgeusia, anorexia, flatulence, cholestasis. Pseudomembranous colitis. *Allergic:* Urticaria, rashes (maculopapular, morbilliform, or erythematous), pruritus (including anal and genital areas), fever, chills, erythema, **angioedema,** serum sickness, joint pain, exfoliative dermatitis, chest tightness, myalgia, erythema multiforme, edema, itching, numbness, chills, **Stevens-Johnson syndrome, anaphylaxis.** *NOTE:* Cross-allergy may be manifested between cephalosporins and penicillins. *Hematologic:* Leukopenia, leukocytosis, lymphocytosis, neutropenia (transient), eosinophilia, thrombocytopenia, thrombocythemia, **agranulocytosis,** granulocytopenia, bone marrow depression, **hemolytic anemia,** pancytopenia, decreased platelet function, **aplastic anemia,** hypoprothrombinemia (may lead to bleeding), thrombocytosis (transient). *CNS:* Headache, malaise, fatigue, vertigo, dizziness, lethargy, confusion, paresthesia, precipitation of **seizures** (especially in clients with impaired renal function). *Hepatic:* Hepatomegaly, hepatitis. Intrathecal use may result in hallucinations, nystagmus, or **seizures.** *Miscellaneous:* Superinfection including oral candidiasis and enterococcal infections, hypotension, sweating, flushing, dyspnea, interstitial pneumonitis.

IV or IM use may result in local swelling, inflammation, cellulitis, paresthesia, burning, phlebitis, thrombophlebitis. IM use may also cause pain and induration, tenderness, increased temperature. Sterile abscesses have been observed following SC use. Nephrotoxicity (↑ BUN with and without ↑ serum creatinine) may occur in clients over 50 and in young children.

**OD Overdose Management:** *Symptoms:* Parenteral use of large doses of cephalosporins may cause seizures, especially in clients with impaired renal function. *Treatment:* If seizures occur, discontinue the drug immediately and give anticonvulsant drugs. Hemodialysis may also be effective.

**Drug Interactions**
*Aminoglycosides* / ↑ Risk of renal toxicity with certain cephalosporins
*Anticoagulants* / Certain cephalosporins ↑ PT
*Bacteriostatic agents* / ↓ Effect of cephalosporins

*Bumetanide* / ↑ Risk of renal toxicity
*Colistimethate* / ↑ Risk of renal toxicity
*Colistin* / ↑ Risk of renal toxicity
*Ethacrynic acid* / ↑ Risk of renal toxicity
*Furosemide* / ↑ Risk of renal toxicity
*Polymyxin B* / ↑ Risk of renal toxicity
*Probenecid* / ↑ Effect of cephalosporins by ↓ excretion by kidneys
*Vancomycin* / ↑ Risk of renal toxicity

**Laboratory Test Interferences:** False + for urinary glucose with Benedict's solution, Fehling's solution, or Clinitest tablets. Enzyme tests (Clinistix, Tes-Tape) are unaffected. False + Coombs' test and urinary 17-ketosteroids.

↑ AST, ALT, total bilirubin, GGTP, LDH, alkaline phosphatase.

**Dosage**
See individual drugs.

## NURSING CONSIDERATIONS

See also *General Nursing Considerations for All Anti-Infectives.*
**Administration/Storage**
1. Parenteral solutions infused too rapidly may cause pain and irritation; infuse over 30 min unless otherwise indicated and assess site frequently.
2. Continue therapy for at least 2–3 days after symptoms of infection have disappeared.
3. For group A beta-hemolytic streptococcal infections, continue therapy for at least 10 days to prevent the development of glomerulonephritis or rheumatic fever.
**Assessment**
1. With hypersensitivity reactions to penicillin, assess for cross-sensitivity to cephalosporins.
2. Many agents in this group of antibiotics are quite expensive. Clients on fixed incomes with limited health benefits may be unable to afford the prescription expense.
3. Document indications for therapy

and symptoms of infection; obtain baseline cultures.

4. Monitor CBC, serum glucose, electrolytes, liver and renal function studies. With renal impairment reduce dose; for dialysis clients, administer after treatment.

5. Drug may cause false positive Coombs' test.

**Interventions**

1. The cephalosporins all have similar sounding and similarly spelled names. Use care when transcribing orders for administration and request clarification as needed.

2. Pseudomembranous colitis may occur. If diarrhea develops, note any fever and report immediately. Continue to monitor VS, I&O, stool C&S, and for lab evidence of electrolyte imbalance.

3. Persistent temperature elevations may be indicative of drug-induced fever.

**Client/Family Teaching**

1. Oral meds should be taken on an empty stomach but, if GI upset occurs, may be administered with meals.

2. Report any symptoms that may necessitate drug withdrawal such as vaginal itching or drainage, fever, or diarrhea.

3. Yogurt or buttermilk (4 oz) may be prescribed daily for diarrhea related to intestinal superinfections (to restore intestinal flora).

4. Report signs of superinfection (black furry tongue, vaginal itching or discharge, and loose, foul-smelling stools). Nystatin may be ordered for secondary infections.

5. Take meds as ordered; report side effects so appropriate therapy may be initiated.

6. Immediately report any abnormal bleeding or bruising.

7. May cause false positive Coombs' test. This would be of concern if being cross-matched for blood transfusions or in newborns whose mothers have taken cephalosporins during pregnancy.

8. Avoid alcohol and alcohol-containing products, as a disulfiram-type reaction may occur with some of the cephalosporins.

**Outcomes/Evaluate**

• Presence/absence of pretreatment symptoms; negative C&S reports
• Resolution of infection
• Symptomatic improvement, i.e., ↓ WBCs, ↓ temperature, improved appetite

# CHOLINERGIC BLOCKING AGENTS

Atropine sulfate
Benztropine mesylate
Biperiden hydrochloride
Dicyclomine hydrochloride
Ipratropium bromide
Propantheline bromide
Scopolamine hydrobromide
Scopolamine transdermal therapeutic system
Trihexyphenidyl hydrochloride

**Action/Kinetics:** The cholinergic blocking agents prevent the neurotransmitter acetylcholine from combining with receptors on the postganglionic parasympathetic nerve terminal (muscarinic site). Effects include reduction of smooth muscle spasms, blockade of vagal impulses to the heart, decreased secretions (e.g., gastric, salivation, bronchial mucus, sweat glands), production of mydriasis and cycloplegia, and various CNS effects. In therapeutic doses, these drugs have little effect on transmission of nerve impulses across ganglia (nicotinic sites) or at the neuromuscular junction. Several anticholinergic drugs abolish or reduce the S&S of Parkinson's disease, such as tremors and rigidity, and result in some improvement in mobility, muscular coordination, and motor performance. These effects may be due to blockade of the effects of acetylcholine in the CNS.

**Uses:** See individual drugs.

**Contraindications:** Glaucoma, adhesions between iris and lens of the eye, tachycardia, myocardial ischemia, unstable CV state in acute hemorrhage, partial obstruction of the GI and biliary tracts, prostatic hypertrophy, renal disease, myasthenia gravis, hepatic disease, paralytic ileus, pyloroduodenal stenosis, pyloric obstruction, intestinal atony, ulcerative colitis, obstructive uropathy. Cardiac clients, especially when there is danger of tachycardia; older persons suffering from atherosclerosis or mental impairment. Lactation.

**Special Concerns:** Use with caution in pregnancy. Infants and young children are more susceptible to the toxic side effects of anticholinergic drugs. Use in children when the ambient temperature is high may cause a rapid increase in body temperature due to suppression of sweat glands. Geriatric clients are particularly likely to manifest anticholinergic side effects and CNS effects, including agitation, confusion, drowsiness, excitement, glaucoma, and impaired memory. Use with caution in hyperthyroidism, CHF, cardiac arrhythmias, hypertension, Down syndrome, asthma, spastic paralysis, blonde individuals, allergies, and chronic lung disease.

**Side Effects:** These are desirable in some conditions and undesirable in others. Thus, the anticholinergics have an antisalivary effect that is useful in parkinsonism. This same effect is unpleasant when the drug is used for spastic conditions of the GI tract. Most side effects are dose-related and decrease when dosage decreases. *GI:* N&V, dry mouth, dysphagia, constipation, heartburn, change in taste perception, bloated feeling, paralytic ileus. *CNS:* Dizziness, drowsiness, nervousness, disorientation, headache, weakness, insomnia, fever (especially in children). Large doses may produce CNS stimulation including tremor and restlessness. Anticholinergic psychoses: ataxia, euphoria, confusion, disorientation, loss of short-term memory, decreased anxiety, fatigue, insomnia, hallucinations, dysarthria, agitation. *CV:* Palpitations. *GU:* Urinary retention or hesitancy,

impotence. *Ophthalmologic:* Blurred vision, dilated pupils, photophobia, cycloplegia, precipitation of acute glaucoma. *Allergic:* Urticaria, skin rashes, **anaphylaxis.** *Other:* Flushing, decreased sweating, nasal congestion, suppression of glandular secretions including lactation. Heat prostration (fever and heat stroke) in presence of high environmental temperatures due to decreased sweating.

**OD** **Overdose Management:** *Symptoms ("Belladonna Poisoning"):* Infants and children are especially susceptible to the toxic effects of atropine and scopolamine. Poisoning (dose-dependent) is characterized by the following symptoms: dry mouth, burning sensation of the mouth, difficulty in swallowing and speaking, blurred vision, photophobia, rash, tachycardia, increased respiration, **increased body temperature** (up to 109°F, 42.7°C), restlessness, irritability, confusion, muscle incoordination, dilated pupils, hot dry skin, **respiratory depression and paralysis,** tremors, **seizures,** hallucinations, and **death.** Treatment ("Belladonna Poisoning"):

• Gastric lavage or induction of vomiting followed by activated charcoal. General supportive measures.

• Anticholinergic effects can be reversed by physostigmine (Eserine), 1–3 mg IV (effectiveness uncertain; thus use other agents if possible). Neostigmine methylsulfate, 0.5–2 mg IV, repeated as necessary.

• If there is excitation, diazepam, a short-acting barbiturate, IV sodium thiopental (2% solution), or chloral hydrate (100–200 mL of a 2% solution by rectal infusion) may be given.

• For fever, cool baths may be used. Keep client in a darkened room if photophobia is manifested.

• Artificial respiration should be instituted if there is paralysis of respiratory muscles.

**Drug Interactions**
*Amantadine* / Additive anticholinergic side effects
*Antacids* / ↓ Absorption of anticholinergics from GI tract

*Antidepressants, tricyclic* / Additive anticholinergic side effects

*Antihistamines* / Additive anticholinergic side effects

*Atenolol* / Anticholinergics ↑ effects of atenolol

*Benzodiazepines* / Additive anticholinergic side effects

*Corticosteroids* / Additive ↑ intraocular pressure

*Cyclopropane* / ↑ Chance of ventricular arrhythmias

*Digoxin* / ↑ Effect of digoxin due to ↑ absorption from GI tract

*Disopyramide* / Potentiation of anticholinergic side effects

*Guanethidine* / Reversal of inhibition of gastric acid secretion caused by anticholinergics

*Haloperidol* / Additive ↑ intraocular pressure

*Histamine* / Reversal of inhibition of gastric acid secretion caused by anticholinergics

*Levodopa* / Possible ↓ effect of levodopa due to ↑ breakdown of levodopa in stomach (due to delayed gastric emptying time)

*MAO inhibitors* / ↑ Effect of anticholinergics due to ↓ breakdown by liver

*Meperidine* / Additive anticholinergic side effects

*Methylphenidate* / Potentiation of anticholinergic side effects

*Metoclopramide* / Anticholinergics block action of metoclopramide

*Nitrates, nitrites* / Potentiation of anticholinergic side effects

*Nitrofurantoin* / ↑ Bioavailability of nitrofurantoin

*Orphenadrine* / Additive anticholinergic side effects

*Phenothiazines* / Additive anticholinergic side effects; also, effects of phenothiazines may ↓

*Primidone* / Potentiation of anticholinergic side effects

*Procainamide* / Additive anticholinergic side effects

*Quinidine* / Additive anticholinergic side effects

*Reserpine* / Reversal of inhibition of gastric acid secretion caused by anticholinergics

*Sympathomimetics* / ↑ Bronchial relaxation

*Thiazide diuretics* / ↑ Bioavailability of thiazide diuretics

*Thioxanthines* / Potentiation of anticholinergic side effects

## Dosage
See individual drugs.

# NURSING CONSIDERATIONS

**Administration/Storage:**   Dosage is often small. To prevent overdosage, check dosage and measure the drug exactly.

**Assessment**

1. Document indications for therapy; assess for asthma, glaucoma, or duodenal ulcer (contraindications for therapy).

2. Note history of renal disease, cardiac problems, or hepatic disease.

3. Determine age; elderly clients, especially those with mental impairment or atherosclerosis, should not receive these drugs.

4. Assess for constipation and urinary retention and tolerance.

**Interventions**

1. If the client complains of a dry mouth, provide frequent mouth care and cold drinks, especially postoperatively. Sugarless hard candies and chewing gum may also be of some benefit.

2. Drugs such as atropine may suppress thermoregulatory sweating; counsel client concerning activity (especially in hot weather) and appropriate clothing. Also, children and infants may exhibit "atropine fever."

**Client/Family Teaching**

1. Certain side effects are to be expected, such as dry mouth or blurred vision, and may have to be tolerated because of the overall beneficial effects of drug therapy. These should be reported so symptoms may be alleviated by reducing the dose or by temporarily stopping the drug.

2. With parkinsonism, do not withdraw abruptly. If the medication is changed, one drug should be withdrawn slowly and the other started in small doses.

## ADDITIONAL NURSING CONSIDERATIONS RELATED TO PATHOLOGIC CONDITIONS FOR WHICH THE DRUG IS ADMINISTERED

CARDIOVASCULAR
**Interventions**
1. Monitor VS and ECG. Assess for any hemodynamic changes and intraventricular conduction blocks.
2. Note any complaints of palpitations.

OCULAR
**Assessment**
1. Determine any previous experience with this class of drugs and the results.
2. Document IOP and assess accommodation and pupillary response.
**Interventions**
1. Note complaints of dizziness or blurred vision; assist with ambulation and institute safety measures.
2. Hold meds and report any complaints of eye pain after instillation.
**Client/Family Teaching**
1. Review methods for instillation of drops or ointment.
2. Vision will be affected by the meds; temporary stinging and blurred vision will occur. Assess response and plan activities for safety.
3. Night vision may be impaired. Photophobia, which may occur, can be relieved by wearing dark glasses.
4. Report any marked changes in vision, eye irritation, or persistent headaches immediately.
5. With large doses, lacrimal secretion may be diminished; may experience dry or "sandy" eyes.

GASTROINTESTINAL
**Client/Family Teaching**
1. Take early enough before a meal (at least 20 min) so that it will be effective when needed.
2. Review printed information related to the prescribed diet; see dietitian for assistance in meal planning and preparation as needed.
3. Gastric emptying times may be prolonged and intestinal transit time lengthened. Drug-induced intestinal paralysis is temporary and should resolve after 1–3 days of therapy.

GENITOURINARY
**Interventions**
1. Assess middle-aged male clients for evidence of urinary retention; may be more pronounced in elderly men with prostatic hypertrophy.
2. Monitor I&O. Palpate abdomen for evidence of bladder distention and assess need for catheterization.
3. Consult with the provider for medication adjustment if impotence occurs; may be drug-related.
**Outcomes/Evaluate**
• Dilation of pupils
• ↓ Bowel motility with improved elimination patterns
• ↑ HR
• ↓ Secretion production
• ↓ Muscle tremors, rigidity, and spasticity

# CORTICOSTEROIDS

*See also the following individual entries:*

Beclomethasone dipropionate
Betamethasone
Betamethasone dipropionate
Betamethasone sodium phosphate
Betamethasone sodium phosphate and Betamethasone acetate
Betamethasone valerate
Budesonide
Corticotropin injection
Corticotropin repository injection
Cortisone acetate
Cosyntropin
Dexamethasone
Dexamethasone acetate
Dexamethasone sodium phosphate
Fludrocortisone acetate
Flunisolide
Fluticasone propionate
Hydrocortisone

Hydrocortisone acetate
Hydrocortisone butyrate
Hydrocortisone cypionate
Hydrocortisone sodium phos-
phate
Hydrocortisone sodium succinate
Hydrocortisone valerate
Methylprednisolone
Methylprednisolone acetate
Methylprednisolone sodium suc-
cinate
Prednisolone
Prednisolone acetate
Prednisolone acetate and
Prednisolone sodium phos-
phate
Prednisolone sodium phosphate
Prednisolone tebutate
Prednisone
Triamcinolone
Triamcinolone acetonide
Triamcinolone diacetate
Triamcinolone hexacetonide

**Action/Kinetics:** The hormones of the adrenal gland influence many metabolic pathways and all organ systems and are essential for survival. These processes include carbohydrate metabolism (e.g., glycogen deposition in the liver and conversion of glycogen to glucose), protein metabolism (e.g., gluconeogenesis, protein catabolism), fat metabolism (e.g., deposition of fatty tissue), and water and electrolyte balance (e.g., fluid retention, excretion of potassium, calcium, and phosphorus).

According to their chemical structure and chief physiologic effect, the corticosteroids fall into two subgroups, which have considerable functional overlap. First are those, like cortisone and hydrocortisone, that mainly regulate the metabolic pathways involving protein, carbohydrate, and fat. This group is often referred to as *glucocorticoids*. In the second group are those, like aldosterone and desoxycorticosterone, that are more specifically involved in electrolyte and water balance. These are often referred to as *mineralocorticoids*. Hormones, such as cortisone and hydrocortisone, although classified as glu-

cocorticoids, possess significant mineralocorticoid activity. Therapeutically, a distinction must be made between physiologic doses used for replacement therapy and pharmacologic doses used to treat inflammatory and other disease states.

The hormones have a marked anti-inflammatory effect because of their ability to inhibit prostaglandin synthesis. These agents also inhibit accumulation of macrophages and leukocytes at sites of inflammation as well as inhibit phagocytosis and lysosomal enzyme release. They aid the organism in coping with various stressful situations (trauma, severe illness). The immunosuppressant effect is thought to be due to a reduction of the number of T lymphocytes, monocytes, and eosinophils. Corticosteroids also decrease binding of immunoglobulin to receptors on the cell surface and inhibit the synthesis and/or release of interleukins which, in turn, decrease T-lymphocyte blastogenesis and reduce the primary immune response.

**Uses:** When used for anti-inflammatory or immunosuppressant therapy, the corticosteroid should possess minimal mineralocorticoid activity. Therapy with glucocorticoids is not curative and in many situations should be considered as adjunctive rather than primary therapy. The following list is not inclusive but provides examples of the physiologic and pharmacologic uses of corticosteroids.

1. **Replacement therapy.** Acute and chronic adrenal insufficiency, including Addison's disease. For replacement therapy, drugs must possess both glucocorticoid and mineralocorticoid effects.

2. **Rheumatic disorders,** including rheumatoid arthritis (including juveniles), other types of arthritis, ankylosing spondylitis, acute and subacute bursitis.

3. **Collagen diseases,** including SLE.

---

✦ = Available in Canada          ***bold italic*** = life threatening side effect

4. **Allergic diseases,** including control of severe allergic conditions as serum sickness, drug hypersensitivity reactions, anaphylaxis.

5. **Respiratory diseases,** including prophylaxis and treatment of bronchial asthma (and status asthmaticus), seasonal or perennial rhinitis.

6. **Ocular diseases,** including severe acute and chronic allergic and inflammatory conditions.

7. **Dermatologic diseases,** including angioedema or urticaria, contact dermatitis, atopic dermatitis, severe erythema multiforme (Stevens-Johnson syndrome).

8. **Diseases of the intestinal tract,** including chronic ulcerative colitis, regional enteritis.

9. **Nervous system,** including acute exacerbations of multiple sclerosis, optic neuritis.

10. **Malignancies,** including leukemias and lymphomas in adults and acute leukemia in children.

11. **Nephrotic syndrome,** including that due to lupus erythematosus or of the idiopathic type.

12. **Hematologic diseases,** including acquired hemolytic anemia, RBC anemia, idiopathic and secondary thrombocytopenic purpura in adults, congenital hypoplastic anemia.

13. **Intra-articular or soft tissue administration,** including acute episodes of synovitis osteoarthritis, rheumatoid arthritis, acute gouty arthritis, bursitis.

14. **Intralesional administration,** including keloids, psoriatic plaques, discoid lupus erythematosus.

**Contraindications:** Suspected infection as these drugs may mask infections. Also peptic ulcer, psychoses, acute glomerulonephritis, herpes simplex infections of the eye, vaccinia or varicella, the exanthematous diseases, Cushing's syndrome, active tuberculosis, myasthenia gravis. Recent intestinal anastomoses, CHF or other cardiac disease, hypertension, systemic fungal infections, open-angle glaucoma. Also, hyperlipidemia, hyperthyroidism or hypothyroidism, osteoporosis, myasthenia gravis, tuberculosis. Lactation (if high doses are used). Inhalation products to relieve acute bronchospasms.

Topically in the eye for dendritic keratitis, vaccinia, chickenpox, other viral disease that may involve the conjunctiva or cornea, and tuberculosis and fungal or acute purulent infections of the eye. Topically in the ear in aural fungal infections and perforated eardrum. Topically in tuberculosis of the skin, herpes simplex, vaccinia, varicella, and infectious conditions in the absence of anti-infective agents.

**Special Concerns:** Use with caution in diabetes mellitus, hypertension, chronic nephritis, thrombophlebitis, convulsive disorders, infectious diseases, renal or hepatic insufficiency, pregnancy. Chronic use may inhibit the growth and development of children or adolescents. Pediatric clients are also at greater risk for developing cataracts, osteoporosis, avascular necrosis of the femoral heads, and glaucoma. Geriatric clients are more likely to develop hypertension and osteoporosis (especially postmenopausal women).

**Side Effects:** Small physiologic doses given as replacement therapy or short-term high-dosage therapy during emergencies rarely cause side effects. Prolonged therapy may cause a Cushing-like syndrome with atrophy of the adrenal cortex and subsequent adrenocortical insufficiency. A steroid withdrawal syndrome may occur following prolonged use; symptoms include anorexia, N&V, lethargy, headache, fever, joint pain, desquamation, myalgia, weight loss, hypotension.

SYSTEMIC.: *Fluid and electrolyte:* Edema, hypokalemic alkalosis, hypokalemia, hypocalcemia, hypotension or shock-like reaction, hypertension, CHF. *Musculoskeletal:* Muscle wasting, muscle pain or weakness, osteoporosis, spontaneous fractures including vertebral compression fractures and fractures of long bones, tendon rupture, aseptic necrosis of femoral and humeral heads. *GI:* N&V, anorexia or increased appetite, diarrhea or constipation, abdominal distention, pancreatitis, gastric irritation, ulcerative esophagitis. *Development or exacerbation of peptic ulcers with the possibility of perforation and hemorrhage; perforation of the small and large bowel,* especially in inflammatory bowel disease. *Endocrine:* Cushing's syndrome (e.g., central obesity, moonface, buffalo hump, enlargement of supraclavicular fat pads), amenorrhea, postmenopausal bleeding, menstrual irregularities, decreased glucose tolerance, hyperglycemia, glycosuria, increased insulin or sulfonylurea requirement in diabetics, development of diabetes mellitus, negative nitrogen balance due to protein catabolism, suppression of growth in children, secondary adrenocortical and pituitary unresponsiveness (especially during periods of stress). *CNS/Neurologic:* Headache, vertigo, insomnia, restlessness, increased motor activity, ischemic neuropathy, EEG abnormalities, *seizures,* pseudotumor cerebri. Also, euphoria, mood swings, depression, anxiety, personality changes, psychoses. *CV:* Thromboembolism, thrombophlebitis, ECG changes (due to potassium deficiency), fat embolism, necrotizing angiitis, cardiac arrhythmias, *myocardial rupture following recent MI,* syncopal episodes. *Dermatologic:* Impaired wound healing, skin atrophy and thinning, petechiae, ecchymoses, erythema, purpura, striae, hirsutism, urticaria, *angioneurotic edema,* acneiform eruptions, allergic dermatitis, lupus erythematosus-like lesions, suppression of skin test reactions, perineal irritation. *Ophthalmic:* Glaucoma, posterior subcapsular cataracts, increased intraocular pressure, exophthalmos. *Miscellaneous:* Hypercholesterolemia, atherosclerosis, aggravation or masking of infections, leukocytosis, increased or decreased motility and number of spermatozoa. **In children:** Suppression of linear growth; reversible pseudobrain tumor syndrome characterized by papilledema, oculomotor or abducens nerve paralysis, visual loss, or headache.

PARENTERAL USE: Sterile abscesses, Charcot-like arthropathy, subcutaneous and cutaneous atrophy, burning or tingling (especially in the perineal area following IV use), scarring, inflammation, paresthesia, induration, hyperpigmentation or hypopigmentation, blindness when used intralesionally around the face and head (rare), transient or delayed pain or soreness, nystagmus, ataxia, muscle twitching, hiccoughs, *anaphylaxis with or without circulatory collapse, cardiac arrest, bronchospasm,* arachnoiditis after intrathecal use, foreign body granulomatous reactions.

INTRA-ARTICULAR: Postinjection flare, Charcot-like arthropathy, tendon rupture, skin atrophy, facial flushing, osteonecrosis. Due to reduction in inflammation and pain, clients may overuse the joint.

INTRASPINAL: Aseptic, bacterial, chemical, cryptococcal, or tubercular meningitis; adhesive arachnoiditis, conus medullaris syndrome.

INTRAOCULAR: Increased ocular pressure, thereby inducing or aggravating simple glaucoma. Stinging, burning, dendritic keratitis (herpes simplex), corneal perforation (especially when the drugs are used for diseases that cause corneal thinning). Posterior subcapsular cataracts, especially in children. Exophthalmos, secondary fungal or viral eye infections.

TOPICAL USE: When used over large areas, when the skin is broken, or with occlusive dressings, may cause atrophy of the epidermis, drying of the skin, or atrophy of the dermal collagen. When used on the face, diffuse thinning and homogenization of the collagen, epidermal thinning, and striae formation. Occasionally, sensitization reaction may occur, which necessitates discontinuation of the drug.

**OD** **Overdose Management:** *Symptoms (Continued Use of Large Doses)—Cushing's Syndrome:* Acne, hypertension, moonface, striae, hirsutism, central obesity, ecchymoses, myopathy, sexual dysfunction, osteoporosis, diabetes, hyperlipidemia, increased susceptibility to infection, peptic ulcer, electrolyte and fluid imbalance. Acute toxicity or death is rare. *Treatment of Chronic Overdose:* Gradually taper the dose of the steroid and frequently monitor lab tests. During periods of stress, steroid supplementation is necessary. Dose should be reduced to the lowest one that will control the symptoms (or discontinue the steroid completely). Recovery of normal adrenal and pituitary function may take up to 9 months. Large, acute overdoses may be treated with gastric lavage, emesis, and general supportive measures.

**Drug Interactions**
*Acetaminophen* / ↑ Risk of hepatotoxicity due to ↑ rate of formation of hepatotoxic acetaminophen metabolite
*Alcohol* / ↑ Risk of GI ulceration or hemorrhage
*Amphotericin B* / Corticosteroids ↑ K depletion caused by amphotericin B
*Aminoglutethimide* / ↓ Adrenal response to corticotropin
*Anabolic steroids* / ↑ Risk of edema
*Antacids* / ↓ Effect of corticosteroids due to ↓ absorption from GI tract
*Antibiotics, broad-spectrum* / Concomitant use may result in emergence of resistant strains, leading to severe infection
*Anticholinergics* / Combination ↑ intraocular pressure; will aggravate glaucoma
*Anticoagulants, oral* / ↓ Effect of anticoagulants by ↓ hypoprothrombinemia; also ↑ risk of hemorrhage due to vascular effects of corticosteroids

*Anticholinesterases* / Corticosteroids may ↓ effect of anticholinesterases when used in myasthenia gravis
*Antidiabetic agents* / Hyperglycemic effect of corticosteroids may necessitate an ↑ dose of antidiabetic agent
*Asparaginase* / ↑ Hyperglycemic effect of asparaginase and the risk of neuropathy and disturbances in erythropoiesis
*Barbiturates* / ↓ Effect of corticosteroids due to ↑ breakdown by liver
*Bumetanide* / Enhanced potassium loss due to potassium-losing properties of both drugs
*Carbonic anhydrase inhibitors* / Corticosteroids ↑ K depletion caused by carbonic anhydrase inhibitors
*Cholestyramine* / ↓ Effect of corticosteroids due to ↓ absorption from GI tract
*Colestipol* / ↓ Effect of corticosteroids due to ↓ absorption from GI tract
*Contraceptives, oral* / Estrogen ↑ anti-inflammatory effect of hydrocortisone by ↓ breakdown by liver
*Cyclophosphoramide* / ↑ Effect of cyclophosphoramide due to ↓ breakdown by liver
*Cyclosporine* / ↑ Effect of both drugs due to ↓ breakdown by liver
*Digitalis glycosides* / ↑ Chance of digitalis toxicity (arrhythmias) due to hypokalemia
*Ephedrine* / ↓ Effect of corticosteroids due to ↑ breakdown by liver
*Estrogens* / ↑ Anti-inflammatory effect of hydrocortisone by ↓ breakdown by liver
*Ethacrynic acid* / Enhanced potassium loss due to potassium-losing properties of both drugs
*Folic acid* / Requirements may ↑
*Furosemide* / Enhanced potassium loss due to potassium-losing properties of both drugs
*Heparin* / Ulcerogenic effects of corticosteroids may ↑ risk of hemorrhage
*Immunosuppressant drugs* / ↑ Risk of infection
*Indomethacin* / ↑ Chance of GI ulceration

*Insulin* / Hyperglycemic effect of corticosteroids may necessitate ↑ dose of antidiabetic agent

*Isoniazid* / ↓ Effect of isoniazid due to ↑ breakdown by liver and ↑ excretion

*Ketoconazole* / ↓ Effect of corticosteroids due to ↑ rate of clearance

*Mexiletine* / ↓ Effect of mexiletine due to ↑ breakdown by liver

*Mitotane* / ↓ Response of adrenal gland to corticotropin

*Muscle relaxants, nondepolarizing* / ↓ Effect of muscle relaxants

*Neuromuscular blocking agents* / ↑ Risk of prolonged respiratory depression or paralysis

*NSAIDs* / ↑ Risk of GI hemorrhage or ulceration

*Phenobarbital* / ↓ Effect of corticosteroids due to ↑ breakdown by liver

*Phenytoin* / ↓ Effect of corticosteroids due to ↑ breakdown by liver

*Potassium supplements* / ↓ Plasma levels of potassium

*Rifampin* / ↓ Effect of corticosteroids due to ↑ breakdown by liver

*Ritodrine* / ↑ Risk of maternal edema

*Salicylates* / Both are ulcerogenic; also, corticosteroids may ↓ blood salicylate levels

*Somatrem, Somatropin* / Glucocorticoids may inhibit effect of somatrem

*Streptozocin* / ↑ Risk of hyperglycemia

*Theophyllines* / Corticosteroids ↑ effect of theophyllines

*Thiazide diuretics* / Enhanced potassium loss due to potassium-losing properties of both drugs

*Tricyclic antidepressants* / ↑ Risk of mental disturbances

*Vitamin A* / Topical vitamin A can reverse impaired wound healing in clients receiving corticosteroids

**Laboratory Test Interferences:** ↑ Urine glucose, serum cholesterol, serum amylase. ↓ Serum potassium, triiodothyronine, serum uric acid. Alteration of electrolyte balance.

## Dosage

Highly individualized, according to both the condition being treated and the client's response. Therapy must not be discontinued abruptly. Except for replacement therapy, treatment should always involve the minimum effective dose and the shortest period of time. If corticosteroids are used for replacement therapy or high doses are used for prolonged periods of time, the dose must be *increased* if surgery is required.

Lotions are considered best for weeping eruptions, especially in areas subject to chafing (axilla, feet, and groin). Creams are suitable for most inflammations; ointments are preferred for dry, scaly lesions.

## NURSING CONSIDERATIONS

### Administration of Oral Corticosteroids

1. Administer PO forms of drug with food to minimize ulcerogenic effect.

2. At frequent intervals, reduce the dose gradually to determine if symptoms of the disease can be effectively controlled by the smaller amount of drug.

3. When treating clients with conditions such as asthma, ulcerative colitis, and rheumatoid arthritis, corticosteroids, given every other day, provide the beneficial effect of the steroid while minimizing pituitary-adrenal suppression. With this therapy, twice the usual daily dose of an intermediate-acting steroid is given every other morning.

4. Local administration of corticosteroids is preferred over systemic therapy to minimize systemic side effects.

5. Discontinue gradually if used chronically.

### Administration of Topical Corticosteroids

1. Cleanse area before applying the medication.

2. Wear gloves, apply sparingly, and rub gently into the area.

3. When prescribed, apply an occlu-

sive dressing (not to be used if an infection is present) to promote hydration of the stratum corneum and increase the absorption of the medication.The following are two methods of applying an occlusive type dressing:

• Apply a large amount of medication to the cleansed area. Cover with a thin, pliable, nonflammable plastic film, which is then sealed to the surrounding tissue with skin tape or held in place with gauze. Change the dressing q 3–4 days.

• Apply a small amount of medication to the area and cover with a damp cloth. Then cover with a thin, pliable, nonflammable plastic film and seal to the surrounding tissue with tape, or hold in place with gauze. Change dressing b.i.d.

**Assessment:** (General)

1. Document indications for therapy, type, onset, and characteristics of symptoms; note underlying cause: adrenal or nonadrenal disorder.

2. Record mental status (i.e., mood, affect, aggression, behavioral changes, depression) and neurologic function.

3. Check for evidence of allergic reactions to corticosteroids or tartrazine, a coloring agent in certain preparations.

4. Monitor ECG, electrolytes, glucose, urinalysis, liver and renal function studies.

5. Document VS and weight. Obtain CXR and PPD if prolonged therapy.

6. Note childhood illnesses and immunization status.

7. List medications taking and identify those that may interact with corticosteroids. These include antidiabetic agents, cardiac glycosides, oral contraceptives, anticoagulants, and drugs influenced by liver enzymes.

8. If female, determine if pregnant.

**Interventions**

TOPICAL CORTICOSTEROIDS

1. Assess for local sensitivity reaction at the site of application.

2. Absorption varies regionally with the highest absorption in scrotal skin and the lowest on the foot. Inflamed skin enhances absorption several-fold.

3. Better action has been noted with the ointment bases than with the lotion or cream vehicles.

4. Observe for signs of infections since corticosteroids tend to mask. Avoid occlusive dressing when an infection is present. Document the site of the infection, the nature of the infection, and characteristics (e.g., redness, swelling, odor, or drainage).

5. With large occlusive dressing, take temperatures q 4 hr. Report if elevated and remove the dressing.

6. Assess for evidence of systemic absorption. Protracted use of large quantities of potent topical corticosteroids to large BSAs may precipitate iatrogenic Cushing's syndrome. Symptoms may include edema and transient inhibition of pituitary-adrenal cortical function as manifested by muscular pain, lassitude, depression, hypotension, and weight loss.

7. Advise family members applying the topical ointment to wash their hands and to wear gloves or to apply with a sterile applicator (e.g., tongue blade).

8. Report erythema, telangiectases, purpura, bruising, pustules, and depressed shiny, wrinkled skin. Prolonged use of potent topical corticosteroids may increase incidence of systemic side effects.

**Interventions**

ORAL CORTICOSTEROIDS

1. When first placed on corticosteroids, check BP b.i.d. until a maintenance dose has been established; report any significant increases.

2. Short-term oral therapy (e.g., 60 mg PO for 5 days) does not require divided doses or titration. With long-term therapy, continuously monitor for symptoms of adrenal insufficiency, which include hypotension, confusion, restlessness, lethargy, weakness, N&V, anorexia, and weight loss; titrate dose to withdraw.

3. Evaluate for increased sodium and fluid retention. Monitor weight

and observe for edema. If noted, adjust the diet to one low in sodium and high in potassium. Anticipate a small weight gain due to increased appetite, but sudden increases are probably due to edema. Edema occurs most frequently with cortisone or desoxycorticosterone acetate and less frequently with the synthetic agents.

4. Assess for SOB, distended neck veins, edema, and easy fatigue; S&S of CHF. Obtain a CXR and ECG.

5. Monitor serum glucose, electrolytes, and platelet counts with long-term therapy. Report any unusual bleeding, bruising, the presence of petechiae, symptoms of diabetes, and any other skin changes.

6. Assess muscles for weakness and wasting; signs of a negative nitrogen balance.

7. Report changes in appearance, especially those resembling Cushing's syndrome (such as rounding of the face, hirsutism, presence of acne, and thinning of the hair and nails) so dosage can be adjusted.

8. With diabetes, may develop hyperglycemia and a change in diet and insulin dosage may be necessary.

9. Assess for signs of depression, lack of interest in personal appearance, complaints of insomnia and anorexia.

10. Discuss the potential for menstrual difficulties and amenorrhea that may be caused by long-term therapy.

11. Observe for S&S of other illnesses as these drugs tend to mask the severity of most illnesses.

12. GI bleeding may occur; periodically test stools for occult blood and monitor hematologic profile.

**Client/Family Teaching**

1. Take the oral medication with food and report any symptoms of gastric distress. To prevent the problem of gastric irritation, may use antacids and eat frequent small meals. If the symptoms persist, diagnostic X rays may be indicated.

2. High doses of glucocorticoids stimulate the stomach to produce excess acid and pepsin and may cause peptic ulcers. Antacids 3–4 times/day may relieve epigastric distress.

3. These agents generally work by inhibiting or decreasing the inflammatory response.

4. Report any changes in mood or affect immediately.

5. Weigh self daily at the same time, wearing clothing of approximately the same weight, and using the same scales. Consistent weight gain may be evidence of fluid retention; initiate caloric management to prevent obesity.

6. Identify foods high in potassium and low in sodium content to prevent electrolyte disturbances. Supplement diet with potassium-rich foods such as citrus juices and bananas. Read labels of canned or processed foods and consult dietician for assistance in shopping, meal planning, and preparation.

7. Eat a diet high in protein to compensate for the loss due to protein breakdown from gluconeogenesis.

8. Exercise daily and consume foods high in calcium to decrease possibility of osteoporosis (due to catabolic bone effects). Consume adequate protein, calcium, and vitamin D to minimize bone loss. On-going bone resorption with depressed bone formation is the cause of osteoporosis.

9. Avoid falls and accidents. Steroids may cause osteoporosis, which makes the bones more susceptible to fractures. Use a night light and a hand rail or other device for support if need to get up at night.

10. Corticosteroids can cause a loss of contraceptive action with oral contraceptives. Keep accurate menstrual records and consider alternative methods of birth control. May also have an adverse effect on sperm production and count.

11. Weight gain, acne, and excess hair growth may occur.

12. Need to gradually withdraw the

medication when therapy has exceeded 7 consecutive days. This should proceed slowly so that the adrenal cortex will gradually be reactivated and take over the production of hormones. Sudden withdrawal may be life-threatening. Any sudden change will provoke symptoms of adrenal insufficiency.

13. With dosage reduction, flare-ups may occur; these are caused by the reduction.

14. With arthritis, do not overuse the joint once injected and painless. Permanent joint damage may result from overuse, because underlying pathology is still present.

15. With diabetes, monitor glucose levels frequently and report changes as insulin dose and diet may require adjustment.

16. Wounds may heal slowly because steroid therapy causes a delay in development of granulation tissue, increasing potential for infection. Observe any healing process for signs of infection and report any injury or postoperative separation of wound or suture line.

17. These drugs mask symptoms of infection and cause immunosuppression. Because antibody production is decreased by corticosteroids, clients are at risk for infection. Must maintain general hygiene and scrupulous cleanliness to avoid infection. Report if sore throat, cough, fever, malaise, or an injury that does not heal occurs. Avoid contact with persons with known contagious diseases.

18. Delay any vaccinations, immunizations, or skin testing while receiving corticosteroid therapy because there is limited immune response.

19. Clients on long-term ophthalmic therapy are prone to developing cataracts, exophthalmus, and increased IOP. Schedule routine ophthalmic exams.

20. Avoid OTC meds, including aspirin and ibuprofen compounds, as well as alcohol, since these may aggravate gastric irritation and bleeding.

21. Carry ID, listing drugs and dosage, condition being treated, and who to contact in the event of an emergency.

**Outcomes/Evaluate**
- Effective wound healing
- Suppression of inflammatory and immune responses or disease manifestation in allergic reactions, autoimmune diseases, and organ transplant recipients
- Serum cortisol levels within desired range in adrenal deficiency states (8 a.m. level 110–520 nmol/L)

**Special Concerns**
1. Check child's height and weight regularly and graph; growth suppression is a hazard of corticosteroid therapy and not prevented by growth hormone administration.
2. Advise parents that large doses of glucocorticoids in children may increase intracranial pressure (pseudotumor cerebri). Report symptoms of this disorder: vertigo, headache, and convulsions. These should disappear once therapy discontinued (under medical supervision).

# DIURETICS, LOOP

*See also the following individual entries:*

> Bumetanide
> Ethacrynate sodium
> Ethacrynic acid
> Furosemide
> Torsemide

See also *Diuretics, Thiazides.*

**Action/Kinetics:** Loop diuretics inhibit reabsorption of sodium and chloride in the proximal and distal tubules and the loop of Henle. Metabolized in the liver and excreted primarily through the urine. Significantly bound to plasma protein.

**Uses:** See individual drugs.

**Contraindications:** Hypersensitivity to loop diruetics or to sulfonylureas. In hepatic coma or severe electrolyte depletion (until condition improves or is corrected). Lactation.

**Special Concerns:** Sudden alterations of electrolytes in hepatic cirrhosis and ascites may precipitate hepatic encephalopathy and coma. SLE may be activated or worsened. Ototoxicity is most common with rapid injection, in severe renal impairment, with doses several times the usual dose, and with concurrent use of other ototoxic drugs. Safety and efficacy of most loop diuretics have not been determined in children or infants.

**Side Effects:** See individual drugs. Excessive diuresis may cause dehydration with the possibility of *circulatory collapse and vascular thrombosis or embolism.* Ototoxicity including tinnitus, hearing impairment, deafness (usually reversible), and vertigo with a sense of fullness are possible. Electrolyte imbalance, especially in clients with restricted salt intake. Photosensitivity. Changes include hypokalemia, hypomagnesemia, and hypocalcemia.

**OD** **Overdose Management:** *Symptoms:* Acute profound water loss, volume and electrolyte depletion, dehydration, decreased blood volume, and *circulatory collapse with possibility of vascular thrombosis and embolism.* *Treatment:* Replace fluid and electrolyte loss. Carefully monitor urine and plasma electrolyte levels. Emesis and gastric lavage may be useful. Supportive measures may include oxygen or artificial respiration.

**Drug Interactions**
*Aminoglycosides /* ↑ Ototoxicity with hearing loss
*Anticoagulants /* ↑ Anticoagulant activity
*Chloral hydrate /* Transient diaphoresis, hot flashes, hypertension, tachycardia, weakness and nausea
*Cisplatin /* Additive ototoxicity
*Digitalis glycosides /* ↑ Risk of arrhythmias due to diuretic-induced electrolyte disturbances
*Lithium /* ↑ Plasma levels of lithium → toxicity
*Muscle relaxants, nondepolarizing /* Effect of muscle relaxants may be either ↑ or ↓, depending on the dose of diuretic

*Nonsteroidal anti-inflammatory drugs /* ↓ Effect of loop diuretics
*Probenecid /* ↓ Effect of loop diuretics
*Salicylates /* Diuretic effect may be ↓ in clients with cirrhosis and ascites
*Sulfonylureas/* Loop diuretics may ↓ glucose tolerance
*Theophyllines /* Action of theophyllines may be ↑ or ↓
*Thiazide diuretics /* Additive effects with loop diuretics → profound diuresis and serious electrolyte abnormalities

**Dosage**
See individual drugs.

## NURSING CONSIDERATIONS

See also *Diuretics, Thiazides.*
**Assessment**
1. Document indications for therapy. Note other agents prescribed and the outcome.
2. Monitor CBC, electrolytes, Mg, Ca, glucose, uric acid, liver and renal function studies.
3. Note any sensitivity to sulfonamides. Furosemide is a derivative and may exhibit cross-reactivity.
4. Determine presence of SLE; drug may worsen condition.
5. Assess auditory function carefully especially when large doses are anticipated or when used concurrently with other ototoxic agents. Ototoxicity is dose related and generally reversible.
**Interventions**
1. Record weights I&O; keep bedpan or urinal within reach. Report absence/decrease in diuresis and note changes in lung sounds.
2. When ambulatory, check for edema in the extremities; if on bed rest, check for edema in the sacral area.
3. Monitor for serum electrolyte levels, pH, and the following *signs of electrolyte imbalance*
• *Hyponatremia* (low-salt syndrome)—characterized by muscle weakness, leg cramps, dryness of

---

✦ = Available in Canada                    ***bold italic*** = life threatening side effect

mouth, dizziness, and GI disturbances.

• *Hypernatremia* (excessive sodium retention)—characterized by CNS disturbances, i.e., confusion, loss of sensorium, stupor, and coma. Poor skin turgor and postural hypotension are not as prominent as when combined deficits of sodium and water exist.

• *Water intoxication* (caused by defective water diuresis)—characterized by lethargy, confusion, stupor, and coma. Neuromuscular hyperexcitability with increased reflexes, muscular twitching, and convulsions if acute.

• *Metabolic acidosis*—characterized by weakness, headache, malaise, abdominal pain, and N&V. Hyperpnea occurs in severe metabolic acidosis. Signs of volume depletion, such as poor skin turgor, soft eyeballs, and a dry tongue may also be observed.

• *Metabolic alkalosis*—characterized by irritability, neuromuscular hyperexcitability, tetany if severe.

• *Hypokalemia (potassium deficiency)*—characterized by muscular weakness, peristalsis failure, postural hypotension, respiratory embarrassment, and cardiac arrhythmias.

• *Hyperkalemia (excess potassium)*—characterized by early signs of irritability, nausea, intestinal colic, and diarrhea; and by later signs of weakness, flaccid paralysis, dyspnea, difficulty speaking, and arrhythmias.

4. With high doses monitor for hyperlipidemia and hyperuricemia; precipitating a gout attack.

5. With liver dysfunction, assess for electrolyte imbalances, which could cause stupor, coma, and death.

6. If receiving enteric-coated potassium tablets, assess for abdominal pain, distention, or GI bleeding; can cause small bowel ulceration. Monitor stool to ensure tablets have not passed through intact.

7. If also receiving antihypertensive drugs, monitor BP. Diuretics potentiate the effects of antihypertensive agents.

8. May precipitate symptoms of diabetes mellitus in clients with latent or mild diabetes. Test urine or perform finger sticks and monitor chemisty studies.

9. If taking digitalis, hyper- or hypokalemia associated with diuretic therapy may potentiate the toxic effects of digitalis and precipitate cardiac arrhythmias.

10. Assess for sore throat, skin rash, and yellowing of the skin or sclera; may be blood dyscrasias.

**Client/Family Teaching**

1. May cause frequent, copious voiding; take in the morning to prevent disruption of sleep. Plan activities to accommodate this occurrence.

2. Take with food or milk to decrease GI upset.

3. Weakness and/or dizziness may occur with diuresis. Use caution in driving a car or operating other hazardous machinery until drug effects apparent. Rise slowly from bed and sit down or lie down if feeling faint or dizzy.

4. The use of alcohol, standing for prolonged periods, and exercise in hot weather may enhance effects of orthostatic hypotension.

5. Ensure adequate hydration; monitor BP and weight; report excessive weight loss or loss of skin turgor.

6. Report if dizziness, nausea, muscle weakness, cramps, or tingling of the extremities occurs.

7. Wear protective clothing, sunscreens, and sunglasses while in the sun, to prevent photosensitivity reactions.

8. Include foods in the diet that are high in potassium, such as citrus, grape, cranberry, apple, pear, and apricot juices; bananas; meat, fish, or fowl; cereals; and tea and cola beverages. This is preferable to taking potassium chloride supplements but potassium supplements are usually prescribed with non-potassium-sparing diuretics. Unless conditions such as gastric ulcer or diabetes exists, encourage to drink a large glass of orange juice daily. Consult dietitian as needed, for assistance in shopping, planning, selecting, and preparing appropriate menus.

9. Avoid all OTC preparations without approval.

**Outcomes/Evaluate**
- Symptomatic relief (↓ weight, ↓ swelling, ↑ diuresis)
- Clinical improvement in S&S associated with CHF and renal failure

# DIURETICS, THIAZIDES

*See also the following individual entries:*

Chlorothiazide
Chlorothiazide sodium
Chlorthalidone
Hydrochlorothiazide
Indapamide

**Action/Kinetics:** Thiazides promote diuresis by decreasing the rate at which sodium and chloride are reabsorbed by the distal renal tubules of the kidney. By increasing the excretion of sodium and chloride, they force excretion of additional water. They also increase the excretion of potassium and, to a lesser extent, bicarbonate, as well as decrease the excretion of calcium and uric acid. Sodium and chloride are excreted in approximately equal amounts. The thiazides do not affect the glomerular filtration rate. Thiazides also have an antihypertensive effect which is attributed to direct dilation of the arterioles, as well as to a reduction in the total fluid volume of the body and altered sodium balance. The thiazide diuretics are related chemically to the sulfonamides. Although devoid of anti-infective activity, the thiazides can cause the same hypersensitivity reactions as the sulfonamides. A large fraction is excreted unchanged in urine.

**Uses:** Edema, CHF, hypertension, pregnancy, and premenstrual tension. Thiazides are used for edema due to CHF, nephrosis, nephritis, renal failure, PMS, hepatic cirrhosis, corticosteroid or estrogen therapy. Hypertension. *Investigational:* Thiazides are used alone or in combination with allopurinol (or amiloride) for prophylaxis of calcium nephrolithiasis. Nephrogenic diabetes insipidus.

**Contraindications:** Hypersensitivity to drug, anuria, renal decompensation. Impaired renal function and advanced hepatic cirrhosis. Do not use indiscriminately in clients with edema and toxemia of pregnancy, even though they may be therapeutically useful, because the thiazides may have adverse effects on the newborn (thrombocytopenia and jaundice).

**Special Concerns:** Geriatric clients may manifest an increased risk of hypotension and changes in electrolyte levels. Administer with caution to debilitated clients or to those with a history of hepatic coma or precoma, gout, diabetes mellitus, or during pregnancy and lactation. Particular care must be exercised when thiazides are administered concomitantly with drugs that also cause potassium loss, such as digitalis, corticosteroids, and some estrogens. Clients with advanced heart failure, renal disease, or hepatic cirrhosis are most likely to develop hypokalemia. May activate or worsen SLE.

**Side Effects:** The following side effects may be observed with most thiazides. See also individual drugs. *Electrolyte imbalance:* Hypokalemia (most frequent) characterized by cardiac arrhythmias. Hyponatremia characterized by weakness, lethargy, epigastric distress, N&V. Hypokalemic alkalosis. *GI:* Anorexia, epigastric distress or irritation, N&V, cramping, bloating, abdominal pain, diarrhea, constipation, jaundice, pancreatitis. *CNS:* Dizziness, lightheadedness, headache, vertigo, xanthopsia, paresthesias, weakness, insomnia, restlessness. *CV:* Orthostatic hypotension, MIs in elderly clients with advanced arteriosclerosis, especially if the client is also receiving therapy with other antihypertensive agents. *Hematologic:* **Agranulocytosis, aplastic or hypoplastic anemia, hemolytic anemia,** leukopenia, thrombocytopenia. *Dermatologic:*

---

Purpura, photosensitivity, photosensitivity dermatitis, rash, urticaria, necrotizing angiitis, vasculitis, cutaneous vasculitis. *Metabolic:* neutropenia, hemolytic anemia. *Endocrine:* Hyperglycemia, glycosuria, hyperuricemia. *Miscellaneous:* Blurred vision, impotence, reduced libido, fever, muscle cramps, muscle spasm, respiratory distress.

**OD** **Overdose Management:** *Symptoms:* Symptoms of plasma volume depletion, including orthostatic hypotension, dizziness, drowsiness, syncope, electrolyte abnormalities, hemoconcentration, hemodynamic changes. Signs of potassium depletion, including confusion, dizziness, muscle weakness, and GI disturbances. Also, N&V, GI irritation, GI hypermotility, CNS effects, cardiac abnormalities, **seizures, hypotension, decreased respiration, and coma.** *Treatment:*

• Induce emesis or perform gastric lavage followed by activated charcoal. Undertake measures to prevent aspiration.

• Electrolyte balance, hydration, respiration, CV, and renal function must be maintained. Cathartics should be avoided, as use may enhance fluid loss.

• Although GI effects are usually of short duration, treatment may be required.

**Drug Interactions**

*Allopurinol* / ↑ Risk of hypersensitivity reactions to allopurinol

*Amphotericin B* / Enhanced loss of electrolytes, especially potassium

*Anesthetics* / Thiazides may ↑ effects of anesthetics

*Anticholinergic agents* / ↑ Effect of thiazides due to ↑ amount absorbed from GI tract

*Anticoagulants, oral* / Anticoagulant effects may be decreased

*Antidiabetic agents* / Thiazides antagonize hypoglycemic effect of antidiabetic agents

*Antigout agents* / Thiazides may ↑ uric acid levels; thus, ↑ dose of antigout drug may be necessary

*Antihypertensive agents* / Thiazides potentiate the effect of antihypertensive agents

*Antineoplastic agents* / Thiazides may prolong leukopenia induced by antineoplastic agents

*Calcium salts* / Hypercalcemia due to renal tubular reabsorption or bone release may be ↑ by exogenous calcium

*Cholestyramine* / ↓ Effect of thiazides due to ↓ absorption from GI tract

*Colestipol* / ↓ Effect of thiazides due to ↓ absorption from GI tract

*Corticosteroids* / Enhanced potassium loss due to potassium-losing properties of both drugs

*Diazoxide* / Enhanced hypotensive effect. Also, ↑ hyperglycemic response

*Digitalis glycosides* / Thiazides produce ↑ potassium and magnesium loss with ↑ chance of digitalis-induced arrhythmias

*Ethanol* / Additive orthostatic hypotension

*Fenfluramine* / ↑ Antihypertensive effect of thiazides

*Furosemide* / Profound diuresis and electrolyte loss

*Guanethidine* / Additive hypotensive effect

*Indomethacin* / ↓ Effect of thiazides, possibly by inhibition of prostaglandins

*Insulin* / ↓ Effect due to thiazide-induced hyperglycemia

*Lithium* / ↑ Risk of lithium toxicity due to ↓ renal excretion; may be used together but use should be carefully monitored

*Loop diuretics* / Additive effect to cause profound diuresis and serious electrolyte losses

*Methenamine* / ↓ Effect of thiazides due to alkalinization of urine by methenamine

*Methyldopa* / ↑ Risk of hemolytic anemia (rare)

*Muscle relaxants, nondepolarizing* / ↑ Effect of muscle relaxants due to hypokalemia

*Norepinephrine* / Thiazides ↓ arterial response to norepinephrine

*Quinidine* / ↑ Effect of quinidine due to ↑ renal tubular reabsorption

*Reserpine* / Additive hypotensive effect

*Sulfonamides* / ↑ Effect of thiazides due to ↓ plasma protein binding

*Sulfonylureas* / ↓ Effect due to thiazide-induced hyperglycemia

*Tetracyclines* / ↑ Risk of azotemia

*Tubocurarine* / ↑ Muscle relaxation and ↑ hypokalemia

*Vasopressors (sympathomimetics)* / Thiazides ↓ responsiveness of arterioles to vasopressors

*Vitamin D* / ↑ Effect of vitamin D due to thiazide-induced hypercalcemia

**Laboratory Test Interferences:** Hypokalemia, hypercalcemia, hyponatremia, hypomagnesemia, hypochloremia, hypophosphatemia, hyperuricemia. ↑ BUN, creatinine, glucose in blood and urine. ↓ Serum PBI levels (no signs of thyroid disturbance). Initial ↑ total cholesterol, LDL cholesterol, and triglycerides.

**Dosage** ———————
See individual drugs.

## NURSING CONSIDERATIONS

### Administration/Storage

1. Clients resistant to one type of thiazide may respond to another.

2. Liquid potassium preparations are bitter. When used, administer with fruit juice or milk to make them more palatable.

3. To minimize electrolyte imbalance, thiazides may be taken every other day or on a 3–5-day basis for treatment of edema.

4. To prevent excess hypotension, reduce the dose of other antihypertensive agents when beginning thiazide therapy.

### Assessment

1. Note any hypersensitivity to the drug. Document indications for therapy and any previous experience with these drugs.

2. Monitor CBC, glucose, electrolytes, Ca, Mg, liver and renal function tests.

3. Note any history of heart disease or gout; check uric acid levels.

4. Determine extent of edema; assess skin turgor, mucous membranes, and lung fields.

5. With cirrhosis monitor serum K to avoid depletion and hepatic encephalopathy.

### Interventions

1. With surgery, stop drug at least 48 hr before procedure. Thiazide inhibits the pressor effects of epinephrine.

2. Potassium chloride supplements should be given only when dietary measures are inadequate. If supplements required, use liquid preparations to avoid ulcerations that may be produced by potassium salts in the solid dosage form. Exceptions include slow-K forms (potassium salt imbedded in a wax matrix) and micro-K forms (microencapsulated potassium salt).

### Client/Family Teaching

1. Administer in the morning so that the major diuretic effect will occur before bedtime.

2. Take with food or milk if GI upset occurs.

3. Eat a diet high in potassium. Include orange juice, bananas, citrus fruits, broccoli, spinach, tomato juice, cucumbers, beets, dried fruits, or apricots. Avoid eating black licorice; may precipitate severe hypokalemia.

4. Rise slowly and dangle legs before standing to minimize orthostatic effects. Sit or lie down if feeling faint or dizzy.

5. With gout, avoid foods high in purines and continue antigout agents as prescribed.

6. With diabetes, monitor finger sticks more frequently as may need to adjust dose of insulin or oral hypoglycemic agent.

7. Alcohol in combination with thiazides causes severe hypotension; avoid.

8. Do not take any other medication (including OTC drugs for asthma,

cough and colds, hay fever, weight control) unless approved.

9. Report any severe weight loss, muscle weakness, cramps, dizziness, or fatigue.

10. Occasionally skin rashes may occur but severe symptoms R/T allergic reactions include acute pulmonary edema, acute pancreatitis, thrombocytopenia, cholestatic jaundice, and hemolytic anemia and should be reported immediately.

**Outcomes/Evaluate**

• Control of hypertension; ↓ BP

• ↑ Urine output; ↓ edema; ↓ weight

• Adequate tissue perfusion as evidenced by warm dry skin and good pulses

• Normal electrolyte levels and fluid balance

# ERYTHROMYCINS

*See also the following individual entries:*

Erythromycin base
Erythromycin estolate
Erythromycin ethylsuccinate
Erythromycin lactobionate
Erythromycin stearate

**Action/Kinetics:** Erythromycins are considered to be macrolide antibiotics.They inhibit protein synthesis of microorganisms by binding reversibly to a ribosomal subunit (50S), thus interfering with the transmission of genetic information and inhibiting protein synthesis. The drugs are effective only against rapidly multiplying organisms. Absorbed from the upper part of the small intestine. Those for PO use are manufactured in enteric-coated or film-coated forms to prevent destruction by gastric acid. Erythromycin is approximately 70% bound to plasma proteins and achieves concentrations in body tissues about 40% of those in the plasma. Diffuses into body tissues; peritoneal, pleural, ascitic, and amniotic fluids; saliva; through the placental circulation; and across the mucous membrane of the tracheo-bronchial tree. Diffuses poorly into spinal fluid, although penetration is increased in meningitis. Alkalinization of the urine (to pH 8.5) increases the gram-negative antibacterial action. **Peak serum levels: PO,** 1–4 hr. **t½:** 1.5–2 hr, *but prolonged in clients with renal impairment.* Partially metabolized by the liver and primarily excreted in bile. Also excreted in breast milk.

**Uses**

1. Upper respiratory tract infections due to *Streptococcus pyogenes* (group a beta-hemolytic streptococci), *Streptococcus pneumoniae,* and *Haemophilus influenzae* (combined with sulfonamides).

2. Mild to moderate lower respiratory tract infections due to *S. pyogenes* and *S. pneumoniae.* Respiratory tract infections due to *Mycoplasma pneumoniae.*

3. Pertussis (whooping cough) caused by *Bordetella pertussis;* may also be used as prophylaxis of pertussis in exposed individuals.

4. Mild to moderate skin and skin structure infections due to *S. pyogenes* and *Staphylococcus aureus.*

5. As an adjunct to antitoxin in diphtheria (caused by *Corynebacterium diphtheriae*), to prevent carriers, and to eradicate the organism in carriers.

6. Intestinal amebiasis due to *Entamoeba histolytica* (PO erythromycin only).

7. Acute pelvic inflammatory disease due to *Neisseria gonorrhoeae.*

8. Erythrasma due to *Corynebacterium minutissimum.*

9. *Chlamydia trachomatis* infections causing urogenital infections during pregnancy, conjunctivitis in the newborn, or pneumonia during infancy. Also, uncomplicated chlamydial infections of the urethra, endocervix, or rectum in adults (when tetracyclines are contraindicated or not tolerated).

10. Nongonococcal urethritis caused by *Ureaplasma urealyticum* when tetracyclines are contraindicated or not tolerated.

11. Legionnaires' disease due to *Legionella pneumophilia*.

12. As an alternative to penicillin (in penicillin-sensitive clients) to treat primary syphilis caused by *Treponema pallidum*.

13. Prophylaxis of initial or recurrent attacks of rheumatic fever in clients allergic to penicillin or sulfonamides.

14. Infections due to *Listeria monocytogenes*.

15. Bacterial endocarditis due to alpha-hemolytic streptococci, Viridans group, in clients allergic to penicillins.

*Investigational:* Infections due to *N. gonorrhoeae,* including uncomplicated urethral, rectal, or endocervical infections and disseminated gonococcal infections (including use in pregnancy). Severe or prolonged diarrhea due to *Campylobacter jejuni*. Genital, inguinal, or anorectal infections due to *Lymphogranuloma venereum*. Chancroid due to *Haemophilus ducreyi*. Primary, secondary, or early latent syphilis due to *T. pallidum*. Erythromycin base used with PO neomycin prior to elective colorectal surgery to reduce wound complications. As an alternative to penicillin to treat anthrax, Vincent's gingivitis, erysipeloid, actinomycosis, tetanus, with a sulfonamide to treat *Nocardia* infections, infections due to *Eikenella corrodens,* and *Borrelia* infections (including early Lyme disease).

**Contraindications:** Hypersensitivity to erythromycin; in utero syphilis.

**Special Concerns:** Use with caution in liver disease and during lactation. Use may result in bacterial and fungal overgrowth (i.e., superinfection).

**Side Effects:** Erythromycins have a low incidence of side effects (except for the estolate salt). *GI* (most common): N&V, diarrhea, cramping, abdominal pain, stomatitis, anorexia, melena, heartburn, pruritus ani, pseudomembranous colitis. *Allergic:* Skin rashes with or without pruritus, bullous fixed eruptions, urticaria, eczema, **anaphylaxis** (rare). *CNS:* Fear, confusion, altered thinking, uncontrollable crying or hysterical laughter, feeling of impending loss of consciousness. *CV:* Rarely, ventricular arrhythmias, including **ventricular tachycardia and torsades de pointes in clients with prolonged QT intervals**. *Miscellaneous:* Superinfection, hepatotoxicity, ototoxicity. *Following topical use:* Itching, burning, irritation, or stinging of skin. Dry, scaly skin.

IV use may result in venous irritation and thrombophlebitis; IM use produces pain at the injection site, with development of necrosis or sterile abscesses.

**OD** **Overdose Management:** *Symptoms:* N&V, diarrhea, epigastric distress, acute pancreatitis (mild), hearing loss (with or without tinnitus and vertigo). *Treatment:* Induce vomiting. General supportive measures. Allergic reactions should be controlled with conventional therapy.

**Drug Interactions**

*Alfentanil* / ↓ Excretion of alfentanil → ↑ effect

*Anticoagulants* / ↑ Anticoagulant effect → possible hemorrhage

*Astemizole* / Serious CV side effects, including torsades de pointes and other ventricular arrhythmias (including QT interval prolongation), cardiac arrest, and death

*Bromocriptine* / ↑ Serum levels of bromocriptine → ↑ pharmacologic and toxic effects

*Carbamazepine* / ↑ Effect (and toxicity requiring hospitalization and resuscitation) of carbamazepine due to ↓ breakdown by liver

*Cyclosporine* / ↑ Effect of cyclosporine due to ↓ excretion (possibly with renal toxicity)

*Digoxin* / Erythromycin ↑ bioavailability of digoxin

*Disopyramide* / ↑ Plasma levels of disopyramide → arrhythmias and ↑ QTc intervals

*Ergot alkaloids* / Acute ergotism manifested by peripheral ischemia

*Lincosamides* / Drugs antagonize each other

*Methylprednisolone* / ↑ Effect of methylprednisolone due to ↓ breakdown by liver

*Penicillin* / Erythromycins either ↓ or ↑ effect of penicillins

*Sodium bicarbonate* / ↑ Effect of erythromycin in urine due to alkalinization

*Terfenadine* / Serious CV side effects, including torsades de pointes and other ventricular arrhythmias (including QT interval prolongation), cardiac arrest, and death

*Theophyllines* / ↑ Effect of theophylline due to ↓ breakdown in liver; ↓ erythromycin levels may also occur

*Triazolam* / ↑ Bioavailability of triazolam → ↑ CNS depression

**Laboratory Test Interferences:** False + or ↑ values of urinary catecholamines, urinary steroids, and AST and ALT.

**Dosage** ————————
See individual drugs.

## NURSING CONSIDERATIONS

See also *General Nursing Considerations for All Anti-Infectives*.

**Administration/Storage:**    Inject deep into muscle mass. Injections are painful and irritating.

**Assessment**
1. Identify allergy to any antibiotics; note allergens.
2. Document type, onset, and characteristics of symptoms, other agents used, and the outcome.
3. Monitor CBC, cultures, liver and renal function studies.
4. Avoid if also prescribed astemizole, seldane, digoxin, and theophyllines, because erythromycins can inhibit cytochrome P-450 and enhance effects of these drugs or cause lethal arrhythmias.

**Client/Family Teaching**
1. Do not administer with or immediately prior to ingestion of fruit juice or other acidic drinks; acidity may decrease drug activity. Con-

sume up to 8 oz of water with each dose and a fluid intake of 2.5 L/day.
2. May take with food to diminish GI upset; however, food decreases the absorption of most erythromycins. Take only as directed and complete entire prescription despite feeling better.
3. If tablets are not coated, take them 2 hr after meals. Stomach acid destroys the erythromycin base thus it must be administered with an enteric coating.
4. Doses of erythromycins should be evenly spaced throughout a 24-hr period.
5. If nausea is intolerable, notify provider so the prescription can be changed to coated tablets that can be taken with meals.
6. Report symptoms of superinfection, i.e., furry tongue, vaginal itching, rectal itching, or diarrhea.
7. Any rash, yellow discoloration of skin or eyes, or irritation of the mouth or tongue should be reported.
8. Drug may increase GI motility with diabetic gastric paresis.
9. With topical use, clean affected area before applying ointment and wash hands before and after treatment.
10. Instill otic solutions at room temperature. Gently pull ear lobe down and back for children under 3 years of age; pull ear lobe up and back when over 3 years of age.
11. Report any evidence of hearing loss, which is usually temporary.

**Outcomes/Evaluate**
- Resolution of infection (negative culture reports, ↓ temperature, wound healing, ↓ WBCs, improved appetite)
- Symptomatic improvement

# ESTROGENS

*See also the following individual entries:*

Diethylstilbestrol diphosphate
Esterified estrogens
Estradiol transdermal system
Estrogens conjugated, oral

Estrogens conjugated, parenteral
Estrogens conjugated, vaginal
Estropipate
Oral Contraceptives

**Action/Kinetics:** The three primary estrogens in the human female are estradiol, estrone, and estriol, which are steroids. Nonsteroidal estrogens include diethylstilbestrol and chlorotrianisene. Estrogens combine with receptors in the cytoplasm of the cell, resulting in an increase in protein synthesis. For example, estrogens are required for development of secondary sex characteristics, development and maintenance of the female genital system and breasts. They also produce effects in the pituitary and hypothalamus. In adult women, estrogens participate in bone maintenance by aiding the deposition of calcium in the protein matrix of bones. They increase elastic elements in the skin, tend to cause sodium and fluid retention, and produce an anabolic effect by enhancing the turnover of dietary nitrogen and other elements into protein. Furthermore, they tend to keep plasma cholesterol at relatively low levels. Natural estrogens have a significant first-pass effect; thus, they are given parenterally. Synthetic derivatives can be given PO and are rapidly absorbed, distributed, and excreted. Estrogens are metabolized in the liver and excreted in urine (major portion) and feces. When given transdermally, the skin metabolizes estradiol only to a small extent.

**Uses:** See individual drugs. Estrogens are used both systemically and vaginally.

**Contraindications:** Breast cancer, except in those clients being treated for metastatic disease. Cancer of the genital tract and other estrogen-dependent neoplasms. Undiagnosed abnormal genital bleeding. History of thrombophlebitis, thrombosis, or thromboembolic disorders associated with previous estrogen use (except when used to treat breast or prostatic cancer). Known or suspected pregnancy. Prolonged therapy in women who plan to become pregnant. Use during lactation. May be contraindicated in clients with blood dyscrasias, hepatic disease, or thyroid dysfunction.

**Special Concerns:** Use with caution, if at all, in those with asthma, epilepsy, migraine, cardiac failure, renal insufficiency, diseases involving calcium or phosphorous metabolism, or a family history of mammary or genital tract cancer. Safety and effectiveness have not been determined in children and should be used with caution in adolescents in whom bone growth is incomplete.

**Side Effects: Systemic use.** Side effects to estrogens are dose dependent. *CV:* Potentially, the most serious side effects involve the CV system. ***Thromboembolism,*** thrombophlebitis, ***MI, pulmonary embolism,*** retinal thrombosis, ***mesenteric thrombosis, subarachnoid hemorrhage, postsurgical thromboembolism.*** Hypertension, edema, ***stroke.*** *GI:* N&V, abdominal cramps, bloating, cholestatic jaundice, colitis, acute pancreatitis, changes in appetite. *Dermatologic:* Most common are chloasma or melasma. Also, erythema multiforme, erythema nodosum, hemorrhagic eruptions, urticaria, dermatitis, photosensitivity. *Hepatic:* Cholestatic jaundice, aggravation of porphyria, benign (most common) or malignant liver tumors. *GU:* Breakthrough bleeding, spotting, changes in amount and/or duration of menstrual flow, amenorrhea during and after use, dysmenorrhea, premenstrual-like syndrome, change in cervical eversion and degree of cervical secretion, cystitis-like syndrome, hemolytic uremic syndrome, endometrial cystic hyperplasia, increased incidence of *Candida* vaginitis. *CNS:* Mental depression, dizziness, changes in libido, chorea, headache, aggravation of migraine headaches, fatigue, nervousness, ***convulsions.*** *Ocular:* Steepening of corneal curvature resulting in intolerance of contact

---

♣ = Available in Canada                    *bold italic* = life threatening side effect

lenses. Optic neuritis or retinal thrombosis, resulting in sudden or gradual, partial or complete loss of vision, double vision, papilledema. *Hematologic:* Increase in prothrombin and blood coagulation factors VII, VIII, IX, and X. Decrease in antithrombin III. *Local:* Pain at injection site, sterile abscesses, postinjection flare, redness and irritation at site of application of transdermal system. *Miscellaneous:* Breast tenderness, enlargement, or secretions. Increased risk of gallbladder disease (with high doses). Premature closure of epiphyses in children. Increased frequency of benign or malignant tumors of the cervix, uterus, vagina, and other organs. Weight gain. Increased risk of congenital abnormalities. Hypercalcemia in clients with metastatic breast carcinoma. In males, estrogens may cause gynecomastia, loss of libido, decreased spermatogenesis, testicular atrophy, and feminization. Prolonged use of high doses may inhibit the function of the anterior pituitary. Estrogen therapy affects many laboratory tests. **Vaginal use.** *GU:* Vaginal bleeding, vaginal discharge, endometrial withdrawal bleeding, serious bleeding in ovariectomized women with endometriosis. *Miscellaneous:* Breast tenderness.

**Drug Interactions**
*Anticoagulants, oral* / ↓ Anticoagulant response by ↑ activity of certain clotting factors
*Anticonvulsants* / Estrogen-induced fluid retention may precipitate seizures. Also, contraceptive steroids ↑ effect of anticonvulsants by ↓ breakdown in liver and ↓ plasma protein binding
*Antidiabetic agents* / Estrogens may impair glucose tolerance and thus change requirements for antidiabetic agent
*Barbiturates* / ↓ Effect of estrogen by ↑ breakdown by liver
*Phenytoin* / See *Anticonvulsants*
*Rifampin* / ↓ Effect of estrogen due to ↑ breakdown by liver
*Succinylcholine* / Estrogens may ↑ effects of succinylcholine

*Tricyclic antidepressants* / Possible ↑ effects of tricyclic antidepressants
**Laboratory Test Interferences:** Alter liver function tests and thyroid function tests. False + urine glucose test. ↓ Serum cholesterol, total serum lipids, pregnanediol excretion, serum folate. ↑ Serum triglyceride levels, thyroxine-binding globulin, sulfobromophthalein retention, prothrombin; factors VII, VIII, IX, X. Impaired glucose tolerance, reduced response to metyrapone.

**Dosage**
PO, IM, SC, vaginal, topical, or by implantation. The dosage of estrogens is highly individualized and is aimed at the minimal effective amount.

## NURSING CONSIDERATIONS
**Administration/Storage**
1. Most PO administered estrogens are metabolized rapidly and, with the exception of chlorotrianisene, must be administered daily.
2. Parenterally administered estrogens are released more slowly from aqueous suspensions or oily solutions. When administered by injection, give slowly and deeply.
3. To avoid continuous stimulation of reproductive tissue, cyclic therapy consisting of 3 weeks on and 1 week off is usually recommended for most uses.
4. To reduce postpartum breast engorgement, give during the first few days after delivery.
**Assessment**
1. Document indications for therapy, type and onset of symptoms. List other agents prescribed and the outcome.
2. Note any history of thromboembolic problems as estrogens enhance blood coagulability; monitor blood coagulation factors and PT.
3. Assess mental status; note any history of depression, migraine headaches, or suicide attempts.
4. Determine any undiagnosed genital bleeding, liver disease, asthma, migraines, epilepsy, or cancer of the endometrium or breast (estrogen-

dependent neoplasms), as these preclude drug therapy.

5. Monitor VS, glucose, triglycerides, electrolytes, liver and renal function studies.

**Client/Family Teaching**

1. Review the dose, form, and frequency of the prescribed agent.

2. Taking oral medications with meals or a light snack will prevent gastric irritation and usually eliminates nausea. With once-a-day therapy, taking it at bedtime may eliminate problems. Nausea, bloating, abdominal cramping, changes in appetite, and vomiting may occur and usually disappear with the continuation of therapy.

3. Report any alterations in mental attitude: depression or withdrawal, insomnia or anorexia, or a lack of attention to personal appearance.

4. With cyclical therapy, take meds for 3 weeks and then omit it for 1 week. Menstruation may then occur, but pregnancy will not occur because ovulation is suppressed. Keep a record of periods and any problems, such as missed menses, unusual vaginal bleeding, spotting, or irregularity. Report immediately if pregnancy is suspected.

5. Breast tenderness, enlargement, or secretion may occur. Perform BSE monthly (usually 2 weeks after menses) and report any continued problems or changes in the breasts.

6. Report immediately if there are leg pains, sudden onset of chest pain, dizziness, SOB, weakness of the arms or legs, or any evidence of numbness (S&S of thromboembolic problems).

7. May develop changes in the curvature of the cornea, making it difficult to wear contact lenses. Consult ophthalmologist if evidenced.

8. Report any skin changes, such as alopecia or discoloration.

9. Estrogen can alter glucose tolerance. Monitor sugars and report any significant increases as dose of antidiabetic medication may need to be changed.

10. Males may develop feminine characteristics or suffer from impotence; these usually disappear once therapy completed.

11. With suppositories, insert high into the vault. If applying a vaginal preparation, it is best done at bedtime. Wear a sanitary napkin when vaginal preparations are being used and avoid the use of tampons. Store suppositories in the refrigerator.

12. Report if estrogen ointments cause systemic reactions.

13. If pregnant and planning to breast-feed the baby, do not take estrogens while breast-feeding. Consult provider for alternative forms of contraception; breast-feeding does not provide any degree of contraception.

14. *Do not smoke.* Attend formal smoking cessation program if unable to quit.

15. Some potential risks, related to endometrial cancer, have been associated with estrogen therapy. Therapy requires close medical follow-up.

**Outcomes/Evaluate**

- Control of estrogen imbalance
- Effective contraceptive agent
- Adjunct in slowing postmenopausal osteoporosis
- Relief of postmenopausal symptoms
- Control of tumor size/spread in metastatic breast and prostate cancer

# FLUOROQUINOLONES

*See also the following individual entries:*

Ciprofloxacin hydrochloride
Enoxacin
Levofloxacin
Lomefloxacin hydrochloride
Norfloxacin
Ofloxacin
Sparfloxacin
Trovafloxacin

**Action/Kinetics:** Synthetic, broad-spectrum antibacterial agents. The fluorine molecule confers increased activity against gram-negative organisms as well as broadens the spectrum against gram-positive organisms. Are bactericidal agents by interfering with DNA gyrase, an enzyme needed for the synthesis of bacterial DNA. Food may delay the absorption of ciprofloxacin, lomefloxacin, and norfloxacin. Ciprofloxacin, levofloxacin, ofloxacin, and trovafloxacin may be given IV; all fluoroquinolones may be given PO.

**Uses:** See individual drugs; these drugs are used for a large number of gram-positive and gram-negative infections.

**Contraindications:** Hypersensitivity to the quinolone group of antibiotics, including cinoxacin and nalidixic acid. Lactation. Use in children less than 18 years of age.

**Special Concerns:** Use lower doses in impaired renal function. There may be differences in CNS toxicity between the various fluoroquinolones. Use may increase the risk of Achilles and other tendon inflammation and rupture.

**Side Effects:** See individual drugs. The following side effects are common to each of the fluoroquinolone antibiotics. *GI:* N&V, diarrhea, abdominal pain or discomfort, dry or painful mouth, heartburn, dyspepsia, flatulence, constipation, pseudomembranous colitis. *CNS:* Headache, dizziness, malaise, lethargy, fatigue, drowsiness, somnolence, depression, insomnia, **seizures,** paresthesia. *Dermatologic:* Rash, photosensitivity, pruritus (except for ciprofloxacin). *Hypersensitivity reactions:* Facial or **pharyngeal edema,** dyspnea, urticaria, itching, tingling, loss of consciousness, **CV collapse.** *Other:* Visual disturbances and ophthalmologic abnormalities, hearing loss, superinfection, phototoxicity, eosinophilia, crystalluria, Achilles and other tendon inflammation and rupture. Fluoroquinolones, except norfloxacin, may also cause vaginitis, syncope, chills, and edema.

**OD** **Overdose Management:** *Symptoms:* Extension of side effects. *Treatment:* For acute overdose, vomiting should be induced or gastric lavage performed. The client should be carefully observed and, if necessary, symptomatic and supportive treatment given. Hydration should be maintained.

**Drug Interactions**
*Antacids* / ↓ Serum levels of fluoroquinolones due to ↓ absorption from the GI tract
*Anticoagulants* / ↑ Effect of anticoagulant
*Antineoplastic agents* / ↓ Serum levels of fluoroquinolones
*Cimetidine* / ↓ Elimination of fluoroquinolones
*Cyclosporine* / ↑ Risk of nephrotoxicity
*Didanosine* / ↓ Serum levels of fluoroquinolones due to ↓ absorption from the GI tract
*Iron salts* / ↓ Serum levels of fluoroquinolones due to ↓ absorption from the GI tract
*Probenecid* / ↑ Serum levels of fluoroquinolones due to ↓ renal clearance
*Sucralfate* / ↓ Serum levels of fluoroquinolones due to ↓ absorption from the GI tract
*Theophylline* / ↑ Plasma levels and ↑ toxicity of theophylline due to ↓ clearance
*Zinc salts* / ↓ Serum levels of fluoroquinolones due to ↓ absorption from the GI tract

**Laboratory Test Interferences:** ↑ ALT, AST. See also individual drugs.

**Dosage** ————————————
See individual drugs.

## NURSING CONSIDERATIONS

See also *General Nursing Considerations for All Anti-Infectives.*

**Assessment**
1. Document type, onset, and characteristics of symptoms.
2. Note any previous experiences with these antibiotics. Discontinue at the first sign of skin rash or other allergic manifestations. Hypersensitivity reactions may occur even following the first dose
3. Assess for soft tissue or extremity injury; note any instability, pain, or swelling.

4. Monitor VS, I&O, CBC, cultures, liver and renal function studies.

5. If receiving anticoagulants and theophyllines, monitor closely as quinolones can cause increased drug levels with toxic drug effects, including increased bleeding or seizures.

**Client/Family Teaching**

1. Take only as directed. Do not take ofloxacin with food; take enoxacin and norfloxacin 1 hr before or 2 hr after meals; ciprofloxacin, lomefloxacin, and sparfloxacin may be taken without regard to meals.

2. Consume liberal amounts of fluids (>2.5 L/day).

3. Do not take any mineral supplements (i.e., iron or zinc) or antacids containing magnesium or aluminum simultaneously or 4 hr before or 2 hr after dosing with fluoroquinolones.

4. Do not perform hazardous tasks until drug effects realized; dizziness may be experienced.

5. Report any persistent, bothersome symptoms. The most frequently reported side effects include N&V and diarrhea.

6. Report symptoms of superinfection (furry tongue, vaginal or rectal itching, diarrhea).

7. Stop drug and report any new onset tendon pain or inflammation as tendon rupture may occur.

8. Wear protective clothing and sunscreens; avoid excessive sunlight or artificial ultraviolet light. Photosensitivity reactions may occur up to several weeks after stopping fluoroquinolone therapy.

**Outcomes/Evaluate**

• Symptomatic improvement
• Resolution of infection ( ↓ WBCs, ↓ temperature, ↑ appetite)
• Negative culture reports

# HISTAMINE H₂ ANTAGONISTS

*See also the following individual entries:*

Cimetidine
Famotidine
Nizatidine
Ranitidine bismuth citrate
Ranitidine hydrochloride

**Action/Kinetics:** Histamine H₂ antagonists are competitive blockers of histamine. As such they inhibit all phases of gastric acid secretion including that caused by histamine, gastrin, and muscarinic agents. Both fasting and nocturnal acid secretion are inhibited. In addition, the volume and hydrogen ion concentration of gastric juice are decreased. Cimetidine, famotidine, and ranitidine have no effect on gastric emptying; cimetidine and famitidine have no effect on lower esophageal pressure. Fasting or postprandial serum gastrin is not affected by famotidine, nizatidine, or ranitidine. Cimetidine is known to affect the cytochrome P-450 drug metabolizing system for other drugs. Ranitidine also affects the P-450 enzyme system, but its effect on elimination of other drugs is not significant. Neither famotidine nor nizatidine affects the P-450 enzyme system.

**Uses:** See individual drugs. Also, these drugs are used as part of combination therapy to treat *Helicobacter pylori*–associated duodenal ulcer and maintenance therapy after healing of the active ulcer.

**Contraindications:** Hypersensitivity.

**Special Concerns:** Use with caution in impaired hepatic and renal function. Symptomatic response to these drugs does not preclude gastric malignancy. Do not use cimetidine, famotidine, and nizatidine during lactation; use ranitidine with caution. Safety and effectiveness have not been established for use in children; use of cimetidine is not recommended in children less than 16 years of age unless benefits outweigh risks.

**Side Effects:** The following side effects are common to all or most of the H₂-histamine antagonists. See individual drugs for complete listing. *GI:* N&V, abdominal discomfort, diarrhea, constipation, hepatocellular effects. *CNS:* Headache, fatigue, somnolence, dizziness, confusion, hallucinations, insomnia. *Dermatologic:* Rash, urticaria, pruritus, alopecia (rare), erythema multiforme (rare). *Hematologic:* Rarely, thrombocytopenia, agranulocytosis, granulocytopenia. *Other:* Gynecomastia, impotence, loss of libido, arthralgia, bronchospasm, transient pain at injection site, cardiac arrhythmias following rapid IV use (rare), arthralgia (rare), ***anaphylaxis*** (rare).

**OD** **Overdose Management:** *Symptoms:* No experience is available for deliberate overdose. *Treatment:* Induce vomiting or perform gastric lavage to remove any unabsorbed drug. Monitor the client and undertake supportive therapy.

**Dosage**

See individual drugs.

## NURSING CONSIDERATIONS
### Administration/Storage
1. May be taken without regard for meals.
2. Stagger doses of antacids if used with cimetidine or ranitidine.
3. Do not take the maximum dose of OTC products for more than 2 weeks continuously without medical supervision.

### Assessment
1. Document symptoms of epigastric or abdominal pain/discomfort, noting onset, duration, intensity, and any previous treatment.
2. Assess for number of reflux occurrences. Chronic treatment usually initiated after two to three recurrences.
3. Monitor CBC, liver and renal function studies.
4. Perform CNS assessment noting level of orientation.
5. Note results of radiographic/endoscopic procedures; document *H. pylori* results.
6. Determine gastric pH; maintain greater than 5.

**Client/Family Teaching**
1. Antacids must be taken as prescribed; do not take within 1 hr of the histamine H$_2$ antagonist.
2. Take meds as prescribed; do not stop if pain subsides or if "feeling better" as drug is necessary to inhibit gastric acid secretion.
3. These agents reduce the secretion of gastric acid and are usually prescribed for 4–8 weeks initially to control symptoms and promote healing.
4. Report any confusion or disorientation immediately.
5. Avoid alcohol, caffeine, aspirin-containing products (cough and cold products), and foods that may cause GI irritation, i.e., harsh spices.
6. Stop 24–72 hr before skin testing begins; may cause false negative response in tests with allergen extracts.
7. Smoking may interfere with drug's action. Stop smoking and do not smoke following the last dose of the day.
8. Any blood-tinged emesis or dark tarry stools as well as dizziness or rash, require immediate reporting.
9. Report for all scheduled follow-up studies; a response to these agents does not preclude gastric malignancy.

**Outcomes/Evaluate**
- Duodenal ulcer healing
- ↓ Gastric irritation/bleeding; ↓ abdominal pain/ discomfort
- Gastric pH > 5
- Stabilization of H&H

## INSULINS

See *Antidiabetic Agents: Hypoglycemic Agents and Insulin.*

## LAXATIVES

*See also the following individual entries:*

Docusate calcium
Docusate potassium
Docusate sodium

Lactulose
Magnesium sulfate
Psyllium hydrophilic muciloid

**Action/Kinetics:** Laxatives act locally, either by specifically stimulating the smooth muscles of the bowel or by changing the bulk or consistency of the stools. Laxatives can be divided into five categories.

1. *Stimulant laxatives:* Substances that chemically stimulate the smooth muscles of the bowel to increase contractions. Drugs include bisacodyl, cascara, danthron, and senna.

2. *Saline laxatives:* Substances that increase the bulk of the stools by retaining water. Includes magnesium salts and sodium phosphate.

3. *Bulk-forming laxatives:* Nondigestible substances that pass through the stomach and then increase the bulk of the stools. Examples are methylcellulose and psyllium.

4. *Emollient and lubricant laxatives:* Agents that soften hardened feces and facilitate their passage through the lower intestine. Examples include docusate and mineral oil.

5. *Miscellaneous:* Includes glycerin suppositories and lactulose.

**Uses:** See individual agents. Short-term treatment of constipation. Prophylaxis in clients who should not strain during defecation, i.e., following anorectal surgery or after MI (fecal softeners or lubricant laxatives). To evacuate the colon for rectal and bowel examinations (certain lubricant, saline, and stimulant laxatives). In conjunction with surgery or anthelmintic therapy. The underlying cause of constipation should be determined since a marked change in bowel habits may be a symptom of a pathologic condition.

**Contraindications:** Severe abdominal pain that *might* be caused by appendicitis, enteritis, ulcerative colitis, diverticulitis, intestinal obstruction. Laxative use in these conditions may cause rupture of the abdomen or intestinal hemorrhage. Undiagnosed abdominal pain. Children under the age of 2. Castor oil is contraindicated during pregnancy as the irritant effects may result in premature labor.

**Side Effects:** *GI:* Excess activity of the colon resulting in nausea, diarrhea, griping, or vomiting. Perianal irritation, bloating, flatulence. *Electrolyte Balance:* Dehydration, disturbance of the electrolyte balance. *Miscellaneous:* Dizziness, fainting, weakness, sweating, palpitations.

*Bulk laxatives:* Obstruction in the esophagus, stomach, small intestine, or rectum. *Stimulant laxatives:* Chronic abuse may lead to malfunctioning colon. *Mineral Oil:* Large doses may cause anal seepage resulting in itching, irritation, hemorrhoids, and perianal discomfort.

Chronic use of laxatives may cause laxative dependency and result in chronic constipation and other intestinal disorders because the client may start to depend on the psychologic effect and physical stimulus of the drug rather than on the body's own natural reflexes.

**Drug Interactions**

*Anticoagulants, oral* / ↓ Absorption of vitamin K from GI tract induced by laxatives may ↑ effects of anticoagulants and result in bleeding
*Digitalis* / Cathartics may ↓ absorption of digitalis
*Tetracyclines* / Laxatives containing Al, Ca, or Mg may ↓ effect of tetracyclines due to ↓ absorption from GI tract

**Dosage**
See individual drugs.

## NURSING CONSIDERATIONS
**Administration**

1. When administering a laxative, note the length of time it takes for the laxative to take effect and give it so that the result of the laxative will not interfere with the client's rest or digestion and absorption of nutrients.

2. Administer laxatives at a temperature that makes them more agreeable.

3. If laxative is to be administered in a liquid, select one that the client finds palatable.

4. If ordered to prepare for a diagnostic exam, check directions carefully to ensure accurate administration.

**Assessment**

1. Determine how long relied on laxatives and the underlying causes; note type of laxative taking and effectiveness.

2. With abdominal pain and discomfort, note exact location and type of discomfort experiencing. R/O other intestinal disorders where laxatives should not be used.

3. Determine stool character and frequency of bowel movements. The client's definition of constipation may determine if, in fact, constipation exists.

4. Note age, state of health, activity level, and general nutritional status.

5. Identify any special restriction or limitation due to illness; may include fluid restriction or sodium-restricted diet.

6. List other drugs that may contribute to constipation (i.e., diuretics, anticholinergics, antihistamines, antidepressants, iron products, and some antihypertensive agents, especially verapamil).

7. Identify recent life-style changes that may contribute to problem.

**Interventions**

1. If hospitalized or ill at home, provide a commode at the bedside. This will promote better bowel function by encouraging client to move about and ensure privacy.

2. Encourage to alter dietary habits to include bulk foods and sufficient fluids to enhance elimination.

3. Discuss need for regular exercise, as well as a reduction of their dependence on laxatives.

**Client/Family Teaching**

1. Have a regular schedule for defecation; keep record of bowel function and response to all laxatives taken.

2. Laxatives reduce the amount of time other drugs remain in the intestine and may diminish effectiveness.

3. If laxative is to be taken in prep for a diagnostic study, review instruc-

tions. If unable to read, find someone in the family or a friend that can review directions to ensure an accurate test.

4. Review techniques that facilitate elimination; sitting with legs slightly elevated and leaning forward to increase abdominal pressure often encourages elimination.

5. Bowel tone will be lost with long-term use of laxatives; bowel movements do not have to occur daily. Use diet to achieve same purpose; two or three prunes a day are preferable to laxatives.

6. Frequent use of any type of enemas may cause damage to the rectum and small bowel as well as inhibit bowel tone and may cause electrolyte abnormalities.

7. Review importance of diet high in fiber foods (and juices such as prune) and daily exercise and benefits in maintaining proper bowel function. Consult dietitian if assistance is needed in meal planning/preparation and food selections.

8. Report if constipation persists because there could be a physiologic problem that requires attention.

9. If pregnant, consult with provider before taking any laxatives to treat constipation.

10. Nursing mothers should avoid laxatives unless prescribed as many are excreted in breast milk and can cause infant diarrhea.

**Outcomes/Evaluate**

• Relief of constipation; evacuation of a soft, formed stool

• Effective colon prep for diagnostic procedures (no stool in bowel)

# NARCOTIC ANALGESICS

*See also the following individual entries:*

Alfentanil hydrochloride
Buprenorphine hydrochloride
Butorphanol tartrate
Codeine phosphate
Codeine sulfate

Dezocine
Fentanyl citrate
Fentanyl transdermal system
Fiorinal
Fiorinal with Codeine
Hydrocodone bitartrate and
    Acetaminophen
Hydromorphone hydrochloride
Levomethadyl acetate hydrochloride
Meperidine hydrochloride
Methadone hydrochloride
Morphine hydrochloride
Morphine sulfate
Nalbuphine hydrochloride
Oxycodone hydrochloride
Oxycodone terephthalate
Oxymorphone hydrochloride
Paregoric
Pentazocine hydrochloride with
    Naloxone hydrochloride
Pentazocine lactate
Percocet
Propoxyphene hydrochloride
Propoxyphene napsylate
Remifentanil hydrochloride
Sufentanil
Tramadol hydrochloride
Tylenol with Codeine

**Action/Kinetics**

Narcotic analgesics are classified as agonists, mixed agonist-antagonists, or partial agonists depending on their activity at opiate receptors. The narcotic analgesics attach to specific receptors located in the CNS (cortex, brain stem, and spinal cord) resulting in various CNS effects. The mechanism is believed to involve decreased permeability of the cell membrane to sodium, which results in diminished transmission of pain impulses. Five categories of opioid receptors have been identified: mu, kappa, sigma, delta, and epsilon. Narcotic analgesics are believed to exert their activity at mu, kappa, and sigma receptors. Mu receptors are thought to mediate supraspinal analgesia, euphoria, and respiratory and physical depression. Pentazocine-like spinal analgesia, miosis, and sedation are mediated by kappa receptors while sigma receptors mediate dysphoria, hallucinations, as well as respiratory and vasomotor stimulation (caused by drugs with antagonist activity). In addition to an alteration of pain perception (analgesia), the drugs, especially at higher doses, induce euphoria, drowsiness, changes in mood, mental clouding, and deep sleep.

The narcotic analgesics also depress respiration. Death by overdosage is almost always the result of respiratory arrest. These drugs cause nausea and emesis due to direct stimulation of the CTZ. They depress the cough reflex, and small doses of narcotic analgesics (e.g., codeine) are found in certain antitussive products. Little effect on BP when the client is in a supine position. Most narcotics decrease the capacity of the client to respond to stress. Morphine and other narcotic analgesics induce peripheral vasodilation, which may result in hypotension. Many narcotic analgesics constrict the pupil, a sign of dependence with such drugs. They also decrease peristaltic motility causing constipation. The constipating effects (e.g., Paregoric) are sometimes used therapeutically in diarrhea. The narcotic analgesics also increase the pressure within the biliary tract. See also individual agents.

**Uses:** See individual drugs. Generally are used to treat pain due to various causes (e.g., MI, carcinoma, surgery, burns, postpartum), as preanesthetic medication, as adjuncts to anesthesia, acute vascular occlusion, diarrhea, and coughs. Methadone is used for heroin withdrawal and maintenance.

**Contraindications:** Asthma, emphysema, kyphoscoliosis, severe obesity, convulsive states as in epilepsy, delirium tremens, tetanus and strychnine poisoning, diabetic acidosis, myxedema, Addison's disease, hepatic cirrhosis, and children under 6 months.

**Special Concerns:** Use with caution in clients with head injury or after head surgery because of morphine's capacity to elevate ICP and mask the pupillary response. Use with caution in the elderly, in the debilitated, in young children, in individuals with increased ICP, in obstetrics, and with clients in shock or during acute alcoholic intoxication.

Use morphine with extreme caution in pulmonary heart disease (cor pulmonale). Deaths following ordinary therapeutic doses have been reported. Use cautiously in prostatic hypertrophy, because it may precipitate acute urinary retention. Use cautiously in clients with reduced blood volume, such as in hemorrhaging clients who are more susceptible to the hypotensive effects of morphine.

Since the drugs depress the respiratory center, give early in labor, at least 2 hr before delivery, to reduce the danger of respiratory depression in the newborn. When given before surgery, give at least 1–2 hr preoperatively so that the danger of maximum depression of respiratory function will have passed before anesthesia is initiated. These drugs may need to be withheld prior to diagnostic procedures so that the physician can use pain to locate dysfunction.

**Side Effects:** *Respiratory:* **Respiratory depression, apnea.** *CNS:* Dizziness, lightheadedness, sedation, lethargy, headache, euphoria, mental clouding, fainting. Idiosyncratic effects including excitement, restlessness, tremors, delirium, insomnia. *GI:* N&V, vomiting, constipation, increased pressure in biliary tract, dry mouth, anorexia. *CV:* Flushing, changes in HR and BP, circulatory collapse. *Allergic:* Skin rashes including pruritus and urticaria. Sweating, *laryngospasm,* edema. *Miscellaneous:* Urinary retention, oliguria, reduced libido, changes in body temperature. Narcotics cross the placental barrier and depress respiration of the fetus or newborn.

DEPENDENCE AND TOLERANCE: All drugs of this group are addictive.

Psychologic and physical dependence and tolerance develop even when clients use clinical doses. Tolerance is characterized by the fact that the client requires shorter periods of time between doses or larger doses for relief of pain. Tolerance usually develops faster when the narcotic analgesic is administered regularly and when the dose is large.

**OD** **Overdose Management:** *Symptoms (Acute Toxicity):* Severe toxicity is characterized by **profound respiratory depression, apnea, deep sleep, stupor or coma, circulatory collapse, seizures, cardiopulmonary arrest, and death.** Less severe toxicity results in symptoms including CNS depression, miosis, respiratory depression, deep sleep, flaccidity of skeletal muscles, hypotension, bradycardia, hypothermia, pulmonary edema, pneumonia, shock. The respiratory rate may be as low as 2–4 breaths/min. The client may be cyanotic. Urine output is decreased, the skin feels clammy, and body temperature decreases. If death occurs, it almost always results from **respiratory depression.** *Symptoms (Chronic Toxicity):* The problem of chronic dependence on narcotics occurs not only as a result of "street" use but is also found often among those who have easy access to narcotics (physicians, nurses, pharmacists). All the principal narcotic analgesics (morphine, opium, heroin, codeine, meperidine, and others) have, at times, been used for nontherapeutic purposes.

The nurse must be aware of the problem and be able to recognize signs of chronic dependence. These are constricted pupils, GI effects (constipation), skin infections, needle scars, abscesses, and itching, especially on the anterior surfaces of the body, where the client may inject the drug.

*Withdrawal signs* appear after drug is withheld for 4–12 hr. They are characterized by intense craving for the drug, insomnia, yawning, sneezing, vomiting, diarrhea, tremors, sweating, mental depression, muscular aches and pains, chills, and anxiety. Although the symptoms of narcotic withdrawal are uncomfortable, they are rarely life-threatening. This is in contrast to the withdrawal syndrome from depressants, where the life of the individual may be endangered because of the possibility of tonic-clonic seizures.

*Treatment (Acute Overdose):* Initial treatment is aimed at combating progressive respiratory depression by maintaining a patent airway and by artificial respiration. Gastric lavage and induced emesis are indicated in case of oral poisoning. The narcotic antagonist naloxone (Narcan), 0.4 mg IV, is effective in the treatment of acute overdosage. Respiratory stimulants (e.g., caffeine) should not be used to treat depression from the narcotic overdosage.

**Drug Interactions**
*Alcohol, ethyl* / Potentiation or addition of CNS depressant effects; concomitant use may lead to drowsiness, lethargy, stupor, respiratory collapse, coma, or death
*Anesthetics, general* / See *Alcohol*
*Antianxiety drugs* / See *Alcohol*
*Antidepressants, tricyclic* / ↑ Narcotic-induced respiratory depression
*Antihistamines* / See *Alcohol*
*Barbiturates* / See *Alcohol*
*Cimetidine* / ↑ CNS toxicity (e.g., disorientation, confusion, respiratory depression, apnea, seizures) with narcotics
*CNS depressants* / See *Alcohol*
*MAO inhibitors* / Possible potentiation of either MAO inhibitor (excitation, hypertension) or narcotic (hypotension, coma) effects; death has resulted
*Methotrimeprazine* / Potentiation of CNS depression
*Phenothiazines* / See *Alcohol*
*Sedative-hypnotics, nonbarbiturate* / See *Alcohol*
*Skeletal muscle relaxants (surgical)* / ↑ Respiratory depression and ↑ muscle relaxation
**Laboratory Test Interferences:** Altered liver function tests. False + or ↑

urinary glucose test (Benedict's). ↑ Plasma amylase or lipase.

**Dosage**
See individual drugs.

## NURSING CONSIDERATIONS
**Administration/Storage**
1. Review list of drugs with which narcotics interact and their associated effects.
2. Request that orders be rewritten at timed intervals as required for continued administration.
3. Record amount of narcotic used on the narcotic inventory sheet, noting drug, the date, the time, the dose, and to whom, or if the drug was wasted; include appropriate witness as necessary, addressing all requirements for documentation.
**Assessment**
1. Document indications for therapy, type and onset of symptoms; differentiate acute vs. chronic syndromes and rate pain levels.
2. Note any prior experience with narcotic analgesics such as an adverse reaction with the drug or category of drugs prescribed.
3. Identify clinical conditions that would precipitate pain syndromes, i.e., cancer, neuropathic as in diabetic neuropathy, postherpetic neuralgia, or musculoskeletal injury.
4. Determine cause and document amount of pain or discomfort, its location, intensity, and duration, frequency of occurrence, and what drug has been effective in the past.
5. Use a pain rating scale (e.g., 0–10) to assess pain quantitatively so clients can accurately describe their level of pain and measure the level of effectiveness of therapy.
6. Obtain baseline VS; generally, if the respiratory rate is less than 12/min or the SBP is less than 90 mm Hg, a narcotic should not be administered unless there is ventilatory support or specific written guidelines, with parameters for administration.
7. Note weight, age, and general body size. Too large a dosage for

---

the client's weight and age can result in serious side effects.

8. Document amount of time elapsed between doses for relief from recurring pain.

9. Note precipitating factors as well as the impact of the pain on the client's ability to function.

10. Document asthma or other conditions that tend to compromise respirations.

11. Determine if pregnant. Narcotics cross the placental barrier and depress fetal respirations; may be contraindicated under certain circumstances.

12. Monitor CBC, electrolytes, liver and renal function studies.

**Interventions**

1. Determine when to use supportive measures, such as relaxation techniques, repositioning, and reassurance to assist in relieving pain.

2. Explore source of pain; use nonnarcotic analgesics when possible. Coadministration (such as with NSAIDs) may increase analgesic effects and permit lower doses of the narcotic.

3. Administer when needed; *prolonging until the maximum amount of pain experienced reduces drugs' effectiveness*.

4. Monitor VS and mental status. During parenteral therapy:

• Monitor for respiratory depression.

• Narcotics depress the cough reflex. Turn q 2 hr; cough and deep breathe to prevent atelectasis. Splinting incisions and painful areas may assist in compliance. Administer narcotic at least 30–60 min prior to activities or painful procedures.

• Monitor for hypotension.

• If HR below 60 beats/min in the adult or 110 beats/min in an infant, withhold and report.

• Observe for decrease in BP, deep sleep, or constricted pupils.

• Assess during meals to prevent choking and aspiration.

• Monitor closely when administered as sedation for a procedure.

• Note effects on mental status. One who has experienced pain, fear, or anxiety may become euphoric and excited. Note dizziness, drowsiness, pupil reactions, or hallucinations.

5. Report if N&V occurs; may need an antiemetic or change in therapy.

6. If taking by mouth, a snack or milk may decrease gastric irritation and lessen nausea.

7. Monitor bowel function; narcotics, especially morphine, can have a depressant effect on the GI tract and may promote constipation. Increase fluid intake to 2.5–3 L/day; consume fruit juices, fruits, and fiber. Increase level and frequency of exercise if tolerated.

8. Narcotics may cause urinary retention. Monitor I&O; palpate abdomen to detect bladder distention; empty bladder q 3–4 hr. Question about difficulty voiding, pain in the bladder area, sensation of not emptying the bladder, dysuria, or any unusual odors.

9. Note difficulty with vision. Check pupillary response to light; report if pupils remain constricted.

10. Monitor mental status. If bedridden, put up side rails and provide safety measures; assist with ambulation, BR, and transfers.

11. Reassure that flushing and a feeling of warmth may occur with therapeutic doses.

12. May perspire profusely; be prepared to bathe; change clothes and linens frequently.

13. Assess for evidence of tolerance and addiction with ATC therapy.

14. With terminal disease states, dependence on drug therapy is not a consideration, whereas *adequate pain control is of the utmost concern*.

**Client/Family Teaching**

1. Drug may become habit forming; explore alternative methods for pain control.

2. Take as prescribed before the pain becomes too severe.

3. Avoid alcohol in any form.

4. Do not take OTC drugs without approval. Many contain small amounts of alcohol and some may

interact unfavorably with the prescribed drug.

5. For fecal impaction, use preventive actions, such as increased fluid intake, increased use of fruit and fruit juices, and a stool softener.

6. Drug can cause drowsiness and dizziness; use caution when operating a motor vehicle or performing other tasks that require mental alertness.

7. Rise slowly from a lying to sitting position and dangle legs before standing, to minimize orthostatic effects.

8. When used as sedation for outpatient procedures, someone must accompany client. Expect a recovery period (to assess for any adverse side effects) of up to several hours before release.

9. Store all drugs in a safe place, out of the reach of children and away from the bedside to prevent accidental overdosage.

10. During prolonged usage, do not stop abruptly; withdrawal symptoms may occur.

11. Determine extent of relief achieved with each dosage (e.g., pain level decreased from a level 5 to a level 2, 20 min after administration of medication). Keep a record of narcotic use for breakthrough pain so that maintenance dose can be adjusted.

12. Review techniques to enhance pain relief such as relaxation techniques, splinting incision, supporting painful areas, and taking medication before strenuous activities and before pain becomes severe.

13. Identify appropriate support groups for assistance with understanding, accepting, and managing chronic pain. Seek locale of regional pain management center.

14. For those with terminal diseases, identify local support groups to provide contact with those experiencing similar symptoms and treatments.

**Outcomes/Evaluate**

• Control of severe pain without altered hemodynamics or impaired level of consciousness

• Absence of acute toxicity, tolerance, or addiction, during short-term therapy

**Special Concerns:** For the elderly, blood levels of narcotic may be higher, resulting in longer periods of pain relief. Assess physical parameters and client complaints carefully before readministering narcotic for short-term pain control on the prescribed as-needed frequency.

# NARCOTIC ANTAGONISTS

*See also the following individual entries:*

> Nalmefene hydrochloride
> Naloxone hydrochloride
> Naltrexone

**Action/Kinetics:** Narcotic antagonists competitively block the action of narcotic analgesics by displacing previously given narcotics from their receptor sites or by preventing narcotics from attaching to the opiate receptors, thereby preventing access by the analgesic. Not effective in reversing the respiratory depression induced by barbiturates, anesthetics, or other nonnarcotic agents. These drugs almost immediately induce withdrawal symptoms in narcotic addicts and are sometimes used to unmask dependence.

## NURSING CONSIDERATIONS

### Assessment

1. Determine etiology of respiratory depression. Narcotic antagonists do not relieve the toxicity of nonnarcotic CNS depressants.

2. Note mental status and VS.

### Interventions

1. Note agent being reversed. If narcotic is long acting or sustained release, repeated doses will be required in order to continue to counteract drug effects. Monitor VS and respirations closely after duration of action of antagonist; additional doses may be necessary.

2. Observe for appearance of with-

drawal symptoms characterized by restlessness, crying out due to sudden loss of pain control, lacrimation, rhinorrhea, yawning, perspiration, vomiting, diarrhea, sweating, writhing, anxiety, pain, chills, and an intense craving for the drug.

3. Observe for symptoms of airway obstruction; if comatose, turn frequently and position on side to prevent aspiration.

4. Maintain a safe, protective environment. Use side rails, supervise ambulation, and use soft supports as needed.

5. If used to diagnose narcotic use or dependence, observe for initial dilation of the pupils, followed by constriction.

6. Anticipate readministration of smaller doses of narcotic (once depressant symptoms reversed) with terminal pain and conditions that warrant narcotic pain management.

**Outcomes/Evaluate**

- Reversal of toxic effects of narcotic analgesic evidenced by ↑ level of consciousness and improved breathing patterns
- Confirmation of narcotic dependence evidenced by withdrawal symptoms

# NASAL DECONGESTANTS

*See also the following individual entries:*

Ephedrine sulfate
Epinephrine hydrochloride
Phenylephrine hydrochloride
Pseudoephedrine hydrochloride

**Action/Kinetics:** The most commonly used agents for relief of nasal congestion are the adrenergic drugs. They act by stimulating alpha-adrenergic receptors, thereby constricting the arterioles in the nasal mucosa; this reduces blood flow to the area, decreasing congestion. However, drugs such as ephedrine and pseudoephedrine also have beta-adrenergic effects. Both topical (sprays, drops)

and oral agents may be used, although oral agents are not as effective.

**Uses: PO.** Nasal congestion due to hay fever, common cold, allergies, or sinusitis. To help sinus or nasal drainage. To relieve congestion of eustachian tubes. **Topical.** Nasal and nasopharyngeal mucosal congestion due to hay fever, common cold, allergies, or sinusitis. With other therapy to decrease congestion around the eustachian tubes. Relieve ear block and pressure pain during air travel.

**Contraindications:** Oral use in severe hypertension or CAD. Use with MAO inhibitors. Oral use of pseudoephedrine and phenylpropanolamine during lactation.

**Special Concerns:** Use with caution in hyperthyroidism, arteriosclerosis, increased intraocular pressure, prostatic hypertrophy, angina, diabetes, ischemic heart disease, hypertension. Also, clients receiving MAO inhibitors may manifest hypertensive crisis following the use of oral nasal decongestants. Use with caution in geriatric clients and during pregnancy and lactation. Rebound congestion may occur after topical use. OTC products containing ephedrine have been abused.

**Side Effects:** *Topical use:* Stinging and burning, mucosal dryness, sneezing, local irritation, rebound congestion (rhinitis medicamentosa). Systemic use may produce the following symptoms. *CV: **CV collapse with hypotension,*** arrhythmias, palpitations, precordial pain, tachycardia, transient hypertension, bradycardia. *CNS:* Anxiety, dizziness, headache, fear, restlessness, tremors, insomnia, tenseness, lightheadedness, drowsiness, psychologic disturbances, weakness, psychoses, hallucinations, *seizures,* depression. *GI:* N&V, anorexia. *Ophthalmologic:* Irritation, photophobia, tearing, blurred vision, blepharospasm. *Other:* Dysuria, sweating, pallor, breathing difficulties, orofacial dystonia.

*NOTE:* Ephedrine may also produce anorexia and urinary retention in men with prostatic hypertrophy.

**OD** **Overdose** **Management:**
*Symptoms:* Somnolence, sedation, *coma,* profuse sweating, *hypotension, shock.* *Severe hypertension,* bradycardia, and rebound hypotension may occur with naphazoline and tetrahydrozoline. *Treatment:* Supportive therapy. IV phentolamine may be used in severe cases.

**Drug Interactions**
*Furazolidone* / ↑ Pressor sensitivity to drugs with both alpha- and beta-adrenergic effects (e.g., ephedrine)
*Guanethidine* / ↑ Effect of direct-acting agents (e.g., epinephrine) and ↓ effect of mixed-acting drugs; also, ↓ hypotensive effect of guanethidine
*MAO inhibitors* / Use with mixed-acting drugs (e.g., ephedrine) → severe headache, hypertension, hyperpyrexia, and possibly hypertensive crisis
*Methyldopa* / ↑ Risk of a pressor response
*Phenothiazines* / May ↓ or reverse action of nasal decongestants
*Reserpine* / ↑ Pressor effect of direct-acting drugs and ↓ effect of mixed-acting drugs
*Theophyllines* / Enhanced toxicity
*Tricyclic antidepressants* / ↑ Pressor effect of direct-acting agents → possibility of dysrhythmias; ↓ pressor effect of mixed-acting drugs
*Urinary acidifiers* / ↑ Excretion of nasal decongestants → ↓ effect
*Urinary alkalinizers* / ↓ Excretion of nasal decongestants → ↑ effect

**Dosage**
See individual drugs.

## NURSING CONSIDERATIONS
**Administration/Storage**
1. Most nasal decongestants are used topically in the form of sprays, drops, or solutions.
2. Solutions may become contaminated with use, resulting in the growth of bacteria and fungi. Thus, the dropper or spray tip should be rinsed in hot water after each use and covered.

3. Use separate equipment with topical administration to prevent the spread of infection. If only one container of medication is available, use an individual dropper for each client and rinse thoroughly with hot water after each use.
4. During administration, have facial tissues and a receptacle available for used tissues.
5. Topical decongestants should not be used longer than 3–5 days and should be used sparingly, especially in infants, children, and clients with CV disease.

**Client/Family Teaching**
1. Blow the nose gently before administering therapy. If unable to blow the nose, clear the nasal passages with a bulb-type aspirator as needed.
2. Review the prescribed method of administration, whether drops, spray, or jelly and the goals of therapy.
3. After completing therapy, rinse the dropper or tip of spray container with hot water. Dry with a tissue and cover, using care not to introduce water into the spray container. Wipe the tip of the nasal jelly tube with a damp tissue and replace the cap.
4. Seek medical assistance if symptoms worsen or do not improve after 3–5 days of therapy.
5. Overuse or misuse of these agents may cause significant medical problems; i.e., a nasal spray used regularly for more than 3 or 4 days may precipitate rebound congestion.
6. Many OTC agents contain sympathomimetics; these should be avoided with hypertension, hyperthyroidism, angina, and insulin-dependent diabetes.

**Outcomes/Evaluate**
- ↓ Nasal congestion
- Resolution of eustachian tube congestion/pain
- ↓ Duration/intensity of allergic manifestations

# NEUROMUSCULAR BLOCKING AGENTS

*See also the following individual entries:*

Atracurium besylate
Cisatracurium besylate
Doxacurium chloride
Mivacurium chloride
Pancuronium bromide
Pipecuronium bromide
Rocuronium bromide
Succinylcholine chloride
Tubocurarine chloride
Vecuronium bromide

**Action/Kinetics:** The drugs fall into two groups, both of which act peripherally: competitive (nondepolarizing) and depolarizing agents. Competitive agents include all of the above listed drugs *except* succinylcholine. They compete with acetylcholine for the receptor site in the muscle cells. The depolarizing agent—succinylcholine—initially excites skeletal muscle and then prevents the muscle from contracting by prolonging the time during which the receptors at the end plate cannot respond to acetylcholine (depolarization during refractory time).

The muscle paralysis caused by the neuromuscular blocking agents is sequential. Therapeutic doses produce muscle depression in the following order: heaviness of eyelids, difficulty in swallowing and talking, diplopia, progressive weakening of the extremities and neck, followed by relaxation of the trunk and spine. The diaphragm (respiratory paralysis) is affected last. The drugs do not affect consciousness, and their use, in the absence of adequate levels of general anesthesia, may be frightening to the client. After IV infusion, flaccid paralysis occurs within a few minutes with maximum effects within about 6 min. Maximal effects last 35–60 min and effective muscle paralysis may last for 25–90 min with complete recovery taking several hours. There is a narrow margin of safety between a therapeutically effective dose causing muscle relaxation and a toxic dose causing respiratory paralysis. **The neuromuscular blocking agents are always administered initially by a physician.** The nurse must be prepared to maintain and monitor respiration until the effect of the drug subsides.

**Uses:** See individual agents. General uses include as an adjunct to general anesthesia to cause muscle relaxation; to reduce the intensity of skeletal muscle contractions in either drug-induced or electrically induced convulsions; to assist in the management of mechanical ventilation.

**Contraindications:** Allergy or hypersensitivity to any of these drugs.

**Special Concerns:** Use with caution in myasthenia gravis; renal, hepatic, endocrine, or pulmonary impairment; respiratory depression; during lactation; and in elderly, pediatric, or debilitated clients. The action may be altered in clients by electrolyte imbalances (especially hyperkalemia), some carcinomas, body temperature, dehydration, renal disease, and in those taking digitalis.

**Side Effects:** *Respiratory paralysis. Severe and prolonged muscle relaxation. CV:* Cardiac arrhythmias, bradycardia, hypotension, cardiac arrest. These side effects are more frequent in neonates and premature infants. *GI:* Excessive salivation during light anesthesia. *Miscellaneous: Bronchospasms, hyperthermia,* hypersensitivity (rare). See also individual agents.

**OD Overdose Management:** *Symptoms:* Decreased respiratory reserve, extended skeletal muscle weakness, prolonged apnea, low tidal volume, sudden release of histamine, *CV collapse. Treatment:* There are no known antidotes.

• Use a peripheral nerve stimulator to monitor and assess client's response to the neuromuscular blocking medication.

• Have anticholinesterase drugs, such as edrophonium, pyridostigmine, or neostigmine available to counteract respiratory depression due to paralysis of skeletal muscles.

These drugs increase the body's production of acetylcholine. To minimize the muscarinic cholinergic side effects, give atropine.

• Correct BP, electrolyte imbalance, or circulating blood volume by fluid and electrolyte therapy. Vasopressors can be used to correct hypotension due to ganglionic blockade.

**Drug Interactions:** The following drug interactions are for nondepolarizing skeletal muscle relaxants. See also succinylcholine.

*Aminoglycoside antibiotics* / Additive muscle relaxation, including prolonged respiratory depression

*Amphotericin B* / ↑ Muscle relaxation

*Anesthetics, inhalation* / Additive muscle relaxation

*Carbamazepine* / ↓ Duration or effect of muscle relaxants

*Clindamycin* / Additive muscle relaxation, including prolonged respiratory depression

*Colistin* / ↑ Muscle relaxation

*Corticosteroids* / ↓ Effect of muscle relaxants

*Furosemide* / ↑ or ↓ Effect of skeletal muscle relaxants (may be dose-related)

*Hydantoins* / ↓ Duration or effect of muscle relaxants

*Ketamine* / ↑ Muscle relaxation, including prolonged respiratory depression

*Lincomycin* / ↑ Muscle relaxation, including prolonged respiratory depression

*Lithium* / ↑ Recovery time of muscle relaxants → prolonged respiratory depression

*Magnesium salts* / ↑ Muscle relaxation, including prolonged respiratory depression

*Methotrimeprazine* / ↑ Muscle relaxation

*Narcotic analgesics* / ↑ Respiratory depression and ↑ muscle relaxation

*Nitrates* / ↑ Muscle relaxation, including prolonged respiratory depression

*Phenothiazines* / ↑ Muscle relaxation

*Pipercillin* / ↑ Muscle relaxation, including prolonged respiratory depression

*Polymyxin B* / ↑ Muscle relaxation

*Procainamide* / ↑ Muscle relaxation

*Procaine* / ↑ Muscle relaxation by ↓ plasma protein binding

*Quinidine* / ↑ Muscle relaxation

*Ranitidine* / Significant ↓ effect of muscle relaxants

*Theophyllines* / Reversal of effects of muscle relaxant (dose-dependent)

*Thiazide diuretics* / ↑ Muscle relaxation due to hypokalemia

*Verapamil* / ↑ Muscle relaxation, including prolonged respiratory depression

**Dosage**
See individual drugs.

## NURSING CONSIDERATIONS
### Assessment
1. Document indications for therapy, desired outcome, and anticipated length of use.
2. Note age and condition; elderly and debilitated clients should not receive drugs in this category.
3. Monitor CBC, electrolytes, CXR, ECG, liver and renal function studies.
4. Note other drugs receiving. Clients requiring neuromuscular blocking agents are often receiving other drugs that may have the effect of prolonging client response to the prescribed neuromuscular blocking agent.
5. Question client concerning changes in vision, ability to chew or to move the fingers.
6. Note initial selective paralysis followed by paralysis in the following sequence: levator muscles of the eyelids, mastication muscles, limb muscles, abdominal muscles, glottis muscles, intercostal muscles, and the diaphragm muscles. Of note is that neuromuscular recovery occurs in the reverse order.

### Interventions
1. Drugs should only be administered in a closely monitored envi-

ronment and generally used only when intubated.

2. Prevent overdosage during infusions by frequent evaluations (q 4 hr) with a peripheral nerve stimulator or by allowing partial return of muscle function.

3. Monitor BP and pulse frequently and respirations and pulmonary status continuously. Cardiac monitor and ventilator alarms should be set and checked frequently.

4. Observe for excessive bronchial secretions or respiratory wheezing; suction to maintain patent airway (ET tube).

5. Perform frequent neurovascular assessments. Prolonged use of neuromuscular blocking agents may cause profound weakness and even paralysis; may precipitate an acute myopathy in some individuals.

6. Observe for drug interactions which may potentiate muscular relaxation and prove fatal.

7. Consciousness and pain thresholds are not affected by neuromuscular blocking agents; clients can still hear, feel, and see while receiving these agents. Avoid any discussions that should not be overheard. Adequate anesthesia and analgesics should be administered for pain or when painful procedures are necessary.

8. Clients requiring prolonged ventilatory therapy should be adequately sedated with analgesics and benzodiazepines. Anxiety levels may be very high, but client cannot communicate this.

9. Administer eye drops and eye patches to protect corneas during prolonged therapy. Explain to client and family why this is done (i.e., because the blink reflex has been suppressed).

10. Avoid use of corticosteroids during prolonged neuromuscular blockade unless benefits outweigh the risks.

11. Perform passive range of motion to prevent loss of function and contractures with prolonged therapy.

**Outcomes/Evaluate**
• Desired level of skeletal muscle paralysis
• Insertion of ET tube/tolerance of mechanical ventilation
• Suppression of twitch response

# NONSTEROIDAL ANTI-INFLAMMATORY DRUGS

*See also the following individual entries:*

> Auranofin
> Aurothioglucose suspension
> Diclofenac potassium
> Diclofenac sodium
> Diflunisal
> Etodolac
> Fenoprofen calcium
> Flurbiprofen
> Flurbiprofen sodium
> Gold sodium thromalate
> Ibuprofen
> Indomethacin
> Indomethacin sodium trihydrate
> Ketoprofen
> Ketorolac tromethamine
> Meclofenamate sodium
> Mefenamic acid
> Nabumetone
> Naproxen
> Naproxen sodium
> Oxaprozin
> Piroxicam
> Sulindac
> Suprofen
> Tolmetin sodium

**Action/Kinetics:** The anti-inflammatory effect is believed to result from the inhibition of the enzyme cyclooxygenase, resulting in decreased prostaglandin synthesis. The agents are effective in reducing joint swelling, pain, and morning stiffness, as well as in increasing mobility in individuals with inflammatory disease. They do not alter the course of the disease, however. Their anti-inflammatory activity is comparable to that of aspirin. The analgesic activity is due, in part, to relief of inflammation. Also, the drugs may inhibit lipoxygenase, inhibit synthesis of leukotrienes, inhibit release of lysosomal enzymes, and inhibit neutrophil aggregation. Rheumatoid factor production may also be inhibited. The antipyretic action occurs by decreasing prostaglandin synthesis in the hypothalamus, resulting in an increase in peripheral blood flow and heat loss as well as promoting sweating. NSAIDs also inhibit miosis induced by prostaglandins during the course of cataract surgery; thus, these drugs are useful for a number of ophthalmic inflammatory conditions.

The NSAIDs differ from one another with respect to their rate of absorption, length of action, anti-inflammatory activity, and effect on the GI mucosa. Most are rapidly and completely absorbed from the GI tract; food delays the rate, but not the total amount, of drug absorbed. These drugs are metabolized in the kidney and are excreted through the urine, mainly as metabolites.

**Uses:** See individual drugs. Generally are used to treat inflammatory disease, including rheumatoid arthritis, osteoarthritis, ankylosing spondylitis, gout, and other musculoskeletal diseases. Treatment of nonrheumatic inflammatory conditions including bursitis, acute painful shoulder, synovitis, tendinitis, or tenosynovitis. Mild to moderate pain including primary dysmenorrhea, episiotomy pain, strains and sprains, postextraction dental pain. Primary dysmenorrhea. Ophthalmically to inhibit intraoperative miosis, for postoperative inflammation after cataract surgery, and for relief of ocular itching due to seasonal allergic conjunctivitis.

**Contraindications:** Most for children under 14 years of age. Lactation. Individuals in whom aspirin, NSAIDs, or iodides have caused hypersensitivity, including acute asthma, rhinitis, urticaria, nasal polyps, bronchospasm, angioedema or other symptoms of allergy or anaphylaxis.

**Special Concerns:** Clients intolerant to one of the NSAIDs may be intolerant to others in this group. Use with caution in clients with a history of GI disease, reduced renal function, in geriatric clients, in clients with intrinsic coagulation defects or those on anticoagulant therapy, in compromised cardiac function, in hypertension, in conditions predisposing to fluid retention, and in the presence of existing controlled infection. The safety and efficacy of most NSAIDs have not been determined in children or in functional class IV rheumatoid arthritis (i.e., clients incapacitated, bedridden, or confined to a wheelchair).

**Side Effects:** *GI (most common):* Peptic or duodenal ulceration and GI bleeding, intestinal ulceration with obstruction and stenosis, reactivation of preexisting ulcers. Heartburn, dyspepsia, N&V, anorexia, diarrhea, constipation, increased or decreased appetite, indigestion, stomatitis, epigastric pain, abdominal cramps or pain, gastroenteritis, paralytic ileus, salivation, dry mouth, glossitis, pyrosis, icterus, rectal irritation, gingival ulcer, occult blood in stool, hematemesis, gastritis, proctitis, eructation, sore or dry mucous membranes, ulcerative colitis, rectal bleeding, melena, *perforation and hemorrhage of esophagus, stomach, duodenum, small or large intestine.* *CNS:* Dizziness, drowsiness, vertigo, headaches, nervousness, migraine, anxiety, mental confusion, aggravation of parkinsonism and epilepsy, lightheadedness, paresthesia, peripheral neuropathy, akathisia, excitation, tremor, *seizures,* myalgia, asthenia, malaise, insomnia, fatigue, drowsiness, confusion, emotional lability, depression, inability to concentrate, psychoses, hallucinations, depersonalization, amnesia, *coma,* syncope. *CV:* CHF, hypotension, hypertension, arrhythmias, peripheral edema and fluid retention, vasodilation, exacerbation of angiitis, palpitations, tachycardia, chest pain, sinus bradycardia, peripheral vascular disease, peripheral edema. *Respiratory:* **Bronchospasm, laryngeal edema,** rhinitis, dyspnea, pharyngitis, hemoptysis, SOB, eosinophilic pneumonitis. *Hematologic:* Bone marrow depression, neutropenia, leukopenia, pancytopenia, eosinophila, thrombocytopenia, granulocytopenia, **agranulocytosis, aplastic anemia, hemolytic anemia,** decreased H&H, hypocoagulability, epistaxis. *Ophthalmologic:* Amblyopia, visual disturbances, corneal deposits, retinal hemorrhage, scotomata, retinal pigmentation changes or degeneration, blurred vision, photophobia, diplopia, iritis, loss of color vision (reversible), optic neuritis, cataracts, swollen, dry, or irritated eyes. *Dermatologic:* Pruritus, skin eruptions, sweating, erythema, eczema, hyperpigmentation, ecchymoses, petechiae, rashes, urticaria, purpura, onycholysis, vesiculobullous eruptions, cutaneous vasculitis, **toxic epidermal necrolysis, angioneurotic edema,** erythema nodosum, **Stevens-Johnson syndrome,** exfoliative dermatitis, photosensitivity, alopecia, skin irritation, peeling, erythema multiforme, desquamation, skin discoloration. *GU:* Menometrorrhagia, menorrhagia, impotence, menstrual disorders, hematuria, cystitis, azotemia, nocturia, proteinuria, UTIs, polyuria, dysuria, urinary frequency, oliguria, pyuria, anuria, renal insufficiency, nephrosis, nephrotic syndrome, glomerular and interstitial nephritis, urinary casts, acute renal failure in clients with impaired renal function, renal papillary necrosis *Metabolic:* Hyperglycemia, hypoglycemia, glycosuria, hyperkalemia, hyponatremia, diabetes mellitus. *Other:* Tinnitus, hearing loss or disturbances, ear pain, deafness, metallic or bitter taste in mouth, thirst, chills, fever, flushing, jaundice, sweating, breast changes, gynecomastia, muscle cramps, dyspnea, involuntary muscle movements, muscle weakness, facial edema, pain, serum sickness, aseptic meningitis, hypersensitivity reactions including asthma, acute respiratory distress, *shock-like syndrome, angioedema,* angiitis, dyspnea, *anaphylaxis.*

*Following ophthalmic use:* Transient burning and stinging upon installation, ocular irritation.

**OD   Overdose Management:** *Symptoms:* CNS symptoms include dizziness, drowsiness, mental confusion, lethargy, disorientation, intense headache, paresthesia, and *seizures.* GI symptoms include N&V, gastric irritation, and abdominal pain. Miscellaneous symptoms include tinnitus, sweating, blurred vision, increased serum creatinine and BUN, and acute renal failure. *Treatment:* There are no antidotes; treatment includes general supportive measures. Since the drugs are acidic, it may be beneficial to alkalinize the urine and induce diuresis to hasten excretion.

**Drug Interactions:**
*Anticoagulants* / Concomitant use results in ↑ PT
*Aspirin* / ↓ Effect of NSAIDs due to ↓ blood levels; also, ↑ risk of adverse GI effects
*Beta-adrenergic blocking agents* / ↓ Antihypertensive effect of blocking agents
*Cimetidine* / ↑ or ↓ Plasma levels of NSAIDs
*Cyclosporine* / ↑ Risk of nephrotoxicity
*Lithium* / ↑ Serum lithium levels
*Loop diuretics* / ↓ Effect of loop diuretics
*Methotrexate* / ↑ Risk of methotrexate toxicity (i.e., bone marrow suppression, nephrotoxicity, stomatitis)
*Phenobarbital* / ↓ Effect of NSAIDs due to ↑ breakdown by liver
*Phenytoin* / ↑ Effect of phenytoin due to ↓ plasma protein binding
*Probenecid* / ↑ Effect of NSAIDs due to ↑ plasma levels
*Salicylates* / Plasma levels of NSAIDs may be ↓ ; also, ↑ risk of GI side effects
*Sulfonamides* / ↑ Effect of sulfonamides due to ↓ plasma protein binding
*Sulfonylureas* / ↑ Effect of sulfonylureas due to ↓ plasma protein binding

**Dosage**
See individual drugs.

## NURSING CONSIDERATIONS
### Administration/Storage
1. Do not take alcohol or aspirin together with NSAIDs.
2. Should GI upset occur, take with food, milk, or antacids.
3. NSAIDs may have an additive analgesic effect when administered with narcotic analgesics, thus permitting lower narcotic dosages.
4. Clients who do not respond clinically to one NSAID may respond to another.
### Assessment
1. Note any allergic responses to aspirin or any other anti-inflammatory agents.
2. Document indications for therapy, type, onset, and characteristics of symptoms.
3. Note location, intensity, and type of pain experienced. Assess joint mobility and ROM.
4. Review indications and dosage prescribed. For anti-inflammatory effects, high doses are required whereas analgesia and pain relief may be achieved with much lower dosages. Identify clients that may require gastric protective benefits of Cytotec.
5. Determine any asthma or nasal polyps; may be exacerbated by NSAIDs.
6. Note age. Children under 14 years of age generally should not receive drugs in this category.
7. Monitor CBC, liver and renal function studies. These agents cause platelet inhibition which is reversible in 24–48 hr, whereas aspirin requires 4–5 days to reverse its antiplatelet effects.
### Client/Family Teaching
1. Take NSAIDs with a full glass of water or milk, with meals, or with a prescribed antacid and remain upright 30 min following administration to reduce gastric irritation or ulcer formation.
2. Consume large quantities of water (2–3 L/day) during therapy.
3. Report any changes in stool consistency or symptoms of GI irritation not relieved by adhering to the prescribed protocol. Sustained GI effects may need to be managed with misoprostol.
4. Regular intake of drug is necessary to sustain anti-inflammatory effects. If desired response not obtained, another drug in this class may provide the desired response.
5. Report any episodes of bleeding, blurred vision or other eye symptoms, tinnitus, skin rashes, purpura, weight gain or edema as well as decreased urine output, fever, or increased joint pain.
6. Use caution in operating machinery or in driving a car; may cause dizziness or drowsiness.
7. Avoid alcohol, aspirin, acetaminophen, and any other OTC preparations without approval because of increased risk for GI bleeding.
8. If diabetic, be aware of hypoglycemic effect of NSAIDs on hypoglycemic agents; dosage of agent and NSAID may need to be adjusted.
9. Record weights periodically and report any significant changes. NSAIDs cause Na and water retention; avoid with chronic heart failure.
10. Notify all providers of the medication being taken to avoid having prescriptions written for drugs that would interact unfavorably with NSAIDs.
### Outcomes/Evaluate
- ↑ Joint mobility and ROM
- ↓ Discomfort and pain
- Improvement in pretreatment symptoms

# OPHTHALMIC CHOLINERGIC (MIOTIC) AGENTS

*See also the following individual entries:*

Physostigmine salicylate
Physostigmine sulfate
Pilocarpine hydrochloride
Pilocarpine nitrate
Pilocarpine ocular therapeutic
    system

**Action/Kinetics:** The ophthalmic cholinergic drugs fall into two classes: direct-acting (carbachol, pilocarpine) and indirect-acting (demecarium, echothiophate, isoflurophate, neostigmine, physostigmine), which inhibit the enzyme acetylcholinesterase. In the treatment of glaucoma, the drugs lead to an accumulation of acetylcholine, which stimulates the ciliary muscles and increases contraction of the iris sphincter muscle. This opens the angle of the eye and results in increased outflow of aqueous humor and consequently in a decrease of intraocular pressure. This effect is of particular importance in narrow-angle glaucoma. The drugs also cause spasms of accommodation.

**Uses:** See individual drugs.

**Contraindications:** *Direct-acting drugs:* Inflammatory eye disease (iritis), asthma, hypertension. *Indirect-acting drugs:* Same as for *direct-acting drugs,* as well as acute-angle glaucoma, history of retinal detachment, ocular hypotension accompanied by intraocular inflammatory processes, intestinal or urinary obstruction, peptic ulcer, epilepsy, parkinsonism, spastic GI conditions, vasomotor instability, severe bradycardia or hypotension, and recent MIs. Lactation.

**Side Effects:** *Local:* Painful contraction of ciliary muscle, pain in eye, blurred vision, spasms of accommodation, darkened vision, failure to accommodate to darkness, twitching, headaches, painful brow. Most of these symptoms lessen with prolonged usage. Iris cysts and retinal detachment (indirect-acting drugs only).

*Systemic:* Systemic absorption of drug may cause nausea, GI discomfort, diarrhea, hypotension, bronchial constriction, and increased salivation.

**Dosage**

See individual drugs.

## NURSING CONSIDERATIONS

**Administration:** Have epinephrine and atropine available for emergency treatment of increased intraocular pressure.

**Assessment**

1. Document indications for therapy, onset and characteristics of symptoms. List other agents prescribed and the outcome.
2. Document complete fundoscopic exam.
3. Review list of drugs and existing medical conditions that may preclude drug therapy to ensure that none are present.
4. Carefully monitor geriatric clients.
5. Hourly tonometric measurements are recommended during initiation of therapy.
6. Assess for redness around the cornea. Epinephrine or phenylephrine hydrochloride (10%) may be ordered with demecarium bromide, echothiophate iodide, or isoflurophate to minimize this kind of reaction.

**Client/Family Teaching**

1. Review why prescribed and the importance of compliance in order to maintain vision by reducing intraocular pressures.
2. Wash hands before and after therapy. Review appropriate method for instilling eye drops or ointment and frequency and duration of therapy.
3. Take eye drops exactly as prescribed. Minimize side effects by taking at least one dose of medication at bedtime.
4. To prevent overflow of solution into the nasopharynx after topical instillation of drops, exert pressure on the nasolacrimal duct for 1–2 min before closing the eyelids.
5. Do not drive for 1–2 hr after instilling cholinergic agents. Night vision may also be impaired.
6. Pain and blurred vision may occur;

should diminish with continued use of the drug.

7. Report any changes in vision, eye irritation, or evidence of severe headaches.

8. Painful eye spasms may be relieved by applying cold compresses.

9. Report for eye exams as scheduled and refill prescriptions as needed.

**Outcomes/Evaluate**

• Improved visual fields and tonometric measurements

• ↓ Intraocular pressures

# ORAL CONTRACEPTIVES: ESTROGEN-PROGESTERONE COMBINATIONS

*See Table 1.*

**General Statement:** There are three types of combination (i.e., both an estrogen and progestin in each tablet) oral contraceptives: (1) monophasic—contain the same amount of estrogen and progestin in each tablet; (2) biphasic—contain the same amount of estrogen in each tablet but the progestin content is lower for the first part of the cycle and higher for the last part of the cycle; (3) triphasic—the estrogen content may be the same or may vary throughout the medication cycle; the progestin content may be the same or varies, depending on the part of the cycle. The purpose of the biphasic and triphasic products is to provide hormones in a manner similar to that occurring physiologically. This is said to decrease breakthrough bleeding during the medication cycle. The other type of oral contraceptive is the progestin-only ("mini-pill") product, which contains a small amount of a progestin in each tablet.

**Action/Kinetics:** The combination oral contraceptives act by inhibiting ovulation due to an inhibition (through negative-feedback mechanism) of LH and FSH, which are required for development of ova. These products also alter the cervical mucus so that it is not conducive to sperm penetration, render the endometrium less suitable for implantation of the blastocyst should fertilization occur, and inhibit enzymes required by sperm to enter the ovum.

The estrogen used in combination oral contraceptives is either ethinyl estradiol or mestranol. Mestranol is demethylated to ethinyl estradiol in the liver. **t½:** 6–20 hr. The progestin used in combination oral contraceptives is either desogestrel, ethynodiol diacetate, levonorgestrel, norethindrone, norethindrone acetate, norgestimate, or norgestrel.

The progestin-only products do not consistently inhibit ovulation. However, these products also alter the cervical mucus and render the endometrium unsuitable for implantation. These products contain either norethindrone or norgestrel. This method of contraception is less reliable than combination therapy.

Although oral contraceptives may be associated with serious side effects, a number of noncontraceptive health benefits have been confirmed. These include increased regularity of the menstrual cycle, decreased incidence of dysmenorrhea, decreased blood loss, decreased incidence of functional ovarian cysts and ectopic pregnancies, and decreased incidence of diseases such as fibroadenomas, fibrocystic disease, acute pelvic inflammatory disease, endometrial cancer, and ovarian cancer.

**Uses:** Contraception, menstrual irregularities, menopausal symptoms. High doses are used for endometriosis and hypermenorrhea. *Investigational:* High doses of Ovral (ethinyl estradiol and norgestrel) have been used as a postcoital contraceptive.

**Contraindications:** Thrombophlebitis, history of deep-vein

---

**Table 1    Combination Oral Contraceptive Preparations Available in the United States**

| Trade Name | Estrogen | Progestin |
|---|---|---|
| | **MONOPHASIC** | |
| Alesse 21-Day and 28-Day | Ethinyl estradiol (20 mcg) | Levonorgestrel (0.1 mg) |
| Brevicon 21-Day and 28-Day | Ethinyl estradiol (35 mcg) | Norethindrone (0.5 mg) |
| Demulen 1/35–21 and 1/35–28 | Ethinyl estradiol (35 mcg) | Ethynodiol diacetate (1 mg) |
| Demulen 1/50–21 and 1/50–28 | Ethinyl estradiol (50 mcg) | Ethynodiol diacetate (1 mg) |
| Desogen (28 day) | Ethinyl estradiol (30 mcg) | Desogestrel (0.15 mg) |
| Genora 0.5/35 21 Day and 28 Day | Ethinyl estradiol (35 mcg) | Norethindrone (0.5 mg) |
| Genora 1/35 21 Day and 28 Day | Ethinyl estradiol (35 mcg) | Norethindrone (1 mg) |
| Genora 1/50 21 Day and 28 Day | Mestranol (50 mcg) | Norethindrone (1 mg) |
| Levlen 21 and 28 | Ethinyl estradiol (30 mcg) | Levonorgestrel (0.15 mg) |
| Levora 0.15/30-21 and -28 | Ethinyl estradiol (30 mcg) | Levonorgestrel (0.15 mg) |
| Loestrin 21 1/20 | Ethinyl estradiol (20 mcg) | Norethindrone acetate (1 mg) |
| Loestrin 21 1.5/30 | Ethinyl estradiol (30 mcg) | Norethindrone acetate (1.5 mg) |
| Loestrin Fe 1/20 (28 day) | Ethinyl estradiol (20 mcg) | Norethindrone acetate (1 mg) |
| Loestrin Fe 1.5/30 (28 day) | Ethinyl estradiol (30 mcg) | Norethindrone acetate (1.5 mg) |
| Lo/Ovral-21 and -28 | Ethinyl estradiol (30 mcg) | Norgestrel (0.3 mg) |
| Modicon 21 and 28 | Ethinyl estradiol (35 mcg) | Norethindrone (0.5 mg) |
| Necon 0.5/35-21 Day and 28 Day | Ethinyl estradiol (35 mcg) | Norethindrone (0.5 mg) |
| Necon 1/35-21 Day and 28 Day | Ethinyl estradiol (35 mcg) | Norethindrone (1 mg) |
| Necon 1/50-21 Day and 28 Day | Mestranol (50 mcg) | Norethindrone (1 mg) |
| N.E.E. 1/35 21 Day and 28 Day | Ethinyl estradiol (35 mcg) | Norethindrone (1 mg) |
| Nelova 0.5/35E 21 Day and 28 Day | Ethinyl estradiol (35 mcg) | Norethindrone (0.5 mg) |
| Nelova 1/35E 21 Day and 28 Day | Ethinyl estradiol (35 mcg) | Norethindrone (1 mg) |
| Nelova 1/50M 21 Day and 28 Day | Mestranol (50 mcg) | Norethindrone (1 mg) |
| Neocon 0.5/35-21 Day and -28 Day | Ethinyl estradiol (35 mcg) | Norethindrone (0.5 mg) |
| Neocon 1/35-21 Day and -28 Day | Ethinyl estradiol (35 mcg) | Norethindrone (1 mg) |
| Neocon 1/50-21 Day and -28 Day | Ethinyl estradiol (50 mcg) | Norethindrone (1 mg) |
| Nordette-21 and -28 | Ethinyl estradiol (30 mcg) | Levonorgestrel (0.15 mg) |

| Trade Name | Estrogen | Progestin |
|---|---|---|
| | **MONOPHASIC** | |
| Norethin 1/35E 21 Day and 28 Day | Ethinyl estradiol (35 mcg) | Norethindrone (1 mg) |
| Norethin 1/50M 21 Day and 28 Day | Mestranol (50 mcg) | Norethindrone (1 mg) |
| Norinyl 1 + 35 21-Day and 28-Day | Ethinyl estradiol (35 mcg) | Norethindrone (1 mg) |
| Norinyl 1 + 50 21-Day and 28-Day | Mestranol (50 mcg) | Norethindrone (1 mg) |
| Norlestrin 1/50 21 Day and 28 Day | Ethinyl estradiol (50 mcg) | Norethindrone (1 mg) |
| Norlestrin 2.5/50 21 Day and 28 Day | Ethinyl estradiol (50 mcg) | Norethindrone (2.5 mg) |
| Ortho-Cept 21 Day and 28 Day | Ethinyl estradiol (30 mcg) | Desogestrel (0.15 mg) |
| Ortho-Cyclen–21 and –28 | Ethinyl estradiol (35 mcg) | Norgestimate (0.25 mg) |
| Ortho Novum 1/35–21 and –28 | Ethinyl estradiol (35 mcg) | Norethindrone (1 mg) |
| Ortho Novum 1/50–21 and –28 | Mestranol (50 mcg) | Norethindrone (1 mg) |
| Ovcon-35 21 Day and 28 Day | Ethinyl estradiol (35 mcg) | Norethindrone (0.4 mg) |
| Ovcon-50 21 Day and 28 Day | Ethinyl estradiol (50 mcg) | Norethindrone (1 mg) |
| Ovral 21 Day and 28 Day | Ethinyl estradiol (50 mcg) | Norgestrel (0.5 mg) |
| Zovia 1/35E-21 and -28 | Ethinyl estradiol (35 mcg) | Ethynodiol diacetate (1 mg) |
| Zovia 1/50E-21 and -28 | Ethinyl estradiol (50 mcg) | Ethynodiol diacetate (1 mg) |
| | **BIPHASIC** | |
| Jenest-28 | Ethinyl estradiol (35 mcg in each tablet) | Norethindrone (10 tablets of 0.5 mg followed by 11 tablets of 1 mg) |
| Necon 10/11 21 Day and 28 Day | Ethinyl estradiol (35 mcg in each tablet) | Norethindrone (10 tablets of 0.5 mg followed by 11 tablets of 1 mg) |
| Nelova 10/11–21 and –28 | Ethinyl estradiol (35 mcg in each tablet) | Norethindrone (10 tablets of 0.5 mg followed by 11 tablets of 1 mg) |
| Necon 10/11–21 and –28 | Ethinyl estradiol (35 mcg in each tablet) | Norethindrone (10 tablets of 0.5 mg followed by 11 tablets of 1 mg) |
| Ortho-Novum 10/11–21 and –28 | Ethinyl estradiol (35 mcg in each tablet) | Norethindrone (10 tablets of 0.5 mg followed by 11 tablets of 1 mg) |

✿ = Available in Canada                    ***bold italic*** = life threatening side effect

**Table 1**  *(continued)*

| Trade Name | Estrogen | Progestin |
|---|---|---|
| | **TRIPHASIC** | |
| Estrostep (21 or 28 days) | Ethinyl estradiol (20, 30, and 35 mcg) | Norethindrone (1 mg in each tablet) |
| Ortho-Novum 7/7/7 (21 or 28 days) | Ethinyl estradiol (35 mcg in each tablet) | Norethindrone (0.5 mg the first 7 days, 0.75 the next 7 days, and 1 mg the last 7 days) |
| Ortho-Tri-Cyclen (21 or 28 days) | Ethinyl estradiol (35 mcg in each tablet) | Norgestimate (0.18 mg the first 7 days, 0.215 mg the next 7 days, and 0.25 mg the last seven days) |
| Tri-Levlen 21 Day and | First 6 days: Ethinyl estradiol (30 mcg) | Levonorgestrel (0.05 mg) |
| Tri-Levlen 28 Day | Next 5 days: Ethinyl estradiol (40 mcg)<br>Last 10 days: Ethinyl estradiol (30 mcg) | Levonorgestrel (0.075 mg)<br>Levonorgestrel (0.125 mg) |
| Tri-Norinyl (21 or 28 day) | Ethinyl estradiol (35 mcg in each tablet) | Norethindrone (0.5 mg the first 7 days, 1 mg the next 9 days, and 0.5 mg the last 5 days) |
| Triphasil 21 (21 or 28 day) | First 6 days: Ethinyl estradiol (30 mcg)<br>Next 5 days: Ethinyl estradiol (40 mcg)<br>Last 10 days: Ethinyl estradiol (30 mcg) | Levonorgestrel (0.05 mg)<br>Levonorgestrel (0.075 mg)<br>Levonorgestrel (0.125 mg) |

All combination oral contraceptives are Rx and Pregnancy category: X.

thrombophlebitis, thromboembolic disorders, cerebral vascular disease, CAD, MI, current or past angina, known or suspected breast cancer or estrogen-dependent neoplasm, endometrial carcinoma, hepatic adenoma or carcinoma, undiagnosed abnormal genital bleeding, known or suspected pregnancy, cholestatic jaundice of pregnancy. Smoking.

**Special Concerns:** Cigarette smoking increases the risk of cardiovascular side effects from use of oral contraceptives. Low estrogen-containing oral contraceptives do not increase the risk of stroke in women. Use with caution in clients with a history of hypertension, preexisting renal disease, hypertension-related diseases during pregnancy, familial tendency to hypertension or its consequences, a history of excessive weight gain or fluid retention during the menstrual cycle; these individuals are more likely to develop elevated BP. Use with caution in clients with asthma, epilepsy, migraine, diabetes, metabolic bone disease, renal or cardiac disease, and a history of mental depression. Use with drugs (e.g., barbiturates, hydantoins, rifampin) that increase the hepatic metabolism of oral contraceptives may result in breakthrough bleeding and an increased risk of pregnancy. Use combination products during lactation only if absolutely necessary; progestin-only products do not appear to have any adverse effects on breastfeeding performance or on the health, growth, or development of the infant.

**Side Effects:** The oral contraceptives have wide-ranging effects. These are particularly important, since the drugs may be given for several years to healthy women. Many authorities have voiced concern about the long-term safety of these agents. Some advise discontinuing therapy after 18–24 months of continuous use. The majority of side effects of oral contraceptives are due to the estrogen component. *CV:* **MI, thrombophlebitis, venous thrombosis with or without embolism, pulmonary embolism, coronary thrombosis, cerebral thrombosis, arterial thromboembolism, mesenteric thrombosis, thrombotic and hemorrhagic strokes, postsurgical thromboembolism, subarachnoid hemorrhage,** elevated BP, hypertension. *CNS:* Onset or exacerbation of migraine headaches, depression. *GI:* N&V, bloating, abdominal cramps. *Ophthalmic:* Optic neuritis, retinal thrombosis, steepening of the corneal curvature, contact lens intolerance. *Hepatic:* **Benign and malignant hepatic adenomas,** focal nodular hyperplasia, **hepatocellular carcinoma,** gallbladder disease, cholestatic jaundice. *GU:* Breakthrough bleeding, spotting, amenorrhea, change in menstrual flow, change in cervical erosion and cervical secretions, **invasive cervical cancer,** bleeding irregularities (more common with progestin-only products), vaginal candidiasis, **ectopic pregnancies in contraceptive failures,** breast tenderness, breast enlargement. *Miscellaneous:* Acute intermittent porphyria, photosensitivity, congenital anomalies, melasma, skin rash, edema, increase or decrease in weight, decreased carbohydrate tolerance, increased incidence of cervical *Chlamydia trachomatis,* decrease in the quantity and quality of breast milk.

**Drug Interactions**
*Acetaminophen* / ↓ Effect of acetaminophen due to ↑ breakdown by liver
*Anticoagulants, oral* / ↓ Effect of anticoagulants by ↑ levels of certain clotting factors (however, an ↑ effect of anticoagulants has also been noted in some clients)
*Antidepressants, tricyclic* / ↑ Effect of antidepressants due to ↓ breakdown by liver
*Benzodiazepines* / ↑ or ↓ Effect of benzodiazepines due to changes in breakdown by liver

*Beta-adrenergic blockers* / ↑ Effect of beta blockers due to ↓ breakdown by liver

*Carbamazepine* / ↓ Effect of oral contraceptives due to ↑ breakdown by liver

*Corticosteroids* / ↑ Effect of corticosteroids due to ↓ breakdown by liver

*Erythromycins* / ↓ Effect of oral contraceptives due to altered enterohepatic absorption

*Griseofulvin* / May ↓ effect of oral contraceptives due to ↑ breakdown

*Hypoglycemics* / Oral contraceptives ↓ effect of hypoglycemics due to their effect on carbohydrate metabolism

*Insulin* / Oral contraceptives may ↑ insulin requirements

*Penicillins, oral* / ↓ Effect of oral contraceptives due to altered enterohepatic absorption

*Phenobarbital* / ↓ Effect of oral contraceptives due to ↑ breakdown by liver

*Phenytoin* / ↓ Effect of oral contraceptives due to ↑ breakdown by liver

*Rifampin* / ↓ Effect of contraceptives due to ↑ breakdown by liver

*Tetracyclines* / ↓ Effect of contraceptives due to altered enterohepatic absorption

*Theophyllines* / ↑ Effect of theophyllines due to ↓ breakdown by liver

*Troleandomycin* / ↑ Chance of jaundice

**Laboratory Test Interferences:** Altered liver and thyroid function tests. ↓ PT, 17-hydroxycorticosteroids, 17-ketosteroids, and 17-ketogenic steroids. ↑ Factors I (prothrombin), VII, VIII, IX, and X. (Therapy with ovarian hormones should be discontinued 60 days before performance of laboratory tests.) ↑ Gamma globulins.

**Dosage** ————————
See *Administration/Storage*.

## NURSING CONSIDERATIONS

See also *Nursing Considerations* for

*Estrogens,* and *Progesterone and Progestins.*

**Administration/Storage**

1. Take tablets at approximately the same time each day (e.g., with a meal or at bedtime).

2. Spotting or breakthrough bleeding may occur for the first 1–2 cycles; if it continues past this time, consult provider.

3. For the initial cycle, an **additional** form of contraception should be used for the first week.

4. The type of oral contraceptive preparation will determine the precise manner in which the drug is taken:

• For the 21-day regimen, 1 tablet is taken daily beginning on day 5 of menses (day 1 is the first day of menstrual flow). No tablets are taken for 7 days.

• For a 28-day regimen, hormone-containing tablets are taken for the first 21 days, followed by 7 days of inert or iron-containing tablets.

• Certain products, including the biphasic and selected triphasic oral contraceptives, are termed *Sunday start.* The first tablet should be taken the Sunday following the beginning of menses (if menses begins on Sunday, the first tablet should be taken that day). *NOTE:* The biphasic and triphasic products have varying amounts of estrogen and/or progestin, depending on the stage of the cycle; the client should understand fully how these preparations are to be taken and which tablets are to be taken at various times during the medication cycle. Often tablets are different shapes and/or colors to help with compliance.

• For progestin-only products, the first tablet is taken on the first day of menses; thereafter, 1 tablet is taken every day of the year.

5. It is recommended that for a woman beginning combination oral contraceptive therapy a product be chosen that contains the least amount of estrogen for that particular client.

6. If it is necessary to switch brands of oral contraceptives, wait 7 days to start the new pack if on a 21-day

regimen or the day after the last tablet if on a 28-day regimen.

7. Non-nursing mothers may begin oral contraceptive therapy at the first postpartum exam (i.e., 4–6 weeks), regardless of whether spontaneous menstruation has occurred. Nursing mothers should not take oral contraceptives until the infant has been weaned.

**Assessment**

1. Document annual physical and internal examinations and Pap smears.
2. Note any previous experience with these agents and the results.
3. Note any family history of breast or uterine cancer or any existing medical condition that may preclude this drug therapy; procure smoking history.

**Client/Family Teaching**

1. Take the tablets exactly as prescribed to prevent pregnancy.
2. If 1 tablet is missed, take as soon as remembered.
3. If 2 tablets have been missed, the dosage must be doubled for the next 2 consecutive days. The regular schedule may then be resumed; use additional contraceptive measures for the remainder of the cycle.
4. If 3 tablets are missed, discontinue the therapy and start a new course as indicated by the type of medication. Alternative contraceptive measures should be used when the tablets are not taken and should be continued for 7 days after a new course has been started.
5. Report any missed menstrual periods. If two consecutive periods are missed, discontinue the therapy until pregnancy has been ruled out.
6. Provide a written list of symptoms that require immediate reporting. If pain in the legs or chest, respiratory distress, an unexplained cough, severe headaches, dizziness, or blurred vision occurs, stop therapy and notify provider immediately.
7. Symptoms of eye pathology, such as headaches, dizziness, blurred vi-

sion, or partial loss of sight, should also be reported immediately.

8. Oral contraceptives decrease the viscosity of cervical mucus, increasing the susceptibility to vaginal infections. These are difficult to treat successfully; therefore, good hygienic practice is essential.
9. If persistent nausea, edema, and skin eruptions develop and last beyond the four cycles, consult with provider for a dose adjustment or for a different combination.
10. Alterations in thought processes, depression, or fatigue should be reported; a preparation with less progesterone activity may be indicated.
11. Androgenic effects, such as weight gain, increased oiliness of the skin, acne, or hirsutism, should also be reported because a change in medication or dosage may be necessary.
12. Do not take tablets longer than 18 months without medical consultation. Report for yearly Pap smear and physical examination; perform BSE (1 week after or 2 weeks before menstrual cycle).
13. Practice another form of contraception if receiving ampicillin, anticonvulsants, phenylbutazone, rifampin, or tetracycline. These may cause intermittent bleeding and the drug interactions could result in an unwanted pregnancy.
14. Contraceptives interfere with the elimination of caffeine. Limit caffeine consumption to prevent insomnia, irritability, tremors, and cardiac irregularities.
15. If breast-feeding infant, another form of contraception should be used until lactation is well established.
16. **Do not smoke.** Attend formal smoking cessation program if unable to quit.
17. Oral contraceptives do not provide any protection against STDs; use appropriate barrier protection with intercourse.

---

✿ = Available in Canada          ***bold italic*** = life threatening side effect

**Outcomes/Evaluate**
- Effective contraception
- Menstrual regularity
- ↓ Menstrual blood loss resulting from hormone imbalances

---

# PENICILLINS

*See also the following individual entries:*

Amoxicillin
Amoxicillin and Potassium clavulanate
Ampicillin oral
Ampicillin sodium parenteral
Ampicillin sodium/Sulbactam sodium
Bacampicillin hydrochloride
Carbenicillin indanyl sodium
Cloxacillin sodium
Dicloxacillin sodium
Methicillin sodium
Mezlocillin sodium
Nafcillin sodium
Oxacillin sodium
Penicillin G, sodium for injection
Penicillin G benzathine and procaine combined
Penicillin G benzathine, parenteral
Penicillin G potassium for injection
Penicillin G procaine suspension, sterile
Penicillin V potassium
Piperacillin sodium
Piperacillin sodium and Tazobactam sodium
Ticarcillin disodium
Ticarcillin disodium and Clavulanate potassium

**Action/Kinetics:** The bactericidal action of penicillins depends on their ability to bind penicillin-binding proteins (PBP-1 and PBP-3) in the cytoplasmic membranes of bacteria, thus inhibiting cell wall synthesis. Some penicillins act by acylation of membrane-bound transpeptidase enzymes, thereby preventing cross-linkage of peptidoglycan chains, which are necessary for bacterial cell wall strength and rigidity. Cell division and growth are inhibited and often ly-sis and elongation of susceptible bacteria occur. Penicillin is most effective against young, rapidly dividing organisms and has little effect on mature resting cells. Depending on the concentration of the drug at the site of infection and the susceptibility of the infectious microorganism, penicillin is either bacteriostatic or bactericidal. Penicillins are distributed throughout most of the body and pass the placental barrier. They also pass into synovial, pleural, pericardial, peritoneal, ascitic, and spinal fluids. Although normal meninges and the eyes are relatively impermeable to penicillins, they are better absorbed by inflamed meninges and eyes. **Peak serum levels, after PO:** 1 hr. **t½:** 30–110 min; protein binding: 20%–98% (see individual agents). Excreted largely unchanged by the urine as a result of glomerular filtration and active tubular secretion.
**Uses:** See individual drugs. Effective against a variety of gram-positive, gram-negative, and anaerobic organisms.
**Contraindications:** Hypersensitivity to penicillins, imipenem, and cephalosporins. PO use of penicillins during the acute stages of empyema, bacteremia, pneumonia, meningitis, pericarditis, and purulent or septic arthritis.
**Special Concerns:** Use of penicillins during lactation may lead to sensitization, diarrhea, candidiasis, and skin rash in the infant. Use with caution in clients with a history of asthma, hay fever, or urticaria. Clients with cystic fibrosis have a higher incidence of side effects with broad spectrum penicillins. Safety and effectiveness of carbenicillin, piperacillin, and the beta-lactamase inhibitor/penicillin combinations (e.g., amoxicillin/potassium clavulanate, ticarcillin/ potassium clavulanate) have not been determined in children less than 12 years of age. The incidence of resistant strains of staphylococci to penicillinase-resistant penicillins is increasing. Use of prolonged therapy may lead to superinfection (i.e., bacterial or fungal

overgrowth of nonsusceptible organisms).

**Side Effects:** Penicillins are potent sensitizing agents; it is estimated that up to 10% of the US population is allergic to the antibiotic. Hypersensitivity reactions are reported to be on the increase in pediatric populations. Sensitivity reactions may be immediate (within 20 min) or delayed (as long as several days or weeks after initiation of therapy). *Allergic:* Skin rashes (including maculopapular and exanthematous), exfoliative dermatitis, erythema multiforme (rarely, ***Stevens-Johnson syndrome***), hives, pruritus, wheezing, ***anaphylaxis,*** fever, eosinophilia, ***angioedema,*** serum sickness, ***laryngeal edema, laryngospasm, prostration, angioneurotic edema, bronchospasm, hypotension, vascular collapse, death.*** *GI:* Diarrhea (may be severe), abdominal cramps or pain, N&V, bloating, flatulence, increased thirst, bitter/unpleasant taste, glossitis, gastritis, stomatitis, dry mouth, sore mouth or tongue, furry tongue, black "hairy" tongue, bloody diarrhea, rectal bleeding, enterocolitis, pseudomembranous colitis. *CNS:* Dizziness, insomnia, hyperactivity, fatigue, prolonged muscle relaxation. Neurotoxicity including lethargy, neuromuscular irritability, ***seizures,*** hallucinations following large IV doses (especially in clients with renal failure). *Hematologic:* Thrombocytopenia, leukopenia, ***agranulocytosis,*** anemia, thrombocytopenic purpura, ***hemolytic anemia,*** granulocytopenia, neutropenia, bone marrow depression. *Renal:* Oliguria, hematuria, hyaline casts, proteinuria, pyuria (all symptoms of interstitial nephritis), nephropathy. Electrolyte imbalance following IV use. *Miscellaneous:* Hepatotoxicity (cholestatic jaundice), superinfection, swelling of face and ankles, anorexia, hyperthermia, transient hepatitis, vaginitis, itchy eyes. IM injection may cause pain and induration at the injection site, ecchymosis, and hematomas. IV use may cause vein irritation, deep vein thrombosis, and thrombophlebitis.

**OD** **Overdose Management:** *Symptoms:* Neuromuscular hyperexcitability, convulsive seizures. Massive IV doses may cause agitation, asterixis, hallucinations, confusion, stupor, multifocal myoclonus, seizures, coma, hyperkalemia, and encephalopathy. *Treatment (Severe Allergic or Anaphylactic Reactions):* Administer epinephrine (0.3–0.5 mL of a 1:1,000 solution SC or IM, or 0.2–0.3 mL diluted in 10 mL saline, given slowly by IV). Corticosteroids should be on hand. In those instances where penicillin is the drug of choice, the physician may decide to use it even though the client is allergic, adding a medication to the regimen to control the allergic response.

**Drug Interactions**
*Aminoglycosides* / Penicillins ↓ effect of aminoglycosides
*Antacids* / ↓ Effect of penicillins due to ↓ absorption from GI tract
*Antibiotics, Chloramphenicol, Erythromycins, Tetracyclines* / ↓ Effect of penicillins
*Anticoagulants* / Penicillins may potentiate pharmacologic effect
*Aspirin* / ↑ Effect of penicillins by ↓ plasma protein binding
*Chloramphenicol* / Either ↑ or ↓ effects
*Erythromycins* / Either ↑ or ↓ effects
*Heparin* / ↑ Risk of bleeding following parenteral penicillins
*Oral contraceptives* / ↓ Effect of oral contraceptives
*Phenylbutazone* / ↑ Effect of penicillins by ↓ plasma protein binding
*Probenecid* / ↑ Effect of penicillins by ↓ excretion
*Tetracyclines* / ↓ Effect of penicillins

**Laboratory Test Interferences:** ↓ Hematocrit, hemoglobin, WBC lymphocytes, serum potassium, albumin, total proteins, uric acid. ↑ Basophils, lymphocytes, monocytes, platelets, serum alkaline phosphatase, serum sodium. ↑ AST, ALT,

---

✦ = Available in Canada　　　　***bold italic*** = life threatening side effect

bilirubin, LDH following semisynthetic penicillins.

## Dosage

See individual drugs. Penicillins are available in a variety of dosage forms for PO, parenteral, inhalation, and intrathecal administration. PO doses must be higher than IM or SC doses because a large fraction of penicillin given PO may be destroyed in the stomach.

## NURSING CONSIDERATIONS

See also *General Nursing Considerations for All Anti-Infectives*.

**Administration/Storage**

1. IM and IV administration of penicillin causes a great deal of local irritation; thus, inject slowly.
2. IM injections are made deeply into the gluteal muscle. IV injections are usually made through the tubing of an IV infusion.

**Assessment:** Assess for allergic reactions; if reaction occurs, stop drug immediately. Allergic reactions are more likely to occur with a history of asthma, hay fever, urticaria, or allergy to cephalosporins.

**Interventions**

1. Detain in an ambulatory care site for at least 20 min after administering to assess for anaphylaxis.
2. Long-acting types of penicillin are for IM use only; may cause emboli, CNS pathology, or cardiac pathology if administered IV.
3. Do not massage repository (long-acting) penicillin products after injection; rate of absorption should not be increased.
4. Rapid administration of IV penicillin may cause local irritation and may precipitate convulsions. With some agents, high-dose therapy may precipitate aplastic anemia.
5. The elderly may be more sensitive to the effects of penicillin than younger people. Use care when calculating the dose based on weight and height.
6. Most penicillins are excreted in breast milk and should be prescribed cautiously to nursing mothers.

**Client/Family Teaching**

1. Review drugs prescribed, method and frequency of administration, side effects, and expected outcome/goals of therapy.
2. Report any S&S of allergic reactions, i.e., rashes, fever, joint swelling, angioneurotic edema, intense itching, and respiratory distress (during therapy and in some cases 7–12 days after therapy). Stop medication when noted and call for help immediately.
3. Oral penicillins may cause GI upset (N&V and diarrhea). Take oral penicillin with a glass of water 1 hr before or 2 hr after meals to minimize binding to foods.
4. Return for repository penicillin injections to complete treatment as scheduled.
5. Complete the entire prescribed course of therapy, even if feeling well. Incomplete therapy will predispose client to development of resistant bacterial strains. With alpha-hemolytic *Streptococcus* infection, must continue with penicillin therapy for a minimum of 10 days, and preferably 14 days, to prevent development of rheumatic fever or glomerulonephritis.
6. Report S&S of superinfections (furry tongue, vaginal or rectal itching, diarrhea).
7. Notify provider if S&S do not improve or get worse after 48–72 hr of therapy.

**Outcomes/Evaluate**

- Symptomatic improvement
- Resolution of infection manifested by ↓ fever, ↓ WBCs, ↑ appetite, and negative culture reports

# PROGESTERONE AND PROGESTINS

*See also the following individual entries:*

> Levonorgestrel implants
> Medroxyprogesterone acetate
> Megestrol acetate
> Oral Contraceptives
> Progesterone gel

**Action/Kinetics:** Progesterone is the primary endogenous progestin. Progesterone inhibits, through positive feedback, the secretion of pituitary gonadotropins; in turn, this prevents follicular maturation and ovulation or alternatively promotes it for the "primed" follicle. It is required to prepare the endometrium for implantation of the embryo. Once implanted, progesterone is required to maintain pregnancy. Progestins inhibit spontaneous uterine contractions; certain progestins may cause androgenic or anabolic effects. Progestins given PO are rapidly absorbed and quickly metabolized in the liver. **Peak levels, after PO:** 1–2 hr. **t½, after PO:** 2–3 hr during the first 6 hr after ingestion; thereafter, 8–9 hr. **After IM,** effective levels can be maintained for 3–6 months with a **t½** of about 10 weeks. **t½, elimination, gel:** 5–20 min. A major portion is excreted in the urine with a small amount in the bile and feces.

**Uses:** Abnormal uterine bleeding, primary or secondary amenorrhea (used with an estrogen), endometriosis. Alone or with an estrogen for contraception. May also be used in combination with an estrogen for endometriosis and hypermenorrhea. Certain types of cancer. AIDS wasting syndrome (megestrol acetate). Infertility (progesterone gel). *NOTE:* Not to be used to prevent habitual abortion or to treat threatened abortion. *Investigational:* Medroxyprogesterone has been used to treat menopausal symptoms.

**Contraindications:** Carcinoma of the breast or genital organs, thromboembolic disease, thrombophlebitis, vaginal bleeding of unknown origin, impaired liver function, cerebral hemorrhage or those with a history of such, missed abortion, as a diagnostic test for pregnancy. Pregnancy, especially during the first 4 months.

**Special Concerns:** Use with caution in case of asthma, epilepsy, depression, migraine, and cardiac or renal dysfunction.

**Side Effects:** See also individual drugs. Occasionally noted with short-term dosage, frequently observed with prolonged high dosage. *CNS:* Depression, insomnia, somnolence. *GU:* Breakthrough bleeding, spotting, amenorrhea, changes in amount and/or duration of menstrual flow, changes in cervical secretions and cervical erosion, breast tenderness or secretions. *Dermatologic:* Allergic rashes with and without pruritus, acne, melasma, chloasma, photosensitivity, local reactions at the site of injection. *Note:* Progesterone is especially irritating at the site of injection, especially aqueous products. *Miscellaneous:* Weight gain or loss, cholestatic jaundice, masculinization of the female fetus, nausea, edema, precipitation of acute intermittent porphyria, pyrexia, hirsutism.

**Laboratory Test Interferences:** Progestins may affect laboratory test results of hepatic function, thyroid, pregnanediol determination, and endocrine function. ↑ Prothrombin and Factors VII, VIII, IX, and X. ↓ Glucose tolerance (especially in diabetic clients).

**Dosage**

See individual drugs. The usual schedule of administration for *functional uterine bleeding, amenorrhea, infertility, dysmenorrhea, premenstrual tension, and contraception* is days 5 through 25 of the menstrual cycle, with day 1 being the first day of menstrual flow.

## NURSING CONSIDERATIONS
### Assessment
1. Identify indications for therapy. Assess for any thrombophlebitis, pulmonary embolism, cardiac, liver, or renal dysfunction, cerebral hemorrhage, breast or genital cancers.
2. Monitor VS, weight, and labs.
3. Note any history of psychic depression or diabetes mellitus.
4. Document last menstrual period and absence of pregnancy.

---

✦ = Available in Canada    ***bold italic*** = life threatening side effect

**Client/Family Teaching**

1. To avoid gastric irritation and nausea, take with a light snack, in the evening. Establish a schedule and take at the same time each day.

2. Gastric distress usually subsides after the first few cycles of the drug; report if these symptoms persist.

3. Report any symptoms of thrombic disorders such as pains in the legs, sudden onset of chest pain, SOB, and coughing for no apparent reason.

4. Weigh at least twice a week and report any unusual weight gain; may indicate the presence of edema.

5. Report any yellowing of the skin or sclera (jaundice) which may necessitate discontinuation of the medication, lab evaluation of liver function, and possibly a dosage change.

6. Report any episodes of unusual bleeding.

7. Progestins may reactivate or worsen a psychic depression. Report any mental status changes and the circumstance of the depression.

8. With diabetes, progesterone may alter glucose tolerance and the dosage of antidiabetic medication may need to be adjusted.

9. Early symptoms of ophthalmic pathology, such as headaches, dizziness, blurred vision, or partial loss of vision, should be reported so that a thorough eye exam can be performed.

10. Stop smoking; if unable, enroll in a formal smoking cessation program.

11. With birth control, injections must be administered every 3 mo to ensure adequate protection.

12. Progestin-only oral contraceptives may be used as early as 3 weeks after delivery in women who partially breast feed and within 6 weeks after delivery in women who fully breast feed.

**Outcomes/Evaluate**

• Control of abnormal menstrual bleeding
• Weight gain with AIDS clients
• Menstrual regularity
• Effective contraceptive agent
• Symptomatic improvement in menstrual pain and flow
• ↓ Size or resolution of ovarian cyst(s)

---

# SKELETAL MUSCLE RELAXANTS, CENTRALLY ACTING

*See also the following individual entries:*

Baclofen
Carisoprodol
Chlorzoxazone
Cyclobenzaprine hydrochloride
Dantrolene sodium
Diazepam
Methocarbamol
Soma Compound
Soma Compound with Codeine
Tizanidine

**Action/Kinetics:** These drugs decrease muscle tone and involuntary movement. Many relieve anxiety and tension as well. Although the precise mechanism of action is unknown, most of these agents depress spinal polysynaptic reflexes. Their beneficial effects may also be attributable to their antianxiety activity. Several of the drugs in this group also manifest analgesic properties.

**Uses:** Musculoskeletal and neurologic disorders associated with muscle spasms, hyperreflexia, and hypertonia, including parkinsonism, tetanus, tension headaches, acute muscle spasms caused by trauma, and inflammation (e.g., low back syndrome, sprains, arthritis, bursitis). They also may be useful in the management of cerebral palsy and multiple sclerosis.

**Side Effects:** See individual drugs.

**OD** **Overdose Management:** *Symptoms:* Often extensions of the side effects. Stupor, ***coma, shock-like syndrome, respiratory depression,*** loss of muscle tone, and impaired deep tendon reflexes may also occur. *Treatment:* Symptomatic. Emesis or gastric lavage (followed by activated charcoal). If necessary, artificial respiration, oxygen administration, pressor agents, and IV fluids may be used. It may be possible to increase the rate of excretion of selected drugs by diuretics (including mannitol), peritoneal dialysis, or hemodialysis.

**Drug Interactions:** Centrally acting muscle relaxants may increase the sedative and respiratory depressant effects of CNS depressants (e.g., alcohol, barbiturates, sedatives and hypnotics, and antianxiety agents).

**Dosage**
See individual agents.

## NURSING CONSIDERATIONS
**Administration**
1. If unable to swallow, crush tablets or empty capsules into a small amount of fruit juice.
2. If skeletal muscle relaxant is to be discontinued after long-term use, taper the dose to prevent rebound spasticity, hallucinations, or other withdrawal symptoms.
3. Determine the lowest dosage to treat symptoms.

**Assessment**
1. Document indications for therapy. List other agents prescribed and the outcome.
2. Note any prior seizures. Some in this category may cause loss of seizure control.
3. Assess extent of musculoskeletal and neurologic disorders associated with muscle spasm. Note muscle stiffness, pain, and extent of ROM.
4. Document baseline mental status exam.

**Interventions**
1. Monitor BP q 4 hr. Supervise ambulation/transfers and ensure safe environment. With these drugs, sedentary or immobilized clients are more prone to hypotension upon ambulation.
2. Monitor urinary output; if too low, evaluate need for drugs to increase excretion rate .
3. Document level of mobility (ROM) and comfort (pain) prior to and following drug administration.
4. Check muscle responses and deep tendon reflexes for evidence of drug overdosage.

**Client/Family Teaching**
1. Take with meals to reduce GI irritation.
2. These drugs may impair mental alertness; do not operate dangerous machinery or drive a car.
3. Do not stop abruptly as this may precipitate withdrawal symptoms, rebound spasticity, and hallucinations.
4. Review additional therapies that may be prescribed for muscle spasm (heat, rest, exercise, physical therapy) and the importance of adhering to the prescribed regimen.
5. Increase fluids and bulk in diet to prevent constipation.
6. Discontinue and report if the urine becomes dark, the skin or sclera appears yellow, or pruritus develops.
7. Avoid alcohol and any other CNS depressants. Antihistamines may produce an additive depressant effect.
8. Report nausea, anorexia, or changes in taste perception if persistent, as nutritional state may become impaired.
9. Report as scheduled for all lab and medical visits so therapy can be evaluated and drug dosage adjusted.

**Outcomes/Evaluate**
• Improvement in extent/intensity of muscle spasm and pain
• ↑ ROM with measurable improvement in muscle tone, mobility, and involuntary movements
• Relief of tension headaches

# SUCCINIMIDE ANTICONVULSANTS

*See also the following individual entries:*

Ethosuximide
Methsuximide
Phensuximide

**Action/Kinetics:** The succinimide derivatives suppress the paroxysmal 3-

cycle/sec spike and wave activity that is associated with lapses of consciousness seen in absence seizures. They apparently do so by depressing the motor cortex and by raising the threshold of the CNS to convulsive stimuli. The drugs are rapidly absorbed from the GI tract.

**Uses:** Primarily absence seizures (petit mal). May be given concomitantly with other anticonvulsants if other types of epilepsy are manifested with absence seizures.

**Contraindications:** Hypersensitivity to succinimides.

**Special Concerns:** Safe use during pregnancy has not been established. Use with caution in clients with abnormal liver and kidney function.

**Side Effects:** *CNS:* Drowsiness, ataxia, dizziness, headaches, euphoria, lethargy, fatigue, insomnia, irritability, nervousness, dream-like state, hyperactivity. Psychiatric or psychologic aberrations such as mental slowing, hypochondriasis, sleep disturbances, inability to concentrate, depression, night terrors, instability, confusion, aggressiveness. Rarely, auditory hallucinations, paranoid psychosis, increased libido, suicidal behavior. *GI:* N&V, hiccoughs, anorexia, diarrhea, gastric distress, weight loss, abdominal and epigastric pain, cramps, constipation. *Hematologic:* Leukopenia, granulocytopenia, eosinophilia, *agranulocytosis,* pancytopenia with or without bone marrow suppression, monocytosis. *Dermatologic:* Pruritus, urticaria, erythema multiforme, lupus erythematosus, *Stevens-Johnson syndrome,* pruritic erythematous rashes, skin eruptions, alopecia, hirsutism, photophobia. *GU:* Urinary frequency, vaginal bleeding, renal damage, microscopic hematuria. *Miscellaneous:* Blurred vision, muscle weakness, hyperemia, hypertrophy of gums, swollen tongue, myopia, periorbital edema.

**OD Overdose Management:** *Symptoms (Acute Overdose):* Confusion, sleepiness, slow shallow respiration, N&V, **CNS depression with coma and respiratory depression,** hypotension, cyanosis, hyper- or hypothermia, absence of reflexes, unsteadiness, flaccid muscles. *Symptoms (Chronic Overdose):* Ataxia, dizziness, drowsiness, confusion, depression, proteinuria, skin rashes, hangover, irritability, poor judgment, N&V, muscle weakness, periorbital edema, hepatic dysfunction, **fatal bone marrow aplasia, delayed onset of coma,** nephrosis, hematuria, casts. *Treatment:* General supportive measures. Charcoal hemoperfusion may be helpful.

**Drug Interactions:** Succinimides may ↑ effects of hydantoins by ↓ breakdown by the liver.

**Dosage**

*Individualized.* See individual agents. Succinimides may be given in combination with other anticonvulsants if two or more types of seizures are present.

## NURSING CONSIDERATIONS

See also *Nursing Considerations* for *Anticonvulsants.*

**Client/Family Teaching**

1. Take as directed and do not stop abruptly; may cause an increase in the severity and frequency of seizures.

2. Caution should be exercised while driving or performing other tasks requiring alertness and coordination; may cause, dizziness, blurred vision, headaches, N&V, and drowsiness, which should subside after several weeks of therapy.

3. Alert family to the possibility of transient personality changes, hypochondriacal behavior, and aggressiveness, which should be reported immediately.

4. Report any increase in frequency of tonic-clonic (grand mal) seizures.

5. Any persistent fever, swollen glands, and bleeding gums should be reported; may signal a blood dyscrasia.

6. May discolor urine pinkish brown.

7. Report for CBC, liver and renal function studies as scheduled.

**Outcomes/Evaluate:** Control or ↓ frequency of seizure activity

# SULFONAMIDES

*See also the following individual entries:*

  Mafenide acetate
  Pediazole
  Sulfacetamide sodium
  Sulfadiazine
  Sulfamethoxazole
  Sulfasalazine
  Sulfisoxazole
  Sulfisoxazole diolamine
  Trimethoprim and
    Sulfamethoxazole

**Action/Kinetics:** Sulfonamides are structurally related to PABA and, as such, competitively inhibit the enzyme dihydropteroate synthetase, which is responsible for incorporating PABA into dihydrofolic acid. Thus, the synthesis of dihydrofolic acid is inhibited, resulting in a decrease in tetrahydrofolic acid, which is required for synthesis of DNA, purines, and thymidine. Thus, sulfonamides are bacteriostatic. Readily absorbed from the GI tract. Distributed throughout all tissues, including the CSF, where concentrations attain 50%–80% of those found in the blood. The sulfonamides are metabolized in the liver and primarily excreted by the kidneys. Small amounts are found in the feces, bile, breast milk, and other secretions.

**Uses: PO, Parenteral.** See individual drugs. Uses include urinary tract infections, chancroid, meningitis caused by *Hemophilus influenzae,* meningogoccal meningitis, rheumatic fever, nocardiosis, trachoma, with pyrimethamine for toxoplasmosis, with quinine sulfate and pyrimethamine for chloroquine-resistant *Plasmodium falciparum,* and with penicillin for otitis media.

  **Ophthalmic.** Conjunctivitis, corneal ulcer, and other superficial ocular infections due to susceptible organisms. Adjunct to systemic sulfonamides to treat trachoma.

  **Vaginal.** Sulfanilamide is used to treat *Candida albicans* vulvovaginitis only.

**Contraindications:** Hypersensitivity reactions to sulfonamides and chemically related drugs (e.g., thiazides, sulfonylureas, loop diuretics, carbonic anhydrase inhibitors, local anesthetics, PABA-containing sunscreens). Use in infants less than 2 years of age, except with pyrimethamine to treat congenital toxoplasmosis. Use at term during pregnancy. Use in premature infants who are nursing or those with hyperbilirubinemia or G6PD deficiency. Group A beta-hemolytic streptococcal infections.

**Special Concerns:** Use with caution, and in reduced dosage, in clients with impaired liver or renal function, intestinal or urinary tract obstructions, blood dyscrasias, allergies, asthma, and hereditary G6PD deficiency. Use with caution if exposed to sunlight or ultraviolet light as photosensitivity may occur. Superinfection is a possibility. Ophthalmic products should be used with caution in clients with dry eye. Safety and efficacy of ophthalmic use in children have not been determined.

**Side Effects: Systemic.** *GI:* N&V, diarrhea, abdominal pain, glossitis, stomatitis, anorexia, pseudomembranous enterocolitis, pancreatitis, hepatitis, **hepatocellular necrosis.** *Allergic:* Rash, pruritus, photosensitivity, erythema nodosum or multiforme, generalized skin eruptions, **Stevens-Johnson syndrome,** conjunctivitis, rhinitis, balanitis. Serum sickness, urticaria, pruritus, exfoliative dermatitis, **anaphylaxis, toxic epidermal necrolysis** with or without corneal damage, periorbital edema, conjunctival and scleral injection, allergic myocarditis, decreased pulmonary function with eosinophila, disseminated lupus erythematosus, periarteritis nodosa, arteritis. *CNS:* Headaches, mental depression, **seizures,** hallucinations, vertigo, insomnia, apathy, ataxia, drowsiness, restlessness. *Renal:* Crystalluria, toxic nephrosis with oliguria and anuria, elevated creatinine. *Hematologic:* **Aplastic anemia,** leukopenia, neutropenia, **agranulocytosis,** thrombocytopenia, hemolytic anemia, methemoglobinemia, purpura, hypoprothrombinemia. *Neurologic:* Peripheral neuropathy, polyneuritis, neuritis, optic neuritis. *Miscellaneous:* Jaundice, tinnitus, arthralgia, superinfection, hearing loss, drug fever, pyrexia, chills, lupus erythematosus phenomenon, transient myopia.

By killing the intestinal flora, the sulfonamides also reduce the bacterial synthesis of vitamin K. This may result in **hemorrhage.** Administration of vitamin K to clients on long-term sulfonamide therapy is recommended.

**Ophthalmic Use.**    Headache, browache. Blurred vision, eye irritation, itching, transient epithelial keratitis, reactive hyperemia, conjunctival edema, burning and transient stinging. Rarely, **Stevens-Johnson syndrome,** exfoliative dermatitis, **toxic epidermal necrolysis,** photosensitivity, fever, skin rash, GI disturbances, and bone marrow depression.

**OD**  **Overdose Management:** *Symptoms:* N&V, anorexia, colic, dizziness, drowsiness, headache, unconsciousness, vertigo, toxic fever. More serious manifestations include **acute hemolytic anemia, agranulocytosis,** acidosis, maculopapular dermatitis, hepatic jaundice, sensitivity reactions, toxic neuritis, **death** (several days after the first dose). *Treatment:* Immediately discontinue the drug.

• Induce emesis or perform gastric lavage, especially if large doses were taken.

• To hasten excretion, alkalinize the urine and force fluids (if kidney function is normal). If there is renal blockage due to sulfonamide crystals, catheterization of the ureters may be needed.

• In the event of agranulocytosis, antibiotic therapy is needed to combat infection.

• To treat severe anemia or thrombocytopenia, blood or platelet transfusions are required.

**Drug Interactions**
*Anticoagulants, oral* / ↑ Effect of anticoagulants due to ↓ plasma protein binding
*Antidiabetics, oral* / ↑ Hypoglycemic effect due to ↓ plasma protein binding
*Cyclosporine* / ↓ Effect of cyclosporine and ↑ nephrotoxicity
*Diuretics, thiazide* / ↑ Risk of thrombocytopenia with purpura
*Indomethacin* / ↑ Effect of sulfonamides due to ↓ plasma protein binding
*Methenamine* / ↑ Chance of sulfonamide crystalluria due to acid urine
*Methotrexate* / ↑ Risk of methotrexate-induced bone marrow suppression
*Phenytoin* / ↑ Effect of phenytoin due to ↓ breakdown in liver
*Probenecid* / ↑ Effect of sulfonamides due to ↓ plasma protein binding
*Salicylates* / ↑ Effect of sulfonamides due to ↓ plasma protein binding
*Silver products* / Incompatible with ophthalmic products
*Uricosuric agents* / Potentiation of uricosuric action
**Laboratory Test Interferences:** False + or ↑ liver function tests (amino acids, bilirubin, BSP), renal function (BUN, NPN, creatinine clearance), blood counts, PT, Coombs' test. False + or ↑ urine glucose (copper reduction methods, such as Benedict's solution or Clinitest), protein, urobilinogen.

**Dosage** ————
See individual drugs.

## NURSING CONSIDERATIONS

See also *General Nursing Considerations for All Anti-Infectives.*
**Administration/Storage**
1. Do not use ophthalmic solutions if they have darkened or contain a precipitate.
2. Care must be taken to avoid contamination of ophthalmic products.
**Assessment**
1. Obtain a thorough nursing and drug history.

2. Note if ever received sulfonamide therapy and the response.

3. Document indications for therapy, type, onset, and characteristics of symptoms. List other agents prescribed and the outcome.

4. Question concerning any conditions that may preclude drug therapy, such as intestinal problems, urinary tract obstructions, G6PD deficiency (may precipitate hemolysis), or allergies.

5. Determine if pregnant; drug may be harmful to developing fetus.

6. Monitor CBC, blood sugars, bleeding times, cultures, liver and renal function studies.

**Interventions**

1. During drug therapy, assess for any of the following reactions that may require drug withdrawal:

• Skin rashes, abdominal pain, anorexia, irritation of the mouth or tingling of the extremities

• Blood dyscrasias (characterized by sore throat, fever, pallor, purpura, jaundice, or weakness)

• Serum sickness (characterized by eruptions of purpuric spots and pain in limbs and joints). Serum sickness may develop 7–10 days after initiation of therapy.

• Early symptoms of Stevens-Johnson syndrome (characterized by high fever, severe headaches, stomatitis, conjunctivitis, rhinitis, urethritis, and balanitis [inflammation of the tip of the penis])

• Jaundice, which may indicate hepatic involvement, with onset 3–5 days after initiation of therapy

• Renal involvement (characterized by renal colic, oliguria, anuria, hematuria, and proteinuria)

• Ecchymosis and hemorrhage (caused by decreased synthesis of vitamin K by intestinal bacteria)

• Hemolytic anemia especially in the elderly

• Behavioral changes or acute mental disturbances

2. Monitor I&O and record. Encourage adequate fluid intake to prevent crystalluria. Observe urinalysis for evidence of crystals. Minimum urine output should be 1.5 L/day. Test urine pH to determine excess acidity. Administration of a particularly insoluble sulfonamide may require alkalinization of urine (usually sodium bicarbonate).

3. If administering long-acting sulfonamides, adequate fluid intake must be maintained for 24–48 hr after the drug has been discontinued.

**Client/Family Teaching**

1. Take drug on time and as prescribed and remain under medical care during course of therapy despite feeling better.

2. Certain sulfonamides may color urine orange-red or brown; not cause for alarm but should be reported.

3. Take with 6–8 oz (180–240 mL) of water and maintain adequate fluid intake for 24–48 hr after discontinuing drug.

4. Drug may cause N&V and loss of appetite. Monitor I&O and try to consume greater than 2.5 L/day of fluids.

5. Test urine pH and report changes in acidity as additional drug therapy may be necessary.

6. Vitamin C may make the urine more acidic and contribute to crystal formation, so avoid.

7. If also taking anticoagulants, be particularly alert to an increase in bleeding tendencies (bruising, cuts that bleed for a longer time than usual, etc.).

8. Avoid prolonged exposure to sunlight; may cause a photosensitivity reaction. Wear protective clothing, sunglasses, and sunscreen when exposed.

9. Report any changes in vision or hearing. With ophthalmic use, report if improvement is not seen within 5–7 days, if the condition worsens, or if pain, redness, itching, or swelling of the eye occurs.

10. Do not perform activities that require mental alertness until drug effects realized.

11. Vaginal intercourse should be

---

avoided when vaginal products are being used.

12. Report for lab studies as scheduled and notify provider if symptoms do not improve or worsen after 48–72 hr.

**Outcomes/Evaluate**

• Negative C&S results (note any organism resistance to sulfonamide)
• Resolution of infection; symptomatic improvement

---

# SYMPATHOMIMETIC DRUGS

*See also the following individual entries:*

Albuterol
Bitolterol mesylate
Brimonidine tartrate
Dobutamine hydrochloride
Dopamine hydrochloride
Ephedrine sulfate
Epinephrine
Epinephrine bitartrate
Epinephrine borate
Epinephrine hydrochloride
Isoetharine hydrochloride
Isoetharine mesylate
Isoproterenol
Isoproterenol hydrochloride
Isoproterenol sulfate
Levarterenol bitartrate
Mephentermine sulfate
Metaproterenol sulfate
Metaraminol bitartrate
Phenylephrine hydrochloride
Phenylpropanolamine hydrochloride
Pirbuterol acetate
Pseudoephedrine hydrochloride
Pseudoephedrine sulfate
Salmeterol xinafoate
Terbutaline sulfate

**Action/Kinetics:** The adrenergic drugs work in two ways: (1) by mimicking the action of norepinephrine or epinephrine by combining with alpha and/or beta receptors (directly acting sympathomimetics) or (2) by causing or regulating the release of the natural neurohormones from their storage sites at the nerve terminals (indirectly acting sympathomimetics). Some drugs exhibit a combination of effects 1 and 2.

Adrenergic stimulation of receptors will manifest the following general effects:

*Alpha-1-adrenergic:* / Vasoconstriction, decongestion, constriction of the pupil of the eye, contraction of splenic capsule, contraction of the trigone-sphincter muscle of the urinary bladder.

*Alpha-2-adrenergic:* / Presynaptic to regulate amount of transmitter released; decrease tone, motility, and secretory activity of the GI tract (possibly involved in hypersecretory response also); decrease insulin secretion.

*Beta-1-adrenergic:* / Myocardial contraction (inotropic), regulation of heartbeat (chronotropic), improved impulse conduction, ↑ lipolysis.

*Beta-2-adrenergic:* / Peripheral vasodilation, bronchial dilation; ↓ tone, motility, and secretory activity of the GI tract; ↑ renin secretion.

**Uses:** See individual drugs.

**Contraindications:**    Tachycardia due to arrhythmias; tachycardia or heart block caused by digitalis toxicity.

**Special Concerns:** Use with caution in hyperthyroidism, diabetes, prostatic hypertrophy, seizures, degenerative heart disease, especially in geriatric clients or those with asthma, emphysema, or psychoneuroses. Also, use with caution in clients with coronary insufficiency, CAD, ischemic heart disease, CHF, cardiac arrhythmias, hypertension, or history of stroke. Asthma clients who rely heavily on inhaled beta-2-agonist bronchodilators may increase their chances of death. Thus, these agents should be used to "rescue" clients but should not be prescribed for regular long-term use. Beta-2 agonists may inhibit uterine contractions.

**Side Effects:** See individual drugs; side effects common to most sympathomimetics are listed. *CV:* Tachycardia, arrhythmias, palpitations, BP changes, anginal pain, precordial pain, pallor, skipped beats, chest tightness, hypertension. *GI:* N&V, heartburn, anorexia, altered taste or bad taste, GI distress, dry mouth, diarrhea. *CNS:* Restlessness, anxiety, tension, insomnia, hyperkinesis, drowsiness, weakness, vertigo, irritability, dizziness, headache, tremors, general CNS stimulation, nervousness, shakiness, hyperactivity. *Respiratory:* Cough, dyspnea, dry throat, pharyngitis, **paradoxical bronchospasm,** irritation. *Other:* Flushing, sweating, **allergic reactions**.

**OD** **Overdose Management:** *Symptoms:* Following inhalation: Exaggeration of side effects resulting in anginal pain, hypertension, hypokalemia, **seizures.** Following systemic use: CV symptoms include bradycardia, tachycardia, palpitations, extrasystoles, **heart block,** elevated BP, chest pain, hypokalemia. CNS symptoms include anxiety, insomnia, tremor, delirium, **convulsions, collapse, and coma.** Also, fever, chills, cold perspiration, N&V, mydriasis, and blanching of the skin. *Treatment:*

• For overdosage due to inhalation: General supportive measures with sedatives given for restlessness. Cautious use of metoprolol or atenolol may be used but these drugs may induce an asthmatic attack in clients with asthma.

• For systemic overdosage: Discontinue or decrease dose. General supportive measures. For overdose due to PO agents, emesis, gastric lavage, or charcoal may be helpful. In severe cases, propranolol may be used but this may cause airway obstruction. Phentolamine may be given to block strong alpha-adrenergic effects.

**Drug Interactions**
*Beta-adrenergic blocking agents /* Inhibit adrenergic stimulation of the heart and bronchial tree; cause bronchial constriction; hypertension, asthma, not relieved by adrenergic agents

*Ammonium chloride /* ↓ Effect of sympathomimetics due to ↑ excretion by kidney
*Anesthetics /* Halogenated anesthetics sensitize heart to adrenergics—causes cardiac arrhythmias
*Anticholinergics /* Concomitant use aggravates glaucoma
*Antidiabetics /* Hyperglycemic effect of epinephrine may necessitate ↑ dosage of insulin or oral hypoglycemic agents
*Corticosteroids /* Chronic use with sympathomimetics may result in or aggravate glaucoma; aerosols containing sympathomimetics and corticosteroids may be lethal in asthmatic children
*Digitalis glycosides /* Combination may cause cardiac arrhythmias
*Furazolidone /* Furazolidone ↑ effects of mixed-acting sympathomimetics
*Guanethidine /* Direct-acting sympathomimetics ↑ effects of guanethidine, while indirect-acting sympathomimetics ↓ effects of guanethidine; also reversal of hypotensive effects of guanethidine
*Lithium /* ↓ Pressor effect of direct-acting sympathomimetics
*MAO inhibitors /* All effects of sympathomimetics are potentiated; symptoms include hypertensive crisis with possible intracranial hemorrhage, hyperthermia, convulsions, coma; death may occur
*Methyldopa /* ↑ Pressor response
*Methylphenidate /* Potentiates pressor effect of sympathomimetics; combination hazardous in glaucoma
*Oxytocics /* ↑ Chance of severe hypertension
*Phenothiazines /* ↑ Risk of cardiac arrhythmias
*Reserpine /* ↑ Risk of hypertension following use of direct-acting sympathomimetics and ↓ effect of indirect-acting sympathomimetics
*Sodium bicarbonate /* ↑ Effect of sympathomimetics due to ↓ excretion by kidney

---

*Theophylline* / Enhanced toxicity (especially cardiotoxicity); also ↓ theophylline levels

*Thyroxine* / Potentiation of pressor response of sympathomimetics

*Tricyclic antidepressants* / ↑ Effect of direct-acting sympathomimetics and ↓ effect of indirect-acting sympathomimetics

**Dosage**

See individual drugs.

## NURSING CONSIDERATIONS

**Administration/Storage:**   Discard colored solutions.

**Assessment**

1. Determine any sensitivity to adrenergic drugs.
2. Note previous experience with drugs in this class and the outcome.
3. Document any history of CAD, tachycardia, endocrine disturbances, or respiratory tract problems.
4. Obtain baseline data regarding general physical condition and hemodynamic status including ECG, VS, and lab data.
5. Document indications for therapy, contributing factors, and anticipated response.

**Interventions**

1. During period of dosage adjustment, closely monitor and record BP and pulse.
2. Monitor I&O and continue to assess VS throughout therapy.

**Client/Family Teaching**

1. Review prescribed drug therapy and printed material regarding potential drug side effects.
2. Take exactly as directed. Do not increase the dosage of drug and do not take more frequently than prescribed. Consult provider if symptoms become more severe.
3. Take early in the day to prevent insomnia.
4. Feelings or symptoms of fear or anxiety may be evident because these drugs mimic the body's stress response.
5. Avoid all OTC preparations without approval.
6. Stop smoking now in order to preserve current lung function. Attend formal smoking cessation classes.

## SPECIAL NURSING CONSIDERATIONS FOR ADRENERGIC BRONCHODILATORS

**Assessment**

1. Obtain history prior to starting the drug therapy.
2. Note any previous experience with this class of drugs.
3. Monitor VS, ABGs (or $O_2$ saturation).
4. Document lung assessment and pulmonary function tests. Note characteristics of cough and sputum production.

**Interventions**

1. Monitor BP and pulse to assess CV response.
2. Observe effects on CNS; if pronounced, adjust dosage and frequency of administration.
3. With status asthmaticus and abnormal ABGs, continue to provide oxygen and ventilating assistance even though the symptoms appear to be relieved by the bronchodilator.
4. To prevent depression of respiratory effort, administer oxygen based on client's clinical symptoms and ABGs or $O_2$ saturations.
5. If three to five aerosol treatments of the same agent have been administered within the last 6–12 hr, with no relief, further evaluation is warranted.
6. If dyspnea worsens after repeated excessive use of the inhaler, paradoxical airway resistance may occur. Be prepared to assist with alternative therapy and respiratory support.

**Client/Family Teaching**

1. Review technique for use and care of prescribed inhalers and respiratory equipment. Rinsing of equipment and of mouth after use is imperative in preventing oral fungal infections. Maintain record of peak flow readings and seek medical attention at identified levels.
2. If postural drainage prescribed, review how to cough productively and show family how to clap and vibrate the chest to promote good respiratory hygiene.
3. Regular, consistent use of the

drug is essential for maximum benefit, but overuse can be life-threatening.

4. To improve lung ventilation and reduce fatigue during eating, start inhalation therapy upon arising in the morning and before meals.

5. A single aerosol treatment is usually enough to control an asthma attack. Overuse of adrenergic bronchodilators may result in reduced effectiveness, possible paradoxical reaction, and death from cardiac arrest.

6. Increased fluid intake will aid in liquefying secretions, facilitating removal.

7. Consult provider if dizziness or chest pain occurs, or if there is no relief when the usual dose is used.

8. Avoid OTC preparations and any other adrenergic meds unless expressly ordered.

9. Consult provider if more than three aerosol treatments in a 24-hr period are required for relief.

10. If using inhalable meds and bronchodilators, use the bronchodilator first and wait 5 min before using the other medication.

11. **Stop smoking,** avoid crowds during "flu seasons," dress warmly in cold weather, receive the pneumonia vaccine and seasonal flu shot, and stay in air conditioning during hot, humid days to prevent exacerbations of illness.

12. Have family/significant other learn CPR.

**Outcomes/Evaluate**

• Knowledge and understanding of illness; compliance with prescribed medication regimen

• A positive clinical response as evidenced by ↓ symptoms for which the therapy was originally prescribed

# TETRACYCLINES

*See also the following individual entries:*

Doxycycline calcium
Doxycycline hyclate
Doxycycline monohydrate
Tetracycline
Tetracycline hydrochloride

**Action/Kinetics:** The tetracyclines inhibit protein synthesis by microorganisms by binding to the ribosomal 50S subunit, thereby interfering with protein synthesis. The drugs block the binding of aminoacyl transfer RNA to the messenger RNA complex. Cell wall synthesis is not inhibited. The drugs are mostly bacteriostatic and are effective only against multiplying bacteria. Well absorbed from the stomach and upper small intestine. Well distributed throughout all tissues and fluids and diffuse through noninflamed meninges and the placental barrier. They become deposited in the fetal skeleton and calcifying teeth. **t½:** 7–18.6 hr (see individual agents) and is increased in the presence of renal impairment. The drugs bind to serum protein (range: 20%–93%; see individual agents). The drugs are concentrated in the liver in the bile and are excreted mostly unchanged in the urine and feces.

**Uses:** See individual drugs. Used mainly for infections caused by *Rickettsia, Chlamydia,* and *Mycoplasma.* Due to development of resistance, tetracyclines are usually not used for infections by common gram-negative or gram-positive organisms. Atypical pneumonia caused by *Mycoplasma pneumoniae.* Adjunct in the treatment of trachoma.

As an alternative to penicillin for uncomplicated gonorrhea or disseminated gonococcal infections, especially with penicillin allergy. Acute pelvic inflammatory disease. Tetracyclines are also useful as an alternative to penicillin for early syphilis.

Although not generally used for gram-positive infections, tetracyclines may be beneficial in anthrax, *Listeria* infections, and actinomycosis. They have also been used in conjunction with quinine sulfate for chloroquine-resistant *Plasmodium falciparum* malaria and as an intracavitary injection to control pleural or pericardial effusions caused by metastatic carcinoma. As an adjunct to amebicides in acute intestinal amebiasis. Used PO to treat uncomplicated endocervical, rectal, or urethral *Chlamydia* infections.

Topical uses include skin granulomas caused by *Mycobacterium marinum;* ophthalmic bacterial infections causing blepharitis, conjunctivitis, or keratitis; and as an adjunct in the treatment of ophthalmic chlamydial infections such as trachoma or inclusion conjunctivitis. As an alternative to silver nitrate for prophylaxis of neonatal gonococcal ophthalmia. Vaginitis. Severe acne.

**Contraindications:** Hypersensitivity. Avoid drug during tooth development stage (last trimester of pregnancy, neonatal period, during breast-feeding, and during childhood up to 8 years) because tetracyclines interfere with enamel formation and dental pigmentation. Never administer intrathecally.

**Special Concerns:** Use with caution and at reduced dosage in clients with impaired kidney function.

**Side Effects:** *GI* (most common): N&V, thirst, diarrhea, anorexia, sore throat, flatulence, epigastric distress, bulky loose stools. Less commonly, stomatitis, dysphagia, black hairy tongue, glossitis, or inflammatory lesions of the anogenital area. Rarely, pseudomembranous colitis. PO dosage forms may cause esophageal ulcers, especially in clients with esophageal obstructive element or hiatal hernia. *Allergic* (rare): Urticaria, pericarditis, polyarthralgia, fever, rash, pulmonary infiltrates with eosinophilia, **angioneurotic edema,** worsening of SLE, **anaphylaxis,** purpura. *Skin:* Photosensitivity, maculopapular and erythematous rashes, exfoliative dermatitis (rare), onycholysis, discoloration of nails. *CNS:* Dizziness, lightheadedness, unsteadiness, paresthesias. *Hematologic:* Eosinophilia, **hemolytic anemia,** neutropenia, thrombocytopenia, thrombocytopenic purpura.

*Hepatic:* Fatty liver, increases in liver enzymes; rarely, hepatotoxicity, hepatitis, hepatic cholestasis. *Miscellaneous:* Candidal superinfections including oral and vaginal candidiasis, discoloration of infants' and children's teeth, bone lesions, delayed bone growth, abnormal pigmentation of the conjunctiva, pseudotumor cerebri in adults and bulging fontanels in infants.

IV administration may cause thrombophlebitis; IM injections are painful and may cause induration at the injection site.

The administration of deteriorated tetracyclines may result in Fanconi-like syndrome characterized by N&V, acidosis, proteinuria, glycosuria, aminoaciduria, polydipsia, polyuria, hypokalemia.

**Drug Interactions**

*Aluminum salts* / ↓ Effect of tetracyclines due to ↓ absorption from GI tract

*Antacids, oral* / ↓ Effect of tetracyclines due to ↓ absorption from GI tract

*Anticoagulants, oral* / IV tetracyclines ↑ hypoprothrombinemia

*Bismuth salts* / ↓ Effect of tetracyclines due to ↓ absorption from GI tract

*Bumetanide* / ↑ Risk of kidney toxicity

*Calcium salts* / ↓ Effect of tetracyclines due to ↓ absorption from GI tract

*Cimetidine* / ↓ Effect of tetracyclines due to ↓ absorption from GI tract

*Contraceptives, oral* / ↓ Effect of oral contraceptives

*Digoxin* / Tetracyclines ↑ bioavailability of digoxin

*Diuretics, thiazide* / ↑ Risk of kidney toxicity

*Ethacrynic acid* / ↑ Risk of kidney toxicity

*Furosemide* /↑ Risk of kidney toxicity

*Insulin* / Tetracyclines may ↓ insulin requirement

*Iron preparations* / ↓ Effect of tetracyclines due to ↓ absorption from GI tract

*Lithium* / Either ↑ or ↓ levels of lithium

*Magnesium salts* / ↓ Effect of tetracyclines due to ↓ absorption from GI tract

*Methoxyflurane* / ↑ Risk of kidney toxicity

*Penicillins* / Tetracyclines may mask bactericidal effect of penicillins

*Sodium bicarbonate* / ↓ Effect of tetracyclines due to ↓ absorption from GI tract

*Zinc salts* / ↓ Effect of tetracyclines due to ↓ absorption from GI tract

**Laboratory Test Interferences:** False + or ↑ urinary catecholamines and urinary protein (degraded); ↑ coagulation time. False – or ↓ urinary urobilinogen, glucose tests (see *Nursing Considerations*). Prolonged use or high doses may change liver function tests and WBC counts.

**Dosage** ———————————
See individual drugs.

## NURSING CONSIDERATIONS

See also *General Nursing Considerations for All Anti-Infectives.*

**Administration/Storage**
1. Do not use outdated or deteriorated drugs as a Fanconi-like syndrome may occur (see *Side Effects*).
2. Discard unused capsules to prevent use of deteriorated medication.
3. Administer IM into large muscle mass to avoid extravasation into subcutaneous or fatty tissue.
4. Administer on an empty stomach at least 1 hr before or 2 hr after meals. Withhold antacids, iron salts, dairy foods, and other foods high in calcium for at least 2 hr after PO administration. Do not administer milk with tetracyclines.

**Assessment**
1. Determine any drug allergens or sensitivity. IM form contains procaine HCl.
2. Document indications for therapy, type, onset, and characteristics of symptoms. List other agents trialed and the outcome.

3. Note any colitis or other bowel problems.
4. If pregnant, document trimester.
5. Monitor VS, weight, CBC, BUN, creatinine, electrolytes, and cultures. Assess for impaired kidney function.

**Interventions**
1. Monitor VS and I&O. Maintain adequate I&O because renal dysfunction may result in drug accumulation, leading to toxicity. With impaired renal function assess for increased BUN, acidosis, anorexia, N&V, weight loss, and dehydration; after therapy latent symptoms may appear.
2. To prevent or treat pruritus ani, cleanse anal area with water several times a day and/or after each bowel movement. Observe for symptoms of enterocolitis, such as diarrhea, pyrexia, abdominal distention, and scanty urine; may need to discontinue drug and try another antibiotic.
3. If GI disturbances occur, avoid antacids that contain calcium, magnesium, or aluminum. May take with a light meal to reduce distress. An alternative would be to reduce the dose but increase the frequency of administration.
4. Assess with IV therapy for N&V, chills, fever, and hypertension resulting from too rapid administration or an excessively high dose; slow rate and report. Observe infant for bulging fontanelle, which may also be caused by a too rapid infusion rate.
5. Side effects such as sore throat, dysphagia, fever, dizziness, hoarseness, and inflammation of mucous membranes candidal superinfections.
6. Assess for altered level of consciousness or other CNS disturbances with impaired hepatic or renal function; may cause hepatic and renal toxicity.
7. May cause onycholysis (loosening or detachment of the nail from the nail bed) or discoloration.

**Client/Family Teaching**
1. Take on a full stomach to enhance absorption. Do not lay down

---

after administration; may precipitate erosive esophagitis.

2. Do not take with milk, cheese, ice cream, yogurt, or other foods or drugs containing calcium. If taken with meals, avoid these foods for 2 hr after administration.

3. Zinc tablets or vitamin preparations containing zinc may interfere with drug absorption. Food sources high in zinc that should be avoided include oysters, fresh and raw; cooked lobster; dry oat flakes; steamed crabs; veal; and liver.

4. Avoid direct or artificial sunlight, which can cause a severe sunburn-like reaction; report if erythema occurs. Wear protective clothing, sunglasses, and a sunscreen if exposed and for up to 3 weeks following therapy.

5. Tetracyclines interfere with formation of tooth enamel and dental pigmentation from the third trimester of pregnancy through age 8.

6. Prevent or treat pruritus ani by cleansing the anal area with water several times a day and/or after each bowel movement.

7. Use alternative method of birth control, as drug may interfere with oral contraceptives; may also cause a vaginal infection.

8. Take only as directed and complete full prescription. Discard any leftover meds to prevent reaction from deteriorated drugs.

**Outcomes/Evaluate**

• Resolution of infection (↓ temperature, ↓ WBCs, ↑ appetite)

• Symptomatic improvement

• Negative cultures; no organism resistance

---

# THEOPHYLLINE DERIVATIVES

*See also the following individual entries:*

Aminophylline
Theophylline

**Action/Kinetics:** Theophyllines stimulate the CNS, directly relax the smooth muscles of the bronchi and pulmonary blood vessels (relieve bronchospasms), produce diuresis, inhibit uterine contractions, stimulate gastric acid secretion, and increase the rate and force of contraction of the heart. The bronchodilator activity of theophyllines is due to direct relaxation of the bronchiolar smooth muscle and pulmonary blood vessels, which relieves bronchospasm. Although the exact mechanism is not known, theophyllines may act by altering the calcium levels of smooth muscle, blocking adenosine receptors, inhibiting the effect of prostaglandins on smooth muscle, and inhibiting the release of slow-reacting substance of anaphylaxis and histamine. Aminophylline releases free theophylline in vivo. Response to the drugs is highly individualized. Theophylline is well absorbed from uncoated plain tablets and PO liquids. *Theophylline salts:* **Onset:** 1–5 hr, depending on route and formulation. **Therapeutic plasma levels:** 10–20 mcg/mL. **t½:** 3–15 hr in nonsmoking adults, 4–5 hr in adult heavy smokers, 1–9 hr in children, and 20–30 hr for premature neonates. An increased t½ may be seen in individuals with CHF, alcoholism, liver dysfunction, or respiratory infections. Because of great variations in the rate of absorption (due to dosage form, food, dose level) as well as its extremely narrow therapeutic range, theophylline therapy is best monitored by determination of the serum levels. If these determinations cannot be obtained, saliva (contains 60% of corresponding theophylline serum levels) determinations can be used. Eighty-five percent to 90% metabolized in the liver and various metabolites, including the active 3-methylxanthine. Theophylline is metabolized partially to caffeine in the neonate. The premature neonate excretes 50% unchanged theophylline and may accumulate the caffeine metabolite. Excretion is through the kidneys (about 10% unchanged in adults).

**Uses:** Prophylaxis and treatment of bronchial asthma. Reversible bronchospasms associated with chronic bronchitis, emphysema, and COPD. *Investigational:* Treatment of neonatal apnea and Cheyne-Stokes respiration.

**Contraindications:** Hypersensitivity to any xanthine, peptic ulcer, seizure disorders (unless on medication), hypotension, CAD, angina pectoris.

**Special Concerns:** Use during lactation may result in irritability, insomnia, and fretfulness in the infant. Use with caution in premature infants due to the possible accumulation of caffeine. Xanthines are not usually tolerated by small children because of excessive CNS stimulation. Geriatric clients may manifest an increased risk of toxicity. Use with caution in the presence of gastritis, alcoholism, acute cardiac diseases, hypoxemia, severe renal and hepatic disease, severe hypertension, severe myocardial damage, hyperthyroidism, glaucoma.

**Side Effects:** Side effects are uncommon at serum theophylline levels less than 20 mcg/mL. At levels greater than 20 mcg/mL, 75% of individuals experience side effects including N&V, diarrhea, irritability, insomnia, and headache. At levels of 35 mcg/mL or greater, individuals may manifest *cardiac arrhythmias,* hypotension, tachycardia, hyperglycemia, *seizures, brain damage, or death. GI:* N&V, diarrhea, anorexia, epigastric pain, hematemesis, dyspepsia, rectal irritation (following use of suppositories), rectal bleeding, gastroesophageal reflux during sleep or while recumbent (theophylline). *CNS:* Headache, insomnia, irritability, fever, dizziness, lightheadedness, vertigo, reflex hyperexcitability, *seizures,* depression, speech abnormalities, alternating periods of mutism and hyperactivity, *brain damage, death. CV:* Hypotension, *life-threatening ventricular arrhythmias,* palpitations, tachycardia, *peripheral vascular collapse,* extrasystoles. *Renal:* Proteinuria, excretion of erythrocytes and renal tubular cells, dehydration due to diuresis, urinary retention (men with prostatic hypertrophy). *Other:* Tachypnea, *respiratory arrest,* fever, flushing, hyperglycemia, antidiuretic hormone syndrome, leukocytosis, rash, alopecia.

*NOTE:* Aminophylline given by rapid IV may produce hypotension, flushing, palpitations, precordial pain, headache, dizziness, or hyperventilation. Also, the ethylenediamine in aminophylline may cause allergic reactions, including urticaria and skin rashes.

**OD** **Overdose Management:** *Symptoms:* Agitation, headache, nervousness, insomnia, tachycardia, extrasystoles, anorexia, N&V, fasciculations, tachypnea, *tonic-clonic seizures.* The first signs of toxicity may be seizures or ventricular arrhythmias. Toxicity is usually associated with parenteral administration but can be observed after PO administration, especially in children. *Treatment:*
• Have ipecac syrup, gastric lavage equipment, and cathartics available to treat overdose if the client is conscious and not having seizures. Otherwise a mechanical ventilator, oxygen, diazepam, and IV fluids may be necessary for the treatment of overdosage.
• For postseizure coma, an airway must be maintained and the client oxygenated. To remove the drug, perform only gastric lavage and give the cathartic and activated charcoal by a large-bore gastric lavage tube. Charcoal hemoperfusion may be necessary.
• Atrial arrhythmias may be treated with verapamil and ventricular arrhythmias may be treated with lidocaine or procainamide.
• IV fluids are used to treat acid-base imbalance, hypotension, and dehydration. Hypotension may also be treated with vasopressors.
• Tepid water sponge bath or a hypothermic blanket is used to treat hyperpyrexia.

- Apnea is treated with artificial respiration.
- Serum levels of theophylline must be monitored until they fall below 20 mcg/mL as secondary rises of theophylline may occur, especially with sustained-release products.

**Drug Interactions**

*Allopurinol* / ↑ Theophylline levels
*Aminogluthethimide* / ↓ Theophylline levels
*Barbiturates* / ↓ Theophylline levels
*Benzodiazepines* / Sedative effect may be antagonized by theophylline
*Beta-adrenergic agonists* / Additive effects
*Beta-adrenergic blocking agents* / ↑ Theophylline levels
*Calcium channel blocking drugs* / ↑ Theophylline levels
*Carbamazepine* / Either ↑ or ↓ theophylline levels
*Charcoal* / ↓ Theophylline levels
*Cimetidine* / ↑ Theophylline levels
*Ciprofloxacin* / ↑ Plasma levels of theophylline with ↑ possibility of side effects
*Corticosteroids* / ↑ Theophylline levels
*Digitalis* / Theophylline ↑ toxicity of digitalis
*Disulfiram* / ↑ Theophylline levels
*Ephedrine and other sympathomimetics* / ↑ Theophylline levels
*Erythromycin* / ↑ Effect of theophylline due to ↓ breakdown by liver
*Ethacrynic acid* / Either ↑ or ↓ theophylline levels
*Furosemide* / Either ↑ or ↓ theophylline levels
*Halothane* / ↑ Risk of cardiac arrhythmias
*Interferon* / ↑ Theophylline levels
*Isoniazid* / Either ↑ or ↓ theophylline levels
*Ketamine* / Seizures of the extensor-type
*Ketoconazole* / ↓ Theophylline levels
*Lithium* / ↓ Effect of lithium due to ↑ rate of excretion
*Loop diuretics* / ↓ Theophylline levels
*Mexiletine* / ↑ Theophylline levels

*Muscle relaxants, nondepolarizing* / Theophylline ↓ effect of these drugs
*Oral contraceptives* / ↑ Effect of theophyllines due to ↓ breakdown by liver
*Phenytoin* / ↓ Theophylline levels
*Propofol* / Theophyllines ↓ sedative effect of propofol
*Quinolones* / ↑ Theophylline levels
*Reserpine* / ↑ Risk of tachycardia
*Rifampin* / ↓ Theophylline levels
*Sulfinpyrazone* / ↓ Theophylline levels
*Sympathomimetics* / ↓ Theophylline levels
*Tetracyclines* / ↑ Risk of theophylline toxicity
*Thiabendazole* / ↑ Theophylline levels
*Thyroid hormones* / ↓ Theophylline levels in hypothyroid clients
*Tobacco smoking* / ↓ Effect of theophylline due to ↑ breakdown by liver
*Troleandomycin* / ↑ Effect of theophylline due to ↓ breakdown by liver
*Verapamil* / ↑ Effect of theophylline

**Laboratory Test Interferences:** ↑ Plasma free fatty acids, bilirubin, urinary catecholamines, ESR. Interference with uric acid tests and tests for furosemide, probenecid, theobromine, and phenylbutazone.

## Dosage

Individualized. Initially, dosage should be adjusted according to plasma level of drug. Usual: 10–20 mcg theophylline/mL plasma. The dose of the various salts should be equivalent based on the content of anhydrous theophylline. See individual agents.

## NURSING CONSIDERATIONS
### Administration/Storage

1. Review list of agents with which theophylline derivatives interact.
2. Dilute drugs and maintain proper infusion rates to minimize problems of overdosage.
3. Wait to initiate PO therapy for at least 4–6 hr after switching from IV therapy.

**Assessment**

1. Assess for any hypersensitivity to xanthine compounds. Note any experience with this class of drugs and the outcome.

2. Document indications for therapy, type, onset, and characteristics of symptoms.

3. Note any history of hypotension, CAD, angina, PUD, or seizure disorders; avoid drug or use very cautiously in these conditions.

4. Assess for cigarette or marijuana use. These induce hepatic metabolism of the drug and require an increase in the drug dosage from 50% to 100%.

5. Assess diet habits which can influence the excretion of theophylline. A high-protein and/or low-carbohydrate diet will cause an increased drug excretion. A low-protein and/or high-carbohydrate diet will cause a decrease in the excretion of theophylline.

6. Assess lung fields closely and describe findings. Note characteristics of the sputum and cough and note ABGs and PFTs.

**Interventions**

1. Monitor BP and pulse and report any significant changes.

2. Observe for S&S of toxicity such as nausea, anorexia, insomnia, irritability, hyperexcitability, or cardiac arrhythmias; monitor serum levels.

3. Observe small children for excessive CNS stimulation; children often are unable to report side effects.

**Client/Family Teaching**

1. To avoid epigastric pain, take with a snack or with meals. Avoid or minimize consumption of charbroiled foods (e.g., burgers).

2. Take ATC and only as prescribed; more is *not* better. Report if nausea, vomiting, GI pain, or restlessness occurs.

3. Do not smoke; may aggravate underlying medical conditions as well as interfere with drug absorption. If unable to quit, attend a smoking cessation program.

4. Protect from acute exacerbations of illness by avoiding crowds, dressing warmly in cold weather, obtaining the pneumonia vaccine and seasonal flu shot, covering mouth and nose so cold air is not directly inhaled, staying in air conditioning during excessively hot and humid weather, maintaining proper diet and nutrition, exercising daily, and taking in adequate fluid.

5. Report early S&S of infections, adverse drug effects, difficulty breathing, and significant peak flow readings.

6. When secretions become thick and tacky, increase intake of fluids, avoiding milk and milk products. This thins secretions and assists in their removal.

7. Learn to pace activity and avoid overexertion at all times.

8. Hold medication and report immediately any side effects or CNS depression in children and infants.

9. Review dietary restrictions and limit intake of xanthine-containing products such as coffee, colas, and chocolate.

10. Identify local support groups that may assist in understanding and coping with chronic respiratory dysfunction.

**Outcomes/Evaluate**

• Knowledge and understanding of disease management; compliance with prescribed regimen

• Improved airway exchange, ↓ wheezing, improved breathing patterns

• Drug levels within therapeutic range (10–20 mcg/mL)

# THYROID DRUGS

*See also the following individual entries:*

Levothyroxin sodium
Liothyronine sodium
Liotrix

**Action/Kinetics:** The thyroid manufactures two active hormones: thyroxine and triiodothyronine, both of

---

which contain iodine. These thyroid hormones are released into the bloodstream, where they are bound to protein. Synthetic derivatives include liothyronine ($T_3$), levothyronine ($T_4$), and liotrix (a 4:1 mixture of $T_4$ and $T_3$).The thyroid hormones regulate growth by controlling protein synthesis and regulating energy metabolism by increasing the resting or basal metabolic rate. This results in increases in respiratory rate; body temperature; CO; oxygen consumption; HR; blood volume; enzyme system activity; rate of fat, carbohydrate, and protein metabolism; and growth and maturation. Excess thyroid hormone causes a decrease in TSH, and a lack of thyroid hormone causes an increase in the production and secretion of TSH. Normally, the ratio of $T_4$ to $T_3$ released from the thyroid gland is 20:1 with about 35% of $T_4$ being converted in the periphery (e.g., kidney, liver) to $T_3$.

**Uses:** Replacement or supplemental therapy in hypothyroidism due to all causes except transient hypothyroidism during the recovery phase of subacute thyroiditis. To treat or prevent euthyroid goiters. With antithyroid drugs for thyrotoxicosis (to prevent goiter or hypothyroidism). Diagnostically to differentiate suspected hyperthyroidism from euthyroidism. The treatment of choice for hypothyroidism is usually $T_4$ because of its consistent potency and its prolonged duration of action although it does have a slow onset and its effects are cumulative over several weeks.

**Contraindications:** Uncorrected adrenal insufficiency, acute MI, hyperthyroidism, and thyrotoxicosis. When hypothyroidism and adrenal insufficiency coexist unless treatment with adrenocortical steroids is initiated first. To treat obesity or infertility.

**Special Concerns:** Geriatric clients may be more sensitive to the usual adult dosage of these hormones. Use with extreme caution in the presence of angina pectoris, hypertension, and other CV diseases, renal insufficiency, and ischemic states. Use with caution during lactation.

**Side Effects:** Thyroid preparations have cumulative effects, and overdosage (e.g., symptoms of hyperthyroidism) may occur. *CV:* Arrhythmias, palpitations, angina, increased HR and pulse pressure, *cardiac arrest,* aggravation of CHF. *GI:* Cramps, diarrhea, N&V, appetite changes. *CNS:* Headache, nervousness, mental agitation, irritability, insomnia, tremors. *Miscellaneous:* Weight loss, hyperhidrosis, excessive warmth, irregular menses, heat intolerance, fever, dyspnea, allergic skin reactions (rare). Decreased bone density in pre- and postmenopausal women following long-term use of levothyroxine.

**OD** **Overdose Management:** *Symptoms:* Signs and symptoms of hyperthyroidism including headache, irritability, sweating, tachycardia, nervousness, increased bowel motility, palpitations, vomiting, psychosis, menstrual irregularities, *seizures,* fever. Production or aggravation of angina or CHF, *shock, arrhythmias, cardiac failure.*

**Drug Interactions**

*Anticoagulants* / ↑ Effect of anticoagulants by ↑ hypoprothrombinemia

*Antidepressants, tricyclic* / ↑ Effect of antidepressants and ↑ effect of thyroid

*Antidiabetic agents* / Hyperglycemic effect of thyroid preparations may necessitate ↑ in dose of antidiabetic agent

*Beta-adrenergic blockers* / ↓ Effect of beta blockers when the hypothyroid state is converted to the euthyroid state

*Cholestyramine* / ↓ Effect of thyroid hormone due to ↓ absorption from GI tract

*Colestipol* / ↓ Effect of thyroid hormone due to ↓ absorption from GI tract

*Corticosteroids* / Thyroid preparations ↑ tissue demands for corticosteroids. Adrenal insufficiency must be corrected with corticosteroids before administering thyroid hor-

mones. In clients already treated for adrenal insufficiency, dosage of corticosteroids must be increased when initiating therapy with thyroid drug
*Digitalis compounds* / ↓ Effect of digitalis, with worsening of arrhythmias or CHF
*Epinephrine* / CV effects ↑ by thyroid preparations
*Estrogens* / May ↑ requirements for thyroid hormone
*Ketamine* / Concomitant use may result in severe hypertension and tachycardia
*Levarterenol* / CV effects ↑ by thyroid preparations
*Phenytoin* / ↑ Effect of thyroid hormone by ↓ plasma protein binding
*Salicylates* / Salicylates compete for thyroid-binding sites on protein
*Theophylline* / ↓ Theophylline clearance in hypothyroid client is returned to normal when euthyroid state is reached
**Laboratory Test Interferences:** Alter thyroid function tests. ↑ PT. ↓ Serum cholesterol. A large number of drugs alter thyroid function tests.

## Dosage
See individual hormone products.

## NURSING CONSIDERATIONS
### Administration/Storage
1. Initiate treatment with small doses that are gradually increased.
2. The dose of medication for a child may be the same as the dosage for an adult.
3. Due to differences from one brand of drug to another, brand interchange is not recommended without consulting with provider or pharmacist. Use caution to prevent overdosage or relapse.
4. Store in a cool, dark place away from moisture and light.
### Assessment
1. Perform a thorough nursing history, documenting onset of symptoms and thyroid function tests.
2. Review all meds currently receiving to be sure none interacts unfavorably with the antithyroid drug; note

especially antidiabetic or anticoagulant therapy.
3. Assess clinical presentation noting any symptoms consistent with hypothyroidism (i.e., fatigue, lethargy, weight gain, puffy face and eyelids, large tongue, cold intolerance, hair loss, and cardiomegaly).
4. Assess general physical condition (age, severity and duration of disease) and note any angina, cardiac problems, or other health problems.
5. Obtain and monitor ECG, labs, and thyroid function studies.
### Interventions
1. Monitor thyroid function studies closely (for reduced $T_3$, $T_4$; ↑radioimmunoassay of TSH).
2. Observe for drug side effects and report complaints of headache, insomnia, and tremors.
3. With anticoagulant therapy observe for purpura or ↑ bleeding. Monitor PT/PTT closely; anticoagulant are potentiated by thyroid preparations.
4. Report any symptoms or history of CAD. Monitor BP, HR, and cardiac rhythms and report if HR exceeds 100 bpm.
5. Note general response to the therapy. Complaints of abdominal cramps, weight gain, edema, dyspnea, palpitations, angina, fatigue, or increased pallor may indicate cardiac problems and further assessment is needed.
6. Monitor weights. Observe for heat intolerance and excessive weight loss.
7. Note agent prescribed; thyroid extracts from hog or sheep do not have as predictable a response as the synthetic agents and may see more reactions. Also, animal derivatives are less stable and will degrade with exposure to moisture.
8. Stop drug therapy 4 weeks before radioimmunoassay.
### Client/Family Teaching
1. Drug must be taken only under medical supervision and must be taken for life.
2. Side effects may not appear for

---

4–6 weeks after the start of therapy or when dosage is increased. Therefore, report any new signs or symptoms.

3. Take in a single morning dose, at the same time each day, to reduce the likelihood of insomnia.

4. Do not substitute or change brands of medication without approval.

5. Record BP, pulse, and weight for review at each visit, to evaluate effectiveness of drug therapy.

6. Any excessive weight loss, palpitations, leg cramps, nervousness, or insomnia requires immediate reporting, as dosage may be too high.

7. Carefully monitor child's growth and chart for provider review.

8. With diabetes, thyroid preparations may require adjustment of insulin dosage. Monitor finger sticks closely and report any significant changes.

9. Certain foods, such as cabbage, turnips, pears, and peaches, are goitrogenic and may alter the requirements for thyroid hormone. Consult dietitian to discuss diet and assist with selecting foods according to increased energy demands resulting from the therapy.

10. Thyroid hormones increase client's toxicity to iodine. Therefore avoid foods high in iodine (dried kelp, iodized salt, saltwater fish/shellfish), multivitamins, dentifrices, and other nonprescription meds containing iodine.

11. Thyroid preparations potentiate the action of anticoagulants; therefore, if receiving anticoagulant therapy, report any excessive bruising or bleeding.

12. Females should keep a record of menstrual cycles and report any significant changes.

13. Children may experience temporary hair loss.

14. After several weeks of therapy, report if irritability, nervousness, and excitability occur; may indicate overdosage.

15. Report as scheduled for follow-up visits and lab tests.

**Outcomes/Evaluate**
• Appropriate weight; normal sleep patterns
• Thyroid function tests within desired range
• Normal metabolism evidenced by ↑ mental alertness, improvement in hair and skin condition, normal growth and development, normal HR, and bowel function

# TRANQUILIZERS/ANTI-MANIC DRUGS/HYPNOTICS

*See also the following individual entries:*

Alprazolam
Barbiturates
Buspirone hydrochloride
Chlordiazepoxide
Clorazepate dipotassium
Diazepam
Estazolam
Flurazepam hydrochloride
Hydroxyzine hydrochloride
Hydroxyzine pamoate
Lithium carbonate
Lithium citrate
Lorazepam
Meprobamate
Midazolam hydrochloride
Oxazepam
Temazepam
Triazolam
Zolpidem tartrate

**Action/Kinetics:** Benzodiazepines are the major antianxiety agents. They are thought to affect the limbic system and reticular formation to reduce anxiety by increasing or facilitating the inhibitory neurotransmitter activity of GABA. Two benzodiazepine receptor subtypes have been identified in the brain—$BZ_1$ and $BZ_2$. Receptor subtype $BZ_1$ is believed to be associated with sleep mechanisms, whereas receptor subtype $BZ_2$ is associated with memory, motor, sensory, and cognitive function. When used for 3–4 weeks for sleep, certain benzodiazepines may cause

REM rebound when discontinued. Meprobamate and the benzodiazepines also possess varying degrees of anticonvulsant activity, skeletal muscle relaxation, and the ability to alleviate tension. The benzodiazepines generally have long half-lives (1–8 days); thus cumulative effects can occur. Several of the benzodiazepines are metabolized to active metabolites in the liver, which prolongs their duration of action. Benzodiazepines are widely distributed throughout the body. Approximately 70%–99% of an administered dose is bound to plasma protein. Metabolites of benzodiazepines are excreted through the kidneys. All tranquilizers have the ability to cause psychologic and physical dependence.

**Uses:** See individual drugs. Depending on the drug, used as antianxiety agents, hypnotics, anticonvulsants, and muscle relaxants.

**Contraindications:** Hypersensitivity, acute narrow-angle glaucoma, psychoses, primary depressive disorder, psychiatric disorders in which anxiety is not a signficiant symptom.

**Special Concerns:** Use with caution in impaired hepatic or renal function and in the geriatric or debilitated client. Use during lactation may cause sedation, weight loss, and possibly feeding difficulties in the infant. Geriatric clients may be more sensitive to the effects of benzodiazepines; symptoms may include oversedation, dizziness, confusion, or ataxia. When used for insomnia, rebound sleep disorders may occur following abrupt withdrawal of certain benzodiazepines.

**Side Effects:** *CNS:* Drowsiness, fatigue, confusion, ataxia, sedation, dizziness, vertigo, depression, apathy, lightheadedness, delirium, headache, lethargy, disorientation, hypoactivity, crying, anterograde amnesia, slurred speech, stupor, *coma,* fainting, difficulty in concentration, euphoria, nervousness, irritability, akathisia, hypotonia, vivid dreams, "glassy-eyed," hysteria, *suicide attempt,* psychosis. Paradoxical excitement manifested by anxiety, acute hyperexcitability, increased muscle spasticity, insomnia, hallucinations, sleep disturbances, rage, and stimulation. *GI:* Increased appetite, constipation, diarrhea, anorexia, N&V, weight gain or loss, dry mouth, bitter or metallic taste, increased salivation, coated tongue, sore gums, difficulty in swallowing, gastritis, fecal incontinence. *Respiratory:* **Respiratory depression and sleep apnea,** especially in clients with compromised respiratory function. *Dermatologic:* Urticaria, rash, pruritus, alopecia, hirsutism, dermatitis, edema of ankles and face. *Endocrine:* Increased or decreased libido, gynecomastia, menstrual irregularities. *GU:* Difficulty in urination, urinary retention, incontinence, dysuria, enuresis. *CV:* Hypertension, hypotension, bradycardia, tachycardia, palpitations, edema, *CV collapse.* *Hematologic:* Anemia, *agranulocytosis,* leukopenia, eosinophilia, thrombocytopenia. *Ophthalmologic:* Diplopia, conjunctivitis, nystagmus, blurred vision. *Miscellaneous:* Joint pain, lymphadenopathy, muscle cramps, paresthesia, dehydration, lupus-like symptoms, sweating, SOB, flushing, hiccoughs, fever, hepatic dysfunction. *Following IM use:* Redness, pain, burning. *Following IV use:* Thrombosis and phlebitis at site.

**OD** **Overdose Management:** *Symptoms:* Severe drowsiness, confusion with reduced or absent reflexes, tremors, slurred speech, staggering, hypotension, SOB, labored breathing, *respiratory depression,* impaired coordination, *seizures,* weakness, slow HR, *coma.* NOTE: Geriatric clients, debilitated clients, young children, and clients with liver disease are more sensitive to the CNS effects of benzodiazepines. *Treatment:* Supportive therapy. In the event of an overdose of a benzodizepine, a benzodiazepine antagonist (flumazenil) should be readily available. Gastric lavage, provided that an ET tube with an inflated cuff is used to prevent aspiration of vomitus. Emesis only if drug ingestion was recent and client is fully conscious. Activated charcoal and saline cathartic may be given after emesis or lavage. Adequate respiratory function must be maintained. Hypotension may be reversed by IV fluids, norepinephrine, or metaraminol. Excitation should **not** be treated with barbiturates.

**Drug Interactions**

*Alcohol* / Potentiation or addition of CNS depressant effects. Concomitant use may lead to drowsiness, lethargy, stupor, respiratory collapse, coma, or death

*Anesthetics, general* / See *Alcohol*

*Antacids* / ↓ Rate of absorption of benzodiazepines

*Antidepressants, tricyclic* / Concomitant use with benzodiazepines may cause additive sedative effect and/or atropine-like side effects

*Antihistamines* / See *Alcohol*

*Barbiturates* / See *Alcohol*

*Cimetidine* / ↑ Effect of benzodiazepines by ↓ breakdown in liver

*CNS depressants* / See *Alcohol*

*Digoxin* / Benzodiazepines ↑ effect of digoxin by ↑ serum levels

*Disulfiram* / ↑ Effect of benzodiazepines by ↓ breakdown in liver

*Erythromycin* / ↑ Effect of benzodiazepines by ↓ breakdown in liver

*Fluoxetine* / ↑ Effect of benzodiazepines due to ↓ breakdown in liver

*Isoniazid* / ↑ Effect of benzodiazepines due to ↓ breakdown in liver

*Ketoconazole* / ↑ Effect of benzodiazepines due to ↓ breakdown in liver

*Levodopa* / Effect may be ↓ by benzodiazepines

*Metoprolol* / ↑ Effect of benzodiazepines due to ↓ breakdown in liver

*Narcotics* / See *Alcohol*

*Neuromuscular blocking agents* / Benzodiazepines may ↑ , ↓ , or have no effect on the action of neuromuscular blocking agents

*Oral contraceptives* / ↑ Effect of benzodiazepines due to ↓ breakdown in liver; or, ↑ rate of clearance of benzodiazepines that undergo glucuronidation (e.g., lorazepam, oxazepam)

*Phenothiazines* / See *Alcohol*

*Phenytoin* / Concomitant use with benzodiazepines may cause ↑ effect of phenytoin due to ↓ breakdown by liver

*Probenecid* / ↑ Effect of selected benzodiazepines due to ↓ breakdown by liver

*Propoxyphene* / ↑ Effect of benzodiazepines due to ↓ breakdown by liver

*Propranolol* / ↑ Effect of benzodiazepines due to ↓ breakdown by liver

*Ranitidine* / May ↓ absorption of benzodiazepines from the GI tract

*Rifampin* / ↓ Effect of benzodiazepines due to ↑ breakdown by liver

*Sedative-hypnotics, nonbarbiturate* / See *Alcohol*

*Theophyllines* / ↓ Sedative effect of benzodiazepines

*Valproic acid* / ↑ Effect of benzodiazepines due to ↓ breakdown by liver

**Laboratory Test Interferences:** ↑ AST, ALT, LDH, alkaline phosphatase.

**Dosage** ─────────────────

See individual drugs.

## NURSING CONSIDERATIONS

### Administration/Storage

1. Persistent drowsiness, ataxia, or visual disturbances may require dosage adjustment.

2. Lower dosage is usually indicated for older clients.

3. GI effects are decreased when drugs are given with meals or shortly afterward.

4. Withdraw drugs gradually.

### Assessment

1. Document indications for therapy, onset of symptoms, and behavioral manifestations. Note any prior treatment for these problems, what was used, for how long, and the outcome.

2. List drugs currently prescribed to ensure none interact unfavorably. Note any adverse reactions to this class of drugs.

3. Assess life-style and general level

of health; note any situations that may contribute to these symptoms.

4. Assess the manner in which client responds to questions and discusses problems.

5. Monitor CBC, liver and renal function studies; assess for blood dyscrasias or impaired function.

6. Review physical and history for any contraindications to therapy.

**Interventions**

1. Document any symptoms consistent with overdosage.

2. Report any complaints of sore throat (other than those caused by NG or ET tubes), fever, or weakness and assess for blood dyscrasias; check CBC.

3. Monitor BP before and after IV dose of antianxiety medication. Keep recumbent for 2–3 hr after IV administration.

4. Administer the lowest possible effective dose, especially if elderly or debilitated.

5. When administered PO to a hospitalized client, remain until drug is swallowed.

6. If client exhibits ataxia, or weakness or lack of coordination when ambulating, provide supervision/assistance. Use side rails once in bed and identify at risk for falls.

7. Note any S&S of cholestatic jaundice: nausea, diarrhea, upper abdominal pain, or the presence of high fever or rash; check LFTs.

8. If yellowing of sclera, skin, or mucous membranes evident (late sign of cholestatic jaundice and biliary tract obstruction), withhold drug and report.

9. If overly sleepy/confused or becomes comatose, withhold drug and report.

10. With suicidal tendencies, anticipate drug will be prescribed in small doses. Report signs of increased depression immediately.

11. If history of alcoholism or if taking excessive quantities of drug, carefully supervise amount of drug prescribed and dispensed. Assess for manifestations of ataxia, slurred speech, and vertigo (symptoms of chronic intoxication and that client may be exceeding recommended dose).

12. Note any evidence of physical or psychologic dependence. Assess frequency and quantity of refills.

**Client/Family Teaching**

1. These drugs may reduce ability to handle potentially dangerous equipment, such as automobiles and other machinery.

2. Take most of the daily dose at bedtime if condition permits, with smaller doses during the waking hours to minimize mental and motor impairment.

3. Avoid alcohol while taking antianxiety agents. Alcohol potentiates the depressant effects of both the alcohol and the medication.

4. Do not take any unprescribed or OTC medications without approval.

5. Arise slowly from a supine position and dangle legs over side of the bed for a few minutes before standing up.

6. If feeling faint sit or lie down immediately and lower the head.

7. Allow extra time to prepare for daily activities to take the necessary precautions before arising, thereby reducing one source of anxiety and stress.

8. Do not stop taking drug suddenly. Any sudden withdrawal after prolonged therapy or after excessive use may cause a recurrence of the preexisting symptoms of anxiety. It may also cause a withdrawal syndrome, manifested by increased anxiety, anorexia, insomnia, vomiting, ataxia, muscle twitching, confusion, and hallucinations. Some clients may develop seizures and convulsions.

9. Identify/practice relaxation techniques that may assist in lowering anxiety levels.

10. These drugs are generally for short-term therapy; follow-up is imperative to evaluate response and the need for continued therapy.

11. Attend appropriate counselling

sessions as condition and length of therapy dictate.

**Outcomes/Evaluate**
- Symptomatic improvement with ↓ frequency in anxiety/tension episodes
- Effective coping
- ↓ Frequency and intensity of muscle spasms and tremor
- Improved sleeping patterns; less frequent early morning awakenings
- Control of seizures
- Control of alcohol withdrawal symptoms

# VACCINES

*See Table 2 and Table 3.*

**General Statement:** Vaccines have played an important role in the health and life span of our population. They have been in use over 200 years, but since World War II, once the importance of disease prevention became evident, research into the area of vaccine development exploded.

Use of a vaccine (or actually contracting the disease) usually renders one temporary or permanent resistance to an infectious disease. Vaccines and toxoids promote the type of antibody production one would see if they had experienced the natural infection. This active immunization involves the direct administration of antigens to the host to cause them to produce the desired antibodies and cell-mediated immunity. These agents may consist of live attenuated agents or killed (inactivated) agents. Immunizations confer this resistance without actually producing the disease.

Passive immunization occurs when immunologic agents are administered. Immunoglobulins and antivenins only offer passive short-term immunity and are usually administered for a specific exposure.

Aggressive pediatric immunization programs have helped reduce preventable infections and death in children worldwide. This focus should continue and be expanded to the adult population, many of whom have missed the natural infection and their past immunizations. A careful immunization history should be documented for every client, regardless of age. When in doubt or if unknown if had infection or immunization, appropriate titers may be drawn. Table 2 lists some of the more common diseases, the general recommended schedule to confer immunization, and the length of immunity conferred; Table 3 outlines the active childhood immunization schedule.

# VITAMINS

**General Statement:** Vitamins are essential, carbon-containing, noncaloric substances that are required for normal metabolism. They are produced by living materials such as plants and animals and they are generally obtained from the diet. Vitamin D is synthesized in the diet to a limited extent and Vitamin B–12 is synthesized in the intestinal tract by bacterial flora.

Vitamins are essential for promoting growth, health, and life. They are necessary for the metabolic processes responsible for transforming foods into tissue or energy. Vitamins are also involved in the formation and maintenance of blood cells, chemicals supporting the nervous system, hormones, and genetic materials. Vitamins do not provide energy because they contain no calories. Yet, some do help convert the calories in fats, carbohydrates, and proteins into usable body energy.

Disease states caused by severe nutritional deficiencies prompted the discovery of vitamins because scientists were able to reverse the signs and symptoms of these disease states with vitamins. Severe deficiencies include scurvy, rickets, pellagra, pernicious anemia, xerophthalmia, beriberi, osteomalacia, infantile hemolytic anemia, and hemorrhagic diseases of the newborn. Moderate

**Table 2    Common Diseases, General Recommended Immunization Schedule, and Length of Immunity**

| DISEASE | IMMUNIZATION SCHEDULE | LENGTH OF IMMUNITY |
|---|---|---|
| Cholera | Two doses 1 week to 1 month apart | 6 months |
| Diphtheria | Given as DPT; four doses at ages 2, 4, 6, and 15–18 months | 10 years |
| Haemophilus influenzae (Hib) | Four doses at ages 2, 4, 6, and 15 months | Unknown |
| Hepatitis B | Three doses: at birth (or initial dose), 1 month later, and 6 months after initial dose | 10 years |
| Influenza | One dose (or two doses of split virus if under 13 years) | 1–3 years |
| Measles | Given as MMR at ages 12–15 months and 4–6 years | Lifetime |
| Meningococcal meningitis | One dose (antibody response requires 5 days); antibiotic prophylaxis (Rifampin 600 mg or 10 mg/kg q 12 hr for four doses should be given to all contacts) | ?Lifetime; not consistently effective in those <2 years of age |
| Mumps | Given as MMR at ages 12–15 months and 4–6 years | Lifetime |
| Pertussis | Given as DPT; four doses at ages 2, 4, 6, and 15–18 months | 10 years |
| Pneumococcus | One dose (0.5 mL) | Approx. 5 years |
| Poliomyelitis | Four doses at ages 2, 4, and 6 months, then at age 4–6 years | Lifetime |

*(continued)*

✿ = Available in Canada          ***bold italic*** = life threatening side effect

**Table 2**  *(continued)*

| DISEASE | IMMUNIZATION SCHEDULE | LENGTH OF IMMUNITY |
|---|---|---|
| Rabies | Postexposure: five doses on days 0, 3, 7, 14, and 28 with the rabies immune globulin; pre-exposure: two doses 1 week apart, third dose 2–3 weeks later | Approx. 2 years |
| Rubella | Given as MMR at ages 12–15 months and 4–6 years | Lifetime |
| Smallpox | One dose; this disease has been eradicated and vaccine is used only with military personnel and lab workers using pox viruses | 3 years |
| Tetanus | Given initially as DPT; four doses at ages 2, 4, 6, and 15–18 months | 10 years; a tetanus booster is required q 10 years |
| VZV (varicellazoster virus; chicken pox) | One dose (0.5 mL) age 12 months to 12 years; two injections of 0.5 mL 4–8 weeks apart in age 13 and older | ?Lifetime |
| Yellow fever | One dose | 10 years |

**Table 3    Active Childhood Immunization Schedule**

|       | #1                   | #2                        | #3                                    | #4           |
|-------|----------------------|---------------------------|---------------------------------------|--------------|
| DPT   | 2 months             | 4 months                  | 6 months                              | 15–18 months |
| OPV   | 2 months             | 4 months                  | 6 months                              | 4–6 years    |
| Hib   | 2 months             | 4 months                  | 6 months                              | 15–18 months |
| MMR   | 12 months            | 4 years                   |                                       |              |
| Hep B | birth or initial dose | 1 month after first dose | 6 months or more after second dose    |              |

✦ = Available in Canada                                    **_bold italic_** = life threatening side effect

vitamin deficiencies may also produce symptoms of impaired health.

Environmental factors and genetic predisposition may influence individual requirements for specific vitamins. Disease processes, growth, hormone balance, and drugs may also alter the dietary requirements and function of vitamins.

Many deficiency states can be traced to special circumstances such as pernicious anemia after gastrectomy; pellagra in corn–eating populations, and scurvy in the elderly subsisting on soft foods (e.g., eggs, bread, milk) while neglecting citrus fruits. Generally, although not common in the United States, vitamin deficiency usually involves multiple rather than single deficiencies and usually can be attributed to poor dietary habits with an inadequate intake of many nutrients, including all vitamins.

There are two categories of vitamins: fat soluble and water soluble. Fat soluble viatmins A, D, E, and K are found in the fat or oil of foods and require digestible fat and bile salts for absorption in the small intestine. The water-soluble vitamins, C and B complex (B-1, B-2, niacin, B-6, folic acid, B-12, pantothenic acid, and biotin) are found in the watery portion of foods and are well absorbed by the GI tract. They are easily lost through overcooking and do not require fat for absorption. Water soluble vitamins mix easily in the blood, are excreted by the kidneys, and only small amounts are stored in the tissues, so regular daily intake is essential. Fat soluble vitamins are stored in the body after binding to specific plasma globulins in fat parts of the body.

Recommended Dietary Allowances (RDAs) are the recommended human vitamin and mineral intake requirements. These were developed by the Food and Nutrition Board, National Research Council of the National Academy of Sciences and have evolved over the past 50 years and are updated every 5 years. They are based on age, height, weight, and gender. These are only estimates of nutrient needs; each client and the surrounding factors warrant individualized evaluation when replacement is being considered.

**Table 4**

| Vitamin | RDA | Physiologic Effects Essential for: |
|---|---|---|
| A (retinol, retinaldehyde, retonic acid) | 1400-6000 IU | growth & development epithelial tissue maintenance; reproduction |
| *B complex:* | | |
| B-1 (thiamine) | 0.3–1.5 mg | energy metabolism: normal nerve function |
| B-2 (riboflavin) | 0.4–1.8 mg | reactions in energy cycle that produce ATP; oxidation of amino acids and hydroxy-acids; oxidation of purines |
| Niacin (nicotinic acid, nicotinamide) | 5–19 mg | synthesis of fatty acids and cholesterol; conversion of phenylalanine to tyrosine |
| B-6 (pyridoxine, pyridoxal, pyridoxamine) | 0.3–2.5 mg | amino acid metabolism; glycogenolysis, Hb synthesis; formation of neurotransmitters; formation of antibodies |

**Table 4**   *(continued)*

| Vitamin | RDA | Physiologic Effects Essential for: |
|---|---|---|
| Folacin (folic acid, pteroylglutamic acid) | 50–800 mcg | DNA synthesis, formation of RBCs in bone marrow with cyanocobalamine |
| B-3 Pantothenic acid (calcium pantothenate, dexpanthenol) | 10 mg | synthesis of sterols, steroid hormones, porphyrins; synthesis and degradation of fatty acids; oxidative metabolism of carbohydrates, gluconeogenesis |
| B-12 (cyanocobalamin, hydroxocobalamin, extrinsic factor) | 0.3–4.0 mcg | DNA synthesis in bone marrow; RBC production with folacin |
| B-7 (Biotin) | No recommendation | synthesis of fatty acids, generation of tricarboxylic acid cycle; formation of purines |
| C (ascorbic acid, ascorbate) | 60 mg | formation of collagen; conversion of cholesterol to bile acids; Protects A and E and polyunsaturated fats from excessive oxidation; absorption and utilization of iron; converts folacin to folinic acid; some role in clotting, adreno-cortical hormones, and resistance to cancer and infections |
| D (calcitriol, cholecalciferol, dihydrotachysterol, ergocalciferol, viosterol) | 400 IU | intestinal absorption and metabolism of calcium and phosphorus as well as renal reabsorption; release of calcium from bone and resorption |
| E (tocopherol) | 4–15 IU | May oppose destruction of Vit. A and fats by oxygen fragments called free radicals; antioxidant; may affect production of prostaglandins which regulate a variety of body processes |
| K (menadione, Phytonadione) | No recommendation | formation of prothrombin and other clotting proteins by the liver |

♣ = Available in Canada     ***bold italic*** = life threatening side effect

**Table 5**

| Vitamin | Effect | Uses |
|---|---|---|
| A (retinoic acid) | reduces formation of comedones; keratin production suppression | acne, psoriasis, ichthyosis, Darier's disease |
| Niacin | reduction of blood cholesterol and triglycerides | hypercholesterolemia, hyperbetalipoproteinemia |
| D (dihydrotachysterol) | maintains calcium and phosphorus levels in bone and blood | hypoparathyroidism |
| C | reduces urine pH; converts methemoglobin to hemoglobin | idiopathic methemoglobin; recurrent UTIs in high risk clients |
| E | reduces endogenous peroxidases | hemolytic anemia in premature infants |
| K | increases liver production of thrombin | warfarin toxicity |

**Table 6    Vitamin Deficiency States**

| Vitamin | Deficiency | Signs & Symptoms |
|---|---|---|
| A | Xerophthalmia | progressive eye changes: night blindness to xerosis of conjunctiva and cornea with scarring |
|  | Keratomalacia | degeneration of epithelial cells with hardening and shrinking |
| B-6 | Beriberi | fatigue, weight loss, weakness, irritability; headaches, insomnia peripheral neuropathy, CHF, cardiomyopathy |
| Niacin | Pellagra | depression, anorexia, beefy red glossitis, cheilosis, dermatitis |
| B-12 | Pernicious anemia | macrocytic, megaloblastic anemia progressive neuropathy R/T progressive demyelination |
| C | Scurvy | joint pain, growth retardation anemia, poor wound healing with increased susceptibility to infection; petechial hemorrhages |
| D | Rickets (child) Osteomalacia (adult) | demineralization of bones and teeth with bone pain and skeletal muscle deformities |
| E | Hemolytic anemia in low birth weight infants | macrocytic anemia; increased hemolysis of RBC's and increased capillarity fragility |
| K | Hemorrhagic disease in newborns | increase tendency to hemorrhage |

# CHAPTER 3
# A–Z Listing of Drugs

## A

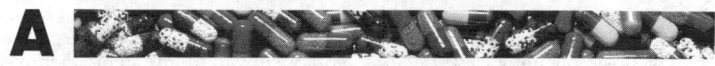

## Abciximab
(ab-**SIX**-ih-mab)
**Pregnancy Category:** C
ReoPro **(Rx)**
**Classification:** Antiplatelet agent

**Action/Kinetics:** Abciximab is the Fab fragment of the chimeric human-murine monoclonal antibody 7E3. It binds to a glycoprotein receptor on human platelets, thus inhibiting platelet aggregation by preventing binding of fibrinogen, von Willebrand factor, and other adhesive molecules to receptor sites on activated platelets. **t½, after IV bolus:** 30 min. Recovery of platelet function: About 48 hr, although drug remains in circulation bound to platelets for up to 10 days. Following IV infusion, free drug levels in the plasma decrease rapidly for about 6 hr and then decline at a slower rate.

**Uses:** Inhibition of platelet aggregation. Adjunct to percutaneous transluminal coronary angioplasty or atherectomy for prophylaxis of acute cardiac ischemic complications in clients at high risk for abrupt closure of the treated coronary vessel. Used with aspirin and heparin. Adjunct with heparin to prevent cardiac ischemic complications in those undergoing PCI; also, for unstable angina clients not responding to conventional therapy when PCI is scheduled within 24 hr.

**Contraindications:** Due to potential for drug-induced bleeding, abciximab is contraindicated as follows: history of CVA (within 2 years) or CVA with significant residual neurologic deficit; active internal bleeding; within 6 weeks of GI or GU bleeding of clinical significance; bleeding diathesis; within 7 days of administration of oral anticoagulants unless the PT is less than 1.2 times control; thrombocytopenia (less than 100,000 cells/μL); within 6 weeks of major surgery or trauma; intracranial neoplasm; arteriovenous malformation or aneurysm; severe uncontrolled hypertension; presumed or documented history of vasculitis; use of IV dextran before atherectomy or intent to use it during atherectomy; hypersensitivity to murine proteins.

**Special Concerns:** Benefits versus risk of increased bleeding should be assessed in clients who weigh less than 75 kg, are 65 years of age or older, have history of GI disease, are receiving thrombolytics, and are receiving heparin. The following conditions are also associated with increased risk of bleeding in angioplasty setting and which may be additive to that of abciximab: atherectomy within 12 hr of onset of symptoms for acute MI, atherectomy lasting more than 70 min, and failed atherectomy. Use with caution when abciximab is used with other drugs that affect hemostasis, including thrombolytics, oral anticoagulants, NSAIDs, dipyridamole, and ticlopidine. Use with caution during lactation. Safety and efficacy have not been determined in children.

**Side Effects:** *CV: Increased bleeding tendencies,* hypotension, bradycardia, atrial fibrillation or flutter, vascular disorder, pulmonary edema, *complete AV block,* supraventricular tachycardia, weak pulse, palpitations,

**A**

intermittent claudication, pericardial effusion, limb embolism, **pulmonary embolism, ventricular arrhythmia.** *GI:* N&V, diarrhea, constipation, ileus. *Hematologic:* Thrombocytopenia, anemia, leukocytosis, hemolytic anemia, petechiae. *CNS:* Hypesthesia, confusion, abnormal thinking, dizziness, **coma, brain ischemia,** insomnia. *Respiratory:* Pleural effusion, pleurisy, pneumonia. *Musculoskeletal:* Myopathy, cellulitis, myalgia. *GU:* Urinary tract infection, urinary retention, abnormal renal function. *Miscellaneous:* Pain, peripheral edema, abnormal vision, development of human antichimeric antibody, dysphonia, pruritus.

## Dosage
• **IV Bolus Followed by IV Infusion**
   *Clients undergoing atherectomy with concomitant use of heparin and aspirin.*
**IV bolus:** 0.25 mg/kg given 10–60 min before the start of atherectomy. This is followed by **continuous IV infusion:** 10 mcg/min for 12 hr.

## NURSING CONSIDERATIONS
### Administration/Storage
**IV** 1. Stop infusion after 12 hr to avoid the effects of prolonged platelet receptor blockade.
2. Stop continuous infusion in clients with failed atherectomy, as there is no evidence the drug is effective in such situations.
3. Discontinue abciximab and heparin if serious bleeding occurs that is not controlled by compression.
4. Preparations of abciximab should not be used if they contain visibly opaque particles.
5. If symptoms of allergic reaction or anaphylaxis occur, the infusion should be stopped immediately and appropriate treatment started. Epinephrine, dopamine, theophylline, antihistamines, and corticosteroids should be available for immediate use.
6. Withdraw drug (2 mg/mL) for bolus administration through a sterile, nonpyrogenic, low-protein-binding 0.2- or 0.22-µm filter into a syringe;

give bolus 10–60 min before procedure.
7. For continuous infusion, withdraw 4.5 mL abciximab through sterile, nonpyrogenic, low-protein-binding 0.2- or 0.22-µm filter into syringe. Inject into 250 mL of 0.9% NSS or D5% and infuse at a rate of 17 mL/hr (10 mcg/min) for 12 hr using a continuous infusion, pump equipped with in-line sterile, nonpyrogenic, low-protein-binding 0.2- or 0.22-µm filter. Any unused drug should be discarded at end of 12-hr infusion.
8. Give drug through a separate IV line with no other medication added to the infusion solution. No incompatibilities have been noted with glass bottles, PVC bags or administration sets.
9. Store vials at 2°C–8°C (36°F–46°F); do not freeze or shake vials.
### Assessment
1. Obtain a thorough nursing history and document indications and goals of therapy.
2. Note any history of CVA, bleeding disorders, recent episodes of bleeding, trauma, or surgery.
3. List other agents prescribed/OTC and when last consumed to determine if any enhance the potential for bleeding.
4. Monitor PT, INR, PTT, CBC, VS, and EKG. Check platelet count 2–4 hr after initial bolus and again in 24 hr.
### Interventions
1. Anticipate client undergoing PTCA and atherectomy will be bolused with abciximab (0.25 mg/kg) 10–60 min before procedure followed by a continuous IV infusion (10 mcg/min) for 12 hr.
2. Insert separate IV lines with saline locks for blood draws.
3. Observe carefully during infusion as anaphylaxis may occur at any time.
4. Administer 325 mg aspirin orally 2 hr before procedure and prepare heparin bolus and infusion for administration as prescribed.
5. Observe for any potential bleeding sites: catheter insertion sites, needle punctures, GI, GU, and retroperitoneal

sites. Remove tape and dressings gently.

6. If serious bleeding develops (not controlled with pressure), stop infusions of abciximab and heparin.

7. Keep on complete bedrest while vascular access sheath is in place. Restrain limb in a straight position, and raise head of bed no more that 30 degrees. Discontinue heparin infusion at least 4 hr before sheath removal. Palpate and monitor distal pulses of involved extremity.

8. Apply pressure for 30 min over femoral artery once sheath is removed. When hemostasis evident, apply a pressure dressing (sandbag) and check frequently for evidence of bleeding. Monitor any hematoma formation for enlargement. Enforce bedrest for 6–8 hr after abciximab infusion is completed and the sheath has been removed.

**Client/Family Teaching**

1. Review indications for therapy, what to expect, clinical management, and the anticipated results.

2. Review risks associated with this therapy, e.g., bleeding from intracranial hemorrhage, which may be lethal, or hematuria or hematemesis, which may require blood and/or platelet transfusions.

3. Drug may cause formation of human antichimeric antibody, which may cause allergic or hypersensitivity reactions, thrombocytopenia, or diminished response on readministration.

**Outcomes/Evaluate:** Prevention of abrupt coronary vessel closure with associated ischemic complications

# Acarbose

(ah-**KAR**-bohs)
**Pregnancy Category:** B
Prandase ✦, Precose **(Rx)**
**Classification:** Antidiabetic agent

**Action/Kinetics:** Acarbose is an oligosaccharide obtained from a fermentation process using the microorganism *Actinoplans utahensis*. Drug causes competitive, reversible inhibition of pancreatic alpha-amylase and membrane-bound intestinal alpha-glucosidase hydrolase enzymes. This causes delayed glucose absorption resulting in a smaller increase in blood glucose following meals. Glycosylated hemoglobin levels are decreased in those with non-insulin-dependent diabetes mellitus. Because mechanism of action is different from sulfonylureas (i.e., enhance insulin secretion), acarbose is additive to effect of sulfonylureas. Approximately 65% of oral dose of acarbose remains in GI tract, which is site of action. Metabolized in GI tract by both intestinal bacteria and intestinal enzymes. Acarbose and metabolites that are absorbed are excreted in the urine.

**Uses:** Used alone, with diet control, to decrease blood glucose in type 2 diabetes mellitus. Also, used with sulfonylurea when diet plus either acarbose or sulfonylurea alone do not control blood glucose adequately.

**Contraindications:** Diabetic ketoacidosis, cirrhosis, inflammatory bowel disease, colonic ulceration, partial intestinal obstruction or predisposition to intestinal obstruction, chronic intestinal diseases associated with marked disorders of digestion or absorption, conditions that may deteriorate as a result of increased gas formation in the intestine. In significant renal dysfunction. Severe, persistent bradycardia. Lactation.

**Special Concerns:** Safety and efficacy have not been determined in children. Acarbose does not cause hypoglycemia; however, sulfonylureas and insulin can lower blood glucose sufficiently to cause symptoms or even life-threatening hypoglycemia.

**Side Effects:** *GI:* Abdominal pain, diarrhea, flatulence. GI side effects may be severe and be confused with paralytic ileus.

**OD** **Overdose Management:** *Symptoms:* Flatulence, diarrhea, abdominal discomfort. *Treatment:* Reduce dose; symptoms will subside.

**Drug Interactions**
*Charcoal* / ↓ Effect of acarbose
*Digestive enzymes* / ↓ Effect of acarbose
*Digoxin* / ↓ Serum digoxin levels
*Insulin* / ↑ Hypoglycemia which may cause severe hypoglycemia
*Sulfonylureas* / ↑ Hypoglycemia which may cause severe hypoglycemia

**Laboratory Test Interferences:** ↑ Serum transaminases (especially with doses greater than 50 mg t.i.d.). Small ↓ in hematocrit. Low plasma B$_6$ levels.

**Dosage** ————————
• **Tablets**
*Type 2 diabetes mellitus.*
Individualized, depending on effectiveness and tolerance. **Initial:** 25 mg (one-half of a 50-mg tablet) t.i.d. with the first bite of each main meal. **Maintenance:** After the initial dose of 25 mg t.i.d., the dose can be increased to 50 mg t.i.d. Some may benefit from 100 mg t.i.d. The dosage can be adjusted at 4- to 8-week intervals. The recommended maximum daily dose is 50 mg t.i.d. for clients weighing less than 60 kg and 100 mg t.i.d. for those weighing more than 60 kg.

## NURSING CONSIDERATIONS

**Administration/Storage**
1. Start with a low dose to reduce GI side effects and to help determine the minimum effective dose.
2. If a dose is missed, the usual dose should be taken at the start of the next main meal.

**Assessment**
1. Document indications for therapy, age at symptom onset, other agents trialed and the outcome.
2. Note any cirrhosis or chronic intestinal diseases with disorders of digestion or absorption.
3. Obtain baseline CBC, HbA1C, blood sugar, electrolytes, urinalysis, liver and renal function tests; assess for B$_6$ deficiency. Monitor HbA1C and LFTs every 3 months.
4. Initiate and titrate acarbose based on blood glucose results. Ideally, a 1-hr postprandial plasma glucose level

should be measured to determine the effective dose.
5. Acarbose may enhance glycemic control with a sulfonylurea, but it may also be used alone.

**Client/Family Teaching**
1. Take drug as prescribed, three times a day with the first bite of main meals.
2. Acarbose delays the digestion of ingested carbohydrates (glucose) and is a treatment in addition to diet and not instead of.
3. Caloric restrictions and weight loss, especially in the obese client, must be continued to control blood sugar and to prevent complications of diabetes; continue regular physical exercise.
4. The most common side effects are of GI origin (abdominal discomfort, diarrhea, gas), and should subside in frequency and intensity with continued use.
5. Do frequent monitoring of glucose (finger sticks) and record to assess the therapeutic response.
6. Loss of glucose control may result when exposed to stress, such as fever, trauma, infection, or surgery. In these instances, temporary insulin may be needed.
7. Candy bars should not be used to counteract hypoglycemia; use glucose tablets or gel or lactose for this purpose.

**Outcomes/Evaluate:** Control of blood sugar with non-insulin-dependent diabetes mellitus

# Acebutolol hydrochloride
(ays-**BYOU**-toe-lohl)
**Pregnancy Category:** B
Apo-Acebutolol ✤, Monitan ✤, Novo-Acebutolol ✤, Nu-Acebutolol ✤, Rhotral ✤, Sectral **(Rx)**
**Classification:** Beta-adrenergic blocking agent

See also *Beta-Adrenergic Blocking Agents.*
**Action/Kinetics:** Predominantly beta-1 blocking activity but will inhibit beta-2 receptors at higher doses. Some intrinsic sympathomi-

metic activity. **t½:** 3–4 hr. Low lipid solubility. **Duration:** 24–30 hr. Metabolized in liver and excreted in urine and bile. Fifteen to 20% excreted unchanged.
**Uses:** Hypertension (either alone or with other antihypertensive agents such as thiazide diuretics). Premature ventricular contractions.
**Additional Contraindications:** Severe, persistent bradycardia.
**Special Concerns:** Dosage not established in children.

**Dosage**
• **Capsules**
*Hypertension.*
**Initial:** 400 mg/day (although 200 mg b.i.d. may be needed for optimum control; **then,** 400–800 mg/day (range: 200–1,200 mg/day).
*Premature ventricular contractions.*
**Initial:** 200 mg b.i.d.; **then,** increase dose gradually to reach 600–1,200 mg/day.
Dosage should not exceed 800 mg/day in geriatric clients. In those with impaired kidney or liver function, decrease dose by 50% when creatinine clearance is 50 mL/min/1.73 m² and by 75% when it is less than 25 mL/min/1.73 m².

**NURSING CONSIDERATIONS**

See also *Nursing Considerations* for *Beta-Adrenergic Blocking Agents,* and *Antihypertensive Agents.*
**Administration/Storage**
1. When discontinued, gradually withdraw drug over a 2-week period.
2. Bioavailability increases in elderly clients; thus, such clients may require lower maintenance doses (no more than 800 mg/day).
3. May be combined with another antihypertensive agent.
4. Reduce dosage with impaired liver and renal function.
**Client/Family Teaching**
1. Drug may cause drowsiness; do not perform tasks that require mental alertness until drug effects realized.

2. May cause an increased sensitivity to cold; dress appropriately.
3. Report any evidence of sudden weight gain, edema, or SOB.
4. Do not stop abruptly without provider approval.
**Outcomes/Evaluate:** ↓ BP; control of PVCs

# Acetaminophen (Apap, Paracetamol)

(ah-**SEAT**-ah-**MIN**-oh-fen)
**Caplets:** Arthritis Foundation Pain Reliever Aspirin Free, Aspirin Free Pain Relief, Aspirin Free Anacid Maximum Strength, Atasol ✿, Atasol Forte ✿, Genapap Extra Strength, Genebs Extra Strength Caplets, Panadol, Panadol Junior Strength, Tapanol Extra Strength, Tylenol Caplets, Tylenol Extended Relief, **Capsules:** Dapacin, Meda Cap, **Elixir:** Aceta, Genapap Children's, Mapap Children's, Oraphen-PD, Ridenol, Silapap Children's, Tylenol Children's, **Gelcaps:** Aspirin Free Anacid Maximum Strength, Tapanol Extra Strength, Tylenol Extra Strength, **Oral Liquid/Syrup:** Atasol ✿, Children's Acetaminophen Elixir Drops ✿, Halenol Children's, Panadol Children's, Pediatrix ✿, Tempra ✿, Tempra 2 Syrup, Tempra Children's Syrup ✿, Tylenol Extra Strength, **Oral Solution:** Acetaminophen Drops, Apacet, Atasol ✿, Children's Acetaminophen Oral Solution ✿, Genapap Infants' Drops, Mapap Infant Drops, Panadol Infants' Drops, Pediatrix ✿, PMS-Acetaminophen ✿, Silapap Infants, Tempra 1, Tylenol Infants' Drops, Uni-Ace, **Oral Suspension:** Tylenol Children's Suspension ✿, Tylenol Infants' Suspension ✿, **Sprinkle Capsules:** Feverall Children's, Feverall Junior Strength, **Suppositories:** Abenol 120, 325, 650 mg ✿, Acephen, Acetaminophen Uniserts, Children's Feverall, Infant's Feverall, Junior Strength Feverall, Neopap, **Tablets:** Aceta, A.F. Anacin ✿, A.F. Anacin Extra Strength ✿, Apo-Acetaminophen ✿, Aspirin Free Pain Relief, Aspirin Free Anacin Maximum Strength, Atasol ✿, Atasol Forte ✿, Extra Strength Acetaminophen ✿, Fem-Etts, Genapap, Genapap Extra Strength, Genebs, Genebs Extra Strength, Mapap

---

Regular Strength, Mapap Extra Strength, Maranox, Meda Tab, Panadol, Redutemp, Regular Strength Acetaminophen ✱, Tapanol Regular Strength, Tapanol Extra Strength, Tempra, Tylenol Regular Strength, Tylenol Extra Strength, Tylenol Junior Strength, Tylenol Tablets 325 mg, 500 mg ✱, **Tablets, Chewable:** Apacet, Children's Chewable Acetaminophen ✱, Children's Genapap, Children's Panadol, Children's Tylenol, Tempra ✱, Tempra 3, Tylenol Chewable Tablets Fruit, Tylenol Junior Strength Chewable Tablets Fruit ✱ **(OTC)**

# Acetaminophen, buffered

(ah-**SEAT**-ah-**MIN**-oh-fen)
Alka-Seltzer, Bromo Seltzer **(OTC)**
**Classification:** Nonnarcotic analgesic, para-aminophenol type

**Action/Kinetics:**    Acetaminophen decreases fever by an effect on the hypothalamus leading to sweating and vasodilation. It also inhibits the effect of pyrogens on the hypothalamic heat-regulating centers. It may cause analgesia by inhibiting CNS prostaglandin synthesis; however, due to minimal effects on peripheral prostaglandin synthesis, acetaminophen has no anti-inflammatory or uricosuric effects. It does not cause any anticoagulant effect or ulceration of the GI tract. The antipyretic and analgesic effects are comparable to those of aspirin.

**Peak plasma levels:** 30–120 min. **t½:** 45 min–3 hr. **Therapeutic serum levels** (analgesia): 5–20 mcg/mL. **Plasma protein binding:** Approximately 25%. Metabolized in the liver and excreted in the urine as glucuronide and sulfate conjugates. However, an intermediate hydroxylated metabolite is hepatotoxic following large doses of acetaminophen.

Acetaminophen is often combined with other drugs, as in Darvocet-N, Parafon Forte, and Tylenol with Codeine.

The extended-relief product uses a bilayer system that allows the outer layer to release acetaminophen rapidly while the inner layer is designed to release the remainder of the dose more slowly. This allows prolonged relief of symptoms.

The buffered product is a mixture of acetaminophen, sodium bicarbonate, and citric acid that effervesces when placed in water. This product has a high sodium content (0.76 g/¾ capful).

**Uses:** Control of pain due to headache, earache, dysmenorrhea, arthralgia, myalgia, musculoskeletal pain, immunizations, teething, tonsillectomy. To reduce fever in bacterial or viral infections. As a substitute for aspirin in upper GI disease, aspirin allergy, bleeding disorders, clients on anticoagulant therapy, and gouty arthritis. *Investigational:* In children receiving diptheria-pertussis-tetanus vaccination to decrease incidence of fever and pain at injection site.

**Contraindications:** Renal insufficiency, anemia. Clients with cardiac or pulmonary disease are more susceptible to toxic effects of acetaminophen.

**Special Concerns:** Evidence indicates that acetaminophen may have to be used with caution in pregnancy. Heavy drinking and fasting may be risk factors for acetaminophen toxicity, especially if larger than recommended doses of acetaminophen are used. As little as twice the recommended dosage, over time, can lead to serious liver damage.

**Side Effects:** Few when taken in usual therapeutic doses. Chronic and even acute toxicity can develop after long symptom-free usage. *Hematologic:* Methemoglobinemia, **hemolytic anemia** , neutropenia, thrombocytopenia, pancytopenia, leukopenia. *Allergic:* Urticarial and erythematous skin reactions, skin eruptions, fever. *Miscellaneous:* CNS stimulation, hypoglycemic coma, jaundice, drowsiness, glossitis.

**OD** **Overdose Management:** *Symptoms:* May be no early specific symptoms. Within first 24 hr: N&V, diaphoresis, anorexia, drowsiness, confusion, liver tenderness, cardiac arrhythmias, low BP, jaundice, acute hepatic and renal failure. Within 24–48 hr, increased AST, ALT, bilibrubin, prothrombin levels. After 72–96 hr, peak hepatotoxicity with death possible due to liver necrosis. *Treatment:* Initially, induction of emesis, gastric lavage, activated charcoal. Oral *N*-acetylcysteine is said to reduce or prevent hepatic damage by inactivating acetaminophen metabolites, which cause liver toxicity.

**Drug Interactions**

*Alcohol, ethyl* / Chronic use of alcohol ↑ toxicity of larger therapeutic doses of acetaminophen

*Barbiturates* / ↑ Potential of hepatotoxicity due to ↑ breakdown of acetaminophen by liver

*Carbamazepine* / ↑ Potential of hepatotoxicity due to ↑ breakdown of acetaminophen by liver

*Charcoal, activated* / ↓ Absorption of acetaminophen when given as soon as possible after overdose

*Diuretics, loop* / ↓ Effect of diuretic due to ↓ renal prostaglandin excretion and ↓ plasma renin activity

*Hydantoins (including Phenytoin)* / ↑ Potential of hepatotoxicity due to ↑ breakdown of acetaminophen by liver

*Isoniazid* / ↑ Potential of hepatotoxicity due to ↑ breakdown of acetaminophen by liver

*Lamotrigene* / ↓ Serum lamotrigene levels → ↓ effect

*Oral contraceptives* / ↑ Breakdown of acetaminophen by liver → ↓ t½

*Propranolol* / ↑ Effect due to ↓ breakdown by liver

*Rifampin* / ↑ Potential of hepatotoxicity due to ↑ breakdown of acetaminophen by liver

*Sulfinpyrazone* / ↑ Potential of hepatotoxicity due to ↑ breakdown of acetaminophen by liver

*AZT* / ↓ Effect of AZT due to ↑ nonhepatic or renal clearance

**Dosage** —————————
• **Caplets, Capsules, Chewable Tablets, Gelcaps, Elixir, Oral Liquid, Oral Solution, Oral Suspension, Sprinkle Capsules, Syrup, Tablets**
*Analgesic, antipyretic.*
**Adults:** 325–650 mg q 4 hr; doses up to 1 g q.i.d. may be used. Daily dosage should not exceed 4 g. **Pediatric:** Doses given 4–5 times/day. **Up to 3 months:** 40 mg/dose; **4–11 months:** 80 mg/dose; **1–2 years:** 120 mg/dose; **2–3 years:** 160 mg/dose; **4–5 years:** 240 mg/dose; **6–8 years:** 320 mg/dose; **9–10 years:** 400 mg/dose; **11 years:** 480 mg/dose. **12–14 years:** 640 mg/dose. **Over 14 years:** 650 mg/dose. *Alternative pediatric dose:* 10–15 mg/kg q 4 hr.
• **Extended Relief Caplets**
*Analgesic, antipyretic.*
**Adults:** 2 caplets (1,300 mg) q 8 hr.
• **Suppositories**
*Analgesic, antipyretic.*
**Adults:** 650 mg q 4 hr, not to exceed 4 g/day for up to 10 days. Clients on long-term therapy should not exceed 2.6 g/day. **Pediatric, 3–11 months:** 80 mg q 6 hr. **1–3 years:** 80 mg q 4 hr; **3–6 years:** 120–125 mg q 4–6 hr, with no more than 720 mg in 24 hr. **6–12 years:** 325 mg q 4–6 hr with no more than 2.6 g in 24 hr. Dosage should be given as needed while symptoms persist.

BUFFERED
*Analgesic, antipyretic.*
**Adult, usual:** 1 or 2 three-quarter capfuls are placed into an empty glass; add half a glass of cool water. May be taken while fizzing or after settling. Can be repeated q 4 hr as required or directed by provider.

—————————
**NURSING CONSIDERATIONS**
**Administration/Storage**
1. Suppositories should be stored below 80°F (27°C).
2. The extended-relief product should be taken with water and should not be crushed, chewed, or dissolved before swallowing.
3. Acetaminophen should not be taken for more than 5 days for pain in children, 10 days for pain in adults, or more than 3 days for fever in adults or children without consulting provider.
4. Bubble gum flavored OTC pediatric products (suspension liquid and

A

chewable tablet) are available for use in children to treat fever and/or pain.

**Assessment**

1. Identify indications for therapy and expected outcomes.
2. If for long-term therapy, monitor CBC, liver and renal function studies.
3. Document presence of fever. Rate pain, noting type, onset, location, duration, and intensity.
4. Check urine for occult blood and albumin to assess for nephritis.

**Client/Family Teaching**

1. Take only as directed and with food or milk to minimize GI upset.
2. Review symptoms of acute toxicity that require immediate reporting such as N&V or abdominal pain. Also, any bluish coloration of the mucosa and nailbeds or complaints of dyspnea, weakness, headache, or vertigo are symptoms of methemoglobinemia caused by anoxia and require immediate attention.
3. Pallor, weakness, and complaints of heart palpitations should be reported as these symptoms may signal the presence of hemolytic anemia.
4. Complaints of dyspnea; rapid, weak pulse; cold extremities; unexplained bleeding, bruising, sore throat, malaise, or feeling clammy or sweaty; or subnormal temperatures may be symptoms of chronic poisoning. Report any unusual complaints and symptoms during drug therapy.
5. Reports of abdominal pain, yellow discoloration of skin and sclera, dark urine, itching, or clay-colored stools may indicate hepatotoxicity.
6. Phenacetin, the major active metabolite of acetaminophen, may cause the urine to become dark brown or wine-colored.
7. Read the labels on all OTC preparations consumed. Many contain acetaminophen and can produce toxic reactions if taken over time with the prescribed drug.
8. Headache and minor pain relievers containing combinations of salicylates, acetaminophen, and caffeine may be no more beneficial than aspirin alone; such combinations may be more dangerous so when in doubt consult provider.
9. Any unexplained pain or fever that persists for longer than 3–5 days requires medical evaluation.

**Outcomes/Evaluate**

• ↓ Fever
• Relief of pain

# Acetazolamide
(ah-set-ah-**ZOE**-la-myd)
**Pregnancy Category:** C
Acetazolam ✸, Apo-Acetazolamide ✸, Dazamide, Diamox, Diamox Sequels, Novo-Zolamide ✸ **(Rx)**

# Acetazolamide sodium
(ah-set-ah-**ZOE**-la-myd)
Diamox **(Rx)**
**Classification:** Anticonvulsant, carbonic anhydrase inhibitor

See also *Anticonvulsants*.

**Action/Kinetics:** Acetazolamide is a sulfonamide derivative possessing carbonic anhydrase inhibitor activity. As an anticonvulsant, beneficial effects may be due to inhibition of carbonic anhydrase in the CNS, which increases carbon dioxide tension resulting in a decrease in neuronal conduction. Systemic acidosis may also be involved. As a diuretic, the drug inhibits carbonic anhydrase in the kidney, which decreases formation of bicarbonate and hydrogen ions from carbon dioxide, thus reducing the availability of these ions for active transport. Use as a diuretic is limited because the drug promotes metabolic acidosis, which inhibits diuretic activity. This may be partially circumvented by giving acetazolamide on alternate days. Acetazolamide also reduces intraocular pressure.

Absorbed from the GI tract and widely distributed throughout the body, including the CNS. Excreted unchanged in the urine. **Tablets: Onset,** 60–90 min; **peak:** 1–4 hr; **duration:** 8–12 hr. **Sustained-release capsules: Onset,** 2 hr; **peak:** 3–6 hr; **duration:** 18–24 hr. **Injection (IV): Onset,** 2 min; **peak:** 15

min; **duration:** 4–5 hr. The drug is eliminated mainly unchanged through the kidneys.
**Uses:** Adjunct in the treatment of edema due to congestive heart failure, drug-induced edema. Absence (petit mal) and unlocalized seizures. Open-angle, secondary, or acute-angle closure glaucoma when delay of surgery is desired to lower intraocular pressure. Prophylaxis or treatment of acute mountain sickness in climbers attempting a rapid ascent or in those who are susceptible to mountain sickness even with gradual ascent.
**Contraindications:** Low serum sodium and potassium levels. Renal and hepatic dysfunction. Hyperchloremic acidosis, adrenal insufficiency, suprarenal gland failure, hypersensitivity to thiazide diuretics, cirrhosis. Chronic use in presence of noncongestive angle-closure glaucoma.
**Special Concerns:** Use with caution in the presence of mild acidosis and advanced pulmonary disease and during lactation. Increasing the dose of acetazolamide does not increase effectiveness and may increase the risk of drowsiness or paresthesia. Safety and efficacy have not been established in children.
**Side Effects:** *GI:* Anorexia, N&V, melena, constipation, alteration in taste, diarrhea. *GU:* Hematuria, glycosuria, urinary frequency, renal colic, renal calculi, crystalluria, polyuria, phosphaturia, decreased or absent libido, impotence. *CNS:* **Seizures,** weakness, malaise, fatigue, nervousness, drowsiness, depression, dizziness, disorientation, confusion, ataxia, tremor, headache, tinnitus, flaccid paralysis, lassitude, paresthesia of the extremities. *Hematologic:* **Bone marrow depression,** thrombocytopenic purpura, thrombocytopenia, **hemolytic anemia,** leukopenia, pancytopenia, agranulocytosis. *Dermatologic:* Pruritus, urticaria, skin rashes, erythema multiforme, **Stevens-Johnson syndrome, toxic epidermal necroly-**

**sis,** photosensitivity. *Other:* Weight loss, fever, acidosis, electrolyte imbalance, transient myopia, hepatic insufficiency. *NOTE:* Side effects similar to those produced by sulfonamides may also occur.
**OD** **Overdose Management:** *Symptoms:* Drowsiness, anorexia, N&V, dizziness, ataxia, tremor, paresthesias, tinnitus. *Treatment:* Emesis or gastric lavage. Hyperchloremic acidosis may respond to bicarbonate. Administration of potassium may also be necessary. Client should be observed carefully with supportive treatment given.
**Drug Interactions**
Also see *Diuretics.*
*Amphetamine /* ↑ Effect of amphetamine by ↑ renal tubular reabsorption
*Cyclosporine /* ↑ Levels of cyclosporine → possible nephrotoxicity and neurotoxicity
*Diflunisal /* Significant ↓ in intraocular pressure with ↑ side effects
*Ephedrine /* ↑ Effect of ephedrine by ↑ renal tubular reabsorption
*Lithium carbonate /* ↓ Effect of lithium by ↑ renal excretion
*Methotrexate /* ↓ Effect of methotrexate due to ↑ renal excretion
*Primidone /* ↓ Effect of primidone due to ↓ GI absorption
*Pseudoephedrine /* ↑ Effect of pseudoephedrine by ↑ renal tubular reabsorption
*Quinidine /* ↑ Effect of quinidine by ↑ renal tubular reabsorption
*Salicylates /* Accumulation and toxicity of acetazolamide (including CNS depression and metabolic acidosis). Also, acidosis due to acetazolamide may ↑ CNS penetration of salicylates

**Dosage** ────────────
• **Extended-Release Capsules, Tablets, IV**
  *Epilepsy.*
**Adults/children:** 8–30 mg/kg/day in divided doses. Optimum daily dosage: 375–1,000 mg (doses higher

---

than 1,000 mg do not increase therapeutic effect).

*Adjunct to other anticonvulsants.*
**Initial:** 250 mg/day; dose can be increased up to 1,000 mg/day in divided doses if necessary.

*Glaucoma, simple open-angle.*
**Adults:** 250–1,000 mg/day in divided doses. Doses greater than 1 g/day do not increase the effect.

*Glaucoma, closed-angle prior to surgery or secondary.*
**Adults, short-term therapy:** 250 mg q 4 hr or 250 mg b.i.d. **Adults, acute therapy:** 500 mg followed by 125–250 mg q 4 hr using tablets. For extended-release capsules, give 500 mg b.i.d. in the morning and evening. IV therapy may be used for rapid decrease in intraocular pressure. **Pediatric:** 5–10 mg/kg/dose IM or IV q 6 hr or 10–15 mg/kg/day in divided doses q 6–8 hr using tablets.

*Acute mountain sickness.*
**Adults:** 250 mg b.i.d.–q.i.d. (500 mg 1–2 times/day of extended-release capsules). During rapid ascent, 1 g/day is recommended.

*Diuresis in CHF.*
**Adults, initial:** 250–375 mg (5 mg/kg) once daily in the morning. If the client stops losing edema fluid after an initial response, the dose should not be increased; rather, medication should be skipped for a day to allow the kidney to recover. The best diuretic effect occurs when the drug is given on alternate days or for 2 days alternative with a day of rest.

*Drug-induced edema.*
**Adults:** 250–375 mg once daily for 1 or 2 days. The drug is most effective if given every other day or for 2 days followed by a day of rest. **Children:** 5 mg/kg/dose PO or IV once daily in the morning.

## NURSING CONSIDERATIONS

See also *Nursing Considerations* for *Anticonvulsants*.
**Administration/Storage**
1. Change over from other anticonvulsant therapy to acetazolamide should be gradual.

2. Acetazolamide tablets may be crushed and suspended in a cherry, chocolate, raspberry, or other sweet syrup. Do not use vehicles containing glycerin or alcohol. As an alternative, 1 tablet may be submerged in 10 mL of hot water and added to 10 mL of honey or syrup.
3. Tolerance after prolonged use may necessitate dosage increase.
4. Do not administer the sustained-release dosage form as an anticonvulsant; it should be used only for glaucoma and acute mountain sickness.
5. When used for prophylaxis of mountain sickness, dosage should be initiated 1–2 days before ascent and should be continued for at least 2 days while at high altitudes.
6. Due to possible differences in bioavailability, brands should not be interchanged.
**IV** 7. IV administration is preferred; IM administration is painful due to alkalinity of solution.
8. For parenteral use, reconstitute each 500-mg vial with at least 5 mL of sterile water for injection. Use parenteral solutions within 24 hr after reconstitution, although reconstituted solutions retain potency for 1 week if refrigerated.
9. Reconstitute each 500-mg vial with at least 5 mL of sterile water for injection. For direct IV use, administer over at least 1 min. For intermittent IV use, further dilute in dextrose or saline solution and infuse over 4–8 hr.
**Assessment**
1. Note indications for therapy, type and onset of symptoms.
2. Review electrolytes, uric acid, and glucose. Note any liver and renal dysfunction prior to administering.
3. List drugs currently prescribed to ensure none interacts unfavorably.
4. With glaucoma, note baseline ophthalmic exam and intraocular pressures and assess for visual effects.
5. Perform a thorough CV and pulmonary assessment in clients with CHF.
**Client/Family Teaching**
1. Taking drug with food may decrease gastric irritation and GI upset.
2. Determine drug effects before

undertaking tasks that require mental alertness.

3. Drug increases the frequency of voiding; take early in the day to avoid interrupting sleep.

4. Take only as directed. If prescribed every other day or with rest days in between (as with CHF), document administration to enhance compliance.

5. Increase fluid intake (2–3 L/day) to prevent crystalluria and stone formation.

6. Warn clients with diabetes that drug may increase blood glucose levels. Monitor levels and report increases because the dose of hypoglycemic agent may require adjustment.

7. Report if nausea, dizziness, rapid weight gain, muscle weakness, or cramps occur as well as any changes in the color and consistency of stools.

8. Report for labs to determine need for potassium replacement.

**Outcomes/Evaluate**

- ↓ Seizure activity
- ↓ Intraocular pressure
- ↓ CHF-associated edema
- Prevention of mountain sickness

## Acetohexamide
(ah-seat-oh-**HEX**-ah-myd)
**Pregnancy Category:** C
Dimelor ✿, Dymelor **(Rx)**
**Classification:** First-generation sulfonylurea

See also *Antidiabetic Agents, Oral.*
**Action/Kinetics: Onset:** 1 hr. **t½:** 1.3 hr for acetohexamide and 6–8 hr for active metabolite. **Duration:** 12–24 hr. Metabolized in the liver to a potent active metabolite. Excreted through the kidney (80%) and feces (10%).
**Additional Side Effects:** Hair loss.

**Dosage**
- **Tablets**
  *Diabetes.*
**Adults, initial:** 250–1,500 mg/day.
**Maintenance:** Adjust dosage until

optimum control is achieved. Doses in excess of 1.5 g/day are not recommended. **Geriatric clients, initial:** 125–250 mg/day; **then,** adjust dosage gradually until desired effect is achieved.

## NURSING CONSIDERATIONS

See *Nursing Considerations for Antidiabetic Agents, Oral.*
**Administration/Storage:** Maintenance doses less than 1 g/day can be given once daily; doses of 1 g or more should be divided, usually before the morning and evening meals.
**Outcomes/Evaluate:** ↓ Glucose levels (HbA1C<8)

## Acetylcysteine
(ah-see-till-**SIS**-tay-een)
**Pregnancy Category:** B
Mucomyst, Mucosil, Parvolex **(Rx)**
**Classification:** Mucolytic

**Action/Kinetics:** Acetylcysteine reduces the viscosity of purulent and nonpurulent pulmonary secretions and facilitates their removal by splitting disulfide bonds. Action increases with increasing pH (peak: pH 7–9).
**Onset, inhalation:** Within 1 min; **by direct instillation:** immediate.
**Time to peak effect:** 5–10 min.
**Uses:** Adjunct in the treatment of acute and chronic bronchitis, emphysema, tuberculosis, pneumonia, bronchiectasis, atelectasis. Routine care of clients with tracheostomy, pulmonary complications after thoracic or CV surgery, or in posttraumatic chest conditions. Pulmonary complications of cystic fibrosis. Diagnostic bronchial asthma. Antidote in acetaminophen poisoning to reduce hepatotoxicity. *Investigational:* As an ophthalmic solution for dry eye.
**Contraindications:** Sensitivity to drug.
**Special Concerns:** Use with caution during lactation, in the elderly, and in clients with asthma.
**Side Effects:** *Respiratory:* Increased incidence of bronchospasm in clients with asthma. Increased amount of

liquefied bronchial secretions, which must be removed by suction if cough is inadequate. Bronchial and tracheal irritation, tightness in chest, bronchoconstriction. *GI:* N&V, stomatitis. *Other:* Rashes, fever, drowsiness, rhinorrhea.

**Drug Interactions:** Acetylcysteine is incompatible with antibiotics and should be administered separately.

## Dosage

• **10% or 20% Solution: Nebulization, Direct Application, or Direct Intratracheal Instillation**

*Nebulization into face mask, tracheostomy, mouth piece.*
1–10 mL of 20% solution or 2–10 mL of 10% solution 3–4 times/day.

*Closed tent or croupette.*
Up to 300 mL of 10% or 20% solution/treatment.

*Direct instillation into tracheostomy.*
1–2 mL of 10%–20% solution q 1–4 hr.

*Percutaneous intratracheal catheter.*
1–2 mL of 20% solution or 2–4 mL of 10% solution q 1–4 hr by syringe attached to catheter.

*Instillation to particular portion of bronchopulmonary tree using small plastic catheter into the trachea.*
2–5 mL of 20% solution instilled into the trachea by means of a syringe connected to a catheter.

*Diagnostic procedures.*
2–3 doses of 1–2 mL of 20% or 2–4 mL of 10% solution by nebulization or intratracheal instillation before the procedure.

*Acetaminophen overdose.*
**Given PO, initial:** 140 mg/kg; **then,** 70 mg/kg q 4 hr for a total of 17 doses.

## NURSING CONSIDERATIONS

### Administration/Storage

1. Use nonreactive plastic, glass, or stainless steel equipment for administration.
2. The 10% solution may be used undiluted.
3. Use either water for injection or saline to dilute the 20% solution.
4. May administer via face mask, face tent, oxygen tent, head tent, or by positive-pressure breathing apparatus.
5. Administer with compressed air for nebulization. Hand nebulizers are contraindicated.
6. After prolonged nebulization, dilute the last fourth of the medication with sterile water for injection to prevent concentration of the medication.
7. The solution may develop a light purple color. This does not affect the action of the medication.
8. Closed bottles of solution remain stable for 2 years when stored at 20°C (68°F). Open bottles should be stored at 2°C–8°C (35°F–46°F) and used within 96 hr. Once opened, record the time and date of opening to prevent use beyond the 96-hr period.
9. Acetylcysteine is incompatible with antibiotics and must be administered separately.
10. Have ET tube available and suction machine at the bedside for removal of increased bronchial secretions.

### Assessment

1. Determine when bronchial spasms occur.
2. Document conditions likely to cause congestion and wheezing.
3. Identify previous approaches (successful and unsuccessful) used in treating symptoms.
4. Determine if a smoker and if currently taking any antibiotics.
5. With acetaminophen overdosage document time. Drug should be administered within 8–10 hr following overdose to protect from hepatoxicity and death. Monitor LFTs and acetaminophen levels.

### Interventions

1. If bronchospasm occurs, have a bronchodilator, such as isoproterenol for aerosol inhalation, readily available.
2. Position to facilitate removal of secretions. If unable to cough up secretions, provide suction.
3. Monitor VS and I&O.
4. Wash face following nebulization treatments; medication may cause the face to become sticky.

5. Administration route for acetaminophen toxicity is oral and will consist of 17 doses.

**Client/Family Teaching**
1. Use only as directed; do not exceed prescribed dosage.
2. Report any unusual changes in color, consistency, or characteristics of sputum.
3. The nauseous odor present when the treatment begins will likely become less noticeable as therapy continues.
4. Avoid any triggers that may stimulate bronchospasm (i.e., cigarette smoke, dust, chemicals, cold air).
5. Promote smoking cessation classes and support groups to help stop smoking.

**Outcomes/Evaluate**
• Improved airway exchange with ↓ viscosity and mobilization and expectoration of secretions
• ↓ Acetaminophen levels and associated liver toxicity

# Acetylsalicylic acid (ASA, Aspirin)

(ah-**SEE**-till-sal-ih-**SILL**-ick **AH**-sid)
**Pregnancy Category:** C
Apo-Asa ✹, Asaphen ✹, Aspergum, Aspirin, Aspirin Regimen Bayer 81 mg with Calcium, Bayer Children's Aspirin, Easprin, Ecotrin Caplets and Tablets, Ecotrin Maximum Strength Caplets and Tablets, Empirin, Entrophen ✹, Excedrin Geltabs, Genprin, Genuine Bayer Aspirin Caplets and Tablets, Halfprin, 8-Hour Bayer Timed-Release Caplets, Maximum Bayer Aspirin Caplets and Tablets, MSD Enteric Coated ASA ✹, Norwich Extra Strength, Novasen ✹, St. Joseph Adult Chewable Aspirin, Therapy Bayer Caplets, ZOR-prin **(OTC)** (Easprin and ZOR-prin are Rx)

# Acetylsalicylic acid, buffered

(ah-**SEE**-till-sal-ih-**SILL**-ick **AH**-sid)
**Pregnancy Category:** C
Alka-Seltzer with Aspirin, Alka-Seltzer with Aspirin (flavored), Alka-Seltzer Extra Strength with Aspirin, Arthritis Pain Formula, Ascriptin Regular Strength, Ascriptin A/D, Bayer Buffered, Buffered Aspirin, Bufferin, Buffex, Cama Arthritis Pain Reliever, Magnaprin, Magnaprin Arthritis Strength Captabs, Tri-Buffered Bufferin Caplets and Tablets **(OTC)**
**Classification:** Nonnarcotic analgesic, antipyretic, anti-inflammatory agent

**Action/Kinetics:** Aspirin manifests antipyretic, anti-inflammatory, and analgesic effects. The antipyretic effect is due to an action on the hypothalamus, resulting in heat loss by vasodilation of peripheral blood vessels and promoting sweating. Prostaglandins have been implicated in the inflammatory process, as well as in mediation of pain. Thus, if levels are decreased, the inflammatory reaction may subside. The anti-inflammatory effects are probably mediated through inhibition of cyclo-oxygenase, which results in a decrease in prostaglandin synthesis and other mediators of the pain response. The mechanism of action for the analgesic effects of aspirin is not known fully but is partly attributable to improvement of the inflammatory condition. Aspirin also produces inhibition of platelet aggregation by decreasing the synthesis of endoperoxides and thromboxanes—substances that mediate platelet aggregation.

Large doses of aspirin (5 g/day or more) increase uric acid secretion, while low doses (2 g/day or less) decrease uric acid secretion. However, aspirin antagonizes drugs used to treat gout.

Rapidly absorbed after PO administration. Is hydrolyzed to the active salicylic acid, which is 70%–90% protein bound. For arthritis and rheumatic disease, blood levels of 150–300 mcg/mL should be maintained. For analgesic and antipyretic, achieve blood levels of 25–50 mcg/mL. For acute rheumatic fever, achieve blood levels of 150–300 mcg/mL. **Therapeutic salicylic acid serum levels:** 150–300 mcg/

mL, although tinnitus occurs at serum levels above 200 mcg/mL and serious toxicity above 400 mcg/mL. **t½:** aspirin, 15–20 min; salicylic acid, 2–20 hr, depending on the dose. Salicylic acid and metabolites are excreted by the kidney. The bioavailability of enteric-coated salicylate products may be poor. The addition of antacids (buffered aspirin) may decrease GI irritation and increase the dissolution and absorption of such products.

Aspirin is found in many combination products including Darvon Compound, Empirin Compound Plain and with Codeine, Equagesic, Fiorinal Plain and with Codeine, Norgesic and Norgesic Forte, and Synalgos DC.

**Uses:** *Analgesic:* Pain arising from integumental structures, myalgias, neuralgias, arthralgias, headache, dysmenorrhea, and similar types of pain. Antipyretic. *Anti-Inflammatory:* Arthritis, osteoarthritis, SLE, acute rheumatic fever, gout, and many other conditions. Mucocutaneous lymph node syndrome (Kawasaki disease). Reduce the risk of recurrent transient ischemic attacks and strokes in men. Decrease risk of death from nonfatal MI in clients who have a history of infarction or who manifest unstable angina; aortocoronary bypass surgery. Gout. May be effective in less severe postoperative and postpartum pain; pain secondary to trauma and cancer. *Investigational:* Chronic use to prevent cataract formation; low doses to prevent toxemia of pregnancy; in pregnant women with inadequate uteroplacental blood flow. Reduce colon cancer mortality (low doses).

**Contraindications:** Hypersensitivity to salicylates. Clients with asthma, hay fever, or nasal polyps have a higher incidence of hypersensitivity reactions. Severe anemia, history of blood coagulation defects, in conjunction with anticoagulant therapy. Salicylates can cause congestive failure when taken in the large doses used for rheumatic diseases. Vitamin K deficiency; 1 week before and af-

ter surgery. In pregnancy, especially the last trimester as the drug may cause problems in the newborn child or complications during delivery. In children or teenagers with chickenpox or flu due to possibility of development of Reye's syndrome.

Controlled-release aspirin is not recommended for use as an antipyretic or short-term analgesic because adequate blood levels may not be reached. Also, controlled-release products are not recommended for children less than 12 years of age and in children with fever accompanied by dehydration.

**Special Concerns:** Use with caution during lactation. Use with caution in the presence of gastric or peptic ulcers, in mild diabetes, erosive gastritis, or bleeding tendencies, in cardiac disease, and in liver or kidney disease. Aspirin products now carry the following labeling: "It is especially important not to use aspirin during the last three months of pregnancy unless specifically directed to do so by a doctor because it may cause problems in the newborn child or complications during delivery."

**Side Effects:** The toxic effects of the salicylates are dose-related. *GI:* Dyspepsia, heartburn, anorexia, nausea, occult blood loss, epigastric discomfort, ***massive GI bleeding, potentiation of peptic ulcer***. *Allergic:* ***Bronchospasm, asthma-like symptoms, anaphylaxis,*** skin rashes, angioedema, urticaria, rhinitis, nasal polyps. *Hematologic:* Prolongation of bleeding time, thrombocytopenia, leukopenia, purpura, shortened erythrocyte survival time, decreased plasma iron levels. *Miscellaneous:* Thirst, fever, dimness of vision.

*NOTE:* Use of aspirin in children and teenagers with flu or chickenpox may result in the development of ***Reye's syndrome***. Also, dehydrated, febrile children are more prone to salicylate intoxication.

**OD** **Overdose Management:** *Symptoms of Mild Salicylate Toxicity (Salicylism):* At serum levels between 150 and 200 mcg/mL. *GI:*

N&V, diarrhea, thirst. *CNS:* Tinnitus (most common), dizziness, difficulty in hearing, mental confusion, lassitude. *Miscellaneous:* Flushing, sweating, tachycardia. Symptoms of salicylism may be observed with doses used for inflammatory disease or rheumatic fever. *Symptoms of Severe Salicylate Poisoning:* At serum levels over 400 mcg/mL. *CNS:* Excitement, confusion, disorientation, irritability, hallucinations, lethargy, stupor, *coma, respiratory failure, seizures.* *Metabolic:* Respiratory alkalosis (initially), respiratory acidosis and metabolic acidosis, dehydration. *GI:* N&V. *Hematologic:* Platelet dysfunction, hypoprothrombinemia, increased capillary fragility. *Miscellaneous:* **Hyperthermia, hemorrhage, CV collapse, renal failure,** hyperventilation, pulmonary edema, tetany, hypoglycemia (late). *Treatment (Toxicity):*
1. If the client has had repeated administration of large doses of salicylates, document and report evidence of hyperventilation or complaints of auditory or visual disturbances (symptoms of salicylism).
2. Severe salicylate poisoning, whether due to overdose or accumulation, will have an exaggerated effect on the CNS and the metabolic system:
• Clients may develop a salicylate jag characterized by garrulous behavior. They may act as if they were inebriated.
• Convulsions and coma may follow.
3. When working with febrile children or the elderly who have been treated with aspirin, maintain adequate fluid intake. These clients are more susceptible to salicylate intoxication if they are dehydrated.
4. The following treatment approaches may be considered for treatment of *acute salicylate toxicity:*
• Initially induce vomiting or perform gastric lavage followed by activated charcoal (most effective if given within 2 hr of ingestion).
• Monitor salicylate levels and acid-base and fluid and electrolyte bal-

ance. If required, administer IV solutions of dextrose, saline, potassium, and sodium bicarbonate as well as vitamin K.
• Seizures may be treated with diazepam.
• Treat hyperthermia if present.
• Alkaline diuresis will enhance renal excretion. Hemodialysis is effective but should be reserved for severe poisonings.
• If necessary, administer oxygen and artificial ventilation

**Drug Interactions**
*Acetazolamide* / ↑ CNS toxicity of salicylates; also, ↑ excretion of salicylic acid if urine kept alkaline
*Alcohol, ethyl* / ↑ Chance of GI bleeding caused by salicylates
*Alteplase, recombinant* / ↑ Risk of bleeding
*PAS* / Possible ↑ effect of PAS due to ↓ excretion by kidney or ↓ plasma protein binding
*Ammonium chloride* / ↑ Effect of salicylates by ↑ renal tubular reabsorption
*ACE inhibitors* / ↓ Effect of ACE inhibitors possibly due to prostaglandin inhibition
*Antacids* / ↓ Salicylate levels in plasma due to ↑ rate of renal excretion
*Anticoagulants, oral* / ↑ Effect of anticoagulant by ↓ plasma protein binding and plasma prothrombin
*Antirheumatics* / Both are ulcerogenic and may cause ↑ GI bleeding
*Ascorbic acid* / ↑ Effect of salicylates by ↑ renal tubular reabsorption
*Beta-adrenergic blocking agents* / Salicylates ↓ action of beta-blockers, possibly due to prostaglandin inhibition
*Charcoal, activated* / ↓ Absorption of salicylates from GI tract
*Corticosteroids* / Both are ulcerogenic; also, corticosteroids may ↓ blood salicylate levels by ↑ breakdown by liver and ↑ excretion
*Dipyridamole* / Additive anticoagulant effects

---

*Furosemide* / ↑ Chance of salicylate toxicity due to ↓ renal excretion; also, salicylates may ↓ effect of furosemide in clients with impaired renal function or cirrhosis with ascites

*Heparin* / Inhibition of platelet adhesiveness by aspirin may result in bleeding tendencies

*Hypoglycemics, oral* / ↑ Hypoglycemia due to ↓ plasma protein binding and ↓ excretion

*Indomethacin* / Both are ulcerogenic and may cause ↑ GI bleeding

*Insulin* / Salicylates ↑ hypoglycemic effect of insulin

*Methionine* / ↑ Effect of salicylates by ↑ renal tubular reabsorption

*Methotrexate* / ↑ Effect of methotrexate by ↓ plasma protein binding; also, salicylates block renal excretion of methotrexate

*Nitroglycerin* / Combination may result in unexpected hypotension

*Nizatidine* / ↑ Serum levels of salicylates

*NSAIDs* / Additive ulcerogenic effects; also, aspirin may ↓ serum levels of NSAIDs

*Phenylbutazone* / Combination may produce hyperuricemia

*Phenytoin* / ↑ Effect of phenytoin by ↓ plasma protein binding

*Probenecid* / Salicylates inhibit uricosuric activity of probenecid

*Sodium bicarbonate* / ↓ Effect of salicylates by ↑ rate of excretion

*Spironolactone* / Aspirin ↓ diuretic effect of spironolactone

*Sulfinpyrazone* / Salicylates inhibit uricosuric activity of sulfinpyrazone

*Sulfonamides* / ↑ Effect of sulfonamides by ↑ blood levels of salicylates

*Valproic acid* / ↑ Effect of valproic acid due to ↓ plasma protein binding

**Laboratory Test Interferences:** False + or ↑ : Amylase, AST, ALT, uric acid, PBI, urinary VMA (most tests), catecholamines, urinary glucose (Benedict's, Clinitest), and urinary uric acid (at high doses) values. False − or ↓ : $CO_2$ content, glucose (fasting), potassium, urinary VMA (Pisano method), and thrombocyte values.

## Dosage

• **Gum, Chewable Tablets, Coated Tablets, Effervescent Tablets, Enteric-Coated Tablets, Suppositories, Tablets, Timed (Controlled) Release Tablets**

*Analgesic, antipyretic.*

**Adults:** 325–500 mg q 3 hr, 325–600 mg q 4 hr, or 650–1,000 mg q 6 hr. As an alternative, the adult chewable tablet (81 mg each) may be used in doses of 4–8 tablets q 4 hr as needed. **Pediatric:** 65 mg/kg/day (alternate dose: 1.5 g/m²/day) in divided doses q 4–6 hr, not to exceed 3.6 g/day. Alternatively, the following dosage regimen can be used: **Pediatric, 2–3 years:** 162 mg q 4 hr as needed; **4–5 years:** 243 mg q 4 hr as needed; **6–8 years:** 320–325 mg q 4 hr as needed; **9–10 years:** 405 mg q 4 hr as needed; **11 years:** 486 mg q 4 hr as needed; **12–14 years:** 648 mg q 4 hr.

*Arthritis, rheumatic diseases.*

**Adults:** 3.2–6 g/day in divided doses.

*Juvenile rheumatoid arthritis.*

60–110 mg/kg/day (alternate dose: 3 g/m²) in divided doses q 6–8 hr. When initiating therapy at 60 mg/kg/day, dose may be increased by 20 mg/kg/day after 5–7 days and by 10 mg/kg/day after another 5–7 days.

*Acute rheumatic fever.*

**Adults, initial:** 5–8 g/day. **Pediatric, initial,** 100 mg/kg/day (3 g/m²/day) for 2 weeks; **then,** decrease to 75 mg/kg/day for 4–6 weeks.

*Transient ischemic attacks in men.*

**Adults:** 650 mg b.i.d. or 325 mg q.i.d. A dose of 300 mg/day may be as effective and with fewer side effects.

*Prophylaxis of MI.*

**Adults:** 300 or 325 mg/day (both solid PO dosage forms–regular and buffered as well as buffered aspirin in solution). The adult chewable tablets be also be used.

*Kawasaki disease.*

**Adults:** 80–180 mg/kg/day during the febrile period. After the fever resolves, the dose may be adjusted to 10 mg/kg/day.

*NOTE:* Doses as low as 80–100 mg/day are being studied for use in unstable angina, MI, and aortocoronary bypass surgery. Aspirin Regimen Bayer 81 mg with Calcium contains 250 mg calcium carbonate (10% of RDA) and 81 mg of acetylsalicylic acid for individuals who require aspirin to prevent recurrent heart attacks and strokes.

## NURSING CONSIDERATIONS
### Administration/Storage
1. Enteric-coated tablets or buffered tablets are better tolerated by some clients.
2. Aspirin should be taken with a full glass of water to prevent lodging of the drug in the esophagus.
3. Have epinephrine available to counteract hypersensitivity reactions should they occur. Asthma caused by hypersensitive reaction to salicylates may be refractory to epinephrine, so antihistamines should also be available for parenteral and PO use.
### Assessment
1. Take a complete drug history and note any evidence of hypersensitivity. Individuals allergic to tartrazine should not take aspirin. Clients who have tolerated salicylates well in the past may suddenly have an allergic or anaphylactoid reaction.
2. If administered for pain, rate and determine the type and pattern of pain, if the pain is unusual, or if it is recurring. Note the effectiveness of aspirin if used in the past for pain control.
3. Note if client has asthma, hay fever, ulcer disease or nasal polyps.
4. Document age; drug is discouraged in those under 12. Assess for chickenpox or the flu.
5. Note any history of peptic ulcers or other conditions that would deter the use of salicylates.
6. Test for blood in the stool and urine and monitor CBC routinely during high-dose and chronic therapy.
7. Determine if diagnostic tests scheduled. Drug causes irreversible platelet effects. Anticipate 4–7 days for the body to replace these once drug discontinued; hence no salicylates one week prior to procedure.
8. Determine any history of bleeding tendencies. Obtain baseline bleeding parameters if prolonged use is anticipated.
9. Review drugs currently prescribed to determine the potential for drug interactions.
10. The therapeutic serum level of salicylate is 150–300 mcg/mL for adult and juvenile rheumatoid arthritis and acute rheumatic fever. Reassure that the higher dosage is necessary for anti-inflammatory effects.
### Client/Family Teaching
1. Take only as directed. To reduce gastric irritation, administer with meals, milk, a full glass of water, or crackers.
2. Do not take salicylates if product is off-color or has a strange odor. Note expiration date.
3. Report any toxic effects: ringing in the ears, difficulty hearing, dizziness or fainting spells, unusual increase in sweating, severe abdominal pain, or mental confusion.
4. Salicylates potentiate the effects of antidiabetic drugs. Monitor glucose levels and report if hypoglycemia occurs.
5. When administering for antipyretic effect, follow temperature administeration parameters.
• Obtain temperature 1 hr after administering to assess outcome.
• Check for marked diaphoresis, and if present, dry client, change linens, provide fluids, and prevent chilling.
6. Cardiac clients on large doses should be alert to symptoms of CHF and report if evident.
7. Tell the dentist and other HCPs you are taking salicylates and why.
8. Before purchasing other OTC

preparations, notify provider and note the quantity used per day.

9. Salicylates should be administered to children only upon specific medical recommendation due to increased risk of Reye's syndrome.

10. If a child refuses to take the medication or vomits it, discuss possibility of using aspirin suppositories or acetaminophen.

11. Children who are dehydrated and who have a fever are especially susceptible to aspirin intoxication from even small amounts of aspirin. Report any gastric irritation and pain; these may be symptoms of hypersensitivity or toxicity.

12. Sodium bicarbonate may decrease the serum level of aspirin, reducing its effectiveness.

13. Report any unusual bruising or bleeding. Large doses may increase PT and should be avoided. Aspirin and NSAIDs may interfere with blood-clotting mechanisms (antiplatelet effects) and are usually discontinued 1 week before surgery to prevent increased risk of bleeding.

14. Avoid indiscriminate use of salicylate drugs.

**Outcomes/Evaluate**

• Relief of pain/discomfort; Improved joint mobility/function
• ↓ Fever
• Prophylaxis of MI/TIA

# Acitretin

(ah-sih-**TREH**-tin)
**Pregnancy Category:** X
Soriatane **(Rx)**
**Classification:** Antipsoriasis product.

**Action/Kinetics:** Retinoic acid derivative that is the main metabolite of etretinate. Mechanism is not known. Absorption optimal when given with food.**t½, terminal:** 49 hr. Extensively metabolized; excreted through feces and urine.

**Uses:** Severe psoriasis, including erythrodermic and generalized pustular types. *Investigational:* Darier's disease, palmoplantar pustulosis, lichen planus, children with lamellar ichthyosis, non-bullous and bullous ichthyosiform erythroderma, Sjö-

gren-Larsson syndrome, lichen sclerosus et atrophicus of the vulva and palmoplantar lichen nitidus.

**Contraindications:** Use during pregnancy or in those who intend to become pregnant during therapy or at any time for at least 3 years following discontinuation of therapy. Use by females who may not use reliable contraception during treatment or for at least 3 years following treatment. Use of ethanol in women either during treatment or for 2 months after cessation of treatment. Lactation.

**Special Concerns:** Use with caution in those with severely impaired liver or kidney function. Safety and efficacy have not been determined in children.

**Side Effects:** *Dermatologic:* Alopecia, skin peeling, dry skin, nail disorder, pruritus, erythematous rash, hyperesthesia, paresthesia, paronychia, skin atrophy, sticky skin, abnormal skin odor, abnormal hair texture, bullous eruption, cold/clammy skin, dermatitis, increased sweating, infection, psoriasis-like rash, purpura, pyogenic granuloma, rash, seborrhea, skin fissures, skin ulceration, sunburn. *CNS:* Rigors, headache, pain, depression, insomnia, somnolence. *GI:* Abdominal pain, nausea, diarrhea, tongue disorder, altered taste, hepatotoxicity. *Ophthalmic:* Xerophthalmia, blurred vision, abnormal vision, blepharitis, irritation, conjunctivitis, corneal epithelial abnormality, decreased night vision, blindness, eye abnormality, eye pain, photophobia. *Musculoskeletal:* Arthralgia, spinal hyperostosis, arthritis, arthrosis, back pain, hypertonia, myalgia, osteodynia, peripheral joint hyperostosis. *Mucous membranes:* Cheilitis, rhinitis, epistaxis, dry mouth, gingival bleeding, gingivitis, increased salivation, stomatitis, thirst, ulcerative stomatitis. *Body as a whole:* Anorexia, edema, fatigue, hot flashes, increased appetite, flushing, sinusitis. *Otic:* Earache, tinnitus.

**Laboratory Test Alterations:** ↑ AST, ALT, GGT, LDH, triglyceride, cholesterol. ↓ HDL.

**Drug Interactions**
*Ethanol* / Possible formation of etretinate which has a longer half-life than acitretin
*Glyburide* / Enhanced clearance of blood glucose
*Methotrexate* / ↑ Risk of hepatotoxicity
*Oral contraceptives, "minipill"* / Acitretin interferes with the contraceptive effect

**Dosage**
• **Capsules**
  *Psoriasis.*
Must individualize dosage. **Initial:** 25 or 50 mg/day given as a single dose with main meal. **Maintenance:** 25 to 50 mg/day.

**NURSING CONSIDERATIONS**
**Administration/Storage:** Terminate therapy when lesions have sufficiently resolved. Treat relapses as described for initial therapy.
**Assessment**
1. Document/photograph condition requiring therapy; note other treatments trialed and outcome.
2. Determine if pregnant. Females must undergo pregnancy testing and receive contraceptive counselling due to risk of fetal abnormalities; limit refills.
3. Monitor lipids and LFTs at 1-2 week intervals until drug response obtained (4-8 weeks).
**Client/Family Teaching**
1. Take with food to enhance absorption.
2. Do not consume vit A supplements; avoid sun lamps and excess sun exposure.
3. Females should avoid all alcohol products during and for 2 mo following therapy.
4. Practice reliable contraception 1 mo prior to and during therapy; avoid pregnancy for at least 3 yrs following therapy due to risk of severe fetal malformations.
5. Tubal ligation and microdose progestin "minipill" products may fail; use alternative forms of birth control.

6. May experience worsening of psoriasis during initial treatment period; may take 2-3 mo to see improvement.
7. Do not donate blood during and for up to 3 yr following therapy.
8. Report any unusual or persistent adverse effects.
**Outcomes/Evaluate:** Healing/clearing of lesions

# Acyclovir (Acycloguanosine)
(ay-**SYE**-kloh-veer, ay-**SYE**-kloh-**GWON**-oh-seen)
**Pregnancy Category:** C
Avirax ✦, Nu-Acyclovir ✦, Zovirax **(Rx)**
**Classification:** Antiviral anti-infective

See also *Antiviral Drugs.*
**Action/Kinetics:** Acyclovir is a synthetic acyclic purine nucleoside analog. It is converted by HSV-infected cells to acyclovir triphosphate, which interferes with HSV DNA polymerase, thereby inhibiting DNA replication. Systemic absorption is slow from the GI tract (although therapeutic levels are reached) and following topical administration. It is preferentially taken up and converted to the active triphosphate form by herpes virus–infected cells. Food does not affect absorption. **Peak levels after PO:** 1.5–2 hr. Widely distributed in tissues and body fluids. The half-life and total body clearance depend on renal function. **t½, PO, creatinine clearance, greater than 80 mL/min/1.73 m²:** 2.5 hr. Metabolites and unchanged drug (up to 85%) are excreted through the kidney. Reduce dosage in clients with impaired renal function. Clients who take acyclovir (600–800 mg/day) with AZT had a significantly prolonged survival rate compared with clients taking only acyclovir.
**Uses: PO.** Initial and recurrent genital herpes in immunocompromised and nonimmunocompromised clients. Prophylaxis of frequently recurrent genital herpes infections in

nonimmunocompromised clients. Treatment of chickenpox in children ranging from 2 to 18 years of age. Acute treatment of herpes zoster (shingles).

**Parenteral.** Initial therapy for severe genital herpes in clients who are not immunocompromised; initial and recurrent mucosal and cutaneous HSV-1 and HSV-2 infections in immunocompromised individuals. Varicella zoster infections (shingles) in immunocompromised clients. HSE in clients over 6 months of age.

**Topical.** Acyclovir decreases healing time and duration of viral shedding in initial herpes genitalis. Limited non-life-threatening mucocutaneous HSV infections in immunocompromised clients. No beneficial effect in recurrent herpes genitalis or in herpes labialis in nonimmunocompromised clients.

*Investigational:* Cytomegalovirus and HSV infection following bone marrow or renal transplantation; herpes simplex ocular infections; herpes simplex proctitis; herpes simplex labialis; herpes simplex whitlow; herpes zoster encephalitis; disseminated primary eczema herpeticum; herpes simplex–associated erythema multiforme; infectious mononucleosis; and varicella pneumonia.

**Contraindications:** Hypersensitivity to formulation. Use in the eye. Use to prevent recurrent HSV infections.

**Special Concerns:** Use with caution during lactation or with concomitant intrathecal methotrexate or interferon. Safety and efficacy of PO form not established in children less than 2 years of age. Prolonged or repeated doses in immunocompromised clients may result in emergence of resistant viruses. Use of oral acyclovir does not eliminate latent HSV and is not a cure.

**Side Effects: PO.** *Short-term treatment of herpes simplex. GI:* N&V, diarrhea, anorexia, sore throat, taste of drug. *CNS:* Headache, dizziness, fatigue. *Miscellaneous:* Edema, skin rashes, leg pain, inguinal adenopathy.

*Long-term treatment of herpes simplex. GI:* Nausea, diarrhea. *CNS:* Headache. *Other:* Skin rash, asthenia, paresthesia.

*Treatment of herpes zoster. GI:* N&V, diarrhea, constipation. *CNS:* Headache, malaise.

*Treatment of chickenpox. GI:* Vomiting, diarrhea, abdominal pain, flatulence. *Dermatologic:* Rash.

**Parenteral (frequency greater than 1%).** *At injection site:* Phlebitis, inflammation. *GI:* N&V. *CNS:* Encephalopathic changes, including lethargy, obtundation, tremors, agitation, confusion, hallucination, *seizures, coma* , jitters, headache. *Miscellaneous:* Skin rashes, urticaria, itching, transient elevation of serum creatinine or BUN (most often following rapid IV infusion), elevation of transaminases.

**Topical.** Transient burning, stinging, pain. Pruritus, rash, vulvitis, local edema. *NOTE:* All of these effects have also been reported with the use of a placebo preparation.

**OD** **Overdose Management:** *Symptoms:* Increased BUN and serum creatinine, *renal failure following parenteral overdose. Treatment:* Hemodialysis (peritoneal dialysis is less effective).

**Drug Interactions**
*Probenecid* / ↑ Bioavailability and half-life of acyclovir → ↑ effect
*Zidovudine* / Severe lethargy and drowsiness

**Dosage** ⸺
- **Capsules, Suspension, Tablets**
   *Initial genital herpes.*
200 mg q 4 hr, 5 times/day for 10 days.
   *Chronic genital herpes.*
400 mg b.i.d., 200 mg t.i.d., or 200 mg 5 times/day for up to 12 months.
   *Intermittent therapy for genital herpes.*
200 mg q 4 hr, 5 times/day for 5 days. Start therapy at the first symptom/sign of recurrence.
   *Herpes zoster, acute treatment.*
800 mg q 4 hr, 5 times/day for 7–10 days.
   *Chickenpox.*

20 mg/kg (of the suspension) q.i.d. for 5 days. A single dose should not exceed 800 mg. Begin therapy at the earliest sign/symptom.

• **IV Infusion**

*Mucosal and cutaneous herpes simplex in immunocompromised clients.*

**Adults:** 5 mg/kg infused at a constant rate over 1 hr, q 8 hr (15 mg/kg/day) for 7 days. **Children less than 12 years of age:** 250 mg/m² infused at a constant rate over 1 hr, q 8 hr for 7 days.

*Varicella-zoster infections (shingles) in immunocompromised clients.*

**Adults:** 10 mg/kg infused at a constant rate over 1 hr, q 8 hr for 7 days (not to exceed 500 mg/m² q 8 hr). **Children less than 12 years of age:** 500 mg/m² infused at a constant rate over at least 1 hr, q 8 hr for 7 days.

*Herpes simplex encephalitis.*

**Adults:** 10 mg/kg infused at a constant rate over at least 1 hr, q 8 hr for 10 days. **Children less than 12 years of age and greater than 6 months of age:** 500 mg/m² infused at a constant rate over at least 1 hr, q 8 hr for 10 days.

• **Topical (5% Ointment)**

**Adults and children:** Lesion should be covered with sufficient amount of ointment (0.5-in. ribbon/4 in.² of surface area) q 3 hr, 6 times/day for 7 days. Initiate treatment as soon as possible after onset of symptoms.

## NURSING CONSIDERATIONS

See also *General Nursing Considerations for All Anti-Infectives*, and *Antiviral Drugs*.

**Administration/Storage**

1. Store ointment in a dry place at room temperature.

2. Both the PO and parenteral dose and/or dosing interval should be adjusted in acute or chronic renal impairment.

3. The suspension may be used to treat varicella zoster infections.

**IV** 4. Prepare IV solution by dissolving the contents of the 500- or 1000-mg vial in 10 or 20 mL sterile water for injection, respectively (final concentration of 50 mg/mL). Infusion concentrations of 7 mg/mL or lower are recommended; thus, the calculated dose must be added to an appropriate IV solution at the correct volume. Reconstituted solution should be used within 12 hr. Bacteriostatic water containing benzyl alcohol or parabens should not be used as it will cause a precipitate.

5. Accompany IV infusion by adequate hydration (3 L/day) to prevent precipitation in renal tubules (crystalluria).

6. The drug for IV infusion only is administered over 1 hr to prevent renal tubular damage; it should not be administered by rapid or bolus IV, IM, or SC injections.

7. If refrigerated, reconstituted solution may show a precipitate, which dissolves at room temperature.

**Assessment**

1. Document indications for therapy and assessment of all skin lesions.

2. Monitor CBC, electrolytes, liver and renal function studies.

3. With chickenpox or herpes zoster, institute appropriate precautions for all susceptible individuals [i.e., pregnant women, immunocompromised clients, and those who have not had chickenpox (may check titer if unknown)].

**Client/Family Teaching**

1. Apply acyclovir ointment in the amount directed with a finger cot or rubber glove to prevent transmission of infection to other body sites.

2. Adequately cover all lesions with topical acyclovir as ordered, but do not exceed dosage or the frequency of application or the length of time for treatment.

3. Report any burning, stinging, itching, and rash if evident when applying acyclovir.

4. Complete all examinations and tests to rule out possible presence of other sexually transmitted diseases.

5. Acyclovir is ineffective for treat-

ment of reinfection; return to provider if HSV recurs.

6. Drug is not a cure, it is only used to help manage symptoms. Acyclovir will not prevent transmission of disease to others or prevent reinfection.

7. Use condoms for sexual intercourse to prevent reinfections while undergoing treatment. Abstain during acute outbreaks (lesions present) and use condoms at all other times.

8. The total dose and dosage schedule differ depending on whether the infection is initial or chronic and whether intermittent therapy regimen is being used. Therefore, following prescribed dosage, dosage combinations (i.e., with AZT) and duration of treatment are extremely important.

9. Consume 2–3 L/day of fluids, especially during parenteral therapy, to prevent renal toxicity and crystalluria.

10. Females should have an annual Pap test; an increased risk of cervical cancer has been associated with genital herpes.

11. Do not exceed recommended dosage and do not share medication with others.

**Outcomes/Evaluate**
• Less severe and less frequent herpes outbreaks
• Crusting and healing of herpetic lesions

---

# Adapalene
(ah-**DAP**-ah-leen)
**Pregnancy Category:** C
Differin **(Rx)**
**Classification:** Topical acne product

**Action/Kinetics:** Adapalene binds to specific retinoic acid receptors which may normalize the differentiation of follicular epithelial cells resulting in decreased microcomedone formation. Trace amounts of the drug are absorbed through the skin.
**Uses:** Topical treatment of acne vulgaris.
**Contraindications:** Hypersensitivity to adapalene or any components of the vehicle gel. Use in those with

sunburn until they are fully recovered.
**Special Concerns:** Use with caution in those who normally have high levels of sun exposure or in those sensitive to the sun. Use with caution with medicated or abrasive soaps and cleaners, with soaps and cosmetics that have a strong drying effect, and with products that have high concentrations of alcohol, stringents, spices, or lime. Also use particular caution with products containing sulfur, resorcinol, or salicylic acid. Use with caution during lactation. Safety and efficacy have not been determined in children less than 12 years of age.
**Side Effects:** *Dermatologic:* Erythema, scaling, dryness, pruritus, burning, pruritus or burning immediately after application, skin irritation, stinging sunburn, acne flares.

**Dosage** ———————————
• **Topical Gel**
*Treatment of acne vulgaris.*
**Adults and children over 12 years of age:** Apply a thin film once a day to affected areas after washing in the evening prior to retiring.

---

## NURSING CONSIDERATIONS
**Administration/Storage**
1. Avoid contact with eyes, lips, and mucous membranes.
2. During early weeks of therapy, acne may worsen due to action of the drug on previously unseen lesions—not a reason to discontinue therapy.
3. Beneficial effects should be seen after 8 to 12 weeks of treatment.
4. Store at controlled room temperatures of 20°C to 25°C (68°F to 77°F).
**Assessment**
1. Document indications for therapy, noting onset, duration, and location of acne lesions.
2. List other agents trialed and the outcome; note any family history with condition.
3. Determine skin type and any sensitivity reactions to soaps, sun, or other agents or conditions.
4. Describe clinical presentation;

use photographs to document baseline presentation and extent of lesions.

**Client/Family Teaching**

1. Apply only as directed and avoid contact with cut, irritated, or sunburned skin. Avoid contact with eyes, lips, and mucous membranes.

2. Excessive application will cause increased peeling, discomfort, and redness.

3. Avoid prolonged sun exposure and weather extremes (i.e., wind, cold). Use sunscreen and protective clothing when exposed.

4. Condition may worsen before improving; do not become discouraged.

5. Expect itching, burning, scaling, and erythema during the first 2 to 4 weeks of therapy; these should lessen with continued use. If severe discomfort is experienced, reduce frequency of application or stop therapy and report.

**Outcomes/Evaluate:** Clearing and healing of acne lesions in 8 to 12 weeks.

# Adenosine
(ah-**DEN**-oh-seen)
**Pregnancy Category:** C
Adenocard, Adenoscan **(Rx)**
**Classification:** Antiarrhythmic

See also *Antiarrhythmic Agents.*

**Action/Kinetics:** Adenosine is found naturally in all cells of the body. It slows conduction time through the AV node, interrupts the reentry pathways through the AV node, and restores normal sinus rhythm in paroxysmal supraventricular tachycardia (including Wolff-Parkinson-White syndrome). It is competitively antagonized by caffeine, theophylline, and dipyridamole. **Onset, after IV:** 34 sec. **t½:** Less than 10 sec (taken up by erythrocytes and vascular endothelial cells). **Duration:** 1–2 min. Exogenous adenosine becomes part of the body pool and is metabolized mainly to inosine and AMP.

**Uses:** Conversion of sinus rhythm of paroxysmal SVT (including that associated with accessory bypass tracts). The phosphate salt is used for symptomatic relief of complications with stasis dermatitis in varicose veins. *Investigational:* With thallium-201 tomography in noninvasive assessment of clients with suspected CAD who cannot exercise adequately prior to being stress-tested. Adenosine is not effective in converting rhythms other than paroxysmal SVT. The phosphate salt has been used to treat herpes infections and to increase blood flow to brain tumors and in porphyria cutanea tarda.

**Contraindications:** Second- or third-degree AV block or sick sinus syndrome (except in clients with a functioning artificial pacemaker). Also, atrial flutter, atrial fibrillation, ventricular tachycardia. History of MI or cerebral hemorrhage.

**Special Concerns:** At time of conversion to normal sinus rhythm, new rhythms (PVC, atrial premature contractions, sinus bradycardia, skipped beats, varying degrees of AV block, sinus tachycardia) lasting a few seconds may occur. Use with caution in clients with asthma. Safety and efficacy as a diagnostic agent have not been determined in clients less than 18 years of age.

**Side Effects:** *CV:* Short lasting first-, second-, or ***third-degree heart block; cardiac arrest*** , sustained ventricular tachycardia, sinus bradycardia, ST-segment depression, sinus exit block, sinus pause, arrhythmias, T-wave changes, hypertension. prolonged asystole, Nonfatal MI, transient increase in BP, ***ventricular fibrillation***. Facial flushing (common), chest pain, sweating, palpitations, hypotension (may be significant). *CNS:* Lightheadedness, dizziness, numbness, headache, blurred vision, apprehension, paresthesia, drowsiness, emotional instability, tremors, nervousness. *GI:* Nausea, metallic taste, tightness in throat. *Respiratory:* SOB or dyspnea (common), urge to

**A**

breathe deeply, chest pressure or discomfort, cough, hyperventilation, nasal congestion. *GU:* Urinary urgency, vaginal pressure. *Miscellaneous:* Pressure in head, burning sensation, neck and back pain, weakness, blurred vision, dry mouth, ear discomfort, pressure in groin, scotomas, tongue discomfort, discomfort (tingling, heaviness) in upper extremities, discomfort in throat, neck, or jaw.

**Drug Interactions**
*Carbamazepine* / ↑ Degree of heart block
*Caffeine* / Competitively antagonizes effect of adenosine
*Digitalis* / Possibility of ventricular fibrillation (rare)
*Dipyridamole* / ↑ Effect of adenosine
*Theophylline* / Competitively antagonizes effect of adenosine

**Dosage** ―――――――――――
• **Rapid IV Bolus Only**
*Antiarrhythmic.*
**Initial:** 6 mg over 1–2 sec. If the first dose does not reverse the SVT within 1–2 min, 12 mg should be given as a rapid IV bolus. The 12-mg dose may be repeated a second time, if necessary. Doses greater than 12 mg are not recommended.
• **IV Infusion Only**
*Diagnostic aid.*
**Adults:** 140 mcg/kg/min infused over 6 min (total dose of 0.84 mg/kg).
• **IM Only**
*Varicose veins.*
**Initial:** 25–50 mg 1–2 times daily until symptoms subside. **Maintenance:** 25 mg 2 or 3 times weekly.

## NURSING CONSIDERATIONS

See also *Nursing Considerations* for *Antiarrhythmic Agents.*
**Administration/Storage**
**IV** 1. Drug can be stored at room temperature; crystallization may result if the drug is refrigerated. If crystals form, they can be dissolved by warming to room temperature. The solution must be clear when administered.

2. Discard any unused portion because the product contains no preservatives.
3. Administer directly into a vein. If it is to be given into an IV line, introduce the drug in the most proximal line and follow with a rapid saline flush.
4. When used as a diagnostic aid, the dose of thallium-201 should be given at the midpoint of the adenosine infusion (i.e., after 3 min).

**Assessment**
1. Document indications for therapy, onset of symptoms, and ECG confirmation of arrhythmia.
2. Monitor rhythm strips closely for evidence of varying degrees of AV block and increased arrhythmias during conversion to sinus rhythm. These are usually only transient.
3. Monitor BP and pulse. Report complaints of numbness, tingling in the arms, blurred vision, or apprehensiveness, as this may be an indication to discontinue drug therapy.
4. Document chest pressure, SOB, heaviness of the arms, palpitations, or dyspnea. Note any history of MI or CVA as drug is contraindicated.
5. In stasis dermatitis carefully assess extremities and note findings.

**Client/Family Teaching**
1. Facial flushing is a common temporary side effect of therapy.
2. Avoid caffeine and note if concurrently prescribed theophylline, digoxin, or dipyridamole.
3. Drug helps restore heart to a normal, slower rhythm.

**Outcomes/Evaluate**
• Conversion of paroxysmal SVT to NSR
• Symptomatic relief when used for stasis dermatitis

# Albendazole
((al-**BEN**-dah-zohl))
**Pregnancy Category:** C
Albenza **(Rx)**
**Classification:** Anthelmintic

――――――――――――――

See also *Anthelmintics.*
**Action/Kinetics:** Albendazole acts by inhibiting tubular polymerization,

resulting in the loss of cytoplasmic microtubules and inability of the cell to function. It is poorly absorbed from the GI tract; absorption can be enhanced by ingesting a meal containing at least 40 g of fat. The drug is rapidly converted to albendazole sulfoxide, the active metabolite. **Peak plasma levels, sulfoxide:** 2–5 hr. **t½, terminal, of sulfoxide:** 8–12 hr. The drug is further metabolized to other metabolites with excretion through the bile, accounting for a portion of elimination.

**Uses:** Treatment of parenchymal neurocysticercosis due to *Taenia solium*. Treatment of cystic hydatid disease of the liver, lung, and peritoneum caused by the larval form of the dog tapeworm, Echinococcus granulosus.

**Contraindications:** Hypersensitivity to benzimidazole compounds.

**Special Concerns:** Use with caution during lactation. Clients should not become pregnant for at least 1 month following termination of albendazole therapy.

**Side Effects:** *GI:* N&V, abdominal pain. *CNS:* Headache, dizziness, vertigo, increased ICP, meningeal signs. *Hematologic:* Leukopenia, granulocytopenia, pancytopenia, agranulocytosis, thrombocytopenia (rare). *Dermatologic:* Reversible alopecia, rash, urticaria. *Miscellaneous:* Fever, allergic reactions, acute renal failure.

**Drug Interactions**
*Cimetidine* / ↑ Levels of albendazole sulfoxide in bile and cystic fluid in hydatid cyst clients
*Dexamethasone* / Possible ↑ plasma levels of albendazole sulfoxide
*Praziquantel* / ↑ Plasma levels of albendazole sulfoxide

**Dosage** ————————————
• **Tablets**
*Hydatid disease.*
**Those weighing 60 kg or more:** 400 mg b.i.d. with meals for a 28-day cycle followed by a 14-day albendazole-free interval, for a total of three cycles. **Those weighing less**

**than 60 kg:** 15 mg/kg/day given in divided doses b.i.d. with meals, up to a maximum of 800 mg/day, using the same duration as for those weighing 60 kg or more.
*Neurocysticercosis.*
**Those weighing 60 kg or more:** 400 mg b.i.d. with meals for 8 to 30 days. **Those weighing less than 60 kg:** 15 mg/kg/day given in divided doses b.i.d. with meals, up to a maximum dose of 800 mg/day, for 8 to 30 days.

## NURSING CONSIDERATIONS

See also *Nursing Considerations* for *Anthelmintics.*

**Administration/Storage:**   Clients being treated for neurocysticercosis should receive corticosteroid and anticonvulsant therapy as needed. PO or IV steroids should be considered for the first week of treatment to prevent cerebral hypertensive episodes.

**Assessment**
1. Document indications for therapy as length of therapy is based on condition requiring treatment.
2. Obtain negative pregnancy test, baseline cultures, and neurologic assessment.
3. Determine baseline CBC and check every 2 weeks during each 28-day cycle.
4. Obtain liver function tests and monitor for significant elevations which may necessitate interruption of drug therapy until enzymes return to baseline.
5. Assess for retinal lesions with cysticercosis. The need for anticysticeral therapy should be weighed against the possibility of retinal damage due to albendazole-induced changes to the retinal lesion.

**Interventions**
1. Anticipate coadministration of PO or IV corticosteroids during the first week of therapy to prevent cerebral hypertensive episodes with anticysticeral therapy.
2. Monitor neurologic status carefully. Steroids and anticonvulsants

**A**

should be administered with neurocysticerosis.

**Client/Family Teaching**

1. Review the prescribed dosage, frequency, and cycle or length of therapy required.
2. Take as directed with food.
3. Use reliable birth control during and for 4–6 weeks following completion of drug therapy; drug may cause fetal harm.
4. Avoid crowds and persons with contagious diseases; report any S&S of infection.

**Outcomes/Evaluate:** Symptomatic improvement with resolution of infective organisms

# Albuterol (Salbutamol)

(al-**BYOU**-ter-ohl)
**Pregnancy Category:** C
Alti-Salbutamol Sulfate ✹, Asmavent ✹, Gen-Salbutamol Sterinebs P.F. ✹, Novo-Salmol Inhaler ✹, PMS-Salbutamol Respirator Solution ✹, Proventil, Proventil HFA—3M, Proventil Repetabs, Rho-Salbutamol ✹, Sabulin ✹, Salbutamol Nebuamp ✹, Ventodisk Disk/Diskhaler ✹, Ventolin, Ventolin Rotacaps, Volmax **(Rx)**
**Classification:** Direct-acting adrenergic (sympathomimetic) agent

See also *Sympathomimetic Drugs.*

**Action/Kinetics:** Albuterol stimulates beta-2 receptors of the bronchi, leading to bronchodilation. Causes less tachycardia and is longer-acting than isoproterenol. Has minimal beta-1 activity. Albuterol sulfate is now available as an inhaler that contains no chlorofluorocarbons (Proventil HFA–3M). **Onset, PO:** 15–30 min; **inhalation,** 5–15 min. **Peak effect, PO:** 2–3 hr; **inhalation,** 60–90 min (after 2 inhalations). **Duration, PO:** 8 hr (up to 12 hr for extended-release); **inhalation,** 3–6 hr. Metabolites and unchanged drug excreted in urine and feces. Tablets not to be used in children less than 12 years of age.

**Uses:** Bronchial asthma; bronchospasm due to bronchitis or emphysema; bronchitis; reversible obstructive pulmonary disease in those 4 years of age and older; exercise-induced bronchospasm. Prophylaxis of bronchial asthma or bronchospasms. Parenteral for treatment of status asthmaticus. *Investigational:* Nebulized albuterol may be useful as an adjunct to treat serious acute hyperkalemia in hemodialysis clients.

**Contraindications:** Aerosol for prevention of exercise-induced bronchospasm is not recommended for children less than 12 years of age. Use during lactation.

**Special Concerns:** Dosage has not been established for the syrup in children less than 2 years of age, for tablets in children less than 6 years of age, and for extended-release tablets in children less than 12 years of age. Albuterol may delay preterm labor.

**Additional Side Effects:** *GI:* Diarrhea, dry mouth, increased appetite, epigastric pain. *CNS:* CNS stimulation, malaise, emotional lability, fatigue, lightheadedness, nightmares, disturbed sleep, aggressive behavior, irritability. *Respiratory:* Bronchitis, epistaxis, hoarseness (especially in children), nasal congestion, increase in sputum. *Hypersensitivity (may be immediate):* Urticaria, *angioedema,* rash, *bronchospasm. Miscellaneous:* Muscle cramps, pallor, teeth discoloration, conjunctivitis, dilated pupils, difficulty in urination, muscle spasm, voice changes, oropharyngeal edema.

**OD** **Overdose Management:** *Symptoms:* Seizures, anginal pain, hypertension, hypokalemia, tachycardia (rate may increase to 200 beats/min).

See *Sympathomimetic Drugs.*

## Dosage

• **Metered Dose Inhaler**
*Bronchodilation.*

**Adults and children over 12 years of age:** 180 mcg (2 inhalations) q 4–6 hr (Ventolin aerosol may be used in children over 4 years of age). In some clients 1 inhalation (90 mcg) q 4 hr may be sufficient.

*Prophylaxis of exercise-induced bronchospasm.*

**Adults and children over 12 years of age:** 180 mcg (2 inhalations) 15 min before exercise.
• **Solution for Inhalation**
*Bronchodilation.*
**Adults and children over 12 years of age:** 2.5 mg t.i.d.–q.i.d. by nebulization (dilute 0.5 mL of the 0.5% solution with 2.5 mL sterile NSS and deliver over 5–15 min).
• **Capsule for Inhalation**
*Bronchodilation.*
**Adults and children over 4 years of age:** 200 mcg q 4–6 hr using a Rotahaler inhalation device. In some clients, 400 mcg q 4–6 hr may be required.
*Prophylaxis of exercise-induced bronchospasm.*
**Adults and children over 12 years:** 200 mcg 15 min before exercise using a Rotahaler inhalation device.
• **Syrup**
*Bronchodilation.*
**Adults and children over 14 years of age:** 2–4 mg t.i.d.–q.i.d., up to a maximum of 8 mg q.i.d. **Children, 6–14 years, initial:** 2 mg (base) t.i.d.–q.i.d.; **then,** increase as necessary to a maximum of 24 mg/day in divided doses. **Children, 2–6 years, initial:** 0.1 mg/kg t.i.d.; **then,** increase as necessary up to 0.2 mg/kg, not to exceed 4 mg t.i.d.
• **Tablets**
*Bronchodilation.*
**Adults and children over 12 years of age, initial:** 2–4 mg (of the base) t.i.d.–q.i.d.; **then,** increase dose as needed up to a maximum of 8 mg t.i.d.–q.i.d. In geriatric clients or those sensitive to beta agonists, start with 2 mg t.i.d.–q.i.d. and then increase dose gradually, if needed, to a maximum of 8 mg t.i.d.–q.i.d. **Children, 6–12 years of age, usual, initial:** 2 mg t.i.d.–q.i.d.; **then,** if necessary, increase the dose in a stepwise fashion to a maximum of 24 mg/day in divided doses.
• **Extended-Release Tablets**
*Bronchodilation.*
**Adults and children over 12 years**

**of age:** 4 or 8 mg (of the base) q 12 hr up to a maximum of 32 mg/day. Clients on regular-release albuterol can be switched to the Repetabs in that a 4-mg extended-release tablet q 12 hr is equivalent to a regular 2-mg tablet q 6 hr.

## NURSING CONSIDERATIONS

See also *Nursing Considerations* for *Sympathomimetic Drugs.*
**Administration/Storage**
1. When given by nebulization, either a face mask or mouthpiece may be used. Compressed air or oxygen with a gas flow of 6–10 L/min should be used, with a single treatment lasting from 5 to 15 min.
2. When given by IPPB, the inspiratory pressure should be from 10 to 20 cm water, with the duration of treatment ranging from 5 to 20 min depending on the client and instrument control.
3. The MDI may also be administered on a mechanical ventilator through an adapter.
4. Extended-release tablets should be taken whole with the aid of liquids; do not chew or crush. The outer coating of Volmax Extended-Release Tablets is not absorbed and is excreted in the feces; the empty outer coating may be observed in the stool.
5. The contents of the MDI container are under pressure. Do not store near heat or open flames and do not puncture the container.
**Assessment**
1. Obtain nursing history and assess CNS status.
2. Document pulmonary function and lung sounds. Note any evidence of anxiety as this may contribute to air hunger.
3. Document symptom characteristics, onset, duration, frequency, and any precipitating factors.
4. Determine if able to self-administer medication.
**Interventions**
1. Maintain a calm, reassuring ap-

proach. Do not leave unattended if acutely short of breath.

2. Instruct how to inhale through nose and exhale with pursed lip or diaphragmatic breathing in order to prolong expiration and keep the airways open longer, thus reducing the work of breathing.

3. Monitor pulmonary status (i.e., breath sounds, VS, peak flow, or ABGs) for effects of the therapy, adjusting the dose or frequency of medication, if needed.

4. Observe for evidence of allergic responses and be prepared to intervene.

**Client/Family Teaching**

1. Take only as directed; do not exceed prescribed dose.

2. Do not put lips around inhaler; go two fingerbreadths away before attempting to activate and inhale. Attend instruction on the correct method for administration.

3. When using albuterol inhalers, do not use other inhalation medication unless specifically prescribed.

4. A spacer used with the MDI may enhance drug dispersion. Always thoroughly rinse mouth and equipment with water following each use to prevent oral fungal infections.

5. Establish dosing regimens that fit life-style, i.e., 1–2 puffs q 6 hr or 4 puffs 4 times/day; the usual dosing is q 4–6 hr with an as-needed order. Record peak flows, call if requiring more puffs more frequently than prescribed or if the dose of drug used previously does not provide relief.

**Outcomes/Evaluate:**    Improved breathing patterns and improved airway exchange

---

# Aldesleukin (Interleukin-2; IL-2)

(al-des-**LOO**-kin)

**Pregnancy Category:** C

Proleukin **(Rx)**

**Classification:** Antineoplastic, miscellaneous

---

See also *Antineoplastic Agents.*

**Action/Kinetics:** Aldesleukin, pro-

duced by recombinant DNA technology, is a human interleukin-2 (IL-2) product. The recombinant form differs from natural IL-2 in that aldesleukin is not glycosylated, the molecule has no N-terminal alanine, the molecule has serine substituted for cysteine at amino acid position 125, and the aggregation state of aldesleukin may be different from that of native IL-2. However, aldesleukin possesses the biologic activity of human native IL-2. Drug effects include activation of cellular immunity with profound lymphocytosis, eosinophilia, and thrombocytopenia; the production of cytokines, including tumor necrosis factor, IL-1, and gamma-interferon; and inhibition of tumor growth. The exact mechanism of action of aldesleukin is not known. The drug reaches high plasma levels after a short IV infusion, and it is rapidly distributed to the extravascular, extracellular space. It is rapidly cleared from the circulation by both glomerular filtration and peritubular extraction; metabolized in the kidneys with little or no active form excreted through the urine. **t½, distribution:** 13 min; **t½, elimination:** 85 min.

**Uses:** Metastatic renal cell carcinoma in adults 18 years of age and older. *Investigational:* Kaposi's sarcoma in combination with AZT, metastatic melanoma in combination with low-dose cyclophosphamide, colorectal cancer and non-Hodgkin's lymphoma often in combination with lymphokine-activated killer cells.

**Contraindications:** Hypersensitivity to IL-2 or any components of the product. Abnormal thallium stress test or pulmonary function tests. Organ allografts. Use in either men or women not practicing effective contraception. Lactation.

Retreatment is contraindicated in those who have experienced the following during a previous course of therapy: sustained ventricular tachycardia; uncontrolled or unresponsive cardiac rhythm disturbances; recurrent chest pain with ECG changes that are consistent with angina or MI; intubation required for more than 72 hr; pericardial tamponade; renal dysfunction requiring dialysis for more than 72 hr; coma or toxic psychosis lasting more than 48 hr; seizures that are repetitive or difficult to control; ischemia or perforation of the bowel; and GI bleeding requiring surgery.

**Special Concerns:** Aldesleukin may worsen symptoms in clients with unrecognized or untreated CNS metastases. Use of medications known to be nephrotoxic or hepatotoxic may further increase toxicity to the kidney and liver caused by aldesleukin. May increase the risk of allograft rejection in transplant clients. Safety and efficacy have not been established in children less than 18 years of age.

**Side Effects:** Side effects are frequent, often serious, and sometimes fatal. Most clients will experience fever, chills, rigors, pruritus, and GI side effects. The frequency and severity of side effects are usually dose-related and schedule-dependent. Incidence of side effects is greater in PS 1 clients than in PS 0 clients. The side effects listed have an incidence of 1% or greater.

*Capillary leak syndrome (CLS):* Results from extravasation of plasma proteins and fluid into the extracellular space with loss of vascular tone. This results in a drop in mean arterial BP within 2–12 hr after the start of treatment and reduced organ perfusion that may be severe and result in death. CLS causes hypotension, hypoperfusion, and extravasation that leads to edema and effusion. *CLS may be associated with supraventricular and ventricular arrhythmias, MI,* angina, respiratory insufficiency requiring intubation, GI bleeding or infarction, renal insufficiency, and changes in mental status.

*CV:* Hypotension (sometimes requiring vasopressor therapy), sinus tachycardia, *arrhythmias (atrial, junctional, supraventricular, ventricular)* , bradycardia, PVCs, premature atrial contractions, myocardial ische-

mia, *MI, cardiac arrest, CHF,* myocarditis, endocarditis, gangrene, *stroke, pericardial effusion, thrombosis. Respiratory:* Pulmonary congestion, dyspnea, pulmonary edema, *respiratory failure,* tachypnea, pleural effusion, wheezing, apnea, pneumothorax, hemoptysis. *GI:* N&V, diarrhea, stomatitis, anorexia, *GI bleeding* (sometimes requiring surgery), dyspepsia, constipation, *intestinal perforation,* intestinal ileus, pancreatitis. *CNS:* Changes in mental status (may be an early indication of bacteremia or early bacterial sepsis), dizziness, sensory dysfunction, disorders of special senses (speech, taste, vision), syncope, motor dysfunction, *coma, seizure. GU:* Oliguria or anuria, proteinuria, hematuria, dysuria, impaired renal function requiring dialysis, urinary retention, urinary frequency. *Hepatic:* Jaundice, ascites, hepatomegaly. *Hematologic:* Anemia, thrombocytopenia, leukopenia, coagulation disorders, leukocytosis, eosinophilia. *Dermatologic:* Pruritus, erythema, rash, dry skin, exfoliative dermatitis, purpura, petechiae, urticaria, alopecia. *Musculoskeletal:* Arthralgia, myalgia, arthritis, muscle spasm. *Electrolyte and other disturbances:* Hypomagnesemia, acidosis, hypocalcemia, hypophosphatemia, hypokalemia, hyperuricemia, hypoalbuminemia, hypoproteinemia, hyponatremia, hyperkalemia, alkalosis, hypoglycemia, hyperglycemia, hypocholesterolemia, hypercalcemia, hypernatremia, hyperphosphatemia. *Miscellaneous:* Fever, chills, pain (abdominal, chest, back), fatigue, malaise, weakness, edema, infection (including the injection site, urinary tract, catheter tip, phlebitis, sepsis), weight gain or weight loss, headache, conjunctivitis, reactions at the injection site, allergic reactions, hypothyroidism.

**OD  Overdose Management:** *Symptoms:* See *Side Effects.* Administration of more than the recommended dose will cause a more rapid onset of toxicities. *Treatment:*

---

Side effects will usually reverse if the drug is stopped, especially because the serum half-life is short. Continuing toxicity is treated symptomatically. Life-threatening side effects have been treated by the IV administration of dexamethasone (which may result in loss of the therapeutic effectiveness of aldesleukin).

**Drug Interactions**

*Aminoglycosides* / ↑ Risk of kidney toxicity

*Antihypertensives* / Potentiate hypotension seen with aldesleukin

*Asparaginase* / ↑ Risk of hepatic toxicity

*Cardiotoxic agents* / ↑ Risk of cardiac toxicity

*Corticosteroids* / Concomitant use may ↓ the antitumor effectiveness of aldesleukin (although the corticosteroids ↓ side effects of aldesleukin)

*Cytotoxic chemotherapy* / ↑ Risk of myelotoxicity

*Doxorubicin* / ↑ Risk of cardiac toxicity

*Hepatotoxic drugs* / ↑ Risk of liver toxicity

*Indomethacin* / ↑ Risk of kidney toxicity

*Methotrexate* / ↑ Risk of hepatic toxicity

*Myelotoxic agents* / ↑ Risk of myelotoxicity

*Nephrotoxic agents* / ↑ Risk of kidney toxicity

**Laboratory Test Interferences:** ↑ BUN, bilirubin, serum creatinine, transaminase, alkaline phosphatase. See also *Electrolyte and other disturbances* under Side Effects.

**Dosage** ————————————————

• **Intermittent IV Infusion**

*Metastatic renal cell carcinoma in adults.*

Each course of treatment consists of two 5-day treatment cycles separated by a rest period. **Adults:** 600,000 IU/kg (0.037 mg/kg) given q 8 hr by a 15-min IV infusion for a total of 14 doses. Following 9 days of rest, repeat schedule for another 14 doses, for a maximum of 28 doses per course. *NOTE:* Due to toxicity, clients may not be able to receive all 28 doses (median number of doses given is 20).

*Retreatment for metastatic renal cell carcinoma.*

Evaluate for a response about 4 weeks after completion of a course of therapy and again just prior to the start of the next treatment course. Give additional courses only if there is evidence of some tumor shrinkage following the last course and retreatment is not contraindicated (see preceding *Contraindications*). Separate each treatment course by at least 7 weeks from the date of hospital discharge.

## NURSING CONSIDERATIONS

See also *Nursing Considerations* for *Antineoplastic Agents*.

**Administration/Storage**

**IV** 1. Dose modification for toxicity should be undertaken by withholding or interrupting a dose rather than reducing the dose to be given.

2. *Permanently discontinue* therapy for the following toxicities:

• CV: Sustained ventricular tachycardia, uncontrolled or unresponsive cardiac rhythm disturbances, recurrent chest pain with ECG changes indicating angina or MI, pericardial tamponade

• Pulmonary: Intubation required for more than 72 hr

• Renal: Renal dysfunction requiring dialysis for more than 72 hr

• CNS: Coma or toxic psychosis lasting more than 48 hr, seizures that are repetitive or difficult to control

• GI: Bowel ischemia, bowel perforation, GI bleeding requiring surgery

3. The guidelines for held doses and subsequent doses of aldesleukin are detailed in the information provided by the manufacturer and should be consulted carefully.

4. Reconstitute vials aseptically with 1.2 mL sterile water for injection. If reconstituted as directed, each milliliter will contain 18 million IU (1.1 mg) of aldesleukin. Such solutions should be clear and colorless to slightly yellow.

5. The vial is for a single use only and any unused portion should be discarded. Drug is not for use with transplant clients, as there is a risk of allograft rejection.

6. During reconstitution, the sterile water for injection should be directed at the side of the vial. The contents should be swirled gently to avoid foaming. *The vial should not be shaken.*

7. The reconstituted drug may be diluted in 50 mL of D5% injection and then infused over 15 min.

8. Plastic bags should be used as this results in more consistent drug delivery. In-line filters should *not* be used when giving aldesleukin.

9. Reconstitution is not to be undertaken using bacteriostatic water for injection or 0.9% NaCL injection due to increased aggregation.

10. Dilution with albumin can alter the pharmacology of aldesleukin. Also, do not mix aldesleukin with other drugs.

11. After reconstitution, the drug is stable for 48 hr if stored at room temperature or 2°C–8°C (36°F–46°F). Administer within 48 hr of reconstitution, bringing the solution to room temperature before infusing. Do not freeze the product.

12. The undiluted drug is stable for 5 days if refrigerated in 1-mL B-D syringes.

13. The drug is compatible with glass, polyvinylchloride (preferred), or polypropylene syringes.

**Assessment**

1. Note any liver or renal dysfunction as well as cardiac, pulmonary, or CNS impairment.

2. The following baseline parameters should be determined prior to initiation of therapy and daily during drug use: CBC, blood chemistries, liver and renal function tests, and CXRs. All clients should have baseline pulmonary function tests with ABGs.

3. Screen with a thallium stress test to document normal ejection fraction and unimpaired wall motion. If minor abnormalities in wall motion of questionable significance are noted, a stress echocardiogram may be useful to exclude significant CAD.

4. Assess for any S&S of infection. Obtain cultures to rule out any potential sources. Preexisting bacterial infections must be treated prior to initiation of aldesleukin therapy, as intensive treatment may cause impaired neutrophil function and an increased risk of disseminated infection leading to sepsis and bacterial endocarditis.

5. All clients with in-dwelling central lines should receive antibiotic prophylaxis against *Saccharomyces aureus.*

**Interventions**

1. Initiate therapy in a closely monitored environment where VS and I&O are assessed often.

2. Cardiac function should be assessed daily by clinical examination and assessment of VS. Clients who have chest pain, murmurs, gallops, irregular rhythm, or palpitations should be further assessed with an ECG examination and CPK evaluation. If there is evidence of cardiac ischemia or CHF, a repeat stress thallium study should be undertaken.

3. Perform daily CV evaluations to identify any early S&S of drug toxicity. Monitor for symptoms of CLS characterized by hypotension and hypoperfusion, altered mental status, and decreased urine output. Mental status changes are usually transient but should be evaluated carefully. Alterations in urinary output may signal renal toxicity.Monitor for evidence of dehydration, liver or renal failure. Be prepared to stop infusion and transport client to ICU for intubation and dialysis if progressive toxicity is evident.

**Client/Family Teaching**

1. Report any persistent abdominal pain or discomfort, unusual bruising or bleeding, fatigue, or increased SOB.

2. Review list of potential drug side effects and note those (dyspnea, palpitations, hemoptysis, confusion,

---

✤ = Available in Canada                    ***bold italic*** = life threatening side effect

chest pain, or impaired vision) requiring immediate medical intervention.

3. Practice reliable contraceptive methods.

4. Avoid any OTC drugs unless specifically ordered.

**Outcomes/Evaluate:** Disease regression with evidence of ↓ tumor size and spread.

# Alendronate sodium
(ay-**LEN**-droh-nayt)
**Pregnancy Category:** C
Fosamax **(Rx)**
**Classification:** Bone growth regulator (biphosphonate)

**Action/Kinetics:** Alendronate binds to bone hydroxyapatite and inhibits osteoclast activity, thereby preventing bone resorption. It appears to reduce fracture risk and reverse the progression of osteoporosis. Alendronate does not inhibit bone mineralization. It is well absorbed orally and is initially distributed to soft tissues, but then quickly redistributed to bone. The drug is not metabolized and is excreted through the urine. However, the **t½, terminal** is believed to be more than 10 years, due to slow release from the skeleton. **Uses:** Prevention and treatment of osteoporosis in postmenopausal women (concomitant estrogen therapy is not recommended due to lack of experience). Prevention of fractures in postmenopausal women with osteoporosis. Paget's disease of bone. **Contraindications:** In hypocalcemia. Those with severe renal insufficiency (creatinine clearance less than 35 mL/min). Lactation. **Special Concerns:** Use with caution in those with upper GI problems, such as dysphagia, symptomatic esophageal diseases, gastritis, duodenitis, or ulcers. Safety and effectiveness have not been determined in children or for use in male osteoporosis. **Side Effects:** *GI:* Abdominal pain, nausea, dyspepsia, constipation, diarrhea, flatulence, acid regurgitation, esophageal ulcer, vomiting, dyspha-

gia, abdominal distention, gastritis. *Miscellaneous:* Musculoskeletal pain, headache, taste perversion, rash and erythema (rare).

**OD** **Overdose Management:** *Symptoms:* Hypocalcemia, hypophosphatemia, upset stomach, heartburn, esophagitis, gastritis, ulcer. *Treatment:* Administration of milk or antacids to bind the drug should be considered.

**Drug Interactions**
*Antacids* / ↓ Absorption of alendronate
*Aspirin* / ↑ Risk of upper GI events
*Calcium supplements* / ↓ Absorption of alendronate
*Ranitidine* / ↑ Bioavailability of alendronate (significance not known)
**Laboratory Test Interferences:** ↓ Serum calcium and phosphate.

**Dosage**
• **Tablets**
*Prevention of osteoporosis in postmenopausal women.*
5 mg once a day in the morning ½ hr before the first food, beverage, or medication of the day with 6–8 oz of plain water.
*Treatment of osteoporosis or prevention of fractures in postmenopausal women with osteoporosis.*
10 mg once a day in the morning ½ hr before the first food, beverage, or medication of the day with 6–8 oz of plain water. Safety of treatment for more than 4 years has not been determined.
*Paget's disease of bone.*
40 mg once a day for 6 months taken as for osteoporosis.

## NURSING CONSIDERATIONS
**Administration/Storage**
1. To facilitate delivery to the stomach and reduce the potential for irritation of the esophagus, the client should not lie down for at least 30 min following administration.
2. Due to possible interference with absorption, at least 30 min should elapse before taking antacids or calcium supplements.
3. Retreatment for Paget's disease

may be considered following a 6-month posttreatment evaluation in clients who have relapsed, based on increases in serum alkaline phosphatase. Retreatment may also be appropriate for those who failed to normalize their serum alkaline phosphatase.

**Assessment**
1. Document indications for therapy: osteoporosis prevention or treatment in postmenopausal women or Paget's disease. Note symptoms, age at onset, and physical changes present.
2. Obtain baseline calcium, liver and renal function studies and correct any calcium or vitamin D deficiencies before starting therapy.
3. Note any history of upper GI problems such as gastritis, dysphagia, duodenitis, or ulcers.
4. Document bone mineral density studies if available and/or skeletal X rays.
5. Assess for fractures and manage appropriately to prevent further injury and loss of function.
6. With Paget's disease, document baseline alkaline phosphatase and monitor periodically during therapy.

**Client/Family Teaching**
1. Take only as prescribed. Benefit will be seen only when each tablet is taken with plain water the first thing in the morning at least 30 min before the first food, beverage, or medication of the day. Waiting longer than 30 min will improve the absorption of alendronate. Taking medication with juice or coffee will markedly reduce the drug's absorption.
2. Do not lie down after taking drug; wait at least 30 min.
3. Take calcium (500 mg) and vitamin D daily, especially if dietary intake or sun exposure is inadequate.
4. Osteoporosis occurs usually after age 40 and is a systemic skeletal disease characterized by low bone mass due to a higher amount of bone resorbed than formed.

**Outcomes/Evaluate**
• Prevention of osteoporosis and bone resorption (↓ bone turnover)
• Inhibition of kyphosis and pain due to bone fracture or deformity
• ↓ Pain; ↓ Serum alkaline phosphatase levels with Paget's disease

# Alfentanil hydrochloride
(al-FEN-tah-nil )
**Pregnancy Category:** C
Alfenta **(C-II) (Rx)**
**Classification:** Narcotic analgesic

See also *Narcotic Analgesics.*
**Action/Kinetics: Onset:** Immediate. **t½:** 1–2 hr (after IV use).
**Uses:** *Continuous infusion:* As an analgesic with nitrous oxide/oxygen to maintain general anesthesia. *Incremental doses:* Adjunct with barbiturate/nitrous oxide/oxygen to maintain general anesthesia. *Anesthetic induction:* As primary agent when ET intubation and mechanical ventilation are necessary. Analgesic component for monitored anesthesia care.
**Contraindications:** Use during labor and in children less than 12 years of age.
**Special Concerns:** Use with caution during lactation.
**Additional Side Effects:** Bradycardia, postoperative confusion, blurred vision, hypercapnia, shivering, and *asystole*. Neonates with respiratory distress syndrome have manifested hypotension with doses of 20 mcg/kg.

**Dosage**
• **IV**
*Continuous infusion, duration 45 min or more.*
**Initial for induction:** 50–75 mcg/kg; **maintenance, with nitrous oxide/oxygen:** 0.5–3 mcg/kg/min (average infusion rate: 1–1.5 mcg/kg/min). Following the induction dose, the infusion rate requirement should be reduced by 30%–50% for the first hour of maintenance.

*Induction of anesthesia, duration 45 min or more.*
**Initial for induction:** 130–245 mcg/kg; **maintenance:** 0.5–1.5 mcg/kg/min. If a general anesthetic is used for maintenance, the concentration of inhalation agents should be reduced by 30%–50% for the first hour.

*Anesthetic adjunct, 30–60 min duration, incremental injection.*
**Initial for induction:** 20–50 mcg/kg; **maintenance:** 5–15 mcg/kg, up to a total dose of 75 mcg/kg.

*Anesthetic adjunct, less than 30 min duration, incremental injection.*
**Initial for induction:** 8–20 mcg/kg; **maintenance:** 3–5 mcg/kg (or 0.5–1 mcg/kg/min, up to a total dose of 8–40 mcg/kg).

*Monitored anesthesia care, less than 30 min duration.*
**Initial for induction:** 3–8 mcg/kg; **maintenance:** 3–5 mcg/kg every 5–20 min to 1 mcg/kg/min, up to a total dose of 3–40 mg/kg.

*NOTE:* If there is a lightening of general anesthesia or the client manifests signs of surgical stress, the rate of administration of alfentanil may be increased to 4 mcg/kg/min or a bolus dose of 7 mcg/kg may be used. If the situation is not controlled following three bolus doses over 5 min, an inhalation anesthetic, a barbiturate, or a vasodilator should be used. If signs of lightening anesthesia are noted within the last 15 min of surgery, a bolus dose of 7 mcg/kg should be given rather than increasing the infusion rate. A potent inhalation anesthetic may be used as an alternative.

## NURSING CONSIDERATIONS

See also *Nursing Considerations* for *Narcotic Analgesics*.
**Administration/Storage**
**IV** 1. Individualize drug dosage for each client and for each use.
• Reduce dosage for elderly or debilitated clients.
• For those who are more than 20% above their ideal body weight, base dosage on lean body weight.

2. A tuberculin syringe or equivalent should be used to administer small volumes of alfentanil.
3. The injectable form may be reconstituted with either NSS, D5%/NSS, RL solution, or D5W. Direct IV administration over 1½–3 min. For continous IV administration dilute 20 cc of alfentanil in 230 mL diluent to provide a solution of 40 mcg/mL.
4. The infusion should be discontinued 10–15 min prior to the end of surgery.
**Assessment**
1. Note any history of drug hypersensitivity.
2. Obtain baseline weight and VS prior to administering.
3. Report any evidence of muscular rigidity before proceeding with the next dose.
4. Assess respiratory and CV status continuously during therapy.
**Client/Family Teaching**
1. Review preoperative teaching and report lack of understanding.
2. May experience dizziness, drowsiness, and orthostatic hypotension.
3. Avoid alcohol or any CNS depressants for at least 24 hr following drug administration.
**Outcomes/Evaluate**
• Induction and maintenance of anesthesia
• Facilitation of intubation and mechanical ventilation

# Alglucerase
(al-**GLOO**-sir-ace)
**Pregnancy Category:** C
Ceredase **(Rx)**
**Classification:** Treatment of Gaucher's disease

**Action/Kinetics:** Gaucher's disease is a rare congenital disorder of lipid metabolism where there is a deficiency in beta-glucocerebrosidase leading to an accumulation of lipid glucocerebroside in the liver, spleen, and bone marrow. Symptoms include an enlarged spleen, increased skin pigmentation, bone lesions, severe anemia, and thrombocytopenia. Alglucerase, which is a modified form of beta-glucocerebrosidase, is derived from human placental tissue; it catalyzes the hydrolysis of the glycolipid glucocerebroside to glucose and ceramide, which is part of the normal degradation pathway for membrane lipids. Following IV infusion, steady-state enzyme levels were observed in 60 min. **t½:** 3.6–10.4 min.

**Uses:** Chronic enzyme replacement in clients with confirmed diagnosis of type I Gaucher's disease who meet the following criteria: moderate to severe anemia, thrombocytopenia with bleeding tendency, significant hepatomegaly or splenomegaly, and bone disease.

**Special Concerns:** Use with caution during lactation. Since alglucerase is derived from human placental tissue, there is always the risk of some viral contamination; however, the drug product has been found to be free from hepatitis B surface antigen and for antigens of HIV (HIV-1).

**Side Effects:** Nausea, vomiting, chills, abdominal discomfort, slight fever.

**Dosage** ─────────────

- **IV Infusion**
  *Gaucher's disease.*

**Initial:** Up to 60 units/kg/infusion with infusions usually given q 2 weeks. Dose is then adjusted downward for maintenance therapy; dosage can be lowered q 3–6 months with some clients responding to doses as low as 1 unit/kg.

───────────────────

**NURSING CONSIDERATIONS**

**Administration/Storage**

**IV** 1. The severity of the disease (and client convenience) may require administration as frequently as every other day or as infrequently as q 4 weeks.

2. Response parameters should be closely monitored as the dose is progressively lowered.

3. Small dosage adjustments (either increased or decreased) may be made to avoid discarding partially used bottles provided that the

monthly administered dosage is not altered.

4. Prior to administration, the drug is diluted with NSS to a final volume not to exceed 100 mL. An in-line particulate filter is recommended for the infusion apparatus.

5. Do not shake the product; shaking may denature the glycoprotein, making it inactive.

6. Discard after opening, as the product does not contain any preservative.

7. Store at 4°C (39°F). Do not use if the bottle shows any discoloration or particulate matter.

**Assessment**

1. Note onset and list symptoms of disease requiring treatment.

2. Obtain baseline CBC and determine laboratory confirmation of type I Gaucher's disease, note presence of anemia, thrombocytopenia with bleeding tendency, enlarged liver and spleen, and any evidence of bone disease (potential for pathologic fractures due to demineralization).

**Client/Family Teaching**

1. May experience "flu-like" symptoms (N&V, fever, chills, and abdominal discomfort) but this is usually only temporary.

2. Drug has been derived from pooled human placental tissue; review potential risks.

3. Report for scheduled visits as the dose is progressively lowered based on response parameters.

**Outcomes/Evaluate**

- ↓ Splenomegaly and hepatomegaly within 6 months of continued alglucerase therapy
- Improved hematologic parameters (e.g., ↑ H&H, erythrocyte, and platelet counts)

# Allopurinol

(al-oh-**PYOUR**-ih-nohl)
**Pregnancy Category:** C
Alloprin ✦, Apo-Allopurinol ✦, Novo-Purol ✦, Zyloprim **(Rx)**
**Classification:** Antigout agent

───────────────────────────────

**A**

**Action/Kinetics:** Allopurinol and its major metabolite, oxipurinol, are potent inhibitors of xanthine oxidase, an enzyme involved in the synthesis of uric acid, without disrupting the biosynthesis of essential purine. This results in decreased levels of uric acid. The drug also increases reutilization of xanthine and hypoxanthine for synthesis of nucleotide and nucleic acid synthesis by acting on the enzyme hypoxanthine-guanine phosphoribosyltransferase. The resultant increases in nucleotides cause a negative feedback to inhibit synthesis of purines and a decrease in uric acid levels. **Peak plasma levels:** 1.5 hr for allopurinol and 4.5 hr for oxipurinol. **Onset:** 2–3 days. **t½ (allopurinol):** 1–3 hr; **t½ (oxipurinol):** 12–30 hr. **Peak serum levels, allopurinol:** 2–3 mcg/mL; **oxipurinol:** 5–6.5 mcg/mL (up to 50 mcg/mL in clients with impaired renal function). **Maximum therapeutic effect:** 1–3 weeks. Well absorbed from GI tract, metabolized in liver, excreted in urine and feces (20%).

**Uses:** Primary or secondary gout (acute attacks, tophi, joint destruction, nephropathy, uric acid lithiasis). Clients with leukemia, lymphoma, or other malignancies in whom drug therapy causes elevations of serum and urinary uric acid. Recurrent calcium oxalate calculi whose daily uric acid excretion exceeds 800 mg/day in males and 750 mg/day in females. *Investigational:* Mixed with methylcellulose as a mouthwash to prevent stomatitis following fluorouracil administration. Reduce the granulocyte suppressant effect of fluorouracil. Prevent ischemic reperfusion tissue damage. Reduce the incidence of perioperative mortality and postoperative arrhythmias in coronary artery bypass surgery. Reduce the rates of *Helicobacter pylori*-induced duodenal ulcers and treatment of hematemesis from NSAID-induced erosive esophagitis. Alleviate pain due to acute pancreatitis. Treatment of American cutaneous leishmaniasis and against *Trypanosoma cruzi.*

Treat Chagas' disease. As an alternative in epileptic seizures refractory to standard therapy.

**Contraindications:** Hypersensitivity to drug. Clients with idiopathic hemochromatosis or relatives of clients suffering from this condition. Children except as an adjunct in treatment of neoplastic disease. Severe skin reactions on previous exposure. To treat asymptomatic hyperuricemia.

**Special Concerns:** Use with caution during lactation. Use with caution in clients with liver or renal disease. In children use has been limited to rare inborn errors of purine metabolism or hyperuricemia as a result of malignancy or cancer therapy.

**Side Effects:** *Dermatologic* (most frequent): Pruritic maculopapular skin rash (may be accompanied by fever and malaise). Vesicular bullous dermatitis, eczematoid dermatitis, pruritus, urticaria, onycholysis, purpura, lichen planus, **Stevens-Johnson syndrome, toxic epidermal necrolysis.** Skin rash has been accompanied by hypertension and cataract development. *Allergy:* Fever, chills, leukopenia, eosinophilia, arthralgia, skin rash, pruritus, N&V, nephritis. *GI:* N&V, diarrhea, gastritis, dyspepsia, abdominal pain (intermittent). *Hematologic:* Leukopenia, eosinophilia, thrombocytopenia, leukocytosis. *Hepatic:* Hepatomegaly, cholestatic jaundice, **hepatic necrosis,** granulomatous hepatitis. *Neurologic:* Headache, peripheral neuropathy, paresthesia, somnolence, neuritis. *CV:* Necrotizing angiitis, hypersensitivity vasculitis. *Miscellaneous:* Ecchymosis, epistaxis, taste loss, arthralgia, acute attacks of gout, fever, myopathy, renal failure, uremia, alopecia.

**Drug Interactions**
*ACE inhibitors* / ↑ Risk of hypersensitivity reactions
*Aluminum salts* / ↓ Effect of allopurinol
*Ampicillin* / ↑ Risk of ampicillin-induced skin rashes
*Anticoagulants, oral* / ↑ Effect of anticoagulant due to ↓ breakdown by liver

*Azathioprine* / ↑ Effect of azathioprine due to ↓ breakdown by liver
*Cyclophosphamide* / ↑ Risk of bleeding or infection due to ↑ myelosuppressive effects of cyclophosphamide
*Iron preparations* / Allopurinol ↑ hepatic iron concentrations
*Mercaptopurine* / ↑ Effect of mercaptopurine due to ↓ breakdown by liver
*Theophylline* / Allopurinol ↑ plasma theophylline levels → possible toxicity
*Thiazide diuretics* / ↑ Risk of hypersensitivity reactions to allopurinol
*Uricosuric agents* / ↓ Effect of oxipurinol due to ↑ rate of excretion
**Laboratory Test Interferences:** ↑ ALT, AST, alkaline phosphatase. ↑ Serum cholesterol. ↓ Serum glucose levels.

**Dosage**
• **Tablets**
*Gout/hyperuricemia.*
**Adults:** 200–600 mg/day, depending on severity (minimum effective dose: 100–200 mg/day). Maximum daily dose should not exceed 800 mg.
*Prevention of uric acid nephropathy during treatment of neoplasms.*
**Adults:** 600–800 mg/day for 2–3 days (with high fluid intake).
*Prophylaxis of acute gout.*
**Initial:** 100 mg/day; increase by 100 mg at weekly intervals until serum uric acid level of 6 mg/100 mL or less is reached.
*Hyperuricemia associated with malignancy.*
**Pediatric, 6–10 years of age:** 300 mg/day either as a single dose of 100 mg t.i.d.; **under 6 years of age:** 150 mg/day in three divided doses.
*Recurrent calcium oxalate calculi.*
200–300 mg/day in one or more doses (dose may be adjusted according to urinary levels of uric acid).
*To ameliorate granulocyte suppressant effect of fluorouracil.*

600 mg/day.
*Reduce perioperative mortality and postoperative arrhythmias in coronary artery bypass surgery.*
300 mg 12 hr and 1 hr before surgery.
*Reduce relapse rates of* H. pylori-*induced duodenal ulcers; treat hematemesis from NSAID-induced erosive gastritis.*
50 mg q.i.d.
*Alleviate pain due to acute pancreatitis.*
50 mg q.i.d.
*Treat American cutaneous leishmaniasis and* T. cruzi.
20 mg/kg for 15 days.
*Treat Chagas' disease.*
600–900 mg/day for 60 days.
*Alternative to treat epileptic seizures refractory to standard therapy.*
300 mg/day, except use 150 mg/day in those less than 20 kg.
• **Mouthwash**
*Prevent fluorouracil-induced stomatitis.*
20 mg in 3% methylcellulose (1 mg/mL).

## NURSING CONSIDERATIONS
### Administration/Storage
1. Keep urine slightly alkaline to prevent the formation of uric acid stones.
2. Transfer from colchicine, uricosuric agents, and/or anti-inflammatory agents to allopurinol should be made gradually by decreasing the dosage of the preceding agents and increasing the dosage of allopurinol until a normal serum uric acid level is achieved.
3. Reduce the dose as follows in impaired renal function: creatinine clearance ($C_{cr}$) less than 10 mL/min: 100 mg 3 times a week; $C_{cr}$, 10 mL/min: 100 mg every other day; $C_{cr}$, 20 mL/min: 100 mg/day; $C_{cr}$, 40 mL/min: 150 mg/day; $C_{cr}$, 60 mL/min: 200 mg/day.
### Assessment
1. Take a complete drug history, noting any medications that may interact unfavorably.
2. Document indications for thera-

---

py, type and onset of symptoms and any history of previous allopurinol use. Note location, severity, and frequency of attacks and any joint deformity.

3. If female and of childbearing age, or if the woman is nursing, allopurinol is contraindicated.

4. Determine any history of idiopathic hemochromatosis.

5. Obtain baseline CBC, uric acid, and liver and renal function studies and monitor during therapy. Anticipate reduced dose with renal dysfunction.

**Client/Family Teaching**

1. Take with food or immediately after meals to lessen potential gastric irritation. At least 10–12 8-oz glasses of fluid should be taken each day to prevent stone formation.

2. Monitor weight if experiencing N&V or other signs of gastric irritation. Keep log and report if persistent weight loss is evident.

3. Skin rashes may start after months of drug therapy. If they are caused by allopurinol, the drug needs to be discontinued.

4. Do not take iron salts while taking allopurinol as high concentrations of iron may occur in the liver.

5. Avoid excessive intake of vitamin C, which may lead to increased potential for the formation of kidney stones.

6. Avoid caffeine and alcoholic beverages. These decrease the effect of allopurinol.

7. Avoid foods high in purine; these may include sardines, roe, salmon, scallops, anchovies, organ meats, and mincemeat.

8. Minimize exposure to ultraviolet light because of the increased risk of cataracts. If vision changes occur, see an ophthalmologist.

**Outcomes/Evaluate**

• ↓ Serum uric acid levels (6 mg/dL)
• ↓ Joint pain and inflammation
• ↓ Frequency of gout attacks
• Inhibition of stomatitis following fluorouracil therapy

# Alpha-1-Proteinase Inhibitor (Human) (Alpha-1-PI)

(**AL**-fah-1-**PROH**-tee-in-ayz)

**Pregnancy Category:** C

Prolastin **(Rx)**

**Classification:** Alpha-1-proteinase inhibitor

**Action/Kinetics:** Alpha-1-PI is the enzyme that is deficient in alpha-1-antitrypsin disease. This disease causes a progressive breakdown of elastin tissues in the alveoli, resulting in emphysema. Often fatal, alpha-1-antitrypsin disease is usually manifested in the third and fourth decades of life. Prolastin is a sterile, lyophilized product obtained from pooled human plasma that is nonreactive for the HIV antibody and the hepatitis B surface antigen. $t^{1/2}$: 4.5 days. **Therapeutic serum levels:** Approximately 80 mg/dL, although such levels may not reflect actual functional alpha-1-PI levels.

**Uses:** Panacinar emphysema due to congenital alpha-1-proteinase deficiency.

**Contraindications:** Clients with PiMZ or PiMS phenotypes of alpha-1-antitrypsin deficiency.

**Special Concerns:** Safety and efficacy for use in children not determined. Use with caution in clients at risk for circulatory overload.

**Side Effects:** Although precautions are taken during the manufacture of this product, it is possible that hepatitis and other infectious viruses may be present. *Miscellaneous:* Delayed fever up to 12 hr following treatment, dizziness, lightheadedness, mild transient leukocytosis.

## Dosage
• **IV Only**

*Panacinar emphysema.*

**Adults:** 60 mg/kg each week at a rate of 0.08 mL/kg/min (or greater).

## NURSING CONSIDERATIONS
**Administration/Storage**

**IV** 1. Administer only via IV. Follow

recommended procedures for reconstitution.

2. When reconstituted, Prolastin is equal to or greater than 20 mg/mL and has a pH of 6.6–7.4.

3. Do not mix the reconstituted drug with other diluents except for normal saline.

4. Immunize clients against hepatitis B prior to using Prolastin. If time does not permit adequate immunization, give a single dose of Hepatitis B Immune Globulin (Human), 0.06 mL/kg IM, at the time of the initial dose of Prolastin.

5. Administer within 3 hr after reconstitution. Do not refrigerate.

6. Store at 2°C–8°C (36°F–46°F); do not freeze.

7. Equipment used and any unused reconstituted alpha-1-PI (human) should be appropriately discarded.

**Assessment**
1. Perform a complete nursing history and lung assessment.

2. Obtain a hepatitis profile. If the client has not received hepatitis B immunization, document and provide appropriate therapy.

**Client/Family Teaching**
1. There is a familial tendency for alpha-1-antitrypsin deficiency; all blood relatives should be screened and provided appropriate counseling.

2. Report weekly for medication administration to maintain an adequate antielastase barrier. Therapy must continue throughout the client's lifetime.

3. Delayed fever may occur within 12 hr and is usually resolved in 24 hr.

4. Report any complaints of lightheadedness or dizziness.

5. Cigarette smoking may accelerate and aggravate condition by causing an increase of elastin secretion.

6. Product is prepared from human plasma; explain the potential associated risks.

**Outcomes/Evaluate**
• ↑ Serum prolastin levels (80 mg/dL)

• Slowing of destructive process on lung tissue
• Family members identified, screened, and counseled

---

# Alprazolam
(al-**PRAYZ**-oh-lam)
**Pregnancy Category:** D
Alti-Alprazolam ✹, Apo-Alpraz ✹, Gen-Alprazolam ✹, Novo-Alprazol ✹, Nu-Alpraz ✹, Xanax, Xanax TS ✹ **(C-IV) (Rx)**
**Classification:** Antianxiety agent

---

See also *Tranquilizers/Antimanic Drugs/Hypnotics.*
**Action/Kinetics: Peak plasma levels: PO,** 8–37 ng/mL after 1–2 hr. **t½:** 12–15 hr. 80% plasma protein bound. Metabolized to alpha-hydroxyalprazolam, an active metabolite. **t½:** 12–15 hr. Excreted in urine.
**Uses:** Anxiety. Anxiety associated with or without agoraphobia. *Investigational:* Agoraphobia with social phobia, depression, PMS.
**Contraindications:** Use with itraconazole or ketoconazole.

**Dosage** ————————
• **Tablets, Concentrate, Solution**
*Anxiety disorder.*
**Adults, initial:** 0.25–0.5 mg t.i.d.; **then,** titrate to needs of client, with total daily dosage not to exceed 4 mg. **In elderly or debilitated: initial;** 0.25 mg b.i.d.–t.i.d.; **then,** adjust dosage to needs of client.
*Antipanic agent.*
**Adults:** 0.5 mg t.i.d.; increase dose as needed up to a maximum of 10 mg/day.
*Agoraphobia with social phobia.*
**Adults:** 2–8 mg/day.
*PMS.*
0.25 mg t.i.d.

## NURSING CONSIDERATIONS

See also *Nursing Considerations* for *Tranquilizers/Antimanic Drugs/Hypnotics.*

---

**Administration/Storage**

1. Do not decrease the daily dose more than 0.5 mg over 3 days if therapy is terminated or the dose decreased.

2. Reduce dosage in elderly and debilitated clients.

**Client/Family Teaching**

1. May take with milk or food to decrease GI upset.

2. Include extra fluids and bulk in the diet to minimize constipation.

3. Use support devices as needed, especially at night, because elderly clients tend to become confused. Store drug away from bedside.

**Outcomes/Evaluate**

• Positive behaviors with phobias

• ↓ Anxiety/restlessness; Control of panic disorder

• Improvement in symptoms of PMS

# Alprostadil (PGE₁)

(al-**PROSS**-tah-dill)
Caverject, Edex, Muse, Prostin VR ✱, Prostin VR Pediatric **(Rx)**
**Classification:** Prostaglandin

**Action/Kinetics:** Alprostadil is the naturally occurring acidic lipid prostaglandin $E_1$. Alprostadil relaxes smooth muscle of the ductus arteriosus leading to increased pulmonary blood flow with increased blood oxygenation and lower body perfusion. Clients with low $pO_2$ values respond best. The drug may also cause vasodilation, inhibit platelet aggregation, and stimulate both intestinal and uterine smooth muscle. When injected intracavernosally, alprostadil relaxes the trabecular cavernous smooth muscles and causes dilation of penile arteries. This results in increased arterial blood flow to the corpus cavernosa and thus swelling and elongation of the penis. **Onset, systemic:** 1.5–3 hr for acyanotic congenital heart disease and 15–30 min for cyanotic congenital heart disease. **Time to peak effect:** 3 hr for coarctation of the aorta and 1.5 hr for interruption of aortic arch. **Duration:** Closure of the ductus arteriosus usually begins

1–2 hr after infusion discontinued. Alprostadil is rapidly metabolized (80% in one pass) by oxidation in the lung, and metabolites are excreted by the kidney.

**Uses:** Diagnosis and treatment of erectile dysfunction (male impotence) due to neurologic, vascular, psychologic, or mixed causes. *Investigational:* Diagnostic peripheral arteriography. Treat atherosclerosis, gangrene, and pain due to peripheral vascular disease. Prostin VR Pediatric is used in newborns with congenital heart defects to maintain patency of the ductus arteriosus.

**Contraindications:** Respiratory distress syndrome. Conditions that predispose to priapism: sickle cell anemia or trait, multiple myeloma, leukemia. In clients with anatomic deformation of the penis or in those with penile implants. Use in women, children, newborns, or men for whom sexual activity is not advisable or is contraindicated. Use for sexual intercourse with a pregnant woman unless a condom is used. Hyaline membrane disease.

**Side Effects:** *Respiratory: Apnea (in 10%–12% of neonates), especially in neonates less than 2 kg at birth;* bronchial wheezing, bradypnea, hypercapnia, respiratory depression. Also, in adults, respiratory infection, flu syndrome, sinusitis, rhinitis, nasal congestion, cough. *CNS:* Fever, *seizures,* hypothermia, jitteriness, lethargy, *cerebral bleeding,* stiffness, hyperextension of the neck, irritability. *CV:* Flushing, especially after intra-arterial dosage, bradycardia, hypotension, tachycardia, edema, *cardiac arrest, CHF, shock, arrhythmias.* GI: Diarrhea, hyperbilirubinemia, gastric regurgitation. *Renal:* Hematuria, anuria. *Skeletal:* Cortical proliferation of long bones. *Hematologic: Disseminated intravascular coagulation,* thrombocytopenia, anemia, bleeding. *Miscellaneous: Sepsis, peritonitis,* hypoglycemia, hypokalemia or hyperkalemia.

*Side effects when used for erectile dysfunction:* Penile pain, prolonged erection, penile fibrosis, hematoma at injection site, penile disorders, including numbness, yeast infection, irritation, sensitivity, phimosis, pruritus, erythema, venous leak, penile skin tear, strange feeling in penis, discoloration of penile head, itch at tip of penis. Painful erection, abnormal ejaculation, penile rash, penile edema, priapism, hematoma, ecchymosis, urethral pain, urethral burning, urethral bleeding or spotting, testicular pain.

**OD** **Overdose Management:** *Symptoms:* **Apnea,** bradycardia, flushing, hypotension, pyrexia. *Treatment:* Reduce rate of infusion if symptoms of hypotension or pyrexia occur; discontinue infusion if symptoms of apnea or bradycardia occur.

**Drug Interactions**
*Cyclosporine* / ↓ Blood levels of cyclosporine
*Heparin, Warfarin* / ↑ Bleeding after intracavernosal injection
**Laboratory Test Interferences:** ↑ Bilirubin. ↓ Glucose, serum calcium. ↑ or ↓ Potassium.

**Dosage** ────────────
• **Continuous IV Infusion or Umbilical Artery**
*Maintain patency of ductus arteriosus.*
**Initial:** 0.05–0.1 mcg/kg/min; **then,** after response achieved, decrease infusion rate to lowest dose that will maintain response (e.g., 0.1–0.05 to 0.025–0.01 mcg/kg/min). *NOTE:* If 0.1 mcg/kg/min is insufficient, dosage can be increased up to 0.4 mcg/kg/min.
• **Intracavernosal**
*Erectile dysfunction due to vascular, psychogenic, or mixed etiology.*
The dose should be individualized for each client by careful titration. **Initial:** 2.5 mcg. If there is a partial response, increase the dose by 2.5 mcg to 5 mcg and then in increments of 5–10 mcg, depending on the erectile response, until a dose is reached that results in an erection suitable for intercourse but not exceeding 1 hr in duration. If there is

no response to the initial 2.5-mcg dose, the second dose may be increased to 7.5 mcg, followed by increments of 5 to 10 mcg. **Maximum dose:** 60 mcg. The drug should not be given more than 3 times/week with at least 24 hr between each dose.
*Erectile dysfunction due to pure neurogenic etiology (spinal cord injury).*
**Initial:** 1.25 mcg. The dose may be increased by 1.25 mcg to 2.5 mcg, followed by an increment of 2.5 mcg to a dose of 5 mcg. The dose may be increased in 5-mcg increments until a dose is reached that produces an erection suitable for intercourse and not exceeding 1 hr in duration.

────────────
**NURSING CONSIDERATIONS**
**Administration/Storage**
1. For use in impotence, the diluent is mixed with alprostadil powder, and the solution is swirled gently. One milliliter of the reconstituted solution contains either 10 or 20 mcg of alprostadil. The solution should be used immediately and not stored or frozen.
2. For treating impotence, alprostadil is injected into the corpus cavernosum using a small, thin needle (½ in., 27- to 30-gauge). The injection site must be cleansed with an alcohol swab. The first injection should be administered in a physician's office.
3. Store ampules at 2°C–8°C (36°F–46°F).
**IV** 4. Administer infusions only in pediatric intensive care facilities.
5. Dilute 500 mcg with either NaCL injection or dextrose injection in volumes appropriate for the infant's fluid intake and suitable for the type of infusion pump available.
6. Use a Y set-up.
7. Discard any unused solutions and prepare a fresh infusion solution q 24 hr.
8. Sterile solutions should be infused for the shortest time and at the lowest dose that will produce the desired effect.

**A**

## Assessment

1. Document indications for therapy, onset of symptoms, and any associated predisposing factors.
2. Document VS and cardiac and respiratory function before administering the medication.
3. Determine if the neonate has restricted pulmonary blood flow. Have a respirator readily available.
4. Note any evidence of bleeding tendencies or sickle cell anemia.
5. With sexual dysfunction, list all medications currently prescribed and those being consumed. Note any reference to alterations in psychosocial balance.

## Interventions

1. Monitor arterial pressure intermittently by umbilical artery catheter, auscultation, Dinemapp or with a Doppler transducer. Obtain written guidelines for arterial pressures; if the arterial pressure falls significantly, decrease the rate of flow immediately and report.
2. Observe infant for apnea, bradycardia, pyrexia, flushing, and hypotension; symptoms of *overdose*. The following guidelines are appropriate.
- If apnea or bradycardia occur, stop infusion, change to the unmedicated solution, and start resuscitation.
- If infant develops pyrexia or hypotension, reduce rate of IV flow and report. Reduce rate until the temperature and BP return to baseline values.
- Report if flushing occurs; this indicates an incorrect intra-arterial placement of the catheter and requires repositioning.
3. If the infant has restricted pulmonary blood flow, monitor ABGs. A positive response to alprostadil is indicated by at least a 10 mm Hg increase in blood $pO_2$.
4. If the infant has restricted systemic blood flow, monitor BP and serum pH. If the infant has acidosis, a positive response to alprostadil would be indicated by an increased pH, an increase in BP, and a decreased ratio of PA pressure to aortic pressure.

5. Monitor neurological status and level of consciousness; report seizures, hyperexcitability, or stiffness as drug must be stopped.
6. Treatment for impotence should be discontinued in clients who develop penile angulation, cavernosal fibrosis, or Peyronie's disease.

## Client/Family Teaching

1. Advise neonates' parents of condition and why drug is indicated; review risks and benefits.
2. With erectile dysfunction, once initial injection response is evaluated, obtain instruction in the method for administration. Review written guidelines to ensure proper administration and dosing.
3. Do not exceed amount or frequency of use.
4. With penile insert, report any foul discharge, pain, or local irritation and rash.
5. Report any unusual drug side effects. Seek immediate attention if an erection lasts longer than 6 hr.
6. When using alprostadil for impotence, report for follow-up to detect signs of penile fibrosis.

## Outcomes/Evaluate

- Improved pulmonary blood flow with ↑ $pO_2$
- Closure of ductus arteriosus 1–2 hr following infusion
- Penile erection with intracavernosal therapy

# Alteplase, recombinant

(**AL**-teh-playz)

**Pregnancy Category:** C

Activase, Activase rt-PA ✷ **(Rx)**

**Classification:** Thrombolytic agent (tissue plasminogen activator)

**Action/Kinetics:** Alteplase, a tissue plasminogen activator, is synthesized by a human melanoma cell line using recombinant DNA technology. This enzyme binds to fibrin in a thrombus, causing a conversion of plasminogen to plasmin. This conversion results in local fibrinolysis and a decrease in circulating fibrinogen. Within 10 min following termination of an infusion, 80% of the alteplase has been cleared from the plasma by the liver. The enzyme activity of alteplase is 580,000 IU/mg. **t½, initial:** 4 min; **final:** 35 min (elimination phase).

**Uses:** Improvment of ventricular function following acute MI, including reducing the incidence of CHF and decreasing mortality. Treat acute ischemic stroke, after intracranial hemorrhage has been excluded by CT scan or other diagnostic imaging. Acute pulmonary thromboembolism. *Investigational:* Unstable angina pectoris.

**Contraindications:** *Acute MI or pulmonary embolism:* Active internal bleeding, history of CVA, within 2 months of intracranial or intraspinal surgery or trauma, intracranial neoplasm, AV malformation or aneurysm, bleeding diathesis, severe uncontrolled hypertension.

*Acute ischemic stroke:* Symptoms of intracranial hemorrhage on pretreatment evaluation, suspected subarachnoid hemorrhage, recent intracranial surgery or serious head trauma, recent previous stroke, history of intracranial hemorrhage, uncontrolled hypertension (above 185 mm Hg systolic or above 110 Hg diastolic) at time of treatment, active internal bleeding, seizure at onset of stroke, intracranial neoplasm, AV malformation or aneurysm, bleeding diathesis.

**Special Concerns:** Use with caution in the presence of recent GI or GU bleeding (within 10 days), subacute bacterial endocarditis, acute pericarditis, significant liver dysfunction, concomitant use of oral anticoagulants, diabetic hemorrhagic retinopathy, septic thrombophlebitis or occluded arteriovenous cannula (at infected site), lactation, mitral stenosis with atrial fibrillation. Since fibrin will be lysed during therapy, careful attention should be given to potential bleeding sites such as sites of catheter insertion and needle puncture sites. Use with caution within 10 days of major surgery (e.g., obstetrics, coronary artery bypass) and in cli-

ents over 75 years of age. Safety and efficacy have not been established in children. *NOTE:* Doses greater than 150 mg have been associated with an increase in intracranial bleeding.

**Side Effects:** *Bleeding tendencies: Internal bleeding* (including the GI and GU tracts and intracranial or retroperitoneal site). Superficial bleeding (e.g., gums, sites of recent surgery, venous cutdowns, arterial punctures). Ecchymosis, epistaxis. *CV:* Bradycardia, hypotension, cardiogenic shock, arrhythmias, *heart failure, cardiac arrest, cardiac tamponade, myocardial rupture,* recurrent ischemia, reinfarction, mitral regurgitation, pericardial effusion, pericarditis, venous thrombosis and embolism, electromechanical dissociation. *Allergic:* Rash, *laryngeal edema, anaphylaxis. GI:* N&V. *Miscellaneous:* Fever, urticaria, pulmonary edema, cerebral edema.

*Due to accelerated infusion: Strokes, hemorrhagic stroke,* nonfatal stroke. Incidence increases with age.

**OD Overdose Management:** *Symptoms:* Bleeding disorders. *Treatment:* Discontinue therapy immediately as well as any concomitant heparin therapy.

**Drug Interactions**
*Abciximab* / ↑ Risk of bleeding
*Acetylsalicylic acid* / ↑ Risk of bleeding
*Dipyridamole* / ↑ Risk of bleeding
*Heparin* / ↑ Risk of bleeding, especially at arterial puncture sites

**Dosage** ————————
• **IV Infusion Only**
*AMI, accelerated infusion.*
**Weight >67 kg:** 100 mg as a 15-mg IV bolus, followed by 50 mg infused over the next 30 min and then 35 mg infused over the next 60 min. **Weight <67 kg:** 15 mg IV bolus, followed by 0.75 mg/kg infused over the next 30 min (not to exceed 50 mg) and then 0.50 mg/kg infused over the next 60 min (not to exceed 35 mg). The safety and efficacy of this regimen have only been evaluated

**A**

using heparin and aspirin concomitantly.

*AMI, 3-hr infusion.*
100 mg total dose subdivided as follows: 60 mg (34.8 million IU) the first hour with 6–10 mg given in a bolus over the first 1–2 min and the remaining 50–54 mg given over the hour; 20 mg (11.6 million IU) over the second hour and 20 mg (11.6 million IU) given over the third hour. **Clients less than 65 kg:** 1.25 mg/kg given over 3 hr, with 60% given the first hour with 6%–10% given by direct IV injection within the first 1–2 min; 20% is given the second hour and 20% during the third hour. Doses of 150 mg have caused an increase in intracranial bleeding.

*Pulmonary embolism.*
100 mg over 2 hr; heparin therapy should be instituted near the end of or right after the alteplase infusion when the partial thromboplastin or thrombin time returns to twice that of normal or less.

*Acute ischemic stroke.*
0.9 mg/kg (maximum of 90 mg) infused over 60 min with 10% of the total dose given as an initial IV bolus over 1 min. Doses greater than 0.9 mg/kg may cause an increased incidence of intracranial hemorrhage. Use with aspirin and heparin during the first 24 hr after onset of symptoms has not been investigated.

## NURSING CONSIDERATIONS
### Administration/Storage
**IV** 1. Alteplase therapy should be initiated as soon as possible after onset of symptoms and within 3 hr after the onset of stroke symptoms.

2. For acute MI, nearly 90% of clients also receive heparin concomitantly with alteplase and either aspirin or dipyridamole during or after heparin therapy.

3. The product must be reconstituted with only sterile water for injection without preservatives immediately prior to use. The reconstituted preparation contains 1 mg/mL and is a colorless to pale yellow transparent solution.

4. Using an 18-gauge needle, the stream of sterile water for injection should be directed into the lyophilized cake. The product should be left undisturbed for several minutes to allow dissipation of any large bubbles.

5. If necessary, the reconstituted solution may be further diluted immediately prior to use in an equal volume of 0.9% NaCL injection or 5% dextrose injection to yield a concentration of 0.5 mg/mL. Dilution should be accomplished by gentle swirling or slow inversion.

6. Either glass bottles or polyvinyl-chloride bags may be used for administration.

7. Alteplase is stable for up to 8 hr following reconstitution or dilution. Stability will not be affected by light.

8. Do not use 50-mg vials if the vacuum is not present (100-mg vials do not contain a vacuum). Reconstitute 50-mg vials with a large-bore needle (e.g., 18 gauge) directing the stream of sterile water for injection into the lyophilized cake. For the 100-mg vial, use the transfer device provided for reconstitution.

9. Use an electronic infusion device for medication administration. Do not add any other medications to the line. Anticipate 3 lines for access (1–alteplase; 1–heparin and other drugs such as lidocaine; 1–blood drawing and transfusions).

10. Lyophilized alteplase should be stored at room temperatures not to exceed 30°C (86°F) or under refrigeration between 2°C–8°C (35°F–46°F).

11. Have available emergency drugs (especially aminocaproic acid) and resuscitative equipment.

### Assessment
1. Note any history of hypertension, internal bleeding, PUD, or recent surgery.

2. Document onset and characteristics of chest pain and/or stroke symptoms and assess throughout therapy.

3. Assess and document overall physical condition; note CV and neurologic findings; obtain weight and ECG.

4. Obtain a drug history and determine what client is currently taking; note any anticoagulants.

5. Obtain baseline hematologic parameters, type and cross, coagulation times, cardiac marker panel, and renal function studies.

**Interventions**

1. Carefully review and follow instructions for drug reconstitution, review contraindications before initiating therapy, and document if accelerated or 3 hr infusion is prescribed.

2. Observe in a closely monitored environment; obtain VS and review and document monitor strips.

3. Anticipate and assess for reperfusion reactions such as:

- Reperfusion arrhythmias usually of short duration. These may include accelerated idioventricular rhythm and sinus bradycardia.
- Reduction of chest pain
- Return of the elevated ST segment to near baseline levels
- Smaller Q waves

4. Check all access sites for any evidence of bleeding.

5. During IV therapy, arterial sticks require 30 min of manual pressure followed by application of a pressure dressing.

6. In the event of any uncontrolled bleeding, terminate the alteplase and heparin infusions and report immediately.

7. Monitor neurologic status and record findings q 15–30 min during infusion.

8. During treatment of stroke, note CT or MRI results.

9. During treatment for pulmonary embolism, ensure that the PTT or PT is no more than twice that of normal before heparin therapy is added.

10. Keep on bed rest and observe for S&S of abnormal bleeding (hematuria, hematemesis, melena, CVA, cardiac tamponade).

11. Obtain appropriate postinfusion laboratory studies (cardiac marker, platelets, H&H, PTT, ECG) as directed.

**Client/Family Teaching**

1. Review the goals of therapy and

inherent risks during acute coronary artery occlusion and/or stroke.

2. To be effective, the therapy should be instituted within 4–6 hr of onset of symptoms of AMI.

3. Encourage family members to learn CPR.

**Outcomes/Evaluate**

- Lysis of thrombi with reperfusion of ischemic cardiac and/or cereberal tissue
- ↓ Infarct size with restoration of coronary perfusion and improved ventricular function (↑ CO, ↓ incidence of CHF, ↓ mortality)

# Altretamine (Hexylmethyl-melamine)

(all-**TRET**-ah-meen)

**Pregnancy Category:** D

Hexalen **(Rx)**

**Classification:** Antineoplastic, miscellaneous

See also *Antineoplastic Agents*.

**Action/Kinetics:** The mechanism of action of altretamine is unknown although metabolism of the drug is required for cytotoxicity. Well absorbed following PO ingestion; undergoes rapid demethylation in the liver, yielding the principal metabolites–pentamethylmelamine and tetramethylmelamine. **Peak plasma levels:** 0.5–3 hr. **t½:** 4.7–10.2 hr. Metabolites are excreted mainly through the kidney.

**Uses:** Used alone in the palliative treatment of persistent or recurrent ovarian cancer after first-line cisplatin- or alkylating agent-based combination therapy.

**Contraindications:** Preexisting bone marrow depression or severe neurologic toxicity, although the drug has been used safely in clients with preexisting cisplatin neuropathies. Lactation.

**Special Concerns:** Safety and effectiveness have not been determined in children. High daily doses may result in gradual onset of N&V.

**Side Effects:** *GI:* N&V (most common). *Neurologic:* Peripheral sensory neuropathy, fatigue, anorexia, seizures. *CNS:* Mood disorders, disorders of consciousness, ataxia, dizziness, vertigo. *Hematologic:* Leukopenia, thrombocytopenia, anemia. *Miscellaneous:* **Hepatic toxicity,** skin rash, pruritus, alopecia.

**Drug Interactions:** Use with MAO inhibitors may cause severe orthostatic hypotension, especially in clients over the age of 60 years.

**Laboratory Test Interferences:** ↑ Serum creatinine, BUN, alkaline phosphatase.

**Dosage** _____

- **Capsules**
  *Ovarian cancer.*
  260 mg/m²/day given either for 14 or 21 consecutive days in a 28-day cycle. The total daily dose is given as four divided doses PO after meals and at bedtime.

## NURSING CONSIDERATIONS

See also *Nursing Considerations* for *Antineoplastic Agents.*

**Assessment**

1. Document onset of symptoms and note all previous therapies.
2. Document baseline neurologic findings.
3. Obtain hematologic and liver function studies prior to initiating drug therapy.

**Interventions**

1. Anticipate neurotoxicity as a side effect of drug therapy. Conduct a neurologic exam prior to starting therapy and updated before each course of altretamine.
2. Administering pyridoxine with altretamine may reduce the severity of the neurotoxic effects.
3. Peripheral blood counts should be monitored monthly, prior to the initiation of each course of therapy and as clinically indicated.

**Client/Family Teaching**

1. Report any adverse symptoms, such as tingling, decreased sensation, dizziness, and N&V. Drug dose

may need to be decreased or therapy discontinued.
2. Practice barrier contraception as drug may cause fetal damage.
3. Report for monthly hematologic studies.

**Outcomes/Evaluate:** Control of tumor growth and spread

---

# Amantadine hydrochloride
(ah-**MAN**-tah-deen)
**Pregnancy Category:** C
Endantadine ✹, Gen-Amantadine ✹, PMS-Amantadine ✹, Symadine, Symmetrel **(Rx)**
**Classification:** Antiviral and antiparkinson agent

---

See also *Antiviral Drugs.*

**Action/Kinetics:** Amantadine is believed to prevent penetration of the virus into cells, possibly by inhibiting uncoating of the RNA virus. The reaction appears to be virus specific for influenza A but not host specific. It may also prevent the release of infectious viral nucleic acid into the host cell. The drug reduces symptoms of viral infections if given within 24–48 hr after onset of illness. For the treatment of parkinsonism, amantadine may increase the release of dopamine from dopaminergic nerve terminals in the substantia nigra of parkinson clients, resulting in an increase in dopamine levels in dopaminergic synapses. The drug decreases extrapyramidal symptoms, including akinesia, rigidity, tremors, excessive salivation, gait disturbances, and total functional disability. Well absorbed from GI tract. **Onset:** 48 hr. **Peak serum concentration:** 0.2 mcg/mL after 1–4 hr. **t½:** Approximately 15 hr; elimination half-life increases two- to threefold when creatinine clearance is less than 40 mL/min/1.73 m². Ninety percent excreted unchanged in urine.

**Uses:** Influenza A viral infections of the respiratory tract (prophylaxis and treatment of high-risk clients with immunodeficiency, CV, metabolic, neuromuscular, or pulmonary disease). Symptomatic treatment of idiopathic parkinsonism and parkinsonism syndrome resulting from encephalitis, carbon monoxide intoxication, drugs, or cerebral arteriosclerosis. Favorable results have been obtained in about 50% of the clients. Improvements can last for up to 30 months, although some clients report that the effect of the drug wears off in 1–3 months. A rest period or an increased dosage may reestablish effectiveness. For parkinsonism, amantadine hydrochloride is usually used concomitantly with other agents, such as levodopa and anticholinergic agents.

Amantadine is recommended for prophylaxis in the following situations:
• Short-term prophylaxis during the course of a presumed outbreak of influenza A
• Adjunct to late immunization in high-risk clients
• To reduce disruption of medical care and to decrease spread of virus in high-risk clients when influenza A virus outbreaks occur
• To supplement vaccination protection in clients with impaired immune responses
• As chemoprophylaxis during flu season for those high-risk clients for whom influenza vaccine is contraindicated due to anaphylactic response to egg protein or prior severe reactions associated with flu vaccination

**Contraindications:** Hypersensitivity to drug.

**Special Concerns:** Use with caution in clients with liver and renal disease, history of epilepsy, CHF, peripheral edema, orthostatic hypotension, recurrent eczematoid dermatitis, or severe psychosis, in clients taking CNS stimulant drugs, to those exposed to rubella, and to nursing mothers. Safe use in lactating mothers and in children less than 1 year has not been established.

**Side Effects:** *GI:* N&V, constipation, anorexia, xerostomia. *CNS:* Depres-

sion, psychosis, **convulsions,** hallucinations, lightheadedness, confusion, ataxia, irritability, anxiety, headache, dizziness, fatigue, insomnia. *CV:* **CHF,** orthostatic hypotension, peripheral edema. *Miscellaneous:* Urinary retention, leukopenia, neutropenia, mottling of skin of the extremities due to poor peripheral circulation (livedo reticularis), skin rashes, visual problems, slurred speech, oculogyric episodes, dyspnea, weakness, eczematoid dermatitis.

**OD** **Overdose Management:** *Symptoms:* Anorexia, N&V, CNS effects. *Treatment:* Gastric lavage or induction of emesis followed by supportive measures. Ensure that client is well hydrated; give IV fluids if necessary. To treat CNS toxicity: IV physostigmine, 1–2 mg given q 1–2 hr in adults or 0.5 mg at 5–10-min intervals (maximum of 2 mg/hr) in children. Sedatives and anticonvulsants may be given if needed; antiarrhythmics and vasopressors may also be required.

**Drug Interactions**
*Anticholinergics* / Additive anticholinergic effects (including hallucinations, confusion), especially with trihexyphenidyl and benztropine
*CNS stimulants* / May ↑ CNS and psychic effects of amantadine; use cautiously together
*Hydrochlorothiazide/triamterene combination* / ↓ Urinary excretion of amantadine → ↑ plasma levels
*Levodopa* / Potentiated by amantadine

**Dosage**
• **Capsules, Syrup**
*Antiviral.*
**Adults:** 200 mg/day as a single or divided dose. **Children, 1–9 years:** 4.4–8.8 mg/kg/day up to a maximum of 150 mg/day in one or two divided doses (use syrup); **9–12 years:** 100 mg b.i.d.
*Prophylactic treatment.*
Institute before or immediately after exposure and continue for 10–21

days if used concurrently with vaccine or for 90 days without vaccine.

*Symptomatic management.*
Initiate as soon as possible and continue for 24–48 hr after disappearance of symptoms. Decrease dose in renal impairment (see package insert). Reduce dose to 100 mg/day for persons with active seizure disorders due to the increased risk of seizure frequency using daily doses of 200 mg.

*Parkinsonism.*
**Use as sole agent, usual:** 100 mg b.i.d., up to 400 mg/day in divided doses, if necesssary. **Use with other antiparkinson drugs:** 100 mg 1–2 times/day.

*Drug-induced extrapyramidal symptoms.*
100 mg b.i.d. (up to 300 mg/day may be required in some). Reduce dose in impaired renal function.

## NURSING CONSIDERATIONS

See also *General Nursing Considerations for All Anti-Infectives*, and *Antiviral Drugs*.

### Administration/Storage
1. Protect capsules from moisture.
2. Therapy should be started for viral illness as soon as possible after symptoms begin and for 24–48 hr after symptoms disappear.

### Assessment
1. Obtain a thorough nursing history and note any evidence of seizures, CHF, and renal insufficiency.
2. With active seizure disorder drug dosage must be reduced to prevent breakthrough seizures. With an increase in seizure activity, take appropriate precautions and ensure that dosage is reduced to 100 mg/day to prevent loss of seizure control.
3. Monitor I&O; observe clients with renal impairment for crystalluria, oliguria, and increased BUN or creatinine levels.
4. With Parkinson's disease, following loss of effectiveness of the drug, benefits may be regained by increasing the dosage or discontinuing the drug for several weeks and then reinstituting it.

### Client/Family Teaching
1. Administer last daily dose several hours before retiring to prevent insomnia.
2. Do not drive a car or work in a situation where alertness is important until drug effects are realized; medication can affect vision, concentration, and coordination.
3. Rise slowly from a prone position because orthostatic hypotension may occur. Lie down if dizzy or too weak to relieve these symptoms.
4. Report diffuse patchy discoloration or mottling of the skin. Discoloration lessens when legs are elevated and usually fades completely within weeks after discontinuing drug.
5. Report any exposure to rubella as drug may increase susceptibility to disease.
6. Susceptible individuals (elderly, immunocompromised) should avoid crowds during "flu" season and receive annual flu shot and pneumonia vaccine.
7. Psychologic changes such as confusion, mental status changes, nervousness, or depression should be reported as well as any persistent, or new symptoms.
8. Avoid alcohol or any other unprescribed OTC products.
9. Clients with parkinsonism should not stop drug abruptly.
10. Clients with seizure disorders should be advised to report any early signs or symptoms of seizure activity as dosage may require adjustment.

### Outcomes/Evaluate
• ↓ Drug-induced extrapyramidal symptoms
• Improved motor control with ↓ tremor
• Influenza A prophylaxis and ↓ spread of infection to high-risk individuals during outbreaks

## Amifostine
((**am**-ih-**FOS**-teen))
**Pregnancy Category:** C
Ethyol **(Rx)**
**Classification:** Cytoprotective drug

**Action/Kinetics:** Amifostine, an organic thiophosphate prodrug, is dephosphorylated by alkaline phosphatase in tissue to the active free thiol metabolite. The thiol metabolite reduces the toxic effects of cisplatin. The abilitiy to protect normal tissues differentially is due to the higher capillary alkaline phosphatase activity, higher pH, and better vascularity of normal tissues compared with tumor tissue. This results in a more rapid generation of the active thiol metabolite as well as greater uptake into tissues. The higher levels of the thiol metabolite in normal tissues binds to, and thus detoxifies, reactive metabolites of cisplatin; the thiol metabolite can also scavange free radicals that may be generated in tissues exposed to cisplatin. Rapidly cleared from the plasma. **t½, distribution:** less than 1 min; **t½, elimination:** about 8 min. The thiol metabolite is further broken down to a disulfide metabolite that is less active.

**Uses:** To decrease cumulative renal toxicity due to repeated use of cisplatin in clients with advanced ovarian cancer and in those with non-small-cell lung cancer.

**Contraindications:** Hypersensitivity to aminothiol compounds or mannitol. Use in hypotensive or dehydrated clients, in those on antihypertensive therapy that cannot be terminated for 24 hr, and in clients receiving chemotherapy for malignancies that are potentially curable (e.g., certain malignancies of germ cell origin). Use during lactation.

**Special Concerns:** Safety has not been determined in clients over 70 years of age or in those with preexisting CV or cerebrovascular conditions, such as ischemic heart disease, arrhythmias, CHF, or history of stroke or transient ischemic attacks. Use with caution in those where N&V or hypotension may be more likely to have serious consequences.

**Side Effects:** *CV:* Transient decrease in BP, hypotension. *GI:* Severe N&V.

*CNS:* Dizziness, somnolence, reversible loss of consciousness (rare). *Hypersensitivity:* Mild skin rash, rigors. *Miscellaneous:* Flushing or feeling of warmth, chills or feeling of coldness, hiccoughs, sneezing, hypocalcemia.

**Drug Interactions:** Amifostine may cause hypotension in clients receiving antihypertensive drugs or other drugs that may potentiate hypotension.

**Dosage** ————————————
• **IV Infusion**
   *Cytoprotective agent used with cisplatin.*
**Initial:** 910 mg/m² given once daily as a 15-min IV infusion, starting within 30 min prior to cisplatin chemotherapy.

## NURSING CONSIDERATIONS
### Administration/Storage
**IV** 1. The 15-min infusion is better tolerated than infusions of longer duration.
2. Keep client supine during administration with BP monitored every 5 min.
3. Give an antiemetic medication, including dexamethasone (20 mg IV) and a serotonin 5HT₃ receptor antagonist, prior to and in conjunction with amifostine.
4. Stop the infusion of amifostine if the systolic BP decreases significantly from baseline values that are listed in the guidelines from the manufacturer. If BP returns to normal within 5 min and the client has no symptoms, the infusion may be restarted so the full dose of amifostine can be given. If the full dose of amifostine cannot be given, the dose for subsequent cycles should be 740 mg/m².
5. Reconstitute by adding 9.5 mL of sterile 0.9% NaCL injection (use of other solutions is not recommended). The reconstituted solution contains 500 mg amifostine/10 mL and is stable for 5 hr at room temperature (25°C; 77°F) or up to 24 hr under refrigeration (2°C–8°C; 36°F–46°F).

**A**

### Assessment

1. Note type of malignancy being managed, onset and duration of symptoms, other agents trialed, and the anticipated dose and length of cisplatin chemotherapy.
2. List drugs currently prescribed to ensure none interact unfavorably.
3. Obtain baseline VS, calcium, and renal function studies and monitor throughout therapy. Ensure that client is not dehydrated or hypotensive.
4. Monitor VS and I&O. Keep supine during 15 min administration of drug and check BP every 5 min during infusion.
5. Administer antiemetics prior to amifostine therapy; evaluate need for further antiemetic administration.
6. Review the manufacturer''s guidelines for interrupting infusion due to decreased SBP and the suggested dose for readmission.

### Client/Family Teaching

1. Explain that drug is given to protect the kidneys during repeated cisplastic chemotherapy.
2. Stop BP medications 24 hr prior to therapy and ensure client is well hydrated.
3. Advise that chills, flushing, dizziness, somnolence, hiccups, and sneezing may occur transiently.

**Outcomes/Evaluate:** ↓ Renal toxicity in clients receiving cisplatin chemotherapy

---

## Amikacin sulfate

(am-ih-**KAY**-sin)
**Pregnancy Category:** D
Amikin **(Rx)**
**Classification:** Antibiotic, aminoglycoside

---

See also *Anti-Infectives,* and *Aminoglycosides.*

**Action/Kinetics:** Derived from kanamycin. Its spectrum is somewhat broader than that of other aminoglycosides, including *Serratia* and *Acinetobacter* species, as well as certain staphylococci and streptococci. Effective against both penicillinase- and non-penicillinase-producing organisms. **Peak therapeutic**

**serum levels: IM,** 16–32 mcg/mL. **t½:** 2–3 hr. Toxic serum levels: >35 mcg/mL (peak measured after 1 hr) and >10 mcg/mL (trough measured before next dose).

**Uses:** Short-term treatment of gram-negative bacterial infections including *Pseudomonas, Escherichia coli, Proteus, Providencia, Klebsiella, Enterobacter, Serratia,* and *Acinetobacter.* For infections due to gentamicin or tobramycin resistant strains of *Providencia rettgeri, P. stuartii, Serratia marcescens,* and *Pseudomonas aeruginosa.*

Infections include bacterial septicemia (including neonatal sepsis); serious infections of the respiratory tract, bones, joints, skin, soft tissue, and CNS (including meningitis); intra-abdominal infections (including peritonitis); burns; postoperative infections (including postvascular surgery). Also, serious complicated and recurrent infections of the urinary tract. May be used as initial therapy in certain situations in the treatment of known or suspected staphylococcal disease. *Investigational:* Intrathecal or intraventricular use. As part of multiple drug regimen for *Mycobacterium avium* complex (commonly seen in AIDS clients).

**Special Concerns:** Use with caution in premature infants and neonates.

### Dosage

• **IM (Preferred) and IV**
**Adults, children, and older infants:** 15 mg/kg/day in two to three equally divided doses q 8–12 hr for 7–10 days; **maximum daily dose:** 15 mg/kg.

*Uncomplicated UTIs.*
250 mg b.i.d.; **newborns:** loading dose of 10 mg/kg followed by 7.5 mg/kg q 12 hr.

*Use in neonates.*
**Initial:** Loading dose of 10 mg/kg; **then,** 7.5 mg/kg q 12 hr. Lower doses may be safer during the first 2 weeks of life.

*Intrathecal or intraventricular use.*
8 mg/24 hr.

*As part of multiple drug regimen for* M. avium complex.
15 mg/kg/day IV in divided doses q 8–12 hr.
*In clients with impaired renal function.*
Normal loading dose of 7.5 mg/kg; **then** monitor administration by serum level of amikacin (35 mcg/mL maximum) or creatinine clearance rates. Duration of treatment: **Usual:** 7–10 days.

## NURSING CONSIDERATIONS

See also *Nursing Considerations* for *Aminoglycosides.*
**Administration/Storage**
**IV** 1. Add 500-mg vial to 200 mL of sterile diluent, such as NSS or D5W.
2. Administer over a 300- to 600-min period for adults.
3. Administer to infants in the amount of prescribed fluid. The IV administration to infants should be over 1–2 hr.
4. Store colorless liquid at room temperature for no longer than 2 years.
5. Potency is not affected if the solution turns a light yellow.
**Assessment**
1. Obtain audiometric assessment with high dosage or prolonged use.
2. Note any vestibular dysfunction and monitor for eighth cranial nerve impairment R/T elevated peak drug levels.
**Outcomes/Evaluate**
• Resolution of infection
• Therapeutic serum drug levels (peak 30–35 mcg/mL; trough < 10 mcg/mL)

————COMBINATION DRUG————

# Amiloride and Hydrochlorothiazide

(ah-**MILL**-oh-ryd, hy-droh-klor-oh-**THIGH**-ah-zyd)
**Pregnancy Category:** C
Alti-Amiloride HCTZ ✶, Ami-Hydro ✶, Apo-Amilzide, Moduretic, Moduret ✶, Novamilor ✶, Nu-Amilzide ✶ **(Rx)**
**Classification:** Antihypertensive

See also *Amiloride,* and *Hydrochlorothiazide.*
**Content:** *Diuretic, potassium-sparing:* Amiloride HCl, 5 mg. *Antihypertensive/diuretic:* Hydrochlorothiazide, 50 mg.
**Uses:** Hypertension or CHF, especially when hypokalemia occurs. Used alone or with other antihypertensive drugs, such as beta-adrenergic blocking drugs and methyldopa.
**Special Concerns:** Use with caution during lactation. Geriatric clients may be more sensitive to the hypotensive and electrolyte effects of this combination; also, age-related decreases in renal function may require a decrease in dosage.

**Dosage**
• **Tablets**
*All uses.*
**Initial:** 1 tablet/day; **then,** dosage may be increased to 2 tablets/day.

## NURSING CONSIDERATIONS

See *Nursing Considerations* for *Antihypertensive Agents* and individual agents.
**Administration/Storage**
1. Take with food.
2. Give the daily dose as a single dose or in divided doses.
3. More than 2 tablets/day are not usually necessary.
4. Maintenance therapy may be intermittent.
**Assessment**
1. Note indications for therapy and assess appropriate parameters.
2. Document age; obtain baseline electrolytes and renal function studies.
**Client/Family Teaching**
1. Take with food.
2. Give the daily dose as a single dose or in divided doses.
3. More than 2 tablets/day are not usually necessary.
4. Maintenance therapy may be intermittent.
**Outcomes/Evaluate**
• Control of hypertension
• Desired diuresis

**A**

# Amiloride hydrochloride
(ah-**MILL**-oh-ryd)
**Pregnancy Category:** B
Midamor **(Rx)**
**Classification:** Diuretic, potassium-sparing

**Action/Kinetics:** Amiloride acts on the distal tubule to inhibit N$^{a+}$, $^{K+}$-ATPase, thereby inhibiting sodium exchange for potassium; this results in increased secretion of sodium and water and conservation of potassium. In the proximal tubule, amiloride inhibits the N$^{a+}$/$^{H+}$ exchange mechanism. The drug also has weak diuretic and antihypertensive activity. **Onset:** 2 hr. **Peak effect:** 6–10 hr. **Peak plasma levels:** 3–4 hr. **Duration:** 24 hr. **t½:** 6–9 hr. Twenty-three percent is bound to plasma protein. Approximately 50% is excreted unchanged by kidney and 40% by the feces unchanged.

**Uses:** Adjunct with thiazides or loop diuretics in the treatment of hypertension or edema due to CHF, hepatic cirrhosis, and nephrotic syndrome to help restore normal serum potassium or prevent hypokalemia. Prophylaxis of hypokalemia in clients who would be at risk if hypokalemia developed (e.g., digitalized clients or clients with significant cardiac arrhythmias). *Investigational:* To reduce lithium-induced polyuria. Aerosolized amiloride may slow the progression of pulmonary function reduction in adults with cystic fibrosis.

**Contraindications:** Hyperkalemia (>5.5 mEq potassium/L). In clients receiving other potassium-sparing diuretics or potassium supplements. Impaired renal function. Diabetes mellitus. Use during lactation.

**Special Concerns:** Use with caution in metabolic or respiratory acidosis; during lactation. Geriatric clients may have a greater risk of developing hyperkalemia. Safety and efficacy have not been determined in children.

**Side Effects:** *Electrolyte:* Hyperkalemia, hyponatremia, and hypochloremia if used with other diuretics. *CNS:* Headache, dizziness, encephalopathy, tremors, paresthesias, mental confusion, insomnia, decreased libido, depression, sleepiness, vertigo, nervousness. *GI:* Nausea, anorexia, vomiting, diarrhea, changes in appetite, gas and abdominal pain, dry mouth, flatulence, abdominal fullness, GI bleeding, GI disturbance, thirst, dyspepsia, heartburn, jaundice, constipation, activation of preexisting peptic ulcer. *Respiratory:* Dyspnea, cough, SOB. *Musculoskeletal:* Weakness; muscle cramps; fatigue; joint, chest and back pain; neck or shoulder ache; pain in extremities. *GU:* Impotence, polyuria, dysuria, bladder spasms, urinary frequency. *CV:* Angina, palpitations, *arrhythmias,* orthostatic hypotension. *Hematologic:* **Aplastic anemia,** neutropenia. *Dermatologic:* Skin rash, itching, pruritus, alopecia. *Miscellaneous:* Visual disturbances, nasal congestion, tinnitus, increased intraocular pressure, abnormal liver function.

**OD** **Overdose Management:** *Symptoms:* Electrolyte imbalance, **dehydration.** *Treatment:* Induce emesis or gastric lavage. Treat hyperkalemia by IV sodium bicarbonate or oral or parenteral glucose with a rapid-acting insulin. Sodium polystyrene sulfonate, oral or by enema, may also be used.

**Drug Interactions**
*ACE inhibitors* / ↑ Risk of significant hyperkalemia
*Digoxin* / Possible ↑ renal clearance and ↓ nonrenal clearance of digoxin. Possible ↑ inotropic effect of digoxin
*Lithium* / ↓ Renal excretion of lithium → ↑ chance of toxicity
*NSAIDs* / ↓ Therapeutic effect of amiloride
*Potassium products* / Hyperkalemia with possibility of cardiac arrhythmias or cardiac arrest
*Spironolactone, Triamterene* / Hyperkalemia, hyponatremia, hypochloremia

**Dosage** ————————
• **Tablets**
   *As single agent or with other diuretics.*

**Adults, initial:** 5 mg/day; 10 mg/day may be necessary in some clients. Doses as high as 20 mg/day may be used, if needed, with careful monitoring of electrolytes.

*Reduce lithium-induced polyuria.* 10–20 mg/day.

*Slow progression of pulmonary function reduction in cystic fibrosis.*
**Adults:** Drug is dissolved in 0.3% saline and delivered by nebulizer.

## NURSING CONSIDERATIONS

See also *Nursing Considerations* for *Diuretics.*
**Assessment**
1. Monitor renal function studies, I&O, and weights.
2. Obtain serum electrolytes. Assess for hyperkalemia and for indications to withdraw drug; cardiac irregularities may be precipitated.
**Client/Family Teaching**
1. Administer with food to reduce chance of GI upset.
2. Avoid potassium supplementation or foods rich in potassium because drug does not promote potassium excretion. Do not take with other potassium-sparing diuretics.
**Outcomes/Evaluate**
• ↓ BP and enhanced diuresis
• Conservation of potassium
• ↓ Lithium-induced polyuria
• Maintenance of pulmonary function with cystic fibrosis

# Aminophylline
(am-in-**OFF**-ih-lin)
**Pregnancy Category:** C
Aminophyllin, Jaa Aminophylline ✸, Phyllocontin, Phyllocontin-350 ✸, Truphyllin **(Rx)**
**Classification:** Bronchodilator

See also *Theophylline Derivatives.*
**Action/Kinetics:** Aminophylline contains 79% theophylline.
**Additional Uses:** Neonatal apnea, respiratory stimulant in Cheyne-Stokes respiration. Parenteral form has been used for biliary colic and as a cardiac stimulant, a diuretic, and an adjunct in treating CHF, although

such uses have been replaced by more effective drugs.
**Special Concerns:** Use with caution when aminophylline and sodium chloride are used with corticosteroids or in clients with edema.
**Additional Side Effects:** The ethylenediamine in the product may cause exfoliative dermatitis or urticaria.

## Dosage
• **Oral Solution, Tablets**
*Bronchodilator, acute attacks, in clients not currently on theophylline therapy.*
**Adults and children up to 16 years of age, loading dose:** Equivalent of 5–6 mg of anhydrous theophylline/kg.
*Bronchodilator, acute attacks, in clients currently receiving theophylline.*
**Adults and children up to 16 years of age:** If possible, a serum theophylline level should be obtained first. Then, base loading dose on the premise that each 0.5 mg theophylline/kg lean body weight will result in a 0.5–1.6-mcg/mL increase in serum theophylline levels. If immediate therapy is needed and a serum level cannot be obtained, a single dose of the equivalent of 2.5 mg/kg of anhydrous theophylline can be given.
*Maintenance in acute attack, based on equivalent of anhydrous theophylline.*
**Young adult smokers:** 4 mg/kg q 6 hr; **healthy, nonsmoking adults:** 3 mg/kg q 8 hr; **geriatric clients or clients with cor pulmonale:** 2 mg/kg q 8 hr; **clients with CHF or liver failure:** 2 mg/kg q 8–12 hr. **Pediatric, 12–16 years:** 3 mg/kg q 6 hr; **9–12 years:** 4 mg/kg q 6 hr; **1–9 years:** 5 mg/kg q 6 hr; **6–12 months:** Use the formula: dose (mg/kg q 8 hr) = (0.05) (age in weeks) + 1.25; **up to 6 months:** Use the formula: dose (mg/kg q 8 hr) = (0.07) (age in weeks) + 1.7.
*Chronic therapy, based on equivalent of anhydrous theophylline.*

---

**A**

**Adults, initial:** 6–8 mg/kg up to a maximum of 400 mg/day in three to four divided doses at 6–8-hr intervals; **then,** dose can be increased in 25% increments at 2–3 day intervals up to a maximum of 13 mg/kg or 900 mg/day, whichever is less. **Pediatric, initial:** 16 mg/kg up to a maximum of 400 mg/day in three to four divided doses at 6–8 hr intervals; **then,** dose may be increased in 25% increments at 2–3 day intervals up to the following maximum doses (without measuring serum theophylline): **16 years and older:** 13 mg/kg or 900 mg/day, whichever is less; **12–16 years:** 18 mg/kg/day; **9–12 years:** 20 mg/kg/day; **1–9 years:** 24 mg/kg/day; **up to 12 months,** Use the following formula: dose (mg/kg/day) = (0.3) (age in weeks) + 8.0.

• **Enteric-Coated Tablets**

*Bronchodilator, chronic therapy, based on equivalent of anhydrous theophylline.*

**Adults, initial:** 6–8 mg/kg up to a maximum of 400 mg/day in three to four divided doses at 6–8-hr intervals; **then,** dose may be increased, if needed and tolerated, by increments of 25% at 2–3 day intervals up to a maximum of 13 mg/kg/day or 900 mg/day, whichever is less, without measuring serum theophylline. **Pediatric, over 12 years of age, initial:** 4 mg/kg q 8–12 hr; **then,** dose may be increased by 2–3 mg/kg/day at 3-day intervals up to the following maximum doses (without measuring serum levels): **16 years and older:** 13 mg/kg/day or 900 mg/day, whichever is less; **12–16 years:** 18 mg/kg/day.

• **Enema**

For use as a bronchodilator for loading doses and for maintenance in acute attacks, see doses for oral solution and tablets.

• **IV Infusion**

*Bronchodilator, acute attacks, for clients not currently on theophylline.*

**Adults and children up to 16 years, loading dose based on anhydrous theophylline:** 5 mg/kg given over a period of 20 min.

*Bronchodilator, acute attack, for clients currently on theophylline.*

**Adults and children up to 16 years, loading dose based on anhydrous theophylline:** If possible, a serum theophylline level should be obtained first. Then, base loading dose on the premise that each 0.5 mg theophylline/kg lean body weight will result in a 0.5–1.6 mcg/mL increase in serum theophylline levels. If immediate therapy is needed and a serum level cannot be obtained, a single dose of the equivalent of 2.5 mg/kg of anhydrous theophylline can be given.

*Maintenance for acute attacks, based on equivalent of anhydrous theophylline.*

**Young adult smokers:** 0.7 mg/kg/hr; **nonsmoking, healthy adults:** 0.43 mg/kg/hr; **geriatric clients or clients with cor pulmonale:** 0.26 mg/kg/hr; **clients with CHF or liver failure:** 0.2 mg/kg/hr. **Pediatric, 12–16 years, nonsmokers:** 0.5 mg/kg/hr; **9–12 years,** 0.7 mg/kg/hr; **1–9 years,** 0.8 mg/kg/hr; **up to 1 year,** Based on the following formula: dose (mg/kg/hr) = (0.008) (age in weeks) + 0.21.

## NURSING CONSIDERATIONS

See also *Nursing Considerations* for *Theophylline Derivatives.*

**Administration/Storage**

1. IM injection is not recommended due to severe, persistent pain at the site of injection.

2. Enteric-coated tablets may be incompletely and slowly absorbed.

3. Enteric-coated tablets are not recommended for children less than 12 years of age.

4. Use of aminophylline suppositories is not recommended due to the possibility of slow and unreliable absorption.

**IV** 5. To avoid hypotension, administer IV doses at a rate not to exceed 25 mg/min.

6. Only the 25 mg/mL injection (which should be further diluted) should be used for IV administration. Use an infusion pump or de-

vice to regulate infusion rates of IV solutions.

7. A minimum of 4–6 hr should elapse when switching from IV infusion to the first dose of PO therapy.

**Assessment**

1. Document indications for therapy, onset, duration, and characteristics of symptoms; note other therapies tried.

2. List medications currently prescribed to ensure that none interact unfavorably.

3. Perform baseline lung assessments and pulmonary function studies; note ABGs and ECG.

4. Monitor pulse and BP closely during IV administration. Aminophylline may cause a transitory lowering of the BP. If this occurs, adjust the dosage of drug and rate of flow.

5. Monitor clients with a history of CAD for chest pain and ECG changes.

6. Report serum levels greater than 20 mcg/mL or symptoms of toxicity.

**Client/Family Teaching**

1. Drug acts by relaxation of muscles of bronchi and pulmonary blood vessels to relieve bronchospasm.

2. Take with a snack or meal to prevent GI upset; avoid coffee, cola, and chocolate.

3. Instruct in pursed-lip and diaphragmatic breathing to help reduce the work of breathing by prolonging expiration and keeping the airways open longer.

4. Report symptoms of toxicity, i.e., N&V, restlessness, convulsions, and arrhythmias.

5. Initiate and stress the importance of smoking cessation with all clients that still smoke.

**Outcomes/Evaluate**

• Improved airway exchange
• ↓ SOB; relief of PND
• Termination of acute asthma attack
• Therapeutic serum drug levels (10–20 mcg/mL)

# Amiodarone hydrochloride

(am-ee-**OH**-dah-rohn)

**Pregnancy Category:** D

Cordarone, Cordarone I.V. ✹ **(Rx)**

**Classification:** Antiarrhythmic, class III

See also *Antiarrhythmic Agents*.

**Action/Kinetics:** The drug blocks sodium channels at rapid pacing frequencies, causing an increase in the duration of the myocardial cell action potential and refractory period, as well as alpha- and beta-adrenergic blockade. The drug decreases sinus rate, increases PR and QT intervals, results in development of U waves, and changes T-wave contour. After IV use, amiodarone relaxes vascular smooth muscle, reduces peripheral vascular resistance (afterload), and increases cardiac index slightly. No significant changes are seen in left ventricular ejection fraction after PO use. Absorption is slow and variable. **Maximum plasma levels:** 3–7 hr after a single dose. **Onset:** Several days up to 1–3 weeks. Drug may accumulate in the liver, lung, spleen, and adipose tissue. **Therapeutic serum levels:** 0.5–2.5 mcg/mL. **t½:** Biphasic: initial t½: 2.5–10 days; final t½: 26–107 days. Effects may persist for several weeks or months after therapy is terminated. Effective plasma concentrations are difficult to predict although concentrations below 1 mg/L are usually ineffective, whereas those above 2.5 mg/L are not necessary. Neither amiodarone nor its metabolite, desethylamiodarone, is dialyzable.

**Uses: Oral.** Use should be reserved for life-threatening ventricular arrhythmias unresponsive to other therapy, such as recurrent ventricular fibrillation and recurrent, hemodynamically unstable ventricular tachycardia.

**IV.** Initial treatment and prophylaxis of frequently recurring ventricular fibrillation and hemodynamically unstable ventricular tachycardia in clients refractory to other therapy. Ventricular tachycardia/ventricular fibrillation clients unable to take PO medication. *Investigational:* Refractory sustained or paroxysmal atrial fibrillation, paroxysmal SVT, symptomatic atrial flutter. Also, low doses in CHF with decreased LV ejection fraction, exercise tolerance and ventricular arrhythmias.

**Contraindications: Parenteral or PO use:** Marked sinus bradycardia due to severe sinus node dysfunction, second- or third-degree AV block, syncope caused by bradycardia (except when used with a pacemaker). Cardiogenic shock (parenteral use only). Lactation.

**Special Concerns:** Safety and effectiveness in children have not been determined. The drug may be more sensitive in geriatric clients, especially in thyroid dysfunction. Carefully monitor the IV product in geriatric clients and in those with severe left ventricular dysfunction.

**Side Effects:** Adverse reactions, some potentially fatal, are common with doses greater than 400 mg/day. *Pulmonary:* Pulmonary infiltrates or fibrosis, interstitial/alveolar pneumonitis, hypersensitivity pneumonitis, alveolitis, pulmonary inflammation or fibrosis, **ARDS (after parenteral use),** lung edema, cough and progressive dyspnea. Oral use may cause a clinical syndrome of cough and progressive dyspnea accompanied by functional, radiographic, gallium scan, and pathologic data indicating pulmonary toxicity. *CV:* **Worsening of arrhythmias, paroxysmal ventricular tachycardia,** proarrhythmias, symptomatic bradycardia, sinus arrest, SA node dysfunction, **CHF,** edema, hypotension (especially with IV use), **cardiac conduction abnormalities, coagulation abnormalities, cardiac arrest (after IV use).** IV use may result in atrial fibrillation, nodal arrhythmia, prolonged QT interval, and sinus bradycardia. *Hepatic:* Abnormal liver function tests, nonspecific hepatic disorders, cholestatic hepatitis, cirrhosis, hepatitis. *CNS:* Malaise, tremor, lack of coordi-

nation, fatigue, ataxia, paresthesias, peripheral neuropathy, abnormal involuntary movements, sleep disturbances, dizziness, insomnia, headache, decreased libido, abnormal gait. *GI:* N&V, constipation, anorexia, abdominal pain, abnormal taste and smell, abnormal salivation. *Ophthalmologic:* Ophthalmic abnormalities, including optic neuropathy and/or optic neuritis (may progress to permanent blindness). Papilledema, corneal degeneration, photosensitivity, eye discomfort, scotoma, lens opacities, macular degeneration. Corneal microdeposits (asymptomatic) in clients on therapy for 6 months or more, photophobia, dry eyes, visual disturbances, blurred vision, halos. *Dermatologic:* Photosensitivity, solar dermatitis, blue discoloration of skin, rash, alopecia, spontaneous ecchymosis, flushing. *Miscellaneous:* Hypothyroidism or hyperthyroidism, vasculitis, flushing, pseudotumor cerebri, epididymitis, thrombocytopenia, angioedema. IV use may cause abnormal kidney function, Stevens-Johnson syndrome, respiratory syndrome, and **shock.**

**OD Overdose Management:** *Symptoms:* Bradycardia, hypotension, **disorders of cardiac rhythm, cardiogenic shock,** AV block, hepatoxicity. *Treatment:* Use supporztive treatment. The cardiac rhythm and BP should be monitored. A beta-adrenergic agonist or a pacemaker is used to treat bradycardia; hypotension due to insufficient tissue perfusion is treated with a vasopressor or positive inotropic agents. There is some evidence that cholestyramine hastens the reversal of side effects by increasing elimination. Drug is not dialyzable.

**Drug Interactions**
*Anticoagulants* / ↑ Anticoagulant effect → bleeding disorders
*Beta-adrenergic blocking agents* / ↑ Chance of bradycardia and hypotension
*Calcium channel blockers* / ↑ Risk of AV block with verapamil or dil-

tiazem or hypotension with all calcium channel blockers

*Cholestyramine* / ↑ Elimination of amiodarone → ↓ serum levels and half-ife

*Cimetidine* / ↑ Serum levels of amiodarone

*Cyclosporine* / ↑ Levels of plasma cyclosporine → elevated creatinine levels (even with ↓ doses of cyclosporine)

*Dextromethorphan* / Chronic use of PO amiodarone (> 2 weeks) impairs metabolism of dextromethorphan

*Digoxin* / ↑ Serum digoxin levels → toxicity

*Disopyramide* / ↑ QT prolongation → possible arrhythmias

*Fentanyl* / Possibility of hypotension, bradycardia, ↓ CO

*Flecainide* / ↑ Plasma levels of flecainide

*Methotrexate* / Chronic use of PO amiodarone (> 2 weeks) impairs metabolism of methotrexate

*Procainamide* / ↑ Serum procainamide levels → toxicity

*Phenytoin* / ↑ Serum phenytoin levels → toxicity; also, ↓ levels of amiodarone

*Quinidine* / Serum quinidine toxicity, including fatal cardiac arrhythmias

*Ritonavir* / ↑ Levels of amiodarone → ↑ risk of amiodarone toxicity

*Theophylline* / ↑ Serum theophylline levels → toxicity (effects may not be seen for 1 week and may last for a prolonged period after drug is discontinued)

**Laboratory Test Interferences:** ↑ AST, ALT, GGT. Alteration of thyroid function tests ( ↑ serum $T_4$, ↓ serum $T_3$).

## Dosage

Due to the drug's side effects, unusual pharmacokinetic properties, and difficult dosing schedule, administer amiodarone in a hospital only by physicians trained in treating life-threatening arrhythmias. Loading doses are required to ensure a reasonable onset of action.

- **IV Infusion**
  *Life-threatening ventricular arrhythmias.*
**Loading dose, rapid:** 150 mg over the first 10 minutes (15 mg/min). **Then, slow loading dose:** 360 mg over the next 6 hr (1 mg/min). **Maintenance dose:** 540 mg over the remaining 18 hr (0.5 mg/min). After the first 24 hr, continue maintenance infusion rate of 0.5 mg/min (720 mg/24 hr). This may be continued with monitoring for 2 to 3 weeks.

Once arrhythmias have been suppressed, the client may be switched to PO amiodarone. The following is intended only as a guideline for PO amiodarone dosage after IV infusion. **IV infusion less than 1 week:** Initial daily dose of PO amiodarone, 800–1,600 mg. **IV infusion from 1 to 3 weeks:** Initial daily dose of PO amiodarone, 600–800 mg. **IV infusion longer than 3 weeks:** Initial daily dose of PO amiodarone, 400 mg.

- **Tablets**
  *Life-threatening ventricular arrhythmias.*
**Loading dose:** 800–1,600 mg/day for 1–3 weeks (or until initial response occurs); **then,** reduce dose to 600–800 mg/day for 1 month. **Maintenance dose:** 400 mg/day (as low as 200 mg/day or as high as 600 mg/day may be needed in some clients).

  *Refractory sustained or paroxysmal atrial fibrillation, paroxysmal SVT.*
**Initial:** 600–800 mg/day for 7 to 10 days; **then,** 200–400 mg/day.

  *LV ejection fraction, exercise tolerance, ventricular arrhythmias with CHF.*
200 mg/day.

## NURSING CONSIDERATIONS

See also *Nursing Considerations* for *Antiarrhythmic Agents*.
### Administration/Storage
1. Correct potassium or magnesium deficiencies before initiation of ther-

**A**

apy since antiarrhythmics may be ineffective or arrhythmogenic in those with hypokalemia.

2. When initiating amiodarone therapy, gradually discontinue other antiarrhythmic drugs.

3. To minimize side effects, determine the lowest effective dose. If side effects occur, reduce the dose.

4. If dosage adjustments are required, monitor the client for an extended period of time due to the long and variable half-life of the drug and the difficulty in predicting the time needed to achieve a new steady-state plasma drug level.

5. Administer daily PO doses of 1,000 mg or more in divided doses with meals.

6. If additional antiarrhythmic therapy is required, the initial dose of such drugs should be about one-half the usual recommended dose.

**IV** 7. For the first rapid loading dose, add 3 mL amiodarone IV (150 mg) to 100 mL D5W for a concentration of 1.5 mg/mL; infuse at a rate of 100 mL/10 min. For the slower loading dose, add 18 mL amiodarone IV (900 mg) to 500 mL of D5W for a concentration of 1.8 mg/mL.

8. IV concentrations of amiodarone greater than 3 mg/mL in D5W cause a high incidence of peripheral vein phlebitis; concentrations of 2.5 mg/mL or less are not as irritating. Thus, for infusions greater than 1 hr, the IV concentration should not exceed 2 mg/mL unless a central venous catheter is used.

9. Because amiodarone adsorbs to PVC, IV infusions exceeding 2 hr must be given in glass or polyolefin bottles containing D5W.

10. Amiodarone IV in D5W is incompatible with aminophylline, cefamandole nafate, cefazolin sodium, mezlocillin sodium, heparin sodium, and sodium bicarbonate.

11. The injection is stored at room temperature and protected from light.

**Assessment**

1. Determine if client is taking any other antiarrhythmic medications.

2. Assess quality of respirations and breath sounds; note cardiac status and CV findings.

3. Note baseline VS and perfusion (skin temperature, color). Document ABGs and assess for circulatory impairment and hypotension.

4. Assess vision before starting therapy.

5. Monitor thyroid studies because drug inhibits conversion of $T_4$ to $T_3$.

6. Determine that baseline CBC, electrolytes, CXR, and liver and renal function studies have been performed.

7. Obtain ECG and document rhythm strips; note EPS findings when available. During administration, observe ECG for increased PR and QRS intervals, increased arrhythmias, and HR below 60 beats/min.

8. Anticipate reduced dosages of digoxin, warfarin, quinidine, procainamide, and phenytoin if administered concomitantly with amiodarone.

**Client/Family Teaching**

1. Report if crystals develop on the skin, producing a bluish color, so dosage can be adjusted.

2. Avoid direct exposure to sunlight. Wear protective clothing, hat, sunglasses, and a sunscreen when exposed.

3. Report all side effects, especially any abnormal swelling, bleeding, or bruising.

4. Complaints of painful breathing, wheezing, fever, coughing, or dyspnea are all symptoms of pulmonary problems and require prompt attention.

5. CNS symptoms such as tremor, lack of coordination, paresthesias, and dizziness should be evaluated.

6. Complaints of headaches, depression, or insomnia as well as any change in behavior such as decreased interest in personal appearance or apparent hallucinations may require a change in drug therapy.

7. Schedule periodic ophthalmic examinations because small yellowbrown granular corneal deposits may develop during prolonged therapy. Visual changes require prompt ophthalmic evaluation.

8. Therapy with this medication requires frequent laboratory studies and close medical evaluation.
**Outcomes/Evaluate**
• Termination and control of life-threatening ventricular arrhythmias
• Serum drug levels within therapeutic range (0.5–2.5 mcg/mL)

―――――COMBINATION DRUG―――――
# Amitriptyline and Perphenazine
(ah-me-**TRIP**-tih-leen, per-**FEN**-ah-zeen)
Apo-Peram ✚, Elavil Plus ✚, Etrafon 2-10 ✚, Etrafon-A ✚, Etrafon-D ✚, Etrafon-F ✚, PMS-Levazine 2/25 ✚, PMS-Levazine 4/25 ✚, Proavil ✚, Triavil 2-10, 2-25, 4-10, 4-25, and 4-50 **(Rx)**
**Classification:** Antidepressant

**Content:** See also information on individual components.
*Antidepressant:* Amitriptyline HCl, 10, 25, or 50 mg. *Antipsychotic:* Perphenazine, 2 or 4 mg.

There are five different strengths of Triavil: Triavil 2–10, Triavil 2–25, Triavil 4–10, Triavil 4–25, and Triavil 4–50. *NOTE:* The first number refers to the number of milligrams of perphenazine and the second number refers to the number of milligrams of amitriptyline.
**Uses:** Depression with moderate to severe anxiety and/or agitation. Depression and anxiety in clients with chronic physical disease. Also schizophrenic clients with symptoms of depression.
**Contraindications:** Use during pregnancy. CNS depression due to drugs. In presence of bone marrow depression. Concomitant use with MAO inhibitors. During acute recovery phase from MI. Use in children.

**Dosage** ―――――――――――――
• **Tablets**
*Antidepressant.*
**Adults, initial:** One tablet of Triavil 2–25 or 4–25 t.i.d.–q.i.d. or 1 tablet of Triavil 4–50 b.i.d. Schizophrenic clients should receive an initial dose of

2 tablets of Triavil 4–50 t.i.d., with a fourth dose at bedtime, if necessary. Initial dosage for geriatric or adolescent clients in whom anxiety dominates is Triavil 4–10 t.i.d.–q.i.d., with dosage adjusted as required. **Maintenance:** One tablet Triavil 2–25 or 4–25 b.i.d.–q.i.d. or 1 tablet Triavil 4–50 b.i.d.

## NURSING CONSIDERATIONS

See also *Nursing Considerations* for *Antidepressants, Tricyclic,* and *Amitriptyline.*
**Administration/Storage**
1. Total daily dosage of Triavil should not exceed 4 of the 4–50 tablets or 8 tablets of all other dosage strengths.
2. The therapeutic effect may take up to several weeks to be manifested.
3. Once a satisfactory response has been observed, reduce the dose to the smallest amount required for relief of symptoms.
**Outcomes/Evaluate:** Relief of symptoms of depression and associated anxiety

# Amitriptyline hydrochloride
(ah-me-**TRIP**-tih-leen)
**Pregnancy Category:** C
Apo-Amitriptyline ✚, Elavil, Levate ✚ **(Rx)**, Novo-Tryptin ✚
**Classification:** Antidepressant, tricyclic

See also *Antidepressants, Tricyclic.*
**Action/Kinetics:** Amitriptyline is metabolized to an active metabolite, nortriptyline. Has significant anticholinergic and sedative effects with moderate orthostatic hypotension. Very high ability to block serotonin uptake and moderate activity with respect to norepinephrine uptake. **Effective plasma levels of amitriptyline and nortriptyline:** Approximately 110–250 ng/mL. **Time to reach steady state:** 4–10 days. **$t^{1/2}$:** 31–46 hr. Up to 1 month may be required for beneficial effects to be

manifested. Amitriptyline is also found in Limbitrol and Triavil.

**Uses:** Relief of symptoms of depression, including depression accompanied by anxiety and insomnia. Chronic pain due to cancer or other pain syndromes. Prophylaxis of cluster and migraine headaches. *Investigational:* Pathologic laughing and crying secondary to forebrain disease, bulimia nervosa, antiulcer agent, enuresis.

**Contraindications:** Use in children less than 12 years of age.

**Dosage** ————————
• **Tablets**
   *Antidepressant.*

**Adults (outpatients):** 75 mg/day in divided doses; may be increased to 150 mg/day. *Alternate dosage:* **Initial,** 50–100 mg at bedtime; **then,** increase by 25–50 mg, if necessary, up to 150 mg/day. **Hospitalized clients: initial,** 100 mg/day; may be increased to 200–300 mg/day. **Maintenance: usual,** 40–100 mg/day (may be given as a single dose at bedtime). **Adolescent and geriatric:** 10 mg t.i.d. and 20 mg at bedtime up to a maximum of 100 mg/day. **Pediatric, 6–12 years:** 10–30 mg (1–5 mg/kg) daily in two divided doses.
   *Chronic pain.*
   50–100 mg/day.
   *Enuresis.*

**Pediatric, over 6 years:** 10 mg/day as a single dose at bedtime; dose may be increased up to a maximum of 25 mg. **Less than 6 years:** 10 mg/day as a single dose at bedtime.
• **IM Only**
   *Antidepressant.*

**Adults:** 20–30 mg q.i.d.; switch to **PO** therapy as soon as possible.

## NURSING CONSIDERATIONS

See also *Nursing Considerations* for *Antidepressants, Tricyclic.*
**Administration/Storage**
1. Initiate increases in dosage in late afternoon or at bedtime.
2. Beneficial antidepressant effects may not be noted for 30 days.

3. Sedative effects may be manifested prior to antidepressant effects.
**Client/Family Teaching**
1. Take with food to minimize gastric upset.
2. Do not drive a car or operate hazardous machinery until drug effects realized; drug causes a high degree of sedation.
3. May take entire dose at bedtime if sedation is manifested during waking hours.
4. Rise slowly from a lying to a sitting position to reduce orthostatic drug effects.
5. Urine may appear blue-green in color; this is harmless.
**Outcomes/Evaluate**
• ↓ Symptoms of depression
• Control of incontinence
• Enhanced pain control with chronic pain management
• Relief of insomnia

# Amlexanox
(am-**LEX**-an-ox)
**Pregnancy Category:** B
Aphthasol **(Rx)**
**Classification:** Aphthous ulcer product.

**Action/Kinetics:** Mechanism not known. May be absorbed through GI tract.
**Uses:** Treat aphthous ulcers in those with normal immune systems.
**Special Concerns:** Use caution during lactation. Safety and efficacy in children have not been determined.
**Side Effects:** Transient pain, burning, or stinging at application site. Contact mucositis, nausea, diarrhea.

**Dosage** ————————
• **Paste**
   *Aphthous ulcers.*

Squeeze about 0.25 inch of paste onto fingertip and, with gentle pressure, dab onto each mouth ulcer. Apply following oral hygiene after breakfast, lunch, dinner, and at bedtime. Start as soon as possible after symptoms of aphthous ulcer noted and continue until ulcer heals.

## NURSING CONSIDERATIONS
### Administration/Storage
1. If significant healing has not occurred within 10 days, consult physician or dentist.
2. Wash hands immediately after applying paste.
### Client/Family Teaching
1. Apply paste as soon as ulcers appear; rinse mouth thoroughly and use after each meal and at bedtime.
2. Place a small amount of paste on fingertip and gently dab onto each oral ulcer.
3. Wash hands after applying; avoid contact with eyes and wash promptly if eye contact occurs.
4. Continue to apply paste until healing takes place. Report if pain or ulcers persist after 10 days.
**Outcomes/Evaluate:** Pain relief; ulcer healing

---

# Amlodipine
(am-**LOH**-dih-peen)
**Pregnancy Category:** C
Norvasc **(Rx)**
**Classification:** Antihypertensive, antianginal (calcium channel blocking agent)

---

See also *Calcium Channel Blocking Agents.*
**Action/Kinetics:** Amlodipine increases myocardial contractility although this effect may be counteracted by reflex activity. CO is increased and there is a pronounced decrease in peripheral vascular resistance. **Peak plasma levels:** 6–12 hr. **t½, elimination:** 30–50 hr. 90% metabolized in the liver to inactive metabolites; 10% excreted unchanged in the urine.
**Uses:** Hypertension alone or in combination with other antihypertensives. Chronic stable angina alone or in combination with other antianginal drugs. Confirmed or suspected Prinzmetal's or variant angina alone or in combination with other antianginal drugs.
**Special Concerns:** Use with caution in clients with CHF and in those with impaired hepatic function or reduced hepatic blood flow. Safety and efficacy have not been determined in children.
**Side Effects:** *CNS:* Headache, fatigue, lethargy, somnolence, dizziness, lightheadedness, sleep disturbances, depression, amnesia, psychosis, hallucinations, paresthesia, asthenia, insomnia, abnormal dreams, malaise, anxiety, tremor, hand tremor, hypoesthesia, vertigo, depersonalization, migraine, apathy, agitation, amnesia. *GI:* Nausea, abdominal discomfort, cramps, dyspepsia, diarrhea, constipation, vomiting, dry mouth, thirst, flatulence, dysphagia, loose stools. *CV:* Peripheral edema, palpitations, hypotension, syncope, bradycardia, unspecified arrhythmias, tachycardia, ventricular extrasystoles, peripheral ischemia, ***cardiac failure,*** pulse irregularity, increased risk of MI. *Dermatologic:* Dermatitis, rash, pruritus, urticaria, photosensitivity, petechiae, ecchymosis, purpura, bruising, hematoma, cold/clammy skin, skin discoloration, dry skin. *Musculoskeletal:* Muscle cramps, pain, or inflammation; joint stiffness or pain, arthritis, twitching, ataxia, hypertonia. *GU:* Polyuria, dysuria, urinary frequency, nocturia, sexual difficulties. *Respiratory:* Nasal or chest congestion, sinusitis, rhinitis, SOB, dyspnea, wheezing, cough, chest pain. *Ophthalmologic:* Diplopia, abnormal vision, conjunctivitis, eye pain, abnormal visual accommodation, xerophthalmia. *Miscellaneous:* Tinnitus, flushing, sweating, weight gain, epistaxis, anorexia, increased appetite, taste perversion, parosmia.

## Dosage
- **Tablets**
  *Hypertension.*
**Adults, usual, individualized:** 5 mg/day, up to a maximum of 10 mg/day. Titrate the dose over 7–14 days.
  *Chronic stable or vasospastic angina.*

---

★ = Available in Canada          ***bold italic*** = life threatening side effect

**Adults:** 5–10 mg, using the lower dose for elderly clients and those with hepatic insufficiency. Most clients require 10 mg.

## NURSING CONSIDERATIONS

See also *Nursing Considerations* for *Calcium Channel Blocking Agents.*

**Administration/Storage**

1. Food does not affect the bioavailability of amlodipine. Thus, may be taken without regard to meals.

2. Elderly clients, small/fragile clients, or those with hepatic insufficiency may be started on 2.5 mg/day. This dose may also be used when adding amlodipine to other antihypertensive therapy.

**Assessment**

1. Note any history of CAD or CHF.

2. Review list of drugs currently prescribed to prevent any unfavorable interactions.

3. Document baseline VS, ECG, CBC, and liver and renal function studies and monitor. Reduce dose with cirrhosis.

**Client/Family Teaching**

1. Take only as directed, once daily.

2. Report any symptoms of chest pain, SOB, dizziness, swelling of extremities, irregular pulse, or altered vision immediately.

**Outcomes/Evaluate**

- Desired BP control
- ↓ Frequency and intensity of anginal episodes

————COMBINATION DRUG————

# Amlodipine and Benazepril hydrochloride

(am-**LOH**-dih-peen, beh-**NAYZ**-eh- prill)

**Pregnancy Category:** C (first trimester), D (second and third trimesters)

Lotrel **(Rx)**

**Classification:** Antihypertensive

See also *Amlodipine,* and *Benazepril hydrochloride.*

**Content:** Lotrel 2.5/10: *Calcium channel blocking agent:* Amlodipine, 2.5 mg. *ACE inhibitor:* Benazepril hydrochloride, 10 mg. Lotrel 5/10 and Lotrel 5/20 contain 5 mg of amlodipine and either 10 or 20 mg of benazepril hydrochloride.

**Action/Kinetics:** The incidence of edema is significantly reduced with this combination product. **Peak plasma levels, benazepril:** 0.5–2 hr (1.5–4 hr for benazeprilat, the active metabolite). **Peak plasma levels, amlodipine:** 6–12 hr. **Elimination t½, benazeprilat:** 10–11 hr; **elimination t½, amlodipine:** 2 days.

**Uses:** Treatment of hypertension. Therapy with this combination is suggested when the client either has failed to achieve the desired antihypertensive effect with either drug alone or has demonstrated inability to achieve an adequate antihypertensive effect with amlodipine without developing edema.

**Contraindications:** Initial treatment of hypertension. Hypersensitivity to amlodipine or benazepril. Lactation.

**Special Concerns:** Discontinue ACE inhibitors as soon as pregnancy is determined. The addition of benazepril to amlodipine should not be expected to provide additional antihypertensive effects in African-Americans, although there will be less edema. Use with caution in those with severe renal disease, in CHF, and in severe hepatic impairment. Safety and efficacy have not been determined in children.

**Side Effects:** See individual drugs. Side effects include angioedema, cough, headache, and edema.

**Dosage**

- **Capsules**

  *Hypertension.*

One 2.5/10 mg, 5/10 mg, or 5/20 mg capsule once daily. In those with severe renal impairment, the recommended initial dose of benazepril is 5 mg (Lotrel is not recommended in these clients). In small, elderly, frail, or hepatically impaired clients, the recommended initial dose of amlodipine (either as monotherapy or in combination) is 2.5 mg.

## NURSING CONSIDERATIONS

See also *Nursing Considerations* for *Antihypertensive Agents, Amlodipine,* and *Benazepril hydrochloride.*

**Assessment**

1. Document indications for therapy, onset, duration of symptoms, and other agents trialed.

2. Obtain baseline ECG, electrolytes, and liver and renal function studies and monitor. Anticipate reduced dosage with organ impairment and with the frail, elderly client.

**Client/Family Teaching**

1. Take exactly as directed, at the same time each day.

2. Review importance of regular exercise, diet, rest, and stress reduction in the overall control of high BP.

3. Avoid alcohol and tobacco use; attend counseling.

4. Practice reliable contraception; stop drug and notify provider if pregnancy is suspected.

5. Report any persistent headaches, cough, or swelling of the extremities.

6. Maintain a record of BP recordings and bring to each provider visit.

**Outcomes/Evaluate:** Desired BP control

---

# Amoxapine

(ah-**MOX**-ah-peen)
**Pregnancy Category:** C
Asendin **(Rx)**
**Classification:** Antidepressant, tricyclic

See also *Antidepressants, Tricyclic.*

**Action/Kinetics:** In addition to its effect on monoamines, this drug also blocks dopamine receptors. Significant anticholinergic effects, moderate sedation, and slight orthostatic hypotensive effect. Metabolized to the active metabolites 7-hydroxy- and 8-hydroxyamoxapine. **Peak blood levels:** 90 min. **Effective plasma levels:** 200–500 ng/mL. **Time to reach steady state:** 2–7

days. **t½:** 8 hr; t½ of major metabolite: 30 hr. Excreted in urine.

**Uses:** Endogenous and reactive depression. Antianxiety agent.

**Contraindications:** Avoid high dose levels in clients with a history of convulsive seizures. During acute recovery period after MI.

**Special Concerns:** Safe use in children under 16 years of age and during lactation not established.

**Additional Side Effects:** Tardive dyskinesia. *Overdosage may cause seizures (common), neuroleptic malignant syndrome,* testicular swelling, impairment of sexual function, and breast enlargement in males and females. Also, renal failure may be seen 2–5 days after overdosage.

**Dosage** ———————
• **Tablets**
  *Antidepressant.*
**Adults, individualized, initial:** 50 mg t.i.d. Can be increased to 100 mg t.i.d. during first week. Do not use doses greater than 300 mg/day unless this dose has been ineffective for at least 14 days. **Maintenance:** 300 mg as a single dose at bedtime. **Hospitalized clients:** Up to 150 mg q.i.d. **Geriatric, initial:** 25 mg b.i.d.–t.i.d. If necessary, increase to 50 mg b.i.d.–t.i.d. after first week. **Maintenance:** Up to 300 mg/day at bedtime.

---

## NURSING CONSIDERATIONS

See also *Nursing Considerations* for *Antidepressants, Tricyclic.*

**Client/Family Teaching**

1. Take with food to minimize gastric upset.

2. Administer entire dose at bedtime if daytime sedation experienced.

3. Report early CNS manifestations of tardive dyskinesia, i.e., slow repetitive movements.

4. Report any side effects R/T overdosage, especially seizures, that require immediate medical care.

**Outcomes/Evaluate**
• Improved coping mechanisms

---

A

• Control of depression; ↓ anxiety levels

# Amoxicillin (amoxycillin)
(ah-mox-ih-**SILL**-in)
Amox ✱, Amoxil, Amoxil Pediatric Drops, Apo-Amoxi ✱, Biomox, Nova-moxin ✱, Nu-Amoxi ✱, Polymox, Polymox Drops, Pro-Amox ✱, Trimox 125, 250, and 500, Wymox **(Rx)**

*NOTE:* Canadian products are all amoxicillin trihydrate.
**Classification:** Antibiotic, penicillin

See also *Anti-Infectives* and *Penicillins.*

**Action/Kinetics:** Semisynthetic broad-spectrum penicillin closely related to ampicillin. Destroyed by penicillinase, acid stable, and better absorbed than ampicillin. From 50% to 80% of a PO dose is absorbed from the GI tract. **Peak serum levels: PO:** 4–11 mcg/mL after 1–2 hr. t½: 60 min. Mostly excreted unchanged in urine.

**Uses:** Gram-positive streptococcal infections including *Streptococcus faecalis, S. pneumoniae,* and non-penicillinase-producing staphylococci. Gram-negative infections due to *Hemophilus influenzae, Proteus mirabilis, Escherichia coli,* and Neisseria gonorrhoeae.

**Special Concerns:** Safe use during pregnancy has not been established.

## Dosage
• **Capsules, Oral Suspension, Chewable Tablets**

*Susceptible infections of ear, nose, throat, GU tract, skin and soft tissues, lower respiratory tract.*
**Adults:** 250–500 mg q 8 hr; **pediatric under 20 kg:** 20–40 (or more) mg/kg/day in three equal doses. The pediatric dose should not exceed the maximum adult dose.

*Prophylaxis of bacterial endocarditis.*
3 g 60 min prior to procedure (dental, oral, or upper respiratory tract) and 1.5 g 6 hr later. Alternatively, ampicillin, 1–2 g (50 mg/kg for children) plus gentamicin, 1.5 mg/kg (2 mg/kg for children) not to exceed 80 mg, both either IM or IV 30 min before procedure followed by amoxicillin, 1.5 g (25 mg/kg for children) 6 hr after initial dose. Amoxicillin may be given as an alternate procedure for GU or GI procedures at a dose of 3 g 1 hr before procedure followed by 1.5 g 6 hr after the initial dose.

*Gonococcal infections.*
3 g with probenecid, 1 g, given as a single dose. In addition, tetracycline, 0.5 mg, q.i.d. for 7 days.

*Gonococcal infection in pregnancy.*
3 g with probenecid, 1 g, given as a single dose. In addition, erythromycin base, 0.5 g q.i.d. for 7 days.

*Disseminated gonococcal infections.*
3 g with probenecid, 1 g, given as a single dose; **then,** 0.5 g q.i.d. for 7 days.

*Acute pelvic inflammatory disease.*
3 g with probenecid, 1 g, given as a single dose. In addition, doxycycline, 100 mg b.i.d. for 10–14 days.

*Sexually transmitted epididymoorchitis.*
3 g with probenecid, 1 g, given as a single dose. In addition, tetracycline, 0.5 g q.i.d. for 10 days.

*Bacterial vaginosis.*
0.5 g q.i.d. for 7 days.

*Chlamydia trachomatis during pregnancy (as an alternative to erythromycin).*
0.5 g t.i.d. for 7 days.

## NURSING CONSIDERATIONS

See also *Nursing Considerations* for *Penicillins.*
**Administration/Storage**
1. Dry powder is stable at room temperature for 18–30 months. Reconstituted suspension is stable for 1 week at room temperature and for 2 weeks at 2°C–8°C (36°F–46°F).
2. Chewable tablets are available for pediatric use. These may be administered with food.
**Client/Family Teaching**
1. Take entire prescription; do not stop when feeling "better" as this creates antibiotic resistance.

2. With school-age child space medication evenly over the 24-hr period. Give suspension or tablet before school, upon arrival home, and at bedtime.

3. Report any unusual rash or lack of response.

**Outcomes/Evaluate**

• Resolution of infection; symptomatic inprovement

• Therapeutic peak serum drug levels (4–11 mcg/mL)

————COMBINATION DRUG————

# Amoxicillin and Potassium clavulanate

(ah-mox-ih-**SILL**-in, poh-**TASS**-ee-um klav-you-**LAN**-ayt)
**Pregnancy Category:** B
Augmentin **(Rx)**
**Classification:** Antibiotic, penicillin

See also *Anti-Infectives* and *Penicillins.*

**Content:** Each '250' Tablet contains: 250 mg amoxicillin and 125 mg potassium clavulanate. Each '500' Tablet contains 500 mg amoxicillin and 125 mg potassium clavulanate.

Each "875" tablet contains: 875 mg amoxicillin, 125 mg potassium clavulanate

Each '125' Chewable Tablet contains 125 mg amoxicillin and 31.25 mg potassium clavulanate. Each 200 Chewable Tablet contains 200 mg amoxicillin and 28.5 mg clavulanate. Each '250' Chewable Tablet contains 250 mg amoxicillin and 62.5 mg potassium clavulanate.

Each 400 Chewable Tablet contains 400 mg amoxicillin and 57 mg potassium clavulanate.

Each 5 mL of the '125' Powder for Oral Suspension contains 125 mg amoxicillin and 31.25 mg potassium clavulanate. Each 5 mL of the 200 Powder for Oral Suspension contains 200 mg amoxicillin and 28.5 mg potassium clavulanate. Each 5 mL of the '250' Powder for Oral Suspension contains 250 mg amoxicillin and 62.5 mg potassium clavulanate.

Each 5 mL of the 400 Powder or the 400 Powder for Oral Suspension contains 400 mg amoxicillin and 57 mg potassium clavulanate.

**Action/Kinetics:** *For details, see amoxicillin.* Potassium clavulanate inactivates lactamase enzymes, which are responsible for resistance to penicillins. Thus, is effective against microorganisms that have manifested resistance to amoxicillin. For potassium clavulanate: **Peak serum levels:** 1–2 hr. **t½:** 1 hr.

**Uses:** For beta-lactamase-producing strains of the following organisms: *Hemophilus influenzae* and *Moraxella catarrhalis* causing lower respiratory tract infections, otitis media, and sinusitis; *Staphylococcus aureus, Escherichia coli,* and *Klebsiella,* causing skin and skin structure infections; *E. coli, Klebsiella,* and *Enterobacter,* causing UTI. *Note:* Mixed infections caused by organisms susceptible to ampicillin and organisms susceptible to amoxicillin/potassium clavulanate should not require an additional antibiotic.

**Dosage** ————

• **Oral Suspension, Chewable Tablets, Tablets**
*Susceptible infections.*
**Adults, usual:** One 500-mg tablet q 12 hr or one 250-mg tablet q 8 hr. Adults unable to take tablets can be given the 125-mg/5 mL or the 250-mg/5 mL suspension in place of the 500-mg tablet or the 200-mg/5 mL or 400-mg/5 mL suspension can be given in place of the 875-mg tablet. **Children less than 3 months old:** 30 mg/kg/day amoxicillin in divided doses q 12 hr. Use of the 125-mg/5 mL suspension is recommended. **Children over 3 months old:** 25 mg/kg/day in divided doses q 12 hr or 20 mg/kg/day in divided doses q 8 hr.
*Respiratory tract and severe infections.*
**Adults:** One 875-mg tablet q 12 hr or one 500-mg tablet q 8 hr. **Children over 3 months old:** 45 mg/kg/day of

amoxicillin in divided doses q 12 hr or 40 mg/kg/day in divided doses q 8 hr (these doses are used in children for otitis media, lower respiratory tract infections, or sinusitis). Treatment duration for otitis media is 10 days.

*Chancroid* (Haemophilus ducreyi infection).

**Adults:** One 500-mg tablet t.i.d. for 7 days (alternative to erythromycin or ceftriaxone).

*Disseminated gonococcal infections.*

Following therapy with an appropriate cephalosporin, (ceftriaxone, ceftizoxime, or cefotaxime) uncomplicated disease therapy may be completed with one 500-mg tablet t.i.d. for 1 week.

## NURSING CONSIDERATIONS

See also *Nursing Considerations* for *Penicillins.*

**Administration/Storage**

1. Both the "250" and "500" tablets contain 125 mg clavulanic acid; therefore, two "250" tablets are not the same as one "500" tablet. Also, the 250-mg tablet and the 250-mg chewable tablet do not contain the same amount of potassium clavulanate and are thus not interchangeable. The 250-mg tablet should not be used until children are over 40 kg.

2. This combination may be taken without regard for meals; however, absorption of clavulanate potassium is enhanced if taken at the beginning of a meal.

3. The reconstituted suspension should be refrigerated and discarded after 10 days.

4. Pediatric formulations are now available in fruit flavors for the oral suspension and chewable tablets. These formulations allow twice-daily dosing, which is more convenient than three-times daily dosing and, importantly, the incidence of diarrhea is significantly reduced.

5. The 200- and 400-mg suspensions and chewable tablets contain aspartame and should not be used by phenylketonurics.

**Client/Family Teaching**

1. Take exactly as directed and complete entire prescription.

2. Report any rash, persistent diarrhea, lack of response or worsening of symptoms after 48–72 hr of therapy.

3. Return as scheduled for follow-up evaluation.

**Outcomes/Evaluate:** Resolution of infection; symptomatic improvement

# Amphetamine sulfate

(am-**FET**-ah-meen)

**Pregnancy Category:** C

Dexedrine ✱ **(C-II) (Rx)**

**Classification:** CNS stimulant

See also *Amphetamines and Derivatives.*

**Action/Kinetics:** After PO, completely absorbed in 3 hr. **Duration: PO,** 4–24 hr; **t½:** 10–30 hr, depending on urinary pH. Excreted in urine. Acidification increases excretion, whereas alkalinization decreases it. For every one unit increase in pH, the plasma half-life will increase by 7 hr.

**Uses:** Attention deficit disorders in children, narcolepsy. A product containing dextroamphetamine sulfate, dextroamphetamine saccharate, amphetamine sulfate, and amphetamine aspartate is available for use in children aged three years and older who have attention deficit disorder with hyperactivity or narcolepsy.

**Special Concerns:** Use in children less than 3 years of age for attention deficit disorders and in children less than 6 years of age for narcolepsy. Not recommended as an appetite suppressant.

**Dosage**

• **Tablets**

*Narcolepsy.*

**Adults:** 5–20 mg 1–3 times/day. **Children over 12 years, initial:** 5 mg b.i.d.; increase in increments of 10 mg/day at weekly intervals until optimum dose is reached. **Children, 6–12 years, initial:** 2.5 mg b.i.d.; increase in increments of 5 mg at weekly intervals until optimum dose is reached (maximum is 60 mg/day).

*Attention deficit disorders in children.*
**3–6 years, initial:** 2.5 mg/day; increase by 2.5 mg/day at weekly intervals until optimum dose is achieved (usual range 0.1–0.5 mg/kg/dose each morning). **6 years and older, initial:** 5 mg 1–2 times/day; increase in increments of 5 mg/week until optimum dose is achieved (rarely over 40 mg/day).

## NURSING CONSIDERATIONS

See also *Nursing Considerations* for *Amphetamines and Derivatives.*
**Administration/Storage:** The peak effects of the drug are observed 2–3 hr after administration. The effects last from 4 to 24 hr.
**Assessment**
1. Review CNS/neurologic status prior to initiating therapy.
2. Document type and onset of symptoms and pretreatment physical assessment data.
3. Determine if pregnant.
4. Obtain and assess baseline weight, CBC, chemistry profile, urinalysis, and ECG.
**Client/Family Teaching**
1. When used for attention deficit disorders or narcolepsy, give the first dose on awakening with an additional one or two doses given at intervals of 4–6 hr. Give the last dose 6 hr before bedtime.
2. Report any changes in mood or affect, including symptoms of impaired mental processes.
3. Do not use caffeine or caffeine-containing products. Avoid any OTC preparations that contain caffeine, phenylpropanolamine, or other agents that affect the CV system; check if unsure.
4. Avoid using heavy machinery or driving a car until drug effects evaluated.
5. Monitor weight and maintain a graph to share at each visit.
6. Drink at least 2.5 L/day of fluids and increase intake of high-fiber foods and fruits to prevent constipation.

7. Chew sugarless gum or candies and rinse the mouth frequently with nonalcoholic mouth rinses to offset dry mouth.
8. Children receiving amphetamines may have their growth retarded. Drug should periodically be discontinued by provider to allow growth to proceed normally and to evaluate the need for continued drug therapy.
**Outcomes/Evaluate**
• Improved attention span
• ↓ Episodes of narcolepsy

# Amphotericin B (Deoxycholate)
(am-foe-**TER**-ih-sin)
**Pregnancy Category:** B
Amphotec, Fungizone ✲, Fungizone Intravenous **(Rx)**

# Amphotericin B Lipid Complex (Amphotericin B Cholesteryl Sulfate Complex)
(am-foe-**TER**-ih-sin)
**Pregnancy Category:** B
Abelcet, AmBisome, Amphotec **(Rx)**
**Classification:** Antibiotic, antifungal

See also *Anti-Infectives.*
**Action/Kinetics:** This antibiotic is produced by *Streptomyces nodosus;* it is fungistatic or fungicidal depending on the concentration of the drug in body fluids and the susceptibility of the fungus. Amphotericin B binds to specific chemical structures—sterols—of the fungal cellular membrane, increasing cellular permeability and promoting loss of potassium and other substances. Liposomal encapsulation or incorporation in a lipid complex can significantly affect the functional properties of the drug compared with those of the unencapsulated or non-lipid-associated drug. The liposomal amphotericin B product causes less nephrotoxicity. Amphotericin B is used either IV or topically. It is highly bound to serum protein (90%) **Peak plasma levels:**

0.5–2 mcg/mL. t½, **initial:** 24 hr; **second phase:** 15 days. Slowly excreted by kidneys.The kinetics of the drug differ in adults and children.

**Uses:** The drug is toxic and should be used only for clients under close medical supervision with progressive or potentially fatal fungal infections. *Systemic: Amphotericin B deoxycholate:* Disseminated North American blastomycosis, cryptococcosis, and other systemic fungal infections, including coccidioidomycosis, histoplasmosis, mucormycosis, sporotrichosis, aspergillosis, disseminated candidiasis, and monilial overgrowth resulting from oral antibiotic therapy. Secondary therapy to treat American mucocutaneous leishmaniasis. *Liposomal Amphotericin B:* Aspergillosis in clients refractory to or intolerant of conventional amphotericin B therapy. *Investigational:* Prophylaxis of fungal infections in clients with bone marrow transplantation. *Topical:* Cutaneous and mucocutaneous infections of *Candida (Monilia)* infections, especially in children, adults, and AIDS clients with thrush.

**Contraindications:** Hypersensitivity to drug unless the condition is life-threatening and amenable only to amphotericin B therapy. Use to treat common forms of fungal diseases showing only positive skin or serologic tests. Use to treat noninvasive forms of fungal disease such as oral thrush, vaginal candidiasis, and esophageal candidiasis in clients with normal neutrophil counts. Lactation.

**Special Concerns:** The bone marrow depressant effects may result in increased incidence of microbial infection, delayed healing, and gingival bleeding. Although used in children, safety and efficacy have not been determined. Use with caution in clients receiving leukocyte transfusions.

**Side Effects: After topical use.** Irritation, pruritus, dry skin. Redness, itching, or burning especially in skin folds. **After IV use.** A*cute reactions occurring 1 to 3 hr after starting IV infusion:* Fever, hypotension, shaking chills, hypotension, anorexia, N&V, headache, tachypnea. Rapid infusion may cause hypotension, hypokalemia, arrhythmias, and **shock.** *GI:* N&V, diarrhea, dyspepsia, stomatitis, anorexia, abdominal cramps, epigastric pain, melena; rarely, GI disorder, *GI hemorrhage,* hematemesis, dyspepsia, enlarged abdomen, hepatomegaly, cholangitis, cholecystitis, hemorrhagic gastroenteritis, acute liver failure, hepatitis, jaundice, veno-occlusive liver disease, hepatic failure. *CNS:* Fever, chills, headache, depressoin, abnormal thinking, malaise, vertigo, leukoencephalopathy; rarely, dizziness, somnolence, agitation, stupor, tremor, anxiety, paresthesia, hallucinations, *seizures,* encephalopathy, extrapyramidal symptoms, peripheral neuropathy, and other neurologic symptoms. *Respiratory:* Respiratory disorder, pneumonia, *respiratory failure.* Acute dyspnea, hypoxia, epistaxis, increased cough, lung disorder, hemoptysis, hyperventilation, hypersensitivity pneumonitis, apnea. Interstitial infiltrates seen in neutropenic clients receiving amphotericin B and leukocyte transfusions. *CV:* Thrombophlebitis, hypotension, hypertension, tachycardia, tachypnea, phlebitis. Rarely, arrhythmias, phlebitis, syncope, ventricular extrasystoles, postural hypotension, supraventricular tachycardia, thrombophlebitis, pleural effusion, hemoptysis, atrial fibrillation, bradycardia, CHF, *ventricular fibrillation, cardiac arrest, cardiac failure, shock, hemorrhage, pulmonary embolus, MI, cardiomyopathy.* *Renal:* Renal damage (including tubular dysfunction), azotemia, hyposthenuria, nephrocalcinosis, renal tubular acidosis, *kidney failure;* rarely, acute renal failure, decreased renal function, anuria, oliguria, hematuria, dysuria, infection. *Hematologic:* Normochromic, normocytic anemia; anemia, coagulation disorder. Rarely, *coagulation defects,* thrombocytopenia, leukopenia, agranulocytosis, eosinophilia, leukocytosis, hypochromic anemia, blood dyscrasias.

*Dermatologic:* Maculopapular rash, pruritus, rash; rarely, exfoliative dermatitis, erythema multiforme, skin disorder. *Hypersensitivity:* Rarely, **bronchospasm, asthma, anaphylactoid reactions,** wheezing. *Ophthalmic/Otic:* Rarely, tinnitus, hearing loss, blurred vision, eye hemorrhage, diplopia, impaired vision. *At injection site:* Venous pain with phlebitis and thrombophlebitis. *Miscellaneous:* Muscle and joint pain, weight loss, infection, sweating, pain, chest pain, back pain, **multiple organ failure, sepsis,** face edema, asthenia, peripheral edema, mucous membrane disorder; rarely, flushing, impotence, myasthenia, arthralgia, myalgia, **After intrathecal use:** Blurred vision, changes in vision, difficulty in urination, numbness, tingling, pain, or weakness.

**Drug Interactions**

*Aminoglycosides* / Additive nephrotoxicity and/or ototoxicity

*Antineoplastic drugs* / ↑ Risk for renal toxicity, bronchospasm, and hypotension

*Corticosteroids, Corticotropin* / ↑ Potassium depletion caused by amphotericin B → cardiac dysfunction

*Cyclosporine* / ↑ Serum creatinine levels

*Digitalis glycosides* / ↑ Potassium depletion caused by amphotericin B → ↑ incidence of digitalis toxicity

*Flucytosine* / ↑ Risk of flucytosine toxicity due to ↑ cellular uptake or ↓ renal excretion

*Nephrotoxic drugs* / ↑ Risk of nephrotoxicity

*Skeletal muscle relaxants, surgical* (e.g., succinylcholine, *d*-tubocurarine) / ↑ Muscle relaxation due to amphotericin B–induced hypokalemia

*Tacrolimus* / ↑ Serum creatinine levels

*Thiazides* / ↑ Electrolyte depletion, especially potassium

*AZT* / ↑ Risk of myelotoxicity and nephrotoxicity

**Laboratory Test Interferences:** ↑ AST, ALT, GGT, LDH, alkaline phosphatase, serum creatinine, BUN, bilirubin, BSP retention values, PT. Hypomagnesemia, hyperkalemia, hypocalcemia, hypercalemia, acidosis, hypoglycemia, hyperglycemia, hypermyalesmia, hyperuricemia, hypophosphatemia.

**Dosage**

• **Amphotericin B deoxycholate, IV**

*Test dose by slow IV infusion.*

1 mg in 20 mL of 5% dextrose injection should be infused over 20 to 30 min to determine tolerance.

*Severe and rapidly progressing fungal infection.*

**Initial:** 0.3 mg/kg over 2 to 6 hr. *Note:* In impaired cardiorenal function or if a severe reaction to the test dose, therapy should be initiated with smaller daily doses (e.g., 5–10 mg). Depending on the status of the client, the dose may be increased gradually by 5–10 mg/day to a final daily dose of 0.5–0.7 mg/kg. The total daily dose should not exceed 1.5 mg/kg.

*Sporotrichosis.*

20 mg/injection. Therapy may be required for up to 9 months.

*Aspergillosis.*

Total dose of 3.6 g or less per day for 11 months or less.

*Rhinocerebral phycomyosis.*

A cumulative dose of 3 g/day.

*Prophylaxis of fungal infections in bone marrow transplants.*

0.1 mg/kg/day.

• **Amphotericin B Deoxycholate Suspension**

*Oral candidiasis.*

Swish the suspension in the mouth and then swallow.

• **Liposomal Amphotericin B**

*All uses.*

**Adults and children, initial:** 3–4 mg/kg/day, as required. May be increased to 6 mg/kg/day if there is no improvement or if the fungal infection has progressed.

*Aspergillosis.*
**Adults and children:** 5 mg/kg/day as a single infusion.

- **Intrathecal, Intraventricular**
  *Fungal meningitis.*
  **Initial:** 0.1 mg; **then,** increase gradually up to 0.5 mg q 48 to 72 hr.
- **Bladder Irritation**
  *Candidal cystitis.*
  5–15 mg/dL instilled periodically or continuously for 5 to 10 days.
- **Topical (Lotion, Cream, Ointment—Each 3%)**
  Apply liberally to affected areas b.i.d.–q.i.d. Depending on the type of lesion, up to 4 weeks of therapy may be necessary.

## NURSING CONSIDERATIONS

See also *General Nursing Considerations For All Anti-Infectives.*
### Administration/Storage
1. Rub creams and lotions into lesion.
2. The cream may cause drying and slight skin discoloration; the lotion and ointment may cause staining of nail lesions, but not skin.
**IV** 3. *Preparation of amphotericin B deoxycholate:* To obtain an initial concentration of 5 mg/mL, rapidly inject 10 mL sterile water for injection (without a bacteriostatic agent) directly into the lyophilized cake, using a sterile 20-gauge needle. The vial should be shaken immediately until the colloidal solution is clear. To obtain the infusion solution of 0.1 mg/mL, further dilute 1:50 with 5% dextrose injection with a pH of 4.2 or above.
4. *Preparation of liposomal amphotericin B:* Shake the vial gently until there is no yellow sediment at the bottom. The appropriate dose is withdrawn from the required number of vials into one or more sterile 20-mL syringes using an 18-gauge needle. The needle is then removed from each syringe filled with liposomal amphotericin B and replaced with a 5-micron filter needle. Each filter needle is used for just one vial. Insert the filter needle on the syringe into an IV bag containing 5% dextrose injec-

tion and empty the syringe contents into the bag. The infusion concentration should be 1 mg/mL. For pediatric clients and those with CV disease, the drug may be diluted with 5% dextrose injection to a final infusion concentration of 2 mg/mL.
5. Strict aseptic technique must be used in preparation because there is no bacteriostatic agent in the medication.
6. Do not use saline solution or distilled water with bacteriostatic agent as a diluent because a precipitate may result. Use sterile water with continuous bladder irrigation.
7. Do not use the initial concentrate if any precipitate is present.
8. An in-line membrane filter with a pore diameter of 1 μm may be used. Since preparation is a colloidal suspension, anything smaller may remove the medication.
9. Protect from light during administration. However, loss of drug activity during administration is likely negligible if the solution is exposed for 8 hr or less.
10. Do not mix other drugs or electrolytes with lipsomal amphotericin B as compatabilities are not known. Flush an existing IV line with 5% dextrose injection before infusion of liposomal amphotericin B (or, a separate infusion line can be used).
11. Minimize local inflammation and danger of thrombophlebitis by administering the solution below the recommended dilution of 0.1 mg.
12. Initiate therapy in the most distal veins. When administered peripherally, changing sites with each dose may decrease phlebitis.
13. Have on hand 200–400 units of heparin sodium, since it may be ordered for the infusion to prevent thrombophlebitis.
14. Administer by slow IV infusion over 6 hr.
15. *Storage/stability of conventional amphotericin B:* Vials should be refrigerated and protected from light. After reconstitution the concentrate may be stored in the dark at room temperature for 24 hr or under refrigeration for 1 week. Any unused

solution should be discarded. Diluted solutions for IV infusion should be used promptly after preparation.

16. *Storage/stability of liposomal amphotericin B:* Prior to admixture, liposomal amphotericin B should be stored at 2°C–8°C (36°F–46°F), without freezing. This product should be kept in the carton until used. The admixed liposomal amphotericin B and 5% dextrose injection may be stored for 15 hr at 2°C–8°C (36°F–46°F) and an additional 6 hr at room temperature. Any unused drug should be discarded.

**Assessment**

1. Assess for any adverse effects and hypersensitivity to any anti-infectives or drugs in the antifungal category.
2. Assess mental status and age.
3. Assess and describe characteristics of any lesions requiring therapy.
4. Review list of drugs currently prescribed to ensure none interact unfavorably.
5. Ensure that baseline CBC, liver and renal function, and laboratory cultures have been performed.

**Interventions**

1. Ensure correct form, liposomal or conventional, as ordered, is prepared correctly for administration.
2. Determine that a 1-mg test dose has been administered (1 mg in 20 mL D5W over 20–30 min) and response.
3. Premedicate with antipyretics, antihistamines, corticosteroids, and/or antiemetic drugs to reduce side effects. Rashes, fevers, and chills may occur frequently with this therapy.
4. Infuse slowly, monitoring VS every 15–30 min during first dose; interrupt for adverse effects.
5. Monitor I&O; report reduction in blood sediment or cloudy urine.
6. Weigh twice weekly and assess for malnutrition or dehydration.
7. Anticipate hypokalemia with concomitant digoxin therapy. Observe for toxicity and muscle weakness and monitor serum potassium and digoxin levels.

8. Intrathecal administration of amphotericin may cause inflammation of the spinal roots; report sensory loss or foot drop.

**Client/Family Teaching**

1. GI effects may be reduced by an antihistamine or antiemetic before drug therapy and by administering the drug before mealtime. If diarrhea develops, try small frequent meals.
2. Report any incidents of anorexia, nausea, vomiting, headache, rashes, fever, or chills.
3. Report any decrease in I&O and extreme weight loss. Advise adequate hydration (2½ L/day) to prevent nephrotoxic effects.
4. Amphotericin therapy usually requires long-term treatments (6–11 weeks) to ensure an adequate response and to prevent any relapse.
5. Neurologic symptoms such as tinnitus, blurred vision, or vertigo should be reported immediately.
6. Guidelines for therapy with creams and lotions:
- Drug does not stain skin when it is rubbed into lesion.
- Any discoloration of fabric caused by cream or lotion may be removed by washing with soap and water.
- Any discoloration of clothing caused by ointment may be removed with a standard cleaning fluid.
- Report any increased worsening of condition, lack or response, itching, burning, or rash at site of local application.
- Do not apply an occlusive dressing as this may promote yeast growth.

**Outcomes/Evaluate**

- Clinical/laboratory evidence of resolution of fungal infection
- Reduction in size/number of lesions
- Symptomatic improvement

# Ampicillin oral

(am-pih-**SILL**-in)
**Pregnancy Category:** B

---

Apo-Ampi ✱, Jaa Amp ✱, Novo-Ampicillin ✱, Nu-Ampi ✱, Omnipen, Penbritin ✱, Polycillin, Polycillin Pediatric Drops, Principen, Pro-Ampi ✱, Taro-Ampicillin ✱, Totacillin **(Rx)**

*NOTE:* The following Canadian drugs are ampicillin trihydrate: Apo-Ampi, Jaa Amp, Nu-Ampi, Pro-Ampi, Taro-Ampicillin.

―――COMBINATION DRUG―――
# Ampicillin with Probenecid
(am-pih-**SILL**-in, proh-**BEN**-ih-sid)
Pro-Biosan ✱, Polycillin-PRB, Probampacin **(Rx)**

# Ampicillin sodium, parenteral
(am-pih-**SILL**-in)
**Pregnancy Category:** B
Ampicin ✱, Omnipen-N, Polycillin-N, Totacillin-N **(Rx)**
**Classification:** Antibiotic, penicillin

See also *Anti-Infectives* and Penicillins.
**Content:** The Powder for Oral Suspension of Ampicillin with Probenecid contains 3.5 g ampicillin and 1 g probenecid per bottle.
**Action/Kinetics:** Synthetic, broad-spectrum antibiotic suitable for gram-negative bacteria. Acid resistant, destroyed by penicillinase. Absorbed more slowly than other penicillins. From 30% to 60% of PO dose absorbed from GI tract. **Peak serum levels: PO:** 1.8–2.9 mcg/mL after 2 hr; **IM,** 4.5–7 mcg/mL. **t½:** 80 min—range 50–110 min. Partially inactivated in liver; 25%–85% excreted unchanged in urine.
**Uses:** Infections of respiratory, GI, and GU tracts caused by *Shigella, Salmonella, Escherichia coli, Hemophilus influenzae, Proteus* strains, *Neisseria gonorrhoeae, N. meningitidis,* and *Enterococcus.* Also, otitis media in children, bronchitis, ratbite fever, and whooping cough. Penicillin G-sensitive staphylococci, streptococci, pneumococci.

**Additional Drug Interactions**
*Allopurinol /* ↑ Incidence of skin rashes
*Ampicillin /* ↓ Effect of oral contraceptives

**Dosage**
• **Ampicillin: Capsules, Oral Suspension; Ampicillin Sodium: IV, IM**
*Respiratory tract and soft tissue infections.*
**PO: 20 kg or more:** 250 mg q 6 hr; **less than 20 kg:** 50 mg/kg/day in equally divided doses q 6–8 hr. **IV, IM: 40 kg or more:** 250–500 mg q 6 hr; **less than 40 kg:** 25–50 mg/kg/day in equally divided doses q 6–8 hr.
*Disseminated gonococcal infections.*
**PO:** 1 g q 6 hr.
*Bacterial meningitis.*
**Adults:** A total of 8–12 g/day given in divided doses q 3–4 hr. **Pediatric:** 100–200 mg/kg/day in divided doses q 3–4 hr.
*Bacterial endocarditis prophylaxis (dental, oral, or upper respiratory tract procedures; GI or GU tract surgery or instrumentation).*
**Adult, IM, IV:** 1–2 g (use 2 g for GI or GU tract surgery) plus gentamicin, 1.5 mg/kg (not to exceed 80 mg) IM or IV, given 30 min before procedure followed by amoxicillin, 1.5 g, 6 hr after initial dose; or, repeat parenteral dose 8 hr after initial dose. **Pediatric:** Ampicillin, 50 mg/kg with gentamicin, 2 mg/kg 30 min prior to procedure followed by amoxicillin, 25 mg/kg, after 6 hr or a parenteral dose of ampicillin is given after 8 hr.
*Septicemia.*
**Adults/children:** 150–200 mg/kg, IV for first 3 days, then IM q 3–4 hr.
• **Ampicillin with Probenecid: Oral Suspension**
*Urethral, endocervical, or rectal infections due to* N. gonorrhoeae.
**Adults:** 3.5 g ampicillin and 1 g probenecid as a single dose.
*Prophylaxis of infection in rape victims.*
3.5 g with 1 g probenecid.

## NURSING CONSIDERATIONS

See also *Nursing Considerations* for *Penicillins*.

**Administration/Storage**

1. For IM use, dilute only with sterile water for injection or bacteriostatic water for injection; use within the hour.

2. If the creatinine clearance is less than 10 mL/min, the dosing interval should be increased to 12 hr.

**IV** 3. After reconstitution for IM or direct IV administration, the solution of sodium ampicillin **must be used within the hour**.

4. For IVPB, ampicillin may be reconstituted with NaCL injection.

5. Give IV injections of reconstituted sodium ampicillin slowly; 2 mL should be given over a period of at least 3–5 min.

6. For administration by IV drip, check compatibility and length of time that drug retains potency in a particular solution.

**Assessment**

1. Document indications for therapy, type, onset, and duration of symptoms.

2. Note history of sensitivity/reactions to this drug or related drugs.

3. Monitor CBC, cultures, liver and renal function studies.

4. When administering IM, tell client it may be painful; rotate and document injection sites.

5. Monitor urinary output and serum potassium levels especially in the elderly.

**Client/Family Teaching**

1. Take medication 1 hr before or 2 hr after meals.

2. Teach person administering drug the appropriate method for administration and storage.

3. Take for the prescribed number of days even if the symptoms subside to prevent drug resistance.

4. Ampicillin chewable tablets should not be swallowed whole.

5. Do not save for future use or share with family members/friends who have similar symptoms.

6. May decrease effectiveness of oral contraceptives; practice alternative method of contraception during therapy.

7. Report any "ampicillin rashes"; a dull, red, itchy, flat or raised rash occurs more often with this drug than with other penicillins and is usually benign. If a late skin rash develops with symptoms of fever, fatigue, sore throat, generalized lymphadenopathy, and enlarged spleen, a heterophil antibody test may be considered to rule out mononucleosis.

**Outcomes/Evaluate**

• Resolution of S&S of infection; symptomatic improvement

• Negative culture reports (note resistance to drug)

————COMBINATION DRUG————

# Ampicillin sodium/ Sulbactam sodium

(am-pih-**SILL**-in/sull-**BACK**-tam)

**Pregnancy Category:** B

Unasyn **(Rx)**

**Classification:** Antibiotic, penicillin

See also *Anti-Infectives* and Penicillins.

**Content:** The Powder for Injection contains either 1 g ampicillin sodium and 0.5 g sulbactam sodium or 2 g ampicillin sodium and 1 g sulbactam sodium.

**Action/Kinetics:** For details, see *Ampicillin oral.* Sulbactam is present in this product because it irreversibly inhibits beta-lactamases, thus ensuring activity of ampicillin against beta-lactamase-producing microorganisms. Thus, sulbactam broadens the antibiotic spectrum of ampicillin to those bacteria normally resistant to it. **Peak serum levels, after IV infusion:** 15 min. **t½, both drugs:** about 1 hr. From 75%–85% of both drugs is excreted unchanged in the urine within 8 hr after administration.

**Uses:** Infections caused by beta-lactamase-producing strains of the following: (a) skin and skin structure infections caused by *Staphylococcus*

**A**

*aureus, Escherichia coli, Klebsiella* species (including *K. pneumoniae*), *Proteus mirabilis, Bacteroides fragilis, Enterobacter* species, and *Acinetobacter calcoaceticus;* (b) intra-abdominal infections caused by *E. coli, Klebsiella* species (including *K. pneumoniae*), *Bacteroides* (including *B. fragilis* and *Enterobacter)* (c) gynecologic infections caused by *E. coli* and *Bacteroides* (including *B. fragilis). NOTE:* Mixed infections caused by ampicillin-susceptible organisms and beta-lactamase-producing organisms are susceptible to this product; thus, additional antibiotics do not have to be used.

**Special Concerns:** Safety and efficacy in children less than 12 years of age have not been established.

**Side Effects:** *At site of injection:* Pain and thrombophlebitis. *GI:* Diarrhea, N&V, flatulence, abdominal distention, glossitis. *CNS:* Fatigue, malaise, headache. *GU:* Dysuria, urinary retention. *Miscellaneous:* Itching, chest pain, edema, facial swelling, erythema, chills, tightness in throat, epistaxis, substernal pain, mucosal bleeding, candidiasis.

**OD** **Overdose Management:** *Symptoms: **Neurologic symptoms, including convulsions.*** *Treatment:* Both ampicillin and sulbactam may be removed by hemodialysis.

**Laboratory Test Interferences:** ↑ AST, ALT, alkaline phosphatase, LDH, creatinine, BUN; also, ↑ basophils, eosinophils, lymphocytes, monocytes, platelets. ↓ Serum albumin and total proteins, H&H, RBCs, WBCs, and platelets. Presence of RBCs and hyaline casts in urine.

**Dosage** ————————————
• **IV, IM**
**Adults:** 1 g ampicillin/0.5 g sulbactam to 2 g ampicillin/1 g sulbactam q 6 hr, not to exceed 4 g sulbactam daily. Doses must be decreased in renal impairment.

## NURSING CONSIDERATIONS

See also *Nursing Considerations* for *Penicillins* and *Ampicillin.*

**Administration/Storage**
1. For IM use, the drug can be reconstituted with sterile water for injection or 0.5% or 2% lidocaine HCl injection.
2. Must use solutions for IM administration within 1 hr of preparation.
**IV** 3. After reconstitution, solutions should stand so that any foaming will dissipate and the vial can be inspected visually to ensure dissolution.
4. For IV use, the drug can be reconstituted with any of the following: 5% dextrose injection, D5%/0.45% saline, 10% invert sugar, RL injection, 0.9% NaCL injection, M/6 sodium lactate injection, or sterile water for injection.
5. For IV use, drug can be given by slow injection over 10–15 min or, if mixed with 50–100 mL of diluent, can be given over 15–30 min.
6. If aminoglycosides are prescribed concomitantly, administer each separately (1 hr apart) because ampicillin will inactivate aminoglycosides.

**Interventions**
1. Reduce dose with impaired renal function.
2. IM injections are extremely painful; follow manufacturer's recommendations for reconstitution and advise to expect some discomfort.
3. If clients develop a skin rash, consider and test for mononucleosis.

**Outcomes/Evaluate**
• Resolution of infection
• Symptomatic improvement

# Amrinone lactate

(**AM**-rih-nohn)
**Pregnancy Category:** C
Inocor **(Rx)**
**Classification:** Cardiac inotropic agent

**Action/Kinetics:** Amrinone causes an increase in CO by increasing the force of contraction of the heart, probably by inhibiting cyclic AMP phosphodiesterase, thereby increasing cellular levels of c-AMP. It reduces afterload and preload by directly relaxing vascular smooth muscle. **Time to peak effect:** 10 min. **t½,**

**after rapid IV:** 3.6 hr; **after IV infusion:** 5.8 hr. **Steady-state plasma levels:** 2.4 mcg/mL by maintaining an infusion of 5–10 mcg/kg/min. **Duration:** 30 min–2 hr, depending on the dose. Excreted primarily in the urine both unchanged and as metabolites. Children have a larger volume of distribution and a decreased elimination half-life.

**Uses:** Congestive heart failure (short-term therapy in clients unresponsive to digitalis, diuretics, and/or vasodilators). Can be used in digitalized clients.

**Contraindications:** Hypersensitivity to amrinone or bisulfites. Severe aortic or pulmonary valvular disease in lieu of surgery. Acute MI.

**Special Concerns:** Safety and efficacy not established in children. Use with caution during lactation.

**Side Effects:** *GI:* N&V, abdominal pain, anorexia. *CV:* Hypotension, ***supraventricular and ventricular arrhythmias.*** *Allergic:* Pericarditis, pleuritis, ascites, allergic reaction to sodium bisulfite present in the product. *Other:* Thrombocytopenia, ***hepatotoxicity,*** fever, chest pain, burning at site of injection.

**OD** **Overdose Management:** *Symptoms:* Hypotension. *Treatment:* Reduce or discontinue drug administration and begin general supportive measures.

**Drug Interactions:** Excessive hypotension when used with disopyramide.

**Dosage** ————————
• **IV**
   *CHF.*
**Initial:** 0.75 mg/kg as a bolus given slowly over 2–3 min; may be repeated after 30 min if necessary. **Maintenance, IV infusion:** 5–10 mcg/kg/min. Daily dose should not exceed 10 mg/kg although up to 18 mg/kg/day has been used in some clients for short periods.

## NURSING CONSIDERATIONS
### Administration/Storage
**IV** 1. Administer undiluted or dilut-

ed in 0.9% or 0.45% saline to a concentration of 1–3 mg/mL. Use diluted solutions within 24 hr.
2. Do not dilute with solutions containing dextrose (glucose) prior to injection. However, the drug may be injected into running dextrose (glucose) infusions through a Y connector or directly into the tubing.
3. Administer loading dose over 2–3 min; may be repeated in 30 min.
4. Solutions should appear clear yellow.
5. Administer solution with an electronic infusion device.
6. Do not administer in an IV line containing furosemide because a precipitate will form.
7. Protect from light and store at room temperature.
### Assessment
1. Determine that baseline VS, CXR, and ECG have been performed.
2. Assess serum potassium levels, CBC, and platelets; report any unusual bruises or bleeding.
3. Document cardiac and pulmonary assessment findings, noting any new-onset $S_3$, rales, or pedal edema.
4. Monitor VS, I&O, weights, and urine output. Document CVP, CO, and PA pressures if Swan Ganz catheter in place.
5. Observe for any hypersensitivity reactions, including pericarditis, pleuritis, or ascites.
6. Identify previous pharmacologic agents used for these symptoms and the results.
### Outcomes/Evaluate
• ↓ Preload and afterload; ↑ CO
• Improvement in S&S of CHF

———————————————

# Amyl nitrite
(**AM**-ill)
**Pregnancy Category:** X
Amyl Nitrite Aspirols, Amyl Nitrite Vaporole **(Rx)**
**Classification:** Coronary vasodilator, antidote for cyanide poisoning

See also *Antianginal Drugs—Nitrates/Nitrites.*

———————————————

**Action/Kinetics:** Believed to act by reducing systemic and PA pressure (afterload) and by decreasing CO due to peripheral vasodilation. Vascular relaxation occurs due to stimulation of intracellular cyclic guanosine monophosphate. As an antidote to cyanide poisoning, amyl nitrite promotes formation of methemoglobin which combines with cyanide to form the nontoxic cyanmethemoglobin. **Onset (inhalation):** 30 sec. **Duration:** 3–5 min. About 33% is excreted through the kidneys.

**Uses:** Prophylaxis or relief of acute attacks of angina pectoris; acute cyanide poisoning. *Investigational:* Diagnostic aid to assess reserve cardiac function.

**Contraindications:** Lactation.

**Special Concerns:** Use of amyl nitrite in children has not been studied. Hypotensive effects are more likely to occur in geriatric clients.

**Dosage**

• **Inhalation**

   *Angina pectoris.*

**Usual:** 0.3 mL (1 container crushed). Usually, 1–6 inhalations from one container produces relief. Dosage may be repeated after 3–5 min.

   *Antidote for cyanide poisoning.*

Administer for 30–60 sec q 5 min until client is conscious; is then repeated at longer intervals for up to 24 hr.

**NURSING CONSIDERATIONS**

See also *Nursing Considerations* for *Antianginal Drugs—Nitrates/Nitrites.*

**Administration/Storage**

1. Administer only by inhalation.

2. Protect containers from light and store at a temperature of 15°C–30°C (59°F–86°F).

3. *Amyl nitrite vapors are highly flammable. Do not use near flame or intense heat.*

**Assessment**

1. List precipitating incidents that precede the onset of chest pain.

2. Document degree, location, radiation, type, and duration of chest pain.

3. Identify cardiac risk factors.

4. With cyanide poisoning, document source and presenting symptoms.

**Client/Family Teaching**

1. Discuss and mutually set goals of therapy.

2. Identify changes in lifestyle that may reduce the need for amyl nitrite.

3. Enclose fabric-covered ampule in a handkerchief or piece of cloth and crush by hand.

4. Sit or lie down during inhalation to avoid hypotension.

5. Drug has a pungent odor, but several deep breaths must nevertheless be taken to attain drug effects.

6. Drug is inactivated when exposed to heat.

7. Always store medication out of reach of children.

8. The medication has the potential for abuse (sexual stimulant) and must be stored appropriately.

**Outcomes/Evaluate**

• Improved tissue perfusion with termination of angina attack

• Antidote for cyanide poisoning

# Anagrelide hydrochloride

(an-**AG**-greh-lyd)

**Pregnancy Category:** C

Agrylin **(Rx)**

**Classification:** Antiplatelet drug

**Action/Kinetics:** May act to reduce platelets by decreasing megakaryocyte hypermaturation. Does not cause significant changes in white cell counts or coagulation parameters. Inhibits platelet aggregation at higher doses than needed to reduce platelet count. **Peak plasma levels:** 5 ng/mL at 1 hr. **t½:** 1.3 hr; **terminal t½:** About 3 days. Metabolized in liver and excreted in urine and feces.

**Uses:** Reduce platelet count in essential thrombocythemia.

**Contraindications:** Lactation.

**Special Concerns:** Use with caution in known or suspected heart disease and in impaired renal or hepatic function. Safety and efficacy have not been determined in those less than 16 years of age.

**Side Effects:** *CV:* CHF, palpitations, chest pain, tachycardia, arrhythmias, angina, postural hypotension, hypertension, cardiovascular disease, vasodilation, migraine, syncope, *MI, cardiomyopathy, complete heart block, fibrillation, CVA, pericarditis, hemorrhage, heart failure,* cardiomegaly, atrial fibrillation. *GI:* Diarrhea, abdominal pain, pancreatitis, gastric/duodenal ulcers, N&V, flatulence, anorexia, constipation, GI distress, *GI hemorrhage,* gastritis, melena, aphthous stomatitis, eructations. *Respiratory:* Rhinitis, epistaxis, respiratory disease, sinusitis, pneumonia, bronchitis, asthma, pulmonary infiltrate, *pulmonary fibrosis, pulmonary hypertension,* dyspnea. *CNS:* Headache, *seizures,* dizziness, paresthesia, depression, somnolence, confusion, insomnia, nervousness, amnesia. *Musculoskeletal:* Arthralgia, myalgia, leg cramps. *Dermatologic:* Pruritus, skin disease, alopecia, rash, urticaria. *Hematologic:* Anemia, thrombocytopenia, ecchymosis, lymphadenoma. *Body as a whole:* Fever, flu symptoms, chills, photosensitivity, dehydration, malaise, asthenia, edema, pain. *Ophthalmic:* Amblyopia, abnormal vision, visual field abnormality, diplopia. *Miscellaneous:* Back pain, tinnitus.

**Laboratory Test Alterations:** ↑ Liver enzymes.

**OD Overdose Management:** *Symptoms:* Thrombocytopenia. *Treatment:* Close clinical monitoring. Decrease or stop dose until platelet count returns to within the normal range.

**Dosage** ─────────────
• **Capsules**
*Essential thrombocythemia.*
**Initial:** 0.5 mg q.i.d. or 1 mg b.i.d. Maintain for one week or more. **Then,** adjust to lowest effective dose to maintain platelet count less than 600,000/mcL. Can increase the dose by 0.5 mg or less/day in any 1 week. **Maximum dose:** 10 mg/day or 2.5 mg in single dose. Most respond at a dose of 1.5 to 3 mg/day.

**NURSING CONSIDERATIONS**
**Assessment**
1. Document etiology, onset, and duration of essential thrombocythemia.
2. Note any CAD, liver or renal dysfunction; document cardiovascular assessment and monitor closely.
3. Monitor VS, CBC, liver and renal function; check platelets every 2 days during first week and then weekly thereafter until stablized.
4. Determine if pregnant; precludes therapy.

**Client/Family Teaching**
1. Take exactly as directed.
2. Drug is used to lower platelet counts. Platelet increases usually occur within 4 days after interruption of therapy.
3. Practice reliable contraception; may cause fetal harm.
4. Report any palpitations, SOB, dizziness, chest or abdominal pain or unusual bleeding.

**Outcomes/Evaluate:** Reduction in platelet counts; ↓ risk of thrombosis

# Anastrozole
((an-**AS**-troh-zohl))
**Pregnancy Category:** D
Arimidex **(Rx)**
**Classification:** Antineoplastic, hormone

See also *Antineoplastic Agents.*
**Action/Kinetics:** Growth of many breast cancers is due to stimulation of estrogen receptors by estrogens. In postmenopausal women the main source of circulating estrogen is conversion of androstenedione to estrone by aromatase in peripheral tissues with further conversion to estradiol. Anastrozole is a nonsteroidal aromatase inhibitor and, as such, significantly decreases serum estradiol levels. It has no effect on formation of adrenal corticosteroids or aldosterone. The drug is well absorbed from the GI tract; food does not affect the extent of absorption. **t½, terminal:** 50 hr. It is metabolized by the liver and both unchanged parent

drug (about 10%) and metabolites are excreted through the urine.

**Uses:** Advanced breast cancer in postmenopausal women with progression of the disease following tamoxifen therapy. *NOTE:* Clients with negative tumor estrogen receptors and those who do not respond to tamoxifen are rarely helped by anastrozole.

**Special Concerns:** Use with caution during lactation. Safety and efficacy have not been determined in children.

**Side Effects:** *GI:* N&V, diarrhea, constipation, abdominal pain, anorexia, dry mouth, increased appetite. *CNS:* Headache, paresthesia, dizziness, depression, somnolence, confusion, insomnia, anxiety, nervousness. *CV:* Hypertension, thromboembolic disease, thrombophlebitis. *Musculoskeletal:* Asthenia, back pain, bone pain, myalgia, arthralgia, pathological fracture. *Respiratory:* Dyspnea, increased cough, pharyngitis, sinusitis, bronchitis, rhinitis. *Dermatologic:* Hot flushes, rash, sweating, hair thinning, pruritus. *GU:* Vaginal hemorrhage, UTI, breast pain, vaginal dryness, vaginal bleeding during first few weeks after changing from hormone therapy. *Hematologic:* Anemia, leukopenia. *Miscellaneous:* Pain, peripheral edema, pelvic pain, chest pain, weight gain or loss, flu syndrome, fever, neck pain, malaise, accidental injury, infection.

**Laboratory Test Alterations:** ↑ GGT, AST, ALT, alkaline phosphatase, total cholesterol, LDL cholesterol.

**Dosage** ————————————
• **Tablets**
  *Advanced breast cancer.*
  1 mg daily.

---

## NURSING CONSIDERATIONS

See also *Nursing Considerations* for *Antineoplastic Agents.*

**Administration/Storage:** Glucocorticoid or mineralocorticoid therapy is not required.

**Assessment**
1. Document disease progression and last tamoxifen therapy.
2. Obtain baseline CBC and liver and renal function studies.
3. Document negative pregnancy test.

**Client/Family Teaching**
1. Take as directed at the same time each day.
2. Use reliable birth control; drug may cause fetal harm and impair fertility.

**Outcomes/Evaluate:** Control of malignant cell proliferation

---

# Anistreplase
(an-ih-**STREP**-layz)
**Pregnancy Category:** C
Eminase **(Rx)**
**Classification:** Thrombolytic enzyme

**Action/Kinetics:** Anistreplase is prepared by acylating human plasma derived from lys-plasminogen and purified streptokinase derived from group C beta-hemolytic streptococci. When prepared, anistreplase is an inactive derivative of a fibrinolytic enzyme although the compound can still bind to fibrin. Anistreplase is activated by deacylation and subsequent release of the anisoyl group in the blood stream. The production of plasmin from plasminogen occurs in both the blood stream and the thrombus leading to thrombolysis. The drug will lyse thrombi obstructing coronary arteries and reduce the size of infarcts. **t½:** 70–120 min.

**Uses:** Management of AMI in adults, resulting in improvement of ventricular function and reduction of mortality. Treatment should be initiated as soon as possible after the onset of symptoms of AMI.

**Contraindications:** Use in active internal bleeding; within 2 months of intracranial or intraspinal surgery; recent trauma, including cardiopulmonary resuscitation; history of CVA; intracranial neoplasm; arteriovenous malformation or aneurysm; known bleeding diathesis; severe, uncontrolled hypertension; severe allergic reactions to streptokinase. **Special Concerns:** Use with caution in nursing mothers. Safety and effectiveness have not been determined in children.

NOTE: The risks of anistreplase therapy may be increased in the following conditions; thus, benefit versus risk must be assessed prior to use. Within 10 days of major surgery (e.g., CABG, obstetric delivery, organ biopsy, previous puncture of noncompressible vessels); cerebrovascular disease; within 10 days of GI or GU bleeding; within 10 days of trauma including cardiopulmonary resuscitation; SBP > 180 mm Hg or DBP > 110 mm Hg; likelihood of left heart thrombus (e.g., mitral stenosis with atrial fibrillation); SBE; acute pericarditis; hemostatic defects including those secondary to severe hepatic or renal disease; pregnancy; clients older than 75 years of age; diabetic hemorrhagic retinopathy or other hemorrhagic ophthalmic conditions; septic thrombophlebitis or occluded arteriovenous cannula at seriously infected site; clients on oral anticoagulant therapy; any condition in which bleeding constitutes a significant hazard or would be difficult to manage due to its location.

**Side Effects:** *Bleeding:* Including at the puncture site (most common), nonpuncture site hematoma, hematuria, hemoptysis, *GI hemorrhage, intracranial bleeding,* gum/mouth hemorrhage, epistaxis, anemia, eye hemorrhage. *CV: Arrhythmias,* conduction disorders, hypotension; *cardiac rupture,* chest pain, emboli (causal relationship to use of anistreplase unknown). *Allergic: Anaphylaxis, bronchospasm,* angioedema, urticaria, itching, flushing, rashes, eosinophilia, delayed purpuric rash which may be associated with arthralgia, ankle edema, mild hematuria, GI symptoms, and proteinuria. *GI:* N&V. *Hematologic:* Thrombocytopenia. *CNS:* Agitation, dizziness, paresthesia, tremor, vertigo. *Respira-*

*tory:* Dyspnea, lung edema. *Miscellaneous:* Chills, fever, headache, shock.

**Drug Interactions:** Increased risk of bleeding or hemorrhage if used with heparin, oral anticoagulants, vitamin K antagonists, aspirin, or dipyridamole.

**Laboratory Test Interferences:** ↑ Transaminase levels, thrombin time, activated PTT, and PT. ↓ Plasminogen and fibrinogen.

## Dosage

**IV only:** 30 units over 2–5 min into an IV line or vein as soon as possible after onset of symptoms.

## NURSING CONSIDERATIONS

See also *Nursing Considerations* for *Alteplase, Recombinant.*

### Administration/Storage

**IV** 1. Reconstitute by slowly adding 5 mL of sterile water for injection. To minimize foaming, gently roll the vial after directing the stream of sterile water against the side of the vial. The vial should not be shaken.

2. The reconstituted solution should be colorless to pale yellow without any particulate matter or discoloration.

3. Do not further dilute the reconstituted solution before administration.

4. Do not add the reconstituted solution to any infusion fluids and no other medications should be added to the vial or syringe containing anistreplase.

5. Discard the solution if not administered within 30 min of reconstitution.

### Assessment

1. Note any history and/or evidence of bleeding.

2. Take a full drug history, noting any aspirin, anticoagulant, or vitamin K antagonist use.

3. Note resistance to the effects of anistreplase, which may be observed if the drug is given more than 5 days after a previous dose, after streptokinase therapy, or after a streptococcal infection.

4. Increased antistreptokinase anti-

body levels between 5 days and 6 months after anistreplase or streptokinase administration may increase the risk of allergic reactions.
5. Obtain baseline hematologic parameters, type and cross, coagulation studies, cardiac marker panel, and renal function studies.

**Interventions**
1. Avoid invasive procedures to minimize bleeding potential. Post bleeding precautions.
2. If an arterial puncture is necessary following use of anistreplase, an upper extremity vessel accessible to manual compression should be used. Apply 30 min of manual pressure followed by application of a pressure dressing. Puncture site should be checked frequently for any evidence of bleeding.
3. Monitor ECG closely and document any reperfusion arrhythmias.

**Client/Family Teaching**
1. Review the goals of therapy and inherent risks during acute coronary artery occlusion.
2. To be effective, the therapy should be instituted as soon as possible after the onset of symptoms of AMI.
3. Encourage family members to learn CPR.

**Outcomes/Evaluate**
• Restoration of blood flow to ischemic cardiac tissue
• ↓ Infarct size; ↓ mortality, and improved ventricular function with AMI

---

# Antihemophilic factor (AHF, Factor VIII)

(an-tie-hee-moh-**FILL**-ick)
**Pregnancy Category:** C
Alphanate, Antihemophilic Factor (Porcine) Hyate:C, Bioclate, Helixate, Hemofil M, Humate-P, Koate-HP, Kogenate, Monoclate-P, Profilate HP, Recombinate **(Rx)**
**Classification:** Hemostatic, systemic

**Action/Kinetics:** Antihemophilic factor either is isolated from pooled normal human blood or is derived from monoclonal antibodies. The potency and purity of preparation

vary but each lot is standardized. Details on the package should be noted. Plasma protein (factor VIII) accelerates abnormally slow transformation of prothrombin to thrombin. **t½:** 9–15 hr. One AHF unit is the activity found in 1 mL of normal pooled human plasma.
**Uses:** Control of bleeding in clients suffering from hemophilia A (factor VIII deficiency and acquired factor VIII inhibitors). These products temporarily replace the missing clotting factor in order to correct or prevent bleeding episodes or to perform surgery. AHF is safe and effective for use in children of all ages, including neonates.
**Contraindications:** Use of monoclonal antibody-derived AHF in clients hypersensitive to bovine, hamster, or mouse protein.
**Special Concerns:** Since AHF is prepared from human plasma, there is a risk of transmitting hepatitis or AIDS. However, the products are carefully prepared and tested.
**Side Effects:** *CNS:* Headache, somnolence, lethargy, fatigue, dizziness. *CV:* Increased bleeding tendency, flushing, slight hypotension, acute hemolytic anemia, hyperfibrinogenemia. *Allergic:* Nausea, fever, hives, chills, urticaria, wheezing, hypotension, chest tightness, stinging at infusion site, hypotension, *anaphylaxis.* *Miscellaneous:* Sore throat, cold feet, taste perversion, nonspecific rash.

Antibodies may form to the mouse protein found in AHF derived from monoclonal antibodies. Approximately 10% of clients develop inhibitors to Factor VIII, which leads to a significantly decreased response. Antihemophilic factor contains traces of blood group A and B isohemagglutins. These may cause *intravascular hemolysis* in clients with types A, B, or AB blood.

*Both hepatitis and AIDS may be transmitted from AHF prepared from human plasma.*

**Dosage**
• **IV Only**
**Individualized,** depending on

severity of bleeding, degree of deficiency, body weight, and presence of inhibitors of factor VIII. *NOTE:* AHF levels may rise 2% for every unit of AHF per kilogram administered. The following formula provides a guide for dosage calculation :Expected Factor VIII increase (in % of normal):AHF/IU administered × 2 ÷ body weight (in kg) Dosages given are only guidelines.

*Prophylaxis of spontaneous hemorrhage.*

Increase AHF levels to about 5% of normal; 30% of normal is the minimum required for hemostasis following surgery and trauma. A single dose of 10 IU/kg (increases of approximately 20%) may be sufficient for mild superficial bleeds or early hemorrhages. Smaller doses may be sufficient for early hemarthrosis.

*Mild hemorrhage.*

Single infusion to achieve AHF levels of at least 30%. Dosage should not be repeated.

*Minor surgery, moderate hemorrhage.*

AHF levels should be raised to 30%–50% of normal. **Initial:** 15–25 IU/kg; **maintenance**, **if necessary:** 10–15 IU/kg q 8–12 hr.

*Severe hemorrhage.*

Increase AHF levels to 80%–100% of normal. **Initial:** 40–50 IU/kg; **maintenance:** 20–25 IU/kg q 8–12 hr.

*Major surgery.*

Raise AHF levels to 80%–100% of normal. Administer 1 hr before surgery; one-half the priming dose may be given 5 hr after the first dose. AHF levels should be maintained at 30% of normal for at least 10–14 days.

*Dental extraction.*

Factor VIII level should be increased to 50% immediately before the procedure.

## NURSING CONSIDERATIONS
### Administration/Storage
**IV** 1. AHF is labile and is inactivated rapidly: within 10 min at 56°C

and within 3 hr at 49°C. Store vials at 2°C–8°C (35°F–46°F). Check expiration date. **Do not freeze.**

2. Warm the concentrate and diluent to room temperature before reconstitution.

3. Place one needle in the concentrate to act as an airway and then aseptically with a syringe and needle add the diluent to the concentrate.

4. Gently agitate or roll the vial containing diluent and concentrate to dissolve the drug. **Do not shake vigorously.**

5. Administer drug within 3 hr of reconstitution, to avoid incubation if contamination occurred during mixing.

6. Do not refrigerate drug after reconstitution, because the active ingredient may precipitate out.

7. Keep reconstituted drug at room temperature during infusion because, at a lower temperature, precipitation of active ingredients may occur.

8. Administer IV only using a plastic syringe (solutions stick to glass syringes). Administer medication at a rate of 2 mL/min although rates up to 10 mL/min can be used if necessary. If the pulse rate increases significantly, the rate of administration should be reduced or discontinued.

9. There are a large number of products available. It is important to note the actual AHF units, which are indicated on the vial.

### Assessment
1. Note blood type. Clients with A, B, and AB are more prone to hemolytic reactions.

2. Determine any recent trauma or injury; assess joints carefully.

3. Document baseline hematologic parameters and factor VIII levels. Monitor H&H and factor levels and perform Coombs' test during therapy.

### Interventions
1. Document baseline VS and monitor q 5–15 min during infusion. If tachycardia and hypotension occur, slow IV and report.

2. Premedicate (usually diphenhy-

**A**

dramine) to reduce allergic reactions.

3. Document I&O. Assess urine for quantity, color, and occult blood.

4. Slow infusion and report if client complains of headaches, flushing, numbness, back pain, visual disturbances, or chest constriction.

**Client/Family Teaching**

1. Review appropriate method for storing and administering AHF at home.

2. If product is prepared from human plasma identify the rare but associated potential risks, such as hepatitis and HIV.

3. Avoid any drugs or OTC agents that may alter clotting (i.e., aspirin, ibuprofen).

4. Determine knowledge concerning disease process and hereditary transmission. Identify and reinforce any areas necessary to ensure compliance with therapy.

5. Reinforce safety measures related to sports, work, risk taking, and sexual activity.

6. Identify local support groups that may assist client to understand and cope with this disease.

**Outcomes/Evaluate**

• Prevention and control of bleeding with hemophilia A

• Promotion of normal clotting mechanisms

• Coagulation times and factor VIII levels within desired range

---

# Antithrombin III (Human)

(an-tee-**THROM**-bin)
**Pregnancy Category:** C
ATnativ, Thrombate III ✱ (Rx)
**Classification:** Antithrombin

**Action/Kinetics:** Antithrombin III (human) is derived from pooled human plasma obtained from healthy donors. It is identical with heparin cofactor I, which is a component of plasma necessary for heparin to exert its anticoagulant effect. Plasma used for antithrombin III (human) has been found to be nonreactive for hepatitis B surface antigen and neg-

ative for antibody to HIV. The drug also undergoes heat treatment for 10 hr to prevent transmittal of viral infections. One unit is the amount of antithrombin III (AT-III) in 1 mL of normal pooled human plasma. Antithrombin III inactivates all coagulation enzymes except factor VIIa and factor XIII.

**Uses:** Hereditary AT-III deficiency in pregnant clients, in clients requiring surgery, and in individuals with thromboembolism.

**Special Concerns:** Safety and effectiveness have not been determined in children. Even though special precautions are taken, individuals may develop S&S of viral infections, including non-A, non-B hepatitis.

**Side Effects:** No side effects have been reported to date.

**Drug Interactions:** The anticoagulant effect of heparin is increased when used concomitantly with AT-III; the dose of heparin should be decreased during AT-III therapy.

**Dosage**

• **IV**

The dose must be individualized depending on the status of the client. Assuming a plasma volume of 40 mL/kg, an initial loading dose may be calculated as follows:

Dosage units = [desired AT-III level (%) − baseline AT-III level (%)] × body weight (kg)/1% (IU/kg)

Administration of 1 IU/kg raises the level of AT-III by 1%–2.1%. The drug may be infused slowly over 5–10 min at a rate of 50 IU (1 mL)/min, not to exceed 100 IU (2 mL)/min.

---

**NURSING CONSIDERATIONS**

**Administration/Storage**

**IV** 1. To reconstitute, dissolve the powder by gently swirling in 10 mL sterile water for injection, 0.9% NaCL injection, or D5% injection. Do not shake the product.

2. After reconstitution, bring the drug to room temperature and administer within 3 hr.

3. After the initial dose (which may increase AT-III levels to 120% of

normal), adjust the dose to maintain AT-III levels greater than 80% of normal.

4. Measure AT-III levels at least b.i.d. initially and until the client is stabilized and then once daily, immediately before the next infusion.

5. Anticipate a loading dose followed by once daily dosing, based on frequent plasma AT-III levels. Dosing recommendations are only guidelines; the exact loading and maintenance doses must be individualized depending on the status of the client, response to therapy, and actual plasma AT-III levels achieved.

**Assessment**

1. Perform a complete nursing history noting any positive family history of venous thrombosis.

2. Determine that AT-III levels have been obtained prior to drug therapy and before each subsequent infusion.

3. Document pretreatment weight.

**Interventions**

1. Observe for dyspnea and elevated BP during IV administration; slow infusion rate and report if evident.

2. Monitor VS closely (q 5–15 min) during infusion.

3. Note early S&S of acute thrombosis. Perform routine vascular checks and monitor AT-III levels.

4. Observe for any evidence of bleeding. Anticipate a reduced dose of heparin when administered concomitantly with AT-III.

5. Anticipate that when AT-III is given for clients with heredity deficiency to control an acute thrombosis or to prevent thrombosis due to surgery or in obstetrics, that levels should be maintained for 2–8 days, depending on the status of the client.

**Client/Family Teaching**

1. Explain the high risk of thrombosis during pregnancy and surgery with hereditary deficiencies because AT-III levels are generally 50% of the level of normal.

2. The disease is inherited; obtain appropriate medical follow-up, counseling, and family planning.

3. Review associated risks of drug therapy; product is derived from pooled human plasma.

**Outcomes/Evaluate**

• Serum AT-III levels > 80% of normal during therapy for high-risk procedures

• Prevention of thrombus formation

# Aprotinin

(ah-**PROH**-tih-nin)

**Pregnancy Category:** B

Trasylol **(Rx)**

**Classification:** Systemic hemostatic

**Action/Kinetics:** Aprotinin, a natural protease inhibitor derived from bovine lung, inhibits plasmin and kallikrein, thereby directly affecting fibrinolysis. It also inhibits the contact phase activation of coagulation which initiates coagulation and promotes fibrinolysis. In addition, aprotinin preserves the adhesive glycoproteins in the platelet membrane, rendering them resistant to damage from the increased plasmin levels and mechanical injury that occur during cardiopulmonary bypass. The net effect is to inhibit both fibrinolysis and turnover of coagulation factors and to decrease bleeding. **t½, IV:** 150 min with a terminal elimination phase half-life of 10 hr. Aprotinin is slowly broken down by lysosomal enzymes, although depending on the dose, up to 9% may be excreted through the urine unchanged.

**Uses:** Prophylactically to reduce perioperative blood loss and the need for blood transfusions in clients undergoing cardiopulmonary bypass surgery in the course of repeat coronary artery bypass graft surgery. In selected cases of primary coronary artery bypass graft surgery where the risk of bleeding is high or where transfusion is unavailable or unacceptable. Use in coronary artery bypass graft is based on the risk of renal dysfunction and the risk of anaphylaxis (i.e., should a second procedure be required).

---

✦ = Available in Canada    *bold italic* = life threatening side effect

**Contraindications:** Hypersensitivity to aprotinin.

**Special Concerns:** All clients should first receive a test dose of aprotinin to assess for potential allergic reactions; caution is required when administering aprotinin (including test doses) to clients who have received the drug previously due to the risk of anaphylaxis. Safety and efficacy have not been determined in children.

**Side Effects:** *CV:* Atrial fibrillation, *MI, heart failure, heart arrest* , atrial flutter, ventricular tachycardia, hypotension, CHF, supraventricular tachycardia, pericarditis, phlebitis, heart block, hemolysis, *CVA, ventricular fibrillation.* Possibly an increased incidence of saphenous vein graft closure in clients undergoing primary or repeat coronary artery bypass graft. *Respiratory:* Pneumonia, respiratory disorder, asthma, apnea, dyspnea, lung edema, pleural effusion, pneumothorax. *GU: Acute kidney failure,* kidney tubular necrosis. *CNS:* Confusion, *convulsions, cerebral embolism. Body as a whole:* Fever, sepsis, *shock, allergic reactions, anaphylaxis. Miscellaneous:* Liver damage.

**Drug Interactions**

*Captopril* / Aprotinin may block the acute hypotensive effect of captopril

*Fibrinolytic drugs* / Aprotinin may inhibit the effects of fibrinolytic drugs

*Heparin* / In the presence of heparin, aprotinin prolongs activated clotting time

**Laboratory Test Interferences:** ↑ Creatinine, transaminases, creatine kinase, PTT, activated clotting time, serum glucose. ↑ Incidence of postoperative renal dysfunction.

**Dosage** ───────

• **IV**

*Coronary bypass graft surgery.*
A 1-mL (1.4-mg or 10,000-KIU) test dose must be given 10 min prior to the loading dose. The test dose is followed by the loading dose using either regimen A or B; the loading dose is then followed by the constant infusion dose. In addition, the "pump prime" dose is added to the priming fluid of the cardiopulmonary bypass circuit by replacing an aliquot of the priming fluid prior to beginning cardiopulmonary bypass. **Regimen A, loading dose:** 280 mg (or 2 million KIU) with 280 mg (or 2 million KIU) into the pump prime volume; **constant infusion dose:** 70 mg/hr (500,000 KIU/hr). **Regimen B, loading dose:** 140 mg (or 1 million KIU) with 140 mg (or 1 million KIU) into the pump prime volume; **constant infusion dose:** 35 mg/hr (250,000 KIU/hr). Total doses greater than 7 million KIU have not been studied.

---

## NURSING CONSIDERATIONS
### Administration/Storage

**IV** 1. Experience with regimen B is limited. Regimen A seems more effective than regimen B in clients given aspirin preoperatively.

2. All IV doses are given through a central line. Do not administer any other drug through the same line.

3. It is important to remember that both regimens include a 1-mL test dose, a loading dose, a dose to be added to the priming fluid of the cardiopulmonary bypass circuit, and a constant infusion dose.

4. The loading dose is given slowly over 20–30 min after induction of anesthesia (but prior to sternotomy) with the client in a supine position.

5. When the loading dose is completed, it is followed by the constant infusion dose which is continued until the client leaves the operating room.

6. Aprotinin is incompatible in vitro with corticosteroids, heparin, tetracyclines, and nutrient solutions containing amino acids or fat emulsion. If these agents must be given, each should be given separately through different venous lines or catheters.

7. The drug should be stored between 2°C and 5°C (36°F–77°F) and prevented from freezing.

### Assessment

1. Determine if client has received

this drug previously because there is an increased risk of anaphylaxis. Anticipate antihistamine administration before the loading dose if this is a re-exposure case.

2. Ensure that client has received a 1-mL test dose 10 min before the loading dose and note results.

**Interventions**

1. Drug may cause increased serum glucose, CPK-MB fractions, transaminase levels, and postoperative renal dysfunction. Monitor and observe client closely.

2. Drug prolongs whole blood clotting time of heparinized blood and lab results may not report true state of anticoagulation. Therefore, an activated clotting time greater than 400–450 sec may in fact lead to inadequate anticoagulation.

3. During cardiopulmonary bypass, administer standard loading doses of heparin. Additional heparin should be administered either in a fixed-dose regimen or based on client weight and duration of cardiopulmonary bypass, since the activated clotting time is not reliable.

4. Coordinate with the lab; a protamine titration test may be useful in determining heparin levels, as this is not altered by aprotinin.

5. Observe client closely for cardiac arrhythmias, hemorrhage, hypotension, and fever, as these are frequent drug-related side effects.

**Outcomes/Evaluate:** ↓ Perioperative blood loss in clients undergoing cardiopulmonary bypass surgery

# Ardeparin sodium

(ar-dee-**PAH**-rin)
**Pregnancy Category:** C
Normiflo **(Rx)**
**Classification:** Anticoagulant, low molecular weight heparin

See also *Anticoagulants*.

**Action/Kinetics:** Binds to and accelerates activity of antithrombin III, thus inhibiting thrombosis by inactivating Factor Xa and thrombin. Also inhibits thrombin by binding to heparin cofactor II. At usual doses, no effect on PT; APTT may not be affected or may be slightly prolonged. Plasma levels of ardeparin can not be measured directly; rather, serine protease activity is used. Well absorbed following SC administration. $t\frac{1}{2}$, **disposition:** 3.3 hr (for ardeparin anti-Xa) and 1.2 hr (for ardeparin anti-IIa).

**Uses:** Prevention of deep vein thrombosis following knee replacement surgery.

**Contraindications:** Use with active major bleeding, hypersensitivity to drug or to pork products, thrombocytopenia associated with a positive *in vitro* test for anti-platelet antibodies in the presence of ardeparin. IM or IV use.

**Special Concerns:** Use with caution during lactation, in hypersensitivity to methylparaben or propylparaben, in those with bleeding diathesis, recent GI bleeding, thrombocytopenia or platelet defects, severe liver disease, hypertensive or diabetic retinopathy, in those undergoing invasive procedures (especially if they are receiving other drugs that interfere with hemostasis), or in severe renal failure. Use with extreme caution in those with a history of heparin-induced thrombocytopenia or in which there is an increased risk of hemorrhage (e.g., bacterial endocarditis, congenital or acquired bleeding disorders, active ulceration or angiodysplastic GI disease, severe uncontrolled hypertension, hemorrhagic stroke, soon after brain, spinal, or ophthalmologic surgery; or, with concomitant treatment with platelet inhibitors). Product contains metasulfite which may cause an allergic reaction in some. Safety and efficacy have not been determined in children.

**Side Effects:** *Bleeding events:* Intraoperative bleeding, postoperative surgical site or nonsurgical site hematoma or hemorrhage, bleeding requiring an invasive procedure; ecchymosis, *GI hemorrhage,* hematemesis, hematuria, melena, petechiae, *rectal hemorrhage, retroperitoneal hemorrhage, CVA,* abnormal stools. *GI:* N&V, constipation. *Allergic reaction:* Maculopapular rash, vesiculobullous rash, urticaria. *CNS:* Confusion, dizziness, headache, insomnia. *Miscellaneous:* Fever, pruritus, anemia, thrombocytopenia, arthralgia, chest pain, dyspnea, reactions at injection site (edema, hypersensitivity, inflammation, pain), peripheral edema.

**Laboratory Test Alterations:** ↑ ALT,AST, serum triglycerides.

**OD Overdose Management:** *Symptoms:* Bleeding at the surgical site or at venipuncture sites. Epistaxis, hematuria, blood in stools, easy bruising, petechiae. *Treatment:* Most bleeding can be controlled by discontinuing drug, applying pressure to site, and replacing volume and hemostatic blood elements as needed. If above is ineffective, can give protamine sulfate (1 mg protamine sulfate neutralizes about 100 anti-Xa units of ardeparin). If bleeding persists about 2 hr after protamine sulfate, draw blood and determine residual anti-Xa levels. Additional protamine sulfate can be given if clinically important bleeding persists or if anti-Xa levels are higher than desired.

**Drug Interactions:** Additive anticoagulant effects if given with other anticoagulants or platelet inhibitors (e.g., aspirin, NSAIDs).

**Dosage** ─────────────
• **SC**
*Prophylaxis of deep vein thrombosis during knee replacement surgery.*
**Adults:** 50 anti-Xa U/kg q 12 hr. Begin treatment evening of day of surgery or following morning and continue for up to 14 days or until client is fully ambulatory, whichever is shorter.

## NURSING CONSIDERATIONS
### Administration/Storage
1. Give by deep (intra-fat) SC injection in abdomen, avoiding navel, anterior aspect of thighs, or outer aspect of upper arms.

2. Before using, inspect visually for particulate matter and discoloration.
3 Store at room temperature, 15°C–30°C (59°F–77°F).

### Assessment
1. Take a complete history; note any conditions that may preclude drug therapy.
2. Drug dosage is based on weight; obtain reliable dry weight.
3. Note any sensitivity to heparin or pork products or metasulfites.
4. Determine any active major bleeding, bleeding disorders, or thrombocytopenia.
5. Monitor CBC, urinalysis, liver and renal function studies.

### Client/Family Teaching
1. Review indications for therapy and how to administer. Therapy consists of 2 injections deep SC q 12 hr while sitting or lying down. May be given in abdomen, avoiding navel, anterior aspect of thighs, or outer aspect of upper arms. Vary administration site with each injection.
2. To minimize bruising, do not rub site after giving injection.
3. Use Tubex® injector and follow printed guidelines for loading and removing Tubex®. Remove air and excess medication from Tubex® unit before injection. Discard used needles safely.
4. Therapy is continued until client is fully ambulatory or for about 14 days.
5. Avoid aspirin and NSAIDs.
6. Report any unusual bruising, bleeding or dizziness.
7. Periodic CBC, FOB (fecal occult blood) and urinalysis will be requested.

**Outcomes/Evaluate:** DVT prophylaxis after TKR

───────────────────────

# Asparaginase
(ah-**SPAIR**-ah-jin-ays)
**Pregnancy Category:** C
Colaspase, Elspar, Kidrolase ✦ (Abbreviation: Lcf-ASP) **(Rx)**
**Classification:** Antineoplastic, miscellaneous

─────────────────────

See also *Antineoplastic Agents.*

**Action/Kinetics:** Asparaginase, derived from *Escherichia coli,* contains the enzyme L-asparagine amidohydrolase, type EC-2. Cell cycle specific ($G_1$ phase). Neoplastic cells are unable to synthesize sufficient asparagine, an amino acid, to meet their metabolic needs. The supply of asparagine is further decreased by the enzyme asparaginase, which breaks down asparagine to aspartic acid and ammonia. Asparaginase interferes with synthesis of DNA, RNA, and protein and is cell-cycle specific for the $G_1$ phase of cell division. **Time to peak plasma levels, after IM:** 14–24 hr. **t½, after IV:** 8–30 hr; **after IM:** 39–49 hr. The drug accumulates in plasma and tissue, and a small amount (1%) appears in CSF. Excretion is unknown. More toxic in adults than in children.

**Uses:** Acute lymphocytic leukemia in children; mostly used in combination with other drugs. Not to be used for maintenance therapy. *Investigational:* Acute myelocytic and myelomonocytic leukemia, chronic lymphocytic leukemia, Hodgkin's and non-Hodgkin's lymphomas, melanosarcoma.

**Contraindications:** Anaphylactic reactions to asparaginase. Pancreatitis or a history of pancreatitis. Lactation.

**Special Concerns:** Use with caution in presence of liver dysfunction. Due to the possibility of an increased risk of hypersensitivity, institute retreatment with great care.

**Side Effects:** *GI:* N&V, anorexia, abdominal cramps, *pancreatitis (sometimes fulminant), acute hemorrhagic pancreatitis. CNS:* Depression, somnolence, coma, confusion, fatigue, agitation, mild to severe hallucinations, headache, irritability, Parkinson–like syndrome with tremor and a progressive increase in muscle tone (rare). *Hematologic:* Marked leukopenia, bone marrow depression (rare). Depression of clotting factors; rarely, *intracranial hemorrhage and fatal bleeding. Hyper-*

*sensitivity:* Skin rashes, urticaria, arthralgia, respiratory distress, *acute anaphylaxis. Renal:* Azotemia, proteinuria (rare), acute renal shutdown, *fatal renal insufficiency. Hepatic:* Hepatotoxicity, fatty changes in the liver. *Miscellaneous:* Hyperglycemia with glucosuria and polyuria. Marked hypoalbuminemia associated with peripheral edema, malabsorption syndrome, *fatal hyperthermia,* chills, fever, mild weight loss.

**Drug Interactions**
*Methotrexate* / Asparaginase ↓ effect of methotrexate
*Prednisone* / Even though used with asparaginase, may cause ↑ toxicity
*Vincristine* / Even though used with asparaginase, may cause ↑ toxicity; ↑ hyperglycemic effect

**Laboratory Test Interferences:** ↑ Blood ammonia, BUN, glucose, uric acid, AST, ALT, alkaline phosphatase, bilirubin (direct and indirect). ↓ Serum albumin, cholesterol (total and esters), plasma fibrinogen. ↑ or ↓ Decreases in total lipids. Interference with interpretation of thyroid function tests.

**Dosage** ————————
• **IV, IM**
*When used as the sole agent for induction.*
**Adults and children:** 200 IU/kg/day **IV** for 28 days.
*Regimen I for acute lymphocytic leukemia in children.*
Prednisone: 40 mg/m²/day PO in three divided doses for 15 days, followed by tapering of dosage as follows: 20 mg/m²/day for 2 days, 10 mg/m²/day for 2 days, 5 mg/m²/day for 2 days, 2.5 mg/m²/day for 2 days, and then discontinue. Vincristine sulfate: 2 mg/m² IV once weekly on days 1, 8, and 15. The maximum single dose should not exceed 2 mg. Asparaginase: 1,000 IU/kg/day IV for 10 successive days beginning on day 22.
*Regimen II for acute lymphocytic leukemia in children.*

---

✦ = Available in Canada          ***bold italic*** = life threatening side effect

Prednisone: 40 mg/m²/day PO in three divided doses for 28 days with the total daily dose to the nearest 2.5 mg; then, discontinue gradually over 14 days. Vincristine sulfate: 1.5 mg/m² IV weekly for four doses on days 1, 8, 15, and 22. The maximum single dose should not exceed 2 mg. Asparaginase: 6,000 IU/m² IM on days 4, 7, 10, 13, 16, 19, 22, 25, and 28.

When remission is obtained with either regimen, appropriate maintenance therapy should be instituted. Asparaginase should not be used for maintenance therapy.

## NURSING CONSIDERATIONS

See also *General Nursing Considerations* for *Antineoplastic Agents*.

### Administration/Storage

1. Undertake an intradermal skin test (0.1 mL of a 20-IU/mL solution) at least 1 hr before initial administration of drug and when 1 week or more has elapsed between treatments. Observe for at least 1 hr for a wheal or erythema that indicates a positive reaction. A negative skin test reaction does not preclude the possibility of an allergic reaction.

2. A desensitization procedure, with increasing amounts of asparaginase, is sometimes carried out in clients hypersensitive to the drug (1 IU, then double dose every 10 min until total dose for day or reaction occurs).

3. Due to the unpredictability of side effects, initiate treatment only in hospitalized clients.

4. Do not use asparaginase as the sole induction agent unless a combined regimen is not possible due to toxicity or because the client is refractory.

5. For IM use, reconstitute by adding 2 mL NaCL injection to the 10,000-unit vial. Use within 8 hr and only if clear. When used IM, give no more than 2 mL at a single injection site.

6. Handle the drug with care because it is a contact irritant.

7. Have emergency equipment readily available during each administration of asparaginase because a severe hypersensitivity reaction is more likely to occur with this drug.

8. Store both the lyophilized product and reconstituted solution at 2°C–8°C (36°F to 46°F). Discard the reconstituted solution after 8 hr (sooner if it is cloudy).

**IV** 9. See administration guidelines.

10. For IV use, reconstitute the 10,000-unit vial with either 5 mL sterile water for injection or NaCL injection. This solution may be given by direct IV administration within 8 hr following reconstitution. For administration by infusion, dilute solutions with NaCL injection or 5% dextrose injection. Infuse within 8 hr and only if the solution is clear. Infuse over at least 30 min.

### Assessment

1. Document indications for therapy and baseline laboratory studies. Drug may cause mild lymphocyte suppression. Nadir: 7–10 days; recovery 14 days.

2. Obtain LFTs, amylase, and lipase levels periodically and check for evidence of pancreatitis.

3. Assess cardiopulmonary function and document ECG and CXR.

### Interventions

1. Anticipate antiemetic administration prior to drug therapy.

2. Administer vincristine and prednisone before asparaginase to reduce the toxic effects.

3. Asparaginase administration 9–10 days before or within 24 hr after methotrexate may reduce the GI and hematologic effects of methotrexate.

4. Weigh weekly and monitor I&O; assess for any evidence of renal failure. Alkalinization of the urine and allopurinol therapy may help prevent urate stone formation.

5. Observe for peripheral edema due to hypoalbuminemia triggered by asparaginase.

6. Monitor for hyperglycemia, glycosuria, and polyuria, all of which may be precipitated by asparaginase. Have IV fluids and regular insulin available to treat hyperglycemia and stop asparaginase.

**Client/Family Teaching**
1. Promptly report any stomach pain and N&V; may be symptoms of pancreatitis.
2. Report any sudden increase in SOB or coughing, feet swelling, frequent urination, increased thirst, or hyperthermia.
3. Consume 2–3 L/day of fluids.
4. Drug may cause drowsiness, even several weeks after administration; therefore, do not drive a car or operate hazardous machinery.
5. Report shakiness or unusual body movements. A Parkinson-like condition may be precipitated by asparaginase.
6. Avoid immunizations and contact with child who has recently taken poliovirus vaccine.
7. Avoid crowds, especially during flu season. Consider pneumoccal vaccine and annual flu shot.
8. Do not take any aspirin-containing compounds or drink alcoholic beverages.

**Outcomes/Evaluate**
• Improved hematologic parameters
• Inhibition of malignant cell proliferation

---

# Astemizole
(ah-**STEM**-ih-zohl)
**Pregnancy Category:** C
Hismanil **(Rx)**
**Classification:** Antihistamine, miscellaneous

See also *Antihistamines*.
**Action/Kinetics:** Low to no sedative, antiemetic, or anticholinergic effects. Absorption decreased up to 60% when taken with food. Metabolized in the liver to both active and inactive metabolites and excreted through the feces. **t½:** About 1.6 days. **Onset:** 2–3 days. **Duration:** Up to several weeks. Over 95% is bound to plasma protein. Mainly excreted through the feces.
**Uses:** Allergic rhinitis, urticaria.
**Contraindications:** Impaired hepatic function.

**Special Concerns:** Safety and efficacy have not been established in children less than 12 years of age. Dose should not exceed 10 mg/day.
**Additional Side Effects:** *Serious CV side effects, including death, cardiac arrest, QT interval prolongation, torsades de pointes and other ventricular arrhythmias* have been observed in clients exceeding the recommended dose of astemizole. Syncope may precede severe arrhythmias. Overdose may be observed with doses as low as 20–30 mg/day.
**Drug Interactions:** Concomitant use of astemizole with erythromycin, itraconazole, or ketoconazole may cause serious CV effects, including death, cardiac arrest, torsades de pointes, and other ventricular arrhythmias (including QT interval prolongation).

**Dosage**
• **Tablets**
**Adults and children over 12 years:** 10 mg once daily. **Children, 6–12 years:** 5 mg daily; **children, less than 6 years:** 0.2 mg/kg/day.

## NURSING CONSIDERATIONS

See also *Nursing Considerations* for *Antihistamines*.
**Administration/Storage:** Do not exceed the recommended dose in an attempt to increase the onset of action.
**Client/Family Teaching**
1. Take medication on an empty stomach at least 2 hr after a meal with no additional food taken for at least 1 hr after taking because food interferes with drug absorption.
2. Do not exceed prescribed dose. Take only as directed; effects may not be noticeable immediately. Usual initial course of therapy is 10 days.
3. Report if S&S unrelieved or any persistent side effects, including depression or weight gain.
4. Advise all providers of drug therapy to prevent any potentially lethal

---

A

drug interactions, as with erythromycin, itraconazole, or ketoconazole.
**Outcomes/Evaluate:** ↓ Congestion and ↓ allergic symptoms

---

# Atenolol

(ah-**TEN**-oh-lohl)
**Pregnancy Category:** C
Apo-Atenol ✦, Gen-Atenolol ✦, Med-Atenolol ✦, Novo-Atenol ✦, Nu-Atenol ✦, Taro-Atenolol ✦, Tenolin ✦, Tenormin **(Rx)**
**Classification:** Beta-adrenergic blocking agent

---

See also *Beta-Adrenergic Blocking Agents.*
**Action/Kinetics:** Predominantly beta-1 blocking activity. Has no membrane stabilizing activity or intrinsic sympathomimetic activity. Low lipid solubility. **Peak blood levels:** 2–4 hr. t½: 6–9 hr. 50% eliminated unchanged in the feces.
**Uses:** Hypertension (either alone or with other antihypertensives such as thiazide diuretics). Angina pectoris due to hypertension, coronary atherosclerosis, and AMI. *Investigational:* Prophylaxis of migraine, alcohol withdrawal syndrome, situational anxiety, ventricular arrhythmias, prophylactically to reduce incidence of supraventricular arrhythmias in coronary artery bypass surgery.
**Special Concerns:** Dosage has not been established in children.

**Dosage** —————————————
• **Tablets**
*Hypertension.*
**Initial:** 50 mg/day, either alone or with diuretics; if response is inadequate, 100 mg/day. Doses higher than 100 mg/day will not produce further beneficial effects. Maximum effects usually seen within 1–2 weeks.
*Angina.*
**Initial:** 50 mg/day; if maximum response is not seen in 1 week, increase dose to 100 mg/day (some clients require 200 mg/day).
*Alcohol withdrawal syndrome.*
50–100 mg/day.
*Prophylaxis of migraine.*

50–100 mg/day.
*Ventricular arrhythmias.*
50–100 mg/day.
*Prior to coronary artery bypass surgery.*
50 mg/day started 72 hr prior to surgery.
Adjust dosage in cases of renal failure to 50 mg/day if creatinine clearance is 15–35 mL/min/1.73 m² and to 50 mg every other day if creatinine clearance is less than 15 mL/min/1.73 m².
• **IV**
*Acute myocardial infarction.*
**Initial:** 5 mg over 5 min followed by a second 5-mg dose 10 min later. Begin treatment as soon as possible after client arrives at the hospital. In clients who tolerate the full 10-mg dose, give a 50-mg tablet 10 min after the last IV dose followed by another 50-mg dose 12 hr later. **Then,** 100 mg/day or 50 mg b.i.d. for 6–9 days (or until discharge from the hospital).

---

# NURSING CONSIDERATIONS

See also *Nursing Considerations* for *Antihypertensive Agents* and *Beta-Adrenergic Blocking Agents.*
**Administration/Storage**
1. For hemodialysis clients, give 50 mg in the hospital after each dialysis. **IV** 2. For IV use, the drug may be diluted in NaCL injection, dextrose injection, or NaCL and dextrose injection.
**Assessment**
1. Document indications for therapy, type, and onset of symptoms.
2. Note any history of diabetes, pulmonary disease, or cardiac failure.
**Client/Family Teaching**
1. With angina, do not stop drug abruptly as this could precipitate an anginal attack.
2. Report any changes in mood or affect, especially severe depression.
3. Drug may enhance sensitivity to cold.
4. With initiation of therapy or change in dosage stress the importance of returning as scheduled for evaluation of response to medication.

## Outcomes/Evaluate

- ↓ BP; ↓ HR
- ↓ Frequency of anginal attacks
- Prevention of reinfarction

# Atorvastatin calcium
((ah-**TORE**-vah-**stah**-tin))
**Pregnancy Category:** X
Lipitor **(Rx)**
**Classification:** Antihyperlipidemic, HMG–CoA reductase inhibitor

See also *Antihyperlipidemic Agents —HMG–CoA Reductase Inhibitors.*
**Action/Kinetics:** Atorvastatin undergoes first-pass metabolism. **t½:** 14 hr. The drug is over 98% bound to plasma proteins. Plasma levels are not affected by renal disease but they are markedly increased with chronic alcoholic liver disease.
**Uses:** Adjunct to diet to reduce elevated total and LDL cholesterol levels in primary hypercholesterolemia (Types IIa and IIb) when the response to diet and other nondrug measures alone have been inadequate.
**Contraindications:** Active liver disease or unexplained persistently high liver function tests. Pregnancy, lactation.
**Special Concerns:** Safety and efficacy have not been determined in children less than 18 years of age.
**Side Effects:** See also *Antihyperlipidemic Agents—HMG–CoA Reductase Inhibitors. GI:* Altered liver function tests (usually within the first 3 months of therapy). *Musculoskeletal:* Myalgia. *Miscellaneous:* Infection, hypersensitivity reactions, photosensitivity.
**Laboratory Test Alterations:** ↑ CPK (due to myalgia).
**Drug Interactions**
*Antacids /* ↓ Atorvastatin plasma levels
*Colestipol /* ↓ Plasma levels of atorvastatin
*Erythromycin /* ↑ Plasma levels of erythromycin
*Oral contraceptives /* ↑ Plasma levels of norethindrone and ethinyl estradiol

## Dosage

- **Tablets**
  *Hyperlipidemia.*
  **Initial:** 10 mg/day; **then,** a dose range of 10–80 mg/day may be used.

# NURSING CONSIDERATIONS

See also *Nursing Considerations* for *Antihyperlipidemic Agents—HMG–CoA Reductase Inhibitors.*
**Administration/Storage**
1. Give as a single dose at any time of the day, with or without food.
2. Determine lipid levels within 2–4 weeks and adjust dosage accordingly.
3. For an additive effect, atorvastatin may be used in combination with a bile acid binding resin. However, atorvastatin should not be used with fibrates.
**Assessment**
1. Document indications for therapy, onset and duration of disease, and other agents and measures trialed.
2. Obtain baseline cholesterol profile and liver function tests.
3. Monitor liver function tests at 6 and 12 weeks after starting therapy and with any dosage change; monitor semiannually thereafter. If ALT or AST exceed 3 times the normal level, reduce dose or withdraw drug therapy. Assess need for liver biopsy if elevations remain after stopping drug therapy.
4. Avoid combination therapy with fibrates.
5. Review dietary habits, weight, and exercise patterns; identify lifestyle changes needed.
**Client/Family Teaching**
1. These drugs help to lower blood cholesterol and fat levels, which have been proven to promote CAD.
2. Drug may be taken with or without food.
3. Continue dietary restrictions of saturated fat and cholesterol, regular exercise and weight loss in the over-

---

✦ = Available in Canada                    ***bold italic*** = life threatening side effect

all goal of lowering serum cholesterol levels. See dietician for additional diet instructions.

4. Report immediately any unexplained muscle pain, weakness, or tenderness, especially if accompanied by fever or malaise.

5. Use UV protection (i.e., sunglasses, sunscreens, protective clothing, and hat) to prevent a photosensitivity reaction.

6. Report for lab studies to evaluate drug effectiveness and for dosage adjustments.

**Outcomes/Evaluate:** Reduction in total and LDL cholesterol levels

---

# Atovaquone
(ah-**TOV**-ah-kwohn)
**Pregnancy Category:** C
Mepron **(Rx)**
**Classification:** Antiprotozoal agent

**Action/Kinetics:** The mechanism of action of atovaquone against *Pneumocystis carinii* is not known. However, in *Plasmodium,* the drug appears to act by inhibiting electron transport resulting in inhibition of nucleic acid and ATP synthesis. The bioavailability of the drug is increased twofold when taken with food. The tablet formulation has been replaced by a suspension, as the latter achieves plasma levels of atovaquone that are 58% higher than those reached using tablets. Plasma levels in AIDS clients are about one-third to one-half the levels achieved in asymptomatic HIV-infected volunteers. **t½:** 2.2 days in AIDS clients due to enterohepatic cycling and eventually fecal elimination. Not metabolized in the liver; over 94% is excreted unchanged in the feces.

**Uses:** Acute oral treatment of mild to moderate *P. carinii* in clients who are intolerant to trimethoprim-sulfamethoxazole. The drug has not been evaluated as an agent for prophylaxis of *P. carinii*. Not effective for concurrent pulmonary diseases such as bacterial, viral, or fungal pneumonia or in mycobacterial diseases.

**Contraindications:** Hypersensitivity to atovaquone or any components of the formulation; potentially life-threatening allergic reactions are possible.

**Special Concerns:** Use with caution during lactation and in elderly clients. There are no efficacy studies in children. GI disorders may limit absorption of atovaquone.

**Side Effects:** Since many clients taking atovaquone have complications of HIV disease, it is often difficult to distinguish side effects caused by atovaquone from symptoms caused by the underlying medical condition. *Dermatologic:* Rash (including maculopapular), pruritus. *GI:* Nausea, diarrhea, vomiting, abdominal pain, constipation, dyspepsia, taste perversion. *CNS:* Headache, fever, insomnia, dizziness, anxiety, anorexia. *Respiratory:* Cough, sinusitis, rhinitis. *Hematologic:* Anemia, neutropenia. *Miscellaneous:* Asthenia, oral monilia, pain, sweating, hypoglycemia, hypotension, hyperglycemia, hyponatremia.

**Drug Interactions:** Since atovaquone is highly bound to plasma proteins (>99.9%), caution should be exercised when giving the drug with other highly plasma protein-bound drugs with narrow therapeutic indices as competition for binding may occur.

**Laboratory Test Interferences:** ↑ ALT, AST, alkaline phosphatase, amylase.

## Dosage
• **Suspension**
**Adults:** 750 mg (5 mL) given with food b.i.d. for 21 days (total daily dose: 1,500 mg).

## NURSING CONSIDERATIONS
### Administration/Storage
1. Take with meals as food significantly enhances absorption. Failure to give the drug with food may result in lower plasma levels and may limit the response to therapy.

2. Dispense drug in a well-closed container and store at 15°C –25°C (59°F –77°F).

### Assessment
1. Document previous therapy for

*P. carinii,* agents used, and outcome.

2. Assess baseline pulmonary status, CBC, and pulmonary culture results.

3. Clients with acute *P. carinii* must be carefully evaluated/screened for other related pulmonary diseases of viral, bacterial, or fungal origin and treated with additional drugs as appropriate.

**Client/Family Teaching**

1. Take only as directed and with meals to enhance absorption.

2. Review drug side effects noting those that require immediate reporting.

3. This is not a cure but alleviates symptoms of *P. carinii.*

4. Do not exceed prescribed dose and do not share medication.

5. Continue precautions for safe sex, as the risk of HIV transmission is not reduced.

6. Identify appropriate support groups and individuals to assist the client/family to understand and cope with disease.

**Outcomes/Evaluate:** Relief of symptoms R/T *Pneumocystis carinii*; three consecutive negative sputum cultures

---

# Atracurium besylate

(ah-trah-**KYOUR**-ee-um)
**Pregnancy Category:** C
Tracrium Injection **(Rx)**
**Classification:** Nondepolarizing skeletal muscle relaxant

---

See also *Neuromuscular Blocking Agents.*

**Action/Kinetics:** Atracurium prevents the action of acetylcholine by competing for the cholinergic receptor at the motor end plate. It may also release histamine, leading to hypotension. **Onset:** Within 2 min. **Peak effect:** 1–2 min. **Duration:** 20–40 min with balanced anesthesia. Recovery from blockade under balanced anesthesia begins about 20–35 min after injection; recovery is usually 95% complete within 60–70 min after injection. **t½:** 20 min.

Recovery occurs more rapidly than recovery from *d*-tubocurarine, metocurine, and pancuronium. Metabolized in the plasma.

**Uses:** Skeletal muscle relaxant during surgery; adjunct to general anesthesia; assist in ET intubation. *Investigational:* Treat seizures due to drugs or electrically induced.

**Contraindications:** In clients with myasthenia gravis, Eaton-Lambert syndrome, electrolyte disorders, bronchial asthma.

**Special Concerns:** Use with caution during labor and delivery and when significant histamine release would be dangerous (e.g., CV disease, asthma). Safety and efficacy have not been determined during lactation. Children up to 1 month of age may be more sensitive to the effects of atracurium. The drug has no known effect on pain threshold or consciousness; use only with adequate anesthesia.

**Additional Side Effects:** *CV:* Flushing, tachycardia. *Dermatologic:* Rash, urticaria, reaction at injection site. *Musculoskeletal:* Prolonged block, inadequate block. *Respiratory:* Dyspnea, laryngospasm. *Hypersensitivity:* Allergic reactions. Other side effects may be due to histamine release and include flushing, erythema, wheezing, urticaria, bronchial secretions, BP and HR changes.

**OD** **Overdose Management:** *Symptoms:* Hypotension, enhanced pharmacologic effects. *Treatment:* CV support. Ensure airway and ventilation. An anticholinesterase reversing agent (e.g., neostigmine, edrophonium, pyridostigmine) with an anticholinergic agent (e.g., atropine, glycopyrrolate) may be used.

**Additional Drug Interactions**

*Acetylcholinesterase inhibitors /* Muscle relaxation is inhibited and neuromuscular block is reversed

*Aminoglycosides /* ↑ Muscle relaxation

*Corticosteroids /* Prolonged weakness

*Enflurane /* ↑ Muscle relaxation

---

Halothane / ↑ Muscle relaxation
Isoflurane / ↑ Muscle relaxation
Lithium / ↑ Muscle relaxation
Phenytoin / ↓ Effect of atracurium
Procainamide / ↑ Muscle relaxation
Quinidine / ↑ Muscle relaxation
Succinylcholine / ↑ Onset and
depth of muscle relaxation
Theophylline / ↓ Effect of atracurium
Trimethaphan / ↑ Muscle relaxation
Verapamil / ↑ Muscle relaxation

## Dosage

• **IV Bolus Only**
Intubation and maintenance of neuromuscular blockade.
**Adults and children over 2 years, initial:** 0.4–0.5 mg/kg as IV bolus; **maintenance:** 0.08–0.1 mg/kg. The first maintenance dose is usually required 20–45 min after the initial dose. Give maintenance doses every 15–25 min under balanced anesthesia, slightly longer under isoflurane or enflurane anesthesia.
Following use of succinylcholine for intubation under balanced anesthesia.
**Initial:** 0.3–0.4 mg/kg; if using potent inhalation anesthetics, further reductions may be required.
Use in neuromuscular disease, severe electrolyte disorders, or carcinomatosis.
Dosage reductions should be considered where potentiation of neuromuscular blockade or difficulty with reversal have been noted.
Use after steady-state enflurane or isoflurane anesthesia established.
0.25–0.35 mg/kg (about ⅓ less than the usual initial dose).
Use in infants 1 month to 2 years of age under halothane anesthesia.
0.3–0.4 mg/kg. More frequent maintenance doses may be required.
• **IV Infusion**
Balanced anesthesia.
**IV infusion:** 9–10 mcg/kg until the level of neuromuscular blockade is reestablished; **then,** rate of infusion is adjusted according to client needs (usually 5–9 mcg/kg/min although some clients may require as little as 2 mcg/kg/min and others as much as 15 mcg/kg/min).

For cardiopulmonary bypass surgery in which hypothermia is induced.
Reduce rate of infusion by 50%.

## NURSING CONSIDERATIONS

See also Nursing Considerations for Neuromuscular Blocking Agents.
### Administration/Storage
**IV** 1. Use only by those skilled in airway management and respiratory support. Equipment and personnel must be available immediately for endotracheal intubation and support of ventilation. Anticholinesterase reversal agents should be immediately available.
2. Reduce initial dose to 0.25–0.35 mg/kg if drug is being used with steady-state enflurane or isoflurane (smaller reductions if halothane is being used).
3. Reduce dosage in clients with myasthenia gravis or other neuromuscular diseases, electrolyte disorders, or carcinomatosis.
4. Infusion solutions are prepared by admixing atracurium with either 5% dextrose injection, 0.9% sodium chloride injection, or 5% dextrose and 0.9% sodium chloride injection. Do not mix with alkaline solutions, including lactated Ringer's injection.
5. Maintenance doses can be given by continuous infusion of a diluted solution to clients 2 years of age to adulthood.
6. Solutions containing 0.2 or 0.5 mg/mL can be stored either under refrigeration or at room temperature for 24 hr without significant loss of potency.
7. To preserve potency, refrigerate the drug at 2°C–8°C (36°F–46°F).
8. IM administration may cause tissue irritation.
9. Drug does not affect consciousness or pain threshold; use concomitant antianxiety agents and analgesics.
10. IV atropine may be used to treat bradycardia due to atracurium.
### Assessment
1. Document indications for therapy, onset, duration, and characteristics of symptoms.
2. Utilize a peripheral nerve stimula-

tor to assess neuromuscular response and recovery.
3. Obtain baseline ECG, VS, and lab studies and monitor. Drug can cause vagal stimulation resulting in bradycardia, hypotension, and cardiac arrhythmias.
4. Document length of therapy; drug should only be used on a short-term basis and in a continuously monitored environment.
5. Client may be fully conscious and aware of surroundings and conversations. Drug does not affect pain or anxiety; administer analgesics and/or antianxiety agents regularly.

**Outcomes/Evaluate**
- Skeletal muscle relaxation
- Facilitation of ET intubation; tolerance of mechanical ventilation
- Control of electrically/pharmacologically induced seizures

# Atropine sulfate
(**AH**-troh-peen)
**Pregnancy Category:** C
Atropair, Atropine-1 Ophthalmic, Atropine Sulfate Ophthalmic, Atropine-Care Ophthalmic, Atropisol Ophthalmic, Dioptic's Atropine ✴, Isopto Atropine Ophthalmic, Minims Atropine ✴ (**Rx**)
**Classification:** Cholinergic blocking agent

See also *Cholinergic Blocking Agents.*
**Action/Kinetics:** Atropine blocks the action of acetylcholine on postganglionic cholinergic receptors in smooth muscle, cardiac muscle, exocrine glands, urinary bladder, and the AV and SA nodes in the heart. Ophthalmologically, atropine blocks the effect of acetylcholine on the sphincter muscle of the iris and the accommodative muscle of the ciliary body. This results in dilation of the pupil (mydriasis) and paralysis of the muscles required to accommodate for close vision (cycloplegia). **Peak effect:** M*ydriasis,* 30–40 min; *cycloplegia,* 1–3 hr. **Recovery:** Up to 12 days. **Duration, PO:** 4–6 hr. **t½:**

2.5 hr. Metabolized by the liver although 30%–50% is excreted through the kidneys unchanged.
**Uses: PO:** Adjunct in peptic ulcer treatment. Irritable bowel syndrome. Adjunct in treatment of spastic disorders of the biliary tract. Urologic disorders, urinary incontinence. During anesthesia to control salivation and bronchial secretions. Has been used for parkinsonism but more effective drugs are available.
  **Parenteral:** Antiarrhythmic, adjunct in GI radiography. Prophylaxis of arrhythmias induced by succinylcholine or surgical procedures. Reduce sinus bradycardia (severe) and syncope in hyperactive carotid sinus reflex. Prophylaxis and treatment of toxicity due to cholinesterase inhibitors, including organophosphate pesticides. Treatment of curariform block. As a preanesthetic or in dentistry to decrease secretions.
  **Ophthalmologic:** Cycloplegic refraction or pupillary dilation in acute inflammatory conditions of the iris and uveal tract. *Investigational:* Treatment and prophylaxis of posterior synechiae; pre- and postoperative mydriasis; treatment of malignant glaucoma.
**Additional Contraindications:** Ophthalmic use: Infants less than 3 months of age, primary glaucoma or a tendency toward glaucoma, adhesions between the iris and the lens, geriatric clients and others where undiagnosed glaucoma or excessive pressure in the eye may be present, in children who have had a previous severe systemic reaction to atropine.
**Special Concerns:** Use with caution in infants, small children, geriatric clients, diabetes, hypo- or hyperthyroidism, narrow anterior chamber angle, individuals with Down syndrome.
**Additional Side Effects:** *Ophthalmologic:* Blurred vision, stinging, increased intraocular pressure, contact dermatitis. Long-term use may cause irritation, photophobia, eczematoid

---

**A**

dermatitis, conjunctivitis, hyperemia, or edema.

**OD** **Overdose Management:** *Treatment of Ocular Overdose:* Eyes should be flushed with water or normal saline. A topical miotic may be necessary.

## Dosage

- **Tablets**

*Anticholinergic or antispasmodic.*
**Adults:** 0.3–1.2 mg q 4–6 hr. **Pediatric, over 41 kg:** same as adult; **29.5–41 kg:** 0.4 mg q 4–6 hr; **18.2–29.5 kg:** 0.3 mg q 4–6 hr; **10.9–18.2 kg:** 0.2 mg q 4–6 hr; **7.3–10.9 kg:** 0.15 mg q 4–6 hr; **3.2–7.3 kg:** 0.1 mg q 4–6 hr.

*Prophylaxis of respiratory tract secretions and excess salivation during anesthesia.*
**Adults:** 2 mg.

*Parkinsonism.*
**Adults:** 0.1–0.25 mg q.i.d.

- **IM, IV, SC**

*Anticholinergic.*
**Adults, IM, IV, SC:** 0.4–0.6 mg q 4–6 hr. **Pediatric, SC:** 0.01 mg/kg, not to exceed 0.4 mg (or 0.3 mg/m²).

*To reverse curariform blockade.*
**Adults, IV:** 0.6–1.2 mg given at the same time or a few minutes before 0.5–2 mg neostigmine methylsulfate (use separate syringes).

*Treatment of toxicity from cholinesterase inhibitors.*
**Adults, IV, initial:** 2–4 mg; **then,** 2 mg repeated q 5–10 min until muscarinic symptoms disappear and signs of atropine toxicity begin to appear. **Pediatric, IM, IV, initial:** 1 mg; **then,** 0.5–1 mg q 5–10 min until muscarinic symptoms disappear and signs of atropine toxicity appear.

*Treatment of mushroom poisoning due to muscarine.*
**Adults, IM, IV:** 1–2 mg q hr until respiratory effects decrease.

*Treatment of organophosphate poisoning.*
**Adults, IM, IV, initial:** 1–2 mg; **then,** repeat in 20–30 min (as soon as cyanosis has disappeared). Dosage may be continued for up to 2 days until symptoms improve.

*Arrhythmias.*

**Pediatric, IV:** 0.01–0.03 mg/kg.

*Prophylaxis of respiratory tract secretions, excessive salivation, succinylcholine- or surgical procedure-induced arrhythmias.*
**Pediatric, up to 3 kg, SC:** 0.1 mg; **7–9 kg:** 0.2 mg; **12–16 kg:** 0.3 mg; **20–27 kg:** 0.4 mg; **32 kg:** 0.5 mg; **41 kg:** 0.6 mg.

- **Ophthalmic Solution**

*Uveitis.*
**Adults:** 1–2 gtt instilled into the eye(s) up to q.i.d. **Children:** 1–2 gtt of the 0.5% solution into the eye(s) up to t.i.d.

*Refraction.*
**Adults:** 1–2 gtt of the 1% solution into the eye(s) 1 hr before refracting. **Children:** 1–2 gtt of the 0.5% solution into the eye(s) b.i.d. for 1–3 days before refraction.

- **Ophthalmic Ointment**

Instill a small amount into the conjunctival sac up to t.i.d.

## NURSING CONSIDERATIONS

See also *Nursing Considerations* for *Cholinergic Blocking Agents.*

### Administration/Storage

1. For ophthalmic use, atropine sulfate is available in 0.5%, 1%, or 2% solutions or 1% ointment.
2. After instillation of the ophthalmic ointment, compress the lacrimal sac by digital pressure for 1–3 min. This tends to decrease systemic effects.
3. Have physostigmine available in the event of overdose.

### Assessment

1. Document indications for therapy and any presenting symptoms.
2. Check for any history of angle-closure glaucoma before ophthalmic administration because atropine may precipitate an acute crisis.
3. Obtain VS and ECG; monitor cardiopulmonary status during IV therapy.

### Client/Family Teaching

1. When used in the eye, vision will be temporarily impaired. Close work, operating machinery, or driving a car should be avoided until drug effects have worn off.

2. Do not blink excessively; wait 5 min before instilling any other drops.

3. Drug impairs heat regulation; avoid strenuous activity in hot environments; wear sunglasses with sun exposure.

4. Males with prostatic hypertrophy may experience urinary retention and hesitancy.

5. Increase fluids and add bulk to diet to diminish constipating effects.

6. Use sugarless candies and gums to decrease dry mouth symptoms.

**Outcomes/Evaluate**

- ↑ HR
- Desired pupillary dilatation
- ↓ GI activity; ↓ Salivation
- Reversal of muscarinic effects of anticholinesterase agents

---

# Auranofin

(or-**AN**-oh-fin)
**Pregnancy Category:** C
Ridaura **(Rx)**
**Classification:** Antiarthritic, oral gold compound

**Action/Kinetics:** Auranofin is a gold-containing (29%) compound for PO administration. It has fewer side effects than injectable gold products. Although the mechanism is not known, auranofin will improve symptoms of rheumatoid arthritis; it is most effective in the early stages of active synovitis and may act by inhibiting sulfhydryl systems. Other possible mechanisms include inhibition of phagocytic activity of macrophages and polymorphonuclear leukocytes, alteration of biosynthesis of collagen, and alteration of the immune response. Gold will not reverse damage to joints caused by disease. Approximately 25% of an oral dose is absorbed. **Plasma t½ of auranofin gold:** 26 days. **Onset:** 3–4 months (up to 6 months in certain clients). Approximately 3 months are required for steady-state blood levels to be achieved. The drug is metabolized and excreted in both the urine and feces.

**Uses:** Adults and children with rheumatoid arthritis that has not responded to other drugs. Up to 6 months may be required for beneficial effects to occur. Auranofin should be part of a total treatment regimen for rheumatoid arthritis, including nondrug treatments.

**Contraindications:** History of gold-induced disorders including necrotizing enterocolitis, pulmonary fibrosis, exfoliative dermatitis, bone marrow aplasia, or other hematologic severe disorders. Use during lactation.

**Special Concerns:** Use with extreme caution in renal or hepatic disease, skin rashes, marked hypertension, compromised cerebral or CV circulation, or history of bone marrow depression (e.g., agranulocytopenia, anemia). Gold dermatitis may be aggravated by exposure to sunlight. Although used in children, a recommended dosage has not been established. Tolerance to gold is often decreased in geriatric clients.

**Side Effects:** *GI:* N&V, diarrhea (common), abdominal pain, metallic taste, stomatitis, glossitis, gingivitis, anorexia, constipation, flatulence, dyspepsia, dysgeusia, melena. Rarely, dysphagia, *GI bleeding, ulcerative enterocolitis.* *Dermatologic:* Skin rashes, pruritus, alopecia, urticaria, angioedema, actinic rash. *Hematologic:* Leukopenia, anemia, thrombocytopenia (with or without purpura), neutropenia, agranulocytosis, eosinophilia, pancytopenia, hypoplastic anemia, *aplastic anemia,* pure red cell aplasia. *Renal:* Proteinuria, hematuria. *Hepatic:* Jaundice (with or without cholestasis, hepatitis with jaundice, *toxic hepatitis,* intrahepatic cholestasis. *Other:* Conjunctivitis, cholestatic jaundice, fever, interstitial pneumonia and fibrosis, peripheral neuropathy.

**OD** **Overdose Management:** *Symptoms:* Rapid appearance of hematuria, proteinuria, thrombocytopenia, granulocytopenia. Also, N&V, diarrhea, fever, urticaria, papu-

---

lovesicular lesions, urticaria, exfoliative dermatitis, pruritus. *Treatment:* Discontinue promptly and give dimercaprol. Supportive therapy should be provided for renal and hematologic symptoms. Treat moderately severe skin and mucous membrane symptoms with topical corticosteroids, oral antihistamines, and anesthetic lotions. Treat severe stomatitis or dermatitis with prednisone, 10–40 mg daily. Treat serious renal, hematologic, pulmonary, and enterocolitic complications with prednisone, 40–100 mg daily in divided doses. The duration of treatment varies, depending on the severity of symptoms and the response to steroids. In acute overdosage, induce emesis or perform gastric lavage immediately.

**Laboratory Test Interferences:** ↑ Liver enzymes.

## Dosage

- **Capsules**

  *Rheumatoid arthritis.*

**Adults, initial:** Either 6 mg/day or 3 mg b.i.d. If response is unsatisfactory after 6 months, increase to 3 mg t.i.d. If response is still inadequate after 3 additional months, the drug should be discontinued. Dosages greater than 9 mg/day are not recommended.

**Children, initial:** 0.1 mg/kg/day; **maintenance:** 0.15 mg/kg/day, not to exceed 0.2 mg/kg/day.

  *Transfer from injectable gold.*

Discontinue injectable gold and begin auranofin at a dose of 6 mg/day.

## NURSING CONSIDERATIONS

**Administration/Storage:** A positive response should be noted after 6 months of therapy.

**Assessment**

1. Review history, note any other severe systemic diseases such as renal, hepatic, or cardiac dysfunction.

2. Document extent of debilitation (functional class), pain level, ROM, and active synovitis.

3. Note onset, course of disease, other agents used, including disease-modifying agents, and the outcome.

4. Inspect skin to determine if there are any skin eruptions.

5. Assess gums and oral mucosa, noting any lesions or treatment needs.

6. Obtain baseline CBC, ESR, X rays, and liver and renal function studies.

7. Clients with diabetes mellitus or CHF should be well controlled before beginning gold therapy.

**Interventions**

1. Determine if a dermal test dose has ever been performed with a gold salt.

2. Monitor and record I&O and weight.

3. If diarrhea develops, monitor electrolytes and report any abnormality.

4. Monitor liver and renal function studies; send urine for protein and blood.

5. Observe for peripheral neuropathy.

6. Encourage to return for follow-up evaluation; provide a 2-week medication supply.

**Client/Family Teaching**

1. Avoid sunlight. If exposure is necessary, wear long sleeves and pants, a hat, glasses, and apply a sunscreen.

2. Practice regular oral hygiene, including regular tooth brushing, daily flossing, checkups and mouth washes, avoiding those with alcohol or other drying ingredients.

3. Report any signs of toxicity (skin rash, pruritus, metallic taste, stomatitis, diarrhea, leukopenia, and thrombocytopenia).

4. Women should use a reliable form of contraception.

5. Skin irritation (puritic dermatitis) and mouth ulcers may persist for months after discontinuing medication.

6. Expect to continue anti-inflammatory doses of NSAIDs for several weeks to months until auranofin takes effect. It may take up to 6 months of therapy before improvement will be noticed.

**Outcomes/Evaluate**

- Improved mobility and ROM
- ↓ Pain, swelling, and stiffness in joints

- Slowing of the progression and degenerative effects of rheumatoid arthritis

# Aurothioglucose suspension

(or-oh-thigh-oh-**GLOO**-kohz)
**Pregnancy Category:** C
Solganol **(Rx)**
**Classification:** Antiarthritic

For additional information regarding aurothioglucose, see *Gold Sodium Thiomalate*.
**Action/Kinetics:** The gold content of aurothioglucose is 50%. **Time to peak effect:** 4–6 hr. **Mean steady-state plasma levels:** 1–6 mc/mL. Is 95%–99% protein bound. **t½, after 11th dose:** Up to 168 days. Seventy percent is excreted in the urine and 30% is excreted through the urine.
**Side Effects:** *GI:* N&V, anorexia, abdominal cramps, metallic taste, gastritis, *ulcerative enterocolitis*, colitis. *Dermatologic:* Dermatitis (papular, vesicular, exfoliative), rash, urticaria, angioedema, chrysiasis. *Renal:* Nephrotic syndrome, glomerulonephritis with proteinuria and hematuria, acute renal failure secondary to acute tubular necrosis, acute nephritis, degeneration of proximal tubular epithelium. *Hematologic:* **Granulocytopenia, panmyelopathy, hemorrhagic diathesis.** *Respiratory:* Inflammation of upper respiratory tract, pharyngitis, tracheitis, bold bronchitis, interstitial pneumonitis, fibrosis. *CNS:* Confusion, hallucinations, *seizures*. *Mucous membranes:* Stomatitis, diffuse glossitis, gingivitis. *Reactions of the nitroid type:* Anaphylactoid symptoms, flushing, fainting, dizziness, sweating, N&V, malaise, headache, weakness. *Ophthalmologic:* Iritis, corneal ulcers, gold deposits in ocular tissues. *Miscellaneous:* Vaginitis.
**OD** **Overdose Management:** *Treatment:* Discontinue and give dimercaprol. Provide supportive therapy for renal and hematologic

symptoms. In acute overdose, induce emesis or gastric lavage immediately.

**Dosage**
- **IM Only**
  *Rheumatoid arthritis.*
**Adults:** *Week 1:* 10 mg; *weeks 2 and 3:* 25 mg; **then,** 25–50 (maximum) mg/week until a total of 0.8–1 g has been administered. If client tolerates the dose and has improved, 50 mg may be given q 3–4 weeks for several months. **Pediatric, 6–12 years:** *Week 1:* 2.5 mg; *weeks 2 and 3:* 6.25 mg; **then,** 12.5 mg/week until a total dose of 200–250 mg has been administered. **Maintenance:** 6.25–12.5 mg q 3–4 weeks.

# NURSING CONSIDERATIONS

See also *Nursing Considerations* for *Gold Sodium Thiomalate*.
**Administration/Storage**
1. Give IM injections only in the upper outer quadrant of the gluteal region using an 18-gauge, 1½-in. needle (or 2 in. for obese clients).
2. To obtain a uniform suspension, shake the vial carefully before the dose is withdrawn.
3. Both the syringe and needle used to withdraw the dose should be dry.
4. The vial can be immersed in warm water to assist with withdrawing the appropriate dose of the suspension.
**Assessment**
1. Document any sensitivity to sesame oil and determine if a dermal test dose has been performed.
2. Monitor CBC, liver and renal function studies. Assess for blood dyscrasias, photosensitivity reactions, hepatic dysfunction, nephrotoxicity, and fibrosis of the lungs (pneumonitis).
3. Client should remain lying down for 10 min after injection and be observed for 15 min following administration for evidence of flushing, dizziness, sweating, and hypotension (nitritoid reaction).
4. Carefully determine dosage and

track until maximum total level is administered.

5. Assess mobility and stress the need to continue anti-inflammatory doses of NSAIDs for several more months.

**Outcomes/Evaluate**
• ↓ Joint pain, swelling, and stiffness with improved ROM
• Slowing of the progression and degenerative effects of rheumatoid arthritis

# Azathioprine
(ay-zah-**THIGH**-oh-preen)
**Pregnancy Category:** D
Imuran **(Rx)**
**Classification:** Immunosuppressant

**Action/Kinetics:** Antimetabolite that is quickly split to form mercaptopurine. To be effective, the drug must be given during the induction period of the antibody response. The precise mechanism in depressing the immune response is unknown, but it suppresses cell-mediated hypersensitivities and alters antibody production. The drug inhibits synthesis of DNA, RNA, and proteins and may interfere with meiosis and cellular metabolism. The mechanism for its effect on autoimmune diseases is not known. Is readily absorbed from the GI tract. The anuric client manifests increased effectiveness and toxicity (up to twofold). **Onset:** 6–8 weeks for rheumatoid arthritis. **t½:** 3 hr.

**Uses:** As an adjunct to prevent rejection in renal homotransplantation. In adult clients meeting criteria for classic or definite rheumatoid arthritis as defined by the American Rheumatism Association. Restrict use to clients with severe, active, and erosive disease that is not responsive to conventional therapy. *Investigational:* Chronic ulcerative colitis, generalized myasthenia gravis, to control the progression of Behçet's syndrome (especially eye disease), Crohn's disease (low doses).

**Contraindications:** Treatment of rheumatoid arthritis in pregnancy or in clients previously treated with alkylating agents. Pregnancy and lactation.

**Special Concerns:** Hematologic toxicity is dose-related and may occur late in the course of therapy; may be more severe in renal transplant clients undergoing rejection. Although used in children, safety and efficacy have not been established.

**Side Effects:** *Hematologic:* Leukopenia, thrombocytopenia, macrocytic anemia, *severe bone marrow depression,* selective erythrocyte aplasia. *GI:* N&V, diarrhea, abdominal pain, steatorrhea. *CNS:* Fever, malaise. *Other: Increased risk of carcinoma,* severe infections (fungal, viral, bacterial, and protozoal), and *hepatotoxicity* are major side effects. Also, skin rashes, alopecia, myalgias, increase in liver enzymes, hypotension, negative nitrogen balance.

**OD** **Overdose Management:** *Symptoms:* Large doses may result in *bone marrow hypoplasia,* bleeding, infection, and death. *Treatment:* Approximately 45% can be removed from the body following 8 hr of hemodialysis.

**Drug Interactions**
*ACE inhibitors* / ↑ Risk of severe leukopenia
*Allopurinol* / ↑ Pharmacologic effect of azathioprine due to ↓ breakdown in liver
*Anticoagulants* / ↓ Effect of anticoagulants
*Corticosteroids* / With azathioprine, it may cause muscle wasting after prolonged therapy
*Cyclosporine* / ↑ Plasma levels of cyclosporine
*Methotrexate* / ↑ Plasma levels of the active metabolite, 6-mercaptopurine
*Tubocurarine* / Azathioprine ↓ effect of tubocurarine and other nondepolarizing neuromuscular blocking agents

**Dosage**
• **Tablets, IV**
*Use in renal homotransplantation.*
**Adults and children, initial:** 3–5 mg/kg (120 mg/m²), 1–3 days before

or on the day of transplantation; **maintenance:** 1–3 mg/kg (45 mg/m²) daily.
*Rheumatoid arthritis, SLE.*
**Adults and children, tablets, initial:** 1 mg/kg (50–100 mg); **then,** increase dose by 0.5 mg/kg/day after 6–8 weeks and thereafter q 4 weeks, up to maximum of 2.5 mg/kg/day; **maintenance:** lowest effective dose. Dosage should be reduced in clients with renal dysfunction.
*Myasthenia gravis.*
2–3 mg/kg/day. However, side effects occur in more than 35% of clients.
*To control progression of Behçet's syndrome.*
2.5 mg/kg/day.
*To treat Crohn's disease.*
75–100 mg/day.

## NURSING CONSIDERATIONS
### Administration/Storage
1. If GI upset occurs, give in divided doses or take with food.
2. When used for rheumatoid arthritis, a therapeutic response may not be observed for 6–8 weeks.
3. Azathioprine may be discontinued abruptly, but delayed effects are possible.
4. When used with allopurinol, reduce the dose of azathioprine by 25%–33% of the usual dose.
**IV** 5. Reconstitute drug (100 mg) with 10 mL of sterile water for injection and use within 24 hr. Further dilution with NSS or dextrose is usually made and infusion time ranges from 5 min to 8 hr.
### Assessment
1. Document indications for therapy and include preassessment data.
2. Assess for drug interactions.
3. Obtain and monitor CBC and liver and renal function studies. Observe for symptoms of hepatic dysfunction. Stop drug and report if client becomes jaundiced or develops abnormal liver function tests.
4. Assess I&O and weigh daily. Report any decreases in urine volume and creatinine clearance or oliguria;

symptoms of kidney transplant rejection.
### Client/Family Teaching
1. Take only as directed and do not skip or stop medication without approval; increase fluid intake.
2. Practice reliable contraception during and for 4 months following therapy.
3. Report any bruising, bleeding, S&S of infection, fever, rash, abdominal pain, yellow eyes or skin, itching, and/or clay-colored stools.
4. In order to prevent transplant rejection the client must take this medication for life.
5. Avoid crowds or contact with any person who has taken oral poliovirus vaccine recently or persons with active infections.
6. When used for rheumatoid arthritis, improvement in joint pain, swelling, and stiffness may take 6–12 weeks. The client should be considered refractory if no beneficial effect is noted after 12 weeks of therapy.
### Outcomes/Evaluate
• Prevention of transplant rejection
• Suppression of cell-mediated immunity
• With RA ↓ joint pain and inflammation with improved mobility

## Azelaic acid
(ah-zih-**LAY**-ic ah-**SID**)
**Pregnancy Category:** B
Azelex **(Rx)**
**Classification:** Antiacne drug

**Action/Kinetics:** Azelaic acid is a dietary constituent found in whole grain cereals and animal products; it can be formed endogenously from longer chain dicarboxylic acids, metabolism of oleic acid, and co-oxidation of monocarboxylic acids. The precise mechanism of action in treating acne is not known, but the drug possesses antimicrobial activity against *Propionibacterium acnes* and *Staphylococcus epidermidis.* Azelaic acid causes a decrease in the thickness of the stratum corneum, a reduction in the number and size of keratohyalin granules, and a reduction in the amount and distribution of filaggrin in epidermal layers. After application, the drug penetrates to the stratum corneum, epidermis, and dermis. A small amount of the drug (4%) is absorbed into the systemic circulation.

**Uses:** Treatment of mild to moderate inflammatory acne vulgaris.

**Contraindications:** Ophthalmic use.

**Special Concerns:** Use with caution during lactation. Safety and efficacy have not been determined in children less than 12 years of age.

**Side Effects:** *Dermatologic:* Pruritus, burning, stinging, tingling, erythema, dryness, rash, peeling, irritation, dermatitis, contact dermatitis, vitiligo depigmentation, small depigmented spots, hypertrichosis, reddening (sign of keratosis pilaris), exacerbation of recurrent herpes labialis (rare). *Miscellaneous:* **Worsening of asthma, allergic reactions.**

**Dosage** ————————
• **Cream**
  *Acne vulgaris.*
Gently but thoroughly massage a thin film into the affected areas b.i.d., in the morning and evening, after the skin is thoroughly washed and patted dry.

## NURSING CONSIDERATIONS
### Administration/Storage
1. The duration of treatment depends on the severity of the acne. The majority of clients improve within 4 weeks.
2. Avoid the use of occlusive dressings or wrappings.
3. Protect the cream from freezing and store between 15°C and 30°C (59°F and 86°F).

### Assessment
1. Document indications for therapy, onset and duration of symptoms, and other agents/therapies trialed.
2. Assess severity of acne and the number of inflammatory lesions. Pretreatment photographs may be useful.

### Client/Family Teaching
1. Use only as directed; after thorough cleansing and drying of skin, massage a small amount of cream into affected areas every morning and every evening. Improvement should be evident within 4 weeks.
2. Wash hands thoroughly before and after use. Keep cream away from mouth, eyes, and other mucous membranes.
3. Do not cover area with any wrappings or occlusive dressings.
4. Cream may cause temporary skin irritation (due to low pH) when applied to broken or inflamed skin; this should subside with continued therapy. If rash is persistent, apply the drug only once a day or stop treatment until symptoms improve. Discontinue treatment if sensitivity or severe irritation develops.
5. Clients with dark complexions should report any alterations in skin color.

**Outcomes/Evaluate:** Clearing and healing of acne and inflammatory lesions

# Azithromycin
(az-**zith**-roh-**MY**-sin)
**Pregnancy Category:** B
Zithromax **(Rx)**
**Classification:** Antibiotic, macrolide

**Action/Kinetics:** Azithromycin is an azalide antibiotic (subclass of macrolides) derived from erythromycin. The drug acts by binding to the 50S ribosomal subunit of susceptible organisms, thus interfering with microbial protein synthesis. Rapidly absorbed and distributed widely throughout the body. Food decreases the absorption of azithromycin. **t½, terminal:** 68 hr. A loading dose will achieve steady-state levels more quickly. Elimination is by biliary excretion of unchanged drug with a small amount being excreted through the kidneys.

**Uses: Adults:** Acute bacterial exacerbations of COPD due to *Hemophilus influenzae, Moraxella catarrhalis,* or *Streptococcus pneumoniae.* Required initial IV therapy in community-acquired pneumonia due to *S. pneumoniae, H. influenzae, M. catarrhalis, Legionella pneumophila,* and *Staphylococcus aureus.* Those who can take PO therapy in community-acquired pneumonia due to *Chlamydia pneumoniae, Mycoplasma pneumoniae, S. pneumoniae,* or *H. influenzae.* Used alone or with rifabutin for prophylaxis of *Mycobacterium avium* complex (MAC) disease in clients with advanced HIV infections. PO for genital ulcer disease in men due to *Haemophilus ducrey.* Initial IV therapy in pelvic inflammatory disease due to *Chlamydia trachomatis, Neisseria gonorrhoeae,* or *Mycoplasma hominis.* As an alternative to first-line therapy to treat streptococcal pharyngitis or tonsillitis due to *Streptococcus pyogenes.* PO for uncomplicated skin and skin structure infections due to *S. aureus, Staphyloccus pyogenes,* or *Streptococcus agalactiae.* Abscesses usually require surgical drainage. PO for urethritis and cervicitis due to *C. trachomatis* or *N. gonorrhoeae.*

**Children:** PO for acute otitis media due to *H. influenzae, M. catarrhalis,* or *S. pneumoniae* in children over 6 months of age. PO for community-acquired pneumonia due to *C. pneumoniae, H. influenzae, M. pneumoniae,* or *S. pneumoniae* in children over 6 months of age. Pharyngitis/tonsillitis due to *S. pyogenes* in children over 2 years of age who cannot use first-line therapy.

**Contraindications:** Hypersensitivity to azithromycin, any macrolide antibiotic, or erythromycin. In clients who are not eligible for outpatient PO therapy (e.g., known or suspected bacteremia, immunodeficiency, functional asplenia, nosocomially acquired infections, geriatric or debilitated clients).

**Special Concerns:** Use with caution in clients with impaired hepatic or renal function and during lactation. Safety and efficacy for acute otitis media have not been determined in children less than 6

months of age or for pharyngitis/tonsillits in children less than 2 years of age. Recommended doses should not be relied upon to treat gonorrhea or syphilis.

**Side Effects:** *GI:* N&V, diarrhea, loose stools, abdominal pain, dyspepsia, flatulence, melena, cholestatic jaundice, pseudomembranous colitis. In children, gastritis, constipation, and anorexia have also been noted. *CNS:* Dizziness, headache, somnolence, fatigue, vertigo. In children, hyperkinesia, agitation, nervousness, insomnia, fever, and malaise have also been noted. *CV:* Chest pain, palpitations, ***ventricular arrhythmias (including ventricular tachycardia and torsades de pointes in clients with prolonged QT intervals observed with other macrolides).*** *GU:* Monilia, nephritis, vaginitis. *Allergic:* Angioedema, photosensitivity, rash, **anaphylaxis.** *Hematologic:* Leukopenia, neutropenia, decreased platelet count. *Miscellaneous:* Superinfection, local IV site reactions. In children, rash, conjunctivitis, and chest pain have been noted.

**Drug Interactions:** See also *Drug Interactions* for *Erythromycins.*
*Aluminum- and magnesium-containing antacids /* ↑ Peak serum levels of azithromycin but not the total amount absorbed
*Carbamazepine /* ↑ Serum levels of carbamazepine due to ↓ metabolism
*Cyclosporine /* ↑ Serum levels of cyclosporine due to ↓ metabolism
*Digoxin /* ↑ Digoxin levels
*Ergot alkaloids /* Acute ergot toxicity, including severe peripheral vasospasm and dysesthesia
*Phenytoin /* ↑ Serum levels of phenytoin due to ↓ metabolism
*Tacrolimus /* Azithromycin may ↑ plasma levels of tacrolimus → ↑ risk of toxicity
*Terfenadine /* ↑ Serum levels of terfenadine due to ↓ metabolism
*Triazolam /* ↓ Clearance of triazolam → ↑ effect

---

*bold italic* = life threatening side effect

**Laboratory Test Interferences:** ↑ Serum CPK, potassium, ALT, GGT, AST, serum alkaline phosphatase, bilirubin, BUN, creatinine, blood glucose, LDH, and phosphate.

## Dosage

• **Capsules, Suspension, Tablets**

*Adults: Mild to moderate acute bacterial exacerbations of COPD, mild community-acquired pneumonia, second-line therapy for pharyngitis/tonsillitis; uncomplicated skin and skin structure infections.*

**Adults and children over 16 years of age:** 500 mg as a single dose on day 1 followed by 250 mg once daily on days 2–5 for a total dose of 1.5 g.

*Nongonococcal urethritis and cervicitis due to* C. trachomatis *or genital ulcer disease due to* H. ducreyi.

1 g given as a single dose.

*Gonococcal urethritis/cervicitis due to* N. gonnorheae.

2 g given as a single dose.

• **Tablets**

*Prophylaxis of* M. avium *complex in advanced HIV infections.*

1,200 mg once a week (two 600-mg tablets).

• **Oral Suspension**

*Pediatric: otitis media or community-acquired pneumonia.*

10 mg/kg (not to exceed 500 mg) on day 1, followed by 5 mg/kg (not to exceed 250 mg/day) on days 2–5.

*Pediatric: pharyngitis/tonsillitis.*

12 mg/kg/day for 5 days, not to exceed 500 mg/day.

• **IV**

*Community-acquired pneumonia.*

500 mg IV as a single daily dose for at least 2 days followed by a single daily dose of 500 mg PO to complete a 7- to 10-day course of therapy.

*Pelvic inflammatory disease.*

500 mg IV as a single daily dose for 1 or 2 days followed by a single daily dose of 250 mg PO to complete a 7-day course of therapy.

## NURSING CONSIDERATIONS

See also *Nursing Considerations* for *Erythromycins*.

### Administration/Storage

1. Give suspension at least 1 hr prior to a meal or at least 2 hr after a meal. Tablets may be taken with or without food, although increased tolerability has been observed if taken with food.

**IV** 2. Infuse IV over 60 min or longer; not to be given as a bolus or IM injection.

3. To obtain a concentration range of 1 to 2 mg/mL, transfer 5 mL of the 100-mg/mL solution into the appropriate amount of any of the following: 0.9% or 0.45% NaCl, D5%W, RL solution, D5%/0.45% NaCl with 20 mEq KCl, D5%/RL solution, D5%/0.3% NaCl, D5%/0.45% NaCl, Normosol-M in D5%, or Normosol-R in D5%.

4. The rate of infusion should be either 1 mg/mL over 3 hr or 2 mg/mL over 1 hr.

5. The reconstituted solution for injection is stable for 24 hr if stored below 30°C (86°F).

### Assessment

1. Determine any history of sensitivity to erythromycins and note any previous experience with macrolide antibiotics.

2. Determine other drugs prescribed as azithromycin may cause an increase in serum concentrations of certain drugs (digoxin, carbamazepine, cyclosporine, dilantin).

3. Obtain documentation that clients with sexually transmitted cervicitis or urethritis are tested for gonorrhea and syphilis at the time of diagnosis. Ensure that appropriate drug therapy is instituted if necessary.

4. Obtain baseline liver and renal function studies and appropriate cultures when warranted.

### Client/Family Teaching

1. Do not administer capsules with meals because food decreases absorption.

2. Avoid ingesting aluminum- or magnesium-containing antacids simultaneously with azithromycin.

3. Notify provider if N&V or diarrhea is excessive.

4. Avoid sun exposure and use protection when necessary.

5. With STDs, encourage sexual partner to seek medical evaluation and treatment to prevent reinfections. Use condoms during intercourse throughout therapy.

**Outcomes/Evaluate:** Resolution of S&S of infection; Negative cultures

---

# Aztreonam for injection
(as-TREE-oh-nam)
**Pregnancy Category:** B
Azactam for Injection **(Rx)**
**Classification:** Monobactam antibiotic

---

See also *Anti-Infectives*.

**Action/Kinetics:** Aztreonam belongs to a class of synthetic antibiotics called *monobactams*. It is bactericidal against gram-negative aerobic pathogens. The drug acts by inhibiting cell wall synthesis due to a high affinity of the drug for penicillin binding protein 3; this results in cell lysis and death. Widely distributed to all body fluids. **Time to peak serum levels:** 0.6–1.3 hr. **t½:** 1.5–2 hr. The t½ is prolonged in clients with impaired renal function. Approximately 60%–75% excreted unchanged in the urine within 8 hr.

**Uses:** Complicated and uncomplicated urinary tract infections (including pyelonephritis and cystitis) due to *Escherichia coli, Klebsiella pneumoniae, Proteus mirabilis, Pseudomonas aeruginosa, Enterobacter cloacae, Klebsiella oxytoca, Citrobacter* species, and *Serratia marcescens*. Lower respiratory tract infections (including bronchitis and pneumonia) due to *E. coli, K. pneumoniae, P. aeruginosa, Hemophilus influenzae, P. mirabilis, Enterobacter* species, and *S. marcescens*. Septicemia due to *E. coli, K. pneumoniae, P. aeruginosa, P. mirabilis, S. marcescens* and *Enterobacter* species. Skin and skin structure infections (including postoperative wounds, ulcers, and burns) caused by *E. coli, P. mirabilis, S. marcescens, Enterobacter* species, *P. aeruginosa, K. pneumoniae,* and *Citrobacter* species. Intra-abdominal infections (including peritonitis) due to *E. coli, Klebsiella* species including *K. pneumoniae, Enterobacter* species including *E. cloacae, P. aeruginosa, Citrobacter* species including *C. freundii,* and *Serratia* species including *S. marcescens*. Gynecologic infections (including endometritis and pelvic cellulitis) due to *E. coli, K. pneumoniae, P. mirabilis,* and *Enterobacter* species including *E. cloacae*. As an adjunct to surgery to manage infections caused by susceptible organisms. As an alternative to spectinomycin in clients with acute uncomplicated gonorrhea who are resistant to penicillin. Concomitant initial therapy with other anti-infective drugs and aztreonam in seriously ill clients is recommended before the causative organism is known and who are at risk for an infection due to gram-positive aerobic pathogens.

**Contraindications:** Allergy to aztreonam. Lactation.

**Special Concerns:** Safety and effectiveness have not been determined in children and infants. Use with caution in clients allergic to penicillins or cephalosporins and in those with impaired hepatic or renal function.

**Side Effects:** *GI:* N&V, diarrhea, abdominal cramps, mouth ulcers, numb tongue, halitosis, pseudomembranous colitis, *Clostridium difficile*-associated diarrhea or GI bleeding. *CNS:* Confusion, **seizures,** vertigo, headache, paresthesia, insomnia, dizziness. *Hematologic:* Anemia, neutropenia, thrombocytopenia, leukocytosis, thrombocytosis, pancytopenia, eosinophilia. *Dermatologic:* Rash, purpura, erythema multiforme, urticaria, petechiae, pruritus, diaphoresis, exfoliative dermatitis, **toxic epidermal necrolysis.** *CV:* Hypotension, transient ECG changes, flushing. *Following parenteral*

---

*use:* Phlebitis and thrombophlebitis after IV use; discomfort and swelling at the injection site after IM use. *Allergic:* **Anaphylaxis,** angioedema, bronchospasm. *Miscellaneous:* Superinfection, weakness, fever, malaise, hepatitis, jaundice, muscle aches, tinnitus, diplopia, nasal congestion, altered taste, sneezing, vaginal candidiasis, vaginitis, breast tenderness, chest pain, numb tongue, wheezing.

**OD** **Overdose Management:** *Treatment:* Hemodialysis or peritoneal dialysis to reduce serum levels.

**Drug Interactions**

*Aminoglycosides* / ↑ Risk of nephrotoxicity and ototoxicity

*Cefoxitin* / Inhibition of activity of aztreonam

*Imipenem* / Inhibition of activity of aztreonam

**Laboratory Test Interferences:** ↑ AST, ALT, alkaline phosphatase, serum creatinine, PT, PTT. Positive Coombs' test.

**Dosage**

- **IM, IV**

    *Urinary tract infections.*
    **Adults:** 0.5–1 g q 8–12 hr, not to exceed 8 g/day. **Children:** 30 mg/kg q 6–8 hr.

    *Moderate to severe systemic infections.*
    1–2 g q 8–12 hr, not to exceed 8 g/day.

    *Severe systemic or life-threatening infections.*
    2 g q 6–8 hr, not to exceed 8 g/day.

    *P. aeruginosa infections in children.*
    50 mg/kg q 4–6 hr.

    *NOTE:* Dose must be reduced in clients with impaired renal function.

# NURSING CONSIDERATIONS

See also *General Nursing Considerations For All Anti-Infectives.*

**Administration/Storage**

1. Continue therapy for at least 48 hr after the client becomes asymptomatic or until lab tests indicate that the infection has been eradicated.

2. For IM use, give the drug in a large muscle mass.

3. Aztreonam is incompatible with cephradine, nafcillin sodium, and metronidazole.

**IV** 4. Use the IV route for doses greater than 1 g or in clients with septicemia.

5. For use as a bolus, dilute the 15-mL vial with 6–10 mL sterile water for injection. For IM use, dilute the 15-mL vial with at least 3 mL of either sterile water for injection, NaCL injection, bacteriostatic water for injection, or bacteriostatic NaCL injection. Final dilution should not exceed 20 mg/mL.

6. An IV bolus injected slowly over 3–5 min may be used to initiate therapy. IV infusion should be given over 20–60 min.

7. IV solutions prepared with 0.9% NaCL injection or D5% injection to which clindamycin, cefazolin, gentamicin, or tobramycin has been added are stable for 48 hr or less at room temperature or 7 days if refrigerated.

**Assessment**

1. Note any allergy to penicillins or cephalosporins.

2. Monitor CBC, liver and renal function studies; reduce dosage with impaired renal function.

3. Monitor renal and auditory function if used with an aminoglycoside (especially if high doses are used or if therapy is prolonged).

**Client/Family Teaching**

1. During therapy a slightly itchy, red rash and nasal congestion may occur.

2. A taste alteration may be experienced during IV therapy; report if eating is impaired.

**Outcomes/Evaluate:** Resolution of infecting organism; Symptomatic improvement

**B**

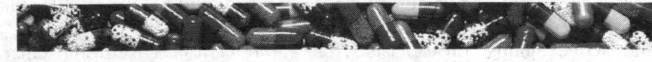

# Bacampicillin hydrochloride
(bah-kam-pih-**SILL**-in)
**Pregnancy Category:** B
Penglobe ✴, Spectrobid **(Rx)**
**Classification:** Antibiotic, penicillin

See also *Anti-Infectives* and Penicillins.

**Action/Kinetics:** Bacampicillin is a semisynthetic, acid-resistant penicillin that is hydrolyzed to the active ampicillin in the GI tract. Food does not affect absorption of the drug. The drug is 98% absorbed from the GI tract and is approximately 20% plasma protein bound. **Peak serum levels:** About 3 times equivalent doses of ampicillin after 0.9 hr. Seventy-five percent is excreted in the urine as active ampicillin within 8 hr.

**Uses:** Upper and lower respiratory tract infections caused by beta-hemolytic streptococcus, *Staphylococcus pyogenes,* pneumococci, non-penicillinase-producing staphylococci, and *Haemophilus influenzae.* UTIs caused by *Escherichia coli, Proteus mirabilis,* and enterococci. Skin infections caused by streptococci and susceptible staphylococci. Acute uncomplicated urogenital infections caused by Neisseria gonorrhoeae.

**Contraindications:** History of penicillin allergy. Concomitant use with disulfiram (Antabuse).

**Drug Interactions:** Bacampicillin should not be used concomitantly with disulfiram.

**Laboratory Test Interferences:** False + reaction to Clinitest, Benedict's solution, and Fehling's solution. ↑ AST.

**Dosage**————————

* **Tablets**
  *Upper respiratory tract infections,*
  *otitis media, UTIs, skin and skin structure infections.*
  **Adults (25 kg or more):** 400 mg q 12 hr; **pediatric:** 25 mg/kg/day in equally divided doses q 12 hr. Dose may be doubled in cases of lower respiratory tract infections, severe infections, or in treating less susceptible organisms.
  *Gonorrhea.*
  **Males and females:** 1.6 g with 1 g probenecid as a single dose. No pediatric dosage has been established.

## NURSING CONSIDERATIONS

See also *General Nursing Considerations for All Anti-Infectives.*
**Client/Family Teaching**
1. Take on an empty stomach.
2. Do not start disulfiram while taking bacampicillin.
3. Diabetics should perform sticks to determine replacement needs.
4. With allopurinol therapy, report any skin rash.
**Outcomes/Evaluate:** Resolution of infection; negative C&S results

# Bacitracin intramuscular
(bass-ih-**TRAY**-sin)
Bacitracin Sterile **(Rx)**

# Bacitracin ointment
(bass-ih-**TRAY**-sin)
Baciguent, Bacitin ✴ **(OTC)**

# Bacitracin ophthalmic ointment
(bass-ih-**TRAY**-sin)
AK-Tracin, Bacitracin Ophthalmic Ointment **(Rx)**
**Classification:** Antibiotic, miscellaneous

See also *Anti-Infectives.*
**Action/Kinetics:** Produced by *Bacillus subtilis.* Interferes with synthesis of cell wall, preventing incor-

poration of amino acids and nucleotides. Is bactericidal, bacteriostatic, and active against protoplasts. Not absorbed from the GI tract. When given parenterally, drug is well distributed in pleural and ascitic fluids. High nephrotoxicity. Systemic use is restricted to infants (see *Uses*). Carefully evaluate renal function prior to, and daily, during use. **Peak plasma levels: IM,** 0.2–2 mcg/mL after 2 hr. From 10% to 40% is excreted in the urine after IM administration.

**Uses: Parenteral:** Limited to the treatment of staphylococcal pneumonia and staphylococcus-induced empyema in infants. **Topical:** Prophylaxis or treatment of infections in minor cuts, wounds, burns, and skin abrasions. As an aid to healing and for treating superficial infections of the skin due to susceptible organisms. **Ophthalmic:** Effective against species of *Staphylococcus, S. aureus, Streptococcus, S. pneumoniae, S. pyogenes, Corynebacterium, Neisseria, N. gonorrhoeae,* and beta-hemolytic streptococci. Topical antibiotics should not be used in deep-seated ocular infections or in those that are likely to become systemic.

**Contraindications:** Hypersensitivity or toxic reaction to bacitracin. Pregnancy. Epithelial herpes simplex keratitis, vaccinia, varicella, mycobacterial eye infections, fungal diseases of the eye.

**Special Concerns:** Ophthalmic ointments may retard corneal epithelial healing. Prolonged or repeated use may result in bacterial or fungal overgrowth of nonsusceptible organisms leading to a secondary infection.

**Side Effects: Parenteral use:** *Nephrotoxicity due to tubular and glomerular necrosis, renal failure;* toxic reactions; N&V. **Topical use:** Allergic contact dermatitis, superinfection. **Ophthalmic use:** Transient burning, stinging, itching, irritation, inflammation, angioneurotic edema, urticaria, vesicular and maculopapular dermatitis.

**Drug Interactions**
*Aminoglycosides /* Additive nephro-toxicity and neuromuscular blocking activity
*Anesthetics /* ↑ Neuromuscular blockade → possible muscle paralysis
*Neuromuscular blocking agents /* Additive neuromuscular blockade → possible muscle paralysis

**Dosage** —————————
• **IM Only**
**Infants, 2.5 kg and below:** 900 units/kg/day in two to three divided doses; **infants over 2.5 kg:** 1,000 units/kg/day in two to three divided doses.
• **Ophthalmic Ointment (500 units/g)**
   *Acute infections.*
½ in. in lower conjunctival sac q 3–4 hr until improvement occurs. Reduce treatment before the drug is discontinued.
   *Mild to moderate infections.*
½ in. b.i.d.–t.i.d.
• **Topical Ointment (500 units/g)**
Apply a small amount equal to the surface area of a fingertip 1–3 times/day after cleaning the affected area. Do not use for more than 1 week.

——————————————

## NURSING CONSIDERATIONS

See also *General Nursing Considerations for All Anti-Infectives*.
**Administration/Storage:** Do not mix bacitracin with glycerin or other polyalcohols that cause drug to deteriorate. When used topically, the affected area may be covered with a sterile bandage.
**Assessment**
1. Document indications for therapy, type, onset, and duration of symptoms.
2. List any previous experiences with this type of infection (especially of ocular origin), agents used, and the outcome.
3. Recurrent ophthalmic infections should be cultured and carefully assessed by an ophthalmologist.
**Interventions**
1. Monitor renal function studies

and maintain adequate I&O with parenteral therapy.
2. Test urine pH daily; pH should be kept at 6 or greater to decrease renal irritation. Have sodium bicarbonate or other alkali available if pH < 6.
3. Do not administer with a topical or systemic nephrotoxic drug.

**Client/Family Teaching**

1. Apply as directed. Cleanse area thoroughly before applying bacitracin as a wet dressing or ointment.
2. Report any lack of response, rash, or unusual symptoms.

**Outcomes/Evaluate**

- Resolution of S&S of infection
- Restoration of skin integrity

## Baclofen

(**BAK**-low-fen)
**Pregnancy Category:** C
Apo-Baclofen ✱, Dom-Baclofen ✱, Gen-Baclofen ✱, Lioresal, Med-Baclofen ✱, Nu-Baclofen ✱, PMS-Baclofen ✱ **(Rx)**
**Classification:** Skeletal muscle relaxant, centrally acting

See also *Skeletal Muscle Relaxants, Centrally Acting*.

**Action/Kinetics:** Related chemically to GABA, an inhibitory neurotransmitter. May cause its effects by combining with the $GABA_B$ receptor subtype. However, the mechanism of action of baclofen is not fully known; is known to inhibit both mono- and polysynaptic spinal reflexes perhaps by hyperpolarization of afferent terminals. May also act at certain brain sites. Has CNS depressant effects. After PO use, baclofen is rapidly and extensively absorbed. **Peak serum levels**, **PO:** 2–3 hr. **Therapeutic serum levels:** 80–400 ng/mL. **t½, PO:** 3–4 hr. **Onset after intrathecal bolus:** 30–60 min; **peak effect after intrathecal bolus:** 4 hr; **duration after intrathecal bolus:** 4–8 hr. **t½ after bolus lumbar injection of 50 or 100 mcg:** 1.5 hr over the first 4 hr. **Onset after intrathecal continuous infusion:** 6–8 hr; **peak effect after intrathecal continuous infusion:** 24–48 hr. Seventy percent to 80% of the drug is eliminated unchanged by the kidney.

**Uses: PO.** Multiple sclerosis (flexor spasms, pain, clonus, and muscular rigidity) and diseases and injuries of the spinal cord associated with spasticity. Not effective for the treatment of cerebral palsy, stroke, parkinsonism, or rheumatic disorders. *Investigational:* Trigeminal neuralgia, tardive dyskinesia, intractable hiccoughs.

**Intrathecal.** Severe spasticity of spinal cord of cerebral origin in clients unresponsive to PO baclofen therapy or who have intolerable CNS side effects. *Investigational:* Reduce spasticity in children with cerebral palsy.

**Contraindications:** Hypersensitivity. PO used to treat rheumatic disorders, spasm resulting from Parkinson's disease, stroke, cerebral palsy. Intrathecal product for IV, IM, SC, or epidural use.

**Special Concerns:** Use during lactation only if potential benefit outweighs the potential risk. Safe use of the oral product for children under 12 years of age and of the intrathecal product for children under 4 years of age has not been established. Use with caution in impaired renal function, in those with autonomic dysreflexia, and where spasticity is used to sustain an upright posture and balance in locomotion. Also, use with caution in those with psychotic disorders, schizophrenia, or confusional states as worsening of these conditions has occurred following PO use. Geriatric clients may be at higher risk for developing CNS toxicity, including mental depression, confusion, hallucinations, and significant sedation. Due to serious, life-threatening side effects after intrathecal use, physicians must be trained and educated in chronic intrathecal infusion therapy. Abrupt drug withdrawal may cause hallucinations and seizures.

**B**

**Side Effects: PO.** *CNS:* Drowsiness, dizziness, lightheadedness, weakness, lethargy, fatigue, confusion, headaches, insomnia, euphoria, excitement, depression, paresthesia, muscle pain, coordination disorder, tremor, ridigity, dystonia, ataxia, strabismus, dysarthria. Hallucinations following abrupt withdrawal. *CV:* Hypotension. Rarely, chest pain, syncope, palpitations. *GI:* N&V, constipation, dry mouth, anorexia, taste disorder, abdominal pain, diarrhea. *GU:* Urinary frequency, enuresis, urinary retention, dysuria, impotence, inability to ejaculate, nocturia. *Ophthalmic:* Nystagmus, miosis, mydriasis, diplopia. *Miscellaneous:* Rash, pruritus, ankle edema, increased perspiration, weight gain, dyspnea, nasal congestion.

**Intrathecal, spasticity of spinal origin.** *CNS:* Dizziness, somnolence, paresthesia, headache, **convulsion,** confusion, speech disorder, coma, **death,** insomnia, anxiety, depression, hallucinations. *GI:* N&V, constipation, dry mouth, diarrhea, anorexia. *GU:* Urinary retention, impotence, urinary incontinence, urinary frequency. *CV:* Hypotension, hypertension. *Miscellaneous:* Accidental injury, asthenia, amblyopia, pain, peripheral edema, dyspnea, hypoventilation, fever, urticaria, anorexia, diplopia, dysautonomia.

**Intrathecal, spasticity of cerebral origin.** *CNS:* Somnolence, headache, **convulsion,** dizziness, paresthesia, abnormal thinking, agitation, coma, speech disorder, tremor. *GI:* N&V, increased salivation, constipation, dry mouth. *GU:* Urinary retention, urinary incontinence, impaired urination. *Miscellaneous:* Hypertonia, hypoventilation, hypotension, back pain, pain, pruritus, peripheral edema, asthenia, chills, pneumonia.

**OD** **Overdose Management:** *Symptoms:* Symptoms after PO use include vomiting, drowsiness, muscular hypotonia, muscle twitching, accommodation disorders, respiratory depression, seizures, coma. Symptoms after intrathecal use include drowsiness, dizziness, lightheadedness, somnolence, respiratory depression, rostral progression of hypotonia, *seizures, loss of consciousness leading to coma (for up to 24 hr).* *Treatment:*
1. After PO use:
• Induce vomiting (only if the client is alert and conscious) followed by gastric lavage.
• If the client is not alert and conscious, undertake only gastric lavage making sure the airway is secured with a cuffed ET tube.
• Maintain an adequate airway.
• Atropine may be used to improve HR, BP, ventilation, and core body temperature.
2. After intrathecal use:
• The residual solution is to be removed from the pump as soon as possible.
• Intubate the client with respiratory depression until the drug is eliminated.
• IV physostigmine (total dose of 1–2 mg given over 5–10 min) may be tried, with caution.
• Consideration can also be given to withdrawing 30–60 mL of CSF to decrease baclofen levels (provided that lumbar puncture is not contraindicated).

**Drug Interactions:** Concomitant use with CNS depressants → additive CNS depression.

**Laboratory Test Interferences:** ↑ AST, alkaline phosphatase, blood glucose.

**Dosage** ————
• **Tablets**
   *Muscle relaxant.*
**Adults, initial:** 5 mg t.i.d. for 3 days; **then,** 10 mg t.i.d. for 3 days, 15 mg t.i.d. for 3 days, and 20 mg t.i.d. Additional increases in dose may be required but should not exceed 20 mg q.i.d.
   *Trigeminal neuralgia.*
50–60 mg/day.
   *Tardive dyskinesia.*
40 mg/day used in combination with neuroleptics.
• **Intrathecal**
   *Initial screening bolus.*

50 mcg/mL given into the intrathecal space by barbotage over a period of not less than 1 min. The client is observed for 4–8 hr for a positive response consisting of a decrease in muscle tone, frequency, and/or severity of muscle spasms. If the response is not adequate, a second bolus dose of 75 mcg/1.5 mL, 24 hr after the first bolus dose, can be given with the client observed for 4–8 hr. If the response is still inadequate, a final bolus screening dose of 100 mcg/2 mL can be given 24 hr later.

*Postimplant dose titration.*
To determine the initial daily dose of baclofen following the implant for intrathecal use, the screening dose that gave a positive response should be doubled and given over a 24-hr period. However, if the effectiveness of the bolus dose lasted for more than 12 hr, the daily dose should be the same as the screening dose but delivered over a period of 24 hr. After the first 24 hr, the dose can be increased slowly by 10%–30% increments only once each 24 hr until the desired effect is reached.

*Maintenance therapy.*
The maintenance dose may need to be adjusted during the first few months of intrathecal therapy. The daily dose may be increased by 10% to no more than 40% daily. If side effects occur, the daily dose may be decreased by 10%–20%. Daily doses for long-term continuous infusion have ranged from 12 to 1,500 mcg (usual maintenance is 300-800 mcg/day). The lowest dose producing optimal control should be used.

*Reduce spasticity of cerebral palsy in children.*
25, 50, or 100 mcg.

## NURSING CONSIDERATIONS

See also *Nursing Considerations* for *Skeletal Muscle Relaxants, Centrally Acting.*
**Administration/Storage**
1. If beneficial effects are not noted, withdraw the drug slowly.
2. Check the manufacturer's manual for specific instructions and precautions for programming the implantable intrathecal infusion pump and refilling the reservoir.
3. Prior to intrathecal implantation of the pump, clients must show a positive response to a bolus dose of baclofen in a screening trial.
4. If there is not a significant clinical response to increases in the daily dose given intrathecally, check the pump for proper function and the catheter for patency.
5. During long-term intrathecal treatment, approximately 10% of clients become tolerant to increasing doses. If this occurs, a drug "holiday" consisting of a gradual decrease of intrathecal baclofen over a 2-week period can be considered. Alternate methods to treat spasticity must be undertaken. After a few days, sensitivity to baclofen may return. However, to avoid possible side effects or overdose, the alternative medication should be discontinued slowly.
6. Filling of the reservoir for intrathecal use must be performed only by fully trained and qualified personnel. Refill intervals must be carefully calculated to avoid depletion of the reservoir.
7. Extreme caution should be used when filling an FDA-approved implantable pump equipped with an injection port (i.e., that allows direct access to the intrathecal catheter). Direct injection into the catheter through the access port may result in a life-threatening overdose of baclofen.
8. For screening purposes, intrathecal baclofen, either 10 mg/20 mL or 10 mg/5 mL, must be diluted with sterile preservative-free NaCL for injection, to a concentration of 50 mcg/mL for bolus administration. For maintenance, baclofen must be diluted with sterile preservative-free NaCL for injection USP for clients who require concentrations other than 500 mcg/mL (i.e., the 10 mg/20 mL

product) or 2,000 mcg/mL (i.e., the 10 mg/5 mL product).

**Assessment**

1. Document indications for therapy; include pretreatment assessments.

2. With epilepsy assess for clinical S&S of disease. Obtain EEG at regular intervals to assess for reduced seizure control.

3. Obtain initial liver and renal function studies.

4. Note if client has diabetes.

5. Clients must be closely monitored in a fully equipped and staffed facility during both the intrathecal screening phase and dose-titration period following the intrathecal implant. Resuscitative equipment should be readily available.

6. Ensure client is free from S&S of infection. Systemic infection may alter response to screening trials and (during pump implantation) may lead to surgical complications and interfere with the pump dosing rate.

7. Assess for level of useful spasticity (e.g., to aid in transfers or to maintain posture) as rigidity is important for gait in some clients.

8. In those who require hypertonicity to stand upright, to maintain balance when walking, or to increase functionality, baclofen may be contraindicated because it interferes with this coping mechanism.

**Interventions**

1. Note any evidence of hypersensitivity reaction and report.

2. Monitor urine output; test for occult blood.

3. If improvement in condition does not occur within 6–8 weeks, the drug should be withdrawn gradually.

4. For clients with an intrathecal pump:

• Calculate pump refill interval carefully to prevent an empty reservoir and the return of severe spasticity.

• The pump reservoir should only be accessed percutaneously, refilled, and programmed by someone specifically trained in this procedure.

• When filling pumps with injection ports that permit direct access to the catheter, use care as an injection directly into the catheter can cause a lethal overdose. And, in this event, immediately remove any residual drug from the pump and follow guidelines for Treatment under Overdose Management.

• When the dose requirements suddenly escalate, assess for catheter kinks or dislodgement.

• When programming for increased dosage, for example at bedtime, the flow rate should be programmed to change 2 hr before the desired effect.

**Client/Family Teaching**

1. Take oral medication with meals or a snack to avoid gastric irritation. Report if GI symptoms are severe or persistent.

2. To prevent constipation, increase fluid intake and roughage in the diet.

3. It may take several weeks of therapy before physical improvement occurs.

4. Monitor weight and I&O; keep a record of the frequency and amounts of each voiding and report any edema.

5. Drug may alter insulin requirements.

6. May cause impotence; report as a change of drug or dosage may be required. Do not discontinue drug abruptly.

7. With the intrathecal pump:

• Once screening trials completed, the "baclofen pump" will be surgically placed in the abdominal wall and attached to an implanted lumbar intrathecal catheter. Demonstrate proper postoperative site care and review S&S of infection that require immediate reporting.

• Maintain a log identifying when the spasms are greatest. This facilitates proper pump programming to ensure optimal control of spasticity and discomfort.

• Identify symptoms that require immediate medical intervention.

• Report as scheduled (usually monthly with maintenance) to ensure proper reservoir drug levels and to prevent loss of effect or air entering the reservoir.

• Drowsiness, dizziness, and lower extremity weakness may occur; report if persistent or progressive as drug dose may require adjustment.

• Those who become refractory to increasing doses may require hospitalization for a "drug holiday." This would consist of a *gradual reduction* of intrathecal baclofen over a 2-week period and alternative therapy with other agents. Sensitivity to baclofen usually returns after several days and may be resumed intrathecally at the initial continuous dose.

**Outcomes/Evaluate**

• Improved muscle tone and involuntary movements; ↓ muscle spasticity and pain

• ↓ Painful/disabling symptoms permitting ↑ functioning level

---

# Beclomethasone dipropionate
(be-kloh-**METH**-ah-zohn)
**Pregnancy Category:** C
**Aerosol Inhaler:** Alti-Beclomethasone Dipropionate ✿, Beclodisk Diskhaler ✿, Becloforte Inhaler ✿, Beclovent, Beclovent Rotacaps or Rotahaler ✿, Vanceril, Vanceril DS **(Rx)**, **Intranasal:** Beclodisk for Oral Inhalation ✿, Beconase AQ Nasal, Beconase Inhalation, Gen-Beclo Aq. ✿, Vancenase AQ 84 mcg Double Strength, Vancenase AQ Forte, Vancenase AQ Nasal, Vancenase Nasal Inhaler **(Rx)**, **Topical:** Propaderm ✿
**Classification:** Glucocorticoid

---

See also *Corticosteroids*.
**Action/Kinetics:** t½: 15 hr. Rapidly inactivated, thereby resulting in few systemic effects.

*NOTE:* If a client is on systemic steroids, transfer to beclomethasone may be difficult because recovery from impaired renal function may be slow.

**Uses:** Relief of symptoms of seasonal or perennial rhinitis in clients not responsive to more conventional therapy, to prevent recurrence of nasal polyps following surgical removal, and to treat allergic or non-allergic (vasomotor) rhinitis (spray formulations). Inhalation therapy for chronic use in bronchial asthma. In glucocorticoid-dependent clients, beclomethasone often permits a decrease in the dosage of the systemic agent. Withdrawal of systemic corticosteroids must be carried out gradually.

**Contraindications:** Status asthmaticus, acute episodes of asthma, hypersensitivity to drug or aerosol ingredients.

**Special Concerns:** Safe use during lactation and in children under 6 years of age not established.

**Side Effects:** *Intranasal:* Headache, pharyngitis, coughing, epistaxis, nasal burning, pain, conjunctivitis, myalgia, tinnitus. Rarely, ulceration of the nasal mucosa and nasal septum perforation.

---

**Dosage**

• **Metered Dose Inhaler**
  *Asthma.*

*Beclovent.* **Adults:** 2 inhalations (total of 84 mcg beclomethasone) t.i.d.–q.i.d. In some clients, 4 inhalations (168 mcg) b.i.d. have been effective. Do not exceed 20 inhalations (840 mcg) daily. **Pediatric, 6–12 years:** 1–2 inhalations (42–84 mcg) t.i.d.–q.i.d. In some, 4 inhalations (168 mcg) b.i.d. have been effective. Do not to exceed 10 inhalations (420 mcg) daily. Dosage has not been determined in children less than 6 years of age.

*Vanceril.* **Adults:** 2 inhalations (total of 168 mcg) b.i.d. In those with severe asthma, start with 6–8 inhalations/day and adjust dose downward as determined by client response. Do not exceed 10 inhalations (840 mcg) daily. **Children, 6–12 years:** 2 inhalations (168 mcg) b.i.d. Do not exceed 5 inhalations (420 mcg) daily. Dosage has not been determined in children less than 6 years of age.

---

*NOTE:* Vanceril DS can be used once daily for treatment of asthma.

In clients also receiving systemic glucocorticosteroids, beclomethasone should be started when client's condition is relatively stable.

- **Nasal Aerosol or Spray**

*Allergic or nonallergic rhinitis, Prophylaxis of nasal polyps.*

**Adults and children over 12 years:** 1 inhalation (42 mcg) in each nostril b.i.d.–q.i.d. (i.e., total daily dose: 168–336 mcg). If no response after 3 weeks, discontinue therapy. **Maintenance, usual:** 1 inhalation in each nostril t.i.d. (252 mcg/day). For nasal polyps, treatment may be required for several weeks or more before a therapeutic effect can be assessed fully. Two sprays of the double-strength product (Vancenase AQ 84 mcg Double Strength) are administered once daily.

Vancenase AQ Forte may be used once daily for treatment of rhinitis.

## NURSING CONSIDERATIONS

See also *Nursing Considerations* for *Corticosteroids.*

### Administration/Storage

1. To administer beclomethasone with an inhaler, use the following procedure and instruct clients to:
- Shake metal canister thoroughly immediately prior to use.
- Exhale as completely as possible.
- Place the mouthpiece of the inhaler into the mouth and tighten their lips around it.
- Inhale deeply through the mouth while pressing the metal canister down with their forefinger.
- Hold their breath for as long as possible.
- Remove mouthpiece.
- Exhale slowly.
2. A minimum of 60 sec must elapse between inhalations.
3. To prevent explosion of contents under pressure, do not store or use near heat or open flame, or throw into a fire or incinerator. Keep secure from children.
4. If the cannister is cold, the therapeutic effect may be decreased.

### Assessment

1. Note any history of sensitivity to corticosteroids or fluorocarbon propellants.
2. Document indications for therapy, pretreatment pulmonary assessments, presenting symptoms, and PFT's.

### Client/Family Teaching

1. Review use, care, and storage of inhaler. Rinse out mouth and wash the mouth piece, spacer, sprayer and dry after each use.
2. A spacer may facilitate administration. With nasal administration aim toward the outer eye and not the septum to decrease nasal irritation. Review video/instruction to ensure proper use.
3. Inhaler is not to be used for acute asthma attacks but should be used regularly to prevent the occurrence of these attacks.
4. Comply with the prescribed drug therapy even though it may take 1–4 weeks for any improvement in respiratory function to be realized.
5. Report signs of adrenal insufficiency (i.e., muscular pain, lassitude, and depression) even if respiratory function has improved. Symptoms such as hypotension and weight loss are indications that the dosage of systemic steroid should be boosted temporarily, and then withdrawn more gradually.
6. More than 1 mg in adults or more than 500 mcg in children may precipitate hypothalamic-pituitary axis depression, resulting in adrenal insufficiency. Do not overuse inhaler or exceed prescribed dosage.
7. Report any symptoms of localized fungal infections in the mouth. Gargling and rinsing after treatments and rinsing of the spacer and/or administration port may help prevent these infections. These must be reported immediately and will require antifungal meds and possibly discontinuation of the drug.
8. If also receiving bronchodilators by inhalation (i.e., Albuterol) use the bronchodilator first to open the airways and then use beclomethasone. This increases the penetration of

steroid and reduces the potential toxicity from inhaled fluorocarbon propellants of both inhalers.

9. For those receiving systemic steroid therapy, initiate beclomethasone therapy *very* slowly, withdrawing the systemic steroids as ordered. The benefit of inhaled steroids is that it requires a much lower dose since it goes to the target organ and does not require weaning. Once systemic steroid withdrawn, provide with a supply of PO glucocorticoids. Take these immediately if subjected to unusual stress; note and report all usage.

10. Carry ID with diagnosis, treatment, and possible need for systemic glucocorticoids, in the event of exposure to unusual stress.

11. Identify and practice relaxation techniques during stressful situations.

**Outcomes/Evaluate**
• Control of asthma
• Relief of rhinitis
• Prophylaxis of nasal polyp recurrence

# Benazepril hydrochloride
(beh-**NAYZ**-eh-prill)
**Pregnancy Category:** D
Lotensin **(Rx)**
**Classification:** Antihypertensive, ACE inhibitor

See also *Angiotensin-Converting Enzyme Inhibitors*

**Action/Kinetics:** Both supine and standing BPs are reduced with mild-to-moderate hypertension and no compensatory tachycardia. Also an antihypertensive effect in clients with low-renin hypertension. Food does not affect the extent of absorption. Almost completely converted to the active benazeprilat, which has greater ACE inhibitor activity. **Onset:** 1 hr. **Duration:** 24 hr. **Peak plasma levels, benazepril:** 30–60 min. **Peak plasma levels, benazeprilat:** 1–2 hr if fasting and 2–4 hr if not fasting. **t½, benazeprilat:** 10–11 hr. **Peak reduction in BP:** 2–4 hr after dosing. **Peak effect with chronic therapy:** 1–2 weeks. Highly bound to plasma protein and excreted through the urine with about 20% of a dose excreted as benazeprilat.

**Uses:** Alone or in combination with thiazide diuretics to treat hypertension.

**Contraindications:** Hypersensitivity to benazepril or any other ACE inhibitor.

**Special Concerns:** Use with caution during lactation. Safety and effectiveness have not been determined in children.

**Side Effects:** *CNS:* Headache, dizziness, fatigue, anxiety, insomnia, nervousness. *GI:* N&V, constipation, abdominal pain, melena. *CV:* Symptomatic hypotension, postural hypotension, syncope, angina pectoris, palpitations, peripheral edema, ECG changes. *Dermatologic:* Dermatitis, pruritus, rash, flushing, diaphoresis. *GU:* Decreased libido, impotence, UTI. *Respiratory:* Cough, asthma, bronchitis, dyspnea, sinusitis, bronchospasm. *Neuromuscular:* Paresthesias, arthralgia, arthritis, asthenia, myalgia. *Hematologic:* Occasionally, eosinophilia, leukopenia, neutropenia, decreased hemoglobin. *Miscellaneous:* Angioedema, which may be associated with involvement of the tongue, glottis, or larynx; hypertonia; proteinuria; hyponatremia; infection.

**Drug Interactions**
*Diuretics* / Excessive ↓ in BP
*Lithium* / ↑ Serum lithium levels with ↑ risk of lithium toxicity
*Potassium-sparing diuretics, potassium supplements* / ↑ Risk of hyperkalemia

**Laboratory Test Interferences:** ↑ Serum creatinine, BUN, serum potassium. ↓ Hemoglobin. ECG changes.

**Dosage**
• **Tablets**
*Clients not receiving a diuretic.*
**Initial:** 10 mg once daily; **maintenance:** 20–40 mg/day given as a single dose or in two equally divided

doses. Total daily doses greater than 80 mg have not been evaluated.

*Clients receiving a diuretic.*
**Initial:** 5 mg/day.
*Creatinine clearance < 30 mL/min/ 1.73 m².* The recommended starting dose is 5 mg/day; **maintenance:** titrate dose upward until BP is controlled or to a maximum total daily dose of 40 mg.

## NURSING CONSIDERATIONS

See also *Nursing Considerations* for *Angiotensin-Converting Enzyme Inhibitors,* and *Antihypertensive Agents.*

**Administration/Storage**
1. Dosage adjustment should be based on measuring peak (2–6 hr after dosing) and trough responses. Consider increasing the dose or give divided doses if once-daily dosing does not provide an adequate trough response.
2. If BP cannot be controlled by benazepril alone, a diuretic can be added.
3. If receiving a diuretic, discontinue the diuretic, if possible, 2–3 days before beginning benazepril therapy.

**Assessment**
1. Note any previous experience with this class of drugs.
2. Review diet, weight loss, exercise, and life-style changes necessary to control BP.
3. Monitor electrolytes, liver and renal function studies.

**Client/Family Teaching**
1. Take only as directed. May be taken with or without food.
2. Avoid concomitant administration of potassium supplements, potassium salt substitutes, or potassium-sparing diuretics; may lead to serum potassium increases.
3. Side effects such as headache, fatigue, dizziness, and cough have been associated with this drug therapy; report if persistent or bothersome.

**Outcomes/Evaluate:** Control of hypertension

# Benzonatate
(ben-**ZOH**-nah-tayt)
**Pregnancy Category:** C
Tessalon Perles **(Rx)**
**Classification:** Antitussive, nonnarcotic

**Action/Kinetics:** Acts peripherally by anesthetizing stretch receptors in the respiratory passages, lungs, and pleura, thus depressing the cough reflex at its source. No effect on the respiratory center in the doses recommended. **Onset:** 15–20 min. **Duration:** 3–8 hr.

**Uses:** Symptomatic relief of cough.

**Contraindications:** Sensitivity to benzonatate or related drugs such as procaine and tetracaine.

**Special Concerns:** Use with caution during lactation. Safety and efficacy have not been determined in children less than 10 years of age.

**Side Effects:** *Hypersensitivity reactions:* **Bronchospasm, laryngospasm, CV collapse.** *GI:* Nausea, GI upset, constipation. *CNS:* Sedation, headache, dizziness, mental confusion, visual hallucinations. *Dermatologic:* Pruritus, skin eruptions. *Miscellaneous:* Nasal congestion, sensation of burning in the eyes, "chilly" sensation, numbness of the chest.

**OD** **Overdose Management:** *Symptoms:* Oropharyngeal anesthesia if capsules are chewed or dissolved in the mouth. CNS stimulation, including restlessness, tremors, and clonic convulsions followed by profound CNS depression. *Treatment:* Evacuate gastric contents followed by copious amounts of activated charcoal slurry. Due to depressed cough and gag reflexes, efforts may be needed to protect against aspiration of gastric contents and orally administered substances. Treat convulsions with a short-acting IV barbiturate. Do not use CNS stimulants. Support of respiration and CV-renal function.

**Dosage**
• **Capsules (Perles)**
*Antitussive.*

**Adults and children over 10 years of age:** 100 mg t.i.d., up to a maximum of 600 mg/day.

## NURSING CONSIDERATIONS
### Assessment
1. Document indications for therapy, onset, duration, and characteristics of symptoms.
2. Note any sensitivity to benzonatate or tetracaine.
3. Not for use during pregnancy.
### Client/Family Teaching
1. Take only as directed and with plenty of fluids. Swallow perles without chewing to avoid the local anesthetic effect on the oral mucosa and to prevent choking.
2. Do not perform tasks that require alertness until drug effects realized.
3. Do not change positions suddenly due to postural effects; take appropriate precautions if dizziness or drowsiness occur.
4. Report if symptoms intensify or do not improve after 5 days.
**Outcomes/Evaluate:** Control of persistent coughing episodes.

---

# Benztropine mesylate
(**BENS**-troh-peen)
**Pregnancy Category:** C
Apo-Benztropine ✱, Cogentin, PMS-Benztropine ✱ **(Rx)**
**Classification:** Synthetic anticholinergic, antiparkinson agent

See also *Cholinergic Blocking Agents.*
**Action/Kinetics:** Synthetic anticholinergic possessing antihistamine and local anesthetic properties. **Onset, PO:** 1–2 hr; **IM, IV:** Within a few minutes. Effects are cumulative; is long-acting (24 hr). Full effects are manifested in 2–3 days. Low incidence of side effects.
**Uses:** Adjunct in the treatment of parkinsonism (all types). To reduce severity of extrapyramidal effects in phenothiazine or other antipsychotic drug therapy (not effective in tardive dyskinesia).
**Special Concerns:** Not recommended for children under 3 years of age. Geriatric and emaciated clients cannot tolerate large doses. Certain drug-induced extrapyramidal symptoms may not respond to benztropine.

### Dosage
• **Tablets**
*Parkinsonism.*
**Adults:** 1–2 mg/day (range: 0.5–6 mg/day).
*Idiopathic parkinsonism.*
**Adults, initial:** 0.5–1 mg/day, increased gradually to 4–6 mg/day, if necessary.
*Postencephalitic parkinsonism.*
**Adults:** 2 mg/day in one or more doses.
*Drug-induced extrapyramidal effects.*
**Adults:** 1–4 mg 1–2 times/day.
• **IM, IV (Rarely)**
*Acute dystonic reactions.*
**Adults, initial:** 1–2 mg; **then,** 1–2 mg PO b.i.d. usually prevents recurrence. Clients can rarely tolerate full dosage.

---

## NURSING CONSIDERATIONS

See also *Nursing Considerations* for *Cholinergic Blocking Agents.*
### Administration/Storage
1. When used as replacement for or supplement to other antiparkinsonism drugs, substitute or add gradually.
2. For difficulty swallowing tablets, the tablets may be crushed and mixed with a small amount of food or liquid.
3. Some may benefit by taking the entire dose at bedtime while others are best treated by taking divided doses, b.i.d.–q.i.d.
4. Initiate therapy with a low dose (e.g., 0.5 mg) and then increase in increments of 0.5 mg at 5–6-day intervals. The maximum daily dose should not exceed 6 mg.
**IV** 5. If administered IV, may give undiluted at a rate of 1 mg over 1 min.
### Assessment
1. Note if phenothiazines or tricyclic

antidepressants are being used; may cause a paralytic ileus.

2. Assess for conditions that would preclude drug therapy.

3. Note age; elderly clients require a lower dosage.

**Interventions**

1. Monitor I&O. Assess for urinary retention and bowel sounds; especially important with limited mobility.

2. Inspect skin at regular intervals for any evidence of skin changes.

3. Observe for extrapyramidal symptoms, i.e., drooling, muscle spasms, shuffling gait, muscle rigidity, and pill rolling before and during therapy.

4. If excitation or vomiting occurs, withdraw drug temporarily and resume at a lower dose.

**Client/Family Teaching**

1. Review goals of therapy (control of parkinsonian symptoms, i.e., improved gait and balance and less rigidity and involuntary movements; control of extrapyramidal symptoms, i.e., less drooling, muscle spasms, shuffling gait, or pill rolling).

2. Use caution when performing tasks that require mental alertness because drug has a sedative effect and may also cause postural hypotension.

3. It usually takes 2–3 days for the drug to exert a desired effect. Take as ordered unless side effects occur; these should be reported. Side effects usually subside with continued use of the drug.

4. Avoid strenuous activity and increased heat exposure. Plan rest periods during the day as ability to tolerate heat will be reduced and heat stroke may occur.

5. Report any difficulty in voiding or inadequate emptying of the bladder.

6. Avoid alcohol and any other CNS depressants.

**Outcomes/Evaluate**

• ↓ Involuntary movements and rigidity with improved gait and balance

• Control of extrapyramidal side effects of antipsychotic agents

# Bepridil hydrochloride
(**BEH**-prih-dill)
**Pregnancy Category:** C
Vascor **(Rx)**
**Classification:** Antianginal, calcium channel blocking drug

See also *Calcium Channel Blocking Agents.*

**Action/Kinetics:** Bepridil inhibits the transmembrane influx of calcium ions into cardiac and vascular smooth muscle. It increases the effective refractory period of the atria, AV node, His-Purkinje fibers, and ventricles. Dilates peripheral arterioles and reduces total peripheral resistance; it reduces HR and arterial pressure at rest and at a given level of exercise. Is rapidly and completely absorbed following PO use. **Onset:** 60 min. **Time to peak plasma levels:** 2–3 hr. Greater than 99% bound to plasma protein. Food does not affect either the peak plasma levels or the extent of absorption. **Therapeutic serum levels:** 1–2 ng/mL. **t½, distribution:** 2 hr; **terminal elimination:** 24 hr. Steady-state blood levels do not occur for 8 days. Metabolized in the liver and metabolites are excreted through both the kidney (70%) and the feces (22%).

**Uses:** Chronic stable angina (classic effort-associated angina) in clients who have failed to respond to other antianginal medications or who are intolerant to such medications. May be used alone or with beta blockers or nitrates. An additive effect occurs if used with propranolol.

**Contraindications:** Clients with a history of serious ventricular arrhythmias, sick sinus syndrome, second- or third-degree heart block (except in the presence of a functioning ventricular pacemaker), hypotension (less than 90 mm Hg systolic), uncompensated cardiac insufficiency, congenital QT interval prolongation, and in those taking other drugs that prolong the QT interval (e.g., quinidine, procainamide, tricyclic antidepressants). Use in clients with

MI during the previous 3 months. During lactation.

**Special Concerns:** Safety and effectiveness have not been determined in children. Use with caution in clients with CHF, left bundle block, sinus bradycardia (less than 50 beats/min), serious hepatic or renal disorders. New arrhythmias can be induced. Geriatric clients may require more frequent monitoring.

**Side Effects:** *CV: Induction of new serious arrhythmias such as torsades de pointes type ventricular tachycardia, prolongation of QTc and QT interval, increased PVC rates, new sustained VT and VT/VF,* sinus tachycardia, sinus bradycardia, hypertension vasodilation, palpitations. *GI:* Nausea (common), dyspepsia, GI distress, diarrhea, dry mouth, anorexia, abdominal pain, constipation, flatulence, gastritis, increased appetite. *CNS:* Nervousness, dizziness, drowsiness, insomnia, depression, vertigo, akathisia, anxiousness, tremor, hand tremor, syncope, paresthesia. *Respiratory:* Cough, pharyngitis, rhinitis, dyspnea, respiratory infection. *Body as a whole:* Asthenia, headache, flu syndrome, fever, pain, superinfection. *Dermatologic:* Rash, skin irritation, sweating. *Miscellaneous:* Tinnitus, arthritis, blurred vision, taste change, loss of libido, impotence, agranulocytosis.

**Drug Interactions**
*Cardiac glycosides* / Exaggeration of the depression of AV nodal conduction
*Digoxin* / Possible ↑ serum digoxin levels
*Potassium-wasting diuretics* / Hypokalemia, which causes an ↑ risk of serious ventricular arrhythmias
*Procainamide* / ↑ Risk of serious side effects due to exaggerated prolongation of the QT interval
*Quinidine* / ↑ Risk of serious side effects due to exaggerated prolongation of the QT interval
*Tricyclic antidepressants* / ↑ Risk of serious side effects due to exaggerated prolongation of the QT interval

**Laboratory Test Interferences:** ↑ ALT, transaminase. Abnormal liver function tests.

**Dosage** ─────────────
• **Tablets**
*Chronic stable angina.*
**Adults, initial:** 200 mg once daily; after 10 days the dosage may be adjusted upward depending on the response of the client (e.g., ability to perform ADL, QT interval, HR, frequency and severity of angina). **Maintenance:** 300 mg/day, not to exceed 400 mg/day. The minimum effective dose is 200 mg.

## NURSING CONSIDERATIONS

See also *Nursing Considerations* for *Calcium Channel Blocking Agents.*
**Assessment**
1. Note antianginal agents used previously and their effects.
2. Monitor VS, CBC, serum electrolytes (especially K), and ECG.
3. List drugs currently prescribed; note any that may prolong the QT interval (e.g., procainamide, quinidine, tricyclic antidepressants).
4. QT intervals should be checked prior to initiating therapy with bepridil, 1 to 3 weeks after beginning therapy, and periodically thereafter; especially after any dosage adjustment. Prolongation of QT intervals may lead to serious ventricular arrhythmias, especially torsades de pointes tachycardia.
5. Note any evidence of AV block, new arrhythmias, or history of MI, and/or implanted ventricular pacemaker.
6. Geriatric clients require more frequent monitoring.
7. If diuretics required, use a potassium-sparing agent.
**Client/Family Teaching**
1. Can be taken with meals or at bedtime if nausea occurs.
2. Take at about the same time each day. If a dose is missed, the next dose should *not* be doubled.

**B**

3. Continue taking nitroglycerin if prescribed.

4. Report any dizziness, chest pain, altered mental status, ↑ SOB, or fainting.

**Outcomes/Evaluate**

• Prophylaxis and control of angina

• Therapeutic levels (1–2 ng/mL)

---

# Beractant

(beh-**RACK**-tant)

Survanta **(Rx)**

**Classification:** Lung surfactant

**Action/Kinetics:** Beractant, derived from natural bovine lung extract, contains phospholipids, fatty acids, neutral lipids, and surfactant-associated proteins (to which colfosceril palmitate, tripalmitin, and palmitic acid are added). The proteins in the product—SP-B and SP-C—are hydrophobic, low molecular weight, and surfactant associated. Beractant replenishes pulmonary surfactant and restores surface activity to the lungs of premature infants to reduce respiratory distress syndrome. Intended for intratracheal use only. Significant improvement is observed in the arterial-alveolar oxygen ratio and mean airway pressure. Significantly decreases the incidence of respiratory distress syndrome, mortality due to respiratory distress syndrome, and air leak complications.

**Uses:** Prevention and treatment ("rescue") of respiratory distress syndrome (hyaline membrane disease) in premature infants.

**Special Concerns:** Beractant can quickly affect oxygenation and lung compliance; thus, it should only be used in a highly supervised setting with immediate availability of physicians experienced with intubation, ventilator management, and general care of premature infants.

**Side Effects:** Commonly, side effects are associated with the dosing procedure and include transient bradycardia, oxygen desaturation, ET tube reflux, vasoconstriction, pallor, hypotension, hypertension, ET tube blockage, hypocarbia, hypercarbia,

and **apnea.** Other symptoms include **intracranial hemorrhage,** rales, moist breath sounds, and nosocomial sepsis.

**OD** **Overdose Management:** *Symptoms:* **Acute airway obstruction.**

**Dosage**

• **Intratracheal Only**

4 mL/kg (100 mg phospholipids/kg birth weight).

## NURSING CONSIDERATIONS

**Administration/Storage**

1. For prevention of respiratory distress syndrome in premature infants weighing less than 1,250 g at birth or with evidence of surfactant deficiency, give as soon as possible, preferably within 15 min of birth.

2. To treat infants with confirmed respiratory distress syndrome and who require mechanical ventilation, give as soon as possible, preferably within 8 hr of birth.

3. Four doses can be given within the first 48 hr of life; doses should be given no sooner than q 6 hr.

4. Refrigerate at 2°C–8°C (36°F–46°F) and warm at room temperature for at least 20 min or in the hand for at least 8 min before administration. Does not have to be reconstituted or sonicated before use. If a prevention dose is required, preparation should begin before the infant is born. Do not warm and then return to the refrigerator for future use more than once.

5. Visually inspect vial before administration for discoloration (beractant is off-white to light brown). If settling occurs during storage, swirl the vial gently (do not shake) to redisperse although some foaming may occur at the surface during handling.

6. Each vial is for single use only; any residual drug should be discarded.

7. Instill beractant through a 5 French end-hole catheter that has been inserted into the ET tube of the infant with the tip of the catheter protruding just beyond the end of the ET tube above the infant's carina. The length of the catheter should be

shortened before inserting it through the ET tube. Do not give into a mainstem bronchus.

8. To ensure homogeneous distribution, divide each dose into four quarter-doses with each quarter-dose given with the infant in a different position—head and body inclined slightly down, head turned to the right; head and body inclined slightly down, head turned to the left; head and body inclined slightly up, head turned to the right; and head and body inclined slightly up, head turned to the left.

9. For the first dose, determine the total dose based on the infant's birth weight and withdraw the entire contents of the vial into the plastic syringe using at least a 20-gauge needle. The premeasured 5 French end-hole catheter is attached to the syringe and the catheter filled with beractant. Discard any excess through the catheter so that only the total dose to be given remains in the syringe. Before giving the drug, proper placement and patency of the ET tube must be ensured (the tube may be suctioned before giving the drug). The infant should be allowed to stabilize before proceeding with dosing.

10. If the first dose is to be used for prevention strategy, give the dose to the stabilized infant as soon as possible after birth (preferably within 15 min). The infant is positioned appropriately and the first quarter-dose is gently injected through the catheter over 2–3 sec. After the first quarter-dose is given, the catheter is removed from the ET tube. To prevent cyanosis, manually ventilate with sufficient oxygen using a hand-bag (ambu type) at a rate of 60 breaths/min with sufficient positive pressure to provide adequate air exchange and chest wall excursion.

11. If rescue strategy is to be undertaken, give the first dose as soon as possible after the infant is placed on a ventilator for management of hyaline membrane disease. Studies have been undertaken in which the infant's ventilator settings were changed to a rate of 60/min (inspiratory time 0.5 sec and $FiO_2$ 1) immediately before instilling the first quarter-dose. The infant is positioned appropriately and the first quarter-dose is gently injected through the catheter over 2–3 sec. The catheter is removed from the ET tube and the infant is returned to the mechanical ventilator.

12. When using both prevention and rescue strategies, the infant is ventilated for 20 sec or until stable. The infant is repositioned for instillation of the next quarter-dose. The remaining quarter-doses are given using the same procedures. After instillation of each quarter-dose, the catheter is removed and the infant is ventilated for 30 sec or until stabilized. After the final quarter-dose is instilled, the catheter is removed without flushing. The infant should not be suctioned for 1 hr after dosing unless signs of significant airway obstruction occur. After the dosing procedure is completed, resume usual ventilator management and clinical care.

13. If repeat doses are necessary, the dose is also 100 mg phospholipids/kg with the dose based on the infant's birth weight (the infant should not be reweighed). Additional doses are determined by evidence of continuing respiratory distress. Give repeat doses no sooner than 6 hr after the preceding dose if the infant remains intubated and requires a $FiO_2$ of at least 30 to maintain a $pO_2$ of less than or equal to 80 torr. Radiographic confirmation of respiratory distress syndrome should be made before giving additional doses to infants who received a prevention dose.

14. Repeat doses are given by the same procedure as described for prevention strategy. However, studies have used different ventilator settings. For repeat doses, the $FiO_2$ was increased by 0.2 or an amount sufficient to prevent cyanosis. The venti-

lator delivered a rate of 30/min with an inspiratory time of less than 1 sec. If the infant's pretreatment rate was greater than or equal to 30, it was left unchanged during instillation. Manual hand-bag ventilation should *not* be used to give repeat doses.

15. Store unopened vials in the refrigerator at 2°C–8°C (36°F–46°F) and protect from light. Store vials in the carton until ready for use.

16. Ross Laboratories offers audiovisual instructional materials concerning administration procedures and dosing requirements.

**Assessment**

1. Note indications for therapy (prevention, rescue, or both).

2. The infant HR, color, chest expansion, facial expression, oximeter readings, and ET tube patency and position should be documented and monitored carefully.

3. Ascertain that the ET tube tip is in the trachea and not in the esophagus or right or left mainstem bronchus, before inserting the 5 French end-hole catheter, to ensure appropriate drug dispersion to all lung areas.

4. Document baseline birth weight, ABGs, CXR, and physical assessment findings.

**Interventions**

1. Follow administration guidelines carefully. Beractant is for intratracheal administration. It should only be administered by trained personnel in a highly supervised environment permitting continuous observation.

2. Auscultate lung fields frequently and avoid suctioning for 1 hr after dosing unless symptoms of significant airway obstruction are evident.

3. Monitor ECG, arterial BP, and transcutaneous oxygen saturation continuously. After beractant treatment, frequent ABGs should be measured to prevent postdosing hyperoxia and hypocarbia.

4. Monitor (during dosing) for any evidence of transient bradycardia and decreased oxygen saturation. If evident, the dosing procedure should be stopped and the infant treated symptomatically until stabilized; then the dosing procedure may be resumed.

5. Observe closely for air leaks and mucous plugs. If mucous plug is unrelieved by suctioning, the ET tube must be replaced immediately.

**Outcomes/Evaluate**

• Improved airway exchange with ↓ pulmonary air leaks

• Oxygen saturation readings between 90% and 95%; improved pulmonary parameters more consistent with survival

• Prevention or successful treatment of respiratory distress syndrome in premature infants

---

# Betamethasone
(bay-tah-**METH**-ah-zohn)
Celestone **(Rx)**

# Betamethasone dipropionate
(bay-tah-**METH**-ah-zohn)
**Topical:** Alphatrex, Betaprolene ✳, Betaprone ✳, Diprolene, Diprolene Glycol ✳, Diprosone, Maxivate, Occlucort ✳, Taro-Sone ✳, Topilene ✳, Topisone ✳ **(Rx)**

# Betamethasone sodium phosphate
(bay-tah-**METH**-ah-zohn)
Betnesol ✳, Celestone Phosphate, Cel-U-Jec **(Rx)**

# Betamethasone sodium phosphate and Betamethasone acetate
(bay-tah-**METH**-ah-zohn)
Celestone Soluspan **(Rx)**

# Betamethasone valerate
(bay-tah-**METH**-ah-zohn)
**Topical:** Betacort ✳, Betaderm ✳, Betatrex, Betnovate ✳, Betnovate-1/2 ✳, Celestoderm-V ✳, Celestoderm-V/2 ✳, Dermabet, Ectosone Mild ✳, Ectosone Regular, Ectosone Scalp Lotion ✳, Prevex B ✳, Rivasone ✳, Valisone, Valisone Reduced Strength, Valnac **(Rx)**
**Classification:** Glucocorticoid

See also *Corticosteroids.*
**Action/Kinetics:** Causes low degree of sodium and water retention, as well as potassium depletion. The injectable form contains both rapid-acting and repository forms of betamethasone (mixture of betamethasone sodium phosphate and betamethasone acetate). Not recommended for replacement therapy in any acute or chronic adrenal cortical insufficiency because it does not have strong sodium-retaining effects. Long-acting. **t½:** over 300 min.
**Additional Uses:** Prevention of respiratory distress syndrome in premature infants.
**Special Concerns:** Safe use during pregnancy and lactation has not been established.

**Dosage** ———————
BETAMETHASONE
• **Syrup, Tablets**
0.6–7.2 mg/day.
BETAMETHASONE SODIUM PHOSPHATE
• **IV, Intra-articular, Intralesional, Soft Tissue Injection**
**Initial:** up to 9 mg/day; **then,** adjust dosage at minimal level to reduce symptoms.
BETAMETHASONE SODIUM PHOSPHATE
AND BETAMETHASONE ACETATE(contains 3 mg/mL each of the acetate and sodium phosphate)
• **IM**
**Initial:** 0.5–9 mg/day (dose ranges are ⅓–½ the PO dose given q 12 hr.)
• **Intra-articular, Intrabursal, Intradermal, Intralesional**
*Bursitis, peritendinitis, tenosynovitis.*
1 mL.
*Rheumatoid arthritis and osteoarthritis.*
0.25–2 mL, depending on size of the joint.
*Foot disorders, bursitis.*
0.25–0.5 mL under heloma durum or heloma molle; 0.5 mL under calcaneal spur or over hallux rigidus or digiti quinti varus. Tenosynovitis or periostitis of cuboid: 0.5 mL.
*Acute gouty arthritis.*

0.5–1 mL.
• **Intradermal**
0.2 mL/cm² not to exceed 1 mL/ week.
BETAMETHASONE DIPROPIONATE, BETAMETHASONE VALERATE
• **Topical Aerosol, Cream, Lotion, Ointment**
Apply sparingly to affected areas and rub in lightly.

## NURSING CONSIDERATIONS

See *Nursing Considerations for Corticosteroids.*
**Administration/Storage:** Avoid injection into deltoid muscle because SC atrophy of tissue may occur.
**Assessment:** Document indications for therapy, type, onset, and duration of symptoms; list agents trialed with the outcome.
**Client/Family Teaching**
1. Report any S&S of infection, i.e., increased fever and any redness, odor, or purulent drainage of wound.
2. Cover topical area to avoid sun burn.
3. Do not overuse joint after injection; this may further injure joint.
4. Record weight; report any sudden weight gain or presence of edema.
**Outcomes/Evaluate**
• ↓ Pain/inflammation; ↑ mobility of extremity
• Prevention of respiratory distress syndrome in premies
• Improved skin integrity; healing of lesions

# Betaxolol hydrochloride
(beh-**TAX**-oh-lohl)
**Pregnancy Category:** C
Betoptic, Betoptic S, Kerlone **(Rx)**
**Classification:** Beta-adrenergic blocking agent

See also *Beta-Adrenergic Blocking Agents.*
**Action/Kinetics:** Inhibits beta-1-adrenergic receptors although beta-2 receptors will be inhibited at high

---

doses. Has some membrane stabilizing activity but no intrinsic sympathomimetic activity. Low lipid solubility. When used in the eye, betaxolol reduces the production of aqueous humor, thus, reducing intraocular pressure. It has no effect on pupil size or accommodation. **t½:** 14–22 hr. Metabolized in the liver with most excreted through the urine; about 15% is excreted unchanged.

**Uses: PO:** Hypertension, alone or with other antihypertensive agents (especially diuretics). **Ophthalmic:** Ocular hypertension and chronic open-angle glaucoma (used alone or in combination with other antiglaucoma drugs).

**Special Concerns:** Use with caution during lactation. Safety and effectiveness have not been determined in children. Geriatric clients are at greater risk of developing bradycardia.

**Dosage** ————————
• **Tablets**
*Hypertension.*
**Initial:** 10 mg once daily either alone or with a diuretic. If the desired effect is not reached, the dose can be increased to 20 mg although doses higher than 20 mg will not increase the therapeutic effect. In geriatric clients the initial dose should be 5 mg/day.
• **Ophthalmic Solution, Suspension**
**Adults:** 1–2 gtt b.i.d. If used to replace another drug, continue the drug being used and add 1 gtt of betaxolol b.i.d. The previous drug should be discontinued the following day. If transferring from several antiglaucoma drugs being used together, adjust one drug at a time at intervals of not less than 1 week. The agents being used can be continued and add 1 gtt betaxolol b.i.d. The next day, another agent should be discontinued. The remaining antiglaucoma drug dosage can be decreased or discontinued depending on the response of the client.

## NURSING CONSIDERATIONS

See also *Nursing Considerations* for *Beta-Adrenergic Blocking Agents* and *Antihypertensive Agents*.

**Administration/Storage**
1. The full antihypertensive effect is usually observed within 7 to 14 days.
2. As the PO dose is increased, the HR decreases.
3. Discontinue PO therapy gradually over a 2-week period.
4. Shake ophthalmic suspension well before use.
5. Store ophthalmic products at room temperature not to exceed 30°C (86°F).

**Outcomes/Evaluate**
• ↓ BP (PO)
• ↓ Intraocular pressure (Ophth)

# Bethanechol chloride
(beh-**THAN**-eh-kohl)
**Pregnancy Category:** C
Duvoid, Myotonachol, PMS-Bethanechol Chloride ✤, Urecholine **(Rx)**
**Classification:** Cholinergic (parasympathomimetic), direct-acting

**Action/Kinetics:** Directly stimulates cholinergic receptors, primarily muscarinic type. This results in stimulation of gastric motility, increases gastric tone, and stimulates the detrusor muscle of the urinary bladder. Produces a slight transient fall of DBP, accompanied by minor reflex tachycardia. The drug is resistant to hydrolysis by acetylcholinesterase, which increases its duration of action. **PO: Onset,** 30–90 min; **maximum:** 60–90 min; **duration:** up to 6 hr. **SC: Onset,** 5–15 min; **maximum:** 15–30 min; **duration:** 2 hr.

**Uses:** Postpartum or postoperative urinary retention, neurogenic atony of the bladder with urinary retention. *Investigational:* Reflux esophagitis in adults and gastroesophageal reflux in infants and children.

**Contraindications:** Hypotension, hypertension, CAD, coronary occlusion, AV conduction defects, vasomotor instability, pronounced bradycardia, peptic ulcer, asthma (latent or active), hyperthyroidism, parkinsonism, epilepsy, obstruction of the bladder, if the strength or integrity of the GI or bladder wall is questionable, peritonitis, GI spastic disease, inflammatory lesions of the GI tract, marked vagotonia. Not to be used IM or IV.

**Special Concerns:** Use with caution during lactation. Safety and effectiveness have not been determined in children.

**Side Effects:** Serious side effects are uncommon with PO dosage but more common following SC use. *GI:* Nausea, diarrhea, salivation, GI upset, involuntary defecation, cramps, colic, belching, rumbling/gurgling of stomach. *CV:* Hypotension with reflex tachycardia, vasomotor response. *CNS:* Headache, malaise. *Other:* Flushing, sensation of heat about the face, sweating, urinary urgency, attacks of asthma, bronchial constriction, miosis, lacrimation.

**OD** **Overdose Management:** *Symptoms:* Early signs include N&V, abdominal discomfort, salivation, sweating, flushing. *Treatment:* Atropine, 0.6 mg SC for adults; a dose of 0.01 mg/kg atropine SC (up to a maximum of 0.4 mg) is recommended for infants and children up to 12 years of age. IV atropine may be used in emergency situations.

**Drug Interactions**
*Cholinergic inhibitors* / Additive cholinergic effects
*Ganglionic blocking agents* / Critical hypotensive response preceded by severe abdominal symptoms
*Procainamide* / Antagonism of cholinergic effects
*Quinidine* / Antagonism of cholinergic effects

**Dosage** ─────────
• **Tablets**
*Urinary retention.*
**Adults, usual:** 10–50 mg t.i.d.–q.i.d. The minimum effective dose can be determined by giving 5–10 mg initially and repeating this dose q 1–2 hr until a satisfactory response is

observed or a maximum of 50 mg has been given.
*Treat reflux esophagitis in adults.*
25 mg q.i.d.
*Gastroesophageal reflex in infants and children.*
3 mg/m²/dose t.i.d.
• **SC**
*Urinary retention.*
**Adults, usual:** 5 mg t.i.d.–q.i.d. The minimum effective dose is determined by giving 2.5 mg initially and repeating this dose at 15–30-min intervals to a maximum of four doses or until a satisfactory response is obtained.
*Diagnosis of reflux esophagitis in adults.*
Two 50-mcg/kg doses 15 min apart.

## NURSING CONSIDERATIONS
### Administration/Storage
1. Administer only PO or SC.
2. Observe closely 30 to 60 min after drug administration for possible severe side effects. Have atropine available during SC therapy to counteract manifestations of acute toxicity.
### Assessment
1. Take a complete nursing history.
2. Note drugs currently prescribed to ensure none interact unfavorably.
3. Assess I&O with urinary tract problems.
4. With GI atony, assess bowel sounds, function and habits.
5. If taking antacids, assess for peptic ulcers.
### Client/Family Teaching
1. Take tablets on an empty stomach (usually, 1 hr before or 2 hr after meals) to avoid N&V. Take exactly as prescribed for maximum effect.
2. With SC therapy, administer 2 hr before eating to reduce the potential for nausea.
3. Report decreased bowel activity when used for GI atony.
4. Any marked decrease in urine output, or any gnawing, aching, burning, or epigastric pain in the left epigastric area should be reported.

**Outcomes/Evaluate**
- Improved bladder tone and function without retention
- ↑ GI tract motility with ↓ abdominal distension

# Bicalutamide

(**buy**-kah-**LOO**-tah-myd)
**Pregnancy Category:** X
Casodex **(Rx)**
**Classification:** Antineoplastic, antiandrogen

See also *Antineoplastic Agents.*

**Action/Kinetics:** A nonsteroidal antiandrogen that competitively inhibits the action of androgens by binding to androgen receptors in the cytosol in target tissues. Well absorbed after PO administration; food does not affect the rate or amount absorbed. Metabolized in the liver, and both parent drug and metabolites are eliminated in the urine and feces. t½: 5.8 days. **Mean steady-state concentration in prostatic cancer:** 8.9 mcg/mL.

**Uses:** In combination therapy with a leutinizing hormone-releasing hormone analog for the treatment of advanced prostate cancer.

**Contraindications:** Pregnancy.

**Special Concerns:** Use with caution in clients with moderate to severe hepatic impairment and during lactation. Safety and efficacy have not been established in children.

**Side Effects:** *GI:* Constipation, N&V, diarrhea, anorexia, dyspepsia, rectal hemorrhage, dry mouth, melena. *CNS:* Dizziness, paresthesia, insomnia, anxiety, depression, decreased libido, hypertonia, confusion, neuropathy, somnolence, nervousness. *GU:* Gynecomastia, nocturia, hematuria, UTI, impotence, urinary incontinence, urinary frequency, impaired urination, dysuria, urinary retention, urinary urgency. *CV:* Hot flashes (most common), hypertension, angina pectoris, CHF. *Metabolic:* Peripheral edema, hyperglycemia, weight loss or gain, dehydration, gout. *Musculoskeletal:* Myasthenia, arthritis, myalgia, leg cramps, pathologic fracture. *Respiratory:* Dyspnea, increased cough, pharyngitis, bronchitis, pneumonia, rhinitis, lung disorder. *Dermatologic:* Rash, sweating, dry skin, pruritus, alopecia. *Hematologic:* Anemia, hypochromic and iron deficiency anemia. *Body as a whole:* General pain, back pain, asthenia, pelvic pain, abdominal pain, chest pain, flu syndrome, edema, neoplasm, fever, neck pain, chills, **sepsis.** *Miscellaneous:* Infection, bone pain, headache, breast pain, diabetes mellitus.

**Drug Interactions:** Bicalutamide may displace coumarin anticoagulants from their protein-binding sites, resulting in an increased anticoagulant effect.

**Laboratory Test Interferences:** ↑ Alkaline phosphatase, creatinine, AST, ALT, bilirubin, BUN, liver enzyme tests. ↓ Hemoglobin, white cell count.

**Dosage**
- **Tablets**
  *Prostatic carcinoma.*
  50 mg (1 tablet) once daily (morning or evening) in combination with an LHRH analog with or without food.

## NURSING CONSIDERATIONS

See also *Nursing Considerations* for *Antineoplastic Agents*

**Administration/Storage**
1. Take Bicalutamide at the same time each day.
2. Start treatment with bicalutamide at the same time as treatment with an LHRH analog.

**Assessment**
1. Note indications for therapy, onset, duration of symptoms, and any other agents/therapies trialed.
2. Monitor liver and renal function studies, CBC, and PSA. (If transaminases increase over two times the upper limit of normal, discontinue drug.)
3. If prescribed warfarin, monitor PT/INR closely as bicalutamide can

displace from its protein binding sites.

**Client/Family Teaching**

1. Take as directed, at the same time each day, with prescribed LHRH analog drug (i.e., goserelin implant or leuprolide depot) .

2. Side effects that require immediate medical care include hemorrhage, urinary retention, yellow skin, fracture, and respiratory distress.

3. Periodic lab studies for PSA, CBC, liver and renal function will be required to assess response to therapy.

**Outcomes/Evaluate**

• Symptomatic improvement
• Reductions of serum PSA and inhibition of tumor growth

# Biperiden hydrochloride
(bye-**PER**-ih-den)
**Pregnancy Category:** C
Akineton Hydrochloride **(Rx)**
**Classification:** Synthetic anticholinergic, antiparkinson agent

See also *Antiparkinson Drugs* and *Cholinergic Blocking Agents.*

**Action/Kinetics:** Tolerance may develop to this synthetic anticholinergic. Tremor may increase as spasticity is relieved. Slight respiratory and CV effects. **Time to peak levels:** 60–90 min. **Peak levels:** 4–5 mcg/L. **t½:** About 18–24 hr.

**Uses:** Parkinsonism, especially of the postencephalitic, arteriosclerotic, and idiopathic types. Drug-induced (e.g., phenothiazines) extrapyramidal manifestations.

**Additional      Contraindications:** Children under the age of 3 years.

**Special Concerns:** Use with caution in older children.

**Additional Side Effects:** Muscle weakness, inability to move certain muscles.

**Dosage**
• **Tablets**
*Parkinsonism.*

**Adults:** 2 mg t.i.d.–q.i.d., to a maximum of 16 mg/day.

   *Drug-induced extrapyramidal effects.*
**Adults:** 2 mg 1–3 times/day. Maximum daily dose: 16 mg.
**Adults:** 2 mg; repeat q 30 min until symptoms improve, but not more than four doses daily. **Pediatric:** 0.04 mg/kg (1.2 mg/m²); repeat q 30 min until symptoms improve, but not more than four doses daily.

## NURSING CONSIDERATIONS

See also *Nursing Considerations* for *Antiparkinson Drugs* and *Cholinergic Blocking Agents.*

**Assessment**

1. Note age; older clients should receive lower doses of biperiden.

2. Record drugs client taking to prevent any unfavorable interactions.

**Interventions**

1. If administered IM, supervise and assist in walking; may cause transient incoordination.

2. If administered IV, have client remain recumbent during and for 15 min after administration. Assist to get up by having them dangle their legs at the bedside prior to standing and walking, to prevent hypotension, syncope, and falling.

**Client/Family Teaching**

1. Take after meals to avoid gastric irritation.

2. Do not use antacids or antidiarrheal for 1–2 hr after taking drug.

3. Record stools; increase intake of fluids, fruit juices, and fiber to avoid constipation.

4. Avoid overheating; drug decreases perspiration.

5. Record I&O; report urinary difficulty.

6. Use sugarless gum or candies and rinse mouth often to control dry mouth effects.

**Outcomes/Evaluate:** Control of drug-induced (phenothiazine) extrapyramidal manifestations (i.e., ↓ muscle rigidity and drooling)

---

# Bismuth subsalicylate, Metronidazole, Tetracycline hydrochloride

**B**

(**BIS**-muth, meh-froh-**NYE**-dah-zohl, teh-trah-**SYE**-kleen)
**Pregnancy Category:** B (Metronidazole), D (Tetracycline)
Helidac **(Rx)**
**Classification:** Agent to treat *Helicobacter pylori* infections

See also *Metronidazole* and *Tetracycline hydrochloride.*

**Action/Kinetics:** The information to follow was derived from each drug being given alone and not in the combination in this product. Bismuth subsalicylate is hydrolyzed in the GI tract to bismuth and salicylic acid. Less than 1% of bismuth from PO doses of bismuth subsalicylate is absorbed into the general circulation. However, more than 80% of salicylic acid is absorbed. Metronidazole is well absorbed from the GI tract. **Peak plasma levels, metronidazole:** 1–2 hr; **t½, elimination:** 8 hr. Metronidazole is metabolized by the liver and is excreted through both the urine (60% to 80%) and the feces (6% to 15%). Tetracyclines are readily absorbed from the GI tract. The relative contributions of systemic versus local antimicrobial activity against *H. pylori* for agents used in eradication therapy have not been determined.

**Uses:** In combination with an $H_2$ antagonist to treat active duodenal ulcer associated with *H. pylori* infection.

**Contraindications:** Use during pregnancy or lactation or in children. Use in renal or hepatic impairment. Hypersensitivity to bismuth subsalicylate, metronidazole or other imidazole derivatives, and any tetracycline. Use in those allergic to aspirin or salicylates. Children and teenagers who have or who are recovering from chicken pox or the flu should not take bismuth subsalicylate due to the possibility of Reye's

syndrome. Tetracyclines should not be used during tooth development in children (i.e., last half of pregnancy, infancy, and childhood to 8 years of age) due to the possibility of permanent tooth discoloration.

**Special Concerns:** Use with caution in elderly clients and in clients with evidence or history of blood dyscrasias. Safety and efficacy have not been determined in children.

**Side Effects:** See also *Metronidazole* and *Tetracyclines* for specific side effects for these drugs. The following side effects were noted when the three drugs were given concomitantly. *GI:* N&V, diarrhea, abdominal pain, melena, anal discomfort, anorexia, constipation. *CNS:* Dizziness, paresthesia, insomnia. *Miscellaneous:* Asthenia, pain, upper respiratory infection.

Excessive doses of bismuth subsalicylate may cause neurotoxicity, which is reversible if therapy is terminated. Large doses of metronidazole have been associated with seizures and peripheral neuropathy (characterized by numbness or paresthesia of an extremity). Metronidazole may exacerbate candidiasis. Tetracycline use may cause superinfection, benign intracranial hypertension (pseudotumor cerebri), and photosensitivity.

**Drug Interactions:** See also *Metronidazole,* and *Tetracyclines.* There may be a decrease in absorption of tetracycline due to the presence of bismuth or calcium carbonate (an excipient in bismuth subsalicylate tablets).

**Dosage** ――――――――――
• **Tablets (Bismuth Subsalicylate, Metronidazole) and Capsules (Tetracycline Hydrochloride)**
*Treatment of H. pylori.*
Each dose includes two pink, round chewable tablets (525 mg bismuth subsalicylate), one white tablet (250 mg metronidazole), and one pale orange and white capsule (500 mg tetracycline hydrochloride). Each dose is taken q.i.d. with meals and at bedtime for 14 days. *NOTE:* Concomitant

therapy with an $H_2$ antagonist is also required.

## NURSING CONSIDERATIONS

See also *Nursing Considerations* for *Metronidazole*, and *Tetracycline hydrochloride*.

**Administration/Storage**

1. Bismuth subsalicylate may cause darkening of the tongue and black stools, do not confuse with melena.

2. The bismuth subsalicylate tablets should be chewed and swallowed. Take Metronidazole and tetracycline whole with 8 oz of water.

3. Ingest adequate fluids, especially with the bedtime dose, in order to decrease the risk of esophageal irritation and ulceration.

4. If a dose is missed, it can be made up by continuing the normal dosage schedule until the medication is gone. Double doses are not to be taken. If more than four doses are missed, contact the provider.

**Assessment**

1. Note clinical presentation and characteristics of symptoms, including onset and duration.

2. Document any allergy to aspirin or salicylates.

3. Determine that women of childbearing age are not pregnant. Do not use in children under 8 years old.

4. Obtain baseline CBC, liver and renal function studies; note any dysfunction.

5. Document serum and/or endoscopic confirmation of organism.

6. Note $H_2$ agent prescribed; therapy requires an $H_2$ antagonist.

**Client/Family Teaching**

1. Review the tablets: 2 pink round chewable (bismuth), 1 white tablet (metronidazole), and 1 pale orange and white capsule (tetracycline). All must be taken 4 times a day with meals and at bedtime for 14 days total. Chew and swallow the pink chewables (bismuth); swallow the others with a full glass of water. Consume plenty of fluids to prevent esophageal irritation. Avoid milk/ dairy products; may alter tetracycline absorption. Take $H_2$ antagonist as prescribed.

2. Do not double up on missed doses; take next dose and continue prescription as directed until completed. Frequent multiple missed doses should be reported.

3. Avoid alcohol during and for 24 hr following completion of therapy.

4. Use additional contraception with birth control pills; tetracycline may lower effectiveness.

5. Avoid prolonged sun exposure to prevent a photosensitivity reaction. Use sunglasses, sun screen, and protective clothing when exposed.

6. Tongue may darken and stools may appear black; this is only temporary. Report any unusual or persistent side effects.

**Outcomes/Evaluate**

- Eradication of *H. pylori* infection
- ↓ Recurrence of duodenal ulcers

# Bisoprolol fumarate

(**BUY**-soh-**proh**-lol)
**Pregnancy Category:** C
Zebeta **(Rx)**
**Classification:** Beta-adrenergic blocking agent

See also *Beta-Adrenergic Blocking Agents*.

**Action/Kinetics:** Inhibits beta-1-adrenergic receptors; at higher doses beta-2 receptors are also inhibited. No intrinsic sympathomimetic activity and no membrane-stabilizing activity. t½: 9–12 hr. Over 90% of PO dose is absorbed. Approximately 50% is excreted unchanged through the urine and the remainder as inactive metabolites; a small amount (less than 2%) is excreted through the feces.

**Uses:** Hypertension alone or in combination with other antihypertensive agents. *Investigational:* Angina pectoris, SVTs, PVCs.

**Special Concerns:** Use with caution during lactation. Safety and efficacy have not been determined in children. Since bisoprolol is rather selective for beta-1 receptors, it may be used with caution in clients with bronchospastic disease who do not respond to, or who cannot tolerate, other antihypertensive therapy.

**Laboratory Test Interferences:** ↑ AST, ALT, uric acid, creatinine, BUN, serum potassium, glucose, and phosphorus. ↓ WBCs and platelets.

**Dosage**
- **Tablets**
  *Antihypertensive.*

Dose must be individualized. **Adults, initial:** 5 mg once daily (in some clients, 2.5 mg/day may be appropriate). **Maintenance:** If the 5-mg dose is inadequate, the dose may be increased to 10 mg/day and then, if needed, to 20 mg once daily. In clients with impaired renal or hepatic function, the initial daily dose should be 2.5 mg with caution used in titrating the dose upward.

## NURSING CONSIDERATIONS

See also *Nursing Considerations* for *Beta-Adrenergic Blocking Agents.*
**Administration/Storage**
1. Food does not affect the bioavailability of bisoprolol; may be given without regard to meals.
2. The half-life of bisoprolol is increased in clients with a creatinine clearance below 40 mL/min and in those with cirrhosis; adjust dose.
3. Bisoprolol is not dialyzable so dose adjustments are not required in clients undergoing hemodialysis.
**Assessment**
1. Document indications for therapy, previous agents used, and the outcome.
2. Monitor CBC, electrolytes, liver and renal function studies. Reduce dose with renal and liver dysfunction.
3. Once baseline parameters have been determined, continue to monitor BP in both arms with client lying, sitting, and standing.
4. Document cardiac rhythm; note any arrhythmias.
**Outcomes/Evaluate**
- ↓ BP; relief of angina
- Stable cardiac rhythm

---COMBINATION DRUG---

# Bisoprolol fumarate and Hydrochlorothiazide

(**BUY**-soh-**proh**-lol, **high**-droh-**klor**-oh-**THIGH**-ah-zyd)
**Pregnancy Category:** C
Ziac **(Rx)**
**Classification:** Antihypertensive

See also *Bisoprolol fumarate* and *Hydrochlorothiazide.*
**Content:** *Beta-adrenergic blocking agent:* Bisoprolol fumarate: 2.5, 5, or 10 mg. *Diuretic/antihypertensive:* Hydrochlorothiazide: 6.25 mg in all tablets.
**Uses:** First-line therapy in mild to moderate hypertension.
**Contraindications:** Use in bronchospastic pulmonary disease, cardiogenic shock, overt CHF, second- or third-degree AV block, marked sinus bradycardia, anuria, hypersensitivity to either drug or to other sulfonamide-derived drugs, during lactation.
**Special Concerns:** Use with caution in clients with peripheral vascular disease, impaired renal or hepatic function, and progressive liver disease and in clients also receiving myocardial depressants or inhibitors of AV conduction such as verapamil, diltiazem, and disopyramide. Elderly clients may be more sensitive to the effects of this drug product. Safety and effectiveness have not been determined in children.
**Side Effects:** See individual drugs. Most commonly, dizziness and fatigue. At higher doses, bisoprolol inhibits beta-2-adrenergic receptors located in bronchial and vascular muscle.
**Drug Interactions**
*Antihypertensives* / Additive effect to decrease BP
*Cyclopropane* / Additive depression of myocardium
*Trichloroethylene* / Additive depression of myocardium

**Dosage**
- **Tablets**
  *Antihypertensive.*
**Adults, initial:** One 2.5/6.25-mg tablet given once daily. If needed,

the dose may be increased q 14 days to a maximum of two 10/6.25-mg tablets given once daily.

## NURSING CONSIDERATIONS

See also *Nursing Considerations* for *Beta-Adrenergic Blocking Agents, Antihypertensive Agents,* and *Diuretics, Thiazides.*

**Administration/Storage**
1. The combination of bisoprolol and hydrochlorothiazide may be substituted for the titrated individual components.
2. If withdrawal is necessary, it should be done gradually over a 2 week period with careful monitoring.
3. Clients whose BP is controlled adequately with 50 mg hydrochlorothiazide but who experience significant potassium loss may achieve similar control of BP without the electrolyte disturbances by using the combination of bisoprolol and hydrochlorothiazide.

**Assessment**
1. Document indications for therapy, other agents used, and the outcome.
2. Determine any sensitivity to drug components.
3. List all drugs prescribed to ensure none interact unfavorably.
4. Obtain baseline electrolytes, liver and renal function studies.
5. Screen client carefully as drug is not for use with bronchospastic pulmonary disease, PVD, diabetes, thyrotoxicosis, compensated cardiac failure, liver or renal disease.
6. Assess ECG to ensure no dysrhythmias (second- or third-degree AV block or bradycardia) that would preclude drug therapy.

**Interventions**
1. Monitor VS carefully; drug will cause a reduction in SBP and DBP and HR. Request parameters for administration (e.g., hold if SBP < 90; HR < 50) when necessary.
2. Monitor I&O and serum electrolytes; observe for S&S of fluid and electrolyte imbalance.
3. To withdraw therapy, taper dosages over 2 weeks to prevent any adverse sequelae.
4. If therapy is to be discontinued in clients receiving both clonidine and Ziac, the Ziac should be withdrawn several days before withdrawal of clonidine.

**Client/Family Teaching**
1. Do not stop abruptly. With CAD, a heart attack or ventricular arrhythmia may be precipitated.
2. Do not perform activities that require mental alertness until drug effects realized.
3. Report S&S of heart failure (↑ SOB, edema, fatigue) as alternative therapy may be indicated.
4. Diabetics should monitor blood sugars carefully as beta blockers may mask symptoms of hypoglycemia.
5. Report any persistent or bothersome side effects.
6. Record BP and pulse regularly and bring to each visit.
7. Continue diet restrictions (e.g., low salt, low fat, low calorie), weight reduction, and a regular exercise routine.

**Outcomes/Evaluate:** Control of BP

# Bitolterol mesylate
(bye-**TOHL**-ter-ohl)
**Pregnancy Category:** C
Tornalate Aerosol **(Rx)**
**Classification:** Bronchodilator

See also *Sympathomimetic Drugs.*
**Action/Kinetics:** Bitolterol is a prodrug in that it is converted by esterases in the body to the active colterol. Colterol combines with beta-2-adrenergic receptors, producing dilation of bronchioles. Minimal beta-1-adrenergic activity. **Onset following inhalation:** 3–4 min. **Time to peak effect:** 30–60 min. **Duration:** 5–8 hr.
**Uses:** Prophylaxis and treatment of bronchial asthma and bronchospasms. Treatment of bronchitis, emphysema, bronchiectasis, and

B

COPD. May be used with theophylline and/or steroids.

**Special Concerns:** Safety has not been established for use during lactation and in children less than 12 years of age. Use with caution in ischemic heart disease, hypertension, hyperthyroidism, diabetes mellitus, cardiac arrhythmias, seizure disorders, or in those who respond unusually to beta-adrenergic agonists. There may be decreased effectiveness in steroid-dependent asthmatic clients. Hypersensitivity reactions may occur.

**Additional Side Effects:** *CNS:* Hyperactivity, hyperkinesia, lightheadedness. *CV:* Premature ventricular contractions. *Other:* Throat irritation.

**Drug Interactions:** Additive effects with other beta-adrenergic bronchodilators.

**Laboratory Test Interferences:** ↑ AST. ↓ Platelets, WBCs. Proteinuria.

**Dosage** ————————

• **Metered Dose Inhaler**
  *Bronchodilation.*

**Adults and children over 12 years:** 2 inhalations at an interval of 1–3 min q 8 hr (if necessary, a third inhalation may be taken). The dose should not exceed 3 inhalations q 6 hr or 2 inhalations q 4 hr.
  *Prophylaxis of bronchospasm.*

**Adults and children over 12 years:** 2 inhalations q 8 hr.

## NURSING CONSIDERATIONS

See also *Nursing Considerations* for *Sympathomimetic Drugs*.

**Administration/Storage**

1. Bitolterol is available in a MDI. The inhaler delivers 0.37 mg bitolterol per actuation.

2. Do not store the medication above 120°F (49°C).

**Client/Family Teaching**

1. With the inhaler in an upright position, breathe out completely in a normal fashion. Breathe in slowly and deeply, squeeze the canister and mouthpiece between the thumb and forefinger to activate the medication. Hold the breath for 10 sec and then slowly exhale. A spacer may facilitate drug dispersion. Review video/instruction for proper administration guidelines.

2. Do not exceed prescribed dosage; seek medical assistance if symptoms worsen.

**Outcomes/Evaluate**

• Improved airway exchange with ↓ airway resistance

• Asthma/bronchospasm prophylaxis

# Bleomycin sulfate

(blee-oh-**MY**-sin)
**Pregnancy Category:** D
Blenoxane (Abbreviation: BLM) **(Rx)**
**Classification:** Antineoplastic, antibiotic

See also *Antineoplastic Agents*.

**Action/Kinetics:** Bleomycin is a mixture of cytotoxic glycopeptide antibiotics isolated from *Streptomyces verticillus*. The action may be due to binding to DNA, inducing lability of the DNA structure and decreasing synthesis of DNA and to a lesser extent RNA and protein. It is most effective in the $G_2$ and M phases of cell division. Drug currently used is mostly a mixture of bleomycin $A_2$ and $B_2$. Relatively low bone marrow depressant activity, localizes in certain tissues, and is an important component of some combination regimens. **Peak plasma levels** (after 4–5 days of therapy): 50 ng/mL. **t½, distribution, after IV:** 10–20 min. **Peak blood levels, after IM:** 30–60 min with levels that are about one-third that of IV. **t½, elimination, $C_{CR}$ less than 35 mL/min:** About 2 hr; half-life increases exponentially as (creatinine clearance) decreases below 35 mL/min. Two-thirds excreted in the urine as active bleomycin.

**Uses:** Palliative treatment of cancers listed, either used alone or in combination. Squamous cell carcinoma of the head and neck, including mouth, tongue, tonsil, nasopharynx, oropharynx, sinus, palate, lip, buccal mucosa, gingiva, epiglottis, skin, and larynx. Carcinoma of the skin, penis, cervix, and vulva. Lymphomas, including Hodgkin's, non-Hodgkin's, reticulum cell sarcoma, and lymphosarcoma. Testicular carcinoma, including embryonal cell, choriocarcinoma, and teratocarcinoma. Sclerosing agent to prevent or treat malignant pleural effusions associated with cancer. *Investigational:* Soft tissue sarcomas, osteosarcoma, malignant effusions (peritoneal, pleural), ovarian tumors. Also for severe, recalcitrant common warts (verruca vulgaris).

**Contraindications:** Lactation. Renal or pulmonary diseases. Pregnancy.

**Special Concerns:** Safety and efficacy have not been determined in children. When used in combination with other antineoplastic drugs, pulmonary toxicity may occur at lower doses.

**Side Effects:** *Pulmonary:* Pneumonitis, ***pulmonary fibrosis, especially in older clients.*** *Hypersensitivity:* In approximately 1% of lymphoma clients, an idiosyncratic reaction manifested by hypotension, fever, chills, mental confusion, and wheezing has been reported. *Integumentary and mucous membranes:* Erythema, rash, striae, vesiculation, hyperpigmentation, skin tenderness, hyperkeratosis, nail changes, alopecia, pruritus, stomatitis, skin toxicity. *GI:* Vomiting, anorexia, weight loss. *Miscellaneous:* Renal and hepatic toxicity.

**Drug Interactions**

*Digoxin* / ↓ Digoxin serum levels
*Filgrastim* / ↑ Risk of pulmonary toxicity
*Phenytoin* / ↓ Phenytoin serum levels

**Dosage** ————————
• **SC, IM, IV**
*Hodgkin's disease.*
**Initial:** 0.25–0.5 units/kg (10–20 units/m² once or twice weekly). **Maintenance:** After a 50% response, give 1 unit/day or 5 units/week given IM or IV. Due to pulmo-

nary toxicity, give doses greater than 400 units with great caution.

*Squamous cell carcinoma, non-Hodgkin's lymphoma, testicular carcinoma.*
0.25–0.5 units/kg (10–20 units/m²) once or twice a week. Due to the possibility of anaphylaxis, lymphoma clients should receive 2 units or less for the first two doses; if no acute reaction occurs, follow the regular dosage schedule.

• **Intrapleural Injection**
*Malignant pleural effusion.*
60 units given as a single bolus dose by a thoracostomy tube following drainage of excess pleural fluid and confirmation of complete lung expansion.

• **Intralesional**
*Warts.*
0.2–0.8 unit (depending on the size) one or more times q 2–4 weeks (up to a maximum total dose of 2 units using a solution of 15 units of sterile bleomycin solution in 15 mL 0.9% saline or water for injection).

## NURSING CONSIDERATIONS

See also *Nursing Considerations* for *Antineoplastic Agents.*

**Administration/Storage**
1. For IM or SC use, reconstitute the drug with 1–5 mL(15-unit vial) or 2–10 mL (30-unit vial) with sterile water for injection, 5% dextrose injection, 0.9% NaCL injection, or bacteriostatic water for injection.
2. For intrapleural use, dissolve 60 units in 50–100 mL of 0.9% NaCL injection and give through a thoracostomy tube following drainage of excess pleural fluid and confirmation of complete lung expansion. The amount of drainage from the chest tube should be as minimal as possible before instillation of bleomycin. Clamp the thoracostomy tube after bleomycin instillation. Move client from the supine to the left and right lateral positions several times during the next 4 hr, followed by removal of the clamp to reestablish suction.

3. Do not reconstitute with 5% dextrose injection or other dextrose-containing dilutions as there is a loss of potency.

4. Hodgkin's disease and testicular tumors should respond within 2 weeks; squamous cell cancers require at least 3 weeks.

5. Bleomycin is stable for 24 hr at room temperature (14 days if refrigerated) in sodium chloride.

**IV** 6. For IV use, reconstitute the contents of the 15- or 30-unit vial with 5 or 10 mL, respectively, of 0.9% NaCL injection. Administer IV slowly over 10 min. Do not reconstitute with 5% dextrose injection or other dextrose-containing dilutions as there is a loss of potency.

**Assessment**
1. Document indications for therapy. Note onset and describe symptoms.
2. Obtain baseline CBC, LFTs, and PFTs. Assess for basilar rales, cough, DOE, and tachypnea, all of which are dose-related symptoms of pulmonary toxicity.
3. Document and avoid adhesive on the skin; drug accumulates in keratin and may discolor epithelium.
4. If receiving digoxin, monitor levels.
5. Clients with lymphoma may be prescribed two test doses of 2 units each initially to assess for idiosyncratic response.
6. Drug may cause mild granulocyte suppression. Nadir: 10 days; recovery: 14 days.

**Client/Family Teaching**
1. Clients with lymphoma may experience symptoms of idiosyncratic reaction (*hypoxia, fever, chills, confusion*).
2. Fever 3–6 hr after treatment is common; take prescribed antipyretics to relieve.
3. Avoid vaccinations during therapy.
4. Practice safe, barrier form of contraception.
5. Report any abnormal oral or skin rashes.
6. Smoking may aggravate pulmonary symptoms.

**Outcomes/Evaluate**
• ↓ Tumor size/spread

• Resolution of recalcitrant common warts

# Bretylium tosylate
(breh-**TILL**-ee-um **TOZ**-ill-ayt)
**Pregnancy Category:** C
Bretylate Parenteral ✶, Bretylol **(Rx)**
**Classification:** Antiarrhythmic, class III

**Action/Kinetics:** Bretylium inhibits catecholamine release at nerve endings by decreasing excitability of the nerve terminal. Initially there is a release of norepinephrine, which may cause tachycardia and a rise in BP; this is followed by a blockade of release of catecholamines. The drug also increases the duration of the action potential and the effective refractory period, which may assist in reversing arrhythmias. **Peak plasma concentration and effect:** 1 hr after IM injection. Antifibrillatory effect within a few minutes after IV use. Suppression of ventricular tachycardia and ventricular arrhythmias takes 20–120 min, whereas suppression of PVCs does not occur for 6–9 hr. **Therapeutic serum levels:** 0.5–1.5 mcg/mL. t½: Approximately 5–10 hr. **Duration:** 6–8 hr. From 0% to 8% is protein bound. Up to 90% of drug is excreted unchanged in the urine after 24 hr.

**Uses:** Life-threatening ventricular arrhythmias that have failed to respond to other antiarrhythmics. Prophylaxis and treatment of ventricular fibrillation. For short-term use only. *Investigational:* Second-line drug (after lidocaine) for advanced cardiac life support during CPR.

**Contraindications:** Severe aortic stenosis, severe pulmonary hypertension.

**Special Concerns:** Safety and efficacy in children have not been established. Dosage adjustment is required in clients with impaired renal function.

**Side Effects:** *CV:* Hypotension (including postural hypotension), transient hypertension, increased frequency of PVCs, bradycardia, precipitation of anginal attacks, initial increase in arrhythmias, sensation of substernal pressure. *GI:* N&V (especially after rapid IV administration), diarrhea, abdominal pain, hiccoughs. *CNS:* Vertigo, dizziness, lightheadedness, syncope, anxiety, paranoid psychosis, confusion, mood swings. *Miscellaneous:* Renal dysfunction, flushing, hyperthermia, SOB, nasal stuffiness, diaphoresis, conjunctivitis, erythematous macular rash, lethargy, generalized tenderness.

**OD** **Overdose Management:** *Symptoms:* Marked hypertension followed by hypotension. *Treatment:* Hypertension can be treated by nitroprusside or another short-acting IV antihypertensive. Hypotension can be treated with appropriate fluid therapy and pressor agents such as norepinephrine or dopamine.

**Drug Interactions**
*Digitoxin, Digoxin* / Bretylium may aggravate digitalis toxicity due to initial release of norepinephrine
*Procainamide, Quinidine* / Concomitant use with bretylium ↓ inotropic effect of bretylium and ↑ hypotension

**Dosage** _____
• **IV**
*Ventricular fibrillation, hemodynamically unstable ventricular tachycardia.*
**Adults:** 5 mg/kg of undiluted solution given rapidly. Can increase to 10 mg/kg if ventricular fibrillation persists; repeat as needed. **Maintenance, IV infusion:** 1–2 mg/min; or, 5–10 mg/kg q 6 hr of diluted drug infused over more than 8 min. **Children:** 5 mg/kg/dose IV followed by 10 mg/kg at 15–30-min intervals for a maximum total dose of 30 mg/kg; **maintenance:** 5–10 mg/kg q 6 hr.
*Other ventricular arrhythmias.*
• **IV Infusion**
5–10 mg/kg of diluted solution over more than 8 min. **Maintenance:** 5–10 mg/kg q 6 hr over a period of 8 min or more or 1–2 mg/min by con-

tinuous IV infusion. **Children:** 5–10 mg/kg/dose q 6 hr.
• **IM**
*Other ventricular arrhythmias.*
**Adults:** 5–10 mg/kg of undiluted solution followed, if necessary, by the same dose at 1–2-hr intervals; **then,** give same dosage q 6–8 hr.

## NURSING CONSIDERATIONS

See also *Nursing Considerations* for *Antiarrhythmic Agents.*
**Administration/Storage**
1. For IM injection, use drug undiluted.
2. Rotate injection sites so that no more than 5 mL of drug is given at any site. This avoids localized atrophy, necrosis, fibrosis, vascular degeneration, or inflammation.
3. Keep supine during therapy or closely observe for postural hypotension.
4. Start on an oral antiarrhythmic medication as soon as possible.
**IV** 5. For IV infusion, bretylium is compatible with 5% dextrose injection, 0.9% NaCl, D5%/ 0.45% NaCl, D5%/0.9% NaCl, D5%/RL, 5% sodium bicarbonate, 20% mannitol, 1/6 molar sodium lactate, RL, CaCL (54.5 mEq/L) in 5% dextrose, and KCL (40 mEq/L) in 5% dextrose.
6. For direct IV, administer undiluted over 15–30 sec; may repeat in 15–30 min if symptoms persist. May further dilute 500 mg in 50 cc and infuse over 10–30 min.
**Assessment**
1. Document indications for therapy, pretreatment ECG, and VS.
2. If taking digitalis, drug may aggravate digitalis toxicity.
**Interventions**
1. Monitor VS and rhythm strips as dose is titrated based on the client's response.
2. To reduce N&V, administer the IV drug slowly over 10 min while supine. Once infusion complete remain supine until the BP has stabilized.
3. Supervise clients once ambulation is permitted because they may

develop lightheadedness and vertigo.

4. Bretylium often causes a fall in supine BP within 1 hr of IV administration. If the SBP falls below 75 mm Hg, anticipate need for pressor agents.

5. If clients develop side effects, stay with them, reassuring and reorienting as needed.

**Outcomes/Evaluate**

• Termination of life-threatening ventricular arrhythmia; stable cardiac rhythm

• Serum drug levels (0.5–1.5 mcg/mL)

# Brimonidine tartrate
(brih-**MOH**-nih-deen)
**Pregnancy Category:** B
Alphagan **(Rx)**
**Classification:** Sympathomimetic

See also *Sympathomimetic Drugs.*

**Action/Kinetics:** Brimonidine tartrate, an alpha-2 adrenergic receptor agonist, reduces aqueous humor production and increases uveoscleral outflow. **Peak plasma levels after intraocular administration:** 1–4 hr. t½, systemic: About 3 hr. Metabolized by the liver and excreted through the urine as unchanged drug and metabolites.

**Uses:** Lower intraocular pressure in open-angle glaucoma or ocular hypertension.

**Contraindications:** Use in clients on MAO inhibitor therapy. Lactation.

**Special Concerns:** Use with caution in those with renal or hepatic impairment; in severe CV disease, depression, cerebral or coronary insufficiency, Raynaud's phenomenon, orthostatic hypotension, or thromboangiitis obliterans. Safety and efficacy have not been determined in children. Benzylkonium chloride, a preservative in the product, may be absorbed by soft contact lenses.

**Side Effects:** *Ophthalmic:* Ocular hyperemia, burning and stinging, blurring, foreign body sensation, conjunctival follicles, ocular allergic reactions, ocular pruritus, corneal staining or erosion, photophobia, eyelid erythema, ocular ache or pain, ocular dryness, tearing, eyelid edema, conjunctival edema, blepharitis, ocular irritation, conjunctival blanching, abnormal vision, lid crusting, conjunctival hemorrhage, conjunctival discharge. *CNS:* Headache, fatigue, drowsiness, dizziness, insomnia, depression, anxiety. *Miscellaneous:* Upper respiratory symptoms, GI symptoms, asthenia, muscle pain, abnormal taste, hypertension, palpitations, nasal dryness, syncope.

**Dosage** —————————————
• **Solution, 0.2%**
*Open-angle glaucoma or ocular hypertension.*
**Adults:** 1 gtt in the affected eye(s) t.i.d., with doses about 8 hr apart.

## NURSING CONSIDERATIONS

See also *Nursing Considerations* for *Sympathomimetic Drugs.*

**Administration/Storage**

1. If soft contact lenses user, wait at least 15 min after instilling drug before inserting soft contact lenses.

2. Store the drug at or below 25°C (77°F).

**Assessment**

1. Document ophthalmic findings and ensure routine screenings.

2. Note if MAO inhibitor ordered as this precludes drug therapy.

**Client/Family Teaching**

1. Wash hands before and after instillation. Use as directed: 1 gtt every 8 hr to affected eye(s).

2. Remove and do not reinsert soft contact lenses for at least 15 min following instillation of drops.

3. Use caution when performing activities that require mental alertness as drug may cause fatigue and drowsiness. Report any unusual or intolerable side effects.

4. Avoid alcohol and any other CNS depressants.

5. Report for follow-up ophthalmic evaluations.

**Outcomes/Evaluate:** Reduction in intraocular pressures

# Bromocriptine mesylate

(broh-moh-**KRIP**-teen)

**Pregnancy Category:** B

Alti-Bromocriptine ✦, Apo-Bromocriptine ✦, Parlodel **(Rx)**

**Classification:** Prolactin secretion inhibitor; antiparkinson agent

**Action/Kinetics:** Bromocriptine is a nonhormonal agent that inhibits the release of the hormone prolactin by the pituitary. Should be used only when prolactin production by pituitary tumors has been ruled out. Its effect in parkinsonism is due to a direct stimulating effect on dopamine type 2 receptors in the corpus striatum. Use for parkinsonism may allow the dose of levodopa to be decreased, thus decreasing the incidence of severe side effects following long-term levodopa therapy. Less than 30% of the drug is absorbed from the GI tract. **Onset, lower prolactin:** 2 hr; **antiparkinson:** 30–90 min; **decrease growth hormone:** 1–2 hr. **Peak plasma concentration:** 1–3 hr. **t½, plasma:** 6–8 hr; **terminal:** 15 hr. **Duration, lower prolactin:** 24 hr (after a single dose); **decrease growth hormone:** 4–8 hr. Significant first-pass effect. Metabolized in liver, excreted mainly through bile and thus the feces.

**Uses:** Short-term treatment of amenorrhea with or without galactorrhea, infertilitiy, or hypogonadism. Alone or as an adjunct in the treatment of acromegaly. As adjunctive therapy with levodopa in the treatment of idiopathic or postencephalitic Parkinson's disease. May provide additional benefit in clients who are taking optimal doses of levodopa, in those who are developing tolerance to levodopa therapy, or in those who are manifesting levodopa "end of dose failure." Clients unresponsive to levodopa are not good candidates for bromocriptine therapy. No longer recommended to suppress postpartum lactation. *Investigational:* Hyperprolactinemia due to pituitary adenoma, neuroleptic malignant syndrome, cocaine dependence, cyclical mastalgia.

**Contraindications:** Sensitivity to ergot alkaloids. Pregnancy, lactation, children under 15 years of age. Peripheral vascular disease, ischemic heart disease.

**Special Concerns:** Geriatric clients may manifest more CNS effects. Use with caution in liver or kidney disease.

**Side Effects:** The type and incidence of side effects depend on the use of the drug. *When used for hyperprolactinemia. GI:* N&V, abdominal cramps, diarrhea, constipation. *CNS:* Headache, dizziness, fatigue, drowsiness, lightheadedness, psychoses. *Other:* Nasal congestion, hypotension; CSF rhinorrhea.

*When used for acromegaly. GI:* N&V, anorexia, dry mouth, dyspepsia, indigestion, GI bleeding. *CNS:* Dizziness, syncope, drowsiness, tiredness, headache, lightheadedness, lassitude, vertigo, sluggishness, paranoia, insomnia, heavy headedness, decreased sleep requirement, delusional psychosis, visual hallucinations. *CV:* Orthostatic hypotension, digital vasospasm, Raynaud's syndrome; rarely, arrhythmias, ventricular tachycardia, bradycardia, vasovagal attack. *Respiratory:* Nasal stuffiness, SOB. *Other:* Potentiation of effects of alcohol, hair loss, paresthesia, tingling of ears, muscle cramps, facial pallor, reduced tolerance to cold.

*When used for parkinsonism. GI:* N&V, abdominal discomfort, constipation, anorexia, dry mouth, dysphagia. *CNS:* Confusion, hallucinations, fainting, drowsiness, dizziness, insomnia, depression, vertigo, anxiety, fatigue, headache, lethargy, nightmares. *GU:* Urinary incontinence, urinary retention, urinary frequency. *Other:* Abnormal involuntary movements, asthenia, visual disturbances, ataxia, hypotension, SOB, edema of feet and ankles, blepharospasm, erythromelalgia, skin mottling, nasal stuffiness, paresthesia, skin rash.

---

✦ = Available in Canada  *bold italic* = life threatening side effect

## Drug Interactions

*Alcohol* / ↑ Chance of GI toxicity; alcohol intolerance

*Antihypertensives* / Additive ↓ BP

*Butyrophenones* / ↓ Effect of bromocriptine because butyrophenones are dopamine antagonists

*Diuretics* / Should be avoided during bromocriptine therapy

*Erythromycins* / ↑ Levels of bromocriptine → ↑ pharmacologic and toxic effects

*Phenothiazines* / ↓ Effect of bromocriptine because phenothiazines are dopamine antagonists

*Sympathomimetics* / ↑ Side effects of bromocriptine, including ventricular tachycardia and cardiac dysfunction

**Laboratory Test Interferences:** ↑ BUN, AST, ALT, GGPT, CPT, alkaline phosphatase, uric acid.

## Dosage

- **Capsules, Tablets**

*For hyperprolactinemic conditions.*

**Adults, initial:** 0.5–2.5 mg/day with meals; **then,** increase dose by 2.5 mg q 3–7 days until optimum response observed (usual: 5–7.5 mg/day; range: 2.5–15 mg/day). For amenorrhea/galactorrhea, do not use for more than 6 months. Side effects may be reduced by temporarily decreasing the dose to ½ tablet 2–3 times/day.

*Parkinsonism.*

**Initial:** 1.25 mg (½ tablet) b.i.d. with meals while maintaining dose of levodopa, if possible. Dosage may be increased q 14–28 days by 2.5 mg/day with meals. The usual dosage range is 10–40 mg/day. Any decrease in dosage should be done gradually in 2.5-mg decrements.

*Acromegaly.*

**Initial:** 1.25–2.5 mg for 3 days with food and on retiring; **then,** increased by 1.25–2.5 mg q 3–7 days until optimum response observed. Usual optimum therapeutic range: 20–30 mg/day, not to exceed 100 mg/day. Clients should be reevaluated monthly and dosage adjusted accordingly.

*Hyperprolactinemia associated with pituitary adenomas.*

**Maintenance:** 0.625–10 mg/day for 6 to 52 months.

## NURSING CONSIDERATIONS

### Administration/Storage

1. Before administering first dose of drug, have client lie down because of the possibility of fainting or dizziness.

2. Use tablets for doses less than 5 mg.

### Assessment

1. Note any sensitivity to ergot alkaloids.

2. Document indications for therapy, onset and type of symptoms, other agents used, and the outcome.

3. Note if female, sexually active and likely to become pregnant.

4. Monitor liver and renal function studies; note any dysfunction.

5. With Parkinson's disease, assess and document baseline physical ability and areas of disability to distinguish between desired response and drug-induced side effects, which may be severe initially before subsiding with therapy. Also note drugs currently in use and their dosage.

### Client/Family Teaching

1. Take with food to minimize GI upset.

2. Drug may cause dizziness, drowsiness, or syncope; lie down if evident and avoid activities that require mental alertness.

3. Report any complaints of fatigue, headache, nausea, drowsiness, cramps, or diarrhea.

4. If using oral contraceptives, use additional nonhormonal method.

5. When menstrual period is missed, the sexually active client should receive pregnancy tests every 4 weeks during period of amenorrhea and after resumption of menses.

6. If pregnancy is likely, withhold drug and report. Pregnancy tests may fail to diagnose early pregnancy and the drug may harm the fetus.

7. Report unusal or persistant side effects.

### Outcomes/Evaluate

- Normal menstrual cycle

- ↓ Growth hormone with acromegaly
- ↓ Muscle rigidity/tremor

# Brompheniramine maleate
(brohm-fen-**EAR**-ah-meen)
**Pregnancy Category:** B
Brombay, Chlorphed, Conjec-B, Cophene-B, Diamine T.D., Dimetane Extentabs, Dimetane-Ten, Histaject Modified, Nasahist B, ND Stat Revised, Oraminic II, Sinusol-B, Veltane (Rx; Dimetane and Dimetane Extentabs are OTC)
**Classification:** Antihistamine, alkylamine type

See also *Antihistamines*.
**Action/Kinetics:** Fewer sedative effects. t½: 25 hr. **Time to peak effect:** 3–9 hr. **Duration:** 4–25 hr.
**Uses:** Allergic rhinitis (oral). Parenterally to treat allergic reactions to blood or plasma; adjunct to treat anaphylaxis; uncomplicated allergic conditions when PO therapy is not possible or is contraindicated.
**Contraindications:** Use in neonates.
**Special Concerns:** Geriatric clients may be more sensitive to the usual adult dose.

## Dosage
- **Liqui-Gels**
  *Allergic rhinitis.*
**Adults and children over 12 years:** 4 mg q 4–6 hr, not to exceed 24 mg/day.
- **IM, IV, SC**
**Adults: usual,** 10 mg (range: 5–20 mg) b.i.d. (maximum daily dose: 40 mg); **pediatric, under 12 years:** 0.5 mg/kg/day (15 mg/m² /day) divided into three or four doses.

## NURSING CONSIDERATIONS

See also *Nursing Considerations* for *Antihistamines*.
**Administration/Storage**
1. For IM or SC use, the drug may be used undiluted or diluted 1:10 with NSS.
**IV** 2. Do not use solutions containing preservatives for IV injection.

3. For IV administration, the 10-mg/mL preparations may be used undiluted or diluted 1:10 with sterile saline for injection. Administer over 1 min.
4. Give IV slowly preferably to a recumbent client.
5. May be added to 0.9% NSS, 5% dextrose, or whole blood for IV administration.
6. The 100-mg/mL preparation is not recommended for IV use.
**Client/Family Teaching**
1. Drug may cause drowsiness.
2. Consume 1.5–2 L of fluids per day to decrease viscosity of secretions.
3. Avoid alcohol.
4. Report any persistent or bothersome side effects and loss of drug responsiveness.
**Outcomes/Evaluate:** Relief of allergic manifestations; ↓ nasal congestion

# Budesonide
(byou-**DES**-oh-nyd)
**Pregnancy Category:** C
Entocort ✦, Pulmicort Nebuamp ✦, Pulmicort Turbuhaler, Rhinocort, Rhinocort Aqua or Turbuhaler ✦ **(Rx)**
**Classification:** Corticosteroid

See also *Corticosteroids*.
**Action/Kinetics:** Budesonide is used intranasally and exerts a direct local anti-inflammatory effect with minimal systemic effects. However, exceeding the recommended dose may result in suppression of hypothalamic-pituitary-adrenal function. t½: 2–3 hr. Metabolism of absorbed drug is rapid.
**Uses:** Treat symptoms of seasonal or perennial allergic rhinitis in both adults and children. Also, nonallergic perennial rhinitis in adults.The Turbuhaler is used for maintenance and prophylaxis of asthma in adults and children 6 years of age and older; also for those requiring oral corticosteroid therapy for asthma.
**Contraindications:** Hypersensitivity to the drug. Untreated localized

nasal mucosa infections. Lactation. Use in children less than 6 years of age or for acute or life-threatening asthma attacks.

**Special Concerns:** Use with caution in clients already on alternate day corticosteroids (e.g., prednisone). Use with caution in clients with active or quiescent tuberculosis infections of the respiratory tract or in untreated fungal, bacterial, or systemic viral infections or ocular herpes simplex. Use with caution in clients with recent nasal septal ulcers, recurrent epistaxis, nasal surgery, or trauma. Exposure to chicken pox or measles should be avoided.

**Side Effects:** *Respiratory:* Nasopharyngeal irritation, nasal irritation, pharyngitis, increased cough, hoarseness, nasal pain, burning, stinging, dryness, epistaxis, bloody mucus, rebound congestion, **bronchial asthma,**, occasional sneezing attacks (especially in children), rhinorrhea, reduced sense of smell, throat discomfort, ulceration of the nasal mucosa, sore throat, dyspnea, localized infections of nose and pharynx with *Candida albicans*, wheezing (rare). *CNS:* Lightheadedness, headache, nervousness. *GI:* Nausea, loss of sense of taste, bad taste in mouth, dry mouth, dyspepsia. *Miscellaneous:* Watery eyes, **immediate and delayed hypersensitivity reactions,** moniliasis, facial edema, rash, pruritus, herpes simplex, alopecia, arthralgia, myalgia, contact dermatitis (rare).

**OD** **Overdose Management:** *Symptoms:* Symptoms of hypercorticism, including menstrual irregularities, acneiform lesions, and cushingoid features (all are rarely seen, however). *Treatment:* Discontinue the drug slowly using procedures that are acceptable for discontinuing oral corticosteroids.

**Dosage** ————————
• **Inhalation Aerosol**
  *Seasonal or perennial rhinitis.*
**Adults and children 6 years of age and older, initial:** 256 mcg/day

given as either 2 sprays in each nostril in the morning and evening or 4 sprays in each nostril in the morning. Doses greater than 256 mcg/day are not recommended. **Maintenance:** Reduce initial dose to the smallest amount necessary to control symptoms; decrease dose q 2–4 weeks as long as desired effect is maintained. If symptoms return, the dose may be increased briefly to the initial dose.
• **Pulmicort Turbuhaler**
  *Prevention or treatment of asthma.*
**Adults:** 200–400 mcg b.i.d. **Children, over 6 years of age:** 200 mcg b.i.d. 200 mcg released with each actuation actually delivers about 160 mcg to the client.

## NURSING CONSIDERATIONS

See also *Nursing Considerations* for *Corticosteroids.*
**Assessment**
1. Note indications for therapy, onset of symptoms, and frequency of occurrence.
2. List drugs currently prescribed to ensure that none interact unfavorably.
**Client/Family Teaching**
1. Review the appropriate method and frequency for administration. A spacer may enhance drug dispersion. Review video/instruction for proper administration guidelines.
2. Rinse mouth and equipment thoroughly after each use to prevent oral fungal infections.
3. Prior to using, clear nasal passages of secretions. If nasal passages are blocked, use a decongestant before using budesonide.
4. Maximum benefit is usually not seen for 3–7 days, although a decrease in symptoms can be seen within 24 hr. Report if no improvement noted within 3 weeks as therapy should be discontinued.
5. Shake canister well before administering. Store valve down and away from areas of high humidity. Once aluminum pouch is opened, use or discard within 6 months.

6. Avoid persons with chicken pox or communicable diseases.

7. Symptoms of hoarseness may be evident but should subside upon completion of therapy.

8. Drug is a steroid; chronic use in excessive amounts may lead to adverse systemic reactions.

9. Identify triggers and avoid irritants to prevent development of symptoms.

**Outcomes/Evaluate:** Relief of nasal congestion and allergic manifestations

# Bumetanide
(byou-**MET**-ah-nyd)
**Pregnancy Category:** C
Bumex, Burinex ✹ **(Rx)**
**Classification:** Loop diuretic

See also *Diuretics, Loop.*

**Action/Kinetics:** Inhibits reabsorption of both sodium and chloride in the proximal tubule as well as the ascending loop of Henle. Possible activity in the proximal tubule to promote phosphate excretion. **Onset, PO:** 30–60 min. **Peak effect, PO:** 1–2 hr. **Duration, PO:** 4–6 hr (dose-dependent). **Onset, IV:** Several minutes. **Peak effect, IV:** 15–30 min. **Duration, IV:** 3.5–4 hr. **t½:** 1–1.5 hr. Metabolized in the liver although 45% excreted unchanged in the urine.

**Uses:** Edema associated with CHF, nephrotic syndrome, hepatic disease. Adjunct to treat acute pulmonary edema. Especially useful in clients refractory to other diuretics. *Investigational:* Treatment of adult nocturia. The drug is not effective in males with prostatic hypertrophy.

**Contraindications:** Anuria. Hepatic coma or severe electrolyte depletion until the condition is improved or corrected. Hypersensitivity to the drug. Lactation.

**Special Concerns:** Safety and efficacy in children under 18 have not been established. Geriatric clients may be more sensitive to the hypotensive and electrolyte effects and are at

greater risk in developing thromboembolic problems and circulatory collapse. SLE may be activated or made worse. Clients allergic to sulfonamides may show cross sensitivity to bumetanide. Sudden changes in electrolyte balance may cause hepatic encephalopathy and coma in clients with hepatic cirrhosis and ascites.

**Side Effects:** *Electrolyte and fluid changes:* Excess water loss, **dehydration,** electrolyte depletion including hypokalemia, hypochloremia, hyponatremia; hypovolemia, thromboembolism, **circulatory collapse.** *Otic:* Tinnitus, reversible and irreversible hearing impairment, deafness, vertigo (with a sense of fullness in the ears). *CV:* **Reduction in blood volume may cause circulatory collapse and vascular thrombosis and embolism, especially in geriatric clients.** Hypotension, ECG changes, chest pain. *CNS:* Asterixis, encephalopathy with preexisting liver disease, vertigo, headache, dizziness. *GI:* Upset stomach, dry mouth, N&V, diarrhea, GI pain. *GU:* Premature ejaculation, difficulty maintaining erection, renal failure. *Musculoskeletal:* Arthritic pain, weakness, muscle cramps, fatigue. *Hematologic:* Agranulocytosis, thrombocytopenia. *Allergic:* Pruritus, urticaria, rashes. *Miscellaneous:* Sweating, hyperventilation, rash, nipple tenderness, photosensitivity, pain following parenteral use.

**OD** **Overdose Management:** *Symptoms:* **Profound loss of water, electrolyte depletion, dehydration, decreased blood volume, circulatory collapse (possibility of vascular thrombosis and embolism).** Symptoms of electrolyte depletion include: anorexia, cramps, weakness, dizziness, vomiting, and mental confusion. *Treatment:* Replace electrolyte and fluid losses and monitor urinary electrolyte levels as well as serum electrolytes. Emesis or gastric lavage. Oxygen or artificial respiration may be necessary. General supportive measures.

**Laboratory Test Interferences:** Alterations in LDH, AST, ALT, alkaline phosphatase, creatinine clearance, total serum bilirubin, serum proteins, cholesterol. Changes in hemoglobin, PT, hematocrit, WBCs, platelet and differential counts, phosphorus, carbon dioxide content, bicarbonate, and calcium. ↑ Urinary glucose and protein, serum creatinine. Also, hyperuricemia, hypochloremia, hypokalemia, azotemia, hyponatremia, hyperglycemia.

**Dosage** ————————
• **Tablets**
**Adults:** 0.5–2 mg once daily; if response is inadequate, a second or third dose may be given at 4–5-hr intervals up to a maximum of 10 mg/day.
• **IV, IM**
**Adults:** 0.5–1 mg; if response is inadequate, a second or third dose may be given at 2–3-hr intervals up to a maximum of 10 mg/day. Initiate PO dosing as soon as possible.

## NURSING CONSIDERATIONS

See also *Nursing Considerations* for *Diuretics, Loop.*
**Administration/Storage**
1. The recommended PO medication schedule is on alternate days or for 3–4 days with a 1–2-day rest period in between.
2. Bumetanide, at a 1:40 ratio of bumetanide:furosemide, may be ordered for clients allergic to furosemide.
3. In severe chronic renal insufficiency, a continuous infusion of bumetanide, 12 mg over 12 hr, may be more effective and cause fewer side effects than intermittent bolus therapy.
4. Reserve IV or IM administration for clients in whom PO use is not practical or in whom absorption from the GI tract is impaired.
**IV** 5. Prepare solutions fresh for IM or IV; use within 24 hr.
6. Ampules may be reconstituted with 5% dextrose in water, 0.9% NaCl, or Ringer's lactate solution.
7. Administer IV solutions slowly over 1–2 min.

**Assessment**
1. Document indications for therapy and pretreatment findings.
2. Note any sulfonamide allergy; may be cross sensitivity.
3. Monitor electrolytes, liver and renal function studies; assess for hypokalemia.
4. Review history; note any hearing impairment, lupus, or thromboembolic events.
5. *NOTE:* 1 mg of bumetanide is equivalent to 40 mg of furosemide.
6. Monitor VS. Rapid diuresis may cause dehydration and circulatory collapse (especially in the elderly). Hypotension may also occur when administered with antihypertensive drugs.
7. Assess hearing and for ototoxicity, especially if receiving other ototoxic drugs
**Client/Family Teaching**
1. Take early in the day to prevent nighttime voidings.
2. Do not perform activities that require mental alertness until drug effects realized.
3. Review dietary requirements such as reduced sodium and high potassium; may see dietitian.
4. Record weights; report any sudden weight gain or evidence of swelling in the hands or feet.
5. Report any unusual side effects.
**Outcomes/Evaluate:** ↓ Peripheral and sacral edema; Enhanced diuresis

# Buprenorphine hydrochloride
(byou-pren-**OR**-feen)
**Pregnancy Category:** C
Buprenex **(C-V) (Rx)**
**Classification:** Narcotic agonist/antagonist

See also *Narcotic Analgesics.*
**Action/Kinetics:** Semisynthetic opiate possessing both narcotic agonist and antagonist activity. It has limited activity at the mu receptor. **IM, onset:** 15 min; **Peak effect:** 1 hr; **Duration:** 6 hr. **t½:** 2–3 hr. May also be given IV with shorter onset and peak effect. Is about equipotent

with naloxone as a narcotic antagonist.

**Uses:** Moderate to severe pain.

**Special Concerns:** Use during lactation only if benefits outweigh risks. Use in children less than 2 years of age has not been established. Use with caution in clients with compromised respiratory function, in head injuries, in impairment of liver or renal function, Addison's disease, prostatic hypertrophy, biliary tract dysfunction, urethral stricture, myxedema, and hypothyroidism. Administration to individuals physically dependent on narcotics may result in precipitation of a withdrawal syndrome.

**Side Effects:** *CNS:* Sedation, dizziness, confusion, headache, euphoria, slurred speech, depression, paresthesia, psychosis, malaise, hallucinations, coma, dysphoria, agitation, seizures. *GI:* N&V, constipation, dyspepsia, loss of appetite, dry mouth. *Ophthalmologic:* Miosis, blurred vision, double vision, conjunctivitis. *CV:* Hypotension, bradycardia, tachycardia, Wenckebach block. *Respiratory:* Decreased respiratory rate, cyanosis, dyspepsia. *Dermatologic:* Sweating, rash, pruritus, flushing. *Other:* Urinary retention, chills, tinnitus.

**Drug Interactions:** Additive CNS depression with alcohol, general anesthetics, antianxiety agents, sedative-hypnotics, phenothiazines, and other narcotic analgesics.

**Dosage**
• **IM, Slow IV**
  *Analgesia.*
**Over 13 years of age:** 0.3 mg q 6 hr. Up to 0.6 mg may be given; doses greater than 0.6 mg not recommended. **Children, 2–12 years of age:** 2–6 mcg/kg q 4–6 hr. Do not give single doses greater than 6 mcg/kg.

## NURSING CONSIDERATIONS

See also *Nursing Considerations* for *Narcotic Analgesics.*

**Administration/Storage**
1. Not all children may clear buprenorphine faster than adults. Thus, fixed interval or "round the clock" dosing should not be undertaken until the proper interdose interval has been established.
2. Some pediatric clients may not need to be remedicated for 6–8 hr.
3. Have naloxone available to reverse drug-induced respiratory depression.
4. Avoid storage in excessive heat and light
**IV** 5. Do not mix buprenorphine with solutions containing diazepam or lorazepam.
6. Buprenorphine may be mixed with solutions containing haloperidol, glycopyrrolate, scopolamine hydrobromide, hydroxyzine chloride, or droperidol.
7. Buprenorphine may be mixed with isotonic saline, RL solution, and D5%/0.9% saline.
8. May be administered undiluted IV, slowly.

**Assessment**
1. Document indications for therapy, onset, location, and intensity of symptoms.
2. Determine any respiratory depression; drug is contraindicated.
3. Report head injuries immediately.
4. If receiving narcotics, observe for withdrawal symptoms.
5. Note any evidence of liver or renal dysfunction, diseases of the biliary tract, or prostatic hypertrophy.

**Client/Family Teaching**
1. Drug may cause drowsiness, dizziness, and orthostatic effects.
2. Cough and deep breathe every 2 hr to prevent atelectasis.
3. Avoid alcohol.

**Outcomes/Evaluate:** Relief of pain

# Bupropion hydrochloride
(byou-**PROH**-pee-on)
**Pregnancy Category:** B
Wellbutrin, Wellbutrin SR, Zyban **(Rx)**
**Classification:** Antidepressant, miscellaneous

**Action/Kinetics:** Bupropion is an antidepressant whose mechanism of action is not known; the drug does not inhibit MAO and it only weakly blocks neuronal uptake of epinephrine, serotonin, and dopamine. The drug exerts moderate anticholinergic and sedative effects, but only slight orthostatic hypotension. **Peak plasma levels:** 2–3 hr. **t½:** 8–24 hr. **Time to steady state:** 1.5–5 days. Significantly metabolized by a first-pass effect through the liver to both active and inactive metabolites. During chronic use the plasma levels of two active metabolites may be higher than bupropion. Excreted through both the urine (87%) and the feces (10%). Zyban is a sustained-release formulation.

**Uses:** Short-term (6 weeks or less) treatment of depression. Aid to stop smoking (may be combined with a nicotine transdermal system).

**Contraindications:** Seizure disorders; presence or history of bulimia or anorexia nervosa due to the higher incidence of seizures in such clients. Concomitant use of an MAO inhibitor. Wellbutrin, Wellbutrin SR, and Zyban all contain bupropion; do not use together.

**Special Concerns:** Use with caution in clients with a history of seizures, cranial trauma, with drugs that lower the seizure threshold, and other situations that might cause seizures (e.g., abrupt cessation of a benzodiazepine). Use with caution and in lower doses in clients with liver or kidney disease and in those with a recent history of MI or unstable heart disease. Assess benefits versus risks during lactation. Safety and efficacy have not been established in clients less than 18 years of age.

**Side Effects:** Listed are side effects with an incidence of 0.1% or greater. *CNS:* Insomnia, abnormal dreams, dizziness, disturbed concentration, nervousness, tremor, dysphoria, somnolence, agitation, abnormal thinking, depression, irritability, CNS stimulation, confusion, decreased libido, decreased memory, depersonalization, emotional lability, hostility, hyperkinesia, hypertonia, hypesthesia, paresthesia, suicidal ideation, vertigo. *GI:* Nausea, dry mouth, constipation, diarrhea, anorexia, mouth ulcer, thirst, increased appetite, dyspepsia, flatulence, vomiting, abnormal liver function, bruxism, dysphagia, gastric reflux, gingivitis, glossitis, jaundice, stomatitis. *CV:* Palpitations, hypertension, flushing, migraine, postural hypotension, hot flashes, *stroke,* tachycardia, vasodilation. *Body as a whole:* Abdominal pain, accidental injury, neck pain, chest pain, facial edema, asthenia, fever, headache, back pain, chills, inguinal hernia, musculoskeletal chest pain, pain, photosensitiviy. *Dermatologic:* Rash, pruritus, urticaria, dry skin, sweating, acne, dry skin. *Musculoskeletal:* Arthralgia, myalgia, leg cramps. *Respiratory:* Rhinitis, bronchitis, increased cough, pharyngitis, sinusitis, epistaxis, dyspnea. *GU:* Urinary frequency, impotence, polyuria, urinary urgency. *Ophthalmic:* Amblyopia, abnormal accommodation, dry eye. *Miscellaneous:* Taste perversion, tinnitus, ecchymosis, edema, increased weight, peripheral edema.

**OD** **Overdose Management:** *Symptoms:* Seizures, hallucinations, loss of consciousness, tachycardia, multiple uncontrolled seizures, bradycardia, fever, muscle rigidity, hypotension, rhabdomyolosis, stupor, coma, respiratory failure, cardiac failure and cardiac arrest prior to death. *Treatment:* Client should be hospitalized. If conscious, syrup of ipecac is given to induce vomiting followed by activated charcoal q 6 hr during the first 12 hr after ingestion. Both ECG and EEG should be monitored for 48 hr and fluid intake must be adequate. If the client is in a stupor, is comatose, or is convulsing, gastric lavage may be undertaken provided intubation of the airway has been performed. Seizures may be treated with IV benzodiazepines and other supportive procedures.

## Drug Interactions

*Alcohol* / Alcohol ↓ seizure threshold; use with bupropion may precipitate seizures

*Amantadine* / Psychotic reactions

*Carbamazepine* / ↑ Bupropion metabolism → ↓ plasma levels

*Cimetidine* / Cimetidine inhibits the metabolism of bupropion

*Fluoxetine* / Panic symptoms and psychotic reactions

*Levodopa* / ↑ Risk of side effects

*MAO inhibitors* / Acute toxicity to bupropion may ↑, especially if used with phenelzine

*Phenobarbital* / ↑ Bupropion metabolism → ↓ plasma levels

*Phenytoin* / ↑ Bupropion metabolism → ↓ plasma levels

*Retonavir* / ↑ Risk of bupropion toxicity

## Dosage

- **Tablets**

  *Antidepressant.*

**Adults, initial:** 100 mg in the morning and evening for the first 3 days; **then,** 100 mg t.i.d., given in the morning, midday, and in the evening (6 hr should elapse between doses). If no response is observed after 4 weeks or longer, the dose may be increased to 450 mg/day with individual doses not to exceed 150 mg. Doses higher than 450 mg should not be administered. The sustained-release dosage form may be used for twice-daily dosing. **Maintenance:** Lowest dose to control depression.

  *Smoking deterrent.*

Begin dosing at 150 mg/day for the first 3 days followed by 150 mg b.i.d. Eight hours or more should elapse between successive doses.

## NURSING CONSIDERATIONS

### Administration/Storage

1. To reduce risk of seizures, the total daily dose should not exceed 450 mg to treat depression or 300 mg as a smoking deterrent; each single dose should not exceed 150 mg, and doses of drug should be increased gradually.

2. Several months of treatment may be necessary to control acute depression.

3. Intitiate treatment while the client is still smoking since about 1 week of treatment is needed to reach steady-state blood levels. A "target quit date," usually in the second week, should be set. Continue treatment for 7 to 12 weeks. If significant progress has not been made by week 7 of treatment, it is not likely the client will stop smoking during this attempt. Thus, discontinue treatment.

### Assessment

1. Document indications for therapy, presenting behaviors, and duration of symptoms.

2. Note any history of seizures, recent MI, bulimia or anorexia nervosa.

3. Determine if client is of child-bearing age and lactating.

4. Monitor weight, ECG, liver and renal function studies; reduce dose with renal and/or liver dysfunction.

5. Assess mental stability and potential for compliance. There are fewer side effects (no CV effects, drug interactions, sedation, and weight gain) with bupropion than with other antidepressants.

6. With tobacco abuse, ensure client is ready to quit; note numbers of cigarettes smoked per day, nicotine content, other failures, and date desired to quit so that treatment can be started 1 week prior to quit date.

### Client/Family Teaching

1. May experience a change in taste perceptions which could result in appetite and weight loss. Record weights and report any significant changes.

2. May cause menstrual irregularities and impotence. Any changes in urinary output should be reported.

3. Beneficial drug effects may not be evident for 5–21 days. Continue taking and do not be discouraged by the delayed response.

4. Dizziness may occur. Do not arise from a supine position sudden-

---

ly. If dizziness occurs during the day, sit down until the sensation subsides and report if persistent.

5. Report for follow-up so that drug therapy and dosage may be evaluated and adjusted as needed.

6. Report any mood swings or suicidal ideations immediately.

7. Drug may cause drowsiness, hyperactivity, GI upset, diarrhea, constipation, and dry mouth. Report if persistent or intolerable.

8. With the sustained-released formulation, for smoking cessation, drug will be started in low dose for b.i.d. consumption. Take last dose 4 to 6 hr before bedtime to prevent insomnia. GlaxoWellcome operates a toll- free number (1-800-u can quit, 822-6784) for assistance and support during withdrawal of nicotine; they can also be reached on the Internet at www.glaxowellcome.com.

**Outcomes/Evaluate**

• Improvement in symptoms of depression such as ↓ fatigue, improved eating and sleeping patterns, and ↑ socialization

• Successful nicotine withdrawal

# Buspirone hydrochloride

(byou-**SPYE**-rohn)

**Pregnancy Category:** B

Apo-Buspirone ✲, BuSpar, Linbuspirone ✲, Nu-Buspirone ✲ **(Rx)**

**Classification:** Nonbenzodiazepine antianxiety agent

**Action/Kinetics:** The mechanism of action is unknown. Not chemically related to the benzodiazepines; no anticonvulsant or muscle relaxant properties. Significant sedation has not been observed. The drug binds to serotonin (5-HT$_{1A}$) and dopamine (D$_2$) receptors in the CNS; it is thus possible that dopamine-mediated neurologic disorders may occur. These include dystonia, Parkinson-like symptoms, akathisia, and tardive dyskinesia. **Peak plasma levels:** 1–6 ng/mL 40–90 min after a single PO dose of 20 mg. **t½:** 2–3 hr. Extensive first-pass metabolism; active and inactive metabolites excreted in the urine and through the feces.

**Uses:** Anxiety disorders, short-term use to relieve symptoms of anxiety due to motor tension, apprehension, autonomic hyperactivity, or hyperattentiveness. Not usually indicated for treatment of anxiety and tension due to stress of everyday living.

**Contraindications:** Psychoses, severe liver or kidney impairment, lactation.

**Special Concerns:** Safety and efficacy in children less than 18 years of age not established. A decrease in dose may be necessary in geriatric clients due to age-related impairment of renal function.

**Side Effects:** *CNS:* Dizziness, drowsiness, insomnia, fatigue, nervousness, excitement, dream disturbances, dysphoria, noise intolerance, euphoria, depersonalization, akathisia, hallucinations, suicidal ideation, seizures, decreased concentration, confusion, anger or hostility, depression. *CV:* Nonspecific chest pain, hypotension, palpitations, tachycardia, syncope, hypertension. *GI:* N&V, diarrhea, constipation, abdominal distress, dry mouth, altered taste, increased appetite, irritable colon. *Ophthalmologic:* Redness and itching of eyes, conjunctivitis, photophobia, eye pain. *Dermatologic:* Skin rash, pruritus, dry skin, edema of face, acne, easy bruising, flushing. *Neurologic:* Paresthesia, tremor, numbness, incoordination. *GU:* Urinary hesitancy or frequency, enuresis, amenorrhea, pelvic inflammatory disease. *Miscellaneous:* Tinnitus, sore throat, nasal congestion, altered smell, muscle aches or pains, skin rash, headache, sweating, hyperventilation, SOB, hair loss, galactorrhea, decreased or increased libido, delayed ejaculation.

**OD** **Overdose Management:** *Symptoms:* Dizziness, drowsiness, N&V, gastric distress, miosis. *Treatment:* Immediate gastric lavage; general symptomatic and supportive measures.

**Drug Interactions:** Use with MAO inhibitors may cause an increase in BP.

**Dosage**
• **Tablets**
**Adults:** 5 mg t.i.d. Dosage may be increased in increments of 5 mg/day q 2–3 days to achieve optimum effects; the total daily dose should not exceed 60 mg. BuSpar is available in a 15-mg tablet that is scored in 5-mg increments and notched in 7.5-mg increments so clients can take the drug b.i.d. rather than t.i.d.

## NURSING CONSIDERATIONS
### Administration/Storage
1. No cross-tolerance with other sedative-hypnotic drugs, including benzodiazepines.
2. Buspirone will not block the withdrawal syndrome, which may occur following cessation of sedative-hypnotics. Thus, withdraw clients on chronic sedative-hypnotic therapy gradually prior to beginning buspirone therapy.
3. To date, no potential for abuse, tolerance, or either physical or psychologic dependence.
4. Up to 2 weeks may be required before beneficial antianxiety effects are manifested.
### Assessment
1. Document indications for therapy and note pretreatment findings.
2. Determine support systems and encourage active family involvement in treatment plan.
3. Assess for any recent benzodiazepine therapy as buspar may be less effective.
4. Document mental status and note age; good agent to use in elderly because of less CNS suppression.
5. Determine causative factor or event that precipitated event.
### Client/Family Teaching
1. Take with food or snack to decrease nausea, which is a common side effect; report if persistant or severe.
2. May cause drowsiness or dizziness. Use caution when operating a motor vehicle or performing tasks that require mental alertness.
3. Avoid the use of alcohol.

4. Do not suddenly stop drug as withdrawal symptoms such as nausea, vomiting, dry mouth, nasal congestion, or sore throat may occur.
5. Report any complaints of weakness, restlessness, nervousness, headaches, or feelings of depression.
6. Report any involuntary, repetitive movements of the face or neck muscles, Parkinson-like symptoms or suicide ideations immediately.
7. Avoid all OTC agents without approval.
**Outcomes/Evaluate:** Relief of agitated depressive symptoms; ↓ anxiety

# Busulfan
(byou-**SUL**-fan)
**Pregnancy Category:** D
Myleran (Abbreviation: Bus) **(Rx)**
**Classification:** Antineoplastic, alkylating agent

See also *Antineoplastic Agents* and *Alkylating Agents*.
**Action/Kinetics:** Busulfan is cell cycle-phase nonspecific and acts predominantly against cells of the granulocytic type and is thought to act by alkylating cellular thiol groups. Cross-linking of nucleoproteins occurs. May cause severe bone marrow depression. Leukocyte count drops during the second or third week. Thus, close medical supervision, including weekly laboratory tests, is mandatory. Resistance may develop and is thought to be due to the altered transport into the cell and/or increased intracellular inactivation. Rapidly absorbed from the GI tract; appears in serum 0.5–2 hr after PO administration. t½: 2.5 hr. Extensively metabolized and excreted in the urine.

Increased appetite and sense of well-being may occur a few days after therapy is started. Sometimes administered with allopurinol to prevent symptoms of clinical gout.
**Uses:** Chronic myelogenous leukemia (granulocytic, myelocytic, mye-

---

loid). Less effective in individuals with chronic myelogenous leukemia who lack the Philadelphia (Ph[1]) chromosome. Not effective in individuals where the disease is in the "blastic" phase.

**Contraindications:** Use during lactation only if benefits outweigh risks.

**Side Effects:** *Hematologic: **Pancytopenia, severe bone marrow hypoplasia,** anemia, leukopenia, thrombocytopenia. *Pulmonary: **Bronchopulmonary dysplasia with interstitial pulmonary fibrosis.** *Ophthalmologic:* Cataracts after prolonged use. *Dermatologic:* Hyperpigmentation, especially in clients with a dark complexion; also, urticaria, erythema multiforme, erythema nodosum, alopecia, porphyria cutanea tarda, excessive dryness and fragility of the skin with anhidrosis, dryness of the oral mucous membranes, cheilosis. *Metabolic:* Syndrome resembling adrenal insufficiency, including symptoms of weakness, severe fatigue, weight loss, anorexia, N&V, and melanoderma (especially after prolonged use). Also, hyperuricemia and hyperuricosuria in clients with chronic myelogenous leukemia. *Miscellaneous:* Cellular dysplasia in various organs, including lymph nodes, pancreas, thyroid, adrenal glands, bone marrow, and liver. Also, gynecomastia, seizures after high doses, cataracts after prolonged use, **hepatotoxicity,** cholestatic jaundice, myasthenia gravis, sterility, **endocardial fibrosis,** and suppression of ovarian function.

**OD**  **Overdose Management:** *Symptoms: **Bone marrow toxicity, CNS stimulation with convulsions and death on the first day.** Treatment:* If ingestion is recent, gastric lavage or induction of vomiting followed by activated charcoal. Hematologic status must be monitored.

**Drug Interactions**
*Cyclophosphamide* / Cardiac tamponade in clients with thalessemia (rare)
*Thioguanine* / ↑ Risk of esophageal varices with abnormal LFTs

**Laboratory Test Interferences:** ↑ Uric acid in blood and urine.

**Dosage**
- **Tablets**
Individualized according to leukocyte count.
   *Chronic myelocytic leukemia.*
**Adults, remission, induction, usual dose:** 4–8 mg/day until leukocyte count falls below 15,000/mm[3]; **maintenance:** 1–3 mg/day. Discontinue therapy if there is a precipitous fall in leukocyte count. **Children, induction:** 0.06–0.12 mg/kg or 1.8 mg/m[2] daily; **maintenance:** dosage is titrated to maintain a leukocyte count of 20,000/mm[3].

## NURSING CONSIDERATIONS

See also *Nursing Considerations* for *Antineoplastic Agents.*

**Administration/Storage:** Do not administer without supervision and availability of facilities for weekly CBCs.

**Assessment**
1. Note previous experience with drug therapy and determine any resistance.
2. Monitor CBC, liver and renal function studies.
3. In clients with chronic myelogenous leukemia note presence of Philadelphia (Ph[1]) chromosome.
4. Document when disease is in "blastic" phase as drug is not effective.
5. Drug may cause moderate to severe granulocyte suppression. Monitor appropriate weekly hematologic profiles. Nadir: 21 days; recovery: 42–56 days.

**Client/Family Teaching**
1. Take at the same time each day.
2. May take on an empty stomach if nausea and vomiting occur. Extra fluid intake may be required during therapy.
3. Report any early symptoms of sore throat or infection; expect weekly CBC studies .
4. Avoid vaccinations and all OTC agents without approval.
5. Any skin rash should be reported immediately; drug may cause increased pigmentation.

6. Increased cough and visual difficulties may be symptoms of toxicity; Report any increased weight loss, fatigue, loss of appetite, or prolonged weakness.

**Outcomes/Evaluate**
• Maintenance of leukocytes at 20,000/mm³
• Absence of blasts on peripheral blood smear; ↓ spleen size

————COMBINATION DRUG————

# Butalbital and Acetaminophen

(byou-**TAL**-bih-tall, ah-**SEAT**-ah-**MIN**-oh-fen)
**Pregnancy Category:** C
Axocet **(Rx)**
**Classification:** Sedative, analgesic

See also *Pentobarbital Sodium* and *Acetaminophen*.
**Content:** Each capsule contains: *Sedative/hypnotic:* Butalbital, 50 mg, and *analgesic:* acetaminophen, 650 mg.
**Uses:** Treatment of tension headaches.
**Contraindications:** Hypersensitivity to butalbital or acetaminophen. Clients with porphyria.
**Special Concerns:** Use with caution as butalbital is habit-forming and has the potential to be abused. Use with caution in geriatric or debilitated clients, those with severe renal or hepatic dysfunction, and clients with acute abdominal conditions. Safety and efficacy have not been determined in children less than 12 years of age.
**Side Effects:** See also *Sedative-hypnotics* and *Acetaminophen*. The most frequently reported side effects are drowsiness, lightheadedness, sedation, dizziness, SOB, N&V, abdominal pain, and an intoxicated feeling.
**Drug Interactions**
*CNS depressants (including alcohol, general anesthetics, narcotic analgesics, sedative-hypnotics, tranquilizers)* / Additive CNS depression

*MAO inhibitors* / MAO inhibitors ↑ the CNS effects of butalbital

**Dosage**
• **Capsules**
*Treatment of tension headaches.*
1 capsule q 4 hr, not to exceed 6 capsules daily.

## NURSING CONSIDERATIONS

See also *Nursing Considerations* for *Acetaminophen* and *Pentobarbital Sodium*.
**Administration/Storage:** Should not be used for extended periods of time due to the potential for development of physical dependence.
**Assessment**
1. Document onset of symptoms, frequency of occurrence, what usually works, and what agents have been used for headaches.
2. Identify triggers; tension headaches usually respond to NSAIDs or acetaminophen if taken at the first symptom.
3. Note any liver or renal dysfunction or acute abdomen; these preclude use of this drug.
4. Determine that appropriate neurologic evaluation has been obtained.
**Client/Family Teaching**
1. Take only as directed and do not exceed 6 capsules daily.
2. Do not drive or perform activities that require mental alertness during therapy.
3. Avoid alcohol and any other CNS depressants.
4. Keep a journal of foods, activities, and any other factors that surround headaches. This may assist to identify triggers.
**Outcomes/Evaluate:** Relief of tension headaches

# Butenafine hydrochloride

(byou-**TEN**-ah-feen)
**Pregnancy Category:** B
Mentax **(Rx)**
**Classification:** Antifungal drug

See also *Anti-Infectives*.

**Action/Kinetics:** Acts by inhibiting epoxidation of squalene, thus blocking the synthesis of ergosterol, an essential component of fungal cell membranes. Depending on the concentration and the fungal species, the drug may be fungicidal. Although applied topically, some of the drug is absorbed into the general circulation.

**Uses:** Treatment of interdigital tinea pedia (athlete's foot) due to *Epidermophyton floccosum, Trichophyton mentagrophytes,* or *T. rubrum.*

**Special Concerns:** Use with caution in clients sensitive to allylamine antifungal drugs as the drugs may be cross-reactive. Use with caution during lactation. Safety and efficacy have not been determined in children less than 12 years of age.

**Side Effects:** *Dermatologic:* Contact dermatitis, burning or stinging, worsening of the condition, erythema, irritation, itching.

**Dosage**
• **Cream, 1%**
  *Athlete's foot.*
Apply the cream to cover the affected area and immediate surrounding skin once daily for 4 weeks or twice daily for 7 days. Review the diagnosis if no beneficial effects are noted after the treatment period.

## NURSING CONSIDERATIONS

See also *General Nursing Considerations for All* Anti-Infectives, .

**Administration/Storage**
1. For external use only; not for ophthalmic, PO, or intravaginal use.
2. Store the drug between 5°C and 30°C (41°F–86°F).

**Assessment:** Document indications for therapy, onset, duration, and characteristics of symptoms; describe clinical presentation.

**Client/Family Teaching**
1. Review appropriate method for site preparation and application of cream; wash hands before and after applying.
2. After bathing, dry feet thoroughly and dry carefully between each toe be-

fore applying. Avoid use of any occlusive dressing.
3. Avoid contact with the eyes, nose, mouth, and other mucous membranes.
4. Do not stop therapy when condition shows improvement; continue for full prescribed time.
5. Report any increased swelling, itching, burning, blistering, drainage, irritation, or lack of improvement.

**Outcomes/Evaluate:** Resolution of fungal infection

## Butoconazole nitrate
(byou-toe-**KON**-ah-zohl)
**Pregnancy Category:** C
Femstat 1 **(Rx)**, Femstat 3 **(OTC)**
**Classification:** Antifungal agent

**Action/Kinetics:** By permeating chitin in the fungal cell wall, butoconazole increases membrane permeability to intracellular substances, leading to reduced osmotic resistance and viability of the fungus. Approximately 5.5% of drug is absorbed following vaginal administration; plasma. $t^{1/2}$: 21–24 hr.

**Uses:** Vulvovaginal fungal infections caused by *Candida* species.

**Contraindications:** Use during first trimester of pregnancy.

**Special Concerns:** Pediatric dosage has not been established. Use with caution during lactation.

**Side Effects:** *GU:* Vaginal burning, vulvar burning or itching, discharge; soreness, swelling, and itching of the fingers.

**Dosage**
• **Vaginal Cream (2%)**
  *During pregnancy, second and third trimesters only.*
One full applicator (about 5 g) of the cream intravaginally at bedtime for 6 days.
  *Nonpregnant.*
One full applicator (about 5 g) intravaginally at bedtime for 3 days (if necessary, may be used for up to 6 days). *NOTE:* Vaginal infections may also be treated by one dose of butoconazole.

## NURSING CONSIDERATIONS
### Administration/Storage
1. During pregnancy, use of a vaginal applicator may be contraindicated.
2. If there is no response, repeat studies to confirm the diagnosis before reinstituting antifungal therapy.
3. Not to be stored above 40°C (104°F).
### Assessment
1. Document onset and symptoms requiring treatment.
2. Determine if pregnant.
3. Obtain appropriate cultures and pretreatment lab studies.
### Client/Family Teaching
1. Review appropriate technique for administration.
2. Use as prescribed and continue during menstrual cycle.
3. Insert cream high into the vagina.
4. Report any irritation or burning.
5. Use of sanitary napkins may prevent soiling and staining of undergarments and clothing.
6. To prevent reinfection, sexual partner should use a condom during intercourse and also seek treatment if symptomatic.
7. If having recurrent vaginal infections and exposed to HIV, consult provider to determine the cause of symptoms. If the symptoms return within 2 months, client may be pregnant or there could be a serious underlying medical cause (e.g., diabetes, HIV infection).
### Outcomes/Evaluate: Eradication of fungal infection; symptomatic improvement

## Butorphanol tartrate
(byou-**TOR**-fah-nohl)
**Pregnancy Category:** C
Stadol, Stadol NS **(C-IV) (Rx)**
**Classification:** Narcotic agonist/antagonist

See also *Narcotic Analgesics*.
**Action/Kinetics:** Has both narcotic agonist and antagonist properties. Analgesic potency is said to be up to 7 times that of morphine and 30–40 times that of meperidine. Overdosage responds to naloxone. After IV use, CV effects include increased PA pressure, pulmonary wedge pressure, LV end-diastolic pressure, system arterial pressure, pulmonary vascular resistance, and increased cardiac work load. **Onset, IM:** 10–15 min; **IV:** rapid; **nasal:** within 15 min. **Duration, IM, IV:** 3–4 hr; **nasal:** 4–5 hr. **Peak analgesia, IM, IV:** 30–60 min; **nasal:** 1–2 hr. **t½, IM:** 2.1–8.8 hr; **nasal:** 2.9–9.2 hr. The half-life is increased up to 25% in clients over 65 years of age. Metabolized in the liver and excreted by the kidney. The drug has about 1/40 the narcotic antagonist activity as naloxone. A metered-dose nasal spray is now available.
**Uses: Parenteral and nasal:** Moderate to severe pain, especially after surgery. **Parenteral:** Preoperative medication (as part of balanced anesthesia). Pain during labor. **Nasal:** Treatment of migraine headaches.
**Contraindications:** Use of the nasal form during labor or delivery.
**Special Concerns:** Safe use during pregnancy, during labor for premature infants, or in children under 18 years not established. Use with extreme caution in clients with AMI, ventricular dysfunction, and coronary insufficiency (morphine or meperidine are preferred). Use in clients physically dependent on narcotics will result in precipitation of a withdrawal syndrome. Geriatric clients may be more sensitive to side effects, especially dizziness.
**Additional Side Effects:** The most common side effects are somnolence, dizziness, N&V. The nasal product commonly causes nasal congestion and insomnia.
**Additional Drug Interactions:** Barbiturate anesthetics may increase respiratory and CNS depression of butorphanol.

**Dosage**
• **IM**
  *Analgesia.*

**Adults, usual:** 2 mg q 3–4 hr, as necessary; **range:** 1–4 mg q 3–4 hr. Single doses should not exceed 4 mg.

*Preoperative/preanesthetic.*
**Adults:** 2 mg 60–90 min before surgery. Individualize dosage.

*Labor.*
**Adults:** 1–2 mg if at full term and during early labor. May be repeated after 4 hr.

• **IV**
*Analgesia.*
**Adults, usual:** 1 mg q 3–4 hr; **range:** 0.5–2 mg q 3–4 hr. **Not recommended for use in children.**

*Balanced anesthesia.*
**Adults:** 2 mg just before induction or 0.5–1 mg in increments during anesthesia. The increment may be up to 0.06 mg/kg, depending on drugs previously given. Total dose range: less than 4 mg to less than 12.5 mg.

*Labor.*
**Adults:** 1–2 mg if at full term and during early labor. May be repeated after 4 hr.

• **Nasal Spray**
*Analgesia.*
**Adults:** 1 spray (1 mg) in one nostril. If pain relief is not reached within 60–90 min, an additional 1 mg may be given. The two-dose sequence may be repeated in 3–4 hr if necessary. In severe pain, 2 mg (1 spray in each nostril) may be given initially followed in 3–4 hr by additional 2-mg doses if needed. **Geriatric clients, initial:** 1 mg; wait 90–120 min before determining if a second 1-mg dose is required.

## NURSING CONSIDERATIONS

See also *Nursing Considerations* for *Narcotic Analgesics.*
### Administration/Storage
1. Give geriatric clients one-half the usual dose at twice the usual interval.
2. With renal/hepatic impairment, increase the initial dosage interval to 6–8 hr with subsequent intervals determined by client response.
3. Have naloxone available for treatment of overdose.
4. Store the nasal product below 86°F (30°C).
**IV** 5. If drug to be administered by direct IV infusion, it may be given undiluted. Administer it at a rate of 2 mg or less over a 3–5-min period of time.
### Assessment
1. Determine if dependent on narcotics; antagonist property of drug may precipitate withdrawal symptoms.
2. Monitor VS and CNS status during therapy.
3. Document any CV problems as morphine may be a preferred drug to use.
**Outcomes/Evaluate:** Relief of pain; termination of migraine headache

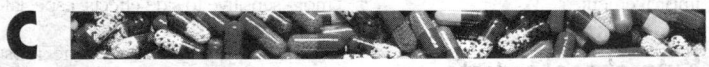

# Caberpoline
(cah-**BER**-goh-leen)
**Pregnancy Category:** B
Dostinex **(Rx)**
**Classification:** Drug to treat hyperprolactinemia

**Action/Kinetics:** Secretion of prolactin occurs through the release of dopamine from tuberofundibular neurons. Cabergoline is a synthetic ergot derivative that is a dopamine receptor agonist at D$_2$ receptors. Inhibits basal and metoclopramide-induced prolactin secretion. **Peak plasma levels:** 2–3 hr. Undergoes a significant first-pass effect. Extensively metabolized in the liver and excreted in both the urine and feces. **t½, elimination:** 63–69 hr.

**Uses:** Treatment of hyperprolactinemia, either idiopathic or due to pituitary adenomas. *Investigational:* Shrink tumors in clients with microprolactinoma or macroprolactinoma. Parkinson's disease. Normalize androgen levels and improve menstrual cyclicity in polycystic ovary syndrome.

**Contraindications:** Uncontrolled hypertension or in pregnancy-induced hypertension (i.e., pre-eclampsia, eclampsia). Hypersensitivity to ergot alkaloids. Lactation. Not to be used to inhibit or suppress physiologic lactation.

**Special Concerns:** Use with caution in those with impaired hepatic function or with other drugs that lower BP. Safety and efficacy have not been determined in children.

**Side Effects:** *GI:* N&V, constipation, abdominal pain, dyspepsia, dry mouth, diarrhea, flatulence, throat irritation, toothache, anorexia, weight loss or gain. *CNS:* Headache, dizziness, somnolence, vertigo, paresthesia, depression, nervousness, anxiety, insomnia. *CV:* Postural hypotension, hypotension, palpitations. *GU:* Breast pain, dysmenorrhea, increased libido. *Body as a whole:* Asthenia, fatigue, syncope, flu-like symptoms, malaise, periorbital edema, peripheral edema, hot flashes. *Miscellaneous:* Nasal stuffiness, abnormal vision, acne, epistaxis, pruritus.

**OD Overdose Management:** *Symptoms:* Nasal congestion, syncope, hallucinations. *Treatment:* Support BP, if necessary.

**Drug Interactions**
*Antihypertensive drugs* / Additive hypotension
*Butyrophenones* / ↓ Effects of cabergoline
*Metoclopramide* / Effects of cabergoline
*Phenothiazines* / Effects of cabergoline
*Thioxanthenes* / Effects of cabergoline

**Dosage** ————
• **Tablets**
*Hyperprolactinemia.*
**Adults, initial:** 0.5 mg twice a week. Dose may be increased by 0.25 mg twice weekly to less than or equal to 1 mg twice a week,

depending on the serum prolactin level. Dosage increases should not occur more often than every 4 weeks.
*Parkinson's disease.*
**Adults:** 7.5 mg/day.
*Improve menstrual cyclicity in polycystic ovary syndrome.*
**Adults:** 0.5 mg/week.

## NURSING CONSIDERATIONS
### Administration/Storage
1. If the client does not respond adequately and higher doses do not result in additional beneficial effects, use the lowest dose that achieved maximal response. Consideration should be given to other approaches.
2. May be discontinued if prolactin levels are normal for 6 months.
3. Efficacy of treatment for > 24 mo has not been determined.

### Assessment
1. Document indications for therapy, onset, duration, and characteristics of symptoms. List other agents trialed and the outcome.
2. Any sensitivity to ergot derivatives precludes drug use, as does lactation and uncontrolled hypertension.
3. Obtain baseline VS, serum prolactin level, and liver and renal function studies; monitor levels and use cautiously with impairment and hypertension.
4. Determine if pregnant; review the risks and do not administer if client plans to become pregnant.
5. With adenomas, review pituitary scans to assess tumor size.
6. With polycystic ovary conditions, review client record of menstrual cycles.

### Client/Family Teaching
1. Take exactly as directed; do not exceed prescribed dose and frequency.
2. Sudden changes in position, especially standing up, may cause dizziness or lightheadedness.
3. Use reliable birth control; report immediately if pregnancy suspected.
4. Report as scheduled for lab work;

drug dosage is dependent on serum prolactin levels with hyperprolactinemic disorders; once prolactin levels are normal for 6 months, drug may be discontinued and levels monitored periodically to determine when or if drug needs to be reinstituted.

**Outcomes/Evaluate**
• ↓ Serum prolactin levels to within desired range (< 20 mcg/L in women; < 15 mcg/L in men)
• Normalization of androgen levels and improved menstrual cycling with polycystic ovary syndrome

# Calcipotriene (Calcipotriol)

(kal-**SIH**-poh-tren)
**Pregnancy Category:** C
Dovonex **(Rx)**
**Classification:** Topical antipsoriatic

**Action/Kinetics:** Calcipotriene is a synthetic vitamin $D_3$ analog. Vitamin $D_3$ receptors are located in skin cells known as keratinocytes. Abnormal growth and production of keratinocytes cause the scaly red patches of psoriasis. Calcipotriene regulates production and development of these skin cells. About 6% of a topically applied dose is absorbed into the systemic circulation where it is converted to inactive metabolites.

**Uses:** Treatment of moderate plaque psoriasis (cream, ointment). Solution is used to control moderately severe scalp psoriasis.

**Contraindications:** Clients with demonstrated hypercalcemia or evidence of vitamin D toxicity. Use on the face. Oral, ophthalmic, intravaginal use.

**Special Concerns:** Side effects are more common in geriatric clients. Use with caution during lactation. Safety and efficacy for use of topical calcipotriene in dermatoses other than psoriasis have not been studied. Safety and efficacy have not been determined in children. Children have a higher ratio of skin surface to body mass; thus, children are at a greater risk than adults of systemic side effects following use of topical medication.

**Side Effects:** *Topical:* Most commonly burning, itching, skin irritation. Also, erythema, dry skin, peeling, rash, worsening of psoriasis, dermatitis, skin atrophy, hyperpigmentation, hypercalcemia, folliculitis. Irritation of lesions and surrounding uninvolved skin. *Systemic:* Transient, rapidly reversible hypercalcemia.

**OD** **Overdose Management:** *Symptoms* Hypercalcemia and other systemic effects. *Treatment:* Discontinue use of the medication until normal calcium levels are restored.

**Dosage**
• **Ointment, Cream, Solution (each 0.005%)**
*Treatment of psoriasis.*
A thin layer is applied to the affected skin b.i.d. and rubbed in gently and completely.

## NURSING CONSIDERATIONS
### Administration/Storage
1. For external use only. Avoid contact with the face and eyes.
2. Safety and efficacy have been shown for use up to 8 weeks.
### Assessment
1. Describe psoriatic lesions requiring therapy; assess extent, location, and size.
2. Monitor calcium levels with extended use.
### Client/Family Teaching
1. Apply a thin layer directly to psoriatic lesions; wash hands before and after application.
2. Use only as directed and do not exceed prescribed dosage; avoid contact with face and eyes.
3. Do not mix or apply at the same time as other topical products.
4. Transient burning and stinging may occur. Avoid use on the face if possible; report if erythema and facial dermatitis occur.
**Outcomes/Evaluate:** Clearing and healing of psoriatic lesions

# Calcitonin-human

(kal-sih-**TOH**-nin)
**Pregnancy Category:** C
**(Rx)**

# Calcitonin-salmon

(kal-sih-**TOH**-nin)
**Pregnancy Category:** C
Calcimar, Caltine ✿, Miacalcin,
Osteocalcin, Salmonine **(Rx)**
**Classification:** Calcium regulator

**Action/Kinetics:** Calcitonins are polypeptide hormones produced in mammals by the parafollicular cells of the thyroid gland. Calcitonin isolated from salmon has the same therapeutic effect as the human hormone, except for a greater potency per milligram and a somewhat longer duration of action. Calcitonin-human is a synthetic product that has the same sequence of amino acids as the naturally occurring calcitonin found in human beings. Calcitonin is ineffective when administered PO. Calcitonin is beneficial in Paget's disease of bone by reducing the rate of turnover of bone; the drug acts to both block initial bone resorption, decreasing alkaline phosphatase levels in the serum and urinary hydroxyproline excretion. Its effectiveness in treating osteoporosis or hypercalcemia is due to decreased serum calcium levels from direct inhibition of bone resorption. Use of the nasal spray for osteoporosis results in significant increases in bone mass density within 6 months. **Time to peak plasma levels, calcitonin-salmon:** 16–25 **min for the injection and 31–39 min for the spray. Duration, calcitonin-salmon: 6–8 hr for hypercalcemia.** t½: 60 min for calcitonin-human and 43 min for calcitonin-salmon. The onset of calcitonin-human in reducing serum alkaline phosphatase level and urinary hydroxyproline excretion in Paget's disease may take 6–24 months. Calcitonin is metabolized to inactive compounds in the kidneys, blood, and peripheral tissues.

**Uses: Injection:** Prevention of progressive loss of bone mass in postmenopausal osteoporosis in women who are more than 5 years past menopause and who have low bone mass compared with women before menopause. Also, for women who cannot or will not take estrogens. Moderate to severe Paget's disease characterized by polyostotic involvement with elevated serum alkaline phosphatase and urinary hydroxyproline excretion. With other therapies for early treatment of hypercalcemic emergencies. *NOTE:* Calcitonin human is now an orphan drug. **Nasal:** Postmenopausal osteoporosis (see above for injection).

**Contraindications:** Allergy to calcitonin-salmon or its gelatin diluent.

**Special Concerns:** Use with caution during lactation. Safe use in children not established.

**Side Effects:** Side effects listed are for calcitonin-salmon. *GI:* N&V, anorexia, epigastric discomfort, salty taste, flatulence, increased appetite, gastritis, diarrhea, dry mouth, abdominal pain, dyspepsia, constipation. *CNS:* Dizziness, paresthesia, insomnia, anxiety, vertigo, migraine, neuralgia, agitation, depression (rare). *CV:* Hypertension, tachycardia, palpitation, bundle branch block, **MI, CVA, thrombophlebitis,** angina pectoris (rare). *Respiratory:* Sinusitis, URTI, pharyngitis, bronchitis, pneumonia, coughing, dyspnea, taste perversion, parosmia, **bronchospasm.** *Musculoskeletal:* Arthrosis, arthritis, polymyalgia rheumatica, stiffness, myalgia. *Dermatologic:* Inflammatory reactions at the injection site, flushing of face or hands, pruritus of ear lobes, edema of feet, skin rash, skin ulceration, eczema, alopecia, increased sweating. *Endocrine:* Goiter, hyperthyroidism. *Ophthalmic:* Abnormal lacrimation, conjunctivitis, eye pain, blurred vision, vitreous floater. *Otic:* Tinnitus, hearing loss, earache. *Hematologic:* Lymphadenopathy, anemia, infection. *Metabolic:* Mild tetanic symptoms, asymptomatic mild hypercalcemia, cholelithiasis, thirst, hepatitis, weight increase. *Miscellaneous:* Flu-like symptoms, fatigue, nocturia, feverish sensation. Use of the nasal spray may cause rhinitis, nasal irritation, redness, nasal sores, back

---

✿ = Available in Canada    ***bold italic*** = life threatening side effect

pain, arthralgia, epistaxis, and headache.

**OD** **Overdose** **Management:**
*Symptoms:* N&V.
**Laboratory Test Interferences:**
Reduction of alkaline phosphatase and 24-hr urinary excretion of hydroxyproline are indicative of successful therapy. Monitor urine for casts (indicative of kidney damage).

### Dosage

- **SC. Calcitonin-Human**
  *Paget's disease.*
**Adults, initial:** 0.5 mg/day; **then,** depending on severity of disease, dosage may range from 0.5 mg 2–3 times/week to 0.25 mg/day.
- **IM, SC. Calcitonin-Salmon**
  *Paget's disease.*
**Adults, initial:** 100 IU/day; **maintenance, usual:** 50 IU/day, every other day, or 3 times/week.
  *Hypercalcemia.*
**Adults, initial:** 4 IU/kg q 12 hr; **then,** increase the dose, if necessary after 1 or 2 days (i.e., if unsatisfactory response), to 8 IU/kg q 12 hr up to a maximum of 8 IU/kg q 6 hr. If the volume to be injected exceeds 2 mL by the SC route, the dose should be given IM with multiple sites used.
  *Postmenopausal osteoporosis.*
**Adults:** 100 IU/day given with calcium carbonate (1.5 g/day) and vitamin D (400 units/day).
- **Nasal Spray. Calcitonin-Salmon**
**Adults:** 200 IU/day, alternating nostrils daily given with calcium carbonate (1.5 g/day) and vitamin D (400 units/day).

## NURSING CONSIDERATIONS
### Administration/Storage
1. Before initiating therapy, determine serum alkaline phosphatase level and urinary hydroxyproline excretion.
2. Repeat the preceding studies at the end of 3 months and q 3–6 months thereafter.
3. The pump for the nasal spray must be activated before use. To do this, hold the bottle upright and the two white side arms depressed toward the bottle six times, until a faint spray is emitted. The pump has been activated once the first faint spray is emitted. The nozzle is then placed firmly into the nostril with the head in the upright position and the pump is depressed toward the bottle. It is not necessary to reactivate the pump before each daily dose.
4. Store calcitonin-salmon injection at a temperature between 2°C and 6°C (36°F and 43°F).
5. *Store the unopened calcitonin nasal spray between 2°C and 8°C (36°F and 43°F).* Once the pump has been activated, it may be stored at room temperature.
6. When being used to treat Paget's disease more than 1 year of therapy may be required to treat neurologic lesions.
7. Check for hypersensitivity reactions before administering either medication. Administer 1 IU intracutaneously in the inner forearm and observe for 15 min to ensure test is negative.
8. Have emergency drugs on hand for immediate use in the event of a hypersensitivity reaction.

### Assessment
1. Note any hypersensitivity to drug or its gelatin diluent.
2. Document indications for therapy, noting baseline assessments and labs.
3. Assess diet and intake of calcium and vitamin D; obtain levels.

### Interventions
1. Perform test dose; note local inflammatory reactions at site; assess for systemic allergic reactions.
2. Observe for hypocalcemic tetany, i.e., muscular fibrillation, twitching, tetanic spasms, and convulsions. Check at least q 10 min for the next 30 min following injection; have IV calcium available.
3. Check for evidence of hypercalcemia and report, i.e., increased thirst, anorexia, polyuria, and N&V.
4. Observe and report facial flushing. Assess for abdominal distress, anorexia, diarrhea, epigastric distress, or changes in taste perception.

Record weights, I&O, and report if symptoms persist.

5. If client has initial good clinical response, then has a relapse, check for antibody formation to serum calcitonin.

**Client/Family Teaching**

1. Identify what to observe for with Pagent's disease and how to assess the response to therapy.

2. Review aseptic methods of reconstituting solution, proper injection technique, and importance of alternating injection sites.

3. With the spray: take with vitamin D (400 IU) and calcium (1,000 mg) daily, alternate nostrils, and do not exceed prescribed dosage.

4. N&V may occur at the onset of therapy, but should subside as treatment continues; report if persists.

5. Report increased urine sediment; have periodic urine tests to assess for kidney damage.

6. Continue regular exercise/activity to minimize bone loss.

7. May take in the evening to minimize flushing.

8. See dietitian for adjustments in the diet.

**Outcomes/Evaluate**

• ↓ Serum calcium, ↓ alkaline phosphatase, and ↓ 24-hr urinary excretion of hydroxyproline

• Promotion of bone formation with ↑ bone mass density

• ↓ Bone pain

• Halt in postmenopausal osteoporosis

# Calcium carbonate

(**KAL**-see-um **KAR**-bon-ayt)
Alka-Mints, Amitone, Antacid Tablets, Apo-Cal ✲, Cal Carb-HD, Calci-Chew, Calciday-667, Calci-Mix, Calcite 500, Calcium 600, Cal-Plus, Calsan ✲, Caltrate ✲, Caltrate 600, Caltrate Jr., Children's Mylanta Upset Stomatch Relief, Chooz, Dicarbosil, Equilet, Extra Strength Antacid, Extra Strength Tums, Florical, Gencalc 600, Maalox Antacid Caplets, Mallamint, Mylanta Lozenges, Nephro-Calci, Os-Cal 500, Os-Cal 500 Chewable, Oysco 500 Chewable, Oyst-Cal 500,

Oystercal 500, Oyster Shell Calcium-500, Tums, Tums Ultra, Webber Calcium Carbonate ✲ **(OTC)**
**Classification:** Calcium salt

See also *Calcium Salts* and *Antacids*.
**Uses:** Mild hypocalcemia, antacid, antihyperphosphatemic.
**Special Concerns:** Dosage has not been established in children.

**Dosage**

• **Chewable Tablets, Tablets, Suspension, Gum, Lozenges, Wafers**
**Adults:** 0.5–1.5 g, as needed.

• **Capsules, Suspension, Tablets, Chewable Tablets**
*Hypocalcemia, nutritional supplement.*
**Adults:** 1.25–1.5 g 1–3 times/day with or after meals.
*Antihyperphosphatemic.*
**Adults:** 5–13 g/day in divided doses with meals.
*NOTE:* The preparation contains 40% elemental calcium and 400 mg elemental calcium/g (20 mEq/g).

• **Florical**
1 capsule or tablet daily (also contains 8.3 mg sodium fluoride per capsule or tablet).

• **Children's Mylanta Upset Stomach Relief Chewable Tablets or Liquid**
*Upset stomach in children.*
1 tablet or 5 mL for children weighing 24–47 pounds (or those aged 2–5 years) and 2 tablets or 10 mL for children weighing 48–95 pounds (or those aged 6–11).

## NURSING CONSIDERATIONS

See also *Nursing Considerations* for *Antacids* and *Calcium Salts*.
**Outcomes/Evaluate**

• Desired serum calcium levels
• ↓ Gastric acidity

# Calcium chloride

(**KAL**-see-um **KLOH**-ryd)
**Pregnancy Category:** C
**(Rx)**
**Classification:** Calcium salt

See also *Calcium Salts*.

**Uses:** Mild hypocalcemia due to neonatal tetany, tetany due to parathyroid deficiency or vitamin D deficiency, and alkalosis. Prophylaxis of hypocalcemia during exchange transfusions. Intestinal malabsorption. Treat effects of serious hyperkalemia as measured by ECG. Cardiac resuscitation after open heart surgery when epinephrine fails to improve weak or ineffective myocardial contractions. Adjunct to treat insect bites or stings to relieve muscle cramping. Depression due to magnesium overdosage. Acute symptoms of lead colic. Rickets, osteomalacia. Reverse symptoms of verapamil overdosage.

**Contraindications:** Use to treat hypocalcemia of renal insufficiency.

**Special Concerns:** Use usually restricted in children due to significant irritation and possible tissue necrosis and sloughing caused by IV calcium chloride.

**Additional Side Effects:** Peripheral vasodilation with moderate decreases in BP. Extravasation can cause severe necrosis, sloughing, or abscess formation following IM or SC use.

**Dosage**
• **IV Only**
  *Hypocalcemia, replenish electrolytes.*
  **Adults:** 0.5–1 g q 1–3 days (given at a rate not to exceed 13.6–27.3 mg/min). **Pediatric:** 25 mg/kg (0.2 mL/kg up to 1–10 mL/kg) given slowly.
  *Magnesium intoxication.*
  0.5 g promptly; observe for recovery before other doses given.
  *Cardiac resuscitation.*
  0.5–1 g IV or 0.2–0.8 g injected into the ventricular cavity as a single dose. **Pediatric:** 0.2 mL/kg.
  *Hyperkalemia.*
  Sufficient amount to return ECG to normal.
  *NOTE:* The preparation contains 27.2% calcium and 272 mg calcium/g (13.6 mEq/g).

## NURSING CONSIDERATIONS

See also *Nursing Considerations* for *Calcium Salts*.

**Administration/Storage**
1. *Never administer IM.*
**IV** 2. May administer undiluted by IV push.

**Outcomes/Evaluate**
• Desired serum calcium levels
• ↓ Magnesium and potassium levels
• Control of twitching and spasm

# Calcium citrate
(**KAL**-see-um **CIH**-trayt)
Citracal, Citracal Liquitab **(OTC)**
**Classification:** Calcium salt

See also *Calcium Salts*.
**Additional Use:** Renal osteodystrophy.
**Special Concerns:** Dosage has not been established in children.

**Dosage**
• **Tablets, Syrup, Effervescent Tablets**
  *Hypocalcemia.*
  **Adults:** 0.9–1.9 g t.i.d.–q.i.d. after meals.
  *Nutritional supplement.*
  3.8–7.1 g/day in three to four divided doses.
  *NOTE:* Contains 21.1% elemental calcium and 211 mg calcium/g (10.5 mEq/g).

## NURSING CONSIDERATIONS

See *Nursing Considerations* for *Calcium Salts*.
**Outcomes/Evaluate:** Restoration of serum calcium levels

# Calcium glubionate
(**KAL**-see-um glue-**BYE**-oh-nayt)
**Pregnancy Category:** C
Neo-Calglucon, Calcium-Sandoz **(OTC)**
**Classification:** Calcium salt

See also *Calcium Salts*.
**Uses:** Hypocalcemia, calcium deficiency, tetany of newborn, hypoparathyroidism, pseudohypoparathyroi-

dism, osteoporosis, rickets, osteomalacia.

**Dosage** ————————————
- **Syrup, Tablets**
  *Dietary supplement.*
  **Adults and children over 4 years:** 15 mL t.i.d.–q.i.d. **Pediatric (under 4 years):** 10 mL t.i.d. **Infants:** 5 mL 5 times/day.
  *Tetany of newborn.*
  On the basis of laboratory tests, usually 50–150 mg/kg/day in three or more divided doses.
  *Other calcium deficiencies.*
  **Adults:** 15–45 mL 1–3 times/day.
  *NOTE:* The preparation contains 115 mg calcium ion/5 mL.

## NURSING CONSIDERATIONS

See *Nursing Considerations* for *Calcium Salts.*
**Outcomes/Evaluate**
- Desired calcium replacement
- Control of twitching and spasm

# Calcium gluceptate (Calcium glucoheptonate)
(**KAL**-see-um **GLUE**-sep-tayt)
**Pregnancy Category:** C
**(Rx)**
**Classification:** Calcium salt

See also *Calcium Salts.*
**Uses:** Mild hypocalcemia due to neonatal tetany, tetany due to parathyroid deficiency or vitamin D deficiency, and alkalosis. Prophylaxis of hypocalcemia during exchange transfusions. Intestinal malabsorption. To replenish electrolytes. Antihypermagnesemic.
**Special Concerns:** Give only IM to infants and children in emergency situations when the IV route is not possible.

**Dosage** ————————————
- **IM**
  *Hypocalcemia.*
  **Adults and children:** 0.44–1.1 g.
- **IV**

*Hypocalcemia.*
**Adults:** 1.1–4.4 g given slowly at a rate not exceeding 36 mg calcium ion/min (2 mL/min). **Pediatric, IV:** 0.44–1.1 g; give as a single dose at a rate not to exceed 36 mg calcium ion/min.
  *Antihypermagnesemic.*
  **Adults:** 1.2–2.4 g given slowly at a rate not to exceed 36 mg calcium ion/min.
  *Exchange transfusions in newborns.*
  0.11 g after every 100 mL blood exchanged.
  *NOTE:* The elemental calcium content is 8.2% and there is 82 mg calcium/g (4.1 mEq/g).

## NURSING CONSIDERATIONS

See also *Nursing Considerations* for *Calcium Salts.*
**Administration/Storage:** In adults if more than 5 mL must be used IM, the IM dose should be given in the gluteal area. For infants, the dose should be given in the lateral thigh.
**Outcomes/Evaluate:** ↑ Calcium and magnesium levels

# Calcium gluconate
(**KAL**-see-um **GLUE**-koh-nayt)
Kalcinate (Rx, injection; OTC, tablets)
**Classification:** Calcium salt

See also *Calcium Salts.*
**Uses:** Mild hypocalcemia due to neonatal tetany, tetany due to parathyroid deficiency or vitamin D deficiency, and alkalosis. Prophylaxis of hypocalcemia during exchange transfusions. Intestinal malabsorption. Adjunct to treat insect bites or stings to relieve muscle cramping. Depression due to magnesium overdosage. Acute symptoms of lead colic. Rickets, osteomalacia. Reverse symptoms of verapamil overdosage. Decrease capillary permeability in allergic conditions, nonthrombocytopenic purpura, and exudative dermatoses (e.g., dermatitis herpetiformis). Pruritus due to certain drugs.

Hyperkalemia to antagonize cardiac toxicity (as long as client is not receiving digitalis).

**Contraindications:** Intramuscular, intramyocardial, or SC use due to severe tissue necrosis, sloughing, and abscess formation.

**Dosage**

• **Chewable Tablets, Tablets**
*Treatment of hypocalcemia.*
**Adults:** 8.8–16.5 g/day in divided doses; **pediatric:** 0.5–0.72 g/kg/day in divided doses.
*Nutritional supplement.*
**Adults:** 8.8–16.5 g/day in divided doses.

• **IV Only**
*Treatment of hypocalcemia.*
**Adults:** 2.3–9.3 mEq (5–20 mL of the 10% solution) as needed (range: 4.65–70 mEq/day). **Children:** 2.3 mEq/kg/day (or 56 mEq/m²/day) given well diluted and slowly in divided doses. **Infants:** No more than 0.93 mEq (2 mL of the 10% solution).
*Emergency elevation of serum calcium.*
**Adults:** 7–14 mEq (15–30.1 mL). **Children:** 1–7 mEq (2.2–15 mL). **Infants:** Less than 1 mEq (2.2 mL). Depending on client response, the dose may be repeated q 1–3 days.
*Hypocalcemic tetany.*
**Children:** 0.5–0.7 mEq/kg (1.1–1.5 mL/kg) t.i.d.–q.i.d. until tetany is controlled. **Infants:** 2.4 mEq/kg/day (5.2 mL/kg/day) in divided doses.
*Hyperkalemia with cardiac toxicity.*
2.25–14 mEq (4.8–30.1 mL) while monitoring the ECG. If needed, the dose can be repeated after 1–2 min.
*Magnesium intoxication.*
**Initial:** 4.5–9 mEq (9.7–19.4 mL). Subsequent dosage based on client response.
*Exchange transfusion.*
**Adults:** 1.35 mEq (2.9 mL) concurrent with each 100 mL citrated blood. **Neonates:** 0.45 mEq (1 mL)/100 mL citrated blood.

• **IM**
*Hypocalcemic tetany.*
**Adults:** 4.5–16 mEq (9.7–34.4 mL) until a therapeutic response is noted.

*Magnesium intoxication.*
**If IV administration is not possible:** 2–5 mEq (4.3–10.8 mL) in divided doses as needed.
*NOTE:* The preparation contains 9% calcium and 90 mg calcium/g (4.5 mEq/g).

## NURSING CONSIDERATIONS

See also *Nursing Considerations* for *Calcium Salts.*
**Administration/Storage**
1. If a precipitate is noted in the syringe, do not use.
2. If a precipitate is noted in the vials or ampules, heat to 80°C (146°F) in a dry heat oven for 1 hr to dissolve. Shake vigorously and allow to cool to room temperature. Do not use if precipitate remains.
**IV** 3. IV rate should not exceed 0.5–2 mL/min.
4. Can be given by intermittent IV infusion at a rate not exceeding 200 mg (19.5 mg calcium ion)/min. Can also be used by continuous IV infusion.
**Outcomes/Evaluate**
• Restoration of serum calcium levels
• ↓ Magnesium and potassium levels

# Calcium lactate
(**KAL**-see-um **LACK**-tayt)
(OTC)
**Classification:** Calcium salt

See also *Calcium Salts.*
**Uses:** Latent hypocalcemic tetany, hyperphosphatemia.

**Dosage**
• **Tablets**
*Treatment of hypocalcemia.*
**Adults:** 7.7 g/day in divided doses with meals. **Pediatric:** 0.34–0.5 g/kg/day in divided doses.
*NOTE:* The preparation contains 13% calcium and 130 mg calcium/g (6.5 mEq/g).

## NURSING CONSIDERATIONS

See *Nursing Considerations* for *Calcium Salts.*
**Outcomes/Evaluate:** Restoration of serum calcium levels

# Capsaicin

(kap-**SAY**-ih-sin)
Zostrix, Zostrix-HP **(Rx)**
**Classification:** Topical analgesic

**Action/Kinetics:** Capsaicin is derived from natural sources from plants of the Solanaceae family. It is believed the drug depletes and prevents the reaccumulation of substance P, thought to be the main mediator of pain impulses from the periphery to the CNS.
**Uses:** Temporary relief of pain due to rheumatoid arthritis and osteoarthritis. Pain following herpes zoster (shingles), painful diabetic neuropathy. *Investigational:* Possible use in psoriasis, vitiligo, intractable pruritus, reflex sympathetic dystrophy, postmastectomy, vulvar vestibulitis, apocrine chromhidrosis, and postamputation and postmastectomy neuroma.
**Special Concerns:** For external use only.
**Side Effects:** *Skin:* Transient burning following application, stinging, erythema. *Respiratory:* Cough, respiratory irritation.

**Dosage**
• **Cream or Lotion, 0.025% or 0.075%**
**Adults and children over 2 years of age:** Apply to affected area no more than 3–4 times/day.

## NURSING CONSIDERATIONS
**Client/Family Teaching**
1. Drug is for external use only. Avoid eyes and broken or irritated skin.
2. Wash hands before and immediately after application.
3. Do not bandage area tightly.
4. Regular use (3–4 times/day) is required for desired response; drug intereferes with substance P (pain neurotransmitter).
5. Report if condition worsens, if symptoms persist > 3 weeks, or if symptoms clear then recur within a few days.
**Outcomes/Evaluate:** Control of pain

# Captopril

(**KAP**-toe-prill)
**Pregnancy Category:** C (first trimester); D (second and third trimesters)
Alti-Captopril ✿, Apo-Capto ✿, Capoten, Gen-Captopril ✿, Med-Captopril ✿, Novo-Captoril ✿, Nu-Capto ✿ **(Rx)**
**Classification:** Antihypertensive, inhibitor of angiotensin synthesis

See also *Angiotensin-Converting Enzyme Inhibitors.*
**Action/Kinetics: Onset:** 15 min. **Peak serum levels:** 30–90 min; presence of food decreases absorption by 30%–40%. **Plasma protein binding:** 25%–30%. **Time to peak effect:** 60–90 min. **Duration:** 6–12 hr. **$t^{1/2}$, normal renal function:** 2 hr; **$t^{1/2}$, impaired renal function:** 3.5–32 hr. More than 95% of absorbed dose excreted in urine (40%–50% unchanged). Food decreases bioavailability of captopril by 30%–40%.
**Uses:** Antihypertensive, step I therapy in clients with normal renal function. Concomitant use with diuretic therapy may, however, cause precipitous hypotension. In combination with diuretics and digitalis in treatment of CHF not responding to conventional therapy. To improve survival following MI in clinically stable clients with LV dysfunction manifested as an ejection fraction of 40% or less. Treatment of diabetic nephropathy (proteinuria > 500 mg/day) in those with type I insulin-dependent diabetes and retinopathy. *Investigational:* Rheumatoid arthritis, hypertensive crisis, neonatal and childhood hypertension, hypertension related to scleroderma renal crisis, diagnosis of anatomic renal artery stenosis, diagnosis of primary aldosteronism, Raynaud's syndrome, hypertension of Takayasu's disease, idiopathic edema, and Bartter's syndrome.
**Contraindications:** Use with a history of angioedema related to previous use of ACE inhibitors.

---

✿ = Available in Canada      ***bold italic*** = life threatening side effect

**Special Concerns:** Use with caution in cases of impaired renal function and during lactation. Use in children only if other antihypertensive therapy has proven ineffective in controlling BP. May cause a profound drop in BP following the first dose.

**Side Effects:** *Dermatologic:* Rash (usually maculopapular) with pruritus and occasionally fever, eosinophilia, and arthralgia. Alopecia, erythema multiforme, photosensitivity, exfoliative dermatitis, *Stevens-Johnson syndrome,* reversible pemphigoid-like lesions, bullous pemphigus, onycholysis, flushing, pallor, scalded mouth sensation. *GI:* N&V, anorexia, constipation or diarrhea, gastric irritation, abdominal pain, dysgeusia, peptic ulcers, aphthous ulcers, dyspepsia, dry mouth, glossitis, pancreatitis. *Hepatic:* Jaundice, cholestasis, hepatitis. *CNS:* Headache, dizziness, insomnia, malaise, fatigue, paresthesias, confusion, depression, nervousness, ataxia, somnolence. *CV:* Hypotension, angina, *MI,* Raynaud's phenomenon, chest pain, palpitations, tachycardia, *CVA, CHF, cardiac arrest,* orthostatic hypotension, rhythm disturbances. *Renal:* Renal insufficiency or failure, proteinuria, urinary frequency, oliguria, polyuria, nephrotic syndrome, interstitial nephritis. *Respiratory:* **Bronchospasm,** cough, dyspnea, asthma, *pulmonary embolism, pulmonary infarction.* *Hematologic:* Agranulocytosis, neutropenia, thrombocytopenia, pancytopenia, *aplastic or hemolytic anemia.* *Other:* Decrease or loss of taste perception with weight loss (reversible), angioedema, asthenia, syncope, fever, myalgia, arthralgia, vasculitis, blurred vision, impotence, hyperkalemia, hyponatremia, myasthenia, gynecomastia, rhinitis, eosinophilic pneumonitis.

**OD** **Overdose Management:** *Symptoms:* Hypotension is the most common with a systolic BP of <80 mm Hg a possibility. *Treatment:* Volume expansion with NSS (IV) is the treatment of choice to restore BP.

**Additional Drug Interactions:** Probenecid increases blood levels of captopril due to decreased renal excretion.

**Laboratory Test Interferences:** False + test for urine acetone.

**Dosage**
• **Tablets**
  *Hypertension.*
**Adults, initial:** 25 mg b.i.d.–t.i.d. If unsatisfactory response after 1–2 weeks, increase to 50 mg b.i.d.–t.i.d.; if still unsatisfactory after another 1–2 weeks, thiazide diuretic should be added (e.g., hydrochlorothiazide, 25 mg/day). Dosage may be increased to 100–150 mg b.i.d.–t.i.d., not to exceed 450 mg/day.

  *Accelerated or malignant hypertension.*
Stop current medication (except for the diuretic) and initiate captopril at a dose of 25 mg b.i.d.–t.i.d. The dose may be increased q 24 hr until a satisfactory response is obtained or the maximum dose reached. Furosemide may be indicated.

  *Heart failure.*
**Initial:** 25 mg t.i.d.; **then,** if necessary, increase dose to 50 mg t.i.d. and evaluate response; **maintenance:** 50–100 mg t.i.d., not to exceed 450 mg/day.

  *NOTE:* For adults, an initial dose of 6.25–12.5 mg (0.15 mg/kg t.i.d. in children) should be given b.i.d.–t.i.d. to clients who are sodium- and water-depleted due to diuretics, who will continue to be on diuretic therapy, and who have renal impairment.

  *Left ventricular dysfunction after MI.*
Therapy may be started as early as 3 days after the MI. **Initial dose:** 6.25 mg; **then,** begin 12.5 mg t.i.d. and increase to 25 mg t.i.d. over the next several days. The target dose is 50 mg t.i.d. over the next several weeks. Other treatments for MI may be used concomitantly (e.g., aspirin, beta blockers, thrombolytic drugs).

  *Diabetic nephropathy.*
25 mg t.i.d. for chronic use. Other antihypertensive drugs (e.g., beta

blockers, centrally-acting drugs, diuretics, vasodilators) may be used with captopril if additional drug therapy is needed to reduce BP.

*Hypertensive crisis.*
**Initial:** 25 mg; **then,** 100 mg 90–120 min later, 200–300 mg/day for 2–5 days (then adjust dose). Sublingual captopril, 25 mg, has also been used successfully.

*Rheumatoid arthritis.*
75–150 mg/day in divided doses.

*NOTE:* For all uses, doses should be reduced in clients with renal impairment.

## NURSING CONSIDERATIONS

See also *Nursing Considerations* for *Angiotensin-Converting Enzyme Inhibitors* and *Antihypertensive Agents.*

**Administration/Storage**
1. Do not discontinue without the provider's consent.
2. Give 1 hr before meals.
3. Discontinue previous antihypertensive medication 1 week before starting captopril, if possible.
4. The tablets can be used to prepare a solution of captopril if desired.

**Assessment**
1. Obtain baseline hematologic, liver and renal function tests.
2. Determine if diuretics, nitroglycerin, or other nitrates prescribed; these may act synergistically with captopril and cause a more pronounced response.
3. Document any ACE intolerance.
4. Determine ability to understand and comply with therapy.
5. Note ejection fraction (at or below 40%) in stable, post-MI clients.
6. Usually very effective in clients with heart failure, diabetes, and arthritis.

**Interventions**
1. Observe for precipitous drop in BP within 3 hr after initial dose if client has been on diuretic therapy and a low-salt diet.
2. If BP falls rapidly, place in a supine position; have saline infusion available.
3. Initially check for proteinuria monthly and for at least 9 months during therapy.
4. Withhold potassium-sparing diuretics; hyperkalemia may result. Be alert to hyperkalemia occurring several months after administration of spironolactone and captopril.

**Client/Family Teaching**
1. Take 1 hr before meals, on an empty stomach; food interferes with drug absorption.
2. Report any fever, skin rash, sore throat, mouth sores, fast or irregular heartbeat, chest pain, or cough.
3. May develop dizziness, fainting, or lightheadedness; these usually disappear once the body adjusts to the medication. Avoid sudden changes in posture to prevent dizziness and fainting.
4. Loss of taste may be experienced for the first 2–3 months and then disappear; report if persists and interferes with nutrition.
5. Carry ID and a list of medications currently prescribed.
6. Call with any questions concerning symptoms or effects of drug therapy; do not stop taking abruptly.
7. Insulin-dependent clients may experience hypoglycemia; monitor blood sugar levels closely.
8. Avoid OTC agents without approval.

**Outcomes/Evaluate**
- ↓ BP
- Improvement in symptoms of CHF (↓ preload, ↓ afterload)
- Improved mortality post-MI

# Carbamazepine
(kar-bah-**MAYZ**-eh-peen)
**Pregnancy Category:** C
Apo-Carbamazepine ✿, Atretol, Depitol, Epitol, Mazepine ✿, Novo-Carbamaz ✿, Nu-Carbamazepine ✿, PMS-Carbamazepine ✿, Taro-Carbamazepine ✿, Tegretol, Tegretol Chewtabs ✿, Tegretol CR ✿, Tegretol XR **(Rx)**

**Classification:** Anticonvulsant, miscellaneous

See also *Anticonvulsants.*

**Action/Kinetics:** Chemically similar to the cyclic antidepressants. It also manifests antimanic, antineuralgic, antidiuretic, anticholinergic, antiarrhythmic, and antipsychotic effects. The anticonvulsant action is not known but may involve depressing activity in the nucleus ventralis anterior of the thalamus, resulting in a reduction of polysynaptic responses and blocking posttetanic potentiation . Due to the potentially serious blood dyscrasias, a benefit-to-risk evaluation should be undertaken before the drug is instituted. **Peak serum levels:** 4–5 hr. **t½** (serum): 12–17 hr with repeated doses. **Therapeutic serum levels:** 4–12 mcg/mL. Metabolized in the liver to an active metabolite (epoxide derivative) with a half-life of 5–8 hr. Metabolites are excreted through the feces and urine.

**Uses:** Partial seizures with complex symptoms (psychomotor, temporal lobe). Tonic-clonic seizures, diseases with mixed seizure patterns or other partial or generalized seizures. Carbamazepine is often a drug of choice due to its low incidence of side effects. For children with epilepsy who are less than 6 years of age for the treatment of partial seizures, generalized tonic-clonic seizures, and mixed seizure patterns and for treating trigeminal neuralgia. To treat pain associated with tic douloureux (trigeminal neuralgia) and glossopharyngeal neuralgia. *Investigational:* Bipolar disorders, unipolar depression, schizoaffective illness, resistant schizophrenia, dyscontrol syndrome associated with limbic system dysfunction, intermittent explosive disorder, PTSD, atypical psychosis. Management of alcohol, cocaine, and benzodiazepine withdrawal symptoms. Restless leg syndrome, nonhereditary chorea in children.

**Contraindications:** History of bone marrow depression. Hypersensitivity to drug or tricyclic antidepressants. Lactation. In clients taking MAO inhibitors. Use for relief of general aches and pains.

**Special Concerns:** Safety and effectiveness have not been established in children less than 6 years of age. Use with caution in glaucoma and in hepatic, renal, CV disease, and a history of hematologic reaction. Use with caution in clients with mixed seizure disorder that includes atypical absence seizures (carbamazepine is not effective and may be associated with an increased frequency of generalized convulsions). Use in geriatric clients may cause an increased incidence of confusion, agitation, AV heart block, syndrome of inappropriate antidiuretic hormone, and bradycardia.

**Side Effects:** *GI:* N&V (common), diarrhea, constipation, gastric distress, abdominal pain, anorexia, glossitis, stomatitis, dryness of mouth and pharynx. *Hematologic:* **Aplastic anemia,** leukopenia, eosinophilia, thrombocytopenia, **agranulocytosis,** leukocytosis, pancytopenia, **bone marrow depression.** *CNS:* Dizziness, drowsiness, disturbances of coordination, headache, fatigue, confusion, speech disturbances, visual hallucinations, depression with agitation, talkativeness, hyperacusis, abnormal involuntary movements, behavioral changes in children. *CV:* CHF, aggravation of hypertension, hypotension, syncope and collapse, edema, recurrence of or primary thrombophlebitis, aggravation of CAD, paralysis and other symptoms of cerebral arterial insufficiency, **arrhythmias (including AV block).** *GU:* Urinary frequency, acute urinary retention, oliguria with hypertension, impotence, renal failure, azotemia, albuminuria, glycosuria, increased BUN, microscopic deposits in urine. *Pulmonary:* Pulmonary hypersensitivity characterized by fever, dyspnea, pneumonitis, or pneumonia. *Dermatologic:* Pruritus, urticaria, photosensitivity, exfoliative dermatitis, erythematous rashes, alterations in pigmentation, alopecia, sweating, purpura, toxic epidermal necrolysis (Lyell's syndrome), **Stevens-Johnson syndrome,** aggravation of disseminated lupus erythematosus, alopecia, erythema nodosum or multiforme. *Ophthalmologic:* Nystagmus, double vision, blurred vision, oculomotor disturbances, conjunctivitis; scattered, punctate lens opacities. *Hepatic:* Abnormal liver function tests, cholestatic or hepatocellular jaundice, hepatitis, acute intermittent porphyria. *Other:* Peripheral neuritis, paresthesias, tinnitus, fever, chills, joint and muscle aches and leg cramps, adenopathy or lymphadenopathy, inappropriate ADH secretion syndrome.

**OD** **Overdose Management:** *Symptoms:* First appear after 1 to 3 hours. Neuromuscular disturbances are the most common. *Pulmonary:* Irregular breathing, **respiratory depression.** *CV:* Tachycardia, hypo- or hypertension, conduction disorders, **shock.** *CNS:* Seizures (especially in small children), impaired consciousness (deep coma possible), **motor restlessness, muscle twitching or tremors, athetoid movements, ataxia, drowsiness, dizziness, nystagmus, mydriasis, psychomotor disturbances, hyperreflexia followed by hyporeflexia, opisthotonos, dysmetria, dizziness, EEG may show dysrhythmias.** *GI:* N&V. *GU:* Anuria, oliguria, urinary retention. *Treatment:* Stomach should be irrigated completely even if more than 4 hr has elapsed following drug ingestion, especially if alcohol has been ingested. Activated charcoal, 50–100 g initially, using a NGT (dose of 12.5 or more g/hr until client is symptom free). Diazepam or phenobarbital may be used to treat seizures (although they may aggravate respiratory depression, hypotension, and coma). Respiration, ECG, BP, body temperature, pupillary reflexes, and kidney and bladder function should be monitored for several days.

If significant bone marrow depression occurs, the drug should be discontinued and daily CBC, platelet and reticulocyte counts determined. Perform bone marrow aspiration and trephine biopsy immediately and repeat often enough to monitor recovery.

**Drug Interactions**

*Acetaminophen* / ↑ Breakdown of acetaminophen → ↓ effect and ↑ risk of hepatotoxicity

*Charcoal* / ↓ Effect of carbamazepine due to ↓ absorption from GI tract

*Cimetidine* / ↑ Effect of carbamazepine due to ↓ breakdown by liver

*Contraceptives, oral* / ↓ Effect of contraceptives due to ↑ breakdown by liver

*Danazol* / ↑ Effect of carbamazepine due to ↓ breakdown by liver

*Desmopressin* / ↑ Effect of desmopressin

*Diltiazem* / ↑ Effect of carbamazepine due to ↓ breakdown by liver

*Doxycycline* / ↓ Effect of doxycycline due to ↑ breakdown by liver

*Erythromycin* / ↑ Effect of carbamazepine due to ↓ breakdown by liver

*Ethosuximide* / ↓ Effect of ethosuximide due to ↑ breakdown by liver

*Felbamate* / Possible ↓ serum levels of either drug

*Fluoxetine* / ↑ Carbamazepine levels → possible toxicity

*Fluvoxamine* / Carbamazepine levels possible toxicity

*Haloperidol* / ↓ Effect of haloperidol due to ↑ breakdown by liver

*Isoniazid* / ↑ Effect of carbamazepine due to ↓ breakdown by liver; also, carbamazepine may ↑ risk of isoniazid-induced hepatotoxicity

*Lithium* / ↑ CNS toxicity

*Lypressin* / ↑ Effect of lypressin

*Macrolide antibiotics* / Effect of carbamazepine due to breakdown by liver

*MAO inhibitors* / Exaggerated side effects of carbamazepine

*Muscle relaxants, nondepolarizing* / Resistance to or reversal of the neuromuscular blocking effects of these drugs

*Nicotinamide* / ↑ Effect of carbamazepine due to ↓ breakdown by liver

*Phenobarbital* / ↓ Effect of carbamazepine due to ↑ breakdown by liver

*Phenytoin* / ↓ Effect of carbamazepine due to ↑ breakdown by liver; also, phenytoin levels may ↑ or ↓

*Primidone* / ↓ Effect of carbamazepine due to ↑ breakdown by liver

*Propoxyphene* / ↑ Effect of carbamazepine due to ↓ breakdown by liver

*Succinimides* / ↓ Effect of succinimides due to ↑ breakdown by the liver

*Terfenadine* / May ↑ carbamazepine levels

*Theophyllines* / ↓ or ↑ Levels of theophylline; ↑ levels of carbamazepine

*Tricyclic antidepressants* / ↓ Effect of tricyclic antidepressants due to ↑ breakdown by liver; also, ↓ levels of tricyclic antidepressants

*Troleandomycin* / ↑ Effect of carbamazepine due to ↓ breakdown by liver

*Valproic acid* / ↓ Effect of valproic acid due to ↑ breakdown by liver; half-life of carbamazepine may be ↑

*Vasopressin* / ↑ Effect of vasopressin

*Verapamil* / ↑ Effect of carbamazepine due to ↓ breakdown by liver

*Warfarin sodium* / ↓ Effect of anticoagulant due to ↑ breakdown by liver

**Dosage** ————————
• **Oral Suspension, Tablets, Chewable Tablets, Extended-Release Tablets**
*Anticonvulsant.*
**Adults and children over 12 years, initial:** 200 mg b.i.d. on day 1 (100 mg q.i.d. of suspension). Increase by 200 mg/day at weekly intervals until best response is attained. Divide total dose and administer q 6–8 hr; the extended-release tablets may be used for twice-daily dosing instead of dosing 3 or 4 times a day. **Maximum dose, children 12–15 years:** 1,000 mg/day; **adults**

**and children over 15 years:** 1,200 mg/day. **Maintenance:** decrease dose gradually to minimum effective level, usually 800–1,200 mg/day. **Children, 6–12 years: initial,** 100 mg b.i.d. on day 1 (50 mg q.i.d. of suspension); **then,** increase slowly, at weekly intervals, by 100 mg/day; dose is divided and given q 6–8 hr. Daily dose should not exceed 1,000 mg. **Maintenance:** 400–800 mg/day. **Children, less than 6 years:** 10–20 mg/kg/day in two to three divided doses; dose can be increased slowly in weekly increments to maintenance levels of 250–300 mg/day (not to exceed 400 mg/day).

*Trigeminal neuralgia.*
**Initial:** 100 mg b.i.d. on day 1 (50 mg q.i.d. of suspension); increase by no more than 200 mg/day, using increments of 100 mg q 12 hr as needed, up to maximum of 1,200 mg/day. **Maintenance: Usual:** 400–800 mg/day (range: 200–1,200 mg/day). Attempt discontinuation of drug at least 1 time q 3 months.

*Restless legs syndrome.*
100–300 mg at bedtime.

*Nonhereditary chorea in children.*
15–25 mg/kg/day.

## NURSING CONSIDERATIONS

See also *Nursing Considerations* for *Anticonvulsants.*

**Administration/Storage**
1. Do not administer for a minimum of 2 weeks after client has received MAO inhibitor drugs.
2. Protect tablets from moisture.
3. Start therapy gradually with the lowest doses of drug to minimize adverse reactions.
4. Add gradually to other anticonvulsant therapy. The other anticonvulsant dosage may be maintained or decreased except for phenytoin, which may need to be increased.
5. If carbamazepine therapy must be discontinued due to side effects, abrupt withdrawal may lead to seizures or status epilepticus.

**Assessment**
1. Document indications for therapy and include pretreatment findings.

With seizures, describe type, frequency, and characteristics.

2. Obtain baseline hematologic, liver, and renal function tests. Do not initiate therapy until significant abnormalities have been ruled out.

3. Review eye exams for evidence of opacities and baseline intraocular pressure measurement.

4. Assess for a history of psychosis; drug may activate symptoms.

**Interventions**

1. CNS depression may impair functions; use side rails if agitated.

2. With high doses, perform weekly CBC's for the first 3 mo, then monthly to assess extent of bone marrow depression.

3. At the first sign of blood dyscrasia, slowly discontinue drug.

4. During dosage adjustment, monitor I&O and VS for evidence of fluid retention, renal failure, or CV complications.

5. Obtain EEG periodically during therapy.

6. Use seizure precautions with quick withdrawal; may precipitate status epilepticus.

**Client/Family Teaching**

1. Take with meals to minimize GI upset.

2. Withhold drug and report if any of the following symptoms occur:

• Fever, sore throat, mouth ulcers, easy bruising, and skin hemorrhages; early signs of bone marrow depression.

• Urinary frequency, retention, reduced output, sexual impotence; early signs of GU dysfunction.

• Symptoms of CHF, fainting, collapse, swelling, blood clot, or cyanosis; CV side effects that require immediate attention.

• Loss of symptom control

3. Use caution in operating an automobile or other dangerous machinery; drug may interfere with vision and coordination.

4. Report any skin eruptions or pigmentation changes.

5. Avoid excessive sunlight; wear protective clothing and sunscreen due to risk of photosensitivity.

6. Use nonhormonal form of birth control.

7. Stress importance of regular lab studies to assess for early organ dysfunction.

**Outcomes/Evaluate**

• Control of refractory seizures
• ↓ Manic/psychotic manifestations
• ↓ Pain with trigeminal neuralgia
• Therapeutic serum drug levels (4–12 mcg/mL)

# Carbenicillin indanyl sodium

(kar-ben-ih-**SILL**-in)
**Pregnancy Category:** B
Geocillin **(Rx)**
**Classification:** Antibiotic, penicillin

See also *Anti-Infectives* and *Penicillins.*

**Action/Kinetics:** The drug is acid stable. **Peak serum levels: PO:** 6.5 mcg/mL after 1 hr. **t½:** 60 min. Rapidly excreted unchanged in urine.

**Uses:** Upper and lower UTIs or bacteriuria due to *Escherichia coli, Proteus vulgaris and P. mirabilis, Morganella morganii, Providencia rettgeri, Enterobacter, Pseudomonas,* and enterococci. Prostatitis due to *E. coli, Streptococcus faecalis* (enterococci), *P. mirabilis,* and *Enterobacter* species.

**Additional Contraindications:** Pregnancy.

**Special Concerns:** Safe use in children not established. Use with caution in clients with impaired renal function.

**Additional Side Effects:** Neurotoxicity in clients with impaired renal function.

**Additional Drug Interactions:** When used in combination with gentamicin or tobramycin for *Pseudomonas* infections, effect of carbenicillin may be enhanced.

**Dosage** ———————
• **Tablets**

---

*UTIs due to* E. coli, Proteus, Enterobacter.
382–764 mg q.i.d.

*UTIs due to* Pseudomonas *and enterococci.*
764 mg q.i.d.

*Prostatitis due to* E. coli, P. mirabilis, Enterobacter, *and enterococci.*
764 mg q.i.d.

## NURSING CONSIDERATIONS

See also *General Nursing Considerations* for *All Anti-Infectives* and *Penicillins.*

**Administration/Storage**
1. Protect from moisture.
2. Store at temperature of 30°C (86°F) or less.

**Interventions**
1. Provide frequent mouth care to minimize nausea and unpleasant aftertaste.
2. With impaired renal function, report any neurotoxicity, manifested by hallucinations, impaired sensorium, muscular irritability, and seizures.
3. Monitor CBC; report any hemorrhagic manifestations, such as ecchymosis, petechiae, and frank bleeding of gums and/or rectum.

**Outcomes/Evaluate**
• Negative C&S results
• Resolution of infection; symptomatic improvement

# Carbidopa
(**KAR**-bih-doh-pah)
Lodosyn **(Rx)**

———COMBINATION DRUG———
# Carbidopa/Levodopa
(**KAR**-bih-doh-pah/**LEE**-voh-doh-pah)
Sinemet-10/100, -25/100, or -25/250, Sinemet CR **(Rx)**
**Classification:** Antiparkinson agent

See also *Levodopa.*
**Content:    Carbidopa/Levodopa:**
Each 10/100 tablet contains: carbidopa, 10 mg, and levodopa, 100 mg.
Each 25/100 tablets contains: carbidopa, 25 mg, and levodopa, 100 mg.
Each 25/250 tablet contains: carbidopa, 25 mg, and levodopa, 250 mg.

Each sustained-release tablet contains: carbidopa, 50 mg, and levodopa, 200 mg.
**Action/Kinetics:** Carbidopa inhibits peripheral decarboxylation of levodopa but not central decarboxylation because it does not cross the blood-brain barrier. Since peripheral decarboxylation is inhibited, this allows more levodopa to be available for transport to the brain, where it will be converted to dopamine, thus relieving the symptoms of parkinsonism. It is recommended that both carbidopa and levodopa be given together (e.g., Sinemet). However, *the dosage of levodopa must be reduced by up to 80% when combined with carbidopa*. This decreases the incidence of levodopa-induced side effects. *NOTE:* Pyridoxine will not reverse the action of carbidopa/levodopa. **t½, carbidopa:** 1–2 hr; when given with levodopa, the t½ of levodopa increases from 1 hr to 2 hr (may be as high as 15 hr in some clients). About 30% carbidopa is excreted unchanged in the urine.
**Uses:** All types of parkinsonism (idiopathic, postencephalitic, following injury to the nervous system due to carbon monoxide and manganese intoxication). Carbidopa alone is used in clients who require individual titration of carbidopa and levodopa. *Investigational:* Postanoxic intention myoclonus. **Warning:** Levodopa must be discontinued at least 8 hr before carbidopa/levodopa therapy is initiated. Also, clients taking carbidopa/levodopa must not take levodopa concomitantly, because the former is a combination of carbidopa and levodopa.
**Contraindications:** History of melanoma. MAO inhibitors should be stopped 2 weeks before therapy. Lactation.
**Special Concerns:** Use during pregnancy only if benefits outweigh risks. Safety and efficacy in children less than 18 years of age have not been determined. Lower doses may be necessary in geriatric clients due to aged-related decreases in peripheral dopa decarboxylase.

**Side Effects:** Because more levodopa reaches the brain, dyskinesias may occur at lower doses with carbidopa/levodopa than with levodopa alone. Clients abruptly withdrawn from levodopa may experience neuroleptic malignant-like syndrome including symptoms of muscular rigidity, hyperthermia, increased serum phosphokinase, and changes in mental status.

**Drug Interactions:** Use with tricyclic antidepressants may cause hypertension and dyskinesia.

**Laboratory Test Interferences:** ↓ Creatinine, BUN, and uric acid.

## Dosage

- **Tablets**

  *Parkinsonism, clients not receiving levodopa.*

  **Initial:** 1 tablet of 10 mg carbidopa/100 mg levodopa t.i.d.–q.i.d. or 25 mg carbidopa/100 mg levodopa t.i.d.; **then,** increase by 1 tablet q 1–2 days until a total of 8 tablets/day is taken. If additional levodopa is required, substitute 1 tablet of 25 mg carbidopa/250 mg levodopa t.i.d.–q.i.d.

  *Parkinsonism, clients receiving levodopa.*

  **Initial:** Carbidopa/levodopa dosage should be about 25% of prior levodopa dosage (levodopa dosage is discontinued 8 hr before carbidopa/levodopa is initiated); **then,** adjust dosage as required. Suggested starting dose is 1 tablet of 25 mg carbidopa/250 mg levodopa t.i.d.–q.i.d. for clients taking more than 1500 mg levodopa or 25 mg carbidopa/100 mg levodopa for clients taking less than 1500 mg levodopa.

- **Sustained-Release Tablets**

  *Parkinsonism, clients not receiving levodopa.*

  1 tablet b.i.d. at intervals of not less than 6 hr. Depending on the response, dosage may be increased or decreased. Usual dose is 2–8 tablets/day in divided doses at intervals of 4–8 hr during waking hours (if divided doses are not equal, the smaller dose should be given at the end of the day).

  *Parkinsonism, clients receiving levodopa.*

  1 tablet b.i.d. Carbidopa is available alone for clients requiring additional carbidopa (i.e., inadequate reduction in N&V); in such clients, carbidopa may be given at a dose of 25 mg with the first daily dose of carbidopa/levodopa. If necessary, additional carbidopa, at doses of 12.5 or 25 mg, may be given with each dose of carbidopa/levodopa.

  *Clients receiving carbidopa/levodopa who require additional carbidopa.*

  In clients taking 10 mg carbidopa/100 mg levodopa, 25 mg carbidopa may be given with the first dose each day. Additional doses of 12.5 or 25 mg may be given during the day with each dose. If the client is taking 25 mg carbidopa/250 mg levodopa, a dose of 25 mg carbidopa may be given with any dose, as needed. The maximum daily dose of carbidopa is 200 mg.

## NURSING CONSIDERATIONS

See also *Nursing Considerations* for *Levodopa.*

**Administration/Storage**

1. Drug dosage must be individualized.

2. Note any potential drug interactions.

3. Do not administer carbidopa/levodopa with levodopa.

4. Administration of the sustained-release form of carbidopa/levodopa with food results in increased availability of levodopa by 50% and increased peak levodopa levels by 25%.

5. The sustained-release form of Sinemet should not be crushed or chewed but can be administered as whole or half tablets.

6. A minimum of 3 days should elapse between dosage adjustments of the sustained-release product.

7. When carbidopa is used as a supplement to carbidopa/levodopa, 1

tablet of carbidopa may be added or omitted per day.

8. If general anesthesia is necessary, continue therapy as long as PO fluids and other medication are allowed. Resume therapy when able to take PO medication.

**Assessment**

1. Assess and document motor function, reflexes, gait, strength of grip, and amount of tremor.

2. Observe extent of tremors, noting muscle weakness, muscle rigidity, difficulty walking, or changing directions. During dosage adjustment period, any involuntary movement may require dosage reduction.

3. Determine usual sleep patterns; assess mental status.

4. Note any history of CV disease, cardiac arrhythmias, or COPD.

5. Elderly clients may require a reduced dosage.

6. Obtain baseline ECG, VS, and respiratory assessment and determine level of bladder function. Monitor BP while supine and standing to detect postural hypotension.

7. Assess need for a drug "holiday" periodically based on decreased drug response

**Client/Family Teaching**

1. Report side effects as dose of drug may need to be reduced or temporarily discontinued. They may be asked to tolerate certain side effects because of the overall benefits gained with therapy.

2. With improvement, client may resume normal activity gradually; with increased activity, other medical conditions must be considered.

3. Antiparkinson drugs should not be withdrawn abruptly. When changing medication, one drug should be withdrawn slowly and the other started in small doses under medical supervision. To facilitate adjustment, take the last dose of levodopa at bedtime and start carbidopa/levodopa upon arising in the morning. Food may alter availability; do not crush or chew sustained-release form of Sinemet. May take as whole or half tablets.

4. Drug may discolor or darken urine and/or sweat.

5. Muscle and eyelid twitching may indicate toxicity and should be reported immediately.

**Outcomes/Evaluate:** Control of parkinsonian symptoms (e.g., improvement in motor function, reflexes, gait, strength of grip, and amount of tremor)

# Carboplatin for Injection
(**KAR**-boh-plah-tin)
**Pregnancy Category:** D
Paraplatin, Paraplatin-AQ ✲ **(Rx)**
**Classification:** Antineoplastic, alkylating agent

See also *Antineoplastic Agents* and *Alkylating Agents*.

**Action/Kinetics:** Related to cisplatin. Acts by producing interstrand DNA cross-links; thought to be cell-cycle nonspecific. **t½, initial:** 1.1–2 hr; **postdistribution:** 2.6–5.9 hr. Not bound to plasma proteins although platinum from carboplatin is irreversibly bound to plasma protein with a slow half-life (5 days). Eliminated unchanged in the urine at a rate related to creatinine clearance.

**Uses:** Initial treatment of advanced ovarian cancer in combination with other chemotherapeutic agents. Palliative treatment of recurrent ovarian cancer either initially or previously treated with chemotherapy, including cisplatin. *Investigational:* Small cell lung carcinoma (in combination with etoposide); advanced or recurrent squamous cell tumors of the head and neck (in combination with fluorouracil); seminoma of testicular cancer; advanced endometrial cancer; relapsed or refractory acute leukemia.

**Additional    Contraindications:** History of severe allergy to mannitol or platinum compounds (including cisplatin). Severe bone marrow depression, significant bleeding, lactation.

**Additional Side Effects:** *Bone marrow suppression* may be severe. Vomiting (common). *Neurologic:* Central neurotoxicity, peripheral neuropathies (more common in ages 65 and over), ototoxicity. *GU:* Nephrotoxicity (including increased BUN and serum creatinine). *Electrolytes:* Loss of calcium, magnesium, potassium, sodium. *Allergic:* Rash, urticaria, pruritus, erythema; **bronchospasm** and hypotension (rare). *Miscellaneous:* Pain, alopecia, asthenia. CV, respiratory, mucosal side effects, ***anaphylaxis.***

**OD** **Overdose Management:** *Symptoms:* ***Bone marrow suppression, hepatic toxicity.*** *Treatment:* Monitor bone marrow and liver function tests. Treat symptomatically.

**Drug Interactions**
*Aluminum /* Carboplatin can react with aluminum (e.g., needles, IV administration sets) → formation of a precipitate and loss of potency
*Phenytoin /* ↓ Serum levels of phenytoin → loss of therapeutic effect

**Laboratory Test Interferences:** ↑ Alkaline phosphatase, AST, total bilirubin.

**Dosage**
• **IV**
*Ovarian cancer, as a single agent.*
360 mg/m² q 4 weeks on day 1. Lower doses are recommended in clients with low creatinine clearances.
*In combination with cyclophosphamide.*
Carboplatin, 300 mg/m² plus cyclophosphamide, 600 mg/m², both on day 1 q 4 weeks for 6 cycles.

## NURSING CONSIDERATIONS

See also *Nursing Considerations* for *Antineoplastic Agents.*
**Administration/Storage**
**IV** 1. Do not repeat single intermittent doses of carboplatin until the neutrophil count is at least 2,000/mm³ and the platelet count is 100,000/mm³.
2. The dose may be escalated by no more than 125% of the starting dose if platelet counts are greater than 100,000/mm³ and neutrophil counts are greater than 2,000/mm³. If platelet counts are less than 50,000/mm³ and neutrophil counts are less than 500/mm³, subsequent doses should be 75% of the prior dose.
3. With impaired kidney function, adjust the dose: $C_{CR}$ of 41–59 mL/min, 250 mg/m² on day 1; $C_{CR}$ of 16–40 mL/min, 200 mg/m². There is no recommended dose if the $C_{CR}$ is less than 15 mL/min.
4. Cisplatin has been confused with carboplatin. Signs should be placed in the storage areas warning of the name mix-ups. Products should not be referred to as "platinum."
5. Do not use with needles or IV administration sets containing aluminum.
6. Immediately before use, reconstitute the drug with either sterile water for injection, D5W, or NaCl injection to a final concentration of 10 mg/mL. May be further diluted to concentrations as low as 0.5 mg/mL with D5W or NaCl injection. The dose is administered by infusion lasting 15 min or longer.
7. Reconstituted solutions are stable for 8 hr at room temperature. Discard after 8 hr as there is no antibacterial preservative in the formulation.
8. Store unopened vials at room temperature, protected from light.
**Assessment**
1. Note any evidence of kidney impairment.
2. Determine history of allergic responses to mannitol or platinum compounds.
3. Document and assess for any neurologic disorders to determine if those occuring at a later date are drug related or exacerbations of a prior condition.
4. Assess CBC for drug-induced anemia, a frequent side effect of carboplatin therapy.
5. Monitor alkaline phosphatase, AST, and total bilirubin.
**Interventions**
1. Premedicate with antiemetics; vomiting is a frequent side effect.

2. Drug dose is based on CBC and creatinine clearance results; reduce dose with impaired liver and/or renal function.

3. With evidence of kidney impairment, initially give 1–2 L of fluids slowly. Use diuretics if overhydration develops.

**Client/Family Teaching**

1. N&V may be experienced.

2. Report if a rash, itching, skin redness, or bronchospasm develops.

3. Maintain adequate fluid intake using favorite fluids, especially those with potassium and calcium, since these electrolytes may be lost in excess with therapy.

4. Report any sore throat, fever, fatigue, breathing problems, or mouth sores; may indicate bone marrow depression, which can be severe with this drug therapy.

**Outcomes/Evaluate:** ↓ Size and spread of tumor; stabilization of malignant process

# Carisoprodol

(kar-eye-so-**PROH**-dohl)

**Pregnancy Category:** C

Soma **(Rx)**

**Classification:** Skeletal muscle relaxant, centrally acting

See also *Skeletal Muscle Relaxants, Centrally Acting.*

**Action/Kinetics:** Does not directly relax skeletal muscles. Sedative effects may be responsible for muscle relaxation. **Onset:** 30 min. **Duration:** 4–6 hr. **Peak serum levels:** 4–7 mcg/mL. **t½:** 8 hr. Metabolized in the liver and excreted in the urine.

**Uses:** As an adjunct to rest, physical therapy, and other measures to treat skeletal muscle disorders including bursitis, low back disorders, contusions, fibrositis, spondylitis, sprains, muscle strains, and cerebral palsy.

**Contraindications:** Acute intermittent porphyria. Hypersensitivity to carisoprodol or meprobamate. Children under 12 years of age.

**Special Concerns:** Use with caution during lactation and in impaired liver or kidney function. May cause GI upset and sedation in infants.

**Side Effects:** *CNS:* Ataxia, dizziness, drowsiness, excitement, tremor, syncope, vertigo, insomnia, irritability, headache, depressive reactions. *GI:* N&V, gastric upset, hiccoughs. *CV:* Flushing of face, postural hypotension, tachycardia. *Allergic reactions:* Pruritus, skin rashes, erythema multiforme, eosinophilia, fever, dizziness, angioneurotic edema, asthmatic symptoms, "smarting" of the eyes, weakness, hypotension, **anaphylaxis**.

**OD** **Overdose Management:** *Symptoms:* Stupor, coma, shock, respiratory depression, and rarely death. *Treatment:* Supportive measures. Diuresis, osmotic diuresis, peritoneal dialysis, hemodialysis. Monitor urinary output to avoid overhydration. Observe client for possible relapse due to incomplete gastric emptying and delayed absorption.

**Drug Interactions**

*Alcohol* / Additive CNS depressant effects

*Antidepressants, tricyclic* / ↑ Effect of carisoprodol

*Barbiturates* / Possible ↑ effect of carisoprodol, followed by inhibition of carisoprodol

*Chlorcyclizine* / ↓ Effect of carisoprodol

*CNS depressants* / Additive CNS depression

*MAO inhibitors* / ↑ Effect of carisoprodol by ↓ breakdown by liver

*Phenobarbital* / ↓ Effect of carisoprodol by ↑ breakdown by liver

*Phenothiazines* / Additive depressant effects

**Dosage**

• **Tablets**

*Skeletal muscle disorders.*

**Adults:** 350 mg q.i.d. (take last dose at bedtime).

## NURSING CONSIDERATIONS

See also *Nursing Considerations* for *Skeletal Muscle Relaxants, Centrally Acting.*

**Assessment**

1. Note any hypersensitivity to meprobamate or carisoprodol.

2. Record extent of skeletal muscular

disorders noting baseline ROM, stiffness, and level of discomfort.
3. Review drugs currently prescribed to ensure no unfavorable interactions.
**Client/Family Teaching**
1. If unable to swallow tablets, mix drug with syrup, chocolate, or a jelly mixture.
2. Administer with food if gastric upset occurs.
3. Report side effects of ataxia, or tremors should they occur.
4. Establish a drug schedule so the last dose is taken at bedtime.
5. Due to the possibility of drug-induced dizziness, drowsiness, and palpitations, use caution when driving or undertaking tasks requiring mental alertness. Report if severe; may necessitate medication discontinuation.
6. Avoid all OTC agents and alcohol.
7. Psychologic dependence may occur.
**Outcomes/Evaluate:** Improvement in skeletal muscle pain and spasticity; ↑ ROM

# Carmustine
(kar-**MUS**-teen)
**Pregnancy Category:** D
BiCNU (Abbreviation: BCNU), Gliadel **(Rx)**
**Classification:** Antineoplastic, alkylating agent

See also *Antineoplastic Agents* and *Alkylating Agents*.
**Action/Kinetics:** Alkylates DNA and RNA, as well as inhibits several enzymes by carbamoylation of amino acids in proteins. It is cell-cycle nonspecific. Not cross-resistant with other alkylating agents. Rapidly cleared from plasma and metabolized. Crosses blood-brain barrier (concentration in CSF at least 50% greater than in plasma). **t½:** 15–30 min. Thirty percent excreted in urine after 24 hr, 60%–70% after 96 hr. Wafers are biodegradable in the brain when implanted into the cavity

after tumor resection. Released carmustine diffuses into the surrounding brain tissue.
**Uses:** *Injection:* Alone or in combination with other antineoplastic agents for palliative treatment of primary (e.g., brain stem glioma, astrocytoma, glioblastoma, ependymoma, medulloblastoma) and metastatic brain tumors, multiple myeloma (in combination with prednisone). Advanced Hodgkin's disease and non-Hodgkin's lymphomas (not the drug of choice) in those who relapse or who fail to respond to primary therapy. *Investigational:* GI cancer, malignant melanoma, mycosis fungoids. *Wafer:* Adjunct to surgery to prolong survival in recurrent glioblastoma multiforme when surgical resection is indicated.
**Special Concerns:** Not recommended for use during lactation. Delayed bone marrow toxicity may be observed. Safety and effectiveness have not been established in children.
**Additional Side Effects:** *GI:* N&V within 2 hr after administration, lasting 4–6 hr. *GU:* Renal failure, azotemia, decrease in kidney size. *Hepatic:* Reversible increases in alkaline phosphatase, bilirubin, and transaminase. *Other:* Rapid IV administration may produce transitory intense flushing of skin and conjunctiva (onset: after 2 hr; duration: 4 hr). ***Pulmonary fibrosis,*** ocular toxicity including retinal hemorrhage.
**Drug Interactions**
*Cimetidine* / Additive bone marrow suppression
*Digoxin* / ↓ Serum levels of digoxin → ↓ effect
*Mitomycin* / Corneal and conjunctival epithelial damage
*Phenytoin* / ↓ Serum levels of phenytoin → ↓ effect
**Dosage**
• **IV**
*In previously untreated clients.*
150–200 mg/m² q 6 weeks as a single dose. Alternate dosing schedule: 75–100 mg/m² on 2 successive days q

6 weeks. Subsequent dosage should be reduced if platelet levels are less than 100,000/mm³ and leukocyte levels are less than 4,000/mm³.

• **Wafer**

*Recurrent glioblastoma multiforme*

Eight wafers placed in the resection cavity if size and shape of the cavity allow. If this is not possible, see the maximum number of wafers allowed.

## NURSING CONSIDERATIONS

See also *Nursing Considerations* for *Antineoplastic Agents*.

**Administration/Storage**

1. Slight overlap of the wafer in the cavity is acceptable. A wafer broken in half may be used; discard wafers broken into more than two pieces.

2. To secure wafers against the cavity surface, oxidized regenerated cellulose may be placed over the wafers.

3. Irrigate resection cavity after wafer placement; dura should be closed in a watertight fashion.

4. Unopened foil pouches of wafers may be kept at ambient room temperature for a maximum of 6 hr. Store at or below −20°C (−4°F).

**IV** 5. Discard vials in which powder has become an oily liquid.

6. Reconstitute powder with absolute ethyl alcohol (provided); then add sterile water. For injection, these dilutions are stable for 24 hr when stored as noted in 13.

7. Stock solutions diluted to 500 mL with 0.9% NaCl for injection or with 5% dextrose for injection are stable for 48 hr when stored as noted in 13.

8. Administer IV over 1–2-hr period; faster injection may produce intense pain and burning at injection site.

9. Check for extravasation if client complains of burning or pain at injection site; discomfort may be from alcohol diluent. If there is no extravasation and burning at injection site experienced, reduce rate of flow.

10. Slow rate of infusion and report if client demonstrates intense flushing of skin and/or redness of conjunctiva.

11. Contact of reconstituted carmustine with skin may result in hyperpigmentation (transient). If contact occurs, wash the skin or mucosa thoroughly with soap and water.

12. *Do not use vial for multiple doses* because there is no preservative in vial.

13. Store unopened vials at 2°C–8°C (36°F–46°F) and protect from light. Store diluted solutions at 4°C (39°F) and protect from light.

**Assessment**

1. Obtain baseline liver and renal functions studies; obtain CBC and monitor up to 6 weeks after drug dose because delayed bone marrow toxicity may develop. Drug causes granulocyte and bone marrow suppression. Nadir: 21 days; recovery: 35–42 days.

2. Document baseline oral and ophthalmic exams and monitor.

**Client/Family Teaching**

1. Report any S&S of fever or infection; increased SOB, abnormal bruising or bleeding.

2. Avoid vaccinations during therapy.

3. Avoid smoking as this enhances pulmonary toxicity.

4. May experience hair loss.

5. Severe flushing after IV dose should subside in 2–4 hr; may also experience N&V 2 hr after infusion.

6. If mouth sores develop, advise provider so a special mouthwash or anesthetic can be prescribed.

**Outcomes/Evaluate**

• ↓ Size of metastatic process

• Platelet counts > 100,000/mm³ and leukocyte counts > 4,000/mm³

# Carteolol hydrochloride

(kar-**TEE**-oh-lohl)

**Pregnancy Category:** C

Cartrol, Ocupress **(Rx)**

**Classification:** Beta-adrenergic blocking agent

See also *Beta-Adrenergic Blocking Agents*.

**Action/Kinetics:** Has both beta-1 and beta-2 receptor blocking activity. It has no membrane-stabilizing activity but does have moderate intrinsic sympathomimetic effects. Low lipid solubility. **t½:** 6 hr. **Duration, ophthalmic use:** 12 hr. Approximately 50%–70% excreted unchanged in the urine.

**Uses: PO.** Hypertension. *Investigational:* Reduce frequency of anginal attacks. **Ophthalmic.** Chronic open-angle glaucoma and intraocular hypertension alone or in combination with other drugs.

**Contraindications:** Severe, persistent bradycardia. Bronchial asthma or bronchospasm, including severe COPD.

**Special Concerns:** Dosage has not been established in children.

**Additional Side Effects: Ophthalmic use.** Transient irritation, burning, tearing, conjunctival hyperemia, edema, blurred or cloudy vision, photophobia, decreased night vision, ptosis, blepharoconjunctivitis, abnormal corneal staining, corneal sensitivity.

**Dosage**
- **Tablets**
  *Hypertension.*
**Initial:** 2.5 mg once daily either alone or with a diuretic. If response is inadequate, the dose may be increased gradually to 5 mg and then 10 mg/day as a single dose. **Maintenance:** 2.5–5 mg once daily. Doses greater than 10 mg/day are not likely to increase the beneficial effect and may decrease the response. Increase the dosage interval in clients with renal impairment.
  *Reduce frequency of anginal attacks.*
10 mg/day.
- **Ophthalmic Solution**
**Usual:** 1 gtt in affected eye b.i.d. If the response is unsatisfactory, concomitant therapy may be initiated.

## NURSING CONSIDERATIONS

See also *Nursing Considerations* for *Beta-Adrenergic Blocking Agents* and *Antihypertensive Agents.*

**Assessment**
1. Document indications for therapy and note baseline findings.
2. Assess renal function; reduce dose with impairment.

**Client/Family Teaching**
1. Do not exceed prescribed dose; may alter desired response.
2. May cause increased sensitivity to cold; dress appropriately.
3. Report any symptoms of bleeding, infection, dizziness, confusion, depression, SOB, weight gain, or rash.
4. Reinforce diet, exercise, and weight reduction.
5. With ophthalmic solution, report any persistent burning, pain, or visual impairment.

**Outcomes/Evaluate**
- ↓ BP; ↓ anginal attacks
- ↓ Intraocular pressure

# Carvedilol
(kar-**VAY**-dih-lol)
**Pregnancy Category:** C
Coreg **(Rx)**
**Classification:** Alpha/beta-adrenergic blocking agent

See also *Adrenergic Blocking Agents.*
**Action/Kinetics:** Has both alpha- and beta-adrenergic blocking activity. Thus, the drug decreases cardiac output, reduces exercise- or isoproterenol-induced tachycardia, reduces reflex orthostatic hypotension, causes vasodilation, and reduces peripheral vascular resistance. Significant beta-blocking activity occurs within 60 min while alpha-blocking action is observed within 30 min. BP is lowered more in the standing than in the supine position. Significantly lowers plasma renin activity when given for at least 4 weeks. Rapidly absorbed after PO administration, but there is a significant first-pass effect. **Terminal t½:** 7–10 hr. Food delays the rate of absorption. Over 98% is bound to plasma protein. Plasma levels average 50% higher in geriatric compared with younger clients. Extensively metabolized in the liver,

with metabolites excreted primarily via the bile into the feces.

**Uses:** Essential hypertension used either alone or in combination with other antihypertensive drugs, especially thiazide diuretics. Used with digitalis, diuretics, and ACE inhibitors to reduce the progression of mild to moderate CHF of ischemic or cardiomyopathic origin. *Investigational:* Angina pectoris, idiopathic cardiomyopathy.

**Contraindications:** Clients with New York Heart Association Class IV decompensated cardiac failure, bronchial asthma, or related bronchospastic conditions, second- or third-degree AV block, sick sinus syndrome (unless a permanent pacemaker is in place), cardiogenic shock, severe bradycardia, drug hypersensitivity. Hepatic impairment. Lactation.

**Special Concerns:** Use with caution in hypertensive clients with CHF controlled with digitalis, diuretics, or an ACE inhibitor. Use with caution in peripheral vascular disease, in surgical procedures using anesthetic agents that depress myocardial function, in diabetics receiving insulin or oral hypoglycemic drugs, in those subject to spontaneous hypoglycemia, or in thyrotoxicosis. Clients with a history of severe anaphylactic reaction to a variety of allergens may be more reactive to repeated challenge while taking beta blockers. Safety and efficacy have not been established in children less than 18 years of age.

**Side Effects:** *CV:* Bradycardia, postural hypotension, dependent or peripheral edema, AV block, extrasystoles, hypertension, hypotension, palpitations, peripheral ischemia, syncope, angina, *cardiac failure,* myocardial ischemia, tachycardia, CV disorder. *CNS:* Dizziness, headache, somnolence, insomnia, ataxia, hypesthesia, paresthesia, vertigo, depression, nervousness, migraine, neuralgia, paresis, amnesia, confusion, sleep disorder, impaired concentration, abnormal thinking, paranoia, emotional lability. *Body as a whole:* Fatigue, viral infection, rash, allergy, asthenia, malaise, pain, injury, fever, infection, somnolence, sweating, *sudden death. GI:* Diarrhea, abdominal pain, bilirubinemia, N&V, flatulence, dry mouth, anorexia, dyspepsia, melena, periodontitis, increased hepatic enzymes, *GI hemorrhage. Respiratory:* Rhinitis, pharyngitis, sinusitis, bronchitis, dyspnea, *asthma, bronchospasm,* pulmonary edema, respiratory alkalosis, dyspnea, respiratory disorder, URTI, coughing. *GU:* UTI, albuminuria, hematuria, frequency of micturition, abnormal renal function, impotence. *Dermatologic:* Pruritus; erythematous, maculopapular, and psoriaform rashes, photosensitivity reaction, exfoliative dermatitis. *Metabolic:* Hypertriglyceridemia, hypercholesterolemia, hyperglycemia, hypovolemia, hyperuricemia, increased weight, gout, dehydration, hypervolemia, glycosuria, hyponatremia, hypokalemia, hyperkalemia, diabetes mellitus. *Hematologic:* Thrombocytopenia, anemia, leukopenia, pancytopenia, purpura, atypical lymphocytes. *Musculoskeletal:* Back pain, arthralgia, myalgia, arthritis, *Otic:* Decreased hearing, tinnitus. *Miscellaneous:* Hot flushes, leg cramps, abnormal vision, *anaphylactoid reaction.*

**OD** **Overdose Management:** *Symptoms:* Severe hypotension, bradycardia, cardiac insufficiency, *cardiogenic shock, cardiac arrest, generalized seizures,* respiratory problems, bronchospasms, vomiting, lapse of consciousness. *Treatment:* Place the client in a supine position and monitor carefully and treat under intensive care conditions. Treatment should continue for a long enough period of time consistent with the 7- to 10-hr half-life of the drug.

• Gastric lavage or induced emesis shortly after ingestion

• For excessive bradycardia, atropine, 2 mg IV. If the bradycardia is resistant to therapy, perform pacemaker therapy.

• To support cardiovascular function, give glucagon, 5–10 mg IV rap-

idly over 30 sec, followed by a continuous infusion of 5 mg/hr. Sympathomimetics (dobutamine, iso-proterenol, epinephrine) may be given.
• For peripheral vasodilation, give epinephrine or norepinephrine with continuous monitoring of circulatory conditions.
• For bronchospasm, give beta sympathomimetics as aerosol or IV or give aminophylline IV.
• In the event of seizures, give a slow IV injection of diazepam or clonazepam.

**Drug Interactions**

*Antidiabetic agents* / The beta-blocking effect may ↑ the hypoglycemic effect of insulin and oral hypoglycemics
*Calcium channel blocking agents* / ↑ Risk of conduction disturbances
*Clonidine* / Potentiation of BP and heart rate lowering effects
*Digoxin* / ↑ Digoxin levels
*Rifampin* / ↓ Plasma levels of carvedilol

**Laboratory Test Interferences:** ↑ ALT, AST, BUN, NPN, alkaline phosphatase. ↓ HDL.

**Dosage** —————————
• **Tablets**
    *Essential hypertension.*
**Initial:** 6.25 mg b.i.d. If this is tolerated, using standing systolic pressure measured about 1 hr after dosing, maintain the dose for 7–14 days. **Then,** increase to 12.5 mg b.i.d., if necessary, based on trough BP, using standing systolic pressure 2 hr after dosing. This dose should be maintained for 7–14 days and can then be adjusted upward to 25 mg b.i.d. if necessary and tolerated. The total daily dose should not exceed 50 mg.
    *Congestive heart failure.*
**Initial:** 3.125 mg b.i.d. for 2 weeks. If this is tolerated, increase to 6.25 mg b.i.d. Dosing is doubled every 2 weeks to the highest tolerated level, up to a maximum of 25 mg b.i.d. in those weighing less than 85 kg and 50 mg b.i.d. in those weighing over 85 kg.

*Angina pectoris.*
25–50 mg b.i.d.
    *Idiopathic cardiomyopathy.*
6.25–25 mg b.i.d.

## NURSING CONSIDERATIONS

See also *Nursing Considerations* for *Antihypertensive Agents* and *Adrenergic Blocking Agents*.
**Administration/Storage**
1. The full antihypertensive effect is seen within 7–14 days.
2. Take with food to slow absorption and decrease the incidence of orthostatic effects.
3. Addition of a diuretic can produce additive effects and exaggerate the orthostatic effect.
**Assessment**
1. Document indications for therapy, type and onset of symptoms, other agents trialed, and the outcome.
2. Note any history or evidence of bronchospastic conditions, asthma, advanced AV block, or severe bradycardia as drug is contraindicated.
3. Obtain baseline CBC and liver and renal function studies.
**Client/Family Teaching**
1. Take as prescribed and with food to decrease adverse side effects.
2. Avoid activities that require mental acuity until drug effects realized.
3. Do not stop abruptly due to beta-blocking activity (especially with ischemic heart disease); notify provider.
4. To prevent orthostatic hypotension, sit or lie until symptoms subside and rise slowly from a sitting or lying position. Concomitant therapy with a diuretic may aggravate the orthostatic drug effects.
5. Decreased lacrimation may be experienced by contact lens wearers.
6. Dosing adjustments will be made every 7–14 days based on standing SBP measured 1 hr after dosing. Keep appointments to evaluate drug response.
**Outcomes/Evaluate**
• Desired reduction of BP

• ↓ Progression of CHF

# Cefaclor

(**SEF**-ah-klor)
**Pregnancy Category:** B
Ceclor, Ceclor CD **(Rx)**
**Classification:** Cephalosporin, second-generation

See also *Anti-Infectives* and *Cephalosporins*.

**Action/Kinetics: Peak serum levels:** 5–15 mcg/mL after 1 hr. **t½: PO,** 36–54 min. Well absorbed from GI tract. From 60% to 85% excreted in urine within 8 hr.

**Uses:** Otitis media due to *Streptococcus pneumoniae, Hemophilus influenzae, Streptococcus pyogenes,* and staphylococci. Upper respiratory tract infections (including pharyngitis and tonsillitis) caused by *S. pyogenes.* Lower respiratory tract infections (including pneumonia) due to *S. pneumoniae, H. influenzae,* and *S. pyogenes.* Skin and skin structure infections due to *Staphylococcus aureus* and *S. pyogenes.* UTIs (including pyelonephritis and cystitis) caused by *Escherichia coli, Proteus mirabilis, Klebsiella,* and coagulase-negative staphylococci. *Extended-release tablets:* Acute bacterial exacerbations of chronic bronchitis due to non-β-lactamase-producing strains of *H. influenzae, Moraxella catarrhalis* (including β-lactamase-producing strains), or *S. pneumoniae.* Secondary bacterial infections of acute bronchitis due to *H. influenzae* (non-β-lactamase-producing strains only), *M. catarrhalis* (including β-lactamase-producing strains), or *S. pneumoniae.* Pharyngitis or tonsillitis due to *S. pyogenes.* Uncomplicated skin and skin structure infections due to *S. aureus* (methicillin-susceptible). *Investigational:* Acute uncomplicated UTIs in select populations using a single dose of 2 g.

**Special Concerns:** Safety for use in infants less than 1 month of age has not been established.

**Additional Side Effects:** Cholestatic jaundice, lymphocytosis.

**Dosage** ⎯⎯⎯⎯⎯⎯
• **Capsules, Oral Suspension**
*All uses.*
**Adults:** 250 mg q 8 hr. Dose may be doubled in more severe infections or those caused by less susceptible organisms. Total daily dose should not exceed 4 g. **Children:** 20 mg/kg/day in divided doses q 8 hr. Dose may be doubled in more serious infections, otitis media, or for infections caused by less susceptible organisms. For otitis media and pharyngitis, the total daily dose may be divided and given q 12 hr. Total daily dose should not exceed 1 g.

• **Tablets, Extended Release**
*Acute bacterial exacerbations, chronic bronchitis, secondary bacterial infections of acute bronchitis.*
500 mg q 12 hr for 7 days.
*Pharyngitis, tonsillits.*
375 mg q 12 hr for 10 days.
*Uncomplicated skin and skin structure infections.*
375 mg q 12 hr for 7–10 days.

## NURSING CONSIDERATIONS

See also *General Nursing Considerations for All Anti-Infectives* and *Cephalosporins.*

**Administration/Storage**
1. Refrigerate the suspension after reconstitution and discard after 2 weeks.
2. The total daily dose for otitis media and pharyngitis can be divided and given q 12 hr.

**Assessment**
1. Document type, onset, and duration of symptoms, and other agents trialed.
2. Note allergic reactions to penicillin; a cross-sensitivity reaction may occur.

**Client/Family Teaching**
1. Take entire prescription as directed; do not stop when feeling better.
2. Report any adverse response or lack of improvement after 48–72 hr.

**Outcomes/Evaluate:** Resolution of infection; symptomatic improvement

# Cefadroxil monohydrate

(sef-ah-**DROX**-ill)
**Pregnancy Category:** B
Duricef **(Rx)**
**Classification:** Cephalosporin, first-generation

See also *Anti-Infectives* and *Cephalosporins.*
**Action/Kinetics: Peak serum levels: PO,** 15–33 mcg/mL after 90 min. **t½: PO,** 70–80 min. Ninety percent of drug is excreted unchanged in urine within 24 hr.
**Uses:** UTIs caused by *Escherichia coli, Proteus mirabilis,* and *Klebsiella.* Skin and skin structure infections due to staphylococci or streptococci. Pharyngitis and tonsillitis due to group A beta-hemolytic streptococci.
**Special Concerns:** Safe use in children not established. Creatinine clearance determinations must be carried out in clients with renal impairment.

**Dosage**
• **Capsules, Oral Suspension, Tablets**
*Pharyngitis, tonsillitis.*
**Adults:** 1 g/day in single or two divided doses for 10 days. **Children:** 30 mg/kg/day in single or two divided doses (for beta-hemolytic streptococcoal infection, dose should be given for 10 days).
*Skin and skin structure infections.*
**Adults:** 1 g/day in single or two divided doses. **Children:** 30 mg/kg/day in divided doses q 12 hr.
*UTIs.*
**Adults:** 1–2 g/day in single or two divided doses for uncomplicated lower UTI (e.g., cystitis). For all other UTIs, the usual dose is 2 g/day in two divided doses. **Children:** 30 mg/kg/day in divided doses q 12 hr.
*For clients with creatinine clearance rates below 50 mL/min.*
**Initial:** 1 g; **maintenance,** 500 mg at following dosage intervals: q 36 hr for creatinine clearance rates of 0–10 mL/min; q 24 hr for creatinine clear-

ance rates of 10–25 mL/min; q 12 hr for creatinine clearance rates of 25–50 mL/min.

## NURSING CONSIDERATIONS

See also *General Nursing Considerations for All Anti-Infectives* and *Cephalosporins.*
**Administration/Storage**
1. Can be given without regard to meals.
2. Shake the suspension well before using.
3. For beta-hemolytic streptococcal infections, continue treatment for 10 days.
**Assessment**
1. Document indications for therapy, type and onset of symptoms, and pretreatment culture results.
2. Note any history of penicillin allergy.
**Client/Family Teaching**
1. Take prescription as directed.
2. Report adverse side effects or lack of response.
**Outcomes/Evaluate**
• Symptomatic improvement
• Negative culture reports

# Cefamandole nafate

(sef-ah-**MAN**-dole)
**Pregnancy Category:** B
Mandol **(Rx)**
**Classification:** Cephalosporin, second-generation

See also *Anti-Infectives* and *Cephalosporins.*
**Action/Kinetics:** Has a particularly broad spectrum of activity. **Peak serum levels: IM,** 12–36 mcg/mL after 30–120 min. **t½: IM,** 60 min; **IV,** 30 min. From 65% to 85% excreted unchanged in urine.
**Uses:** Infections of the urinary tract, lower respiratory tract, bones, joints, skin, and skin structures. Mixed infections of the respiratory tract, skin, and in pelvic inflammatory disease. Peritonitis, septicemia, prophylaxis in surgery. Also, with amino-

glycosides in gram-positive or gram-negative sepsis.

**Special Concerns:** Safety and effectiveness have not been determined in infants less than 1 month of age.

**Additional Side Effects:** Hypoprothrombinemia leading to bleeding and/or bruising; cholestatic jaundice, decreased creatinine clearance in clients with prior renal impairment.

**Additional Drug Interactions:** Concomitant use with ethanol produces a disulfiram-type reaction and hypotension.

**Dosage** ——————————
• **IV or Deep IM Injection Only**
In gluteus or lateral thigh to minimize pain.
*Infections.*
**Adults, usual:** 0.5–1 g q 4–8 hr. **Infants and children:** 50–100 mg/kg/day in equally divided doses q 4–8 hr.
*Severe infections.*
**Adults:** Up to 2 g q 4 hr. **Infants and children:** Up to 150 mg/kg/day (not to exceed adult dose) divided for infections as in the above.
*Preoperative.*
**Adults, initial:** 1–2 g 30–60 min prior to surgery; **then,** 1–2 g q 6 hr for 1–2 days (3 days for prosthetic arthroplasty). For cesarean section, give the first dose just prior to surgery or just after the cord has been clamped. **Pediatric (3 months and older):** 50–100 mg/kg/day in divided doses, using same schedule as for adults.
*Impaired renal function.*
**Initial:** 1–2 g; then a maintenance dosage is given, depending on creatinine clearance, according to schedule provided by manufacturer.

## NURSING CONSIDERATIONS

See also *General Nursing Considerations for All Anti-Infectives* and *Cephalosporins.*
**Administration/Storage**
**IV** 1. Review package insert for details on how to reconstitute drug.
2. Reconstituted solutions are stable for 24 hr at room temperature; 96 hr when stored in the refrigerator.

Cefamandole solutions reconstituted with dextrose or NaCl are stable for 6 mo when frozen immediately after reconstitution.
3. Carbon dioxide gas forms when reconstituted solutions are kept at room temperature. This gas does not affect the activity of the antibiotic and may be dissipated or used to aid in the withdrawal of the contents of the vial.
4. Follow manufacturer guidelines for dosage with impaired renal function.
5. Use separate IV fluid containers and separate injection sites for each drug when administered concomitantly with another antibiotic such as an aminoglycoside.
6. For direct IV administration, dilute 1 g in 10 mL of solution and administer over 3–5 min. May be further diluted and administered over 15–30 min.
7. Peripheral IV site *must* be changed every 2–3 days to prevent phlebitis.
**Client/Family Teaching**
1. Avoid alcohol and any OTC products containing alcohol as a disulfiram-type reaction may occur.
2. Immediately report any evidence of increased bruising or bleeding as well as any yellow discoloration of skin, eyes, or stool.
**Outcomes/Evaluate:** Resolution of infection

———————————————

# Cefazolin sodium
(sef-**AYZ**-oh-lin)
**Pregnancy Category:** B
Ancef, Kefzol, Zolicef **(Rx)**
**Classification:** Cephalosporin, first-generation

———————————————

See also *Anti-Infectives* and *Cephalosporins.*
**Action/Kinetics: Peak serum concentration: IM** 17–76 mcg/mL after 1 hr. **t½: IM, IV:** 90–130 min. From 80% to 100% excreted unchanged in urine.
**Uses:** Infections of the urinary tract, biliary tract, respiratory tract, bones, joints, soft tissue, and skin. Endo-

carditis, septicemia, prophylaxis in surgery.

**Special Concerns:** Safety in infants under 1 month of age has not been determined.

**Additional Side Effects:** When high doses are used in renal failure clients: extreme confusion, *tonic-clonic seizures,* mild hemiparesis.

**Dosage** _____

• **IM, IV Only**

*Mild infections due to gram-positive cocci.*

**Adults:** 250–500 mg q 8 hr.

*Mild to moderate infections.*

**Children over 1 month:** 25–50 mg/kg/day in three to four doses.

*Moderate to severe infections.*

**Adults:** 0.5–1 g q 6–8 hr.

*Acute, uncomplicated UTIs.*

**Adults:** 1 g q 12 hr. *For severe infections,* up to 100 mg/kg/day may be used.

*Endocarditis, septicemia.*

**Adults:** 1–1.5 g q 6 hr (rarely, up to 12 g/day).

*Pneumococcal pneumonia.*

**Adults:** 0.5 g q 12 hr.

*Preoperative.*

**Adults:** 1 g 30–60 min prior to surgery.

*During surgery.*

**Adults:** 0.5–1 g.

*Postoperative.*

**Adults:** 0.5–1 g q 6–8 hr for 24 hr (may be given up to 5 days, especially in open heart surgery or prosthetic arthroplasty).

*Impaired renal function.*

**Initial:** 0.5 g; **then,** maintenance doses are given, depending on creatinine clearance, according to schedule provided by manufacturer.

## NURSING CONSIDERATIONS

See also *General Nursing Considerations for All Anti-Infectives* and *Cephalosporins.*

### Administration/Storage

**IV** 1. Dissolve solute by shaking vial.

2. Follow manufacturer guidelines for dosage with renal dysfunction.

3. For direct IV administration, dilute dose in 10 mL of sterile water and infuse over 3–5 min. For intermittent use, further dilute 500 mg to 1 g in 50–100 mL NSS or D5%/W and administer over 30–60 min. Assess carefully for phlebitis.

4. Discard reconstituted solution after 24 hr at room temperature and after 96 hr when refrigerated.

**Assessment:** Document indications for therapy, type and onset of symptoms, and culture results.

**Outcomes/Evaluate**

• Resolution of infection
• Negative culture reports

# Cefepime hydrochloride

(SEF-eh-pim)

**Pregnancy Category:** B

Maxipime **(Rx)**

**Classification:** Cephalosporin

See also *Cephalosporins.*

**Action/Kinetics:** Antibacterial activity against both gram-negative and gram-positive pathogens, including those resistant to other β-lactam antibiotics. High affinity for the multiple penicillin-binding proteins that are essential for cell wall synthesis. **Peak serum levels, after IV:** 78 mcg/mL. **t½, terminal:** 2 hr. About 85% of the drug is excreted unchanged in the urine.

**Uses:** Uncomplicated and complicated UTIs (including pyelonephritis) caused by *Escherichia coli* or *Klebsiella pneumoniae;* when the infection is severe or caused by *E. coli, K. pneumoniae,* or *Proteus mirabilis;* when the infection is mild to moderate, including infections associated with concurrent bacteremia with these microorganisms. Uncomplicated skin and skin structure infections caused by *Staphylococcus aureus* (methicillin-susceptible strains only) or *Streptococcus pyogenes.* Moderate to severe pneumonia due to *Streptococcus pneumoniae,* including cases associated with concurrent bacteremia, *Pseudomonas aeruginosa, K. pneumoniae,* or *Enterobacter* species. Monotherapy for empiric treatment of febrile neutropenia.

**Contraindications:** Use in those who have had an immediate hypersensitivity reaction to cefepime, cephalosporins, pencillins, or any other β-lactam antibiotics.

**Special Concerns:** Use with caution during lactation. Safety and efficacy have not been determined in children less than 12 years of age.

**Side Effects:** See *Cephalosporins*. The most common side effects include rash, phlebitis, pain, and/or inflammation.

**Laboratory Test Alterations:** ↑ ALT, AST, alkaline phosphatase, BUN, creatinine, potassium, total bilirubin. ↓ Hematocrit, neutrophils, platelets, WBCs. ↑ or ↓ Calcium, phosphorus. Positive Coombs' test. Abnormal PTT, PT.

**Drug Interactions**
*Aminoglycosides* / ↑ Risk of nephrotoxicity and ototoxicity
*Furosemide* / ↑ Risk of nephrotoxicity

**Dosage**
- **IM, IV**

*Mild to moderate uncomplicated or complicated UTIs, including pyelonephritis, due to* E. coli, K. pneumoniae, *or* P. mirabilis.

**Adults and children over 12 years:** 0.5–1 g IV or IM (for *E. coli* infections) q 12 hr for 7–10 days.

*Severe uncomplicated or complicated UTIs, including pyelonephritis, due to* E. coli *or* K. pneumoniae.

**Adults and children over 12 years:** 2 g IV q 12 hr for 10 days.

*Moderate to severe pneumonia due to* S. pneumoniae, P. aeruginosa, K. pneumoniae, *or* Enterobacter *species.*

**Adults and children over 12 years:** 1–2 g IV q 12 hr for 10 days.

*Moderate to severe uncomplicated skin and skin structure infections due to* S. aureus *or* S. pyogenes.

**Adults and children over 12 years:** 2 g IV q 12 hr for 10 days.

*Febrile neutropenia.*

2 g IV q 8 hr for 7 days, or until resolution of neutropenia.

## NURSING CONSIDERATIONS

See also *Nursing Considerations* for *Cephalosporins*.

**Administration/Storage**

1. To reconstitute for IM use, dilute with 0.9% NaCl injection, 5% dextrose injection, 0.5% or 1% lidocaine HCl or bacteriostatic water for injection with parabens or benzyl alcohol.

**IV** 2. Adjust the dose (see package insert) for impaired renal function ($C_{CR}$ less than 60 mL/min).

3. To reconstitute for IV use, dilute with 50–100 mL of 0.9% NaCl injection, 5% and 10% dextrose injection, M/6 sodium lactate injection, 5% dextrose and 0.9% NaCl injection, RL and 5% dextrose injection, or Normosol-R or Normosol-M in 5% dextrose injection and administer over 30 min. Cefepime is compatible at concentrations of 1–40 mg/mL with the above solutions.

4. Solutions of cefepime should not be added to ampicillin at a concentration of 40 mg/mL and should not be added to aminophylline, gentamicin, metronidazole, netilmicin sulfate, tobramycin, or vancomycin. If necessary, each of these antibiotics can be given separately.

5. Protect the reconstituted drug from light and store at a room temperature of 20°C–25°C (68°F–77°F) for 24 hr or refrigerated at 2°C–8°C (36°F–46°F) for 7 days.

**Assessment**

1. Document indications for therapy, onset, location, duration, and characteristics of symptoms. List other agents prescribed and the outcome.

2. Note any previous sensitivity to penicillin, cephalosporins, or other antibiotics.

3. Obtain baseline CBC, liver and renal function studies, and cultures.

4. Anticipate reduced dosing with renal dysfunction.

5. List other agents prescribed; aminoglycosides and furosemide may increase the risk of nephrotoxicity or ototoxicity.

**Client/Family Teaching**
1. Must perform regular dosing to maintain therapeutic serum levels.
2. Drug may cause a positive Coombs' test.
3. Pain and inflammation may occur at infusion site; may experience a rash.
4. Report any prolonged or persistent diarrhea; an overgrowth of colon flora may have occurred and requires additional therapy.

**Outcomes/Evaluate:** Symptomatic improvement with resolution of infective organism

---

## Cefixime oral

(seh-**FIX**-eem)
**Pregnancy Category:** B
Suprax **(Rx)**
**Classification:** Cephalosporin, third-generation

See also *Anti-Infectives* and *Cephalosporins*.

**Action/Kinetics:** Stable in the presence of beta-lactamase enzymes. **Peak serum levels:** 2–6 hr. **t½:** averages 3–4 hr. About 50% excreted unchanged in the urine and approximately 10% in the bile.

**Uses:** Uncomplicated UTIs caused by *E. coli* and *P. mirabilis.* Otitis media due to *H. influenzae* (beta-lactamase positive and negative strains), *Moraxella catarrhalis,* and *S. pyogenes.* Pharyngitis and tonsillitis caused by *S. pyogenes.* Acute bronchitis and acute exacerbations of chronic bronchitis caused by *S. pneumoniae* and *H. influenzae* (beta-lactamase positive and negative strains). Uncomplicated cervical or urethral gonorrhea due to *N. gonorrhoeae* (both penicillinase- and non-penicillinase-producing strains).

**Special Concerns:** Safe use in infants less than 6 months old has not been established.

**Additional Side Effects:** *GI:* Flatulence. *Hepatic:* Elevated alkaline phosphatase levels. *Renal:* Transient increases in BUN or creatinine.

**Additional Laboratory Test Interference:** False + test for ketones using nitroprusside test.

**Dosage**
• **Oral Suspension, Tablets**
**Adults:** Either 400 mg once daily or 200 mg q 12 hr. **Children:** Either 8 mg/kg once daily or 4 mg/kg q 12 hr. Clients on renal dialysis or in whom $C_{CR}$ is 21–60 mL/min, the dose should be 75% of the standard dose (i.e., 300 mg/day). If the $C_{CR}$ is less than 20 mL/min, the dose should be 50% of the standard dose (i.e., 200 mg/day).
  *Uncomplicated gonorrhea.* One 400-mg tablet.

## NURSING CONSIDERATIONS

See also *Nursing Considerations* for *Cephalosporins.*

**Administration/Storage**
1. Continue therapy for at least 10 days when treating *S. pyogenes.*
2. Give the adult dose to children older than 12 years or weighing more than 50 kg.
3. Treat otitis media using the suspension as higher blood levels are achieved compared with the tablet given at the same dose.
4. Once reconstituted, keep the suspension at room temperature where it maintains potency for 14 days.

**Assessment**
1. Note any prior sensitivity to cephalosporins or penicillins.
2. Anticipate reduced dose with impaired renal function.
3. Use suspension in children and when treating otitis media.

**Client/Family Teaching**
1. May cause GI upset; report any bothersome side effects, especially persistent diarrhea.
2. Once-a-day dosing should be taken at the same time each day; prescription cost may be prohibitive.
3. May alter results of urine glucose and ketone testing; do finger sticks for more accurate results.
4. Consult provider if child's condition

C

does not improve or deteriorates after 48–72 hr.

5. Return as scheduled to assess response to therapy.

**Outcomes/Evaluate:** Resolution of infection; symptomatic improvement

# Cefoperazone sodium
(sef-oh-**PER**-ah-zohn)
**Pregnancy Category:** B
Cefobid **(Rx)**
**Classification:** Cephalosporin, third-generation

See also *Anti-Infectives* and *Cephalosporins.*

**Action/Kinetics: Peak serum levels:** 73–153 mcg/mL. **t½:** 102–156 min. Approximately 30% excreted unchanged in the urine.

**Uses:** Infections of skin, skin structures, urinary tract, and respiratory tract. Intra-abdominal infections including peritonitis. Bacterial septicemia, pelvic inflammatory disease, endometritis, other infections of the female genital tract.

**Special Concerns:** Use with caution in hepatic disease or biliary obstruction. Safety and effectiveness have not been determined in children.

**Additional Side Effects:** Hypoprothrombinemia resulting in bleeding and/or bruising.

**Additional Drug Interactions:** Concomitant use with ethanol may cause an Antabuse-like reaction.

## Dosage
• **IM, IV**
**Adults, usual:** 2–4 g/day in divided doses q 12 hr (up to 12–16 g/day has been used in severe infections or for less sensitive organisms).

*NOTE:* This drug is significantly excreted in the bile; thus, the daily dose should not exceed 4 g in hepatic disease or biliary obstruction.

## NURSING CONSIDERATIONS

See also *Nursing Considerations* for *Cephalosporins.*

**Administration/Storage**
**IV** 1. Dilute each gram in 20–40 mL of solution and infuse over 15–30 min.

2. Following reconstitution, allow the solution to stand for dissipation of any foaming and to determine if complete solubilization has occurred. Vigorous shaking may be necessary to dissolve higher concentrations.

3. Reconstituted drug may be frozen; however, after thawing, discard any unused portion.

4. Protect the unreconstituted powder from light and store in refrigerator.

5. If used for neonates, do not reconstitute cefoperazone with diluents containing benzyl alcohol.

**Assessment**
1. Note any penicillin sensitivity. Assess for bruising, hematuria, black stools, or other evidence of bleeding.

2. Obtain baseline coagulation studies and monitor; drug may cause hypoprothrombinemia. Assess need for prophylactic vitamin K administration (usually 10 mg/week).

3. With skin lesions, inspect lesions closely, noting size, location, and extent of involvement.

4. Assess for excessive alcohol use. Reduce dose with liver or biliary tract disease.

**Client/Family Teaching**
1. Avoid alcohol and any alcohol-containing products during and for 72 hr after last dose; an Antabuse-like reaction may occur.

2. Report any unusual bruising or bleeding.

**Outcomes/Evaluate**
• ↓ Size and number of skin lesions; wound healing
• Resolution of infection

# Cefotaxime sodium
(sef-oh-**TAX**-eem)
**Pregnancy Category:** B
Claforan **(Rx)**
**Classification:** Cephalosporin, third-generation

See also *Anti-Infectives* and *Cephalosporins*.
**Action/Kinetics: t½:** 1 hr. From 20% to 36% is excreted unchanged in the urine.
**Uses:** Infections of the GU tract, lower respiratory tract (including pneumonia), skin, skin structures, bones, joints, and CNS (including ventriculitis and meningitis). Intra-abdominal infections (including peritonitis), gynecologic infections (including endometritis, pelvic cellulitis, pelvic inflammatory disease), septicemia, bacteremia, and prophylaxis in surgery. Used with aminoglycosides for gram-positive or gram-negative sepsis where the causative agent has not been identified.

The IV route is preferable for clients with severe or life-threatening infections; for clients after surgery; or for those manifesting malnutrition, trauma, malignancy, heart failure, or diabetes, especially if shock is present or possible.

**Dosage**
• **IV, IM**
  *Uncomplicated infections.*
**Adults:** 1 g q 12 hr.
  *Moderate to severe infections.*
**Adults:** 1–2 g q 8 hr.
  *Septicemia.*
**Adults, IV:** 2 g q 6–8 hr.
  *Life-threatening infections.*
**Adults, IV:** 2 g q 4 hr up to 12 g/day.
  *Gonorrhea.*
**Adults, IM:** Single dose of 1 g.
  *Preoperative prophylaxis.*
**Adults:** 1 g 30–90 min prior to surgery.
  *Cesarean section.*
**IV:** 1 g when the umbilical cord is clamped; **then,** give 1 g 6 and 12 hr after the first dose.
**Pediatric, 1 month to 12 years, IM, IV:** 50–180 mg/kg/day in four to six divided doses; **1–4 weeks, IV:** 50 mg/kg q 8 hr; **0–1 week, IV:** 50 mg/kg q 12 hr. *NOTE:* Use adult dose in children 50 kg or over.

## NURSING CONSIDERATIONS

See also *Nursing Considerations* for *Cephalosporins*.
**Administration/Storage**
1. Continue treatment for a minimum of 10 days for group A beta-hemolytic streptococcal infections to minimize the risk of glomerulonephritis or rheumatic fever.
2. For IM use, reconstitute with sterile water for injection or bacteriostatic water for injection. Inject deeply into large muscle. Divide doses of 2 g and administer into different sites.
**IV** 3. Discontinue IV administration of other solutions during administration of cefotaxime. Do not mix cefotaxime with aminoglycosides for continuous IV infusion; each should be given separately.
4. Cefotaxime is maximally stable at a pH of 5–7; solutions should not be prepared with diluents having a pH greater than 7.5 (e.g., sodium bicarbonate injection).
5. Add recommended amount of diluent, shake to dissolve, and observe for particles or discoloration of solution. Do not administer if particles are present or if solution is discolored. The normal color of solution ranges from light yellow to amber.
6. For direct IV administration, mix 1 or 2 g cefotaxime with 10 mL sterile water for injection and administer over 3–5 min. For intermittent administration, further dilute in 50–100 mL of solution and infuse over 30 min.
7. After reconstitution, the drug remains stable for 24 hr at room temperature, 5 days refrigerated, and 13 weeks frozen. Thaw frozen samples at room temperature before use. Do not refreeze unused portions.
8. Store dry cefotaxime below 30°C (86°F) and protect from excess heat and light to prevent darkening.
**Assessment**
1. With joint infections, assess extent of ROM and freedom of movement.
2. With gynecologic infections,

determine extent of infection and duration of symptoms.

3. Monitor lab studies and review culture results to determine any organism resistance; reduce dose with renal dysfunction.

**Client/Family Teaching**

1. Review drugs prescribed, their side effects, and the expected outcome of therapy.

2. Complete course of therapy as prescribed despite feeling better.

3. Review appropriate technique and frequency for administration and proper storage. Inspect injection site for pain and redness; IM administration may cause thrombophlebitis.

4. Record I&O; report any reduction in urinary output as well as any persistent diarrhea.

5. Avoid alcohol in any form; a disulfiram-type reaction may occur.

**Outcomes/Evaluate**

• Resolution of infection; symptomatic improvement

• Negative culture reports

# Cefotetan disodium

(sef-oh-**TEE**-tan)
**Pregnancy Category:** B
Cefotan **(Rx)**
**Classification:** Cephalosporin, second-generation

See also *Anti-Infectives* and *Cephalosporins*.

**Action/Kinetics:** Administered parenterally only. t½: 3–4.6 hr. From 50% to 80% is excreted unchanged in the urine.

**Uses:** Infections of the urinary tract, lower respiratory tract, skin and skin structures, bones, and joints. Also gynecologic and intra-abdominal infections. Prophylaxis of postoperative infections (e.g., due to abdominal or vaginal hysterectomy, transurethral surgery, GI or biliary tract surgery, cesarean section).

The IV route is preferred for clients with bacterial septicemia, bacteremia, or other severe or life-threatening infections. The IV route is also preferred for poor-risk clients as the

result of malnutrition, surgery, diabetes, trauma, heart failure, malignancy, or if shock is present or impending.

**Special Concerns:** Safety and effectiveness have not been determined in children.

**Additional Side Effects:** Concomitant use with ethanol produces a disulfiram-type reaction and hypotension.

**Additional Laboratory Test Interference:** May affect measurement of creatinine levels by the Jaffe reaction.

**Dosage** ─────────────

• **IV or IM**

*Usual infections.*

**Adults:** 1–2 g q 12 hr for 5–10 days.

*UTIs.*

**Adults:** Either 0.5 g q 12 hr, or 1–2 g q 12–24 hr.

*Severe infections.*

**Adults, IV:** 2 g q 12 hr.

*Life-threatening infections.*

**Adults, IV:** 3 g q 12 hr.

*Prophylaxis of postoperative infection.*

**Adults, IV:** 1–2 g 30–60 min prior to surgery.

## NURSING CONSIDERATIONS

See also *Nursing Considerations* for *Cephalosporins*.

**Administration/Storage**

1. Must be administered parenterally; not absorbed from the GI tract.

2. For IM use, reconstitute with sterile water for injection, NSS, bacteriostatic water for injection, or 0.5%–1% lidocaine HCl.

3. Give IM injections well within a large muscle (e.g., the gluteus maximus).

**IV** 4. Direct IV administration may be completed over 3–5 min following reconstitution (1 g in 10 mL of sterile water for injection). May further dilute in 50–100 mL D5%/W or NSS and infuse over 30–60 min.

5. Reconstituted solutions maintain potency for 24 hr at room temperature, for 96 hr if refrigerated, and for 1 week if frozen.

6. Do not mix cefotetan with solutions containing aminoglycosides.

**Assessment**
1. Note any penicillin sensitivity or excessive alcohol use.
2. Monitor renal function and coagulation studies as drug may cause hypoprothrombinemia; assess for bruising, hematuria, black stools, or other evidence of bleeding.
3. Evaluate need for prophylactic vitamin K administration (usually 10 mg/week).
4. Expect reduced dose with impaired renal function; depending on $C_{CR}$.

**Client/Family Teaching**
1. Avoid alcohol ingestion during and for 72 hr after therapy; an Antabuse-like reaction may occur.
2. Report any unusual diarrhea, bruising/bleeding, or decreased urine output.

**Outcomes/Evaluate**
• Resolution of infection with symptomatic improvement
• Surgical infection prophylaxis

---

# Cefoxitin sodium

(seh-**FOX**-ih-tin)
**Pregnancy Category:** B
Mefoxin **(Rx)**
**Classification:** Cephalosporin, second-generation

---

See also *Anti-Infectives* and *Cephalosporins*.
**Action/Kinetics:** Broad-spectrum cephalosporin that is penicillinase- and cephalosporinase-resistant and is stable in the presence of beta-lactamases. **Peak serum concentration:** IM, 20–30 min. t½: IM, IV, 41–65 min; 85% of drug excreted unchanged in urine after 6 hr.
**Uses:** Infections of the urinary tract (including gonorrhea), bones, joints, lower respiratory tract (including lung abscesses and pneumonia), skin, and skin structures. Intra-abdominal infections (including intra-abdominal abscesses and peritonitis), gynecologic infections (including pelvic inflammatory disease, pelvic cellulitis, and endometritis),

septicemia, and prophylaxis in surgery. Oral bacterial *Eikenella corrodens* infections. *NOTE:* Many gram-negative infections resistant to certain cephalosporins and penicillins respond to cefoxitin.
**Additional Side Effects:** Higher doses have caused increased incidence of eosinophilia and increased AST levels in children over 3 months of age.
**Additional Laboratory Test Interference:** High concentrations may interfere with the measurement of creatinine by the Jaffe method.

**Dosage** ⎯⎯⎯⎯⎯⎯⎯⎯
• **IM, IV**
*Uncomplicated infections (cutaneous, pneumonia, urinary tract).*
**Adults, IV, IM:** 1 g q 6–8 hr.
*Severe infections.*
**Adults, IV:** 1 g q 4 hr or 2 g q 6–8 hr.
*Gas gangrene.*
**Adults, IV:** 2 g q 4 hr or 3 g q 6 hr.
*Gonorrhea.*
**Adults:** 2 g IM with 1 g probenecid PO.
*Prophylaxis in surgery.*
**Adults, IV, IM:** 2 g 30–60 min before surgery followed by 2 g q 6 hr after first dose for 24 hr only (72 hr for prosthetic arthroplasty).
*Cesarean section, prophylaxis.*
2 g **IV** when cord is clamped; **then,** give two additional doses IV or IM 4 and 8 hr later. Subsequent doses may be given q 6 hr for no more than 1 day.
*Transurethral prostatectomy, prophylaxis.*
1 g before surgery; **then,** 1 g q 8 hr for up to 5 days.
*Impaired renal function.*
**Initial:** 1–2 g; **then,** follow maintenance schedule provided by manufacturer.
*Infections.*
**Children over 3 months:** 80–160 mg/kg/day in four to six divided doses. Total daily dosage should not exceed 12 g.
*Prophylaxis.*
**Children:** 30–40 mg/kg q 6 hr.

---

## NURSING CONSIDERATIONS

See also *Nursing Considerations* for *Cephalosporins*.

**Administration/Storage**

1. For IM injections, lidocaine hydrochloride 0.05% (without epinephrine) may be prescribed as a diluent, to reduce pain at injection site.

**IV** 2. For direct IV administration dilute 1 g in 10 mL sterile water and infuse over 3–5 min. For intermittent administration, further dilute in 50–100 mL of solution and infuse over 15–30 min.

3. Do not administer cefoxitin rapidly, as it is irritating to veins. Do not mix with other antibiotics.

4. Reconstituted solutions are white to light amber; color does not affect potency. Consult pharmacist if unsure.

5. Reconstituted solutions are stable for 24 hr at room temperature, 1 week in the refrigerator, and 26 weeks when frozen.

6. Store drug vials below 30°C (86°F).

**Interventions**

1. Monitor I&O, withhold medication, and report any significant reduction in urinary output.

2. Assess infusion site for pain and redness; may cause thrombophlebitis.

**Outcomes/Evaluate**

• Resolution of infection
• Surgical infection prophylaxis

# Cefpodoxime proxetil
(sef-poh-**DOX**-eem)
**Pregnancy Category:** B
Vantin **(Rx)**
**Classification:** Cephalosporin, second-generation

See also *Anti-Infectives* and *Cephalosporins*.

**Action/Kinetics:** From 29% to 33% is excreted unchanged in the urine.

**Uses:** Acute, community-acquired pneumonia due to *Streptococcus pneumoniae* or *Hemophilus influenzae* (only non-β-lactamase-producing strains). Acute bacterial exacerba-

tion of chronic bronchitis caused by *S. pneumoniae*, non-beta-lactamase-producing *H. influenzae*, or *M. catarrhalis*. Acute otitis media caused by *S. pneumoniae, H. influenzae* (including beta-lactamase-producing strains), and *Moraxella catarrhalis*. Pharyngitis or tonsillitis due to *Streptococcus pyogenes*. Acute, uncomplicated urethral and cervical gonorrhea caused by *Neisseria gonorrhoeae* (including penicillinase-producing strains). Acute, uncomplicated anorectal infections in women due to *N. gonorrhoeae* (including penicillinase-producing strains). Uncomplicated skin and skin structure infections due to *Staphylococcus aureus* (including penicillinase-producing strains) or *S. pyogenes*. Uncomplicated UTIs (cystitis) due to *Escherichia coli, Klebsiella pneumoniae, Proteus mirabilis,* or *Staphyloccus saprophyticus*.

**Dosage**

• **Tablets, Suspension**
*Acute community-acquired pneumonia.*
**Adults and children over 13 years:** 200 mg q 12 hr for 14 days.
*Acute bacterial exacerbations of chronic bronchitis.*
**Adults and children over 13 years:** 200 mg q 12 hr for 10 days.
*Uncomplicated gonorrhea (men and women) and rectal gonococcal infections (women).*
**Adults and children over 13 years:** Single dose of 200 mg.
*Skin and skin structure infections.*
**Adults and children over 13 years:** 400 mg q 12 hr for 7–14 days.
*Pharyngitis, tonsillitis.*
**Adults and children over 13 years:** 100 mg q 12 hr for 5–10 days.
**Children, 6 months–12 years:** 5 mg/kg (maximum of 100 mg/dose) q 12 hr (maximum daily dose: 200 mg) for 5–10 days.
*Uncomplicated UTIs.*
**Adults and children over 13 years:** 100 mg q 12 hr for 7 days.
*Acute otitis media.*
**Children, 6 months–12 years:** 5 mg/kg (maximum of 200 mg/dose) q

12 hr or 10 mg/kg q 24 hr for 10 days. The maximum daily dose should not exceed 400 mg.

## NURSING CONSIDERATIONS

See also *General Nursing Considerations for All Anti-Infectives* and *Cephalosporins*.

### Administration/Storage

1. In severe renal impairment ($C_{CR} <$ 30 mL/min), increase the dosing interval to q 24 hr. If on hemodialysis, use a dosage frequency of 3 times/week after hemodialysis. Dosage adjustment is not required with cirrhosis.

2. May use the following formula to estimate $C_{CR}$ (mL/min): males: weight (kg) × (140 − age)/72 × serum creatinine (mg/100 mL); females: 0.85 × male value.

3. Prepare suspension by adding a total of 58 mL of distilled water to the 50 mg/mL product or 57 mL of distilled water to the 100 mg/5 mL product. Tap the bottle gently to loosen the powder, then add 25 mL of water and shake vigorously for 15 sec to wet the powder. Add the remainder of the water and shake the bottle vigorously for 3 min or until all particles are suspended. Shake the reconstituted suspension well before using.

4. After reconstitution, store suspension in the refrigerator; any unused portion should be discarded after 14 days.

### Assessment

1. Note any reactions to cephalosporins or penicillins as cross-sensitivity can occur.

2. Document source of infection; obtain baseline cultures.

3. Note any renal dysfunction; alter dosage if evident.

4. Obtain serologic test for syphilis with gonorrhea treatment.

5. Monitor VS and I&O; persistent diarrhea should be evaluated for other causes, such as *C. difficile*.

6. Discontinue therapy and report if seizures occur.

### Client/Family Teaching

1. Take with food to enhance absorption and to diminish GI upset.

2. Report any persistent N&V or diarrhea as drug or dosage may require adjustment.

3. If receiving treatment for gonorrhea, have partner tested and treated and use barrier contraception to prevent reinfections. Drug is not effective against syphilis; all partners should be tested so that appropriate treatment may be provided.

### Outcomes/Evaluate

• Resolution of infection
• Symptomatic improvement

# Cefprozil

(**SEF**-proh-zill)

**Pregnancy Category:** B

Cefzil **(Rx)**

**Classification:** Cephalosporin, second-generation

See also *Anti-Infectives* and *Cephalosporins*.

**Action/Kinetics:** Sixty percent is recovered in the urine unchanged.

**Uses:** Pharyngitis and tonsillitis due to *Streptococcus pyogenes*. Acute bacterial sinusitis due to *Streptococcus pneumoniae, Staphylococcus aureus, Haemophilus influenzae,* and *Morazella catarrhalis*. Otitis media caused by *S. pneumoniae, H. influenzae,* and *M. catarrhalis*. Uncomplicated skin and skin structure infections due to *S. aureus* (including penicillinase-producing strains) and *S. pyogenes*. Secondary bacterial infection of acute bronchitis and acute bacterial exacerbation of chronic bronchitis due to *S. pneumoniae, H. influenzae* (beta-lactamase positive and negative strains), and M. catarrhalis.

## Dosage

• **Suspension, Tablets**
  *Pharyngitis, tonsillitis, acute sinusitis.*

**Adults and children over 13 years of age:** 500 mg q 24 hr for at least 10 days (especially for *S. pyogenes* infections). **Children, 2–12 years of age:** 7.5 mg/kg q 12 hr for at least 10 days (especially for *S. pyogenes* infections).

*Secondary bacterial infections of acute bronchitis and acute bacterial exacerbation of chronic bronchitis.*
**Adults and children over 13 years of age:** 500 mg q 12 hr for 10 days.

*Uncomplicated skin and skin structure infections.*
**Adults and children over 13 years of age:** Either 250 mg q 12 hr, 500 mg q 24 hr, or 500 mg q 12 hr (all for a duration of 10 days).

*Otitis media.*
**Infants and children 6 months–12 years:** 15 mg/kg q 12 hr for 10 days.

## NURSING CONSIDERATIONS

See also *General Nursing Considerations for All Anti-Infectives* and *Cephalosporins*.
**Administration/Storage**
1. With impaired renal function ($C_{CR}$ of 0–30 mL/min), give 50% of the usual dose at standard intervals.
2. After reconstitution, refrigerate suspension; discard any unused portion after 14 days.
**Assessment:** Reduce dose with impaired renal function; monitor I&O and VS.
**Outcomes/Evaluate**
• Symptomatic improvement
• Resolution of infection

# Ceftazidime

(sef-**TAY**-zih-deem)
**Pregnancy Category:** B
Ceptaz ✿, Fortaz, Tazicef, Tazidime **(Rx)**
**Classification:** Cephalosporin, third-generation

See also *Anti-Infectives* and *Cephalosporins*.
**Action/Kinetics:** Only for IM or IV use. **t½:** 2–3 hr. From 80% to 90% is excreted unchanged in the urine.
**Uses:** Bacterial septicemia. Infections of the lower respiratory tract, skin and skin structures, bones and joints, CNS (including meningitis), and urinary tract. Also, intra-abdominal (including peritonitis) and gynecologic infections (including endometritis, pelvic cellulitis). Use with aminoglycosides, clindamycin, or vancomycin in severe or life-threatening infections or in the immuno-compromised client.
**Special Concerns:** A sodium carbonate formulation should be used if the drug is indicated for children less than 12 years of age.

## Dosage

• **IM, IV**
*Usual infections.*
**Adults:** 1 g q 8–12 hr.
*UTIs, uncomplicated.*
**Adults, IM, IV:** 0.25 g q 12 hr.
*UTIs, complicated.*
**Adults, IM, IV:** 0.5 g q 8–12 hr.
*Uncomplicated pneumonia, skin and skin structure infections.*
**Adults, IM, IV:** 0.5–1 g q 8 hr.
*Bone and joint infections.*
**Adults, IV:** 2 g q 12 hr.
*Serious gynecologic or intra-abdominal infections, meningitis, severe or life-threatening infections (especially in immunocompromised clients).*
**Adults, IV:** 2 g q 8 hr.
*Pseudomonal lung infections in cystic fibrosis clients.*
**IV:** 30–50 mg/kg q 8 hr, not to exceed 6 g/day. **Neonates, 0–4 weeks, IV:** 30 mg/kg q 12 hr. **Infants and children, 1 month–12 years, IV:** 30–50 mg/kg q 8 hr not to exceed 6 g/day.

## NURSING CONSIDERATIONS

See also *General Nursing Considerations for All Anti-Infectives* and *Cephalosporins*.
**Administration/Storage**
1. Ceftazidime must be administered parenterally, because it is not absorbed from the GI tract.
2. For IM administration, reconstitute in sterile water for injection, bacteriostatic water for injection, or 0.5%–1% lidocaine HCl injection.
3. If administering IM, use large muscle mass and inject deeply.
**IV** 4. The IV route is preferred for clients with bacterial septicemia,

peritonitis, bacterial meningitis, or other severe or life-threatening infections. Also, IV should be used for clients considered to be poor risks due to malnutrition, surgery, diabetes, trauma, heart failure, malignancy, or if shock is present or imminent.

5. For direct IV administration, reconstitute 1 g in 10 mL sterile water for injection and administer over 3–5 min.

6. For intermittent administration, further dilute in 50–100 mL of solution and administer over 30–60 min. It is compatible with 0.9% NaCl injection, Ringer's injection, RL injection, 5% or 10% dextrose injection, M/6 sodium lactate injection, 5% dextrose and 0.225%, 0.45%, or 0.9% NaCl injection, 10% invert sugar in water for injection. Sodium bicarbonate injection should not be used for reconstitution; however, a sodium carbonate formulation should be used for children less than 12.

7. For use as an IV infusion, the 1- or 2-g infusion pack is reconstituted with 100 mL sterile water for injection (or a compatible IV solution).

8. Do not add ceftazidime to solutions containing aminoglycosides.

**Assessment**

1. Note any penicillin allergy.

2. Obtain renal function studies; reduce dose with impaired function (see package insert).

**Outcomes/Evaluate**

• Resolution of infection
• Negative culture reports

# Ceftibuten
(sef-**TYE**-byou-ten)
**Pregnancy Category:** B
Cedax **(Rx)**
**Classification:** Cephalosporin

See also *Cephalosporins,*

**Action/Kinetics:** Resistant to beta-lactamase. Has the broadest gram-negative spectrum of any of the current PO cephalosporins. Is well absorbed from the GI tract. Food delays the time to peak serum concentration, lowers the peak cencentration, and decreases the total amount of drug absorbed. **Peak serum levels:** 2 to 3 hours. **t½:** 2 hr. Excreted in the urine.

**Uses:** Acute bacterial exacerbations of chronic bronchitis due to *Haemophilus influenzae* (including beta-lactamase-producing strains), *Moraxella catarrhalis* (including beta-lactamase-producing strains), and penicillin-susceptible strains of *Streptococcus pneumoniae.* Acute bacterial otitis media due to *H. influenzae, M. catarrhalis,* and *Staphylococcus pyogenes.* Pharyngitis and tonsillitis due to S. pyogenes.

**Special Concerns:** Although ceftibuten has been approved for pharyngitis or tonsillitis, only penicillin has been shown to be effective in preventing rheumatic fever. Not approved to treat urinary infections.

**Side Effects:** See *Cephalosporins.* Ceftibuten is usually well tolerated. The most common side effect is diarrhea.

**Dosage**

• **Capsules, Oral Suspension**
*All uses.*

**Adults and children over 12 years of age**: 400 mg once daily for 10 days. The maximum daily dose is 400 mg. Adjust the dose in clients with a creatinine clearance ($C_{cr}$) less than 50 mL/min as follows. If the $C_{cr}$ is between 30 and 49 mL/min, the recommended dose is 4.5 mg/kg or 200 mg once daily. If the $C_{cr}$ is between 5 and 29 mL/min, the recommended dose is 2.25 mg/kg or 100 mg once daily. In clients undergoing hemodialysis 2 or 3 times/week, a single 400-mg dose of ceftibuten capsules or a single dose of 9 mg/kg (maximum of 400 mg) of PO suspension can be given at the end of each hemodialysis session.

*Children: pharyngitis, tonsillitis, acute bacterial otitis media.*
9 mg/kg, up to a maximum of 400 mg daily, for a total of 10 days. Give children over 45 kg the maximum daily dose of 400 mg.

## NURSING CONSIDERATIONS

See also *Nursing Considerations* for *Cephalosporins*.

### Administration/Storage

1. The pediatric suspension is available as either 90 mg/5 mL or 180 mg/5 mL.

2. Follow the directions for mixing ceftibuten suspension carefully, depending on the final concentration and the bottle size. First, tap bottle to loosen the powder; then add the appropriate amount of water in two portions, shaking well after each portion.

3. After mixing, the suspension may be kept for 14 days under refrigeration. Keep the container tightly closed and shake well before each use. Discard any unused drug after 14 days.

### Assessment

1. Document type, onset, duration, and characteristics of symptoms.

2. Obtain cultures and renal function studies; reduce dose with impaired function.

3. Review conditions requiring treatment as drug is only approved for chronic bronchitis, bacterial otitis media, and pharyngitis or tonsillitis, with limitations based on the infective organisms.

### Client/Family Teaching

1. Suspension must be consumed on an empty stomach, at least 2 hr before or 1 hr after a meal.

2. Complete entire prescription; do not stop despite feeling better.

3. Diarrhea may occur; report if persistent.

4. Return for F/U (e.g., ear check, throat culture, X ray) to evaluate response to therapy.

### Outcomes/Evaluate

• Resolution of underlying infection
• Symptomatic improvement

---

# Ceftizoxime sodium

(sef-tih-**ZOX**-eem)
**Pregnancy Category:** B
Cefizox **(Rx)**
**Classification:** Cephalosporin, third-generation

See also *Anti-Infectives* and *Cephalosporins*.

**Action/Kinetics:** t½: Approximately 1–2 hr. Approximately 80% excreted unchanged in the urine.

**Uses:** Infections of the urinary tract, lower respiratory tract, skin, skin structures, bones, and joints. Intra-abdominal infections, septicemia, meningitis (caused by *Haemophilus influenzae* or *Streptococcus pneumoniae*), gonorrhea (including uncomplicated cervical and urethral gonorrhea caused by *Neisseria*). Pelvic inflammatory disease caused by *Neisseria gonorrhoeae, Escherichia coli,* or Streptococcus agalactiae.

**Additional Side Effects:** Transient increased levels of eosinophils, AST, ALT, and CPK have been seen in children over 6 months of age.

### Dosage

• **IM, IV**

*Uncomplicated urinary tract and other infections.*

**Adults:** 0.5 g q 12 hr.

*Severe or resistant infections.*

**Adults:** 1 g q 8 hr or 2 g q 8–12 hr.

*Life-threatening infections.*

**Adults:** Up to 3–4 g q 8 hr.

*Pelvic inflammatory disease.*

2 g q 8 hr IV (doses up to 2 g q 4 hr have been used).

• **IV**

*Uncomplicated gonorrhea.*

**Adults:** 1 g as a single dose **IM. Pediatric, over 6 months:** 50 mg/kg q 6–8 hr up to 200 mg/kg/day (not to exceed the maximum adult dose).

*Impaired renal function.*

**Initial, IM, IV:** 0.5–1 g; **then,** use maintenance schedule in package insert.

---

## NURSING CONSIDERATIONS

See also *General Nursing Considerations for All Anti-Infectives* and *Cephalosporins*.

### Administration/Storage

1. For IM doses of 2 g, divide the dose equally and give in different large muscle masses.

**IV** 2. For direct IV administration, reconstitute 1 g in 10 mL sterile water and give slowly over 3–5 min.

3. For intermittent administration, further dilute in 50–100 mL of D5W or NSS and infuse over 30 min.

4. Reconstituted solutions are stable at room temperature for 8 hr and for 48 hr if refrigerated.

**Outcomes/Evaluate**

- Negative culture reports
- Resolution of S&S of infection

# Ceftriaxone sodium
(sef-try-**AX**-ohn)
**Pregnancy Category:** B
Rocephin **(Rx)**
**Classification:** Cephalosporin, third-generation

See also *Anti-Infectives* and *Cephalosporins.*

**Action/Kinetics:** t½: Approximately 6–8 hr. Significantly protein bound. One-third to two-thirds excreted unchanged in the urine.

**Uses:** Infections of the lower respiratory tract, urinary tract, skin, skin structures, bones, joints, abdomen. Also, uncomplicated gonorrhea (cervical, urethral, rectal) including both penicillinase- and non-penicillinase-producing strains of *Neisseria gonorrhoeae* and pharyngeal gonorrhea caused by non-penicillinase-producing strains of *N. gonorrhoeae.* Pelvic inflammatory disease, pediatric meningitis, prophylaxis of infections in surgery, bacterial septicemia. Acute bacterial otitis media. *Investigational:* Neurologic complications, arthritis, and carditis associated with Lyme disease (infection caused by *Borrelia burgdorferi)* in clients refractory to penicillin G.

**Additional Side Effects:** Increase in serum creatinine, presence of casts in the urine, alteration of PTs (rare).

**Dosage**

- **IV, IM**

*General infections.*
**Adults, usual:** 1–2 g/day in single or divided doses q 12 hr, not to exceed 4 g/day. Maintain therapy for 4–14 days, depending on the infec-

tion. **Pediatric:** *Other than meningitis:* 50–75 mg/kg/day not to exceed total daily dose of 2 g given in divided doses q 12 hr.

*Meningitis.*
**Pediatric:** 100 mg/kg/day, not to exceed total daily dose of 4 g given once daily or in equally divided doses q 12 hr for 7–14 days.

*Prophylaxis of infection in surgery.*
1 g 30–120 min prior to surgery.

*Uncomplicated gonorrhea.*
**Adults, IM:** 125 mg as a single dose plus doxycycline.

*Pharyngeal gonorrhea due to non-penicillinase-producing strains of* N. gonorrhoeae.
250 mg as a single IM dose.

*Gonococcal infections in children.*
**Less than 45 kg:** 125 mg given once. **Infants:** 25–50 mg/kg/day not to exceed 125 mg IV or IM in a single daily dose for 7 days.

*Gonococcal infection during pregnancy.*
**Adults:** 250 mg as a single IM dose plus erythromycin.

*Disseminated gonococcal infection.*
**Adults:** 1 g IM or IV q 24 hr.

*Gonococcal meningitis or endocarditis.*
**Adults:** 1–2 g IV q 12 hr for 10–14 days (meningitis) or 4 weeks (endocarditis).

*Gonococcal ophthalmia.*
**Adults and children over 20 kg:** 1 g given as a single IM dose.

*Acute pelvic inflammatory disease.*
250 mg IM plus doxycycline or tetracycline.

*Lyme disease.*
**IV:** 2–4 g/day for 14 days. Dosage adjustment is not required for renal or hepatic impairment; however, monitor blood levels in dialysis clients.

*Acute bacterial otitis media.*
**IM:** Single dose of 50 mg/kg, not to exceed 1 g.

---

## NURSING CONSIDERATIONS

See also *General Nursing Considerations for All Anti-Infectives* and *Cephalosporins*.

### Administration/Storage

1. IM injections should be deep into the body of a large muscle.

**IV** 2. IV infusions should contain concentrations of 10–40 mg/mL. Reconstitute 500 mg in 4.8 mL of sterile water, NSS, or D5W. Then further dilute in 50–100 mL D5W or NSS and infuse over 30–60 min.

3. Do not mix drug with other antibiotics.

4. Stability of solutions for IM or IV use varies depending on the diluent used; check package insert carefully.

5. Maintain dosage for at least 2 days after symptoms of infection have disappeared (usual course of therapy is 4–14 days, although complicated infections may require longer therapy).

6. Continue dosage for at least 10 days when treating *Streptococcus pyogenes* infections.

### Assessment

1. Document indications for therapy and include pretreatment findings.

2. Note any history of GI disease, especially colitis; use drug cautiously.

3. Note any penicillin reactions.

4. Monitor coagulation studies; drug may alter PTs. Use vitamin K (10 mg/week) prophylactically if bleeding occurs.

### Outcomes/Evaluate

• Resolution of S&S of infection
• Negative culture reports

---

## Cefuroxime axetil

(sef-your-**OX**-eem)
**Pregnancy Category:** B
Ceftin **(Rx)**

## Cefuroxime sodium

(sef-your-**OX**-eem)
**Pregnancy Category:** B
Kefurox, Zinacef **(Rx)**
**Classification:** Cephalosporin, second-generation

See also *Anti-Infectives* and *Cephalosporins*.

**Action/Kinetics:** Cefuroxime axetil is used PO, whereas cefuroxime sodium is used either IM or IV. **IM, IV: t½,** 1–2 hr; 66%–100% is excreted unchanged in the urine. t½ will be prolonged in clients with renal failure.

**Uses: PO (axetil).** Pharyngitis, tonsillitis, otitis media, sinusitis, acute bacterial exacerbations of chronic bronchitis and secondary bacterial infections of acute bronchitis, uncomplicated UTIs, uncomplicated skin and skin structure infections, uncomplicated gonorrhea (urethral and endocervical) caused by non-penicillinase-producing strains of *Neisseria gonorrhoeae*. Early Lyme disease due to *Borrelia burgdorferi*. The suspension is indicated for children from 3 months to 12 years to treat pharyngitis, tonsillitis, acute bacterial otitis media, and impetigo.

**IM, IV (sodium).** Infections of the urinary tract, lower respiratory tract (including pneumonia), skin and skin structures, bones, and joints. Septicemia, meningitis, uncomplicated and disseminated gonococcal infections due to penicillinase- or non-penicillinase-producing strains of *N. gonorrhoeae* in men and women. Mixed infections in which several organisms have been identified. Prophylaxis of postoperative infections in surgical procedures such as vaginal hysterectomy.

**Additional Side Effects:** Decrease in H&H.

**Additional Laboratory Test Interference:** False – reaction in the ferricyanide test for blood glucose.

### Dosage

• **Tablets (Cefuroxime Axetil)**
*Pharyngitis, tonsillits.*
**Adults and children over 13 years:** 250 mg q 12 hr for 10 days. **Children:** 125 mg q 12 hr for 10 days.

*Acute bacterial exacerbations of chronic bronchitis and secondary bacterial infections of acute bronchitis, uncomplicated skin and skin structure infections.*
**Adults and children over 13 years:** 250 or 500 mg q 12 hr for 10

days (5 days for secondary bacterial infections of acute bronchitis).

*Uncomplicated UTIs.*
**Adults and children over 13 years:** 125 or 250 mg q 12 hr for 7–10 days. **Infants and children less than 12 years:** 125 mg b.i.d.

*Acute otitis media.*
**Children:** 250 mg b.i.d. for 10 days.

*Uncomplicated gonorrhea.*
**Adults and children over 13 years:** 1,000 mg as a single dose.

*Early Lyme disease.*
500 mg/day for 20 days.
• **Suspension (Cefuroxime Axetil)**

*Pharyngitis, tonsillitis.*
**Children, 3 months to 12 years:** 20 mg/kg/day in 2 divided doses, not to exceed 500 mg total dose/day, for 10 days.

*Acute otitis media, impetigo.*
**Children, 3 months to 12 years:** 30 mg/kg/day in 2 divided doses, not to exceed 1,000 mg total dose/day, for 10 days.
• **IM, IV (Cefuroxime Sodium)**

*Uncomplicated infections, including urinary tract, pneumonia, disseminated gonococcal, skin and skin structure.*
**Adults:** 750 mg q 8 hr. **Pediatric, over 3 months:** 50–100 mg/kg/day in divided doses q 6–8 hr (not to exceed adult dose for severe infections).

*Severe or complicated infections; bone and joint infections.*
**Adults:** 1.5 g q 8 hr. **Pediatric, over 3 months:** *bone and joint infections,* **IV:** 150 mg/kg/day in divided doses q 8 hr (not to exceed adult dose).

*Life-threatening infections or those due to less susceptible organisms.*
**Adults:** 1.5 g q 6 hr.

*Bacterial meningitis.*
**Adults:** Up to 3 g q 8 hr. **Pediatric, over 3 months, initial, IV:** 200–240 mg/kg/day in divided doses q 6–8 hr; **then,** after clinical improvement, 100 mg/kg/day.

*Gonorrhea (uncomplicated).*
1.5 g as a single IM dose given at two different sites together with 1 g PO probenecid.

*Prophylaxis in surgery.*
**Adults, IV:** 1.5 g 30–60 min before surgery; if procedure is of long duration, **IM, IV,** 0.75 g q 8 hr.

*Open heart surgery, prophylaxis.*
**IV:** 1.5 g when anesthesia is initiated; **then,** 1.5 g q 12 hr for a total of 6 g.

## NURSING CONSIDERATIONS

See also *General Nursing Considerations for All Anti-Infectives* and *Cephalosporins.*

**Administration/Storage**

1. Cefuroxime axetil for PO use is available in tablet and suspension forms. Tablets should be swallowed whole and not crushed, as the crushed tablet has a strong, bitter, persistent taste.

2. To reconstitute the suspension, loosen the powder by shaking the bottle. Add the appropriate amount of water (depending on bottle size). Invert the bottle and shake vigorously.

3. The tablet and suspension are not bioequivalent and are not substitutable on a milligram-per-milligram basis.

4. For IM use, inject deep into a large muscle mass.

**IV** 5. Use IV route for severe or life-threatening infections such as septicemia or in poor-risk clients, especially in presence of shock.

6. For direct IV, reconstitute 750 mg with 8 mL sterile water and give over 3–5 min. For intermittent IV administration, further dilute in 100 mL of dextrose or saline solution and infuse over 30 min.

7. For direct intermittent IV administration, slowly inject the drug over 3 to 5 min, or give in tubing through which the client receives other IV solutions. For intermittent IV infusion with a Y-type administration set, the dose can be given in the tubing through which the client is receiving other medications; however, during drug infusion, discontinue administration of other solutions.

For continuous IV infusion, the drug may be added to 0.9% NaCl injection, 5% or 10% dextrose injection, 5% dextrose and 0.45% or 0.9% NaCl, and M/6 sodium lactate injection.

8. Do not add cefuroxime sodium to solutions of aminoglycosides; if both drugs are required, each should be given separately.

9. Prior to reconstitution, protect the drug from light. The powder and reconstituted drug may darken without affecting potency.

10. Continue therapy for at least 10 days in infections due to *Streptococcus pyogenes.*

**Assessment**

1. Document indications for therapy and note baseline assessments.

2. Assess for any clinical and lab evidence of anemia and renal dysfunction. Reduce dose with impaired renal function.

**Client/Family Teaching**

1. Take tablets and/or suspension with food to enhance absorption.

2. Report S&S of anemia (SOB, dizziness, pale skin, etc.) immediately.

3. Crushed tablets have a distinctive bitter taste even when hidden in foods. If intolerable, report so alternative drug therapy may be instituted.

**Outcomes/Evaluate**

• Resolution of S&S of infection
• Normal H&H
• Surgical infection prophylaxis

---

# Cellulose sodium phosphate

(**SELL**-you-lohs)
**Pregnancy Category:** C
Calcibind (**Rx**)
**Classification:** Calcium-binding agent

**Action/Kinetics:** A synthetic, nonabsorbable compound that is not soluble in water. The sodium ion exchanges for calcium; the cellulose phospate-bound calcium (from both dietary and endogenous sources) is then excreted in the feces. Urinary calcium is decreased while urinary phosphorus and oxalate are increased.

**Uses:** Decrease incidence of new renal stone formation in absorptive hypercalciuria Type I. Diagnostic test for causes of hypercalciuria other than hyperabsorption.

**Contraindications:** Primary or secondary hyperparathyroidism, hypocalcemia, hypomagnesemia, enteric hyperoxaluria, osteoporosis, osteomalacia, osteitis, low intestinal absorption or renal excretion of calcium, when hypercalciuria is due to mobilization from bones. Children under age 16.

**Special Concerns:** Use with caution in CHF or ascites.

**Side Effects:** *GI:* Diarrhea, dyspepsia, loose bowel movements. *Other:* Hyperparathyroid bone disease, hyperoxaluria, hypomagnesiuria, loss of copper, zinc, iron. Long-term use may cause hyperoxaluria and hypomagnesiuria.

**Dosage**

• **Powder**

*Urinary calcium greater than 300 mg/day.*

5 g with each meal.

*Urinary calcium less than 150 mg/day.*

2.5 g with breakfast and lunch and 5 g with dinner.

## NURSING CONSIDERATIONS

### Administration/Storage

1. Monitor parathyroid hormone levels at least once between 2 weeks and 3 mo after therapy has been initiated.

2. A moderate calcium intake is recommended.

3. Mix each dose with water, juice, or soft drink, and take within 30 min of the meal.

4. Magnesium gluconate supplements may be given as follows:

• 1.5 g before breakfast and at bedtime for those receiving 15 g cellulose daily.

• 1 g, as in the preceding, with 10 g cellulose daily.

• To avoid binding, give magnesium either 1 hr before or 1 hr after cellulose.

5. Stop treatment if urinary oxalate is

greater than 55 mg/day with moderate dietary oxalate restriction.
6. Magnesium, iron, and other trace-metal supplements may be ordered.

**Assessment:** Document indications for therapy; note baseline labs and any history of CHF or ascites.

**Client/Family Teaching**
1. Take with meals to maximize the uptake of dietary calcium.
2. Avoid calcium-containing foods such as milk, cheese, or ice cream.
3. Avoid eating spinach and dark green vegetables, rhubarb, chocolate, and brewed tea since all of these contain oxalates, which may lead to calcium stone formation.
4. Avoid vitamin C as it is metabolized to oxalate; avoid salt and lightly salted foods.
5. Drink plenty of fluids; the urinary output should be 2 L/day.

**Outcomes/Evaluate**
• ↓ Urinary calcium
• Prophylaxis in new renal stone formation

# Cephalexin hydrochloride monohydrate
(sef-ah-**LEX**-in)
**Pregnancy Category:** B
Keftab **(Rx)**

# Cephalexin monohydrate
(sef-ah-**LEX**-in)
**Pregnancy Category:** B
Apo-Cephalex ✿, Biocef, Dom-Cephalexin ✿, Keflex, Novo-Lexin ✿, Nu-Cephalex ✿, PMS-Cephalexin ✿, STCC-Cephalexin ✿ **(Rx)**
**Classification:** Cephalosporin, first-generation

See also *Anti-Infectives* and *Cephalosporins*.

**Action/Kinetics: Peak serum levels: PO,** 9–39 mcg/mL after 1 hr. **t½, PO:** 30–72 min. Absorption delayed in children. The HCl monohydrate does not require conversion in the stomach before absorption. Ninety percent of drug excreted unchanged in urine within 8 hr.

**Uses:** Respiratory tract infections caused by *Streptococcus pneumoniae* and group A β-hemolytic streptococci. Otitis media due to *S. pneumoniae, Hemophilus influenzae, Moraxella catarrhalis* (use monohydrate only), staphylococci, and streptococci. Genitourinary tract infections (including acute prostatitis) due to *Escherichia coli, Proteus mirabilis,* and *Klebsiella.* Bone infections caused by *P. mirabilis* and staphylococci. Skin and skin structure infections due to staphylococci and streptococci.

**Special Concerns:** Safety and effectiveness of the HCl monohydrate have not been determined in children.

**Additional Side Effects:** Nephrotoxicity, cholestatic jaundice.

**Dosage** ⎯⎯⎯⎯⎯⎯⎯⎯⎯⎯
• **Capsules, Oral Suspension, Tablets**
  *General infections.*
**Adults, usual:** 250 mg q 6 hr up to 4 g/day. **Pediatric:** *Monohydrate,* 25–50 mg/kg/day in four equally divided doses.
  *Infections of skin and skin structures, streptococcal pharyngitis, uncomplicated cystitis, over 15 years.*
**Adults:** 500 mg q 12 hr. Large doses may be needed for severe infections or for less susceptible organisms. For streptococcal pharyngitis in children over 1 year and for skin and skin structure infections, the total daily dose should be divided and given q 12 hr. In severe infections, the dose should be doubled.
  *Otitis media.*
**Pediatric:** 75–100 mg/kg/day in four divided doses.

## NURSING CONSIDERATIONS

See also *General Nursing Considerations for All Anti-Infectives* and *Cephalosporins*.

**Administration/Storage**
1. After reconstitution, refrigerate; discard any unused drug after 14 days.

---

✿ = Available in Canada                    ***bold italic*** = life threatening side effect

2. If the total daily dose is more than 4 g, undertake parenteral drug therapy.

3. Continue treatment for at least 10 days for beta-hemolytic streptococcal infections.

4. Dosage may have to be reduced with impaired renal function or increased for severe infections. Drug action can be prolonged by concurrent administration of PO probenecid.

### Client/Family Teaching
1. Take with meals for GI upset.
2. Consume 2–3 L/day of fluids to prevent dehydration.
3. Report any changes in elimination patterns, yellow discoloration of the skin or eyes, or a lack of response.

### Outcomes/Evaluate
- Resolution of infection
- Symptomatic improvement

---

# Cephalothin sodium
(sef-**AL**-oh-thin)
**Pregnancy Category:** B
Ceporacin ✱, Keflin ✱, Keflin Neutral
**(Rx)**
**Classification:** Cephalosporin, first-generation

---

See also *Anti-Infectives* and *Cephalosporins*.

**Action/Kinetics:** Poorly absorbed from GI tract; must be given parenterally. **Peak serum levels: IM,** 6–21 mcg/mL after 30 min. **t½, IM, IV:** 30–60 min. Fifty-five percent to 90% excreted unchanged in urine. Its low nephrotoxicity, ototoxicity, and neurotoxicity make the drug suitable for clients with impaired renal function.

**Uses:** Infections of the GU tract, GI tract, respiratory tract, skin, soft tissues, bones, and joints. Meningitis, septicemia (including endocarditis), and prophylaxis in surgery.

**Additional Side Effects:** Nephrotoxicity, severe phlebitis, hemolytic anemia, increased PT.

**Laboratory Test Interferences:** Large doses may produce false + results in urinary protein tests that use sulfosalicylic acid.

## Dosage
- **Deep IM, IV**

*General infections.*
**Adults, usual:** 0.5–1 g q 4–6 hr. **Pediatric:** 80–160 mg/kg/day in divided doses.

*UTIs, uncomplicated pneumonia, furunculosis with cellulitis.*
**Adults:** 0.5 g q 6 hr (for severe infections increase the dose to 1 g or give 0.5 g q 4 hr).

*Life-threatening infections.*
**Adults:** 2 g q 4 hr (up to 12 g/day for bacteremia, septicemia).

*Preoperative and during surgery.*
**Adults:** 1–2 g 30–60 min prior to surgery and during surgery. **Pediatric:** Prophylaxis in surgery: 20–30 mg/kg using adult schedule.

*Postoperative.*
**Adults:** 1–2 g q 6 hr for 24 hr.

*Impaired renal function.*
**Initial:** 1–2 g; **then,** use manufacturer's guidelines for maintenance doses.

---

## NURSING CONSIDERATIONS

See also *General Nursing Considerations for All Anti-Infectives* and *Cephalosporins*.

### Administration/Storage
**IV** 1. For direct IV administration, add a small needle into larger veins.
2. Dilute according to directions on package insert. For direct IV administration, dilute 1 g in 10 mL of solution and infuse over 3–5 min. For intermittent IV administration further dilute 1 g in 50 mL of dextrose or saline solution and infuse over 15–30 min.
3. Dissolve precipitate by warming vial in hand and shaking. Do not overheat.
4. For prolonged IV infusion, replace the medication with a freshly prepared solution every 24 hr to ensure stability.
5. Discard reconstituted solution after 12 hr at room temperature and after 96 hr when refrigerated.

### Assessment
1. Monitor PT and assess for bleeding. May administer vitamin K (10 mg/week) if bleeding occurs.

2. Assess for allergic reactions; monitor I&O and renal function studies; alter dose and follow manufacturer's guidelines with impaired renal function.

**Outcomes/Evaluate**
- Resolution of infection
- Surgical infection prophylaxis

## Cephapirin sodium
(sef-ah-**PIE**-rin)
**Pregnancy Category:** B
**(Rx)**
**Classification:** Cephalosporin, first-generation

See also *Anti-Infectives* and *Cephalosporins*.
**Action/Kinetics: Peak serum levels:** **IM,** 9.4 mcg/mL after 30 min. **t½, IM, IV:** 21–47 min. Virtually entirely excreted in the urine within 6 hr, with 41%–60% excreted unchanged.
**Uses:** Infections of the respiratory tract, urinary tract, skin, and skin structures. Septicemia, endocarditis, osteomyelitis, prophylaxis in surgery.
**Special Concerns:** Before use in children less than 3 months, assess benefits versus risks.
**Laboratory Test Interferences:** Increase in serum bilirubin.

**Dosage** ─────────────
- **IM, IV only**
  *General infections.*
  **Adults:** 0.5–1 g q 4–6 hr up to 12 g/day for serious or life-threatening infections.
    *Preoperatively.*
  **Adults:** 1–2 g 30–60 min before surgery.
    *During surgery.*
  **Adults:** 1–2 g.
    *Postoperatively.*
  **Adults:** 1–2 g q 6 hr for 24 hr. **Pediatric, over 3 months:** 40–80 mg/kg/day in four equally divided doses.

In clients with impaired renal function, a dose of 7.5–15 mg/kg q 12 hr may be adequate.

**NURSING CONSIDERATIONS**

See also *General Nursing Considerations for All Anti-Infectives* and *Cephalosporins*.
**Administration/Storage**
1. Concurrent administration with probenecid may inhibit excretion of cephapirin.
**IV** 2. For direct IV administration reconstitute 1 g in 10 mL of solution and infuse over 3–5 min. For intermittent infusions, further dilute in 50–100 mL of solution and infuse over 15–20 min.
3. Discard after 12 hr when kept at room temperature and after 10 days when refrigerated at 4°C (39°F).
**Assessment:** Note any previous antibiotic reactions; reduce dose with impaired renal function.
**Outcomes/Evaluate**
- Resolution of infection
- Surgical infection prophylaxis

## Cephradine
(**SEF**-rah-deen)
**Pregnancy Category:** B
Anspor, Velosef **(Rx)**
**Classification:** Cephalosporin, first-generation

See also *Anti-Infectives* and *Cephalosporins*.
**Action/Kinetics:** Similar to cephalexin. Rapidly absorbed PO or IM (30 min–2 hr); 60%–90% excreted after 6 hr. **Peak serum levels: PO,** 8–24 mcg/mL after 30–60 min; **IM,** 5.6–13.6 mcg/mL after 1–2 hr. **t½:** 42–120 min; 80%–95% excreted in urine unchanged.
**Uses:** Infections of the respiratory tract (including lobar pneumonia, tonsillitis, pharyngitis), urinary tract (including prostatitis and enterococcal infections), skin, skin structures, and bone. Otitis media, septicemia, prophylaxis in surgery, following cesarean section to prevent infection. In severe infections, therapy is usually initiated parenterally.
**Special Concerns:** Safe use during pregnancy, of the parenteral form in

infants under 1 month of age, and of the PO form in children less than 9 months of age have not been established.

**Additional Laboratory Test Interference:** False + reactions using sulfosalicylic acid for urinary protein tests. High concentrations may interfere with measurement of creatinine by the Jaffe method.

**Dosage**

• **Capsules, Oral Suspension**

*Skin and skin structures, respiratory tract infections.*

**Adults, usual:** 250 mg q 6 hr or 500 mg q 12 hr.

*Lobar pneumonia.*

**Adults:** 500 mg q 6 hr or 1 g q 12 hr.

*Uncomplicated UTIs.*

**Adults, usual:** 500 mg q 12 hr.

*More serious infections and prostatitis.*

500 mg q 6 hr or 1 g q 12 hr (severe, chronic infections may require up to 1 g q 6 hr).

**Pediatric, over 9 months:** 25–50 mg/kg/day in equally divided doses q 6–12 hr (75–100 mg/kg/day for otitis media).

• **Deep IM, IV**

*General infections.*

**Adults:** 2–4 g/day in equally divided doses q.i.d.

*Surgical prophylaxis.*

**Adults:** 1 g 30–90 min before surgery; **then,** 1 g q 4–6 hr for one to two doses (or up to 24 hr postoperatively).

*Cesarean section, prophylaxis.*

**IV:** 1 g when the umbilical cord is clamped; **then,** give two additional 1-g doses **IV or IM** 6 and 12 hr after the initial dose. **Pediatric, over 1 year:** 50–100 mg/kg/day in equally divided doses q.i.d.

## NURSING CONSIDERATIONS

See also *General Nursing Considerations for All Anti-Infectives* and *Cephalosporins*.

**Administration/Storage**

1. Administer oral medication without regard to meals.

2. Carefully inject into muscle; sterile abscesses from accidental SC injection have occurred.

3. Rotate injection sites.

**IV** 4. Dilute according to directions on package insert. Protect from excessive heat and light before and after reconstitution.

5. For direct IV administration dilute 1 g in 10 mL of D5W or NSS; infuse over 3–5 min. For intermittent infusions further reconstitute in 50–100 mL of dextrose or saline solution and infuse over 30–60 min. Discontinue other IV solutions during IV administration of cephalosporins. Do not mix with lactated Ringer's solution.

6. A slightly yellow solution may be retained for use; if unsure, consult with pharmacist.

7. To ensure stability, replace medication infusion solution during prolonged IV administration q 10 hr.

8. Discard reconstituted solution after 10 hr at room temperature and after 48 hr when refrigerated at 5°C (41°F).

**Assessment:** Note any previous penicillin reaction; reduce dose with renal dysfunction.

**Outcomes/Evaluate**

• Resolution of S&S of infection
• Infection prophylaxis in surgery
• Negative culture reports

# Cetirizine hydrochloride
(seh-**TIH**-rah-zeen)
**Pregnancy Category:** B
Reactine ✦, Zyrtec **(Rx)**
**Classification:** Antihistamine

See also *Antihistamines.*

**Action/Kinetics:** A potent $H_1$-receptor antagonist. A mild bronchodilator that protects against histmine-induced bronchospasm; negligible anticholinergic and sedative activity. Rapidly absorbed after PO administration; however, food delays the time to peak serum levels but does not decrease the total amount of drug absorbed. Poorly penetrates the CNS, but high levels are distributed to the skin. **t½:** 8.3 hr (longer in elderly clients and in those with impaired liver or renal function). Excreted mostly unchanged (70%) in the urine; 10% is excreted in the feces.

**Uses:** Relief of symptoms associated with seasonal allergic rhinitis due to ragweed, grass, and tree pollens; perennial allergic rhinitis due to allergens such as dust mites, animal dander, and molds. Chronic idiopathic urticaria.

**Contraindications:** Lactation. In those hypersensitive to hydroxyzine.

**Special Concerns:** Due to the possibility of sedation, use with caution in situations requiring mental alertness. Safety and efficacy have not been determined in children less than 12 years of age.

**Side Effects:** See *Antihistamines*. The most common side effects are somnolence, dry mouth, fatigue, pharyngitis, and dizziness.

**OD** **Overdose Management:** *Symptoms*: Somnolence. *Treatment*: Symptomatic and supportive. Dialysis is not effective in removing the drug from the body.

**Dosage** ─────────
• **Tablets**
*Seasonal or perennial allergic rhinitis, chronic urticaria.*
**Adults and children over 6 years of age, initial:** Depending on the severity of the symptoms, 5 or 10 mg (most common initial dose) once daily. In clients with decreased renal function ($C_{CR}$: 11–31 mL/min), in hemodialysis clients ($C_{CR}$ less than 7 mL/min), and in those with impaired hepatic function, the dose is 5 mg once daily.

**NURSING CONSIDERATIONS**

See also *Nursing Considerations* for *Antihistamines*.
**Assessment**
1. Document type, onset, and characteristics of symptoms; note triggers.
2. Note any hypersensitivity to hydroxyzine.
**Client/Family Teaching**
1. May take with or without food; time of administration may be varied depending on client needs.

2. Use caution when performing activities that require mental alertness until drug effects realized; may cause drowsiness.
3. Drug may cause dry mouth and fatigue; report adverse effects that inhibit compliance with therapy.
4. Avoid alcohol or any other CNS depressants.
5. Review allergens that trigger symptoms, e.g., ragweed, dust mites, molds, animal dander, etc., and instruct in how to control and avoid contact.
**Outcomes/Evaluate**
• Symptom relief with seasonal and perennial allergic rhinitis
• ↓ Occurrence, duration, and severity of hives; ↓ pruritus

# Chenodiol
# (Chenodeoxycholic acid)
(kee-noh-**DYE**-ohl)
**Pregnancy Category:** X
Chenix **(Rx)**
**Classification:** Naturally occurring human bile acid

**Action/Kinetics:** Chenodiol, by reducing hepatic synthesis of cholesterol and cholic acid, replaces both cholic and deoxycholic acids in the bile acid pool. This effect helps desaturation of biliary cholesterol and leads to dissolution of radiolucent cholesterol gallstones. Is ineffective on calcified gallstones or on radiolucent bile pigment stones. Fifty percent of clients have stone recurrence within 5 years. The drug also increases LDLs and inhibits absorption of fluid from the colon. Is well absorbed following PO administration. Metabolized by bacteria in the colon to lithocholic acid, most of which is excreted in the feces.

**Uses:** In radiolucent cholesterol gallstones where surgery is a risk due to age or systemic disease. Ineffective in some; has potential liver toxicity. Best results in thin females with a serum cholesterol not higher than 227 mg/dL and who have a small number of radiolucent cholesterol gallstones.

**Contraindications:** Known hepatic dysfunction or bile ductal abnormalities. Colon cancer. Pregnancy or in those who may become pregnant.

**Special Concerns:** Safety and efficacy in lactation and in children have not been established.

**Side Effects:** Hepatotoxicity including increased ALT in one-third of clients, intrahepatic cholestasis. *GI:* Diarrhea (common), anorexia, constipation, dyspepsia, flatulence, heartburn, cramps, epigastric distress, N&V, abdominal pain. *Hematologic:* Decreased white cell count. ***Chenodiol may contribute to colon cancer in susceptible clients.***

**Drug Interactions**

*Antacids, aluminum* / ↓ Effect of chenodiol due to ↓ absorption from GI tract

*Cholestyramine* / See *Antacids*

*Clofibrate* / ↓ Effect of chenodiol due to ↑ biliary cholesterol secretion

*Colestipol* / See *Antacids*

*Estrogens, oral contraceptives* / ↓ Effect of chenodiol due to ↑ biliary cholesterol secretion

**Dosage** ⸺⸺⸺⸺

• **Tablets**

*Radiolucent cholesterol gallstones.*

**Adults, initial:** 250 mg b.i.d. for 2 weeks; **then,** increase by 250 mg/week until maximum tolerated or recommended dose is reached (13–16 mg/kg/day in two divided doses morning and night with milk or food). *NOTE:* Doses less than 10 mg/kg are usually ineffective and may result in increased risk of cholecystectomy.

**NURSING CONSIDERATIONS**

**Assessment**

1. Document type and onset of symptoms, and any previous therapy utilized.

2. List drugs currently prescribed; note any potential interactions.

3. Test for pregnancy.

4. Obtain liver and renal function

studies and serum cholesterol; monitor for stone dissolution.

**Client/Family Teaching**

1. Drug may need to be taken for 24 mo before gallstones are dissolved; gallstones may recur even after successful treatment.

2. Immediately report any severe, sudden upper quadrant pain that radiates to the shoulder, nonspecific abdominal pain, nausea, or vomiting; may indicate gallstone complications.

3. Avoid pregnancy during therapy; report any possibility of conception. Oral contraceptives may decrease the effectiveness of chenodiol; practice alternative methods of birth control.

4. Stress importance of periodic LFTs and cholecystograms or gallbladder ultrasonography to evaluate the effectiveness of the drug therapy.

5. Consult with provider if antacids are needed; most have an aluminum base that absorbs the drug.

6. Report any incidence of diarrhea; this may be drug related and can be relieved by changes in dosage or with antidiarrheal agents.

7. Discuss drug relationship to colon cancer and potential risks.

**Outcomes/Evaluate:** Dissolution of radiolucent cholesterol gallstones

# Chloral hydrate

(**KLOH**-ral **HY**-drayt)

**Pregnancy Category:** C

Aquachloral Supprettes, Novo-Chlorhydrate ✹, PMS-Chloral Hydrate ✹ **(C-IV) (Rx)**

**Classification:** Nonbenzodiazepine, nonbarbiturate sedative-hypnotic

**Action/Kinetics:** Chloral hydrate is metabolized to trichloroethanol, which is the active metabolite causing CNS depression. Produces only slight hangover effects and is said not to affect REM sleep. High doses lead to severe CNS depression, as well as depression of respiratory and vasomotor centers (hypotension). Both psychologic and physical dependence develop. **Onset:** Within 30 min. **Duration:** 4–8 hr. **t½, tri-**

**chloroethanol:** 7–10 hr. Readily absorbed from the GI tract and distributed to all tissues; passes the placental barrier and appears in breast milk. Metabolites excreted by kidney.

**Uses:** Short-term hypnotic. Daytime sedative and sedation prior to EEG procedures. Preoperative sedative and postoperative as adjunct to analgesics. Prevent or reduce symptoms of alcohol withdrawal.

**Contraindications:** Marked hepatic or renal impairment, severe cardiac disease, lactation. PO use in clients with esophagitis, gastritis, or gastric or duodenal ulcer.

**Special Concerns:** Use by nursing mothers may cause sedation in the infant. A decrease in dose may be necessary in geriatric clients due to age-related decrease in both hepatic and renal function.

**Side Effects:** *CNS:* Paradoxical paranoid reactions. Sudden withdrawal in dependent clients may result in "chloral delirium." ***Sudden intolerance to the drug following prolonged use may result in respiratory depression, hypotension, cardiac effects, and possibly death.*** *GI:* N&V, diarrhea, bad taste in mouth, gastritis, increased peristalsis. *GU:* Renal damage, decreased urine flow and uric acid excretion. *Miscellaneous:* Skin reactions, hepatic damage, allergic reactions, leukopenia, eosinophilia.

Chronic toxicity is treated by gradual withdrawal and rehabilitative measures such as those used in treatment of the chronic alcoholic. Poisoning by chloral hydrate resembles acute barbiturate intoxication; the same supportive treatment is indicated (see *Barbiturates* ).

**Drug Interactions**
*Anticoagulants, oral* / ↑ Effect of anticoagulants by ↓ plasma protein binding
*CNS depressants* / Additive CNS depression; concomitant use may lead to drowsiness, lethargy, stupor, respiratory collapse, coma, or death

*Furosemide (IV)* / Concomitant use results in diaphoresis, tachycardia, hypertension, flushing
**Laboratory Test Interferences:** ↑ 17-Hydroxycorticosteroids. Interference with fluorescence tests for catecholamines and copper sulfate test for glucose.

**Dosage** —————————
• **Capsules, Syrup**
*Daytime sedative.*
**Adults:** 250 mg t.i.d. after meals.
*Preoperative sedative.*
**Adults:** 0.5–1.0 g 30 min before surgery.
*Hypnotic.*
**Adults:** 0.5–1 g 15–30 min before bedtime. **Pediatric:** 50 mg/kg (1.5 g/m²) at bedtime (up to 1 g may be given as a single dose).
*Daytime sedative.*
**Pediatric:** 8.3 mg/kg (250 mg/m²) up to a maximum of 500 mg t.i.d. after meals.
*Premedication prior to EEG procedures.*
**Pediatric:** 20–25 mg/kg.
• **Suppositories, Rectal**
*Daytime sedative.*
**Adults:** 325 mg t.i.d. **Pediatric:** 8.3 mg/kg (250 mg/m²) t.i.d.
*Hypnotic.*
**Adults:** 0.5–1 g at bedtime. **Pediatric:** 50 mg/kg (1.5 g/m²) at bedtime (up to 1 g as a single dose).

—————————————————

## NURSING CONSIDERATIONS

See also *Nursing Considerations* for *Pentobarbital Sodium.*
**Administration/Storage**
1. PO: give capsules after meals with a full glass of water. Give the syrup with half a glass of juice, water, or ginger ale.
2. PO syrups have an unpleasant taste, which can be reduced by chilling the syrup before administration.
3. Have emergency drugs and equipment available should the client require supportive, physiologic treatment of acute poisoning.
**Assessment**
1. Document indications for therapy

and evaluate sleep habits and patterns and life-style.

2. Assess mental status and response to stimuli. Monitor level and pattern of alertness and compare with the premedication history.

3. Observe respiratory and cardiac responses; document evidence of vasomotor depression and dilatation of cutaneous blood vessels.

4. Note any history of cardiac disease, liver or renal dysfunction. Drug is metabolized to an alcohol component. Monitor liver and renal function studies for evidence of impairment.

5. Report any psychologic and physical dependence; symptoms resemble those of acute alcoholism, but with more severe gastritis.

**Client/Family Teaching**

1. Take only as directed.

2. Store away from the bedside.

3. Avoid activities that require mental alertness. Offer measures to promote comfort and relaxation. To protect from injury, assist with ambulation, use side rails, place call bell within reach, and use a night light.

4. Stress that drug is for short-term use only; may cause psychologic and physical dependence.

5. Review other methods to enhance sleep, i.e., no caffeine, increased exercise, muscle relaxation exercises, no daytime napping.

6. Review list of drug side effects, noting those that require immediate attention.

**Outcomes/Evaluate**

- Desired level of sedation
- ↓ Alcohol withdrawal symptoms
- Improved sleep patterns

# Chlorambucil

(klor-**AM**-byou-sill)

**Pregnancy Category:** D

Leukeran (Abbreviation: CHL) **(Rx)**

**Classification:** Antineoplastic, alkylating agent

See also *Antineoplastic Agents* and *Alkylating Agents*.

**Action/Kinetics:** Cell-cycle nonspecific; is also cytotoxic to nonproliferating cells and has immunosuppressant activity. Forms an unstable ethylenimmonium ion which binds (alkylates) with intracellular substances such as nucleic acids. The cytotoxic effect is due to cross-linking of strands of DNA and RNA and inhibition of protein synthesis. Is rapidly absorbed from the GI tract. **Peak plasma levels:** 1 hr. Plasma t½: 1.5 hr. 99% bound to plasma proteins, especially albumin. Extensively metabolized by the liver and at least one metabolite is active. Fifteen to 60% is excreted through the urine 24 hr after drug administration, and 40% is bound to tissues, including fat.

**Uses:** Palliation in chronic lymphocytic leukemia, malignant lymphomas (including lymphosarcoma), giant follicular lymphomas, and Hodgkin's disease. *Investigational:* Uveitis and meningoencephalitis associated with Behcet's disease. With a corticosteroid for idiopathic membranous nephropathy. Rheumatoid arthritis. Possible alternative to MOPP in combination with vinblastine, procarbazine, and prednisone.

**Special Concerns:** Use during lactation only if benefits outweigh risks. Safety and efficacy have not been established in children. The drug is carcinogenic in humans and may be both mutagenic and teratogenic in humans. It also affects fertility. May be cross-hypersensitivity with other alkylating agents.

**Additional Side Effects:** *Hepatic:* Hepatotoxicity with jaundice. *Pulmonary:* **Pulmonary fibrosis,** bronchopulmonary dysplasia. *CNS:* Children with nephrotic syndrome have an increased risk of seizures. *Miscellaneous:* Keratitis, drug fever, sterile cystitis, interstitial pneumonia, peripheral neuropathy. Cross-sensitivity (skin rashes) may occur with other alkylating agents.

**OD** **Overdose Management:** *Symptoms:* Pancytopenia (reversible), ataxia, agitated behavior, *clonic-tonic seizures. Treatment:* General supportive measures. Blood profiles should be carefully monitored; blood transfusions may be required.

**Laboratory Test Interferences:** ↑ Uric acid levels in serum and urine.

**Dosage**

• **Tablets**

*Leukemia, lymphomas.*

Individualized according to response of client. **Adults, children, initial dose:** 0.1–0.2 mg/kg (or 4–10 mg) daily in single or divided doses for 3–6 weeks; **maintenance:** 0.03–0.1 mg/kg/day depending on blood counts.

*Alternative for chronic lymphocytic leukemia.*

**Initial:** 0.4 mg/kg; **then,** repeat this dose every 2 weeks increasing by 0.1 mg/kg until either toxicity or control of condition is observed.

*Nephrotic syndrome, immunosuppressant.*

**Adults, children:** 0.1–0.2 mg/kg body weight daily for 8–12 weeks.

*Uveitis and meningoencephalitis associated with Behcet's disease.*

0.1 mg/kg/day.

*Idiopathic membranous nephropathy.*

0.1–0.2 mg/kg/day every other month, alternating with a corticosteroid for 6 months duration.

*Rheumatoid arthritis.*

0.1–0.3 mg/kg/day.

**NURSING CONSIDERATIONS**

See also *Nursing Considerations* for *Antineoplastic Agents.*

**Administration/Storage:** Store at 15°C–25°C (59°F–77°F) in a dry place.

**Assessment**

1. Document indications for therapy, noting pretreatment lab and physical assessment findings.

2. Drug may cause severe granulocyte and lymphocyte suppression. Nadir: 21 days; recovery: 42–56 days.

**Client/Family Teaching**

1. Take 1 hr before breakfast or 2 hr after the evening meal.

2. Consume 2–3 L/day of fluids to decrease urate crystals.

3. Review side effects; skin rash may result from cross-sensitivity with other alkylating agents and should be reported.

4. Drug is carcinogenic and may also be mutagenic and teratogenic; practice reliable birth control.

**Outcomes/Evaluate**

• Positive tumor response evidenced by ↓ tumor size/spread; suppression of malignant cell proliferation

• Immunosuppressant activity

# Chloramphenicol

(klor-am-**FEN**-ih-kohl)
Chloromycetin (Cream and Otic), Mychel, Pentamycetin ✦, PMS-Chloramphenicol ✦ **(Rx)**

# Chloramphenicol ophthalmic

(klor-am-**FEN**-ih-kohl)
AK Chlor, Chloromycetin Ophthalmic, Chloroptic Ophthalmic, Chloroptic S.O.P. Ophthalmic, Diochloram ✦, Ophtho-Chloram ✦ **(Rx)**

# Chloramphenicol sodium succinate

(klor-am-**FEN**-ih-kohl)
Chloromycetin Injection ✦, Chloromycetin Sodium Succinate, Mychel-S, Novo-Chorocap ✦ **(Rx)**
**Classification:** Anti-infective

See also *Anti-Infectives.*

**Action/Kinetics:** Interferes with or inhibits protein synthesis in bacteria by binding to 50S ribosomal subunits. Therapeutic serum concentrations: *peak,* 10–20 mcg/mL; *trough:* 5–10 mcg/mL (less for neonates). **Peak serum concentration: IM,** 2 hr. **t½:** 4 hr. Metabolized in the liver; 75%–90% of drug excreted in urine within 24 hr, as parent drug (8%–12%) and inactive metabolites.

The drug is mostly bacteriostatic. Well absorbed from the GI tract and is distributed to all parts of the body, including CSF, pleural, and ascitic fluids; saliva; milk; and aqueous and vitreous humors.

**Uses:** *Not to be used for trivial infections, prophylaxis of bacterial infections, or to treat colds, flu, or throat infections.* **Systemic Use.** Treatment of choice for typhoid fever but not for typhoid carrier state. Serious infections caused by *Salmonella, Rickettsia, Chlamydia,* and lymphogranuloma-psittacosis group. Meningitis due to *Haemophilus influenzae.* Brain abscesses due to *Bacteroides fragilis.* Cystic fibrosis anti-infective. Meningococcal or pneumococcal meningitis. **Topical Use.** Otitis externa. Prophylaxis of infection in minor cuts, wounds, skin abrasions, burns; promote healing in superficial infections of the skin. **Ophthalmic Use.** Superficial ocular infections due to *Staphylococcus aureus; Streptococcus* species, including *S. pneumoniae; Escherichia coli, H. influenzae, H. aegyptius, H. ducreyi, Klebsiella* species, *Neisseria* species, *Enterobacter* species, *Moraxella* species, and *Vibrio* species. Should be used only for serious ocular infections for which less dangerous drugs are either contraindicated or ineffective.

**Contraindications:** Hypersensitivity to chloramphenicol; pregnancy, especially near term and during labor; lactation. Avoid simultaneous administration of other drugs that may depress bone marrow. Ophthalmically in the presence of dendritic keratitis, vaccinia, varicella, mycobacterial or fungal eye infections, or following removal of a corneal foreign body. Topical products should not be used near or in the eye.

**Special Concerns:** Use with caution in clients with intermittent porphyria or G6PD deficiency. To avoid gray syndrome, use with caution and in reduced doses in premature and full-term infants. Ophthalmic ointments may retard corneal epithelial healing.

**Side Effects:** *Hematologic* (most serious): ***Aplastic anemia, hypoplastic anemia,*** thrombocytopenia, granulocytopenia, ***hemolytic anemia,*** pancytopenia, hemoglobinuria (paroxysmal nocturnal). *Hematologic studies should be undertaken before and every 2 days during therapy. GI:* N&V, diarrhea, glossitis, stomatitis, unpleasant taste, enterocolitis, pruritus ani. *Allergic:* Fever, angioedema, macular and vesicular rashes, urticaria, hemorrhages of the skin, intestine, bladder, mouth. ***Anaphylaxis.*** *CNS:* Headache, delirium, confusion, mental depression. *Neurologic:* Optic neuritis, peripheral neuritis. *Following topical use:* Burning, itching, irritation, redness of skin. Hypersensitive clients may exhibit ***angioneurotic edema,*** urticaria, vesicular and maculopapular dermatoses. *Miscellaneous:* Superinfection. Jaundice (rare). Herxheimer-like reactions when used for typhoid fever (may be due to release of bacterial endotoxins). ***Gray syndrome in infants:*** Rapid respiration, ashen gray color, failure to feed, abdominal distention with or without vomiting, progressive pallid cyanosis, vasomotor collapse, death. Can be reversed when drug is discontinued. *NOTE: Neonates should be observed closely, since the drug accumulates in the bloodstream and the infant is thus subject to greater hazards of toxicity.*

**After ophthalmic use:** Temporary blurring of vision, stinging, itching, burning, redness, irritation, swelling, decreased vision, persistent or worse pain.

**Drug Interactions**

*Acetaminophen* / ↑ Effect of chloramphenicol due to ↑ serum levels

*Anticoagulants, oral* / ↑ Effect of anticoagulants due to ↓ breakdown by liver

*Antidiabetics, oral* / ↑ Effect of antidiabetics due to ↓ breakdown by liver

*Barbiturates* / ↑ Effect of barbiturates due to ↓ breakdown by liver; also, ↓ serum levels of chloramphenicol

*Chymotrypsin* / Chloramphenicol will inhibit chymotrypsin
*Cyclophosphamide* / Delayed or ↓ activation of cyclophosphamide
*Iron preparations* / ↑ Serum iron levels
*Penicillins* / Either ↑ or ↓ effect when combined to treat certain microorganisms
*Phenytoin* / ↑ Effect of phenytoin due to ↓ breakdown by liver; also, chloramphenicol levels may be ↑ or ↓
*Rifampin* / ↓ Effect of chloramphenicol due to ↑ breakdown by liver
*Vitamin B$_{12}$* / ↓ Response to vitamin B$_{12}$ when treating pernicious anemia

Dosage ─────────────
• **IV: Chloramphenicol**
**Adults:** 50 mg/kg/day in four equally divided doses q 6 hr. Can be increased to 100 mg/kg/day in severe infections, but dosage should be reduced as soon as possible. **Neonates and children with immature metabolic function:** 25 mg/kg once daily in divided doses q 12 hr. **Neonates, less than 2 kg:** 25 mg/kg once daily. **Neonates, over 2 kg, over 7 days of age:** 50 mg/kg/day q 12 hr in divided doses. **Neonates, over 2 kg, from birth to 7 days of age:** 50 mg/kg once daily. **Children:** 50–75 mg/kg/day in divided doses q 6 hr (50–100 mg/kg/day in divided doses q 6 hr for meningitis). *NOTE:* Carefully follow dosage for premature and newborn infants less than 2 weeks of age because blood levels differ significantly from those of other age groups.
• **Chloramphenicol Sodium Succinate—IV Only**
Same dosage as chloramphenicol (see the preceding). Switch to **PO** as soon as possible.
• **Chloramphenicol Ophthalmic Ointment 1%**
0.5-in. ribbon placed in lower conjunctival sac q 3–4 hr for acute infections and b.i.d.–t.i.d. for mild to moderate infections.

• **Chloramphenicol Ophthalmic Solution 0.5%**
1–2 gtt in lower conjunctival sac 2–6 times/day (or more for acute infections).
• **Chloramphenicol Otic Solution 0.5%**
2–3 gtt in ear t.i.d.
• **Chloramphenicol Topical Cream 1%**
Apply 1–4 times/day.

─────────────

# NURSING CONSIDERATIONS

See also *General Nursing Considerations for All Anti-Infectives.*
**Administration/Storage**
1. When used topically for skin infections, a sterile bandage may be used.
2. To instill in the eye, place the head back and place medication in the conjunctival sac; close eyes. Apply light finger pressure on the lacrimal sac for 1 min.
3. To avoid contamination, the tip of the ophthalmic products should not touch any surface.
4. Contact lenses should not be worn if treating bacterial conjunctivitis. If contact lenses are required, do not insert the lenses for at least 15 min after using any solutions that contain benzalkonium chloride (may be absorbed by the lens).
**IV** 5. Administer IV as a 10% solution over at least a 60-sec interval. Reconstitute 1 g in 10 mL of water for injection or 5% dextrose injection. May further dilute in 50–100 mL of dextrose or saline solution and infuse over 30–60 min.
**Assessment**
1. Note any hypersensitivity, or previous reaction to other agents.
2. Document type, onset, and duration of symptoms; list other agents prescribed. If receiving drugs that cause bone marrow depression, use of chloramphenicol is contraindicated.
3. If nursing, transmission of the drug to breast milk can result in the infant also receiving the drug; infants have underdeveloped capacity to metabolize chloramphenicol.

─────────────

4. If diabetic and taking oral hypoglycemic agents, may need insulin during chloramphenicol therapy.

5. Arrange for frequent hematologic studies to detect early signs of bone marrow depression; may also develop weeks to months following drug therapy.

6. Reduce dose with impaired renal function and in newborn infants.

**Interventions**

1. Note drugs that enhance chloramphenicol; monitor closely for evidence of severe toxicity with concurrent therapy.

2. Avoid repeated courses of therapy; drug is highly toxic.

3. Monitor for the development of any of the following; discontinue drug and report:

• *Bone marrow depression* characterized by weakness, fatigue, sore throat, and bleeding.

• *Optic neuritis* characterized by bilaterally reduced visual acuity.

• *Peripheral neuritis* characterized by pain and disturbance of sensation.

• Development of *gray syndrome* in premature and newborn infants, characterized by rapid respiration, failure to feed, abdominal distention with or without vomiting, loose green stools, progressive cyanosis, and vasomotor collapse.

4. Assess for toxic and irritative effects, such as N&V, unpleasant taste, diarrhea, and perineal irritation following PO administration. Differentiation of drug-induced diarrhea from that caused by a superinfection is critical and may be accomplished by assessment and analysis of all presenting symptoms.

**Client/Family Teaching**

1. Take 1 hr before or 2 hr after meals; if GI upset occurs, may be taken with food.

2. Take at regularly spaced intervals *around the clock.*

3. Avoid alcohol during therapy.

4. Do not take salicylates or NSAIDs.

5. Report any signs of hypersensitivity; e.g., itching and rash.

6. Report any sore throat or any unusual fatigue, bruising, or bleeding as drug may need to be discontinued.

7. Ophthalmic solutions may cause blurred vision immediately after instillation; this should clear.

8. During IV administration a bitter taste may be experienced; should subside after several minutes.

**Outcomes/Evaluate**

• Resolution of infection

• Therapeutic drug level (peak 10–20 mcg/mL; trough 5–10 mcg/mL)

# Chlordiazepoxide

(klor-dye-**AYZ**-eh-**POX**-eyed)

**Pregnancy Category:** D

Apo-Chlordiazepoxide ✹, Corax ✹, Libritabs, Librium, Lipoxide, Medillium ✹, Mitran, Novo-Poxide ✹, Reposans-10 **(C-IV) (Rx)**

**Classification:** Antianxiety agent, benzodiazepine

See also *Tranquilizers, Antimanic Drugs, and Hypnotics.*

**Action/Kinetics: Onset: PO,** 30–60 min; **IM,** 15–30 min (absorption may be slow and erratic); **IV,** 3–30 min. **Peak plasma levels (PO):** 0.5–4 hr. **Duration:** t½: 5–30 hr. Is metabolized to four active metabolites: desmethylchlordiazepoxide, desmethyldiazepam, oxazepam, and demoxepam. Has less anticonvulsant activity and is less potent than diazepam.

**Uses:** Anxiety, acute withdrawal symptoms in chronic alcoholics. Sedative-hypnotic. Preoperatively to reduce anxiety and tension. Tension headache. Antitremor agent (PO). Antipanic (parenteral).

**Additional Side Effects:** Jaundice, acute hepatic necrosis, hepatic dysfunction.

**Laboratory Test Interferences**

1. *Interference with test methods:* ↑ 17-Hydroxycorticosteroids, 17-ketosteroids.

2. *Caused by pharmacologic effects:* ↑ Alkaline phosphatase, bilirubin, serum transaminase, porphobilinogen. ↓ PT (clients on Coumarin).

**Dosage**

- **Capsules, Tablets**
  *Anxiety and tension.*
  **Adults:** 5–10 mg t.i.d.–q.i.d. (up to 20–25 mg t.i.d.–q.i.d. in severe cases). Reduce dose to 5 mg b.i.d.–q.i.d. in geriatric or debilitated clients. **Pediatric, over 6 years, initial,** 5 mg b.i.d.–q.i.d. May be increased to 10 mg b.i.d.–q.i.d.
  *Preoperatively.*
  **Adults:** 5–10 mg t.i.d.–q.i.d. on day before surgery.
  *Alcohol withdrawal/sedative-hypnotic.*
  **Adults:** 50–100 mg; may be increased to 300 mg/day; **then,** reduce to maintenance levels.
- **IM, IV (not recommended for children under 12 years)**
  *Acute/severe agitation, anxiety.*
  **Initial:** 50–100 mg; **then,** 25–50 mg t.i.d.–q.i.d.
  *Preoperatively.*
  **Adults:** 50–100 mg IM 1 hr before surgery.
  *Alcohol withdrawal.*
  **Adults:** 50–100 mg IM or IV; repeat in 2–4 hr if necessary. Dosage should not exceed 300 mg/day.
  *Antipanic.*
  **Adults, initial:** 50–100 mg; dose may be repeated in 4–6 hr if needed.

## NURSING CONSIDERATIONS

See also *Nursing Considerations* for *Tranquilizers, Antimanic Drugs, and Hypnotics.*

**Administration/Storage**

1. **IM:** Prepare solution immediately before administration by adding diluent, which is provided, to ampule. Shake until dissolved. Discard any unused solution. Inject slowly into upper, outer quadrant of gluteal muscle.

**IV** 2. Prepare immediately before administration by diluting with 5 mL of sterile water for injection or sterile 0.9% NaCl solution. Inject directly into vein over 1-min period. Do not add to IV infusion because of instability of drug. Do not use IV solution for IM administration.

**Assessment**

1. Document indications for therapy and pretreatment symptoms.
2. Maintain a quiet, supervised environment; keep recumbent for 3 hr following parenteral administration.
3. Obtain liver function studies if impairment is suspected.

**Client/Family Teaching**

1. Take with food and as directed.
2. Consume extra fluids and bulk to minimize constipating effects.
3. Use caution, may cause dizziness and drowsiness.
4. Avoid all OTC agents, alcohol, and any other CNS depressants without approval.

**Outcomes/Evaluate**

- ↓ Tremors; ↓ anxiety
- Sedation; control of panic episodes
- ↓ Alcohol withdrawal symptoms

# Chloroquine hydrochloride
(**KLOR**-oh-kwin)
Aralen HCl **(Rx)**

# Chloroquine phosphate
(**KLOR**-oh-kwin)
Aralen Phosphate, Novo-Chloroquine ✹ **(Rx)**
**Classification:** 4-Aminoquinoline, antimalarial, amebicide

See also *Antimalarial Drugs, 4-Aminoquinolines.*
**Special Concerns:** Use during pregnancy only if benefits outweigh risks.
**Additional Side Effects:** Chloroquine may exacerbate psoriasis and precipitate an acute attack.
**Drug Interactions**
*Cimetidine* / ↓ Oral clearance rate and metabolism of chloroquine
*Kaolin* / ↓ Effect of chloroquine due to ↓ absorption from GI tract
*Magnesium trisilicate* / ↓ Effect of chloroquine due to ↓ absorption from GI tract

---

✹ = Available in Canada                 ***bold italic*** = life threatening side effect

**C**

**Dosage**
- **Tablets (Chloroquine Phosphate)**

*Acute malarial attack.*
**Adults, Day 1:** 1 g (600 mg base); **then,** 500 mg (300 mg base) 6 hr later. **Days 2 and 3:** 500 mg/day (300 mg base/day). **Children, Day 1:** 10 mg base/kg; **then,** 5 mg base/kg 6 hr later. **Days 2 and 3:** 5 mg base/kg/day.

*Suppression (prophylaxis) of malaria.*
**Adults:** 500 mg/week (300 mg base/week) on same day each week. If therapy has not been initiated 14 days before exposure, an initial loading dose of 1 g (600 mg base) may be given in 500-mg doses 6 hr apart. **Children:** 5 mg base/kg/week, not to exceed the adult dose of 300 mg of the base, given on same day each week. If therapy has not been initiated 14 days before exposure, an initial loading dose of 10 mg/kg of the base may be given in two divided doses 6 hr apart.

*Extraintestinal amebiasis.*
**Adults:** 1 g (600 mg base) given as 250 mg q.i.d. for 2 days; **then,** 500 mg (300 mg base) given as 250 mg b.i.d. for 2–3 weeks (combine with an intestinal amebicide). **Children:** 10 mg/kg (not to exceed 500 mg) daily for 3 weeks.

- **IM (Chloroquine Hydrochloride)**

*Acute malarial attack.*
**Adults, initial:** 200–250 mg (160–200 mg base); repeat dosage in 6 hr if necessary. Total daily dose in first 24 hr should not exceed 1 g (800 mg base). Begin PO therapy as soon as possible. **IM, SC. Children and infants:** 6.25 mg/kg (5 mg base/kg) repeated in 6 hr; dose should not exceed 12.5 mg/kg/day (10 mg base/kg/day).

*Extraintestinal amebiasis.*
**Adults:** 200–250 mg/day (160–200 mg of the base) for 10–12 days. Begin PO therapy as soon as possible. **Children:** 7.5 mg/kg/day for 10–12 days.

- **IV Infusion (Chloroquine Hydrochloride)**

*Acute malarial attack.*
**Adults, initial:** 16.6 mg/kg over 8 hr; **then,** 8.3 mg/kg q 6–8 hr by continuous infusion.

---

## NURSING CONSIDERATIONS

See also *Nursing Considerations* for *Antimalarial Drugs, 4-Aminoquinolines.*

**Assessment**
1. Document indications for therapy and onset of symptoms.
2. Determine any history of psoriasis; drug may exacerbate condition and precipitate an acute attack.
3. Note drugs currently prescribed to prevent any unfavorable interactions.

**Client/Family Teaching**
1. Take only as directed; complete prescribed course of therapy.
2. To minimize GI upset, take with food.
3. Avoid activities that require mental alertness until drug effects realized; drug may cause dizziness.
4. Avoid direct sun exposure; wear protective clothing, sunglasses, and sunscreens.
5. Urine may be discolored dark yellow or reddish brown.
6. Review appropriate methods for protection against mosquitoes, i.e., long pants and long-sleeved shirts, repellents, and netting or screens.
7. Avoid ingestion of alcohol in any form.

**Outcomes/Evaluate**
- Symptomatic improvement
- Negative culture reports
- Malarial prophylaxis

---

# Chlorothiazide
(klor-oh-**THIGH**-ah-zyd)
**Pregnancy Category:** C
Diurigen, Diuril **(Rx)**

# Chlorothiazide sodium
(klor-oh-**THIGH**-ah-zyd)
**Pregnancy Category:** C
Sodium Diuril **(Rx)**
**Classification:** Diuretic, thiazide type

See also *Diuretics, Thiazides*.

**Action/Kinetics: Onset:** 2 hr for PO, 15 min for IV; **Peak effect:** 4 hr for PO, 30 min for IV; **Duration:** 6–12 hr. **t½:** 45–120 min. Incompletely absorbed from the GI tract. Produces a greater diuretic effect if given in divided doses. Also found in Diupres.

**Special Concerns:** Geriatric clients may be more sensitive to the usual adult dose.

**Additional Side Effects:** Hypotension, renal failure, renal dysfunction, interstitial nephritis. Following IV use: Alopecia, hematuria, exfoliative dermatitis, toxic epidermal necrolysis, erythema multiforme, ***Stevens-Johnson syndrome.***

**Dosage**

• **Oral Suspension, Tablets, IV**
  *Diuretic.*
**Adults:** 0.5–2 g 1–2 times/day either PO or IV (reserved for clients unable to take PO medication or in emergencies). Some clients may respond to the drug given 3–5 days each week.
  *Antihypertensive.*
**Adults, IV, PO:** 0.5–1 g/day in one or more divided doses. **Pediatric, 6 months and older, PO:** 22 mg/kg/day (10 mg/lb/day) in two divided doses; **6 months and younger, PO:** 33 mg/kg/day (15 mg/lb/day) in two divided doses. Thus, children up to 2 years of age may be given 125–375 mg/day in two doses while children 2–12 years of age may be given 375 mg–1 g/day in two doses. IV use in children is not recommended.

**NURSING CONSIDERATIONS**

See also *Nursing Considerations* for *Diuretics, Thiazides,* and *Antihypertensive Agents*.

**Administration/Storage**
1. Do not give SC or IM.
**IV** 2. IV use not recommended for children; should be reserved for adults in emergency situations or those unable to take medication PO.
3. To obtain an isotonic solution for injection, add 18 mL sterile water for injection to 500 mg powder and administer over 5 min.
4. Avoid simultaneous administration of whole blood or derivatives.
5. IV solution is compatible with NaCL or dextrose solutions.
6. Discard unused reconstituted solutions after 24 hr.

**Assessment:** List drugs currently prescribed; note any sulfa allergy.

**Client/Family Teaching**
1. May cause orthostatic hypotension; use caution when rising or changing positions.
2. Follow high-potassium diet, if prescribed.
3. Use sun screens (avoid ones with PABA), sunglasses, and protective clothing to diminish drug's photosensitivity effects.
4. Avoid alcohol and any OTC agents without provider approval.

**Outcomes/Evaluate**
• ↓ BP
• Enhanced diuresis with ↓ edema

# Chlorpheniramine maleate

(klor-fen-**EAR**-ah-meen)
**Pregnancy Category:** B
**Syrup, Tablets, Chewable Tablets:** Aller-Chlor, Allergy, Chlo-Amine, Chlor-Trimeton Allergy 4 Hour, Chlor-Tripolon ✿ **(OTC), Extended-release Tablets:** Chlor-Trimeton 8 Hour and 12 Hour **(OTC), Injectable:** Chlorpheniramine maleate **(Rx)**
**Classification:** Antihistamine, alkylamine type

See also *Antihistamines*.
**Action/Kinetics:** Moderate anticholinergic and low sedative activity. **Onset:** 15–30 min **t½:** 21–27 hr. **Time to peak effect:** 6 hr. **Duration:** 3–6hr.
**Uses:** *PO:* Allergic rhinitis. *IM, SC:* Allergic reactions to blood and plasma and adjunct to anaphylaxis therapy.
**Contraindications:** IV or intradermal use. Not recommended for children under 6 years of age.
**Special Concerns:** Geriatric clients may be more sensitive to the adult

dose. Parenteral route not recommended for neonates.

## Dosage
• **Syrup, Tablets, Chewable Tablets**
**Adults and children over 12 years:** 4 mg q 6 hr, not to exceed 24 mg in 24 hr. **Pediatric, 6–12 years:** 2 mg (break 4-mg tablets in half) q 4–6 hr, not to exceed 12 mg in 24 hr. **2–6 years:** 1 mg (¼ of a 4-mg tablet) q 4–6 hr.
• **Extended-Release Tablets**
**Adults and children over 12 years:** 8 mg q 8–12 hr or 12 mg q 12 hr, not to exceed 24 mg in 24 hr.
• **IM, SC**
**Adults and children over 12 years:** 5–40 mg for uncomplicated allergic reactions; 10–20 mg for amelioration of allergic reactions to blood or plasma or to treat anaphylaxis. Maximum dose per 24 hr: 40 mg.

## NURSING CONSIDERATIONS

See also *Nursing Considerations* for *Antihistamines.*
**Client/Family Teaching**
1. Absorption is delayed if given with food.
2. May cause drowsiness; use caution.
3. Avoid alcohol in any form.
4. Anticipate dry mouth and use appropriate remedies.
**Outcomes/Evaluate:** ↓ Nasal congestion and associated allergic manifestations

---

# Chlorpromazine
(klor-**PROH**-mah-zeen)
Thorazine **(Rx)**

# Chlorpromazine hydrochloride
(klor-**PROH**-mah-zeen)
Apo-Chlorpromazine ✤, Chlorprom ✤, Chlorpromanyl ✤, Largactil ✤, Novo–Chlorpromazine ✤, Ormazine, Thorazine, Thor-Prom **(Rx)**
**Classification:** Antipsychotic, dimethylamino-type phenothiazine

See also *Antipsychotic Agents, Phenothiazines.*
**Action/Kinetics:** Has significant antiemetic, hypotensive, and sedative effects; moderate to strong anticholinergic effects and weak to moderate extrapyramidal effects. **Peak plasma levels:** 2–3 hr after both PO and IM administration. **t½** (after IV, IM): **Initial,** 4–5 hr; **final,** 3–40 hr. Extensively metabolized in the intestinal wall and liver; certain of the metabolites are active. **Steady-state plasma levels** (in psychotics): 10–1,300 ng/mL. After 2–3 weeks of therapy, plasma levels decline, possibly because of reduction in drug absorption and/or increase in drug metabolism.
**Uses:** Acute and chronic psychoses, including schizophrenia; manic phase of manic-depressive illness. Acute intermittent porphyria. Preanesthetic, adjunct to treat tetanus, intractable hiccoughs, severe behavioral problems in children, neuroses, and N&V. Treatment of choreiform movements in Huntington's disease.
**Special Concerns:** Use during pregnancy only if benefits outweigh risks. PO dosage for psychoses and N&V has not been established in children less than 6 months of age.
**Additional Drug Interactions**
*Epinephrine* / Chlorpromazine ↓ peripheral vasoconstriction and may reverse action of epinephrine
*Norepinephrine* / Chlorpromazine ↓ pressor effect and eliminates bradycardia due to norepinephrine
*Valproic acid* / ↑ Effect of valproic acid due to ↓ clearance

## Dosage
• **Tablets, Extended-Release Capsules, Oral Concentrate, Syrup**
*Psychotic disorders.*
**Adults and adolescents:** 10–25 mg (of the base) b.i.d.–q.i.d.; dosage may be increased by 20–50 mg/day q 3–4 days as needed. Or, 30–300 mg (of the base) using the extended-release capsules 1–3 times/day (the 300-mg extended-release capsules are used only in severe neuropsychi-

atric situations). **Pediatric:** 0.55 mg/
kg (15 mg/m²) q 4–6 hr.
*N&V.*
**Adults and adolescents:** 10–25 mg
(of the base) q 4 hr; dosage may be
increased as needed. **Pediatric:** 0.55
mg/kg (15 mg/m²) q 4–6 hr.
*Preoperative sedation.*
**Adults and adolescents:** 25–50 mg
(of the base) 2–3 hr before surgery.
**Pediatric:** 0.55 mg/kg (15 mg/m²)
2–3 hr before surgery.
*Hiccoughs or porphyria.*
**Adults and adolescents:** 25–50 mg
(of the base) t.i.d.–q.i.d.
• **IM**
*Severe psychoses.*
**Adults:** 25–50 mg (of the base)
repeated in 1 hr if needed; **then,** repeat the dose q 3–4 hr as needed
and tolerated (the dose may be increased gradually over several days).
**Pediatric, over 6 months:** 0.55
mg/kg (15 mg/m²) q 6–8 hr as needed.
*N&V.*
**Adults:** 25 mg (base) as a single
dose; **then,** increase to 25–50 mg q
3–4 hr as needed until vomiting
ceases. **Pediatric:** 0.55 mg/kg q 6–8
hr as needed.
*N&V during surgery.*
**Adults:** 12.5 mg (base) as a single
dose; repeat in 30 min if needed. **Pediatric,** 0.275 mg/kg; repeat in 30
min if needed.
*Preoperative sedative.*
**Adults:** 12.5–25 mg (base) 1–2 hr
before surgery. **Pediatric:** 0.55 mg/
kg 1–2 hr before surgery.
*Hiccoughs.*
**Adults:** 25–50 mg (base) t.i.d.–q.i.d.
*Porphyria.*
**Adults:** 25 mg (base) q 6–8 hr until
client can take PO therapy.
*Tetanus.*
**Adults:** 25–50 mg (base) t.i.d.–q.i.d.
(dose can be increased as needed
and tolerated).
• **IV**
*N&V during surgery.*
**Adults:** 25 mg (base) diluted to 1
mg/mL with 0.9% NaCl injection giv-
en at a rate of no more than 2 mg/2

min. **Pediatric:** 0.275 mg/kg diluted
to 1 mg/mL with 0.9% NaCl injection
given at a rate of no more than 1 mg
q 2 min.
*Tetanus.*
**Adults:** 25–50 mg (base) diluted to 1
mg/mL with 0.9% NaCl injection and
given at a rate of 1 mg/min. **Pediatric:**
0.55 mg/kg diluted to 1 mg/mL with
0.9% NaCl injection and given at a rate
of 1 mg/2 min.
• **Suppositories**
*N&V.*
**Adults and adolescents:** 50–100
mg q 6–8 hr as needed up to a maximum of 400 mg/day. **Pediatric:** 1
mg/kg q 6–8 hr as needed (do not use
the 100-mg suppository in children).

## NURSING CONSIDERATIONS

See also *Nursing Considerations* for
*Antipsychotic Agents, Phenothia-
zines.*
**Administration/Storage**
1. The maximum daily PO and
parenteral dose for adults and adolescents should be 1 g of the base.
2. Swallow sustained-release capsules whole.
3. The concentrate (to be used in
hospitals only) can be mixed with 60
mL or more of fruit or tomato juice,
orange or simple syrup, milk, carbonated drinks, coffee, tea, water, or
semisolid foods (e.g., soup, pudding).
4. When administering the drug IM,
select a large, well-developed muscle
mass. Use the dorsogluteal site or
rectus femoris in adults and the vastus lateralis in children; rotate injection
sites.
5. The maximum IM dose should be
40 mg/day for children up to 5 years
of age and 75 mg/day for children
5–12 years of age.
6. Solutions of chlorpromazine may
cause contact dermatitis; avoid getting
solution on hands or clothing.
7. Slight discoloration of injection or
PO solutions will not affect the action
of the drug.
**IV** 8. When used IV in children for
tetanus, dilute the preparation to 1

mg/mL and give at a rate of 1 mg/2 min.

9. Discard solutions with marked discoloration. Consult with pharmacist if unsure of drug potency.

**Assessment**

1. Note any seizure disorders; drug may be contraindicated.

2. Obtain baseline CBC, liver and renal function studies.

3. Assess male clients for S&S of prostatic hypertrophy.

**Client/Family Teaching**

1. Review side effects; report any extrapyramidal symptoms, especially tardive dyskinesia.

2. Urine may become discolored pinkish to brown.

3. Protect self during sun exposure; exposed skin surfaces may develop pigmentation changes.

4. Use caution when performing activities that require mental alertness.

5. Avoid alcohol and any other CNS depressants; may potentiate orthostatic hypotension.

6. Perform frequent toothbrushing and flossing to discourage oral fungal infections.

7. Report any unusual bruising or bleeding, fever, sore throat, or malaise.

8. Avoid temperature extremes; drug may impair body's ability to regulate temperature.

9. Therapeutic psychologic effects may require 7–8 weeks of therapy.

**Outcomes/Evaluate**

- ↓ Psychotic/manic manifestations
- Control of N&V
- Cessation of hiccoughs
- Sedation; control of muscular twitching

# Chlorpropamide

(klor-**PROH**-pah-myd)

**Pregnancy Category:** C

Apo-Chlorpropamide ✦, Diabinese, Novo–Propamide ✿ **(Rx)**

**Classification:** Sulfonylurea, first-generation

See also *Antidiabetic Agents: Hypoglycemic Agents and Insulin.*

**Action/Kinetics:** May be effective in clients who do not respond well to other antidiabetic agents. **Onset:** 1 hr. **t½:** 35 hr. **Time to peak levels:** 2–4 hr. **Duration:** Up to 60 hr (due to slow excretion). Eighty percent metabolized in liver; 80%–90% excreted in the urine.

**Additional Use:** *Investigational:* Neurogenic diabetes insipidus.

**Special Concerns:** If the client is susceptible to fluid retention or has impaired cardiac function, frequent monitoring is necessary.

**Additional Side Effects:** Side effects are frequent. Severe diarrhea, occasionally accompanied by bleeding in the lower bowel. Relieve severe GI distress by dividing total daily dose in half. In older clients, hypoglycemia may be severe. Inappropriate ADH secretion, leading to hyponatremia, water retention, low serum osmolality, and high urine osmolality.

**Additional Drug Interactions**

*Ammonium chloride* / ↑ Effect of chlorpropamide due to ↓ excretion by kidney

*Disulfiram* / More likely to interact with chlorpropamide than other oral antidiabetics

*Probenecid* / ↑ Effect of chlorpropamide

*Sodium bicarbonate* / ↓ Effect of chlorpropamide due to ↑ excretion by kidney

**Dosage** ———————
- **Tablets**

  *Diabetes.*

**Adults, middle-aged clients, mild to moderate diabetes, initial:** 250 mg/day as a single or divided dose; **geriatric, initial:** 100–125 mg/day. **All clients, maintenance:** 100–250 mg/day as single or divided doses. Severe diabetics may require 500 mg/" day; doses greater than 750 mg/day are not recommended.

  *Neurogenic diabetes insipidus.*
**Adults:** 200–500 mg/day.

## NURSING CONSIDERATIONS

See also *Nursing Considerations* for *Hypoglycemic Agents (Including Sulfonylureas).*

## Assessment

1. Elderly clients tend to be more sensitive to hypoglycemic agents and exhibit more side effects.
2. Determine if pregnant; drug is contraindicated.
3. Obtain baseline CBC, HbA1C, and LFTs.
4. Assess for cardiac dysfunction or fluid retention. Monitor I&O, serum electrolytes, and urine osmolality.

**Client/Family Teaching**
1. Record weight and BP.
2. Report any confusion, dizziness, depression, or nausea; these may be symptoms of inappropriate ADH secretion.
3. Review weight loss, diet, and exercise guidelines.

**Outcomes/Evaluate:** Normalization of serum glucose levels

# Chlorthalidone

(klor-**THAL**-ih-dohn)
**Pregnancy Category:** B
Apo-Chlorthalidone ✹, Hygroton, Novo-Thalidone ✹, Thalitone, Uridon ✹ **(Rx)**
**Classification:** Diuretic, thiazide

See also *Diuretics, Thiazides.*
**Action/Kinetics: Onset:** 2–3 hr. **Peak effect:** 2–6 hr. **Duration:** 24–72 hr. **t½:** 40 hr. Bioavailability may be dose-dependent.
**Additional Use:** To potentiate and reduce dosage of other antihypertensive agents.
**Special Concerns:** Geriatric clients may be more sensitive to the usual adult dose.
**Additional Side Effects:** Exfoliative dermatitis, toxic epidermal necrolysis.

## Dosage

• **Tablets**
   *Edema.*
**Adults, initial:** 50–100 mg/day (30–60 mg Thalitone) or 100–200 mg (60 mg Thalitone) on alternate days. Some clients require 150 or 200 mg (90–120 mg Thalitone). **Maximum daily dose:** 200 mg (120 mg Thali-

tone). **Pediatric:** All uses, 2 mg/kg (60 mg/m²) 3 times/week.
   *Hypertension.*
**Adults, initial:** Single dose of 25 mg (15 mg Thalitone); if response is not sufficient, dose may be increased to 50 mg (30 mg Thalitone). For additional control, increase the dose to 100 mg/day (except Thalitone) or a second antihypertensive drug may be added to the regimen. **Maintenance:** Determined by client response. *NOTE:* Doses greater than 25 mg/day are likely to increase potassium excretion but not cause further benefit in sodium excretion or BP reduction.

## NURSING CONSIDERATIONS

See *Nursing Considerations* for *Diuretics, Thiazides and Antihypertensive Agents.*
**Administration/Storage**
1. Initiate with the lowest possible dose. Maintenance doses may be lower than initial doses.
2. Doses higher than 25 mg/day will increase potassium excretion but will not cause further benefit in sodium excretion or reduction of BP.
**Assessment**
1. Note indications for therapy, other agents trialed, and the outcome.
2. Monitor CBC, electrolytes, glucose, BUN, and creatinine.
**Client/Family Teaching:** Take in the morning with food.
**Outcomes/Evaluate**
• Enhanced diuresis; ↓ edema
• ↓ BP

# Chlorzoxazone

(klor-**ZOX**-ah-zohn)
Paraflex, Parafon Forte DSC, Remular-S **(Rx)**
**Classification:** Muscle relaxant, centrally acting

See also *Skeletal Muscle Relaxants, Centrally Acting.*
**Action/Kinetics:** Inhibits polysynaptic reflexes at both the spinal cord and subcortical areas of the brain.

Effects may also be due to sedation. **Onset:** 1 hr. **Time to peak blood levels:** 1–2 hr. **Peak serum levels:** 10–30 mcg/mL (after 750-mg dose). **Duration:** 3–4 hr. **t½:** 1 hr. Metabolized in the liver and inactive metabolites excreted in the urine.

**Uses:** As adjunct to rest, physical therapy, and other approaches for treatment of acute, painful musculoskeletal conditions (e.g., muscle spasms, sprains, muscle strain).

**Special Concerns:** Use during pregnancy only if benefits clearly outweigh risks. Use with caution in clients with known allergies or a history of allergic reactions to drugs.

**Side Effects:** *CNS:* Dizziness, drowsiness, malaise, lightheadedness, overstimulation. *Dermatologic:* Allergic-type skin rashes, petechiae, ecchymoses (rare). *GI:* GI upset, GI bleeding (rare). *Allergic Reactions:* **Angioneurotic edema, anaphylaxis** (rare). *Miscellaneous:* Discoloration of urine, liver damage.

**OD Overdose Management:** *Symptoms:* N&V, diarrhea, drowsiness, dizziness, lightheadedness, headache, malaise, sluggishness. May be followed by marked loss of muscle tone (voluntary movement may be impossible), decreased or absent deep tendon reflexes, respiratory depression, decreased BP. *Treatment:* Supportive.

**Dosage** ⎯⎯⎯⎯⎯⎯⎯⎯⎯⎯
• **Tablets**
*Skeletal muscle disorders.*
**Adults:** 250–750 mg t.i.d.–q.i.d. with meals and at bedtime; **pediatric:** 125–500 mg t.i.d.–q.i.d. (or 20 mg/kg in three to four divided doses daily).

## NURSING CONSIDERATIONS

See also *Nursing Considerations* for *Skeletal Muscle Relaxants, Centrally Acting.*
**Assessment**
1. Document indications for therapy; note pretreatment findings.
2. During physical exam test for weakness, stiffness, ROM, reflexes;

with low-back pain, perform rectal exam and note sphincter tone.
3. Obtain baseline liver and renal function studies; assess for dysfunction.

**Client/Family Teaching**
1. May take with food if GI upset occurs.
2. May be mixed with food or beverages for administration to children.
3. Do not operate dangerous machinery or drive a car until drug effects evident; causes drowsiness.
4. Drug may cause urine to have an orange or purple-red color when exposed to the air.
5. Review importance of RICE (rest, ice, compression, and elevation) in the setting of an acute injury.
6. Do not overuse extremity during therapy; drug may mask pathology.
7. Return to provider in 3 weeks if no improvement in symptoms.
**Outcomes/Evaluate:** Relief of musculoskeletal spasm and pain

# Cholestyramine resin
(koh-less-**TEER**-ah-meen)
Alti-Cholestyramine Light ✦, Lo-Cholest, Novo-Cholaine Light ✦, PMS-Cholestyramine ✦, Prevalite, Questran, Questran Light **(Rx)**
**Classification:** Hypocholesterolemic agent, bile acid sequestrant

**Action/Kinetics:** Binds sodium cholate (bile salts) in the intestine; thus, the principal precursor of cholesterol is not absorbed due to formation of an insoluble complex, which is excreted in the feces. Decreases cholesterol and LDL and either has no effect or increases triglycerides, VLDL, and HDL. Also, itching is relieved as a result of removing irritating bile salts. The antidiarrheal effect results from the binding and removal of bile acids. **Onset, to reduce plasma cholesterol:** Within 24–48 hr, but levels may continue to fall for 1 yr; **to relieve pruritus:** 1–3 weeks; **relief of diarrhea associated with bile acids:** 24 hr. Cholesterol levels return to pretreatment levels 2–4 weeks after discontinuance. Fat-soluble vitamins (A, D, K) and possibly folic acid may have to be administered IM during long-term therapy because cholestyramine binds these vitamins in the intestine.

**Uses:** Adjunct to reduce elevated serum cholesterol in primary hypercholesterolemia in those who do not respond adequately to diet. Pruritus associated with partial biliary obstruction. Diarrhea due to bile acids. *Investigational:* Antibiotic-induced pseudomembranous colitis (i.e., due to toxin produced by *Clostridium difficile*), digitalis toxicity, treatment of chlordecone (Kepone) poisoning, treatment of thyroid hormone overdose.

**Contraindications:** Complete obstruction or atresia of bile duct.

**Special Concerns:** Use during pregnancy only if benefits outweigh risks. Use with caution during lactation and in children. Long-term effects and efficacy in decreasing cholesterol levels in pediatric clients are not known. Geriatric clients may be more likely to manifest GI side effects as well as adverse nutritional effects. Caution should be exercised by phenylketonurics as Prevalite contains 14.1 mg phenylalanine per 5.5-g dose.

**Side Effects:** *GI:* Constipation (may be severe), N&V, diarrhea, heartburn, GI bleeding, anorexia, flatulence, belching, abdominal distention, abdominal pain or cramping, loose stools, indigestion, aggravation of hemorrhoids, rectal bleeding or pain, black stools, bleeding duodenal ulcer, peptic ulceration, GI irritation, dysphagia, dental bleeding, hiccoughs, sour taste, pancreatitis, diverticulitis, cholescystitis, cholelithiasis. Fecal impaction in elderly clients. Large doses may cause steatorrhea. *CNS:* Migraine or sinus headaches, dizziness, anxiety, vertigo, insomnia, fatigue, lightheadedness, syncope, drowsiness, femoral nerve pain, paresthesia. *Hypersensitivity:* Urticaria, dermatitis, asthma, wheezing, rash. *Hematologic:* Increased PT, ecchymosis, anemia. *Musculoskeletal:* Muscle or joint pain, backache, arthritis, osteoporosis. *GU:* Hematuria, dysuria, burnt odor to urine, diuresis. *Other:* Bleeding tendencies (due to hypoprothrombinemia). Deficiencies of vitamins A and D. Uveitis, weight loss or gain, osteoporosis, swollen glands, increased libido, weakness, SOB, edema, swelling of hands/feet; hyperchloremic acidosis in children, rash and irritation of the skin, tongue, and perianal area.

**OD** **Overdose Management:** *Symptoms:* GI tract obstruction.

**Drug Interactions**

*Anticoagulants, PO* / ↓ Anticoagulant effect due to ↓ absorption from GI tract

*Aspirin* / ↓ Absorption of aspirin from GI tract

*Clindamycin* / ↓ Absorption of clindamycin from GI tract

*Clofibrate* / ↓ Absorption of clofibrate from GI tract

*Digitalis glycosides* / ↓ Effect of digitalis due to ↓ absorption from the GI tract

*Furosemide* / ↓ Absorption of furosemide from GI tract

*Gemfibrozil* / ↓ Bioavailability of gemfibrozil

*Glipizide* / ↓ Serum glipizide levels

*Hydrocortisone* / ↓ Effect of hydrocortisone due to ↓ absorption from GI tract

*Imipramine* / ↓ Absorption of imipramine from GI tract

*Iopanoic acid* / Results in abnormal cholecystography

*Lovastatin* / Effects may be additive

*Methyldopa* / ↓ Absorption of methyldopa from GI tract

*Nicotinic acid* / ↓ Absorption of nicotinic acid from GI tract

*Penicillin G* / ↓ Effect of penicillin G due to ↓ absorption from GI tract

*Phenytoin* / ↓ Absorption of phenytoin from GI tract

*Phosphate supplements* / ↓ Absorption of phosphate supplements from GI tract

*Piroxicam* / ↑ Elimination

*Propranolol* / ↓ Effect of propranolol due to ↓ absorption from GI tract

*Tetracyclines* / ↓ Effect of tetracyclines due to ↓ absorption from GI tract

*Thiazide diuretics* / ↓ Effect of thiazides due to ↓ absorption from GI tract

*Thyroid hormones* / ↓ Effect of thyroid hormones due to ↓ absorption from GI tract

*Tolbutamide* / ↓ Absorption of tolbutamide from GI tract

*Ursodiol* / ↓ Effect of ursodiol due to ↓ absorption from GI tract

*Vitamins A, D, E, K* / Malabsorption of fat-soluble vitamins

*NOTE:* These drug interactions may also be observed with colestipol.

**Laboratory Test Interferences:** Liver function abnormalities.

### Dosage
**• Powder**

**Adults, initial:** 1 g 1–2 times/day. Dose is individualized. **Maintenance:** 2–4 packets or scoopfuls/day (8–16 g anhydrous cholestyramine resin) mixed with 60–180 mL water or noncarbonated beverage. The recommended dosing schedule is b.i.d. but it can be given in one to six doses/day. Maximum daily dose: 6 packets or scoopfuls.

## NURSING CONSIDERATIONS
### Administration/Storage
1. Always mix powder with 60–180 mL water or noncarbonated beverage before administering because resin may cause esophageal irritation or blockage. Highly liquid soups or pulpy fruits such as applesauce or crushed pineapple may also be used.
2. After placing contents of 1 packet of resin on the surface of 4–6 oz of fluid, allow it to stand without stirring for 2 min, occasionally twirling the glass, and then stir slowly (to prevent foaming) to form a suspension.
3. Avoid inhaling the powder while mixing as it may be irritating to mucous membranes.

4. Cholestyramine may interfere with the absorption of other drugs taken orally; thus, take other drug(s) 1 hr before or 4–6 hr after cholestyramine.

### Assessment
1. Document type and onset of symptoms, and other agents trialed.
2. Determine onset of pruritus and note bile acid level.
3. Monitor CBC, cholesterol profile, and liver and renal function studies.
4. Vitamins A, D, E, K, and folic acid will need to be administered in a water-miscible form during long-term therapy.
5. Assess skin and eyes for evidence of jaundice or bile deposits.

### Client/Family Teaching
1. Other prescribed medications should be taken at least 1 hr before or 4 hr after taking antihyperlipidemic medication. These drugs interfere with the absorption and desired effects of other medications.
2. Review constipating effects of drug and ways to control: daily exercise, fluid intake of 2.5–3 L/day, increased intake of citrus fruits, fruit juices, and high-fiber foods; also, a stool softener may help. If persistent constipation, despite efforts to avoid, a change in dosage or drug may be indicated.
3. Clients with high cholesterol levels should follow dietary restrictions of fat and cholesterol as well as smoking cessation, alcohol reduction, and regular exercise.
4. Report tarry stools or abnormal bleeding as supplemental vitamin K (10 mg/week) may be necessary. CBC, PT, and renal function tests should be done routinely.
5. If diarrhea develops, stop constipation measures, record I&O, and weight and report.
6. Pruritus may subside 1–3 weeks after taking the drug but may return after the medication is discontinued. Corn starch or oatmeal baths may also assist to alleviate symptoms.

### Outcomes/Evaluate
• Control of pruritus
• ↓ Serum cholesterol levels
• ↓ Diarrheal stools

• ↓ Bile acid levels

# Chorionic gonadotropin (HCG)

(kor-ee-**ON**-ik go-**NAD**-oh-troh-pin)

**Pregnancy Category:** X

A.P.L., Chorex-5 and -10, Choron 10, Gonic, Pregnyl, Profasi, Profasi HP ✦ **(Rx)**

**Classification:** Gonadotropic hormone

**Action/Kinetics:** The actions of HCG, produced by the trophoblasts of the fertilized ovum and then by the placenta, resemble those of LH. In males, HCG stimulates androgen production by the testes, the development of secondary sex characteristics, and testicular descent when no anatomic impediment is present. In women, HCG stimulates progesterone production by the corpus luteum and completes expulsion of the ovum from a mature follicle. HCG has not been demonstrated to be effective as an adjunct to treat obesity; there is no significant evidence that HCG causes a more attractive or "normal" distribution of fat or that it decreases hunger and discomfort due to calorie-restricted diets.

**Uses:** *Males:* Prepubertal cryptorchidism, hypogonadism due to pituitary insufficiency. *Females:* Infertility not due to primary ovarian failure (used with menotropins).

**Contraindications:** Precocious puberty, prostatic cancer or other androgen-dependent neoplasm, hypersensitivity to drug. Development of precocious puberty is cause for discontinuance of therapy. Pregnancy.

**Special Concerns:** Since HCG increases androgen production, drug should be used with caution in clients in whom androgen-induced edema may be harmful (epilepsy, migraines, asthma, cardiac or renal diseases). Use with caution during lactation. Safety and efficacy have not been shown in children less than 4 years of age.

**Side Effects:** *CNS:* Headache, irritability, restlessness, depression, fatigue, aggressive behavior. *GU:* Precocious puberty, ovarian hyperstimulation syndrome, ovarian malignancy (rare), *enlargement of preexisting ovarian cysts with possible rupture.* *Miscellaneous:* Edema, gynecomastia, pain at injection site, fluid retention, arterial thromboembolism.

## Dosage

• **IM Only**

*Prepubertal cryptorchidism, not due to anatomic obstruction.*

Various regimens including (1) 4,000 USP units 3 times/week for 3 weeks; (2) 5,000 USP units every other day for 4 injections; (3) 15 injections over a period of 6 weeks of 500–1,000 USP units/injection; (4) 500 USP units 3 times/week for 4–6 weeks; may be repeated after 1 month using 1,000 USP units.

*Hypogonadotropic hypogonadism in males.*

The following regimens may be used: (1) 500–1,000 USP units 3 times/week for 3 weeks; **then,** same dose twice weekly for 3 weeks; (2) 4,000 USP units 3 times/week for 6–9 months; then, 2,000 USP units 3 times/week for 3 more months; (3) 1,000–2,000 USP units 3 times/week.

## NURSING CONSIDERATIONS

### Administration/Storage

1. Reconstituted solutions are stable for 1–3 months, depending on manufacturer, when stored at 2°C–8°C (35°F–46°F).

2. Have emergency drugs and equipment available in the event of an acute allergic response.

### Assessment

1. Document indications for therapy, symptom onset, and clinical presentation.

2. Note any drug sensitivity.

3. Assess prepubescent male for appearance of secondary sex characteristics, as drug is contraindicated.

---

✦ = Available in Canada     ***bold italic*** = life threatening side effect

**Client/Family Teaching**
1. Review indications for therapy and the anticipated results.
2. May cause pain at injection site.
3. Record daily weights and report extent of edema; edema is common.
4. Delayed menses, excessive menstrual bleeding, pain in the pelvic region, weakness, and fatigue are S&S of ectopic pregnancy; report immediately.
5. Discuss possibility of multiple births when used with menotropins.
6. With corpus luteum deficiency, if bleeding occurs after day 15 of therapy, hold drug and report.
7. Report headache, easy fatigue, and restlessness; if increasingly irritable, depressed, and changes in attention to physical appearance occur, the drug may have to be withdrawn.
8. Gynecomastia may develop in young males; offer emotional support. Report the beginning of secondary sex characteristics, as this is an indication of sexual precocity and the drug should be withdrawn
9. With cryptorchidism, examine weekly for testicular descent.
10. Return for follow-up visits to monitor the effectiveness of drug therapy.

**Outcomes/Evaluate**
• Testicular descent
• Functional spermatozoa
• ↑ Progesterone → ovum release
• Sexual maturation

# Ciclopirox olamine
(sye-kloh-**PEER**-ox)
**Pregnancy Category:** B
Loprox **(Rx)**
**Classification:** Broad-spectrum topical antifungal

**Action/Kinetics:** At lower concentrations the drug blocks the transport of amino acids into the cell, whereas at higher concentrations the cell membrane of the fungus is altered so that intracellular material leaks out. May also inhibit synthesis of RNA, DNA, and protein in growing fungal cells. A small amount of drug is absorbed through the skin; it also penetrates to the sebaceous glands and dermis as well as into the hair.
**Uses:** Effective against dermatophytes, yeast, *Malassezia furfur, Trichophyton rubrum, T. mentagrophytes, Epidermophyton floccosum, Microsporum canis,* and *Candida albicans* that cause tinea pedis, tinea corporis, tinea cruris, tinea versicolor, candidiasis.
**Contraindications:** Use in or around the eyes.
**Special Concerns:** Safety and efficacy in lactation and in children under 10 years of age not established.
**Side Effects:** *Dermatologic:* Irritation, redness, burning, pain, skin sensitivity, pruritus at application site.

**Dosage** —————————
• **Lotion (1%), Topical Cream (1%)**
Massage gently into the affected area and surrounding skin morning and evening. If there is no improvement after 4 weeks, diagnosis should be reevaluated.

## NURSING CONSIDERATIONS
**Assessment**
1. Document indications for therapy, onset and duration of symptoms.
2. Describe lesion presentation and obtain scrapings.
**Client/Family Teaching**
1. Cleanse skin with soap and water and dry thoroughly. Apply cream with a glove; wash hands before and after therapy.
2. Avoid occlusive dressings or wrappings; adult incontinence pads/diapers are occlusive.
3. Even if symptoms have improved, use for the full prescribed time.
4. Change shoes and socks at least once daily. Shoes should be well-fitted and ventilated.
5. Report any evidence of blistering, burning, itching, oozing, redness, or swelling.
**Outcomes/Evaluate**
• Resolution of infection; wound healing
• Symptomatic improvement

# Cidofovir

(sih-**DOF**-oh-veer)

**Pregnancy Category:** C

Vistide **(Rx)**

**Classification:** Antiviral drug

See also *Antiviral Drugs.*

**Action/Kinetics:** A nucleotide analog that suppresses CMV replication by selective inhibition of viral DNA synthesis. Must be administered with probenecid.

**Uses:** Treatment of CMV retinitis in clients with AIDS.

**Contraindications:** History of severe hypersensitivity to probenecid or other sulfa-containing drugs. Use by direct intraocular injection.

**Special Concerns:** Safety and efficacy have not been determined for children or for treatment of other CMV infections, including pneumonitis, gastroenteritis, congenital or neonatal CMV disease, or CMV disease in non-HIV-infected clients. Increased risk of ocular hypotony in those with preexisting diabetes. Use in clients with a baseline serum creatinine greater than 1.5 mg/dL or creatinine clearances of 55 mL/min or less only when potential benefits outweigh potential risks.

**Side Effects:** *Renal/GU:* Nephrotoxicity, Fanconi's syndrome and decreases in serum bicarbonate associated with renal tubular damage, proteinuria, elevated serum creatinine, glycosuria, hematuria, urinary incontinence, UTI. *GI:* N&V, diarrhea, anorexia, abdominal pain, colitis, constipation, tongue discoloration, dyspepsia, dysphagia, flatulence, gastritis, hepatomegaly, abnormal liver function tests, melena, oral candidiasis, rectal disorder, stomatitis, aphthous stomatitis, mouth ulceration, dry mouth. *CNS:* Headache, asthenia, amnesia, anxiety, confusion, *convulsions,* depression, dizziness, abnormal gait, hallucinations, insomnia, neuropathy, paresthesia, somnolence. *CV:* Hypotension, postural hypotension, pallor, syncope, tachycardia, vasodi-

lation. *Hematologic:* Neutropenia, granulocytopenia, thrombocytopenia, anemia. *Respiratory:* Asthma, bronchitis, coughing, dyspnea, hiccup, increased sputum, lung disorder, pharyngitis, pneumonia, rhinitis, sinusitis. *Dermatologic:* Alopecia, rash, acne, skin discoloration, dry skin, herpes simplex, pruritus, rash, sweating, urticaria. *Musculoskeletal:* Arthralgia, myasthenia, myalgia. *Metabolic:* Edema, dehydration, weight loss. *Ophthalmic:* Ocular hypotony, amblyopia, conjunctivitis, eye disorder, iritis, retinal detachment, uveitis, abnormal vision. *Miscellaneous:* Allergic reactions, facial edema, malaise, back pain, chest pain, neck pain, *sarcoma, sepsis,* fever, infections, chills.

**Laboratory Test Alterations:** ↑ AST, ALT, alkaline phosphatase. Hyperglycemia, hyperlipemia, hypocalcemia, hypokalemia.

**Drug Interactions**

*Amphotericin B* / ↑ Risk of nephrotoxicity

*Aminoglycosides* / ↑ Risk of nephrotoxicity

*Foscarnet* / Risk of nephrotoxicity

*Pentamidine, IV* / ↑ Risk of nephrotoxicity

*Zidovudine* / ↓ Clearance of zidovudine

## Dosage

- **IV Infusion**

    *CMV retinitis.*

**Induction:** 5 mg/kg given once weekly for 2 consecutive weeks as an IV infusion at a constant rate over 1 hr. **Maintenance:** 5 mg/kg given once q 2 weeks as an IV infusion at a constant rate over 1 hr. With each dose of cidofovir, probenecid, 2 g PO, must be given 3 hr prior to the cidofovir dose and 1 g PO given at 2 hr and again at 8 hr after completion of the 1-hr cidofovir infusion. Also, with each dose of cidofovir, the client should receive a total of 1 L of 0.9% NaCl solution IV over a 1- to 2-hr period just before the cidofovir infusion. If the client can tolerate it, give

C

*bold italic* = life threatening side effect

a second liter of 0.9% NaCl solution either at the start of the cidofovir infusion or immediately afterward and infuse over a 1- to 3-hr period. If serum creatinine increases by 0.3 to 0.4 mg/dL, reduce the dose of cidofovir from 5 to 3 mg/kg. Discontinue cidofovir if the serum creatinine increases by 0.5 mg/dL or more or if there is development of 3+ or more proteinuria.

## NURSING CONSIDERATIONS

See also *Nursing Considerations* for *Antiviral Drugs*.

**Administration/Storage**

**IV** 1. A full course of probenecid and IV saline prehydration must be taken with each dose of cidofovir.

2. Use probenecid after a meal or with an antiemetic to decrease nausea due to the probenecid.

3. Prior to administration, dilute cidofovir in 100 mL of 0.9% NaCl solution; administer over 1 hr.

4. Admixtures may be stored at 2°C–8°C (36°F–46°F) for no more than 24 hr. Bring refrigerated admixtures to room temperature prior to use.

**Assessment**

1. Document indications, onset, duration, and characteristics of symptoms.

2. Note sensitivity to probenecid or sulfa drugs; note ophthalmic findings.

3. Monitor CBC, renal function studies, and urinalysis.

4. To minimize potential for nephrotoxicity, ensure prehydration with IV NSS and probenecid administration with each cidofovir infusion

**Client/Family Teaching**

1. This is not a cure but controls symptoms. Retinitis may progress as well as other CMV symptoms; must have regular medical and ophthalmic exams.

2. Stop AZT or decrease its dose by 50% on cidofovir administration days; probenecid inhibits AZT clearance.

3. Complete full probenecid course with each cidofovir dose; take after

meals or use antiemetics to decrease nausea.

4. Women should use reliable contraception during and for 1 month following therapy. Men should practice barrier contraception during and for 3 months following therapy. Infertility may result; identify if candidates for sperm/egg harvesting.

**Outcomes/Evaluate:** Control of symptoms of CMV retinitis

# Cimetidine
(sye-**MET**-ih-deen)

**Pregnancy Category:** B
Apo-Cimetidine ✸, Novo-Cimetine ✸, Nu-Cimet ✸, Peptol ✸, Tagamet **(Rx)**, Tagamet HB **(OTC)**

**Classification:** Histamine H₂ receptor blocking agent

See also *Histamine H₂ Antagonists*.

**Action/Kinetics:** Reduces postprandial daytime and nighttime gastric acid secretion by about 50%–80%. May increase gastromucosal defense and healing in acid-related disorders (e.g., stress-induced ulcers) by increasing production of gastric mucus, increasing mucosal secretion of bicarbonate and gastric mucosal blood flow as well as increasing endogenous mucosal synthesis of prostaglandins. It also inhibits cytochrome P-450 and P-448, which will affect metabolism of drugs. Also possesses antiandrogenic activity and will increase prolactin levels following an IV bolus injection. Well absorbed from GI tract. **Peak plasma level, PO:** 45–90 min. **Time to peak effect, after PO:** 1–2 hr. **Peak plasma levels, after PO use:** 0.7–3.2 mcg/mL (after a 300 mg dose; **after IV:** 3.5–7.5 mcg/mL. **Protein binding:** 13%–25%. **Duration, nocturnal:** 6–8 hr; **basal:** 4–5 hr. **t½:** 2 hr, longer in presence of renal impairment. After PO use, most metabolized in liver; after parenteral use, about 75% of drug excreted unchanged in the urine.

**Uses: Rx.** Treatment and maintenance of active duodenal ulcers. Short-term (6 weeks) treatment of benign gastric ulcers (in rare cases,

healing has occurred). As part of multidrug regimen to eradicate *Helicobacter pylori.* Management of gastric acid hypersecretory states (Zollinger-Ellison syndrome, systemic mastocytosis). Gastroesophageal reflux disease, including erosive esophagitis. Prophylaxis of upper GI bleeding in critically ill hospitalized clients. *Investigational:* Prior to surgery to prevent aspiration pneumonitis, secondary hyperparathyroidism in chronic hemodialysis clients, prophylaxis of stress-induced ulcers, hyperparathyroidism, dyspepsia, herpes virus infections, tinea capitis, hirsute women, chronic idiopathic urticaria, dermatologic anaphylaxis, acetaminophen overdosage, warts, colorectal cancer.

**OTC:** Relief of symptoms of heartburn, acid indigestion, and sour stomach.

**Contraindications:** Children under 16, lactation. Cirrhosis, impaired liver and renal function.

**Special Concerns:** In geriatric clients with impaired renal or hepatic function, confusion is more likely to occur. Not recommended for children less than 16 years of age.

**Side Effects:** *GI:* Diarrhea, pancreatitis (rare), hepatitis, hepatic fibrosis. *CNS:* Dizziness, sleepiness, headache, confusion, delirium, hallucinations, double vision, dysarthria, ataxia. Severely ill clients may manifest agitation, anxiety, depression, disorientation, hallucinations, mental confusion, and psychosis. *CV:* Hypotension and arrhythmias following rapid IV administration. *Hematologic:* Agranulocytosis, thrombocytopenia, **hemolytic or aplastic anemia,** granulocytopenia. *GU:* Impotence (high doses for prolonged periods of time), gynecomastia (long-term treatment). *Dermatologic:* Exfoliative dermatitis, erythroderma, erythema multiforme. *Musculoskeletal:* Arthralgia, reversible worsening of joint symptoms with preexisting arthritis (including gouty arthritis). *Other:* Hypersensitivity reactions, pain at injection site, myalgia, rash, cutaneous vasculitis, peripheral neuropathy, galactorrhea, alopecia, bronchoconstriction.

**Drug Interactions**

*Antacids* / ↓ Effect of cimetidine due to ↓ absorption from GI tract

*Anticholinergics* / ↓ Effect of cimetidine due to ↓ absorption from GI tract

*Benzodiazepines* / ↑ Effect of benzodiazepines due to ↓ breakdown by liver

*Beta-adrenergic blocking drugs* / ↑ Effect of beta blockers due to ↓ breakdown by liver

*Caffeine* / ↑ Effect of caffeine due to ↓ breakdown by liver

*Calcium channel blockers* / ↑ Effect of calcium channel blockers due to ↓ breakdown by liver

*Carbamazepine* / ↑ Effect of carbamazepine due to ↓ breakdown by liver

*Carmustine* / Additive bone marrow depression

*Chloroquine* / ↑ Effect of chloroquine due to ↓ breakdown by liver

*Chlorpromazine* / ↓ Effect of chlorpromazine due to ↓ absorption from GI tract

*Digoxin* / ↓ Serum levels of digoxin

*Flecainide* / ↑ Effect of flecainide

*Fluconazole* / ↓ Effect of fluconazole due to ↓ absorption from GI tract

*Fluorouracil* / ↑ Serum levels of fluorouracil following chronic cimetidine use

*Indomethacin* / ↓ Effect of indomethacin due to ↓ absorption from GI tract

*Iron salts* / ↓ Effect of iron due to ↓ absorption from GI tract

*Ketoconazole* / ↓ Effect of ketoconazole due to ↓ absorption from GI tract

*Labetalol* / ↑ Effect of labetalol due to ↓ breakdown by liver

*Lidocaine* / ↑ Effect of lidocaine due to ↓ breakdown by liver

*Metoclopramide* / ↓ Effect of cimetidine due to ↓ absorption from GI tract

C

*Metoprolol* / ↑ Effect of metoprolol due to ↓ breakdown by liver

*Metronidazole* / ↑ Effect of metronidazole due to ↓ breakdown by liver

*Moricizine* / ↑ Effect of moricizine due to ↓ breakdown by liver

*Narcotics* / Possible ↑ toxic effects (respiratory depression) of narcotics

*Pentoxifylline* / ↑ Effect of pentoxifylline due to ↓ breakdown by liver

*Phenytoin* / ↑ Effect of phenytoin due to ↓ breakdown by liver

*Procainamide* / ↑ Effect of procainamide due to ↓ excretion by kidney

*Propafenone* / ↑ Effect of propafenone due to ↓ breakdown by liver

*Propranolol* / ↑ Effect of propranolol due to ↓ breakdown by liver

*Quinidine* / ↑ Effect of quinidine due to ↓ breakdown by liver

*Quinine* / ↑ Effect of quinine due to ↓ breakdown by liver

*Succinylcholine* / ↑ Neuromuscular blockade → respiratory depression and extended apnea

*Sulfonylureas* / ↑ Effect of sulfonylureas due to ↓ breakdown by liver

*Tacrine* / ↑ Effect of tacrine due to ↓ breakdown by liver

*Tetracyclines* / ↓ Effect of tetracyclines due to ↓ absorption from GI tract

*Theophyllines* / ↑ Effect of theophyllines due to ↓ breakdown by liver

*Tocainide* / ↓ Effect of tocainide

*Triamterene* / ↑ Effect of triamterene due to ↓ breakdown by liver

*Tricyclic antidepressants* / ↑ Effect of tricyclic antidepressants due to ↓ breakdown by liver

*Valproic acid* / ↑ Effect of valproic acid due to ↓ breakdown by liver

*Warfarin* / ↑ Effect of anticoagulant due to ↓ breakdown by liver

## Dosage

• **Tablets, Oral Solution**

*Duodenal ulcers, short-term.*

**Adults:** 800 mg at bedtime. Alternate dosage: 300 mg q.i.d. with meals and at bedtime for 4–6 weeks (administer with antacids, staggering the dose of antacids) or 400 mg

b.i.d. (in the morning and evening). **Maintenance:** 400 mg at bedtime.

*Active benign gastric ulcers.*

**Adults:** 800 mg at bedtime (preferred regimen) or 300 mg q.i.d. with meals and at bedtime for no more than 8 weeks.

*Pathologic hypersecretory conditions.*

**Adults:** 300 mg q.i.d. with meals and at bedtime up to a maximum of 2,400 mg/day for as long as needed.

*Erosive gastroesophageal reflux disease.*

**Adults:** 800 mg b.i.d. or 400 mg q.i.d. for 12 weeks. Use beyond 12 weeks has not been determined.

*Heartburn, acid indigestion, sour stomach (OTC only).*

200 mg with water as symptoms present up to b.i.d.

*Dyspepsia.*

**Adults:** 400 mg b.i.d.

*Prophylaxis of aspiration pneumonitis.*

**Adults:** 400–600 mg 60–90 min before anesthesia.

*Primary hyperparathyroidism, secondary hyperparathyroidism in chronic hemodialysis clients.*

Up to 1 g/day.

• **IM, IV, IV Infusion**

*Hospitalized clients with pathologic hypersecretory conditions or intractable ulcers or those unable to take PO medication.*

**Adults:** 300 mg IM or IV q 6–8 hr. If an increased dose is necessary, administer 300 mg more frequently than q 6–8 hr, not to exceed 2,400 mg/day.

*Prophylaxis of upper GI bleeding.*

**Adults:** 50 mg/hr by continuous IV infusion. If creatinine clearance is less than 30 mL/min, use one-half the recommended dose. Treatment beyond 7 days has not been studied.

*Prophylaxis of aspiration pneumonitis.*

**Adults:** 300 mg IV 60–90 min before induction of anesthetic.

## NURSING CONSIDERATIONS

See also *Nursing Considerations* for *Histamine H₂ Antagonists*.

## Administration/Storage

1. Do not use the OTC product continuously for more than 2 weeks except under medical supervision.

2. If antacids are used, stagger dose with that of cimetidine; antacids (but not food) decrease cimetidine absorption.

3. Administer PO medication with meals and with a snack at bedtime.

4. In renal dysfunction, a dose of 300 mg PO or IV q 12 hr may be necessary. The dose may be given, with caution, q 8 hr if needed.

5. For IM use, give undiluted.

**IV** 6. For IV injections, dilute 300 mg in 0.9% NaCl injection (or other compatible solution) to a total volume of 20 mL. Inject over at least 2 min.

7. For intermittent IV infusion, dilute 300 mg in at least 50 mL of dextrose or saline solution and infuse over 15–20 min.

8. For continuous IV infusion, give a loading dose of 150 mg (by intermittent IV infusion); then, administer 37.5 mg/hr (900 mg/day) in 0.9% NaCl injection, 5% or 10% dextrose injection, 5% sodium bicarbonate injection, RL solution, or as part of TPN. Is stable for 24 hr at room temperature if mixed with these diluents.

9. May be diluted in 100–1,000 mL; if the volume for a 24-hr infusion is less than 250 mL, use a volumetric pump.

10. Do *not* introduce drugs or additives to cimetidine solutions in plastic containers.

11. Cimetidine is incompatible with aminophylline and barbiturates in IV solutions and in the same syringe with pentobarbital sodium and a pentobarbital sodium/atropine sulfate combination.

12. Do not expose premixed single-dose product to excessive heat; store at 15°C–30°C (59°F–86°F).

## Assessment

1. Note general client condition. Those receiving radiation therapy or myelosuppressive drugs may have additional side effects.

2. Review long list of drug interactions; list drugs prescribed to ensure none interact unfavorably.

3. Document indications for therapy, type/onset of symptoms, and anticipated length of therapy.

4. Assess location, characteristics, extent of abdominal pain; note blood in emesis, stool, or gastric aspirate.Maintain gastric pH above 5 to enhance mucosal healing.

5. Document radiologic and/or endoscopic findings.

6. Nonitor CBC, I&O, electrolytes, liver and renal function studies, especially for the elderly, severely ill, or those with renal impairment.

## Client/Family Teaching

1. Take with meals and/or a snack at bedtime. Avoid antacids 1 hr before or after dose; establish schedule to assure compliance.

2. Take entire prescription even if symptoms disappear.

3. Review dietary modifications, especially if being treated for GI problems; consult dietitian as needed.

4. Do not perform tasks that require mental alertness until drug effects realized.

5. Report if gynecomastia or galactorrhea occurs.

6. Report if abdominal pain, bloody stools, or other S&S of reactivated ulcer are evident.

7. Avoid alcohol, caffeine, spicy foods, and aspirin-containing products; may enhance GI irritation.

8. Do not smoke after the last dose of cimetidine to ensure optimal suppression of nocturnal gastric acid secretion. Attend smoking cessation program if unable to quit.

9. Report any new symptoms of confusion/mood swings; more common among the elderly.

10. Note any increased susceptibility to infections; may develop agranulocytosis, thrombocytopenia, or anemia; obtain periodic hematologic evaluations.

11. If diarrhea develops, maintain adequate hydration, monitor fre-

quency and severity, and report if persistent.

12. Report any skin rashes or skin changes.

13. Drug may alter response to skin tests with allergenic extracts. Provider may stop drug 48–72 hr prior to skin testing.

**Outcomes/Evaluate**

* ↓ Abdominal pain; ulcer healing
* Control of acid hypersecretion
* Prophylaxis of GI bleeding

## Cinoxacin

(sin-**OX**-ah-sin)
**Pregnancy Category:** B
Cinobac Pulvules **(Rx)**
**Classification:** Urinary anti-infective

See also *Anti-Infectives.*

**Action/Kinetics:** Related chemically to nalidixic acid. Acts by inhibiting DNA replication, resulting in a bactericidal action. Rapidly absorbed after PO administration; a 500-mg dose results in a urine concentration of 300 mcg/mL during the first 4-hr period and 100 mcg/mL during the second 4-hr period. Within 24 hr, 97% is excreted in the urine, 60% unchanged. **Mean serum t½:** 1.5 hr. Food decreases peak serum levels by approximately 30% but not the total amount absorbed.

**Uses:** Initial and recurrent UTIs caused by *Escherichia coli, Proteus mirabilis, P. vulgaris, Klebsiella,* and *Enterobacter* species. Prevents UTIs for up to 5 months in women with a history of UTIs. *NOTE:* Cinoxacin is ineffective against *Pseudomonas,* staphylococci, and enterococci infections. Prophylaxis of UTIs.

**Contraindications:** Hypersensitivity to cinoxacin or other quinolones. Infants and prepubertal children. Anuric clients. Lactation.

**Special Concerns:** Use with caution in clients with hepatic or kidney disease. Safety and efficacy in children less than 18 years of age have not been determined.

**Side Effects:** *GI:* N&V, anorexia, abdominal cramps and pain, diarrhea, altered sensation of taste. *CNS:* Headache, dizziness, insomnia, drowsiness, confusion, nervousness. *Hypersensitivity:* Rash, pruritus, urticaria, edema, angioedema, eosinophilia, **anaphylaxis (rare)**, toxic epidermal necrolysis (rare), erythema multiforme, **Stevens-Johnson syndrome**. *Other:* Tingling sensation, photophobia, perineal burning, tinnitus, thrombocytopenia.

**OD** **Overdose Management:** *Symptoms:* Anorexia, N&V, epigastric distress, diarrhea, headache, dizziness, insomnia, photophobia, tinnitus, and a tingling sensation. *Treatment:* Well hydrate the client to prevent crystalluria. Maintain an airway and support ventilation and perfusion. VS, blood gases, and serum electrolytes should be meticulously monitored. Decrease absorption by giving activated charcoal.

**Drug Interactions:** Probenecid ↓ excretion of cinoxacin → ↓ concentration in the urine.

**Laboratory Test Interferences:** ↑ BUN, AST, ALT, serum creatinine, and alkaline phosphatase. ↓ Hematocrit/hemoglobin.

## Dosage

* **Capsules**

    *UTIs.*

    **Adults:** 1 g/day in two to four divided doses for 7–14 days. *In clients with impaired renal function:* **Initial,** 500 mg; **then,** dosage schedule based on creatinine clearance (see package insert).

    *Prophylaxis of UTIs in women.* 250 mg at bedtime for up to 5 months.

## NURSING CONSIDERATIONS

See also *General Nursing Considerations for All Anti-Infectives.*

**Assessment:** Obtain baseline liver and renal function studies; hold if anuric.

**Client/Family Teaching**

1. Take exactly as directed.

2. Consume 2–3 L/day of fluids to ensure adequate hydration.

3. Acidic fluids enhance drug action (cranberry, prune juice); limit intake

of alkaline products (milk, bicarbonate).
4. Avoid sun; use sunscreens, protective clothing, and sunglasses to limit photosensitivity reaction.
**Outcomes/Evaluate**
• ↓ S&S of UTI (dysuria, frequency)
• Recurrent UTI prophylaxis

# Ciprofloxacin hydrochloride
(sip-row-**FLOX**-ah-sin)
**Pregnancy Category:** C
Ciloxan Ophthalmic, Cipro, Cipro Cystitis Pack, Cipro I.V. **(Rx)**
**Classification:** Fluoroquinolone anti-infective

See also *Fluoroquinolones.*
**Action/Kinetics:** Effective against both gram-positive and gram-negative organisms. Rapidly and well absorbed following PO administration. Food delays absorption of the drug. **Maximum serum levels:** 2–4 mcg/mL 1–2 hr after dosing. **t½:** 4 hr for PO use and 5–6 hr for IV use. Avoid peak serum levels above 5 mcg/mL. About 40%–50% of a PO dose and 50%–70% of an IV dose is excreted unchanged in the urine.
**Uses: Systemic.** UTIs caused by *Escherichia coli, Enterobacter cloacae, Citrobacter diversus, Citrobacter freundii, Klebsiella pneumoniae, Proteus mirabilis, Providencia rettgeri, Pseudomonas aeruginosa, Morganella morganii, Serratia marcescens, Serratia epidermidis,* and *Streptococcus faecalis.* Uncomplicated cervical and urethral gonorrhea due to *Neisseria gonorrhoeae.* Chancroid due to *Haemophilus ducreyi*; uncomplicated or disseminated gonococcal infections.
Mild to moderate chronic bacterial prostatitis due to *E. coli* or *P. mirabilis.*
Mild to moderate sinusitis due to *S. pneumoniae, H. influenzae,* or *M. catarrhalis.*
Lower respiratory tract infections caused by *E. coli, E. cloacae, K. pneumoniae, P. mirabilis, P. aeruginosa, Haemophilus influenzae, H. parainfluenzae,* and *Streptococcus pneumoniae.*
Bone and joint infections due to *E. cloacae, P. aeruginosa,* and *S. marcescens.*
Skin and skin structure infections caused by *E. coli, E. cloacae, Citrobacter freundii, M. morganii, K. pneumoniae, P. aeruginosa, P. mirabilis, Proteus vulgaris, Providencia stuartii, Staphylococcus pyogenes, Staphylococcus epidermidis,* and penicillinase- and non-penicillinase-producing strains of *Staphylococcus aureus.*
Infectious diarrhea caused by enterotoxigenic strains of *E. coli.* Also, *Campylobacter jejuni, Shigella flexneri,* and *Shigella sonnei.*
Typhoid fever (enteric fever) due to *Salmonella typhi.* Efficacy in eradicating the chronic typhoid carrier state has not been shown.
IV as empirical therapy in febrile neutropenia.
*Investigational:* Clients, over 14 years of age, with cystic fibrosis who have pulmonary exacerbations due to susceptible microorganisms. Malignant external otitis. In combination with rifampin and other tuberculostatics for tuberculosis.
**Ophthalmic.** Superficial ocular infections due to *Staphylococcus* species (including *S. aureus*), *Streptococcus* species (including *S. pneumoniae, S. pyogenes*), *E. coli, H. ducreyi, H. influenzae, H. parainfluenzae, K. pneumoniae, N. gonorrhoeae, Proteus* species, *Klebsiella* species, *Acinetobacter calcoaceticus, Enterobacter aerogenes, P. aeruginosa, S. marcescens, Chlamydia trachomatis, Vibrio* species, and *Providencia* species.
**Contraindications:** Hypersensitivity to quinolones. Use in children. Lactation. Ophthalmic use in the presence of dendritic keratitis, varicella, vaccinia, and mycobacterial and fungal eye infections and after

removal of foreign bodies from the cornea.

**Special Concerns:** Safety and effectiveness of ophthalmic, PO, or IV use have not been determined in children.

**Additional Side Effects**

See also *Side Effects* for *Fluoroquinolones.*

*GI:* N&V, abdominal pain/discomfort, diarrhea, dry/painful mouth, dyspepsia, heartburn, constipation, flatulence, pseudomembranous colitis, oral candidiasis, *intestinal perforation,* anorexia, GI bleeding, bad taste in mouth. *CNS:* Headache, dizziness, fatigue, lethargy, malaise, drowsiness, restlessness, insomnia, nightmares, hallucinations, tremor, lightheadedness, irritability, confusion, ataxia, mania, weakness, psychotic reactions, depression, depersonalization, seizures. *GU:* Nephritis, hematuria, cylindruria, renal failure, urinary retention, polyuria, vaginitis, urethral bleeding, acidosis, renal calculi, interstitial nephritis, vaginal candidiasis. *Skin:* Urticaria, photosensitivity, hypersensitivity, flushing, erythema nodosum, cutaneous candidiasis, hyperpigmentation, rash, paresthesia, edema (of lips, neck, face, conjunctivae, hands), angioedema, toxic epidermal necrolysis, exfoliative dermatitis, *Stevens-Johnson syndrome. Ophthalmic:* Blurred or disturbed vision, double vision, eye pain, nystagmus. *CV:* Hypertension, syncope, angina pectoris, palpitations, atrial flutter, *MI, cerebral thrombosis,* ventricular ectopy, *cardiopulmonary arrest,* postural hypotension. *Respiratory:* Dyspnea, *bronchospasm, pulmonary embolism, edema of larynx or lungs,* hemoptysis, hiccoughs, epistaxis. *Hematologic:* Eosinophilia, pancytopenia, leukopenia, anemia, leukocytosis, *agranulocytosis,* bleeding diathesis. *Miscellaneous:* Superinfections; fever; chills; tinnitus; joint pain or stiffness; back, neck, or chest pain; flare-up of gout; flushing; worsening of myasthenia gravis; *hepatic necrosis;* cholestatic jaundice; hearing loss, dysphasia.

*After ophthalmic use:* Irritation, burning, itching, angioneurotic edema, urticaria, maculopapular and vesicular dermatitis, crusting of lid margins, conjunctival hyperemia, bad taste in mouth, corneal staining, keratitis, keratopathy, allergic reactions, photophobia, decreased vision, tearing, lid edema. Also, a white, crystalline precipitate in the superficial part of corneal defect (onset within 1–7 days after initiating therapy; lasts about 2 weeks and does not affect continued use of the medication).

**Additional Drug Interactions**

*Azlocillin* / ↓ Excretion of ciprofloxacin → possible ↑ effect

*Caffeine* / ↓ Excretion of caffeine → ↑ pharmacologic effects

*Cyclosporine* / ↑ Nephrotoxic effect of cyclosporine

*Hydantoins* / ↓ Phenytoin serum levels

*Theophylline* / Should not be taken with ciprofloxacin

**Laboratory Test Interferences:** ↑ ALT, AST, alkaline phosphatase, serum bilirubin, LDH, serum creatinine, BUN, serum gamma-glutamyltransferase, serum amylase, uric acid, blood monocytes, potassium, PT, triglycerides, cholesterol. ↓ H&H. Either ↑ or ↓ blood glucose, platelets.

**Dosage**

• **Tablets**

*UTIs.*

250 mg (mild to moderate) to 500 mg (severe/complicated) q 12 hr for 7–14 days.

*Mild to moderate chronic bacterial prostatitis.*

**Adults:** 500 mg b.i.d. for 28 days.

*Mild to moderate sinusitis.*

**Adults:** 500 mg b.i.d. for 10 days.

*Urethral or cervical gonococcal infections, uncomplicated.*

250 mg in a single dose.

*Infectious diarrhea.*

500 mg q 12 hr for 5–7 days.

*Skin, skin structures, lower respiratory tract, bone and joint infections.*

500 mg (mild to moderate) to 750 mg (severe or complicated) q 12 hr for 7–14 days. Treatment may be required for 4–6 weeks in bone and joint infections.

*Typhoid fever.*
500 mg (mild to moderate) q 12 hr for 10 days.

*Chancroid* (H. ducreyi infection).
500 mg b.i.d. for 3 days.

*Disseminated gonococcal infections.*
500 mg b.i.d. to complete a full week of therapy after initial treatment with ceftriaxone, 1 g IM or IV q 24 hr for 24–48 hr after improvement begins.

*Uncomplicated gonococcal infections.*
500 mg in a single dose plus doxycycline.

*NOTE:* Dose must be reduced with a creatinine clearance (C_CR) less than 50 mL/min. The PO dose should be 250–500 mg q 12 hr if the C_CR is 30–50 mL/min and 250–500 mg q 18 hr (IV: 200–400 mg q 18–24 hr) if the C_CR is 5–29 mL/min. If the client is on hemodialysis or peritoneal dialysis, the PO dose should be 250–500 mg q 24 hr after dialysis.

• **Cipro Cystitis Pack**
*Uncomplicated UTI infections.*
100 mg b.i.d. for 3 days. The pack contains six 100-mg tablets of ciprofloxacin and is intended to increase compliance.

• **IV Infusion**
*UTIs.*
200 mg (mild to moderate) to 400 mg (severe or complicated) q 12 hr for 7–14 days.

*Skin, skin structures, respiratory tract, bone and joint infections.*
400 mg (for mild to moderate infections) q 12 hr for 7–14 days.

• **Ophthalmic Solution**
*Acute infections.*
**Initial,** 1–2 gtt q 15–30 min; **then,** reduce dosage as infection improves.
*Moderate infections.*
1–2 gtt 4–6 (or more) times/day.

## NURSING CONSIDERATIONS

See also *Nursing Considerations for All Anti-infectives* and *Fluoroquinolones.*

### Administration/Storage
1. Although food delays absorption of the drug, it may be taken with or without meals; recommended dosing time is 2 hr after a meal.
2. Clients on theophylline or probenecid require close observation and potential medication adjustments.
3. Do not administer to children.
4. Following instillation of the ophthalmic solution, apply light finger pressure to the lacrimal sac for 1 min.
**IV** 5. Reconstitute the IV solution dose to 0.5–2 mg/mL and give over a period of 60 min. To minimize discomfort and irritation, slowly infuse a dilute solution into a large vein.
6. The IV product can be diluted with 0.9% NaCl injection or 5% dextrose injection. Such dilutions are stable up to 14 days at refrigerated or room temperatures; do not freeze.
7. Ciprofloxin in admixture is incompatible with aminophylline, amoxicillin sodium, amoxicillin sodium/potassium clavulanate, clindamycin, and mezlocillin.

### Assessment
1. Note indications for therapy; obtain cultures prior to use.
2. Determine age. Not for use in children under 18 as irreversible collagen destruction has occurred.
3. Note meds currently prescribed. Fatal reactions have been reported with concurrent administration of IV ciprofloxacin and theophylline.

### Client/Family Teaching
1. Take 2 hr after meals; food may delay absorption, as will antacids containing magnesium or aluminum.
2. Drink 2–3 L/day of fluids to keep the urine acidic and to minimize the risk of crystalluria.
3. May cause dizziness; use caution in any activity that requires mental alertness or coordination.
4. Report any persistent GI symp-

toms such as diarrhea, vomiting, or abdominal pain.
5. Review side effects; note those that should be reported immediately.
6. Return as scheduled for follow-up evaluation and labs.

**Outcomes/Evaluate**
• Symptomatic improvement; ↓ fever, ↓ WBCs, ↑ appetite
• Negative culture reports

# Cisapride
(**SISS**-ah-pryd)
**Pregnancy Category:** C
Prepulsid ✷, Propulsid **(Rx)**
**Classification:** GI drug

**Action/Kinetics:** Cisapride is a GI prokinetic agent. Acts by enhancing release of acetylcholine at the myenteric plexus, resulting in increased strength of esophageal peristalsis and an increase in lower esophageal sphincter pressure. Also increases gastric emptying time. Rapidly absorbed. **Onset:** 30–60 min. **Peak plasma levels:** 1–1.5 hr. **Terminal t½:** 6–12 hr (up to 20 hr following IV use). Metabolized in the liver with less than 10% excreted unchanged through the urine and feces.

**Uses:** Symptomatic treatment of clients with nocturnal heartburn due to gastroesophageal reflux disease (GERD).

**Contraindications:** Use when an increase in GI motility could be harmful (i.e., in the presence of GI hemorrhage, mechanical obstruction, perforation). Concomitant use with clarithromycin, erythromycin, fluconazole, itraconazole, ketoconazole, IV miconazole, or troleandomycin.

**Special Concerns:** Use with caution during lactation. Safety and efficacy have not been demonstrated in children. Steady-state plasma levels are generally higher in older clients as a result of increased elimination half-life although doses used are similar to those in younger adults. The increased rate of gastric emptying time due to cisapride could affect the rate of absorption of other drugs.

**Side Effects:** *GI:* Diarrhea, abdominal pain, nausea, constipation, flatulence, dyspepsia, vomiting, dry mouth. *CNS:* Headache, insomnia, anxiety, nervousness, dizziness, depression, tremor, **seizures,** extrapyramidal effects, somnolence, migraine. *CV:* Palpitation, sinus tachycardia, tachycardia. ***Rarely, serious cardiac arrhythmias, including ventricular arrhythmias and torsades de pointes associated with QT prolongation*** (usually in those taking antifungal drugs and other multiple medications and who had preexisting cardiac disease or arrhythmia risk factors). *Respiratory:* Rhinitis, sinusitis, coughing, pharyngitis, URTI. *GU:* UTI, increased frequency of urination, vaginitis. *Hepatic:* Hepatitis, elevated liver enzymes. *Musculoskeletal:* Arthralgia, back pain, myalgia. *Hematologic:* Thrombocytopenia, leukopenia, ***aplastic anemia, pancytopenia,*** granulocytopenia (rare). *Miscellaneous:* Pain, fever, viral infection, rash, pruritus, abnormal vision, chest pain, fatigue, dehydration, edema.

**OD** **Overdose Management:** *Symptoms:* One case of overdose included symptoms of retching, borborygmi, flatulence, stool and urinary frequency. *Treatment:* Gastric lavage or activated charcoal. Observe client closely. Provide general supportive treatment.

**Drug Interactions**
*Alcohol* / Possible ↑ sedative effect
*Anticholinergics* / ↓ Effect of cisapride
*Anticoagulants* / ↑ Coagulation times
*Benzodiazepines* / Possible ↑ sedative effect
*Cimetidine* / ↑ Peak plasma levels of cisapride; also ↑ GI absorption of cimetidine
*Clarithromycin* / ↑ Cisapride plasma levels due to ↓ metabolism, resulting in prolonged QT intervals and possibility of ventricular arrhythmias and torsades de pointes
*Erythromycin* / ↑ Cisapride plasma levels due to ↓ metabolism, resulting in prolonged QT intervals and

possibility of ventricular arrhythmias and torsades de pointes

*Fluconazole* / ↑ Cisapride plasma levels due to ↓ metabolism, resulting in prolonged QT intervals and possibility of ventricular arrhythmias and torsades de pointes

*Itraconazole* / ↑ Cisapride plasma levels due to ↓ metabolism, resulting in prolonged QT intervals and possibility of ventricular arrhythmias and torsades de pointes

*Ketoconazole* / ↑ Cisapride plasma levels due to ↓ metabolism, resulting in prolonged QT intervals and possibility of ventricular arrhythmias and torsades de pointes

*Miconazole (IV)* / ↑ Cisapride plasma levels due to ↓ metabolism, resulting in prolonged QT intervals and possibility of ventricular arrhythmias and torsades de pointes

*Ranitidine* / ↑ GI absorption of ranitidine

*Troleandomycin* / ↑ Cisapride plasma levels due to ↓ metabolism, resulting in prolonged QT intervals and possibility of ventricular arrhythmias and torsades de pointes

**Dosage** ⎯⎯⎯⎯⎯⎯
• **Suspension, Tablets**
*GERD.*
**Adults, initial:** 10 mg q.i.d. at least 15 min before meals and at bedtime. May need to increase in some clients to 20 mg q.i.d. 15 min before meals and at bedtime.

**NURSING CONSIDERATIONS**

**Administration/Storage:** Protect the tablets from moisture; protect the 20-mg tablets from light.

**Assessment**

1. Document type, onset, and characteristics of symptoms.
2. List drugs currently prescribed; drug causes increased gastric emptying. Note any conditions that may preclude this therapy.
3. Monitor coagulation times closely if receiving anticoagulants; adjust accordingly.

**Client/Family Teaching**

1. Take at least 15 min before meals and at bedtime.
2. In addition to relieving symptoms of esophageal reflux, the drug increases gastric emptying time; plan administration of additional medications accordingly.
3. Avoid alcohol and benzodiazepines; may potentiate sedative effects.
4. Review most frequently experienced effects (e.g., headaches, abdominal pain, nausea, rhinitis, and constipation); report if persistent or intolerable.

**Outcomes/Evaluate:** Relief of heart burn associated with GERD

# Cisatracurium besylate

(sis-ah-trah-**KYOU**-ree-um)
**Pregnancy Category:** B
Nimbex **(Rx)**
**Classification:** Neuromuscular blocking agent

See also *Neuromuscular Blocking Agents.*

**Action/Kinetics:** As a nondepolarizing neuromuscular blocking agent, the drug binds competitively to cholinergic receptors on the motor end-plate, resulting in antagonism of the action of acetylcholine and therefore neuromuscular blockade. The neuromuscular blocking potency of cisatracurium is about three times greater than that for atracurium. Compared with other neuromuscular blocking agents, cisatracurium is considered to be both intermediate onset and duration. **Time to maximum blockade:** 2 min. **Time to recovery:** Approximately 55 min. Continuous infusion for up to 3 hr may be undertaken without tachyphylaxis or cumulative neuromuscular blockade. The time required for recovery following successive maintenance doses does not change with the number of doses given, provided that partial recovery is allowed to occur between doses. Onset, duration, and recovery are faster in children. About 95% of a dose is excreted as metabolites and unchanged drug (10%) in the urine and 4% is eliminated through the feces. Laudanosine, a major biologically active metabolite with no neuromuscular activity, may cause transient hypotension and cerebral excitatory effects (in high doses).

**Uses:** Neuromuscular blocking agent for in-patients and out-patients as an adjunct to general anesthesia, to facilitate tracheal intubation, and to cause skeletal muscle relaxation during surgery or mechanical ventilation in the intensive care unit.

**Contraindications:** Hypersensitivity to cisatracurium or other bis-benzylisoquinolinium agents or hypersensitivity to benzyl alcohol. Use for rapid-sequence ET intubation due to its intermediate onset of action.

**Special Concerns:** Since the drug has no effect on consciousness, pain threshold, or cerebration, administration should not be undertaken before unconsciousness. May cause a profound effect in those with myasthenia gravis or the myasthenic syndrome. Burn clients may require higher doses. Onset time is faster (about 1 min) and recovery is slower (by about 1 min) in clients with impaired hepatic function. The time to maximum blockage is about 1 min slower in geriatric clients and in those with impaired renal function. Use with caution during lactation. Safety and efficacy have not been determined in children less than 2 years of age.

**Side Effects:** Bradycardia, hypotension, flushing, bronchospasm, rash.

**OD   Overdose   Management:** *Symptoms:* Neuromuscular blockade beyond the time needed for surgery and anesthesia. *Treatment:* Maintain a patent airway and control ventilation until recovery of normal function is assured. Once recovery begins, facilitate the process by using neostigmine or edrophonium with an anticholinergic drug. Do not give these anti-

dotes when complete blockade is evident.

**Drug Interactions**

*Aminoglycosides* / ↑ Effect of cisatracurium
*Bacitracin* / ↑ Effect of cisatracurium
*Carbamazepine* / Resistance to neuromuscular blockage → slightly shorter duration.
*Clindamycin* / ↑ Effect of cisatracurium
*Colistin, sodium colistimethate* / ↑ Effect of cisatracurium
*Enflurane/nitrous oxide/oxygen* / ↑ Duration of cisatracurium
*Isoflurane/nitrous oxide/oxygen* / ↑ Duration of cisatracurium
*Lincomycin* / ↑ Effect of cisatracurium
*Lithium* / ↑ Effect of cisatracurium
*Local anesthetics* / ↑ Effect of cisatracurium
*Magnesium salts* / ↑ Effect of cisatracurium
*Phenobarbital* / Resistance to neuromuscular blockade → slightly shorter duration
*Polymyxins* / ↑ Effect of cisatracurium
*Procainamide* / ↑ Effect of cisatracurium
*Quinidine* / ↑ Effect of cisatracurium
*Succinylcholine* / Time to onset of maximum block of cisatracurium is about 2 min faster
*Tetracyclines* / ↑ Effect of cisatracurium

**Dosage** ————————
• **IV Bolus**
   *Neuromuscular blockade.*
**Adults, initial:** Depending on the desired time to intubation and the anticipated length of surgery, either 0.15 or 0.2 mg/kg is used. These doses are components of a propofol/nitrous oxide/oxygen induction-intubation technique. **Maintenance during prolonged surgery:** 0.03 mg/kg given 40–50 min following an initial dose of 0.15 mg/kg and 50–60 min following an initial dose of 0.2 mg/kg.

**Children, 2–12 years of age:** 0.1 mg/kg over 5–10 sec during either halothane or opioid anesthesia. When given during stable opioid/nitrous oxide/oxygen anesthesia, 0.1 mg/kg produces maximum effects in about 2.8 min and a clinically effective blockade for 28 min.

• **IV Infusion**
*Neuromuscular blockade during extended surgery or use in the intensive care unit.*
In the operating room or intensive care unit, following an initial bolus dose, a diluted solution can be given by continuous infusion to both adults and children over 2 years of age. The rate of administration is dependent on the response of the client determined by peripheral nerve stimulation. An infusion rate of 3 mcg/kg/min can be used to counteract rapid spontaneous recovery of neuromuscular blockade. Thereafter, an infusion rate of 1–2 mcg/kg/min is usually adequate to maintain blockade. Reduce the infusion rate by 30%–40% when given during stable isoflurane or enflurane anesthesia.

## NURSING CONSIDERATIONS

See also *Nursing Considerations* for *Neuromuscular Blocking Agents.*
**Administration/Storage**
**IV** 1. Due to slower times of onset in geriatric clients and those with impaired renal function, extend the interval between administration of the drug and intubation.
2. Spontaneous recovery following infusion will proceed at a rate comparable to that following administration of a bolus dose.
3. Cisatracurium is acidic; thus, it may not be compatible with alkaline solutions with a pH greater than 8.5 (e.g., barbiturate solutions).
4. Cisatracurium is compatible with 5% dextrose injection, 0.9% NaCl injection, 5% dextrose and 0.9% NaCl injection, sufentanil, alfentanil hydrochloride, fentanyl, midazolam hydrochloride, and droperidol. The drug is not compatible with propofol or ketorolac for Y-site administration.
5. Refrigerate vials at 2°C–8°C (36°F–46°F) and protect from light. Once removed from the refrigerator, use vials within 21 days, even if rerefrigerated.
6. Cisatracurium diluted in 5% dextrose injection, 0.9% NaCl injection, or D5%/0.9% NaCl injection may be refrigerated or stored at room temperature for 24 hr without significant loss of potency. Dilutions to 0.1 or 0.2 mg/mL in D5%/RL injection may be refrigerated for 24 hr. Due to chemical instability, do not dilute cisatracurium in RL injection.
**Assessment**
1. Document indications for therapy, other agents trialed, and anticipated duration of therapy.
2. Note any hypersensitivity to benzyl alcohol.
3. Obtain baseline neurologic assessment and note findings.
**Interventions**
1. To be administered only by those trained in administration of neuromuscular blocking agents.
2. Client requires constant monitoring and respiratory support.
3. Medicate with analgesics for pain and agents for anxiety based on assessed need.
4. Utilize a peripheral nerve stimulator to evaluate response to therapy and to ensure partial recovery between doses.
**Outcomes/Evaluate**
• Facilitation of ET intubation
• Skeletal muscle relaxation

# Cisplatin
(sis-**PLAH**-tin)
Platinol-AQ (Abbreviation: CDDP)
**(Rx)**
**Classification:** Antineoplastic, alkylating agent

See also *Antineoplastic Agents.*
**Action/Kinetics:** Binds to DNA and causes production of intrastrand cross-links and formation of DNA

adducts. The drug is cell-cycle non-specific. **t½, plasma:** 20–30 min. **Terminal t½, blood cells:** 36–47 days. Incomplete urinary excretion (only 35%–51% after 5 days). Concentrates in liver, kidneys, and large and small intestines, with low penetration of CNS. The drug is over 90% bound to plasma protein.

**Uses:** Palliative therapy. Combination therapy in metastatic testicular tumors and for metastatic ovarian tumors (e.g., with cyclophosphamide) in those who have received appropriate surgical or radiotherapeutic procedures. Single agent in metastatic ovarian tumors as secondary therapy in those refractory to standard therapy who have not previously received cisplatin. Single agent in transitional cell bladder cancer that is no longer amenable to surgery or radiotherapy.

**Additional    Contraindications:** Lactation. Preexisting renal impairment, myelosuppression, impaired hearing, history of allergic reactions to platinum compounds.

**Additional Side Effects:** *Renal:* Severe cumulative renal toxicity, including renal tubular damage and renal insufficiency. *Electrolytes:* Low levels of calcium, magnesium, potassium, phosphate, and sodium. *Neurologic:* Seizures, taste loss, peripheral neuropathies. Neurotoxicity may occur 4–7 months after prolonged therapy. *Otic:* Ototoxicity characterized by tinnitus, especially in children. *Ophthalmologic:* Papilledema, cerebral blindness, optic neuritis. High doses have resulted in blurred vision and altered color perception. *Miscellaneous:* **Anaphylactic reactions,** hyperuricemia.

**Additional Drug Interactions**
*Aminoglycosides* / Cumulative nephrotoxity
*Anticonvulsants* / Plasma levels of anticonvulsants may become subtherapeutic
*Loop diuretics* / Additive ototoxicity
*Phenytoin* / ↓ Effect of phenytoin due to ↓ plasma levels
**Laboratory Test Interferences:** ↑ Plasma iron levels. Nephrotoxicity results in ↑ serum uric acid, BUN, and creatinine and ↓ creatinine clearance.

**OD  Overdose    Management:** *Symptoms:* Liver and kidney failure, deafness, ocular toxicity (including retinal detachment), significant myelosuppression, intractable N&V, neuritis, death. *Treatment:* General supportive measures.

## Dosage

• **IV only**
  *Metastatic testicular tumors.*
20 mg/m²/day for 5 days/cycle.
  *Metastatic ovarian tumors.*
Cisplatin: 75–100 mg/m² once every 4 weeks/cycle. Cyclophosphamide: 600 mg/m² once every 4 weeks on day 1. Administer cisplatin and cyclophosphamide sequentially.
  *Advanced bladder cancer.*
50–70 mg/m² per cycle once q 3–4 weeks, depending on prior radiation or chemotherapy. For those heavily pretreated, give an initial dose of 50 mg/m²/cycle repeated q 4 weeks.
  *NOTE:* Repeat courses should not be administered until (1) serum creatinine is below 1.5 mg/dL and/or the BUN is below 25 mg/dL; (2) platelets are equal to or greater than 100,000/mm³ and leukocyte count is equal to or greater than 4,000/mm³; and (3) auditory activity is within the normal range.

## NURSING CONSIDERATIONS

See also *Nursing Considerations* for *Antineoplastic Agents.*
### Administration/Storage
**IV** 1. Add dosage recommended from vial to 2 L of 5% dextrose in one-half or one-third NSS containing 37.5 g mannitol. Infuse over a period of 6–8 hr. Furosemide is ordered by some practitioners instead of mannitol. Maintain adequate hydration and urinary output for 24 hr following infusion.
2. Before administration of cisplatin, hydrate client with 1–2 L of IV fluid over a period of 8–12 hr.
3. Do *not* use any equipment with aluminum for preparing or administer-

ing because a black precipitate will form and loss of potency will occur.
4. Platinol-AQ is a sterile, multidose vial without preservatives. Unopened containers should be stored at 15°C–25°C (59°F–77°F), protected from light. Once opened, solution is stable for 28 days protected from light, or 7 days under fluorescent lights.
5. Cisplatin has been confused with carboplatin. Place signs/label warnings of the name mix-ups. Do not refer to as "platinum."
6. Have emergency equipment available if anaphylactic reaction to cisplatin occurs.

**Assessment**
1. Document indications for therapy and anticipated results. Identify previous treatments (XRT, chemotherapy) and the outcome.
2. Obtain audiometry testing before therapy and before subsequent doses to ensure hearing has not been affected.
3. *During therapy monitor client closely for:*
• Facial edema, bronchoconstriction, tachycardia, and shock.
• Tremors that may progress to seizures due to hypomagnesemia.
• Tetany, confusion, or signs of hypocalcemia associated with hypomagnesemia; monitor calcium and magnesium levels.
4. Hydrate well to prevent urate deposits and monitor I&O for 24 hr after treatment.
5. Obtain baseline CBC, uric acid, liver and renal function tests. Cisplatin may cause severe cumulative renal toxicity; additional doses of cisplatin should not be administered until renal function has returned to baseline value and usually not more frequently than every 3–4 weeks. Assess for mild granulocyte suppression. Nadir: 14 days; recovery: 21 days.

**Client/Family Teaching**
1. Report any numbness, tingling, swelling, or joint pain.
2. Avoid vaccinations.

3. Report any ringing in ears, difficulty hearing, edema of lower extremities, and decreased urination.
4. Avoid alcohol and salicylates as these may increase gastric bleeding.
5. Use reliable birth control; may cause infertility. Identify candidates for egg/sperm harvesting if children desired.
**Outcomes/Evaluate:** ↓ Tumor size; suppression of malignant cell proliferation

# Cladribine injection
(**KLAD**-rih-bean)
**Pregnancy Category:** D
Leustatin **(Rx)**
**Classification:** Antineoplastic drug

See also *Antineoplastic Agents.*
**Action/Kinetics:** By inhibiting both DNA synthesis and repair, toxicity occurs to both actively dividing and quiescent lymphocytes and monocytes. The drug results in accumulation of 2-chloro-2'-deoxy-beta-D-adenosine monophosphate (2-CdAMP), which is subsequently converted to the active triphosphate deoxynucleotide (2-CdATP). Cells with high deoxycytidine kinase and low deoxynucleotidase activities (as in lymphocytes and monocytes) will be selectively killed as toxic deoxynucleotides accumulate intracellularly. **t½:** 5.4 hr. Excreted mainly through the urine.
**Uses:** Hairy cell leukemia as defined by clinically significant anemia, neutropenia, thrombocytopenia, or disease-related symptoms. *Investigational:* Advanced cutaneous T-cell lymphomas; chronic lymphocytic leukemia; non-Hodgkin's lymphomas; acute myeloid leukemia; autoimmune hemolytic anemia; mycosis fungoides or the Sezary syndrome.
**Contraindications:** Lactation.
**Special Concerns:** Use with caution in clients with known or suspected renal or hepatic insufficiency. Benzyl alcohol, a constituent of the 7-day infusion solution, has been associated with a fatal "gasping syn-

drome" in premature infants. Although used in children, safety and efficacy have not been established.

**Side Effects:** *Hematologic:* Neutropenia, anemia, thrombocytopenia, prolonged depression of $CD_4$ counts, prolonged bone marrow hypocellularity. *Body as a whole:* Fever, infections (including septicemia, pneumonia), fatigue, chills, asthenia, diaphoresis, malaise, trunk pain. *GI:* Nausea, decreased appetite, vomiting, diarrhea, constipation, abdominal pain. *CV:* Edema, tachycardia, purpura, petechiae, epistaxis. *CNS:* Headache, dizziness, insomnia. *Dermatologic:* Rashes, reactions at injection site, pruritus, pain, erythema. *Respiratory:* Abnormal breath sounds, cough, abnormal chest sounds, SOB. *Musculoskeletal:* Myalgia, arthralgia. *Following IV injection:* Redness, swelling pain, thrombosis, phlebitis.

**OD** **Overdose Management:** *Symptoms:* Irreversible neurologic toxicity (paraparesis/quadriparesis), *acute nephrotoxicity, severe bone marrow suppression.* *Treatment:* Discontinue infusion of the drug. Institute appropriate supportive measures as there is no antidote for cladribine.

**Dosage** —————
• **IV infusion**
  *Hairy cell leukemia.*
A single course given by continuous infusion for 7 consecutive days at a dose of 0.09 mg/kg/day.

## NURSING CONSIDERATIONS

See also *Nursing Considerations* for *Antineoplastic Agents.*
**Administration/Storage**
**IV** 1. If neurotoxicity or renal toxicity occur, delay or discontinue drug therapy.
2. Aseptic technique and proper environmental precautions must be observed; drug product does not contain any antimicrobial preservative.
3. To prepare a single daily dose, 0.09 mg/kg or 0.09 mL/kg of cladribine is added to an infusion bag containing 500 mL of 0.9% NaCl

injection. The use of 5% dextrose is not recommended due to increased degradation of the drug. Admixtures of cladribine are stable for at least 24 hr at room temperature under normal room fluorescent light in Baxter Viaflex PVC infusion containers.
4. To prepare the 7-day infusion, mix the drug only with bacteriostatic 0.9% NaCl injection (benzyl alcohol preserved). To minimize the risk of microbial contamination, pass both the cladribine and diluent through a sterile 0.22-µm disposable hydrophilic syringe filter as each solution is being introduced into the infusion reservoir. The calculated dose of cladribine (0.09 mg/kg or mL/kg for 7 days) is first added to the infusion reservoir through the sterile filter; then, a calculated amount of bacteriostatic 0.9% NaCl injection is run through the filter to bring the total volume of the solution to 100 mL. After completing the preparation of the solution, clamp the line, disconnet and discard the filter. Aseptically aspirate air bubbles from the reservoir as necessary using the syringe and a dry second sterile filter assembly. Admixtures for the 7-day infusion are stable in Pharmacia Deltic medication cassettes.
5. Adherence to the recommended diluents and infusion systems is advised due to limited availability of compatibility data.
6. Do not mix solutions containing cladribine with other IV drugs or additives or infuse simultaneously in a common IV line.
7. Refrigerate unopened vial at 2°C–8°C (36°F–46°F) and protect from light. Although freezing does not affect the solution, a precipitate may form at low temperatures. The drug may be resolubilized by allowing the solution to warm naturally to room temperature and by shaking vigorously. The solution is not to be heated or microwaved. Once thawed, do not refreeze the solution.
8. Once diluted, promptly inject or store in the refrigerator for no more than 8 hr prior to administration.

9. Vials of cladribine are for single use only; discard any unused portion in an appropriate manner.

**Assessment**

1. Document symptom onset; note other therapies trialed.

2. Reconstituted infusion solution contains benzyl alcohol.

3. Client should be infection free prior to administration. Fevers during the first 1–2 months following therapy should be evaluated (e.g., labs, cultures, X rays) to determine need for antibiotics.

4. High dose drug therapy may precipitate acute nephrotoxity and delayed neurotoxity (from demyelination).

5. With large tumor burdens, use allopurinol to empirically treat hyperuricemia and tumor lysis syndrome.

6. Obtain baseline CBC, liver and renal function studies. Monitor hematologic profile closely for 4–8 weeks after therapy; blood transfusions and to a lesser extent platelet transfusions may be required due to cladribine's severe myelosuppressive effects.

**Client/Family Teaching**

1. The recommended dosing requires a continuous infusion for 7 consecutive days.

2. Report any evidence of abnormal bleeding, pain, or fever.

3. Nausea may be relieved with chlorpromazine; report if evident.

4. Fever and fatigue are common side effects but should be reported if prolonged or debilitating. Schedule activities to include frequent rest periods.

5. Drug is teratogenic; women should practice a safe form of contraception.

6. Bone marrow aspiration and biopsy will be repeated after treatment to confirm pharmacologic response.

**Outcomes/Evaluate**

• Normalization of hematologic profile (i.e., Hb > 12 g/dL; Plts > 100,000; ANC > 1,500 x 10⁶/L)

• Absence of hairy cells in peripheral blood and bone marrow

• Inhibition of pathologic and clinical disease progression

# Clarithromycin

(klah-**rith**-roh-**MY**-sin)

**Pregnancy Category:** C

Biaxin **(Rx)**

**Classification:** Antibiotic, macrolide

See also *Anti-Infectives*.

**Action/Kinetics:** Clarithromycin is a macrolide antibiotic that acts by binding to the 50S ribosomal subunit of susceptible organisms, thus interfering with or inhibiting microbial protein synthesis. Rapidly absorbed from the GI tract although food slightly delays the onset of absorption and the formation of the active metabolite but does not affect the extent of the bioavailability. **Peak serum levels:** When fasting, 2 hr for the tablet and 3 hr for the suspension. **Steady-state peak serum levels:** 1 mcg/mL within 2–3 days after 250 mg q 12 hr and 2–3 mcg/mL after 500 mg q 12 hr. Clarithromycin and 14-OH clarithromycin (active metabolite) are readily distributed to body tissues and fluids. **t½, elimination:** 3–7 hr (depending on the dose) for clarithromycin and 5–6 hr for 14-OH clarithromycin. Up to 30% of a dose is excreted unchanged in the urine.

**Uses:** Mild to moderate infections caused by susceptible strains of the following. **Adults.** Pharyngitis/tonsillitis due to *Streptococcus pyogenes* Acute maxillary sinusitis or acute bacterial exacerbaton of chronic bronchitis due to *Sreptococcus pneumoniae, Haemophilus influenzae,* and *Moraxella catarrhalis.* The active metabolite, 14-OH clarithromycin, has significant activity (twice the parent compound) against *H. influenzae.* Pneumonia due to *Mycoplasma pneumoniae, S. pneumoniae,* or *Chlamydia pneumoniae.* Uncomplicated skin and skin structure infections due to *Staphylococcus aureus* or *S. pyogenes.* Treatment of disseminated mycobacterial infections due to *Mycobacterium avium* (commonly seen in AIDS clients) and *M. intracellulare.* Prevention of disseminated *M. avium* complex in individuals with advanced HIV.

Used with omeprazole or ranitidine bismuth citrate (Tritec) for the eradication of *Helicobacter pylori* infection in clients with active duodenal ulcers associated with *H. pylori* infection also with amoxicillin and lansoprazole for the same purpose.

**Children.** Pharyngitis or tonsillitis due to *S. pyogenes.* Acute maxillary sinusitis or acute otitis media due to *S. pneumoniae, H. influenzae,* and *M. catarrhalis.* Uncomplicated skin and skin structure infections due to *S. aureus* or *S. pyogenes.* Disseminated mycobacterial infections due to *M. avium* or *M. intracellulare.* Prevention of disseminated *M. avium* complex disease in clients with advanced HIV infection. Community-acquired pneumonia caused by *M. pneumoniae, Chlamydia pneumoniae,* and *S. pneumoniae.*

**Contraindications:** Hypersensitivity to clarithromycin, other macrolide antibiotics, or erythromycin. Clients taking astemizole, terfenadine, cisapride, or pimozide.

**Special Concerns:** Use with caution in severe renal impairment with or without concomitant hepatic impairment and during lactation. Safety and effectiveness in children less than 6 months of age have not been determined. Safety has not been determined in MAC clients less than 20 months of age.

**Side Effects:** *GI:* Diarrhea, nausea, abnormal taste, dyspepsia, abdominal discomfort or pain, pseudomembranous colitis, glossitis, stomatitis, oral moniliasis, vomiting. *CNS:* Headache, dizziness, behavioral changes, confusion, depersonalization, disorientation, hallucinations, insomnia, nightmares, vertigo. *Allergic:* Urticaria, mild skin eruptions and, rarely, **anaphylaxis and Stevens-Johnson syndrome.** *Hepatic:* Hepatocellular cholestatic hepatitis with or without jaundice, increased liver enzymes, **hepatic failure.** *Miscellaneous:* Hearing loss (usually reversible), alteration of sense of smell (usually with taste perversion).

In children, the most common side effects are diarrhea, vomiting, abdominal pain, rash, and headache.

**Drug Interactions**
*See also Drug Interactions* for *Erythromycins.*
*Anticoagulants* / ↑ Anticoagulant effects
*Astemizole* / Combination not to be used in clients who have preexisting cardiac abnormalities or electrolyte disturbances
*Carbamazepine* / ↑ Blood levels of carbamazepine
*Cisapride* / Possibility of serious cardiac arrhythmias, including ventricular tachycardia, ventricular fibrillation, torsade de pointes, and QT prolongation
*Cyclosporine* ↑ Levels of cyclosporine → ↑ risk of nephrotoxicity and neurotoxicity
*Digoxin* / ↑ Plasma levels of digoxin due to ↓ metabolism of digoxin by the gut flora
*Ergot alkaloids* / Acute ergot toxicity, including severe peripheral vasospasm and dysesthesia
*Omeprazole* / ↑ Plasma levels of omeprazole, clarithromycin, and 14-OH-clarithromycin
*Pimozide* / ↑ Risk of sudden death; do not use together
*Tacrolimus* / ↑ Plasma tacrolimus levels → ↑ risk of toxicity
*Terfenadine* / ↑ Plasma levels of the active acid metabolite of terfenadine; ↑ risk of cardiac arrhythmias, including QT interval prolongation
*Theophylline* / ↑ Serum levels of theophylline
*Triazolam* / ↑ Risk of somnolence and confusion
*AZT* / ↓ Steady-state AZT levels in HIV-infected clients; however, peak serum AZT levels may be ↑ or ↓
**Laboratory Test Interferences:** ↑ ALT, AST, GGT, alkaline phosphatase, LDH, total bilirubin, BUN, serum creatinine, PT. ↓ WBC count.

**Dosage**

• **Tablets, Oral Suspension**

*Pharyngitis, tonsillitis.*

250 mg q 12 hr for 10 days.

*Acute exacerbation of chronic bronchitis due to* S. pneumoniae *or* M. catarrhalis; *pneumonia due to* S. pneumoniae *or* M. pneumoniae; *skin and skin structure infections.*

250 mg q 12 hr for 7–14 days.

*Acute maxillary sinusitis, acute exacerbation of chronic bronchitis due to* H. influenzae.

500 mg q 12 hr for 7–14 days.

*Disseminated* M. avium *complex or prophylaxis of* M. avium *complex.*

**Adults:** 500 mg b.i.d.; **children:** 7.5 mg/kg b.i.d. up to 500 mg b.i.d.

*NOTE:* The usual daily dose for children is 15 mg/kg q 12 hr for 10 days.

*Community-acquired pneumonia in children.*

15 mg/kg/day of the suspension, divided and given q 12 hr for 10 days.

*Active duodenal ulcers associated with* H. pylori *infection.*

Clarithromycin, 500 mg t.i.d., with omeprazole, 40 mg, each morning for 2 weeks. **Then,** omeprazole is given alone at a dose of 20 mg/day for 2 more weeks. Or, clarithromycin, 500 mg t.i.d., with ranitidine bismuth citrate, 400 mg b.i.d., for 2 weeks. **Then,** ranitidine bismuth citrate is given alone at a dose of 400 mg b.i.d. for 2 more weeks or, clarithromycin 500 mg, plus lansoprazole, 30 mg, and amoxicillin, 1 g b.i.d. for 2 weeks.

## NURSING CONSIDERATIONS

See also *Nursing Considerations* for *Erythromycins.*

**Administration/Storage**

1. May be given with or without food, and both tablets and suspension can be given with milk. Food delays both the onset of absorption and the formation of 14-OH clarithromycin (the active metabolite).

2. Consider decreased doses or prolonging the dosing interval in cli-ents with severe renal impairment with or without coexisting impaired hepatic function.

3. Shake the reconstituted suspension well before each use; use within 14 days and do not refrigerate.

**Assessment**

1. Note any sensitivity to erythromycin or any of the macrolide antibiotics.

2. Document type, severity, onset, and duration of symptoms.

3. List drugs currently prescribed to prevent any interactions.

4. Obtain baseline CBC, liver and renal function studies, and cultures when indicated.

**Client/Family Teaching**

1. May take with or without meals; food delays onset of absorption. Drug may cause a bitter taste.

2. Report any persistent diarrhea; an antibiotic-associated colitis may be precipitated by *C. difficile* and require alternative management.

3. Report if no symptom improvement after 48–72 hr.

**Outcomes/Evaluate**

• Symptomatic improvement

• Negative follow-up cultures

# Clemastine fumarate

(kleh-**MAS**-teen)

**Pregnancy Category:** B

Antihist-1 **(OTC)**, Tavist **(Rx)**

**Classification:** Antihistamine

See also Antihistamines.

**Action/Kinetics:** Moderate sedative effects, high anticholinergic activity, and moderate to high antiemetic effects. **Peak blood levels:** 2–4 hr. **Peak effects:** 5–7 hr. **Duration:** 10–12 hr (up to 24 hr in some clients). Metabolized in the liver and excreted through the urine.

**Uses:** Allergic rhinitis. Urticaria and angioedema.

**Contraindications:** Use in newborns or premature infants. Lactation. Treatment of lower respiratory tract symptoms, including asthma. Use with monoamine oxidase (MAO) inhibitors.

---

♣ = Available in Canada                    ***bold italic*** = life threatening side effect

**Special Concerns:** Use with caution in clients with narrow angle glaucoma, stenosing peptic ulcer, pyloroduodenal obstruction, symptomatic prostatic hypertrophy, and bladder neck obstruction. Use with caution in clients 60 years of age and older and in those with a history of bronchial asthma, increased intraocular pressure, hyperthyroidism, CV disease, and hypertension. Safety and efficacy have not been determined in children less than 12 years of age.

**Side Effects:** *CNS:* Drowsiness (common), sedation, sleepiness, dizziness, incoordination, fatigue, confusion, restlessness, excitation, nervousness, tremor, irritability, insomnia, euphoria, paresthesia, blurred vision, diplopia, vertigo, tinnitus, acute labyrinthitis, hysteria, neuritis, *convulsions. GI:* Epigastric distress, anorexia, N&V, diarrhea, constipation. *CV:* Hypotension, headache, palpitations, tachycardia, extrasystoles. *Respiratory:* Thickening of bronchial secretions, tightness of chest, wheezing, nasal stuffiness. *Hematologic:* Hemolytic anemia, thrombocytopenia, agranulocytosis. *GU:* Urinary frequency, difficulty in urination, urinary retention, early menses.

**Dosage** —————————————
- **Syrup, Tablets**
  *Allergic rhinitis.*
**Adults and children over 12 years of age, initial:** 1.34 mg (1 mg clemastine) b.i.d., up to a maximum dose of 8.04 mg (60 mL of syrup or 6 tablets) daily. **Children, aged 6 to 12 years of age, initial:** 0.67 mg (0.5 mg clemastine) b.i.d., up to a maximum of 4.02 mg (3 mg) daily. Use only the syrup in children.
  *Urticaria and angioedema.*
**Adults and children over 12 years of age, initial:** 2.68 mg (use tablet) 1–3 times/day, not to exceed 8.04 mg (6 tablets) daily. **Children, aged 6 to 12 years, initial:** 1.34 mg (use syrup only) b.i.d., not to exceed 4.02 mg daily.

## NURSING CONSIDERATIONS

See also *Nursing Considerations* for Antihistamines.

**Administration/Storage:** The syrup should be stored below 77°F (25°C) in a tight, amber glass bottle. Tablets should be stored at room temperatures between 15°C and 30°C (59°F–86°F) in a tight, light-resistant container.

**Assessment**
1. Document onset, duration, and characteristics of symptoms; list triggers.
2. Determine any evidence or history of asthma, BPH, HTN, PUD, or glaucoma.
3. Obtain baseline CBC, VS, ECG, ENT, and cardiopulmonary assessment.

**Client/Family Teaching**
1. Take as directed; do not exceed prescribed dose.
2. Do not perform activities that require mental alertness until drug effects realized; dizziness and drowsiness may occur.
3. Avoid alcohol and any other CNS depressants.
4. Use sugarless gum and candy or sips of water for dry mouth symptoms. Report any intolerable side effects or loss of symptom control.

**Outcomes/Evaluate:** Relief of allergic manifestations.

# Clindamycin hydrochloride hydrate
(klin-dah-**MY**-sin)
Cleocin Hydrochloride, Dalacin C ✲ **(Rx)**

# Clindamycin palmitate hydrochloride
(klin-dah-**MY**-sin)
Cleocin Pediatric, Dalacin C Palmitate ✲ **(Rx)**

# Clindamycin phosphate
(klin-dah-**MY**-sin)
**Pregnancy Category:** B (vaginal cream, topical gel, lotion, solution) Cleocin Vaginal Cream, Cleocin Phosphate, Cleocin T, Clinda-Derm,

C/T/S, Dalacin C Phosphate ✤,
Dalacin T Topical ✤, Dalacin Vaginal
Cream ✤ (Rx)
**Classification:** Antibiotic, clindamy-
cin and lincomycin

See also *Anti-Infectives*.
**Action/Kinetics:** A semisynthetic
antibiotic that suppresses protein
synthesis by microorganism by binding to ribosomes (50S subunit) and
preventing peptide bond formation. Is
both bacteriostatic and bactericidal.
**Peak serum concentration: PO,** 4
mcg/mL after 300 mg; **IM,** 4.9 mcg/
mL after 300 mg; **IV,** 14.7 mcg/mL
after 300 mg. **t½:** 2.4–3 hr. In serious
infections the rate of IV administration
is adjusted to maintain appropriate
serum drug concentrations: 4–6
mcg/mL.
**Uses:** Should not be used for trivial
infections. **Systemic.** Serious respiratory tract infections (e.g., empyema, lung abscess, pneumonia)
caused by staphylococci, streptococci, and pneumococci. Serious skin
and soft tissue infections, septicemia, intra-abdominal infections, pelvic inflammatory disease, female
genital tract infections. May be the
drug of choice for *Bacteroides fragilis*. In combination with aminoglycosides for mixed aerobic and anaerobic bacterial infections. Staphylococ-
ci-induced acute hematogenous
osteomyelitis. Adjunct to surgery for
chronic bone/joint infections. *Investigational:* Alternative to sulfonamides in combination with pyrimethamine in the acute treatment of
CNS toxoplasmosis in AIDS clients. In
combination with primaquine to
treat *Pneumocystis carinii* pneumonia.
Chlamydial infections in women.
Bacterial vaginosis due to *Gardnerella vaginalis*. **Topical Use.** Used
topically for inflammatory acne vulgaris. Vaginally to treat bacterial vaginosis. *Investigational:* Treatment of
rosacea (lotion used).

**Contraindications:** Hypersensitivity to either clindamycin or lincomycin.
Use in treating viral and minor bacterial infections or in clients with a his-

tory of regional enteritis, ulcerative
colitis, or antibiotic-associated colitis. Lactation.
**Special Concerns:** Use with caution in infants up to 1 month of age,
in clients with GI disease, liver or renal disease, or a history of allergy or
asthma. Safety and efficacy of topical
products have not been established in
children less than 12 years of age.
**Side Effects:** *GI:* N&V, diarrhea,
bloody diarrhea, abdominal pain, GI
disturbances, tenesmus, flatulence,
bloating, anorexia, weight loss,
esophagitis. Nonspecific colitis,
pseudomembranous colitis (may be
severe). *Allergic:* Morbilliform rash
(most common). Also, maculopapular
rash, urticaria, pruritus, fever, hypotension. Rarely, polyarteritis, anaphylaxis, erythema multiforme. *Hematologic:* Leukopenia, neutropenia,
eosinophilia, thrombocytopenia,
***agranulocytosis***. *Miscellaneous:* Superinfection. Also sore throat, fatigue, urinary frequency, headache.
*Following IV use:* Thrombophlebitis, erythema, pain, swelling.
*Following IM use:* Pain, induration,
sterile abscesses.
*Following topical use:* Erythema,
irritation, dryness, peeling, itching,
burning, oiliness of skin.
*Following vaginal use:* Cervicitis,
vaginitis, vulvar irritation, urticaria,
rash.
*NOTE:* The injection contains benzyl alcohol, which has been associated with ***a fatal "gasping syndrome"*** in infants.
**Drug Interactions**
*Antiperistaltic antidiarrheals (opi-
ates, Lomotil)* / ↑ Diarrhea due to ↓
removal of toxins from colon
*Ciprofloxacin HCl* / Additive antibacterial activity
*Erythromycin* / Cross-interference
→ ↓ effect of both drugs
*Kaolin (e.g., Kaopectate)* / ↓ Effect
due to ↓ absorption from GI tract
*Neuromuscular blocking agents* / ↑
Effect of blocking agents
**Laboratory Test Interferences:** ↓
Levels of AST, ALT, NPN, alkaline

phosphatase, bilirubin, BSP retention, and ↓ platelet count.

## Dosage

• **PO only: Capsules, Oral Solution**
**Adults: Clindamycin HCl, Clindamycin palmitate HCl:** 150–450 mg q 6 hr, depending on severity of infection. **Pediatric: Clindamycin HCl hydrate:** 8–20 mg/kg/day divided into three to four equal doses; clindamycin palmitate HCl: 8–25 mg/kg/day divided into three to four equal doses. **Children less than 10 kg:** Minimum recommended dose is 37.5 mg t.i.d.

• **IV**
**Clindamycin phosphate. Adults:** 0.6–2.7 g/day in two to four equal doses depending on severity of infection.
*Life-threatening infections.*
4.8 g. **Pediatric over 1 month:** 15–40 mg/kg/day in three to four equal doses depending on severity of infections.
*Severe infections.*
No less than 300 mg/day, regardless of body weight.
*Acute pelvic inflammatory disease.*
**IV:** 600 mg q.i.d. plus gentamicin, 2 mg/kg IV; **then,** gentamicin, 1.5 mg/kg t.i.d. IV. IV therapy should be continued for 2 days after client improves. The 10–14-day treatment cycle should be completed using clindamycin, **PO:** 450 mg q.i.d.

• **Topical Gel, Lotion, or Solution**
Apply thin film b.i.d. to affected areas. One or more pledgets may also be used.

• **Vaginal Cream (2%)**
One applicatorful (containing about 100 mg clindamycin phosphate), preferably at bedtime, for 7 consecutive days.

## NURSING CONSIDERATIONS

See also *General Nursing Considerations for All Anti-Infectives.*
**Administration/Storage**
1. Shake the lotion well just before using.

2. Reduce dosage in severe renal impairment.
3. Single IM injections greater than 600 mg are not advisable. Inject deeply into muscle to prevent induration, pain, and sterile abscesses.
4. Do not refrigerate; otherwise, solution may become thickened.
**IV** 5. Give parenteral clindamycin only to hospitalized clients.
6. Dilute IV injections to maximum concentration of 12 mg/mL, with no more than 1,200 mg administered in 1 hr.
7. Administer IV over a period of 20–60 min, depending on dose and therapeutic serum concentration to be attained.
**Assessment**
1. Document indications for therapy, type and onset of symptoms.
2. Auscultate lungs and note extent of respiratory tract infections.
3. Describe skin and soft tissue infections; note complaints indicative of pelvic inflammatory disease or intra-abdominal infections.
4. Obtain baseline cultures, liver and renal function studies. Note any history of liver or renal disease, allergies, or GI problems.
5. With IV therapy, observe for hypotension; keep in bed for 30 min following infusion. Advise that a bitter taste may be evident.
6. Observe for drug interactions caused by concurrent administration of neuromuscular blocking agents. Be alert to hypotension, bronchospasms, cardiac disturbances, hyperthermia, and respiratory depression.
7. Observe closely for:
• Skin rash; most frequently reported side effect
• Renal and/or hepatic impairment and newborns for organ dysfunction
• GI disturbances, such as abdominal pain, diarrhea, anorexia, N&V, bloody or tarry stools, and excessive flatulence. Discontinuation of drug may be indicated.
**Client/Family Teaching**
1. Take PO medication with a full glass of water to prevent esophageal ulceration. Take on an empty stomach

to ensure optimum absorption. May take with food if GI upset occurs.

2. Report any side effects such as persistent vomiting, diarrhea, fever, or abdominal pain and cramping.

3. Pseudomembranous colitis may occur 2–9 days or several weeks after initiation of therapy. Fluids, electrolytes, protein supplements, systemic corticosteroids, and oral antibiotics may be needed; report immmediately. Do not use antiperistaltic agents if diarrhea occurs because these can prolong or aggravate condition. Kaolin will reduce absorption of antibiotic; if prescribed, take 3 hr before antibiotic

4. The vaginal cream contains mineral oil, which may weaken latex or rubber products, such as condoms or vaginal contraceptive diaphragms. Use of such products is not recommended for 72 hr following treatment.

5. Do not engage in intercourse when using the vaginal cream as this may enhance irritation.

6. Do not use any acne or topical mercury preparations containing a peeling agent in affected area; severe irritation may occur.

**Outcomes/Evaluate**
- Resolution of infection
- Symptomatic improvement
- Therapeutic drug levels with IV therapy (4–6 mcg/mL)

# Clobetasol propionate
(kloh-**BAY**-tah-sohl)
**Pregnancy Category:** C
Temovate **(Rx)**
**Classification:** Corticosteroid, topical

See also *Corticosteroids*.

**Action/Kinetics:** Has anti-inflammatory, antipruritic, and vasoconstrictive effects.

**Uses:** Relief of inflammatory and pruritic dermatoses.

**Contraindications:** Use in children less than 12 years old, use for more than 2 weeks, to treat rosacea or perioral dermatitis, and use on face, groin, axillae.

**Special Concerns:** May suppress hypothalamic-pituitary-adrenal (HPA)axis at doses as low as 2 g/day. Use with caution during lactation.

**Side Effects:** *Dermatologic:* Burning sensation, stinging, irritation, pruritus, erythema, folliculitis, cracking and fissuring of the skin, skin atrophy, numbness of fingers, telangiectasia. *Miscellaneous:* Cushing's syndrome.

## Dosage
- **Topical gel**
  *Dermatoses.*

Apply thin layer to affected skin b.i.d. and rub in gently and completely. Use no more than 50 g/week.

## NURSING CONSIDERATIONS
### Administration/Storage
1. Do not use with occlusive dressings.
2. Do not refrigerate.

### Assessment
1. Document onset, location, and characteristics of symptoms or photograph; note other agents trialed and outcome.
2. Drug is a potent corticosteroid for short term use; assess for S&S of HPA axis suppression using ACTH stimulation test, a.m. cortisol, and urinary free cortisol test.

### Client/Family Teaching
1. Apply thin layer to affected area and gently rub in. Use only as directed, externally, and avoid contact with eyes.
2. Wash hands before and after application. Do not cover, wrap, or bandage treatment area.
3. Report any failure to heal as this may indicate an allergic contact dermatitis from agent.
4. If skin infections develop, may also need antifungal or antibacterial agent; report if evident.
5. Report any severe burning, stinging, swelling, numbness, or lack of response.

**Outcomes/Evaluate:** Relief of inflammation and pruritic skin manifestations

---

***bold italic*** = life threatening side effect

# Clofazimine

(kloh-**FAYZ**-ih-meen)
**Pregnancy Category:** C
Lamprene **(Rx)**
**Classification:** Leprostatic

**Action/Kinetics:** Inhibits mycobacterial growth (is bactericidal) and binding to mycobacterial DNA in *Mycobacterium leprae.* Is also an anti-inflammatory by controlling erythema nodosum leprosum reactions. Cross-resistance with rifampin or dapsone is not observed. Concentrated in fatty tissues and the reticuloendothelial system. **Average serum levels:** 0.7 mcg/mL after 100 mg/day and 1 mcg/mL after 300 mg/day. **t½:** 70 days. Excreted in the feces via the bile, as well as in sputum, sweat, and sebum.

**Uses:** Lepromatous leprosy (including dapsone-resistant leprosy and leprosy complicated by erythema nodosum leprosum). In combination with other drugs to prevent resistance in multibacillary leprosy.

**Special Concerns:** Use with caution in clients with abdominal pain or diarrhea. Use during lactation only if benefits outweigh risks. Safety and efficacy have not been determined in children.

**Side Effects:** *GI:* N&V, diarrhea, abdominal or epigastric pain, GI intolerance, GI bleeding, intestinal obstruction, anorexia, constipation, liver enlargement, eosinophilic enteritis, taste disorder. *Dermatologic:* Pink to brownish black pigmentation of skin in nearly all clients, ichthyosis, dryness of skin, pruritus, rash, erythroderma, acneiform eruptions, monilial cheilosis. *Ophthalmologic:* Pigmentation of conjunctiva and cornea (due to clofazimine crystals), phototoxicity, decreased vision, eye irritation, burning, itching, or dryness. *CNS:* Headache, dizziness, drowsiness, neuralgia, fatigue, depression, giddiness. Depression due to skin discoloration. *Miscellaneous:* Jaundice, weight loss, hepatitis, anemia, **thromboembolism,** bone pain, edema, cystitis, fever, vascular pain, lymphadenopathy, eosinophilia, hypokalemia. Discoloration of urine, feces, sweat, or sputum.

**OD** **Overdose Management:** *Treatment:* Gastric lavage or induction of vomiting. General supportive measures.

**Laboratory Test Interferences:** ↑ AST, serum bilirubin, albumin, blood sugar, ESR.

**Dosage**

• **Capsules**

*Leprosy resistant to dapsone.*
100 mg/day together with one or more other leprostatic drugs for a period of 3 years; **maintenance:** clofazimine alone, 100 mg/day.

*Erythema nodosum leprosum.*
Dosage depends on severity of symptoms, but doses greater than 200 mg/day are not recommended. Goal is 100 mg/day.

## NURSING CONSIDERATIONS
### Administration/Storage

1. Give with one or more other leprostatic agents to prevent the development of resistance to each drug.

2. Clinical improvement can usually be seen after 1–3 months and is clearly evident within 6 months.

3. When treating dapsone-sensitive multibacillary leprosy, give clofazimine with at least two other antileprosy drugs for at least 2 years or until negative skin smears are obtained. Monotherapy with one of the antileprosy drugs can then be instituted.

4. Store capsules below 30°C (86°F) and protect from moisture.

### Client/Family Teaching

1. Take as directed and with food to minimize GI irritation. Should be taken with one or more leprostatic agent to prevent drug resistance.

2. Report any increased GI distress, depression, and/or unusual side effects immediately.

3. Although reversible, clofazimine will cause pink to brownish black skin discoloration, which may persist after therapy.

4. Do not be alarmed; all body fluids become discolored during therapy.

5. Oil baths and frequent lotion

application may minimize itchy, dry skin formation.

**Outcomes/Evaluate**
- Symptomatic improvement
- ↓ Size and number of skin lesions

# Clofibrate
(kloh-**FYE**-brayt)
**Pregnancy Category:** C
Atromid-S, Claripex ✤, Novo–Fibrate ✤ **(Rx)**
**Classification:** Antihyperlipidemic agent

**Action/Kinetics:** Clofibrate decreases triglycerides and VLDL; cholesterol and LDL are decreased less predictably and less effectively. The mechanism is not known with certainty but may be due to increased catabolism of VLDL to LDL and decreased synthesis of VLDL by the liver. Cholesterol formation is inhibited early in the biosynthetic chain; excretion of neutral streoids is increased. **Peak plasma levels:** 3–6 hr. **t½, plasma:** 15 hr. **Therapeutic effect: Onset,** 2–5 days; **maximum effect:** 3 weeks. Triglycerides return to pretreatment levels 2–3 weeks after therapy is terminated. Clofibrate is hydrolyzed to the active *p*-chlorophenoxyisobutyric acid which is further metabolized and excreted in the urine. The drug may concentrate in fetal blood. LFTs should be performed during therapy.

**Uses:** Dysbetalipoproteinemia (type III hyperlipidemia) not responding to diet. Hyperlipidemia (types IV and V) with a risk of abdominal pain and pancreatitis not responding to diet.

**Contraindications:** Impaired hepatic or renal function, primary biliary cirrhosis, lactation, pregnancy, children.

**Special Concerns:** Use with caution in clients with gout and peptic ulcer. Reduced dosage may be required in geriatric clients due to age-related decreases in renal function.

**Side Effects:** *GI:* Nausea, dyspepsia, weight gain, gastritis, vomiting, bloating, flatulence, abdominal distress, stomatitis, loose stools, diarrhea, hepatomegaly, cholelithiasis, gallstones. *CNS:* Headaches, dizziness, fatigue, weakness, drowsiness. *CV:* Changes in blood-clotting time, arrhythmias, increased or decreased angina, intermittent claudication, thromboembolic events, thrombophlebitis, swelling and phlebitis at xanthoma site, pulmonary embolism. *Skeletal muscle:* Asthenia, arthralgia, myalgia, weakness, muscle cramps, aches. *GU:* Impotence, dysuria, hematuria, decreased urine output, decreased libido, proteinuria. *Hematologic:* Anemia, leukopenia, eosinophilia. *Dermatologic:* Allergic reactions, including urticaria, skin rash, dry skin, pruritus, dry brittle hair, alopecia. *Other:* Dyspnea, polyphagia, flu-like symptoms, ***noncardiovascular death.***

**Drug Interactions**
*Anticoagulants* / Clofibrate ↑ anticoagulant effect by ↓ plasma protein binding
*Antidiabetics (sulfonylureas)* / Clofibrate ↑ effect of antidiabetics
*Furosemide* / Exaggerated diuretic response
*Insulin* / Clofibrate ↑ effect of insulin
*Probenecid* / ↑ Therapeutic and toxic effects of clofibrate due to ↓ breakdown by liver and ↓ kidney excretion
*Ursodiol* / ↑ Risk of gallstone formation

**Laboratory Test Interferences:** ↑ AST, ALT, thymol turbidity, CPK, BSP retention. Proteinuria.

## Dosage
- **Capsules**
  *Antihyperlipidemic.*
**Adults:** 500 mg q.i.d. Therapeutic response may take several weeks to become apparent. Drug must be administered on a continuous basis because lowered levels of cholesterol and other lipids will return to elevated state within several weeks after administration is stopped. Discontin-

---

ue after 3 months if response is poor.

## NURSING CONSIDERATIONS

**Assessment:** Obtain baseline CBC, liver and renal function studies; document cholesterol profile and pregnancy test if appropriate.

**Client/Family Teaching**

1. If GI upset occurs, take with food. Nausea usually decreases with continued therapy or reduced dosage.

2. Anticoagulant dosage is reduced if clofibrate is instituted; report any abnormal bleeding.

3. Report symptoms of hypoglycemia because of possible drug interactions with oral antidiabetic agents.

4. Use contraception during and for several months after drug therapy if pregnancy is planned; drug may be teratogenic.

5. Review potential risks of drug therapy (e.g., gallstones, tumors); report any side effects so therapy can be evaluated.

6. Stress importance of adhering to dietary restrictions, daily exercise, and weight loss in the overall management of high cholesterol.

**Outcomes/Evaluate:** Significant ↓ in serum cholesterol and triglyceride levels

## Clomiphene citrate

(KLOH-mih-feen)

Clomid, Milophene, Serophene **(Rx)**

Classification: Ovarian stimulant

**Action/Kinetics:** Combines with estrogen receptors, thus decreasing the number of available receptor sites. Through negative feedback, the hypothalamus and pituitary are thus stimulated to increase secretion of LH and FSH. Under the influence of increased levels of these hormones, an ovarian follicle develops, followed by ovulation and corpus luteum development. Most women ovulate after the first course of therapy. Further treatment may be inadvisable if pregnancy fails to occur after ovulatory responses. Readily absorbed from the GI tract and excreted in the feces. **t½:** 5–7 days. **Time to peak effect:** 4–10 days after the last day of treatment for ovulation. **Uses:** To treat ovulatory failure in women desiring pregnancy and whose partners are fertile and potent. Normal liver function and normal levels of endogenous estrogen are necessary criteria to clomiphene use. Therapy is ineffective in clients with ovarian or pituitary failure. *Investigational:* Male infertility (controversial).

**Contraindications:** Pregnancy, liver disease or history thereof, abnormal bleeding of undetermined origin. Ovarian cysts or enlargement not due to polycystic ovarian syndrome. Uncontrolled thyroid or adrenal dysfunction, organic intracranial lesion (e.g., pituitary tumor). The absence of neoplastic disease should be established before treatment is initiated.

**Special Concerns:** Multiple births are possible.

**Side Effects:** *Ovarian:* Ovarian overstimulation and/or enlargement and subsequent symptoms resembling those of PMS. *Ophthalmologic:* Blurred vision, spots, or flashes, probably due to intensification of after images. Although cause and effect have not been established, the following have been noted in users of clomiphene: posterior capsular cataract, detachment of the posterior vitreous, spasm of retinal arteriole, and thrombosis of temporal arteries of retina. *GI:* Abdominal distention, pain, bloating, or soreness; N&V. *GU:* Abnormal uterine bleeding, breast tenderness. *CNS:* Insomnia, nervousness, headache, depression, fatigue, lightheadedness, dizziness. *Other:* Hot flashes, increased urination, allergic dermatitis, weight gain, alopecia (reversible).

**Laboratory Test Interferences:** ↑ Serum thyroxine, thyroxine-binding globulin, BSP retention.

## Dosage

• **Tablets**

   *First course.*

50 mg/day for 5 days. Therapy may be initiated at any time in clients

who have had no recent uterine bleeding.

*Second course.*

Same dosage if ovulation has occurred. In absence of ovulation, dose may be increased to 100 mg/day for 5 days. This course may be started as early as 30 days after the previous one.

## NURSING CONSIDERATIONS

### Administration/Storage

1. If the client has had recent uterine bleeding, start the therapy on the fifth day of the cycle.

2. Most clients will respond following the first course of therapy. Further therapy is not recommended if pregnancy does not result following three ovulatory responses.

### Assessment

1. Obtain menstrual history and any history of abnormal bleeding of undetermined origin; note previous therapy.

2. Note history of hepatic dysfunction; document LFTs and abdominal ultrasound.

3. Determine if pregnant.

### Client/Family Teaching

1. Take basal body temperature and chart on graph to determine if ovulation has occurred; usually 4–10 days after treatment.

2. Take at the same time each day.

3. Discontinue drug and report if pain in the pelvic area or abdominal distention occurs; may indicate ovarian enlargement, presence of an ovarian cyst or rupture.

4. Stop drug if blurred vision or spots or flashes in the eyes occur; the retina may be affected. Report for an ophthalmologic exam.

5. Avoid performing hazardous tasks involving body coordination or mental alertness; drug may cause lightheadedness, dizziness, or visual disturbances.

6. Stop drug and report if pregnancy is suspected; drug may have teratogenic effects.

7. Potential for multiple pregnancy exists.

### Outcomes/Evaluate

• ↑ Levels of FSH and LH
• Ovulation → pregnancy

# Clomipramine hydrochloride

(kloh-**MIP**-rah-meen)
**Pregnancy Category:** C
Anafranil, Apo–Clomipramine ✲, Gen-Clomipramine ✲, Novo-Clopamine ✲ **(Rx)**
**Classification:** Antidepressant, tricyclic

See also *Antidepressants, Tricyclic.*

**Action/Kinetics:** Significant anticholinergic and sedative effects as well as moderate orthostatic hypotension. Significant serotonin uptake blocking activity and moderate blocking activity for norepinephrine. t½: 19–37 hr. **Effective plasma levels:** 80–100 ng/mL. **Time to reach steady state:** 7–14 days. Metabolized to the active desmethylclomipramine.

**Uses:** Obsessive-compulsive disorder in which the obsessions or compulsions cause marked distress, significantly interfere with social or occupational activities, or are time-consuming. Panic attacks and cataplexy associated with narcolepsy.

**Contraindications:** To relieve symptoms of depression.

**Special Concerns:** Safety has not been established for use during lactation or in children less than 10 years of age.

**Additional Side Effects:** Hyperthermia, especially when used with other drugs. Increased risk of *seizures.* Aggressive reactions, asthenia, anemia, eructation, failure to ejaculate, laryngitis, vestibular disorders, muscle weakness.

### Dosage

• **Capsules**

**Adult, initial:** 25 mg/day; **then,** increase gradually to approximately 100 mg during the first 2 weeks (depending on client tolerance). The dose may then be increased slowly to

---

✲ = Available in Canada          ***bold italic*** = life threatening side effect

a maximum of 250 mg/day over the next several weeks. **Adolescents, children, initial:** 25 mg/day; **then,** increase gradually during the first 2 weeks to a maximum of 100 mg or 3 mg/kg, whichever is less. The dose may then be increased to a maximum daily dose of 3 mg/kg or 200 mg, whichever is less. **Maintenance, adults and children:** Adjust the dose to the lowest effective dose with periodic reassessment to determine need for continued therapy.

## NURSING CONSIDERATIONS

See also *Nursing Considerations* for *Antidepressants, Tricyclic.*

### Administration/Storage
1. Initially, divide the daily dosage and give with meals to reduce GI side effects.
2. After the optimum dose is determined, the total daily dose can be given at bedtime to minimize daytime sedation.
3. For all ages, adjust to the lowest effective dose and evaluate periodically to determine need for continued treatment.
4. Although efficacy of clomipramine has not been determined after 10 weeks of therapy, clients have successfully used it for up to 1 year without loss of beneficial effects.

### Assessment
1. Document indications for therapy and baseline behavioral findings.
2. List drugs currently prescribed, those used previously for this disorder, and the outcome.

### Client/Family Teaching
1. Take only as directed.
2. Rise slowly to prevent orthostatic drug effects, i.e., dizziness from ↓ BP.
3. Report symptoms of depression.
4. Fluids and lozenges may relieve symptoms of dry mouth.
5. Anticipate 2–3 weeks of therapy before desired effect.

**Outcomes/Evaluate:** Control of obsessive-compulsive behaviors that interfere with normal social or occupational functioning

# Clonazepam
(kloh-**NAY**-zeh-pam)
Alti-Clonazepam ✴, Apo-Clonazepam ✴, Dom-Clonazepam ✴, Klonopin ✴, Nu-Clonazepam ✴, PMS–Clonazepam ✴, Rivotril ✴ **(C-IV) (Rx)**
**Classification:** Anticonvulsant, miscellaneous

See also *Anticonvulsants.*

**Action/Kinetics:** Benzodiazepine derivative which increases presynaptic inhibition and suppresses the spread of seizure activity. **Peak plasma levels:** 1–2 hr. **t½:** 18–60 hr. **Therapeutic serum levels:** 20–80 ng/mL. More than 80% bound to plasma protein; metabolized almost completely in the liver to inactive metabolites, which are excreted in the urine.

Even though a benzodiazepine, clonazepam, is used only as an anticonvulsant. However, contraindications, side effects, and so forth are similar to those for diazepam.

**Uses:** Absence seizures (petit mal) including Lennox-Gastaut syndrome, akinetic and myoclonic seizures. Some effectiveness in clients resistant to succinimide therapy. *Investigational:* Parkinsonian dysarthria, acute manic episodes of bipolar affective disorder, leg movements (periodic) during sleep, adjunct in treating schizophrenia, neuralgias, multifocal tic disorders.

**Contraindications:** Sensitivity to benzodiazepines. Severe liver disease, acute narrow-angle glaucoma. Pregnancy.

**Special Concerns:** Effects on lactation not known.

**Additional Side Effects:** In clients in whom different types of seizure disorders exist, clonazepam may elicit or precipitate **grand mal seizures.**

**Drug Interactions**
*CNS depressants* / Potentiation of CNS depressant effect of clonazepam
*Phenobarbital* / ↓ Effect of clonazepam due to ↑ breakdown by liver

*Phenytoin* / ↓ Effect of clonazepam due to ↑ breakdown by liver

*Valproic acid* / ↑ Chance of absence seizures

## Dosage

- **Tablets**

*Seizure disorders.*

**Adults, initial:** 0.5 mg t.i.d. Increase by 0.5–1 mg/day q 3 days until seizures are under control or side effects become excessive; **maximum:** 20 mg/day. **Pediatric up to 10 years or 30 kg:** 0.01–0.03 mg/kg/day in two to three divided doses up to a maximum of 0.05 mg/kg/day. Increase by increments of 0.25–0.5 mg q 3 days until seizures are under control or maintenance of 0.1–0.2 mg/kg is attained.

*Parkinsonian dysarthria.*

**Adults:** 0.25–0.5 mg/day.

*Acute manic episodes of bipolar affective disorder.*

**Adults:** 0.75–16 mg/day.

*Periodic leg movements during sleep.*

**Adults:** 0.5–2 mg nightly.

*Adjunct to treat schizophrenia.*

**Adults:** 0.5–2 mg/day.

*Neuralgias.*

**Adults:** 2–4 mg/day.

*Multifocal tic disorders.*

**Adults:** 1.5–12 mg/day.

## NURSING CONSIDERATIONS

See also *Nursing Considerations* for *Tranquilizers, Antimanic Drugs, Hypnotics,* and *Anticonvulsants.*

**Administration/Storage**

1. Approximately one-third of clients show some loss of anticonvulsant activity within 3 months; adjustment of dose may reestablish effectiveness.

2. Adding clonazepam to existing anticonvulsant therapy may increase the depressant effects.

3. Divide the daily dose into three equal doses; if doses cannot be divided equally, give the largest dose at bedtime.

**Assessment**

1. Document indications for thera-

py, onset/cause of symptoms, other agents prescribed, and the outcome.

2. Obtain baseline CBC, liver and renal function studies.

**Outcomes/Evaluate:** ↓ Number and frequency of recurrent seizures

# Clonidine hydrochloride

(**KLOH**-nih-deen)

**Pregnancy Category:** C

Apo-Clonidine ✹; Catapres; Catapres-TTS-1, -2, and -3; Dixarit ✹; Duraclon, Novo-Clonidine ✹, Nu-Clonidine ✹ **(Rx)**

**Classification:** Antihypertensive, centrally acting antiadrenergic

See also *Antihypertensive Agents.*

**Action/Kinetics:** Stimulates alpha-adrenergic receptors of the CNS, which results in inhibition of the sympathetic vasomotor centers and decreased nerve impulses. Thus, bradycardia and a fall in both SBP and DBP occur. Plasma renin levels are decreased, while peripheral venous pressure remains unchanged. Few orthostatic effects. Although NaCl excretion is markedly decreased, potassium excretion remains unchanged. Tolerance to the drug may develop. **Onset, PO:** 30–60 min; **transdermal:** 2–3 days. **Peak plasma levels, PO:** 3–5 hr; **transdermal:** 2–3 days. **Maximum effect, PO:** 2–4 hr. **Duration, PO:** 12–24 hr; **transdermal:** 7 days (with system in place). **t½:** 12–16 hr. Approximately 50% excreted unchanged in the urine; 20% excreted through the feces.

The transdermal dosage form contains the following levels of drug: Catapres-TTS-1 contains 2.5 mg clonidine (surface area 3.5 cm²), with 0.1 mg released daily; Catapres-TTS-2 contains 5 mg clonidine (surface area 7 cm²), with 0.2 mg released daily; and Catapres-TTS-3 contains 7.5 mg clonidine (surface area 10.5 cm²), with 0.3 mg released daily.

Epidural use causes analgesia at presynaptic and postjunctional alpha-2-adrenergic receptors in the spinal cord due to prevention of pain signal transmission to the brain. **t½, distribution, epidural:** 19 min; **elimination:** 22 hr.

**Uses:** *Oral, Transdermal:* Mild to moderate hypertension. A diuretic or other antihypertensive drugs, or both, are often used concomitantly. *Investigational:* Alcohol withdrawal, atrial fibrillation, attention deficit hyperactivity disorder, constitutional growth delay in children, cyclosporine-associated nephrotoxicity, diabetic diarrhea, Gilles de la Tourette's syndrome, hyperhidrosis, hypertensive emergencies, mania, menopausal flushing, opiate detoxification, diagnosis of pheochromocytoma, postherpetic neuralgia, psychosis in schizophrenia, reduce allergen-induced inflammatory reactions in extrinsic asthma, restless leg syndrome, facilitate smoking cessation, ulcerative colitis.

*Epidural:* With opiates for severe pain in cancer clients not relieved by opiate analgesics alone. Most effective for neuropathic pain.

**Contraindications:** Epidurally: Presence of an injection site infection, clients on anticoagulant therapy, in bleeding diathesis, administration above the C4 dermatome. For obstetric, postpartum, or perioperative pain.

**Special Concerns:** Use with caution in presence of severe coronary insufficiency, recent MI, cerebrovascular disease, or chronic renal failure. Use with caution during lactation. Safe use in children not established. Geriatric clients may be more sensitive to the hypotensive effects; a decreased dosage may also be necessary in these clients due to age-related decreases in renal function. For children, restrict epidural use to severe intractable pain from malignancy that is not responsive to epidural or spinal opiates or other analgesic approaches.

**Side Effects:** *CNS:* Drowsiness (common), sedation, confusion, dizziness, headache, fatigue, malaise, nightmares, nervousness, restlessness, anxiety, mental depression, increased dreaming, insomnia, hallucinations, delirium, agitation. *GI:* Dry mouth (common), constipation, anorexia, N&V, parotid pain, weight gain, hepatitis, parotitis, ileus, pseudoobstruction, abdominal pain. *CV:* CHF, severe hypotension, Raynaud's phenomenon, abnormalities in ECG, palpitations, tachycardia and bradycardia, postural hypotension, conduction disturbances, sinus bradycardia, *CVA. Dermatologic:* Urticaria, skin rashes, sweating, **angioneurotic edema,** pruritus, thinning of hair, alopecia, skin ulcer. *GU:* Impotence, urinary retention, decreased sexual activity, loss of libido, nocturia, difficulty in urination, UTI. *Respiratory:* Hypoventilation, dyspnea. *Musculoskeletal:* Muscle or joint pain, leg cramps, weakness. *Other:* Gynecomastia, increase in blood glucose (transient), increased sensitivity to alcohol, chest pain, tinnitus, hyperaesthesia, pain, infection, thrombocytopenia, syncope, blurred vision, withdrawal syndrome, dryness of mucous membranes of nose; itching, burning, dryness of eyes; skin pallor, fever.

*Transdermal products:* Localized skin reactions, pruritus, erythema, allergic contact sensitization and contact dermatitis, localized vesiculation, hyperpigmentation, edema, excoriation, burning, papules, throbbing, blanching, generalized macular rash.

*NOTE:* Rebound hypertension may be manifested if clonidine is withdrawn abruptly.

**OD** **Overdose Management:** *Symptoms:* Hypotension, bradycardia, respiratory and CNS depression, hypoventilation, hypothermia, apnea, miosis, agitation, irritability, lethargy, **seizures, cardiac conduction defects, arrhythmias,** transient hypertension, diarrhea, vomiting. *Treatment:* Maintain respiration; perform gastric lavage followed by activated charcoal. Magnesium sulfate may be used to hasten the rate of transport through the GI tract. IV atropine sulfate (0.6 mg for adults; 0.01 mg/kg for children), epinephrine, tolazoline, or dopamine to treat persistent bradycardia. IV fluids and elevation of the legs are used to reverse hypotension; if unresponsive to these measures, dopamine (2–20 mcg/kg/min) or tolazoline (1 mg/kg IV, up to a maximum of 10 mg/dose) may be used. To treat hypertension, diazoxide, IV furosemide, or an alpha-adrenergic blocking drug may be used.

**Drug Interactions**

*Alcohol* / ↑ Depressant effects
*Beta-adrenergic blocking agents* / Paradoxical hypertension; also, ↑ severity of rebound hypertension following clonidine withdrawal
*CNS depressants* / ↑ Depressant effect
*Levodopa* / ↓ Effect of levodopa
*Local anesthetics* / Epidural clonidine → prolonged duration of epidural local anesthetics
*Prazosin* / ↓ Antihypertensive effect of clonidine
*Narcotic analgesics* / Potentiation of hypotensive effect of clonidine
*Tolazoline* / Blocks antihypertensive effect
*Tricyclic antidepressants* / Blocks antihypertensive effect
*Verapamil* / ↑ Risk of AV block and severe hypotension

**Laboratory Test Interferences:** Transient ↑ blood glucose, serum phosphatase, and serum CPK. Weakly + Coombs' test. Alteration of electrolyte balance.

**Dosage**
- **Tablets**
  *Hypertension.*
  **Initial:** 100 mcg b.i.d.; **then,** increase by 100–200 mcg/day until desired response is attained; **maintenance:** 200–600 mcg/day in divided doses (maximum: 2400 mcg/day). Tolerance necessitates increased dosage or concomitant administration of a diuretic. Gradual increase of dosage after initiation minimizes side effects. **Pediatric:** 50–400 mcg b.i.d.
  *NOTE:* In hypertensive clients unable to take PO medication, cloni-

dine may be administered sublingually at doses of 200–400 mcg/day.
  *Alcohol withdrawal.*
  300–600 mcg q 6 hr.
  *Atrial fibrillation.*
  75 mcg 1–2 times/day with or without digoxin.
  *Attention deficit hyperactivity disorder.*
  5 mcg/kg/day for 8 weeks.
  *Constitutional growth delay in children.*
  37.5–150 mcg/m²/day.
  *Diabetic diarrhea.*
  100–600 mcg q 12 hr.
  *Gilles de la Tourette syndrome.*
  150–200 mcg/day.
  *Hyperhidrosis.*
  250 mcg 3–5 times/day.
  *Hypertensive urgency (diastolic > 120 mm Hg).*
  **Initial:** 100–200 mcg; **then,** 50– 100 mcg q hr to a maximum of 800 mcg.
  *Menopausal flushing.*
  100–400 mcg/day.
  *Withdrawal from opiate dependence.*
  15–16 mcg/kg/day.
  *Diagnosis of pheochromocytoma.*
  300 mcg.
  *Postherpetic neuralgia.*
  200 mcg/day.
  *Psychosis in schizophrenia.*
  Less than 900 mcg/day.
  *Reduce allergen-induced inflammation in extrinsic asthma.*
  150 mcg for 3 days or 75 mcg/1.5 mL saline by inhalation.
  *Restless leg syndrome.*
  100–300 mcg/day, up to 900 mcg/day.
  *Facilitate cessation of smoking.*
  150–400 mcg/day.
  *Ulcerative colitis.*
  300 mcg t.i.d.
- **Transdermal**
  *Hypertension.*
  **Initial:** Use 0.1-mg system; **then,** if after 1–2 weeks adequate control has not been achieved, can use another 0.1-mg system or a larger system. The antihypertensive effect may not be seen for 2–3 days. The system should be changed q 7 days.

*Cyclosporine-associated nephrotoxicity.*
100–200 mcg/day.
*Diabetic diarrhea.*
0.3 mg/24 hr patch (1 or 2 patches/week).
*Menopausal flushing.*
100 mcg/24-hr patch.
*Facilitate cessation of smoking.*
200 mcg/24-hr patch.

* **Epidural infusion**
*Analgesia.*
**Initial:** 30 mcg/hr. Dose may then be titrated up or down, depending on pain relief and side effects.

## NURSING CONSIDERATIONS

See also *Nursing Considerations* for *Antihypertensive Agents.*

### Administration/Storage

1. It may take 2–3 days to achieve effective blood levels using the transdermal system. Therefore, any prior drug dosage should be reduced gradually.
2. Clients with severe hypertension may require other antihypertensive drug therapy in addition to transdermal clonidine.
3. If the drug is to be discontinued, it should be done gradually over a period of 2–4 days.
4. Do not use a preservative when given epidurally.
5. Store the injection at controlled room temperature. Discard any unused portion.

### Assessment

1. Document indications for therapy, onset, type of symptoms, and previous treatments.
2. Obtain baseline CBC, liver and renal function studies.
3. Note occupation; drug may interfere with the ability to work.
4. List drugs currently prescribed to prevent any interactions. With propranolol, observe for a paradoxical hypertensive response. With tolazoline or TCA, be aware that these may block the antihypertensive action of clonidine; clonidine dosage may need to be increased
5. Note evidence of alcohol, drug, or nicotine addiction. These agents

usually work well for BP control in this group of clients (especially the once-a-week patch).
6. Initially, monitor BP closely. BP decreases occur within 30–60 min after administration and may persist for 8 hr. Note any fluctuations to determine whether to use clonidine alone or concomitantly with a diuretic. A stable BP reduces orthostatic effects with postural changes.

### Client/Family Teaching

1. With the transdermal system, apply to a hairless area of skin, such as upper arm or torso. Change the system q 7 days and use a different site with each application.
2. If the drug is taken PO, take the last dose of the day at bedtime to ensure overnight control of BP.
3. Do not engage in activities that require mental alertness, such as operating machinery or driving a car; may cause drowsiness.
4. Do not change regimen or discontinue drug abruptly or without medical supervision. If withdrawn, it must be done gradually to prevent rebound hypertension.
5. Record weight daily, in the morning, in clothing of the same weight, to determine if there is edema caused by sodium retention. Any fluid retention should disappear after 3–4 days.
6. Clonidine may reduce the effect of levodopa; report any increase in the S&S of Parkinson's disease previously controlled with levodopa.
7. Report any depression that may be precipitated by the drug, especially with history of mental depression.

### Outcomes/Evaluate

* ↓ BP; ↓ menopausal S&S
* Control of withdrawal symptoms
* Control of neuropathic pain

# Clopidogrel bisulfate
(kloh-**PID**-oh-grel)
**Pregnancy Category:** B
Plavix **(Rx)**
**Classification:** Antiplatelet drug

**Action/Kinetics:** Inhibits platelet aggregation by inhibiting binding of adenosine diphosphate (ADP) to its platelet receptor and subsequent ADP-mediative activation of glycoprotein GPIIb/IIIa complex. Drug modifies receptor irreversibly; thus, platelets are affected for remainder of their lifespan. Also inhibits platelet aggregation caused by agonists other than ADP by blocking amplification of platelet activation by released ADP. Rapidly absorbed from GI tract; food does not affect bioavailability. **Peak plasma levels:** About 1 hr. Extensively metabolized in liver; about 50% excreted in urine and 46% in feces. **t½, elimination:** 8 hr.

**Uses:** Reduction of MI, stroke, and vascular death in clients with atherosclerosis documented by recent stroke, MI, or established peripheral arterial disease.

**Contraindications:** Lactation. Active pathological bleeding such as peptic ulcer or intracranial hemorrhage.

**Special Concerns:** Use with caution in those at risk of increased bleeding from trauma, surgery, or other pathological conditions. Safety and efficacy have not been determined in children.

**Side Effects:** *CV:* Edema, hypertension, ***intracranial hemorrhage***. *GI:* Abdominal pain, dyspepsia, diarrhea, nausea, hemorrhage, ulcers (peptic, gastric, duodenal). *CNS:* Headache, dizziness, depression. *Body as a whole:* Chest pain, accidental injury, flu-like symptoms, pain, fatigue. *Respiratory:* Upper respiratory tract infection, dyspnea, rhinitis, bronchitis, coughing. *Hematologic:* Purpura, epistaxis. *Musculoskeletal:* Arthralgia, back pain. *Dermatologic:* Disorders of skin/appendages, rash, pruritus. *Miscellaneous:* Urinary tract infection.

**Laboratory Test Alteration:** Hypercholesterolemia.

**Drug Interactions**
*NSAIDs* / ↑ Risk of occult blood loss
*Warfarin* / Clopidogrel prolongs bleeding time; safety of use with warfarin not established

**Dosage**
- **Tablets**
*Reduction of atherosclerotic events.*
**Adults:** 75 mg once daily with or without food.

## NURSING CONSIDERATIONS
**Administration/Storage:** Dosage adjustment is not necessary for geriatric clients or those with renal disease.

**Assessment**
1. Document atherosclerotic event (MI, stroke) or established peripheral arterial disease requiring therapy.
2. Assess for any active bleeding as with ulcers or intracranial bleeding.

**Client/Family Teaching**
1. Take exactly as directed; may take without regard to food.
2. Avoid OTC agents especially aspirin and NSAIDs.
3. Report any unusual bruising or bleeding; advise others esp. dentist of prescribed therapy, before surgery or new meds added.
4. Drug should be discontinued 7 days prior to elective surgery.

**Outcomes/Evaluate**
- Inhibition of platelet aggregation
- Reduction of atherosclerotic events

# Clorazepate dipotassium
(klor-**AYZ**-eh-payt)
**Pregnancy Category:** D
Apo-Clorazepate ✦, Gen-Xene, Novo–Clopate ✦, Tranxene-SD, Tranxene-T **(C-IV) (Rx)**
**Classification:** Antianxiety agent, benzodiazepine type; anticonvulsant

See also *Tranquilizers.*
**Action/Kinetics: Peak plasma levels:** 1–2 hr. **t½:** 30–100 hr. Hydrolyzed in the stomach to desmethyldiazepam, the active metabolite. Oxazepam is also an active metabolite. **t½, desmethyldiazepam:** 30–100 hr; **t½, oxazepam:** 5–15 hr. **Time to peak plasma levels:** 0.5–2 hr. Significantly bound to plasma pro-

tein and slowly excreted by the kidneys.

**Uses:** Anxiety, tension. Acute alcohol withdrawal, as adjunct in treatment of seizures. Adjunct for treating partial seizures.

**Additional Contraindications:** Depressed clients, nursing mothers.

**Special Concerns:** Use with caution with impaired renal or hepatic function.

**Dosage**

• **Extended-Release Tablets, Tablets**

*Anxiety.*

**Initial:** 7.5–15 mg b.i.d.–q.i.d.; **maintenance:** 15–60 mg/day in divided doses. **Elderly or debilitated clients, initial:** 7.5–15 mg/day. **Alternative.** Single daily dosage: **Adult, initial,** 15 mg; **then,** 11.25–22.5 mg once daily.

*Acute alcohol withdrawal.*

**Day 1, initial:** 30 mg; **then,** 15 mg b.i.d.–q.i.d. the first day; **day 2:** 45–90 mg in divided doses; **day 3:** 22.5–45 mg in divided doses; **day 4:** 15–30 mg in divided doses. Thereafter, reduce to 7.5/day and discontinue as soon as possible. Maximum daily dose: 90 mg.

*Partial seizures.*

**Adults and children over 12 years, initial:** 7.5 mg t.i.d.; increase no more than 7.5 mg/week to maximum of 90 mg/day. **Children (9–12 years), initial:** 7.5 mg b.i.d.; increase by no more than 7.5 mg/week to maximum of 60 mg/day. Not recommended for children under 9 years of age.

## NURSING CONSIDERATIONS

See also *Nursing Considerations* for *Tranquilizers.*

**Assessment**

1. Note any evidence of depression.
2. With excessive alcohol intake, determine time of last drink.

**Client/Family Teaching**

1. Avoid activities that require mental alertness until drug effects realized.
2. Avoid alcohol and any other CNS depressants.

**Outcomes/Evaluate**

• ↓ Anxiety and tension
• ↓ Symptoms of alcohol withdrawal
• Control of seizures

# Clotrimazole

(kloh-**TRY**-mah-zohl)

**Pregnancy Category:** C (systemic use); B (topical/vaginal use)

Canesten ✦, Canestin 1 ✦, Canestin 3 ✦, Clotrimaderm ✦, FemCare, Gyne-Lotrimin, Lotrimin, Lotrimin AF, Mycelex, Mycelex-7, Mycelex-G, Mycelex OTC, Myclo-Derm ✦, Myclo-Gyne ✦, Neo-Zol **(OTC) (Rx)**

**Classification:** Antifungal

See also *Anti-Infectives.*

**Action/Kinetics:** Depending on concentration, may be fungistatic or fungicidal. Acts by inhibiting the biosynthesis of sterols, resulting in damage to the cell wall and subsequent loss of essential intracellular elements due to altered permeability. May also inhibit oxidative and peroxidative enzyme activity and inhibit the biosynthesis of triglycerides and phospholipids by fungi. When used for *Candida albicans,* the drug inhibits transformation of blastophores into the invasive mycelial form. Poorly absorbed from the GI tract and metabolized in the liver to inactive compounds that are excreted through the feces. **Duration:** up to 3 hr.

**Uses:** Broad-spectrum antifungal effective against *Malassezia furfur, Trichophyton rubrum, Trichophyton mentagrophytes, Epidermophyton floccosum, Microsporum canis, C. albicans. Oral troche:* Oropharyngeal candidiasis. Reduce incidence of oropharyngeal candidiasis in clients who are immunocompromised due to chemotherapy, radiotherapy, or steroid therapy used for leukemia, solid tumors, or kidney transplant. *Topical OTC products:* Topically to treat tinea pedis, tinea cruris, and tinea corporis. *Topical prescription products:* Same as OTC plus candidiasis and tinea versicolor. *Vaginal products:* Vulvovaginal candidiasis.

**Contraindications:** Hypersensitivity. First trimester of pregnancy.
**Special Concerns:** Use with caution during lactation. Safety and effectiveness for PO use in children less than 3 years of age has not been determined.
**Side Effects:** *Skin:* Irritation including rash, stinging, pruritus, urticaria, erythema, peeling, blistering, edema. *Vaginal:* Lower abdominal cramps; urinary frequency; bloating; vaginal irritation, itching or burning; dyspareunia. *Hepatic:* Abnormal liver function tests. *GI:* N&V following use of troche.

**Dosage**
• **Troche**
  *Treatment of oropharyngeal candidiasis.*
One troche (10 mg) 5 times/day for 14 consecutive days.
  *Prophylaxis of oropharyngeal candidiasis.*
One troche t.i.d. for duration of chemotherapy or until maintenance doses of steroids are instituted.
• **Topical Cream, Lotion, Solution (each 1%)**
Massage into affected skin and surrounding areas b.i.d. in morning and evening for 7 consecutive days. Diagnosis should be reevaluated if no improvement occurs in 4 weeks.
• **Vaginal Tablets**
One 100-mg tablet/day at bedtime for 7 days. One 500-mg tablet can be inserted once at bedtime.
• **Vaginal Cream (1%)**
5 g (one full applicator)/day at bedtime for 7 consecutive days.
• **Vaginal Inserts and Clotrimazole, 1%**
  *Vaginal yeast infections.*
Insert daily for 3 consecutive days.

## NURSING CONSIDERATIONS

See also *General Nursing Considerations for All Anti-Infectives.*
**Administration/Storage**
1. Store Mycelex-G vaginal cream at 2°C–30°C (36°F–86°F). Do not store Mycelex-G 100-mg vaginal tablets above 35°C (95°F); store the 500-mg vaginal tablets below 30°C (86°F).
2. Slowly dissolve the troche in the mouth.
3. Do not allow topical products to come in contact with the eyes.
**Client/Family Teaching**
1. Review goals of therapy; appropriate method for administration. Wash hands before and after treatments. Unless otherwise directed, apply only after cleaning the affected area.
2. With vaginal infections, do not engage in intercourse; or, to prevent reinfection, have partner wear a condom.
3. To prevent staining of clothes, use a sanitary napkin with vaginal tablets or cream.
4. If exposed to HIV and recurrent vaginal yeast infections occur, seek prompt medical intervention to determine cause of the symptoms.
**Outcomes/Evaluate**
• Eradication of fungal infection
• Symptomatic improvement

# Cloxacillin sodium
(klox-ah-**SILL**-in)
**Pregnancy Category:** B
Apo-Cloxi ✿, Cloxapen, Novo-Cloxin ✿, Nu-CLoxi ✿, Orbenin ✿, Taro-Cloxacillin ✿, Tegopen **(Rx)**
**Classification:** Antibiotic, penicillin

See also *Anti-Infectives* and *Penicillins.*
**Action/Kinetics:** Resistant to penicillinase and is acid stable. **Peak plasma levels:** 7–15 mcg/mL after 30–60 min. **t½:** 30 min. Protein binding: 88%–96%. Well absorbed from GI tract. Mostly excreted in urine, but some excreted in bile.
**Uses:** Infections caused by penicillinase-producing staphylococci, including pneumococci, group A beta-hemolytic streptococci, and penicillin G-sensitive staphylococci.

**Dosage**
• **Capsules, Oral Solution**

---

✿ = Available in Canada          ***bold italic*** = life threatening side effect

*Skin and soft tissue infections, mild to moderate URTIs.*

**Adults and children over 20 kg:** 250 mg q 6 hr; **pediatric, less than 20 kg:** 50 mg/kg/day in divided doses q 6 hr.

*Lower respiratory tract infections or disseminated infections.*

**Adults and children over 20 kg:** 0.5 g q 6 hr; **pediatric, less than 20 kg:** 100 (or more) mg/kg/day in divided doses q 6 hr. Alternatively, a dose of 50–100 mg/kg/day (up to a maximum of 4 g/day) divided q 6 hr may be used for infants and children.

## NURSING CONSIDERATIONS

See also *Nursing Considerations* for *Penicillins*.

**Administration/Storage**
1. Add amount of water stated on label in two portions; shake well after each addition.
2. Shake well before pouring each dose.
3. Refrigerate reconstituted solution and discard unused portion after 14 days.

**Assessment:** Note any sensitivity to penicillin; obtain baseline CBC, LFTs, and cultures.

**Client/Family Teaching**
1. Review appropriate guidelines for administration; include frequency and amount. Shake well before using; refrigerate; discard any left after 14 days.
2. Take as directed, 1 hr before or 2 hr after meals; food interferes with absorption of drug.
3. Complete prescription despite feeling better.

**Outcomes/Evaluate**
- Eradication of infection
- ↓ Fever, ↓ WBCs, ↑ appetite

## Clozapine

(KLOH-zah-peen)
**Pregnancy Category:** B
Clozaril **(Rx)**
**Classification:** Antipsychotic

**Action/Kinetics:** Interferes with the binding of dopamine to both D-1 and D-2 receptors; more active at limbic than at striatal dopamine receptors. Thus, is relatively free from extrapyramidal side effects and does not induce catalepsy. Also acts as an antagonist at adrenergic, cholinergic, histaminergic, and serotonergic receptors. Increases the amount of time spent in REM sleep. Food does not affect the bioavailability of clozapine. **Peak plasma levels:** 2.5 hr. **Average maximum concentration at steady state:** 122 ng/mL plasma after 100 mg b.i.d. Highly bound to plasma proteins. **t½:** 12 hr. Metabolized in the liver to inactive compounds and excreted through the urine (50%) and feces (30%).

**Uses:** Severely ill schizophrenic clients who do not respond adequately to conventional antipsychotic therapy, either because of ineffectiveness or intolerable side effects from other drugs. Due to the possibility of development of agranulocytosis and seizures, avoid continued use in clients failing to respond.

**Contraindications:** Myeloproliferative disorders. Use with other agents known to suppress bone marrow function. Severe CNS depression or coma due to any cause. Lactation.

**Special Concerns:** Use with caution in clients with known CV disease, prostatic hypertrophy, narrow angle glaucoma, hepatic or renal disease.

**Side Effects:** *Hematologic: Agranulocytosis,* leukopenia, neutropenia, eosinophilia. *CNS: Seizures* (appear to be dose dependent), drowsiness or sedation, dizziness, vertigo, headache, tremor, restlessness, nightmares, hypokinesia, akinesia, agitation, akathisia, confusion, rigidity, fatigue, insomnia, hyperkinesia, weakness, lethargy, slurred speech, ataxia, depression, anxiety, epileptiform movements. *CV:* Orthostatic hypotension (especially initially), tachycardia, syncope, hypertension, angina, chest pain, *cardiac abnormalities,* changes in ECG. *Neuroleptic malignant syndrome: Hyperpyrexia,* muscle rigidity, altered mental status, irregular pulse or BP, tachycardia, diaphoresis, cardiac dysrhythmias.

*GI:* Constipation, nausea, heartburn, abdominal discomfort, vomiting, diarrhea, anorexia. *GU:* Urinary abnormalities, incontinence, abnormal ejaculation, urinary frequency or urgency, urinary retention. *Musculoskeletal:* Muscle weakness, pain (back, legs, neck), muscle spasm, muscle ache. *Respiratory:* Dyspnea, SOB, throat discomfort, nasal congestion. *Miscellaneous:* Salivation, sweating, visual disturbances, fever (transient), dry mouth, rash, weight gain, numb or sore tongue.

**OD** **Overdose Management:** *Symptoms:* Drowsiness, delirium, tachycardia, **respiratory depression,** hypotension, hypersalivation, **seizures, coma.** *Treatment:* Establish an airway and maintain with adequate oxygenation and ventilation. Give activated charcoal and sorbitol. Monitor cardiac status and VS. General supportive measures.

**Drug Interactions**
*Anticholinergic drugs* / Additive anticholinergic effects
*Antihypertensive drugs* / Additive hypotensive effects
*Benzodiazepines* / Possible respiratory depression and collapse
*Digoxin* / ↑ Effect of digoxin due to ↓ binding to plasma protein
*Epinephrine* / Clozapine may reverse effects if epinephrine is given for hypotension
*Warfarin* / ↑ Effect of warfarin due to ↓ binding to plasma protein

**Dosage** ————————
• **Tablets**
*Schizophrenia.*
**Adults, initial:** 25 mg 1–2 times/day; **then,** if drug is tolerated, the dose can be increased by 25–50 mg/day to a dose of 300–450 mg/day at the end of 2 weeks. Subsequent dosage increments should occur no more often than once or twice a week in increments not to exceed 100 mg. **Usual maintenance dose:** 300–600 mg/day (although doses up to 900 mg/day may be required in

some clients). Total daily dose should not exceed 900 mg.

---

**NURSING CONSIDERATIONS**
**Administration/Storage**
1. Clozapine is available through independent "Clozaril treatment systems" based on a plan developed by physicians and pharmacists to ensure safe use of the drug with respect to weekly blood monitoring, data reporting, and drug dispensing. Prescriptions are limited to 1-week supplies, and the drug may only be dispensed following receipt, by the pharmacist, of weekly WBC test results that fall within the established limits. All weekly blood test results must be reported by participating pharmacists to the Clozaril National Registry.
2. If drug is effective, seek the lowest maintenance doses possible to maintain remission.
3. If termination of therapy is planned, gradually reduce the dose over a 1–2-week period. If cessation of therapy is abrupt due to toxicity, observe client carefully for recurrence of psychotic symptoms.
4. Clozapine therapy may be initiated immediately upon discontinuation of other antipsychotic medication; however, a 24-hr "washout period" is desirable.
**Assessment**
1. Document indications for therapy; assess behavioral manifestations. List other therapies trialed and the outcome.
2. Note history of seizure disorder.
3. Document baseline VS and ECG; report any irregular pulse, tachycardia, hyperpyrexia, or hypotension.
4. Obtain CBC and LFTs prior to initiating therapy. If WBCs fall below 2,000/mm³ or granulocyte counts fall below 1,000/mm³, the drug should be discontinued. Such clients should *not* be restarted on clozapine therapy.
5. Periodically reassess to determine continued need for therapy.

---

**Client/Family Teaching**
1. Take only as directed; do not stop abruptly.
2. Report immediately symptoms of lethargy, weakness, fever, sore throat, malaise, mucous membrane ulceration, or other signs of infection.
3. Rinse mouth frequently and perform regular oral care to minimize potential for candidiasis.
4. Avoid driving or other potentially hazardous activity due to possibility of seizures.
5. Because of orthostatic hypotension, especially during initial dosing, use care when rising from a supine or sitting position.
6. Avoid hot showers or baths and hot weather exposure.
7. Report if pregnancy occurs or desire to become pregnant during therapy.
8. Do not breast-feed.
9. Do not take any prescription drugs, OTC drugs, or alcohol.
10. Stress importance of weekly WBC to assess for agranulocytosis. These are reported to a national registry and must be completed before additional prescriptions will be issued and filled.

**Outcomes/Evaluate**
• Improved behavior patterns with ↓ agitation, ↓ hyperactivity, and ↓ delusions, paranoia, and hallucinations
• Improved coping behaviors and thought patterns

# Codeine phosphate
(**KOH**-deen)
**Pregnancy Category:** C
Paveral ✱ (C-II) (Rx)

# Codeine sulfate
(**KOH**-deen )
**Pregnancy Category:** C
(C-II) (Rx)
**Classification:** Narcotic analgesic, morphine type

See also *Narcotic Analgesics.*
**Action/Kinetics:** Resembles morphine pharmacologically but produces less respiratory depression and N&V. Moderately habit-forming and constipating. Dosages over 60 mg often cause restlessness and excitement and irritate the cough center. However, in lower doses, it is a potent antitussive and is an ingredient in many cough syrups. **Onset:** 10–30 min. **Peak effect:** 30–60 min. **Duration:** 4–6 hr. **t½:** 3–4 hr. Codeine is two-thirds as effective PO as parenterally.
**Uses:** Relief of mild to moderate pain. Antitussive to relieve chemical or mechanical respiratory tract irritation. In combination with aspirin or acetaminophen to enhance analgesia.
**Contraindications:** Premature infants or during labor when delivery of a premature infant is expected.
**Special Concerns:** May increase the duration of labor. Use with caution and reduce the initial dose in clients with seizure disorders, acute abdominal conditions, renal or hepatic disease, fever, Addison's disease, hypothyroidism, prostatic hypertrophy, ulcerative colitis, urethral stricture, following recent GI or GU tract surgery, and in the young, geriatric, or debilitated clients.
**Additional Drug Interactions:** Combination with chlordiazepoxide may induce coma.

**Dosage** ─────────────
• **Solution, Tablets, IM, IV, SC**
*Analgesia.*
**Adults:** 15–60 mg q 4–6 hr, not to exceed 360 mg/day. **Pediatric, over 1 year:** 0.5 mg/kg q 4–6 hr. IV should not be used in children.
*Antitussive.*
**Adults:** 10–20 mg q 4–6 hr, up to maximum of 120 mg/day. **Pediatric, 2–6 years:** 2.5–5 mg PO q 4–6 hr, not to exceed 30 mg/day; **6–12 years:** 5–10 mg q 4–6 hr, not to exceed 60 mg/day.

## NURSING CONSIDERATIONS

See also *Nursing Considerations* for *Narcotic Analgesics.*
**Client/Family Teaching**
1. Take only as directed. Tylenol or

aspirin act synergistically with codeine and are usually given together.

2. Increase intake of fluids, fruits, and fiber to diminish drug's constipating effects.

3. Drug may cause dizziness and drowsiness.

4. Avoid alcohol/CNS depressants.

5. Report altered mental patterns.

6. If taking codeine syrups to suppress coughs, discourage from overuse. Productive coughing is suppressed and may result in additional congestion.

**Outcomes/Evaluate**

• Relief of pain

• Control of coughing with improved sleeping patterns

----COMBINATION DRUG----

# Codeine phosphate and guaifenesin

(**KOH**-deen **FOS**-fayt, gwye-**FEN**-eh-sin)

**Pregnancy Category:** C

Brontex **(C-III) (Rx)**

**Classification:** Antitussive/expectorant

See also *Codeine Phosphate* and *Guaifenesin*.

**Content:** *Antitussive:* codeine phosphate, 10 mg/tablet or 20 mL. *Expectorant:* Guaifenesin, 300 mg/tablet or 20 mL.

**Uses:** Relief of cough due to a cold or inhaled irritants. To loosen mucus and thin bronchial secretions.

**Contraindications:** Asthma, during labor and delivery. Use of tablets in children less than 12 years of age and use of the liquid in children less than 6 years of age.

**Special Concerns:** Use with caution in clients with severe CNS depression, respiratory depression, acute alcoholism, chronic pulmonary disease, acute abdominal conditions, seizure disorders, fever, hypothyroidism, Addison's disease, ulcerative colitis, prostatic hypertrophy, following recent GI or urinary tract surgery, and in significant renal or hepatic dysfunction, in the very young and elderly, and during lactation.

**Side Effects:** *CNS:* CNS depression, lightheadedness, dizziness, sedation, headache, euphoria or dysphoria, transient hallucinations, disorientation, visual disturbances, *seizures.* *CV:* Tachycardia, bradycardia, palpitations, syncope, faintness, orthostatic hypotension, circulatory depression. *GI:* N&V, stomach pain, constipation, biliary tract spasm, increased colonic motility in those with ulcerative colitis. *GU:* Oliguria, urinary retention. *Allergic:* Pruritus, urticaria, *angioneurotic edema, laryngeal edema, anaphylaxis.* *Miscellaneous:* Flushing of the face, sweating, weakness.

**Drug Interactions:** Additive CNS depression if used with alcohol, sedatives, antianxiety agents, and MAO inhibitors

**Dosage**

• **Oral Solution, Tablets**

*Cough/colds, bronchial congestion.*

**Adults and children over 12 years of age:** One tablet q 4 hr or 20 mL (4 teaspoonfuls) q 4 hr. **Children, 6–12 years of age:** 10 mL (2 teaspoonfuls) q 4 hr.

## NURSING CONSIDERATIONS

See also *Nursing Considerations* for *Narcotic Analgesics* and *Guaifenesin*.

**Assessment**

1. Document indications for therapy, onset and duration of symptoms, other agents used, and the outcome.

2. Note asthma or any conditions that would preclude drug use.

**Client/Family Teaching**

1. Take as directed with a full glass of water.

2. Report if cough fails to respond; do not increase dose.

3. Do not engage in any activities that require mental or physical alertness until drug effects realized; may cause dizziness and drowsiness.

4. Drug may cause orthostatic hypo-

tension; rise slowly from a sitting or lying position.

5. Avoid alcohol, CNS depressants, sedatives, or antidepressants without approval.

6. Supervise children's activities (i.e., bike riding, games, swings).

7. Drug is for short-term use only; report if symptoms do not subside or get worse after 48 hr.

**Outcomes/Evaluate:** Relief of cough

# Colchicine
(**KOHL**-chih-seen)
**Pregnancy Category:** C (oral use); D (parenteral use)
**(Rx)**
**Classification:** Antigout agent

**Action/Kinetics:** Colchicine is not uricosuric. It may reduce the crystal-induced inflammation by reducing lactic acid production by leukocytes (resulting in a decreased deposition of sodium urate), by inhibiting leukocyte migration, and by reducing phagocytosis. May also inhibit the synthesis of kinins and leukotrienes. **t½, plasma:** 10–60 min. **Onset, IV:** 6–12 hr; **PO:** 12 hr. **Time to peak levels, PO:** 0.5–2 hr. It concentrates in leukocytes (t½, about 46 hr). Colchicine is metabolized in the liver and mainly excreted in the feces with 10%–20% excreted unchanged through the urine.

**Uses:** Prophylaxis and treatment of acute attacks of gout. *Investigational:* To slow progression of chronic progressive multiple sclerosis, to decrease frequency and severity of fever and to prevent amyloidosis in familiar Mediterranean fever, primary biliary cirrhosis, hepatic cirrhosis, adjunct in the treatment of primary amyloidosis, Behcet's disease, pseudogout due to chondrocalcinosis, refractory idiopathic thrombocytopenic purpura, progressive systemic sclerosis, dermatologic disorders including dermatitis herpetiformis, psoriasis, palmoplantar pustulosis, and pyoderma associated with Crohn's disease.

**Contraindications:** Blood dyscrasias. Serious GI, hepatic, cardiac, or renal disorders.

**Special Concerns:** Use with caution during lactation. Dosage has not been established for children. Geriatric clients may be at greater risk of developing cumulative toxicity. Use with extreme caution for elderly, debilitated clients, especially in the presence of chronic renal, hepatic, GI, or CV disease. May impair fertility.

**Side Effects:** The drug is toxic; thus clients must be carefully monitored. *GI:* N&V, diarrhea, abdominal cramping. *Hematologic: **Aplastic anemia, agranulocytosis,*** or thrombocytopenia following long-term therapy. *Miscellaneous:* Peripheral neuritis, purpura, myopathy, neuropathy, alopecia, reversible azoospermia, dermatoses, hypersensitivity, thrombophlebitis at injection site (rare), liver dysfunction. If such symptoms appear, discontinue drug at once and wait at least 48 hr before reinstating drug therapy.

**OD** **Overdose Management:** *Symptoms (Acute Intoxication):* Characterized at first by violent GI tract symptoms such as N&V, abdominal pain, and diarrhea. The latter may be profuse, watery, bloody, and associated with severe fluid and electrolyte loss. Also, burning of throat and skin, hematuria and oliguria, rapid and weak pulse, general exhaustion, muscular depression, and CNS involvement. *Death is usually caused by respiratory paralysis. Treatment (Acute Poisoning):* Gastric lavage, symptomatic support, including atropine and morphine, artificial respiration, hemodialysis, peritoneal dialysis, and treatment of shock.

**Drug Interactions**
*Acidifying agents* / Inhibit the action of colchicine
*Alkalinizing agents* / Potentiate the action of colchicine
*CNS depressants* / Clients on colchicine may be more sensitive to CNS depressant effect of these drugs

*Sympathomimetic agents* / Enhanced by colchicine

*Vitamin B$_{12}$* / Colchicine may interfere with absorption from the gut

**Laboratory Test Interferences:** Alters liver function tests. ↑ Alkaline phosphatase, AST. False + for hemoglobin or RBCs in urine.

## Dosage

- **Tablets**

*Acute attack of gout.*

**Adults, initial:** 1–1.2 mg followed by 0.5–1.2 mg q 1–2 hr until pain is relieved or nausea, vomiting, or diarrhea occurs. **Total amount required:** 4–8 mg.

*Prophylaxis for gout.*

**Adults:** 0.5–0.65 mg/day for 3–4 days a week if the client has less than one attack per year or 0.5–0.65 mg/day if the client has more than one attack per year.

*Prophylaxis for surgical clients.*

**Adults:** 0.5–0.65 mg t.i.d. for 3 days before and 3 days after surgery.

- **IV Only**

*Acute attack of gout.*

**Adults, initial:** 2 mg; **then,** 0.5 mg q 6 hr until pain is relieved; give no more than 4 mg in a 24-hr period. Some physicians recommend a single IV dose of 3 mg while others recommend no more than 1 mg for the initial dose, followed by 0.5 mg once or twice daily, if needed. If pain recurs, 1–2 mg/day may be given for several days; however, colchicine should not be given by any route for at least 7 days after a full course of IV therapy (i.e., 4 mg).

*Prophylaxis or maintenance of recurrent or chronic gouty arthritis.*

0.5–1 mg 1–2 times/day. However, PO colchicine is preferred (usually with a uricosuric drug).

## NURSING CONSIDERATIONS

### Administration/Storage

1. Store in tight, light-resistant containers.

**IV** 2. Parenterally, give only IV; SC or IM causes severe local irritation.

3. For parenteral administration, may administer undiluted or may dilute in 10–20 mL of NSS without a bacteriostatic agent or with sterile water. Administer over 2–5 min.

4. Do not administer turbid solutions.

5. Not compatible with dextrose-containing solutions.

### Assessment

1. Determine symptom onset; any other attacks, the frequency of these attacks, and any preventative therapy prescribed, i.e., allopurinol.

2. Note age and general physical condition.

3. Document joint involvement, noting pain, swelling, and degree of mobility; may need to aspirate for definitive diagnosis.

4. Monitor CBC, joint X ray, uric acid levels, and renal and hepatic function studies.

### Client/Family Teaching

1. If prescribed for use in acute attacks take at the first sign of an impending attack to diminish its severity. Stop uricosuric agent (if prescribed) during acute attack.

2. Start or increase dosage of colchicine as prescribed; at the first sign of joint pain or other symptom of impending gout attack. The maximum dose is 10 tablets or 10 mg in 24 hr; do not exceed. It usually takes 12–48 hr for relief of symptoms.

3. Acute episodes may be precipitated by aspirin or foods high in purine.

4. Stop drug and report if nausea, vomiting, or diarrhea develops; these may be early signs of toxicity. With severe diarrhea, medication (paregoric) may be needed.

5. Report any evidence of liver dysfunction (yellow discoloration of eyes, skin, or stool). LFTs may be scheduled during long-term use.

6. Women should use contraception.

7. Consume 3–3.5 L/day of fluids to enhance excretion.

8. NSAIDs may help with pain and inflammation; use as prescribed.

---

**Outcomes/Evaluate**
- ↓ Joint pain and swelling
- Prophylaxis of acute gout attacks

# Colestipol hydrochloride
(koh-**LESS**-tih-poll)
Colestid **(Rx)**
**Classification:** Hypocholesterolemic, bile acid sequestrant

**Action/Kinetics:** Colestipol, an anion exchange resin, binds bile acids in the intestine, forming an insoluble complex excreted in the feces. The loss of bile acids results in increased oxidation of cholesterol to bile acids and a decrease in LDL and serum cholesterol. Does not affect (or may increase) triglycerides or HDL and may increase VLDL. Not absorbed from the GI tract. **Onset:** 1–2 days; **maximum effect:** 1 month. Return to pretreatment cholesterol levels after discontinuance of therapy: 1 month.
**Uses:** As adjunctive therapy in hyperlipoproteinemia (types IIA and IIB) to reduce serum cholesterol in clients who do not respond adequately to diet. *Investigational:* Digitalis toxicity.
**Contraindications:** Complete obstruction or atresia of bile duct.
**Special Concerns:** Use during pregnancy only if benefits outweigh risks. Use with caution during lactation and in children. Children may be more likely to develop hyperchloremic acidosis although dosage has not been established. Clients over 60 years of age may be at greater risk of GI side effects and adverse nutritional effects.
**Side Effects:** *GI:* Constipation (may be severe and accompanied by fecal impaction), N&V, diarrhea, heartburn, GI bleeding, anorexia, flatulence, steatorrhea, abdominal distention/cramping, bloating, loose stools, indigestion, rectal bleeding/pain, black stools, hemorrhoidal bleeding, *bleeding duodenal ulcer, peptic ulceration,* ulcer attack, GI irritation, dysphagia, dental bleeding/caries, hiccoughs, sour taste, pancreatitis, diverticulitis, cholecystitis, cholelithiasis. *CV:* Chest pain, angina, tachycardia (rare). *CNS:* Migraine or sinus headache, anxiety, vertigo, dizziness, lightheadedness, insomnia, fatigue, tinnitus, syncope, drowsiness, femoral nerve pain, paresthesia. *Hematologic:* Ecchymosis, anemia, beeding tendencies due to hypoprothrombinemia. *Allergic:* Urticaria, dermatitis, asthma, wheezing, rash. *Musculoskeletal:* Backache, muscle/joint pain, arthritis. *Renal:* Hematuria, burnt odor to urine, dysuria, diuresis. *Miscellaneous:* Uveitis, fatigue, weight loss or gain, increased libido, swollen glands, SOB, edema, weakness, swelling of hands/feet, osteoporosis, calcified material in biliary tree and gall bladder, hyperchloremic acidosis in children.
**Drug Interactions**
See *Cholestyramine.*

**Dosage**
- **Oral Granules**
  *Antihyperlipidemic.*
  **Adults, initial:** 5 g 1–2 times/day; **then,** can increase 5 g/day at 1–2-month intervals. **Total dose:** 5–30 g/day given once or in two to three divided doses.
- **Tablets**
  **Adults, initial:** 2 g 1–2 times/day. Dose can be increased by 2 g, once or twice daily, at 1–2-month intervals. **Total dose:** 2–16 g/day given once or in divided doses.
  *Digitalis toxicity.*
  10 g followed by 5 g q 6–8 hr.

## NURSING CONSIDERATIONS

See also *Nursing Considerations* for *Cholestyramine.*
**Administration/Storage**
1. If compliance is good and side effects acceptable but the desired effect is not obtained with 2–16 g/day using the tablets, combined therapy or alternative treatment should be considered.
2. Granules are available in an orange-flavored product.
**Client/Family Teaching**
1. Take 30 min before meals, preferably with the evening meal, since cholesterol synthesis is increased during the evening hours. Take

other drugs 1 hr before or 4 hr after colestipol to reduce interference with their absorption.

2. Never take dose in dry form. Always mix granules with 90 mL or more of fruit juice, milk, water, carbonated beverages, applesauce, soup, cereal, or pulpy fruit before administering to disguise unpalatable taste and to prevent resin from causing esophageal irritation or blockage.

3. Rinse glass with a small amount of additional beverage to ensure the total amount of the drug is taken.

4. Tablets should be swallowed whole (i.e., they should not be cut, crushed, or chewed); may be taken with water or other fluids.

5. Consume adequate amounts of fluids, fruits, and fiber to diminish constipating drug effects.

6. Continue to follow dietary restrictions of fat and cholesterol, regular exercise program, smoking cessation, and weight reduction in the overall goal of cholesterol reduction.

7. Serum cholesterol level will return to pretreatment levels within 1 month if drug is discontinued.

**Outcomes/Evaluate:** ↓ LDL cholesterol level

# Colfosceril palmitate (Dipalmitoylphosphatidyl choline, DPPC)

(kohl-**FOSS**-sir-ill)

Exosurf Neonatal **(Rx)**

**Classification:** Lung surfactant

**Action/Kinetics:** Contains dipalmitoylphosphatidylcholine (DPPC), which reduces surface tension in the lungs, as well as cetyl alcohol, which acts as a spreading agent for DPPC on the air–fluid surface. Also contains tyloxapol, which is a nonionic surfactant that assists in dispersion of DPPC and cetyl alcohol, and NaCL to adjust osmolality. The drug can rapidly affect oxygenation and lung compliance. DPPC is reabsorbed from the alveoli into lung tis-

sue where it is broken down and reutilized for further phospholipid synthesis and secretion.

**Uses:** Prophylaxis of respiratory distress syndrome in infants with birth weights of less than 1,350 g and in infants with birth weights greater than 1,350 g who manifest pulmonary immaturity. Treatment of infants who have developed respiratory distress syndrome. Such infants should be on mechanical ventilation and should have been diagnosed as having respiratory distress syndrome.

**Special Concerns:** Use of colfosceril should be undertaken only by medical personnel trained and experienced in airway and clinical management of unstable premature infants. Although colfosceril is effective in reducing mortality due to premature birth, infants may still develop severe complications resulting in either death or survival but with permanent handicaps. Benefits versus risks should be carefully assessed before using colfosceril in infants weighing 500–700 g.

**Side Effects:** *Respiratory:* ***Pulmonary hemorrhage, pulmonary air leak (pneumothorax, pneumomediastinum, pneumopericardium, pulmonary interstitial emphysema), mucous plugs in the ET tube, apnea,*** congenital pneumonia, nosocomial pneumonia. *CV:* ***Intraventricular hemorrhage,*** patent ductus arteriosus, hypotension, bradycardia, tachycardia, exchange transfusion, persistent fetal circulation. *Changes in blood gases:* Fall or rise in oxygen saturation, fall or rise in transcutaneous $pO_2$, fall or rise in transcutaneous $pCO_2$. *Miscellaneous:* ***Necrotizing enterocolitis,*** major anomalies, hyperbilirubinemia, gagging, thrombocytopenia, ***seizures.***

**Dosage**

- **Intratracheal**

  *Prophylaxis.*

  5 mL/kg (as two 2.5-mL/kg half-doses) as soon as possible after birth. A second and third dose should be given 12 and 24 hr later to infants

who are still on mechanical ventilation.

*Rescue treatment.*
5 mL/kg (as two 2.5-mL/kg half-doses) as soon as possible after the diagnosis of respiratory distress syndrome is confirmed. A second 5-mL/kg dose is given after 12 hr to infants who are still on mechanical ventilation. The safety and effectiveness of additional doses are not known.

## NURSING CONSIDERATIONS
### Administration/Storage
1. Reconstitute according to the manufacturer's directions immediately prior to use with the diluent provided (preservative-free sterile water for injection). The reconstituted product is a milky white suspension.
2. The reconstituted suspension should be uniformly dispersed before administration. If the vial contains large flakes or particulate matter, do not use.
3. Five different-sized ET tube adapters are provided with each vial of colfosceril. The adapters are clean but not sterile. Use adapters according to the instructions provided by the manufacturer.
4. Colfosceril is administered directly into the trachea through the side-port on the special ET tube adapter without interruption of mechanical ventilation.
5. Each half-dose is given slowly over 1–2 min in small bursts timed with inspiration.
6. The first 2.5-mL/kg dose is given with the infant in the midline position; after the first half-dose is given, the infant's head and torso are first turned 45° to the right for 30 sec and then 45° to the left for 30 sec while continuing mechanical ventilation. This allows for gravity to help with lung distribution of the drug.
7. Refluxing of colfosceril into the ET tube may occur if the drug is given rapidly. If reflux is noted, stop drug administration and increase the peak inspiratory pressure on the ventilator by 4–5 cm water until the ET tube clears.
8. Undertake colfosceril administration only by experienced neonatologists and other individuals experienced at neonatal intubation and ventilatory management.

### Assessment
1. Review indications for drug therapy to ensure that infant meets criteria and document as rescue or prophylactic treatment.
2. The infant's color, chest expansion, facial expression, oximeter readings, HR, and ET tube patency and position should be documented and monitored carefully before and during colfosceril dosing.
3. Ascertain that the ET tube tip is in the trachea and not in the esophagus or right or left mainstem bronchus to ensure drug dispersion to all lung areas.
4. Document baseline weight, ABGs, VS, CXR, and physical assessment findings.

### Interventions
1. Confirm brisk and symmetrical chest movement and equal breath sounds in the two axillae with each mechanical inspiration prior to and at the conclusion of each dosing.
2. Infant should be suctioned before administration of the drug but not for 2 hr after colfosceril administration (unless clinically necessary).
3. Continuous monitoring of ECG, arterial BP, and transcutaneous oxygen saturation must be undertaken during dosing. After either prophylactic or rescue treatment, frequent ABGs should be measured to prevent postdosing hyperoxia and hypocarbia.
4. The volume of the 5-mL/kg dose may cause a transient impairment of gas exchange due to physical blockage of the airway. Infants may show a decrease in oxygen saturation during dosing, especially if they are on low ventilator settings prior to dosing. If evident, increase the $FiO_2$ and peak inspiratory pressure on the ventilator by 4–5 cm water for 1–2 min.

5. If chest expansion improves significantly after dosing, reduce the peak ventilator inspiratory pressure immediately. Failure to do this may cause lung overdistention and fatal pulmonary air leak.

6. If the infant becomes pink and transcutaneous oxygen saturation is more than 95%, reduce the FiO$_2$ in small but repeated steps until saturation is 90%–95%. Failure to do this may cause hyperoxia.

7. If arterial or transcutaneous CO$_2$ levels are less than 30 mm Hg, reduce the ventilator rate immediately; otherwise may result in significant hypocarbia, which reduces cerebral blood flow.

8. After dosing, confirm the position of the ET tube by listening for equal breath sounds in both axillae. Pay particular attention to chest expansion, skin color, transcutaneous O$_2$ saturation, and ABGs (samples should be taken frequently); remain at the bedside for at least 30 min after dosing.

9. Observe for air leaks and mucous plugs. If mucous plug is unrelieved by suctioning, replace the ET tube immediately.

**Outcomes/Evaluate**

• Oxygen saturation between 90% and 95%; pulmonary parameters more consistent with survival

• ↓ Pulmonary air leaks and prevention of alveolar collapse

---

# Collagenase
(koh-**LAJ**-eh-nace)
Biozyme-C, Santyl **(Rx)**
Classification: Topical enzyme

**Action/Kinetics:** Digests collagen, thus, effectively removing tissue debris. Assists in the formation of granulation tissue and subsequent epithelialization of dermal ulcers and severely burned areas. May also reduce the incidence of hypertrophic scarring. Collagen in healthy tissue or newly formed granulation is not affected.

**Uses:** Reduces pus, odor, necrosis, and inflammation in chronic dermal ulcers and severely burned areas.

**Contraindications:** Local or systemic hypersensitivity to collagenase.

**Side Effects:** No allergic sensitivity or toxic reactions have been noted.

**Drug Interactions:** Detergents, benzalkonium chloride, hexachlorophene, nitrofurazone, tincture of iodine, and certain heavy metal ions used in some antiseptics (e.g., mercury, silver) inhibit the activity of collagenase.

**Dosage** ─────────────
• **Ointment**
  *Chronic dermal ulcers, burns.*
Apply once daily (more frequently if the dressing becomes soiled).

---

## NURSING CONSIDERATIONS
### Administration/Storage

1. If any of the agents listed under drug interactions have been used, clean the area thoroughly with repeated washings using NSS before collagenase ointment is applied.

2. Before applying the ointment, cleanse the site and other material by gently rubbing with a gauze pad saturated with hydrogen peroxide or Dakin's solution followed by sterile NSS.

3. If infection is present, apply a topical antibiotic powder to the lesion before collagenase is applied. If the infection does not respond, discontinue collagenase therapy until the infection is in remission.

4. Apply collagenase to deep lesions using a wooden tongue depressor or spatula; for shallow lesions, a sterile gauze pad may be applied to the area and properly secured.

5. Crosshatching thick eschar with a #10 blade allows more surface area for the collagenase to come in contact with necrotic tissue. Remove as much loosened debris as possible with forceps and scissors.

---

*bold italic* = life threatening side effect

6. Remove all excess ointment each time the dressing is changed.

7. Terminate therapy when debridement of necrotic tissue is complete and granulation tissue is well established.

8. The action of the enzyme may be stopped by applying Burrow's solution (pH 3.6–4.4) to the lesion.

**Assessment:** Document underlying cause and assess area to be treated, noting wound size, depth, color, presence of eschar, any evidence of drainage, swelling, or odor and determine wound stage.

**Client/Family Teaching**

1. Review the procedure for tissue preparation (described under *Administration*) and collagenase application.

2. Note importance of frequent position changes, methods to reduce pressure to bony prominences, proper body alignment, proper skin care, adequate nutrition, and clean, dry linens in the overall goal to reduce the size and spread of the disrupted tissue, whether from an ulcer or from a burn.

3. Return for follow-up evaluations to determine the effectiveness of therapy and to assess for any evidence of infection.

**Outcomes/Evaluate**

- Formation of granulation tissue
- Wound reepithelialization

————COMBINATION DRUG————

# Conjugated estrogens and Medroxyprogesterone acetate

(**KON**-jyou-**gay**-ted **ES**- troh-jens meh-**drox**-see-proh-**JESS**-ter-ohn)
**Pregnancy Category:** X
PremPro **(Rx)**
**Classification:** Hormones

See also *Conjugated estrogens* and *Medroxyprogesterone acetate.*

**Content:** Each tablet contains: conjugated estrogens, 0.625 mg, and medroxyprogesterone acetate, 2.5 mg.

**Uses:** Moderate to severe vasomotor symptoms associated with menopause in women with an intact uterus. Vulvular and vaginal atrophy. Prevention of osteoporosis.

**Contraindications:** Known or suspected pregnancy, including use for missed abortion or as a diagnostic test for pregnancy. Known or suspected cancer of the breast or estrogen-dependent neoplasia. Undiagnosed abnormal genital bleeding. Active or past history of thrombophlebitis, thromboembolic disease, or stroke. Liver dysfunction or disease. Lactation.

**Special Concerns:** Estrogens reportedly increase the risk of endometrial carcinoma in postmenopausal women. Use with caution in conditions aggravated by fluid retention, including asthma, epilepsy, migraine, and cardiac or renal dysfunction. Estrogens may cause significant increases in plasma triglycerides that may cause pancreatitis and other complications in clients with familial defects of lipoprotein metabolism.

**Side Effects:** See individual drug entries.

**Drug Interactions:** See individual drug entries.

**Dosage** ————

- **Tablets**

   *Vasomotor symptoms due to menopause, vulvar and vaginal atrophy, prevention of osteoporosis.*
   One tablet daily.

## NURSING CONSIDERATIONS

See also *Nursing Considerations* for *Conjugated estrogens* and *Medroxyprogesterone acetate.*

**Assessment**

1. Document indications for therapy (hormone replacement for menopausal symptoms or osteoporosis prevention), onset and duration of symptoms, and anticipated length of therapy.

2. Note any history or experience with replacement therapy.

3. Evaluate for any active or past conditions that may preclude drug therapy: liver dysfunction, throm-

bophlebitis, thromboembolic disorders, cancer of the breast or estrogen-dependent neoplasia, or any undiagnosed abnormal vaginal bleeding.

**Client/Family Teaching**
1. Take only as directed; two cards are provided, marked cards 1 and 2.
2. Stress importance of follow-up exams to assess need for continued therapy. When used for treating vasomotor symptoms or vulval and vaginal atrophy, reevaluate every 3–6 mo to determine if treatment is still necessary.
3. When used to prevent osteoporosis, monitor closely for signs of endometrial cancer. Diagnostic procedures should be undertaken to rule out malignancy in the event of persistent or recurring abnormal vaginal bleeding.

**Outcomes/Evaluate**
• Osteoporosis prophylaxis
• ↓ Menopausal symptoms

---

# Corticotropin injection (ACTH, Adrenocorticotropic hormone)

(kor-tih-koh-**TROH**-pin)
**Pregnancy Category:** C
ACTH, Acthar **(Rx)**

# Corticotropin repository injection (ACTH gel, Corticotropin gel)

(kor-tih-koh-**TROH**-pin)
**Pregnancy Category:** C
ACTH-80, Acthar Gel (H.P.) ✱, H.P. Acthar Gel **(Rx)**
**Classification:** Anterior pituitary hormone

---

See also *Corticosteroids*.

**Action/Kinetics:** The hormone stimulates the functional adrenal cortex to secrete its entire spectrum of hormones, including the corticosteroids. Thus, the overall physiologic effects of corticotropin are similar to

those of cortisone. Since the latter is more easily obtainable, is more predictable, and has more prolonged activity, it is usually used for therapeutic purposes. Corticotropin is, however, useful for the diagnosis of Addison's disease and other conditions in which the functionality of the adrenal cortex is to be determined. *Corticotropin cannot elicit a hormonal response from a nonfunctioning adrenal gland.* **Peak plasma levels (corticotropin injection):** 1 hr. **t½:** 15 min. The repository injection contains ACTH in a gelatin base to delay the rate of absorption and increase the duration. **Duration** (repository form): Up to 3 days.

**Uses:** Diagnosis of adrenal insufficiency syndromes, nonsuppurative thyroiditis, hypercalcemia associated with cancer, tuberculous meningitis with subarachnoid block or impending block (with tuberculostatic drugs). *Investigational:* Infant spasm, multiple sclerosis. For same diseases as glucocorticosteroids.

**Additional Contraindications:** Cushing's syndrome, psychotic or psychopathic clients, active tuberculosis, active peptic ulcers. Lactation.

**Special Concerns:** Use with caution in clients who have diabetes and hypotension.

**Additional Side Effects:** In the treatment of myasthenia gravis, corticotropin may cause severe muscle weakness 2–3 days after initiation of therapy. Equipment for respiratory assistance must be on hand for such emergencies. Muscle strength returns and increases 2–7 days after cessation of treatment, and improvement lasts for about 3 months.

**Laboratory Test Interferences:** ↓ I¹³¹ uptake and suppress skin test reactions. False ↓ levels of estradiol and estriol using the Brown method. False – estrogens using colorimetric or fluorometric tests.

**Dosage**
• **Injection: SC, IM, or Slow IV Drip**

---

*Most uses.*
**Highly individualized. Usual, using aqueous solution IM or SC:** 20 units q.i.d. **IV:** 10–25 units of aqueous solution in 500 mL 5% dextrose injection over period of 8 hr. Infants and young children require larger dose per body weight than do older children or adults.

*Acute exacerbation of multiple sclerosis.*
**IM:** 80–120 units/day for 2–3 weeks.

*Infantile spasms.*
**IM:** 20–40 units/day or 80 units every other day for 3 months (or 1 month after cessations of seizures).

• **Repository Gel: IM, SC**
40–80 units q 24–72 hr. A dose of 12.5 units q.i.d. causes little metabolic disturbance; 25 units q.i.d. causes definite metabolic alterations.

As a general rule, clients are started on 10–12.5 units q.i.d. If no clinical effect is noted in 72–96 hr, dosage is increased by 5 units every few days to a final maximum of 25 units q.i.d.

## NURSING CONSIDERATIONS

See also *Nursing Considerations* for *Corticosteroids.*

### Administration/Storage
**IV** Check label carefully for IV administration. *The label must say that the product is for IV use.* IV administration should be slow, taking 8 hr.

### Assessment
1. Document indications for therapy, noting type and onset of symptoms.
2. Before administering IV corticotropin, make sure that the client allergic to porcine proteins has been tested for any sensitivity to the brand of corticotropin to be used.
3. Potassium requirements will be increased during IV administration of ACTH; monitor serum potassium and sodium levels.
4. Report mental status changes such as exaggerated euphoria and nervousness or complaints of insomnia and depression. Administer sedatives as needed.

5. Monitor BP, I&O, and weight; report any marked changes.
6. Plot and record growth and height in children regularly; drug may inhibit growth.

### Client/Family Teaching
1. Drug may mask S&S of infection.
2. Increased stress may require an increased dosage.
3. Avoid vaccinations during therapy.
4. Avoid alcohol, salicylates, and NSAIDs.
5. Report any unusual bruising or bleeding.
6. Do not discontinue abruptly; drug should be tapered.

### Outcomes/Evaluate
• Adrenal cortex function
• ↓ Serum calcium levels
• ↑ Muscle strength with MS

# Cortisone acetate (Compound E)
(**KOR**-tih-zohn)
Cortone ✶, Cortone Acetate, Cortone Acetate Sterile Suspension **(Rx)**
**Classification:** Corticosteroid, glucocorticoid-type

See also *Corticosteroids.*
**Action/Kinetics:** Possesses both glucocorticoid and mineralocorticoid activity. Short-acting. **t½, plasma:** 30 min; **t½, biologic:** 8–12 hr.
**Uses:** Replacement therapy in chronic cortical insufficiency. Short-term (due to strong mineralocorticoid effect) for inflammatory or allergic disorders. Sterile suspension: Congenital adrenal hyperplasia in children.
**Special Concerns:** Use during pregnancy only if benefits outweigh risks.

### Dosage
• **Tablets, Injection**
*Initial or during crisis.*
25–300 mg/day. Decrease gradually to lowest effective dose.
*Anti-inflammatory.*
25–150 mg/day, depending on severity of the disease.
*Acute rheumatic fever.*

200 mg b.i.d. day 1, thereafter, 200 mg/day.

*Addison's disease.*
**Maintenance:** 0.5–0.75 mg/kg/day.

## NURSING CONSIDERATIONS

See also *Nursing Considerations* for *Corticosteroids*.
**Administration/Storage:** Single course of therapy should not exceed 6 weeks. Rest periods of 2–3 weeks are indicated between treatments.
**Outcomes/Evaluate**
• Replacement with insufficiency
• Relief of allergic manifestations
• Normal plasma cortisol levels (138–635 nmol/L at 8 a.m.)

# Cosyntropin
(koh-**SIN**-troh-pin)
**Pregnancy Category:** C
Cortrosyn, Synacthen Depot ✽ **(Rx)**
**Classification:** ACTH derivative, synthetic

See also *Corticosteroids*.
**Action/Kinetics:** A synthetic ACTH derivative that causes effects similar to those of ACTH, although fewer hypersensitivity reactions have been noted. The activity of 0.25 mg cosyntropin is equal to 25 units of ACTH.
**Uses:** Diagnosis of adrenocortical insufficiency.

## Dosage
• **IM, SC**
**Adults, usual:** 0.25 mg dissolved in sterile saline. Range: 0.25–0.75 mg.
**Pediatric, under 2 years:** 0.125 mg IM.
• **IV**
**Adults:** 0.25 mg given over a 2-min period.
• **IV Infusion**
**Adults:** 0.25 mg given at a rate of 0.04 mg/hr over a 6-hr period.

## NURSING CONSIDERATIONS

See also *Nursing Considerations* for *Corticosteroids*.

**Administration/Storage**
1. For IM use, dissolve drug (usually 0.25 mg) in sterile saline.
**IV** 2. When given by IV infusion, 0.25 mg cosyntropin is added to dextrose or NSS and given at a rate of 0.04 mg/hr over 6 hr.
**Outcomes/Evaluate:** Type of adrenal gland insufficiency (i.e., primary or secondary)

# Cromolyn sodium (Sodium cromoglycate)
(**CROH**-moh-lin)
**Pregnancy Category:** B
Crolom, Gastrocrom, Intal, Nalcrom ✽, Nasalcrom, Novo–Cromolyn ✽, Opticrom ✽, PMS–Sodium Chromoglycate ✽, Rynacrom ✽, Vistacrom ✽ **(OTC)and (Rx)**
**Classification:** Antiasthmatic, antiallergic drug

**Action/Kinetics:** Acts locally to inhibit the degranulation of sensitized mast cells that occurs after exposure to certain antigens. Prevents the release of histamine, slow-reacting substance of anaphylaxis, and other endogenous substances causing hypersensitivity reactions. When effective, reduces the number and intensity of asthmatic attacks as well as decreasing allergic reactions in the eye. The drug has no antihistaminic, anti-inflammatory, or bronchodilator effects and has no role in terminating an acute attack of asthma. After inhalation, some of the drug is absorbed systemically. **t½:** 81 min; from lungs: 60 min. About 50% excreted unchanged through the urine and 50% through the bile. When used in the eye, approximately 0.03% is absorbed. **Onset, ophthalmic:** Several days. **Onset, nasal:** Less than 1 week. **Time to peak effect, nasal:** Up to 4 weeks.
**Uses:** *Inhalation:* Prophylactic and adjunct in the management of severe bronchial asthma in selected clients. Prophylaxis of exercise-induced bronchospasms and bron-

chospasms due to allergens, cold dry air, or environmental pollutants. *Ophthalmologic:* Conjunctivitis, including vernal keratoconjunctivitis, vernal conjunctivitis, and vernal keratitis. *Nasal, OTC:* Prophylaxis and treatment of allergic rhinitis. *PO:* Mastocytosis (improves symptoms including diarrhea, flushing, headaches, vomiting, urticaria, nausea, abdominal pain, and itching). *Investigational:* PO to treat food allergies.

**Contraindications:** Hypersensitivity. Acute attacks and status asthmaticus. Due to the presence of benzalkonium chloride in the product, soft contact lenses should not be worn if the drug is used in the eye. For mastocytosis in premature infants.

**Special Concerns:** Dosage of the ophthalmic product has not been established in children less than 4 years of age; dosage of the nasal product has not been established in children less than 6 years of age. Use with caution for long periods of time, in the presence of renal or hepatic disease, and during lactation.

**Side Effects:** *Respiratory: Bronchospasm, laryngeal edema (rare),* cough, eosinophilic pneumonia. *CNS:* Dizziness, drowsiness, headache. *Allergic:* Urticaria, rash, angioedema, serum sickness, *anaphylaxis. Other:* Nausea, urinary frequency, dysuria, joint swelling and pain, lacrimation, swollen parotid gland.

**Following nebulization:** Sneezing, wheezing, itching, nose bleeds, burning, nasal congestion. **Following nasal solution:** Burning, stinging, irritation of nose; sneezing, nose bleeds, headache, bad taste in mouth, postnasal drip. **Following ophthalmic use:** Stinging and burning after use. Also, conjunctival injection, watery or itchy eyes, dryness around the eye, puffy eyes, eye irritation, styes.

**Following PO use:** *GI:* Diarrhea, taste perversion, spasm of esophagus, flatulence, dysphagia, burning of mouth and throat. *CNS:* Headache, dizziness, fatigue, migraine, paresthesia, anxiety, depression, psychosis, behavior changes, insomnia, hallucinations, lethargy, lightheadedness after eating. *Dermatologic:* Flushing, angioedema, urticaria, skin burning, skin erythema. *Musculoskeletal:* Arthralgia, stiffness and weakness in legs. *Miscellaneous:* Altered liver function test, dyspnea, dysuria, polycythemia, neutropenia.

## Dosage
- **Capsules or Metered Dose Inhaler**
  *Prophylaxis of bronchial asthma.*
  **Adults:** 20 mg q.i.d. at regular intervals. Adjust dosage as required.
  *Prophylaxis of bronchospasm.*
  **Adults:** 20 mg as a single dose just prior to exposure to the precipitating factor. If used chronically, 20 mg q.i.d, up to a maximum of 160 mg/day.
- **Ophthalmic Solution**
  *Allergic ocular disorders.*
  **Adults and children over 4 years:** 1–2 gtt of the 4% solution in each eye 4–6 times/day at regular intervals.
- **Nasal Spray (OTC)**
  *Allergic rhinitis.*
  **Adults and children over 6 years:** 5.2 mg in each nostril 3–4 times/day at regular intervals (e.g., q 4–6 hr). May be used up to 6 times/day.
- **Oral Capsules**
  *Mastocytosis.*
  **Adults:** 200 mg q.i.d. 30 min before meals and at bedtime. **Pediatric, term to 2 years:** 20 mg/kg/day in four divided doses; should be used in this age group only in severe incapacitating disease where benefits outweigh risks. **Pediatric, 2–12 years:** 100 mg q.i.d. 30 min before meals and at bedtime. If relief is not seen within 2–3 weeks, dose may be increased, but should not exceed 40 mg/kg/day for adults and children over 2 years of age and 30 mg/kg/day for children 6 months–2 years.

## NURSING CONSIDERATIONS
### Administration/Storage
1. Continue corticosteroid dosage

when initiating cromolyn therapy. If improvement occurs, taper the steroid dosage slowly. May have to reinstitute steroids if cromolyn inhalation is impaired, in times of stress, or in adrenocortical insufficiency.

2. One drop of ophthalmic solution contains 1.6 mg cromolyn sodium.

3. Protect ophthalmic solution from direct sunlight and, once opened, discard after 4 weeks.

4. The ophthalmic solution contains benzylkonium chloride; therefore, soft contact lenses should not be worn during treatment.

**Client/Family Teaching**

1. Institute only after acute episode is over, when airway is clear and able to inhale adequately.

2. When administered by Spinhaler, the following guidelines should be used:

• Puncture and load the capsule into the Spinhaler.

• Inhale and exhale fully; then introduce the mouthpiece between the lips.

• Tilt head back and inhale deeply and rapidly through the inhaler. This causes the propeller to turn rapidly and to supply more medication in one breath.

• Remove inhaler, hold breath a few seconds, and exhale slowly.

• Repeat this procedure until the powder is completely administered.

• Do not wet powder with breath while exhaling.

• Taking a sip of water or rinsing the mouth immediately before and after using the Spinhaler will diminish the throat irritation and/or cough.

• Replace Spinhaler every 6 months.

3. Continue prescribed medications; may take up to 4 weeks for frequency of asthmatic attacks to decrease.

4. With exposure bronchoconstriction, use inhaler within 10–15 min prior to exposure of precipitating agent (i.e., exercise, antigen, environmental pollutants) for best results.

5. Use a peak expiratory flow meter to monitor asthma control; establish level to seek medical assistance.

6. Do not discontinue medication abruptly. Rapid withdrawal of the drug may precipitate an asthmatic attack, and concomitant corticosteroid therapy may require adjustment.

7. When used in the *eye*:

• Do not wear soft contacts until medically cleared.

• Drug may sting on application, but this should subside.

**Outcomes/Evaluate**

• ↓ Frequency of asthmatic attacks

• Prevention of exposure-induced bronchoconstriction

• Control of symptoms of mastocytosis (↓ diarrhea, N&V, headache, flushing, and abdominal pain)

• Relief of ocular and/or nasal allergic manifestations

# Cyanocobalamin (Vitamin B$_{12}$)

(sye-**an**-oh-koh-**BAL**-ah-min)
**Pregnancy Category:** C
**Nasal gel:** Ener-B, Nascobal **(OTC).**,
**Parenteral:** Berubigen, Kaybovite-1000, Redisol, Rubramin ✿, Rubramin PC **(OTC) (Rx)**

# Cyanocobalamin crystalline

(sye-**an**-oh-koh-**BAL**-ah-min)
**Pregnancy Category:** C
Crystamine, Crystl 1000, Cyanoject, Cyomin, Rubesol-1000, Vitamin B$_{12}$
**Classification:** Vitamin B$_{12}$

**Action/Kinetics:** Cyanocobalamin (vitamin B$_{12}$), a cobalt-containing vitamin, can be isolated from liver and is identical to that of the antianemic factor of liver. Required for hematopoiesis, cell reproduction, nucleoprotein and myelin synthesis. Plasma vitamin B$_{12}$ levels: 150–750 pg/mL.

Intrinsic factor is required for adequate absorption of PO vitamin B$_{12}$, and in pernicious anemia and malabsorption diseases intrinsic factor is administered simultaneously. Rapidly absorbed following IM or SC administration. Following absorption, vitamin $B_{12}$ is carried by plasma proteins to the liver where it is stored until required for various metabolic functions.

Products containing less than 500 mcg vitamin $B_{12}$ are nutritional supplements and are not to be used for the treatment of pernicious anemia. **t½:** 6 days (400 days in the liver). **Time to peak levels, after PO:** 8–12 hr.

**Uses:** Nutritional vitamin $B_{12}$ deficiency, including cancer of the bowel or pancreas, sprue, total or partial gastrectomy, accompanying folic acid deficiency, GI surgery or pathology, gluten enteropathy, fish tapeworm infestation, bacterial overgrowth of the small intestine. Oral products should not be used to treat pernicious anemia. Also, in conditions with an increased need for vitamin $B_{12}$ such as thyrotoxicosis, hemorrhage, malignancy, pregnancy, and in liver and kidney disease. Vitamin $B_{12}$ is particularly suitable for the treatment of clients allergic to liver extract.

*Investigational:* Diagnosis of vitamin $B_{12}$ deficiency.

*NOTE:* Folic acid is not a substitute for vitamin $B_{12}$ although concurrent folic acid therapy may be required.
**Contraindications:** Hypersensitivity to cobalt, Leber's disease.
**Special Concerns:** Use with caution in clients with gout.
**Side Effects:** Manifested following parenteral use. *Allergic:* Urticaria, itching, exanthema, ***anaphylaxis, shock, death.*** *CV: **Peripheral vascular thrombosis,*** CHF, ***pulmonary edema.*** *Other:* Polycythemia vera, optic nerve atrophy in clients with hereditary optic nerve atrophy, diarrhea, hypokalemia, body feels swollen.

*NOTE:* Benzyl alcohol, which is present in certain products, may cause ***a fatal "gasping syndrome"*** in premature infants.
**Drug Interactions**
*Alcohol* / ↓ Vitamin $B_{12}$ absorption
*Chloramphenicol* / ↓ Response to vitamin $B_{12}$ therapy

*Cholestyramine* / ↓ Vitamin $B_{12}$ absorption
*Cimetidine* / ↓ Digestion and release of vitamin $B_{12}$
*Colchicine* / ↓ Vitamin $B_{12}$ absorption
*Neomycin* / ↓ Vitamin $B_{12}$ absorption
*PAS* / ↓ Vitamin $B_{12}$ absorption
*Potassium, timed-release* / ↓ Vitamin $B_{12}$ absorption
**Laboratory Test Interferences:** Antibiotics may interfere with the microbiologic assay for serum and erythrocyte vitamin $B_{12}$.

## Dosage

CYANOCOBALAMIN
• **Tablets, Extended-Release Tablets**
*Nutritional supplement.*
**Adults:** 1 mcg/day (up to 25 mcg for increased requirements). The RDA is 2 mcg/day. **Pediatric, up to 1 year:** 0.3 mcg/day; **over 1 year:** 1 mcg/day.
*Nutritional deficiency.*
25–250 mcg/day.
• **Nasal gel**
*Nutritional deficiency.*
500 mcg/0.1 mL weekly given intranasally.
CYANOCOBALAMIN CRYSTALLINE
• **IM, Deep SC**
*Addisonian pernicious anemia.*
**Adults:** 100 mcg/day for 6–7 days; **then,** 100 mcg every other day for seven doses. If improvement is noted along with a reticulocyte response, 100 mcg q 3–4 days for 2–3 weeks; **maintenance, IM:** 100 mcg once a month for life. Give folic acid if necessary.
*Vitamin $B_{12}$ deficiency.*
**Adults:** 30 mcg daily for 5–10 days; **then,** 100–200 mcg/month. Doses up to 1,000 mcg have been recommended. **Pediatric, for hematologic signs:** 10–50 mcg/day for 5–10 days followed by 100–250 mcg/dose q 2–4 weeks. **Pediatric, for neurologic signs:** 100 mcg/day for 10–15 days; **then,** 1–2 times/week for several months (can possibly

be tapered to 250–1,000 mcg/month by 1 year).

*Diagnosis of vitamin B₁₂ deficiency.*

**Adults:** 1 mcg/day IM for 10 days plus low dietary folic acid and vitamin B₁₂. Loading dose for the Schilling test is 1,000 mcg given IM.

## NURSING CONSIDERATIONS
### Administration/Storage
1. Protect cyanocobalamin crystalline injection from light. Do not freeze.
2. With pernicious anemia, the drug cannot be administered PO.
### Assessment
1. Document indications for therapy, type and onset of symptoms.
2. Determine if allergic to cobalt.
3. Note if prescribed chloramphenicol; this drug antagonizes the hematopoietic response to vitamin B₁₂.
4. Perform a baseline assessment of peripheral pulses and assess for neuropathy.
5. Monitor CBC, potassium, and B₁₂ levels if being treated for megaloblastic anemia.
6. With pernicious anemia and malabsorption syndromes, intrinsic factor should be administered simultaneously.
### Client/Family Teaching
1. With pernicious anemia, vitamin B₁₂ replacement *must* be taken for life.
2. When repository vitamin B₁₂ is used, it provides medication for 4 weeks.
3. The stinging, burning sensation that may occur after injection is transitory.
4. If vitamin B₁₂ therapy is the result of dietary deficiency, identify foods (such as meats, especially liver, fermented cheeses, egg yolks, and seafood) high in B₁₂ and review diet.
5. Avoid alcohol; interferes with drug absorption.
6. Report any symptoms of urticaria, itching, and evidence of anaphylaxis immediately.

7. If diarrhea occurs, record the frequency, quantity, and consistency of stools. If severe or persists, a change in drug may be required.
### Outcomes/Evaluate
• Cause of B₁₂ deficiency state
• Symptomatic improvement
• Plasma vitamin B₁₂ levels of 350–750 pg/mL

# Cyclobenzaprine hydrochloride
(sye-kloh-**BENZ**-ah-preen)
**Pregnancy Category:** B
Alti-Cyclobenzaprine ✚, Apo-Cyclobenzaprine ✚, Flexeril, Novo–Cycloprine ✚, Nu-Cyclobenzaprine ✚, PMS-Cyclobenzaprine ✚ **(Rx)**
**Classification:** Skeletal muscle relaxant, centrally acting

See also *Skeletal Muscle Relaxants, Centrally Acting.*

**Action/Kinetics:** Related to the tricyclic antidepressants; possesses both sedative and anticholinergic properties. Thought to inhibit reflexes by reducing tonic somatic motor activity. **Onset:** 1 hr. **Time to peak plasma levels:** 4–6 hr. **Therapeutic plasma levels:** 20–30 ng/mL. **Duration:** 12–24 hr. **t½:** 1–3 days. Highly bound to plasma protein. Inactive metabolites are excreted in the urine.

**Uses:** Adjunct to rest and physical therapy for relief of muscle spasms associated with acute and/or painful musculoskeletal conditions. Not indicated for the treatment of spastic diseases or for cerebral palsy. *Investigational:* Adjunct in the treatment of fibrositis syndrome.

**Contraindications:** Hypersensitivity. Arrhythmias, heart block or conduction disturbances, CHF, or during acute recovery phase of MI. Hyperthyroidism. Concomitant use of MAO inhibitors or within 14 days of their discontinuation.

**Special Concerns:** Safe use during lactation and in children under age 15 has not been established. Due to atropine-like effects, use with caution in situations where cholinergic blockade is not desired (e.g., history of urinary retention, angle-closure glaucoma, increased intraocular pressure). Geriatric clients may be more sensitive to cholinergic blockade.

**Side Effects:** Since cyclobenzaprine resembles tricyclic antidepressants, side effects to these drugs should also be noted. *GI:* Dry mouth, N&V, constipation, dyspepsia, unpleasant taste, anorexia, diarrhea, GI pain, gastritis, thirst, flatulence, ageusia, paralytic ileus, discoloration of tongue, stomatitis, parotid swelling. *CNS:* Drowsiness, dizziness, fatigue, asthenia, blurred vision, nervousness, headache, **convulsions,** ataxia, vertigo, dysarthria, paresthesia, hypertonia, tremors, malaise, abnormal gait, delusions, Bell's palsy, alteration in EEG patterns, extrapyramidal symptoms. Psychiatric symptoms include: confusion, insomnia, disorientation, depressed mood, abnormal sensations, anxiety, agitation, abnormal thinking or dreaming, excitement, hallucinations. *CV:* Tachycardia, syncope, **arrhythmias,** vasodilation, palpitations, hypotension, edema, chest pain, hypertension, MI, heart block, stroke. *GU:* Urinary frequency or retention, impaired urination, dilation of urinary tract, impotence, decreased or increased libido, testicular swelling, gynecomastia, breast enlargement, galactorrhea. *Dermatologic:* Sweating, skin rashes, urticaria, pruritus, photosensitivity, alopecia. *Musculoskeletal:* Muscle twitching, weakness, myalgia. *Hematologic:* Purpura, bone marrow depression, leukopenia, eosinophilia, thrombocytopenia. *Hepatic:* Abnormal liver function, hepatitis, jaundice, cholestasis. *Miscellaneous:* Tinnitus, diplopia, peripheral neuropathy, increase and decrease of blood sugar, weight gain or loss, **edema of the face and tongue,** inappropriate ADH syndrome, dyspnea.

**OD** **Overdose Management:** *Symptoms:* Temporary confusion, disturbed concentration, transient visual hallucinations, agitation, hyperactive reflexes, muscle rigidity, vomiting, **hyperpyrexia.** Also, drowsiness, hypothermia, tachycardia, **cardiac arrhythmias such as bundle branch block, ECG evidence of impaired conduction,** CHF, dilated pupils, **seizures, severe hypotension,** stupor, **coma,** paradoxical diaphoresis. *Treatment:* In addition to the treatment outlined in , for physostigmine salicylate, 1–3 mg IV may be used to reverse symptoms of severe cholinergic blockade.

**Drug Interactions:** *NOTE:* Because of the similarity of cyclobenzaprine to tricyclic antidepressants, the drug interactions for tricyclics should also be consulted.

*Anticholinergics* / Additive anticholinergic side effects
*CNS depressants* / Additive depressant effects
*Guanethidine* / Cyclobenzaprine may block effect
*MAO inhibitors* / Hypertensive crisis, severe convulsions
*Tricyclic antidepressants* / Additive side effects

**Dosage** ———————————
• **Tablets**
  *Skeletal muscle disorders.*
**Adults:** 20–40 mg/day in three to four divided doses (usual: 10 mg t.i.d.), up to a maximum of 60 mg/day in divided doses.

## NURSING CONSIDERATIONS

See also *Nursing Considerations* for *Skeletal Muscle Relaxants, Centrally Acting.*
**Administration/Storage**
1. Use only for 2–3 weeks.
2. If taking an MAO inhibitor, do not administer cyclobenzaprine for at least 2 weeks after discontinuing the MAO inhibitor.
**Assessment**
1. Document indications for therapy, extent of acute or painful muscu-

loskeletal condition, evidence of weakness, DTRs, and ROM. Review RICE (rest, ice, compression, and elevation) with acute injury to reduce swelling and recovery time.

2. Note any hypersensitivity or spastic diseases; drug is contraindicated.

3. Check for evidence of cardiac arrhythmias. Note history of recent MI.

4. Obtain baseline ECG, CBC and liver profile.

**Client/Family Teaching**

1. Report any unusual fatigue, sore throat, unexplained fever, easy bruising or bleeding; may indicate a blood dyscrasia.

2. Report nausea or abdominal pain, itchy skin, or evidence of yellow sclera or skin; may indicate hepatic toxicity.

3. Symptoms of dry mouth, blurred vision, dizziness, tachycardia, or urinary retention should also be reported and therapy evaluated.

4. Due to drug-induced drowsiness, dizziness, and/or blurred vision, observe caution if performing activities that require mental alertness.

5. Notify provider if S&S do not improve within 2–3 weeks of therapy.

**Outcomes/Evaluate:** Relief of musculoskeletal spasms and pain; ↑ ROM

# Cyclophosphamide

(sye-kloh-**FOS**-fah-myd)

**Pregnancy Category:** D

Cytoxan, Cytoxan Lyophilized, Neosar, Procytox ✦ (Abbreviation: CYC) **(Rx)**

**Classification:** Antineoplastic, alkylating agent

See also *Antineoplastic Agents* and *Alkylating Agents.*

**Action/Kinetics:** Metabolized in the liver to both active antineoplastic alkylating agents and inactive metabolites. The active metabolites alkylate nucleic acids, thus interfering with the growth of neoplastic and normal tissues. The cytotoxic action is due to cross-linking of strands of DNA and RNA and inhibition of protein synthesis. Also possesses immunosuppressive activity. **t½:** 3–12 hr, but remnants of drug and/or metabolites detectable in serum after 72 hr; in children, the **t½** averages 4.1 hr. Metabolites are excreted through the urine with up to 25% of cyclophosphamide excreted unchanged. Cyclophosphamide is also excreted in milk.

**Uses:** Often used in combination with other antineoplastic drugs. *Malignancies:* Malignant lymphomas (Stages III and IV, Ann Arbor Staging System), Hodgkin's disease, lymphocytic lymphoma (nodular or diffuse), mixed-cell-type lymphoma, histiocytic lymphoma, Burkitt's lymphoma, multiple myeloma, neuroblastoma (disseminated), adenocarcinoma of the ovary, retinoblastoma, carcinoma of the breast. *Leukemias:* Chronic lymphocytic and granulocytic leukemia, acute myelogenous and monocytic leukemia, acute lymphoblastic leukemia in children. *Other:* Mycosis fungoides, nephrotic syndrome in children. *Investigational:* Rheumatic diseases including rheumatoid arthritis and lupus erythematosus, Wegemer's granulomatosis, multiple sclerosis, polyarteritis nodosa, polymyositis (use with corticosteroids), severe neuropsychiatric lupus erythematosus.

**Contraindications:** Lactation. Severe bone marrow depression.

**Special Concerns:** Use with caution in clients with thrombocytopenia, leukopenia, previous radiation therapy, bone marrow infiltration of tumor cells, previous therapy causing cytotoxicity, and impaired liver and kidney function. May interfere with wound healing.

**Additional Side Effects:** Acute hemorrhagic cystitis. *Bone marrow depression* appears frequently during days 9–14 of therapy. Alopecia occurs more frequently than with other drugs. *Secondary neoplasia (especially of urinary bladder), pulmonary fibrosis,*

---

✦ = Available in Canada                    ***bold italic*** = life threatening side effect

***cardiotoxicity,*** darkening of skin or fingernails. Interference with oogenesis and spermatogenesis.

**OD Overdose Management:** *Treatment:* General supportive measures. Dialysis.

**Drug Interactions**

*Allopurinol* / ↑ Chance of bone marrow toxicity

*Anticoagulants* / ↑ Effect of anticoagulants

*Chloramphenicol* / ↓ Metabolism of cyclophosphamide to active metabolites → ↓ pharmacologic effect

*Digoxin* / ↓ Serum digoxin levels

*Doxorubicin* / ↑ Cardiotoxicity due to doxorubicin

*Insulin* / ↑ Hypoglycemia

*Phenobarbital* / ↑ Rate of metabolism of cyclophosphamide in liver

*Quinolone antibiotics* / ↓ Antimicrobial effect of quinolones

*Succinylcholine* / ↑ Neuromuscular blockade due to ↓ cholinesterase activity

*Thiazide diuretics* / ↑ Chance of leukopenia

**Laboratory Test Interferences:** ↑ Uric acid in blood and urine; false + Pap test; ↓ serum pseudocholinesterase. Suppression of certain skin tests.

**Dosage**

• **IV**

*Malignancies.*

**Initial, with no hematologic deficiency:** 40–50 mg/kg in divided doses over 2–5 days. *Alternative therapy:* 10–15 mg/kg q 7–10 days or 3–5 mg/kg twice weekly.

• **Tablets**

*Malignancies.*

**Initial and maintenance:** 1–5 mg/kg depending on client tolerance. Attempt to maintain leukocyte count at 3,000–4,000/mm³. Adjust dosage for kidney or liver disease.

*Nephrotic syndrome in children.* 2.5–3 mg/kg/day for 60–90 days.

## NURSING CONSIDERATIONS

See also *Nursing Considerations* for *Antineoplastic Agents.*

**Administration/Storage**

1. Prepare PO solution by dissolving injectable cyclophosphamide in aromatic elixir.

2. The initial loading dose may need to be reduced by one-third to one-half in clients who have previously received cytotoxic drugs or radiation therapy.

**IV** 3. IV/IM: Dissolve 100 mg cyclophosphamide in appropriate amount (depending on vial strength) sterile water for injection.

4. Solutions may be given IV, IM, intraperitoneally, or intrapleurally. May be infused IV with 5% dextrose injection, 5% dextrose and 0.9% NaCl injection, 5% dextrose and Ringer's injection, RL injection, 0.45% NaCl injection, or 1/6M sodium lactate injection.

5. Store reconstituted solution at room temperature for 24 hr or for 6 days if refrigerated at 2°C–8°C (36°F–46°F).

**Assessment**

1. Note any prior radiation or chemotherapy; dose requires reduction.

2. Assess skin condition and integrity noting evidence of breakdown; may interfere with wound healing.

3. Monitor for cardiotoxicity: increased SOB, rales, increased coughing, or tachycardia. Obtain periodic CXR and pulmonary function tests.

4. Check for dysuria and hematuria; monitor urinalysis with specific gravity to assess for syndrome of inappropriate antidiuretic hormone (SIADH).

5. Monitor CBC; may cause granulocyte suppression. Nadir: 14 days; recovery: 17–21 days.

**Client/Family Teaching**

1. Take PO meds on an empty stomach; may take with meals if GI upset occurs.

2. Increase fluid intake before, during, and for 24 hr after therapy.

3. Take in the morning so kidneys can eliminate drug before bedtime; void frequently. Stay well hydrated to help prevent hemorrhagic cystitis due to excessive urinary drug concentrations.

4. May discolor skin and nails.

5. Report any unusual bruising, bleeding, or fever.
6. Avoid vaccinations during therapy.
7. With alopecia, hair should grow back when drug is stopped or when a maintenance dosage is given.
8. Drug may cause a false positive Pap test. May also cause sterility and menstrual irregularities; identify candidates for egg/sperm harvesting.
9. Practice reliable contraception (both sexes) during therapy.
10. S&S of hypoglycemia may be precipitated by drug interactions with insulin; monitor sugars closely and consult with provider for insulin dosage adjustment.
11. Report any evidence of injury or delayed wound healing.
12. May suppress skin test response for *Candida*, mumps, trichophyton, and purified protein derivative.

**Outcomes/Evaluate**
• Improved hematologic parameters
• ↓ Tumor size and spread

# Cycloserine
(sye-kloh-**SEE**-reen)
**Pregnancy Category:** C
Seromycin **(Rx)**
**Classification:** Antitubercular agent for retreatment regimens

**Action/Kinetics:** Produced by a strain of *Streptomyces orchidaceus* or *Garyphalus lavendulae*. Acts by inhibiting cell wall synthesis by interfering with the incorporation of the amino acid alanine. Well absorbed from the GI tract and widely distributed in body tissues. **Time to peak plasma levels:** 3–8 hr. CSF levels are similar to those in plasma. **t½:** 10 hr. From 60% to 70% is excreted unchanged in urine.

**Uses:** With other drugs to treat active pulmonary and extrapulmonary tuberculosis only when primary therapy cannot be used. To treat UTIs when other therapy has failed or if the organism has demonstrated sensitivity.

**Contraindications:** Hypersensitivity to cycloserine, epilepsy, depres-sion, severe anxiety, psychosis, severe renal insufficiency, and alcoholism. Lactation.

**Special Concerns:** Safe use during pregnancy and in children has not been established.

**Side Effects:** *CNS:* Drowsiness, headache, mental confusion, tremors, vertigo, loss of memory, psychoses (possibly with **suicidal tendencies)**, character changes, hyperirritability, aggression, increased reflexes, **seizures,** paresthesias, paresis, coma. Neurotoxic effects depend on blood levels of cycloserine. Hence, frequent determinations of cycloserine blood levels are indicated, especially during the initial period of therapy. *Other:* Sudden development of CHF, skin rashes, increased transaminase.

**OD** **Overdose Management:** *Symptoms:* CNS depression, including drowsiness, mental confusion, headache, vertigo, paresthesias, dysarthrias, hyperirritability, psychosis, paresis, **seizures,** and **coma.** *Treatment:* Supportive therapy. Charcoal may be more effective than emesis or gastric lavage. Hemodialysis may be used for life-threatening toxicity. Pyridoxine may treat neurotoxic effects.

**Drug Interactions**
*Ethanol* / ↑ Risk of epileptic episodes
*Isoniazid* / ↑ Risk of cycloserine CNS side effects (especially dizziness)

**Dosage**
• **Capsules**
**Adults, initially:** 250 mg q 12 hr for first 2 weeks; **then,** 0.5–1 g/day in divided doses based on blood levels. Dosage should not exceed 1 g/day. **Pediatric:** 10–20 mg/kg/day, not to exceed 0.75–1 g/day. *NOTE:* Pyridoxine, 200–300 mg/day may prevent neurotoxic effects.

## NURSING CONSIDERATIONS

See also *General Nursing Considerations for All Anti-Infectives.*

### Assessment

1. Note any evidence of depression, anxiety, seizures, or excessive alcohol use. Report any psychotic or neurologic reactions that may necessitate temporary drug withdrawal.
2. Monitor I&O; observe for any S&S of CHF with high-dose therapy.
3. Monitor liver and renal function studies and cycloserine levels throughout therapy (<25–30 mcg/mL).

### Client/Family Teaching

1. May cause drowsiness and dizziness; do not perform tasks that require mental alertness; report if symptoms persist.
2. Consume 2–3 L/day of fluids.
3. Avoid alcohol.
4. Immediately report any SOB, skin rashes, or overt behavioral changes, especially suicide ideations.

### Outcomes/Evaluate

• Negative sputum cultures for acid-fast bacilli
• Improved CXR and pulmonary function studies

# Cyclosporine

(sye-kloh-**SPOR**-een)
**Pregnancy Category:** C
Neoral, Sandimmune, Sandimmune I.V. ✷, Sandimmune Neoral ✷ **(Rx)**
**Classification:** Immunosuppressant

**Action/Kinetics:** Thought to act by inhibiting the immunocompetent lymphocytes in the $G_0$ or $G_1$ phase of the cell cycle. T-lymphocytes are specifically inhibited; both the T-helper cell and the T-suppressor cell may be affected. Also inhibits interleukin 2 or T-cell growth factor production and release. Absorption from the GI tract is incomplete and variable. Children often require larger PO doses than adults, which may be due to the smaller absorptive surface area of their intestines. **Peak plasma levels:** 3.5 hr. Food may both delay and impair drug absorption. $t^{1/2}$: Approximately 19 hr for adults and 7 hr in children. Metabolized by the liver; inactive metabolites are excreted mainly through the bile.

Neoral immediately forms a microemulsion in an aqueous environment. This product has better bioequivalency; thus, Sandimmune and Neoral are not bioequivalent and cannot be used interchangeably without medical supervision. **Time to peak blood levels:** 1.5–2 hr. Food decreases the amount of drug absorbed.

**Uses:** Prophylaxis of rejection in kidney, liver, and heart allogeneic transplants. Sandimmune is always to be taken with adrenal corticosteroids while Neoral has been used in combination with azathioprine and corticosteroids. Neoral microemulsion: In combination with methotrexate for severe, active rheumatoid arthritis which has not responded to methotrexate alone. Neoral microemulsion: Severe recalcitrant plaque psoriasis. Sandimmune: Treatment of chronic rejection in clients previously treated with other immunosuppressants. Sandimmune has been used in children as young as 6 months with no unusual side effects. *Investigational:* Aplastic anemia, myasthenia gravis, atopic dermatitis, Crohn's disease, Graves ophthalmology, severe psoriasis, multiple sclerosis, polymyositis, Behcet's disease, biliary cirrhosis, corneal transplantation (or other diseases of the eye which have an autoimmune component), dermatomyositis, insulin-dependent diabetes mellitus, lichen planus, lupus nephritis, nephrotic syndrome, pemphigus and pemphigoid, psoriatic arthritis, pulmonary sarcoidosis, pyoderma gangrenosum, rheumatoid arthritis, ulcerative colitis, uveitis.

**Contraindications:** Hypersensitivity to cyclosporine or polyoxyethylated castor oil. Lactation. Use of potassium-sparing diuretics.

**Special Concerns:** Use with caution in clients with impaired renal or hepatic function. Safety and efficacy have not been established in children. Clients with malabsorption may not achieve therapeutic levels following PO use.

**Side Effects:** *GI:* N&V, diarrhea, gum hyperplasia, anorexia, gastritis, hiccoughs, peptic ulcer, abdominal discomfort, upper GI bleeding, pancreatitis, constipation, mouth sores, difficulty in swallowing. *Hematologic:* Leukopenia, lymphoma, thrombocytopenia, microangiopathic hemolytic anemia syndrome. *Allergic:* **Anaphylaxis (rare).** *CV:* Hypertension, edema, **MI.** *CNS:* Headache, tremor, confusion, fever, **seizures,** anxiety, depression, weakness, lethargy, ataxia, hallucinations, mania, encephalopathy, sleep disturbances. *GU:* Renal dysfunction, glomerular capillary thrombosis, nephrotoxicity. *Miscellaneous:* Hepatotoxicity, acne, hirsutism, flushing, paresthesia, sinusitis, gynecomastia, conjunctivitis, brittle fingernails, hearing loss, tinnitus, hyperglycemia, hyperkalemia, hyperuricemia, muscle pain, infections (including fungal, viral), *Pneumocystis carinii* pneumonia, hematuria, blurred vision, cramps, weight loss, chest and joint pain, night sweats, hair breaking, pruritus, tingling, hypomagnesemia in some clients with seizures, infectious complications.

**OD Overdose Management:** *Symptoms:* Transient hepatotoxicity and nephrotoxicity. *Treatment:* Induction of vomiting (up to 2 hr after ingestion). General supportive measures.

**Drug Interactions**

*Allopurinol* / ↑ Plasma levels of cyclosporine due to ↓ breakdown by liver

*Aminoglycosides* / ↑ Risk of nephrotoxicity

*Amiodarone* / ↑ Blood levels of cyclosporine → ↑ risk of nephrotoxicity

*Amphotericin B* / ↑ Risk of nephrotoxicity

*Azathioprine* / ↑ Immunosuppression due to suppression of lymphocytes → possible infection and malignancy

*Bromocriptine* / ↑ Plasma level of cyclosporine due to ↓ breakdown by liver

*Carbamazepine* / ↓ Plasma level of cyclosporine due to ↑ breakdown by liver

*Cimetidine* / ↑ Risk of nephrotoxicity

*Clarithromycin* / ↑ Plasma levels of cyclosporine due to ↓ breakdown by liver

*Colchicine* / Severe side effects, including GI, hepatic, renal, and neuromuscular toxicity

*Corticosteroids* / ↑ Immunosuppression due to suppression of lymphocytes → possible infection and malignancy

*Cyclophosphamide* / ↑ Immunosuppression due to suppression of lymphocytes → possible infection and malignancy

*Danazol* / ↑ Plasma level of cyclosporine due to ↓ breakdown by liver

*Digoxin* / ↑ Digoxin levels due to ↓ clearance; also, ↓ volume of distribution of digoxin → toxicity

*Diltiazem* / ↑ Plasma level of cyclosporine due to ↓ breakdown by liver → possible nephrotoxicity

*Diuretics, potassium-sparing* / ↑ Risk of hyperkalemia

*Erythromycin* / ↑ Plasma level of cyclosporine due to ↓ breakdown by liver and ↓ biliary excretion → possible nephrotoxicity

*Fluconazole* / ↑ Plasma level of cyclosporine due to ↓ breakdown by liver → possible nephrotoxicity

*Imipenem-cilastatin* / ↑ Plasma level of cyclosporine due to ↓ breakdown by liver → CNS toxicity

*Isoniazid* / ↓ Plasma level of cyclosporine due to ↑ breakdown by liver

*Itraconazole* / ↑ Plasma level of cyclosporine due to ↓ breakdown by liver

*Ketoconazole* / ↑ Plasma level of cyclosporine due to ↓ breakdown by liver; also, ↑ risk of nephrotoxicity

*Lovastatin* / ↑ Plasma levels of lovastatin due to ↓ clearance; also, ↑ risk of myositis

*Melphalan* / ↑ Risk of nephrotoxicity

*Methylprednisolone* / ↑ Risk of convulsions

*Metoclopramide* / ↑ Plasma level of cyclosporine due to ↓ breakdown by liver

*Nafcillin* / ↓ Plasma level of cyclosporine due to ↑ breakdown by liver

*Nephrotoxic drugs* / Additive nephrotoxicity

*Nicardipine* / ↑ Plasma level of cyclosporine due to ↓ breakdown by liver → possible nephrotoxicity

*Nifedipine* / ↑ Risk of gingival hyperplasia

*Nondepolarizing muscle relaxants* / ↑ Neuromuscular blockade

*NSAIDs* / ↑ Risk of nephrotoxicity

*Octreotide* / ↓ Plasma level of cyclosporine due to ↑ breakdown by liver

*Oral contraceptives* / ↑ Plasma level of cyclosporine due to ↓ breakdown by liver

*Phenobarbital* / ↓ Plasma level of cyclosporine due to ↑ breakdown by liver

*Phenytoin* / ↓ Plasma level of cyclosporine due to ↑ breakdown by liver

*Prednisolone* / ↑ Plasma level of cyclosporine due to ↓ breakdown by liver

*Probucol* / ↓ Bioavailability of cyclosporine → ↓ clinical effect

*Ranitidine* / ↑ Risk of nephrotoxicity

*Rifampin* / ↓ Plasma level of cyclosporine due to ↑ breakdown by liver

*Sulfamethoxazole and/or trimethoprim* / ↑ Risk of nephrotoxicity; also, ↓ serum levels of cyclosporine → possible rejection

*Tacrolimus* / ↑ Risk of nephrotoxicity

*Ticlopidine* / ↓ Plasma level of cyclosporine due to ↑ breakdown by liver

*Trimethoprim with sulfamethoxazole* / ↑ Risk of nephrotoxicity

*Vancomycin* / ↑ Risk of nephrotoxicity

*Verapamil* / ↑ Immunosuppression

**Laboratory Test Interferences:** ↑ Serum creatinine, BUN, total bilirubin, alkaline phosphatase, serum potassium. Possibly ↑ cholesterol, LDL, and apolipoprotein B.

## Dosage
- **Capsules, Oral Solution**
  *Immunosuppressant.*
**Adults and children, initial:** 15 mg/kg/day given 4–12 hr before transplantation; there is a trend to use lower initial doses of 10–14 mg/kg/day. The dose should be continued postoperatively for 1–2 weeks followed by 5% decrease in dose per week to maintenance dose of 5–10 mg/kg/day (some have used a dose of 3 mg/kg/day successfully). Compared with Sandimmune, lower maintenance doses of Neoral may be sufficient. In converting from Sandimmune to Neoral, start Neoral with the same daily Sandimmune dose (i.e., 1:1 dose conversion); then, adjust Neoral dosage to attain the preconversion cyclosporine blood trough concentration.
- **IV (only in clients unable to take PO medication)**
  *Immunosuppressant.*
**Adults:** 5–6 mg/kg/day 4–12 hr prior to transplantation and postoperatively until client can be switched to PO dosage. *NOTE:* Steroid therapy must be used concomitantly.

  *Investigational uses.*
Oral doses ranging from 1 to 10 mg/kg/day.

## NURSING CONSIDERATIONS
### Administration/Storage
1. Sandimmune and Neoral are not bioequivalent and should not be used interchangeably without the supervision of someone experienced in immunosuppressive therapy.
2. May dilute the PO solution with milk, chocolate milk, orange or apple juice immediately before administering. Do not store PO solutions in the refrigerator; contents should be used within 2 months after being opened. At colder temperatures, Neoral may gel or a light flocculation or formation of a light sediment might occur. This

does not affect the product or dosing schedule. Warming to room temperature will reverse these effects.

3. Due to variable absorption of the PO solution, monitor blood levels.

4. Clients with malabsorption from the GI tract may not achieve appropriate blood levels.

**IV** 5. Dilute the IV concentrate 1 mL (50 mg) in 20–100 mL 0.9% NaCl injection or 5% dextrose injection; give IV infusion slowly over 2–6 hr.

6. Protect IV solution from light.

7. The polyoxyethylated castor oil found in the concentrate for IV infusion may cause phthalate stripping from PVC.

8. Due to possibility of anaphylaxis, monitor clients receiving IV cyclosporine closely for 30 min at the start of therapy. Have epinephrine (1:1,000) readily available for treating anaphylaxis.

**Assessment**

1. Document indications for therapy; note any previous treatment with immunosuppressants. List drugs currently taking and note any potential interactions. Anticipate concomitant administration of adrenal corticosteroids.

2. Monitor VS, CBC, cyclosporine levels, liver and renal function studies. Drug may increase BP, serum potassium, lipid, and uric acid levels.

3. Differentiate nephrotoxicity from rejection using criteria provided by the manufacturer.

**Client/Family Teaching**

1. Review importance of following the written guidelines for medication therapy explicitly. Drug must be taken throughout one's lifetime to prevent transplant rejection.

2. Because this drug is so important in preventing rejection, a written list of all possible drug side effects and those which need to be reported will be provided.

3. Taking the drug with food may reduce nausea and GI upset. If PO form unpalatable, mix with milk or juice in a glass container to mini-

mize container adherence. Measure dose accurately and take immediately after mixing.

4. Do not stop abruptly; must be discontinued gradually.

5. Record BP, I&O, and daily weights. Report any persistent diarrhea and N&V.

6. Avoid crowds and persons with infectious illnesses.

7. Practice reliable birth control.

8. Use nystatin swish and swab to prevent development of thrush. Frequent oral care and dental exams should be routine.

9. May develop acne and hirsutism; report as dermatology referral may be needed.

10. Yellow discoloration of eyes, skin, or stools; fever; other signs of hepatotoxicity require immediate reporting.

11. Report increased fatigue, malaise, unexplained bleeding or bruising, or hematuria.

**Outcomes/Evaluate**

• Prevention of transplant rejection; improved organ function

• Cyclosporine trough levels (100–200 ng/mL)

---

# Cyproheptadine hydrochloride

(sye-proh-**HEP**-tah-deen)
**Pregnancy Category:** B
Periactin, PMS–Cyproheptadine ✤
**(Rx)**
**Classification:** Antihistamine, piperidine-type

See also *Antihistamines.*

**Action/Kinetics:** Moderate anticholinergic activity and low sedative effects. **Onset:** 15–30 min. **Duration:** 3–6 hr.

**Uses:** Hypersensitivity reactions: Perennial and seasonal allergic rhinitis, vasomotor rhinitis, allergic conjunctivitis, uncomplicated allergic skin reactions of urticaria and angioedema, allergic reactions to blood or plasma, cold urticaria, adjunct to treat anaphylaxis, dermographism. *Investigational:* Stimulate appetite in anorexia nervosa and for cachexia associated with cancer. Vascular cluster headaches.

**Additional Contraindications:** Glaucoma, urinary retention.

**Special Concerns:** Geriatric clients may be more sensitive to the usual adult dose.

**Additional Side Effects:** Increased appetite.

**Laboratory Test Interferences:** ↑ Serum amylase and prolactin if given with thyroid-releasing hormone.

**Dosage** —————————
- **Syrup, Tablets**
  *Hypersensitivity reactions.*

**Adults, initial:** 4 mg q 8 hr; **then,** 4–20 mg/day, not to exceed 0.5 mg/kg/day. **Pediatric, 2–6 years:** 2 mg q 8–12 hr, not to exceed 12 mg/day; **6–14 years:** 4 mg q 8–12 hr, not to exceed 16 mg/day.

  *Appetite stimulant.*

**Adults:** 4 mg t.i.d. with meals. **Pediatric, 6–14 years, initial:** 2 mg t.i.d.–q.i.d. with meals; **then,** reduce dose to 4 mg t.i.d. **Pediatric, 2–6 years, initial:** 2 mg t.i.d. with meals; **then,** dose may be increased to a total of 8 mg/day.

## NURSING CONSIDERATIONS

See also *Nursing Considerations* for *Antihistamines.*

**Administration/Storage:** Do not give for more than 6 months to adults and 3 months to children for appetite stimulation.

**Outcomes/Evaluate**
- ↓ Allergic manifestations
- Weight gain
- Relief of cluster headaches

---

# Cysteamine bitartrate
(**SIS**-tee-ah-meen)
**Pregnancy Category:** C
Cystagon **(Rx)**
**Classification:** Urinary tract product

**Action/Kinetics:** Lowers cystine levels of cells in cystinosis, which is an inherited defect of lysosomal transport. In those with cystinosis, cystine transport out of lysosomes is abnormal, resulting in the formation of crystals which damage the kidney. Other tissues are damaged as well, including the retina, muscles, and CNS. Acts within the cell to convert cystine into both cysteine and cysteine-cysteamine mixed disulfide, which can leave the lysosome in those with cystinosis.

**Uses:** Management of nephropathic cystinosis in adults and children.

**Contraindications:** Hypersensitivity to cysteamine or penicillamine. Use during lactation.

**Side Effects:** *CNS:* Lethargy, somnolence, depression, encephalopathy, *seizures,* headache, ataxia, confusion, tremor, hyperkinesia, dizziness, jitteriness, nervousness, abnormal thinking, emotional lability, hallucinations, nightmares. *GI:* N&V, anorexia, abdominal pain (may be severe), diarrhea, bad breath, dyspepsia, constipation, gastroenteritis, duodenitis, duodenal ulceration. *Hematologic:* Reversible leukopenia, anemia. *Miscellaneous:* Decreased hearing, fever, rash, dehydration, hypertension, urticaria.

**OD Overdose Management:** *Symptoms:* Extension of side effects, respiratory symptoms. *Treatment:* Support the cardiovascular and respiratory systems. Hemodialysis may be effective in removing the drug from the body.

**Laboratory Test Interferences:** Abnormal LFTs.

**Dosage** —————————
- **Capsules**
  *Nephropathic cystinosis.*

**Initial:** New clients should be started on one-fourth to one-sixth of the maintenance dose. The dose is then raised gradually over 4–6 weeks to avoid intolerance. **Maintenance, children up to age 12 years:** 1.3 g/m²/day (of the free base) given in four divided doses. **Maintenance, children over 12 years and over 110 lb:** 2 g/day in four divided doses.

## NURSING CONSIDERATIONS
### Administration/Storage
1. Initiate therapy in children and adults promptly after the diagnosis has been confirmed by increased white cell cystine levels.
2. Do not give intact cysteamine capsules to children less than 6 years of age due to the possibility of aspiration. Sprinkle contents of the capsule over food.
3. The goal is to keep leukocyte cystine levels less than 1 nmol/½ cystine/mg protein 5–6 hr following administration of cysteamine. Those with intolerance to cysteamine can still get a beneficial effect if cystine levels are less than 2 nmol/½ cystine/mg protein. To achieve this level, the dose of cysteamine may be increased to a maximum of 1.95 g/m²/day.
4. Cystinotic clients taking cysteamine HCl or phosphocysteamine solutions may be transferred to equimolar doses of cysteamine bitartrate capsules. Clients being transferred should have their white cell cystine levels measured in 2 weeks and every 3 months thereafter.

### Assessment: 
Obtain baseline CBC, liver and renal function tests, $C_{Cr}$ and white cell cystine levels; repeat levels 5–6 hr after drug administered.

### Client/Family Teaching
1. Take only as directed. May be given with electrolyte and mineral replacements, vitamin D, and thyroid hormone to manage renal tubular Fanconi syndrome.
2. Report rash; provider will withhold drug until cleared and then reinstitute at a lower dose with gradual increases to therapeutic dose. This may also have to be done if CNS or GI side effects occur.
3. Obtain labs to assess for leukocyte cystine levels, abnormal liver function, or reversible leukopenia.

### Outcomes/Evaluate
• Prevention of organ damage R/T cystine accumulation
• White cell cystine levels of <1 nmol/½ cystine/mg protein

# Cytarabine (ARA-C, Cytosine arabinoside)
(sye-**TAIR**-ah-been)
**Pregnancy Category:** D
Cytosar ✸, Cytosar-U **(Rx)**
**Classification:** Antineoplastic, antimetabolite

C

See also *Antineoplastic Agents.*

**Action/Kinetics:** Acts by inhibiting DNA polymerase as well as by being incorporated into both DNA and RNA. Is cell-phase specific, acting in the S phase and also blocking the progression of cells from the $G_1$ phase to the S phase. May also decrease the immune response. After PO administration, is rapidly broken down by the GI mucosa and liver, resulting in systemic availability of less than 20%. **t½, after IV:** distribution, 10 min; elimination, 1–3 hr. Metabolized in the liver to uracil arabinoside, which is excreted in the urine. Crosses blood-brain barrier. Eighty percent eliminated in urine in 24 hr.

**Uses:** Induction and maintenance of remission in acute myelocytic leukemia in adults and children, acute lymphocytic leukemia, chronic myelocytic leukemia, erythroleukemia, and meningeal leukemia. In combination with other drugs for non-Hodgkin's lymphoma in children. *Investigational:* Hodgkin's lymphomas, myelodysplastic syndrome.

**Contraindications:** Lactation. Use with caution in impaired hepatic function.

**Special Concerns:** Anaphylaxis has occurred, causing acute cardiopulmonary arrest. Use with caution in clients with impaired renal function.

**Additional Side Effects:** "Cytarabine syndrome" (6–12 hr following drug administration) manifested by bone pain, fever, myalgia, maculopapular rash, conjunctivitis, chest pain, or malaise. Nephrotoxicity, neuritis, skin ulceration, sepsis, acute pancreatitis (in clients previ-

---

✸ = Available in Canada                    ***bold italic*** = life threatening side effect

ously treated with l-asparaginase), pneumonia, hyperuricemia. Thrombophlebitis at injection site.

The incidence of side effects (N&V for several hours) is higher in clients receiving rapid IV injection than in those receiving drug by IV infusion. Intrathecal administration may result in systemic side effects including N&V, fever, and rarely neurotoxicity and paraplegia.

**OD** **Overdose Management:** *Symptoms:* CNS toxicity. *Treatment:* General supportive measures.

**Drug Interactions:** Absorption of digoxin may be impaired when cytarabine is used with other antineoplastics.

## Dosage

*NOTE:* Cytarabine is frequently used in combination with other drugs; thus, dosage varies and must be carefully checked.

• **IV Infusion**

*Acute myelocytic leukemia, acute lymphocytic leukemia.*

100–200 mg/m² as a continuous infusion over 24 hr or in divided doses (by rapid injection) for 5–10 days; repeat q 2 weeks.

*Acute nonlymphocytic leukemia (in combination with other drugs).*

100 mg/m²/day by continuous IV infusion (days 1–7) or 100 mg/m² q 12 hr (days 1–7).

*Refractory acute leukemia.*

**IV:** 3 g/m² q 12 hr for 4–12 doses; repeat at 2–3-wk intervals.

• **Intrathecal**

*Meningeal leukemia.*

**Usual:** 30 mg/m² q 4 days with hydrocortisone sodium succinate and methotrexate, each at a dose of 15 mg/m², until CSF findings are normal, followed by one additional dose.

*NOTE:* The drug should be discontinued if platelet level falls to 50,000/mm³ or less or polymorphonuclear granulocyte level falls to 1,000/mm³ or less.

## NURSING CONSIDERATIONS

See also *Nursing Considerations* for *Antineoplastic Agents.*

**Administration/Storage**

1. Cytarabine may be given SC, IV infusion, or IV injection. It is ineffective PO.

2. Do not use benzyl alcohol for reconstitution if the drug is to be used intrathecally; use 0.9% saline or Elliott's B solution.

**IV** 3. Reconstitute the 100-mg vial of cytarabine with 5 mL bacteriostatic water for injection with benzyl alcohol (0.9%) to yield a solution containing 20 mg/mL. Reconstitute the 500-mg vial with 10 mL of bacteriostatic water for injection with benzyl alcohol (0.9%) to yield a solution containing 50 mg/mL cytarabine.

4. To administer direct IV, reconstitute the 100-mg vial and administer over 1–3 min. May be further diluted into 100 mL of D5W or NSS and infused over 30 min.

5. Store reconstituted solution at room temperature and use within 48 hr. Discard if hazy.

6. Have appropriate resuscitative drugs and equipment readily available in the event of anaphylaxis.

**Assessment**

1. Determine baseline CBC, uric acid, platelets, and liver and renal function. Note any history of impaired hepatic function.

2. Document any previous therapy for leukemia and the results. Observe closely for the development of "cytarabine syndrome" 6–12 hr following administration *(see Additional Side Effects).*

3. Systemic toxicity may result from intrathecal use of cytarabine.

4. Obtain hematologic parameters to interrupt therapy; drug causes severe granulocyte and platelet toxicity. Nadir: 10 days; recovery: 21 days.

**Client/Family Teaching**

1. Report any unusual bruising, bleeding, fever, or S&S of anemia ( fatigue, SOB, dizziness).

2. Consume 2–3 L/day of fluids to prevent renal damage from hyperuricemia related to cell lysis. Alkalinization of the urine may enhance uric acid excretion.

3. Report any inflammation of the

eye, which may require treatment with steroid eye drops.

4. Avoid vaccinations during therapy.

5. Use birth control during and for at least 4 months following therapy.

**Outcomes/Evaluate**

• ↓ Tumor size and spread

• Improved hematologic parameters; evidence of disease remission

# Cytomegalovirus Immune Globulin Intravenous, Human (CMV-IGIV)

(**sigh**-toh-**meg**-ah-loh-**VIGH**-rus im-**MYOUN GLOB**-you-lin)

**Pregnancy Category:** C

CytoGam **(Rx)**

**Classification:** Attenuation of CMV in kidney transplant clients

**Action/Kinetics:** This purified product is obtained from pooled adult human plasma that has been selected for high titers of antibody for CMV. When reconstituted, each milliliter contains 50 mg of immunoglobulin that is primarily IgG with trace amounts of IgA and IgM; albumin is also present. In individuals exposed to CMV, the immune globulin can increase the relevant antibodies to levels that prevent or reduce the incidence of serious CMV disease.

**Uses:** Attenuation of primary CMV disease for kidney transplant recipients who are seronegative for CMV and who receive a kidney from a CMV seropositive donor. (*NOTE:* There is a 50% decrease in primary CMV disease in renal transplant clients given this product.)

**Contraindications:** Use in clients with a history of a prior severe reaction to this product or other human immunoglobulin preparations.

**Special Concerns:** Individuals with selective immunoglobulin (Ig) A deficiency may develop antibodies to IgA and could develop anaphylactic reactions to subsequent administration of blood products that contain IgA.

**Side Effects:** Usually minor and often due to the rate of infusion; the infusion schedule should be adhered to closely. *GI:* N&V. *Body as a whole:* Flushing, chills, fever. *Musculoskeletal:* Muscle cramps, back pain. *Respiratory:* Wheezing. Hypotension and allergic reactions such as ***angioneurotic edema*** and ***anaphylactic shock*** are possible but have not been observed.

**OD** **Overdose Management:** *Symptoms:* Major effects would be those related to volume overload. Also possible are anaphylaxis and a drop in BP. *Treatment:* Discontinue the infusion immediately and have epinephrine and diphenhydramine available for treatment of acute allergic symptoms.

**Drug Interactions:** The antibodies present in this product may interfere with the immune response to live virus vaccines, including measles, mumps, and rubella. Thus, such vaccinations should be deferred until at least 3 months after administration of CMV immune globulin or revaccination may be required.

**Dosage**

• **IV**

*Prevention of rejection of kidney transplants.*

The maximum total dose/infusion is 150 mg/kg given according to the following schedule:

| | Within: |
|---|---|
| 72 hr of transplant: | 150 mg/kg |
| 2–8 weeks of transplant: | 100 mg/kg |
| 12–16 weeks of transplant: | 50 mg/kg |

The rate of infusion for the initial dose is 15 mg/kg/hr. If no side effects occur after 30 min, the rate may be increased to 30 mg/kg/hr. If no side effects occur after a subsequent 30-min period, the dose may be increased to 60 mg/kg/hr at a volume not to exceed 7.5 mL/hr. **This rate of infusion must not be exceeded.** For subsequent doses, the rate of infusion is 15 mg/kg/hr for 15 min. If no side effects occur, increase the rate to 30 mg/kg/hr for 15 min and then increase to a maximum rate of 60 mg/kg/hr at a volume not to exceed 7.5 mL/hr. **This rate of infusion must not be exceeded.**

## NURSING CONSIDERATIONS
### Administration/Storage

**IV** 1. The reconstituted solution should be colorless and translucent. Do not use solution if turbid.

2. After removing tab portion of the vial cap, the rubber stopper is cleaned with 70% alcohol or equivalent. Reconstitute the lyophilized powder with 50 mL of sterile water for injection using a double-ended transfer needle or large syringe. When using a double-ended transfer needle, insert one end first into the vial of water. The lyophilized powder is supplied in an evacuated vial; thus, the water should transfer by suction. To avoid foaming, do not shake the vial. After the water is transferred into the evacuated vial, the residual vacuum should be released to hasten dissolution. Rotate the container gently to wet all the undissolved powder. Allow 30 min for complete dissolution of the powder.

3. This product does not contain a preservative. After reconstitution, enter the vial only once and begin the infusion within 6 hr and complete within 12 hr of reconstitution.

4. Administer drug through a separate IV line using a constant infusion pump. If this is not possible, the drug may be "piggybacked" into a preexisting line that contains either NaCl injection or one of the following dextrose solutions (with or without NaCl added): 2.5%, 5%, 10%, or 20% dextrose in water. If used with a preexisting line, do not dilute the drug more than 1:2 with any of the solutions. See *Dosage* for administration guidelines.

5. If minor side effects occur, slow or temporarily interrupt the infusion.

### Assessment

1. Determine any previous experience with human immunoglobulin preparations.

2. Document any IgA deficiency as these clients may experience anaphylactic reactions with subsequent exposures to IgA products.

3. Follow infusion dosing schedules carefully and assess closely during each rate change. Monitor VS continuously; if side effects develop, slow infusion rate (or interrupt) and notify provider.

### Client/Family Teaching

1. If client is seronegative for CMV and receives a seropositive donor kidney, CMV disease may develop.

2. Identify side effects that would indicate an acute allergic reaction and warrant immediate medical attention.

3. Do not receive any vaccinations for a least 3 mo following therapy; may require revaccination. Antibodies in suspension may interfere with the immune response to live virus vaccines.

4. In order to prevent transmission of infectious agents/hepatitis virus from one client to another, sterile disposable syringes and needles should be used; do not reuse.

5. Identify support groups that may assist family to cope with chronic disease condition.

**Outcomes/Evaluate:** CMV prophylaxis in renal transplant recipients

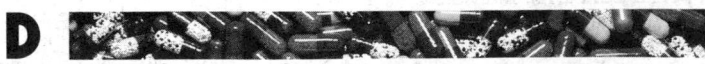

# Dacarbazine
(dah-**KAR**-bah-zeen)
**Pregnancy Category:** C
DTIC ✦, DTIC-Dome, Imidazole Carboxamide (Abbreviation: DTIC)
**(Rx)**

**Classification:** Antineoplastic, alkylating agent

See also *Antineoplastic Agents* and *Alkylating Agents.*

**Action/Kinetics:** Mechanisms of action: alkylation by an activated carbonium ion, antimetabolite to inhibit DNA and RNA synthesis, and alkylation by combining with protein sulfhydryl groups. Is cell-cycle nonspecific. **t½, biphasic, initial,** 19 min; **terminal,** 5 hr. The t½ is increased to 55 min and 7.2 hr in those with renal and hepatic dysfunction. Drug probably localizes in liver. Limited amounts (14% of plasma level) enter CSF. Approximately 40% of drug excreted in urine unchanged within 6 hr. Secreted through the kidney tubules rather than filtered through the glomeruli.

**Uses:** Metastatic malignant melanoma. Hodgkin's disease (with other agents). *Investigational:* In combination with cyclophosphamide and vincristine for malignant pheochromocytoma; in combination with tamoxifen for metastatic malignant melanoma.

**Contraindications:** Lactation.

**Special Concerns:** Dosage not established in children.

**Additional Side Effects:** *Hematologic:* Hemopoietic depression, especially *leukopenia and thrombocytopenia which may cause death.* *GI:* N&V (more than 90% of clients within 1 hr after initial administration, which persists for 12–48 hr), anorexia, diarrhea. *Dermatologic:* Erythematous and urticarial rashes, photosensitivity reactions, alopecia, facial flushing, paresthesia. *Miscellaneous:* Flulike syndrome, including fever, myalgia, and malaise. Hepatotoxicity, hypersensitivity, *anaphylaxis.*

**OD** **Overdose Management:** *Treatment:* Monitor blood cell counts; supportive treatment.

**Laboratory Test Interferences:** ↑ AST, ALT, and other enzymes.

**Dosage** ————————
• **IV Only**
*Malignant melanoma.*
2–4.5 mg/kg/day for 10 days; may be repeated at 4-week intervals; or

250 mg/m²/day for 5 days; may be repeated at 3-week intervals.
*Hodgkin's disease.*
150 mg/m²/day for 5 days; or, 375 mg/m² on day 1, with other drugs and repeated q 15 days.

## NURSING CONSIDERATIONS

See also *Nursing Considerations* for *Antineoplastic Agents.*

**Administration/Storage**
**IV** 1. Avoid extravasation.
2. Reconstitute with sterile water for injection—9.9 mL for the 100-mg vials and 19.7 mL for the 200-mg vials for a final concentration of 10 mg/mL. Drug can be given by IV push over 1-min period. May further dilute with 5% dextrose injection or NaCl injection and given (preferred) over 15–30 min.
3. Protect dry vials from light and store at 2°C–8°C (36°F–46°F).
4. Reconstituted solutions are stable for up to 72 hr at 4°C (39°F) or for 8 hr at 20°C (68°F). More dilute solutions for IV infusions are stable for 24 hr when stored at 2°C–8°C (36°F–46°F).

**Assessment**
1. Ascertain how fluid status is to be handled (fast for 4–6 hr before treatment to reduce emesis or have fluids up to 1 hr before administration to minimize dehydration following treatment).
2. Administer antiemetic before and throughout therapy. Have phenobarbital and/or prochlorperazine available for palliation of vomiting following treatment.
3. Monitor client and labs closely for evidence of bone marrow depression, liver or renal toxicity, or hypersensitivity reaction. Anticipitate mild granulocyte toxicity. Nadir: 10 days; recovery: 21 days.

**Client/Family Teaching**
1. To minimize adverse GI effects, antiemetics, fasting, and limited fluid intake (4–6 hr preceding treatment) have been suggested. After the first

1–2 days of therapy, vomiting should cease as tolerance develops.

2. Report any flu-like symptoms (fever, aches, fatigue) that may occur. Usually occurs 1 week after treatment and may persist for 1–3 weeks. Acetaminophen may assist to relieve symptoms.

3. Avoid prolonged exposure to sun or ultraviolet light and wear protective clothing as photosensitivity reaction may occur.

4. Prepare for hair loss.

5. Practice contraception during and for several months following therapy.

**Outcomes/Evaluate:** ↓ Tumor size/spread with suppression of malignant cell proliferation

# Dactinomycin
(dack-tin-oh-**MY**-sin)
**Pregnancy Category:** C
Actinomycin D, Cosmegen **(Rx)**
**Classification:** Antineoplastic, antibiotic

See also *Antineoplastic Agents.*

**Action/Kinetics:** Chromopeptide antibiotic produced by *Streptomyces parvullus.* Acts by intercalating into the purine-pyrimidine base pair, thereby inhibiting synthesis of messenger RNA. Is cell-cycle nonspecific, although the maximum number of cells are destroyed in the $G_1$ phase. Cleared from the blood within 2 min and concentrated in nucleated cells. **t½:** 36 hr. Does not cross the blood-brain barrier and is excreted mainly unchanged.

During therapy, leukocyte counts should be performed daily, and platelet counts q 3 days. Frequent liver and kidney function tests are recommended. Appearance of toxic manifestations may be delayed by several weeks. Irreversible bone marrow depression may occur in clients with preexisting renal, hepatic, or bone marrow impairment. The drug is corrosive to soft tissue.

**Uses:** In combination with vincristine, surgery, and/or irradiation for treatment of Wilms' tumor (nephroblastoma) and its metastases. In combination with methotrexate to treat metastatic and nonmetastatic choriocarcinoma. In combination with cyclophosphamide, doxorubicin, and vincristine to treat rhabdomyosarcoma. Nonseminomatous testicular carcinoma. With cyclophosphamide and radiotherapy to treat Ewing's sarcoma. In combination with radiotherapy to treat sarcoma botryoides. Endometrial carcinoma. *Investigational:* Ovarian cancer, Kaposi's sarcoma, osteosarcoma, malignant melanoma.

**Contraindications:** Concurrent infection with chickenpox or herpes zoster (death may result). Lactation. Infants less than 6–12 months of age.

**Special Concerns:** When used with X-ray therapy, erythema is seen in normal skin and the buccal and pharyngeal mucosa.

**Additional Side Effects:** *Anaphylaxis.* Due to corrosiveness, extravasation causes severe damage to soft tissues. Hypocalcemia. When combined with radiation, increased severity of skin reactions, GI toxicity, and *bone marrow depression.*

**Laboratory Test Interferences:** Interferes with bioassay tests used to determine antibacterial drug levels.

**Dosage**
• **IV**
   *Carcinomas.*

**Adults, usual:** 0.5 mg/m²/week for 3 weeks; or, 0.01–0.015 mg/kg/day for a maximum of 5 days q 4–6 weeks. Dose is individualized. **Pediatric:** 10–15 mcg/kg (0.45 mg/m²) daily for 5 days; **alternatively,** a total dose of 2.4 mg/m² over 1 week. Total daily dosage for both adults and children should not exceed 15 mcg/kg over a 5-day period. Course of treatment may be repeated after 3 weeks unless contraindicated due to toxicity. If no toxicity, second course can be given after 3 weeks.

• **Isolation Perfusion**
   *Ewing's sarcoma/sarcoma botryoides.*

0.05 mg/kg for pelvis and lower extremities and 0.035 mg/kg for upper extremities.

## NURSING CONSIDERATIONS

See also *Nursing Considerations* for *Antineoplastic Agents*.

**Administration/Storage**

**IV** 1. For IV use, available in a lyophilized dactinomycin-mannitol mixture that turns a gold color upon reconstitution with sterile water. Use only sterile water without a preservative to reconstitute drug for IV use, as it will precipitate. Do not expose solutions to direct sunlight.

2. Exercise extreme care in reconstituting and administering dactinomycin so that the dust or vapors are not inhaled or come in contact with skin or mucous membranes. Take special care to prevent contact with the eyes. Prepare under a laminar flow hood.

3. *The drug is extremely corrosive*. It is most safely administered through the tubing of a running IV (e.g., 5% dextrose or NaCl). May be given directly into the vein, but the needle used to draw up the solution should be discarded and another sterile needle attached, before injection, to prevent SC reaction and thrombophlebitis.

4. Discard any portion of the solution not used.

5. For direct IV administration, reconstitute 0.5-mg vial with 1.1 mL of sterile water for injection and infuse at a rate of 500 mcg/min. May be further diluted in 50 mL of D5%/W or NSS and infused over 10–15 min.

**Assessment**

1. Determine if pregnant, lactating, or infected with herpes, all of which contraindicate therapy.

2. Interferes with bioassay test used to measure antibacterial drug levels; monitor response to antibiotic therapy carefully. Dactinomycin inhibits the action of penicillin; do not use for infection.

3. Monitor CBC, uric acid, liver and renal function studies. Drug may cause severe granulocyte and platelet toxicity. Nadir: 10 days; recovery 21–28 days.

**Client/Family Teaching**

1. Report erythema of the skin, which can lead to desquamation and sloughing, particularly in areas previously affected by radiation. Erythema may be noted in normal skin and buccal and pharyngeal mucosa; use topical viscous xylocaine as needed.

2. Consume 2–3 L/day of fluids to prevent dehydration and urate crystal formation; may need allopurinol therapy if inadequate fluid intake.

3. May be administered intermittently if N&V persist even when an antiemetic is given.

4. Report any unusual bruising, bleeding, fever, stomatitis, or persistent diarrhea; dose may require adjustment.

5. Avoid vaccinations.

6. Practice contraception during and for 4 weeks following therapy.

7. May experience hair loss 7–10 days after therapy.

**Outcomes/Evaluate:** ↓ Tumor size/spread and suppression of malignant cell proliferation

# Dalteparin sodium injection

(**DAL**-tih-**pair**-in)
**Pregnancy Category:** B
Fragmin **(Rx)**
**Classification:** Anticoagulant

**Action/Kinetics:** Dalteparin, a low molecular weight heparin, is prepared through depolymerization of sodium heparin from porcine intestinal mucosa. Acts by increasing the inhibition of factor Xa and thrombin by antithrombin. Causes a significant change in platelet aggregation, fibrinolysis, or global clotting tests (e.g., PT, APTT, or thrombin time). **Peak plasma levels:** 4 hr. **t½, SC:** 3–5 hr. The t½ is increased in those with chronic renal insufficiency requiring hemodialysis.

**D**

**Uses:** To prevent deep vein thrombosis (DVT) in clients undergoing abdominal surgery who are at risk for thromboembolic complications (i.e., pulmonary embolism). High risk includes obesity, general anesthesia more than 30 min, malignancy, history of DVT or pulmonary embolism, age 40 and over. *Investigational:* Systemic anticoagulation in venous and arterial thromboembolic complications.

**Contraindications:** Active major bleeding or thrombocytopenia. Known hypersensitivity to heparin or pork products. IM use.

**Special Concerns:** Cannot be used interchangeably with unfractionated heparin or other low molecular weight heparins. Use with extreme caution in those with a history of heparin-induced thrombocytopenia. Use with caution in clients with an increased risk of hemorrhage, including those with severe uncontrolled hypertension, bacterial endocarditis, congenital or acquired bleeding disorders, active ulceration and angiodysplastic GI disease, or hemorrhagic stroke or shortly after brain, spinal, or ophthalmologic surgery. Also, use with caution in clients with bleeding diathesis, severe liver or kidney disease, hypertensive or diabetic retinopathy, and recent GI bleeding. Use with caution during lactation. Safety and efficacy have not been determined in children.

**Side Effects:** *CV: Hemorrhage,* hematoma at injection site, wound hematoma, reoperation due to bleeding, postoperational transfusions. *Hematologic:* Thrombocytopenia. *Hypersensitivity:* Allergic reactions, including pruritus, rash, fever, injection site reaction, bulleous eruption, skin necrosis (rare), *anaphylaxis. Miscellaneous:* Pain at injection site.

**OD Overdose Management:** *Symptoms:* Hemorrhagic complications. *Treatment:* Slow IV protamine sulfate (1%) at a dose of 1 mg protamine sulfate for every 100 anti-Xa IU of fragmin given. A second infusion protamine sulfate, 0.5 mg for every 100 anti-Xa IU of fragmin, may be given if the APTT measured 2–4 hr after the first infusion of protamine sulfate remains prolonged. Care should be taken not to give an overdose of protamine sulfate.

**Drug Interactions:** Increased anticoagulant effect, and therefore increased risk of bleeding or hemorrhage, when used with oral anticoagulants or other platelet inhibitors.

**Laboratory Test Interferences:** ↑ Serum transaminases (AST, ALT).

**Dosage** ————————
• **SC Only**
*Prevention of DVT in abdominal surgery.*
**Adults:** 2,500 IU each day starting 1–2 hr prior to surgery and repeated once daily for 5–10 days postoperatively. High-risk clients: 5,000 IU the night before surgery and repeated once daily for 5–10 days. In malignancy: 2,500 IU 1–2 hr before surgery followed by 2,500 IU 12 hr later and 5,000 IU once daily for 5–10 days.
*Systemic anticoagulation.*
200 IU/kg SC daily or 100 IU/day b.i.d.

## NURSING CONSIDERATIONS

See also *Nursing Considerations* for *Anticoagulants.*

**Administration/Storage**
1. Available in single-dose prefilled syringes affixed with a 27-gauge × ½-inch needle.
2. Before withdrawing the drug, inspect the vial visually for particulate matter or discoloration.
3. Do not mix with other infusions or injections unless compatibility data are known.
4. Store the drug at controlled room temperature of 20°C–25°C (68°F–77°F).

**Assessment**
1. Determine any sensitivity to heparin or pork products.
2. Note any evidence of active major bleeding, any bleeding disorders, or thrombocytopenia.
3. List criteria for inclusion (i.e., over 40, obese, prolonged general anesthesia, additional risk factors).

**Client/Family Teaching**
1. Review indications for therapy, self-administration technique, and how to rotate sites.
2. Give by deep SC injection while sitting or lying down. May give in a U-shape area around the navel, the upper outer side of the thigh, or the upper outer quadrangle of the buttock. Change injection site daily.
3. If the area around the navel or thigh is used, a fold of skin must be lifted, using the thumb and forefinger, while giving the injection.
4. Insert the entire length of the needle at a 45–90-degree angle.
5. Therapy may last for 5–10 days after surgery.
6. Periodic CBC with platelets, PTT, PT, and stool for occult blood will be performed.
**Outcomes/Evaluate:** DVT prophylaxis

# Danaparoid sodium
(dah-**NAP**-ah-royd)
**Pregnancy Category:** B
Orgaran **(Rx)**
**Classification:** Anticoagulant, glycosaminoglycan

See also *Anticoagulants*.
**Action/Kinetics:** A low molecular weight sulfated glycosaminoglycans obtained from porcine mucosa. Prevents fibrin formation in the coagulation pathway via thrombin generation inhibition by anti-Xa and anti-IIa effects. Minimal effect on clotting assays, fibrinolytic activity, or bleeding time. 100% bioavailable with SC use. **t½:** About 24 hr. Excreted primarily through the kidneys.
**Uses:** Prophylaxis of postoperative deep vein thrombosis (DVT) in clients undergoing elective hip replacement surgery. *Investigational:* Thromboembolism, anticoagulation during hemodialysis, hemofiltration during CV operation, and increased risk of thrombosis during pregnancy.
**Contraindications:** Use in hemophilia, idiopathic thrombocytopenic purpura, active major bleeding state

(including hemorrhagic stroke in the acute phase), and type II thrombocytopenia associated with a positive in vitro test for antiplatelet antibody in the presence of danaparoid. Hypersensitivity to pork products. IM use.
**Special Concerns:** Cannot be dosed interchangeably (unit for unit) with either heparin or low molecular weight heparins. Use with extreme caution in disease states where there is an increased risk of hemorrhage, including severe uncontrolled hypertension, acute bacterial endocarditis, congenital or acquired bleeding disorders, active ulcerative and angiodysplastic GI disease, nonhemorrhagic stroke, postoperative indwelling epidural catheter use, and shortly after brain, spinal, or ophthalmologic surgery. Use with caution during lactation and in those with severely impaired renal function. Use with caution in clients receiving oral anticoagulants or platelet inhibitors. Safety and efficacy have not been determined in children.
**Side Effects:** *CV:* Intraoperative blood loss, postoperative blood loss. *GI:* N&V, constipation. *CNS:* Insomnia, headache, dizziness. *Dermatologic:* Rash, pruritus. *GU:* UTI, urinary retention. *Miscellaneous:* Fever, pain at injection site, peripheral edema, joint disorder, edema, asthenia, anemia, pain, infection.
**OD Overdose Management:** *Symptoms:* Bleeding disorders, including hemorrhage. *Treatment:* Protamine sulfate partially neutralizes the anti-Xa activity of the drug; however, there is no evidence that protamine sulfate will reduce severe nonsurgical bleeding. For serious bleeding, discontinue danaparoid and give blood or blood product transfusions as needed.

**Dosage**
• **SC only**
*Prophylaxis of DVT in hip replacement surgery.*
**Adults:** 750 anti-Xa units b.i.d. SC, beginning 1 to 4 hr preoperatively

and then not sooner than 2 hr post-operatively. Continue treatment throughout the postoperative period until the risk of deep vein thrombosis has decreased. Average duration of treatment is 7 to 10 days, up to 14 days.

## NURSING CONSIDERATIONS

See also *Nursing Considerations* for *Anticoagulants.*

**Administration/Storage:** Protect from light and store at 2°C–30°C (36°F–86°F).

**Assessment**
1. Note any pork or sulfite sensitivity.
2. Assess for any medical conditions that may preclude drug use (i.e., active hemorrhagic disease, bleeding dyscrasias, ITTP, etc.).
3. Monitor VS, I&O, CBC, PT, PTT, INR, and renal function studies; note any urinary retention or altered VS.

**Client/Family Teaching**
1. Drug is used to prevent the formation of blood clots, especially in the legs. Usually given once before surgery and then every 12 hr thereafter for 7 to 10 days.
2. To administer, lie down and grasp a fold of skin on the abdomen between the thumb and forefinger. Insert the entire length of the needle straight in; use a 25- to 26-gauge needle to minimize tissue trauma. Hold the skin fold throughout the injection; do not rub or massage area after administration; rotate sites with each injection.
3. Alternate administration between the left and right anterolateral and left and right posterolateral abdominal walls.
4. Report any unusual bruising or bleeding, acute onset of SOB, itching, rash, chest pain, and leg edema immediately.

**Outcomes/Evaluate:** DVT prophylaxis

---

# Danazol
(**DAN**-ah-zohl)
Cyclomen ✱, Danocrine **(Rx)**
**Classification:** Synthetic androgen (gonadotropin inhibitor)

**Action/Kinetics:** Inhibits the release of gonadotropins (FSH and LH) by the anterior pituitary; thus, inhibits synthesis of sex steroids and competitively inhibits binding of steroids to their cytoplasmic receptors in target tissues. In women this action arrests ovarian function, induces amenorrhea, and causes atrophy of normal and ectopic endometrial tissue. Has weak androgenic effects. **Onset, fibrocystic disease:** 4 weeks. **Time to peak effect, amenorrhea and anovulation:** 6–8 weeks; **fibrocystic disease:** 2–3 months to eliminate breast pain and tenderness and 4–6 months for elimination of nodules. **t½:** 4.5 hr. **Duration:** Ovulation and cyclic bleeding usually resume 60–90 days after cessation of therapy.

**Uses:** Endometriosis amenable to hormonal management in clients who cannot tolerate or who have not responded to other drug therapy. Fibrocystic breast disease. Hereditary angioedema in males and females. *Investigational:* Gynecomastia, menorrhagia, precocious puberty, idiopathic immune thrombocytopenia, lupus-associated thrombocytopenia, and autoimmune hemolytic anemia.

**Contraindications:** Undiagnosed genital bleeding; markedly impaired hepatic, renal, and cardiac function; pregnancy and lactation.

**Special Concerns:** Use with caution in children treated for hereditary angioedema due to the possibility of virilization in females and precocious sexual development in males. Geriatric clients may have an increased risk of prostatic hypertrophy or prostatic carcinoma. Use with caution in conditions aggravated by fluid retention (e.g., epilepsy, migraine, cardiac, or renal dysfunction).

**Side Effects:** *Androgenic:* Acne, decrease in breast size, oily hair and skin, weight gain, deepening of voice and hair growth, clitoral hypertrophy, testicular atrophy. *Estrogen deficiency:* Flushing, sweating, vaginitis, nervousness, changes in emotions. *GI:* N&V, constipation, gastroenteritis. *Hepatic:* Jaundice, dysfunction. *CNS:* Fatigue, tremor, headache, dizziness, sleep problems, paresthesia of extremities, anxiety, depression, appetite changes. *Musculoskeletal:* Muscle cramps or spasms, joint swelling or lock-up, pain in back, legs, or neck. *Miscellaneous:* Allergic reactions (skin rashes and rarely nasal congestion), hematuria, increased BP, chills, pelvic pain, carpal tunnel syndrome, hair loss, change in libido.

**Drug Interactions**
*Insulin* / Danazol ↑ insulin requirements
*Warfarin* / Danazol ↑ PT in warfarin-stabilized clients

**Dosage** —————————
• **Capsules**
*Endometriosis.*
400 mg b.i.d. (moderate to severe) or 100–200 mg b.i.d. (mild) for 3–6 months (up to 9 months may be required in some clients). Begin therapy during menses, if possible, to be sure that client is not pregnant.
*Fibrocystic breast disease.*
50–200 mg b.i.d. beginning on day 2 of menses. Begin therapy during menses to assure client is not pregnant.
*Hereditary angioedema.*
**Initial:** 200 mg b.i.d.–t.i.d.; after desired response, decrease dosage by 50% (or less) at 1–3-month intervals. Treat subsequent attacks by giving up to 200 mg/day. No more than 800 mg/day should be given to adults.

## NURSING CONSIDERATIONS

**Administration/Storage:** Breast pain and tenderness in fibrocystic disease are usually relieved within 30 days and eliminated in 2–3 months; elimination of nodularity requires 4–6 months of uninterrupted therapy. Treatment may be reinstituted if symptoms recur (50% of clients have recurring symptoms within 6 months).

**Assessment**
1. Note reports of endometrial pain, breast pain, tenderness, and the presence of any nodules.
2. Determine any undiagnosed vaginal bleeding; note onset, frequency, extent, and precipitating factors.
3. Obtain baseline CBC, renal and liver function studies; determine if pregnant.
4. Identify factors that trigger angioedema (usually C-1 inhibitor deficiency).

**Client/Family Teaching**
1. Take with meals to decrease GI upset.
2. Virilization may occur with drug therapy (e.g., abnormal hair growth, acne, reduced breast size, increased skin oiliness, enlarged clitoris, voice deepening); report so dosage can be adjusted. Hypoestrogenic side effects usually disappear once discontinued; ovulation will resume in 60–90 days.
3. Wear cotton underwear and pay careful attention to hygiene to diminish danazol-induced vaginitis.
4. Practice birth control; continue breast self-exams and report changes
5. Clients with a history of epilepsy, migraines, and cardiac or renal dysfunction may develop fluid retention; report as drug may need to be stopped.
6. Several months of therapy may be required before any improvements noted.

**Outcomes/Evaluate**
• ↓ Endometrial pain (3–6 mo)
• ↓ Breast pain ( 2–3 mo)

# Dantrolene sodium
(**DAN**-troh-leen)
**Pregnancy Category:** C (parenteral use)
Dantrium, Dantrium IV **(Rx)**
**Classification:** Muscle relaxant, centrally acting

See also *Skeletal Muscle Relaxants, Centrally Acting.*
**Action/Kinetics:** Not related to other skeletal muscle relaxants. Acts

---

directly on skeletal muscle, probably by dissociating the excitation-contraction coupling mechanism as a result of interference of release of calcium from the sarcoplasmic reticulum. This results in a decreased force of reflex muscle contraction and a reduction of hyperreflexia, spasticity, involuntary movements, and clonus. Effectiveness in malignant hyperthermia is due to an inhibition of release of calcium from the sarcoplasmic reticulum. This results in prevention or reduction of the increased myoplasmic calcium ion concentration that activates the acute catabolic processes associated with malignant hyperthermia. Absorption is slow and incomplete, but consistent. **Peak plasma levels:** 4–6 hr. **t½: PO,** 9 hr after a dose of 100 mg; **t½: IV,** 4–8 hr. Significant plasma protein binding.

**Uses: PO:** Muscle spasticity associated with severe chronic disorders, such as multiple sclerosis, cerebral palsy, spinal cord injury, and stroke. Preoperatively to prevent or reduce the development of signs of malignant hyperthermia. To prevent recurrence following a malignant hyperthermia crisis. **IV:** Malignant hyperthermia due to hypermetabolism of skeletal muscle. Preoperatively or postoperatively to prevent or reduce the development of signs of malignant hyperthermia in susceptible clients. *Investigational:* Exercise-induced muscle pain, heat stroke, and neuroleptic malignant syndrome.

**Contraindications:** Orally in active hepatitis or cirrhosis, where spasticity is used to sustain upright posture and balance in locomotion or to obtain or maintain increased function, and to treat skeletal muscle spasm due to rheumatic disease. Pregnancy, lactation, or children under 5 years of age.

**Special Concerns:** Use with caution in clients with impaired pulmonary function, especially those with obstructive pulmonary disease; severely impaired cardiac function due to myocardial disease; and a history of previous liver disease or dysfunction.

**Side Effects: Following PO use:** Side effects are dose-related and decrease with usage. *Fatal* and nonfatal **hepatotoxicity.** *CNS:* Drowsiness, dizziness, weakness, malaise, lightheadedness, headaches, insomnia, seizures, speech disturbances, fatigue, confusion, depression, nervousness. *GI:* Diarrhea (common), anorexia, constipation, GI bleeding, dysphagia, gastric irritation, abdominal cramps. *Musculoskeletal:* Backache, myalgia. *Dermatologic:* Rash (acne-like), photosensitivity, pruritus, urticaria, hair growth, sweating, eczematoid eruption. *CV:* BP changes, phlebitis, tachycardia. *GU:* Urinary retention, increased urinary frequency, urinary incontinence, hematuria, crystalluria, nocturia, impotence. *Ophthalmic:* Visual disturbances, diplopia. *Miscellaneous:* Chills, fever, tearing, feeling of suffocation, alteration of taste, **pleural effusion with pericarditis.**

**Following IV use:** Pulmonary edema, **thrombophlebitis,** urticaria, erythema.

**OD** **Overdose Management:** *Symptoms:* Extension of side effects. *Treatment:* Immediate gastric lavage. Maintain airway and have artificial resuscitation equipment available. Large quantities of IV fluids to prevent crystalluria. Monitor ECG.

**Drug Interactions:** ↓ Plasma protein binding of dantrolene when used with either clofibrate or warfarin

**Dosage** ————————
• **Capsules**
*Spastic conditions.*
**Adults, initial:** 25 mg once daily; **then,** increase to 25 mg b.i.d.–q.i.d.; dose may then be increased by 25-mg increments up to 100 mg b.i.d.–q.i.d. (doses in excess of 400 mg/day not recommended). **Pediatric: initial,** 0.5 mg/kg b.i.d.; **then,** increase to 0.5 mg/kg t.i.d.–q.i.d.; dose may then be increased by increments of 0.5 mg/kg to 3 mg/kg b.i.d.–q.i.d. (doses should not exceed 400 mg/day).

*Malignant hyperthermia, preoperatively.*
**Adults and children:** 4–8 mg/kg/day in three to four divided doses 1–2 days before surgery with the last dose given 3 to 4 hr before surgery.
*Postmalignant hyperthermic crisis.*
**Adults and children:** 4–8 mg/kg/day in four divided doses for 1–3 days.

• **IV Infusion**
*Malignant hyperthermia, crisis treatment.*
**Adults and children, initial:** 2.5 mg/kg 60 min prior to surgery and infused over 1 hr. Additional IV dantrolene may be given during anesthesia and surgery, depending on symptoms.

• **IV Push**
*Malignant hyperthermia, crisis treatment.*
**Initial:** At least 1 mg/kg; continue administration until symptoms decrease or a cumulative dose of 10 mg/kg has been administered.

## NURSING CONSIDERATIONS

See also *Nursing Considerations* for *Skeletal Muscle Relaxants, Centrally Acting.*
**Administration/Storage**
1. When administered PO, the drug can be mixed with fruit juice or other liquids.
2. With spasticity, beneficial effects may take up to a week; discontinue after 6 weeks if none are evident.
3. Due to potential hepatotoxicity, long-term benefits must be evaluated for each client.
**IV** 4. For IV use, reconstitute powder by adding 60 mL of sterile water for injection to each 20-mg vial.
5. Protect reconstituted solutions from light and use within 6 hr. Store reconstituted solutions at controlled room temperatures of 15°C–30°C (59°F–86°F).
**Assessment**
1. Note mental status and general appearance.

2. Monitor CBC, liver and renal function studies; hepatic dysfunction more likely in women over 35 years of age.
3. Assess lung and heart sounds regularly during therapy; note any changes. Note any evidence of impaired pulmonary function, cardiac disorders, active hepatitis or cirrhosis, or history of any benign or malignant breast tumors; dantrolene may increase incidence of mammary tumors.
4. Note extent of client's muscle spasticity, involuntary movements, and clonus. Determine if spasticity is necessary to sustain an upright posture or for mobility as drug should be avoided.
5. Obtain and monitor VS, I&O, electrolytes, and ECG during acute therapy.
**Client/Family Teaching**
1. Do not operate dangerous machinery or drive a car; drug causes drowsiness.
2. If double vision occurs, reassure that this and many of the other bothersome side effects associated with drug therapy may lessen with continued use.
3. Report any increased muscle weakness or impaired physical ability. Several weeks of therapy may be required before improvements in condition will be noted; report any insomnia or depression.
4. Report any marked changes in BP and any evidence of diarrhea or blood in the urine or stool. Also, if slurred speech, drooling, inability to perform usual physical functions, or enuresis develops, drug may require withdrawal.
5. Avoid alcohol and any other CNS depressants.
6. Use protection to prevent photosensitivity reactions.
7. Females should have mammograms and perform BSE to detect any lumps; drug has the potential to cause these. Most important in women with a family history of malignant or benign breast tumors.

8. Males may develop impotence; report if evident.

9. With malignant hyperthermia, carry appropriate identification and notify all providers.

**Outcomes/Evaluate**
- ↓ Muscle spasticity and/or pain
- ↓ exercise-induced muscle pain
- ↓ Temperature (R/T hypermetabolism of skeletal muscle)

---

# Dapiprazole hydrochloride
(dah-**PIP**-rah-zol)
**Pregnancy Category:** B
Rev-Eyes **(Rx)**
**Classification:** Ophthalmic alpha-adrenergic blocking agent

**Action/Kinetics:** Produces miosis by blocking the alpha-adrenergic receptors on the dilator muscle of the iris. No significant action on ciliary muscle contraction; thus, there are no changes in the depth of the anterior chamber of the thickness of the lens. Does not alter the intraocular pressure either in normal eyes or in eyes with elevated IOP. The rate of pupillary constriction may be slightly slower in clients with brown irides than in clients with blue or green irides.

**Uses:** To reverse diagnostic mydriasis induced by adrenergic (e.g., phenylephrine) or parasympatholytic (e.g., tropicamide) agents.

**Contraindications:** Acute iritis or other conditions where miosis is not desirable. To reduce intraocular pressure or to treat open-angle glaucoma.

**Special Concerns:** Use with caution during lactation. Safety and effectiveness have not been determined in children. The drug may cause difficulty in adaptation to dark and may reduce the field of vision.

**Side Effects:** *Ophthalmic:* Conjunctival injection lasting 20 min, burning on instillation, ptosis, lid erythema, itching, lid edema, chemosis, corneal edema, punctate keratitis, photophobia, tearing and blurring of vi-

sion, dryness of eyes. *Miscellaneous:* Headaches, browache.

**Dosage**
- **Ophthalmic Solution**
  *Reverse mydriasis.*
2 gtt followed in 5 min by 2 more gtt applied to the conjunctiva of the eye after ophthalmic examination.

## NURSING CONSIDERATIONS
**Administration/Storage**

1. Do not use more frequently than once a week.

2. To prepare the solution, remove and discard aluminum seals and rubber plugs from the drug and diluent vials. Pour the diluent into the drug vial; remove the dropper assembly from its sterile wrapping and attach to the drug vial. Shake container for several minutes to ensure adequate mixing.

3. Store reconstituted eye drops at room temperature for 21 days. Discard any solution that is not clear and colorless.

**Assessment**

1. Determine any hypersensitivity to alpha-adrenergic blocking agents.

2. Note eye color. Pupillary constriction may be slightly slower in clients with brown irides as opposed to those with blue or green irides.

**Client/Family Teaching:** May cause burning on instillation. Use care; may impair adaptation to dark and reduce field of vision.

**Outcomes/Evaluate:** Reversal of drug-induced mydriasis (constriction of pupils)

---

# Dapsone (DDS, Diphenylsulfone)
(**DAP**-sohn)
**Pregnancy Category:** C
Avlosulfon ✶ **(Rx)**
**Classification:** Sulfone, leprostatic

**Action/Kinetics:** Has both bacteriostatic and bactericidal activity, especially against *Mycobacterium leprae* (Hansen's bacillus). Thought to act similarly to sulfonamides in that it interferes with the metabolism of the infectious organism. Widely distributed throughout the body. **Peak plasma levels:** 4–8 hr. Doses of 200 mg/day for 8 days will lead to a plateau plasma level of 0.1–7 mcg/mL. From 70% to 90% is bound to plasma proteins. **t½:** About 28 hr. Acetylated in the liver and metabolites excreted in the urine. However, excretion is slow and constant blood levels can be maintained with usual dosage.

**Uses:** Lepromatous and tuberculoid types of leprosy, dermatitis herpetiformis. *Investigational:* Relapsing polychondritis, prophylaxis of malaria, inflammatory bowel disease, leishmaniasis, *Pneumocystis carinii* pneumonia, rheumatoid arthritis, lupus erythematosus, bites of the brown recluse spider.

**Contraindications:** Advanced amyloidosis of kidneys. Lactation.

**Side Effects:** *Hematologic:* ***Hemolytic anemia, agranulocytosis,*** methemoglobinemia. *GI:* N&V, anorexia, abdominal discomfort. *CNS:* Headache, insomnia, vertigo, paresthesia, psychoses, peripheral neuropathy. *Dermatologic:* Photosensitivity, lupus-like syndrome. *Hypersensitivity:* Severe skin reactions including exfoliative dermatitis, erythema multiforme, toxic erythema, urticaria, erythema nodosum, toxic erythema, toxic epidermal necrolysis, morbilliform and scarlatiniform reactions. *Sulfone syndrome:* ***Potentially fatal hypersensitivity reaction*** , including symptoms of fever, malaise, jaundice with ***hepatic necrosis,*** exfoliative dermatitis, lymphadenopathy, methemoglobinemia, and ***hemolytic anemia.*** *Renal:* Nephrotic syndrome, renal papillary necrosis, albuminuria. *Miscellaneous:* Muscle weakness, blurred vision, tinnitus, male infertility, fever, tachycardia, mononucleosis-type syndrome, pulmonary eosinophilia, pancreatitis.

A leprosy-reactional state may occur in large numbers of clients during therapy with dapsone. Type 1 occurs soon after therapy is initiated. Clients manifest an enhanced delayed hypersensitivity syndrome, leading to swelling of existing nerve and skin lesions with possible neuritis. However, this is not an indication to discontinue therapy. Steroids, analgesics, and surgical decompression of swollen nerve trunks may be used to reduce symptoms. Type 2 occurs in nearly 50% of clients during the first year of therapy. Symptoms include fever, erythematous skin nodules, joint swelling, neuritis, orchitis, malaise, depression, iritis, or epistaxis. Usually therapy is continued with the use of analgesics, steroids, or clofazimine to suppress the reaction.

**OD   Overdose   Management:** *Symptoms:* N&V, hyperexcitability (up to 24 hr after ingestion of an overdose). Methemoglobin-induced depression, ***seizures,*** severe cyanosis, headache, hemolysis. *Treatment:* Gastric lavage. In normal and methemoglobin-reductase deficient clients, give methylene blue, 1–2 mg/kg by slow IV (may need to be repeated if methemoglobin reaccumulates). In nonemergencies, methylene blue may be given PO, 3–5 mg/kg/4–6 hr.

**Drug Interactions**

*Charcoal, activated* / ↓ Absorption of dapsone from GI tract
*Didanosine* / Possible therapeutic failure of dapsone → increased infection
*Para-aminobenzoic acid* / ↓ Effect of dapsone
*Probenecid* / ↑ Effect of dapsone due to inhibition of renal excretion
*Pyrimethamine* / ↑ Risk of hematologic reactions
*Rifampin* / ↓ Effect of dapsone due to ↑ plasma clearance
*Trimethoprim* / ↑ Serum levels of both drugs → pharmacologic and toxic effects of both

**Laboratory Test Interferences:** Altered liver function tests.

Dosage ───────────
• **Tablets**
  *Leprosy.*
**Adults:** 50–100 mg/day. Initiate and

continue the full dose without interruption.

*Leprosy, bacteriologically negative tuberculoid and indeterminate type.*
**Adults:** 100 mg/day with rifampin, 600 mg/day for 6 months; **then,** continue for a minimum of 3 years.

*Leprosy, lepromatous and borderline clients.*
100 mg/day for at least 2 years with rifampin, 600 mg/day. A third antileprosy drug may be added such as clofazimine, 50–100 mg/day or ethionamide, 250–500 mg/day. Dapsone is continued for up to 10 years until skin scrapings and biopsies are negative for 1 year.

*Dermatitis herpetiformis.*
**Adults, initial:** 50 mg/day; dosage may be increased to 300 mg/day or higher, if necessary. **Maintenance:** Reduce dosage to minimum maintenance dose as soon as possible; maintenance dosage may be reduced or eliminated in clients on a gluten-free diet. Dosage should be correspondingly less in children.

---

## NURSING CONSIDERATIONS

See also *General Nursing Considerations for All Anti-Infectives.*

### Administration/Storage
1. For tuberculoid and indeterminate clients, continue dosage for at least 3 years.
2. For lepromatous clients, full dosage may be necessary for life.
3. Carefully evaluate possible resistance to dapsone, especially if lepromatous or borderline lepromatous clients relapse. If there is no response to dapsone therapy within 3–6 months, dapsone resistance can be confirmed.

### Assessment
1. Note indications for therapy; onset of symptoms. Document size, extent, and location of lesions.
2. Observe clients with other concurrent chronic conditions closely; anticipate reduced dosage of sulfones.
3. Increase dosage slowly during initiation period; determine if client to receive hematinics.

4. Monitor CBC, liver and renal function studies. Assess for anemia; report if WBCs < 4,500/mm$^3$; RBC < 2,500,000/mm$^3$ or if it remains low during first 6 weeks of therapy.

### Client/Family Teaching
1. Take exactly as ordered.
2. Follow prescribed diet (e.g., gluten-free) and see dietitian as needed for instruction.
3. Lactating mothers should report cyanosis of nursing infant; this indicates high sulfone levels, and drug withdrawal may be indicated.
4. Report any evidence of psychoses, GI disturbances, lepra reaction, headaches, dizziness, lethargy, severe malaise, tinnitus, paresthesias, deep aches, neuralgic pains, and ocular disturbances.
5. Report allergic dermatitis (usually appears before week 10 of therapy); may develop into fatal exfoliative dermatitis.
6. Lab studies and follow-up visits are needed to evaluate drug effectiveness.
7. Identify local support groups that may assist client to understand and cope with this chronic disease.

### Outcomes/Evaluate
• ↓ Size and extent of lesions
• ↓ Inflammation and ulceration of mucous membranes
• Malaria prophylaxis

---COMBINATION DRUG---

# Darvocet-N 50 and Darvocet-N 100
(**DAR**-voh-set)
**(Rx)**
**Classification:** Analgesic

---

See also *Acetaminophen* and *Propoxyphene.*

**Content:** *Nonnarcotic analgesic:* Acetaminophen, 325 (Darvocet-N 50) or 650 mg (Darvocet-N 100). *Analgesic:* Propoxyphene napsylate, 50 or 100 mg.

**Uses:** Mild to moderate pain (may be used if fever is present).

**Special Concerns:** Use during pregnancy only if benefits outweigh risks. Safety and a suitable dosage regimen have not been established in children. Increased dosing intervals should be considered in geriatric clients.

**Dosage**
• **Tablets**
*Analgesia.*
Two Darvocet-N 50 tablets or 1 Darvocet-N 100 tablet q 4 hr, not to exceed 600 mg/day of propoxyhene napsylate. Reduce total daily dose in impaired hepatic or renal function.

**NURSING CONSIDERATIONS**

See *Nursing Considerations* for *Acetaminophen* and *Propoxyphene Napsylate*.
**Assessment:** Document indications for therapy, type, duration, and onset of symptoms. Anticipate reduced dose with renal and hepatic dysfunction.
**Outcomes/Evaluate:** ↓ Pain and discomfort

————*COMBINATION DRUG*————

# Darvon Compound 65
(**DAR**-von)
**(Rx)**
**Classification:** Analgesic

See also *Acetylsalicylic Acid* and *Propoxyphene.*
**Content:** Darvon Compound 65: *Analgesic:*Propoxyphene HCl, 65 mg. *Nonnarcotic analgesic:* Aspirin, 389 mg. *CNS stimulant:* Caffeine, 32.4 mg.
**Uses:** Mild to moderate pain, with or without accompanying fever.
**Special Concerns:** Use during pregnancy only if benefits outweigh risks.

**Dosage**
• **Capsules**
*Analgesia.*
One capsule q 4 hr. Total daily dose of propoxyphene HCl should not exceed 390 mg. Decrease total daily dosage in hepatic or renal impairment.

**NURSING CONSIDERATIONS**

See also *Nursing Considerations* for *Acetylsalicylic Acid* and *Propoxyphene Napsylate.*
**Assessment:** Document indications for therapy, onset and type of symptoms; reduce dose with renal or liver dysfunction.
**Client/Family Teaching**
1. Use caution when performing tasks that require mental alertness; may cause dizziness and sedation.
2. Do *NOT* ingest alcohol.
3. Keep out reach of children.
4. Psychologic and physical dependence may occur.
**Outcomes/Evaluate:** ↓ Pain and discomfort

# Daunorubicin
(daw-noh-**ROO**-bih-sin)
**Pregnancy Category:** D
Cerubidine (Abbreviation: DNR) **(Rx)**

# Daunorubicin Citrate Liposomal
(daw-noh-**ROO**-bih-sin)
**Pregnancy Category:** D
DaunoXome **(Rx)**
**Classification:** Antineoplastic, antibiotic

See also *Antineoplastic Agents.*
**Action/Kinetics:** An anthracycline antibiotic produced by *Streptomyces coeruleorubidus* or *S. peucetius*. The liposomal product contains an aqueous solution of the citrate salt of daunorubicin encapsulated within lipid vesicles which are composed of a lipid bilayer of distearoylphosphatidylcholine and cholesterol. Most active in the S phase of cell division but is not cell-cycle specific. Inhibits synthesis of nucleic acid by inserting into the double helix of DNA. Also possesses immunosuppressive, cytotoxic, and antimitotic activity. Rapidly cleared from the plasma. The liposomal preparation helps protect daunorubicin from chemical and enzymatic breakdown; also, it minimizes protein binding

and decreases uptake by normal tissues. Is released from the liposomal preparation over time and improves selectivity for solid tumors. Metabolized to the active daunorubicinol. $t^{1/2}$: daunorubicin (nonliposomal product), 18.5 hr; daunorubicinol, 27 hr. $t^{1/2}$, elimination: 4.4 hr for liposomal form. Drug rapidly taken up by heart, kidneys, lung, liver, and spleen. Chiefly excreted in bile (40%) and unchanged in urine (25%). Does not pass blood-brain barrier.

**Uses:** Acute nonlymphocytic leukemia in adults (myelogenous, erythroid, monocytic). When combined with cytarabine, effectiveness is increased. Acute lymphocytic leukemia in children (increased effectiveness when combined with vincristine and prednisone). The lioposomal product is a first-line cytotoxic therapy for advanced HIV-associated Kaposi's sarcoma. *Investigational:* Ewing's sarcoma, chronic myelocytic leukemia, neuroblastoma, non-Hodgkin's lymphomas, Wilms' tumor.

**Special Concerns:** Not recommended for use during lactation. Use with caution in preexisting heart disease or bone marrow depression, renal or hepatic failure. Safety and effectiveness have not been determined in children or geriatric clients.

**Side Effects:** *For the liposomal product. CNS:* Fatigue, headache, neuropathy, malaise, dizziness, depression, insomnia, amnesia, anxiety, ataxia, confusion, seizures, emotional lability, abnormal gait, hallucinations, hyperkinesia, hypertonia, meningitis, somnolence, abnormal thinking, tremors. *Hematologic:* Myelosuppression, especially of the granulocytic series. Neutropenia. *CV:* Cardiomyopathy associated with a decrease in left ventricular ejection fraction (especially in clients who have received prior anthracyclines or who have preexisting cardiac disease). Also, hot flushes, hypertension, palpitation, syncope, tachycardia. *GI:* Nausea, diarrhea, anorexia, abdominal pain, vomiting, stomatitis, constipation, increased appetite, dysphagia, *GI hemorrhage*, gastritis, gingival bleeding, hemorrhoids, hepatomegaly, melena, dry mouth, tooth caries. *Respiratory:* Cough, dyspnea, rhinitis, sinusitis, hemoptysis, hiccoughs, pulmonary infiltration, increased sputum. *Musculoskeletal:* Rigors, back pain, myalgia, arthralgia. *Dermatologic:* Alopecia, pruritus, foliculitis, seborrhea, dry skin. *GU:* Dysuria, nocturia, polyuria. *Ophthalmic:* Abnormal vision, conjunctivitis, eye pain. *Otic:* Deafness, ear pain, tinnitus. *Miscellaneous:* Fever, allergic reactions, sweating, chest pain, edema, taste perversion, tenesmus, flu-like symptoms, opportunitistic infections, inflammation at injection site, lymphadenopathy, splenomegaly, dehydration, thirst. Back pain, flushing, and chest tightness have been reported within the first 5 min of the infusion.

**Additional Side Effects:** *Myocardial toxicity: Potentially fatal CHF, especially if total dosage exceeds 550 mg/m$^2$ for adults, 300 mg/m$^2$ for children more than 2 years of age, and 10 mg/kg for children less than 2 years of age.* Mucositis (3–7 days after administration), red-colored urine, hyperuricemia. Severe tissue necrosis if extravasation occurs. Cross-resistance with doxorubicin (produced by similar microorganism) and vinca alkaloids. Hyperuricemia may occur due to lysis of leukemic cells; give allopurinol as a precaution, before starting antileukemic therapy.

**OD** **Overdose Management:** *Symptoms:* Granulocytopenia, fatigue, N&V. Also, extension of side effects.

**Dosage** ――――――――――

• **IV Infusion of Daunorubicin**
*Acute nonlymphocytic leukemia.*

**Adults:** Daunorubicin, 45 mg/m$^2$/day on days 1, 2, and 3 of first course and days 1 and 2 of additional courses; *cytosine arabinoside (Ara-c),* 100 mg/m$^2$/day, by IV infusion, for 7 days during first course and for 5 days during any additional courses of treatment. Some recommend reducing the dose of daunorubicin to 30 mg/m² in clients 60 years of age and older. Up to three courses may be required.

*Acute lymphocytic leukemia.*
**Adults:** Daunorubicin, 45 mg/m², IV, on days 1, 2, and 3; vincristine, IV, on days 1, 8, and 15; prednisone, PO, 40 mg/m²/day for days 1–22 and then taper between days 22 and 29; and, L-asparaginase, IV, 500 IU/kg/day on days 22–32.

*Acute lymphocytic leukemia.*
**Children:** Daunorubicin, 25 mg/m², and vincristine, 1.5 mg/m², each IV, on day 1 every week with prednisone, 40 mg/m², PO, daily. Usually four courses will induce remission. *NOTE:* Calculate the dose on the basis of milligrams per kilogram if the child is less than 2 years of age or if the body surface is less than 0.5 m².

*Acute nonlymphocytic leukemia.*
**Geriatric clients:** 30 mg/m² on days 1, 2, and 3 of the first course and days 1 and 2 of the second course in combination with cytarabine.

• **IV infusion of Daunorubicin Citrate Liposomal**

*Advanced HIV-associated Kaposi's sarcoma.*
40 mg/m² given over 1 hr. Dose is repeated q 2 weeks. This regimen is continued until there is progression of the disease or other complications of HIV disease preclude continued therapy.

Reduce dosage for renal or hepatic disease. Recommended dose for liposomal product: three-fourths of normal dose if serum bilirubin is 1.2 to 3 mg/dL; one-half of normal dose if serum bilirubin is less than 3 mg/dL and serum creatinine is greater than 3 mg/dL.

## NURSING CONSIDERATIONS

See also *Nursing Considerations* for *Antineoplastic Agents.*
**Administration/Storage**
**IV** 1. Dilute in vial with 4 mL sterile water for injection USP. Agitate

gently until dissolved (solution contains 5 mg daunorubicin/mL). Withdraw desired dose into syringe containing 10–15 mL isotonic saline; inject into tubing of rapidly flowing 5% glucose or NSS IV and administer over 3–5 min. May further dilute in 50 mL of D5W or NSS and infuse over 10–15 min (or in 100 mL of solution and infuse over 30–45 min).

2. *Never administer daunorubicin IM or SC.*

3. Reconstituted solution stable for 24 hr at room temperature; for 48 hr when refrigerated. Protect from sunlight.

4. Do not mix with other drugs or heparin.

5. Extravasation may cause severe local tissue necrosis.

6. Dilute the liposomal product 1:1 with 5% dextrose injection before use. Do not use an in-line filter for IV infusion.

7. Refrigerate the liposomal product at 2°C–8°C (36°F–46°F). Do not store the reconstituted solution for longer than 6 hr; do not freeze; protect from light.

**Assessment**
1. Assess during and following therapy for myocardial toxicity, manifested by changes in baseline ECG, edema, dyspnea, and cyanosis. A 30% decrease in QRS voltage and a reduction in the systolic ejection fraction may be early signals of cardiomyopathy. Clients with a cardiac history who receive doses above 550 mg/m² are more susceptible to CHF.

2. Follow appropriate guidelines for dose adjustment in liver dysfunction (e.g., bilirubin 1.2–3.0 mg%, give 75% of dose; bilirubin greater than 3.0 mg%, give 50% of dose).

3. Drug may precipitate hyperuricemia; administer allopurinol.

4. Monitor liver and renal function studies and hematologic profile as drug may cause severe granulocyte and platelet toxicity; allow bone marrow recovery before subsequent treatments. Nadir: 10 days; recovery: 21– 28 days.

**Client/Family Teaching**
1. Report any S&S of cardiac toxicity (i.e., increased SOB, increased fatigue, and edema).
2. Report if mouth ulcers or pain interferes with eating.
3. Urine may appear red for several days following therapy; this is not blood.
4. Consume 1.5–2 L/day of fluids. Record I&O and report any altered elimination patterns.
5. Avoid alcohol and foods high in purines.
6. Practice contraception during and for at least 1 month following therapy.
7. Avoid vaccinations.
8. Anticipate hair loss; should grow back in about 5 weeks following therapy.

**Outcomes/Evaluate:** Suppression of malignant cell proliferation

# Deferoxamine mesylate
(deh-fer-**OX**-ah-meen)
**Pregnancy Category:** C
Desferal **(Rx)**
**Classification:** Heavy metal antagonist (iron chelator)

**Action/Kinetics:** Deferoxamine, a complex organic molecule, binds to free iron, iron of ferritin, and hemosiderin forming ferrioxamine, which is a water-soluble chelate excreted by the kidneys (urine is a reddish color) as well as in the feces via the bile. Iron is not removed from hemoglobin, myoglobin, or cytochromes. Must be given parenterally for systemic activity. Adequate renal function is necessary for effectiveness. **t½, IV:** 60 min. Rapidly metabolized by plasma enzymes and excreted in the urine.

**Uses:** Adjunct in treatment of acute iron intoxication. Chronic iron overload including thalassemia. *Investigational:* Accumulation of aluminum in bone in renal failure and in encephalopathy due to aluminum. May be helpful in Alzheimer's disease and some cancers.

**Contraindications:** Severe renal disease, anuria. Do *not* use to treat primary hemochromatosis.

**Special Concerns:** Use in pregnancy only if clearly necessary. Use with caution for clients with pyelonephritis. Should not be used in children under the age of 3 years unless mobilization of 1 mg iron/day or more can be shown. Use deferoxamine and ascorbic acid with caution in geriatric clients due to a greater risk of cardiac decompensation.

**Side Effects: Following long-term therapy.** *Allergic:* Rash, itching, wheal formation, **anaphylaxis.** *GI:* Abdominal discomfort, diarrhea. *Ophthalmologic:* Blurred vision. Rarely, impaired peripheral, night, or color vision; cataracts, decreased visual acuity, retinal pigmentation abnormalities. *Other:* Dysuria, leg cramps, fever, tachycardia, high-frequency hearing loss. **Following rapid IV use.** Hypotension, urticaria, erythema. **Following SC use.** Local pain, erythema, swelling, pruritus, skin irritation.

**Dosage** ⎯⎯⎯⎯
• **IM, IV, SC**
  *Acute iron intoxication.*
**Adults and children over 3 years of age, IM (preferred), initial:** 1 g; **then,** 0.5 g q 4 hr for two doses; if necessary, then give 0.5 g q 4–12 hr, not to exceed 6 g/day. **IV infusion** (*only in emergencies such as CV collapse:*) Same as IM at a rate not to exceed 15 mg/kg/hr. Begin IM therapy as soon as possible.
  *Chronic iron overload.*
**IM:** 0.5–1.0 g/day; **SC:** 1–2 g (20–40 mg/kg/day) given by mini-infusion pump over an 8–24-hr period; **IV:** 2 g (given separately but at same time as each unit of blood and in addition to IM administration); IV rate not to exceed 15 mg/kg/hr.

## NURSING CONSIDERATIONS
### Administration/Storage
1. Dissolve deferoxamine mesylate by adding 2 mL of sterile water to each ampule.
2. Pain and induration may occur at IM injection site.
3. Have epinephrine available to treat allergic reactions. With iron

intoxication or acidosis, have emergency equipment available.

**IV** 4. For IV administration use physiologic saline, glucose in water, or RL solution and administer *slowly* at a rate not exceeding 15 mg/kg/hr.

5. Discard dissolved drug if not used within 1 week. Protect from light and store above 25°C (77°F).

**Assessment**

1. Document indications for therapy, onset of symptoms, and any evidence of pyelonephritis.

2. In poisoning, note time and amount ingested and type of preparation. Document early S&S of iron toxicity: abdominal pain, emesis, and bloody diarrhea; and late S&S: decreased level of consciousness, metabolic acidosis, and shock.

3. Monitor serum iron, total iron-binding capacity, ferritin, and urinary iron excretion levels. Report if anuric as chelated iron is excreted by the kidneys. Conduct renal function studies; determine if pregnant.

4. Drug is oto and ocular toxic; obtain baseline exams.

**Client/Family Teaching**

1. Pain and induration may occur at administration site.

2. Drug may give the urine a reddish color due to the chelated iron.

3. With a history of pyelonephritis, report development of hematuria or pain; may be caused by a deferoxamine-induced disease exacerbation.

4. Report any sudden hearing loss or complaints of visual disturbances such as changes in color vision or altered visual acuity; may be drug induced. Report for periodic ophthalmologic and audiometric exams.

5. Practice reliable birth control.

**Outcomes/Evaluate**

• Relief of symptoms of iron toxicity
• ↓ Serum iron levels

# Delavirdine mesylate

(deh-lah-**VIR**-deen)
**Pregnancy Category:** C
Rescriptor **(Rx)**

**Classification:** Antiviral drug, reverse transcriptase inhibitor

See also *Antiviral Drugs.*

**Action/Kinetics:** Non-nucleoside reverse transcriptase inhibitor that binds directly to reverse transcriptase and blocks RNA-dependent and DNA-dependent DNA polymerase activities. Effect is additive if used with other antiviral drugs. Delavirdine may confer cross-resistance to other non-nucleoside reverse transcriptase inhibitors when used alone or in combination. Rapidly absorbed. **Peak plasma levels:** About 1 hr. Extensively bound to plasma albumin. Converted to inactive metabolites which are excreted in urine and feces. It inhibits its own metabolism.

**Uses:** Treatment of HIV-1 infections in combination with appropriate antiretroviral agents.

**Special Concerns:** Use with caution in impaired hepatic function. Safety and efficacy in combination with other antiretroviral drugs have not been determined in HIV-1-infected clients less than 16 years of age.

**Side Effects:** *Body as a whole:* Headache, fatigue, asthenia, allergic reaction, chest pain, chills, general or local edema, fever, flu syndrome, lethargy, malaise, neck rigidity, general or local pain, trauma. *CV:* Bradycardia, migraine, pallor, palpitation, postural hypotension, syncope, tachycardia, vasodilation. *CNS:* Abnormal coordination, agitation, amnesia, anxiety, change in dreams, cognitive impairment, confusion, decreased libido, depression, disorientation, dizziness, emotional lability, hallucinations, hyperesthesia, hyperreflexia, hypesthesia, impaired coordination, insomnia, mania, nervousness, neuropathy, nightmares, paralysis, paranoia, paresthesia, restlessness, somnolence, tingling, tremor, vertigo, weakness. *GI:* N&V, diarrhea, anorexia, aphthous stomatitis, bloody stool, colitis, constipation,

**D**

appetite decreased or increased, diarrhea, duodenitis, dry mouth, diverticulitis, dyspepsia, dysphagia, fecal incontinence, flatulence, enteritis, esophagitis, gastritis, gagging, gastroesophageal reflux, GI bleeding or disorder, gingivitis, gum hemorrhage, increased saliva, increased thirst, mouth ulcer, abdominal cramps/distention/pain, lip edema, hepatitis (nonspecified), pancreatitis, rectal disorder, sialadenitis, stomatitis, tongue edema, ulceration. *Dermatologic:* Skin rashes, maculopapular rash, pruritus, angioedema, dermal leukocytoblastic vasculitis, dermatitis, desquamation, diaphoresis, dry skin, erythema, erythema multiforme, folliculitis, fungal dermatitis, alopecia, nail disorder, petechial rash, seborrhea, skin disorder, skin nodule, **Stevens-Johnson syndrome,** vesiculobullous rash, sebaceous cyst. *GU:* Breast enlargement, kidney calculi, epididymitis, hematuria, hemospermia, impotence, kidney pain, metrorrhagia, nocturia, polyuria, proteinuria, vaginal moniliasis. *Musculoskeletal:* Back pain, neck rigidity, arthritis or arthralgia of single or multiple joints, bone disorder or pain, leg cramps, muscle weakness, myalgia, tendon disorder, tenosynovitis, tetany, muscle cramps. *Respiratory:* Upper respiratory infection, bronchitis, chest congestion, cough, dyspnea, epistaxis, laryngismus, pharyngitis, rhinitis, sinusitis. *Hematologic:* Anemia, bruises, ecchymosis, eosinophilia, granulocytosis, neutropenia, pancytopenia, petechiae, purpura, spleen disorder, thrombocytopenia. *Ophthalmic:* Nystagmus, blepharitis, conjunctivitis, diplopia, dry eyes, photophobia. *Miscellaneous:* Alcohol intolerance, peripheral edema, weight increase or decrease, taste perversion, tinnitus, ear pain.

**Laboratory Test Alteration:** ↑ ALT, AST, bilirubin, GGT, lipase, serum alkaline phosphatase, serum amylase, serum creatinine phosphatase, serum creatinine. Bilirubinemia, hyperkalemia, hyperuricemia, hypo-calcemia, hyponatremia, hypophosphatemia

**Drug Interactions**

*Antacids* / ↓ Absorption of delavirdine; separate doses by 1 hr

*Anticonvulsants* / ↓ Plasma levels of delavirdine due to ↑ hepatic metabolism

*Astemizole* / Possible serious or life-threatening side effects of astemizole due to ↓ metabolism

*Benzodiazpines* / Possible serious or life-threatening side effects of benzodiazepines due to ↓ metabolism

*Calcium channel blockers, dihydropyridine-type* / Possible serious or life-threatening side effects of calcium channel blocker due to ↓ metabolism

*Cisapride* / Possible serious or life-threatening side effects of cisapride due to ↓ metabolism

*Clarithromycin* / Significant ↑ in amount absorbed of both drugs; possible serious side effects

*Dapsone* / Possible serious or life-threatening side effects of dapsone due to ↓ metabolism

*Didanosine* / ↓ Absorption of both drugs; separate administration by at least 1 hr

*Ergot derivatives* / Possible serious or life-threatening side effects of ergot due to ↓ metabolism

*Fluoxetine* / ↑ Trough levels of delavirdine by 50%

*Indinavir* / ↑ Levels of indinavir due to ↓ metabolism; possible serious side effects

*Quinidine* / Possible serious or life-threatening side effects of quinidine due to ↓ metabolism

*Rifabutin, Rifampin* / ↓ Plasma levels of delavirdine due to ↑ hepatic metabolism

*Saquinavir* / ↑ Levels of saquinavir due to ↓ metabolism; possible serious side effects

*Terfenadine* / Possible serious or life-threatening side effects of terfenadine due to ↓ metabolism

*Warfarin* / Possible serious or life-threatening side effects of warfarin due to ↓ metabolism

**Dosage**
- **Tablets**

*HIV-1 infection.*

400 mg (4-100 mg tablets) t.i.d. in combination with other antiretroviral therapy.

## NURSING CONSIDERATIONS
### Administration/Storage
1. Give with or without food.
2. In achlorhydria, take with an acidic beverage (e.g., orange or cranberry juice).

### Assessment
1. Document disease onset/exposure times, likelihood of transmission, and disease characteristics such as stage of infection, viral load.
2. List drugs prescribed to ensure none interact unfavorably.
3. Monitor CBC, LFTs, viral load, CD$_4$ counts.
4. Assess lifestyle and potential to resume risky behaviors.

### Client/Family Teaching
1. Take as directed, with or without food. Take antacids 1 hr before or 1 hr after drug ingestion.
2. Tablets may be dispersed with water prior to consumption. To prepare, add 4 tablets to at least 3 ounces of water and allow to stand for a few minutes. Stir until a uniform dispersion occurs and consume promptly. Rinse glass and swallow rinse to ensure entire dose is taken.
3. Always administer with other antiretroviral therapy. Drug is not a cure for HIV; may continue to acquire opportunistic infections.
4. Rash on upper body and arms may necessitate interruption of therapy. Report especially if accompanied by fever, blistering, myalgia, eye or mouth lesions.
5. Avoid OTC agents without approval.
6. Continue barrier contraception; drug does not reduce risk of transmission.

### Outcomes/Evaluate: Post-exposure prophylaxis; ↓ viral load

# Desipramine hydrochloride
(dess-**IP**-rah-meen)

Alti-Desipramine ✦, Apo-Desipramine ✦, Dom-Desipramine ✦, Norpramin, Novo-Desipramine ✦, Nu-Desipramine ✦, Pertofrane ✦, PMS-Desipramine ✦ **(Rx)**

**Classification:** Antidepressant, tricyclic

See also *Antidepressants, Tricyclic.*

**Action/Kinetics:** Slight anticholinergic and sedative effects and slight ability to cause orthostatic hypotension. **Effective plasma levels:** 125–300 ng/mL. t½: 12–24 hr. **Time to reach steady state:** 2–11 days. Response usually seen within the first week.

**Uses:** Symptoms of depression. Bulimia nervosa. To decrease craving and depression during cocaine withdrawal. To treat severe neurogenic pain. Cataplexy associated with narcolepsy. Attention deficit disorders with or without hyperactivity in children over 6 years of age.

**Contraindications:** Use in children less than 12 years of age.

**Special Concerns:** Safe use during pregnancy has not been established. Safety and efficacy have not been established in children.

**Additional Side Effects:** Bad taste in mouth, hypertension during surgery.

**Dosage**
- **Tablets**

*Antidepressant.*

**Initial:** 100–200 mg/day in single or divided doses. **Maximum daily dose:** 300 mg in severely ill clients. **Maintenance:** 50–100 mg/day. **Geriatric clients:** 25–50 mg/day in divided doses up to a maximum of 150 mg/day. **Adolescents and geriatric clients:** 25–50 mg/day in divided doses up to a maximum of 150 mg.

*Cocaine withdrawal.*

50–200 mg/day.

---

## NURSING CONSIDERATIONS

See also *Nursing Considerations* for *Antidepressants, Tricyclic.*

**Administration/Storage**

1. Initiate treatment in a hospital setting for those requiring 300 mg/day.

2. Give maintenance doses for at least 2 months following a satisfactory response.

3. Give single daily dose or any dosage increases at bedtime to reduce daytime sedation.

**Outcomes/Evaluate**

• ↓ Perceived depression; ↑ self-worth

• Relief of neurogenic pain

• Therapeutic levels (125–300 ng/mL)

# Desmopressin acetate

(des-moh-**PRESS**-in)

**Pregnancy Category:** B

DDAVP, DDAVP Nasal Solution ✿, Octostim ✿, Rhinyle Nasal Solution ✿, Stimate **(Rx)**

**Classification:** Antidiuretic hormone, synthetic

**Action/Kinetics:** A synthetic analog of arginine vasopressin which possesses antidiuretic activity but is devoid of vasopressor and oxytocic effects. Acts to increase absorption of water in the kidney by increasing permeability of cells in the collecting ducts. **Onset:** 1 hr. **Peak, intranasal:** 1–5 hr.; **peak, PO:** 4–7 hr. **Duration:** 8–20 hr. **t½:** initial, 8 min; final: 75 min. Effect ceases abruptly. It also increases factor VIII levels (**onset:** 30 min; **peak:** 1.5–2 hr) and von Willebrand's factor activity. **Time to reach maximum plasma levels, after PO or intranasal:** 0.9–1.5 hr.

**Uses: DDAVP.** Primary noctural enuresis (intranasal only), central cranial DI (intranasal, oral, parenteral), hemophilia A with factor VIII levels greater than 5% (intranasal, parenteral), von Willebrand's disease (type I) with factor VIII levels greater than 5% (intranasal, parenteral). **Stimate.** Hemophilia A with factor VIII levels greater than 5%,

von Willebrand's disease with factor VIII levels greater than 5%.

*Investigational:* Chronic autonomic failure (nocturnal polyuria, overnight weight loss, morning postural hypotension).

**Contraindications:** Hypersensitivity to drug. Use for treatment of hemophilia A with factor VIII levels less than or equal to 5%, treatment of hemophilia B or in clients who have factor VIII antibodies. Treatment of severe classic von Willebrand's disease (type I) and when an abnormal molecular form of factor VIII antigen is present. Use for type IIB von Willebrand's disease. Parenteral administration for DI in infants under 3 months and intranasal administration in infants less than 11 months. Nephrogenic DI, polyuria due to psychogenic DI, renal disease, hypercalcemia, hyperkalemia, or administration of demeclocycline or lithium.

**Special Concerns:** Safety for use during lactation not established. Use with caution and with restricted fluid intake in infants due to an increased risk of hyponatremia and water intoxication. Geriatric clients may have a greater risk of developing hyponatremia and water intoxication. Use with caution in clients with coronary artery insufficiency and/or hypertensive CV disease. Use cautiously with other pressor agents. Safety and efficacy have not been determined in children less than 12 years of age (parenteral) or less than 2 months of age (intranasal) with DI.

**Side Effects: DDAVP.** *Intranasal:* Transient headaches, nausea, nasal congestion, rhinitis, facial flushing, asthenia, chills, conjunctivitis, cough, dizziness, epistaxis, eye edema, GI disorder, lacrimation, nosebleed, nostril pain, sore throat, URIs. *Parenteral:* Mild abdominal pain, facial flushing, transient headache, nausea, vulval pain, BP changes, burning pain, edema, local erythema, *anaphylaxis (rare).*

**Stimate.** *Intranasal:* Agitation, balanitis, chest pain, chills, dizziness, dyspepsia, edema, insomnia, itch or light-sensitive eyes, pain, palpitations, somnolence, tachycardia, vomiting, warm feeling.

**OD** **Overdose Management:** *Symptoms:* Headache, abdominal cramps, facial flushing, dyspnea, fluid retention, mucous membrane irritation. *Treatment:* Reduce dose, decrease frequency of administration, or withdraw the drug depending on the severity of the condition.

**Drug Interactions:** Chlorpropamide, clofibrate, and carbamazepine may potentiate the effects of desmopressin.

**Dosage**
- **SC, Direct IV**
  *Neurogenic DI.*
**Adults:** 0.5–1 mL/day in two divided doses, adjusted separately for an adequate diurnal rhythm of water turnover. If switching from intranasal to IV, the comparable IV antidiuretic dose is about ¹⁄₁₀ the intranasal dose.
  *Hemophilia A, von Willebrand's disease (type I).*
**Adults:** 0.0003 mg/kg diluted in 50 mL 0.9% NaCl injection infused IV over 15–30 min; dose may be repeated, if necessary. **Pediatric, 3 months or older, weighing 10 kg or less, IV:** 0.0003 mg/kg diluted in 10 mL of 0.9% NaCl injection and given over 15–30 min; repeat if necessary. **Pediatric, 3 months or older, weighing 10 kg or more, IV:** 0.0003 mg/kg diluted in 50 mL of 0.9% NaCl injection and given over 15–30 min; repeat if necessary.
- **Intranasal**
  *Neurogenic DI.*
**Adults:** 0.1–0.4 mL/day, either as a single dose or divided into two to three doses (usual: 0.2 mL/day in two divided doses). Adjust morning and evening doses separately for an adequate diurnal rhythm of water turnover. **Children, 3 months to 12 years:** 0.05–0.3 mL/day, either as a single dose or two divided doses.
  *Nocturnal enuresis.*
**Age 6 years and older, initial:** 0.02 mg (0.2 mL) at bedtime with one-

half the dose in each nostril; if no response, the dose may be increased to 0.04 mg.
  *Hemophilia A and type I von Willenbrand's disease.*
**In clients weighing 50 kg or more:** One spray per nostril (total dose of 300 mcg). **In clients weighing less than 50 kg:** Given as a single spray of 150 mcg. The drug may be given 2 hr prior to minor surgery in the same doses as described above.
  *Renal concentration capacity test.*
**Adults:** 0.040 mg (0.020 mg in each nostril) given any time during the day. **Children, 3–12 years:** 0.020 mg given in the morning.
- **Tablets**
  *Central cranial DI.*
**Adults, initial:** 0.05 mg b.i.d.; adjust individually to optimum therapeutic dose and adjust each dose for an adequate diurnal rhythm of water turnover. Total daily dose should be increased or decreased (range 0.1–1.2 mg divided b.i.d.–t.i.d.) as needed to obtain adequate antidiuresis. **Children, initial:** 0.05 mg. Careful restriction of fluid intake in children is required to prevent hyponatremia and water intoxication.

## NURSING CONSIDERATIONS
### Administration/Storage
1. Measure the dosage exactly because the drug is potent.
2. Note the three graduation marks on the soft flexible plastic nasal tube: 0.2, 0.1, and 0.05 mL. The 0.05-level is not designated by number. Cleanse and dry the tube appropriately.
3. Stimate nasal spray pump can only deliver 0.1 mL (150 mcg). The pump must be primed prior to the first use by pressing down four times. Discard the bottle after 25 (150 mcg) doses since the amount delivered thereafter may be significantly less than 150 mcg.
4. Refrigerate Stimate nasal spray although the product will be stable for

up to 3 weeks when stored at room temperature. DDAVP Nasal Spray needs no refrigeration.

5. If used for hemophilia A or von Willebrand's disease, do not use it more often than q 2 days as tachyphylaxis may occur.

6. To determine the renal concentration capacity in adults, the urine voided within 1 hr after drug administration is discarded; the two subsequent urines collected within 8 hr are saved and tested for osmolality. In children, osmolality is measured on urine voided during 3–5 hr after drug administration. Clients should drink only small amounts of fluid during the test day.

**IV** 7. For direct IV administration (with neurogenic DI) give each dose over 1 min. With hemophilia, may dilute drug in 50 mL of NSS and infuse over 15–30 min.

8. Refrigerate the solution and injection at 4°C (39.2°F).

**Assessment**

1. Monitor CBC, calcium, blood sugar, electrolytes, and appropriate factor levels.

2. Observe for early S&S of water intoxication (drowsiness, headache, and vomiting, excessive fluid consumption, weight gain, and/or seizures). Adjust fluid intake to avoid water intoxication and hyponatremia; if excessive retention, may treat with a diuretic.

3. With hemophilia, monitor BP and HR closely during IV therapy.

4. With neurogenic DI, monitor urine osmolarity and volume; weigh daily; assess for edema and evidence of dehydration.

5. Monitor duration of sleep. The amount of sleep, together with the client's daily I&O provide parameters to estimate the clinical response to drug therapy with enuresis.

**Client/Family Teaching**

1. If spray is prescribed, instruct in appropriate administration technique using the special catheter provided. Insert tip of catheter into nose and blow on the other end of the catheter to deliver the medication deep into the nasal cavity. (A syringe filled with air may be used in children and comatose persons; rinse after use).

2. Review recommendations concerning fluid intake. Measure I&O and keep an accurate record of fluid status. Report any symptoms of water intoxication and hyponatremia.

3. Notify provider at the earliest signs of trouble, such as a decrease in urinary output, the development of headaches, or severe nasal congestion. The latter two can be mistaken for an upper respiratory infection.

4. Avoid alcohol in any form.

5. Tolerance may develop over time and response may be diminished.

**Outcomes/Evaluate**

• Prevention of hemorrhage
• Control of nocturnal enuresis
• Desired antidiuretic effects (↓ urine volume, ↑ urine osmolarity, and relief of polydipsia) with DI

---

# Dexamethasone
(dex-ah-**METH**-ah-zohn)

**Oral:** Decadron, Deronil ✸, Dexameth, Dexamethasone Intensol, Dexasone ✸, Dexone, Hexadrol **(Rx)**.
**Topical:** Aeroseb-Dex, Decaderm. **(Rx), Ophthalmic:** Maxidex Ophthalmic **(Rx)**
**Classification:** Glucocorticoid, synthetic

---

See also *Corticosteroids*.

**Action/Kinetics:** Long-acting. Low degree of sodium and water retention. Diuresis may ensue when clients are transferred from other corticosteroids to dexamethasone. Not recommended for replacement therapy in adrenal cortical insufficiency. **t½:** 110–210 min.

**Additional Uses:** In acute allergic disorders, PO dexamethasone may be combined with dexamethasone sodium phosphate injection and used for 6 days. To test for adrenal cortical hyperfunction. Cerebral edema due to brain tumor, craniotomy, or head injury. *Investigational:* Diagnosis of depression. Antiemetic in cisplatin-induced vomiting. Prophylaxis or treatment of acute mountain sickness. Decrease hearing loss in bacterial meningitis. Bronchopulmonary dysplasia in preterm infants. Hirsutism.

**Special Concerns:** Use during pregnancy only if benefits outweigh risks.

**Additional Drug Interactions:** Ephedrine ↓ effect of dexamethasone due to ↑ breakdown by the liver.

**Dosage**

• **Oral Concentrate Tablets, Elixir**

*Most uses.*

**Initial:** 0.75–9 mg/day; **maintenance:** gradually reduce to minimum effective dose (0.5–3 mg/day).

*Suppression test for Cushing's syndrome.*

0.5 mg q 6 hr for 2 days for 24-hr urine collection (or 1 mg at 11 p.m. with blood withdrawn at 8 a.m. for blood cortisol determination).

*Suppression test to determine cause of pituitary ACTH excess.*

2 mg q 6 hr for 2 days (for 24-hr urine collection).

*Acute allergic disorders or acute worsening of chronic allergic disorders.*

**Day 1:** Dexamethasone sodium phosphate injection, 4–8 mg IM. **Days 2 and 3:** Two 0.75-mg dexamethasone tablets b.i.d. **Day 4:** One 0.75-mg dexamethasone tablet b.i.d. **Days 5 and 6:** One 0.75-mg dexamethasone tablet. **Day 7:** No treatment. **Day 8:** Follow-up visit to physician.

• **Topical Aerosol, Cream**

Apply sparingly as a light film to affected area b.i.d.–t.i.d.

• **Ophthalmic Suspension**

1–2 gtt in the conjunctival sac q hr during day and q 2 hr during night until a satisfactory response obtained; **then,** 1 gtt q 4 hr and finally 1 gtt q 6–8 hr.

**NURSING CONSIDERATIONS**

See also *Nursing Considerations* for *Corticosteroids.*

**Outcomes/Evaluate**

• Status of adrenal cortical function
• ↓ Symptoms of allergic response
• ↓ Cerebral edema

# Dexamethasone acetate

(dex-ah-**METH**-ah-zohn)

Dalalone D.P., Dalalone L.A., Decadron-LA, Decaject-L.A., Dexasone L.A., Dexone LA, Solurex LA **(Rx)**

**Classification:** Glucocorticoid, synthetic

See also *Corticosteroids.*

**Action/Kinetics:** Practically insoluble and provides the prolonged activity suitable for repository injections, although it has a prompt onset of action. Not for IV use.

**Special Concerns:** Use during pregnancy only if benefits outweigh risks.

**Dosage**

• **Repository Injection, IM**

8–16 mg q 1–3 weeks, if necessary.

• **Intralesional**

0.8–1.6 mg.

• **Soft Tissue and Intra-articular**

4–16 mg repeated at 1–3-week intervals.

**NURSING CONSIDERATIONS**

See *Nursing Considerations* for *Corticosteroids.*

**Outcomes/Evaluate**

• ↓ Inflammation
• Symptomatic improvement

# Dexamethasone sodium phosphate

(dex-ah-**METH**-ah-zohn)

**Systemic:** Dalalone, Decadron Phosphate, Decaject, Dexasone, Dexone, Hexadrol Phosphate, R.O.-Dexone ✦, Solurex **(Rx)**. **Inhaler:** Decadron Phosphate Respihaler **(Rx)**. **Nasal:** Decadron Phosphate Turbinaire **(Rx)**. **Ophthalmic:** AK-Dex, Decadron Phosphate Ophthalmic, Diodex ✦, Maxidex, PMS-Dexamethasone Sodium Phosphate ✦, Spersadex ✦ **(Rx)**. **Otic:** AK-Dex,

Decadron, I-Methasone **(Rx)**. **Topical:** Decadron Phosphate **(Rx)**
**Classification:** Glucocorticoid, synthetic

---

See also *Corticosteroids*.
**Action/Kinetics:** Has a rapid onset and a short duration of action.
**Additional Uses:** For IV or IM use in emergency situations when dexamethasone cannot be given PO. Intranasally for nasal polyps, allergic or inflammatory nasal conditions.
**Contraindications:** Acute infections, persistent positive sputum cultures of *Candida albicans*. Lactation.
**Special Concerns:** Use during pregnancy only if benefits outweigh risks.
**Side Effects:** *Following inhalation:* Nasal and nasopharyngeal irritation, burning, dryness, stinging, headache.

**Dosage** ————
• **IM, IV**
*Most uses.*
**Range:** 0.5–9 mg/day (⅓–½ the PO dose q 12 hr).
*Cerebral edema.*
**Adults, initial:** 10 mg IV; **then,** 4 mg IM q 6 hr until maximum effect obtained (usually within 12–24 hr). Switch to PO therapy (1–3 mg t.i.d.) as soon as feasible and then slowly withdraw over 5–7 days.
*Shock, unresponsive.*
**Initial:** either 1–6 mg/kg IV or 40 mg IV; **then,** repeat IV dose q 2–6 hr as long as necessary.
• **Intralesional, Intra-articular, Soft Tissue Injections**
0.4–6 mg, depending on the site (e.g., small joints: 0.8–1 mg; large joints: 2–4 mg; soft tissue infiltration: 2–6 mg; ganglia: 1–2 mg; bursae: 2–3 mg; tendon sheaths: 0.4–1 mg.
• **Metered Dose Inhaler**
*Bronchial asthma.*
**Adults, initial:** 3 inhalations (84 mcg dexamethasone/inhalation) t.i.d.–q.i.d.; **maximum:** 3 inhalations/dose; 12 inhalations/day. **Pediatric: initial,** 2 inhalations t.i.d.–q.i.d.; **maximum:** 2 inhalations/dose; 8 inhalations/day.

• **Intranasal**
*Allergies, nasal polyps.*
**Adults:** 2 sprays (total of 168 mcg dexamethasone) in each nostril b.i.d.–t.i.d. (maximum: 12 sprays/day); **pediatric, 6–12 years:** 1–2 sprays (total of 84–168 mcg dexamethasone) in each nostril b.i.d. (maximum: 8 sprays/day).
• **Ophthalmic Ointment**
Instill a small amount of the ointment into the conjunctival sac t.i.d.–q.i.d. As response is obtained, reduce the number of applications.
• **Ophthalmic Solution**
Instill 1–2 gtt into the conjunctival sac q hr during the day and q 2 hr at night until response obtained; **then,** reduce to 1 gtt q 4 hr and later 1 gtt t.i.d.–q.i.d. may control symptoms.
• **Otic Solution**
3–4 gtt into the ear canal b.i.d.–t.i.d.
• **Topical Cream**
Apply sparingly to affected areas and rub in.

## NURSING CONSIDERATIONS

See also *Nursing Considerations* for *Corticosteroids*.
**Administration/Storage**
1. For intranasal use, some are controlled using 1 spray in each nostril b.i.d.
**IV** 2. For IV administration may give undiluted over 1 min. Do not use preparation containing lidocaine IV.
**Outcomes/Evaluate**
• Improved airway exchange
• Relief of allergic manifestations
• Suppression of inflammatory response; enhanced tissue perfusion

---

# Dexchlorpheniramine maleate

(dex-klor-fen-**EAR**-ah-meen)
**Pregnancy Category:** B
Polaramine **(Rx)**
**Classification:** Antihistamine, alkylamine type

---

See also *Antihistamines*.
**Action/Kinetics:** Minimal sedative and moderate anticholinergic effects. **Duration:** 8 hr.

**Special Concerns:** Extended-release tablets should not be used in children. Geriatric clients may be more sensitive to the usual adult dose.

**Dosage**
• **Syrup, Tablets**
**Adults:** 2 mg q 4–6 hr. **Pediatric, 5–12 years:** 1 mg q 4–6 hr; **2–5 years:** 0.5 mg q 4–6 hr.
• **Extended-Release Tablets**
**Adults and children over 12 years:** 4–6 mg at bedtime or q 8–10 hr. **Children, 6–12 years:** 4 mg/day, taken preferably at bedtime.

## NURSING CONSIDERATIONS

See also *Nursing Considerations* for *Antihistamines.*
**Outcomes/Evaluate:** Symptomatic relief; ↓ allergic manifestations

# Dexrazoxane
(dex-rah-**ZOX**-ayn)
**Pregnancy Category:** C
Zinecard **(Rx)**
**Classification:** Antidote

**Action/Kinetics:** A derivative of EDTA that is a potent chelating agent. It readily penetrates cell membranes, although its mechanism of action as a cardioprotective agent when using anthracyclines (e.g., doxorubicin) is not known. However, the drug may act by interfering with iron-mediated free-radical generation that may be responsible, in part, for anthracycline-induced cardiomyopathy. **t½, elimination:** Approximately 2.5 hr. Metabolized in the liver and both unchanged drug and metabolites are excreted through the urine. Not bound to plasma proteins.
**Uses:** To reduce the incidence and severity of cardiomyopathy associated with doxorubicin administration in women with metastatic breast cancer and who have received a cumulated doxorubicin dose of 300 mg/m² and who need additional doxorubicin therapy.

**Contraindications:** Use with the initiation of doxorubicin therapy, as there is evidence it may interfere with the antitumor efficacy of the regimen (i.e., fluorouracil, doxorubicin, cyclophosphamide). Use with chemotherapy regimens that do not contain an anthracycline. Lactation.
**Special Concerns:** Safety and efficacy have not been determined in children.
**Side Effects:** *NOTE:* The side effects listed may be due to the fluorouracil, doxorubicin, cyclophosphamide regimen. *GI:* N&V, anorexia, stomatitis, diarrhea, esophagitis, dysphagia. *CNS:* Fatigue, malaise, fever, neurotoxicity. *Dermatologic:* Alopecia, streaking/erythema, extravasation, urticaria, recall skin reaction. *CV:* **Hemorrhage,** phlebitis. *Hematologic:* Leukopenia, thrombocytopenia, granulocytopenia. *Miscellaneous:* Pain on injection, **sepsis.**
**OD Overdose Management:** *Symptoms:* Extensions of the side effects, including myelosuppression. *Treatment:* Supportive care, including treatment of infections, fluid regulation, maintenance of nutrition, treatment of myelosuppression. Peritoneal dialysis or hemodialysis may be helpful in removing the drug.
**Drug Interactions:** Dexrazoxane may increase the myelosuppression caused by chemotherapeutic drugs.
**Laboratory Test Interferences:** Marked interference with hepatic or renal function tests.

**Dosage**
• **Slow IV Push or Rapid IV Infusion from a Bag**
*Prevent doxorubicin cardiomyopathy.*
The recommended dosage ratio of dexrazoxane-doxorubicin is 10:1 (i.e., 500 mg/m² dexrazoxane to 50 mg/m² doxorubicin).

## NURSING CONSIDERATIONS
### Administration/Storage
**IV** 1. Reconstitute with 0.167 M

(M/6) sodium lactate injection, to give a concentration of 10 mg/mL.

2. The reconstituted solution may be diluted with either 0.9% NaCl injection or 5% dextrose injection to a concentration range of 1.3–5 mg/mL.

3. Do not mix with other drugs.

4. Do not give doxorubicin prior to the IV injection of dexrazoxane; give doxorubicin within 30 min after beginning the infusion of dexrazoxane.

5. Use caution in the handling and preparation of reconstituted dexrazoxane; use gloves. If the drug or solution comes in contact with the skin or mucous membranes, wash immediately with soap and water.

6. Store the powder for injection at controlled room temperatures of 15°C–30°C (59°F–86°F). The reconstituted and diluted solutions are stable for 6 hr at controlled room temperature or under refrigeration of 2°C–8°C (36°F–46°F). Discard unused solutions.

**Assessment**

1. Note dose of prescribed doxorubicin therapy.

2. Monitor CBC and observe for increased myelosuppression.

3. Perform baseline cardiac assessment, noting any evidence of rales, $S_3$ gallop, PND, increased DOE, or cardiomegaly on X ray or ECG. Assess carefully for any altered cardiac function as cardiomyopathy may still occur.

**Outcomes/Evaluate:** ↓ Incidence/severity of doxorubicin-induced cardiomyopathy

# Dextroamphetamine sulfate

(dex-troh-am-**FET**-ah-meen)
**Pregnancy Category:** C
Dexedrine, Oxydess II, Spancap No. 1 **(C-II) (Rx)**
**Classification:** Central nervous system stimulant, amphetamine type

See also *Amphetamines and Derivatives.*

**Action/Kinetics:** Has stronger CNS effects and weaker peripheral action than does amphetamine; thus, dextroamphetamine manifests fewer undesirable CV effects. After PO administration, completely absorbed in 3 hr. **Duration: PO,** 4–24 hr; **t½, adults:** 10–12 hr; **children:** 6–8 hr. Excreted in urine. Acidification will increase excretion, while alkalinization will decrease it.

**Uses:** Attention deficit disorders in children, narcolepsy.

**Additional     Contraindications:** Lactation. Use for obesity.

**Special Concerns:** Use of extended-release capsules for attention deficit disorders in children less than 6 years of age and the elixir or tablets for attention deficit disorders in children less than 3 years of age is not recommended. Dosage for narcolepsy has not been determined in children less than 6 years of age.

**Dosage** ————————
• **Tablets**
   *Attention deficit disorders in children.*
**3–5 years, initial:** 2.5 mg/day; increase by 2.5 mg/day at weekly intervals until optimum dose is achieved (usual range 0.1–0.5 mg/kg/dose each morning). **6 years and older, initial:** 5 mg 1–2 times/day; increase in increments of 5 mg/week until optimum dose is achieved (rarely over 40 mg/day).
   *Narcolepsy.*
**Adults:** 5–60 mg in divided doses daily. **Children over 12 years, initial:** 10 mg/day; increase in increments of 10 mg/day at weekly intervals until optimum dose is reached. **Children, 6–12 years, initial:** 5 mg/day; increase in increments of 5 mg/week until optimum dose is reached (maximum is 60 mg/day).
• **Extended-Release Capsule**
   *Attention deficit disorders.*
**Children, 6 years and older:** 5–15 mg/day.
   *Narcolepsy.*
**Adults:** 5–30 mg/day. **Children, 6–12 years:** 5–15 mg/day; **12 years and older:** 10–15 mg/day.

## NURSING CONSIDERATIONS

See also *Nursing Considerations* for *Amphetamines and Derivatives.*

**Administration/Storage**

1. Long-acting products may be used for once-a-day dosing in attention deficit disorders and narcolepsy.

2. When tablets or the elixir are used for attention deficit disorders or narcolepsy, give the first dose upon awakening with one or two additional doses given at intervals of 4–6 hr. If possible, give the last dose 6 hr before bedtime.

3. If receiving an MAO inhibitor, wait 14 days after stopping before initiating dextroamphetamine.

**Client/Family Teaching**

1. Take last dose at least 6 hr before bedtime to ensure adequate rest.

2. Avoid activities that require alertness until drug effects realized.

**Outcomes/Evaluate**

• Improved attention span and concentration levels

• ↓ Daytime sleeping

---

# Dextromethorphan hydrobromide

(dex-troh-meth-**OR**-fan)

Balminil DM Children ✢, Balminil DM Syrup ✢, Benylin DM, Benylin DM for Children, Calmylin #1 ✢, Children's Hold, Delsym, Drixoral Cough Liquid Caps ✢, Formula 44 Adult/Pediatric ✢, Hold DM, Koffex DM Children ✢, Koffex DM Syrup ✢, Pertussin CS, Pertussin ES, Robidex Syrup ✢, Robitussin Cough Calmers, Robitussin Pediatric, St. Joseph Cough Suppressant, Scot-Tussin DM Cough Chasers, Sucrets Cough Control, Suppress, Triaminic DM ✢, Trocal, Vick's Formula 44, Vick's Formula 44 Pediatric Formula **(OTC)**

**Classification:** Nonnarcotic antitussive

---

**Action/Kinetics:** Selectively depresses the cough center in the medulla. Dextromethorphan 15–30 mg is equal to 8–15 mg codeine as an antitussive. Does not produce physical dependence or respiratory depression. Well absorbed from GI tract. **Onset:** 15–30 min. **Duration:** 3–6 hr. The sustained liquid contains dextromethorphan plistirex equivalent to 30 mg dextromethorphan hydrobromide per 5 mL.

**Uses:** Symptomatic relief of nonproductive cough due to colds or inhaled irritants.

**Contraindications:** Persistent or chronic cough or when cough is accompanied by excessive secretions. Use during first trimester of pregnancy unless directed otherwise by physician. Use in children less than 2 years of age.

**Special Concerns:** Use with caution in clients with nausea, vomiting, high fever, rash, or persistent headache.

**Side Effects:** *CNS:* Dizziness, drowsiness. *GI:* N&V, stomach pain.

**OD** **Overdose Management:** *Symptoms:* **Adults:** Dysphoria, slurred speech, ataxia, altered sensory perception. **Children:** Ataxia, ***convulsions, respiratory depression.*** *Treatment:* Treat symptoms and provide support.

**Drug Interactions:** Use with MAO inhibitors may cause nausea, hypotension, hyperpyrexia, myoclonic leg jerks, and coma.

**Dosage**

• **Capsules, Liquid, Lozenges, Syrup, Concentrate, Tablets**

*Antitussive.*

**Adults and children over 12 years:** 10–30 mg q 4–8 hr, not to exceed 120 mg/day; **pediatric, 6–12 years:** either 5–10 mg q 4 hr or 15 mg q 6–8 hr, not to exceed 60 mg/day; **pediatric, 2–6 years:** either 2.5–7.5 mg q 4 hr or 7.5 mg q 6–8 hr of the syrup, not to exceed 30 mg/day.

• **Sustained-Release Suspension**

*Antitussive.*

**Adults:** 60 mg q 12 hr. **Pediatric, 6–12 years:** 30 mg q 12 hr, not to exceed 60 mg/day; **pediatric, 2–6 years:** 15 mg q 12 hr, not to exceed 30 mg/day.

---

## NURSING CONSIDERATIONS
### Administration/Storage
1. Increasing the dose of dextromethorphan will not increase its effectiveness but will increase the duration of action.
2. Do not give lozenges to children under 6 years of age.

### Assessment
1. Note length of time cough present. Document sputum production and characteristics. If the cough persists beyond several weeks, do not give dextromethorphan.
2. Determine presence of nausea, vomiting, persistent headaches, or a high fever.
3. If pregnant, determine trimester; drug is contraindicated in the first trimester.

### Client/Family Teaching
1. Avoid tasks that require mental alertness until drug effects realized.
2. Avoid alcohol in any form.
3. Add humidity to a dry environment.
4. Increase fluids to decrease viscosity of secretions.
5. Cigarette smoke, dust, and chemical fumes are irritants that may aggravate condition.
6. Symptoms that persist for more than a week require medical intervention; record onset, triggers, characteristics of secretions, and response to therapy.

**Outcomes/Evaluate:** Control of cough with improved sleep patterns

---

# Dextrose and electrolytes
(**DEX**-trohs)
Pedialyte, Rehydralyte, Resol **(Rx)**
**Classification:** Electrolyte replenisher

**Action/Kinetics:** These oral products contain varying amounts of sodium, potassium, chloride, citrate, and dextrose (Lytren and Resol contain 20 g/L whereas Pedialyte and Rehydralyte contain 25 g/L). In addition, Resol contains magnesium, calcium, and phosphate. **Time to peak effect:** 8–12 hr.
**Uses:** Diarrhea. Prophylaxis and treatment of electrolyte depletion in

diarrhea or in continuing fluid loss. Maintenance of hydration.
**Contraindications:** Anuria, oliguria. Severe dehydration including severe diarrhea (IV therapy is necessary for prompt replacement of fluids and electrolytes). Malabsorption of glucose. Severe and sustained vomiting when the client is unable to drink. Intestinal obstruction, perforated bowel, paralytic ileus.
**Special Concerns:** Use with caution in premature infants.
**Side Effects:** Overhydration indicated by puffy eyelids. Hypernatremia, vomiting (usually shortly after treatment has started).

### Dosage
- **Oral Solution**
  *Mild dehydration.*
**Adults and children over 10 years, initial:** 50 mL/kg over 4–6 hr; **maintenance:** 100–200 mL/kg over 24 hr until diarrhea stops.
  *Moderate dehydration.*
**Adults and children over 10 years, initial:** 100 mL/kg over 6 hr; **maintenance:** 15 mL/kg q hr until diarrhea stops.
  *Moderate to severe dehydration.*
**Pediatric, 2–10 years, initial:** 50 mL/kg over the first 4–6 hr followed by 100 mL/kg over the next 18–24 hr; **less than 2 years, initial:** 75 mL/kg during the first 8 hr and 75 mL/kg during the next 16 hr.

---

## NURSING CONSIDERATIONS
### Administration/Storage
1. Give no more than 1,000 mL/hr to adults and no more than 100 mL/20 min to children.
2. Adjust the amount and rate of solution depending on need, thirst, and response.
3. Assist infants and small children in drinking the solution slowly and frequently in small quantities and, if necessary, feed by a spoon.
4. Do not dilute rehydration solutions with water.

### Client/Family Teaching
1. Soft foods such as bananas, cereal, cooked peas, beans, and potatoes should be given to maintain nutrition.

2. Report if fluid output exceeds intake, if there is no weight gain, or if clinical symptoms of dehydration persist.

3. If vomiting occurs after PO therapy is initiated, continue therapy but give small amounts, frequently and slowly.

4. If dehydration is severe, seek medical attention immediately. IV fluids and electrolytes should be started since the onset of action of PO solution is too slow. Oral solution can be used later for maintenance.

**Outcomes/Evaluate**

• Adequate hydration
• Prevention of electrolyte depletion

---

# Dezocine

(**DEZ**-oh-seen)
**Pregnancy Category:** C
Dalgan **(Rx)**
**Classification:** Narcotic agonist-antagonist analgesic

See also *Narcotic Analgesics.*

**Action/Kinetics:** Dezocine is a parenteral narcotic analgesic possessing both agonist and antagonist activity. Similar to morphine with respect to analgesic potency and onset and duration of action. Less risk of abuse due to the mixed agonist-antagonist properties of the drug. The narcotic antagonist activity is greater than that of pentazocine. **Onset:** Approximately 30 min after IM and approximately 15 min after IV. **Peak effect:** 30–150 min. **Peak plasma levels:** 10–38 ng/mL after a 10-mg dose. **Duration:** 2–4 hr. **t½, after IV:** 2.4 hr. Approximately two-thirds of a dose is excreted in the urine mostly as the glucuronide conjugate.

**Uses:** Analgesic when use of a narcotic is desirable.

**Contraindications:** Lactation. Individuals dependent on narcotics. SC administration.

**Special Concerns:** Elderly clients are at an increased risk for altered respiratory patterns and mental changes.

**Side Effects:** *CNS:* Sedation (common), dizziness, vertigo, confusion, anxiety, crying, sleep disturbances, delusions, headache, depression, delirium. *Respiratory:* Respiratory depression, atelectasis. *CV:* Hypotension, irregular heart or pulse, hypertension, chest pain, pallor, thrombophlebitis. *GI:* N&V, dry mouth, constipation, abdominal pain, diarrhea. *Dermatologic:* Reactions at the injection site, pruritus, rash, erythema. *EENT:* Diplopia, blurred vision, congestion in ears, tinnitus. *GU:* Urinary frequency, retention, or hesitancy. *Miscellaneous:* Sweating, chills, edema, flushing, low hemoglobin, muscle cramps or aches, muscle pain, slurred speech.

**OD** **Overdose Management:** *Treatment:* Naloxone IV with appropriate supportive measures including oxygen, IV fluids, vasopressors, and artificial respiration.

**Drug Interactions:** Additive depressant effect when used with general anesthetics, sedatives, antianxiety drugs, hypnotics, alcohol, and other opiate analgesics.

**Dosage** ――――――――――

• **IM**
   *Analgesia.*
**Adults:** 5–20 mg (usual is 10 mg) as a single dose; dose may be repeated q 3–6 hr with dosage adjusted, if necessary, depending on the status of the client.

• **IV**
   *Analgesia.*
**Adults:** 2.5–10 mg (usual initial dose is 5 mg) repeated q 2–4 hr.

## NURSING CONSIDERATIONS

See also *Nursing Considerations* for *Narcotic Analgesics.*

**Administration/Storage**

1. The maximum single dose should not exceed 20 mg and the maximum daily dose should not exceed 120 mg.

2. Dezocine can be stored at room temperature protected from light.

---

Do not use solution if it contains a precipitate.

**Assessment**

1. Note any sulfite; drug contains sodium metabisulfite. Monitor for evidence of allergic reaction.

2. Determine any history or current use of opiate drugs; may precipitate an acute withdrawal syndrome.

3. Document location, onset, duration, and intensity of pain; note alleviating factors.

4. Note any evidence of impaired renal or liver function; anticipate reduced dose with dysfunction.

5. Assess for any evidence of head injury or increased ICP. If administered with CNS depressants, reduce the dose of one or both agents.

6. Geriatric clients should receive reduced doses and be individually evaluated for subsequent dose levels.

**Client/Family Teaching**

1. Do not drive or operate dangerous machinery until drug effects have worn off.

2. Avoid alcohol and the use of any unprescribed sedatives, hypnotics, or antianxiety agents.

**Outcomes/Evaluate:** Effective pain control, as evidenced by ↑ activity, improved appetite, and reports of relief

---

# Diazepam

(dye-**AYZ**-eh-pam)

**Pregnancy Category:** D

Apo-Diazepam ✲, Diastat, Diazemuls ✲, Diazepam Intensol, Dizac, E Pam ✲, Meval ✲, Novo-Dipam ✲, PMS-Diazepam ✲, Valium, Valium Roche ✲, Vivol ✲ **(C-IV) (Rx)**

**Classification:** Antianxiety agent, anticonvulsant, skeletal muscle relaxant

---

See also *Tranquilizers.*

**Action/Kinetics:** The skeletal muscle relaxant effect of diazepam may be due to enhancement of GABA-mediated presynaptic inhibition at the spinal level as well as in the brain stem reticular formation. **Onset: PO,** 30–60 min; **IM,** 15–30 min; **IV,** more rapid. **Peak plasma levels: PO,** 0.5–2 hr; **IM,** 0.5–1.5; **IV,** 0.25

hr. **Duration:** 3 hr. **t½:** 20–50 hr. Metabolized in the liver to the active metabolites desmethyldiazepam, oxazepam, and temazepam. Diazepam and metabolites are excreted through the urine. Diazepam is 97%–99% bound to plasma protein.

**Uses:** Anxiety, tension (more effective than chlordiazepoxide), alcohol withdrawal, muscle relaxant, adjunct to treat seizure disorders, antipanic drug. Used prior to gastroscopy and esophagoscopy, preoperatively and prior to cardioversion. In dentistry to induce sedation. Treatment of status epilepticus. Relief of skeletal muscle spasm due to inflammation of muscles or joints or trauma; spasticity caused by upper motor neuron disorders such as cerebral palsy and paraplegia; athetotis; and stiff-man syndrome. Relieve spasms of facial muscles in occlusion and temporomandibular joint disorders. IV: Status epilepticus, severe recurrent seizures, and tetanus. Rectal gel: Treat epilepsy in those with stable regimens of anticonvulsant drugs who require intermittent diazepam to control increased seizure activity.

**Additional Contraindications:** Narrow-angle glaucoma, children under 6 months, lactation, and parenterally in children under 12 years.

**Special Concerns:** When used as an adjunct for seizure disorders, diazepam may increase the frequency or severity of clonic-tonic seizures, for which an increase in the dose of anticonvulsant medication is necessary. Safety and efficacy of parenteral diazepam have not been determined in neonates less than 30 days of age. Prolonged CNS depression has been observed in neonates, probably due to inability to biotransform diazepam into inactive metabolites.

**Additional Drug Interactions**

Diazepam potentiates antihypertensive effects of thiazides and other diuretics.

Diazepam potentiates muscle relaxant effects of *d*-tubocurarine and gallamine.

*Fluoxetine* / ↑ half-life of diazepam.
*Isoniazid* / ↑ half-life of diazepam.
*Ranitidine* / ↓ GI absorption of diazepam.

## Dosage

### • Tablets, Oral Solution

*Antianxiety, anticonvulsant, adjunct to skeletal muscle relaxants.*
**Adults:** 2–10 mg b.i.d.–q.i.d. **Elderly, debilitated clients:** 2–2.5 mg 1–2 times/day. May be gradually increased to adult level. **Pediatric, over 6 months, initial:** 1–2.5 mg (0.04–0.2 mg/kg or 1.17–6 mg/m²) b.i.d.–t.i.d.
*Alcohol withdrawal.*
**Adults:** 10 mg t.i.d.–q.i.d. during the first 24 hr; **then,** decrease to 5 mg t.i.d.–q.i.d. as required.
*Anticonvulsant.*
**Adults:** 15–30 mg once daily.

### • Rectal Gel

*Anticonvulsant.*
**Over 12 years:** 0.2 mg/kg. **Children, 6–11 years:** 0.3 mg/kg; **2–5 years:** 0.5 mg/kg. If required, a second dose can be given 4 to 12 hr after the first dose. Do not treat more than five episodes per month or more than one episode every 5 days. Adjust dose downward in elderly or debilitated clients to reduce ataxia or oversedation.

### • IM, IV

*Preoperative or diagnostic use.*
**Adults:** 10 mg IM 5–30 min before procedure.
*Adjunct to treat skeletal muscle spasm.*
**Adults, initial:** 5–10 mg IM or IV; **then,** repeat in 3–4 hr if needed (larger doses may be required for tetanus).
*Moderate anxiety.*
**Adults:** 2–5 mg IM or IV q 3–4 hr if necessary.
*Severe anxiety, muscle spasm.*
**Adults:** 5–10 mg IM or IV q 3–4 hr, if necessary.
*Acute alcohol withdrawal.*
**Initial:** 10 mg IM or IV; **then,** 5–10 mg q 3–4 hr.
*Preoperatively.*

**Adults:** 10 mg IM prior to surgery.
*Endoscopy.*
**IV:** 10 mg or less although doses up to 20 mg can be used; **IM:** 5–10 mg 30 min prior to procedure.
*Cardioversion.*
**IV:** 5–15 mg 5–10 min prior to procedure.
*Tetanus in children.*
**IM, IV, over 1 month:** 1–2 mg, repeated q 3–4 hr as necessary; **5 years and over:** 5–10 mg q 3–4 hr.

### • IV

*Status epilepticus.*
**Adults, initial:** 5–10 mg; **then,** dose may be repeated at 10–15-min intervals up to a maximum dose of 30 mg. Dosage may be repeated after 2–4 hr. **Children, 1 month–5 years:** 0.2–0.5 mg q 2–5 min, up to maximum of 5 mg. Can be repeated in 2–4 hr. **5 years and older:** 1 mg q 2–5 min up to a maximum of 10 mg; dose can be repeated in 2–4 hr, if needed.

*NOTE:* Elderly or debilitated clients should not receive more than 5 mg parenterally at any one time.

## NURSING CONSIDERATIONS

See also *Nursing Considerations* for *Tranquilizers.*

### Administration/Storage

1. Mix the Intensol solution with beverages such as water, soda, and juices or soft foods such as applesauce or puddings. Use only the calibrated dropper provided to withdraw the medication. Once the medication is withdrawn and mixed, use immediately.
2. Except for the deltoid muscle, absorption from IM sites is slow and erratic.
**IV** 3. The IV route is preferred in the convulsing client.
4. Dizac, which is an emulsified injection, should only be given IV; it is not to be given IM or SC.
5. Parenteral administration may cause bradycardia, respiratory or cardiac arrest; have emergency equipment and drugs available.

---

6. Diazepam interacts with plastic; therefore, introducing diazepam into plastic containers or administration sets will decrease availability of the drug.

7. To reduce reactions at the IV site, give diazepam slowly (5 mg/min); avoid small veins or intra-arterial administration. For pediatric use, give the IV solution slowly over a 3-min period at a dose not exceeding 0.25 mg/kg. The initial dose can be repeated after 15–30 min.

8. Due to the possibility of precipitation and instability, do not infuse diazepam. Do not mix or dilute with other solutions or drugs in the syringe or infusion container.

**Assessment**

1. Document indications for therapy and time frame for anticipated results.

2. Determine any depression or drug abuse. Avoid simultaneous use of CNS depressants.

3. Anticipate a gradual reduction of drug to avoid withdrawal symptoms such as anxiety, tremors, anorexia, insomnia, weakness, headache, and N&V.

4. Monitor CBC, platelets, liver and renal function studies.

5. Review anxiety level and identify any contributing factors.

6. Elderly clients may experience adverse reactions more quickly than younger clients; use a lower dose in this group.

**Client/Family Teaching**

1. Drug may cause dizziness and drowsiness. Avoid activities that require mental alertness until drug effects realized.

2. Avoid alcohol and any other CNS depressants.

3. Notify provider if pregnancy suspected.

**Outcomes/Evaluate**
- ↓ Anxiety/tension episodes
- Control alcohol withdrawal
- Control of status epilepticus
- Relief of muscle spasms
- Effective sedation

# Diazoxide IV
(dye-az-**OX**-eyed)
**Pregnancy Category:** C
Hyperstat IV **(Rx)**
**Classification:** Antihypertensive, direct action on vascular smooth muscle

See also *Antihypertensive Agents* and *Diazoxide Oral*.

**Action/Kinetics:** Exerts a direct action on vascular smooth muscle to cause arteriolar vasodilation and decreased peripheral resistance. **Onset:** 1–5 min. **Time to peak effect:** 2–5 min. **Duration** (variable): usual, 3–12 hr. Excreted through the kidney (50% unchanged).

**Uses:** May be the drug of choice for hypertensive crisis (malignant and nonmalignant hypertension) in hospitalized adults and children. Often given concomitantly with a diuretic. Especially suitable for clients with impaired renal function, hypertensive encephalopathy, hypertension complicated by LV failure, and eclampsia. Ineffective for hypertension due to pheochromocytoma.

**Contraindications:** Hypersensitivity to drug or thiazide diuretics. Treatment of compensatory hypertension due to aortic coarctation or AV shunt. Dissecting aortic aneurysm.

**Special Concerns:** A decrease in dose may be necessary in geriatric clients due to age-related decreases in renal function. If given prior to delivery, fetal or neonatal hyperbilirubinemia, thrombocytopenia, or altered carbohydrate metabolism may result. Use with caution during lactation and in clients with impaired cerebral or cardiac circulation.

**Side Effects:** *CV:* Hypotension (may be severe enough to cause shock), sodium and water retention, especially in clients with impaired cardiac reserve, *atrial or ventricular arrhythmias, cerebral or myocardial ischemia,* marked ECG changes with possibility of *MI*, palpitations, bradycardia, SVT, chest discomfort or nonanginal chest tightness. *CNS:*

Cerebral ischemia manifested by unconsciousness, *seizures,* paralysis, confusion, numbness of the hands. Headache, dizziness, weakness, drowsiness, lightheadedness, somnolence, lethargy, euphoria, weakness of short duration, apprehension, anxiety, malaise, blurred vision. *Respiratory:* Tightness in chest, cough, dyspnea, sensation of choking. *GI:* N&V, diarrhea, anorexia, parotid swelling, change in sense of taste, salivation, dry mouth, ileus, constipation, acute pancreatitis (rare). *Other:* Hyperglycemia (may be serious enough to require treatment), sweating, flushing, sensation of warmth, transient neurologic findings due to alteration in regional blood flow to the brain, hyperosmolar coma in infants, tinnitus, hearing loss, retention of nitrogenous wastes, acute pancreatitis, back pain, increased nocturia, lacrimation, hypersensitivity reactions, papilledema, hirsutism, decreased libido. Pain, cellulitis without sloughing, warmth or pain along injected vein, phlebitis at injection site, extravasation.

**OD** **Overdose Management:** *Symptoms:* Hypotension, excessive hyperglycemia. *Treatment:* Use the Trendelenburg maneuver to reverse hypotension.

**Drug Interactions**
*Anticoagulants, oral* / ↑ Effect of oral anticoagulants due to ↓ plasma protein binding
*Nitrites* / ↑ Hypotensive effect
*Phenytoin* / Diazoxide ↓ anticonvulsant effect of phenytoin
*Reserpine* / ↑ Hypotensive effect
*Sulfonylureas* / Destablization of the client resulting in hyperglycemia
*Thiazide diuretics* / ↑ Hyperglycemic, hyperuricemic, and antihypertensive effect of diazoxide
*Vasodilators, peripheral* / ↑ Hypotensive effect
**Laboratory Test Interferences:** False + or ↑ uric acid.

**Dosage** ———————
• **IV Push (30 sec or less)**
*Hypertensive crisis.*

**Adults:** 1–3 mg/kg up to a maximum of 150 mg; may be repeated at 5–15-min intervals until adequate BP response obtained. Drug may then be repeated at 4–24-hr intervals for 4–5 days or until oral antihypertensive therapy can be initiated. **Pediatric:** 1–3 mg/kg (30–90 mg/m²) using the same dosing intervals as adults.

Repeated use can result in sodium and water retention; therefore, a diuretic may be needed to avoid CHF and for maximum reduction of BP.

## NURSING CONSIDERATIONS

See also *Nursing Considerations* for *Antihypertensive Agents* and *Diazoxide oral.*

**Administration/Storage**
**IV** 1. Do not administer IM or SC. Medication is highly alkaline.
2. Ensure patency and inject rapidly (30 sec) undiluted into a peripheral vein to maximize response.
3. Assess site for signs of irritation or extravasation. If extravasation occurs, apply ice packs.
4. Protect from light, heat, and freezing.
5. Have a sympathomimetic drug, such as norepinephrine, to treat severe hypotension should it occur.
6. Protect ampules from light and store between 2°C and 30°C (36°F and 86°F).

**Assessment**
1. Assess for hypersensitivity to thiazide diuretics, sulfa drugs, or diazoxide.
2. With diabetics, can cause serious elevations in blood sugar levels. Note complaints of sweating, flushing, or evidence of hyperglycemia and be prepared to treat
3. Obtain uric acid level and assess for evidence of hyperuricemia.
4. Monitor BP frequently until stabilized, then every hour thereafter until crisis resolved. Obtain final BP upon arising, prior to ambulation. Keep in a recumbent position during and for 30 min after injection to avoid orthostatic hypotension, for

8–10 hr if furosemide is also administered.

**Outcomes/Evaluate:** Significant reduction in BP during hypertensive crisis

---

**D**

# Diazoxide oral

(dye-az-**OX**-eyed)
**Pregnancy Category:** C
Proglycem **(Rx)**
**Classification:** Insulin antagonist, hypotensive agent

---

**Action/Kinetics:** Related to the thiazide diuretics. It inhibits the release of insulin from beta islet cells of the pancreas, leading to an increase in blood glucose levels. Effect is dose related. Causes sodium, potassium, uric acid, and water retention. Other effects include increased pulse rate, increased serum uric acid levels, increased serum free fatty acids, decreased para-aminohippuric acid clearance from the kidneys (little effect on GFR). **Onset:** 1 hr. **t½:** 28 hr (up to 53 hr in clients with anuria). **Duration:** 8 hr. The drug is over 90% bound to plasma proteins. Metabolized in the liver although 50% is excreted through the kidneys unchanged.

**Uses:** Management of hypoglycemia due to hyperinsulinism, including inoperable islet cell adenoma or carcinoma or extrapancreatic malignancies in adults. In children, for treatment of hyperinsulinemia due to leucine sensitivity , islet cell hyperplasia, nesidioblastosis, extrapancreatic malignancy, islet cell adenoma or adenomatosis. The drug is used parenterally as an antihypertensive agent (see *Diazoxide* ).

**Contraindications:** Functional hypoglycemia, hypersensitivity to diazoxide or thiazides.

**Special Concerns:** Infants are particularly prone to development of edema. Use with extreme caution in clients with history of gout and in those in whom edema presents a risk (cardiac disease).

**Side Effects:** *CV:* Sodium and fluid retention (common); precipitation of CHF in clients with compromised cardiac reserve, palpitations, increased HR, hypotension, transient hypertension, chest pain (rare). *Metabolic:* Hyperglycemia, glycosuria, **diabetic ketoacidosis, hyperosmolar nonketotic coma.** *GI:* N&V, diarrhea, transient taste loss, anorexia, ileus, abdominal pain. *CNS:* Weakness, headache, insomnia, extrapyramidal symptoms, dizziness, paresthesia, fever, malaise, anxiety, polyneuritis. *Hematologic:* Thrombocytopenia with or without purpura, eosinophilia, neutropenia, decreased hemoglobin/hematocrit, excessive bleeding, decreased IgG. *Dermatologic:* Skin rashes, hirsutism, herpes, loss of hair from scalp, monilial dermatitis, pruritus. *GU:* Hematuria, decrease in urine production, nephrotic syndrome (reversible), azotemia, albuminuria. *Ophthalmologic:* Blurred or double vision, lacrimation, transient cataracts, ring scotoma, subconjunctival hemorrhage. *Other:* Pancreatitis, **pancreatic necrosis,** galactorrhea, gout, premature aging of bone, polyneuritis, enlargement of lump in breast.

**OD** **Overdose Management:** *Symptoms:* Hypotension; excessive hyperglycemia. *Treatment:* Insulin to treat hyperglycemia; use Trendelenburg maneuver to reverse hypotension.

**Drug Interactions**
*Alpha-adrenergic blocking agents* / ↓ Effect of diazoxide
*Anticoagulants, oral* / ↑ Effect of anticoagulant due to ↓ plasma protein binding
*Antihypertensives* / Excessive ↓ BP due to additive effects
*Phenothiazines* / ↑ Effects of diazoxide, including hyperglycemia
*Phenytoin* / ↓ Effect of phenytoin due to ↑ breakdown by liver
*Sulfonylureas* / ↓ Effect of both drugs
*Thiazide diuretics* / ↑ Hyperglycemic and hyperuricemic effects; hypotension may occur.
**Laboratory Test Interferences:** ↑ Serum uric acid, AST, alkaline phosphatase; ↓ creatinine clearance.

**Dosage**
- **Capsules, Oral Suspension**
  *Diabetes.*

Dosage is individualized on the basis of blood glucose level and response of client. **Adults and children, usual, initial:** 1 mg/kg q 8 hr (adjust according to response); **maintenance:** 3–8 mg/kg/day divided into two or three equal doses q 8–12 hr. **Infants and newborns, initial:** 3.3 mg/kg q 8 hr (adjust according to response); **maintenance:** 8–15 mg/kg/day divided into two or three equal doses q 8–12 hr.

## NURSING CONSIDERATIONS
**Administration/Storage:**
1. Blood glucose levels and urinary glucose and ketones must be monitored carefully until stabilized, which usually takes 1 week. Have available insulin and IV fluids to counteract possible ketoacidosis. Discontinue if a satisfactory effect has not been established within 2–3 weeks.
2. Take on a regular basis with no doses skipped and no extra doses taken.
3. Protect the suspension from light.
**Assessment**
1. Document indications for therapy and time frame for anticipated results. Note sensitivity to thiazides.
2. Determine any history of gout or CAD.
3. Monitor BP for potentiation of antihypertensive effect if currently taking an antihypertensive agent.
4. With overdosage of drug, observe closely for the first 7 days until blood sugar level is again within normal limits (80–110 mg/100 mL).
5. Review list of drug side effects to determine if clinical presentations may be drug related.
**Client/Family Teaching**
1. Report unusual bruising or bleeding; may require drug discontinuation.
2. With history of CHF, observe carefully for fluid retention; could precipitate heart failure.

3. If excessive hair growth develops, should subside once drug discontinued.
**Outcomes/Evaluate:** Control of hypoglycemia with restoration of glucose levels

**D**

# Diclofenac potassium
(dye-**KLOH**-fen-ack)
**Pregnancy Category:** B
Cataflam **(Rx)**

# Diclofenac sodium
(dye-**KLOH**-fen-ack)
**Pregnancy Category:** B
Apo-Diclo ✿, Apo-Diclo SR ✿, Novo–Difenac ✿, Novo–Difenac SR ✿, Nu-Diclo ✿, Taro-Diclofenac ✿, Voltaren, Voltaren Ophtha ✿, Voltaren Ophthalmic, Voltaren SR ✿, Voltaren-XR **(Rx)**
**Classification:** Nonsteroidal anti-inflammatory analgesic

See also *Nonsteroidal Anti-Inflammatory Drugs.*
**Action/Kinetics:** Available as both the potassium (immediate-release) and sodium (delayed-release) salts. *Immediate-release product.* **Onset:** 30 min. **Peak plasma levels:** 1 hr. **Duration:** 8 hr. *Delayed-release product.* **Peak plasma levels:** 2–3 hr. **t½:** 1–2 hr. For all dosage forms, food will affect the rate, but not the amount, absorbed from the GI tract. Metabolized in the liver and excreted by the kidneys.
**Uses:** *PO, Immediate-release:* Analgesic, primary dysmenorrhea. *PO, Immediate- or Delayed-release:* Rheumatoid arthritis, osteoarthritis, ankylosing spondylitis. *PO, Delayed-release:* Osteoarthritis, rheumatoid arthritis. *Investigational:* Mild to moderate pain, juvenile rheumatoid arthritis, acute painful shoulder, sunburn. *Ophthalmic:* Postoperative inflammation following cataract extraction.
**Contraindications:** Wearers of soft contact lenses.
**Special Concerns:** Use with caution during lactation. Safety and effectiveness has not been deter-

mined in children. When used ophthalmically, may cause increased bleeding of ocular tissues in conjunction with ocular surgery. Healing may be slowed or delayed.

**Side Effects:** *Following ophthalmic use:* Keratitis, increased intraocular pressure, ocular allergy, N&V, anterior chamber reaction, viral infections, transient burning and stinging on administration. When used with soft contact lenses, may cause ocular irritation, including redness and burning.

**Dosage** ——————————————
- **Immediate-Release    Tablets, Delayed-Release Tablets**

*Analgesia, primary dysmenorrhea.*
**Adults:** 50 mg t.i.d. of immediate-release tablets. In some, an initial dose of 100 mg followed by 50-mg doses may achieve better results. After the first day, the total daily dose should not exceed 150 mg.

*Rheumatoid arthritis.*
**Adults:** 100–200 mg/day in divided doses (e.g., 50 mg t.i.d. or q.i.d.; 75 mg b.i.d. of the sodium salt). For chronic therapy, use extended-release tablets, 100 mg once or twice daily, not to exceed 225 mg/day.

*Osteoarthritis.*
**Adults:** 100–150 mg/day in divided doses (e.g., 50 mg b.i.d. or t.i.d.; 75 mg b.i.d. of the sodium salt). For chronic therapy, use extended-release tablets, 100 mg/day. Doses greater than 200 mg/day have not been evaluated.

*Ankylosing spondylitis.*
**Adults:** 25 mg q.i.d. with an extra 25-mg dose at bedtime, if necessary. Doses greater than 125 mg/day have not been evaluated.
- **Ophthalmic Solution**

1 gtt of the 0.1% solution in the affected eye q.i.d. beginning 24 hr after cataract surgery and for 2 weeks thereafter.

## NURSING CONSIDERATIONS

See also *Nursing Considerations* for *Nonsteroidal Anti-Inflammatory Drugs.*

**Administration/Storage:** Up to 3 weeks may be required for beneficial effects to be realized when used for rheumatoid arthritis or osteoarthritis.

**Assessment**
1. Assess for redness, infection, pain, or vision changes with ophthalmic therapy.
2. With arthritis, assess joints for inflammation, ROM, and loss of function.
3. Monitor CBC, liver and renal function studies; test stool for occult blood with long-term therapy.
4. Ensure that drug is administered in high enough doses for anti-inflammatory effect when needed and in the lower doses for an analgesic effect.

**Client/Family Teaching**
1. May be taken with meals, a full glass of water or milk if GI upset occurs.
2. Do not crush or chew delayed-release tablets.
3. Limit intake of sodium, monitor weights, and report any evidence of edema or unusual weight gain.
4. Clients with diabetes should monitor blood sugar levels closely as drug may alter response to antidiabetic agents.
5. Avoid alcohol and OTC products.
6. Maintain fluid intake of 2 L/day.
7. Report any changes in stools.

**Outcomes/Evaluate**
- Relief of joint pain and inflammation with improved mobility
- Control of eye inflammation

## Dicloxacillin sodium

(dye-klox-ah-**SILL**-in)
**Pregnancy Category:** B
Dycill, Dynapen, Pathocil **(Rx)**
**Classification:** Antibiotic, penicillin

See also *Anti-Infectives* and *Penicillins.*

**Action/Kinetics:** Penicillinase-resistant and acid-resistant. **Peak serum levels: IM, PO,** 4–20 mcg/mL after 1 hr. **t½:** 40 min. Chiefly excreted in urine.

**Uses:** Resistant staphylococcal infections. To initiate therapy in any suspected staphylococcal infection. Infections due to Streptococcus pneumoniae.

**Contraindications:** Treatment of meningitis.

**Dosage**
- **Capsules, Oral Suspension**
  *Skin and soft tissue infections, mild to moderate URTIs.*

**Adults and children over 40 kg:** 125 mg q 6 hr; **pediatric:** 12.5 mg/kg/day in four equal doses given q 6 hr.

*Lower respiratory tract infections or disseminated infections.*

**Adults and children over 40 kg:** 250 mg q 6 hr, up to a maximum of 4 g/day; **pediatric:** 12–25 mg/kg/day in four equal doses given q 6 hr. Dosage not established for the newborn.

## NURSING CONSIDERATIONS

See also *General Nursing Considerations for All Anti-Infectives* and *Penicillins.*

**Administration/Storage**

1. To prepare PO suspension, shake container to loosen powder, measure water for reconstitution as indicated on label, add half of the water, and immediately shake vigorously because usual handling may cause lumps. Add the remainder of the water and again shake vigorously.
2. Shake well before pouring each dose.
3. The reconstituted PO solution is stable for 7 days at room temperature, 10 days if refrigerated, and 21 days if frozen.

**Assessment:** Note indications for therapy, onset and duration of symptoms. Obtain cultures when indicated.

**Client/Family Teaching:** Take at least 1 hr before meals or no sooner than 2–3 hr after a meal with a full glass of water.

**Outcomes/Evaluate:** Symptomatic relief; negative cultures with resolution of infection

# Dicyclomine hydrochloride
(dye-**SYE**-kloh-meen)

**Pregnancy Category:** C

Antispas, A-Spas, Bentyl, Bentylol ✿, Byclomine, Dibent, Di-Cyclonex, Dilomine, Di-Spaz, Formulex ✿, Or-Tyl **(Rx)**

**Classification:** Cholinergic blocking agent

See also *Cholinergic Blocking Agents.*

**Action/Kinetics: t½, initial:** 1.8 hr; **secondary:** 9–10 hr.

**Uses:** Hypermotility and spasms of GI tract associated with irritable colon and spastic colitis, mucous colitis.

**Additional Contraindications:** Use for peptic ulcer.

**Special Concerns:** Lower doses may be needed in elderly clients due to confusion, agitation, excitement, or drowsiness.

**Additional Side Effects:** Brief euphoria, slight dizziness, feeling of abdominal distention. **Use of the syrup in infants less than 3 months of age:** *Seizures,* syncope, respiratory symptoms, fluctuations in pulse rate, *asphyxia,* muscular hypotonia, ***coma.***

**Dosage**
- **Capsules, Syrup, Tablets**
  *Hypermotility and spasms of GI tract.*

**Adults:** 10–20 mg t.i.d.–q.i.d.; **then,** may increase to total daily dose of 160 mg if side effects do not limit this dosage. **Pediatric, 6 years and older, capsules or tablets:** 10 mg t.i.d.–q.i.d.; adjust dosage to need and incidence of side effects. **Pediatric, 6 months–2 years, syrup:** 5–10 mg t.i.d.–q.i.d.; **2 years and older:** 10 mg t.i.d.–q.i.d. The dose should be adjusted to need and incidence of side effects.

- **IM**
  *Hypermotility and spasms of GI tract.*

**Adults:** 20 mg q 4–6 hr. **Not for IV use.**

---

✿ = Available in Canada          ***bold italic*** = life threatening side effect

## NURSING CONSIDERATIONS

See also *Nursing Considerations* for *Cholinergic Blocking Agents*.
**Administration/Storage:** Can be administered to clients with glaucoma.
**Assessment**
1. Document indications for therapy, onset and duration of symptoms.
2. List other agents trialed and the outcome.
3. Determine any presence of PUD.
**Outcomes/Evaluate:** Restoration of normal bowel function and GI motility

---

# Didanosine (ddI, dideoxyinosine)

(die-**DAN**-oh-seen)
**Pregnancy Category:** B
Videx **(Rx)**
**Classification:** Antiviral

---

See also *Antiviral Agents*.
**Action/Kinetics:** Didanosine is a nucleoside analog of deoxyadenosine. After entering the cell, it is converted to the active dideoxyadenosine triphosphate (ddATP) by cellular enzymes. Due to the chemical structure of ddATP, its incorporation into viral DNA leads to chain termination and therefore inhibition of viral replication. ddATP also inhibits viral replication by interfering with the HIV–RNA-dependent DNA polymerase by competing with the natural nucleoside triphosphate for binding to the active site of the enzyme. Didanosine has shown in vitro antiviral activity in a variety of HIV-infected T cell and monocyte/macrophage cell cultures. Is broken down quickly at acidic pH; therefore, PO products contain buffering agents to increase the pH of the stomach. Food decreases the rate of absorption. **t½, elimination:** 1.6 hr for adults and 0.8 hr for children. Metabolized in the liver and excreted mainly through the urine.
**Uses:** Advanced HIV infection in adult and pediatric (over 6 months of age) clients who are intolerant of AZT therapy or who have demonstrated decreased effectiveness of AZT therapy. Use in adults with HIV infection who have received prolonged AZT therapy. Treatment of HIV infection when antiretroviral therapy is indicated. AZT should be considered as initial therapy for the treatment of advanced HIV infection, unless contraindicated, since this drug prolongs survival and decreases the incidence of opportunistic infections. May be used as monotherapy for the treatment of AIDS.
**Contraindications:** Lactation.
**Special Concerns:** Use with caution in renal and hepatic impairment and in those on sodium-restricted diets. Opportunistic infections and other complications of HIV infection may continue to develop; thus, keep clients under close observation.
**Side Effects:** Commonly pancreatitis and peripheral neuropathy (manifested by distal numbness, tingling, or pain in the feet or hands). Neuropathy occurs more frequently in clients with a history of neuropathy or neurotoxic drug therapy.
**In adults.** *GI:* Diarrhea, abdominal pain, N&V, anorexia, dry mouth, ileus, colitis, constipation, eructation, flatulence, gastroenteritis, *GI hemorrhage,* oral moniliasis, stomatitis, mouth sores, sialadenitis, *stomach ulcer hemorrhage,* melena, oral thrush, liver abnormalities. *CNS:* Headache, *tonic-clonic seizures,* abnormal thinking, anxiety, nervousness, twitching, confusion, depression, acute brain syndrome, amnesia, aphasia, ataxia, dizziness, hyperesthesia, hypertonia, incoordination, *intracranial hemorrhage,* paralysis, paranoid reaction, psychosis, insomnia, sleep disorders, speech disorders, tremor. *Hematologic:* Leukopenia, granulocytopenia, thrombocytopenia, microcytic anemia, *hemorrhage,* ecchymosis, petechiae. *Dermatologic:* Rash, pruritus, herpes simplex, skin disorder, sweating, eczema, impetigo, excoriation, erythema. *Musculoskeletal:* Asthenia, myopathy, arthralgia, arthritis, myalgia, muscle atrophy, decreased strength, hemiparesis, neck rigidity, joint disorder, leg cramps.

*CV:* Chest pain, hypertension, hypotension, migraine, palpitation, peripheral vascular disorder, syncope, vasodilation, arrhythmias. *Body as a whole:* Chills, fever, infection, allergic reaction, pain, abscess, cellulitis, cyst, dehydration, malaise, flu syndrome, numbness of hands and feet, weight loss, alopecia. *Respiratory:* Pneumonia, dyspnea, asthma, bronchitis, increased cough, rhinitis, rhinorrhea, epistaxis, laryngitis, decreased lung function, pharyngitis, hypoventilation, sinusitis, rhonchi, rales, congestion, interstitial pneumonia, respiratory disorders. *Ophthalmic:* Blurred vision, conjunctivitis, diplopia, dry eye, glaucoma, retinitis, photophobia, strabismus. *Otic:* Ear disorder, otitis (externa and media), ear pain. *GU:* Impotency, kidney calculus, kidney failure, abnormal kidney function, nocturia, urinary frequency, vaginal hemorrhage. *Miscellaneous:* Peripheral edema, sarcoma, hernia, hypokalemia, lymphoma-like reaction.

**In children.** *GI:* Diarrhea, N&V, liver abnormalities, abdominal pain, stomatitis, mouth sores, pancreatitis, anorexia, increase in appetite, constipation, oral thrush, melena, dry mouth. *CNS:* Headache, nervousness, insomnia, dizziness, poor coordination, lethargy, neurologic symptoms, **seizures.** *Hematologic:* Ecchymosis, **hemorrhage,** petechaie, leukopenia, granulocytopenia, thrombocytopenia, anemia. *Dermatologic:* Rash, pruritus, skin disorder, eczema, sweating, impetigo, excoriation, erythema. *Musculoskeletal:* Arthritis, myalgia, muscle atrophy, decreased strength. *Body as a whole:* Chills, fever, asthenia, pain, malaise, failure to thrive, weight loss, flu syndrome, alopecia, dehydration. *CV:* Vasodilation, arrhythmia. *Respiratory:* Cough, rhinitis, dyspnea, asthma, rhinorrhea, epistaxis, pharyngitis, hypoventilation, sinusitis, rhonchi, rales, congestion, pneumonia. *Ophthalmic:* Photophobia, strabismus, visual impairment. *Otic:* Ear pain,

otitis. *Miscellaneous:* Urinary frequency, diabetes mellitus, diabetes insipidus, liver abnormalities.

**OD** **Overdose** **Management:** *Symptoms:* Pancreatitis, peripheral neuropathy, diarrhea, hyperuricemia, hepatic dysfunction. *Treatment:* There are no antidotes; treatment should be symptomatic.

**Drug Interactions**
*Ketoconazole* / ↓ Absorption of ketoconazole due to gastric pH change caused by buffering agents in didanosine
*Pentamidine (IV)* / ↑ Risk of pancreatitis
*Quinolone antibiotics* / ↓ Plasma levels of quinolone antibiotics
*Ranitidine* / ↓ Absorption of ranitidine due to gastric pH change caused by buffering agents in didanosine
*Tetracyclines* / ↓ Absorption of tetracyclines from the stomach due to the buffering agents in didanosine
**Laboratory Test Interferences:** ↑ AST, ALT, alkaline phosphatase, bilirubin, uric acid, amylase.

**Dosage**
• **Chewable/Dispersible Buffered Tablets, Buffered Powder for Oral Solution, Powder for Pediatric Oral Solution**
**Adults, initial, weight over 60 kg:** 200 mg q 12 hr (with 250 mg buffered powder q 12 hr). **Weight less than 60 kg:** 125 mg q 12 hr (with 167 mg buffered powder q 12 hr). **Pediatric, BSA 1.1–1.4 m²:** Two 50-mg tablets q 12 hr or 125 mg of the pediatric powder q 12 hr; **BSA 0.8–1.0 m²:** One 50- and one 25-mg tablet q 12 hr or 94 mg of the pediatric powder q 12 hr. **BSA 0.5–0.7 m²:** Two 25-mg tablets q 12 hr or 62 mg of the pediatric powder q 12 hr. **BSA less than 0.4 m²:** One 25-mg tablet q 12 hr or 31 mg of the pediatric powder q 12 hr.

## NURSING CONSIDERATIONS

See also *Nursing Considerations* for *Antiviral Agents.*

## Administration/Storage

1. Administer on an empty stomach.

2. To prevent gastric acid degradation, adult and pediatric (over 1 year) clients should take a 2-tablet dose. Pediatric clients under 12 months of age should receive a 1-tablet dose.

3. To prepare the buffered powder for PO solution, mix with 4 oz of drinking water; do not mix the powder with fruit juice or other acid-containing beverages. Stir the mixture until the powder dissolves completely (about 2–3 min). Consume the entire solution immediately.

4. To prepare the powder for pediatric oral solution, the dry powder must be mixed with purified water to an initial concentration of 20 mg/mL. The resulting solution is then mixed with antacid to a final concentration of 10 mg/mL. This admixture must be shaken thoroughly prior to use and may be stored in a tightly closed container in the refrigerator for up to 30 days.

## Assessment

1. Document all previous experience with AZT therapy; list reasons for transfer to didanosine.

2. Monitor CBC, CD$_4$ counts/viral load, liver and renal function studies.

3. Anticipate reduced dose with liver and renal impairment. Note baseline VS and weight.

## Client/Family Teaching

1. Food decreases the rate of drug absorption; take on empty stomach.

2. Do not swallow tablets whole. Tablets may be chewed or crushed thoroughly before taking or dispersed in at least 1 oz of drinking water (stir thoroughly and drink immediately).

3. Report any symptoms of neuropathy (numbness, burning, or tingling in the hands or feet); drug should be discontinued until symptoms subside. May tolerate a reduced dose once these symptoms resolved.

4. Report any abdominal pain and N&V immediately; may be clinical signs of pancreatitis. Stop drug and report; resume only after pancreatitis has been ruled out.

5. With sodium-restricted diets, sodium content is more in the single-dose packet than in the two-tablet dose.

6. Increase fluid intake; report S&S of diarrhea or hyperuricemia; dosage may require adjustment.

7. Any changes in vision should be evaluated by an ophthalmologist. Get retinal exams every 6 mo to rule out depigmentation with children.

8. Avoid alcohol and any other drugs that may exacerbate the toxicity of didanosine.

9. Remind that didanosine is not a cure, but it alleviates the symptoms of HIV infections; may continue to acquire opportunistic infections.

10. Didanosine *does not* reduce the risk of transmission of HIV to others through sexual contact or blood contamination; use appropriate precautions.

11. Identify local support groups that may assist client/family to understand and cope with disease.

**Outcomes/Evaluate:** Control of symptoms of AIDS, ARC, and opportunistic infections in clients with HIV who are intolerant or have clinically deteriorated during therapy with AZT

# Diethylstilbestrol diphosphate

(dye-eth-ill-still-**BESS**-trohl)
**Pregnancy Category:** X
Honvol ✶, Stilphostrol (Abbreviation: DES) **(Rx)**
**Classification:** Estrogen, synthetic, nonsteroidal

See also *Estrogens* and *Antineoplastic Agents.*

**Action/Kinetics:** Synthetic estrogen, which competes with androgen receptors, thereby preventing androgen from inducing further growth of the neoplasm. Also binds to cytoplasmic receptor protein. The estrogen-receptor complex translocates to the nucleus, where metabolic alterations ensue. Metabolized in the liver.

**Uses:** Palliative treatment of inoperable, progressive prostatic cancer. Postcoital contraceptive (emergency use only).

**Contraindications:** Known or suspected breast cancer, estrogen-dependent neoplasia, active thrombophlebitis, thromboembolic disease, markedly impaired liver function. **Not to be used during pregnancy because of the possibility of vaginal cancer in female offspring.** The diphosphate is not to be used to treat any disorder in women.

**Special Concerns:** Use with caution in presence of hypercalcemia, epilepsy, migraine, asthma, cardiac and renal disease. Use with caution in children in whom bone growth is incomplete.

**Side Effects:** *CV: **Thrombophlebitis, pulmonary embolism, cerebral thrombosis,*** neuro-ocular lesions. *GI:* N&V, anorexia. *CNS:* Headaches, malaise, irritability. *Skin:* Allergic rash, itching. *GU:* Gynecomastia, changes in libido. *Other:* Porphyria, backache, pain and sterile abscess at injection site, postinjection flare.

**Dosage** ————————————
* **Tablets**
  *Palliative treatment of prostatic carcinoma.*
  50 mg t.i.d. up to 200 mg t.i.d., not to exceed 1 g/day.
* **IV**
  *Palliative treatment of prostatic carcinoma.*
  500 mg (in 250 mL 5% dextrose or saline) on day 1 followed by 1 g (in 250–500 mL 5% dextrose or saline) daily for 5 days. **Maintenance, IV:** 250–500 mg 1–2 times/week. Maintenance dose may also be given PO.

## NURSING CONSIDERATIONS

See also *Nursing Considerations* for *Antineoplastic Agents* and *Estrogens*.

**Administration/Storage**

**IV** 1. Administer slowly by IV drip (20–30 gtt/min for first 10–15 min); then adjust for a total administration period of 1 hr.

2. Solution is stable for 5 days at room temperature if stored away from direct light. Do not use if cloudy or if a precipitate has formed.

**Assessment**

1. Document indications for therapy and onset of symptoms. Do not use the diphosphate to treat any disorder in women.

2. Note any history of thrombophlebitis, thromboembolic conditions, or impaired liver function.

3. Withhold and report high serum calcium levels; effect of the steroid and osteolytic metastases may result in hypercalcemia. Monitor closely (VS, weights, and I&O) once drug-induced hypercalcemia is corrected. Promote a high fluid intake to minimize hypercalcemia.

4. Assess client with poor cardiac function for edema; monitor ECG.

5. Determine if pregnant; not given during pregnancy because of the high incidence of genital tumors in offspring.

6. May prevent gynecomastia in men by administering low doses of radiation prior to initiating therapy.

**Client/Family Teaching**

1. Take with solid foods; may relieve nausea.

2. Report any ↑ N&V, lethargy, insomnia, anorexia, visual changes, SOB, or painful swelling of breasts or extremities.

3. With poor cardiac function, record daily weights and and check for edema.

4. Do not smoke.

5. Withdrawal bleeding may occur if drug stopped suddenly in females.

6. May alter amount of antidiabetic agent required.

7. May cause photosensitivity reaction; use protection.

**Outcomes/Evaluate:** Inhibition of malignant cell proliferation

————COMBINATION DRUG————

# Difenoxin hydrochloride with Atropine sulfate
(dye-fen-**OX**-in, **AH**-troh-peen)

---

**Pregnancy Category:** C
Motofen **(Rx)**
**Classification:** Antidiarrheal

See also *Cholinergic Blocking Agents.*

**Content:** Each tablet contains: *Antidiarrheal:* Difenoxin HCl, 1 mg. *Anticholinergic:* Atropine sulfate, 0.025 mg.

**Action/Kinetics:** Difenoxin is related chemically to meperidine; thus, atropine sulfate is incorporated to prevent deliberate overdosage. Difenoxin is the active metabolite of diphenoxylate and is effective at one-fifth the dosage of diphenoxylate. Slows intestinal motility by a local effect on the GI wall. **Peak plasma levels:** 40–60 min. The drug and its inactive metabolites are excreted through both the urine and feces.

**Uses:** Management of acute nonspecific diarrhea and acute episodes of chronic functional diarrhea.

**Contraindications:** Diarrhea caused by *Escherichia coli, Salmonella,* or *Shigella;* pseudomembranous colitis caused by broad-spectrum antibiotics; jaundice; children less than 2 years of age.

**Special Concerns:** Use with caution in ulcerative colitis, liver and kidney disease, lactation, and in clients receiving dependence-producing drugs or in those who are addiction prone. Safety and effectiveness in children less than 12 years of age have not been determined.

**Side Effects:** *GI:* N&V, dry mouth, epigastric distress, constipation. *CNS:* Lightheadedness, dizziness, drowsiness, headache, tiredness, nervousness, confusion, insomnia. *Ophthalmic:* Blurred vision, burning eyes.

**OD** **Overdose Management:** *Symptoms:* Initially include dry skin and mucous membranes, hyperthermia, flushing, and tachycardia. These are followed by hypotonic reflexes, nystagmus, miosis, lethargy, coma, and *respiratory depression* (may occur up to 30 hr after overdose taken). *Treatment:* Naloxone may be used to treat respiratory depression.

**Drug Interactions**
*Antianxiety agents* / Potentiation or addition of CNS depressant effects
*Barbiturates* / Potentiation or addition of CNS depressant effects
*Ethanol* / Potentiation or addition of CNS depressant effects
*MAO inhibitors* / Precipitation of hypertensive crisis
*Narcotics* / Potentiation or addition of CNS depressant effects

**Dosage**
• **Tablets**
**Adults, initial:** 2 tablets (2 mg difenoxin); **then,** 1 tablet (1 mg difenoxin) after each loose stool or 1 tablet q 3–4 hr as needed. Total dose during a 24-hr period should not exceed 8 mg (i.e., 8 tablets).

## NURSING CONSIDERATIONS

**Administration/Storage:** Treatment beyond 48 hr is usually not necessary for acute diarrhea or acute exacerbation of functional diarrhea and generally not recommended if clinical improvement is not noted.

**Assessment**
1. Note the onset, characteristics, and frequency of diarrhea; identify precipitating factors, e.g., travel, stress, food, medication regimens.
2. Assess for evidence of dehydration (weakness, weight loss, poor skin turgor, higher temperature, rapid weak pulse, or decreased urinary output) or electrolyte imbalance (weakness, irritability, anorexia, nausea, and dysrhythmias).
3. Send stool for analysis; C&S.
4. Monitor liver function studies; may precipitate hepatic coma with abnormal liver function.
5. Contains atropine sulfate.
6. May precipitate hypertensive crisis with MAO inhibitors.
7. With overdose, hospitalize, since latent (12–30 hr later) respiratory depression may occur.

**Client/Family Teaching**
1. Do not perform tasks that require mental alertness until drug effects are realized.

2. Take only as directed; do not share.

3. Chew sugarless gum; use sugarless candy or ice chips for dry mouth. Report any swelling of gums or extremity numbness.

4. Keep out of child's reach; may be fatal if ingested.

5. Do *not* take if breast feeding.

6. Avoid alcohol or any other unprescribed CNS depressants.

7. May take 24–36 hr before effects are evident. Record the number, frequency, and characteristics of the stools; report if symptoms persist for more than 5 days.

**Outcomes/Evaluate:** ↓ Frequency and number of diarrheal stools

# Diflunisal

(dye-**FLEW**-nih-sal)
**Pregnancy Category:** C
Apo-Diflunisal ✤, Dolobid, Novo-Diflunisal ✤, Nu-Diflunisal ✤ **(Rx)**
**Classification:** Nonsteroidal analgesic, anti-inflammatory, antipyretic

**Action/Kinetics:** Diflunisal is a salicylic acid derivative although it is not metabolized to salicylic acid. Mechanism not known; may be an inhibitor of prostaglandin synthetase. **Onset:** 20 min (analgesic, antipyretic). **Peak plasma levels:** 2–3 hr. **Peak effect:** 2–3 hr. **Duration:** 4–6 hr **t½:** 8–12 hr. Ninety-nine percent protein bound. Metabolites excreted in urine.

**Uses:** Analgesic, rheumatoid arthritis, osteoarthritis, ankylosing spondylitis, psoriatic arthritis, musculoskeletal pain. Prophylaxis and treatment of vascular headaches.

**Contraindications:** Hypersensitivity to diflunisal, aspirin, or other anti-inflammatory drugs. Acute asthmatic attacks, urticaria, or rhinitis precipitated by aspirin. During lactation and in children less than 12 years of age.

**Special Concerns:** Use with caution in presence of ulcers or in clients with a history thereof, in clients with hypertension, compromised cardiac function, or in conditions leading to

fluid retention. Use with caution in only first two trimesters of pregnancy. Geriatric clients may be at greater risk of GI toxicity.

**Side Effects:** *GI:* Nausea, dyspepsia, GI pain and bleeding, diarrhea, vomiting, constipation, flatulence, peptic ulcer, eructation, anorexia. *CNS:* Headache, fatigue, fever, malaise, dizziness, somnolence, insomnia, nervousness, vertigo, depression, paresthesias. *Dermatologic:* Rashes, pruritus, sweating, **Stevens-Johnson syndrome,** dry mucous membranes, erythema multiforme. *CV:* Palpitations, syncope, edema. *Other:* Tinnitus, asthenia, chest pain, hypersensitivity reactions, **anaphylaxis,** dyspnea, dysuria, muscle cramps, thrombocytopenia.

**OD** **Overdose Management:** *Symptoms:* Drowsiness, N&V, diarrhea, tachycardia, hyperventilation, stupor, disorientation, diminished urine output, **coma, cardiorespiratory arrest.** *Treatment:* Supportive measures. To empty the stomach, induce vomiting, or perform gastric lavage. Hemodialysis may not be effective since the drug is significantly bound to plasma protein.

**Drug Interactions**

*Acetaminophen /* ↑ Plasma levels of acetaminophen

*Antacids /* ↓ Plasma levels of diflunisal

*Anticoagulants /* ↑ PT

*Furosemide /* ↓ Hyperuricemic effect of furosemide

*Hydrochlorothiazide /* ↑ Plasma levels and ↓ hyperuricemic effect of hydrochlorothiazide

*Indomethacin /* ↓ Renal clearance of indomethacin → ↑ plasma levels

*Naproxen /* ↓ Urinary excretion of naproxen and metabolite

**Dosage**

• **Tablets**

*Mild to moderate pain.*

**Adults, initial:** 1,000 mg; **then,** 250–500 mg q 8–12 hr.

*Rheumatoid arthritis, osteoarthritis.*

**Adults:** 250–500 mg b.i.d. Doses in excess of 1,500 mg/day are not recommended. For some, an initial dose of 500 mg followed by 250 mg q 8–12 hr may be effective. Reduce dosage with impaired renal function.

## NURSING CONSIDERATIONS

**Administration/Storage:** Maximum relief occurs in 2–3 weeks when used for the pain and swelling of arthritis. Serum salicylate levels are not used as a guide to dosage or toxicity because the drug is not hydrolyzed to salicylic acid.

**Assessment**

1. Note any hypersensitivity to salicylates or other NSAIDs.
2. Determine any history of peptic ulcers, hypertension, or compromised cardiac function.
3. Check for pregnancy; avoid drug or use with extreme caution during the first two trimesters.
4. Give in high enough doses for anti-inflammatory effects when needed and use the lower dose for analgesic effects.
5. With long-term therapy, monitor CBC, liver and renal function studies.

**Client/Family Teaching**

1. May be given with water, milk, or meals to reduce gastric irritation. Do not crush or chew tablets.
2. Report unusual bruising or bleeding; may inhibit platelet aggregation which is reversible with drug discontinuation. Do not give with acetaminophen or aspirin.
3. May cause dizziness or drowsiness; use care when operating machinery or driving.
4. Report stool color changes or diarrhea; can cause an electrolyte imbalance or GI bleed.
5. Must take on a regular basis to sustain the anti-inflammatory effect of the drug.
6. Report for medical follow-up; drug needs to be adjusted according to age, condition, and changes in disease activity.

**Outcomes/Evaluate**

• ↓ Pain and inflammation; ↑ joint mobility
• Prevention of vascular headaches

# Digitoxin
(dih-jih-**TOX**-in)
**Pregnancy Category:** C
Crystodigin, Digitaline ✦ **(Rx)**
**Classification:** Cardiac glycoside

See also *Cardiac Glycosides.*
**Action/Kinetics:** Most potent of the digitalis glycosides. Slow onset makes it unsuitable for emergency use. Almost completely absorbed from GI tract. **Onset: PO,** 1–4 hr; maximum effect: 8–12 hr. **t½:** 5–9 days; **Duration:** 2 weeks. Significant protein binding (over 90%). Metabolized by the liver and excreted as inactive metabolites through the urine. **Therapeutic serum levels:** 14–26 ng/mL. Withhold drug and check with provider if serum level exceeds 35 ng/mL, indicating toxicity.
**Uses:** Maintenance in CHF.
**Special Concerns:** Digitalis tablets may not be suitable for small children; thus, other digitalis products should be considered.
**Additional Drug Interactions**
*Aminoglutethimide* / ↓ Effect of digitoxin due to ↑ breakdown by liver
*Barbiturates* / ↓ Effect of digitoxin due to ↑ breakdown by liver
*Diltiazem* / May ↑ serum levels of digitoxin
*Phenylbutazone* / ↓ Effect of digitoxin due to ↑ breakdown by liver
*Phenytoin* / ↓ Effect of digitoxin due to ↑ breakdown by liver
*Quinidine* / May ↑ serum levels of digitoxin
*Rifampin* / ↓ Effect of digitoxin due to ↑ breakdown by liver
*Verapamil* / May ↑ serum levels of digitoxin

**Dosage** ————————
• **Tablets**
   *Digitalizing (loading) dose: Rapid.*
**Adults:** 0.6 mg followed by 0.4 mg in 4–6 hr; **then,** 0.2 mg q 4–6 hr until therapeutic effect achieved.
   *Digitalizing (loading) dose: Slow.*
**Adults:** 0.2 mg b.i.d. for 4 days.
   *Digitalizing (loading) dose: children.*

After the neonatal period, the doses are as follows: **Under one year:** 0.045 mg/kg/day divided into three, four, or more doses with 6 hr between doses; **one to two years:** 0.04 mg/kg/day divided into three, four, or more doses with 6 hr between doses; **over two years:** 0.03 mg/kg/day (0.75 mg/m²) divided into three, four, or more doses with 6 hr between doses.

*Maintenance dose: PO.*
**Adults:** 0.05–0.3 mg/day (**usual:** 0.15 mg/day). **Children:** Give one-tenth of the digitalizing dose.

## NURSING CONSIDERATIONS

See also *Nursing Considerations* for *Cardiac Glycosides*.
**Administration/Storage**
1. Incompatible with acids and alkali.
2. Protect from light.
3. Premature/immature infants are especially sensitive to digitoxin; carefully determine lowered dose.
**Outcomes/Evaluate**
• Control of S&S of CHF
• Digitoxin level (14–26 ng/mL)

# Digoxin
(dih-**JOX**-in)
**Pregnancy Category:** A
Lanoxicaps, Lanoxin, Novo–Digoxin
✦ (Rx)
**Classification:** Cardiac glycoside

See also *Cardiac Glycosides*.
**Action/Kinetics:** Action prompter and shorter than that of digitoxin. **Onset: PO,** 0.5–2 hr; **time to peak effect:** 2–6 hr. **Duration:** Over 24 hr. **Onset, IV:** 5–30 min; **time to peak effect:** 1–4 hr. **Duration:** 6 days. **t½:** 30–40 hr. **Therapeutic serum level:** 0.5–2.0 ng/mL. From 20% to 25% is protein bound. Serum levels above 2.5 ng/mL indicate toxicity. Fifty percent to 70% is excreted unchanged by the kidneys. Bioavailability depends on the dosage form: tablets (60%–80%), capsules (90%–100%), and elixir (70%–85%). Thus, changing dosage

forms may require dosage adjustments.
**Uses:** May be drug of choice for CHF because of rapid onset, relatively short duration, and ability to be administered PO or IV.
**OD** **Overdose Management:** *Treatment:* See *Digoxin immune Fab.*
**Additional Drug Interactions**
1. The following drugs increase serum digoxin levels, leading to possible toxicity: Aminoglycosides, amiodarone, anticholinergics, benzodiazepines, captopril, diltiazem, erythromycin, esmolol, flecainide, hydroxychloroquine, ibuprofen, indomethacin, nifedipine, quinidine, quinine, tetracyclines, tolbutamide, verapamil.
2. Disopyramide may alter the pharmacologic effect of digoxin.
3. Penicillamine decreases serum digoxin levels.

**Dosage** ─────────────
• **Capsules**
*Digitalization: Rapid.*
**Adults:** 0.4–0.6 mg initially followed by 0.1–0.3 mg q 6–8 hr until desired effect achieved.
*Digitalization: Slow.*
**Adults:** A total of 0.05–0.35 mg/day divided in two doses for a period of 7–22 days to reach steady-state serum levels. **Pediatric.** Digitalizing dosage is divided into three or more doses with the initial dose being about one-half the total dose; doses are given q 4–8 hr. **Children, 10 years and older:** 0.008–0.012 mg/kg. **5–10 years:** 0.015–0.03 mg/kg. **2–5 years:** 0.025–0.035 mg/kg. **1 month–2 years:** 0.03–0.05 mg/kg. **Neonates, full-term:** 0.02–0.03 mg/kg. **Neonates, premature:** 0.015–0.025 mg/kg.
*Maintenance.*
**Adults:** 0.05–0.35 mg once or twice daily. **Premature neonates:** 20%–30% of total digitalizing dose divided and given in two to three daily doses. **Neonates to 10 years:** 25%–35% of the total digitalizing dose divided

and given in two to three daily doses.

• **Elixir, Tablets**
*Digitalization: Rapid.*
**Adults:** A total of 0.75–1.25 mg divided into two or more doses each given at 6–8-hr intervals.
*Digitalization: Slow.*
**Adults:** 0.125–0.5 mg/day for 7 days. **Pediatric.** (Digitalizing dose is divided into two or more doses and given at 6–8-hr intervals.) **Children, 10 years and older, rapid or slow:** Same as adult dose. **5–10 years:** 0.02–0.035 mg/kg. **2–5 years:** 0.03–0.05 mg/kg. **1 month–2 years:** 0.035–0.06 mg/kg. **Premature and newborn infants to 1 month:** 0.02–0.035 mg/kg.
*Maintenance.*
**Adults:** 0.125–0.5 mg/day. **Pediatric:** One-fifth to one-third the total digitalizing dose daily. *NOTE:* An alternate regimen (referred to as the "small-dose" method) is 0.017 mg/kg/day. This dose causes less toxicity.

• **IV**
*Digitalization.*
**Adults:** Same as tablets. **Maintenance:** 0.125–0.5 mg/day in divided doses or as a single dose. **Pediatric:** Same as tablets.

## NURSING CONSIDERATIONS

See also *Nursing Considerations* for *Cardiac Glycosides.*
**Administration/Storage**
1. Lanoxicaps gelatin capsules are more bioavailable than tablets. Thus, the 0.05-mg capsule is equivalent to the 0.0625-mg tablet; the 0.1-mg capsule is equivalent to the 0.125-mg tablet, and the 0.2-mg capsule is equivalent to the 0.25-mg tablet.
2. Differences in bioavailability have been noted between products; monitor clients when changing from one product to another.
3. Protect from light.
**IV** 4. Give IV injections over 5 min (or longer) either undiluted or diluted fourfold or greater with sterile water for injection, 0.9% NaCl injection, RL injection, or 5% dextrose injection.

**Client/Family Teaching**
1. Check with provider when to hold digoxin, i.e., HR below 50–60 or above 120.
2. Report S&S of digoxin toxicity: abdominal pain, N&V, visual disturbances, irregular heart beat.
3. Continue Na-restricted, low-fat diet.
**Outcomes/Evaluate**
• Control of S&S of CHF ( ↑ CO, ↓ HR, ↓ SOB)
• Serum level (0.5–2.0 ng/mL)

# Digoxin Immune Fab (Ovine)
(dih-**JOX**-in)
**Pregnancy Category:** C
Digibind **(Rx)**
**Classification:** Digoxin antidote

**Action/Kinetics:** Digoxin immune Fab are antibodies that bind to digoxin. In cases of digoxin toxicity, the antibodies bind to digoxin and the complex is excreted through the kidneys. As serum levels of digoxin decrease, digoxin bound to tissue is released into the serum to maintain equilibrium and this is then bound and excreted. The net result is a decrease in both tissue and serum digoxin. **Onset:** Less than 1 min. Improvement in signs of toxicity occurs within 30 min. **t½:** 15–20 hr (after IV administration). Each vial contains 38 mg of pure digoxin immune Fab, which will bind approximately 0.5 mg digoxin or digitoxin.
**Uses:** Life-threatening digoxin or digitoxin toxicity or overdosage. Symptoms of toxicity include severe sinus bradycardia, second- or third-degree heart block which does not respond to atropine, ventricular tachycardia, ventricular fibrillation.
*NOTE:* Cardiac arrest can be expected if a healthy adult ingests more than 10 mg digoxin or a healthy child ingests more than 4 mg. Also, steady-state serum concentrations of digoxin greater than 10 ng/mL or potassium concentrations greater than 5 mEq/L as a result

of digoxin therapy require use of digoxin immune Fab.

**Special Concerns:** Use with caution during lactation. Use in infants only if benefits outweigh risks. Clients sensitive to products of sheep origin may also be sensitive to digoxin immune Fab. Skin testing may be appropriate for high-risk clients.

**Side Effects:** *CV:* Worsening of CHF or low CO, atrial fibrillation (all due to withdrawal of the effects of digoxin). *Other:* Hypokalemia. Rarely, hypersensitivity reactions occur, including fever and *anaphylaxis.*

**Dosage**
• **IV**

Dosage depends on the serum digoxin concentration. A large dose has a faster onset but there is an increased risk of allergic or febrile reactions. The package insert should be carefully consulted. **Adults, usual:** Six vials (228 mg) is usuallly enough to reverse most cases of toxicity. **Children, less than 20 kg:** A single vial (38 mg) should be sufficient.

## NURSING CONSIDERATIONS
### Administration/Storage
**IV** 1. Reconstitute the lyophilized material with 4 mL of sterile water for injection to give a concentration of 10 mg/mL. If small doses are required (e.g., in infants), can be further diluted with 36 mL sterile isotonic saline to obtain a concentration of 1 mg/mL.

2. Administer over a 30-min period through a 0.22-μm membrane filter; may use a bolus injection if immediate danger of cardiac arrest.

3. Use reconstituted antibody immediately. May store for up to 4 hr at 2°C–8°C (36°F–46°F).

4. The total number of vials of antibody needed can be determined by dividing the total body load (in mg) by the amount of digoxin bound by each vial (0.6 mg).

5. If acute digoxin ingestion results in severe symptoms and a serum concentration is not known, 800 mg (20 vials) of digoxin immune Fab may be given. Monitor for volume overload in small children.

6. Administer to infants with a tuberculin syringe.

### Assessment
1. Determine amount, time of drug ingestion, and serum digoxin level.

2. If previous reaction suspected or high-risk client, perform skin testing: Prepare a 10-mL solution (0.1 mL of drug in 9.9 mL NSS); perform intradermal injection or scratch test. Administer 0.1 mL intradermally or perform a scratch test by placing 1 drop of solution on the skin and making a scratch through the drop with a sterile needle; assess site in 20 min. *Do not* use if reaction is positive: urticarial wheal with erythematous surrounding skin.

3. Do not administer to those with known allergy to sheep proteins.

4. Monitor VS and cardiac rhythm. Assess for electrolyte imbalance; note hypokalemia or evidence of increased CHF.

5. Wait several days for redigitalization to ensure complete elimination of digibind. Digoxin levels will take 5–7 days to stabilize following treatment, although improvement in S&S of toxicity should be evident in 30 min.

### Outcomes/Evaluate
• Resolution of digoxin toxicity
• Controlled cardiac rhythm

# Dihydroergotamine mesylate
(dye-hy-droh-er-**GOT**-ah-meen)
**Pregnancy Category:** X
D.H.E. 45, Dihydroergotamine (DHE) Sandoz ✿, Migranal Nasal Spray **(Rx)**
**Classification:** Alpha-adrenergic blocking agent

**Action/Kinetics:** Manifests alpha-adrenergic receptor blocking activity as well as a direct stimulatory action on vascular smooth muscle of peripheral and cranial blood vessels, resulting in vasoconstriction, thus preventing the onset of a migraine attack. Manifests greater adrenergic blocking activity, less pronounced vasoconstriction, less N&V, and less oxytocic properties than does ergotamine. More effective when given early in the course of a migraine attack. **Onset: IM,** 15–30 min; **IV, <5 min. Duration: IM, 3–4 hr. t½: initial, 1.4 hr; final,** 18–22 hr. Metabolized in liver and excreted in feces with less than 10% excreted through the urine.

**Uses:** To prevent or abort migraine, migraine variant, histaminic cephalalgia (cluster headaches). Especially useful when rapid effect is desired or when other routes of administration are not possible.

**Contraindications:** Lactation. Pregnancy. Peripheral vascular disease, coronary heart disease, hypertension, impaired hepatic or renal function, sepsis, hypersensitivity, malnutrition, severe pruritus, presence of infection.

**Special Concerns:** Safety and efficacy have not been determined in children. Geriatric clients may be more affected by peripheral vasoconstriction that results in hypothermia. Prolonged administration may cause ergotism and gangrene.

**Side Effects:** *CV:* Precordial pain, transient tachycardia or bradycardia. Large doses may cause increased BP, vasoconstriction of coronary arteries, and bradycardia. *GI:* N&V, diarrhea. *Other:* Numbness and tingling of fingers and toes, muscle pain in extremities, weakness in legs, localized edema, and itching. *Prolonged use:* Gangrene, ergotism.

**OD** **Overdose Management:** *Symptoms:* N&V, pain in limb muscles, tachycardia or bradycardia, precordial pain, numbness and tingling of fingers and toes, weakness of the legs, hypertension or hypotension, localized edema, S&S of ischemia due to vasoconstriction of peripheral arteries and arterioles. Symptoms of ischemia include the feet and hands becoming cold, pale, and numb;

muscle pain, gangrene. Occasionally confusion, depression, drowsiness, and *seizures. Treatment:* Maintain adequate circulation. IV nitroglycerin and nitroprusside to treat vasospasm. IV heparin and low molecular weight dextran to minimize thrombosis.

**Drug Interactions**
*Beta-adrenergic blockers* / ↑ Peripheral ischemia resulting in cold extremities and possibly peripheral gangrene
*Macrolide antibiotics* / Acute ergotism resulting in peripheral ischemia
*Nitrates* / ↑ Bioavailability of hydroergotamine and ↓ anginal effects of nitrates

**Dosage** ─────────────
• **IM**
*Suppress vascular headache.*
**Adults, initial:** 1 mg at first sign of headache; repeat q hr for a total of 3 mg (not to exceed 6 mg/week).
• **IV**
*Suppress vascular headache.*
Similar to IM but to a maximum of 2 mg/attack or 6 mg/week.
• **Nasal spray**
*Acute migraine headaches.*
0.5 mg spray in each nostril followed in 15 min by a second 0.5 mg spray in each nostil (i.e., total of 2 mg).

─────────────────────────

## NURSING CONSIDERATIONS
**Administration/Storage:** Adjust dosage if client complains of severe headaches; use this dose when subsequent headaches begin.
**Assessment**
1. Obtain a thorough nursing, diet, and drug history; note any contributing factors (i.e., cigarette smoking, alcohol ingestion, OTC agents, and stress).
2. Do not take with nitrates or if any sensitivity to ergotamine.
3. Determine severity and characteristics of headaches; note what agents relieved them.
4. Assess for pregnancy; has an oxytocic effect.
5. Note any history of liver or renal

dysfunction, hypertension, PVD, or CAD.

**Client/Family Teaching**
1. Take at the onset of migraine; drug is most effective when administered early in an attack.
2. Seek bed rest in a darkened room for 1–2 hr after drug ingestion.
3. Practice alternative methods for dealing with stress, such as relaxation techniques.
4. Report any evidence of cold extremities and numbness or tingling immediately, to avoid gangrene.
5. Take only as directed and do not stop abruptly.
6. Keep a headache diary; list foods, events, activities surrounding onset.

**Outcomes/Evaluate:** Relief of migraine headaches

# Diltiazem hydrochloride
(dill-**TIE**-ah-zem)
**Pregnancy Category:** C
Alti-Diltiazem ✦, Apo-Diltiaz ✦, Cardizem, Cardizem CD, Cardizem Injectable, Cardizem Lyo-Ject, Cardizem-SR, Dilacor XR, Diltiazem HCl Extended Release, Gen-Diltiazem ✦, Novo-Diltiazem ✦, Nu-Diltiaz ✦, Tiazac **(Rx)**
**Classification:** Calcium channel blocking agent (antianginal, antihypertensive)

See also *Calcium Channel Blocking Agents.*

**Action/Kinetics:** Decreases SA and AV conduction and prolongs AV node effective and functional refractory periods. The drug also decreases myocardial contractility and peripheral vascular resistance. **Tablets: Onset,** 30–60 min; **time to peak plasma levels:** 2–3 hr; t½, **first phase:** 20–30 min; **second phase:** about 3–4.5 hr (5–8 hr with high and repetitive doses); **duration:** 4–8 hr. **Extended-Release Capsules: Onset,** 2–3 hr; **time to peak plasma levels:** 6–11 hr; t½: 5–7 hr; **duration:** 12 hr. **Therapeutic serum levels:** 0.05–0.2 mcg/mL.

Metabolized to desacetyldiltiazem, which manifests 25%–50% of the activity of diltiazem. Excreted through both the bile and urine.

**Uses: Tablets:** Vasospastic angina (Prinzmetal's variant). Chronic stable angina (classic effort-associated angina), especially in clients who cannot use beta-adrenergic blockers or nitrates or who remain symptomatic after clinical doses of these agents. **Sustained-Release Capsules:** Essential hypertension, angina. **Parenteral:** Atrial fibrillation or flutter. Paroxysmal SVT. Cardizem Lyo-Ject is used on an emergency basis for atrial fibrillation or atrial flutter. *Investigational:* Prophylaxis of reinfarction of nonQ wave MI; tardive dyskinesia, Raynaud's syndrome.

**Contraindications:** Hypotension. Second- or third-degree AV block and sick sinus syndrome except in presence of a functioning ventricular pacemaker. Acute MI, pulmonary congestion. Lactation.

**Special Concerns:** Safety and effectiveness in children have not been determined. The half-life may be increased in geriatric clients. Use with caution in hepatic disease and in CHF. Abrupt withdrawal may cause an increase in the frequency and duration of chest pain. Use with beta blockers or digitalis is usually well tolerated, although the effects of coadministration cannot be predicted (especially in clients with left ventricular dysfunction or cardiac conduction abnormalities).

**Side Effects:** *CV:* AV block, bradycardia, CHF, hypotension, syncope, palpitations, peripheral edema, *arrhythmias,* angina, tachycardia, *abnormal ECG, ventricular extrasystoles. GI:* N&V, diarrhea, constipation, anorexia, abdominal discomfort, cramps, dry mouth, dysgeusia. *CNS:* Weakness, nervousness, dizziness, lightheadedness, headache, depression, psychoses, hallucinations, disturbances in sleep, somnolence, insomnia, amnesia, abnormal

---

✦ = Available in Canada          ***bold italic*** = life threatening side effect

dreams. *Dermatologic:* Rashes, dermatitis, pruritus, urticaria, erythema multiforme, **Stevens-Johnson syndrome.** *Other:* Photosensitivity, joint pain or stiffness, flushing, nasal or chest congestion, dyspnea, SOB, nocturia/polyuria, sexual difficulties, weight gain, paresthesia, tinnitus, tremor, asthenia, gynecomastia, gingival hyperplasia, petechiae, ecchymosis, purpura, bruising, hematoma, leukopenia, double vision, epistaxis, eye irritation, thirst, alopecia, **bundle branch block,** abnormal gait, hyperglycemia.

**Additional Drug Interactions**
*Anesthetics* / ↑ Risk of depression of cardiac contractility, conductivity, and automaticity as well as vascular dilation
*Carbamazepine* / ↑ Effect of diltiazem due to ↓ breakdown by liver
*Cimetidine* / ↑ Bioavailability of diltiazem
*Cyclosporine* / ↑ Effect of cyclosporine possibly leading to renal toxicity
*Digoxin* / ↑ Serum digoxin levels are possible
*Lithium* / ↑ Risk of neurotoxicity
*Ranitidine* / ↑ Bioavailability of diltiazem
*Theophyllines* / ↑ Risk of pharmacologic and toxicologic effects of theophyllines

**Laboratory Test Interferences:** ↑ Alkaline phosphatase, CPK, LDH, AST, ALT.

**Dosage** —————
• **Tablets**
   *Angina.*
**Adults, initial:** 30 mg q.i.d. before meals and at bedtime; **then,** increase gradually to total daily dose of 180–360 mg (given in three to four divided doses). Increments may be made q 1–2 days until the optimum response is attained.
• **Capsules, Sustained-Release**
   *Angina.*
**Cardizem CD: Adults, initial:** 120 or 180 mg once daily. Up to 480 mg/ day may be required. Dosage adjust-

ments should be carried out over a 7–14-day period.
**Dilacor XR: Adults, initial:** 120 mg once daily; **then,** dose may be titrated, depending on the needs of the client, up to 480 mg once daily. Titration may be carried out over a 7–14-day period.
   *Hypertension.*
**Cardizem CD: Adults, initial:** 180–240 mg once daily. Maximum antihypertensive effect usually reached within 14 days. Usual range is 240–360 mg once daily.
**Cardizem SR: Adults, initial:** 60–120 mg b.i.d.; **then,** when maximum antihypertensive effect is reached (approximately 14 days), adjust dosage to a range of 240–360 mg/day.
**Dilacor XR: Adults, initial:** 180–240 mg once daily. Usual range is 180–480 mg once daily. The dose may be increased to 540 mg/day with little or no increased risk of side effects.
**Tiazac: Adults, initial:** 120–240 mg once daily. Usual range is 120–360 mg once daily, although doses up to 540 mg once daily have been used.
• **IV Bolus**
   *Atrial fibrillation/flutter; paroxysmal SVT.*
**Adults, initial:** 0.25 mg/kg (average 20 mg) given over 2 min; **then,** if response is inadequate, a second dose may be given after 15 min. The second bolus dose is 0.35 mg/kg (average 25 mg) given over 2 min. Subsequent doses should be individualized. Some clients may respond to an initial dose of 0.15 mg/kg (duration of action may be shorter).
• **IV Infusion**
   *Atrial fibrillation/flutter.*
**Adults:** 10 mg/hr following IV bolus dose(s) of 0.25 mg/kg or 0.35 mg/ kg. Some clients may require 5 mg/ hr while others may require 15 mg/ hr. Infusion may be maintained for 24 hr.
• **Cardizem Lyo-Ject**
   *Atrial fibrillation/atrial flutter.*
Delivery system consists of a dual-chamber, prefilled, calibrated syringe containing 25 mg of diltiazem hy-

drochloride in one chamber and 5 mL of diluent in the other chamber.

## NURSING CONSIDERATIONS

See also *Nursing Considerations* for *Calcium Channel Blocking Agents*.

**Administration/Storage**

1. Sublingual nitroglycerin may be taken concomitantly for acute angina. Diltiazem may also be taken together with long-acting nitrates.

2. Clients taking other forms of diltiazem can be safely switched to Dilacor XR at the nearest equivalent total daily dose. Titration to larger or smaller doses may be necessary.

3. Use with beta blockers or digitalis is usually well tolerated, but the combined effects cannot be predicted, especially with cardiac conduction abnormalities or LV dysfunction.

**IV** 4. May be administered by direct IV over 2 min or as an infusion (see *Dosage*). For IV infusion, drug may be mixed with NSS, 5% dextrose, or 5% dextrose and 0.45% NaCl.

5. The infusion may be maintained for up to 24 hr; beyond 24 hr is not recommended.

6. The injection should be refrigerated at 2°C–8°C (36°F–46°F). May be stored at room temperature for 1 mo; then, discard any remaining solution.

**Assessment**

1. Document indications for therapy, symptom onset, and any previous treatments.

2. Note any edema or CHF; review ECG for evidence of AV block.

3. Monitor liver and renal function studies; reduce dose with impaired function.

4. The plasma drug half-life may be prolonged in the elderly; monitor closely.

**Client/Family Teaching:**

1. Take the sustained-release capsules on an empty stomach. Do not open, chew, or crush sustained-release capsules; they should be swallowed whole.

2. May cause drowsiness or dizziness.

3. Rise slowly from a lying to a sitting and to a standing position; drug may cause postural hypotension.

4. Report any persistent and bothersome side effects including constipation, unusual tiredness, or weakness.

5. Continue carrying short-acting nitrites (nitroglycerin) at all times and use as directed.

6. Continue diet (low fat and low Na), regular exercise, and decreased intake of caffeine, tobacco, and alcohol.

**Outcomes/Evaluate**

• ↓ Frequency and intensity of vasospastic anginal attacks

• ↓ BP; stable cardiac rhythm

# Dimenhydrinate

(dye-men-**HY**-drih-nayt)

**Pregnancy Category:** B

**Oral Liquid, Syrup, Tablets, Chewable Tablets:** Apo-Dimenhydrinate ✽, Calm-X, Dimentabs, Dramamine, Gravol ✽, Marmine, Motion-Aid, PMS-Dimenhydrinate ✽, Travamine, Travel Tabs ✽, Traveltabs ✽, Triptone **(OTC). Injection:** Dimenhydrinate Injection ✽, Dinate, Dramanate, Dramilin, Dymenate, Gravol ✽, Hydrate, Marmine, Reidamine **(Rx)**

**Classification:** Antihistamine, antiemetic

See also *Antihistamines* and *Antiemetics*.

**Action/Kinetics:** Contains both diphenhydramine and chlorotheophylline. Antiemetic mechanism not known, but it does depress labyrinthine and vestibular function. May mask ototoxicity due to aminoglycosides. Possesses anticholinergic activity. **Duration:** 3–6 hr.

**Uses:** Motion sickness, especially to relieve nausea, vomiting, or dizziness. Treat vertigo.

**Special Concerns:** Use of the injectable form is not recommended in neonates. Geriatric clients may be more sensitive to the usual adult dose.

**D**

**Dosage**
• **Elixir, Syrup, Tablets, Chewable Tablets**
  *Motion sickness.*
  **Adults:** 50–100 mg q 4 hr, not to exceed 400 mg/day. **Pediatric, 6–12 years:** 25–50 mg q 6–8 hr, not to exceed 150 mg/day; **2–6 years:** 12.5–25 mg q 6–8 hr, not to exceed 75 mg/day.
• **IM, IV**
  **Adults:** 50 mg as required. **Pediatric, over 2 years:** 1.25 mg/kg ($37.5$ mg/m$^2$) q.i.d., not to exceed 300 mg/day.
• **IV**
  **Adults:** 50 mg in 10 mL sodium chloride injection given over 2 min; may be repeated q 4 hr as needed. **Pediatric:** 1.25 mg/kg ($37.5$ mg/m$^2$) in 10 mL of 0.9% sodium chloride injection given slowly over 2 min; may be repeated q 6 hr, not to exceed 300 mg/day.

## NURSING CONSIDERATIONS

See also *Nursing Considerations* for *Antihistamines* and *Antiemetics.*
**Assessment:** Document indications for therapy and symptom onset; assess for vestibular damage when administered with antihistamines.
**Client/Family Teaching**
1. Avoid activities that require mental alertness until drug effects realized.
2. May alter skin testing results.
**Outcomes/Evaluate:** Prevention of N&V and control of vertigo R/T motion sickness

---

# Dimercaprol
(dye-mer-**KAP**-rohl)
**Pregnancy Category:** C
BAL In Oil **(Rx)**
**Classification:** Chelating agent for heavy metals

**Action/Kinetics:** Forms a chelate by binding sulfhydryl groups with arsenic, mercury, lead, and gold, thus increasing both urinary and fecal excretion of the metals. Because the drug has a higher affinity for the metal than it does for sulfhydryl groups on protein in the body, BAL reverses enzyme inhibition by regenerating free sulfhydryl groups. To be fully effective, administer 1–2 hr after exposure. **Peak plasma concentration: IM,** 30–60 min. Mostly distributed to extracellular fluid. **Time to peak levels:** 30–60 min. Rapidly metabolized to inactive product and completely excreted in urine and feces in 4 hr.
**Uses:** Acute arsenic, mercury, and gold poisoning. With EDTA in acute lead poisoning. Not effective for chronic mercury poisoning.
**Contraindications:** Iron, cadmium, silver, uranium, or selenium poisoning. Hepatic or renal insufficiency, except postarsenical jaundice.
**Special Concerns:** Use during pregnancy only if poisoning is life-threatening. Use with caution in clients with G6PD deficiency and during lactation. Of questionable value in bismuth or antimony poisoning.
**Side Effects:** *CV:* Most common including hypertension and tachycardia (dose dependent). *GI:* N&V, salivation, abdominal pain, burning feeling of the lips, mouth and throat. *CNS:* Anxiety, weakness, restlessness, headache. *Other:* Constriction and pain in the throat, chest, or hands; sweating of the hands and forehead, conjunctivitis, blepharal spasm, lacrimation, salivation, rhinorrhea, tingling of hands, burning feeling in the penis, sterile abscesses, local pain at injection site. Children may also develop fever. *At high doses dimercaprol may cause coma or convulsions* and metabolic acidosis.
**OD** **Overdose Management:** *Symptoms:* Doses exceeding 5 mg/kg usually result in vomiting, convulsions, and stupor. *Treatment:* Reduce dose; symptoms usually subside within 6 hr.
**Drug Interactions:** Dimercaprol may increase the toxicity of cadmium, iron, selenium, or uranium salts.
**Laboratory Test Interferences:** Iodine-131 thyroidal uptake ↓ during and immediately after dimercaprol therapy.

## Dosage
- **Deep IM Only**

*Mild arsenic and gold poisoning.*
**Adults:** 2.5 mg/kg q.i.d. for 2 days; then, b.i.d. on the third day, and once daily thereafter for 10 days.

*Severe arsenic or gold poisoning.*
**Adults:** 3 mg/kg q 4 hr for days 1 and 2; q.i.d. on day 3; b.i.d. for 10 more days.

*Mercury poisoning, mild.*
**Adults, initial:** 5 mg/kg; **then,** 2.5 mg/kg 1 or 2 times/day for 10 days. Alternate dosing regimen: 2.5 mg/kg q 4 hr on day 1, q 6 hr on day 2, q 12 hr on day 3, and thereafter, once daily for the next 10 days or until recovery occurs.

*Mercury poisoning, severe.*
**Adults:** 5 mg/kg for the first dose followed by 2.5 mg/kg q 3 hr for the first 24 hr; **then,** 2 mg/kg q 4 hr on day 2; 3 mg/kg q 6 hr on day 3; and 3 mg/kg q 12 hr for the next 10 days or until recovery.

*Mild lead encephalopathy.*
**Adults:** 4 mg/kg alone initially; **then,** 3 mg/kg q 4 hr in combination with calcium EDTA administered in a separate site. Treatment should be continued for 2–7 days only if the blood level at the end of the first course of combined BAL-CaEDTA therapy exceeds 80–90 mcg/dL.

*Severe lead encephalopathy.*
**Adults:** 4 mg/kg alone initially; **then,** 4 mg/kg q 4 hr in combination with calcium EDTA administered in a separate site. Treatment should be continued for 2–7 days and repeated after an interval of 2 days for 5 additional days only if the blood lead level at the end of the first course of combined BAL-CaEDTA therapy exceeds 80–90 mcg/dL.

*Lead toxicity in symptomatic children, acute encephalopathy.*
75 mg/m² q 4 hr (up to 450 mg/m² in 24 hr). After the first dose, give calcium EDTA, 1,500 mg/m² over a 24-hr period in divided doses q 4 hr at a separate IM site; maintain treatment for 5 days and after an interval of 2 days, the treatment may be repeated for 5 additional days.

*Lead toxicity in children, other symptoms.*
50 mg/m² q 4 hr. After the first dose, give calcium EDTA, 1,000 mg/m² over a 24-hr period in divided doses q 4 hr at a separate IM site; maintain treatment for 5 days and after an interval of 2 days, the treatment may be repeated for 5 more days if the lead levels are still high.

## NURSING CONSIDERATIONS
### Administration/Storage
1. Initiate therapy and other supportive treatment as soon as possible.
2. Check if a local anesthetic may be given with IM injection to minimize pain at the injection site.
3. Inject deeply into muscle and massage after injection. Do not allow the fluid to come in contact with the skin; may cause a skin reaction.
4. Wait at least 24 hr after the last dose of dimercaprol before administering iron therapy.

### Assessment
1. Document exposure/ingestion, noting form, type, and quantity.
2. Assess I&O, increase fluid intake; monitor urinary pH; keep urine alkaline to protect kidneys during drug therapy.
3. Determine if pregnant.
4. Monitor VS, liver and renal function studies, and levels of toxic substance.
5. Reassure that adverse GI or CNS symptoms during therapy will pass within 30–90 min.
6. Drug imparts a strong, unpleasant garlic-like odor to client's breath; offer mouth rinses.

**Outcomes/Evaluate:** Enhanced excretion of metals with relief of toxic symptoms during acute poisonings

# Dinoprostone (PGE₂)
(**die**-noh-**PROS**-tohn)
**Pregnancy Category:** C
Cervidil, Prepidil Gel, Prostin E₂ **(Rx)**
**Classification:** Obstetrical drug (induction of labor)

**D**

**Action/Kinetics:** Either the gel or vaginal insert provides $PGE_2$, which interacts with prostaglandin receptor to produce changes in the consistency, dilatation, and effacement of the cervix. May also stimulate the smooth muscle of the GI tract, causing vomiting and diarrhea. Extensively metabolized in the lungs on first pass through the pulmonary circulation. Metabolites are excreted through the kidneys. $t\frac{1}{2}$: 2.5–5 min.

**Uses:** Ripening of an unfavorable cervix in pregnant women at or near term with a medical or obstetric need for induction of labor.

**Contraindications:** Use when oxytocic drugs are contraindicated or when prolonged uterine contractions are inappropriate (e.g., history of cesarean section or major uterine surgery), presence of cephalopelvic disproportion, history of difficult labor and/or traumatic delivery, grand multiparae with six or more previous term pregnancies, non-vertex presentation, hyperactive or hypertonic uterine patterns, fetal distress where delivery is not imminent, obstetric emergencies when surgical intervention may be favored. Also, use is contraindicated in ruptured membranes, hypersensitivity to prostaglandins or constituents of the gel, placenta previa or unexplained vaginal bleeding during current pregnancy, or when vaginal delivery is contraindicated (e.g., vasa previa or active herpes genitalis). Use in conjunction with oxytocic agents.

**Special Concerns:** Uterine rupture is possible when high-tone uterine contractions are sustained. Use with caution in clients with asthma or a history thereof, glaucoma, increased intraocular pressure, or impaired hepatic or renal function.

**Side Effects: Gel:** *Maternal:* Uterine contractile abnormality, GI effects, back pain, warm feeling in vagina, fever, premature rupture of membranes, uterine rupture. *Fetal:* Abnormality in fetal HR, bradycardia, deceleration, *fetal depression.* Extraamniotic administration has resulted in amnionitis and *intrauterine fetal sepsis.*

**Vaginal Insert:** Uterine hyperstimulation with or without fetal distress, fetal distress without hyperstimulation, fever, N&V, diarrhea, abdominal pain.

**OD** **Overdose Management:** *Symptoms:* Uterine hypercontractility, uterine hypertonus. *Treatment:* Symptoms may be relieved by changing maternal position, giving oxygen to the mother, or the use of beta-adrenergic drugs to treat hyperstimulation.

**Drug Interactions:** Dinoprostone may increase the action of other oxytocics.

**Dosage** —————————————
• **Gel**
**Initial:** 0.5 mg. If there is no cervical/uterine response, repeat doses of 0.5 mg may given q 6 hr. The maximum cumulative dose for 24 hr is 1.5 mg dinoprostone.
• **Vaginal Insert**
One insert (10 mg), designed to release approximately 0.3 mg dinoprostone/hr over a 12-hr period. The insert should be removed upon onset of active labor or 12 hr after insertion.
• **Vaginal Suppositories**
20 mg repeated every 3–5 hr; dose adjusted according to client response.

## NURSING CONSIDERATIONS
### Administration/Storage
1. Bring gel to room temperature just prior to administration.
2. Avoid contact with the skin; wash hands thoroughly with soap and water after administration.
3. The gel is intended for endocervical placement; do not administer above the level of the internal os. The degree of cervical effacement will regulate shielded catheter size to be used (20-mm catheter for no effacement and 10-mm catheter for 50% effacement).
4. Administer gel by sterile technique and introduce just below the level of the internal os.
5. Keep supine for at least 15–30 min after administration.
6. If desired response is obtained from the initial dose, the recom-

mended interval before giving oxytocin is 6–12 hr. A dosing interval of at least 30 min is recommended following removal of the dinoprostone vaginal insert.

7. The insert is placed transversely in the posterior fornix of the vagina immediately after removal from the foil package. Insertion does not require sterile conditions. Do not use insert without its retrieval system.

8. Insert may be placed in the vagina with a minimal amount of water-miscible lubricant. Prevent excess contact or coating with the lubricant, thus preventing optimal swelling and release of the drug.

9. The gel has a shelf life of 24 months when stored under refrigeration of 2°C–8°C (36°F–46°F). Store the insert in a freezer between –20°C and –10°C (–4°F and –14°F). When stored in a freezer, the insert is stable for up to 3 years.

**Assessment**

1. Document calculated and ultrasound-derived due date; note feto-pelvic relationships.

2. Examine cervix to determine degree of effacement (shortening of cervical canal); this regulates the size of the shielded endocervical catheter used.

3. Document system used, time of insertion, and dosing intervals. Insert must be removed with retrieval system after 12 hr or at the onset of active labor.

4. Carefully monitor uterine contractions, fetal heart tones, cervical dilation and effacement by visual assessment, auscultation and electronic fetal monitoring.

5. Continuous monitoring of uterine activity and fetal status should be undertaken with history of hypertonic uterine contractility or tetanic uterine contractions. Monitor for uterine rupture with sustained high-tone myometrial contractions.

**Client/Family Teaching**

1. Explain purpose of therapy and anticipated outcome.

2. Gel may produce increased vaginal warmth.

3. Must remain supine for 30 min after gel insertion.

**Outcomes/Evaluate:** Desired cervical presentation to facilitate induction of labor

# Diphenhydramine hydrochloride

(dye-fen-**HY**-drah-meen)

**Pregnancy Category:** B

Allerdryl ✦, AllerMax, AllerMax Allergy & Cough Formula, Banophen Caplets, Benadryl, Benadryl Allergy, Benadryl Allergy Ultratabs, Benadryl Dye-Free Allergy, Benadryl Dye-Free Allergy Liqui Gels, Diphen AF, Diphen Cough, Diphenhist, Genahist, Hyrex-in-50, Nytol ✦, Nytol Extra Strength ✦, PMS-Diphenhydramine ✦, Scheinpharm Diphenhydramine ✦, Scot-Tussin DM, Siladryl, Tusstat **(OTC and Rx). Sleep-Aids:** Dormin, Miles Nervine, Nighttime Sleep Aid, Nytol, Sleep-eze 3, Sleep-Eze D ✦, Sleep-well 2-nite, Sominex **(OTC)**

**Classification:** Antihistamine, ethanolamine-type; antiemetic

See also *Antihistamines, Antiemetics,* and *Antiparkinson Drugs.*

**Action/Kinetics:** High sedative, anticholinergic, and antiemetic effects.

**Uses:** Hypersensitivity reactions, motion sickness (PO only), parkinsonism, nighttime sleep aid (PO only), antitussive (syrup only).

**Contraindications:** Topically to treat chickenpox, poison ivy, or sunburn. Topically on large areas of the body or on blistered or oozing skin.

**Dosage**

• **Capsules, Chewable Tablets, Elixir, Liquid, Syrup, Tablets**

*Antihistamine, antiemetic, anti-motion sickness, parkinsonism.*

**Adults:** 25–50 mg t.i.d.–q.i.d.; **pediatric, over 10 kg:** 12.5–25 mg t.i.d.–q.i.d. (or 5 mg/kg/day not to exceed 300 mg/day or 150 mg/m²/day).

*Sleep aid.*

**Adults and children over 12 years:** 50 mg at bedtime.
  *Antitussive (Syrup only).*
**Adults:** 25 mg q 4 hr, not to exceed 100 mg/day; **pediatric, 6-12 years:** 12.5-25 mg q 4 hr, not to exceed 50 mg/day; **pediatric, 2-6 years:** 6.25 mg q 4 hr, not to exceed 25 mg/day.
• **IV, Deep IM**
  *Parkinsonism.*
**Adults:** 10-50 mg up to 100 mg if needed (not to exceed 400 mg/day); **pediatric:** 1.25 mg/kg (or 37.5 mg/m²) q.i.d., not to exceed a total of 300 mg/day.

## NURSING CONSIDERATIONS

See also *Nursing Considerations* for *Antihistamines, Antiemetics,* and *Anti-parkinson Drugs.*
**Administration/Storage**
1. When using for motion sickness, give the full prophylactic dose 30 min prior to travel and preferably 1-2 hr before exposures that precipitate sickness.
2. Take similar doses with meals and at bedtime.
3. Do not use more than 2 weeks to treat insomnia.
**IV** 4. For IV administration, may give undiluted with each 25 mg over at least 1 min.
**Client/Family Teaching**
1. May cause drowsiness; use caution until drug effects realized.
2. Use protection; may cause photosensitivity reaction.
3. Use sugarless gum/candy to diminish dry mouth effects.
4. Avoid alcohol and any other CNS depressants unless prescribed.
**Outcomes/Evaluate**
• ↓ Allergic manifestations
• Relief of nausea
• Promotion of sleep
• Relief of dyskinesias/extrapyramidal symptoms with parkinsonism

———*COMBINATION DRUG*———

# Diphenoxylate hydrochloride with Atropine sulfate

(dye-fen-**OX**-ih-layt, **AH**-troh-peen)

**Pregnancy Category:** C
Lofene, Logen, Lomanate, Lomodix, Lomotil, Lonox, Low-Quel **(C-V) (Rx)**
**Classification:** Antidiarrheal agent, systemic

See also *Cholinergic Blocking Agents.*
**Content:** Each tablet or 5 mL of liquid contains: *Antidiarrheal:* Diphenoxylate HCl, 2.5 mg. *Anticholinergic:* Atropine sulfate, 0.025 mg.
**Action/Kinetics:** Chemically related to the narcotic analgesic drug meperidine but without the analgesic properties. Inhibits GI motility and has a constipating effect. May aggravate diarrhea due to organisms that penetrate the intestinal mucosa (e.g., *Escherichia coli, Salmonella, Shigella)* or in antibiotic-induced pseudomembranous colitis. High doses over prolonged periods may cause euphoria and physical dependence. The product also contains small amounts of atropine sulfate which will prevent abuse by deliberate overdosage. **Onset:** 45-60 min. **t½, diphenoxylate:** 2.5 hr; **diphenoxylic acid:** 12-24 hr. **Duration:** 2-4 hr. Metabolized in the liver to the active diphenoxylic acid and excreted through the urine.
**Uses:** Symptomatic treatment of chronic and functional diarrhea. Also, diarrhea associated with gastroenteritis, irritable bowel, regional enteritis, malabsorption syndrome, ulcerative colitis, acute infections, food poisoning, postgastrectomy, and drug-induced diarrhea. Therapeutic results for control of acute diarrhea are inconsistent. Also used in the control of intestinal passage time in clients with ileostomies and colostomies.
**Contraindications:** Obstructive jaundice, liver disease, diarrhea associated with pseudomembranous enterocolitis after antibiotic therapy or enterotoxin-producing bacteria, children under the age of 2.
**Special Concerns:** Use with caution during lactation, when anticholinergics may be contraindicated, and in advanced hepatic-renal disease or abnormal renal functions. Children

(especially those with Down syndrome) are susceptible to atropine toxicity. Children and geriatric clients may be more sensitive to the respiratory depressant effects of diphenoxylate. Dehydration, especially in young children, may cause a delayed diphenoxylate toxicity.

**Side Effects:** *GI:* N&V, anorexia, abdominal discomfort, paralytic ileus, megacolon. *Allergic:* Pruritus, ***angioneurotic edema,*** swelling of gums. *CNS:* Dizziness, drowsiness, malaise, restlessness, headache, depression, numbness of extremities, ***respiratory depression, coma.*** *Topical:* Dry skin and mucous membranes, flushing. *Other:* Tachycardia, urinary retention, hyperthermia.

**OD** **Overdose Management:** *Symptoms:* Dry skin and mucous membranes, flushing, ***hyperthermia,*** mydriasis, restlessness, tachycardia followed by miosis, lethargy, hypotonic reflexes, nystagmus, ***coma, severe (and possibly fatal) respiratory depression.*** *Treatment:* Gastric lavage, induce vomiting, establish a patent airway, and assist respiration. Activated charcoal (100 g) given as a slurry. IV administration of a narcotic antagonist. Administration may be repeated after 10–15 min. Observe client and readminister antagonist if respiratory depression returns.

**Drug Interactions**
*Alcohol* / Additive CNS depression
*Antianxiety agents* / Additive CNS depression
*Barbiturates* / Additive CNS depression
*MAO inhibitors* / ↑ Chance of hypertensive crisis
*Narcotics* / ↑ Effect of narcotics

**Dosage** ———————
• **Oral Solution, Tablets**
**Adults, initial:** 2.5–5 mg (of diphenoxylate) t.i.d.–q.i.d.; **maintenance:** 2.5 mg b.i.d.–t.i.d. **Pediatric, 2–12 years:** 0.3–0.4 mg/kg/day (of diphenoxylate) in divided doses.

**NURSING CONSIDERATIONS**
See also *Nursing Considerations* for *Difenoxin Hydrochloride with Atropine sulfate.*

**Administration/Storage**
1. For liquid preparations, use only the plastic dropper supplied by the manufacturer to measure dosage.
2. If clinical improvement is not evident after 10 days with a maximum dose of 20 mg/day, further use will not likely control symptoms.

**Assessment**
1. Document indications for therapy, onset, duration of symptoms, and other agents trialed.
2. Determine fluid and electrolyte status. Dehydration in young children may cause a delayed diphenoxylate toxicity.
3. Review culture reports to determine if drug is appropriate if not effective within 24–36 hr after administration.
4. Note any hepatic or renal dysfunction.
5. Assess for abdominal distension and toxic megacolon.

**Client/Family Teaching:** Take only as prescribed; do not exceed dosage, report lack of response. May cause drowsiness; use caution.

**Outcomes/Evaluate:** Control of diarrhea

---

# Dipyridamole
(dye=peer-**ID**-ah-mohl))
**Pregnancy Category:** B
Apo-Dipyridamole FC ✿, Apo-Dipyridamole SC ✿, Novo-Dipiradol ✿, Persantine **(Rx)**
**Classification:** Platelet adhesion inhibitor

---

**Action/Kinetics:** In higher doses may act by several mechanisms, including inhibition of red blood cell uptake of adenosine, itself an inhibitor of platelet reactivity; inhibition of platelet phosphodiesterase, which leads to accumulation of cAMP within platelets; direct stimulation of release of prostacyclin or prostaglandin $D_2$; and/or inhibition of thromboxane A$_2$ formation. Dipyridamole prolongs platelet survival time in clients with valvular heart disease and has maintained platelet count in open heart surgery. Also causes coronary vasodilation which may be due to inhibition of adenosine deaminase in the blood, thus allowing accumulation of adenosine which is a potent vasodilator. Vasodilation may also be caused by delaying the hydrolysis of cyclic 3',5'-adenosine monophosphate as a result of inhibition of the enzyme phosphodiesterase. Incompletely absorbed from the GI tract. **Peak plasma levels, after PO:** 45–150 min. **t½, after PO: initial,** 40–80 min; **terminal,** 10–12 hr. Metabolized in the liver and mainly excreted in the bile.

**Uses:** Orally as an adjunct to coumarin anticoagulants in preventing post-operative thromboembolic complications of cardiac valve replacement. Used IV as an alternative to exercise in thallium myocardial perfusion imaging for the evaluation of CAD in those who cannot exercise adequately. *Investigational:* Alone or as an adjunct to treat angina, to prevent graft occlusion in those undergoing arterial reconstructive bypass surgery, intralingual bypass grafts, and to prevent deterioration of coronary vessel patency after percutaneous transluminal angioplasty. Use with aspirin for preventing migraine headaches, MI, to reduce platelet aggregation at the carotid endarterectomy, to slow progression of peripheral occlusive arterial disease, to reduce incidence of DVT, to reduce the number of platelets deposited on dacron aortofemoral artery grafts, and TIAs.

*NOTE:* Not effective for the treatment of acute episodes of angina and is not a substitute for the treatment of angina pectoris.

**Special Concerns:** Use with caution in hypotension and during lactation. Safety and efficacy have not been determined in children less than 12 years of age.

**Side Effects: After PO use.** *GI:* GI intolerance, N&V, diarrhea. *CNS:* Dizziness, headache, syncope. *CV:* Peripheral vasodilation, flushing. Rarely, angina pectoris or aggravation of angina pectoris (usually at the beginning of therapy). *Miscellaneous:* Weakness, rash, pruritus.

**After IV use.** Most common side effects (1% or greater) are listed. *GI:* Nausea, dyspepsia. *CNS:* Headache, dizziness, paresthesia, fatigue. *CV:* Chest pain, angina pectoris, ECG abnormalities (ST-T changes, extrasystoles, tachycardia), precipitation of acute myocardial ischemia in clients with CAD, hypotension, flushing, blood pressure lability, hypertension. *Miscellaneous:* Dyspnea, unspecified pain.

**OD** **Overdose Management:** *Symptoms:* Hypotension of short duration. *Treatment:* Use of a vasopressor may be beneficial. Due to the high percentage of protein binding of dipyridamole, dialysis is not likely to be beneficial.

**Dosage** —————
• **Tablets**
*Adjunct in prophylaxis of thromboembolism after cardiac valve replacement.*
**Adults:** 75–100 mg q.i.d. as an adjunct to warfarin therapy.
*Prevention of thromboembolic complications in other thromboembolic disorders.*
**Adults:** 150–400 mg/day in combination with another platelet-aggregation inhibitor (e.g., aspirin) or an anticoagulant.
• **IV**
*Adjunct to thallium myocardial perfusion imaging.*
Adjust the dose according to body weight. Recommended dose is 0.142 mg/kg/min infused over 4 min. Total dose should not exceed 60 mg.

**NURSING CONSIDERATIONS**
**Administration/Storage**
**IV** 1. When used IV, to prevent irritation, dilute the injection in at least a 1:2 ratio with 0.45% NaCl injection, 0.9% NaCl injection, or 5% dextrose injection. The total volume should be 20 to 50 mL.

2. With imaging, give thallium-201 within 5 min following the IV dipyridamole injection.

3. Do not mix with other drugs in the same syringe or infusion container.

**Assessment**

1. Document indications for therapy, type, onset, duration, and characteristics of symptoms.

2. List all drugs currently prescribed to ensure none interact unfavorably.

3. Document mental status, skin color, and cardiopulmonary findings.

4. Monitor VS, ECG, CBC, PT, PTT, and INR.

**Client/Family Teaching**

1. Drug helps prevent clots by inhibiting platelet stickiness.

2. Avoid alcohol and tobacco due to hypotensive vasoconstrictive effects; and any other unprescribed drugs including aspirin without approval.

3. Drug may cause dizziness and lightheadedness; change positions slowly.

4. Try small frequent meals if nausea or gastric distress is experienced.

5. Report any increased chest pain, skin rash, fainting or severe headaches.

**Outcomes/Evaluate**

• CAD evaluation with thallium imaging

• Prevention of thromboembolism

# Dirithromycin
(die-**rih**-throw-**MY**- sin)
**Pregnancy Category:** C
Dynabac **(Rx)**
**Classification:** Antibiotic, macrolide

**Action/Kinetics:** Rapidly absorbed and converted during intestinal absorption to the active erythromycylamine. Distributed throughout the body, including the lungs, GI tract, skin, soft tissues, and GU tract. Erythromycylamine acts by binding to the 50S ribosomal subunits of microorganisms, resulting in inhibition of protein synthesis. t½: 2–36 hr. From 81% to 97% of erythromycylamine is excreted in the feces via the bile.

**Uses:** Acute bacterial exacerbations of chronic bronchitis due to *Moraxella catarrhalis* or *Streptococcus pneumoniae.* Secondary bacterial infections of acute bronchitis due to *M. catarrhalis* or *S. pneumoniae.* Community-acquired pneumonia due to *Legionella pneumophila, Mycoplasma pneumoniae,* or *S. pneumoniae.* Pharyngitis or tonsillitis due to *Streptococcus pyogenes.* Uncomplicated infections of the skin and skin structures due to Staphylococcus aureus.

**Contraindications:** Hypersensitivity to erythromycin or any other macrolide antibiotic. Use in children less than 12 years of age. Use in clients with known, suspected, or potential bacteremias since serum levels of the drug are not high enough in the serum to be effective. Use for the empiric treatment of acute bacterial exacerbations of chronic or secondary bacterial infections of acute bronchitis or for empiric treatment of uncomplicated skin and skin structure infections.

**Special Concerns:** Although dirithromycin eradicates *S. pyogenes* from the nasopharynx, data are lacking as to its effectiveness in preventing rheumatic fever. Use with caution during lactation. Safety and efficacy have not been determined in children less than 12 years of age.

**Side Effects:** *GI: **Pseudomembranous colitis,*** abdominal pain, nausea, diarrhea, vomiting, dyspepsia, GI disorder, flatulence, abnormal stools, constipation, dry mouth, gastritis, gastroenteritis, mouth ulceration, taste perversion, thirst. *CNS:* Headache, dizziness, vertigo, insomnia, anxiety, depression, nervousness, paresthesia, somnolence. *CV:* Palpitation, vasodilation, syncope. *GU:* Dysmenorrhea, urinary frequency, vaginal moniliasis, vaginitis. *Dermatologic:* Rash, pruritus, urticaria, sweating. *Respiratory:* Increased cough, dyspnea, hyperventilation. *Miscellaneous:* Nonspecific pain, asthenia, anorexia, dehydration, edema, epistaxis, eye disorder, fever, flu syndrome, hemoptysis, malaise, peripheral edema, *allergic reaction,* amblyopia, eye disorder, myalgia, neck pain, tinnitus, tremor.

**OD   Overdose   Management:** *Symptoms:* N&V, epigastric distress, diarrhea. *Treatment:* Treat symptoms.

**Drug Interactions**
*Antacids /* Slightly ↑ absorption of dirithromycin
*$H_2$ Antagonists /* Slightly ↑ absorption of dirithromycin
*Terfendine /* Possible serious cardiac dysrhythmias

**Laboratory Test Interferences:** ↑ ALT, AST, alkaline phosphatase, potassium, CPK, bands, segs, basophils, eosinophils, platelet count, total bilirubin, creatinine, GGT, leukocyte count, lymphocytes, monocytes, phosphorus, uric acid. ↓ Bicarbonate, albumin, chloride, hematocrit, hemoglobin, seg neutrophils, phosphorus, platelet count, total protein.

**Dosage** ───────────
• **Tablets, Enteric-Coated**
*Acute bacterial exacerbations of chronic bronchitis. Secondary bacterial infection of acute bronchitis.*
**Adults and children over 12 years of age:** 500 mg once a day for 7 days.
*Community-acquired pneumonia.*
**Adults and children over 12 years of age:** 500 mg once a day for 14 days.
*Pharyngitis or tonsillitis.*
**Adults and children over 12 years of age:** 500 mg once a day for 10 days.
*Uncomplicated skin and skin structure infections.*
**Adults and children over 12 years of age:** 500 mg once a day for 7 days.

## NURSING CONSIDERATIONS

See also *General Nursing Considerations for All Anti-infectives.*
**Assessment**
1. Document indications for therapy, type, onset, and duration of symptoms.

2. Obtain cultures for C&S initially; assess for any superinfections.
3. Does not appear to cause CV problems; use caution/avoid use with terfenadine.

**Client/Family Teaching**
1. Take as prescribed with food or within 1 hr of eating.
2. Do not crush, cut, or chew enteric-coated tablets.
3. Report new diarrhea; drug alters normal colon flora, permitting clostridia overgrowth; requires stopping drug and symptom management.

**Outcomes/Evaluate**
• Resolution of infection
• Negative culture reports

# Disopyramide phosphate
(dye-so-**PEER**-ah-myd)
**Pregnancy Category:** C
Norpace, Norpace CR, Rythmodan ✱, Rythmodan-LA ✱ **(Rx)**
**Classification:** Antiarrhythmic, class IA

**Action/Kinetics:** Decreases the rate of diastolic depolarization (phase 4), decreases the upstroke velocity (phase 0), increases the action potential duration (of normal cardiac cells), and prolongs the refractory period (phases 2 and 3). Weak anticholinergic effects; fewer side effects than quinidine. Does not affect BP significantly; can be used in digitalized and nondigitalized clients. **Onset:** 30 min. **Peak plasma levels:** 2 hr. **Duration:** average of 6 hr (range 1.5–8 hr). t½: 4–10 hr. **Therapeutic serum levels:** 2–4 mcg/mL. Do not use serum levels to adjust the dose because of variance in protein binding and potential toxicity of unbound drug. **Protein binding:** 40%–60%. Bioavailability of the controlled-release capsules appears to be similar to that of the immediate-release capsules. Both unchanged drug (50%) and metabolites (30%) are excreted through the urine. Approximately 15% is excreted through the bile.
**Uses:** Life-threatening ventricular arrhythmias (e.g., sustained ventricular tachycardia). Not been shown to improve survival in clients with ven-

tricular arrhythmias. *Investigational:* Paroxysmal SVT.

**Contraindications:** Hypersensitivity to drug. Cardiogenic shock, heart failure, heart block (especially pre-existing second- and third-degree AV block if no pacemaker is present), congenital QT prolongation, asymptomatic ventricular premature contractions, sick sinus syndrome, glaucoma, urinary retention, myasthenia gravis. Use of controlled-release capsules in clients with severe renal insufficiency. Lactation.

**Special Concerns:** Safe use during childhood, labor, and delivery has not been established. Use with caution in Wolff-Parkinson-White syndrome or bundle branch block. Decrease dosage in impaired hepatic function. Geriatric clients may be more sensitive to the anticholinergic effects of this drug. The drug may be ineffective in hypokalemia and toxic in hyperkalemia.

**Side Effects:** *Increased risk of death when used in clients with non-life-threatening cardiac arrhythmias. CV:* Hypotension, CHF, *worsening of arrhythmias,* edema, weight gain, cardiac conduction disturbances, SOB, syncope, chest pain, AV block, *severe myocardial depression (with hypotension and increased venous pressure). Anticholinergic:* Dry mouth, urinary retention, constipation, blurred vision, dry nose, eyes, and throat. *GU:* Urinary frequency and urgency, urinary retention, impotence, dysuria. *GI:* Nausea, pain, flatulence, anorexia, diarrhea, vomiting, severe epigastric pain. *CNS:* Headache, nervousness, dizziness, fatigue, depression, insomnia, psychoses. *Dermatologic:* Rash, dermatoses, itching. *Other:* Fever, respiratory problems, gynecomastia, *anaphylaxis,* malaise, muscle weakness, numbness, tingling, angle-closure glaucoma, hypoglycemia, reversible cholestatic jaundice, symptoms of lupus erythematosus (usually in clients switched to disopyramide from procainamide).

**OD** **Overdose Management:** *Symptoms:* Apnea, loss of consciousness, *cardiac arrhythmias* (widening of QRS complex and QT interval, conduction disturbances), hypotension, bradycardia, anticholinergic symptoms, *loss of spontaneous respiration, death. Treatment:* Induction of vomiting, gastric lavage, or a cathartic followed by activated charcoal. Monitor ECG. IV isoproterenol, IV dopamine, cardiac glycosides, diuretics, intra-aortic balloon counterpulsation, artificial respiration, hemodialysis. Use endocardial pacing to treat AV block and neostigmine to treat anticholinergic symptoms.

**Drug Interactions**
*Anticoagulants* / ↓ PT after discontinuing disopyramide
*Beta-adrenergic blockers* / Possible ↓ clearance of disopyramide; sinus bradycardia, hypotension
*Digoxin* / ↑ Serum digoxin levels (may be beneficial)
*Erythromycin* / ↑ Disopyramide levels → arrhythmias and ↑ QTc intervals
*Phenytoin* / ↓ Effect due to ↑ breakdown by liver; ↑ anticholinergic effects
*Quinidine* / ↑ Disopyramide serum levels or ↓ quinidine levels
*Rifampin* / ↓ Effect due to ↑ breakdown by liver

**Laboratory Test Interferences:** ↑ Creatinine, BUN, cholesterol, triglycerides, and liver enzymes.

**Dosage** ――――――――――――
• **Immediate-Release Capsules**
  *Antiarrhythmic.*
**Adults, initial loading dose:** 300 mg of immediate-release capsule (200 mg if client weighs less than 50 kg); **maintenance:** 400–800 mg/day in four divided doses (usual: 150 mg q 6 hr). **For clients less than 50 kg, maintenance:** 100 mg q 6 hr. **Children, less than 1 year:** 10–30 mg/kg/day in divided doses q 6 hr; **1–4 years of age:** 10–20 mg/kg/day in divided doses q 6 hr; **4–12 years of age:** 10–15 mg/kg/day in divided

doses q 6 hr; **12–18 years of age:** 6–15 mg/kg/day in divided doses q 6 hr.

*Severe refractory tachycardia.*

Up to 400 mg q 6 hr may be required.

*Cardiomyopathy.*

Do not administer a loading dose; give 100 mg q 6 hr of immediate-release or 200 mg q 12 hr for controlled-release.

• **Extended-Release Capsules**

*Antiarrhythmic, maintenance only.*

**Adults:** 300 mg q 12 hr (200 mg q 12 hr for body weight less than 50 kg).

*NOTE:* For all uses, decrease dosage in clients with renal or hepatic insufficiency.

*Moderate renal failure or hepatic failure.*

100 mg q 6 hr (or 200 mg/12 hr of sustained-release form).

*Severe renal failure.*

100 mg q 8–24 hr depending on severity (with or without an initial loading dose of 150 mg).

## NURSING CONSIDERATIONS

See also *Nursing Considerations* for *Antiarrhythmic Agents.*

**Administration/Storage**

1. Administer drug only after ECG assessment has been done.

2. Use with other antiarrhythmics (e.g., class IA or propranolol) should be reserved for life-threatening arrhythmias unresponsive to a single agent.

3. Do not use the controlled-release capsule for initial dosage. These are intended for maintenance therapy.

4. When being transferred from the regular PO capsule, give the first controlled-release capsule 6 hr after the last regular dose.

5. For children, a 1–10-mg/mL suspension may be made; add contents of the immediate-release capsule (do NOT use the controlled-release capsule) to cherry syrup. Syrup is stable for 1 month if refrigerated; shake thoroughly before use and dispense in an amber bottle.

**Assessment**

1. Document indications for therapy, type and onset of symptoms.

2. If taking other antiarrhythmic agents, identify and document response.

3. Assess for drug hypersensitivity.

4. Note any urine dribbling, frequency, or sensation of bladder fullness; may worsen with disopyramide. This is particularly important in men with prostatic hypertrophy and in elderly clients who have had prior urinary tract problems; palpate bladder if hesitancy is severe.

5. Obtain ECG, liver and renal function studies; check serum potassium levels and correct if low.

6. Monitor for hypotensive effect; clients with poor LV function are more likely to develop hypotension.

7. If receiving drug in the hospital, monitor ECG for QRS widening, QT prolongation, or first-degree heart block. Hold drug and report if evident.

**Client/Family Teaching**

1. Take at the same time each day.

2. Increase intake of fruit juices and bulk foods to prevent constipation.

3. For dry mouth, use frequent mouth rinses, sugarless gum/hard candy.

4. Avoid alcohol in any form.

5. Report symptoms of CHF (edema, cough, sudden weight gain, increased SOB).

6. Change positions slowly; avoid hot showers, temperature extremes, exposure to the sun, or prolonged standing.

7. Report any mental status changes or confusion.

**Outcomes/Evaluate:** Control of ventricular arrhythmias; stable cardiac rhythm

# Disulfiram

(dye-**SUL**-fih-ram)
Antabuse **(Rx)**
**Classification:** Treatment of alcoholism

**Action/Kinetics:** Produces severe hypersensitivity to alcohol. Inhibits liver enzymes that participate in the normal degradation of alcohol. This results in accumulation of acetaldehyde in the blood. High levels of acetaldehyde produce a series of symptoms referred to as the disulfiram-alcohol reaction or syndrome. The specific symptoms are listed under *Side Effects*. The symptoms vary individually, are dose-dependent with respect to both alcohol and disulfiram, and persist for periods ranging from 30 min to several hours. A single dose of disulfiram may be effective for 1–2 weeks. **Onset:** May be delayed up to 12 hr because disulfiram is initially localized in fat stores.

**Uses:** To prevent further ingestion of alcohol in chronic alcoholics. Should be given only to cooperating clients fully aware of the consequences of alcohol ingestion.

**Contraindications:** Alcohol intoxication. Severe myocardial or occlusive coronary disease. Use of paraldehyde or alcohol-containing products such as cough syrups. If client is exposed to ethylene dibromide.

**Special Concerns:** Use in pregnancy only if benefits outweigh risks. Use with caution in narcotic addicts or clients with diabetes, goiter, epilepsy, psychosis, hypothyroidism, hepatic cirrhosis, or nephritis.

**Side Effects: In the absence of alcohol,** the following symptoms have been reported: Drowsiness (most common), headache, restlessness, fatigue, psychoses, peripheral neuropathy, dermatoses, hepatotoxicity, metallic or garlic taste, arthropathy, impotence. **In the presence of alcohol,** the following symptoms may be manifested. *CV:* Flushing, chest pain, palpitations, tachycardia, hypotension, syncope, arrhythmias, *CV collapse, MI, acute CHF. CNS:* Throbbing headaches, vertigo, weakness, uneasiness, confusion, unconsciousness, *seizures, death. GI:* Nausea, severe vomiting, thirst. *Respiratory:* Respiratory difficulties, dyspnea, hyperventilation, *respirato-*

*ry depression. Other:* Throbbing in head and neck, sweating. In the event of an Antabuse-alcohol interaction, measures should be undertaken to maintain BP and treat shock. Oxygen, antihistamines, ephedrine, and/or vitamin C may also be used.

**Drug Interactions**
*Anticoagulants, oral* / ↑ Effect of anticoagulants by ↑ hypoprothrombinemia
*Barbiturates* / ↑ Effect of barbiturates due to ↓ breakdown by liver
*Chlordiazepoxide, diazepam* / ↑ Effect of chlordiazepoxide or diazepam due to ↓ plasma clearance
*Isoniazid* / ↑ Side effects of isoniazid (especially CNS)
*Metronidazole* / Acute toxic psychosis or confusional state
*Paraldehyde* / Concomitant use produces Antabuse-like effect
*Phenytoin* / ↑ Effect of phenytoin due to ↓ breakdown by liver
*Tricyclic antidepressants* / Acute organic brain syndrome

**Dosage** ─────────────
• **Tablets**
  *Alcoholism.*
**Adults, initial (after alcohol-free interval of 12–48 hr):** 500 mg/day for 1–2 weeks; **maintenance: usual,** 250 mg/day (range: 120–500 mg/day). Dose should not exceed 500 mg/day.

────────────────────────

**NURSING CONSIDERATIONS**
**Client/Family Teaching**
1. Tablets can be crushed or mixed with liquid.
2. Disulfiram should never be given without client's knowledge.
3. CNS side effects should lessen with continued therapy.
4. Ingesting 30 mL of 100-proof alcohol (e.g., one shot) may cause severe symptoms (within 15 min; lasting several hours) and possibly death. Avoid alcohol in any form, in foods, sauces, or other medications, such as cough syrups or tonics; avoid vinegar, paregoric, skin products, linaments, or lotions containing

alcohol. Read all food labels before consuming.

5. May feel tired, experience drowsiness and headaches, and develop a metallic or garlic-like taste; should subside after 2 weeks of therapy.

6. May have occasional impotence, usually transient. Discuss with provider before discontinuing drug.

7. Report if skin eruptions occur; an antihistamine may be prescribed.

8. Carry identification card stating "taking disulfiram" and describing symptoms and treatment if a disulfiram reaction occurs. Include provider and phone number. (Cards may be obtained from the Wyeth-Ayerst Laboratories, P.O. Box 8299, Philadelphia, PA 19101-1245; attention: Professional Services.)

9. Attend local support group meetings, e.g., Alcoholics Anonymous (AA) and Al-Anon, to gain the support, structure, referral, and encouragement that may help to obtain an alcohol-free life.

**Outcomes/Evaluate:** Freedom from alcohol and its effects with resultant sobriety

# Divalproex sodium
(dye-**VAL**-proh-ex)
Depakote, Epival ✦ **(Rx)**

See *Valproic Acid.*

# Dobutamine hydrochloride
(doh-**BYOU**-tah-meen)
**Pregnancy Category:** B
Dobutrex **(Rx)**
**Classification:** Sympathomimetic drug, direct-acting; cardiac stimulant

See also *Sympathomimetic Drugs.*

**Action/Kinetics:** Stimulates beta-1 receptors (in the heart), increasing cardiac function, CO, and SV, with minor effects on HR. Decreases afterload reduction although SBP and pulse pressure may remain unchanged or increase (due to increased CO). Also decreases elevated ventricular filling pressure and helps AV node conduction. **Onset:** 1–2 min. **Peak effect:** 10 min. t½: 2 min. **Therapeutic plasma levels:** 40–190 ng/mL. Metabolized by the liver and excreted in urine.

**Uses:** Short-term treatment of cardiac decompensation in adults secondary to depressed contractility due to organic heart disease or cardiac surgical procedures. *Investigational:* Congenital heart disease in children undergoing diagnostic cardiac catheterization.

**Contraindications:** Idiopathic hypertrophic subaortic stenosis.

**Special Concerns:** Safe use during childhood or after AMI not established.

**Side Effects:** *CV:* Marked increase in HR, BP, and *ventricular ectopic activity,* precipitous drop in BP, premature ventricular beats, anginal and nonspecific chest pain, palpitations. *Hypersensitivity:* Skin rash, pruritus of the scalp, fever, eosinophilia, *bronchospasm. Other:* Nausea, headache, SOB, fever, phlebitis, and local inflammatory changes at the injection site.

**OD** **Overdose Management:** *Symptoms:* Excessive alteration of BP, anorexia N&V, tremor, anxiety, palpitations, headache, SOB, anginal and nonspecific chest pain, *myocardial ischemia, ventricular fibrillation or tachycardia. Treatment:* Reduce the rate of administration or discontinue temporarily until the condition stabilizes. Establish an airway, ensuring oxygenation and ventilation. Initiate resuscitative measures immediately. Treat severe ventricular tachyarrhythmias with propranolol or lidocaine.

**Additional Drug Interactions:** Concomitant use with nitroprusside causes ↑ CO and ↓ pulmonary wedge pressure.

**Dosage** ————
• **IV Infusion**
**Adults, individualized, usual:** 2.5–15 mcg/kg/min (up to 40 mcg/kg/min). Rate of administration and duration of therapy depend on re-

sponse of client, as determined by HR, presence of ectopic activity, BP, and urine flow.

## NURSING CONSIDERATIONS

See also *Nursing Considerations* for *Sympathomimetic Drugs*.

**Administration/Storage**

**IV** 1. Reconstitute solution according to manufacturers directions; takes place in two stages.

2. Before administration, the solution is diluted further according to the fluid needs of the client. This more dilute solution should be used within 24 hr. Solutions that can be used for further dilution include 5% dextrose injection, D5%/0.45% NaCl injection, D5%/0.9% NaCl injection, 10% dextrose injection, Isolyte M with 5% dextrose injection, RL injection, D5%/RL, Normosol-M in D5W, 20% Osmitrol in water for injection, 0.9% NaCl injection, and sodium lactate injection.

3. The more concentrated solution may be refrigerated for 48 hr or stored at room temperature for 6 hr. After dilution (in glass or Viaflex containers), the solution is stable for 24 hr at room temperature.Dilute solutions may darken; does not affect potency when used within designated time spans.

4. Drug is incompatible with alkaline solutions. Do not give with agents or diluents containing both sodium bisulfite and ethanol. Is physically incompatible with hydrocortisone sodium succinate, cefazolin, cefamandole, neutral cephalothin, penicillin, sodium ethacrynate, and heparin sodium.

5. Drug is compatible when given through same tubing with dopamine, lidocaine, tobramycin, verapamil, nitroprusside, potassium chloride, and protamine sulfate.

6. Give using an electronic infusion device. Carefully reconstitute and calculate dosage according to weight and desired response.

**Assessment:** Ensure that client is adequately hydrated prior to infusion.

**Interventions**

1. Monitor CVP to assess vascular volume and right-sided cardiac pumping efficiency. Normal range 5–10 cm water (1–7 mm Hg). Elevated CVP may indicate disruption of CO, as in pump failure or pulmonary edema; low CVP may indicate hypovolemia.

2. Monitor PAWP to assess the pressures in the left atrium and ventricle and to measure the efficiency of CO; usual range is 6–12 mm Hg.

3. Monitor ECG and BP continuously during drug administration; review written parameters for SBP and titrate infusion.

4. Record I&O.

5. Monitor glucose in diabetics; increased insulin may be needed.

**Outcomes/Evaluate**

- ↑ CO; ↑ urine output
- SBP > 90 mm Hg

# Docetaxel
(doh-seh-**TAX**-ell)
**Pregnancy Category:** D
Taxotere **(Rx)**
**Classification:** Antineoplastic, miscellaneous

See also *Antineoplastic Agents*.

**Action/Kinetics:** Prepared with a precursor extracted from the yew plant. Effect is due to disruption of the microtubular network in cells that is required for mitotic and interphase cellular functions. **t½, 3 phases:** 4 min, 36 min, and 11.1 hr. Metabolized in the liver, and metabolites and small amounts of unchanged drug are excreted through both the feces (75%) and urine (6%).

**Uses:** Locally advanced or metastatic breast cancer in those who have progressed during anthracycline-based therapy or have relapsed during anthracycline-based adjuvant therapy.

**Contraindications:** Severe hypersensitivity to docetaxel or to other drugs formulated with polysorbate

---

✦ = Available in Canada                 **bold italic** = life threatening side effect

80. Use in those with neutrophil counts less than 1,500 cells/mm³, in those with bilirubin greater than the upper limit of normal (ULN), or in those with AST or ALT greater than 1.5 times the ULN. Lactation.

**Special Concerns:** The incidence of treatment-related mortality is increased in clients with abnormal liver function and in those receiving higher doses. Safety and efficacy have not been determined in children less than 16 years of age.

**Side Effects:** *Hematologic:* Neutropenia (virtually in 100% of clients given 100 mg/m²). Leukopenia, thrombocytopenia, anemia, febrile neutropenia. *GI:* N&V, diarrhea, stomatitis, abdominal pain, constipation, ulcer, esophagitis, **GI hemorrhage,** intestinal obstruction, ileus. *CV:* Fluid retention (even with premedication), hypotension, atrial fibrillation, **DVT,** ECG abnormalities, thrombophlebitis, **pulmonary embolism, heart failure,** syncope, tachycardia, sinus tachycardia, atrial flutter, dysrhythmia, unstable angina, pulmonary edema, hypertension (rare). *Respiratory:* Dyspnea, **acute pulmonary edema, ARDS.** *Dermatologic:* Reversible cutaneous reactions characterized by a rash, including localized eruptions on the hands, feet, arms, face, or thorax, and usually associated with pruritus. Nail changes, alopecia. *Hypersensitivity:* Flushing, localized skin reactions. Severe hypersensitivity reactions characterized by hypotension, bronchospasm, or generalized rash/erythema. *Musculoskeletal:* Myalgia, arthralgia. *Neurologic:* Paresthesia, dysesthesia, pain in those with anthracycline-resistant breast cancer. Distal extremity weakness. *Reactions at infusion site:* Hyperpigmentation, inflammation, redness or dryness of the skin, phlebitis, extravasation, mild swelling of the vein. *Miscellaneous:* **Septic death, nonseptic death,** infections, fever in absence of infections, asthenia, diffuse pain, chest pain, renal insufficiency, confusion.

**Drug Interactions:** The metabolism of docetaxel may be modified by drugs that inhibit, induce, or are metabolized by the cytochrome P4503A4 system, including cyclosporine, erythromycin, ketoconazole, terfenidine, and troleandomycin.

## Dosage
• **IV**

*Breast cancer.*
60–100 mg/m² given IV over 1 hr q 3 weeks. Reduce the dose to 75 mg/m² or discontinue therapy in those who are dosed initially at 100 mg/m² and who experience febrile neutropenia, neutrophils less than 500/mm³ for more than 1 week, severe or cumulative cutaneous reactions, or severe peripheral neuropathy. Those who are dosed at 60 mg/m² and do not experience these symptoms may tolerate higher doses.

## NURSING CONSIDERATIONS

See also *Nursing Considerations* for *Antineoplastic Agents.*

### Administration/Storage

**IV** 1. To reduce severity of fluid retention and hypersensitivity reactions, premedicate with PO corticosteroids (e.g., dexamethasone, 16 mg/day) for 5 days starting 1 day prior to therapy.

2. Vials should stand at room temperature for about 5 min before using. Both the injection concentrate and the diluent vials contain an overfill. The 20-mg vial contains 23.6 mg and the 80-mg vial contains 94.4 mg of the drug. Only the final concentration of 10 mg/mL, prepared with the supplied diluent, should be used for preparing doses. Using the entire content of the vial for each 20- or 80-mg dose may result in a significant overdose when multiple vials are used.

3. The diluted concentrate of 10 mg/mL is then used to prepare the solution for infusion. Withdraw the required amount of docetaxel using a calibrated syringe. Inject into a 250-mL infusion bag or bottle of either 0.9% NaCl injection or 5% dextrose injection to produce a final concentration of 0.3–0.9 mg/mL; administer as a 1-hr IV

infusion. If doses greater than 240 mg are required, use more solution so that the concentration to be infused does not exceed 0.9 mg/mL.

4. Protect the drug from light and refrigerate at 2°C–8°C (36°F–46°F). The premixed solution is stable for 8 hr. Do not store in PVC bags.

**Assessment**

1. Document indications for therapy, disease onset, previous agents used, and the outcome.

2. Note any previous experience with this drug. If previous hypersensitivity, do not rechallenge.

3. List other drugs prescribed to ensure none interact unfavorably.

4. Monitor CBC and LFTs. Drug causes bone marrow suppression. Nadir: 8 days.

**Client/Family Teaching**

1. May experience a rash 1 week after treatment; this should subside.

2. Prepare for hair loss.

3. Report any evidence of infection, fever, or illness. Avoid crowds and people with contagious diseases.

**Outcomes/Evaluate:** Control of metastatic process

---

# Docusate calcium (Dioctyl calcium sulfosuccinate)

(**DEW**-kyou-sayt)
**Pregnancy Category:** C
Albert Docusate ✸, DC Softgels, PMS Docusate Calcium ✸, Pro-Cal-Sof, Sulfalax Calcium, Surfak ✸, Surfak Liquigels **(OTC)**

# Docusate potassium (Dioctyl potassium sulfosuccinate)

(**DEW**-kyou-sayt)
**Pregnancy Category:** C
Dialose, Diocto-K **(OTC)**

# Docusate sodium (Dioctyl sodium sulfosuccinate)

(**DEW**-kyou-sayt)

**Pregnancy Category:** C
Colace, Diocto, Dioeze, Disonate, DOK, DOS Softgel, D-S-S, Modane Soft, PMS-Docusate Sodium ✸, Regulax SS, Regulex ✸, Selax ✸, Soflax ✸ **(OTC)**
**Classification:** Laxative, emollient

See also *Laxatives.*

**Action/Kinetics:** Acts by lowering the surface tension of the feces and promoting penetration by water and fat, thus increasing the softness of the fecal mass. Not absorbed systemically and does not seem to interfere with the absorption of nutrients. A microenema formulation is available for clients aged 3 and older. **Onset:** 24–72 hr.; **onset, microenema formulation:** 15 min.

**Uses:** To lessen strain of defecation in persons with hernia or CV diseases or other diseases in which straining at stool should be avoided. Megacolon or bedridden clients. Constipation associated with dry, hard stools. The microemulsion formulation is indicated for relief of occasional constipation in children over the age of 3 years.

**Contraindications:** Nausea, vomiting, abdominal pain, and intestinal obstruction.

**Drug Interactions:** Docusate may ↑ absorption of mineral oil from the GI tract.

**Dosage** ——————
Docusate calcium
• **Capsules**
**Adults:** 240 mg/day until bowel movements are normal; **pediatric, over 6 years:** 50–150 mg/day.
Docusate potassium
• **Capsules**
**Adults:** 100–300 mg/day; **pediatric, over 6 years:** 100 mg at bedtime.
Docusate sodium
• **Capsules, Oral Liquid, Syrup, Tablets**
**Adults and children over 12 years:** 50–500 mg; **pediatric, under 3 years:** 10–40 mg; **3–6 years:** 20–60 mg; **6–12 years:** 40–120 mg.
• **Rectal Solution**

---

*Flushing or retention enema.*
**Adults:** 50–100 mg.

## NURSING CONSIDERATIONS

See also *Nursing Considerations* for *Laxatives.*

**Client/Family Teaching**

1. May administer PO solutions of docusate with milk or fruit juices to help mask bitter taste.
2. Drink a glass of water with each PO dose.
3. When used in enemas, add 50–100 mg (5–10 mL) to a retention or flushing enema.
4. Because docusate salts are minimally absorbed, it may require 1–3 days to soften fecal matter.

**Outcomes/Evaluate:** Elimination of a soft, formed stool; ↓ straining

---

# Dolasetron mesylate

(dohl-**AH**-seh-tron)
**Pregnancy Category:** B
Anzemet **(Rx)**
**Classification:** Antinauseant/antiemetic, serotonin 5-HT$_3$ antagonist

**Action/Kinetics:** Selective serotonin 5-HT$_3$ antagonist that prevents N&V by inhibiting released serotonin from combining with receptors on vagal efferents that initiate vomiting reflex. May also cause acute, usually reversible, PR and QT$_c$ prolongation and QRS widening, perhaps due to blockade of sodium channels by active metabolite of dolasetron. Well absorbed from GI tract. Metabolized to active hydrodolasetron: **peak plasma levels:** 1 hr; t½: 8.1 hr. Food does not affect bioavailability. Hydrodolasetron is excreted through urine and feces. Is eliminated more quickly in children than in adults.

**Uses:** Prevention of N&V associated with moderately-emetogenic cancer chemotherapy (initially and repeat courses). Prevention of postoperative N&V.

**Special Concerns:** Use with caution during lactation and in those who have or may develop prolongation of cardiac conduction intervals, including QT$_c$. These include clients with hypokalemia or hypomagnesemia, those taking diuretics with potential for electrolyte abnormalities, in congenital QT syndrome, those taking anti-arrhythmic drugs or other drugs which lead to QT prolongation, and cumulative high dose anthracycline therapy. Safety and efficacy in children less than 2 years of age have not been determined.

**Side Effects: Chemotherapy clients.** Headache, fatigue, diarrhea, bradycardia, dizziness, pain, tachycardia, dyspepsia, chills, shivering. **Postoperative clients.** Headache, hypotension, dizziness, fever, pruritus, oliguria, hypertension, tachycardia. **Chemotherapy or postoperative clients.** *CV:* Hypotension, edema, peripheral edema, peripheral ischemia, thrombophlebitis, phlebitis. *GI:* Constipation, dyspepsia, abdominal pain, anorexia, pancreatitis, taste perversion. *CNS:* Flushing, vertigo, paresthesia, tremor, ataxia, twitching, agitation, sleep disorder, depersonalization, confusion, anxiety, abnormal dreaming. *Dermatologic:* Rash, increased sweating. *Hematologic:* Hematuria, epistaxis, anemia, purpura, hematoma, thrombocytopenia. *Hypersensitivity:* Rarely, **anaphylaxis,** facial edema, urticaria. *Musculoskeletal:* Myalgia, arthralgia. *Respiratory:* Dyspnea, bronchospasm. *GU:* Dysuria, polyuria, acute renal failure. *Ophthalmic:* Abnormal vision, photophobia. *Miscellaneous:* Tinnitus.

**Laboratory Test Alteration:** ↑ PTT, AST, ALT, alkaline phosphatase. Prolonged prothrombin time.

**Drug Interactions:** There is the potential for dolasetron to interact with other drugs that prolong the QT$_c$ interval.

**Dosage**
• **Tablets**
*Prevention of N&V during chemotherapy.*
**Adults:** 100 mg within 1 hr before chemotherapy. **Children, 2 to 16 years:** 1.8 mg/kg within 1 hr before

chemotherapy, up to a maximum of 100 mg.

*Prevention of postoperative N&V.*
**Adults:** 100 mg within 2 hr before surgery. **Children, 2 to 16 years:** 1.2 mg/kg within 2 hr before surgery, up to a maximum of 100 mg.

• **IV**
*Prevention of N&V during chemotherapy.*
**Adults:** 1.8 mg/kg as a single dose about 30 min before chemotherapy. Alternatively, a fixed dose of 100 mg can be given over 30 seconds. **Children, 2 to 16 years:** 1.8 mg/kg as a single dose about 30 min before chemotherapy, up to a maximum of 100 mg.

*Prevention of postoperative N&V.*
**Adults:** 12.5 mg given as a single dose. **Children, 2 to 16 years:** 0.35 mg/kg, up to a maximum of 12.5 mg. For adults and children, give about 15 min before cessation of anesthesia or as soon as nausea and vomiting presents.

**Note:** For children, injection may be mixed with apple or apple-grape juice and used for oral dosing. When injection is used PO, recommended dose for prevention of cancer chemotherapy N&V is 1.8 mg/kg (up to a maximum of 100 mg) and dose for prevention of postoperative N&V is 1.2 mg/kg (up to a maximum of 100 mg). Diluted injection may be kept up to 2 hr at room temperature before use.

## NURSING CONSIDERATIONS
### Administration/Storage
**IV** 1. Injection can be safely infused as rapidly as 100 mg/30 seconds. May also be diluted to 50 mL with 0.9% NaCl injection, 5% dextrose injection, D5/0.45% NaCl, D5%/RL injection, lactated Ringer's injection, and 10% mannitol injection. Dilutions are given over 15 min. Diluted product is stable for 24 hr (48 hr if refrigerated).
2. Do not mix injection with any other drugs.

3. Flush infusion line before and after administration of dolasetron.
4. Inspect visually for particulate matter and discoloration before using.
5. Store injection at controlled room temperature protected from light.

**Assessment**
1. Note indications for therapy.
2. List drugs prescribed to ensure none interact unfavorably.
3. Monitor CBC, electrolytes, Mg and ECG.
4. Give 1 hr before chemo or 2 hrs before surgery to gain desired effect.
5. With children, calculate appropriate dose (cancer chemo or postop N&V); may administer orally with apple or apple-grape juice.

**Outcomes/Evaluate:** Inhibition of cancer chemotherapy induced or postop N&V

# Donepezil hydrochloride
(dohn-**EP**-eh-zil)
**Pregnancy Category:** C
Aricept **(Rx)**
**Classification:** Psychotherapeutic drug for Alzheimer's disease

**Action/Kinetics:** A decrease in cholinergic function may be the cause of Alzheimer's disease. Donepezil is a cholinesterase inhibitor and exerts its effect by enhancing cholinergic function by increasing levels of acetylcholine. There is no evidence that the drug alters the course of the underlying dementing process. Well absorbed from the GI tract. **Peak plasma levels:** 3–4 hr. Food does not affect the rate or extent of absorption. Metabolized in the liver, and both unchanged drug and metabolites are excreted in the urine and feces.

**Uses:** Treatment of mild to moderate dementia of the Alzheimer's type.
**Contraindications:** Hypersensitivity to piperidine derivatives.
**Special Concerns:** Use with caution in clients with a history of asthma or obstructive pulmonary disease. Safety and efficacy have not been determined for use in children.

**Side Effects:** *NOTE:* Side effects with an incidence of 1% or greater are listed. *GI:* N&V, diarrhea, anorexia, fecal incontinence, GI bleeding, bloating, epigastric pain. *CNS:* Insomnia, dizziness, depression, abnormal dreams, somnolence. *CV:* Hypertension, vasodilation, atrial fibrillation, hot flashes, hypotension, bradycardia. *Body as a whole:* Headache, pain (in various locations), accident, fatigue, influenza, chest pain, toothache. *Musculoskeletal:* Muscle cramps, arthritis, bone fracture. *Dermatologic:* Diaphoresis, urticaria, pruritus. *GU:* Urinary incontinence, nocturia, frequent urination. *Respiratory:* Dyspnea, sore throat, bronchitis. *Ophthalmic:* Cataract, eye irritation, blurred vision. *Miscellaneous:* Dehydration, syncope, ecchymosis, weight loss.

**OD** **Overdose Management:** *Symptoms:* Cholinergic crisis characterized by severe N&V, salivation, sweating, bradycardia, hypotension, respiratory depression, collapse, convulsions, increased muscle weakness (may cause death if respiratory muscles are involved). *Treatment:* Atropine sulfate at an initial dose of 1–2 mg IV with subsequent doses based on the response. General supportive measures.

**Drug Interactions**
*Anticholinergic drugs* / The cholinesterase inhibitor activitiy of donepezil interferes with the activity of anticholinergics
*Bethanechol* / Synergistic effect
*NSAIDs* / ↑ Gastric acid secretion → ↑ risk of active or occult GI bleeding
*Succinylcholine* / ↑ Muscle relaxant effect

**Dosage** ————
• **Tablets**
*Alzheimer's disease.*
**Initial:** 5 mg. Use of a 10-mg dose did not provide a clinical effect greater than the 5-mg dose; however, in some clients, 10 mg daily may be superior. Do not increase the dose to 10 mg until clients have been on a daily dose of 5 mg for 4 to 6 weeks.

## NURSING CONSIDERATIONS

**Administration/Storage:** Store at controlled room temperatures from 15°C to 30°C (59°F to 86°F).

**Assessment**
1. Document onset/duration, other agents trialed, and the outcome.
2. Describe clinical presentation.
3. Note any history of asthma or COPD.
4. Obtain baseline ECG and lab values.

**Client/Family Teaching**
1. Take in the evening, just prior to bedtime.
2. May take with or without food.
3. Report any irregular pulse or dizzy spells, lack of response or worsening of symptoms.

**Outcomes/Evaluate:** Improved cognitive functioning with Alzheimer's.

————*COMBINATION DRUG*————

# Donnatal Capsules, Elixir, Tablets

(**DON**-nah-tal)
**Pregnancy Category:** C
**(Rx)**
**Classification:** Anticholinergic

**Content:** Each tablet, capsule, or 5 mL elixir contains: *Anticholinergic:* Atropine sulfate, 0.0194 mg. *Anticholinergic:* Hyoscyamine sulfate, 0.1037 mg. *Anticholinergic:* Scopolamine hydrobromide, 0.0065 mg. *Sedative:* Phenobarbital, 16.2 mg. *NOTE:* The Extentabs contain three times the amount of drugs found in tablets.

**Uses:** Possibly effective as an adjunct in the treatment of irritable colon, spastic colon, mucous colitis, and acute enterocolitis. Has also been used in the treatment of duodenal ulcer.

**Special Concerns:** It is not known with certainty whether or not anticholinergic drugs aid in the healing in duodenal ulcer or decrease the rate of recurrence or prevent complications.

**Dosage** ————
• **Tablets, Capsules, Extentabs, Elixir**
**Adults, usual:** 1–2 tablets or capsules t.i.d.–q.i.d. (or one Extentab q 12

hr). If the elixir is used, **adult, usual:** 5–10 mL t.i.d.–q.i.d. **Pediatric:** Use elixir as follows: **4.5–9.0 kg:** 0.5 mL q 4 hr or 0.75 mL q 6 hr; **9.1–13.5 kg:** 1.0 mL q 4 hr or 1.5 mL q 6 hr; **13.6–22.6 kg:** 1.5 mL q 4 hr or 2.0 mL q 6 hr; **22.7–33.9 kg:** 2.5 mL q 4 hr or 3.75 mL q 6 hr. **34.0–45.3 kg:** 3.75 mL q 4 hr or 5 mL q 6 hr; **45.4 kg:** 5 mL q 4 hr or 7.5 mL q 6 hr.

## NURSING CONSIDERATIONS

See also *Nursing Considerations* for *Cholinergic Blocking Agents* and *Barbiturates*.
**Outcomes/Evaluate:** Relief of abdominal pain; improved bowel motility

# Dopamine hydrochloride
(**DOH**-pah-meen)
**Pregnancy Category:** C
Intropin **(Rx)**
**Classification:** Sympathomimetic, direct- and indirect-acting; cardiac stimulant and vasopressor

See also *Sympathomimetic Drugs.*
**Action/Kinetics:** Dopamine is the immediate precursor of epinephrine in the body. Exogenously administered, it produces direct stimulation of beta-1 receptors and variable (dose-dependent) stimulation of alpha receptors (peripheral vasoconstriction). Will cause a release of norepinephrine from its storage sites . These actions result in increased myocardial contraction, CO, and SV, as well as increased renal blood flow and sodium excretion. Exerts little effect on DBP and induces fewer arrhythmias than are seen with isoproterenol. **Onset:** 5 min. **Duration:** 10 min. **t½:** 2 min. Does not cross the blood-brain barrier. Metabolized in liver and excreted in urine.
**Uses:** Cardiotonic shock due to MI, trauma, endotoxic septicemia, open heart surgery, renal failure, and chronic cardiac decompensation (as in CHF). Clients most likely to respond include those in whom urine flow,

myocardial function, and BP have not deteriorated significantly. Best responses are observed when the time is short between onset of symptoms of shock and initiation of dopamine and volume correction. *Investigational:* COPD, CHF, respiratory distress syndrome in infants.
**Additional Contraindications:** Pheochromocytoma, uncorrected tachycardia or arrhythmias. Pediatric clients.
**Special Concerns:** Use with caution during lactation. Safety and efficacy have not been established in children. Dosage may have to be adjusted in geriatric clients with occlusive vascular disease.
**Additional Side Effects:** *CV:* Ectopic heartbeats, tachycardia, anginal pain, palpitations, vasoconstriction, hypotension, hypertension. Infrequently: aberrant conduction, bradycardia, widened QRS complex. *Other:* Dyspnea, headache, mydriasis. Infrequently, piloerection, azotemia, polyuria. High doses may cause mydriasis and ventricular arrhythmia. Extravasation may result in necrosis and sloughing of surrounding tissue.
**OD Overdose Management:** *Symptoms:* Extravasation. *Treatment:* To prevent sloughing and necrosis, infiltrate as soon as possible with 10–15 mL of 0.9% NaCl solution containing 5–10 mg phentolamine using a syringe with a fine needle. Infiltrate liberally throughout the ischemic area.
**Additional Drug Interactions**
*Diuretics* / Additive or potentiating effect
*Phenytoin* / Hypotension and bradycardia
*Propranolol* / ↓ Effect of dopamine

**Dosage**
• **IV Infusion**
  *Shock.*
**Initial:** 2–5 mcg/kg/min; **then,** increase in increments of 1–4 mcg/kg/min at 10–30-min intervals until desired response is obtained.

---

***bold italic*** = life threatening side effect

*Severely ill clients.*
**Initial:** 5 mcg/kg/min; **then,** increase rate in increments of 5–10 mcg/kg/min up to 20–50 mcg/kg/min as needed.
*NOTE:* Dopamine is a potent drug. Be sure to dilute the drug before administration. The drug should not be given as a bolus dose.

## NURSING CONSIDERATIONS

See also *Nursing Considerations* for *Sympathomimetic Drugs.*
**Administration/Storage**
**IV** 1. Must be diluted before use—see package insert.
2. For reconstitution use dextrose or saline solutions: 200 mg/250 mL for a concentration of 0.8 mg/mL or 800 mcg/mL; 400 mg/250 mL for a concentration of 1.6 mg/mL or 1,600 mcg/mL. Alkaline solutions such as 5% sodium bicarbonate, oxidizing agents, or iron salts will inactivate dopamine.
3. Dilute solution stable for 24 hr at room temperature; dilute just prior to administration. Protect from light.
4. To prevent overloading system with excess fluid, may use more concentrated solutions with higher doses.
5. Administer using an electronic infusion device. Carefully reconstitute and calculate dosage.
6. When discontinuing, gradually decrease dose; sudden cessation may cause marked hypotension.
**Assessment:** Determine that client is hydrated prior to initiating infusion.
**Interventions**
1. Monitor VS, I&O, and ECG; titrate infusion to maintain SBP as ordered.
2. Be prepared to monitor CVP and pulmonary artery wedge pressures.
3. Report any ectopy, palpitations, anginal pain, or vasoconstriction.
**Outcomes/Evaluate**
• SBP > 90; ↑ urine output
• Improved organ perfusion

# Dornase alfa recombinant
(**DOR**-nace **AL**-fah)

**Pregnancy Category:** B
Pulmozyme **(Rx)**
**Classification:** Drug for Cystic Fibrosis

**Action/Kinetics:** This drug is a highly purified solution of recombinant human deoxyribonuclease I (rhDNase), an enzyme that selectively cleaves DNA. It is produced by genetically engineered Chinese hamster ovary cells that contain DNA encoded for the native human protein, deoxyribonuclease (DNase). The amino acid sequence is identical to that of the native human enzyme. Cystic fibrosis (CF) clients have viscous purulent secretions in the airways that contribute to reduced pulmonary function and worsening of infection. These secretions contain high concentrations of extracellular DNA released by degenerating leukocytes that accumulate as a result of infection. Dornase alfa hydrolyzes the DNA in sputum of CF clients, thereby reducing sputum viscoelasticity and reducing infections.
**Uses:** In CF clients in conjunction with standard therapy to decrease the frequency of respiratory infections that require parenteral antibiotics and to improve pulmonary function.
**Contraindications:** Known sensitivity to dornase alfa or products from Chinese hamster ovary cells.
**Special Concerns:** Safety and effectiveness of daily use have not been demonstrated in clients less than 5 years of age, in those with forced vital capacity (FVC) of less than 40% of predicted, or for longer than 12 months. Use with caution during lactation.
**Side Effects:** *Respiratory:* Pharyngitis, voice alteration, and laryngitis are the most common. Also, *apnea,* bronchiectasis, bronchitis, change in sputum, cough increase, dyspnea, hemoptysis, lung function decrease, nasal polyps, pneumonia, pneumothorax, rhinitis, sinusitis, sputum increase, wheezing. *Body as a whole:* Abdominal pain, asthenia, fever, flu syndrome, malaise, sepsis, weight loss. *GI:* Intestinal obstruction, gall

bladder disease, liver disease, pancreatic disease. *Miscellaneous:* Rash, urticaria, chest pain, conjunctivitis, diabetes mellitus, hypoxia.

## Dosage
- **Inhalation Solution**
  *Cystic fibrosis.*
One 2.5-mg single-dose ampule inhaled once daily using a recommended nebulizer (see what follows). Older clients and clients with baseline FVC above 85% may benefit from twice daily dosing.

## NURSING CONSIDERATIONS
### Administration/Storage
1. Approved nebulizers include the disposable jet nebulizer Hudson T U-draft II, disposable jet nebulizer Marquest Acorn II in conjunction with a Pulmo-Aide compressor, and the reusable PARI LC Jet+ nebulizer in conjunction with the PARI PRONEB compressor. Safety and efficacy have been demonstrated with only these nebulizers.
2. Do not dilute or mix with other drugs in nebulizer. Mixing could lead to adverse physicochemical or functional changes in dornase alfa.
3. Must be stored in the refrigerator at 2°C–8°C (36°F–46°F) in the protective foil pouch and protected from strong light.
4. Refrigerate when transported and do not expose to room temperature for a total time of 24 hr.
5. Discard if solution is cloudy or discolored.
6. Product does not contain a preservative; thus, once opened, entire ampule must be used or discarded.
### Assessment
1. Document age of CF symptom onset, other therapies trialed, and outcome.
2. Drug is produced by genetically engineered Chinese hamster ovary cells; assess for sensitivity.
3. Monitor PFTs.
### Client/Family Teaching
1. Drug is administered by inhalation of an aerosol mist generated by a compressed air-driven nebulizer system; review dose, frequency, and method for inhalation. Ensure familiarity with use, care, and storage of equipment and drug.
2. Must be performed on a daily schedule to obtain full pharmacologic benefits. Must continue standard therapies for CF, e.g., chest PT, antibiotics, bronchodilators, oral and inhaled corticosteroids, enzyme supplements, vitamins, and analgesics during dornase alfa therapy.
3. Report symptoms that require immediate medical intervention: severe rashes, itching, respiratory distress, fever. Learn CPR.
4. Identify support groups that may assist to cope with this disease.
### Outcomes/Evaluate
- ↓ Respiratory tract infectious exacerbations; ↓ sputum viscosity
- Improved PFTs

# Dorzolamide hydrochloride ophthalmic solution
(dor-**ZOH**-lah-myd)
**Pregnancy Category:** C
Trusopt **(Rx)**
**Classification:** Carbonic anhydrase inhibitor

**Action/Kinetics:** Decreases aqueous humor secretion in the ciliary processes of the eye by inhibiting carbonic anhydrase. Occurs by decreasing the formation of bicarbonate ions with a reduction in sodium and fluid transport and a subsequent decrease in intraocular pressure. The drug may reach the systemic circulation, where it and the metabolite are excreted through the urine. The drug and metabolite also accumulate in RBCs.
**Uses:** Elevated intraocular pressure (IOP) in those with ocular hypertension or open-angle glaucoma.
**Contraindications:** Use with severe renal impairment ($C_{Cr}$ < 30 mL/min) or in soft contact lens wearers as the preservative (benzalko-

nium chloride) may be absorbed by the lenses. Lactation.

**Special Concerns:** Dorzolamide is a sulfonamide and, as such, may cause similar systemic reactions, including side effects and allergic reactions, as sulfonamides. Use with caution in hepatic impairment. Due to additive effects, concurrent use of dorzolamide with systemic carbonic anhydrase inhibitors is not recommended. Safety and efficacy have not been determined in children. It is possible geriatric clients may show greater sensitivity to the drug.

**Side Effects:** *Ophthalmic:* Conjunctivitis, lid reactions, bacterial keratitis (due to contamination by concurrent corneal disease). Ocular burning, stinging, or discomfort immediately following administration. Also, superficial punctate keratitis, ocular allergic reaction, blurred vision, tearing, dryness, photophobia, iridocyclitis (rare). *Miscellaneous:* Acid-base and electrolyte disturbances (i.e., similar to systemic use of carbonic anhydrase inhibitors). Also, bitter taste following instillation, headache, nausea, asthenia, fatigue. Rarely, skin rashes, urolithiasis.

**Dosage**
• **Ophthalmic Solution**
    *Increased intraocular pressure.*
    **Adults:** 1 gtt in the affected eye(s) t.i.d.

**NURSING CONSIDERATIONS**

**Administration/Storage:** Protect from light and store at 15°C–30°C (59°F–86°F).

**Assessment:** Document visual symptoms and baseline IOP. Note any sensitivity to sulfonamides or impaired renal function.

**Client/Family Teaching**
1. Do not let dispenser tip come in contact with eye or surrounding structures as contamination may result.
2. Use only as prescribed. Report any evidence of conjunctivitis or ocular or lid reaction. Burning or stinging may accompany administra-

tion and a bitter taste may also be noted.
3. May be used with other topical ophthalmic drugs. If more than one is being used, give them at least 10 min apart.
4. Do not administer drops while wearing contact lenses as they may absorb solution preservative.
**Outcomes/Evaluate:** ↓ IOP

# Doxacurium chloride
(dox-ah-**KYOUR**-ee-um **KLOR**-ide)
**Pregnancy Category:** C
Neuromax, Nuromax ✱ **(Rx)**
**Classification:** Neuromuscular blocking agent

See also *Neuromuscular Blocking Agents.*

**Action/Kinetics:** Binds to cholinergic receptors on the motor end-plate to block the action of acetylcholine, resulting in a blockade of neuromuscular transmission. Up to 3 times more potent than pancuronium and up to 12 times more potent than metocurine. The time to maximum neuromuscular blockade during balanced anesthesia is dose-dependent and ranges from 9.3 min (following doses of 0.025 mg/kg) to 3.5 min (following doses of 0.08 mg/kg). The time to 25% recovery from blockade following balanced anesthesia ranges from 55 min for doses of 0.025 mg/kg to 160 min for doses of 0.08 mg/kg. **t½, elimination:** Dose-dependent, ranging from 86 to 123 min. The half-life is prolonged in kidney transplant clients. Children require higher doses on a mg/kg basis than adults to achieve the same level of blockade. Also, the onset, time, and duration of block are shorter in children than adults. The blockade may be reversed by anticholinesterase agents. Excreted unchanged through the urine and bile.
**Uses:** Adjunct to general anesthesia to provide skeletal muscle relaxation during surgery. Skeletal muscle relaxation for ET intubation or to facilitate mechanical ventilation.

**Special Concerns:** Use with caution during lactation. Safety and effectiveness have not been determined in children less than 2 years of age. The duration of action may be up to twice as long for clients over 60 years of age and those who are obese (more than 30% more than ideal body weight for height). Malignant hyperthermia may occur in any client receiving a general anesthetic. A profound effect may be noted in clients with neuromuscular diseases such as myasthenia gravis and the myasthenic syndrome.

**Side Effects:** *Neuromuscular:* Skeletal muscle weakness, *profound and prolonged skeletal muscle paralysis causing respiratory insufficiency and apnea;* difficulty in reversing the neuromuscular blockade. *CV:* Hypotension, flushing, *ventricular fibrillation, MI. Respiratory:* Wheezing, *bronchospasm. Dermatologic:* Urticaria, reaction at injection site. *Miscellaneous:* Fever, diplopia.

**OD Overdose Management:** *Symptoms:* Prolonged neuromuscular block. *Treatment:* Maintain a patent airway and use controlled ventilation if necessary until recovery of normal neuromuscular function. Once recovery begins, it can be facilitated by giving neostigmine, 0.06 mg/kg.

**Drug Interactions**
*Aminoglycosides* / ↑ Effect of doxacurium
*Bacitracin* / ↑ Effect of doxacurium
*Carbamazepine* / ↑ Onset of effects and ↓ the duration of action of doxacurium
*Clindamycin* / ↑ Effect of doxacurium
*Colistin* / ↑ Effect of doxacurium
*Enflurane* / ↓ Amount of doxacurium necessary to cause blockade and ↑ the duration of action
*Halothane* / ↓ Amount of doxacurium necessary to cause blockade and ↑ the duration of action
*Isoflurane* / ↓ Amount of doxacurium necessary to cause blockade and ↑ the duration of action

*Lincomycin* / ↑ Effect of doxacurium
*Lithium* / ↑ Effect of doxacurium
*Local anesthetics* / ↑ Effect of doxacurium
*Magnesium salts* / ↑ Effect of doxacurium
*Phenytoin* / ↑ Onset of effects and ↓ the duration of action of doxacurium
*Polymyxins* / ↑ Effect of doxacurium
*Procainamide* / ↑ Effect of doxacurium
*Quinidine* / ↑ Effect of doxacurium
*Sodium colistimethate* / ↑ Effect of doxacurium
*Tetracyclines* / ↑ Effect of doxacurium

**Dosage**
• **IV Only**
*As a component of thiopental/narcotic induction-intubation, to produce neuromuscular blockade of long duration.*
**Adults, initial:** 0.05 mg/kg.
*If administered during steady-state enflurane, halothane, or isoflurane anesthesia.*
Reduce dose by one-third. **Children:** 0.03 mg/kg for blockade lasting about 30 min or 0.05 mg/kg for blockade lasting about 45 min when used during halothane anesthesia. Maintenance doses are required more frequently in children.
*Used with succinylcholine to facilitate ET intubation.*
**Initial:** 0.025 mg/kg will provide approximately 60 min of effective blockade. **Maintenance doses:** Required about 60 min after an initial dose of 0.025 mg/kg or 100 min after an initial dose of 0.05 mg/kg during balanced anesthesia. Maintenance doses between 0.005–0.01 mg/kg provide an average of 30 min and 45 min, respectively, of additional neuromuscular blockade.

## NURSING CONSIDERATIONS

See also *Nursing Considerations* for *Neuromuscular Blocking Agents.*

---

## Administration/Storage

**IV** 1. Individualize the dose for each client.

2. Reduce the dose in debilitated clients, those with neuromuscular disease, severe electrolyte abnormalities, and carcinomatosis.

3. Dose may need to be increased in burn clients.

4. The dose for obese clients is determined using the ideal body weight (IBW), calculated as follows:
- For men: IBW (kg) = (106 + [6 × inches in height above 5 feet])/2.2
- For women: IBW (kg) = (106 + [5 × inches in height above 5 feet])/2.2

5. May not be compatible with alkaline solutions with a pH more than 8 (e.g., barbiturates).

6. May be mixed with 5% dextrose injection, D5%/0.9% NaCl injection, 0.9% NaCl injection, RL injection, and D5%/ RL injection. The drug is also compatible with alfentanil, fentanyl, and sufentanil.

7. Doxacurium diluted 1:10 with 5% dextrose injection or 0.9% NaCl injection is stable for 24 hr if stored in polypropylene syringes at 5°C–25°C (41°F–77°F). However, when diluted, immediate use is preferable. Discard any unused diluted portion after 8 hr at room temperature.

## Assessment

1. Determine any history of neuromuscular disease (e.g., myasthenia gravis).

2. List drugs prescribed.

3. Obtain baseline weight, VS, and serum electrolyte levels.

## Interventions

1. To be administered only by those experienced with skeletal muscle relaxants, in a controlled, monitored environment.

2. Use a peripheral nerve stimulator to monitor drug response and recovery; have antagonist available.

3. Do not administer before unconsciousness (to avoid client stress); doxacurium has no effect on consciousness, pain threshold, or cerebration. Determine need and administer medications for anxiety, pain, and sedation.

4. Explain all procedures and pro-vide emotional support. Reassure they will be able to talk and move once the drug effects are reversed.

5. Position for comfort and for proper body alignment. Turn and perform mouth and eye care frequently.

6. Provide continuous ventilatory support. Ventilator alarms should be set and on at all times.

7. Explain direction of recovery, i.e., facial muscles, diaphragm, legs, arms, and torso. Residual weakness and respiratory difficulty may slow recovery.

## Outcomes/Evaluate

- Skeletal muscle relaxation
- Facilitation of ET intubation; tolerance of mechanical ventilation
- Suppression of twitch response

# Doxazosin mesylate
(dox-**AYZ**-oh-sin)

**Pregnancy Category:** B

Cardura, Cardura-1, -2, -3 ✹ **(Rx)**

**Classification:** Antihypertensive

**Action/Kinetics:** Blocks the alpha-1 (postjunctional) adrenergic receptors resulting in a decrease in systemic vascular resistance and a corresponding decrease in BP. **Peak plasma levels:** 2–3 hr. **Peak effect:** 2–6 hr. Significantly bound (98%) to plasma proteins. Metabolized in the liver to active and inactive metabolites, which are excreted through the feces and urine. **t½:** 22 hr.

**Uses:** Alone or in combination with diuretics, calcium channel blockers, or beta blockers to treat hypertension. Treatment of BPH.

**Contraindications:** Clients allergic to prazosin or terazosin.

**Special Concerns:** Use with caution during lactation, in impaired hepatic function, or in those taking drugs known to influence hepatic metabolism. Safety and effectiveness have not been demonstrated in children. Due to the possibility of severe hypotension, do not use the 2-, 4-, and 8-mg tablets for initial therapy.

**Side Effects:** *CV:* Dizziness (most frequent), syncope, vertigo, lightheadedness, edema, palpitation, arrhythmia, postural hypotension, tachycardia, peripheral ischemia. *CNS:* Fatigue, headache, paresthesia, kinetic disorders, ataxia, somnolence, nervousness, depression, insomnia. *Musculoskeletal:* Arthralgia, arthritis, muscle weakness, muscle cramps, myalgia, hypertonia. *GU:* Polyuria, sexual dysfunction, urinary incontinence, urinary frequency. *GI:* Nausea, diarrhea, dry mouth, constipation, dyspepsia, flatulence, abdominal pain, vomiting. *Respiratory:* Fatigue or malaise, rhinitis, epistaxis, dyspnea. *Miscellaneous:* Rash, pruritus, flushing, abnormal vision, conjunctivitis, eye pain, tinnitus, chest pain, asthenia, facial edema, generalized pain, slight weight gain.

**OD** **Overdose Management:** *Symptoms:* Hypotension. *Treatment:* IV fluids.

**Dosage** ———————————
• **Tablets**
*Hypertension.*
**Adults: initial,** 1 mg once daily at bedtime; **then,** depending on the response (client's standing BP both 2–6 hr and 24 hr after a dose), the dose may be increased to 2 mg/day. A maximum of 16 mg/day may be required to control BP.
*Benign prostatic hyperplasia.*
**Initial:** 1 mg once daily. **Maintenance:** Depending on the urodynamics and symptoms, dose may be increased to 2 mg daily and then 4–8 mg once daily (maximum recommended dose). The recommended titration interval is 1–2 weeks.

## NURSING CONSIDERATIONS
### Administration/Storage
1. To minimize the possibility of severe hypotension, limit initial dosage to 1 mg/day.
2. Increasing the dose higher than 4 mg/day increases the possibility of severe syncope, postural dizziness, vertigo, and postural hypotension.
### Assessment
1. Note any allergy to prazosin or terazosin; drug is a quinazoline derivative.

2. Assess liver function and BP.
3. When used for BPH, numerically score severity.
### Client/Family Teaching
1. Take once daily at bedtime; do not stop abruptly.
2. Record BP and weight; check for edema.
3. Rise slowly to a sitting position before attempting to stand to prevent postural hypotension. Postural effects are most likely to occur 2–6 hr after a dose.
4. Driving and hazardous tasks should be avoided for 24 hr after first dose until effects are evident.
5. Report if S&S do not improve after several weeks of therapy as drug dosage may need adjustment.
### Outcomes/Evaluate
• ↓ BP
• ↓ Nocturnal dysuria

# Doxepin hydrochloride
(**DOX**-eh-pin)
Alti-Doxepin ✦, Apo-Doxepin ✦, Novo-Doxepin ✦, Rho-Doxepin ✦, Sinequan, Triadapin ✦, Zonalon ✦
**(Rx)**
**Classification:** Antidepressant, tricyclic

See also *Antidepressants, Tricyclic.*
**Action/Kinetics:** Metabolized to the active metabolite, desmethyldoxepin. Moderate anticholinergic effects and orthostatic hypotension; high sedative effects. **Minimum effective plasma level of both doxepin and desmethyldoxepin:** 100–200 ng/mL. **Time to reach steady state:** 2–8 days. **t½:** 8–24 hr.
**Uses:** Depression. Antianxiety agent, depression accompanied by anxiety and insomnia, depression in clients with manic-depressive illness. Depression or anxiety due to organic disease or alcoholism. Chronic, severe neurogenic pain. PUD. Dermatologic disorders including chronic urticaria, angioedema, and nocturnal pruritus due to atopic eczema.

**Additional Contraindications:** Glaucoma or a tendency for urinary retention.

**Special Concerns:** Safety has not been determined in pregnancy. Not recommended for use in children less than 12 years of age.

**Additional Side Effects:** Doxepin has a high incidence of side effects, including a high degree of sedation, decreased libido, extrapyramidal symptoms, dermatitis, pruritus, fatigue, weight gain, edema, paresthesia, breast engorgement, insomnia, tremor, chills, tinnitus, and photophobia.

**Dosage** ————

- **Capsules, Oral Concentrate**

  *Antidepressant, mild to moderate anxiety or depression.*
  **Adults:** 25 mg t.i.d. (or up to 150 mg can be given at bedtime); **then,** adjust dosage to individual response (usual optimum dosage: 75–150 mg/day).
  **Geriatric clients, initially:** 25–50 mg/day; dose can be increased as needed and tolerated.
  *Severe symptoms.*
  **Initial:** 50 mg t.i.d.; **then,** gradually increase to 300 mg/day.
  *Emotional symptoms with organic disease.*
  25–50 mg/day.
  *Antipruritic.*
  10–30 mg at bedtime.

- **Cream 5%**

  Apply a thin film q.i.d. with at least a 3–4 hr interval between applications.

## NURSING CONSIDERATIONS

See also *Nursing Considerations* for *Antidepressants, Tricyclic.*

**Administration/Storage**

1. Oral concentrate is to be diluted with 4 oz water, fruit juice, or milk just before ingestion. Do not mix the concentrate with carbonated beverages or grape juice.

2. The antianxiety effect is manifested rapidly; however, it may take 2 to 3 weeks to observe the optimum antidepressant effect.

**Assessment**

1. Document type, onset and characteristics of symptoms.

2. List any other prescribed therapy for this problem and the outcome.

3. Document clinical presentation and attempt to identify any factors that may be contributing to this disorder.

**Client/Family Teaching**

1. Beneficial effects may take up to 3 weeks.

2. Do not perform activities that require mental alertness until drug effects realized.

3. Avoid alcohol and any other CNS depressants.

**Outcomes/Evaluate**

- ↓ Symptoms of anxiety and depression
- Improved sleeping patterns
- Control of chronic neurogenic pain
- Relief of nocturnal pruritus

# Doxorubicin hydrochloride (ADR)

(dox-oh-**ROO**-bih-sin)
**Pregnancy Category:** D
Adriamycin PFS, Adriamycin RDF, Rubex **(Rx)**

# Doxorubicin hydrochloride liposomal

**Pregnancy Category:** D
Doxil **(Rx)**
**Classification:** Antineoplastic, anthracycline antibiotic

See also *Antineoplastic Agents.*

**Action/Kinetics:** Produced by *Streptomyces peucetius.* Cell-cycle specific for the S phase of cell division. Antineoplastic activity may be due to binding to DNA by intercalating between base pairs resulting in inhibition of synthesis of DNA and RNA by template disordering and steric obstruction. The liposomal product is produced with surface-bound methoxypolyethylene in order to protect liposomes from detection by mononuclear phagocytes and to increase blood circulation time. It is believed the liposomes are able to penetrate altered and often compromised vasculature of tumors. Conventional doxorubicin is significantly bound to tissue and plasma proteins whereas the liposomal product is confined mostly to the vascular fluid and does not bind to plasma proteins. Metabolized in the liver to the active doxorubicinol as well as inactive metabolites, which are excreted through the bile. **t½, doxorubicin, conventional: triphasic:** 12 min, 3.3 hr, and 29.6 hr. **t½, liposomes:** About 55 hr.

**Uses: Conventional doxorubicin:** Acute lymphoblastic leukemia, acute myeloblastic leukemia, Wilms' tumor, soft tissue and osteogenic sarcomas, neuroblastoma, cancer of the breast, ovaries, lungs, bladder, and thyroid, lymphomas (Hodgkin's and non-Hodgkin's), bronchogenic carcinoma (especially small cell histologic type) and gastric carcinoma. **Liposomal product:** AIDS-related Kaposi's sarcoma in clients where the disease has progressed on prior combination therapy or in those who are intolerant of such therapy. *Investigational (conventional):* Cancer of the head and neck, cervix, liver, pancreas, prostate, testes, and endometrium.

**Contraindications:** Malignant melanoma, cancer of the kidney, large bowel carcinoma, brain tumors and metastases to the CNS (not responsive to doxorubicin therapy). Initiation of therapy in those with marked myelosuppression induced by previous treatment with other drugs or with radiotherapy. Use in preexisting heart disease. Previous treatment with complete cumulative doses of doxorubicin or daunorubicin.

**Additional Contraindications:** Lactation. Depressed bone marrow or cardiac disease. IM or SC use.

**Special Concerns:** Use with caution in impaired hepatic function and necrotizing colitis. Cardiotoxicity may be more frequent in children.

**Additional Side Effects:** *Myocardial toxicity:* Potentially fatal **CHF.** *Infusion reactions liposomal product:* Flushing, SOB, facial swelling, headache, chills, back pain, tightness in chest and throat, hypotension. *GI:* N&V, mucositis (stomatitis, esophagitis), anorexia, diarrhea. *Ulceration and necrosis of the colon.* *Dermatologic:* Reversible complete alopecia, hyperpigmentation of nail beds and dermal creases (especially in children), onycholysis, recall of skin reaction to prior radiotherapy, palmar-plantar erythrodysesthesia (swelling, pain, erythema, and desquamation of the skin on the hands and feet). *Local:* Severe cellulitis, vesication, and tissue necrosis if the drug is extravasated. Erythematous streaking along the vein next to injection site. *Hypersensitivity:* Fever, chills, urticaria, cross-sensitivity with lincomycin, **anaphylaxis.** *Hematologic:* Myelosuppression. *Ophthalmic:* Conjunctivitis, lacrimation.

**OD** **Overdose Management:** *Symptoms:* Mucositis, leukopenia, thrombocytopenia, pancytopenia. Increased risk of **cardiomyopathy** and subsequent **CHF** with chronic overdosage. *Treatment:* If the client is myelosuppressed, antibiotics and platelet and granulocyte transfusions may be necessary. Treat symptoms of mucositis. Treat CHF with digitalis preparations and diuretics as well as peripheral vasodilators.

**Drug Interactions**
*Barbiturates* / ↑ Plasma clearance of doxorubicin
*Cyclophosphamide* / ↑ Risk of hemorrhagic cystitis
*Digoxin* / ↓ Digoxin plasma levels and renal excretion
*6-Mercaptopurine* / ↑ Risk of hemorrhagic cystitis

**Dosage**
- **IV Only**
- **Conventional Doxorubicin**
**Adults, highly individualized:** 60–75 mg/m² as a single injection q 21 days, or 25–30 mg/m² for 3 successive

days q 4 weeks, or 20 mg/m² q week. Total dose should not exceed 550 mg/m² (440 mg/m² in clients with previous chest irradiation or medications increasing cardiotoxicity). **Pediatric:** 30 mg/m² on 3 successive days q 4 weeks. Use reduced dosage in clients with hepatic dysfunction, depending on serum bilirubin level. If bilirubin is 1.2–3 mg/100 mL, give 50% of usual dose; if it is greater than 3 mg/100 mL, give 25% of usual dose.

- **Liposomal Doxorubicin**
**Adults:** 20 mg/m² over 30 min once q 3 weeks, as long as the client responds satisfactorily and tolerates the drug. For clients with hepatic dysfunction, use the same dosing schedule as conventional doxorubicin.

## NURSING CONSIDERATIONS

See also *Nursing Considerations* for *Antineoplastic Agents.*
### Administration/Storage
**IV** 1. Initiate while hospitalized. Give drug by slow IV into the tubing of a running IV infusion of NaCl injection or 5% dextrose injection; attached to a butterfly needle inserted into a large vein. Avoid veins over joints or in extremities with compromised venous or lymphatic drainage. Although infusion rate depends on vein size, do not administer in less than 3 to 5 min.
2. Reconstitute conventional drug with saline to give a final concentration of 2 mg/mL (e.g., dilute 10-mg vial with 5 mL) and administered over 3–5 min. The reconstituted solution is stable for 24 hr at room temperature and 48 hr if stored at 2°C–8°C (36°F–46°F). The liposomal product is diluted, up to 90 mg, in 250 mL of 5% dextrose injection prior to administration. Do not use in-line filters. Refrigerate diluted liposomal doxorubicin at 2°C–8°C (36°F–46°F). Short-term freezing (less than 1 month) should not affect the liposomal product.
3. If the powder or solution comes in contact with the skin or mucous membranes, wash with soap and water thoroughly.

4. *Do not administer SC or IM because severe necrosis of tissue may result.* To minimize danger of extravasation, inject as directed above. Monitor carefully; stinging, burning, or edema may indicate extravasation. Stop infusion and change sites to avoid tissue necrosis.
5. Be prepared with an injectable corticosteroid for local infiltration and flood site with NSS. Examine area frequently for ulceration that may necessitate early wide excision followed by plastic surgery.
6. Do not give the liposomal product as a bolus injection or as an undiluted solution. Rapid infusion may increase the risk of infusion-related events.
7. Do not mix conventional doxorubicin with heparin, dexamethasone sodium phosphate, or cephalothin because a precipitate may form. Mixing with aminophylline or 5-fluorouracil will result in a change from red to blue-purple indicating decomposition. Do not mix liposomal doxorubicin with other drugs and do not use with any diluent other than 5% dextrose injection. Liposomal doxorubicin is a translucent, red liposomal dispersion.
8. Check package insert carefully for alternate dosing regimens for liposomal doxorubicin in clients with palmar-plantar erythrodysesthesia, hematologic toxicity, or stomatitis.
### Assessment
1. Observe for cardiac arrhythmias, ST segment depression, sinus tachycardia, and/or respiratory difficulties indicative of cardiac toxicity. Have dexrazoxane available to prevent drug-induced cardiomyopathy. Assess for late-onset (up to 6 mo) CHF.
2. Administer antiemetics 30–45 min before therapy and ATC as needed.
3. Monitor VS and I&O; encourage fluid intake of 2–3 L/day. Anticipate allopurinol administration and alkalinization of urine to decrease urate stone formation.
4. Monitor CBC, uric acid, liver and renal function studies; drug may cause granulocyte toxicity. Nadir: 14 days; recovery: 21 days.

**Client/Family Teaching**

1. If medication reactivates previous radiotherapy damage, such as erythema, edema, and desquamation; symptoms should disappear after 7 days.

2. Consume 2–3 L/day of fluids.

3. Urine will turn red-brown for 1–2 days; this is not blood.

4. Nail beds may become discolored.

5. Any hair lost should grow back 2–3 months after therapy.

6. Report any flu-like symptoms; drug causes severe myelosuppression.

7. Avoid vaccinations.

8. Practice contraception during and for 4 months after therapy.

9. Report mouth ulcers; stomatitis may occur 5–10 days after dose and last for 3–7 days. A special mouth rinse may help decrease symptoms.

**Outcomes/Evaluate:** Inhibition of malignant cell proliferation

---

# Doxycycline calcium
(dox-ih-**SYE**-kleen)
**Pregnancy Category:** D
Vibramycin **(Rx)**

# Doxycycline hyclate
(dox-ih-**SYE**-kleen)
**Pregnancy Category:** D
Alti-Doxycycline ✤, Apo-Doxy ✤, Apo-Doxy-Tabs ✤, Doryx, Doxy 100 and 200, Doxy-Caps, Doxycin ✤, Doxychel Hyclate, Doxytec ✤, Novo-Doxylin ✤, Nu-Doxycycline ✤, Rho-Doxycyline ✤, Vibramycin, Vibramycin IV, Vibra-Tabs, Vivox **(Rx)**

# Doxycycline monohydrate
(dox-ih-**SYE**-kleen)
**Pregnancy Category:** D
Monodox, Vibramycin **(Rx)**
**Classification:** Antibiotic, tetracycline

See also *Anti-Infectives* and *Tetracyclines.*

**Action/Kinetics:** More slowly absorbed, and thus more persistent, than other tetracyclines. Preferred for clients with impaired renal function for treating infections outside the urinary tract. From 80% to 95% is bound to serum proteins. **t½:** 14.5–22 hr; 30%–40% excreted unchanged in urine.

**Additional Uses:** Orally for uncomplicated gonococcal infections in adults (except anorectal infections in males); acute epididymo-orchitis caused by *Neisseria gonorrhoeae* and *Chlamydia trachomatis;* gonococcal arthritis-dermatitis syndrome; nongonococcal urethritis caused by *C. trachomatis* and *Ureaplasma urealyticum.* Prophylaxis of malaria due to *Plasmodium falciparum* in short-term travelers (< 4 months) to areas with chloroquine- or pyrimethamine-sulfadoxine-resistant strains.

**Contraindications:** Prophylaxis of malaria in pregnant individuals and in children less than 8 years old. Use during the last half of pregnancy and in children up to 8 years of age (tetracycline may cause permanent discoloration of the teeth). Lactation.

**Special Concerns:** Safety for IV use in children less than 8 years of age has not been established.

**Additional Drug Interactions:** Carbamazepine, phenytoin, and barbiturates ↓ effect of doxycycline by ↑ breakdown of doxycycline by the liver.

**Dosage** ————————
• **Capsules, Delayed-Release Capsules, Oral Suspension, Syrup, Tablets, IV**
*Infections.*
**Adult: First day,** 100 mg q 12 hr; **maintenance:** 100–200 mg/day, depending on severity of infection. **Children, over 8 years (45 kg or less): First day,** 4.4 mg/kg in 1–2 doses; **then,** 2.2–4.4 mg/kg/day in divided doses depending on severity of infection. Children over 45 kg should receive the adult dose.
*Acute gonorrhea.*
200 mg at once given PO; **then,** 100 mg at bedtime on first day, followed by 100 mg b.i.d. for 3 days. Alterna-

tively, 300 mg immediately followed in 1 hr with 300 mg.

*Syphilis (primary/secondary).*
300 mg/day in divided PO doses for 10 days.

*C. trachomatis infections.*
100 mg b.i.d. PO for minimum of 7 days.

*Prophylaxis of "traveler's diarrhea."*
100 mg/day given PO.

*Prophylaxis of malaria.*
**Adults:** 100 mg PO once daily; **children, over 8 years of age:** 2 mg/kg/day up to 100 mg/day.

• **IV**

*Endometritis, parametritis, peritonitis, salpingitis.*
100 mg b.i.d. with 2 g cefoxitin, IV, q.i.d. continued for at least 4 days or 2 days after improvement observed. This is followed by doxycycline, PO, 100 mg b.i.d. for 10–14 days of total therapy.

*NOTE:* The Centers for Disease Control have established treatment schedules for STDs.

## NURSING CONSIDERATIONS

See also *General Nursing Considerations for All Anti-Infectives* and for *Tetracyclines.*

### Administration/Storage

1. Prophylaxis for malaria can begin 1–2 days before travel begins, during travel, and for 4 weeks after leaving the malarious area.

2. The powder for suspension expires 12 months from date of issue.

3. Solution is stable for 2 weeks when stored in refrigerator.

**IV** 4. Follow directions on vial for dilution. Concentrations should be no lower than 0.1 mg/mL and no higher than 1.0 mg/mL.

5. During infusion protect solution from light.

6. Complete administration of solutions diluted with NaCl injection, D5W, Ringer's injection, and 10% invert sugar within 12 hr.

7. Complete administration of solutions diluted with RL injection or D5%/RL within 6 hr.

### Client/Family Teaching

1. May take with food; take with a full glass of water to prevent esophageal ulceration.

2. Avoid direct exposure to sunlight and wear protective clothing and sunscreens when exposed .

3. With STDs advise that partner be tested and treated. Use condoms until medically cleared.

4. Take entire prescription; do not stop if symptoms subside.

### Outcomes/Evaluate

• Resolution of infection
• Symptomatic improvement

# Dronabinol (Delta-9-tetrahydro-cannabinol)

(droh-**NAB**-ih-nohl)
**Pregnancy Category:** C
Marinol **(C-II) (Rx)**
**Classification:** Antinauseant

**Action/Kinetics:** As the active component in marijuana, significant psychoactive effects may occur. (See *Side Effects.*) In therapeutic doses, the drug also causes conjunctival injection and an increased HR. Antiemetic effect may be due to inhibition of the vomiting center in the medulla. **Peak plasma levels:** 2–3 hr. Significant first-pass effect. The 11-hydroxytetrahydrocannabinol metabolite is active. **t½, biphasic:** 4 hr and 25–36 hr. **t½, 11-hydroxy-THC:** 15–18 hr. Metabolized in the liver and mainly excreted in the feces. Cumulative toxicity using clinical doses may occur. Highly bound to plasma proteins and may thus displace other protein-bound drugs.

**Uses:** Nausea and vomiting associated with cancer chemotherapy, especially in clients who have not responded to other antiemetic treatment. To stimulate appetite and prevent weight loss in AIDS clients.

**Contraindications:** Nausea and vomiting from any cause other than cancer chemotherapy. Lactation. Hypersensitivity to sesame oil.

**Special Concerns:** Monitor pediatric and geriatric clients carefully due to an increased risk of psychoactive effects. Use with caution in clients with hypertension, occasional hypotension, syncope, tachycardia; those with a history of substance abuse, including alcohol abuse or dependence; clients with mania, depression, or schizophrenia (the drug may exacerbate these illnesses); clients receiving sedatives, hypnotics, or other psychoactive drugs (due to the potential for additive or synergistic CNS effects).

**Side Effects:** *CNS:* Side effects are due mainly to the psychoactive effects of the drug and, in addition to those listed in the preceding, include dizziness, muddled thinking, coordination difficulties, irritability, weakness, headache, ataxia, cannabinoid "high," paresthesia, hallucinations, visual distortions, depersonalization, confusion, nightmares, disorientation, and confusion. *CV:* Palpitations, tachycardia, vasodilation, facial flush, hypotension. *GI:* Abdominal pain, N&V, diarrhea, dry mouth, fecal incontinence, anorexia. *Respiratory:* Cough, rhinitis, sinusitis. *Other:* Asthenia, conjunctivitis, myalgias, tinnitus, speech difficulty, vision difficulties, chills, headache, malaise, sweating, elevated hepatic enzymes.

*Symptoms of Abstinence Syndrome:* An abstinence syndrome has been reported following discontinuation of doses greater than 210 mg/day for 12–16 days. Symptoms include irritability, insomnia, and restlessness within 12 hr; within 24 hr, symptoms include "hot flashes," sweating, rhinorrhea, loose stools, hiccoughs, and anorexia. Disturbed sleep may occur for several weeks.

**OD** **Overdose Management:** *Symptoms:* Extension of the pharmacologic effects. Symptoms of mild overdose include: drowsiness, euphoria, heightened sensory awareness, altered time perception, reddened conjunctiva, dry mouth, and tachycardia. Symptoms of moderate toxicity include impaired memory, depersonalization, mood alteration,

urinary retention, and reduced bowel motility. Severe intoxication includes decreased motor coordination, lethargy, slurred speech, and postural hypotension. Seizures may occur in clients with existing seizure disorders. Hallucinations, psychotic episodes, *respiratory depression* , and *coma* have been reported. *Treatment:* Clients with depressive, hallucinatory, or psychotic reactions should be placed in a quiet environment and provided supportive treatment, including reassurance. Diazepam (5–10 mg PO) may be used for extreme agitation. Hypotension usually responds to IV fluids and Trendelenburg position. In unconscious clients with a secure airway, administer activated charcoal (30–100 g in adults and 1–2 g/kg in children); this may be followed by a saline cathartic.

**Drug Interactions**
*Amphetamine* / Additive hypertension, tachycardia, possibly cardiotoxicity
*Anticholinergics* / Additive or super-additive tachycardia; drowsiness
*CNS depressants* / Additive CNS depressant effects
*Cocaine* / See *Amphetamine*
*Antidepressants, tricyclic* / Additive tachycardia, hypertension, drowsiness
*Ethanol* / During subchronic dronabinol use, lower and delayed peak alcohol blood levels
*Sympathomimetics* / See *Amphetamine*
*Theophylline* / Possible increased metabolism of theophylline

**Dosage**
• **Capsules**
*Antiemetic.*
**Adults and children, initial:** 5 mg/m² 1–3 hr before chemotherapy; **then,** 5 mg/m² q 2–4 hr for a total of four to six doses/day. If ineffective, this dose may be increased by 2.5 mg/m² to a maximum of 15 mg/m²/dose. However, the incidence of

serious psychoactive side effects increases dramatically at these higher dose levels.

*Appetite stimulation.*
**Initial:** 2.5 mg b.i.d. before lunch and dinner. If unable to tolerate 5 mg/day, reduce the dose to 2.5 mg/day as a single evening or bedtime dose. If side effects are absent or minimal and an increased effect is desired, the dose may be increased to 2.5 mg before lunch and 5 mg before dinner (or 5 mg at lunch and 5 mg after dinner). The dose may be increased to 20 mg/day in divided doses. The incidence of side effects increases at higher doses.

## NURSING CONSIDERATIONS
### Administration/Storage
1. Due to its CNS effects, use only when the client can be under close supervision.
2. Due to abuse potential, prescriptions should be limited to one course of chemotherapy (i.e., several days) and reordered as needed to ensure benefit of therapy.
### Assessment
1. Note any allergy to sesame oil or seeds.
2. Document onset of symptoms; assess if N&V may be caused by anything other than chemotherapy.
3. List other agents trialed.
4. Assess for symptoms of abstinence syndrome which may be seen following discontinuation of doses greater than 210 mg/day for 12–16 days.
### Client/Family Teaching
1. Take 1–3 hr before chemotherapy.
2. Avoid sudden position changes; dizziness may occur.
3. Do not drive or perform hazardous tasks requiring mental acuity.
4. Potential for psychoactive symptoms, visual distortions, and mental confusion; these may be minimized by a quiet, supportive environment.
5. Keep out of child's reach; do not share with anyone, regardless of symptoms.
### Outcomes/Evaluate
• Relief of chemotherapy-induced N&V

• ↑ Appetite; ↓ weight loss

# Droperidol
(droh-**PER**-ih-dol)
**Pregnancy Category:** C
Inapsine **(Rx)**
**Classification:** Antipsychotic, butyrophenone; antianxiety agent

**Action/Kinetics:** Causes sedation, alpha-adrenergic blockade, peripheral vascular dilation; has antiemetic properties. For other details, see *Haloperidol*, and *Phenothiazines*. **Onset** (after IM, IV): 3–10 min. **Peak effect:** 30 min. **Duration:** 2–4 hr, although alteration of consciousness may last up to 12 hr. t½: 2.2 hr. Metabolized in the liver and excreted in both the feces and urine.
**Uses:** Preoperatively; induction and maintenance of anesthesia. To relieve N&V and reduce anxiety in diagnostic procedures or surgery. Neuroleptic analgesia. Antiemetic in cancer chemotherapy (used IV).
**Special Concerns:** Use with caution during lactation; in the elderly, debilitated, or poor risk client; and in renal or hepatic impairment. Safety for use during labor has not been established. Safety and efficacy have not been established in children less than 2 years of age.
**Side Effects:** *CNS:* Postoperative drowsiness (common), restlessness, hyperactivity, anxiety, dizziness, postoperative hallucinations; extrapyramidal symptoms (e.g., akathisia, dystonia, oculogyric crisis). *CV:* Hypotension and tachycardia (common), increase in BP (when combined with fentanyl or other parenteral analgesics). *Respiratory:* **Respiratory depression (when combined with fentanyl), laryngospasm, bronchospasm.** *Miscellaneous:* Chills, shivering.
**Drug Interactions**
*Anesthetics, conduction (e.g., spinal)* / Peripheral vasodilation and hypotension
*CNS depressants* / Additive or potentiating effects
*Narcotic analgesics* / ↑ Respiratory depressant effects

## Dosage

• **IM**

*Preoperatively.*

**Adults:** 2.5–10 mg 30–60 min before surgery (modify dosage in elderly, debilitated); **pediatric, 2–12 years,** 88–165 mcg/kg.

*Diagnostic procedures.*

**Adults:** 2.5–10 mg 30–60 min before procedure; **then,** if necessary, **IV,** 1.25–2.5 mg.

• **IV**

*Adjunct to general anesthesia.*

**Adults:** 0.28 mg/kg with analgesic or anesthetic; **maintenance:** 1.25–2.5 mg (total dose).

• **IV (Slow) or IM**

*Adjunct to regional anesthesia.*

**Adults:** 2.5–5 mg.

## NURSING CONSIDERATIONS

See also *Nursing Considerations* for *Antipsychotic Agents and Phenothiazines.*

**Administration/Storage**

**IV** 1. May be administered by direct IV slowly over 1 min; may also be reconstituted in 250 mL of D5W or NSS and administered slowly via infusion control device as prescribed.

2. At a concentration of 1 mg/50 mL, droperidol is stable for 7–10 days in glass bottles with 5% dextrose injection, RL injection, and 0.9% NaCl injection. Droperidol is stable for 7 days in PVC bags containing 5% dextrose injection or 0.9% NaCl injection.

3. If used with Innovar injection (fentanyl plus droperidol), consider the dose of droperidol in the injection.

4. Droperidol is compatible at a concentration of 2.5 mg/mL for 15 min when combined in a syringe with the following: atropine sulfate, butorphanol tartrate, chlorpromazine hydrochloride, diphenhydramine hydrochloride, fentanyl citrate, glycopyrrolate, hydroxyzine hydrochloride, meperidine hydrochloride, morphine sulfate, perphenazine, promazine hydrochloride, promethazine hydrochloride, and scopolamine hydrobromide.

5. A precipitate will form if droperidol is mixed with barbiturates.

**Interventions**

1. Keep on bedrest; supervise activities and ambulation until VS stable. Drug causes orthostatic hypotension and drowsiness

2. Assess for extrapyramidal S&S; may use anticholinergics as needed.

**Outcomes/Evaluate**

• ↓ Procedure anxiety

• Control of N&V

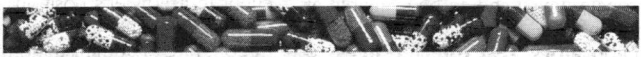

# Edetate disodium (EDTA)

(**ED**-eh-tayt)

**Pregnancy Category:** C

Disotate, Endrate **(Rx)**

**Classification:** Heavy metal chelator.

**Action/Kinetics:** Has a great affinity for calcium, forming a soluble chelate in the blood which is excreted through the urine. This leads to a lowering of serum calcium and a mobilization of calcium stores, especially from bone. When used to treat digitalis toxicity, edetate disodium exerts a negative inotropic effect on the heart and thus the chronotropic and inotropic effects of digitalis on the heart are antagonized. Also forms chelates with magnesium, zinc, and other trace elements. When used ophthalmically, calcified corneal deposits are dissolved from the conjunctiva, corneal epithelium, and anterior layers of the stroma.

**Uses:** Hypercalcemia. Ventricular arrhythmias associated with digitalis toxicity. *Investigational:* Ophthalmically to treat corneal calcium deposits, eye burns from calcium hydroxide, and eye injury by zinc chloride.

**Contraindications:** Anuria. Ventricular arrhythmias. To treat arteriosclerosis, atherosclerotic vascular disease, lead poisoning, or renal calculi by retrograde irrigation.

**Special Concerns:** Use during pregnancy only if the benefits clearly outweigh the risks. Use with extreme caution in digitalized clients as EDTA and calcium may reverse the desired effect of digitalis. Use with caution in clients with heart disease (e.g., CHF) or hypokalemia.

**Side Effects:** *Metabolic:* Electrolyte imbalance including hypocalcemia, hypokalemia, hypomagnesemia, hyperuricemia may occur during treatment. *CV:* Decrease in both systolic and diastolic pressure, thrombophlebitis, anemia. *GI:* N&V, diarrhea. *CNS:* Headache, numbness, circumoral paresthesia, fever. *Other:* Exfoliative dermatitis, nephrotoxicity, *reticuloendothelial system damage with hemorrhagic tendencies. Rapid injection may produce hypocalcemic tetany and convulsions, respiratory arrest, and severe arrhythmias.*

**OD** **Overdose Management:** *Symptoms:* Precipitous drop in calcium. *Treatment:* IV calcium gluconate which should be available at all times.

**Laboratory Test Interferences:** ↓ Alkaline phosphatase levels.

**Dosage** ─────────
• **IV**
   *Hypercalcemia, digitalis toxicity.*
Individualized and depending on degree of hypercalcemia. **Adults, usual:** 50 mg/kg over 24 hr (up to 3 g/day may be prescribed); dose may be repeated for 5 consecutive days followed by a 2-day rest period with repeated courses, if needed, up to 15 doses. **Pediatric:** 40 mg/kg over 24 hr up to a maximum of 70 mg/kg/day. An alternative dosing regimen is 15–50 mg/kg/day, to a maximum of

3 g/day followed by a 5-day rest period between courses.
• **Ophthalmic**
   *Calcium deposits, calcium hydroxide burns.*
**Adults and children:** 0.35%–1.85% solution as an irrigation for 15–20 min.
   *Zinc chloride injury.*
**Adults and children:** 1.7% solution as an irrigation for 15 min.

## NURSING CONSIDERATIONS
### Administration/Storage
1. There is no ophthalmic product available in the U.S.; however, the injection can be used to prepare the ophthalmic dosage form.
**IV** 2. Check label on vial carefully to determine that drug is disodium edetate and not calcium disodium edetate.
3. For use in adults, dilute medication in 500 mL of 5% dextrose solution or isotonic saline solution. For pediatric use, dissolve in either 5% dextrose injection or 0.9% NaCl injection; the final concentration should not exceed 3%.
4. Repeated use of the same vein may result in thrombophlebitis. Greater solution dilution and slower infusion reduce the incidence of thrombophlebitis if the same vein must be used.
5. Infuse slowly over 3–4 hr, with client in a Fowler's position. Do not exceed recommended dose, concentration, rate of administration, or cardiac reserve of the client.
### Assessment
1. Document indications for therapy, symptom onset, and anticipated results.
2. Use cautiously with heart disease, seizures, and/or tuberculosis.
3. Monitor calcium, magnesium, electrolytes, urinalysis, and renal function studies.
4. Transitory hypotension may occur; place supine until BP stabilized.
5. Be alert to a generalized systemic reaction that may occur from 4 to 8 hr after drug infusion (usually subsides within 12 hr). Provide supportive care should fever, chills, back pain,

vomiting, muscle cramps, or urinary urgency occur.

6. With lead toxicity, notify local health department; identify source and need for further investigation.

**Client/Family Teaching**

1. Review goals of therapy and frequency of administration.

2. May cause hypoglycemia with diabetes; consult provider concerning management of diabetes (i.e., reduce insulin dosage or increase food intake).

3. Report any unusual bruising or bleeding.

**Outcomes/Evaluate**

• ↓ Calcium; ↓ digoxin levels

• Lead levels < 50 mcg/dL

• Dissolution of corneal deposits

# Edrophonium chloride

(ed-roh-**FOH**-nee-um)

**Pregnancy Category:** C

Enlon, Reversol, Tensilon **(Rx)**

————COMBINATION DRUG————

# Edrophonium chloride and Atropine sulfate

(ed-roh-**FOH**-nee-um)

**Pregnancy Category:** C

Enlon-Plus **(Rx)**

**Classification:** Cholinesterase inhibitor, indirectly-acting

See also *Neostigmine* and *Atropine Sulfate.*

**Action/Kinetics:** By increasing the duration of action at the motor end plate, edrophonium causes a transient increase in muscle strength in myasthenia gravis clients and either no change or a slight weakness in muscle strength in clients with other disorders. Atropine has been added to edrophonium to counteract the muscarinic side effects that will occur due to edrophonium (e.g., increased secretions, bradycardia, bronchoconstriction). **Onset: IM,** 2–10 min; **IV,** <1 min. **Duration: IM,** 5–30 min; **IV,** 10 min. Eliminated through the kidneys.

**Uses: Edrophonium:** Differential diagnosis of myasthenia gravis. Adjunct to evaluate requirements for treating myasthenia gravis. Adjunct to treat respiratory depression due to curare and similar nondepolarizing agents such as gallamine, pancuronium, and tubocurarine.

**Edrophonium and Atropine:** To antagonize or reverse nondepolarizing neuromuscular blocking agents. Adjunct to treat respiratory depression caused by overdosage of curare.

**Contraindications:** Edrophonium combined with atropine in the differential diagnosis of myasthenia gravis.

**Special Concerns:** Edrophonium combined with atropine is not effective against depolarizing neuromuscular blocking agents.

**Dosage**

• **Edrophonium, IV**

*Differential diagnosis of myasthenia gravis.*

**IV, Adults:** 2 mg initially over 15–30 sec; with needle in place, wait 45 sec; if no response occurs after 45 sec inject an additional 8 mg. If a cholinergic reaction is obtained following 2 mg (muscarinic side effects, skeletal muscle fasciculations, increased muscle weakness), test is discontinued and atropine, 0.4–0.5 mg, is given IV. The test may be repeated in 30 min. **Pediatric, up to 34 kg, IV:** 1 mg; if no response after 45 sec, can give up to 5 mg. **Pediatric, over 34 kg, IV:** 2 mg; if no response after 45 sec, can give up to 10 mg in 1-mg increments q 30–45 sec. **Infants:** 0.5 mg. If IV injection is not feasible, IM can be used.

*To evaluate treatment needs in myasthenic clients.*

1 hr after PO administration of drug used to treat myasthenia, give edrophonium IV, 1–2 mg. (*NOTE:* Response will be myasthenic in undertreated clients, adequate in controlled clients, and cholinergic in overtreated clients.)

*Curare antagonist.*
**Slow IV:** 10 mg over 30–45 sec to detect onset of cholinergic reaction; repeat if necessary to maximum of 40 mg. Should not be given before use of curare, gallamine, or tubocurarine.

• **Edrophonium, IM**
*Differential diagnosis of myasthenia gravis.*
**Adults:** 10 mg; if hyperreactivity occurs, retest after 30 min with 2 mg IM to rule out false negative. **Pediatric, up to 34 kg:** 2 mg; **more than 34 kg:** 5 mg. (There is a 2–10-min delay in reaction with IM route.)

• **Edrophonium and Atropine, IV**
**Adults:** 0.5–1 mg/kg edrophonium and 0.007–0.014 mg/kg atropine.

## NURSING CONSIDERATIONS

See also *Nursing Considerations* for *Neostigmine* and *Atropine Sulfate*.
**Administration/Storage**
**IV** 1. Do not give edrophonium before curare or curare-like drugs.
2. Have IV atropine sulfate available to use as an antagonist.
3. When atropine is combined with edrophonium, monitor carefully; assisted or controlled ventilation should be undertaken.
4. Recurarization has not been noted following satisfactory reversal with edrophonium and atropine.
**Assessment**
1. Document therapy indications.
2. List drugs currently prescribed.
3. Note any history of asthma, seizures, CAD, or hyperthyroidism.
**Interventions**
1. Monitor closely during drug administration; effects last up to 30 min.
2. Monitor VS and I&O at least q 4 hr.
3. Document any increased salivation, bronchial spasm, bradycardia, and cardiac arrhythmia; especially important with the elderly.
4. When administered as an antidote for curare, assess for each dose effect; do not administer the next dose unless prior effects have been

observed. Larger doses may potentiate effects.
5. Evaluate respiratory effort and provide assisted ventilation prn.
6. During cholinergic crisis, monitor state of consciousness closely.
**Outcomes/Evaluate**
• With myasthenia gravis (transient ↑ muscle strength, improved gait)
• Curare antagonist
• Reversal of respiratory depression
• Differentiation of myasthenic from cholinergic crisis

# Enalapril maleate
(en-**AL**-ah-prill)
**Pregnancy Category:** D
Apo-Enalapril ✶, Vasotec, Vasotec I.V., Vasotec Oral ✶ **(Rx)**
**Classification:** Angiotensin-converting enzyme inhibitor

See also *Angiotensin-Converting Enzyme Inhibitors*.
**Action/Kinetics:** Converted in the liver by hydrolysis to the active metabolite, enalaprilat. The parenteral product is enalaprilat injection. **Onset, PO:** 1 hr; **IV,** 15 min. **Time to peak action, PO:** 4–6 hr; **IV,** 1–4 hr. **Duration, PO:** 24 hr; **IV,** About 6 hr. Approximately 50%–60% is protein bound. t½, enalapril, **PO:** 1.3 hr; **IV,** 15 min. t½, **enalaprilat, PO:** 11 hr. Excreted through the urine (half unchanged) and feces; over 90% of enalaprilat is excreted through the urine.
**Uses:** Alone or in combination with a thiazide diuretic for the treatment of hypertension (step I therapy). As adjunct with digitalis and diuretic in acute and chronic CHF. *Investigational:* Hypertension in children, hypertension related to scleroderma renal crisis, diabetic nephropathy, asymptomatic left ventricular dysfunction following MI. Enalaprilat may be used for hypertensive emergencies (effect is variable).
**Special Concerns:** Use with caution during lactation. Safety and effectiveness have not been determined in children.

**Side Effects:** *CV:* Palpitations, hypotension, chest pain, angina, ***CVA, MI,*** orthostatic hypotension, disturbances in rhythm, tachycardia, ***cardiac arrest,*** orthostatic effects, atrial fibrillation, bradycardia. *GI:* N&V, diarrhea, abdominal pain, alterations in taste, anorexia, dry mouth, constipation, dyspepsia, glossitis, ileus, melena, stomatitis. *CNS:* Insomnia, headache, fatigue, dizziness, paresthesias, nervousness, sleepiness, ataxia, confusion, depression, vertigo. *Hepatic:* Hepatitis, hepatocellular or cholestatic jaundice, pancreatitis, elevated liver enzymes, hepatic failure. *Respiratory:* Bronchitis, cough, dyspnea, bronchospasm, upper respiratory infection, pneumonia, pulmonary infiltrates, asthma, ***pulmonary embolism and infarction, pulmonary edema.*** *Renal:* Renal dysfunction, oliguria, UTI, transient increases in creatinine and BUN. *Hematologic:* Rarely, neutropenia, thrombocytopenia, bone marrow depression, decreased H&H in hypertensive or CHF clients. Hemolytic anemia, including hemolysis, in clients with G6PD deficiency. *Dermatologic:* Rash, pruritus, alopecia, flushing, erythema multiforme, exfoliative dermatitis, photosensitivity, urticaria, increased sweating, pemphigus, ***Stevens-Johnson syndrome,*** herpes zoster, toxic epidermal necrolysis. *Other:* Angioedema, asthenia, impotence, blurred vision, fever, arthralgia, arthritis, vasculitis, eosinophilia, tinnitus, syncope, myalgia, rhinorrhea, sore throat, hoarseness, conjunctivitis, tearing, dry eyes, loss of sense of smell, hearing loss, peripheral neuropathy, anosmia, myositis, flank pain, gynecomastia.

**Additional Drug Interactions:** Rifampin may ↓ the effects of enalapril. Do not discontinue without first reporting to the provider.

**Dosage** ———————
• **Tablets (Enalapril)**
*Antihypertensive in clients not taking diuretics.*

**Initial:** 5 mg/day; **then,** adjust dosage according to response (range: 10–40 mg/day in one to two doses).
*Antihypertensive in clients taking diuretics.*
**Initial:** 2.5 mg. Since hypotension may occur following the initiation of enalapril, the diuretic should be discontinued, if possible, for 2–3 days before initiating enalapril. If BP is not maintained with enalapril alone, diuretic therapy may be resumed.
*Adjunct with diuretics and digitalis in heart failure.*
**Initial:** 2.5 mg 1–2 times/day; **then,** depending on the response, 5–20 mg/day in two divided doses. Dose should not exceed 40 mg/day. Dosage must be adjusted in clients with renal impairment or hyponatremia.
*In clients with impaired renal function.*
**Initial:** 5 mg/day if $C_{CR}$ ranges between 30 and 80 mL/min and serum creatinine is less than 3 mg/dL; 2.5 mg/day if $C_{CR}$ is less than 30 mL/min and serum creatinine is more than 3 mg/dL and in dialysis clients on dialysis days.
*Renal impairment or hyponatremia.*
**Initial:** 2.5 mg/day if serum sodium is less than 130 mEq/L and serum creatinine is more than 1.6 mg/dL. The dose may be increased to 2.5 mg b.i.d. and then 5 mg b.i.d. or higher if required; dose is given at intervals of 4 or more days. Maximum daily dose is 40 mg.
*Asymptomatic LV dysfunction following MI.*
2.5–20 mg/day beginning 72 hr or longer after onset of MI. Therapy is continued for 1 year or longer.
*NOTE:* Dosage should be decreased in clients with a $C_{CR}$ less than 30 mL/min and a serum creatinine level greater than 3 mg/dL.
• **IV (Enalaprilat)**
*Hypertension.*
1.25 mg over a 5-min period; repeat q 6 hr.

**E**

*Antihypertensive in clients taking diuretics.*

**Initial:** 0.625 mg over 5 min; if an adequate response is seen after 1 hr, administer another 0.625-mg dose. Thereafter, 1.25 mg q 6 hr.

*Clients with impaired renal function.*

Give enalapril, 1.25 mg q 6 hr for clients with a $C_{CR}$ more than 30 mL/min and an initial dose of 0.625 mg for clients with a $C_{CR}$ less than 30 mL/min. If there is an adequate response, an additional 0.625 mg may be given after 1 hr; thereafter, additional 1.25-mg doses can be given q 6 hr. For dialysis clients, the initial dose is 0.625 mg q 6 hr.

## NURSING CONSIDERATIONS

See also *Nursing Considerations* for *Angiotensin-Converting Enzyme Inhibitors* and *Antihypertensive Agents*.

**Administration/Storage**

1. To convert from IV to PO therapy in clients on a diuretic, begin with 2.5 mg/day for clients responding to a 0.625-mg IV dose. Thereafter, 2.5 mg/day may be given.

2. Anticipate lowered dose if receiving diuretics or with impaired renal function.

**IV** 3. To convert from PO to IV therapy in clients not on a diuretic, use the recommended IV dose (i.e., 1.25 mg/6 hr). To convert from IV to PO therapy, begin with 5 mg/day.

4. Following IV administration, first dose peak effect may take 4 hr (whether or not on a diuretic). For subsequent doses, the peak effect is usually within 15 min.

5. Give enalaprilat as a slow IV infusion (over 5 min) either alone or diluted up to 50 mL with an appropriate diluent. Any of the following can be used: 5% dextrose injection, D5%/RL , Isolyte E, 0.9% NaCl, D5%/0.9% NaCl.

6. When used initially for heart failure, observe for at least 2 hr after the initial dose and until BP has stabilized for an additional hour. If possible, reduce dose of diuretic.

**Assessment**

1. Document indications for therapy, presenting symptoms, other agents trialed, and the outcome.

2. Record baseline ECG, VS, and weight.

3. Monitor CBC, electrolytes, liver and renal function studies.

**Client/Family Teaching**

1. Use caution, may cause orthostatic effects and dizziness.

2. Maintain a healthy diet; limit intake of caffeine; avoid alcohol, salt substitutes, or high-Na and high-K foods.

3. Report any weight loss that may result from the loss of taste or rapid weight gain that may result from fluid overload.

4. Any flu-like symptoms should be reported immediately.

**Outcomes/Evaluate**

- ↓ BP
- ↓ Preload and afterload with CHF

------COMBINATION DRUG------

# Enalapril maleate and Hydrochlorothiazide

(en-**AL**-ah-prill, **high**-droh-**KLOR**oh-**THIGH**-ah-zyd)
**Pregnancy Category:** D
Vaseretic **(Rx)**
**Classification:** Antihypertensive

See also *Enalapril maleate* and *Hydrochlorothiazide*.

**Content:** *ACE inhibitor:* Enalapril, 5 mg or 10 mg. *Diuretic:* Hydrochlorothiazide, 12.5 mg or 25 mg.

**Uses:** Combination therapy for hypertension.

**Contraindications:** Use for initial therapy of hypertension. Anuria or severe renal dysfunction. History of angioedema related to use of ACE inhibitors. Lactation.

**Special Concerns:** Excessive hypotension may be observed in clients with severe salt or volume depletion such as those treated with diuretics or on dialysis. Significant hypotension may also be seen with severe CHF, with or without associated renal insufficiency. A significant fall in BP may result in MI or CVA in clients with ischemic heart or cerebrovascular disease. Safety and effectiveness have not been established in children.

## Dosage
• **Tablets**
**Adults:** 1–2 tablets once daily.

## NURSING CONSIDERATIONS

See also *Nursing Considerations* for *Antihypertensive Agents* and individual agents.

### Administration/Storage
1. Individualize the dose determined by the titration of the individual components. Once the client has been successfully titrated with the individual components, Vaseretic (1 or 2 of the 10–25 tablets) may be given once daily if the titrated doses are the same as those in the fixed combination.
2. Do not exceed 2 tablets/day.
3. If being treated with hydrochlorothiazide, hypotension may occur following the initial dose of enalapril. Thus, if possible, discontinue the diuretic 2–3 days before beginning therapy with enalapril. If diuretic cannot be discontinued, use an initial dose of 2.5 mg enalapril under close medical supervision for at least 2 hr and until BP has stabilized for another 1 hr.
4. The usual dose of Vaseretic is recommended for clients with a $C_{CR}>$ 30 mL/min.

### Assessment
1. Monitor BP, CBC, electrolytes, liver and renal function.
2. Note any evidence of heart failure, cerebrovascular disease, angioedema, gout, elevated cholesterol levels, or diabetes.

### Client/Family Teaching
1. Take as directed and do not stop abruptly.
2. Avoid activities that require mental alertness until drug effects realized.
3. Avoid alcohol, xanthines, potassium supplements or salt substitutes, potassium-sparing drugs, and OTC agents without approval.
**Outcomes/Evaluate:** Control of hypertension

# Enoxacin
(ee-**NOX**-ah-sin)
**Pregnancy Category:** C
Penetrex **(Rx)**
**Classification:** Antibacterial, fluoroquinolone derivative

See also *Fluoroquinolones*.
**Action/Kinetics:** The drug inhibits certain isozymes of the cytochrome P-450 hepatic microsomal enzyme system, resulting in alterations of metabolism of some drugs. **Peak plasma levels:** 0.83 mcg/mL 1–3 hr after a 200-mg dose and 2 mcg/mL 1–3 hr after a 400-mg dose. Mean peak plasma levels are 50% higher in geriatric clients than in young adults. Diffuses into the cervix, fallopian tubes, and myometrium at levels 1–2 times those seen in plasma and into kidney and prostate at levels 2–4 times those seen in plasma. **t½:** 3–6 hr. More than 40% excreted unchanged through the urine.
**Uses:** To treat uncomplicated urethral or cervical gonorrhea due to *Neisseria gonorrhoeae*. To treat uncomplicated UTIs due *Escherichia coli, Staphylococcus epidermidis,* or *S. saprophyticus;* for complicated UTIs due to *E. coli, Klebsiella pneumoniae, Proteus mirabilis, Pseudomonas aeruginosa, S. epidermidis,* or *Enterobacter cloacae.* Not effective for syphilis.
**Contraindications:** Lactation.
**Special Concerns:** Safety and efficacy have not been determined in children less than 18 years of age. Dosage adjustment is not required in elderly clients with normal renal function. Not efficiently removed by hemodialysis or peritoneal dialysis.
**Additional Side Effects:** *GI:* Anorexia, bloody stools, gastritis, stomatitis. *CNS:* Confusion, nervousness, anxiety, tremor, agitation, my-

oclonus, depersonalization, hypertonia. *Dermatologic:* Toxic epidermal necrolysis, **Stevens-Johnson syndrome,** urticaria, hyperhidrosis, mycotic infection, erythema multiforme. *CV:* Palpitations, tachycardia, vasodilation. *Respiratory:* Dyspnea, cough, epistaxis. *GU:* Vaginal moniliasis, urinary incontinence, renal failure. *Hematologic:* Eosinophilia, leukopenia, increased or decreased platelets, decreased hemoglobin, leukocytosis. *Miscellaneous:* Glucosuria, pyuria, increased or decreased potassium, asthenia, back or chest pain, myalgia, arthralgia, purpura, vertigo, unusual taste, tinnitus, conjunctivitis.

**Additional Drug Interactions**
*Bismuth subsalicylate* / Bioavailability of enoxacin is ↓ when bismuth subsalicylate is given within 1 hr; should not use together
*Digoxin* / ↓ Serum digoxin levels
**Laboratory Test Interferences:** ↑ ALT, AST, alkaline phosphatase, bilirubin. Proteinuria, albuminuria.

## Dosage

- **Tablets**
  *Uncomplicated gonorrhea.*
  **Adults:** 400 mg for one dose.
  *Uncomplicated UTIs, cystitis.*
  **Adults:** 200 mg q 12 hr for 7 days.
  *Complicated UTIs.*
  **Adults:** 400 mg q 12 hr for 14 days.

## NURSING CONSIDERATIONS

See also *General Nursing Considerations for All Anti-Infectives* and for *Fluoroquinolones.*
**Administration/Storage:** Adjust the dose if $C_{CR}$ is 30 mL (or less)/min/ 1.73 m². After a normal initial dose, use a 12-hr interval and one-half the recommended dose.
**Assessment**
1. Note any sensitivity to quinolones.
2. Identify source of infection; obtain cultures.
3. Obtain CBC, liver and renal function studies; reduce dose with renal dysfunction.

**Client/Family Teaching**
1. Take only as directed; 1 hr before or 2 hr after meals.
2. Increase fluid intake to prevent crystallization.
3. Avoid high intake of alkaline foods (dairy products) and drugs (antacids).
4. With STDs, inform partners so thay can receive treatment, to prevent reinfections.
**Outcomes/Evaluate**
- Resolution of infection
- Relief of pain and burning R/T UTI

# Enoxaparin injection

(ee-**nox**-ah-**PAIR**-in)
**Pregnancy Category:** B
Lovenox **(Rx)**
**Classification:** Anticoagulant, low molecular weight heparin

**Action/Kinetics:** The drug is characterized by a higher ratio of anti–factor Xa to anti–factor IIa activity than unfractionated heparin. **t½, elimination:** 4.5 hr after SC use. **Duration:** 12 hr following a 40-mg dose. Excreted mainly through the urine.
**Uses:** Prophylaxis of deep vein thrombosis (DVT), which may lead to pulmonary embolism, after hip or knee replacement surgery or abdominal surgery in those at risk for thromboembolic complications. Unstable angina and non-Q-wave MI. *Investigational:* Systemic anticoagulation, secondary prophylaxis for thromboembolic recurrence.
**Contraindications:** In clients with active major bleeding; thrombocytopenia associated with a positive in vitro test for antiplatelet antibody in the presence of enoxaparin; or in those with hypersensitivity to enoxaparin, heparin, or pork products. IM use. Interchangeable (unit for unit) use with unfractionated heparin or other low molecular weight heparins.
**Special Concerns:** Use with caution during lactation. Use with extreme caution in clients with a histo-

ry of heparin-induced thrombocytopenia and in conditions with increased risk of hemorrhage (e.g., bacterial endocarditis, congenital or acquired bleeding disorders, active ulcer and angiodysplastic GI disease, hemorrhagic stroke, or shortly after brain, spinal, or ophthalmic surgery). Use with caution in clients with a bleeding diathesis, uncontrolled arterial hypertension, a history of recent GI ulceration and hemorrhage, or in clients receiving oral anticoagulants and/or platelet inhibitors. Elderly clients and those with renal insufficiency may have delayed elimination of the drug. Safety and efficacy have not been determined in children.

**Side Effects:** *Hematologic:* Thrombocytopenia, thrombocythemia, ***hemorrhage,*** hypochromic anemia, ecchymosis. *At site of injection:* Mild local irritation, pain, hematoma, erythema. *GI:* Nausea. *CNS:* Confusion. *Miscellaneous:* Fever, pain, edema, peripheral edema.

**OD** **Overdose Management:** *Symptoms:* ***Hemorrhagic complications.*** *Treatment:* Slow IV injection of protamine sulfate (1% solution). Give 1 mg protamine sulfate to neutralize 1 mg enoxaparin injection. A second infusion of 0.5 mg protamine sulfate may be given if the APTT measured 2–4 hr after the first infusion remains prolonged. However, even with higher doses of protamine sulfate, the APTT may remain more prolonged than under normal conditions. Care should be taken to avoid overdosage with protamine sulfate.

**Laboratory Test Interferences:** ↑ AST, ALT.

**Dosage** ———————
- **SC**

  *Clients undergoing hip or knee replacement.*

**Adults:** 30 mg b.i.d. with the initial dose given not more than 24 hr after surgery for 7–10 days (usually).

  *Abdominal surgery.*

**Adults:** 40 mg once daily, with the initial dose given 2 hr prior to surgery.

**Duration:** 7–10 days, up to 12 days.

  *Systemic anticoagulation.*

1 mg/kg b.i.d.

  *Thromboembolic recurrence/prophylaxis.*

40 mg once daily.

## NURSING CONSIDERATIONS

See also *Nursing Considerations* for *Anticoagulants.*

**Administration/Storage**

1. Give only by deep SC when client is lying down; do *not* give IM.
2. Continue treatment throughout the postsurgical period until the risk of DVT has decreased.
3. Do not mix with other injections or infusions.
4. Discard any unused solution.
5. Do *not* interchange (unit for unit) with unfractionated heparin or other low molecular weight heparins.
6. The injection is clear colorless to pale yellow; store at temperatures < 25°C (<77°F). Do not freeze.

**Assessment**

1. Note any history of heparin or pork product sensitivity or disorders that may preclude drug therapy.
2. Document baseline hematologic parameters, liver function, and coagulation studies and monitor. Drug may cause significant, nonsymptomatic increases in SGOT and SGPT.
3. Monitor VS; observe for early S&S of abnormal bleeding. Any unexplained fall in hematocrit or BP should lead to a search for a bleeding site.
4. Monitor clients with renal dysfunction and the elderly closely.
5. Report any evidence of a thromboembolic event.

**Client/Family Teaching**

1. Lie down during self-administration; use prefilled syringes and administer at the same time each day.
2. Alternate administration between the left and right anterolateral and left and right posterolateral abdominal wall.

---
♣ = Available in Canada        ***bold italic*** = life threatening side effect

3. Introduce the entire length of the needle into a skin fold held between the thumb and forefinger; hold throughout the injection. To minimize bruising, do not rub the injection site.

4. May experience mild discomfort, irritation, and hematoma at injection site. Report any unusual bruising or bleeding.

**Outcomes/Evaluate**
• DVT prophylaxis following surgery
• Thromboembolic occurrence/recurrence prophylaxis

# Ephedrine sulfate
(eh-**FED**-rin)
**Pregnancy Category:** C
**Nasal decongestants:** Kondon's Nasal, Pretz-D, Vatronol Nose Drops **(OTC). Systemic:** Ephed II **(Rx:** Injection; **OTC:** Oral dosage forms)
**Classification:** Adrenergic agent, direct- and indirect-acting

See also *Sympathomimetic Drugs* and *Nasal Decongestants*.

**Action/Kinetics:** Releases norepinephrine from synaptic storage sites. Has direct effects on alpha, beta-1, and beta-2 receptors, causing increased BP due to arteriolar constriction and cardiac stimulation, bronchodilation, relaxation of GI tract smooth muscle, nasal decongestion, mydriasis, and increased tone of the bladder trigone and vesicle sphincter. It may also increase skeletal muscle strength, especially in myasthenia clients. Significant CNS effects include stimulation of the cerebral cortex and subcortical centers. Hepatic glycogenolysis is increased, but not as much as with epinephrine. More stable and longer-lasting than epinephrine. Rapidly and completely absorbed following parenteral use. **Onset, IM:** 10–20 min; **PO:** 15–60 min; **SC:** < 20 min. **Duration, IM, SC:** 30–60 min; **PO:** 3–5 hr. **t½, elimination:** About 3 hr when urine is at a pH of 5 and about 6 hr when urinary pH is 6.3. Excreted mostly unchanged through the urine (rate dependent on urinary pH—increased in acid urine).

**Uses:** Bronchial asthma and reversible bronchospasms associated with obstructive pulmonary diseases. Nasal congestion in vasomotor rhinitis, acute sinusitis, hay fever, and acute coryza. Parenterally to treat narcolepsy and depression. Parenterally as a vasopressor to treat shock. In acute hypotension states, especially that associated with spinal anesthesia and Stokes-Adams syndrome with complete heart block.

**Additional Contraindications:** Angle closure glaucoma, anesthesia with cyclopropane or halothane, thyrotoxicosis, diabetes, obstetrics where maternal BP is greater than 130/80. Lactation.

**Special Concerns:** Geriatric clients may be at higher risk to develop prostatic hypertrophy. May cause hypertension resulting in intracranial hemorrhage; may also cause anginal pain in clients with coronary insufficiency or ischemic heart disease.

**Additional Side Effects:** *CNS:* Nervousness, shakiness, confusion, delirium, hallucinations. Anxiety and nervousness following prolonged use. *CV:* Precordial pain, **excessive doses may cause hypertension sufficient to result in cerebral hemorrhage**. *GU:* Difficult and painful urination, urinary retention in males with prostatism, decrease in urine formation. *Miscellaneous:* Pallor, respiratory difficulty, hypersensitivity reactions. *Abuse:* Prolonged abuse can cause an anxiety state, including symptoms of paranoid schizophrenia, tachycardia, poor nutrition and hygiene, dilated pupils, cold sweat, and fever.

**Additional Drug Interactions**
*Dexamethasone* / Ephedrine ↓ effect of dexamethasone
*Diuretics* / Diuretics ↓ response to sympathomimetics
*Furazolidone* / ↑ Pressor effect → possible hypertensive crisis and intracranial hemorrhage
*Guanethidine* / ↓ Effect of guanethidine by displacement from its site of action

*Halothane* / Serious arrhythmias due to sensitization of the myocardium to sympathomimetics by halothane

*MAO Inhibitors* / ↑ Pressor effect → possible hypertensive crisis and intracranial hemorrhage

*Methyldopa* / Effect of ephedrine ↓ in methyldopa-treated clients

*Oxytocic drugs* / Severe persistent hypertension

## Dosage

• **Capsules**

*Bronchodilator, systemic nasal decongestant, CNS stimulant.*

**Adults:** 25–50 mg q 3–4 hr. **Pediatric:** 3 mg/kg (100 mg/m²) daily in four to six divided doses.

• **SC, IM, Slow IV**

*Bronchodilator.*

**Adults:** 12.5–25 mg; subsequent doses determined by client response. **Pediatric:** 3 mg/kg (100 mg/m²) daily divided into four to six doses SC or IV.

*Vasopressor.*

**Adults:** 25–50 mg (IM or SC) or 5–25 mg (by slow IV push) repeated at 5- to 10-min intervals, if necessary. Absorption following IM is more rapid than following SC use. **Pediatric (IM):** 16.7 mg/m² q 4–6 hr.

• **Topical (0.25% Spray)**

*Nasal decongestant.*

**Adults and children over 6 years:** 2–3 gtt of solution or small amount of jelly in each nostril q 4 hr. Do not use topically for more than 3 or 4 consecutive days. Do not use in children under 6 years of age unless ordered by provider.

## NURSING CONSIDERATIONS

See also *Nursing Considerations* for *Sympathomimetic Drugs* and *Nasal Decongestants.*

### Administration/Storage

1. Tolerance may develop; however, temporary cessation of therapy restores the original response to the drug.

**IV** 2. May administer 10 mg IV undiluted over at least 1 min.

3. Use only clear solutions and discard any unused solution with IV therapy. Protect against exposure to light; drug is subject to oxidation.

### Assessment

1. Document indications for therapy, type and onset of symptoms.

2. Assess mental status and pulmonary function; monitor ECG and VS. If administered for hypotension, monitor BP until stabilized.

3. If used for prolonged periods, assess for drug resistance. Rest without medication for 3–4 days, then resume; will usually respond to the drug again.

4. Monitor I&O. Elderly men may have difficulty and pain on urination.

### Client/Family Teaching

1. Notify provider if SOB is unrelieved by medication and accompanied by chest pain, dizziness, or palpitations. Report any elevated or irregular pulse.

2. With males, report any difficulty with voiding; may be drug-induced urinary retention.

3. Report any signs of depression, lack of interest in personal appearance, or complaints of insomnia or anorexia.

4. Avoid OTC drugs and alcohol.

### Outcomes/Evaluate

• Improved airway exchange
• ↓ Nasal congestion/mucus
• ↑ BP
• Control of narcolepsy

# Epinephrine

(ep-ih-**NEF**-rin)

**Pregnancy Category:** C

Adrenalin Chloride Solution, Bronkaid Mist, Bronkaid Mistometer ✦, EpiE-Z Pen, EpiE-Z Pen Jr., Epipen, Epipen Jr., Primatene Mist Solution, Sus-Phrine (Both Rx and OTC)

# Epinephrine bitartrate

(ep-ih-**NEF**-rin)

**Pregnancy Category:** C

Asthmahaler Mist, Bronitin Mist, Bronkaid Mist Suspension, Epitrate, Primatene Mist Suspension **(OTC)**

---

✦ = Available in Canada     ***bold italic*** = life threatening side effect

# Epinephrine borate

(ep-ih-**NEF**-rin)
**Pregnancy Category:** C
Epinal Ophthalmic Solution **(Rx)**

# Epinephrine hydrochloride

(ep-ih-**NEF**-rin)
**Pregnancy Category:** C
Adrenalin Chloride, AsthmaNefrin, Epifrin, Glaucon, microNefrin, Nephron, S-2 Inhalant, Vaponefrin (Both Rx and OTC)
**Classification:** Adrenergic agent, direct-acting

See also *Sympathomimetic Drugs* and *Nasal Decongestants*.

**Action/Kinetics:** Causes marked stimulation of alpha, beta-1, and beta-2 receptors, causing sympathomimetic stimulation, pressor effects, cardiac stimulation, bronchodilation, and decongestion. It crosses the placenta but not the blood-brain barrier. **Extreme caution must be taken never to inject 1:100 solution intended for inhalation—injection of this concentration has caused death. SC: Onset,** 6–15 min; **duration:** <1–4 hr. **Inhalation: Onset,** 1–5 min; **duration:** 1–3 hr. **IM, Onset:** variable; duration: <1–4 hr. Ineffective when given PO.

**Uses:** Cardiac arrest, Stokes-Adams syndrome, low CO following ECB. To prolong the action of local anesthetics. As a hemostatic during ocular surgery; treatment of conjunctival congestion during surgery; to induce mydriasis during surgery; treat ocular hypertension during surgery. Topically to control bleeding. Acute bronchial asthma, bronchospasms due to emphysema, chronic bronchitis, or other pulmonary diseases. Treatment of anaphylaxis, angioedema, anaphylactic shock, drug-induced allergic reactions, transfusion reactions, insect bites or stings. As an adjunct in the treatment of open-angle glaucoma (may be used with miotics, beta blockers, hyperosmotic agents, or carbonic anhydrase inhibitors). To produce mydriasis; to treat conjunctivitis. *NOTE:* Autoinjectors are available for emergency self-administration of first aid for anaphylactic reactions due to insect stings or bites, foods, drugs, and other allergens as well as idiopathic or exercise-induced anaphylaxis.

**Additional Contraindications:** Narrow-angle glaucoma. Use when wearing soft contact lenses (may discolor lenses). Aphakia. Lactation.

**Special Concerns:** May cause anoxia in the fetus. Safety and efficacy of ophthalmic products have not been determined in children; administer parenteral epinephrine to children with caution. Syncope may occur if epinephrine is given to asthmatic children. Administration of the SC injection by the IV route may cause severe or fatal hypertension or cerebrovascular hemorrhage. Epinephrine may temporarily increase the rigidity and tremor of parkinsonism. Use with caution and in small quantities in the toes, fingers, nose, ears, and genitals or in the presence of peripheral vascular disease as vasoconstriction-induced tissue sloughing may occur.

**Additional Side Effects:** *CV: **Fatal ventricular fibrillation, cerebral or subarachnoid hemorrhage,*** obstruction of central retinal artery. ***A rapid and large increase in BP may cause aortic rupture, cerebral hemorrhage, or angina pectoris.*** *GU:* Decreased urine formation, urinary retention, painful urination. *CNS:* Anxiety, fear, pallor. Parenteral use may cause or aggravate disorientation, memory impairment, psychomotor agitation, panic, hallucinations, **suicidal or homicidal tendencies,** schizophrenic-type behavior. *Miscellaneous:* Prolonged use or overdose may cause elevated serum lactic acid with severe metabolic acidosis. *At injection site:* Bleeding, urticaria, wheal formation, pain. Repeated injections at the same site may cause necrosis from vascular constriction. *Ophthalmic:* Transient stinging or burning when administered, conjunctival hyperemia, brow ache, headache, blurred vision, photophobia, allergic lid reaction, ocular hypersensitivity, poor night vision, eye ache, eye pain. Prolonged ophthalmic use may cause deposits of pigment in the cornea, lids, or conjunctiva. When used for glaucoma in aphakic clients, reversible cystoid macular edema.

**Additional Drug Interactions**
*Beta-adrenergic blocking agents* / Initial effectiveness in treating glaucoma of this combination may ↓ over time
*Chymotrypsin* / Epinephrine, 1:100, will inactivate chymotrypsin in 60 min

**Laboratory Test Interferences:** False + or ↑ BUN, fasting glucose, lactic acid, urinary catecholamines, glucose (Benedict's). ↓ Coagulation time. The drug may affect electrolyte balance.

**Dosage**

- **Metered Dose Inhaler**
*Bronchodilation.*
**Adults and children over 4 years of age:** 0.2–0.275 mg (1 inhalation) of the Aerosol or 0.16 mg (1 inhalation) of the Bitartrate Aerosol; may be repeated after 1–2 min if needed. At least 3 hr should elapse before subsequent doses. Dosage not established in children less than 4 years of age.
- **Inhalation Solution**
*Bronchodilation.*
**Adults and children over 6 years of age:** 1 inhalation of the 1% solution (of the base); may be repeated after 1–2 min.
- **IM, IV, SC**
*Bronchodilation using the solution (1:1,000).*
**Adults:** 0.3–0.5 mg SC or IM repeated q 20 min–4 hr as needed; dose may be increased to 1 mg/dose. **Infants and children (except premature infants and full-term newborns):** 0.01 mg/kg (0.3 mg/m²) SC up to a maximum of 0.5 mg/dose; may be repeated q 15 min for two doses and then q 4 hr as needed.

*Bronchodilation using the sterile suspension (1:200).*
**Adults:** 0.5–1.5 mg SC. **Infants and children, 1 month–12 years:** 0.025 mg/kg SC; **children less than 30 kg:** 0.75 mg as a single dose.
*Anaphylaxis.*
**Adults:** 0.2–0.5 mg SC q 10–15 min as needed, up to a maximum of 1 mg/dose if needed. **Pediatric:** 0.01 mg/kg (0.3 mg/m²) up to a maximum of 0.5 mg/dose; may be repeated q 15 min for two doses and then q 4 hr as needed.
- **Autoinjector, IM**
*First aid for anaphylaxis.*
The autoinjectors deliver a single dose of either 0.3 mg or 0.15 mg (for children) of epinephrine. In cases of a severe reaction, repeat injections may be necessary.
*Vasopressor.*
**Adults, IM or SC, initial:** 0.5 mg repeated q 5 min if needed; **then,** give 0.025–0.050 mg IV q 5–15 min as needed. **Adults, IV, initial:** 0.1–0.25 mg given slowly. May be repeated q 5–15 min as needed. Or, use IV infusion beginning with 0.001 mg/min and increasing the dose to 0.004 mg/min if needed. **Pediatric, IM, SC:** 0.01 mg/kg, up to a maximum of 0.3 mg repeated q 5 min if needed. **Pediatric, IV:** 0.01 mg/kg/5–15 min if an inadequate response to IM or SC administration is observed.
*Cardiac stimulant.*
**Adults, intracardiac or IV:** 0.1–1 mg repeated q 5 min if needed. **Pediatric, intracardiac or IV:** 0.005–0.01 mg/kg (0.15–0.3 mg/m²) repeated q 5 min if needed; this may be followed by IV infusion beginning at 0.0001 mg/kg/min and increased in increments of 0.0001 mg/kg/min up to a maximum of 0.0015 mg/kg/min.
*Adjunct to local anesthesia.*
**Adults and children:** 0.1–0.2 mg in a 1:200,000–1:20,000 solution.
*Adjunct with intraspinal anesthetics.*
**Adults:** 0.2–0.4 mg added to the anesthetic spinal fluid.
- **Solution**

E

*Antihemorrhagic, mydriatic.*
**Adults and children, intracameral or subconjunctival:** 0.01%–0.1% solution.
*Topical antihemorrhagic.*
**Adults and children:** 0.002%–0.1% solution.
*Nasal decongestant.*
**Adults and children over 6 years of age:** Apply 0.1% solution as drops or spray or with a sterile swab as needed.

• **Borate Ophthalmic Solution, Hydrochloride Ophthalmic Solution**
*Glaucoma.*
**Adults:** 1–2 gtt into affected eye(s) 1–2 times/day. Determine frequency of use by tonometry. Dosage has not been established in children.

## NURSING CONSIDERATIONS

See also *Nursing Considerations* for *Sympathomimetic Drugs* and *Nasal Decongestants.*
**Administration/Storage**
1. Briskly massage site of SC or IM injection to hasten drug action. Do not expose epinephrine to heat, light, or air, as this causes deterioration of the drug.
2. Discard solution if reddish brown and after expiration date.
3. With sodium bisulfite as a preservative in the topical preparation, there may be slight stinging after administration.
4. Do not use the topical preparation in children under 6 years of age.
5. Ophthalmic use may result in discomfort, which decreases over time.
6. The ophthalmic preparation is not for injection or intraocular use.
7. If ophthalmic glaucoma product is used with a miotic, instill the miotic first.
8. Keep the ophthalmic product tightly sealed and protected from light. Store at 2°C–4°C (36°F–75°F). Discard the solution if it becomes discolored or contains a precipitate.
**IV** 9. *Never administer* 1:100 solution IV. Use 1:1,000 solution for IV administration.
10. Use a tuberculin syringe to measure epinephrine; parenteral doses are small and the drug is potent, errors in measurement may be disastrous.
11. For direct IV administration to adults, the drug must be well diluted as a 1:1,000 solution; inject quantities of 0.05–0.1 mL of solution cautiously taking about 1 min for each injection; note response (BP and pulse). Dose may be repeated several times if necessary. May be further diluted in D5W or NSS.
**Assessment**
1. Note history of sulfite sensitivity.
2. Document indications for therapy; describe type and onset of symptoms and anticipated results.
3. Assess cardiopulmonary function.
4. During IV therapy, continuously monitor ECG, BP, and pulse until desired effect achieved. Then take VS every 2–5 min until condition has stabilized; once stable, monitor BP q 15–30 min.
5. Note any symptoms of shock such as cold, clammy skin, cyanosis, and loss of consciousness.
**Client/Family Teaching**
1. Review method for administration carefully. When prescribed for anaphylaxis, administer autoinjector immediately and then seek further medical care.
2. Report any increased restlessness, chest pain, or insomnia as dosage adjustment may be necessary.
3. Limit intake of caffeine, as with colas, coffee, tea, and chocolate; avoid OTC drugs without provider approval.
4. Rinse mouth after MDI use.
5. Ophthalmic solution may burn on administration; this should subside. These preparations may stain contact lens.
6. Use caution when performing activities that require careful vision; ophthalmic solution may diminish visual fields, cause double vision, and alter night vision.
**Outcomes/Evaluate**
• Restoration of cardiac activity
• Improved CO with EC bypass
• ↓ IOP
• Reversal of S&S of anaphylaxis

- Improved airway exchange
- Hemostasis with ocular surgery

# Epoetin alfa recombinant
(ee-POH-ee-tin)
**Pregnancy Category:** C
Epogen, Eprex ✹, Procrit **(Rx)**
**Classification:** Recombinant human erythropoietin

**Action/Kinetics:** Epoetin alfa is a 165-amino-acid glycoprotein made by recombinant DNA technology; it has the identical amino acid sequence and same biologic effects as endogenous erythropoietin (which is normally synthesized in the kidney and stimulates RBC production). Epoetin alfa will elevate or maintain the RBC level, decreasing the need for blood transfusions. **t½:** 4–13 hr in clients with chronic renal failure. **Peak serum levels after SC:** 5–24 hr.

**Uses:** Treatment of anemia associated with chronic renal failure, including clients on dialysis (end-stage renal disease) or not on dialysis. AZT-induced anemia in HIV-infected clients. Treatment of anemia in clients with nonmyeloid malignancies (Procrit only). Reduce allogeneic blood transfusions in surgery clients. *Investigational:* Pruritus associated with renal failure.

**Contraindications:** Uncontrolled hypertension. Hypersensitivity to mammalian cell-derived products or to human albumin. Use in chronic renal failure clients who need severe anemia corrected. To treat anemia in HIV-infected or cancer clients due to factors such as iron or folate deficiencies, hemolysis, or GI bleeding. Anemic clients willing to donate autologous blood.

**Special Concerns:** Safety and efficacy have not been established in children or in clients with a history of seizures or underlying hematologic disease (e.g., hypercoagulable disorders, myelodysplastic syndromes, sickle cell anemia). Use with caution in clients with porphyria, during lac-

tation, and preexisting vascular disease. Increased anticoagulation with heparin may be required in clients on epoetin alfa undergoing hemodialysis.

**Side Effects: In Chronic Renal Failure Clients (symptoms may be due to the disease).** *CV:* Hypertension, tachycardia, edema, *MI, CV accident,* TIA, clotted vascular access. *CNS:* Headache, fatigue, dizziness, *seizures. GI:* Nausea, diarrhea, vomiting, worsening of porphyria. *Allergic reactions:* Skin rashes, urticaria, *anaphylaxis. Miscellaneous:* SOB, hyperkalemia, arthralgias, myalgia, chest pain, skin reaction at administration site, asthenia.

**In AZT-Treated HIV-Infected Clients.** *CNS:* Pyrexia, fatigue, headache, dizziness, *seizures. Respiratory:* Cough, respiratory congestion, SOB. *GI:* Diarrhea, nausea. *Miscellaneous:* Rash, asthenia, reaction at injection site, allergic reactions.

**In Cancer Clients.** *CNS:* Pyrexia, fatigue, dizziness. *GI:* Diarrhea, nausea, vomiting. *Musculoskeletal:* Asthenia, paresthesia, trunk pain. *Miscellaneous:* Edema, SOB, URI.

**In Surgery Clients.** *CNS:* Pyrexia, insomnia, headache, dizziness, anxiety. *GI:* N&V, constipation, diarrhea, dyspepsia. *CV:* Hypertension, DVT, edema. *Miscellaneous:* Reaction at injection site, skin pain, pruritus, UTI.

**OD** **Overdose Management:** *Symptoms:* Polycythemia. *Treatment:* Withhold drug until hematocrit returns to the target range.

**Dosage** ─────────
- **IV, SC**
  *Chronic renal failure.*
**IV, initial (dialysis or nondialysis clients), SC (nondialysis clients), initial:** 50–100 U/kg 3 times/week. The rate of increase of hematocrit depends on both dosage and client variation. **Maintenance:** Individualize (usual: 25 U/kg 3 times/week). However, doses of 75–150 U/kg/week have maintained hematocrits

of 36%–38% for up to 6 months in nondialysis clients.

*AZT-treated, HIV infections.*

**IV, SC, initial:** 100 U/kg 3 times/ week for 8 weeks (in clients with serum erythropoietin levels less than or equal to 500 mU/mL who are receiving less than or equal to 4,200 mg/week of AZT). If a satisfactory response is obtained, the dose can be increased by 50–100 U/kg 3 times/ week. The response should be evaluated q 4–8 weeks thereafter with dosage adjusted by 50–100 U/kg increments 3 times/week. If clients have not responded to 300 U/kg 3 times/week, it is likely they will not respond to higher doses.

*Cancer clients on chemotherapy (Procrit only).*

**Initial, SC:** 150 units/kg 3 times/ week. Treatment of clients with highly elevated erythropoietin levels (> 200 mU/mL) is not recommended. If response is not satisfactory after 8 wks, the dose may be increased up to 300 units/kg 3 times/week. Clients not responding at this level are not likely to respond at higher levels. If the hematocrit exceeds 40%, the dose should be withheld until the hematocrit falls to 36%. When treatment is resumed, reduce the dose by 25%.

*NOTE:* The dose should be individualized for clients on dialysis. The median dose is 75 units/kg 3 times/week (range 12.5–525 units/ kg 3 times/week).

*Surgery to reduce allogeneic blood transfusions.*

**SC:** 300 U/kg/day for 10 days before surgery, on the day of surgery, and for 4 days after surgery. Alternative: 600 U/kg SC once a week 21, 14, and 7 days before surgery plus a fourth dose on the day of surgery. Iron supplementation is required at the time of epoetin therapy and continuing throughout the course of therapy.

## NURSING CONSIDERATIONS
### Administration/Storage

1. During hemodialysis, clients may require increased anticoagulation with heparin to prevent clotting of the artificial kidney.

2. Determine hematocrit twice weekly until it has stabilized in the target range and the maintenance dose of epoetin alfa has been determined. Do not adjust more often than once a month, unless clinically indicated. Also, after any dosage adjustment, monitor the hematocrit twice weekly for 2–6 weeks.

3. If the hematocrit approaches 36%, decrease the dose to maintain the suggested target hematocrit range. If the decrease in dose does not stop the rise in hematocrit and it exceeds 35%, temporarily withhold doses until the hematocrit begins to decrease; then, reinitiate therapy at a lower dose. Then, determine maintenance doses individually.

4. If the hematocrit increases by more than 4 points in a 2-week period, decrease the dose immediately. After reducing the dose, monitor the hematocrit twice weekly for 2–6 weeks; make further adjustments in dosage individually using the range outlined in the maintenance dose.

5. If the hematocrit does not increase by 5–6 points after 8 weeks of therapy and iron stores are adequate, increase the dose incrementally. Further increases may be made at 4–6-week intervals until a desired response is observed.

6. Do *not* shake; shaking will denature the glycoprotein, making it biologically inactive.

7. Do not use vials showing particulate matter or discoloration.

8. Withdraw only one dose per vial; discard any unused portion. The product contains no preservative.

9. Store at 2°C–8°C (36°F–46°F).

10. Do not give with any other drug solutions. However, at the time of SC administration, the drug may be admixed in a syringe with bacteriostatic 0.9% NaCl injection with benzyl alcohol, 0.9%, at a 1:1 ratio. The benzyl alcohol acts as a local anesthetic that may reduce discomfort at the SC injection site.

## Assessment

1. Note any hypersensitivity to mammalian cell-derived products or human albumin.

2. Determine CBC and iron stores. Transferrin saturation should be at least 20% and serum ferritin should be at least 200 ng/mL. Provide supplemental iron to increase or maintain transferrin saturation to levels required to support stimulation of erythropoiesis by epoetin alfa.

3. With HIV, note when AZT therapy was instituted, the onset and cause of anemia.

4. Assess BP; control hypertension.

5. Monitor renal function studies, electrolytes, phosphorous and uric acid levels; especially with chronic renal failure.

## Client/Family Teaching

1. Over 95% of clients with chronic renal failure manifested significant increases in hematocrit and nearly all were transfusion-independent within 2 months after beginning epoetin alfa therapy; drug does not cure renal disease and desired drug response may take as long as 6 weeks.

2. Supplemental iron is administered to enhance the effects of epoetin alfa.

3. Report as scheduled for lab studies as drug dose is adjusted based on these results.

4. Review list of drug side effects; report any persistent and/or bothersome ones and practice contraception during therapy.

5. Must continue to follow prescribed dietary and dialysis recommendations; schedule activities to permit rest periods.

6. Do not perform any tasks that require mental alertness until drug effects realized (especially during the first 3 mo of therapy).

## Outcomes/Evaluate

- ↑ Hematocrit
- Relief of symptoms of anemia
- ↓ Need for allogeneic blood transfusions

# Epoprostenol sodium

(eh-poh-**PROST**-en-ohl)

**Pregnancy Category:** B

Flolan **(Rx)**

**Classification:** Antihypertensive, miscellaneous

See also *Antihypertensive Agents*.

**Action/Kinetics:** Acts by direct vasodilation of pulmonary and systemic arterial vascular beds and by inhibition of platelet aggregation. IV infusion in clients with pulmonary hypertension results in increases in cardiac index and SV and decreases in pulmonary vascular resistance, total pulmonary resistance, and mean systemic arterial pressure. Is rapidly hydrolyzed at the neutral pH of the blood as well as by enzymatic degradation. Metabolites are less active than the parent compound. **t½:** 6 min.

**Uses:** Long-term IV treatment of primary pulmonary hypertension in New York Heart Association Class III and Class IV clients.

**Contraindications:** Chronic use in those with CHF due to severe LV systolic dysfunction and in those who develop pulmonary edema during dose ranging.

**Special Concerns:** Abrupt withdrawal or sudden large decreases in the dose may cause rebound pulmonary hypertension. Use caution in dose selection in the elderly due to the greater frequency of decreased hepatic, renal, or cardiac function, as well as concomitant disease or other drug therapy. Use with caution during lactation. Safety and efficacy have not been determined in children.

**Side Effects:** Side effects have been classified as those occurring during acute dose ranging, those as a result of the drug delivery system, and those occurring during chronic dosing.

**Those occurring during acute dose ranging.** *CV:* Flushing, hypotension, bradycardia, tachycardia. *GI:* N&V, abdominal pain, dyspepsia. *CNS:* Headache, anxiety, nervousness, agitation, dizziness, hypesthesia, paresthesia. *Miscellaneous:* Chest pain, musculoskeletal pain, dyspnea, back pain, sweating.

**Those occurring as a result of the drug delivery system.** *Due to the chronic indwelling catheter:* Local infection, pain at the injection site, sepsis, infections.

**Those occurring during chronic dosing.** *CV:* Flushing, tachycardia. *GI:* N&V, diarrhea. *CNS:* Headache, anxiety, nervousness, tremor, dizziness, hypesthesia, hyperesthesia, paresthesia. *Musculoskeletal:* Jaw pain, myalgia, nonspecific musculoskeletal pain. *Miscellaneous:* Flu-like symptoms, chills, fever, sepsis.

**OD** **Overdose Management:** *Symptoms:* Flushing, headache, hypotension, tachycardia, nausea, vomiting, diarrhea. *Treatment:* Reduce dose of epoprostenol.

**Drug Interactions**
*Anticoagulants* / Possible ↑ risk of bleeding
*Antiplatelet drugs* / Possible ↑ risk of bleeding
*Diuretics* / Additional ↓ in BP
*Vasodilators* / Additional ↓ in BP

**Dosage** ───────────────
• **Chronic IV Infusion**
  *Pulmonary hypertension.*
**Acute dose ranging:** The initial chronic infusion rate is first determined. The mean maximum dose that did not elicit dose-limiting pharmacologic effects was 8.6 ng/kg/min. **Continuous chronic infusion, initial:** 4 ng/kg/min less than the maximum-tolerated infusion rate determined during acute dose ranging. If the maximum-tolerated infusion rate is less than 5 ng/kg/min, start the chronic infusion at one-half the maximum-tolerated infusion rate. **Dosage adjustments:** Changes in the chronic infusion rate are based on persistence, recurrence, or worsening of the symptoms of primary pulmonary hypertension. If symptoms require an increase in infusion rate, increase by 1–2 ng/kg/min at intervals (at least 15 min) sufficient to allow assessment of the clinical response. If a decrease in infusion rate is necessary, gradually make 2-ng/kg/min decrements every 15 min or longer until the dose limiting effects resolve. Abrupt withdrawal or sudden large reductions in infusion rates are to be avoided.

## NURSING CONSIDERATIONS

See also *Nursing Considerations* for *Antihypertensive Agents.*
**Administration/Storage**
**IV** 1. Chronic administration is delivered continuously by a permanent indwelling central venous catheter and an ambulatory infusion pump (see package insert for requirements for the infusion pump). Unless contraindicated, give anticoagulant therapy to decrease the risk of pulmonary thromboembolism or systemic embolism.
2. Do not dilute reconstituted solutions or administer with other parenteral solutions or medications.
3. Check package insert carefully to make 100 mL of a solution with the appropriate final concentration of drug and for infusion delivery rates for doses equal to or less than 16 ng/kg/min based on client weight, drug delivery rate, and concentration of solution to be used.
4. Protect unopened vials from light and store at 15°C–25°C (59°F–77°F). Protect reconstituted solutions from light and refrigerate at 2°C–8°C (36°F–46°F) for no more than 40 hr.
5. Do not freeze reconstituted solutions; discard any solution refrigerated for more than 48 hr.
6. A single reservoir of reconstituted solution can be given at room temperature for 8 hr; alternatively, it can be used with a cold pouch and given for up to 24 hr. Do not expose solution to sunlight.
**Assessment**
1. Perform a full cardiopulmonary assessment. Based on symptoms, determine New York Heart Association functional class (III or IV). Note agents previously used and the outcome.

2. Determine mental status and ability to handle medication preparation and IV administration; or identify someone in the home that can and is willing to perform this function on a regular basis and/or initiate home infusion referral.

3. Determine that a permanent indwelling central venous catheter is available for continuous ambulatory delivery once dose ranging has been completed.

4. Assess central venous access site for any evidence of infection, discharge, odor, erythema, or swelling.

5. Consult manufacturer's guidelines for dosage and delivery rate based on client weight for acute dose ranging.

**Client/Family Teaching**

1. Drug helps reduce RV and LV afterload and increases CO and SV, thereby improving symptoms of SOB, fatigue, and exercise intolerance.

2. Administered continuously through an indwelling catheter to the heart by a portable external infusion pump; may be needed for years to help control symptoms.

3. Proper site care and pump maintenance as well as appropriate reconstitution for desired drug concentration, proper storage, protection from light, pouch filling, pump settings, and accessing VAD are imperative to safe therapy.

4. Review written guidelines for drug preparation, infusion, dose reduction, storage, and administration and site inspection and care; pump maintenance, programming, trouble shooting, and care.

5. When drug is reconstituted and administered at room temperature, the pump must be programmed to administer pouch contents in 8 hr, whereas if drug is reconstituted and refrigerated at 2°C–8°C (36°F–46°F) it may be administered over 24 hr.

6. Side effects that indicate excessive dosing and require a reduction in dosage and reporting include tachycardia, headache, N&V, diarrhea, hypotension.

7. Brief interruptions in therapy may cause rapid deterioration in condition.

**Outcomes/Evaluate:** Improvement in exercise capacity; ↓ dyspnea and fatigue

———COMBINATION DRUG———

# Equagesic
(eh-kwah-**JEE**-sik)
**(Rx)**
**Classification:** Analgesic

See also *Acetylsalicylic Acid* and *Meprobamate*.

**Content:** *Nonnarcotic Analgesic:* Aspirin, 325 mg. *Antianxiety agent:* Meprobamate, 200 mg. See also information on individual components.

**Uses:** Treatment (short-term only) of pain due to musculoskeletal disease accompanied by anxiety and tension.

**Additional Contraindications:** Pregnancy. Children under 12 years of age. Use for longer than 4 months.

**Dosage**
• **Tablets**
  *Pain due to musculoskeletal disease.*
**Adults:** 1–2 tablets t.i.d.–q.i.d.

## NURSING CONSIDERATIONS

See also *Nursing Considerations* for *Acetylsalicylic Acid* and *Meprobamate*.
**Outcomes/Evaluate:** Relief of pain; ↓ anxiety and tension

# Erythromycin base
(eh-**rih**-throw-**MY**-sin)
**Pregnancy Category:** B (A/T/S, Erymax, Staticin, and T-Stat are C)
**Capsules/Tablets:** Alti-Erythromycin ✦, Apo-Erythro Base ✦, Apo-Erythro-EC ✦, Diomycin ✦, E-Base Caplets, E-Base Tablets, E-Mycin, Erybid ✦, Eryc, Ery-Tab, Erythro-Base ✦, Erythromid ✦, Erythromycin Base Film-Tabs, Novo–Rythro EnCap ✦, PCE Dispertab, PMS-Erythromycin ✦, Ro-

bimycin Robitabs. **Gel, topical:**A/T/S, Erygel. **Ointment, topical:** Aknemycin. **Ointment, ophthalmic:** Ilotycine Ophthalmic, **Pledgets:** Erycette, T-Stat. **Solution:** Del-Mycin, Eryderm 2%, Erymax, Erythra-Derm, Staticin, Theramycin Z, T-Stat **(Rx)**
**Classification:** Antibiotic, erythromycin

See also *Erythromycins* and *Anti-Infective Agents.*

**Uses:** See *Erythromycins.* **Ophthalmic solution:** Treatment of ocular infections (along with PO therapy) due to *Streptococcus pneumoniae, Staphylococcus aureus, S. pyogenes, Corynebacterium* species, *Haemophilus influenzae,* and *Bacteroides* infections. Also prophylaxis of ocular infections due to *Neisseria gonorrhoeae* and *Chlamydia trachomatis.* **Topical solution:** Acne vulgaris. **Topical ointment:** Prophylaxis of infection in minor skin abrasions; treatment of superficial infections of the skin. Acne vulgaris.

**Contraindications:** Use of topical preparations in the eye or near the nose, mouth, or any mucous membrane. Ophthalmic use in dendritic keratitis, vaccinia, varicella, myobacterial infections of the eye, fungal diseases of the eye. Use with steroid combinations following uncomplicated removal of a corneal foreign body.

**Special Concerns:** Use of other drugs for acne may result in a cumulative irritant effect.

**Additional Side Effects:** *When used topically:* Erythema, desquamation, burning sensation, eye irritation, tenderness, dryness, pruritus, oily skin, generalized urticaria.

**Drug Interactions:** Antagonism has been observed when topical erythromycin is used with clindamycin.

**Dosage** ————————
• **Delayed-Release Capsules, Enteric-Coated Tablets, Delayed-Release Tablets, Film-Coated Tablets, Suspension**
*Respiratory tract infections due to* Mycoplasma pneumoniae.

500 mg q 6 hr for 5–10 days (up to 3 weeks for severe infections).
*URTIs (mild to moderate) due to* S. pyogenes and S. pneumoniae.
250–500 mg q.i.d. (or 20–50 mg/kg/day in divided doses) for 10 days.
*URTIs due to* H. influenzae.
Erythromycin ethylsuccinate, 50 mg/kg/day, plus sulfisoxazole, 150 mg/kg/day, given together for 10 days.
*Lower respiratory tract infections (mild to moderate) due to* S. pyogenes and S. pneumoniae.
250–500 mg q.i.d. (or 20–50 mg/kg/day in divided doses) for 10 days.
*Intestinal amebiasis due to* Entamoeba histolytica.
**Adults:** 250 mg q.i.d. for 10–14 days; **pediatric:** 30–50 mg/kg/day in divided doses for 10–14 days.
*Legionnaire's disease.*
500–1,000 mg q.i.d. for 3 weeks (or 1–4 g/day in divided doses).
Bordetella pertussis.
500 mg q.i.d. for 10 days (or 40–50 mg/kg/day in divided doses for 5–14 days).
*Infections due to* Corynebacterium diphtheriae.
500 mg q.i.d. for 10 days.
*Erythrasma.*
250 mg t.i.d. for 3 weeks.
*Primary syphilis.*
20 g in divided doses over 10 days.
*Chlamydial infections.*
**Infants:** 50 mg/kg/day in four divided doses for 14 (conjunctivitis) to 21 (pneumonia) days; **adults:** 500 mg q.i.d. for 7 days or 250 mg q.i.d. for 14 days for urogenital infections.
*Mild to moderate skin and skin structure infections due to* S. pyogenes and S. aureus.
250–500 mg q 6 hr (or 50 mg/kg/day in divided doses—to a maximum of 4 g/day) for 10 days.
Listeria monocytogenes *infections.*
500 mg q 12 hr (or 250 mg q 6 hr), up to maximum of 4 g/day.
*Pelvic inflammatory disease, acute* N. gonorrhoeae.
Erythromycin lactobionate, 500 mg IV q 6 hr for 3 days; **then,** 250 mg erythromycin base q 6 hr for 7 days. Al-

ternatively for pelvic inflammatory disease, 500 mg PO q.i.d. for 10–14 days.

*Prophylaxis of initial or recurrent rheumatic fever.*
250 mg b.i.d.

*Bacterial endocarditis due to alpha-hemolytic streptococcus.*
**Adults:** 1 g 2 hr prior to the procedure; **then,** 500 mg 6 hr after the initial dose. **Pediatric,** 20 mg/kg 2 hr prior to the procedure; **then,** 10 mg/kg 6 hr after the initial dose.

*Pneumonia of infancy, conjunctivitis of the newborn, and urogenital infections during pregnancy due to C. trachomatis.*
500 mg q.i.d. for 7 days (or 250 mg q.i.d. for 14 days).

*Nongonococcal urethritis due to* Ureaplasma urealyticum.
500 mg q.i.d. for at least 7 days.

*Erythrasma due to* Corynebacterium minutissimum.
250 mg t.i.d. for 21 days.

• **Ophthalmic Ointment**
*Mild to moderate infections.*
0.5-in. ribbon b.i.d.–t.i.d.
*Acute infections.*
0.5 in. q 3–4 hr until improvement is noted.
*Prophylaxis of neonatal gonococcal or chlamydial conjunctivitis.*
0.2–0.4 in. into each conjunctival sac.

• **Topical Gel (2%), Ointment (2%), Solution (2%)**
Clean the affected area and apply, using fingertips or applicator, morning and evening, to affected areas. If no improvement is seen after 6 to 8 weeks, discontinue therapy.

## NURSING CONSIDERATIONS

See also *Nursing Considerations* for *Erythromycins*.
**Administration/Storage:** The topical gel is prepared by adding 3 mL of ethyl alcohol to the vial and immediately shaking to dissolve erythromycin. This solution is added to the gel and stirred until it appears ho-

mogenous (1–1.5 min). Refrigerate the gel.
**Assessment**
1. Document indications for therapy, type and onset of symptoms.
2. Assess for sensitivity reactions.
3. Obtain cultures, CBC, wound documentation, and appropriate diagnostic studies.
**Client/Family Teaching**
1. Continue entire prescription; do not stop if symptoms subside. Return for follow-up once completed.
2. Report any unusual or intolerable side effects or lack of response.
3. Take on an empty stomach; the delayed-release forms of the base can be taken without regard for meals.
4. Do not wash ophthalmic ointment from the eyes.
5. Before applying the topical solution, wash, rinse, and dry the affected areas. Wash hands before and after application.
6. A sterile bandage may be used with the topical ointment.
7. The topical and ophthalmic products are for external use only.
**Outcomes/Evaluate**
• Negative C&S results
• Symptomatic improvement
• Desired infection prophylaxis

# Erythromycin estolate
(eh-**rih**-throw-**MY**-sin)
**Pregnancy Category:** B
Ilosone, Novo-Rythro Estolate ✦ **(Rx)**
**Classification:** Antibiotic, erythromycin

See also *Erythromycins*.
**Action/Kinetics:** Most active form of erythromycin, with relatively long-lasting activity.
**Uses:** See *Erythromycins*.
**Additional Contraindications:** Cholestatic jaundice or preexisting liver dysfunction. Treatment of chronic disorders such as acne, furunculosis, or prophylaxis of rheumatic fever.
**Additional Side Effects:** Hepatotoxicity.

**Dosage**
• **Capsules, Suspension, Tablets**
See *Erythromycin base.* Similar blood levels are achieved using erythromycin base, estolate, or stearate.

## NURSING CONSIDERATIONS

See also *Nursing Considerations* for *Erythromycins.*
**Assessment**
1. Document indications for therapy, duration and onset of symptoms.
2. Note evidence of liver failure.
**Client/Family Teaching**
1. Shake suspension well before using; do not store for more than 2 weeks at room temperature.
2. Chew or crush chewable tablets.
3. May take without regard to meals.
**Outcomes/Evaluate:** Resolution of infection

# Erythromycin ethylsuccinate
(eh-**rih**-throw-**MY**-sin)
**Pregnancy Category:** B
Apo-Erythro-ES, E.E.S. 200 and 400, E.E.S. Granules, EryPed, EryPed 200, EryPed 400, EryPed Drops, Erythro-ES ✤, Novo-Rythro Ethylsuccinate ✤ **(Rx)**
**Classification:** Antibiotic, erythromycin

See also *Erythromycins.*
**Uses:** See *Erythromycins.*
**Additional Contraindications:** Pre-existing liver disease.

**Dosage**
• **Oral Suspension, Tablets, Chewable Tablets**
See *Erythromycin base. NOTE:* 400 mg of erythromycin ethylsuccinate will achieve the same blood levels of erythromycin as 250 mg of the base, estolate, or stearate forms.
   *Hemophilus influenzae infections.*
Erythromycin ethylsuccinate, 50 mg/kg/day with sulfisoxazole, 150 mg/kg/day, both for a total of 10 days.

## NURSING CONSIDERATIONS

See also *Nursing Considerations* for *Erythromycins.*

**Client/Family Teaching**
1. Take without regard to meals.
2. Chew or crush chewable tablets.
3. Refrigerate oral suspension; store for 1 week maximum.
**Outcomes/Evaluate:** Resolution of infection

# Erythromycin lactobionate
(eh-**rih**-throw-**MY**-sin)
**Pregnancy Category:** B
Erythrocin I.V. ✤, Erythrocin Lactobionate IV **(Rx)**
**Classification:** Antibiotic, erythromycin

See also *Erythromycins.*
**Uses:** For seriously ill or vomiting clients with infections caused by susceptible organisms; acute pelvic inflammatory disease due to gonorrhea. Legionnaire's disease.
**Additional Side Effects:** Transient deafness.
**Additional Drug Interactions:** Do not add drugs to IV solutions of erythromycin lactobionate.

**Dosage**
• **IV**
**Adults and children:** 15–20 mg/kg/day up to 4 g/day in severe infections.
   *Acute pelvic inflammatory disease caused by gonorrhea.*
500 mg q 6 hr for 3 days followed by 250 mg erythromycin stearate, **PO,** q 6 hr for 7 days.
   *Legionnaire's disease.*
1–4 g/day in divided doses. Change to PO therapy as soon as possible.

## NURSING CONSIDERATIONS

See also *Nursing Considerations* for *Erythromycins.*
**Administration/Storage**
**IV** 1. Sterile water for injection is the preferred diluent. However, 5% dextrose injection or D5%/RL may also be used if buffered with 4% sodium bicarbonate injection.
2. For intermittent IV administration, may be further diluted in 100 to 250

mL of D5W or NSS and infused over 20–60 min.

3. The initial reconstituted solution is stable for 2 weeks if refrigerated or for 24 hr at room temperature and if final diluted solution used within 8 hr. Use the reconstituted piggyback vial within 24 hr if stored in the refrigerator or 8 hr if stored at room temperature.

4. If reconstituted solution is frozen, it can be stored for 30 days. Once thawed, use within 8 hr. Do not refreeze thawed solutions.

**Assessment**

1. Obtain CBC and cultures.

2. Assess for hearing deficits.

**Outcomes/Evaluate:** Resolution of infection; negative cultures

# Erythromycin stearate

(eh-**rih**-throw-**MY**-sin)
**Pregnancy Category:** B
Apo-Erythro-S ✿, Eramycin, Novo-Rythro Stearate ✿, Nu-Erythromycin-S ✿ **(Rx)**
**Classification:** Antibiotic, erythromycin

See also *Erythromycins.*
**Uses:** See *Erythromycins.*
**Additional Side Effects:** Causes more allergic reactions (e.g., skin rash and urticaria) than other erythromycins. Hepatotoxicity.

**Dosage**
• **Tablets, Film Coated**
See *Erythromycin base.* Similar blood levels are achieved using erythromycin base, estolate, or stearate forms.

## NURSING CONSIDERATIONS

See also *Nursing Considerations* for *Erythromycins.*
**Client/Family Teaching**
1. Take on an empty stomach; food decreases absorption.
2. Report lack of effect or evidence of allergic reaction, i.e., rash or itching.
**Outcomes/Evaluate:** Resolution of infection

# Esmolol hydrochloride

(**EZ**-moh-lohl)
**Pregnancy Category:** C
Brevibloc **(Rx)**
**Classification:** Beta-adrenergic blocking agent

See also *Beta-Adrenergic Blocking Agents.*
**Action/Kinetics:** Preferentially inhibits beta-1 receptors. Rapid onset (<5 min) and a short duration of action. Has no membrane-stabilizing or intrinsic sympathomimetic activity. Low lipid solubility. **t½:** 9 min. Rapidly metabolized by esterases in RBCs.
**Uses:** Supraventricular tachycardia or arrhythmias, sinus tachycardia.
**Special Concerns:** Dosage has not been established in children.
**Additional Side Effects:** *Dermatologic:* Inflammation at site of infusion, flushing, pallor, induration, erythema, burning, skin discoloration, edema. *Other:* Urinary retention, midscapular pain, asthenia, changes in taste.
**Additional Drug Interactions**
*Digoxin* / Esmolol ↑ digoxin blood levels
*Morphine* / Morphine ↑ esmolol blood levels

**Dosage**
• **IV Infusion**
*SVT.*
**Initial:** 500 mcg/kg/min for 1 min; **then,** 50 mcg/kg/min for 4 min. If after 5 min an adequate effect is not achieved, repeat the loading dose followed by a maintenance infusion of 100 mcg/kg/min for 4 min. This procedure may be repeated, increasing the maintenance infusion by 50 mcg/kg/min increments (for 4 min) until the desired HR or lowered BP is approached. **Then,** omit the loading infusion and reduce incremental infusion rate from 50 to 25 mcg/kg/min or less. The interval between titrations may be increased from 5 to 10 min.

E

---

Once the HR has been controlled, the client may be transferred to another antiarrhythmic agent. Reduce the infusion rate of esmolol by 50% 30 min after the first dose of the alternative antiarrhythmic agent. If satisfactory control is observed for 1 hr after the second dose of the alternative agent, the esmolol infusion may be stopped.

## NURSING CONSIDERATIONS

See also *Nursing Considerations* for *Beta-Adrenergic Blocking Agents.*

### Administration/Storage

**IV** 1. Infusions may be necessary for 24–48 hr.
2. Not for direct IV push administration.
3. Do not dilute concentrate with sodium bicarbonate.
4. To minimize irritation and thrombophlebitis, do not infuse concentrations greater than 10 mg/mL.
5. Diluted esmolol (concentration of 10 mg/mL) is compatible with D5%/W, D5%/RL, D5%/ Ringer's injection, D5%/0.9% NaCl, D5%/ 0.45% NaCl, 0.45% NaCl, RL, potassium chloride (40 mEq/L) in D5 injection, 0.9% NaCl, and 0.45% NaCl.

### Assessment

1. Note indications for therapy, type, onset, and characteristics of symptoms.
2. Document and monitor cardiopulmonary assessments, ECG, and VS. Assess for hypotension or bradycardia.
3. Administer in a monitored environment; wean according to guidelines.

### Outcomes/Evaluate

• Suppression of SVT
• Restoration of stable rhythm

# Estazolam

(es-**TAYZ**-oh-lam)
**Pregnancy Category:** X
ProSom **(C-IV) (Rx)**
**Classification:** Hypnotic, benzodiazepine

See also *Tranquilizers, Antimanic Drugs, and Hypnotics.*

**Action/Kinetics: Peak plasma levels:** 2 hr. **t½:** 10–24 hr. The clearance is increased in smokers compared with nonsmokers. Metabolized in the liver and excreted mainly in the urine. Two metabolites—4'-hydroxy estazolam and 1-oxo-estazolam—have minimal pharmacologic activity although at the levels present they do not contribute significantly to the hypnotic effect.

**Uses:** Short-term use for insomnia characterized by difficulty in falling asleep, frequent awakenings, and/or early morning awakenings.

**Contraindications:** Pregnancy. Use during labor and delivery and during lactation.

**Special Concerns:** Use with caution in geriatric or debilitated clients, in those with impaired renal or hepatic function, in those with compromised respiratory function, and in those with depression or who show suicidal tendencies. Safety and efficacy have not been determined in children less than 18 years of age.

### Dosage
• **Tablets**
**Adults:** 1 mg at bedtime (although some clients may require 2 mg). The initial dose in small or debilitated geriatric clients is 0.5 mg. Prolonged use is not recommended or necessary.

## NURSING CONSIDERATIONS

See also *Nursing Considerations* for *Tranquilizers, Antimanic Drugs, and Hypnotics.*

### Assessment

1. Note history of depression, suicidal tendencies, or respiratory problems.
2. Monitor liver and renal function studies; reduce dose in geriatric and debilitated clients and those with impaired renal and hepatic function.
3. Identify underlying cause(s) for insomnia; investigate alternative nonpharmacologic methods for sleep inducement.
4. Drug may enhance the duration and quality of sleep for up to 12 weeks; assess need for continued therapy after this period.

**Client/Family Teaching**
1. Identify symptoms that require immediate reporting.
2. Practice contraception; discontinue drug before becoming pregnant.
3. Do not perform tasks that require mental alertness until drug effects are realized; ability to drive or operate dangerous machinery may be impaired.
4. Avoid alcohol and do not take any OTC drugs without consent; smoking may alter drug absorption.
5. Take only as directed; may cause psychologic and physical dependence.
6. Do not stop abruptly; after prolonged treatment, withdraw gradually.
7. Identify any contributing factors; review alternative methods for sleep induction.
**Outcomes/Evaluate:** Enhanced duration and quality of sleep

# Esterified estrogens
(es-**TER**-ih-fyd **ES**-troh-jens)
**Pregnancy Category:** X
Estratab, Menest, Neo-Estrone ✦ **(Rx)**
**Classification:** Estrogen, natural

See also *Estrogens.*
**Action/Kinetics:** This product is a mixture of sodium salts of sulfate esters of natural estrogenic substances: 75%–85% estrone sodium sulfate and 6%–15% equilin sodium sulfate. Less potent than estrone.
**Uses:** Replacement therapy in primary ovarian failure, following castration, or hypogonadism. Inoperable, progressing prostatic or breast carcinoma (in postmenopausal women and selected men). Moderate to severe vasomotor symptoms, atrophic vaginitis, and kraurosis vulvae due to menopause.

**Dosage**
• **Tablets**
*Moderate to severe vasomotor symptoms, atrophic vaginitis, or kraurosis vulvae due to menopause.*

0.3–1.25 mg/day given cyclically for short-term use. Adjust dose to the lowest effective level and discontinue as soon as possible.
*Hypogonadism.*
2.5–7.5 mg/day in divided doses for 20 days, followed by a 10-day rest period. If menses does not occur by the end of this period of time, repeat dosage schedule. The number of courses of estrogen required to produce bleeding varies, depending on the responsiveness of the endometrium. If bleeding occurs before the end of the 10-day period, a 20-day estrogen-progestin cycle should be started with 2.5–7.5 mg/day of estrogen with a progestin added the last 5 days. If bleeding occurs before the end of this regimen, discontinue therapy and resume on day 5 of bleeding.
*Primary ovarian failure, castration.*
1.25 mg/day given cyclically.
*Prostatic carcinoma, inoperable and progressing.*
1.25–2.5 mg t.i.d. Effectiveness can be determined using phosphatase determinations and symptomatic improvement.
*Breast carcinoma, inoperable and progressing, in selected men and postmenopausal women.*
10 mg t.i.d. for at least 3 months.

## NURSING CONSIDERATIONS

See *Nursing Considerations for Estrogens.*
**Assessment:** Document indications for therapy; note type, onset, and characteristics of symptoms.
**Outcomes/Evaluate**
• Stimulation of menses
• Relief of postmenopausal S&S
• Suppression of tumor growth and spread
• Osteoporosis prophylaxis

# Estradiol transdermal system
(ess-trah-**DYE**-ohl)

**Pregnancy Category:** X
Alora, Climara, Estraderm, Estring,
FemPatch, Vivelle **(Rx)**
**Classification:** Estrogen

See also *Estrogens.*
**Action/Kinetics:** This transdermal
system allows a constant low dose
of estradiol to directly reach the systemic circulation. The system over-
comes certain problems associated
with PO use, including first-pass hepatic metabolism, GI upset, and induction of liver enzymes. The system is available in various surface
areas, release rates, and total estradiol content (the package insert
should be carefully consulted). The
patches are made either with a
reservoir and a rate-controlling
membrane or using a matrix where
estradiol is embedded in the adhesive,
allowing for a translucent, small,
thin patch.
**Uses:** Vasomotor symptoms due to
menopause, including hot flashes,
night sweats, and vaginal burning,
itching, and dryness. Female hypogonadism or castration; atrophic
vaginitis or kraurosis vulvae due to
menopause; primary ovarian failure;
prevention of osteoporosis.
**Side Effects:** Skin irritation, URTI,
headache, breast tenderness.

**Dosage** ————————
• **Dermal System**
*Menopausal symptoms.*
**Initial:** One 0.05-mg system applied
to the skin twice weekly (if using
Alora, Estraderm, or Vivelle) or once
a week (if using Climara). Adjust
dose as necessary to control symptoms. Taper or discontinue dose at 3-
to 6-month intervals. Alora is available
in 0.05-, 0.75-, and 0.1-mg dosage
strengths. Climara and Estraderm are
available in strengths to release 0.05
or 0.1 mg/24 hr. Vivelle is available in
strengths to release 0.0375, 0.05,
0.075, or 0.1 mg/24 hr.
*Prevention of osteoporosis.*
**Initial:** 0.05 mg/day as soon as possible after menopause. Adjust dosage to control concurrent menopausal symptoms.

## NURSING CONSIDERATIONS

See also *Nursing Considerations* for
*Estrogens.*
**Client/Family Teaching**
1. If taking oral estrogens, stop the
pills and wait 1 week before applying
the system.
2. Without a hysterectomy, the system
is usually used for 3 weeks, followed by 1 week of rest. May be
used continuously in those without an
intact uterus.
3. Place the system on a clean, dry
area of the skin on the trunk of the
body (preferably the abdomen).
Avoid using areas with excessive
amounts of hair. Also may use on
the hip or buttock. Do not apply to
the breasts or the waistline.
4. Rotate application site; date
patch. Allow at least a 1-week interval between reapplication to a particular site.
5. Apply system immediately after
the pouch is opened and the protective liner is removed. Firmly press in
place with the palm for approximately 10 sec. Ensure good contact,
especially around the edges. If system
falls, reapply the same system or
place a new one and follow the
same schedule.
6. Weight gain may occur; report if
marked or if symptoms of edema
develop.
7. Stop smoking; this increases risk of
thromboembolic problems.
8. Addition of a progestin for 7 or
more days may reduce the incidence
of endometrial hyperplasia.
**Outcomes/Evaluate**
• Relief of menopausal symptoms
• Therapeutic estrogen levels

# Estramustine phosphate sodium
(es-trah-**MUS**-teen)
Emcyt **(Rx)**
**Classification:** Antineoplastic, hormonal agent, alkylating agent

See also *Antineoplastic Agents.*
**Action/Kinetics:** Estramustine is a
water-soluble drug that combines

estradiol and mechlorethamine (a nitrogen mustard). The estradiol facilitates uptake into cells containing the estrogen receptor while the nitrogen mustard acts as an alkylating agent. Chronic estramustine administration results in plasma levels and effects of estradiol similar to those of conventional estradiol therapy. Well absorbed from the GI tract and dephosphorylated before reaching the general circulation. Metabolites include estromustine, estrone, and estradiol. **t½:** 20 hr. Major route of excretion is in the feces.

**Uses:** Palliative treatment of metastatic and/or progressive prostatic carcinoma.

**Contraindications:** Active thrombophlebitis or thromboembolic disease unless the tumor mass is causing the thromboembolic disorder. Allergy to nitrogen mustard or estrogen.

**Special Concerns:** Use with caution in presence of cerebrovascular disease, CAD, diabetes, hypertension, CHF, impaired liver or kidney function, and metabolic bone diseases associated with hypercalcemia.

**Additional Side Effects:** *CV: MI, CVA,* thrombosis, CHF, increased BP, thrombophlebitis, leg cramps, edema. *Respiratory: Pulmonary embolism,* dyspnea, upper respiratory discharge, hoarseness. *GI:* Flatulence, burning sensation of throat, thirst. *CNS:* Emotional lability, insomnia, anxiety, lethargy, headache. *Dermatologic:* Easy bruising, flushing, peeling of skin or fingertips. *Miscellaneous:* Chest pain, tearing of eyes, leg cramps, breast tenderness or enlargement, decreased glucose tolerance.

**OD** **Overdose Management:** *Symptoms:* Extensions of the side effects. *Treatment:* Gastric lavage; treat symptoms. Monitor blood counts and liver profiles for at least 6 weeks.

**Drug Interactions:** Drugs or food containing calcium may ↓ absorp-

tion of estramustine phosphate sodium.

**Laboratory Test Interferences:** ↑ Bilirubin, AST, LDH. ↓ Glucose tolerance. Abnormal hematologic tests for leukopenia and thrombocytopenia.

**Dosage**
• **Capsules**
14 mg/kg/day in three to four divided doses (range: 10–16 mg/kg/day) or 600 mg (base)/m² daily in three divided doses. One 140-mg capsule is taken for each 10 kg or 22 lb of body weight. Treat for 30–90 days before assessing beneficial effects; continue therapy as long as the drug is effective. Some clients have taken doses from 10 to 16 mg/kg/day for more than 3 years.

## NURSING CONSIDERATIONS

See also *Nursing Considerations* for *Antineoplastic Agents.*

**Administration/Storage:** Store capsules in the refrigerator at 2°C–8°C (36°F–46°F), although they may be kept at room temperature up to 48 hr without affecting potency.

**Assessment**
1. Note any allergy to nitrogen mustard or estrogen.
2. Assess diabetics for hyperglycemia, increased fatigue, weakness; glucose tolerance may be decreased.
3. Monitor CBC, electrolytes, liver and renal function studies.
4. Assess for symptoms of hypercalcemia: insomnia, lethargy, anorexia, N&V, coma, and vascular collapse.
5. Assess serum calcium levels (normal: 4.5–5.5 mEq/L). The effect of the steroid and osteolytic metastases may result in hypercalcemia.

**Client/Family Teaching**
1. Take capsules with water 1 hr before or 2 hr after meals. Do not take milk, milk products, and calcium-rich foods and drugs simultaneously with estramustine.
2. Check BP and record; elevations may occur.
3. Consume 2–3 L/day of fluids to minimize hypercalcemia.

4. Report symptoms of hypercalcemia (chest pain, SOB, swelling or redness and pain in an extremity).

5. Impotence resulting from previous estrogen therapy may be reversed.

6. Drug may cause genetic mutation; consider sperm/egg harvesting; practice contraceptive measures to prevent teratogenesis.

**Outcomes/Evaluate:** ↓ Size and spread of prostatic carcinoma

# Estrogens conjugated, oral (conjugated estrogenic substances)

(**ES**-troh-jens)
**Pregnancy Category:** X
C.E.S. ✿, Congest ✿, Conjugated Estrogens C.S.D. ✿, Premarin **(Rx)**

# Estrogens conjugated, parenteral

**Pregnancy Category:** X
(**ES**-troh-jens)
Premarin IV **(Rx)**

# Estrogens conjugated, vaginal

(**ES**-troh-jens)
**Pregnancy Category:** X
**Classification:** Estrogen, natural

See also *Estrogens* and *Esterified Estrogens*.

**Action/Kinetics:** Contains 50%–65% sodium estrone sulfate and 20%–35% sodium equilin sulfate.

**Uses: PO:** Moderate to severe vasomotor symptoms due to menopause, atrophic vaginitis, kraurosis vulvae, female hypogonadism, primary ovarian failure, female castration. Palliation in mammary cancer in men or postmenopausal women; prostatic carcinoma (inoperable and progressive). Prophylaxis of osteoporosis.

**Parenteral:** Abnormal bleeding due to imbalance of hormones and in the absence of disease.

**Vaginal:** Atrophic vaginitis and kraurosis vulvae associated with menopause.

**Special Concerns:** Use of estrogen replacement therapy for prolonged periods of time may increase the risk of fatal ovarian cancer and may also have a higher risk of breast cancer.

## Dosage

• **Tablets**

*Moderate to severe vasomotor symptoms due to menopause.*

1.25 mg/day given cyclically. If the client has not menstruated in 2 or more months, begin therapy on any day; if, however, the client is menstruating, begin therapy on day 5 of bleeding.

*Primary ovarian failure, female castration.*

1.25 mg/day given cyclically. Adjust dose to lowest effective level.

*Atrophic vaginitis or kraurosis vulvae associated with menopause.*

0.3–1.25 mg/day (higher doses may be necessary, depending on the response) given cyclically.

*Hypogonadism in females.*

2.5–7.5 mg/day in divided doses for 20 days, followed by a 10-day rest period. If menses does not occur by the end of this period of time, repeat the dosage schedule. The number of courses of estrogen required to produce bleeding varies, depending on the responsiveness of the endometrium. If bleeding occurs before the end of the 10-day period, start a 20-day estrogen-progestin cycle with 2.5–7.5 mg/day of estrogen with a progestin added the last 5 days. If bleeding occurs before the end of this regimen, discontinue therapy and resume on day 5 of bleeding.

*Palliation of mammary carcinoma in men or postmenopausal women.*

10 mg t.i.d. for at least 90 days.

*Palliation of prostatic carcinoma.*

1.25–2.5 mg t.i.d. Effectiveness can be measured by phosphatase determinations and symptomatic improvement.

*Prophylaxis of osteoporosis.*

0.625 mg/day given cyclically.

• **IM, IV**

*Abnormal bleeding.*

25 mg; repeat after 6–12 hr if necessary.

• **Vaginal Cream**

½–2 g daily given for 3 weeks on and 1 week off. Repeat as needed. Attempt to taper the dose or discontinue the medication at 3- to 6-month intervals.

## NURSING CONSIDERATIONS

See also *Nursing Considerations* for *Estrogens*.

### Administration/Storage

1. For all uses, except palliation of mammary and prostatic carcinoma and prevention of postpartum breast engorgement, oral conjugated estrogens are best administered cyclically—3 weeks of hormone therapy and 1 week off.

2. When used vaginally, insert the cream high into the vagina (two-thirds the length of the applicator).

**IV** 3. Parenteral solutions of conjugated estrogens are compatible with NSS, invert sugar solutions, and dextrose solutions.

4. Parenteral solutions are incompatible with acid solutions, ascorbic acid solutions, and protein hydrolysates.

5. Use reconstituted parenteral solutions within a few hours after mixing if kept at room temperatures. Put the date and time of reconstitution on the solution label.

6. If solution is refrigerated, it will remain stable for 60 days.

7. IV use is preferred over IM as it induces a more rapid response.

8. Administer IV premarin slowly to prevent flushing.

### Assessment

1. Document indications for therapy, type, onset, and duration of symptoms.

2. Review potential risks R/T to the development of breast and fatal ovarian cancers with prolonged therapy.

3. Monitor serum phosphatase levels with prostatic cancer.

### Outcomes/Evaluate

• Inhibition of malignant proliferation
• Control of abnormal uterine bleeding
• Osteoporosis prophylaxis
• Relief of menopausal symptoms

# Estropipate (Piperazine estrone sulfate)

(es-troh-**PIE**-payt)

**Pregnancy Category:** X

Ogen, Ogen Vaginal Cream, Ortho-Est **(Rx)**

**Classification:** Estrogen, semisynthetic

See also *Estrogens*.

**Action/Kinetics:** Contains solubilized crystalline estrone stabilized with piperazine.

**Uses: PO:** Vasomotor symptoms, atrophic vaginitis, or kraurosis vulvae associated with menopause. Primary ovarian failure, female castration, female hypogonadism. Prevention of osteoporosis.

**Vaginal:** Atrophic vaginitis and kraurosis vulvae associated with menopause.

**Contraindications:** Use during pregnancy.

### Dosage

• **Tablets**

*Moderate to severe vasomotor symptoms; atrophic vaginitis or kraurosis vulvae due to menopause.*

0.625–5 mg/day for short-term therapy (give cyclically). May also be used continuously. The lowest dose that will control symptoms should be selected.

*Hypogonadism, primary ovarian failure, castration.*

1.25–7.5 mg/day for first 3 weeks; **then,** rest period of 8–10 days. A PO progestin can be given during the third week if withdrawal bleeding does not occur.

*Prevention of osteoporosis.*

0.625 mg/day for 25 days of a 31-day cycle per month.

• **Vaginal Cream**

2–4 g (containing 3–6 mg estropipate) daily (depending on severity of condition) for 3 weeks followed by a 1-week rest period. Attempt to taper the dose or discontinue the medication at 3- to 6-month intervals.

## NURSING CONSIDERATIONS

See also *Nursing Considerations* for *Estrogens*.

**Administration/Storage**

1. Administration should be cyclic—3 weeks on the medication and 1 week off.

2. Attempts should be made to taper or discontinue the medication at 3- to 6-month intervals.

3. When used to relieve vasomotor symptoms, cyclic administration is initiated on day 5 of bleeding if menstruating. If the client has not menstruated within the last 2 months (or more), cyclic administration may be initiated at any time.

**Client/Family Teaching**

1. Take medications at the same time each day.

2. Nausea during PO therapy may be relieved by consuming solid foods.

3. Report any evidence of thromboembolic S&S (headache, blurred vision, pain, swelling or tenderness in the extremities); fluid retention (weight gain, swelling of extremities); hepatic dysfunction (yellowing of skin or eyes, itching, dark urine, clay-colored stools); changes in mental status or any unusual bleeding.

4. With vaginal preparations, administer at bedtime, remaining recumbent for 30 min; protect clothing and bed linens by using a sanitary pad. To deliver cream, the end of the applicator (after the appropriate amount is introduced) should be inserted into the vagina and the plunger pushed all the way down.

5. Between uses the plunger of the applicator should be pulled out of the barrel and washed in warm, soapy water. Do not put in hot or boiling water.

6. Do not smoke.

7. Drug may cause increased pigmentation of skin. Wear protective clothing and sunscreens with any exposure; avoid prolonged exposures.

8. Stop drug and report if pregnant.

**Outcomes/Evaluate**

- Relief of menopausal symptoms
- Stimulation of menses
- Restoration of hormonal balance

# Ethacrynate sodium
(eth-ah-**KRIH**-nayt)
**Pregnancy Category:** B
Sodium Edecrin **(Rx)**

# Ethacrynic acid
(eth-ah-**KRIH**-nik **AH**-sid)
**Pregnancy Category:** B
Edecrin **(Rx)**
**Classification:** Diuretics, loop

See also *Loop Diuretics*.

**Action/Kinetics:** Inhibits the reabsorption of sodium and chloride in the loop of Henle; it also decreases reabsorption of sodium and chloride and increases potassium excretion in the distal tubule. Also acts directly on the proximal tubule to enhance excretion of electrolytes. Large quantities of sodium and chloride and smaller amounts of potassium and bicarbonate ion are excreted during diuresis. **Onset: PO,** 30 min; **IV,** Within 5 min. **Peak: PO,** 2 hr; **IV,** 15–30 min. **Duration: PO,** 6–8 hr. **IV,** 2 hr. **t½, after PO:** 60 min. Metabolites are excreted through the urine. Diuresis and electrolyte loss are more pronounced with ethacrynic acid than with thiazide diuretics. Is often effective in clients refractory to other diuretics. Careful monitoring of the diuretic effects is necessary.

**Uses:** Of value with resistant to less potent diuretics. CHF, acute pulmonary edema, edema associated with nephrotic syndrome, ascites due to idiopathic edema, lymphedema, malignancy. Short-term use for ascites as a result of malignancy, lymphedema, or idiopathic edema; also, for short-term use in pediatric clients (except infants) with congenital heart disease. *Investigational.*

**Ethacrynic acid:** Single injection into the eye to treat glaucoma (effective for a week or more). **Ethacrynate sodium:** Hypercalcemia, bromide intoxication, and with mannitol in ethylene glycol poisoning.

**Contraindications:** Pregnancy (usually), lactation, use in neonates. Anuria and severe renal damage.

**Special Concerns:** Geriatric clients may be more sensitive to the usual adult dose. To be used with caution in diabetic clients and those with hepatic cirrhosis (who are particularly susceptible to electrolyte imbalance). Monitor gout clients carefully. Safety and efficacy of oral use in infants and IV use in children have not been established.

**Side Effects:** *Electrolyte imbalance:* Hypokalemia, hyponatremia, hypochloremic alkalosis, hypomagnesemia, hypocalcemia. *GI:* Anorexia, nausea, vomiting, diarrhea (may be sudden watery, profuse diarrhea), acute pancreatitis, abdominal discomfort or pain, jaundice, *GI bleeding or hemorrhage,* dysphagia. *Hematologic:* Severe neutropenia, thrombocytopenia, *agranulocytosis,* rarely Henoch-Schoenlein purpura in clients with rheumatic heart disease. *CNS:* Apprehension, confusion, vertigo, headache. *Body as a whole:* Fever, chills, fatigue, malaise. *Otic:* Sense of fullness in the ears, tinnitus, irreversible hearing loss. *Miscellaneous:* Hematuria, acute gout, abnormal liver function tests in seriously ill clients on multiple drug therapy including ethacrynic acid, blurred vision, rash, local irritation and pain following parenteral use, hyperuricemia, hyperglycemia.

*Ethacrynic acid may cause death in critically ill clients refractory to other diuretics.* These include (a) clients with severe myocardial disease who also received digitalis and who developed acute hypokalemia with fatal arrhythmias and (b) those with severely decompensated hepatic cirrhosis with ascites, with or without encephalopathy, who had electrolyte imbalances with death due to intensification of the electrolyte effect.

**OD** **Overdose Management:** *Symptoms:* Profound water loss, electrolyte depletion (causes dizziness, weakness, mental confusion, vomiting, anorexia, lethargy, cramps), dehydration, reduction of blood volume, *circulatory collapse (possibility of vascular thrombosis and embolism).* *Treatment:* Replace electrolytes and fluid and monitor urine output and serum electrolyte levels. Induce emesis or perform gastric lavage. Artificial respiration and oxygen may be needed. Treat other symptoms.

**Dosage**
ETHACRYNATE SODIUM
• **IV**
**Adults:** 50 mg (base) (or 0.5–1 mg/kg); may be repeated in 2–4 hr, although only one dose is usually needed. A single 100-mg dose IV has also been used.
ETHACRYNIC ACID
• **Tablets**
**Adults, initial:** 50–200 mg/day in single or divided doses to produce a gradual weight loss of 2.2–4.4 kg/day (1–2 lb/day). The dose can be increased by 25–50 mg/day if needed. **Maintenance:** Usually 50–200 mg (up to a maximum of 400 mg) daily may be required in severe, refractory edema. If used with other diuretics, the initial dose should be 25 mg with increments of 25 mg. **Pediatric, initial:** 25 mg/day; can increase by 25 mg/day if needed. **Maintenance:** Adjust dose to needs of client. Dosage for infants has not been determined.

## NURSING CONSIDERATIONS

See also *Nursing Considerations* for *Diuretics, Loop.*

**Administration/Storage**
1. When used PO, administer after meals.
2. Due to local pain and irritation, do not give SC or IM.
3. Ammonium chloride or arginine

chloride may be prescribed for those at a higher risk of developing metabolic acidosis.

**IV** 4. Reconstitute powder for injection by adding 50 mL of 5% dextrose injection or NaCl injection.

5. Intermittent IV administration should be slowly over a 30-min period given either directly or through IV tubing. For direct IV, may give at a rate of 10 mg/min.

6. When reconstituted with 5% dextrose injection, the resulting solution may be hazy or opalescent. Do not use such solutions. Do not mix this solution with whole blood or its derivatives.

7. If a second IV injection is necessary, a different site should be used to prevent thrombophlebitis.

8. Use reconstituted solutions within 24 hr; discard any unused solution.

**Assessment**

1. Document indications for therapy, other agents trialed, and outcome.

2. Note history of diabetes or cirrhosis.

3. Establish lack of anuria.

4. Monitor electrolytes, CBC, liver and renal function studies.

5. With prolonged therapy, obtain audiometric assessment.

**Interventions**

1. Monitor VS, I&O, and weight. Note excessive diuresis or weight loss; electrolyte imbalance may develop quickly.

2. With rapid excessive diuresis, assess for pain in calves, pelvic area, or the chest; rapid hemoconcentration may cause thromboembolic effects.

3. Drug should be withdrawn if severe, watery diarrhea presents. Test for occult blood in urine and stools.

4. Observe for vestibular disturbances. Do not administer concomitantly with any other ototoxic agent. Hearing loss is most common following high dosing or rapid IV administration.

5. Monitor serum potassium levels; determine need for supplementary potassium.

6. Since drug has such a profound effect on sodium excretion, dietary salt restriction is not necessary; if sodium is restricted, hyponatremia may result.

**Outcomes/Evaluate**

• Enhanced diuresis
• ↓ Edema (↑ weight loss)
• ↓ Abdominal girth R/T ascites

# Ethambutol hydrochloride

(eh-**THAM**-byou-tohl)
Etibi ✦, Myambutol **(Rx)**
**Classification:** Primary antitubercular agent

**Action/Kinetics:** Inhibits the synthesis of metabolites resulting in impairment of cell metabolism, arrest of multiplication, and ultimately cell death. Is active against *Mycobacterium tuberculosis,* but not against fungi, other bacteria, or viruses. Readily absorbed after PO administration. Widely distributed in body tissues except CSF. **Peak plasma concentration:** 2–5 mcg/mL after 2–4 hr. t½: 3–4 hr. About 65% of metabolized and unchanged drug excreted in urine and 20%–25% unchanged drug excreted in feces. Drug accumulates in clients with renal insufficiency.

**Uses:** Pulmonary tuberculosis in combination with other tuberculostatic drugs. Use only in conjunction with at least one other antituberculostatic.

**Contraindications:** Hypersensitivity to ethambutol, preexisting optic neuritis, and in children under 13 years of age.

**Special Concerns:** Use with caution and in reduced dosage in clients with gout and impaired renal function and in pregnant women.

**Side Effects:** *Ophthalmologic:* Optic neuritis, decreased visual acuity, loss of color (green) discrimination, temporary loss of vision or blurred vision. *GI:* N&V, anorexia, abdominal pain. *CNS:* Fever, headache, dizziness, confusion, disorientation, malaise, hallucinations. *Allergic:* Pruritus, dermatitis, **anaphylaxis.** *Miscellaneous:* Peripheral neuropathy (numbness, tingling), precipitation of gout, thrombocytopenia, joint pain, toxic epidermal necrolysis. Renal damage.

Also **anaphylactic shock,** peripheral neuritis (rare), hyperuricemia, and decreased liver function. Adverse symptoms usually appear during the early months of therapy and disappear thereafter. Periodic renal and hepatic function tests as well as uric acid determinations are recommended.

**Drug Interactions:** Aluminum may delay and decrease the absorption of ethambutol.

**Dosage** ⎯⎯⎯⎯⎯⎯⎯⎯⎯
• **Tablets**

**Adults, initial treatment:** 15 mg/kg/day until maximal improvement noted; **for retreatment:** 25 mg/kg/day as a single dose with at least one other tuberculostatic drug; **after 60 days:** 15 mg/kg/day.

**NURSING CONSIDERATIONS**

See also *General Nursing Considerations for All Anti-Infectives.*

**Assessment**

1. Note indications for therapy, onset and duration of symptoms, other treatments, and outcomes.

2. Obtain a visual acuity test before ethambutol therapy. Document no preexisting visual problems (especially if dose exceeds 15 mg/kg/day).

3. Monitor CBC, cultures, liver and renal function studies.

4. With positive AFB cultures, identify close contacts and advise treatment.

**Client/Family Teaching**

1. Take as prescribed to prevent any relapses or complications.

2. Consume 2–3 L/day of fluids to ensure adequate hydration.

3. Avoid aluminum-based antacids; may interfere with drug absorption.

4. Obtain periodic vision testing during therapy (q 1–2 months); report any vision changes that may indicate optic neuritis. Ocular side effects generally disappear within weeks to several months after completion of therapy.

5. Practice reliable birth control;

stop drug and report if pregnancy is suspected.

**Outcomes/Evaluate**
• Negative sputum cultures
• Resolution of infection (↓ fever, WBC, sputum; improved CXR)

# Ethosuximide
(eth-oh-**SUCKS**-ih-myd)
Zarontin **(Rx)**
**Classification:** Anticonvulsant, succinimide type

⎯⎯⎯⎯⎯⎯⎯⎯⎯⎯⎯⎯

See also *Anticonvulsants* and *Succinimides.*

**Action/Kinetics: Peak serum levels:** 3–7 hr. **t½, adults:** 40–60 hr; **t½, children:** 30 hr. Steady serum levels reached in 7–10 days. **Therapeutic serum levels:** 40–100 mcg/mL. Not bound to plasma protein. Metabolized in the liver. Both inactive metabolites and unchanged drug are excreted in the urine.

**Uses:** Absence (petit mal) seizures.

**Additional Drug Interactions:** Both isoniazid and valproic acid may ↑ the effects of ethosuximide.

**Dosage** ⎯⎯⎯⎯⎯⎯⎯⎯⎯
• **Capsules, Syrup**
*Absence seizures.*

**Adults and children over 6 years, initial:** 250 mg b.i.d.; the dose may be increased by 250 mg/day at 4–7-day intervals until seizures are controlled or until total daily dose reaches 1.5 g. **Children under 6 years, initial:** 250 mg/day; dosage may be increased by 250 mg/day every 4–7 days until control is established or total daily dose reaches 1 g.

**NURSING CONSIDERATIONS**

See also *Nursing Considerations* for *Anticonvulsants* and *Succinimides.*

**Administration/Storage:** May be given with other anticonvulsants when other forms of epilepsy are present.

**Client/Family Teaching**

1. Take with meals to minimize GI upset.

2. Do not engage in hazardous activities while on drug therapy.

3. Do not stop abruptly; may precipitate withdrawal seizures.

4. Report loss of seizure control.

5. Need lab studies q 3 mo to assess uric acid levels, hematologic, liver, and renal function.

**Outcomes/Evaluate**
• Control of petit mal seizures
• Therapeutic serum drug levels (40–100 mcg/mL)

# Etidronate disodium (oral)

(eh-tih-**DROH**-nayt)
**Pregnancy Category:** B
Didronel **(Rx)**

# Etidronate disodium (parenteral)

(eh-tih-**DROH**-nayt)
**Pregnancy Category:** C
Didronel IV **(Rx)**
**Classification:** Bone growth regulator, antihypercalcemic

**Action/Kinetics:** Slows bone metabolism, thereby decreasing bone resorption, bone turnover, and new bone formation; it also reduces bone vascularization. Renal tubular reabsorption of calcium is not affected. **Absorption:** Dose-dependent; after 24 hr, one-half of absorbed drug is excreted unchanged. Absorption is affected by food or preparations containing divalent ions. **Onset:** 1 month for Paget's disease and within 24 hr for hypercalcemia. The drug remaining in the body is adsorbed to bone, where therapeutic effects for Paget's disease persist 3–12 months after discontinuation of the drug. **Plasma t½:** 6 hr. Approximately 50% excreted unchanged in the urine; unabsorbed drug is excreted through the feces.

**Uses: PO:** Paget's disease (osteitis deformans), especially of the polyostotic type accompanied by pain and increased urine levels of hydroxyproline and serum alkaline phosphatase. Heterotopic ossification due to spinal cord injury or total hip replacement. **Parenteral:** Hypercalcemia of malignancy inadequately managed by dietary modification or oral hydration or which persists after adequate hydration is restored. *Investigational:* Postmenopausal osteoporosis.

**Contraindications:** Enterocolitis, fracture of long bones, hypercalcemia of hyperparathyroidism. Serum creatinine greater than 5 mg/dL.

**Special Concerns:** Use with caution in the presence of renal dysfunction and during lactation. Safety and efficacy have not been established in children.

**Side Effects:** *GI:* Nausea, diarrhea, constipation, ulcerative stomatitis. *Bones:* Increased incidence of bone fractures and increased or recurrent bone pain. Drug should be discontinued if fracture occurs and not restarted until healing takes place. *Allergy:* Angioedema, rash, pruritus, urticaria. *Electrolytes:* Hypophosphatemia, hypomagnesemia. *Miscellaneous:* Metallic taste, abnormal hepatic function, fever, fluid overload, dyspnea, convulsions. Symptoms of rachitic syndrome have been reported in children receiving 10 mg or more/kg daily for long periods (up to 1 year) to treat heterotopic ossification or soft tissue calcification.

**OD** **Overdose Management:** *Symptoms:* Following PO ingestion, hypocalcemia may occur. Rapid IV administration may cause renal insufficiency. *Treatment:* Gastric lavage following PO ingestion. Treat hypocalcemia by giving calcium IV.

**Drug Interactions:** Products containing calcium or other multivalent cations ↓ absorption of etidronate

**Dosage**
• **Tablets**
*Paget's disease.*
**Adults, initial:** 5–10 mg/kg/day for 6 months or less; or, 11–20 mg/kg for a maximum of 3 months. Reserve doses above 10 mg/kg when lower doses are ineffective, when there is a need for suppression of increased bone turnover, or when a prompt

decrease in CO is needed. Do not exceed doses of 20 mg/kg/day. Another course of therapy may be instituted after rest period of 3 months if there is evidence of active disease process.

*Heterotopic ossification due to spinal cord injury.*
**Adults:** 20 mg/kg/day for 2 weeks; **then** 10 mg/kg/day for 10 weeks. Treatment should be initiated as soon as possible after the injury, preferably before evidence of heterotopic ossification.

*Heterotopic ossification complicating total hip replacement.*
**Adults:** 20 mg/kg/day for 30 days preoperatively; **then,** 20 mg/kg/day for 90 days postoperatively.

- **IV Infusion**
*Hypercalcemia due to malignancy.*
7.5 mg/kg/day for 3 successive days. If necessary, a second course of treatment may be instituted after a 7-day rest period. The safety and effectiveness of more than two courses of therapy has not been determined. Etidronate tablets may be started the day after the last infusion at a dose of 20 mg/kg/day for 30 days (treatment may be extended to 90 days if serum calcium levels are normal). Use for more than 90 days is not recommended.

## NURSING CONSIDERATIONS
### Administration/Storage
1. Administer as a single dose (if GI upset occurs, divide dose) with juice or water 2 hr before meals.
2. There are no indications to date that etidronate will affect mature heterotopic bone.
**IV** 3. Dilute IV dose in at least 250 mL of sterile NSS and administer over a 2-hr period.
4. May experience a metallic taste during IV administration.
5. The diluted solution shows no loss of drug for 48 hr if stored between 15°C and 30°C (59°F and 86°F).

### Assessment
1. Document indications for therapy.
2. Note any evidence of renal dysfunction. Monitor uric acid, alkaline phosphatase, urinary hydroxyproline excretion, electrolytes, magnesium, phosphate, calcium, and renal function studies.
3. Determine if pregnant.
### Client/Family Teaching
1. Maintain a well-balanced diet with adequate intake of calcium and vitamin D; may refer to dietitian.
2. Do not eat for 2 hr after taking medication. Foods high in calcium (e.g., milk, milk products) and vitamins with mineral supplements (e.g., aluminum, calcium, iron, or magnesium) may decrease absorption. If GI upset with single dose, may divide dose.
3. Report any S&S of hypercalcemia, i.e., lethargy, N&V, anorexia, tremors, and bone pain.
4. Obtain lab studies as scheduled: with Paget's disease, levels of urinary hydroxyproline excretion and serum alkaline phosphatase reductions indicate a beneficial therapeutic response. Levels usually decrease 1–3 months after initiation of therapy.
5. With hypercalcemia, serum calcium levels show drug response and need for continued therapy. Reduction usually occurs in 2–8 days in hypercalcemia R/T bone metastasis. Therapy may be repeated only after 7 days of rest; risk for hypocalcemia greatest 3 days after IV therapy.
### Outcomes/Evaluate
- Suppression of bone resorption
- ↓ Serum calcium levels
- ↓ Pain with Paget's disease

**E**

# Etodolac
(ee-toh-**DOH**-lack)
**Pregnancy Category:** C
Lodine **(Rx)**
**Classification:** Nonsteroidal anti-inflammatory drug

---

See also *Nonsteroidal Anti-Inflammatory Drugs.*

**Action/Kinetics:** Etodolac is a NSAID in a class called the pyranocarboxylic acids. **Time to peak levels:** 1–2 hr. **Onset of analgesic action:** 30 min; **duration:** 4–12 hr. **t½:** 7.3 hr. The drug is metabolized by the liver and metabolites are excreted through the kidneys.

**Uses:** Acute and chronic treatment of osteoarthritis, mild to moderate pain. Treatment of rheumatoid arthritis.

**Contraindications:** Clients in whom etodolac, aspirin, or other NSAIDs have caused asthma, rhinitis, urticaria, or other allergic reactions. Use during lactation, during labor and delivery, and in children.

**Special Concerns:** Use with caution in impaired renal or hepatic function, heart failure, those on diuretics, and in geriatric clients. Safety and effectiveness have not been determined in children.

**Additional Side Effects:** *GI:* Diarrhea, gastritis, thirst, ulcerative stomatitis, anorexia. *CNS:* Nervousness, depression. *CV:* Syncope. *Respiratory:* Asthma. *Dermatologic:* Angioedema, vesiculobullous rash, cutaneous vasculitis with purpura, hyperpigmentation. *Miscellaneous:* Jaundice, hepatitis.

**OD** **Overdose Management:** *Symptoms:* N&V, drowsiness, lethargy, epigastric pain, *anaphylaxis.* Rarely, hypertension, acute renal failure, respiratory depression. *Treatment:* Since there are no antidotes, treatment is supportive and symptomatic. If discovered within 4 hr, emesis followed by activated charcoal and an osmotic cathartic may be tried.

**Additional Drug Interactions**
*Cyclosporine* / ↑ Serum levels of cyclosporine due to ↓ renal excretion; ↑ risk of cyclosporine-induced nephrotoxicity
*Digoxin* / ↑ Serum levels of digoxin due to ↓ renal excretion
*Lithium* / ↑ Serum levels of lithium due to ↓ renal excretion

*Methotrexate* / ↑ Serum levels of methotrexate due to ↓ renal excretion

**Laboratory Test Interferences:** False + reaction for urinary bilirubin and for urinary ketones (using the dip-stick method). ↑ Liver enzymes, serum creatinine. ↑ Bleeding time.

**Dosage** —————————
• **Capsules, Tablets**
*Osteoarthritis.*
**Adults, initial:** 800–1,200 mg/day in divided doses; **then,** adjust dose within the range of 600–1,200 mg/day in divided doses (400 mg b.i.d.–t.i.d.; 300 mg b.i.d., t.i.d., or q.i.d.; 200 mg t.i.d. or q.i.d.). Total daily dose should not exceed 1,200 mg.
*Acute pain.*
**Adults:** 200–400 mg q 6–8 hr as needed, not to exceed 1,200 mg/day. For clients weighing less than 60 kg, the dose should not exceed 20 mg/kg.
*Rheumatoid arthritis.*
**Adults:** 500 mg b.i.d.

## NURSING CONSIDERATIONS

See also *Nursing Considerations* for *Nonsteroidal Anti-Inflammatory Drugs.*

**Administration/Storage:** The capsules should be protected from moisture.

**Assessment**
1. Note any previous experience with NSAIDs or acetylsalicylic acid and the results.
2. Document indications for therapy (i.e., analgesic or anti-inflammatory), include onset of symptoms and status of ROM.
3. With long-term therapy, obtain baseline CBC with bleeding parameters, liver and renal function studies, and stool for occult blood and monitor periodically.
4. Determine any history of heart disease or cardiac failure.
5. Note age and weight of client and if currently prescribed diuretics.

**Outcomes/Evaluate:** Control of pain and inflammation with improved joint mobility

# Etomidate
(eh-**TOM**-ih-dayt)
**Pregnancy Category:** C
Amidate **(Rx)**
**Classification:** General anesthetic and adjunct to general anesthesia

**Action/Kinetics:** Is a hypnotic with no analgesic activity. Appears to act like GABA and is thought to exert its mechanism by depressing the activity of the brain stem reticular system. Minimal CV and respiratory depressant effects. **Onset:** 1 min. **Duration:** 3–5 min. **t½:** 75 min. Rapidly metabolized in the liver with inactive metabolites excreted mainly through the urine.
**Uses:** Induction of general anesthesia. As a supplement to nitrous oxide during short surgical procedures. *Investigational:* Prolonged sedation of critically ill or ventilator-dependent clients (is an increased risk of acute insufficiency and mortality).
**Special Concerns:** Use with caution during lactation. Safety and efficacy have not been established in children less than 10 years of age.
**Side Effects:** *Skeletal muscle:* Myoclonic skeletal muscle movements, tonic movements. *Respiratory:* Apnea of short duration, hyperventilation or hypoventilation, ***laryngospasm.*** *CV:* Either hypertension or hypotension; tachycardia or bradycardia; arrhythmias. *GI:* Postoperative N&V. *Miscellaneous:* Eye movements, averting movements, hiccoughs, snoring.

**Dosage** —————————
• **IV Only**
    *Induction of anesthesia.*
**Adults and children over 10 years of age:** 0.2–0.6 mg/kg (usual: 0.3 mg/kg) injected over 30–60 sec.

## NURSING CONSIDERATIONS
**Administration/Storage**
1. Lower doses may be used as adjuncts to supplement less potent general anesthetics such as nitrous oxide.
2. Etomidate may be used following preanesthetic medications.
3. Protect from extreme heat and freezing.
**Interventions**
1. Nausea and vomiting likely to occur postoperatively; have equipment (suction, emesis basins, washcloths, etc.) available to manage.
2. Monitor during immediate postoperative period for hypo/hypertension, tachy/bradycardia; treat symptomatically.
**Outcomes/Evaluate:** Desired anesthetic level

# Etoposide (VP-16–213)
(eh-**TOH**-poh-syd)
**Pregnancy Category:** D
Etopophos, VePesid **(Rx)**, Etoposide Phosphate
**Classification:** Antineoplastic, miscellaneous

See also *Antineoplastic Agents.*
**Action/Kinetics:** Acts as a mitotic inhibitor at the $G_2$ portion of the cell cycle to inhibit DNA synthesis. At high doses, cells entering mitosis are lysed, whereas at low doses, cells will not enter prophase. **t½:** biphasic, initial, 1.5 hr; final, 4–11 hr. **Effective plasma levels:** 0.3–10 mcg/mL. Poor CNS penetration. Eliminated through both the urine and bile unchanged and as liver metabolites. Is water soluble.
**Uses:** With combination therapy to treat refractory testicular tumors and small cell lung cancer. *Investigational:* Alone or in combination to treat acute monocytic leukemia, non-Hodgkin's lymphoma, Hodgkin's disease, AIDS-associated Kaposi's sarcoma, Ewing's sarcoma. Also, choriocarcinoma; hepatocellular carcinoma; nonsmall cell lung, breast, endometrial, and gastric cancers; acute lymphocytic leukemia; soft tissue carcinoma; rhabdomyosarcoma.
**Contraindications:** Lactation.
**Special Concerns:** Safety and efficacy in children have not been estab-

lished. Severe myelosuppression may occur.

**Additional Side Effects:** *Anaphylactic-type reactions,* hypotension, peripheral neuropathy, somnolence.

### Dosage
- **IV**

  *Testicular carcinoma.*

  50–100 mg/m²/day on days 1–5 or 100 mg/m²/day on days 1, 3, and 5 q 3–4 weeks (i.e., after recovery from toxic effects). Used in combination with other agents.

  *Small cell lung carcinoma.*

  35 mg/m²/day for 4 days to 50 mg/m²/day for 5 days, repeated q 3–4 weeks.

- **Capsules**

  *Small cell lung carcinoma.*

  70 mg/m² (rounded to the nearest 50 mg) daily for 4 days to 100 mg/m² (rounded to the nearest 50 mg) daily for 5 days; repeat q 3–4 weeks.

  *NOTE:* Etopophos is given in higher concentrations than VePesid. Doses above are for VePesid.

## NURSING CONSIDERATIONS

See also *Nursing Considerations* for *Antineoplastic Agents.*

### Administration/Storage
1. Store capsules at 2°C–8°C (36°F–46°F); do not freeze.

**IV** 2. For IV use, dilute drug with either 5% dextrose or 0.9% NaCl for a final concentration of 0.2 or 0.4 mg/mL (5-mL vial in 250 or 500 mL of IV solution).

3. A slow IV infusion of VePesid over 30–60 min will decrease the chance of hypotension. Do not give by rapid IV push. Etoposide can be given over a period of 5 min.

4. Wear gloves when preparing this medication; if drug comes in contact with the skin or mucosa, wash the area immediately and thoroughly with soap and water.

5. Diluted solutions with a final concentration of 0.2 mg/mL are stable for 96 hr at room temperature; final concentrations of 0.4 mg/mL are stable for 48 hr at room temperature.

### Assessment
1. Assess nutritional status. Pretreat with antiemetic; drug may cause N&V.

2. Monitor CBC, liver and renal function studies; may cause granulocyte and platelet suppression. Nadir: 14 days; recovery: 21 days.

3. Determine if pregnant.

4. May cause increased uric acid levels.

5. Assess for signs of infection and bleeding; occurs more often with this drug than with most antineoplastic agents.

6. With infusions, stress bed rest and supervise ambulation as orthostatic hypotension may occur. Record BP during infusions and at least twice a day with PO therapy; note any significant decreases.

7. Be prepared to treat anaphylactic reactions.

### Client/Family Teaching
1. Report any flu-like symptoms; drug combination therapy may cause severe myelosuppression.

2. Consume 2–3 L/day of fluids to prevent kidney damage.

3. May feel fatigued and sleepy during and after drug administration; schedule activities to ensure adequate rest.

4. Report any tingling sensations or numbness—signs of peripheral neuropathy.

5. Report if N&V impair intake.

6. Practice reliable contraception.

### Outcomes/Evaluate
- ↓ Malignant cell proliferation
- Improved hematologic parameters with leukemia

**F**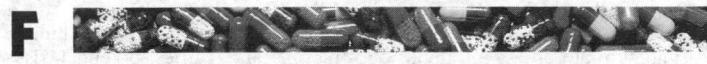

# Factor IX Complex (Human)

(**FAK**-tor 9)
**Pregnancy Category:** C
AlphaNine SD, Benefix, Konyne 80,
Hemonyne, Mononine, Profilnine SD,
Proplex T **(Rx)**
**Classification:** Hemostatic, systemic

**Action/Kinetics:** This product causes an increase in factor IX levels, thus minimizing hemorrhage in those with factor IX deficiency. Factors II, VII, and X may also be increased. **t½:** 22 hr. The mean increase in circulating factor IX after IV infusion is 0.67–1.15 IU/dL rise per IU/kg body weight.

**Uses:** To prevent or control bleeding in clients with factor IX deficiency, especially hemophilia B and Christmas disease. Factor VII deficiency (Proplex T only). Hemophilia A with inhibitors to factor VIII.

**Contraindications:** Factor VII deficiency, except for Proplex T. Use when fresh frozen plasma is effective. Liver disease with suspected intravascular coagulation or fibrinolysis. Hypersensitivity to mouse proteins.

**Special Concerns:** Assess benefit versus risk prior to use in liver disease or elective surgery.

**Side Effects:** *CV: DIC, thrombosis. High doses may cause MI, venous or pulmonary thrombosis.* Miscellaneous: Chills, fever. *Symptoms due to rapid infusion:* N&V, headache, fever, chills, tingling, flushing, urticaria, and changes in BP or pulse rate. Most of these side effects disappear when rate of administration is slowed.

The preparation also contains trace amounts of blood groups A and B and isohemagglutinins, which may cause intravascular hemolysis when administered in large amounts to clients with blood groups A, B, and AB.

Although careful screening is undertaken, both hepatitis and AIDS may be transmitted using factor IX Complex since it is derived from pooled human plasma.

**Drug Interactions:** ↑ Risk of thrombosis if administered with aminocaproic acid.

## Dosage
• **IV**
  *Factor IX deficiency.*
**Individualized,** depending on severity of bleeding, degree of deficiency, body weight, and level of factor required. Minimum factor IX level required in surgery or following trauma is 25% of normal, which is maintained for 1 week after surgery. As a guide in determining the units required to raise blood level percentages of factor IX, use the following formula for human-derived factor IX:
  1 unit/kg × body weight (kg) × desired increase (% of normal).
For recombinant factor IX, use the following formula:
  1.2 IU/kg × body weight (kg) × desired increase (% of control).
  *Factor VII deficiency (Proplex T only).*
To determine the units needed to raise blood level percentages, use the following:
  0.5 unit/kg × body weight (kg) × desired increase (% of normal).
The dose may be repeated q 4–6 hr. The package insert should be checked carefully as a guideline for doses for various factor deficiencies.
  *Factor VII deficiency (hemophilia A) — Proplex T or Konyne 80 only.*
Use dosage levels approximating 75 IU/kg.
  *Bleeding in hemophilia A with factor VIII inhibitors.*
75 IU/kg.

## NURSING CONSIDERATIONS
**Administration/Storage**
**IV** 1. The rate of administration

---

varies with the product. As a general guideline, infuse about 100–200 IU/min at a rate of 2–3 mL/min, not to exceed 3 mL/min.

2. Store at 2°C–8°C (36°F–46°F).

3. Avoid freezing diluent provided with drug.

4. Discard 2 years after date of manufacture.

5. Before reconstitution, warm diluent to room temperature but not above 40°C (104°F).

6. Agitate the solution gently until powder is dissolved.

7. Administer within 3 hr of reconstitution to avoid incubation in case contamination occurred during preparation.

8. Do not refrigerate after reconstitution; active ingredient may precipitate out.

**Assessment**

1. Document any previous experience/treatment with factor replacement and outcome.

2. Obtain weight, height, and blood type.

3. Note any S&S of liver disease (i.e., urticaria, fever, pruritus, anorexia, N&V); monitor LFTs.

4. Monitor CBC, coagulation, and factor assay levels.

**Interventions**

1. Monitor BP and pulse q 30 min during infusion.

2. Report increased bleeding and joint swelling; use rest, ice, and elevation with affected joints.

3. Reduce flow rate and report if a tingling sensation, headache, chills, or fever occur.

4. Avoid aminocaproic acid administration; may precipitate clot formation.

5. Assess for DIC if factor IX level is increased above 50% of normal. At 50% or greater, there is an increased risk for the development of a thromboembolic event and/or DIC.

6. Make sure client has received hepatitis B vaccine.

7. Monitor I&O; test urine for occult blood. Hemolytic reactions are more pronounced in clients with A, B, and AB type blood.

**Client/Family Teaching**

1. Product is prepared from human plasma and carries potential risks (i.e., hepatitis, AIDS).

2. Avoid contact sports and any activities that may lead to injury or excessive jostling.

3. Report any evidence of uncontrolled bleeding or joint swelling.

4. Ensure family members are screened and genetically counseled; disease is hereditary.

5. Avoid aspirin-containing products.

6. Identify local support groups that may assist to cope with this disease.

**Outcomes/Evaluate**

- Prevention of hemorrhage
- Factor levels within desired range

# Famciclovir

(fam-**SY**-kloh-veer)

**Pregnancy Category:** B

Famvir **(Rx)**

**Classification:** Antiviral agent

See also *Antiviral Agents.*

**Action/Kinetics:** Undergoes rapid biotransformation to the active compound penciclovir. Inhibits viral DNA synthesis and therefore replication in HSV types 1 (HSV-1) and 2 (HSV-2) and varicella-zoster virus. Penciclovir is further metabolized to inactive compounds that are excreted through the urine. **t½:** 2 hr following IV administration and 2.3 hr following PO use. Half-life increased in renal insufficiency.

**Uses:** Management of acute herpes zoster (shingles). Treatment of recurrent herpes simplex (genital herpes) and to prevent outbreaks of recurrent genital herpes.

**Contraindications:** Use during lactation.

**Special Concerns:** The dose should be adjusted in clients with creatinine clearance less than 60 mL/min. Safety and efficacy have not been determined in children less than 18 years of age.

**Side Effects:** *GI:* N&V, diarrhea, constipation, anorexia, abdominal pain, dyspepsia, flatulence. *CNS:*

Headache, dizziness, paresthesia, somnolence, insomnia. *Body as a whole:* Fatigue, fever, pain, rigors. *Musculoskeletal:* Back pain, arthralgia. *Respiratory:* Pharyngitis, sinusitis, upper respiratory infection. *Dermatologic:* Pruritus; signs, symptoms, and complications of zoster and genital herpes.

**Drug Interactions**
*Digoxin* / ↑ Levels of digoxin
*Probenecid* / Probenecid ↑ plasma levels of penciclovir
*Theophylline* / ↑ Levels of penciclovir

**Dosage**
- **Tablets**
  *Herpes zoster infections.*

500 mg q 8 hr for 7 days. Dosage reduction is recommended in clients with impaired renal function: for $C_{CR}$ of 40–59 mL/min, the dose should be 500 mg q 12 hr; for $C_{CR}$ of 20–39 mL/min, the dose should be 500 mg q 24 hr; for $C_{CR}$ less than 20 mL/min, the dose should be 250 mg q 48 hr. For hemodialysis clients, the recommended dose is 250 mg given after each dialysis treatment.
  *Recurrent genital herpes.*

125 mg b.i.d. for 5 days. Should be taken within 6 hr of symptoms or lesion onset. Dosage reduction is as follows for those with impaired renal function: for $C_{CR}$ of 40 mL/min or greater, use the recommended dose of 125 mg b.i.d.; for $C_{CR}$ of 20–39 mL/min, the dose should be 125 mg q 24 hr; for $C_{CR}$ less than 20 mL/min, the dose should be 125 mg q 48 hr. For hemodialysis clients, the recommended dose is 125 mg given after each dialysis treatment.
  *Prevent outbreaks of genital herpes.*

250 mg b.i.d.

## NURSING CONSIDERATIONS

See also *Nursing Considerations* for *Antiviral Agents.*

**Administration/Storage**
1. Initiate therapy as soon as herpes zoster is diagnosed and at the first symptoms of genital herpes.
2. Therapy is most useful if started within the first 48 hr of appearance of rash.
3. Effect greatest in those over 50 years of age.
4. May be taken without regard for meals.

**Assessment**
1. Document onset of symptoms, location, extent of lesions; note duration and frequency of recurrence.
2. Initiate as soon as diagnosis is confirmed.
3. Monitor CBC and renal function studies. Anticipate reduced dosage with renal dysfunction; follow dosing guidelines.

**Client/Family Teaching**
1. Review frequency, amount of drug to consume, and duration of therapy.
2. Side effects frequently associated with therapy include diarrhea, nausea, headaches, and fatigue; report if intolerable.
3. When lesions are open and draining, carrier is extremely contagious and should avoid any exposure or outside contact unless confirmed that the person(s) have had the chickenpox and are not pregnant.

**Outcomes/Evaluate**
- Resolution of herpetic lesions
- ↓ Duration of neuralgia

# Famotidine
(fah-**MOH**-tih-deen)
**Pregnancy Category:** B
Apo-Famotidine ✦, Gen-Famotidine ✦, Novo-Famotidine ✦, Nu-Famotidine ✦, Pepcid, Pepcid AC Acid Controller, Pepcid IV **(Rx)** (Pepcid AC is OTC)
**Classification:** Histamine $H_2$ receptor antagonist

See also *Histamine $H_2$ Antagonists.*
**Action/Kinetics:** Competitive inhibitor of histamine $H_2$ receptors leading to inhibition of gastric acid secretion. Both basal and nocturnal gastric acid secretion and secretion

stimulated by food or pentagastrin are inhibited. **Peak plasma levels:** 1–3 hr. **t½:** 2.5–3.5 hr. **Onset:** 1 hr. **Duration:** 10–12 hr. Does not inhibit the cytochrome P-450 system in the liver; thus, drug interactions due to inhibition of liver metabolism are not expected to occur. From 25% to 30% of a PO dose is eliminated through the kidney unchanged; from 65% to 70% of an IV dose is excreted through the kidney unchanged.

**Uses: Rx:** Treatment of active duodenal ulcers. Maintenance therapy for duodenal ulcer, at reduced dosage, after active ulcer has healed. Pathologic hypersecretory conditions such as Zollinger-Ellison syndrome or multiple endocrine adenomas. GERD, including erosive esophagitis. Treatment of benign gastric ulcer. *Investigational:* Prevent aspiration pneumonitis, for prophylaxis of stress ulcers, prevent acute upper GI bleeding, as part of multidrug therapy to eradicate *Helicobacter pylori.*

**OTC:** Relief of and prevention of the symptoms of heartburn, acid indigestion, and sour stomach.

**Contraindications:** Cirrhosis of the liver, impaired renal or hepatic function, lactation.

**Special Concerns:** Safety and efficacy in children have not been established.

**Side Effects:** *GI:* Constipation, diarrhea, N&V, anorexia, dry mouth, abdominal discomfort. *CNS:* Dizziness, headache, paresthesias, depression, anxiety, confusion, hallucinations, insomnia, fatigue, sleepiness, agitation, **grand mal seizure,** psychic disturbances. *Skin:* Rash, acne, pruritus, alopecia, urticaria, dry skin, flushing. *CV:* Palpitations. *Musculoskeletal:* Arthralgia, asthenia, musculoskeletal pain. *Hematologic:* Thrombocytopenia. *Other:* Fever, orbital edema, conjunctival injection, bronchospasm, tinnitus, taste disorders, decreased libido, impotence, pain at injection site (transient).

**Drug Interactions**
*Antacids* / ↓ Absorption of famotidine from the GI tract
*Diazepam* / ↓ Absorption of diazepam from the GI tract

**Dosage**
• **Oral Suspension, Tablets**
*Duodenal ulcer, acute therapy.*
**Adults:** 40 mg once daily at bedtime or 20 mg b.i.d. Most ulcers heal within 4 weeks and it is rarely necessary to use the full dosage for 6–8 weeks.
*Duodenal ulcer, maintenance therapy.*
**Adults:** 20 mg once daily at bedtime.
*Benign gastric ulcers, acute therapy.*
**Adults:** 40 mg at bedtime.
*Hypersecretory conditions.*
**Adults, individualized, initial:** 20 mg q 6 hr; **then,** adjust dose to response, although doses of up to 160 mg q 6 hr may be required for severe cases.
*Gastroesophageal reflux disease.*
**Adults:** 20 mg b.i.d. for 6 weeks. For esophagitis with erosions and ulcerations, give 20 or 40 mg b.i.d. for up to 12 weeks.
*Prophylaxis of upper GI bleeding.*
**Adults:** 20 mg b.i.d.
*Prophylaxis of stress ulcers.*
**Adults:** 40 mg/day.
*Relief of and prevention of heartburn, acid indigestion, and sour stomach (OTC).*
**Adults and children over 12 years of age, for relief:** 10 mg (1 tablet) with water. **For prevention:** 10 mg 1 hr before eating a meal that may cause symptoms. **Maximum dose:** 20 mg/24 hr. Not to be used continuously for more than 2 weeks unless medically prescribed.
• **IM, IV, IV Infusion**
*Hospitalized clients with hypersecretory conditions, duodenal ulcers, gastric ulcers; clients unable to take PO medication.*
**Adults:** 20 mg IV q 12 hr.
*Before anesthesia to prevent aspiration of gastric acid.*
**Adults:** 40 mg IM or PO.

## NURSING CONSIDERATIONS

See also *Nursing Considerations* for *Histamine H₂ Antagonists*.

**Administration/Storage**

1. Use antacids concomitantly if needed.

2. If $C_{CR}$ is less than 10 mL/min, can reduce the dose to 20 mg at bedtime or increase the interval between doses to 36–48 hr.

**IV** 3. For IV injection, dilute 2 mL (containing 10 mg/mL) with 0.9% NaCl injection to a total volume of 5–10 mL; give over at least a 2-min period.

4. For IV infusion, dilute 2 mL (20 mg) with 100 mL of 5% dextrose and infuse over 15–30 min.

5. A solution is stable for 48 hr at room temperature when added to or diluted with water for injection, 0.9% NaCl injection, 5% or 10% dextrose injection, RL injection, or 5% sodium bicarbonate injection.

6. Stable when mixed with various TPN solutions. Length of stability depends on the solution.

**Assessment**

1. Document reasons for therapy, type, onset, and duration of symptoms.

2. Note location, extent, and characteristics of abdominal pain.

3. Review upper GI findings; note modifications trialed with GERD.

4. Assess mental status.

5. Check for occult blood in stools and gastric secretions; note presence of *H. pylori* antibodies.

6. Assess for history of seizures.

7. If pregnant, list benefits versus risks.

8. Note hepatic or renal dysfunction; review CBC and assess for bleeding.

**Client/Family Teaching**

1. Drug may cause dizziness, headaches, and anxiety; use caution and report if symptoms persist.

2. Increasing lack of concern for personal appearance, depression, or sleeplessness warrants medical assessment.

3. Report any diarrhea, constipation, loss of appetite, easy bruising,or fatigue.

4. Avoid alcohol, aspirin-containing products, OTC cough and cold products, smoking, and foods that increase GI irritation (i.e., caffeine, black pepper, harsh spices).

5. Report a reduction in urinary output; may need a change in dosage.

**Outcomes/Evaluate**

- ↓ Abdominal pain
- Prophylaxis of stress ulcers
- Control of hypersecretion of acid
- Duodenal ulcer healing
- Control of symptoms of GERD

**F**

# Felbamate

(**FELL**-bah-mayt)

**Pregnancy Category:** C

Felbatol **(Rx)**

**Classification:** Anticonvulsant, miscellaneous (second-line therapy)

See also *Anticonvulsants*.

*NOTE:* In August 1994 it was recommended that felbamate treatment be discontinued for epilepsy clients due to several cases of aplastic anemia. Revised labeling states, "...Felbatol should only be used in patients whose epilepsy is so severe that the risk of aplastic anemia is deemed acceptable in light of the benefits conferred by its use..."

**Action/Kinetics:** Mechanism not known. Felbamate may reduce seizure spread and increase seizure threshold. Has weak inhibitory effects on both GABA and benzodiazepine receptor binding. Well absorbed after PO use. **Terminal t½:** 20–23 hr. Trough blood levels are dose dependent. From 40% to 50% excreted unchanged in the urine.

**Uses:** Alone or as part of adjunctive therapy for the treatment of partial seizures with and without generalization in adults with epilepsy. As an adjunct in the treatment of partial and generalized seizures associated with Lennox-Gastaut syndrome in children. The drug should be used only as second-line therapy.

**Contraindications:** Preexisting liver pathology.

**Special Concerns:** Use with caution in clients who are hypersensitive to carbamates. Aplastic anemia and acute liver failure have been observed in a few clients. Use with caution during lactation. Safety and efficacy have not been established in children other than those with Lennox-Gastaut syndrome.

**Side Effects:** May differ depending on whether the drug is used as monotherapy or adjunctive therapy in adults or for Lennox-Gastaut syndrome in children. *CNS:* Insomnia, headache, anxiety, somnolence, dizziness, nervousness, tremor, abnormal gait, depression, paresthesia, ataxia, stupor, abnormal thinking, emotional lability, agitation, psychologic disturbance, aggressive reaction, hallucinations, euphoria, *suicide attempt,* migraine. *GI:* Dyspepsia, vomiting, constipation, diarrhea, dry mouth, nausea, anorexia, abdominal pain, hiccoughs, esophagitis, increased appetite. *Respiratory:* Upper respiratory tract infection, rhinitis, sinusitis, pharyngitis, coughing. *CV:* Palpitation, tachycardia, SVT. *Body as a whole:* Fatigue, weight decrease or increase, facial edema, fever, chest pain, pain, asthenia, malaise, flu-like symptoms, *anaphylaxis. Ophthalmologic:* Miosis, diplopia, abnormal vision. *GU:* Urinary incontinence, intramenstrual bleeding, UTI. *Hematologic: Aplastic anemia,* purpura, leukopenia, lymphadenopathy, leukopenia, leukocytosis, thrombocytopenia, granulocytopenia, positive antinuclear factor test, *agranulocytosis,* qualitative platelet disorder. *Dermatologic:* Pruritus, urticaria, bullous eruption, buccal mucous membrane swelling, *Stevens-Johnson syndrome. Miscellaneous:* Otitis media, *acute liver failure,* taste perversion, hypophosphatemia, myalgia, photosensitivity, substernal chest pain, dystonia, allergic reaction.

**Drug Interactions**
*Carbamazepine* / Felbamate ↓ steady-state carbamazepine levels

and ↑ steady-state carbamazepine epoxide (metabolite) levels. Also, carbamazepine → 50% ↑ in felbamate clearance
*Phenytoin* / Felbamate ↑ steady-state phenytoin levels necessitating a 40% decrease in phenytoin dose. Also, phenytoin ↑ felbamate clearance
*Valproic acid* / Felbamate ↑ steady-state valproic acid levels

**Laboratory Test Interferences:** ↑ ALT, AST, gamma-glutamyl transpeptidase, LDH, alkaline phosphatase, CPK. Hypophosphatemia, hypokalemia, hyponatremia.

**Dosage** ——————
- **Suspension, Tablets**
  *Monotherapy, initial therapy.*
  **Adults over 14 years of age, initial:** 1,200 mg/day in divided doses t.i.d.–q.i.d. The dose may be increased in 600-mg increments q 2 weeks to 2,400 mg/day based on clinical response and thereafter to 3,600 mg/day, if needed.
  *Conversion to monotherapy.*
  **Adults:** Initiate at 1,200 mg/day in divided doses t.i.d.–q.i.d. Reduce the dose of concomitant antiepileptic drugs by ⅓ at initiation of felbamate therapy. At week 2, the felbamate dose should be increased to 2,400 mg/day while reducing the dose of other antiepileptic drugs up to another ⅓ of the original dose. At week 3, increase the felbamate dose to 3,600 mg/day and continue to decrease the dose of other antiepileptic drugs as indicated by response.
  *Adjunctive therapy.*
  **Adults:** Add felbamate at a dose of 1,200 mg/day in divided doses t.i.d.–q.i.d. while reducing current antiepileptic drugs by 20%. Further decreases of concomitant antiepileptic drugs may be needed to minimize side effects due to drug interactions. The dose of felbamate can be increased by 1,200-mg/day increments at weekly intervals to 3,600 mg/day.
  *Lennox-Gastaut syndrome in children, aged 2–14 years.*

As an adjunct, add felbamate at a dose of 15 mg/kg/day in divided doses t.i.d.–q.i.d. while decreasing present antiepileptic drugs by 20%. Further decreases in antiepileptic drug dosage may be needed to minimize side effects due to drug interactions. The dose of felbamate may be increased by 15-mg/kg/day increments at weekly intervals to 45 mg/kg/day.

## NURSING CONSIDERATIONS

See also *Nursing Considerations* for *Anticonvulsants*.

**Administration/Storage**
1. Shake suspension well before using.
2. Store in a tightly closed container at room temperature away from heat, direct sunlight, or moisture and away from children.
3. Most side effects seen during adjunctive therapy are resolved as the dose of concomitant antiepileptic drugs is decreased.

**Assessment**
1. Document type, location, duration, and characteristics of seizures.
2. Determine if monotherapy or adjunctive therapy is needed.
3. List drugs prescribed to ensure none interact unfavorably and to determine need for dosage adjustments.
4. Inform of potentially lethal side effects R/T aplastic anemia with this therapy.
5. Monitor CBC, liver and renal function studies.

**Client/Family Teaching**
1. Take only as prescribed; store appropriately to prevent loss of effectiveness.
2. Avoid activities that require mental alertness until drug effects realized.
3. Side effects include anorexia, vomiting, insomnia, nausea, and headaches; report if persistent or bothersome.
4. Report any changes in mental status or loss of seizure control; dosage is determined by clinical response.

5. Do not stop taking due to possibility of increasing seizure frequency.
6. Seizure control benefit should far outweigh the potential for development of aplastic anemia; assess risk.
**Outcomes/Evaluate:** Control of seizures

# Felodipine
(feh-**LOHD**-ih-peen)
**Pregnancy Category:** C
Plendil, Renedil ✜ **(Rx)**
**Classification:** Calcium channel blocking agent

See also *Calcium Channel Blocking Agents*.
**Action/Kinetics: Onset after PO:** 120–300 min. **Peak plasma levels:** 2.5–5 hr. Over 99% bound to plasma protein. **t½, elimination:** 11–16 hr. Metabolized in the liver.
**Uses:** Treatment of mild to moderate hypertension, alone or with other antihypertensives.
**Contraindications:** Use during lactation.
**Special Concerns:** Use with caution in clients with CHF or compromised ventricular function, especially in combination with a beta-adrenergic blocking agent. Use with caution in impaired hepatic function or reduced hepatic blood flow. Felodipine may cause a greater hypotensive effect in geriatric clients. Safety and effectiveness have not been determined in children.
**Side Effects:** *CV:* Significant hypotension, syncope, angina pectoris, peripheral edema, palpitations, AV block, *MI, arrhythmias,* tachycardia. *CNS:* Dizziness, lightheadedness, headache, nervousness, sleepiness, irritability, anxiety, insomnia, paresthesia, depression, amnesia, paranoia, psychosis, hallucinations. *Body as a whole:* Asthenia, flushing, muscle cramps, pain, inflammation, warm feeling, influenza. *GI:* Nausea, abdominal discomfort, cramps, dyspepsia, diarrhea, constipation, vomiting, dry mouth, flatulence. *Dermatologic:* Rash, dermatitis, urticaria,

pruritus. *Respiratory:* Rhinitis, rhinorrhea, pharyngitis, sinusitis, nasal and chest congestion, SOB, wheezing, dyspnea, cough, bronchitis, sneezing, respiratory infection. *Miscellaneous:* Anemia, gingival hyperplasia, sexual difficulties, epistaxis, back pain, facial edema, erythema, urinary frequency or urgency, dysuria.

**Additional Drug Interactions**
*Cimetidine* / ↑ Bioavailability of felodipine
*Digoxin* / ↑ Peak plasma levels of digoxin
*Fentanyl* / Possible severe hypotension or ↑ fluid volume
*Ranitidine* / ↑ Bioavailability of felodipine

**Dosage**
• **Tablets, Extended Release**
*Hypertension.*
**Initial:** 5 mg once daily (2.5 mg in clients over 65 years of age and in those with impaired liver function); **then:** adjust dose according to response, usually at 2-week intervals with the usual dosage range being 2.5–10 mg once daily. Doses greater than 10 mg increase the rate of peripheral edema and other vasodilatory side effects.

## NURSING CONSIDERATIONS

See also *Nursing Considerations* for *Calcium Channel Blocking Agents.*
**Administration/Storage:** Bioavailability is not affected by food. It is increased more than twofold when taken with doubly concentrated grapefruit juice when compared with water or orange juice.
**Assessment**
1. Document onset of symptoms, other agents used, and outcome.
2. Note history of heart failure or compromised ventricular function.
3. List drugs currently prescribed; note any potential interactions.
4. During dosage adjustments, monitor BP closely in clients over 65 or with impaired hepatic function.
**Client/Family Teaching**
1. Swallow tablets whole; do not chew or crush.
2. Do not stop abruptly; abrupt

withdrawal may cause an increased frequency and duration of chest pain.
3. Avoid activities that require mental alertness until drug effects are realized.
4. Rise slowly from a lying position and dangle feet before standing to minimize postural effects.
5. Practice frequent careful oral hygiene to minimize the incidence and severity of drug-induced gingival hyperplasia.
**Outcomes/Evaluate:** Control of hypertension

# Fenoldopam mesylate
(feh-**NOL**-doh-pam)
**Pregnancy Category:** B
Corlopam **(Rx)**
**Classification:** Drug for hypertensive emergency

**Action/Kinetics:** Rapid-acting vasodilator that is an agonist for $D_1$-like dopamine receptors and $\alpha_2$-adrenoreceptors. Causes vasodilation in coronary, renal, mesenteric, and peripheral arteries; vascular beds do not respond uniformly. **$t\frac{1}{2}$, elimination:** About 5 min in mild to moderate hypertensives. **Steady-state levels:** About 20 min. Metabolized in liver and most is excreted in urine.
**Uses:** Hypertensive emergencies.
**Contraindications:** Use with beta-blockers or in those with sulfite sensitivity.
**Special Concerns:** Use with caution during lactation and in those with glaucoma or intraocular hypertension. Safety and efficacy have not been determined in children.
**Side Effects:** *CV:* Tachycardia, hypotension, flushing, ST-T abnormalities, postural hypotension, extrasystoles, palpitations, bradycardia, **heart failure, ischemic heart disease, MI,** angina pectoris. *Body as a whole:* Headache, sweating, back pain, non-specific chest pain, pyrexia, limb cramp. *CNS:* Nervousness, anxiety, insomnia, dizziness. *GI:* N&V, abdominal pain or fullness, constipation, diarrhea. *Respiratory:* Nasal

congestion, dyspnea, upper respiratory disorder. *Hematologic:* Leukocytosis, bleeding. *Miscellaneous:* Reaction at injection site, urinary tract infection, oliguria.

**Laboratory Test Alteration:** ↑ Creatinine, BUN, serum glucose, transaminase, LDH. Hypokalemia.

**Dosage** ——————————

• **Constant IV infusion**
*Hypertensive emergency.*
Rate of infusion is individualized according to body weight and to desired speed and extent of effect. See package insert for table of infusion rates. Doses range from 0.025 mcg/kg/min–0.3 mcg/kg/min for a body weight of 40 kg to 0.094 mcg/kg/min–1.13mcg/kg/min for a body weight of 150 kg.

## NURSING CONSIDERATIONS
### Administration/Storage
**IV** 1. Do not use a bolus dose.
2. Most of the effect of a given infusion is reached in 15 min.
3. Initial dose is titrated up or down no more often than every 15 min, and less frequently as desired BP is approached. Recommended increments for titration are 0.05–0.1 mcg/kg/min.
4. Initial doses of 0.03–0.1 mcg/kg/min have been associated with less reflex tachycardia than higher doses (greater than 0.3 mcg/kg/min).
5. Administer using a calibrated mechanical infusion pump that can deliver desired infusion rate accurately and reliably.
6. Infusion may be discontinued abruptly or tapered gradually prior to discontinuation.
7. Transition to PO therapy can be started any time after BP is stablized during fenoldopam infusion.
8. Dilute ampule concentrate in 0.9% NaCl injection or 5% dextrose injection for a final concentration of 40 mcg/mL (i.e., add 4 mL of the concentrate to 1,000 mL; 2 mL of the concentrate to 500 mL; or, 1 mL of the concentrate to 250 mL). Each mL of concentrate contains 10 mg of drug. Each ampule is for single use only.
9. Store ampules at 2°C–30°C 36°F–86°F).
10. The diluted solution is stable under normal light and temperature for 24 hr or less. Discard any diluted solution that is not used within 24 hr of preparation.

**Assessment**
1. Document clinical presentation, onset, and duration of symptoms.
2. Note any glaucoma, sulfite sensitivity, or I.O. (intraocular) hypertension.
3. Monitor VS, ECG, liver and renal function studies. Obtain weight.
4. List drugs prescribed to ensure none interact unfavorably; avoid use with beta–blockers.
5. Assess for physical conditions that may have precipitated event; evaluate life-style changes needed.

**Outcomes/Evaluate:** Significant reduction in BP during hypertensive crisis

# Fenoprofen calcium
(fen-oh-**PROH**-fen)
**Pregnancy Category:** B
Fenopron, Nalfon **(Rx)**
**Classification:** Nonsteroidal antiinflammatory analgesic

See also *Nonsteroidal Anti-Inflammatory Drugs.*

**Action/Kinetics: Peak serum levels:** 1–2 hr. **Peak effect:** 2–3 hr. **Duration:** 4–6 hr. **t½:** 2–3 hr. **antiarthritic:** Within 2 days; **maximum effect:** 2–3 weeks. Ninety-nine percent protein bound. Food (but not antacids) delays absorption and decreases the total amount absorbed.

**Uses:** Rheumatoid arthritis, osteoarthritis, mild to moderate pain. *Investigational:* Juvenile rheumatoid arthritis, prophylaxis of migraine, migraine due to menses, sunburn.

**Contraindications:** Use in pregnancy and children less than 12 years of age.

**Additional Contraindications:** Renal dysfunction.

**Special Concerns:** Safety and efficacy in children have not been established.

**Additional Side Effects:** *GU:* Dysuria, hematuria, cystitis, interstitial nephritis, nephrotic syndrome. Overdosage has caused tachycardia and hypotension.

## Dosage

- **Capsules, Tablets**
  *Rheumatoid and osteoarthritis.*
  **Adults:** 300–600 mg t.i.d.–q.i.d. Adjust dose according to response of client.
  *Mild to moderate pain.*
  **Adults:** 200 mg q 4–6 hr. Maximum daily dose for all uses: 3,200 mg.

## NURSING CONSIDERATIONS

See also *Nursing Considerations* for *Nonsteroidal Anti-Inflammatory Drugs.*

**Administration/Storage:** Those over 70 years of age generally require half the usual adult dose.

**Assessment**

1. Document indications for therapy, type, onset, and duration of symptoms.
2. Perform periodic ophthalmic and auditory tests with chronic therapy.
3. Monitor CBC, PT/PTT, liver and renal function during chronic therapy.

**Client/Family Teaching**

1. Take 30 min before or 2 hr after meals; food decreases absorption.
2. With swallowing difficulty, the tablets can be crushed and the contents mixed with applesauce or other similar foods.
3. Avoid aspirin and OTC agents.
4. If vomiting or diarrhea occurs, monitor appetite, and weight; report if persistent.
5. Report any unusual bruising or bleeding, oozing of blood from the gums, nosebleeds, sore throat, or fever.
6. Report increased headaches, sleepiness, dizziness, nervousness, weakness, or fatigue.
7. Report evidence of liver toxicity, such as jaundice, right upper quadrant abdominal pain, or a change in the color and consistency of stools.

**Outcomes/Evaluate:** ↓ Joint pain and inflammation with ↑ mobility

# Fentanyl citrate
(**FEN**-tah-nil)
**Pregnancy Category:** C
Actiq, Fentanyl Oralet, Sublimaze **(C-II) (Rx)**
**Classification:** Narcotic analgesic, morphine type

See also *Narcotic Analgesics.*

**Action/Kinetics:** Similar to those of morphine and meperidine. **IV. Onset:** 7–8 min. **Peak effect:** Approximately 30 min. **Duration:** 1–2 hr, **t½:** 1.5–6 hr. When the oral lozenge (transmucosal administration) is sucked, fentanyl citrate is absorbed through the mucosal tissues of the mouth and GI tract. **Peak effect, transmucosal:** 20–30 min. Actiq resembles a lollipop; sucking provides a rapid onset of action. Faster-acting and shorter duration than morphine or meperidine.

**Uses: Parenteral:** Preanesthetic medication, induction, and maintenance of anesthesia of short duration and immediate postoperative period. Supplement in general or regional anesthesia. Combined with droperidol for preanesthetic medication, induction of anesthesia, or as adjunct in maintenance of general or regional anesthesia. Combined with oxygen for anesthesia in high-risk clients undergoing open heart surgery, orthopedic procedures, or complicated neurologic procedures.

**Oral (transmucosal):** Anesthetic premedication in children and adults in an operating room setting. To induce conscious sedation before diagnostic or medical procedures (use only in closely monitored situations due to the risk of hypoventilation). Actiq is used for severe pain associated with cancer treatment in those already using an opiate but experience breakthrough pain.

**Contraindications:** The transmucosal form is contraindicated in children who weigh less than 15 kg, for the treatment of acute or chronic pain (safety for this use not established), and for doses in excess of 15 mcg/kg in children and in excess of 5 mcg/kg (maximum of 400 mcg) in adults. Use outside the hospital setting is contraindicated. Myasthenia gravis and other conditions in which muscle relaxants should not be used. Clients particularly sensitive to respiratory depression. Use during labor.

**Special Concerns:** Safety and effectiveness have not been determined in children less than 2 years of age. Use with caution and at reduced dosage in poor-risk clients, children, the elderly, and when other CNS depressants are used. Use of the transmucosal form carries a risk of hypoventilation that may result in death.

**Additional Side Effects:** Skeletal and thoracic muscle rigidity, especially after rapid IV administration. Bradycardia, *seizures,* diaphoresis.

**Additional Drug Interactions:** ↑ Risk of CV depression when high doses of fentanyl are combined with nitrous oxide or diazepam.

**Dosage** ⎯⎯⎯⎯⎯⎯⎯⎯⎯⎯

• **IM, IV**

*Preoperatively.*
**Adults:** 0.05–0.1 mg IM 30–60 min before surgery.

*Adjunct to anesthesia, induction.*
**Adults:** 0.002–0.05 mg/kg IV, depending on length and depth of anesthesia desired; **maintenance:** 0.025–0.1 mg/kg when indicated.

*Adjunct to regional anesthesia.*
**Adults:** 0.05–0.1 mg IM or IV over 1–2 min when indicated.

*Postoperatively.*
**Adults:** 0.05–0.1 mg IM q 1–2 hr for control of pain.

*As general anesthetic with oxygen and a muscle relaxant.*
0.05–0.1 mg/kg (up to 0.15 mg/kg may be required).

*Children, induction and maintenance of anesthesia.*
**Pediatric, 2–12 years:** 2–3 mcg/kg.

*Children, general anesthetic.*
0.05–0.1 mg/kg with oxygen and a muscle relaxant when attenuation of the responses to surgical stress is important (e.g., open heart surgery).

• **Transmucosal (Oral Lozenge)**
Individualize according to weight, age, physical status, general condition and medical status, underlying pathology, use of other drugs, type of anesthetic to be used, and the type and length of the surgical procedure. Doses of 5 mcg/kg are equivalent to IM fentanyl, 0.75–1.25 mcg/kg. Clients receiving more than 5 mcg/kg should be under the direct observation of medical personnel. Children may require up to 15 mcg/kg, provided their body weight is not less than 10 kg. Clients over 65 years of age should receive a dose from 2.5 to 5 mcg/kg. The maximum dose for adults and children, regardless of weight, is 400 mcg.

## NURSING CONSIDERATIONS

See also *Nursing Considerations* for *Narcotic Analgesics.*

**Administration/Storage**

1. Protect drug from light. Protect transmucosal product from freezing and moisture; store below 30°C (86°F).

2. Oral form is supplied as a raspberry-flavored lozenge mounted on a handle and comes in strengths of 200, 300, and 400 mcg.

3. The foil overwrap of the oral form is to be removed just prior to administration. After removing the plastic overcap, instruct client to place the transmucosal unit in the mouth and to suck (not chew) it. After consumed or client shows signs of respiratory depression, the unit is removed from the mouth by the handle. If any of the medication remains, separate the matrix from the handle using a twisting motion. The drug matrix is then flushed down the toilet. If any drug matrix remains on the handle, it may be removed by running the handle under warm water. The drug-free handle should be

disposed of according to institutional protocol. During the disposal process, the drug matrix should not come in contact with the skin, eyes, or mucous membranes. Hands should be washed thoroughly when finished.

4. Give the transmucosal product 20–40 min prior to time for the desired effect.

5. Consider lower doses of the transmucosal form with head injury, CV or pulmonary disease, liver dysfunction, or hepatic disease.

6. When using the transmucosal form, client must be attended to at all times by an individual skilled in airway management and resuscitative techniques. Have naloxone available in the event of an overdose.

**IV** 7. Direct IV infusions may be given, undiluted, over a period of 2–3 min.

**Assessment**

1. Document indications for therapy, anticipated time frame, and any previous use.

2. Note any neurovascular or pulmonary disease.

**Client/Family Teaching**

1. Rise slowly; may experience orthostatic hypotension. Drug causes dizziness and drowsiness.

2. Avoid alcohol and any other CNS depressant for at least 24 hr.

3. Reinforce that transmucosal agent is not candy with children; it is a very potent medication.

4. Recall or memory may be suppressed so may not fully recall events surrounding procedure. Assure that procedure was done, answer any questions; this is normal with this medication.

**Outcomes/Evaluate**

• Desired analgesia/relaxation
• Conscious sedation

# Fentanyl Transdermal System

(FEN-tah-nil)
**Pregnancy Category:** C
Duragesic-25, -50, -75, and -100 **(C-II) (Rx)**

**Classification:** Narcotic analgesic, morphine type

See also *Narcotic Analgesics* and *Fentanyl citrate.*

**Action/Kinetics:** The system provides continuous delivery of fentanyl for up to 72 hr. The amount of fentanyl released from each system each hour depends on the surface area (25 mcg/hr is released from each 10 cm²). Each system also contains 0.1 mL of alcohol/10 cm²; the alcohol enhances the rate of drug flux through the copolymer membrane and also increases the permeability of the skin to fentanyl. Following application of the system, the skin under the system absorbs fentanyl, resulting in a depot of the drug in the upper skin layers, which is then available to the general circulation. After the system is removed, the residual drug in the skin continues to be absorbed so that serum levels fall 50% in about 17 hr. Metabolized in the liver and excreted mainly in the urine.

**Uses:** Restrict use for the management of severe chronic pain that cannot be managed with less powerful drugs. Only use on clients already on and tolerant to narcotic analgesics and who require continuous narcotic administration.

**Contraindications:** Use for acute or postoperative pain (including out-patient surgeries). To manage mild or intermittent pain that can be managed by acetaminophen-opioid combinations, NSAIDs, or short-acting opioids. Hypersensitivity to fentanyl or adhesives. ICP, impaired consciousness, coma, medical conditions causing hypoventilation. Use during labor and delivery. Use of initial doses exceeding 25 mcg/hr, use in children less than 12 years of age and clients under 18 years of age who weigh less than 50 kg. Lactation.

**Special Concerns:** Use with caution in clients with brain tumors and bradyarrhythmias, as well as in elderly, cachectic, or debilitated individuals. Safety and efficacy have not been determined in children.

**Additional Side Effects:** Sustained hypoventilation.

Dosage
───────────────
- **Transdermal System**
  *Analgesia.*

**Adults, usual initial:** 25 mcg/hr unless the client is tolerant to opioids (Duragesic-50, -75, and -100 are intended for use only in clients tolerant to opioids). Initial dose should be based on (1) the daily dose, potency, and characteristics (i.e., pure agonist, mixed agonist/antagonist) of the drug the client has been taking; (2) the reliability of the relative potency estimates used to calculate the dose as estimates vary depending on the route of administration; (3) the degree, if any, of tolerance to narcotics; and (4) the general condition and status of the client.

To convert clients from PO or parenteral opioids to the transdermal system, the following method should be used: (1) the previous 24-hr analgesic requirement should be calculated; (2) convert this amount to the equianalgesic PO morphine dose; (3) find the calculated 24-hr morphine dose and the corresponding transdermal fentanyl dose using the table provided with the product; and (4) initiate treatment using the recommended fentanyl dose. The dose may be increased no more frequently than 3 days after the initial dose or q 6 days thereafter. The ratio of 90 mg/24 hr of PO morphine to 25 mcg/hr increase in transdermal fentanyl dose should be used to base appropriate dosage increments on the daily dose of supplementary opioids.

If the dose of the fentanyl transdermal system exceeds 300 mcg/hr, it may be necessary to change clients to another narcotic analgesic. In such cases, the transdermal system should be removed and treatment initiated with one-half the equianalgesic dose of the new opioid 12–18 hr later.

The dose of the new analgesic should be titrated based on the level of pain reported by the client.

## NURSING CONSIDERATIONS

See also *Nursing Considerations* for *Narcotic Analgesics* and *Fentanyl citrate.*

**Administration/Storage**
1. Multiple systems may be used if the delivery rate needs to exceed 100 mcg/hr.
2. Do not undertake initial evaluation of the maximum analgesic effect until 24 hr after the system is applied.
3. If required, a short-acting analgesic may be used for the first 24 hr (i.e., until analgesic efficacy is reached with the transdermal system).
4. Clients may continue to require periodic supplemental doses of a short-acting analgesic to treat breakthrough pain.
5. If opioid therapy is to be discontinued, a gradual decrease in dose is recommended to minimize S&S of abrupt narcotic withdrawal.

**Assessment**
1. Document indications for therapy, previous agents used, and outcome.
2. Rate pain level at various times throughout the day to ensure adequate dosing. Determine that dose required is based on conversion guidelines provided by manufacturer.
3. Note increased ICP or brain tumors.

**Client/Family Teaching**
1. Apply the system to a nonirritated and nonirradiated fatty, flat surface of the skin, preferably on the upper torso. If needed, clip hair (not shaved) from the site prior to application.
2. Use only clear water, if needed, to cleanse the site prior to application. Do not use soaps, oils, lotions, alcohol, or other agents that might irritate the skin. Allow the skin to dry completely prior to applying the system.

If liquid comes in contact with the skin, use clear water only to remove.
3. Remove the system from the sealed package and apply immediately by pressing firmly in place (for 10–20 sec) with the palm of the hand. *Never cut or open the system.* Ensure complete contact of the system, especially around the edges. Date and time patches and tape securely to avoid any confusion or dislodgement.
4. Keep each system in place for 72 hr; if additional analgesia is required, a new system can be applied to a different skin site after removal of the previous system.
5. Fold systems removed from a skin site so that the adhesive side adheres to itself; flush down the toilet immediately after removal. Keep systems out of the reach of children.
6. Dispose of any unused systems as soon as they are no longer needed by removing them from their package and flushing down the toilet. Follow appropriate institutional guidelines for disposing of controlled substances during hospitalization.
7. Note time and frequency of short-acting analgesic use for breakthrough pain. Report if use exceeds expected needs; transdermal dosage may require adjustment.
8. Use only as prescribed; do not stop suddenly.
**Outcomes/Evaluate:** Adequate pain control

# Ferrous fumarate
(**FAIR**-us **FYOU**-mar-ayt)
Femiron, Feostat, Feostat Drops and Suspension, Fumasorb, Fumerin, Hemocyte, Ircon, Nephro-Fer, Palafer ✹, Palafer Pediatric Drops ✹, Span-FF **(OTC)**
**Classification:** Antianemic, iron

See also *Antianemic Drugs.*
**Action/Kinetics:** Better tolerated than ferrous gluconate or ferrous sulfate. Contains 33% elemental iron.

**Dosage**
• **Extended-Release Capsules**

*Prophylaxis.*
**Adults:** 325 mg/day.
*Anemia.*
**Adults:** 325 mg b.i.d. Capsules are not recommended for use in children.
• **Oral Solution, Oral Suspension, Tablets, Chewable Tablets**
*Prophylaxis.*
**Adults:** 200 mg/day. **Pediatric:** 3 mg/kg/day.
*Anemia.*
**Adults:** 200 mg t.i.d.–q.i.d. **Pediatric:** 3 mg/kg t.i.d., up to 6 mg/kg/day, if needed.

## NURSING CONSIDERATIONS

See *Nursing Considerations* for *Antianemic Drugs.*
**Outcomes/Evaluate:** Restoration of iron stores

# Ferrous gluconate
(**FAIR**-us **GLUE**-kon-ayt)
Apo-Ferrous Gluconate ✹, Fergon, Ferralet, Ferralet Slow Release, Simron **(OTC)**
**Classification:** Antianemic, iron

See also *Antianemic Drugs.*
**Uses:** Particularly indicated for clients who cannot tolerate ferrous sulfate because of gastric irritation. Preparation contains 11.6% elemental iron.

**Dosage**
• **Capsules, Tablets**
*Prophylaxis.*
**Adults:** 325 mg/day. **Pediatric, 2 years and older:** 8 mg/kg/day.
*Anemia.*
**Adults:** 325 mg q.i.d. Can be increased to 650 mg q.i.d. if needed and tolerated. **Pediatric, 2 years and older:** l6 mg/kg t.i.d.
• **Elixir, Syrup**
*Prophylaxis.*
**Adults:** 300 mg/day. **Pediatric, 2 years and older:** 8 mg/kg/day.
*Anemia.*
**Adults:** 300 mg q.i.d. Can be increased to 600 mg q.i.d. as needed and tolerated. **Pediatric, 2 years and older:** 16 mg/kg t.i.d. The

provider must determine dosage for children less than 2 years of age.

## NURSING CONSIDERATIONS

See *Nursing Considerations* for *Antianemic Drugs*.
**Outcomes/Evaluate**
• Restoration of serum iron stores
• H&H within desired range

# Ferrous sulfate
(**FAIR**-us **SUL**-fayt)
Apo-Ferrous Sulfate ✿, Feosol, Fer-in-Sol, Fer-Iron, Ferrodan ✿, Fero-Gradumet, Ferospace, Feratab, Mol-Iron, PMS Ferrous Sulfate ✿ **(OTC)**

# Ferrous sulfate, dried
(**FAIR**-us **SUL**-fayt)
Feosol, Fer-in-Sol, Ferralyn Lanacaps, Ferra-TD, Slow-Fe **(OTC)**
**Classification:** Antianemic, iron

See also *Antianemic Drugs*.
**Action/Kinetics:** Least expensive, most effective iron salt for PO therapy. Ferrous sulfate products contain 20% elemental iron, whereas ferrous sulfate dried products contain 30% elemental iron. The exsiccated form is more stable in air.

**Dosage**
Ferrous sulfate
• **Extended-Release Capsules**
**Adults:** 150–250 mg 1–2 times/day. This dosage form is not recommended for children.
• **Elixir, Oral Solution, Tablets, Enteric-coated Tablets**
*Prophylaxis.*
**Adults:** 300 mg/day. **Pediatric:** 5 mg/kg/day.
*Anemia.*
**Adults:** 300 mg b.i.d. increased to 300 mg q.i.d. as needed and tolerated. **Pediatric:** 10 mg/kg t.i.d. The enteric-coated tablets are not recommended for use in children.
• **Extended-Release Tablets**
**Adults:** 525 mg 1–2 times/day. This dosage form is not recommended for use in children.
Ferrous sulfate, dried

• **Capsules**
*Prophylaxis.*
**Adults:** 300 mg/day. **Pediatric:** 5 mg/kg/day.
*Anemia.*
**Adults:** 300 mg b.i.d. up to 300 mg q.i.d. as needed and tolerated. **Pediatric:** 10 mg/kg t.i.d.
• **Tablets**
*Prophylaxis.*
**Adults:** 200 mg/day. **Pediatric:** 5 mg/kg/day.
*Anemia.*
**Adults:** 200 mg t.i.d. up to 200 mg q.i.d. as needed and tolerated. **Pediatric:** 10 mg/kg t.i.d.
• **Extended-Release Tablets**
**Adults:** 160 mg 1–2 times/day. This dosage form is not recommended for use in children.

## NURSING CONSIDERATIONS

See *Nursing Considerations* for *Antianemic Drugs*.
**Outcomes/Evaluate**
• Restoration of serum iron levels
• Resolution of S&S of anemia

# Fexofenadine hydrochloride
(fex-oh-**FEN**-ah-deen)
**Pregnancy Category:** C
Allegra **(Rx)**
**Classification:** Antihistamine

See also *Antihistamines*.
**Action/Kinetics:** Fexofenadine, a metabolite of terfenadine, is an $H_1$-histamine receptor blocker. Low to no sedative or anticholinergic effects.
**Onset:** Rapid. **Peak plasma levels:** 2.6 hr. **t½, terminal:** 14.4 hr. Approximately 90% of the drug is excreted through the feces (80%) and urine (10%) unchanged.
**Uses:** Seasonal allergic rhinitis in adults and children 12 years of age and older.
**Special Concerns:** Use with care during lactation. Safety and efficacy have not been determined in children less than 12 years of age.

---

✿ = Available in Canada          ***bold italic*** = life threatening side effect

**Side Effects:** *CNS:* Drowsiness, fatigue. *GI:* Nausea, dyspepsia. *Miscellaneous:* Viral infection (flu, colds), dysmenorrhea, sinusitis, throat irritation.

**Drug Interactions:** No differences in side effects or the QTc interval were observed when fexofenadine was given with either erythromycin or ketoconazole.

**Dosage** ————————
• **Capsules**
  *Seasonal allergic rhinitis.*
**Adults and children over 12 years of age:** 60 mg b.i.d. In clients with decreased renal function, the initial dose should be 60 mg once daily.

## NURSING CONSIDERATIONS

See also *Nursing Considerations* for *Antihistamines.*
**Assessment**
1. Document onset, duration, and characteristics of symptoms; identify triggers if known.
2. Note other agents trialed, length of use, and outcome.
3. Assess for renal dysfunction; reduce dose if evident.
**Client/Family Teaching**
1. Take exactly as directed; do not exceed prescribed dosage.
2. May experience headaches, sore throat, nausea, and dysmenorrhea.
3. Report if symptoms intensify or do not improve after 48 hr of therapy.
4. Identify and avoid triggers.
**Outcomes/Evaluate:** Control of symptoms of seasonal allergic rhinitis

# Filgrastim
(fill-**GRASS**-tim)
**Pregnancy Category:** C
Neupogen **(Rx)**
**Classification:** Human granulocyte colony-stimulating factor (G-CSF)

**Action/Kinetics:** Is a human granulocyte colony stimulating factor (G-CSF) produced by recombinant DNA technology by *Escherichia coli* that has been inserted with the human G-CSF gene. Endogenous G-CSF is a glycoprotein that is produced by monocytes, fibroblasts, and other endothelial cells and that regulates the production of neutrophils in the bone marrow. Has minimal effects, either in vivo or in vitro, on the production of other hematopoietic cell types. Filgrastim has an amino acid sequence that is identical to the natural sequence predicted from human DNA sequence analysis except there is an N-terminal methionine that is required for expression in *E. coli*. IV infusion of 20 mcg/kg over 24 hr resulted in a mean serum level of 48 ng/mL, whereas SC administration of 11.5 mcg/kg resulted in a maximum serum level of 49 ng/mL within 2–8 hr. **t½, elimination:** 3.5 hr.

**Uses:** To decrease the incidence of infection, as manifested by febrile neutropenia, in clients with nonmyeloid malignancies who are receiving myelosuppressive anticancer drugs, which are associated with severe neutropenia with fever. To reduce the duration of neutropenia in clients with nonmyeloid malignancies undergoing myeloablative chemotherapy followed by bone marrow transplantation. To reduce infection in severe chronic neutropenia (e.g., congenital, cyclical, or idiopathic neutropenia) after other diseases have been ruled out. For the mobilization of hematopoietic progenitor cells into the peripheral blood for leukapheresis collection. *Investigational:* Use in AIDS, aplastic anemia, hairy cell leukemia, myelodysplasia, drug-induced and congenital agranulocytosis, and alloimmune neonatal neutropenia.

**Contraindications:** Hypersensitivity to proteins derived from *E. coli*. The safety and effectiveness of filgrastim given simultaneously with cytotoxic chemotherapy have not been determined; thus, filgrastim should not be given 24 hr before to 24 hr after cytotoxic chemotherapy.

**Special Concerns:** Use with caution during lactation. Use with caution in any malignancy with myeloid characteristics since the drug may act as a growth factor for any tumor type. Filgrastim does not cause any greater incidence of toxicity in children than in adults. Safety and efficacy have not been determined in neonates and clients with autoimmune neutropenia of infancy. The safety and effectiveness of chronic filgrastim therapy have not been determined. Hypersensitivity reactions usually occur within 30 min after administration and are more frequent in clients receiving the drug IV.

**Side Effects: When used for myelosuppressive therapy.** *Musculoskeletal:* Medullary bone pain, skeletal pain. *GI:* N&V, diarrhea, anorexia, stomatitis, constipation, peritonitis. *Hypersensitivity:* Skin rash, facial edema, wheezing, dyspnea, hypotension, tachycardia. *Hematologic:* Leukocytosis; greater risk of thrombocytopenia and anemia. *Respiratory:* Dyspnea, cough, chest pain, sore throat. *Body as a whole:* Alopecia, neutropenic fever, fever, fatigue, headache, skin rash, mucositis, generalized weakness, unspecified pain. *CV:* Decreased BP (transient), cutaneous vasculitis, hypertension, ***arrhythmias, MI.***

**When used for severe chronic neutropenia.** *Musculoskeletal:* Mild to moderate bone pain, abdominal/flank pain, arthralgia, osteoporosis. *Hematologic:* Thrombocytopenia, epistaxis (associated with thrombocytopenia), anemia, myelodysplasia or myeloid leukemia. *Dermatologic:* Exacerbation of certain skin conditions (e.g., psoriasis), rash, alopecia. *Miscellaneous:* Palpable splenomegaly, hepatomegaly, monosomy, reaction at injection site, cutaneous vasculitis, hematuria, proteinuria.

**When used for bone marrow transplantation.** *GI:* N&V, stomatitis, peritonitis. *CV:* Hypertension, capillary leak syndrome (rare). *Miscellaneous:* Rash, renal insufficiency, erythema nodosum.

**When used for peripheral blood progenitor cell collection.** *Hematologic:* Decreased platelet counts, anemia, increase in neutrophil count, WBC count greater than 100,000/mm³. *Miscellaneous:* Mild to moderate musculoskeletal symptoms, medullary bone pain, headache, increases in alkaline phosphatase.

**Laboratory Test Interferences:** ↑ Uric acid, LDH, alkaline phosphatase.

**Dosage** ——————————
• **SC, IV**
*Myelosuppressive chemotherapy.*
**Initial:** 5 mcg/kg/day as a single injection, either as a SC bolus, by short IV infusion (15–30 min), or by continuous SC or IV infusion (over a 24-hr period). The dose may be increased in increments of 5 mcg/kg for each chemotherapy cycle depending on the duration and severity of the absolute neutrophil count (ANC) nadir. The dose should be given daily for up to 2 weeks, until ANC has reached 10,000/mm³ following the expected chemotherapy-induced neutrophil nadir.
*Severe chronic neutropenia.*
5 mcg/kg/day SC for idiopathic and cyclic disease; 6 mcg/kg/day SC for congenital disease.
*Bone marrow transplantation.*
10 mcg/kg/day given as an IV infusion of 4 or 24 hr or as a continuous 24-hr SC infusion.
*NOTE:* During the period of neutrophil recovery, the daily dose should be titrated against the neutrophil response as follows:
1. When ANC is greater than 1,000/mm³ for 3 consecutive days, reduce the dose of filgrastim to 5 mcg/kg/day. If ANC decreases to less than 1,000/mm³ at any time during the 5-mcg/kg/day dosage, increase filgrastim to 10 mcg/kg/day.
2. If ANC remains greater than 1,000/mm³ for 3 more consecutive days, discontinue filgrastim.
3. If ANC decreases to less than 1,000/mm³, resume filgrastim at 5 mcg/kg/day.
*Peripheral blood progenitor cell collection.*

F

---

10 mcg/kg/day SC, either as a bolus or a continuous infusion. Filgrastim should be given at least 4 days before the first leukapheresis procedure and continued until the last leukapheresis.

## NURSING CONSIDERATIONS
### Administration/Storage
1. Discontinue therapy if the ANC is greater than $10,000/mm^3$ after the expected chemotherapy-induced neutrophil nadir.
2. For myelosuppressive therapy or bone marrow transplantation, give no earlier than 24 hr after cytotoxic chemotherapy and in the 24 hr before administration of chemotherapy.
3. Discontinuing therapy usually results in a 50% decrease in circulating neutrophils within 1–2 days with a return to pretreatment levels in 1–7 days.
4. Do not freeze; store in the refrigerator at 2°C–8°C (36°F–46°F). Prior to use, can be at room temperature for a maximum of 24 hr. Discard if left at room temperature for more than 24 hr.
5. Solution should be clear and colorless.
6. Do not shake.
7. Use only one dose from each vial; do not reenter the vial.
8. Compatible with glass, PVC, or plastic syringes.
**IV** 9. May be diluted in 5% dextrose. When diluted to concentrations between 5 and 15 mcg/mL, protect from adsorption to plastic materials by adding human albumin to a final concentration of 2 mg/mL.
10. The following drugs are incompatible as an admixture with filgrastim: amphotericin B, cefonicid, cefoperazone, cefotaxime, cefoxitin, ceftizoxime, ceftriaxone, cefuroxime clindamycin, dactinomycin, etoposide, fluorouracil, furosemide, heparin, mannitol, metronidazole, methylprednisolone, mezlocillin, mitomycin, prochlorperazine, piperacillin, and thiotepa.

### Assessment
1. Determine sensitivity to *E. coli*-derived products.
2. Document indications for therapy (i.e., chemotherapy-induced neutropenia, myelopsuppressive therapy for bone marrow transplantation, leukapheresis) and expected time frame for administration.
3. Monitor CBC and platelet counts twice weekly during therapy.
4. Note last dose of cytotoxic agent and determine ANC nadir. Do not administer from 24 hr before to 24 hr after cytotoxic chemotherapy.

### Client/Family Teaching
1. Demonstrate appropriate technique for administration. Review written guidelines concerning dose, administration time, drug storage, storing, handling, and discarding of syringes.
2. Do not shake container; only enter the vial once, then discard.
3. "Flu-like" symptoms (N&V and aching; bone pain) may be side effects of drug therapy. Take at bedtime, with prescribed analgesics, and report if persistent.
4. Record daily temperatures; report evidence of infection or any unusual bruising or bleeding.
5. Avoid crowds and persons with infectious diseases.

### Outcomes/Evaluate
- Prevention of infection
- ↓ Duration of neutropenia
- Improved neutrophil counts
- Mobilization of progenitor cells into peripheral blood

# Finasteride
(fin-**AS**-teh-ride)
**Pregnancy Category:** X
Propecia, Proscar **(Rx)**
**Classification:** Androgen hormone inhibitor

**Action/Kinetics:** Is a specific inhibitor of steroid 5-alpha-reductase, the enzyme that converts testosterone to the active 5-alpha-dihydrotestosterone (DHT). The reduced plasma level of DHT results in regression of prostate tissue and decreased scalp levels. Well absorbed after PO administration. **Elimination $t^{1/2}$:** 6 hr in clients 45–60 years of age and 8 hr in clients over 70 years of age. Slow accumulation after multiple dosing. Metabolized in the liver and excreted through both the urine and feces.

**Uses:** Treatment of symptomatic benign prostatic hyperplasia. There is rapid regression of the enlarged prostate gland in most clients; however, less than 50% of clients show an increase in urine flow and improvement of symptoms of benign prostatic hyperplasia when treated for 12 months. Male pattern baldness (vertex and anterior midscalp). *Investigational:* Adjuvant monotherapy following radical prostatectomy, prevention of the progression of first-stage prostate cancer, acne, and hirsutism.

**Contraindications:** Hypersensitivity to finasteride or any excipient in the product. Use during pregnancy, during lactation, and in children.

**Special Concerns:** Use with caution in clients with impaired liver function.

**Side Effects:** *GU:* Impotence, decreased libido, decreased volume of ejaculate. *Miscellaneous:* Breast tenderness and enlargement, hypersensitivity reactions (including skin rash and swelling of the lips).

**Laboratory Test Interferences:** ↓ Serum PSA levels.

**Dosage** —————————————
• **Tablets**
  *Benign prostatic hyperplasia.*
5 mg/day, with or without meals.
  *Androgenetic alopecia.*
**Males:** 1 mg once a day with or without meals.

## NURSING CONSIDERATIONS
### Administration/Storage
1. At least 6–12 months of therapy may be required in some to determine whether a beneficial response has been achieved for benign prostatic hyperplasia.
2. Daily use for three months or longer is necessary to observe beneficial effects.
3. Continued use is required to

sustain beneficial effects for hair growth. Withdrawal leads to reversal of effects within 12 months.
4. Women who are pregnant or may become pregnant should not handle crushed finasteride tablets as there is potential for drug absorption and subsequent potential risk to the male fetus. Also, when the male's sexual partner is or may become pregnant, exposure of semen to his partner should be avoided or drug use discontinued.
5. Do not adjust dosage in the elderly or in those with impaired renal function.

### Assessment
1. Note indications for therapy, include onset, characteristics of clinical presentation, and any associated family history.
2. Determine that a urologic exam has been performed to rule out other conditions similar to BPH (e.g., prostate cancer, infection, stricture, hypotonic bladder, neurogenic disorders).
3. Monitor LFTs and PSA. May cause a decrease in PSA levels (prostate-specific antigen: a blood screening study to detect prostate cancer) even in the presence of prostate cancer.
4. Schedule regular digital rectal exams to assess prostate gland.
5. Not for use in females.
6. With liver impairment monitor closely; drug is metabolized by the liver.
7. Not all clients show a response to finasteride. Assess clients with a large residual urinary volume or severely diminished urinary flow for obstructive uropathy; these may not be candidates for finasteride therapy.
8. May obtain pre-treatment photos to assess/gauge response.
9. Ensure that history and physical exam completed.
### Client/Family Teaching
1. The following symptoms of BPH should show improvement with continued drug therapy: hesitancy, feelings of incomplete bladder emp-

tying, interruption of urinary stream, impairment of size and force of urinary stream, and terminal urinary dribbling. May take 6–12 months of continued therapy before a beneficial effect is evident

2. Use barrier contraception; drug may cause male fetal abnormalities. If pregnancy occurs, either discontinue finasteride or avoid exposure of partner to semen (use a condom).

3. BPH symptoms return upon discontinuation of drug.

4. Take once a day with or without meals as directed. More than prescribed dose will not increase hair growth but may cause adverse symptoms. May take 3 mg or more before any response noted.

5. If partner is pregnant or may become pregnant, avoid partner exposure to semen. Drug may cause damage to male fetus; either stop drug or use a condom to prevent semen exposure.

6. Decreased volume of ejaculate may occur but does not interfere with sexual function. Impotence and decreased libido may also occur.

7. Report as scheduled for F/U labs, checkups and prostate exams. Any unusual side effects should be reported promptly.

8. Interruption of therapy will reverse effects within 12 months

**Outcomes/Evaluate**

• ↓ Size of enlarged prostate gland
• Symptomatic improvement
• Regrowth of hair with male pattern baldness

————COMBINATION DRUG————

# Fiorinal
(fee-**OR**-in-al)
**(Rx)**

# Fiorinal with Codeine
(fee-**OR**-in-al, **KOH**-deen)
**Pregnancy Category:** C
**(C-III) (Rx)**
**Classification:** Analgesic

See also *Narcotic Analgesics, Acetylsalicylic Acid,* and *Barbiturates.*
**Content:** Each Fiorinal capsule or tablet contains:

*Nonnarcotic analgesic:* Aspirin, 325 mg.
*Sedative barbiturate:* Butalbital, 50 mg.
*CNS stimulant:* Caffeine, 40 mg.
In addition to the above, Fiorinal with Codeine capsules contain codeine phosphate, 7.5 mg (No. 1), 15 mg (No. 2), or 30 mg (No. 3).
**Uses:** Fiorinal is indicated for tension headaches. Fiorinal with Codeine is indicated as an analgesic for all types of pain.

**Dosage** ————
• **Capsules, Tablets**
FIORINAL
1–2 tablets or capsules q 4 hr, not to exceed 6 tablets or capsules/day.
FIORINAL WITH CODEINE
**Initial:** 1–2 capsules; **then,** dose may be repeated, if necessary, up to maximum of 6 capsules/day.

## NURSING CONSIDERATIONS

See *Nursing Considerations* for *Acetylsalicylic Acid* and *Narcotic Analgesics.*
**Assessment**
1. Document pain level, onset, location, and duration of symptoms.
2. List agents previously used and the outcome.
**Outcomes/Evaluate**
• Control of pain
• Relief of tension headaches

# Flavoxate hydrochloride
(flay-**VOX**-ayt)
**Pregnancy Category:** B
Urispas **(Rx)**
**Classification:** Urinary tract antispasmodic

**Action/Kinetics:** Relieves muscle spasms of the urinary tract by relaxing the detrusor muscle by cholinergic blockade and also by a direct effect. Also has local anesthetic and analgesic effects. Well absorbed from GI tract; 10%–30% is excreted in urine.
**Uses:** Symptomatic relief of urinary tract irritation, dysuria, urgency, nocturia, suprapubic pain, incontinence associated with cystitis, pro-

statitis, urethritis, urethrocystitis, and other urinary tract disorders. Compatible for use with urinary tract germicides.

**Contraindications:** Obstructive disorders of urinary tract, including pyloric or duodenal obstructions, obstructive intestinal lesions, ileus, achalasia, obstructive uropathies of the lower urinary tract, and GI hemorrhage.

**Special Concerns:** Use with caution in glaucoma and during lactation. Confusion is more likely to occur in geriatric clients. Safety and effectiveness have not been determined in children less than 12 years of age.

**Side Effects:** *GI:* N&V, xerostomia. *CNS:* Drowsiness, headache, vertigo, nervousness, mental confusion (especially in the elderly). *CV:* Tachycardia, palpitations. *Hematologic:* Eosinophilia, leukopenia. *Ophthalmologic:* Blurred vision, increased ocular tension, accommodation disturbances. *Other:* Urticaria, skin rashes, fever, dysuria.

**Dosage**
• **Tablets**
**Adults and children over 12 years:** 100 or 200 mg t.i.d.–q.i.d. Dose may be reduced when symptoms improve.

## NURSING CONSIDERATIONS

See also *Nursing Considerations* for *Cholinergic Blocking Agents*.
**Client/Family Teaching**
1. Do not drive a car or operate hazardous machinery; may cause drowsiness and blurred vision.
2. Practice good oral hygiene. Relieve dryness of mouth with ice chips or hard candy. Ensure adequate hydration.
3. Avoid strenuous exercise; body's heat-regulating mechanism may be altered and sweating inhibited.
4. Report any persistent, bothersome, or new symptoms.
**Outcomes/Evaluate**
• Relief of urinary tract discomfort

• Normal elimination patterns

# Flecainide acetate
(fleh-**KAY**-nyd)
**Pregnancy Category:** C
Tambocor **(Rx)**
**Classification:** Antiarrhythmic, class IC

See also *Antiarrhythmic Agents.*
**Action/Kinetics:** The antiarrhythmic effect is due to a local anesthetic action, especially on the His-Purkinje system in the ventricle. Drug decreases single and multiple PVCs and reduces the incidence of ventricular tachycardia. **Peak plasma levels:** 3 hr.; **steady state levels:** 3–5 days. **Effective plasma levels:** 0.2–1 mcg/mL (trough levels). **t½:** 20 hr (12–27 hr). Forty percent is bound to plasma protein. Approximately 30% is excreted in urine unchanged. Impaired renal function decreases rate of elimination of unchanged drug. Food or antacids do not affect absorption.
**Uses:** Life-threatening arrhythmias manifested as sustained ventricular tachycardia. Prevention of paroxysmal supraventricular tachycardias (PSVT) and paroxysmal atrial fibrillation or flutter (PAF) associated with disabling symptoms but not structural heart disease. Antiarrhythmic drugs have not been shown to improve survival in clients with ventricular arrhythmias.
**Contraindications:** Cardiogenic shock, preexisting second- or third-degree AV block, right bundle branch block when associated with bifascicular block (unless pacemaker is present to maintain cardiac rhythm). Recent MI. Cardiogenic shock. Chronic atrial fibrillation. Frequent premature ventricular complexes and symptomatic nonsustained ventricular arrhythmias. Lactation.
**Special Concerns:** Use with caution in sick sinus syndrome, in clients with a history of CHF or MI, in disturbances of potassium levels, in clients with permanent pacemakers or

temporary pacing electrodes, renal and liver impairment. Safety and efficacy in children less than 18 years of age are not established. The incidence of proarrhythmic effects may be increased in geriatric clients.

**Side Effects:** *CV: **New or worsened ventricular arrhythmias, increased risk of death in clients with non-life-threatening cardiac arrhythmias,** new or worsened CHF, palpitations, chest pain, sinus bradycardia, sinus pause, sinus arrest, **ventricular fibrillation, ventricular tachycardia that cannot be resuscitated,** second- or third-degree AV block, tachycardia, hypertension, hypotension, bradycardia, angina pectoris. CNS:* Dizziness, faintness, syncope, lightheadedness, neuropathy, unsteadiness, headache, fatigue, paresthesia, paresis, hypoesthesia, insomnia, anxiety, malaise, vertigo, depression, *seizures,* euphoria, confusion, depersonalization, apathy, morbid dreams, speech disorders, stupor, amnesia, weakness, somnolence. *GI:* Nausea, constipation, abdominal pain, vomiting, anorexia, dyspepsia, dry mouth, diarrhea, flatulence, change in taste. *Ophthalmic:* Blurred vision, difficulty in focusing, spots before eyes, diplopia, photophobia, eye pain, nystagmus, eye irritation, photophobia. *Hematologic:* Leukopenia, thrombocytopenia. *GU:* Decreased libido, impotence, urinary retention, polyuria. *Musculoskeletal:* Asthenia, tremor, ataxia, arthralgia, myalgia. *Dermatologic:* Skin rashes, urticaria, exfoliative dermatitis, pruritus, alopecia. *Other:* Edema, dyspnea, fever, *bronchospasm,* flushing, sweating, tinnitus, swollen mouth, lips, and tongue.

**OD** **Overdose Management:** *Symptoms:* Lengthening of PR interval; increase in QRS duration, QT interval, and amplitude of T wave; decrease in HR and contractility; conduction disturbances; hypotension; *respiratory failure* or *asystole. Treatment:* Charcoal will remove unabsorbed drug up to 90 min after drug ingestion. Administration of dopamine, dobutamine, or isoproterenol. Artificial respiration.

Intra-aortic balloon pumping, transvenous pacing (to correct conduction block). Acidification of the urine may be beneficial, especially in those with an alkaline urine. Due to the long duration of action of the drug, treatment measures may have to be continued for a prolonged period of time.

**Drug Interactions**
*Acidifying agents* / ↑ Renal excretion of flecainide
*Alkalinizing agents* / ↓ Renal excretion of flecainide
*Amiodarone* / ↑ Plasma levels of flecainide
*Cimetidine* / ↑ Bioavailability and renal excretion of flecainide
*Digoxin* / ↑ Digoxin plasma levels
*Disopyramide* / Additive negative inotropic effects
*Propranolol* / Additive negative inotropic effects; also, ↑ plasma levels of both drugs
*Smoking (Tobacco)* / ↑ Plasma clearance of flecainide
*Verapamil* / Additive negative inotropic effects

**Dosage**
- **Tablets**
  *Sustained ventricular tachycardia.*
  **Initial:** 100 mg q 12 hr; **then,** increase by 50 mg b.i.d. q 4 days until effective dose reached. **Usual effective dose:** 150 mg q 12 hr; dose should not exceed 400 mg/day.
  *PSVT, PAF.*
  **Initial:** 50 mg q 12 hr; **then,** dose may be increased in increments of 50 mg b.i.d. q 4 days until effective dose reached. Maximum recommended dose: 300 mg/day. *NOTE:* For PAF clients, increasing the dose from 50 to 100 mg b.i.d. may increase efficacy without a significant increase in side effects.
  *NOTE:* For clients with a $C_{CR}$ less than 35 mL/min/1.73 m$^2$, the starting dose is 100 mg once daily (or 50 mg b.i.d.). For less severe renal disease, the initial dose may be 100 mg q 12 hr.

## NURSING CONSIDERATIONS

See also *Nursing Considerations* for *Antiarrhythmic Agents*.

**Administration/Storage**

1. For most situations, start therapy in a hospital setting (especially in clients with symptomatic CHF, sustained ventricular arrhythmias, compensated clients with significant myocardial dysfunction, or sinus node dysfunction).
2. In renal impairment, increase the dose at intervals greater than 4 days. Monitor carefully for adverse toxic effects.
3. The chance of toxic effects increases if the trough plasma levels exceed 1 mcg/mL.
4. If being transferred to flecainide from another antiarrhythmic, at least two to four plasma half-lives should elapse for the drug being discontinued before initiating flecainide therapy.
5. Dosing at 8-hr intervals may benefit some.
6. To minimize toxicity, may reduce dose once the arrhythmia is controlled.

**Assessment**

1. Document physical assessment findings. Review history, echocardiograms, and ECGs for evidence of CHF, ventricular arrhythmias, sinus node dysfunction, or abnormal ejection fractions.
2. Monitor VS, ECG, CXR, electrolytes, liver and renal function studies. Assess ECG for increased arrhythmias or AV block. Preexisting hypo- or hyperkalemia may alter drug effects; should be corrected. Monitor for labile BP.
3. Concomitant administration with disopyramide, propranolol, or verapamil will promote negative inotropic effects.
4. Check pacing thresholds of clients with pacemakers; adjust before and 1 week following drug therapy.

**Client/Family Teaching**

1. Take at the dose and prescribed frequency. Report changes in elimination.
2. Report any bruising or increased bleeding tendencies, dyspnea, edema, or chest pain.
3. Keep appointments so that drug effectiveness can be monitored carefully.
4. Report adverse CNS effects, such as dizziness, visual disturbances, headaches, nausea, or depression.
5. Obtain urinary pH to detect alkalinity or acidity. Alkalinity of the urine decreases renal excretion and acidity increases renal excretion, which in turn affects the rate of drug elimination.

**Outcomes/Evaluate**

• Termination of lethal ventricular arrhythmias; stable cardiac rhythm
• Therapeutic serum (trough) drug levels (0.2–1.0 mcg/mL)

# Floxuridine

(flox-**YOUR**-ih-deen)
**Pregnancy Category:** D
FUDR **(Rx)**
**Classification:** Antineoplastic, antimetabolite

See also *Antineoplastic Agents*.

**Action/Kinetics:** Cell-cycle specific for the S phase of cell division. Rapidly metabolized to fluorouracil. The drug inhibits DNA and RNA synthesis. Crosses blood-brain barrier. t½: 5–20 min. From 60% to 80% of fluorouracil is excreted as respiratory $CO_2$ (8–12 hr); small amount (15%) excreted in urine (1–6 hr).

**Uses:** Intra-arterially as palliative treatment of GI adenocarcinoma metastatic to the liver (especially in clients incurable by surgery or other treatment). Used in clients with disease limited to an area capable of infusion by a single artery. *Investigational:* Cancer of the breast, ovaries, cervix, bladder, kidney, and prostate.

**Contraindications:** If client is at poor risk, including depressed bone marrow function, nutritionally poor, or potentially serious infections. Lactation. Should not be used during pregnancy unless benefits clearly outweigh risks.

**Additional Side Effects:** Esophagopharyngitis, myocardial ischemia, angina, acute cerebellar syndrome, photophobia, lacrimation, decreased vision. Complications of intra-arterial administration are arterial aneurysm, arterial ischemia, arterial thrombosis, bleeding at catheter site, occluded, displaced, or leaking catheters, embolism, fibromyositis, infection at catheter site, thrombophlebitis.

**Laboratory Test Interferences:** ↑ Excretion of 5-hydroxyindoleacetic acid. ↑ Serum transaminase and bilirubin, LDH, alkaline phosphatase. ↓ Plasma albumin.

## Dosage

• **Intra-arterial Infusion**

0.1–0.6 mg/kg/day by continuous infusion over 24 hr. Infusion is continued until a response or toxicity occurs (usually for 14–21 days with a rest period of 2 weeks between courses of therapy).

## NURSING CONSIDERATIONS

See also *Nursing Considerations* for *Antineoplastic Agents*.

**Administration/Storage**

1. Higher doses (0.4–0.6 mg) are best given by hepatic artery infusion because the liver metabolizes the drug, reducing the possibility of systemic toxicity.

2. Give until adverse effects are manifested. Resume therapy after adverse effects have subsided. WBC nadir: 1 week. Platelet nadir: 10 days.

3. Use an infusion pump to overcome pressure in the large arteries and to assure a uniform rate of infusion.

4. Reconstitute each vial with 5 mL sterile water to yield a 100-mg/mL concentration. This may be further reconstituted in D5W or NSS and infused intra-arterially.

5. Store reconstituted vials in the refrigerator at 2°C–8°C (36°F–46°F) for no longer than 2 weeks.

**Outcomes/Evaluate:** Suppression of metastatic processes

# Fluconazole

(flew-**KON**-ah-zohl)
**Pregnancy Category:** C
Diflucan, Diflucan-150 ✸ **(Rx)**
**Classification:** Antifungal agent

**Action/Kinetics:** Inhibits the enzyme cytochrome P-450 in the organism, which results in a decrease in cell wall integrity and extrusion of intracellular material, leading to death. Apparently does not affect the cytochrome P-450 enzyme in animals or humans. **Peak plasma levels:** 1–2 hr. **t½:** 30 hr, which allows for once daily dosing. Penetrates all body fluids at steady state. Bioavailability is not affected by agents that increase gastric pH. Eighty percent of the drug is excreted unchanged by the kidneys.

**Uses:** Oropharyngeal and esophageal candidiasis. Serious systemic candidal infection (including UTIs, peritonitis, and pneumonia). Cryptococcal meningitis. Maintenance therapy to prevent cryptococcal meningitis in AIDS clients. Vaginal candidiasis. To decrease the incidence of candidiasis in clients undergoing a bone marrow transplant who receive cytotoxic chemotherapy or radiation therapy. Treatment of cryptococcal meningitis and candidal infections in children.

**Contraindications:** Hypersensitivity to fluconazole.

**Special Concerns:** Use with caution if client shows hypersensitivity to other azoles. Care should be used when fluconazole is prescribed during lactation. The effectiveness of the drug has not been adequately assessed in children.

**Side Effects: Following single doses.** *GI:* Nausea, abdominal pain, diarrhea, dyspepsia, taste perversion. *CNS:* Headache, dizziness. *Other:* Angioedema, *anaphylaxis (rare)*.

**Following multiple doses.** Side effects are more frequently reported in HIV-infected clients than in non-HIV-infected clients. *GI:* N&V, abdominal pain, diarrhea, **serious hepatic reactions.** *CNS:* Headache, **seizures.** *Dermatologic:* Skin rash, exfoliative skin disorders (including **Stevens-Johnson syndrome,** and toxic epidermal necrolysis), alopecia. *Hematologic:* Leukopenia, thrombocytopenia. *Other:* Hypercholesterolemia, hypertriglyceridemia, hypokalemia.

**Drug Interactions**

*Cimetidine* / ↓ Plasma levels of fluconazole

*Cyclosporine* / Fluconazole may ↑ cyclosporine levels in renal transplant clients with or without impaired renal function

*Hydrochlorothiazide* / ↑ Plasma levels of fluconazole due to ↓ renal clearance

*Glipizide* / ↑ Plasma levels of glipizide due to ↓ breakdown by the liver

*Glyburide* / ↑ Plasma levels of glyburide due to ↓ breakdown by the liver

*Phenytoin* / Fluconazole ↑ plasma levels of phenytoin

*Rifampin* / ↓ Plasma levels of fluconazole due to ↑ breakdown by the liver

*Theophylline* / ↑ Plasma levels of theophylline

*Tolbutamide* / ↑ Plasma levels of tolbutamide due to ↓ breakdown by the liver

*Warfarin* / ↑ PT

*Zidovudine* / ↑ Plasma levels of AZT

**Laboratory Test Interferences:** ↑ AST, serum transaminase (especially if used with isoniazid, oral hypoglycemic agents, phenytoin, rifampin, valproic acid).

**Dosage** ————————

• **Tablets, Oral Suspension, IV**

*Vaginal candidiasis.*

150 mg as a single oral dose.

*Oropharyngeal or esophageal can-didiasis.*

**Adults, first day:** 200 mg; **then,** 100 mg/day for a minimum of 14 days (for oropharyngeal candidiasis) or

21 days (for esophageal candidiasis). Up to 400 mg/day may be required for esophageal candidiasis. **Children, first day:** 6 mg/kg; **then,** 3 mg/kg once daily for a minimum of 14 days (for oropharyngeal candidiasis) or 21 days (for esophageal candidiasis).

*Candidal UTI and peritonitis.*

50–200 mg/day.

*Systemic candidiasis (e.g., candidemia, disseminated candidiasis, and pneumonia).*

Optimal dosage and duration in adults have not been determined although doses up to 400 mg/day have been used. **Children:** 6–12 mg/kg/day.

*Acute cryptococcal meningitis.*

**Adults, first day:** 400 mg; **then,** 200 mg/day (up to 400 mg may be required) for 10 to 12 weeks after CSF culture is negative. **Children, first day:** 12 mg/kg; **then,** 6 mg/kg once daily for 10 to 12 weeks after CSF culture is negative.

*Maintenance to prevent relapse of cryptococcal meningitis in AIDS clients.*

**Adults:** 200 mg once daily. **Pediatric:** 6 mg/kg once daily.

*Prevention of candidiasis in bone marrow transplant.*

400 mg once daily. In clients expected to have severe granulocytopenia (less than 500 neutrophils/mm$^3$), fluconazole should be started several days before the anticipated onset of neutropenia and continued for 7 days after the neutrophil count rises about 1,000 cells/mm$^3$. In clients with renal impairment, an initial loading dose of 50–400 mg can be given; daily dose is based then on creatinine clearance.

————————————

## NURSING CONSIDERATIONS

See also *General Nursing Considerations for All Anti-Infectives.*

**Administration/Storage**

1. The daily dose is the same for PO and IV administration.

2. Usually, a loading dose of twice the daily dose is recommended for the

first day of therapy in order to obtain plasma levels close to the steady state by the second day of therapy.
3. Due to a long half-life, once daily dosing (either IV or PO) is possible.
4. To prevent relapse, maintenance therapy is usually required in clients with AIDS, cryptococcal meningitis, or recurrent oropharyngeal candidiasis.
5. Shake the oral suspension well before using. Store the reconstituted suspension at 5°C–30°C (4° F–86°F). Discard any unused drug after 2 weeks. Do not freeze the suspension.
**IV** 6. Do not use the IV solution if cloudy or precipitated or if seal not intact.
7. Do not exceed a continuous IV infusion rate of 200 mg/hr.
8. Do not add supplementary medication to the IV bag.

**Assessment**
1. Note any sensitivity to azoles or similar drugs.
2. Determine if HIV infected; may place client at increased risk for side effects.
3. Obtain baseline cultures, liver and renal function studies. Clients who develop abnormal LFTs should be closely monitored for the development of more serious liver toxicity.

**Client/Family Teaching**
1. Review goals of therapy and appropriate method and schedule for medication administration and lab studies. Take as directed.
2. Report any rash or persistent side effects (especially if immunocompromised); drug may need to be discontinued.

**Outcomes/Evaluate**
• Elimination of pathogenic fungi
• Candida prophylaxis in transplant recipients

# Flucytosine
(flew-SYE-toe-seen)
**Pregnancy Category:** C
Ancobon **(Rx)**
**Classification:** Antibiotic, antifungal

**Action/Kinetics:** Less toxic than amphotericin B. Monitor liver, renal, and hematopoietic systems closely. Appears to penetrate the fungal cell membrane and , after metabolism, acts as an antimetabolite interfering with nucleic acid and protein synthesis. Well absorbed from the GI tract and distributed to the joints, aqueous humor, peritoneal and other body fluids and tissues. **Peak plasma concentration:** 2–6 hr. **Therapeutic serum concentration:** 20–25 mcg/mL. t½: 2–5 hr, higher in presence of impaired renal function. Eighty percent to 90% of the drug is excreted unchanged in urine.

**Uses:** Serious systemic fungal infections by susceptible strains of *Candida* (e.g., endocarditis, septicemia, UTIs) or *Cryptococcus* (pulmonary or UTIs, meningitis, septicemia).

**Contraindications:** Hypersensitivity to drug. Lactation.

**Special Concerns:** Safety and effectiveness have not been determined in children. Use with extreme caution in clients with kidney disease or history of bone marrow depression. The bone marrow depressant effects may cause an increased incidence of microbial infection, gingival bleeding, and delayed healing.

**Side Effects:** *GI:* N&V, diarrhea, abdominal pain, dry mouth, anorexia, duodenal ulcer, GI hemorrhage, ulcerative colitis. *Hematologic:* Anemia, leukopenia, thrombocytopenia, *aplastic anemia, agranulocytosis,* pancytopenia, eosinophilia. *CNS:* Headache, vertigo, confusion, sedation, hallucinations, paresthesia, parkinsonism, psychosis, pyrexia. *Hepatic:* Hepatic dysfunction, jaundice, elevation of hepatic enzymes, increase in bilirubin. *GU:* Increase in BUN and creatinine, azotemia, crystalluria, renal failure. *Respiratory:* Chest pain, dyspnea, *respiratory arrest. Dermatologic:* Pruritus, rash, urticaria, photosensitivity. *Other:* Ataxia, hearing loss, peripheral neuropathy, weakness, hypoglycemia, fatigue, *cardiac arrest,* hypokalemia.

**OD** **Overdose Management:** *Symptoms (serum levels > 100 mcg/mL):* N&V, diarrhea, leukopenia, thrombocytopenia, hepatitis. *Treatment:* Prompt induction of vomiting or gastric lavage. Adequate fluid intake (by IV if necessary). Monitor blood, liver, and kidney parameters frequently. Hemodialysis will quickly decrease serum levels.

**Drug Interactions**
*Amphotericin B* / ↑ Effect and toxicity of flucytosine due to kidney impairment
*Cytosine* / Inactivates antifungal effect of flucytosine

**Dosage**
• **Capsules**
**Adult and children:** 50–150 mg/kg/day in four divided doses. Clients with renal impairment receive lower dosages.

## NURSING CONSIDERATIONS

See also *General Nursing Considerations for All Anti-Infectives.*
**Assessment**
1. Obtain cultures, CBC, liver and renal function studies and monitor; reduce dose with impaired renal function
2. Describe clinical presentation.
**Client/Family Teaching**
1. Reduce or avoid nausea by administering capsules a few at a time over a 15-min period.
2. Report as scheduled for weekly cultures to determine that strains have not become resistant. A strain is considered resistant if the MIC value is greater than 100.
3. Report any volume reduction, blood, sediment, or cloudiness in the urine.
4. Side effects that interfere with dosing should be reported.
**Outcomes/Evaluate**
• Resolution of fungal infection
• Therapeutic drug levels (20–25 mcg/mL)

# Fludarabine phosphate

(floo-**DAIR**-ah-bean)
**Pregnancy Category:** D
Fludara **(Rx)**

**Classification:** Antineoplastic, antimetabolite

See also *Antineoplastic Agents.*
**Action/Kinetics:** Rapidly dephosphorylated to 2-fluoro-ara-A and then phosphorylated within the cell by the enzyme deoxycytidine kinase to the active 2-fluoro-ara-ATP. This compound inhibits DNA polymerase alpha, ribonucleotide reductase, and DNA primase, resulting in inhibition of DNA synthesis. **t½, 2-fluoro-ara-A:** About 10 hr. Approximately 23% of a dose of fludarabine is excreted in the urine as unchanged 2-fluoro-ara-A.
**Uses:** Chronic lymphocytic leukemia in individuals who have not responded to at least one standard alkylating agent-containing regimen. *Investigational:* Non-Hodgkin's lymphoma, macroglobulinemic lymphoma, prolymphocytic leukemia or prolymphocytoid variant of chronic lymphocytic leukemia, mycosis fungoides, hairy cell leukemia, Hodgkin's disease.
**Contraindications:** Lactation.
**Special Concerns:** Use with caution in clients with renal insufficiency. The safety and effectiveness of fludarabine in children and in previously untreated or nonrefractory chronic lymphocytic leukemia clients have not been established. Fludarabine produces dose-dependent toxic effects. An increased risk of toxicity is possible in geriatric clients, in renal insufficiency, and in bone marrow impairment.
**Side Effects:** *Hematologic:* Neutropenia, thrombocytopenia, anemia. *Tumor lysis syndrome:* Hyperuricemia, hyperphosphatemia, hypocalcemia, hyperkalemia, hematuria, metabolic acidosis, urate crystalluria, renal failure. Flank pain and hematuria may signal the onset of the syndrome. *GI:* N&V, anorexia, stomatitis, diarrhea, GI bleeding. *CNS:* Malaise, fatigue, weakness, agitation, confusion, coma. *Neuromuscular:* Peripheral neuropathy, paresthesia, myal-

F

gia. *Respiratory:* Pneumonia, dyspnea, cough, interstitial pulmonary infiltrate. *GU:* Dysuria, urinary infection, hematuria. *Miscellaneous:* Edema (common), skin rashes, fever, chills, **serious opportunistic infections,** pain, visual disturbances, hearing loss.

**OD** **Overdose Management:** *Symptoms:* Irreversible CNS toxicity including delayed blindness, **coma, and death.** Severe thrombocytopenia and neutropenia. *Treatment:* Discontinue administration of the drug and treat symptoms. The hematologic profile should be monitored.

**Dosage**
• **IV**
**Adults, usual:** 25 mg/m² given over a period of 30 min for 5 consecutive days. A 5-day course of therapy should be initiated every 28 days.

## NURSING CONSIDERATIONS

See also *Nursing Considerations* for *Antineoplastic Agents.*

**Administration/Storage**
**IV** 1. Dose may be decreased or delayed based on presence of hematologic or neurotoxicity.
2. After a maximal response noted, give three additional cycles, then discontinue drug.
3. Reconstitute the lyophilized product with 2 mL of sterile water for injection, USP. Each milliliter of the resulting solution will contain 25 mg fludarabine with the final pH ranging from 7.2 to 8.2. This may then be diluted in 100 or 125 mL of 5% dextrose injection, or 0.9% NaCl, and administered over 30 min.
4. Use reconstituted fludarabine within 8 hr as it contains no preservatives.
5. If solution comes in contact with the skin or mucous membranes, wash thoroughly with soap and water. Rinse eyes thoroughly with plain water.
6. Store the product under refrigeration at 2°C–8°C (36°F–46°F).

**Assessment**
1. Document indications for therapy; note previous agents used and outcome.

2. Document baseline CNS assessment; high doses may precipitate neurotoxicity.
3. Monitor hematologic and renal function studies. Nadir: 5–25 days.
**Client/Family Teaching**
1. Report any evidence of flank pain or hematuria; may precede a tumor lysis syndrome.
2. Practice barrier birth control.
3. Report any evidence of infection (sore throat, fever) or any abnormal bruising or bleeding.
**Outcomes/Evaluate:** Hematologic improvement; control of malignant process

# Fludrocortisone acetate
(flew-droh-**KOR**-tih-sohn)
**Pregnancy Category:** C
Florinef **(Rx)**
**Classification:** Mineralocorticoid

See also *Corticosteroids.*
**Action/Kinetics:** Produces marked sodium retention and inhibits excess adrenocortical secretion. Supplementary potassium may be indicated.
**Uses:** Addison's disease and adrenal hyperplasia.
**Contraindications:** Use systemically as an anti-inflammatory.

**Dosage**
• **Tablets**
*Addison's disease.*
0.1–0.2 mg/day to 0.1 mg 3 times/ week, usually in conjunction with hydrocortisone or cortisone.
*Salt-losing adrenogenital syndrome.*
0.1–0.2 mg/day.

## NURSING CONSIDERATIONS

See *Nursing Considerations* for *Corticosteroids.*
**Assessment**
1. Document clinical presentation and onset of symptoms.
2. Obtain baseline cortisol test, Na and K levels.
**Client/Family Teaching**
1. Addison's disease will require lifetime replacement therapy. Do not

stop drug abruptly; may precipitate Addison's crisis.

2. Review dietary recommendations of high-potassium, low-sodium diet.

**Outcomes/Evaluate:** Control of symptoms during adrenal cortical hypofunction

# Flumazenil
(floo-**MAZ**-eh-nill)
**Pregnancy Category:** C
Anexate ✹, Romazicon **(Rx)**
**Classification:** Benzodiazepine receptor antagonist

**Action/Kinetics:** Antagonizes the effects of benzodiazepines on the CNS by competitively inhibiting their action at the benzodiazepine recognition site on the GABA/benzodiazepine receptor complex. Does not antagonize the CNS effects of ethanol, general anesthetics, barbiturates, or opiates. Depending on the dose, there will be partial or complete antagonism of sedation, impaired recall, and psychomotor impairment. **Onset of reversal:** 1–2 min. **Peak effect:** 6–10 min. The duration of reversal is related to the plasma levels of the benzodiazepine and the dose of flumazenil. **Distribution t½, initial:** 7–15 min; **terminal t½:** 41–79 min. Metabolized in the liver with 90%–95% excreted through the urine and 5%–10% excreted in the feces. Hepatic impairment prolongs the half-life of the drug. Ingestion of food results in a 50% increase in clearance of flumazenil.

**Uses:** Complete or partial reversal of benzodiazepine-induced depression of the ventilatory responses to hypercapnia and hypoxia. Situations include cases where general anesthesia has been induced or maintained by benzodiazepines, where sedation has been produced by benzodiazepines for diagnostic and therapeutic procedures, and for the management of benzodiazepine overdosage.

**Contraindications:** Use in clients given a benzodiazepine for control of intracranial pressure or status epilepticus. In clients manifesting signs of serious cyclic antidepressant overdose. Use during labor and delivery or in children as the risks and benefits are not known. To treat benzodiazepine dependence or for the management of protracted benzodiazepine abstinence syndrome. Use until the effects of neuromuscular blockade have been fully reversed.

**Special Concerns:** The reversal of benzodiazepine effects may be associated with the onset of seizures in certain high-risk clients (e.g., concurrent major sedative-hypnotic drug withdrawal, recent therapy with repeated doses of parenteral benzodiazepines, myoclonic jerking or seizure activity prior to administration of flumazenil in cases of overdose, and concurrent cyclic antidepressant overdosage). Use with caution in clients with head injury as the drug may precipitate seizures or alter cerebral blood flow in clients receiving benzodiazepines. Use with caution in clients with alcoholism and other drug dependencies due to the increased frequency of benzodiazepine tolerance and dependence. Use with caution during lactation.

Flumazenil may precipitate a withdrawal syndrome if the client is dependent on benzodiazepines. Flumazenil may cause panic attacks in clients with a history of panic disorder.

Use with caution in mixed-drug overdosage as toxic effects (e.g., cardiac dysrhythmias, convulsions) may occur (especially with cyclic antidepressants).

**Side Effects:** *Deaths* have occurred in clients receiving flumazenil, especially in those with serious underlying disease or in those who have ingested large amounts of nonbenzodiazepine drugs (usually cyclic antidepressants) as part of an overdose.

---

*Seizures* are the most common serious side effect noted.

*CNS:* Dizziness, vertigo, ataxia, anxiety, nervousness, tremor, palpitations, insomnia, dyspnea, hyperventilation, abnormal crying, depersonalization, euphoria, increased tears, depression, dysphoria, paranoia, delirium, difficulty concentrating, *seizures,* somnolence, stupor, speech disorder. *GI:* N&V, hiccoughs, dry mouth. *CV:* Sweating, flushing, hot flushes, *arrhythmias (atrial, nodal, ventricular extrasystoles),* bradycardia, tachycardia, hypertension, chest pain. *At injection site:* Pain, thrombophlebitis, rash, skin abnormality. *Body as a whole:* Headache, increased sweating, asthenia, malaise, rigors, shivering, paresthesia. *Ophthalmologic:* Abnormal vision including visual field defect and diplopia; blurred vision. *Otic:* Transient hearing impairment, tinnitus, hyperacusis.

## Dosage

• **IV Only**

*To reverse conscious sedation or in general anesthesia.*

**Adults, initial:** 0.2 mg (2 mL) given IV over 15 sec. If the desired level of consciousness is not reached after waiting an additional 45 sec, a second dose of 0.2 mg (2 mL) can be given and repeated at 60-sec intervals, up to a maximum total dose of 1 mg (10 mL). Most clients will respond to doses of 0.6–1 mg. To treat resedation, give no more than 1 mg (given as 0.2 mg/min) at any one time and give no more than 3 mg in any 1 hr.

*Management of suspected benzodiazepine overdose.*

**Adults, initial:** 0.2 mg (2 mL) given IV over 30 sec; a second dose of 0.3 mg (3 mL) can be given over another 30 sec. Further doses of 0.5 mg (5 mL) can be given over 30 sec at 1-min intervals up to a total dose of 3 mg (although some clients may require up to 5 mg given slowly as described). If the client has not responded 5 min after receiving a cumulative dose of 5 mg, the major cause of sedation is probably not due to benzodiaze-

pines and additional doses of flumazenil are likely to have no effect. For resedation, repeated doses may be given at 20-min intervals; no more than 1 mg (given as 0.5 mg/min) at any one time and no more than 3 mg in any 1 hr should be administered.

## NURSING CONSIDERATIONS
### Administration/Storage

**IV** 1. Must individualize dosage. Give only the smallest amount that is effective. The 1-min wait between individual doses in the dose-titration recommended for general uses may be too short for high-risk clients as it takes 6–10 min for any single dose of flumazenil to reach full effects. Thus, slow the rate of administration in high-risk clients.

2. A major risk is resedation; the duration of effect of a long-acting or a large dose of a short-acting benzodiazepine may exceed that of flumazenil. If there is resedation, give repeated doses at 20-min intervals as needed.

3. Best given as a series of small injections to allow the provider to control reversal of sedation to desired end point and to decrease possibility of side effects.

4. Reduce the dose to 40%–60% of normal with severe hepatic dysfunction.

5. Give through a freely running IV infusion into a large vein to minimize pain at the injection site.

6. Doses larger than a total of 3 mg do not reliably produce additional effects.

7. Flumazenil is compatible with 5% dextrose in water, RL, and NSS solutions. If flumazenil is drawn into a syringe or mixed with any of these solutions, discard after 24 hr.

8. For optimum sterility, keep in the vial until just before use.

9. Before administering, have a secure airway and IV access; awaken clients gradually.

### Assessment
1. Note any history of seizure disorder or panic attacks.
2. Determine    type,    time,    and

amount of drug ingested; especially note any tricyclic antidepressant or mixed-drug overdose.

3. Document liver dysfunction; subsequent doses require adjustment.

4. Assess for evidence of head injury or increased ICP.

5. Note evidence of sedative or benzodiazepine dependence, alcohol abuse, or recent use of either; drug may precipitate withdrawal symptoms.

**Interventions**

1. The effects of flumazenil usually wear off before the effects of many benzodiazepines. Observe closely for resedation, depressed respirations, or other residual benzodiazepine effects for up to 2 hr after administration.

2. Flumazenil is intended as an adjunct to, not a substitute for, proper management of the airway, assisted breathing, circulatory access and support, use of lavage and charcoal, and adequate clinical evaluation. Prior to giving flumazenil, proper measures should be undertaken to secure an airway for ventilation and IV access. Be prepared for clients attempting to withdraw ET tubes or IV lines due to confusion and agitation following awakening; awakening should be gradual.

3. Drug should be used with caution in the ICU due to increased risk of unrecognized benzodiazepine dependence; may produce convulsions in benzodiazepine-dependent clients.

4. Not intended to be used to diagnose benzodiazepine-induced sedation in the ICU. Failure to respond may be masked by metabolic disorders, traumatic injury, or other drugs.

5. Incorporate seizure precautions; increased risk for seizures with large overdoses of cyclic antidepressants and with long-term benzodiazepine sedation.

6. Drug-associated convulsions may be treated with benzodiazepines, phenytoin, or barbiturates. (Higher doses of benzodiazepines may be needed.)

7. Do not use until the effects of neuromuscular blockade have been fully reversed.

8. Flumazenil does not consistently reverse amnesia. Therefore, clients may not remember instructions during the postprocedure period; provide written instructions.

**Client/Family Teaching**

1. Do not undertake any activities requiring complete alertness and do not operate hazardous machinery or a motor vehicle until at least 18–24 hr after discharge and until it has been determined that no residual sedative effects of benzodiazepines remain. Memory and judgment may be impaired.

2. Avoid alcohol or nonprescription drugs for 18–24 hr after administration of flumazenil or if the effects of the benzodiazepines persist.

**Outcomes/Evaluate:** Reversal of benzodiazepine sedative/psychomotor effects

# Flunisolide
(flew-**NISS**-oh-lyd)
**Pregnancy Category:** C
**Inhalation:** AeroBid, Bronalide Aerosol ✦ **(Rx), Intranasal:** Nasalide, Nasarel, Rhinalar ✦ **(Rx)**
**Classification:** Corticosteroid

See also *Corticosteroids*.

**Action/Kinetics:** Minimal systemic effects with intranasal use. Significant first-pass after inhalation; rapidly metabolized. Several days may be required for full beneficial effects. $t\frac{1}{2}$: 1.8 hr.

**Uses: Inhalation:** Prophylaxis and treatment of bronchial asthma in combination with other therapy. Not used when asthma can be relieved by other drugs, in clients where systemic corticosteroid treatment is infrequent, and in nonasthmatic bronchitis. **Intranasal:** Seasonal or perennial rhinitis, especially if other treatment has proven unsatisfactory.

**Contraindications:** Active or quiescent TB, especially of the respiratory tract. Untreated fungal, bacterial, systemic viral infections. Ocular herpes simplex. Use until healing occurs following recent ulceration of nasal septum, nasal surgery, or trauma. Lactation.

**Special Concerns:** Safety and effectiveness in children less than 6 years of age have not been determined.

**Additional Side Effects:** *Respiratory:* Hoarseness, coughing, throat irritation; *Candida* infections of nose, larynx, and pharynx. *After intranasal use:* Nasopharyngeal irritation, stinging, burning, dryness, headache. *GI:* Dry mouth. Systemic corticosteroid effects, especially if recommended dose is exceeded.

## Dosage

- **Inhalation**
  *Bronchial asthma.*
**Adults:** 2 inhalations (total of 500 mcg flunisolide) in a.m. and p.m., not to exceed 4 inhalations b.i.d. (i.e., total daily dose of 2,000 mcg). **Pediatric, 6–15 years:** 2 inhalations in the morning and evening, with total daily dose not to exceed 1,000 mcg.

- **Intranasal**
  *Rhinitis.*
**Adults, initial:** 50 mcg (2 sprays) in each nostril b.i.d.; may be increased to 2 sprays t.i.d. up to maximum daily dose of 400 mcg (i.e., 8 sprays in each nostril). **Pediatric, 6–14 years, initial:** 25 mcg (1 spray) in each nostril t.i.d. or 50 mcg (2 sprays) in each nostril b.i.d., up to maximum daily dose of 200 mcg (i.e., 4 sprays in each nostril). **Maintenance, adults, children:** Smallest dose necessary to control symptoms. Some clients (approximately 15%) are controlled on 1 spray in each nostril daily.

## NURSING CONSIDERATIONS

See also *Nursing Considerations* for *Corticosteroids.*
**Administration/Storage**
1. When initiating the inhalant in clients receiving systemic cortico-steroids, use aerosol concomitantly with the systemic steroid for 1 week. Then, slowly withdraw the systemic corticosteroid over several weeks.
2. If nasal congestion present, use a decongestant before administration to ensure drug reaches site of action.
3. If beneficial effects do not occur within 3 weeks, discontinue therapy. Improvement of symptoms usually is evident within a few days.
**Client/Family Teaching**
1. Use a demonstrator and instruct client and family how to administer nasal spray or inhalant.
2. Gargle and rinse mouth with water after inhalation to prevent alterations in taste and to maintain adequate oral hygiene. Report any symptoms of fungal infections.
3. Mild nasal bleeding may occur; this is usually transient.
**Outcomes/Evaluate**
- Improved airway exchange
- ↓ Allergic manifestations

# Fluorouracil (5-Fluorouracil, 5-FU)

(flew-roh-**YOUR**-ah-sill)
**Pregnancy Category:** X
Adrucil, Efudex, Fluoroplex (Abbreviation: 5-FU) **(Rx)**
**Classification:** Antineoplastic, antimetabolite

See also *Antineoplastic Agents.*
**Action/Kinetics:** Pyrimidine antagonist that inhibits the methylation reaction of deoxyuridylic acid to thymidylic acid. Thus, synthesis of DNA and, to a lesser extent, RNA is inhibited. Cell-cycle specific for the S phase of cell division. **t½, initial:** 5–20 min; **final:** 20 hr. From 60% to 80% eliminated as respiratory $CO_2$ (8–12 hr); small amount (15%) excreted unchanged in urine (1–6 hr). Highly toxic; initiate use in hospital. When used topically, the following response occurs:
- Early inflammation: erythema for several days (minimal reaction)
- Severe inflammation: burning, stinging, vesiculation

• Disintegration: erosion, ulceration, necrosis, pain, crusting, reepithelialization

• Healing: within 1–2 weeks with some residual erythema and temporary hyperpigmentation

**Uses: Systemic:** Palliative management of certain cancers of the rectum, stomach, colon, pancreas, and breast. In combination with levamisole for Dukes' stage C colon cancer after surgical resection. In combination with leucovorin for metastatic colorectal cancer. *Investigational:* Cancer of the bladder, ovaries, prostate, cervix, endometrium, lung, liver, head, and neck. Also, malignant pleural, peritoneal, and pericardial effusions. **Topical (as solution or cream):** Multiple actinic or solar keratoses. Superficial basal cell carcinoma. *Investigational:* Condylomata acuminata (1% solution in 70% ethanol or the 5% cream).

**Additional Contraindications: Systemic:** Clients in poor nutritional state, with severe bone marrow depression, severe infection, or recent (4-week-old) surgical intervention. Lactation. To be used with caution in clients with hepatic or liver dysfunction.

**Special Concerns:** Safety and efficacy of topical products have not been established in children. Occlusive dressings may result in increased inflammation in adjacent normal skin when topical products are used.

**Additional Side Effects: Systemic:** Esophagopharyngitis, myocardial ischemia, angina, acute cerebellar syndrome, photophobia, lacrimation, decreased vision. Also, arterial thrombosis, arterial ischemia, arterial aneurysm, bleeding or infection at site of catheter, thrombophlebitis, embolism, fibromyositis, abscesses. **Topical:** D*ermatologic:* Pain, pruritus, hyperpigmentation, irritation, inflammation, burning at site of application, scarring, soreness, allergic contact dermatitis, tenderness, scaling, swelling, suppuration, alopecia, photosensitivity, urticaria. *CNS:* Insomnia, irritability. *GI:* Stomatitis, medicinal taste. *Miscellaneous:* Lacrimation, telangiectasia, toxic granulation.

**OD Overdose Management:** *Symptoms:* N&V, diarrhea, GI ulceration, GI bleeding, thrombocytopenia, *agranulocytosis,* leukopenia. *Treatment:* Monitor hematologically for at least 4 weeks.

**Drug Interactions:** Leucovorin calcium ↑ toxicity of fluorouracil.

**Laboratory Test Interferences:** ↑ Alkaline phosphatase, LDH, serum bilirubin, and serum transaminase.

**Dosage** ──────────────

• **IV**

*Palliative management of selected carcinomas.*

**Individualize dosage. Initial:** 12 mg/kg/day for 4 days, not to exceed 800 mg/day. If no toxicity seen, administer 6 mg/kg on days 6, 8, 10, and 12. Discontinue therapy on day 12 even if there are no toxic symptoms. **Maintenance:** Repeat dose of first course q 30 days or when toxicity from initial course of therapy is gone; or, give 10–15 mg/kg/week as a single dose. Do not exceed 1 g/week. **If client is debilitated or is a poor risk:** 6 mg/kg/day for 3 days; if no toxicity, give 3 mg/kg on days 5, 7, and 9 (daily dose should not exceed 400 mg).

*Metastatic colorectal cancer.*

Leucovorin, **IV,** 200 mg/m²/day for 5 days followed by fluorouracil, **IV,** 370 mg/m²/day for 5 days. Repeat q 28 days to maximize response and to prolong survival.

*Dukes' stage C colon cancer after surgical resection.*

See *Levamisole.*

• **Cream, Topical Solution**

*Actinic or solar keratoses.*

Apply 1%–5% cream or solution to cover lesion 1–2 times/day for 2–6 weeks.

*Superficial basal cell carcinoma.*

F

Apply 5% cream or solution to cover lesion b.i.d. for 3–6 weeks (up to 10–12 weeks may be required).

## NURSING CONSIDERATIONS

See also *Nursing Considerations* for *Antineoplastic Agents*.

### Administration/Storage

1. Apply with fingertips, nonmetallic applicator, or rubber gloves. Wash hands immediately thereafter.
2. Avoid contact with eyes, nose, and mouth.
3. Limit occlusive dressings to lesions; cause increased inflammatory reactions in normal skin.
4. Complete healing of keratoses may require 2 months.
**IV** 5. Further dilution not needed; solution may be injected directly into the vein with a 25-gauge needle over 1–2 min.
6. Drug can be diluted in D5W or NSS and administered by IV infusion for periods of 30 min–8 hr. This method produces less systemic toxicity than rapid injection.
7. Do not mix with other drugs or IV additives.
8. If precipitate forms, resolubilize by heating to 60°C (140°F) with vigorous shaking. Allow to return to room temperature and allow air to settle out before withdrawing and administering medication.
9. Solution may discolor slightly during storage, but potency and safety are not affected.
10. Store in a cool place (10°C–27°C, or 50°F–80°F). Do not freeze. Excessively low temperature causes precipitation. Do not expose the solution to light.

### Assessment

1. Observe for intractable vomiting, stomatitis, and diarrhea; early signs of toxicity indicating immediate discontinuation of drug.
2. Hydrate well before and after therapy. Give antiemetics 1 hr before therapy.
3. Protect and supervise ambulation if symptoms of cerebellar dysfunction occur (altered balance, dizziness, or weakness).

4. Prevent exposure to strong sunlight and other ultraviolet rays; these intensify skin reactions.
5. Hair loss and mouth lesions may occur but are usually transient.
6. Use precautions and strict asepsis when WBC count is below 2,000/mm³.
7. Discontinue if WBC and platelet counts are depressed below 3,500/mm³ and 100,000/mm³, respectively. Nadir: 10–20 days; recovery: 30 days.

### Client/Family Teaching

1. Review and demonstrate appropriate method for topical administration.
2. Affected area may appear much worse before healing takes place in 1–2 months.
3. Drink plenty of fluids (2–3 L/day) during therapy.
4. Both men and women should practice barrier contraception during systemic therapy.
5. Avoid exposure to sunlight. If exposed, wear protective clothing, sunglasses, and sunscreen.
6. Hair loss and mouth sores may occur but are usually transient with parenteral therapy.

### Outcomes/Evaluate

- Control of malignant process
- Reepithelialization of skin lesion

# Fluoxetine hydrochloride
(flew-**OX**-eh-teen)

**Pregnancy Category:** B

Apo-Fluoxetine ✱, Dom-Fluoxetine ✱, Novo-Fluoxetine ✱, Nu-Fluoxetine ✱, PMS-Fluoxetine ✱, Prozac, STCC-Fluoxetine ✱ **(Rx)**

**Classification:** Antidepressant, miscellaneous

**Action/Kinetics:** Not related chemically to tricyclic, tetracyclic, or other antidepressants. Effect thought to be due to inhibition of uptake of serotonin into CNS neurons. Slight to no anticholinergic, sedative, or orthostatic hypotensive effects. Also binds to muscarinic, histaminergic, and alpha-1-adrenergic receptors, accounting for many of the side effects. Metabolized in the liver to norfluoxetine, a metabolite with equal potency to fluoxetine. Norfluoxetine is further metabolized by the liver to inactive metabolites that are excreted by the kidneys. **Time to peak plasma levels:** 6–8 hr. **Peak plasma concentrations:** 15–55 ng/mL. **t½, fluoxetine:** 2–7 days; **t½, norfluoxetine:** 7–9 days. **Time to steady state:** 2–4 weeks. Active drug maintained in the body for weeks after withdrawal.

**Uses:** Depression, obsessive-compulsive disorders (as defined in the current edition of DSM), bulimia nervosa. *Investigational:* Many (see *Dosage*).

**Contraindications:** Use with or within 14 days of discontinuing an MAO inhibitor.

**Special Concerns:** Use with caution during lactation and in clients with impaired liver or kidney function. Safety and efficacy have not been determined in children. A lower initial dose may be necessary in geriatric clients. Use in hospitalized clients, use for longer than 5–6 weeks for depression, or use for more than 13 weeks for obsessive-compulsive disorder has not been studied adequately.

**Side Effects:** A large number of side effects have been reported for this drug. Listed are those with a reported frequency of greater than 1%. *CNS:* Headache (most common), activation of mania or hypomania, insomnia, anxiety, nervousness, dizziness, fatigue, sedation, decreased libido, drowsiness, lightheadedness, decreased ability to concentrate, tremor, disturbances in sensation, agitation, abnormal dreams. Although less frequent than 1%, *some clients may experience seizures or attempt suicide. GI:* Nausea (most common), diarrhea, vomiting, constipation, dry mouth, dyspepsia, anorexia, abdominal pain, flatulence, alteration in taste, gastroenteritis, increased appetite. *CV:* Hot flashes, palpitations. *GU:* Sexual dysfunction, impotence, anorgasmia, frequent urination, in-

fection of the urinary tract, dysmenorrhea. *Respiratory:* Upper respiratory tract infections, pharyngitis, cough, dyspnea, rhinitis, bronchitis, nasal congestion, sinusitis, sinus headache, yawn. *Skin:* Rash, pruritus, excessive sweating. *Musculoskeletal:* Muscle, joint, or back pain. *Miscellaneous:* Flu-like symptoms, asthenia, fever, chest pain, allergy, visual disturbances, blurred vision, weight loss, bacterial or viral infection, limb pain, chills.

**Drug Interactions**

*Alprazolam* / ↑ Alprazolam levels and ↓ psychomotor performance

*Buspirone* / ↓ Effects of buspirone; worsening of obsessive-compulsive disorder

*Carbamazepine* / ↑ Serum levels of carbamazepine → toxicity

*Clozapine* / ↑ Serum clozapine levels

*Dextromethorphan* / Possibility of hallucinations

*Diazepam* / Fluoxetine ↑ half-life of diazepam → excessive sedation or impaired psychomotor skills

*Haloperidol* / ↑ Serum levels of haloperidol

*Lithium* / ↑ Serum levels of lithium → possible neurotoxicity

*MAO inhibitors* / MAO inhibitors should be discontinued 14 days before initiation of fluoxetine therapy due to the possibility of symptoms resembling a neuroleptic malignant syndrome or fatal reactions

*Phenytoin* / Fluoxetine may ↑ phenytoin levels

*Tricyclic antidepressants* / ↑ Pharmacologic and toxicologic effects of tricyclics due to ↓ breakdown by liver

*Tryptophan* / Symptoms of CNS toxicity (headache, sweating, dizziness, agitation, aggressiveness) or peripheral toxicity (N&V)

*Warfarin* / ↑ Bleeding diathesis with unaltered PT

**Dosage**
- **Capsules, Liquid**
  *Antidepressant.*

---

**Adults, initial:** 20 mg/day in the morning. If clinical improvement is not observed after several weeks, the dose may be increased to a maximum of 80 mg/day in two equally divided doses.

*Obsessive-compulsive disorder.*
**Initial:** 20 mg/day in the morning. If improvement is not significant after several weeks, the dose may be increased. **Usual dosage range:** 20–60 mg/day; the total daily dosage should not exceed 80 mg.

*Treatment of bulimia nervosa.*
60 mg/day given in the morning. May be necessary to titrate up to this dose over several days.

*Alcoholism.*
40–80 mg/day.

*Anorexia nervosa, bipolar II affective disorder, trichotillomania.*
20–80 mg/day.

*Attention deficit hyperactivity disorder, obesity, schizophrenia.*
20–60 mg/day.

*Borderline personality disorder.*
5–80 mg/day.

*Cataplexy and narcolepsy, Tourette's syndrome.*
20–40 mg/day.

*Kleptomania.*
60–80 mg/day.

*Migraine, chronic daily headaches, tension headaches.*
20 mg every other day to 40 mg/day.

*Posttraumatic stress disorder.*
10–80 mg/day.

*Premenstrual syndrome, recurrent syncope.*
20 mg/day.

*Levodopa-induced dyskinesia.*
40 mg/day.

*Social phobia.*
10–60 mg/day.

## NURSING CONSIDERATIONS
### Administration/Storage
1. Divide doses greater than 20 mg/day and give in the morning and at noon.
2. If doses lower than 20 mg are necessary, the drug may be emptied from the capsule into cranberry, orange, or apple juice; this should not be refrigerated (is stable for 2 weeks). *NOTE:* A liquid preparation (20 mg/5 mL) is also available.
3. The maximum therapeutic effect may not be observed until 4 weeks after beginning therapy.
4. Elderly clients, clients taking multiple medications, and those with liver or kidney dysfunction should take lower or less frequent doses.
5. When used for obsessive-compulsive disorders, therapy has been continued for over 6 months. However, reassess periodically to determine if continued drug therapy is needed.

### Assessment
1. Document indications for therapy, type and onset of symptoms.
2. Review drugs currently prescribed; note any that may interact unfavorably.
3. Determine if pregnant or lactating.
4. Obtain baseline liver and renal function studies; anticipate reduced dose with hepatic and/or renal insufficiency.
5. Periodically reassess client to determine need for continued therapy.

### Client/Family Teaching
1. Use caution when driving or performing tasks that require mental alertness; drug may cause drowsiness and/or dizziness.
2. Report any side effects, especially rashes, hives, increased anxiety, and loss of appetite.
3. Take medication at the specific times designated as nervousness and insomnia may occur.
4. It usually takes 1 month to note any significant benefits from therapy. Do not become discouraged and discontinue the medication before benefits are attained.
5. Avoid alcohol; do not take any OTC medications without approval.
6. Any thoughts of suicide or evidence of increased suicide ideations should be reported immediately.
7. Use reliable birth control during therapy.

### Outcomes/Evaluate
• ↓ Symptoms of depression, as evidenced by improved sleeping and

eating patterns, ↓ fatigue, and ↑ social involvement and activity
• Control of repetitive behavioral manifestations
• Improvement of symptoms for which drug prescribed

## Fluphenazine decanoate

(flew-**FEN**-ah-zeen)
Modecate Decanoate ✦, PMS-Fluphenazine ✦, Prolixin Decanoate, Rho-Fluphenazine Decanoate ✦ **(Rx)**

## Fluphenazine enanthate

(flew-**FEN**-ah-zeen)
Moditen Enanthate ✦, Prolixin Enanthate **(Rx)**

## Fluphenazine hydrochloride

(flew-**FEN**-ah-zeen)
Apo-Fluphenazine ✦, Permitil, Prolixin, Moditen HCl ✦, PMS-Fluphenazine ✦ **(Rx)**
**Classification:** Antipsychotic, piperazine-type phenothiazine

See also *Antipsychotic Agents, Phenothiazines*.
**Action/Kinetics:** High incidence of extrapyramidal symptoms and a low incidence of sedation, anticholinergic effects, antiemetic effects, and orthostatic hypotension. The enanthate and decanoate esters dramatically increase the duration of action. *Decanoate:* **Onset,** 24–72 hr; **peak plasma levels,** 24–48 hr; **t½** (approximate), 14 days; **duration,** up to 4 weeks. *Enanthate:* **Onset,** 24–72 hr; **peak plasma levels,** 48–72 hr; **t½** (approximate), 3.6 days; **duration,** 1–3 weeks.

Fluphenazine hydrochloride can be cautiously administered to clients with known hypersensitivity to other phenothiazines.

Fluphenazine enanthate may replace fluphenazine hydrochloride if desired response occurs with hypersensitivity reaction to fluphenazine.
**Uses:** Psychotic disorders. Adjunct to tricyclic antidepressants for chronic pain states (e.g., diabetic neuropathy, and clients trying to withdraw from narcotics).

**Dosage**

Fluphenazine hydrochloride is administered **PO and IM.** Fluphenazine enanthate or decanoate is administered **SC and IM.**

*Hydrochloride.*

• **Elixir, Oral Solution, Tablets**

*Psychotic disorders.*

**Adults and adolescents, initial:** 2.5–10 mg/day in divided doses q 6–8 hr; **then,** reduce gradually to maintenance dose of 1–5 mg/day (usually given as a single dose, not to exceed 20 mg/day). **Geriatric, emaciated, debilitated clients, initial:** 1–2.5 mg/day; **then,** dosage determined by response. **Pediatric:** 0.25–0.75 mg 1–4 times/day.

*Hydrochloride.*

• **IM**

*Psychotic disorders.*

**Adults and adolescents:** 1.25–2.5 mg q 6–8 hr as needed. Maximum daily dose: 10 mg. Elderly, debilitated, or emaciated clients should start with 1–2.5 mg/day.

*Decanoate.*

• **IM, SC**

*Psychotic disorders.*

**Adults, initial:** 12.5–25 mg; **then,** the dose may be repeated or increased q 1–3 weeks. The usual maintenance dose is 50 mg/1–4 weeks. Maximum adult dose: 100 mg/dose. **Pediatric, 12 years and older:** 6.25–18.75 mg/week; the dose can be increased to 12.5–25 mg given q 1–3 weeks. **Pediatric, 5–12 years:** 3.125–12.5 mg with this dose being repeated q 1–3 weeks.

*Enanthate.*

• **IM, SC**

*Psychotic disorders.*

**Adults and adolescents:** 25 mg; dose can be repeated or increased q 1–3 weeks. For doses greater than 50 mg, increases should be made in increments of 12.5 mg. Maximum adult dose: 100 mg.

## NURSING CONSIDERATIONS

See also *Nursing Considerations* for *Antipsychotic Agents, Phenothiazines.*

### Administration/Storage

1. Protect all forms of medication from light.
2. Store at room temperature and avoid freezing.
3. Color of parenteral solution may vary from colorless to light amber. Do not use solutions that are darker than light amber.
4. Do not mix the hydrochloride concentrate with any beverage containing caffeine, tannates (e.g., tea), or pectins (e.g., apple juice) due to a physical incompatibility.
5. Give the short-acting form when beginning phenothiazine therapy. Consider the decanoate and enanthate forms after the response to the drug has been evaluated and for those who demonstrate compliance problems.

### Assessment

1. Document indications for therapy, onset and duration of symptoms, other treatments utilized, and the outcome.
2. Note age, mental status, and physical condition. Elderly and debilitated clients are at increased risk for acute extrapyramidal symptoms.

### Client/Family Teaching

1. Review administration techniques; determine if client able to assume responsibility for self-medication.
2. Review written guidelines concerning side effects that should be reported and when to return for follow-up. Stress the importance of psychotherapy.

### Outcomes/Evaluate

- Improved behavior patterns with ↓ agitation, ↓ paranoia and withdrawal
- Control of tics

# Flurazepam hydrochloride

(flur-**AYZ**-eh-pam)
Apo-Flurazepam ✽, Dalmane, Dura-pam, Novo-Flupam ✽, PMS-Flu-razepam ✽, Somnol ✽, Som Pam ✽
**(C-IV) (Rx)**

**Classification:** Benzodiazepine seda-tive-hypnotic

See also *Tranquilizers, Antimanic Drugs, and Hypnotics.*

**Action/Kinetics:** Combines with benzodiazepine receptors, which are part of the benzodiazepine-GABA receptor-chloride ionophore complex. Results in enhanced inhibitory action of GABA leading to interference of transmission of nerve impulses in the reticular activating system. **Onset:** 17 min. The major active metabolite, *N*-desalkyl-flu-razepam, is active and has a t½ of 47–100 hr. **Time to peak plasma levels, flurazepam:** 0.5–1 hr; **active metabolite:** 1–3 hr. **Duration:** 7–8 hr. **Maximum effectiveness:** 2–3 days (due to slow accumulation of active metabolite). Significantly bound to plasma protein. Elimination is slow because metabolites remain in the blood for several days. Exceeding the recommended dose may result in development of tolerance and dependence.

**Uses:** Insomnia (all types). Flurazepam is increasingly effective on the second or third night of consecutive use and for one or two nights after the drug is discontinued.

**Contraindications:** Hypersensitivity. Pregnancy or in women wishing to become pregnant. Depression, renal or hepatic disease, chronic pulmonary insufficiency, children under 15 years.

**Special Concerns:** Use during the last few weeks of pregnancy may result in CNS depression of the neonate. Use during lactation may cause sedation and feeding problems in the infant. Geriatric clients may be more sensitive to the effects of flurazepam.

**Side Effects:** *CNS:* Ataxia, dizziness, drowsiness/sedation, headache, disorientation. Symptoms of stimulation including nervousness, apprehension, irritability, and talkativeness. *GI:* N&V, diarrhea, gastric upset or pain, heartburn, constipation. *Miscellaneous:* Arthralgia, chest pains, or palpitations. Rarely, symptoms of

allergy, SOB, jaundice, anorexia, blurred vision.
**Drug Interactions**
*Cimetidine* / ↑ Effect of flurazepam due to ↓ breakdown by liver
*CNS depressants* / Addition or potentiation of CNS depressant effects—drowsiness, lethargy, stupor, respiratory depression or collapse, coma, and possible death
*Disulfiram* / ↑ Effect of flurazepam due to ↓ breakdown by liver
*Ethanol* / Additive depressant effects up to the day following flurazepam administration
*Isoniazid* / ↑ Effect of flurazepam due to ↓ breakdown by liver
*Oral contraceptives* / Either ↑ or ↓ effect of benzodiazepines due to effect on breakdown by liver
*Rifampin* / ↓ Effect of benzodiazepines due to ↑ breakdown by liver
**Laboratory Test Interferences:** ↑ Alkaline phosphatase, bilirubin, serum transaminases.

**Dosage**
• **Capsules**
**Adults:** 15–30 mg at bedtime; 15 mg for geriatric and/or debilitated clients.

## NURSING CONSIDERATIONS

See also *Nursing Considerations* for *Tranquilizers, Antimanic Drugs, and Hypnotics.*
**Assessment**
1. Document indications for therapy, symptom onset, other agents prescribed, and the results.
2. Anticipate short-term therapy. Attempt to identify and address causative factors.
**Client/Family Teaching**
1. Use caution in driving or operating machinery until daytime sedative effects are evaluated. Report persistent morning "hangover."
2. With simple insomnia, try warm baths, warm drinks, soft music, white noise simulator, and other relaxation methods to induce sleep.
3. Avoid ingestion of alcohol.
4. Report tolerance and any symp-

toms of psychologic and/or physical dependence. Drug is for short-term therapy; continued use causes a tolerance and a decrease in drug responsiveness.
5. Keep a diary of foods, activities, and events for at least 5 days to determine if there are any relationships to insomnia condition.
**Outcomes/Evaluate:** Improved sleeping patterns and less frequent awakenings

# Flurbiprofen
(flur-**BIH**-proh-fen)
**Pregnancy Category:** B
Alti-Flurbiprofen ✹, Ansaid, Apo-Flurbiprofen ✹, Froben ✹, Froben SR ✹, Novo-Flurprofen ✹, Nu-Flurbiprofen ✹ **(Rx)**

# Flurbiprofen sodium
(flur-**BIH**-proh-fen)
**Pregnancy Category:** C
Flurbiprofen Sodium Ophthalmic, Ocufen **(Rx)**
**Classification:** Nonsteroidal antiinflammatory drug, ophthalmic and systemic use.

See also *Nonsteroidal Anti-Inflammatory Drugs.*
**Action/Kinetics:** By inhibiting prostaglandin synthesis, flurbiprofen reverses prostaglandin-induced vasodilation, leukocytosis, increased vascular permeability, and increased intraocular pressure. Also inhibits miosis occurring during cataract surgery. **PO form, time to peak levels:** 1.5 hr; t½: 5.7 hr.
**Uses: Ophthalmic:** Prevention of intraoperative miosis. **PO:** Rheumatoid arthritis, osteoarthritis. *Investigational:* Inflammation following cataract surgery, uveitis syndromes. Topically to treat cystoid macular edema. Primary dysmenorrhea, sunburn, mild to moderate pain.
**Contraindications:** Dendritic keratitis.
**Special Concerns:** Use with caution in clients hypersensitive to aspirin or other NSAIDs and during lacta-

tion. Wound healing may be delayed with use of the ophthalmic product. Acetylcholine chloride and carbachol may be ineffective when used with ophthalmic flubiprofen. Safety and efficacy in children have not been established.

**Additional Side Effects:** *Ophthalmic:* Ocular irritation, transient stinging or burning following use, delay in wound healing. Increased bleeding of ocular tissues in conjunction with ocular surgery.

**Dosage**
- **Ophthalmic Drops**

Beginning 2 hr before surgery, instill 1 gtt q 30 min (i.e., total of 4 gtt of 0.03% solution).
- **Tablets**

*Rheumatoid arthritis, osteoarthritis.*
**Adults, initial:** 200–300 mg/day in divided doses b.i.d.–q.i.d.; **then,** adjust dose to client response. Doses greater than 300 mg/day are not recommended.

*Dysmenorrhea.*
50 mg q.i.d.

## NURSING CONSIDERATIONS

See also *Nursing Considerations* for *Nonsteroidal Anti-Inflammatory Drugs.*

**Administration/Storage:** Use a dose of 300 mg only for initiating therapy or for treating acute exacerbations of the disease.

**Assessment**
1. Document indications for therapy.
2. Assess ROM of involved extremity, noting any discoloration, swelling, crepitus, or warmth.
3. Prior to eye surgery, carefully follow the prescribed dosing intervals.

**Client/Family Teaching**
1. May take tablets with food to decrease GI upset.
2. Review appropriate method of administering eye medication. Avoid rubbing eyes after medication administered; report any stinging, burning, or irritation immediately.
3. Report delays in wound healing.
4. Muscle-strengthening exercises should be performed daily.

**Outcomes/Evaluate**
- ↓ Pain and inflammation with ↑ joint mobility
- ↓ Optic inflammation
- ↓ Abnormal pupillary contractions

# Flutamide
(**FLOO**-tah-myd)
**Pregnancy Category:** D
Euflex ✦, Eulexin **(Rx)**
**Classification:** Antineoplastic, hormonal agent

See also *Antineoplastic Agents.*

**Action/Kinetics:** Acts either to inhibit uptake of androgen or to inhibit nuclear binding of androgen in target tissues. Thus, the effect of androgen is decreased in androgen-sensitive tissues. Rapidly metabolized to active (alpha-hydroxylated derivative) and inactive metabolites in the liver and mainly excreted in the urine. **t½ of active metabolite:** 6 hr (8 hr in geriatric clients). Ninety-four percent to 96% is bound to plasma proteins.

**Uses:** In combination with leuprolide acetate (i.e., a LHRH agonist) to treat stage $D_2$ metastatic prostatic carcinoma as well as locally confined stage $B_2$-C prostate cancer.

**Contraindications:** Use during pregnancy.

**Side Effects:** Side effects are listed for treatment of flutamide with LHRH agonist. *GU:* Loss of libido, impotence. *CV:* Hot flashes, hypertension. *GI:* N&V, diarrhea, GI disturbances, anorexia. *CNS:* Confusion, depression, drowsiness, anxiety, nervousness. *Hematologic:* Anemia, leukopenia, thrombocytopenia, **hemolytic anemia,** macrocytic anemia, methemoglobinemia. *Hepatic:* Hepatitis, cholestatic jaundice, hepatic encephalopathy, **hepatic necrosis.** *Dermatologic:* Rash, injection site irritation, erythema, ulceration, bullous eruptions, **epidermal necrolysis.** *Miscellaneous:* Gynecomastia, edema, neuromuscular symptoms, pulmonary symptoms, GU symptoms, malignant breast tumors.

**OD** **Overdose Management:** *Symptoms:* Breast tenderness, gynecomastia, increases in AST. Also possible are ataxia, anorexia, vomiting, decreased respiration, lacrimation, sedation, hypoactivity, and piloerection. *Treatment:* Induce vomiting if client is alert. Frequently monitor VS and observe closely.

**Laboratory Test Interferences:** ↑ AST, ALT, serum creatinine, SGGT, BUN, bilirubin

**Dosage**

• **Capsules**

*Locally confined stage B₂-C and stage D₂ metastatic cancer of the prostate.*

250 mg (2 capsules) t.i.d. q 8 hr for a total daily dose of 750 mg.

**NURSING CONSIDERATIONS**

See also *Nursing Considerations* for *Antineoplastic Agents*.

**Administration/Storage**

1. For stage B₂-C prostatic cancer, start flutamide and the LHRH agonist 8 weeks prior to initiating radiation therapy and continue during radiation therapy.

2. For maximum benefit in stage D₂ metastatic prostatic cancer, start flutamide and the LHRH agonist together and continue until disease progression.

**Assessment**

1. Document indications for therapy, agents previously used, and the outcome.

2. Administer with an LHRH agonist (such as leuprolide acetate).

3. Monitor CBC and LFTs during long-term therapy.

**Client/Family Teaching**

1. Take flutamide and the LHRH agonist (leuprolide) at the same time.

2. Drug therapy should not be interrupted or discontinued without consulting the provider.

3. Hot flashes, impotence, and diarrhea are all potential side effects of drug therapy; report if persistent or bothersome.

4. Male sexual problems may be drug induced (impotence, decreased

libido, gynecomastia). Counseling may be indicated.

5. Compliance may be a problem if diarrhea experienced. Manage diarrhea by cutting down on dairy products, drinking plenty of fluids, not using laxatives, using antidiarrheal products, and eating smaller, more frequent meals high in dietary fibers.

**Outcomes/Evaluate**

• ↓ Production of testosterone

• Control of metastatic processes

# Fluticasone propionate

(flu-**TIH**-kah-sohn)

**Pregnancy Category:** C

Flonase, Flovent **(Rx)**

**Classification:** Corticosteroid

See also *Corticosteroids*.

**Action/Kinetics:** Following intranasal use, a small amount is absorbed into the general circulation. **Onset:** Approximately 12 hr. **Maximum effect:** May take several days. Absorbed drug is metabolized in the liver and excreted in the urine.

**Uses:** Maintenance treatment of asthma in adults and children over four years of age. To manage seasonal and perennial allergic rhinitis in adults and children over four years of age.

**Contraindications:** Use for nonallergic rhinitis. Use following nasal septal ulcers, nasal surgery, or nasal trauma until healing has occurred.

**Special Concerns:** Safety and efficacy in children less than 12 years of age have not been determined. Clients on immunosuppressant drugs, such as corticosteroids, are more susceptible to infections. Use with caution, if at all, in active or quiescent tuberculosis infections; untreated fungal, bacterial, or systemic viral infections; or ocular herpes simplex. Use with caution during lactation.

**Side Effects:** *Allergic:* Rarely, immediate hypersensitivity reactions or contact dermatitis. *Respiratory:* Epistaxis, nasal burning, blood in nasal mucus, pharyngitis, irritation of nasal mucous membranes, sneezing, runny nose, nasal dryness, sinusitis, nasal congestion, bronchitis, nasal ulcer, nasal septum excoriation. *CNS:* Headache, dizziness. *Ophthalmologic:* Eye disorder, cataracts, glaucoma, increased intraocular pressure. *GI:* N&V, xerostomia. *Miscellaneous:* Unpleasant taste, urticaria. High doses have resulted in hypercorticism and adrenal suppression.

### Dosage

• **Metered Dose Inhaler**
*Treatment of asthma.*
**Adults and children over 4 years of age, initial:** 100 mcg b.i.d. For oral steroid sparing, the recommended dose is 1,000 mcg b.i.d.
• **Nasal Spray**
*Allergic rhinitis.*
**Adults and children over 4 years of age, initial:** One 50-mcg spray in each nostril once a day, for a total daily dose of 100 mcg/day. Maximum dose is two sprays (200 mcg) in each nostril once a day.
• **Ointment, Cream**
Apply sparingly to affected area 2–4 times daily.

## NURSING CONSIDERATIONS

See also *Nursing Considerations* for *Corticosteroids.*
**Administration/Storage**
1. Effectiveness depends on regular use.
2. Store the spray at 4°C–30°C (39°F–86°F).
**Assessment**
1. Document indications for therapy, note onset, duration of symptoms, and other agents trialed.
2. Examine for evidence of nasal septal ulcers; note turbinate findings.
3. Determine if immunocompromised or actively infected.
**Client/Family Teaching**
1. Review the technique for administration and demonstrate.
2. Take at regular intervals to ensure effectiveness; do not exceed prescribed dose, it may take several days to achieve full benefits.
3. Do not interrupt therapy if side

effects evident; notify provider as drug may require slow withdrawal. The dosage should also be slowly reduced if S&S of hypercorticism or adrenal suppression occur.
4. Report if S&S of adrenal insufficiency (depression, lassitude, joint and muscle pain) evident; especially when replacing systemic corticosteroids with topical.
5. Use adequate humidity, especially during winter months when dry heat may aggravate mucosa.
6. Avoid persons with active infections. Report exposure to chicken pox or measles. (If not immunized or previously infected with the disease, Varicella or Immune Globulin prophylaxis may be administered to high-risk clients on long-term therapy).
7. Height and weight will be monitored periodically in adolescents to detect any evidence of growth suppression.
8. Identify triggers that aggravate asthma (dust, pollen, smoke, chemicals, pets). Use peak flow meter; mark key zones to help manage asthma.
**Outcomes/Evaluate**
• Control of asthma
• ↓ Symptoms of allergic rhinitis

# Fluvastatin sodium
(flu-vah-**STAH**-tin)
**Pregnancy Category:** X
Lescol **(Rx)**
**Classification:** Antihyperlipidemic agent

See also *Antihyperlipidemic Agents—HMG-CoA Reductase Inhibitors.*
**Action/Kinetics:** $t\frac{1}{2}$: 1.2 hr. Undergoes extensive first-pass metabolism. Significantly bound (greater than 98%) to plasma protein. Metabolized in the liver with 90% excreted through the feces and 5% through the urine.
**Uses:** Adjunct to diet for the reduction of elevated total and LDL cholesterol levels in clients with primary hypercholesterolemia. The lipid-lowering effects of fluvastatin are enhanced

when it is combined with a bile-acid binding resin or with niacin. To slow the progression of coronary atherosclerosis in coronary heart disease.

**Special Concerns:** Use with caution in clients with severe renal impairment.

**Side Effects:** Side effects listed are those most common with fluvastatin. A complete list of possible side effects is provided under *Antihyperlipidemic Agents—HMG-CoA Reductase Inhibitors. GI:* N&V, diarrhea, abdominal pain or cramps, constipation, flatulence, dyspepsia, tooth disorder. *Musculoskeletal:* Muscle cramps or pain, back pain, arthropathy. *CNS:* Headache, dizziness, insomnia. *Respiratory:* Upper respiratory infection, rhinitis, cough, pharyngitis, sinusitis, bronchitis. *Miscellaneous:* Rash, pruritus, fatigue, influenza, allergy, accidental trauma.

**Dosage** ———————

• **Capsules**
*Antihyperlipidemic to slow progression of coronary atherosclerosis.* **Adults:** 20 mg once daily at bedtime. **Dose range:** 20–40 mg/day as a single dose in the evening. Splitting the 40-mg dose into a twice-daily regimen results in a modest improvement in LDL cholesterol.

## NURSING CONSIDERATIONS

See also *Nursing Considerations* for *Antihyperlipidemic Agents—HMG-CoA Reductase Inhibitors.*

**Administration/Storage**
1. Maximum reductions of LDL cholesterol are usually seen within 4 weeks; order periodic lipid determinations during this time, with dosage adjusted accordingly.
2. To avoid fluvastatin binding to a bile-acid binding resin (if given together), give the fluvastatin at bedtime and the resin at least 2 hr before.

**Assessment**
1. Monitor LFTs and total cholesterol profile every 3 to 6 months.
2. Evaluate on a standard cholesterol-lowering diet before giving flu-

vastatin. Continue diet during treatment.

**Client/Family Teaching**
1. May be taken with or without food but is usually consumed with the evening meal.
2. These drugs are used to help lower blood cholesterol and fat levels, which have been proven to promote CAD.
3. Must continue dietary restrictions of saturated fat and cholesterol and regular exercise programs in addition to drug therapy in the overall goal of lowering serum cholesterol levels.

**Outcomes/Evaluate:** ↓ Triglycerides, LDL, and total cholesterol levels

# Fluvoxamine maleate
(flu-**VOX**-ah-meen)
**Pregnancy Category:** C
Luvox **(Rx)**
**Classification:** Selective serotonin-uptake inhibitor

**Action/Kinetics:** Mechanism in obsessive-compulsive disorders is likely due to inhibition of serotonin reuptake in the CNS. Produces few if any anticholinergic, sedative, or orthostatic hypotensive effects. **Maximum plasma levels:** 3–8 hr. About 80% if bound to plasma proteins. t½: 13.6–15.6 hr. **Peak plasma concentration:** 88–546 ng/mL. **Time to reach steady state:** 3–8 hr. Elderly clients manifest higher mean plasma levels and a decreased clearance. Metabolized in the liver and excreted through the urine.

**Uses:** Obsessive-compulsive disorder (as defined in DSM-III-R) for adults, adolescents, and children. *Investigational:* Treatment of depression.

**Contraindications:** Concomitant use with astemizole or terfenadine. Alcohol ingestion. Use with MAO inhibitors or within 14 days of discontinuing treatment with a MAO inhibitor. Lactation.

---

**Special Concerns:** Use with caution in clients with a history of mania, seizure disorders, and liver dysfunction and in those with diseases that could affect hemodynamic responses or metabolism. Safety and efficacy have not been determined in children less than 18 years of age.

**Side Effects:** Side effects listed occur at an incidence of 0.1% or greater. *CNS:* Somnolence, insomnia, nervousness, dizziness, tremor, anxiety, hypertonia, agitation, decreased libido, depression, CNS stimulation, amnesia, apathy, hyperkinesia, hypokinesia, manic reaction, myoclonus, psychoses, fatigue, malaise, agoraphobia, akathisia, ataxia, *convulsion,* delirium, delusion, depersonalization, drug dependence, dyskinesia, dystonia, emotional lability, euphoria, extrapyramidal syndrome, unsteady gait, hallucinations, hemiplegia, hostility, hypersomnia, hypochondriasis, hypotonia, hysteria, incoordination, increased libido, neuralgia, paralysis, paranoia, phobia, sleep disorders, stupor, twitching, vertigo. *GI:* Nausea, dry mouth, diarrhea, constipation, dyspepsia, anorexia, vomiting, flatulence, toothache, tooth caries, dysphagia, colitis, eructation, esophagitis, gastritis, gastroenteritis, **GI hemorrhage,** GI ulcer, gingivitis, glossitis, hemorrhoids, melena, rectal hemorrhage, stomatitis. *CV:* Palpitations, hypertension, postural hypotension, vasodilation, syncope, tachycardia, angina pectoris, bradycardia, **cardiomyopathy,** CV disease, cold extremities, conduction delay, **heart failure, MI,** pallor, irregular pulse, ST segment changes. *Respiratory:* Upper respiratory infection, dyspnea, yawn, increased cough, sinusitis, asthma, bronchitis, epistaxis, hoarseness, hyperventilation. *Body as a whole:* Headache, asthenia, flu syndrome, chills, malaise, edema, weight gain or loss, dehydration, hypercholesterolemia, allergic reaction, neck pain, neck rigidity, photosensitivity, **suicide attempt.** *Dermatologic:* Excessive sweating, acne, alopecia, dry skin, eczema, exfoliative dermatitis, furunculosis, seborrhea, skin discoloration, urticaria. *Musculoskeletal:* Arthralgia, arthritis, bursitis, generalized muscle spasm, myasthenia, tendinous contracture, tenosynovitis. *GU:* Delayed ejaculation, urinary frequency, impotence, anorgasmia, urinary retention, anuria, breast pain, cystitis, delayed menstruation, dysuria, female lactation, hematuria, menopause, menorrhagia, metrorrhagia, nocturia, polyuria, PMS, urinary incontinence, UTI, urinary urgency, impaired urination, **vaginal hemorrhage,** vaginitis. *Hematologic:* Anemia, ecchymosis, leukocytosis, lymphadenopathy, thrombocytopenia. *Ophthalmic:* Amblyopia, abnormal accommodation, conjunctivitis, diplopia, dry eyes, eye pain, mydriasis, photophobia, visual field defect. *Otic:* Deafness, ear pain, otitis media. *Miscellaneous:* Taste perversion or loss, parosmia, hypothyroidism, hypercholesterolemia, dehydration.

**OD** **Overdose Management:** *Treatment:* Establish an airway and maintain respiration as needed. Monitor VS and ECG. Activated charcoal may be as effective as emesis or lavage in removing the drug from the GI tract. Since absorption in overdose may be delayed, measures to reduce absorption may be required for up to 24 hr.

**Drug Interactions**
*Astemisole* / ↑ Risk of severe cardiovascular effects, including QT prolongation, ventricular tachycardia, and torsades de pointes (may be fatal)
*Beta-adrenergic blockers* / Possible ↑ effects on BP and HR
*Carbamazepine* / ↑ Risk of carbamazepine toxicity
*Cloxapine* / ↑ Risk of orthostatic hypotension and seizures
*Diazepam* / ↑ Effect of diazepam due to ↓ clearance
*Diltiazem* / ↑ Risk of bradycardia
*Haloperidol* / ↑ Serum levels of haloperidol
*Lithium* / ↑ Risk of seizures
*MAO inhibitors* / Serious and possibly fatal reactions, including hyperthermia, rigidity, myoclonus, rapid

fluctuations of VS, changes in mental status (agitation, delirium, coma)

*Methadone* / ↑ Risk of methadone toxicity

*Midazolam* / ↑ Effect of midazolam due to ↓ clearance

*Sumatriptan* / ↑ Risk of weakness, hyperreflexia, incoordination

*Terfenadine* / ↑ Risk of severe cardiovascular effects, including QT prolongation, ventricular tachycardia, and torsades de pointes (may be fatal)

*Theophylline* / ↑ Risk of theophylline toxicity (decrease dose by one-third the usual daily maintenance dose)

*Triazolam* / ↑ Effect of triazolam due to ↓ clearance

*Tricyclic antidepressants* / Significant ↑ in plasma levels of tricyclic antidepressants

*Tryptophan* / ↑ Risk of central toxicity (headache, sweating, dizziness, agitation, aggressiveness, worsening of obsessive-compulsive disorder) or peripheral toxicity (N&V)

*Warfarin* / ↑ Plasma levels of warfarin

**Dosage** ————————
• **Tablets**
*Obsessive-compulsive disorder.*
**Adults, initial:** 50 mg at bedtime; **then,** increase the dose in 50-mg increments q 4–7 days, as tolerated, until a maximum benefit is reached, not to exceed 300 mg/day. **Children and adolescents:** 25 mg at bedtime; **then,** increase the dose in 25-mg increments q 4–7 days until a maximum benefit is reached, not to exceed 200 mg/day.

**NURSING CONSIDERATIONS**
**Administration/Storage**
1. If total daily dose exceeds 100 mg, give in two divided doses. If the doses are unequal, give the larger dose at bedtime.
2. Initial and incremental doses may need to be lower in geriatric clients.

3. Use lowest effective dose; assess periodically to determine need for continued treatment.
4. Use for more than 10 weeks has not been evaluated.
**Assessment**
1. Document indications for therapy and presenting or described behaviorial manifestations.
2. List agents currently prescribed to ensure none interact unfavorably.
3. Note history of mania, seizure disorders, or liver dysfunction.
4. Monitor ECG, CBC, and liver and renal function studies.
**Client/Family Teaching**
1. Take only as directed, usually at bedtime, do not exceed dosage.
2. May cause dizziness and drowsiness. Do not perform activities that require mental or physical alertness until drug effects realized.
3. Report any rash, hives, or unusual itching; increased depression or suicide ideations
4. Avoid alcohol and any other prescriptions or OTC agents without provider approval.
5. Practice reliable birth control.
6. Report for scheduled appointments so response to therapy, dosage, and need for continued therapy can be determined.
**Outcomes/Evaluate**
• Reduction in excessive, repetitive behaviors
• Control of persistent, recurrent thoughts, ideas, impulses, or images

# Folic acid
(**FOH**-lik **AH**-sid)
**Pregnancy Category:** A
Apo-Folic ✽, Foldine ✽, Folvite, Novo-Folacid ✽ **(Rx) (OTC)**
**Classification:** Vitamin B complex

**Action/Kinetics:** Folic acid (which is converted to tetrahydrofolic acid) is necessary for normal production of RBCs and for synthesis of nucleoproteins. Tetrahydrofolic acid is a cofactor in the biosynthesis of purines and thymidylates of nucleic acids. Megaloblastic and macrocytic anemias in folic acid deficiency are believed to be due to impairment of thymidylate synthesis. Natural sources of folic acid include liver, dried beans, peas, lentils, whole-wheat products, asparagus, beets, broccoli, brussels sprouts, spinach, and oranges. Synthetic folic acid is absorbed from the GI tract even if the client suffers from malabsorption syndrome. **Peak plasma levels after an oral dose:** 1 hr. It is stored in the liver.

**Uses:** Treatment of megaloblastic anemias due to folic acid deficiency (e.g., tropical and nontropical sprue, pregnancy, infancy or childhood, nutritional causes). Diagnosis of folate deficiency.

**Contraindications:** Use in aplastic, normocytic, or pernicious anemias (is ineffective). Folic acid injection that contains benzyl alcohol should not be used in neonates or immature infants.

**Special Concerns:** Daily folic acid doses of 0.1 mg or greater may obscure pernicious anemia. Prolonged folic acid therapy may cause decreased vitamin $B_{12}$ levels.

**Side Effects:** *Allergic:* Skin rash, itching, erythema, general malaise, respiratory difficulty due to bronchospasm. *GI:* Nausea, anorexia, abdominal distention, flatulence, bitter or bad taste (in those taking 15 mg/day for 1 month). *CNS:* In doses of 15 mg daily, altered sleep patterns, irritability, excitement, difficulty in concentration, overactivity, depression, impaired judgment, confusion.

**Drug Interactions**
*Aminosalicylic acid* / ↓ Serum folate levels
*Corticosteroids (chronic use)* / ↑ Folic acid requirements
*Methotrexate* / Is a folic acid antagonist
*Oral contraceptives* / ↑ Risk of folate deficiency
*Phenytoin* / Folic acid ↑ seizure frequency; also, phenytoin ↓ serum folic acid levels.
*Pyrimethamine* / Folic acid ↓ effect of pyrimethamine in toxoplasmosis; also, pyrimethamine is a folic acid antagonist
*Sulfonamides* / ↓ Absorption of folic acid
*Triamterene* / ↓ Utilization of folic acid as it is a folic acid antagonist
*Trimethoprim* / ↓ Utilization of folic acid as it is a folic acid antagonist

**Dosage**
• **Tablets**
*Dietary supplement.*
**Adults and children:** 100 mcg/day (up to 1 mg in pregnancy); may be increased to 500–1,000 mcg if requirements increase.
*Treatment of deficiency.*
**Adults, initial:** 250–1,000 mcg/day until a hematologic response occurs; **maintenance:** 400 mcg/day (800 mcg during pregnancy and lactation). **Pediatric, initial:** 250–1,000 mcg/day until a hematologic response occurs. **Maintenance, infants:** 100 mcg/day; **children up to 4 years:** 300 mcg/day; **children 4 years and older:** 400 mcg/day.
• **IM, IV, Deep SC**
*Treatment of deficiency.*
**Adults and children:** 250–1,000 mcg/day until a hematologic response occurs.
*Diagnosis of folate deficiency.*
**Adults, IM:** 100–200 mcg/day for 10 days plus low dietary folic acid and vitamin $B_{12}$.

## NURSING CONSIDERATIONS
### Administration/Storage
1. Given PO; if there is severe malabsorption, give either IV or SC.
2. Regardless of age, the dosage should never be less than 0.1 mg/day.
**IV** 3. Folic acid will remain stable in solution if the pH is kept above 5.
4. May be administered IM, by direct IV push or added to infusions. When given IV, the rate should not exceed 5 mcg/min.
5. When parenteral forms are used, have drugs and equipment available to treat anaphylactic reactions.
### Assessment
1. Document baseline CBC, reticu-

locytes, MCV, and serum folate and $B_{12}$ levels.

2. Review drugs prescribed; oral contraceptives, trimethoprim, hydantoins, and alcohol may cause increased body loss of folic acid.

**Client/Family Teaching**

1. Take only as directed.

2. Dietary sources of folic acid include dark green leafy vegetables, beans, fortified breads, and cereals. Prolonged cooking destroys folate in vegetables.

3. Drug may discolor urine a deep yellow.

4. U.S. Public Health Service recommends that all women of childbearing age consume 0.4 mg of folic acid to reduce the risk of neural tube birth defects. Folic acid may prevent the development of spina bifida or anencephaly, which occur during the first month of pregnancy.

**Outcomes/Evaluate**

• Desired hematologic response

• Reversal in symptoms of folic acid deficiency and megaloblastic anemia

• Prophylaxis of newborn neural tube defects

---

# Follitropin alfa

(fol-ih-**TROH**-pin **AL**-fah)
**Pregnancy Category:** X
Gonal-F **(Rx)**

# Follitropin beta

(fol-ih-**TROH**-pin **BAY**-tah)
**Pregnancy Category:** X
Follistim **(Rx)**
**Classification:** Ovarian stimulant, gonadotropin

---

**Action/Kinetics:** Both products are human FSH prepared by recombinant DNA technology. When given with HCG, products stimulate ovarian follicular growth in women who do not have primary ovarian failure. Steady state plasma levels reached within 4 to 5 days. Increased body weight or body mass index (BMI) results in a decrease in rate of absorption. Increased risk of multiple births.

**Uses:** Induction of ovulation and pregnancy in anovulatory infertile clients where cause of infertility is functional. To stimulate development of multiple follicles in ovulatory clients undergoing in-vitro fertilization.

**Contraindications:** Use in primary ovarian failure; uncontrolled thyroid or adrenal dysfunction; in presence of any cause of infertility other than anovulation; tumor of ovary, breast, uterus, hypothalamus, or pituitary gland; abnormal vaginal bleeding of undetermined origin; ovarian cysts or enlargement not due to polycystic ovary syndrome; pregnancy; use in children; hypersensitivity to products.

**Special Concerns:** Use with caution during lactation.

**Side Effects:** *CV:* Intravascular thrombosis and embolism causing venous thrombophlebitis, ***pulmonary embolism,*** pulmonary infarction, stroke, arterial occlusion (leading to loss of limb). *Pulmonary:* Atelectasis, acute respiratory distress syndrome, exacerbation of asthma. *Ovarian hyperstimulation syndrome:* Ovarian enlargement, abdominal pain/distention, N&V, diarrhea, dyspnea, oliguria, ascites, pleural effusion, hypovolemia, electrolyte imbalance, hemoperitoneum, thromboembolic events. *Hypersensitivity:* Febrile reaction, chills, musculoskeletal aches, joint pains, malaise, headache, fatigue. *GI:* N&V, diarrhea, abdominal cramps, bloating. *Dermatologic:* Dry skin, body rash, hair loss, hives. *Miscellaneous:* Ovarian cysts, pain, swelling, headache, irritation at site of injection, breast tenderness.

**Dosage** —————————

FOLLITROPIN ALFA

• **SC only**

*Ovulation induction.*

**Initial, first cycle:** 75 IU/day. An incremental adjustment up to 37.5 IU may be considered after 14 days; further increases can be made, if

---

needed, every 7 days. To complete follicular development and effect ovulation in absence of an endogenous LH surge, give 5,000 units of HCG 1 day after last dose of follitropin alfa. Withold HCG if serum estradiol is greater than 2,000 pg/mL. Base initial dose in subsequent cycles on response in the preceding cycle. Doses greater than 300 IU/day are not recommended routinely. As in initial cycle, HCG at a dose of 5,000 is given 1 day after last dose of follitropin alfa.

*Follicle stimulation.*

Initiate on day 2 or 3 of the follicular phase at a dose of 150 IU/day, until sufficient follicular development is achieved. Usually, therapy does not exceed 10 days. In those undergoing in vitro fertilization whose endogenous gonadotropin levels are suppressed, initiate follitropin alfa at a dose of 225 IU/day. Consider dosage adjustments after 5 days based on client response; adjust subsequent dosage every 3 to 4 days and by less than 75 to 150 IU additional drug at each adjustment, not to exceed 450 IU/day. Once follicular development is achieved, give HCG, 5,000–10,000 units, to cause final follicular maturation in preparation for oocyte retrieval.

FOLLITROPIN BETA
• **SC, IM**
*Ovulation induction.*

Use stepwise, gradually increasing dosage regimen. **Initial:** 75 IU/day for up to 14 days; increase by 37.5 IU at weekly intervals until follicular growth or serum estradiol levels indicate response. Maximum daily dose: 300 IU. Treat until ultrasonic visualization or serum estradiol levels indicate pre-ovulatory conditions greater than or equal to normal values. Then, give HCG 5,000–10,000 IU.

*Follicle stimulation.*

**Initial:** 150–225 IU for first 4 days of treatment. Dose may be adjusted based on ovarian response. Daily maintenance doses from 75–300 IU (however, doses from 375–600 IU have been used) for 6 to 12 days are usually sufficient. Maximum daily dose: 600 IU. When sufficient number of follicles of adequate size are present, induce final maturation by giving HCG, 5,000–10,000 IU. Oocyte retrieval is undertaken 34–36 hr later.

## NURSING CONSIDERATIONS
### Administration/Storage
1. For follitropin alfa or follitropin beta:
• Store vials in refrigerator or at room temperature and protect from light.
• Use immediately after reconstitution; discard unused drug.
2. For follitropin alfa, dissolve powder from one or more vials in 0.5–1 mL of sterile water for injection. Concentration should not exceed 225 IU/0.5 mL.
3. For follitropin beta, inject 1 mL of 0.45% NaCl injection into the vial. Do not shake but gently swirl until the solution is clear. It usually dissolves immediately.
4. When using either drug, if ovaries are abnormally enlarged on last day of therapy, withhold HCG to reduce risk of ovarian hyperstimulation syndrome.

### Assessment
1. Document history, physical exam including gynecologic and endocrine evaluation, and indications for therapy.
2. Obtain serum hormonal levels, gonadotropin levels, pregnancy test, CBC, lytes, thyroid and adrenal function studies; document neurovascular assessments (esp.; peripheral pulses).
3. Determine partner's fertility potential.

### Interventions
1. Obtain urinary estrogen excretion levels daily. If greater than 100 mcg or if daily estriol excretion exceeds 50 mcg, *withhold HCG* and report; these signal impending hyperstimulation syndrome.
2. If hospitalized for hyperstimulation, perform following interventions:
• Place client on bed rest.
• Monitor I&O; weigh daily.

- Monitor urine sp. gravity, serum and urine lytes.
- Assess for hemoconcentration. May need heparin to prevent hypercoagulability.
- Increase fluid intake; replace electrolytes.
- Provide analgesics for comfort.

3. Monitor for respiratory distress or exacerbation of asthma.

4. Report any unexplained fever, ovarian enlargement, or complaints of abdominal pain.

**Client/Family Teaching**

1. Dose is individualized. Alfa is given SC in the abdomen or upper thigh at 45 ° angle; beta is given SC or IM with IM administered in upper outer buttocks muscle at 90° angle.

2. Report any pain, coolness, or pale bluish color of an extremity (signs of arterial bloodclot).

3. Fever or development of lower abdominal pain may be result of overstimulation of ovaries that has caused cysts to form, loss of fluid into peritoneum, or bleeding; report immediately. Need exam for this at least every other day during drug therapy and for 2 weeks thereafter; hospitalization is necessary if evident.

4. Take basal body temperature and graph.

5. Signs that indicate ovulation include increase in basal body temperature, and increase in appearance and volume of cervical mucus.

6. Engage in daily intercourse from day before HcG is administered until ovulation occurs.

7. If symptoms indicate overstimulation of ovaries, significant ovarian enlargement may have occurred. Report and abstain from intercourse because of increased risk of ovarian cyst rupture.

8. Pregnancy usually occurs 4–6 weeks after completion of therapy. Multiple births may occur.

**Outcomes/Evaluate:** Induction of ovulation; pregnancy

# Foscarnet sodium
(fos-**KAR**-net)
**Pregnancy Category:** C
Foscavir **(Rx)**
**Classification:** Antiviral agent

See also *Antiviral Agents*.

**Action/Kinetics:** Inhibits replication of all known herpes viruses by selective inhibition at the pyrophosphate binding site on virus-specific DNA polymerases and reverse transcriptases at levels that do not affect cellular DNA polymerases. Active against herpes simplex virus mutants deficient in thymidine kinase. CMV strains resistant to ganciclovir may be sensitive to foscarnet; viral reactivation of CMV occurs after termination of foscarnet therapy. The latent state of any of the human herpes viruses is not sensitive to foscarnet. Believed to accumulate in human bone and has variable penetration into the CSF. **t½, plasma:** About 3 hr. Approximately 80%–90% of IV foscarnet is excreted unchanged through the urine.

**Uses:** Treatment of CMV retinitis in clients with AIDS. Treatment of acyclovir-resistant HSV infections in immunocompromised clients. With ganciclorvir in those who have relapsed after monotherapy with either drug.

**Special Concerns:** Use with caution during lactation and in clients with impaired renal function (the effects of the drug have not been determined in clients with a creatinine clearance less than 50 mL/min or serum creatinine more than 2.8 mg/dL). Use with caution with drugs that alter serum calcium levels as foscarnet decreases serum levels of ionized calcium. Safety and effectiveness have not been determined in children, for the treatment of other CMV infections such as pneumonitis or gastroenteritis, for congenital or neonatal CMV disease, and in non-immunocompromised clients. Transient changes in electrolytes may increase the risk of cardiac disturbances and seizures. Side effects such as renal impairment, electrolyte abnormalities, and seizures may contribute to client death. The drug is not a cure for HSV infections and relapse occurs in most clients. Repeated treatment has led to the development of viral resistance.

**Side Effects:** *GU:* Renal impairment (most common), albuminuria, dysuria, polyuria, urinary retention, urethral disorder, UTIs, *acute renal failure,* nocturia, hematuria, glomerulonephritis, urinary frequency, toxic nephropathy, nephrosis, urinary incontinence, pyelonephritis, renal tubular disorders, urethral irritation, uremia, perineal pain in women, penile inflammation. *Metabolic/Electrolyte:* Hypocalcemia, hypokalemia, hypomagnesemia, hypophosphatemia, hyponatremia, hyperphosphatemia, hypercalcemia, acidosis, thirst, decreased weight, dehydration, glycosuria, diabetes mellitus, abnormal glucose tolerance, hypochloremia, hypervolemia, hypoproteinemia. *Hematologic:* Anemia (one-third of clients), granulocytopenia, neutropenia, leukopenia, thrombocytopenia, platelet abnormalities, thrombosis, WBC abnormalities, lymphadenopathy, coagulation disorders, decreased coagulation factors, decreased prothrombin, hypochromic anemia, pancytopenia, hemolysis, leukocytosis, cervical lymphadenopathy, lymphopenia. *Body as a whole:* Fever, fatigue, asthenia, pain, infection, rigors, malaise, sepsis, death, back or chest pain, cachexia, flu-like symptoms, edema, bacterial or fungal infections, abscess, moniliasis, leg edema, peripheral edema, hypothermia, syncope, substernal chest pain, ascites, *malignant hyperpyrexia,* herpes simplex, viral infections, toxoplasmosis. *CNS:* Headache, dizziness, *seizures (including tonic-clonic),* tremor, ataxia, dementia, stupor, meningitis, aphasia, abnormal coordination, EEG abnormalities, vertigo, coma, encephalopathy, dyskinesia, extrapyramidal disorders, hemiparesis, paraplegia, speech disorders, tetany, cerebral edema, depression, confusion, anxiety, insomnia, somnolence, amnesia, aggressive reaction, nervousness, agitation, hallucinations, impaired concentration, emotional liability, psychosis, *suicide attempt,* delirium, sleep disorders, personality disorders. *Peripheral nervous system:* Hypesthesia, neuropathy, sensory disturbances, generalized spasms, abnormal gait, hyperesthesia, hypertonia, hyperkinesia, vocal cord paralysis, hyporeflexia, hyperreflexia, neuralgia, neuritis, peripheral neuropathy. *Musculoskeletal:* Arthralgia, myalgia, involuntary muscle contractions, leg cramps, arthrosis, synovitis, torticollis. *GI:* N&V, diarrhea, anorexia, abdominal pain, dry mouth, dysphagia, dyspepsia, rectal hemorrhage, constipation, melena, flatulence, pancreatitis, ulcerative stomatitis, enteritis, glossitis, enterocolitis, proctitis, stomatitis, tenesmus, pseudomembranous colitis, gastroenteritis, oral leukoplakia, oral hemorrhage, rectal disorders, colitis, duodenal ulcer, hematemesis, paralytic ileus, ulcerative proctitis, tongue ulceration, esophageal ulceration. *Hepatic:* Abnormal hepatic function, cholecystitis, cholelithiasis, hepatitis, hepatosplenomegaly, cholestatic hepatitis, jaundice. *CV:* Hypertension, palpitations, sinus tachycardia, first degree AV block, nonspecific ST-T segment changes, hypotension, flushing, cerebrovascular disorder, *cardiomyopathy, cardiac failure, cardiac arrest,* bradycardia, arrhythmias, extrasystole, atrial fibrillation, phlebitis, superficial thrombophlebitis of arm, mesenteric vein thrombophlebitis. *Respiratory:* Cough, dyspnea, pneumonia, sinusitis, rhinitis, pharyngitis, respiratory insufficiency, pulmonary infiltration, *pulmonary embolism,* pneumothorax, hemoptysis, stridor, bronchospasm, laryngitis, bronchitis, respiratory depression, pleural effusion, *pulmonary hemorrhage,* pneumonitis. *Ophthalmic:* Visual field defects, nystagmus, periorbital edema, eye pain, conjunctivitis, diplopia, blindness, retinal detachment, mydriasis, photophobia. *Ear:* Deafness, earache, tinnitus, otitis. *Dermatologic:* Increased sweating, rash, skin ulceration, pruritus, seborrhea, erythematous rash, maculopapular rash, facial edema, skin discoloration, acne, alopecia, dermatitis, anal pruritus, genital pruritus, aggravated psoriasis, psoriaform rash, skin disorders, dry skin, urticaria, skin hypertrophy, verruca. *Miscellaneous:* Epistaxis, taste perversions, pain or inflammation at injection site, lymphoma-like disorder, sarcoma, **malignant lymphoma,** ADH disorders, decreased gonadotropins, gynecomastia.

**OD** **Overdose Management:** *Symptoms:* Extensions of the preceding side effects. Of most concern are development of *seizures,* renal function impairment, paresthesias in limbs or periorally, and electrolyte disturbances especially involving calcium and phosphate. *Treatment:* Monitor the client for S&S of electrolyte imbalance and renal impairment. Symptomatic treatment. Hemodialysis and hydration may be of some benefit.

**Drug Interactions**
*Aminoglycosides* / ↓ Elimination of foscarnet → ↑ risk of renal impairment
*Amphotericin B* / ↓ Elimination of foscarnet → ↑ risk of renal impairment
*AZT* / ↑ Risk of anemia
*Didanosine* / Elimination of foscarnet risk of renal impairment
*Pentamidine, IV* / ↓ Elimination of foscarnet → ↑ risk of renal impairment; also, pentamidine causes hypocalcemia
**Laboratory Test Interferences:** ↑ Alkaline phosphatase, AST, ALT, LDH, BUN, creatine phosphokinase, serum creatinine. ↓ Creatinine clearance. Abnormal X-ray. Abnormal A-G ratio.

**Dosage**
• **IV Infusion**
  *CMV retinitis in AIDS.*
**Individualized, initial, normal renal function:** Either 60 mg/kg over

a minimum of 1 hr q 8 hr or 90 mg/kg q 12 hr for 2–3 weeks, depending on the response. **Maintenance:** 90–120 mg/kg/day (depending on renal function) given as an IV infusion over 2 hr. Most clients should be started on the 90-mg/kg/day dose; however, increasing the dose to 120 mg/kg/day should be considered due to progression of retinitis.

*Acyclovir-resistant HSV infections in immunocompromised clients.*
**Initial:** 40 mg/kg for clients with normal renal function given IV at a constant rate over a minimum of 1 hr q 8 or 12 hr for 2 to 3 weeks or until lesions are healed. **Maintenance:** See dose for CMV retinitis.

## NURSING CONSIDERATIONS
### Administration/Storage
**IV** 1. To avoid local irritation, infuse only into veins with adequate blood flow to allow rapid dilution and distribution.
2. The rate of infusion must be no more than 1 mg/kg/min using controlled IV infusion either by a central venous line or a peripheral vein. Do not give by rapid or bolus IV injection.
3. If using a central venous catheter for infusion, the standard 24-mg/mL solution may be used without dilution. However, if a peripheral vein catheter is used, dilute the 24-mg/mL solution to 12 mg/mL with D5W or NSS to avoid vein irritation. Use diluted solutions within 24 hr of first entry into sealed bottle.
4. To minimize potential for renal impairment, hydrate during drug administration; establish and maintain diuresis.
5. Adjust dose in renal impairment using dosing guide provided with the drug.
6. Do not give any other drug or supplement through the same catheter. Foscarnet is incompatible with 30% dextrose, amphotericin B, and calcium-containing solutions (e.g., RL and TPN). Other incompatibilities include acyclovir sodium, di-

azepam, digoxin, diphenhydramine, dobutamine, droperidol, ganciclovir, gentamicin, haloperidol, isoethionate, leucovorin, midazolam, morphine sulfate, pentamidine, phenytoin, prochlorperazine, trimethoprim/sulfamethoxazole, trimetrexate, and vancomycin. A precipitate can result if foscarnet is given at the same time as divalent cations.

7. Store drug at room temperatures of 15°C–30°C (59°F–86°F). Do not freeze. Concentrations of 12 mg/mL in NSS are stable for 30 days at 5°C (41°F).

**Assessment**

1. Document indications for therapy.
2. Determine confirmation of CMV retinitis by indirect ophthalmoscopy.
3. Note any history of cardiac or neurologic dysfunction.
4. Monitor CBC, electrolytes, calcium, phosphorus, magnesium, and liver and renal function studies.

**Interventions**

1. Due to the possibility of decreased renal function, determine baseline $C_{CR}$ at 2–3 times/week during induction therapy, and at least once every 1–2 weeks during maintenance therapy. This is especially true in geriatric clients who commonly have decreased GFRs.
2. Monitor I&O and VS; ensure well hydrated.
3. Observe for possibility of chelation of divalent metal ions, which will alter serum levels of electrolytes; levels of electrolytes, calcium, magnesium, and creatinine should be monitored closely.
4. Observe for any seizure activity; use seizure precautions.
5. Follow dilution and administration guidelines carefully. Ideally, product should be prepared daily, under a biologic hood, by the pharmacist. Refer to home infusion program for home therapy.

**Client/Family Teaching**

1. Foscarnet is not a cure for CMV retinitis; may continue to experience progression of condition during or following treatment.

2. Report for scheduled ophthalmic exams.
3. Report any evidence of numbness of the extremities, paresthesias, or perioral tingling as these are symptoms of hypocalcemia. Stop infusion and notify provider to correct imbalance before resuming the infusion.

**Outcomes/Evaluate:** Ophthalmic evidence of successful treatment of CMV retinitis

---

# Fosfomycin tromethamine
(fos-foh-**MY**-sin)
**Pregnancy Category:** B
Monurol **(Rx)**
**Classification:** Anti-infective, antibiotic

---

See also *Anti-Infective Agents.*

**Action/Kinetics:** Bactericidal drug that inactivates enzyme enolpyruvyl transferase, irreversibly blocking condensation of uridine diphosphate-N-acetylglucosamine with p-enolpyruvate. This is one of first steps in bacterial wall synthesis. Also reduces adherence of bacteria to uroepithelial cells. Rapidly absorbed from GI tract and converted to fosfomycin. **Maximum serum levels:** 2 hr. **t½, elimination:** 5.7 hr. Excreted unchanged in both urine and feces.

**Uses:** Treatment of uncomplicated urinary tract infections (acute cystitis) in women due to *Escherichia coli* and *Enterococcus faecalis.*

**Contraindications:** Lactation.

**Special Concerns:** Safety and efficacy have not been determined in children 12 years and younger.

**Side Effects:** *GI:* Diarrhea, nausea, dyspepsia, abdominal pain, abnormal stools, anorexia, constipation, dry mouth, flatulence, vomiting. *CNS:* Headache, dizziness, insomnia, migraine, nervousness, paresthesia, somnolence. *GU:* Vaginitis, dysmenorrhea, dysuria, hematuria, menstrual disorder. *Respiratory:* Rhinitis, pharyngitis. *Miscellaneous:* Asthenia, back pain, pain, rash, ear disorder, fever, flu syndrome, infection, lym-

phadenopathy, myalgia, pruritus, skin disorder.
**Drug Interactions**
*Metoclopramide* / ↓ serum levels and urinary excretion of fosfomycin.
**Laboratory Test Interferences:** ↑ ALT, AST, eosinophil count, bilirubin, alkaline phosphatase. ↓ Hematocrit, hemoglobin. ↑ or ↓ WBC, platelet count.

**Dosage**
• **Sachet**
*Acute cystitis.*
**Women, 18 years and older:** One sachet of fosfomycin mixed with water before ingesting.

## NURSING CONSIDERATIONS

See also *Nursing Considerations* for *Anti-Infective Agents*.
**Administration/Storage**
1. Pour entire contents of single-dose sachet into 3 to 4 oz water and stir to dissolve. Do not use hot water. Take immediately after dissolving in water.
2. Can be taken with or without food.
3. Do not use more than one single dose to treat single episode of acute cystitis.
4. Symptoms should improve within 2 to 3 days; if not improved, contact health care provider.
5. Store at controlled room temperature.
**Assessment**
1. Note onset, duration, frequency of occurrence, and characteristics of symptoms.
2. Obtain urine for C&S before and after therapy.
**Client/Family Teaching**
1. May be taken with or without food.
2. Use only one single dose to treat each episode of cystitis. Each packet contains 3 Gm of fosfomycin.
3. Do not take dry, always mix with 3 to 4 oz water and stir to dissolve before ingesting.
4. Report if symptoms do not improve by third day after therapy;

should see improvement in 2–3 days.
**Outcomes/Evaluate:** Resolution of UTI; symptomatic improvement

# Fosinopril sodium
(foh-**SIN**-oh-prill)
**Pregnancy Category:** D
Monopril **(Rx)**
**Classification:** Angiotensin-converting enzyme inhibitor

See also *Angiotensin-Converting Enzyme Inhibitors*.
**Action/Kinetics: Onset:** 1 hr. **Time to peak serum levels:** About 3 hr. Metabolized in the liver to the active fosinoprilat. Significantly bound to plasma proteins. t½: 12 hr for fosinoprilat (prolonged in impaired renal function) following IV administration. **Duration:** 24 hr. Approximately 50% excreted through the urine and 50% in the feces. Food decreases the rate, but not the extent, of absorption of fosinopril.
**Uses:** Alone or in combination with other antihypertensive agents (especially thiazide diuretics) for the treatment of hypertension. Adjunct in treating CHF in clients not responding adequately to diuretics and digitalis.
**Contraindications:** Use during lactation.
**Side Effects:** *CV:* Orthostatic hypotension, chest pain, hypotension, palpitations, angina pectoris, ***CVA, MI,*** rhythm disturbances, hypertensive crisis, claudication. *CNS:* Headache, dizziness, fatigue, confusion, memory disturbance, tremors, drowsiness, mood change, insomnia, vertigo, sleep disturbances. *GI:* N&V, diarrhea, abdominal pain, constipation, dry mouth, dysphagia, taste disturbance, abdominal distention, flatulence, heartburn, appetite changes, weight changes. *Respiratory:* Cough, sinusitis, ***bronchospasm,*** asthma, pharyngitis, laryngitis. *Hematologic:* Leukopenia, eosinophilia, decreases in hemoglobin (mean of 0.1 g/dL) or hematocrit, neutropenia. *Dermatologic:* Diaphoresis, photosensitivity,

flushing, pruritus, rash, urticaria. *Body as a whole:* Angioedema, muscle cramps, syncope, myalgia, arthralgia, edema, weakness, musculoskeletal pain. *GU:* Decreased libido, sexual dysfunction, renal insufficiency, urinary frequency. *Miscellaneous:* Paresthesias, hepatitis, pancreatitis, syncope, tinnitus, gout, lymphadenopathy, rhinitis, epistaxis, vision disturbances, eye irritation, laryngitis.

**Laboratory Test Interferences:** Transient ↓ H&H. False low measurement of serum digoxin levels with DigiTab RIA Kit for Digoxin.

**Dosage** ───────────────
• **Tablets**
  *Hypertension.*
**Initial:** 10 mg once daily; **then,** adjust dose depending on BP response at peak (2–6 hr after dosing) and trough (24 hr after dosing) blood levels. **Maintenance:** Usually 20–40 mg/day, although some clients manifest beneficial effects at doses up to 80 mg.
  *In clients taking diuretics.*
Discontinue diuretic 2–3 days before starting fosinopril. If diuretic cannot be discontinued, use an initial dose of 10 mg fosinopril.
  *Congestive heart failure.*
**Initial:** 10 mg once daily; **then,** following initial dose, observe the client for at least 2 hr for the presence of hypotension or orthostasis (if either is present, monitor until BP stabilizes). An initial dose of 5 mg is recommended in heart failure with moderate to severe renal failure or in those who have had significant diuresis. The dose is increased over several weeks, not to exceed a maximum of 40 mg daily (usual effective range is 20–40 mg once daily).

## NURSING CONSIDERATIONS

See also *Nursing Considerations* for *Angiotensin-Converting Enzyme Inhibitors* and *Antihypertensive Agents*.
**Administration/Storage**
1. If antihypertensive effect decreases at the end of the dosing interval with once-daily dosing, consider b.i.d. administration.
2. If also taking a diuretic, discontinue the diuretic 2–3 days prior to beginning fosinopril therapy. If BP is not controlled, reinstitute the diuretic. If the diuretic cannot be discontinued, give an initial dose of fosinopril of 10 mg.
3. Do not adjust the dose of fosinopril in renal insufficiency except as noted in Dosage.
**Outcomes/Evaluate**
• ↓ BP
• Control of symptoms of CHF

# Fosphenytoin sodium
(**FOS**-fen-ih-toyn)
**Pregnancy Category:** D
Cerebyx **(Rx)**
**Classification:** Anticonvulsant
───────────────

See also *Anticonvulsants* and *Phenytoin.*
**Action/Kinetics:** Fosphenytoin is a prodrug of phenytoin; thus, its anticonvulsant effects are due to phenytoin. For every millimole of fosphenytoin administered, 1 mmol of phenytoin is produced. **t½, fosphenytoin:** 15 min after IV infusion. **Peak plasma levels, after IM:** 30 min. Significantly bound (95% to 99%) to plasma protein. Fosphenytoin displaces phenytoin from plasma protein binding sites. Fosphenytoin is better tolerated at the infusion site than is phenytoin (i.e., pain and burning associated with IV phenytoin is decreased). The IV infusion rate for fosphenytoin is three times faster than for IV phenytoin. IM use results in systemic phenytoin concentrations that are similar to PO phenytoin, thus allowing interchangeable use. Phenytoin derived from fosphenytoin is extensively metabolized in the liver and excreted in the urine.
**Uses:** Short-term parenteral use for the control of generalized convulsive status epilepticus and prophylaxis and treatment of seizures occurring during neurosurgery. It can be substituted, short term, for PO phe-

nytoin when PO administration is not possible.

**Contraindications:** Hypersensitivity to fosphenytoin, phenytoin, or other hydantoins. Use in clients with sinus bradycardia, SA block, second- and third-degree AV block, and Adams-Stokes syndrome. Use to treat absence seizures. Use during lactation.

**Special Concerns:** The safety and efficacy of fosphenytoin have not been determined for longer than 5 days. The safety has not been determined in pediatric clients. After administration of fosphenytoin to those with renal and/or hepatic dysfunction or in those with hypoalbuminemia, fosphenytoin clearance to phenytoin may be increased without a similar increase in phenytoin clearance, thus increasing the potential for serious side effects.

**Side Effects:** See *Phenytoin*. The most common side effects include ataxia, dizziness, headache, nystagmus, paresthesia, pruritus, and somnolence.

**Laboratory Test Alteration:** See *Phenytoin*.

**Drug Interactions:** See *Phenytoin*.

**Dosage** ⸻

*NOTE:* Doses of fosphenytoin are expressed as phenytoin sodium equivalents (PE = phenytoin sodium equivalent). Thus, adjustments in the recommended doses should not be made when substituting fosphenytoin for phenytoin sodium or vice versa.

• **IV**
*Status epilepticus.*
**Loading dose:** 15–20 mg PE/kg given at a rate of 100–150 mg PE/min. The loading dose is followed by maintenance doses of either fosphenytoin or phenytoin, either PO or parenterally.

• **IM, IV**
*Nonemergency loading and maintenance dosing.*
**Loading dose:** 15–20 mg PE/kg given at a rate of 100–150 mg PE/min.
**Maintenance:** 4–6 mg PE/kg/day.

*Temporary substitution for PO phenytoin.*
Use the same daily PO dose of phenytoin in milligrams given at a rate not to exceed 150 mg PE/min.

## NURSING CONSIDERATIONS

See also *Nursing Considerations* for *Anticonvulsants* and *Phenytoin*.

**Administration/Storage**

1. Fosphenytoin can be substituted for PO phenytoin sodium therapy at the same total daily dose.

2. Phenytoin capsules as Dilantin are approximately 90% bioavailable by the PO route and fosphenytoin (available as Cerebyx) is 100% bioavailable by both the IM and IV routes. Thus, plasma phenytoin may increase modestly when IM or IV fosphenytoin (as Cerebyx) is subtituted for PO phenytoin sodium therapy.

3. Do not use IM fosphenytoin to treat status epilepticus because therapeutic phenytoin concentrations may not be reached as quickly as with IV administration.

4. Do not use vials that develop particulate matter.

5. Do not store at room temperature for more than 48 hr. Store under refrigeration at 2°C–8°C (36°F–46°F).

**IV** 6. Prior to IV infusion fosphenytoin must be diluted in 5% dextrose or 0.9% saline solution to obtain a concentration ranging from 1.5 to 25 mg/PE (phenytoin sodium equivalents)/mL.

7. Due to risk of hypotension, do not administer at a rate greater than 150 PE/min.

8. Because the full antiepileptic effect of phenytoin (given as either fosphenytoin or parenteral phenytoin) is not known immediately, other measures to control status epilepticus (e.g., use of an IV benzodiazepine) will be necessary.

**Assessment**

1. Document type, onset, and characteristics of seizures; note other agents trialed and outcome.

2. Fosphenytoin converts to phe-

nytoin and may be administered IV or IM; it's prescribed and dispensed in PE.

3. Monitor ECG, albumin, CBC, and liver and renal function studies. During IV administration, continously monitor ECG, BP, and respirations.

4. Do not use with bradycardia or any type of heart block; may cause atrial and ventricular conduction depression.

5. A waiting period is recommended before ordering laboratory tests for phenytoin plasma levels: 2 hr following IV infusion and 4 hr following IM injection.

**Client/Family Teaching**
1. Review goals of therapy; drug is generally for short-term use.
2. Report any swollen lymph glands.
3. May experience dizziness, drowsiness, itching, and tingling of groin and face. Presence of REMs, gait and speech impairment may indicate toxicity.
4. If rash appears, stop therapy and report. If mild, therapy may be resumed once rash has cleared. If rash recurs, do not reuse this class of drugs.

**Outcomes/Evaluate**
• Control of convulsions
• Seizure prophylaxis during surgery
• Short-term substitution for PO phenytoin

# Furosemide
(fur-**OH**-seh-myd)
**Pregnancy Category:** C
Apo-Furosemide ✦, Furoside ✦, Lasix, Myrosemide, Novo-Semide ✦, Uritol ✦ **(Rx)**
**Classification:** Loop diuretic

See also *Diuretics, Loop.*
**Action/Kinetics:** Inhibits the reabsorption of sodium and chloride in the proximal and distal tubules as well as the ascending loop of Henle; this results in the excretion of sodium, chloride, and, to a lesser degree, potassium and bicarbonate ions. The resulting urine is more acid. Diuretic

action is independent of changes in clients' acid-base balance. Has a slight antihypertensive effect. **Onset: PO, IM:** 30–60 min; **IV:** 5 min. **Peak: PO, IM:** 1–2 hr; **IV:** 20–60 min. **t½:** About 2 hr after PO use. **Duration: PO, IM:** 6–8 hr; **IV:** 2 hr. Metabolized in the liver and excreted through the urine. May be effective for clients resistant to thiazides and for those with reduced GFRs.

**Uses:** Edema associated with CHF, nephrotic syndrome, hepatic cirrhosis, and ascites. IV for acute pulmonary edema. Furosemide can be used orally to treat hypertension in conjunction with spironolactone, triamterene, and other diuretics *except* ethacrynic acid. *Investigational:* Hypercalcemia.

**Contraindications: Never use with ethacrynic acid.** Anuria, hypersensitivity to drug, severe renal disease associated with azotemia and oliguria, hepatic coma associated with electrolyte depletion. Lactation.

**Special Concerns:** Use with caution in premature infants and neonates due to prolonged half-life in these clients (dosing interval must be extended). Geriatric clients may be more sensitive to the usual adult dose. Allergic reactions may be seen in clients who show hypersensitivity to sulfonamides.

**Side Effects:** *Electrolyte and fluid effects:* Fluid and electrolyte depletion leading to dehydration, hypovolemia, thromboembolism. Hypokalemia and hypochloremia may cause metabolic alkalosis. Hyperuricemia, azotemia, hyponatremia. *GI:* Nausea, oral and gastric irritation, vomiting, anorexia, diarrhea (especially in children) or constipation, cramps, pancreatitis, jaundice, ischemic hepatitis. *Otic:* Tinnitus, hearing impairment (may be reversible or permanent), reversible deafness. Usually following rapid IV or IM administration of high doses. *CNS:* Vertigo, headache, dizziness, blurred vision, restlessness, paresthesias, xanthopsia. *CV:* Orthostatic hypotension, thrombophlebitis, chronic aortitis. *Hematologic:* Anemia, thrombocytopenia, neutropenia, leukopenia, *agranulocytosis,* purpura. **Rarely, *aplastic anemia.*** *Allergic:* Rashes, pruritus, urticaria, photosensitivity, exfoliative dermatitis, vasculitis, erythema multiforme. *Miscellaneous:* Interstitial nephritis, fever, weakness, hyperglycemia, glycosuria, exacerbation of, aggravation of or worsening of SLE, increased perspiration, muscle spasms, urinary bladder spasm, urinary frequency.

*Following IV use:* Thrombophlebitis, *cardiac arrest. Following IM use:* Pain and irritation at injection site, *cardiac arrest.*

Because this drug is resistant to the effects of pressor amines and potentiates the effects of muscle relaxants, it is recommended that the PO drug be discontinued 1 week before surgery and the IV drug 2 days before surgery.

**OD** **Overdose Management:** *Symptoms:* Profound water loss, electrolyte depletion (manifested by weakness, anorexia, vomiting, lethargy, cramps, mental confusion, dizziness), decreased blood volume, *circulatory collapse (possibly vascular thrombosis and embolism).* *Treatment:* Replace fluid and electrolytes. Monitor urine electrolyte output and serum electrolytes. Induce emesis or perform gastric lavage. Oxygen or artificial respiration may be needed. Treat symptoms.

**Additional Drug Interactions**
*Charcoal* / ↓ Absorption of furosemide from the GI tract
*Clofibrate* / Enhanced diuretic effect
*Hydantoins* / Hydantoins ↓ the diuretic effect of furosemide
*Propranolol* / Furosemide may cause ↑ plasma levels of propranolol

**Dosage** —————————
• **Oral Solution, Tablets**
*Edema.*
**Adults, initial:** 20–80 mg/day as a single dose. For resistant cases, dosage can be increased by 20–40 mg q 6–8

hr until desired diuretic response is attained. Maximum daily dose should not exceed 600 mg. **Pediatric, initial:** 2 mg/kg as a single dose; **then,** dose can be increased by 1–2 mg/kg q 6–8 hr until desired response is attained (up to 5 mg/kg may be required in children with nephrotic syndrome; maximum dose should not exceed 6 mg/kg). A dose range of 0.5–2 mg/kg b.i.d. has also been recommended.

*Hypertension.*
**Adults, initial:** 40 mg b.i.d. Adjust dosage depending on response.

*CHF and chronic renal failure.*
**Adults:** 2–2.5 g/day.

*Antihypercalcemic.*
**Adults:** 120 mg/day in one to three doses.

• **IV, IM**
*Edema.*
**Adults, initial:** 20–40 mg; if response inadequate after 2 hr, increase dose in 20-mg increments. **Pediatric, initial:** 1 mg/kg given slowly; if response inadequate after 2 hr, increase dose by 1 mg/kg. Doses greater than 6 mg/kg should not be given.

*Antihypercalcemic.*
**Adults:** 80–100 mg for severe cases; dose may be repeated q 1–2 hr if needed.

• **IV**
*Acute pulmonary edema.*
**Adults:** 40 mg slowly over 1–2 min; if response inadequate after 1 hr, give 80 mg slowly over 1–2 min. Concomitant oxygen and digitalis may be used.

*CHF, chronic renal failure.*
**Adults:** 2–2.5 g/day. For IV bolus injections, the maximum should not exceed 1 g/day given over 30 min.

*Hypertensive crisis, normal renal function.*
**Adults:** 40–80 mg.

*Hypertensive crisis with pulmonary edema or acute renal failure.*
**Adults:** 100–200 mg.

## NURSING CONSIDERATIONS

See also *Nursing Considerations* for *Diuretics, Loop.*

**Administration/Storage**

1. Give 2–4 days/week.
2. Food decreases the bioavailability of furosemide and ultimately the degree of diuresis.
3. Slight discoloration resulting from light does not affect potency. However, do not dispense discolored tablets or injection.
4. If used with other antihypertensives, reduce the dose of other agents by at least 50% when furosemide is added in order to prevent an excessive drop in BP.
5. Store in light-resistant containers at room temperature (15°C–30°C, or 59°F–86°F).
6. In CHF or chronic renal failure, oral and parenteral doses of 2–2.5 g/day (or higher) are well tolerated.
**IV** 7. Give IV injections slowly over 1–2 min.
8. If used IV, do not mix with solutions with a pH below 5.5. After pH adjustment, furosemide can be mixed with NaCl injection, RL injection, and 5% dextrose injection and infused at a rate not to exceed 4 mg/min, to prevent ototoxicity.
9. A precipitate may form if mixed with gentamicin, netilmicin, or milrinone in either 5% dextrose or 0.9% NaCl.

**Assessment**

1. When more than 40 mg/day is required, give in divided doses, i.e., 40 mg PO b.i.d.
2. With renal impairment or if receiving other ototoxic drugs, observe for ototoxicity.
3. Assess closely for signs of vascular thrombosis and embolism, particularly in the elderly.

4. Monitor electrolytes; observe for S&S of hypokalemia.
5. With rapid diuresis, observe for dehydration and circulatory collapse; monitor BP and pulse.
6. With chronic use, assess for thiamine deficiency.

**Client/Family Teaching**

1. Take in the morning on an empty stomach to enhance absorption and to avoid interruption of sleep. Time administration to participate in social activities and not have to get up during the night to void frequently.
2. Immediately report any muscle weakness, dizziness, numbness, or tingling.
3. Drug may cause orthostatic hypotension.
4. Sorbitol in the solution vehicle may result in diarrhea, especially in children.
5. Monitor weights; report any gains of > 3 lb/day or > 10 lb/week.
6. Consult provider before taking aspirin for any reason. Salicylate intoxication occurs at lower levels than normal because of competition at the renal excretory sites.
7. Use sunscreens and protective clothing when sun exposed to minimize the effects of drug-induced photosensitivity.
8. Supplement diet with vegetables and fruits high in potassium if oral supplements are not prescribed. Those on a salt-restricted diet should not increase salt intake; NSAIDs and alpha blockers may also cause sodium retention with resultant edema.

**Outcomes/Evaluate**

- Enhanced diuresis
- Resolution of pulmonary edema
- ↓ Dependent edema
- ↓ Serum calcium levels

# Gabapentin
(gab-ah-PEN-tin)
**Pregnancy Category:** C
Neurontin **(Rx)**
**Classification:** Anticonvulsant

See also *Anticonvulsants.*

**Action/Kinetics:** Anticonvulsant mechanism is not known. Food has no effect on the rate and extent of absorption; however, as the dose increases, the bioavailability decreases. **t½:** 5–7 hr. Excreted unchanged through the urine.

**Uses:** In adults as an adjunct in the treatment of partial seizures with and without secondary generalization.

**Special Concerns:** Use during lactation only if benefits outweigh risks. Plasma clearance is reduced in geriatric clients and in those with impaired renal function. Safety and efficacy have not been determined in children less than 12 years of age.

**Side Effects:** Side effects listed are those with an incidence of 0.1% or greater.

*CNS:* Most commonly: somnolence, ataxia, dizziness, and fatigue. Also, nystagmus, tremor, nervousness, dysarthria, amnesia, depression, abnormal thinking, twitching, abnormal coordination, headache, ***convulsions (including the possibility of precipitation of status epilepticus),*** confusion, insomnia, emotional lability, vertigo, hyperkinesia, paresthesia, decreased/increased/absent re-flexes, anxiety, hostility, CNS tumors, syncope, abnormal dreaming, aphasia, hypesthesia, ***intracranial hemorrhage,*** hypotonia, dysesthesia, paresis, dystonia, hemiplegia, facial paralysis, stupor, cerebellar dysfunction, positive Babinski sign, decreased position sense, subdural hematoma, apathy, hallucinations, decreased or loss of libido, agitation depersonalization, euphoria, "doped-up" sensation, ***suicidal tendencies,*** psychoses. *GI:* Most commonly: N&V. Also, dyspepsia, dry mouth and throat, constipation, dental abnormalities, increased appetite, abdominal pain, diarrhea, anorexia, flatulence, gingivitis, glossitis, gum hemorrhage, thirst, stomatitis, taste loss, unusual taste, increased salivation, gastroenteritis, hemorrhoids, bloody stools, fecal incontinence, hepatomegaly. *CV:* Hypertension, vasodilation, hypotension, angina pectoris, peripheral vascular disorder, palpitation, tachycardia, migraine, murmur. *Musculoskeletal:* Myalgia, fracture, tendinitis, arthritis, joint stiffness or swelling, positive Romberg test. *Respiratory:* Rhinitis, pharyngitis, coughing, pneumonia, epistaxis, dyspnea, apnea. *Dermatologic:* Pruritus, abrasion, rash, acne, alopecia, eczema, dry skin, increased sweating, urticaria, hirsutism, seborrhea, cyst, herpes simplex. *Body as a whole:* Weight increase, back pain, peripheral edema, asthenia, facial edema, allergy, weight decrease, chills. *GU:* Hematuria, dysuria, frequent urination, cystitis, urinary retention, urinary incontinence, vaginal hemorrhage, amenorrhea, dysmenorrhea, menorrhagia, breast cancer, inability to climax, abnormal ejaculation, impotence. *Hematologic:* Leukopenia, decreased WBCs, purpura, anemia, thrombocytopenia, lymphadenopathy. *Ophthalmologic:* Diplopia, amblyopia, abnormal vision, cataract, conjunctivitis, dry eyes, eye pain, visual field defect, photophobia, bilateral or unilateral ptosis, eye hemorrhage, hordeolum, eye twitching. *Otic:* Hearing loss, earache, tinnitus, inner ear infection, otitis, ear fullness.

**OD** **Overdose Management:** *Symptoms:* Double vision, slurred speech, drowsiness, lethargy, diarrhea. *Treatment:* Hemodialysis.

**Drug Interactions**
*Antacids* / Antacids ↓ bioavailability of gabapentin
*Cimetidine* / Cimetidine ↓ renal excretion of gabapentin

**Laboratory Test Interferences:** False + reading with Ames N-Multistix SG dipstick test for urinary protein.

## Dosage

• **Capsules**
*Anticonvulsant.*

**Adults:** Dose range of 900–1,800 mg/day in three divided doses. Titration to an effective dose can begin on day 1 with 300 mg followed by 300 mg b.i.d. on day 2 and 300 mg t.i.d. on day 3. If necessary, the dose may be increased to 300–400 mg t.i.d., up to 1,800 mg/day. In clients with a creatinine clearance of 30–60 mL/min, the dose is 300 mg b.i.d.; if the creatinine clearance is 15–30 mL/min, the dose is 300 mg/day; if the creatinine clearance is less than 15 mL/min, the dose is 300 mg every other day.

## NURSING CONSIDERATIONS

See also *Nursing Considerations* for *Anticonvulsants*.

**Administration/Storage**
1. Do not exceed 12 hr between doses using the t.i.d. daily regimen.
2. If gabapentin is discontinued or an alternate anticonvulsant is added to the regimen, do gradually over a 1-week period.
3. The first dose on day 1 may be taken at bedtime to minimize somnolence, dizziness, fatigue, and ataxia.

**Assessment**
1. Document type and onset of symptoms, any other agents prescribed, and the outcome.
2. List other drugs prescribed to ensure that none interact unfavorably.
3. Obtain baseline renal function studies; reduce dose in the elderly and with impaired renal function.
4. When drug therapy is discontinued or supplemental therapy is added, do so gradually over at least 1 week.

**Client/Family Teaching**
1. May be taken with or without food. Do not stop abruptly.
2. Avoid antacids 1 hr before or 2 hr after taking drug.
3. Drug may cause dizziness, fatigue, drowsiness, ataxia, and nystagmus. Do not perform any activities that require mental alertness until full drug effects are realized.
4. Report any new or unusual symptoms.

**Outcomes/Evaluate:** Control of seizure activity

# Gallium nitrate
(**Gal**-ee-um **NIGH**-trayt)
**Pregnancy Category:** C
Ganite **(Rx)**
**Classification:** Antihypercalcemic agent

**Action/Kinetics:** Produces a hypocalcemic effect by inhibiting calcium resorption from bone, perhaps by reducing increased bone turnover. After infusion, steady state is reached in 24–48 hr. **Plasma levels:** 1,134–2,399 ng/mL. Not metabolized by the liver or kidney and is excreted through the kidneys.

**Uses:** Cancer-related hypercalcemia that is not responsive to adequate hydration and where there are symptoms of hypercalcemia.

**Contraindications:** Severe renal impairment (serum creatinine > 2.5 mg/dL). Lactation.

**Special Concerns:** Safety and effectiveness have not been determined in children.

**Side Effects:** *Metabolic:* Hypocalcemia, transient hypophosphatemia, decreased serum bicarbonate (possibly secondary to mild respiratory alkalosis). *GU:* Increased BUN and creatinine. *Hematologic:* Anemia (relationship to drug itself not certain), leukopenia. *GI:* N&V, diarrhea, constipation. *CNS:* Lethargy, confusion, fever, paresthesia, dreams and hallucinations. *CV:* Tachycardia, edema of lower extremities, hypotension. *Respiratory:* Dyspnea, rales and rhonchi, pulmonary infiltrates, pleural effusion. *Ophthalmic:* Acute optic neuritis, visual impairment. *Miscellaneous:* Decreased hearing, hypothermia, skin rash, acute renal failure.

**OD** **Overdose Management:** *Symptoms:* N&V, increased risk of renal insufficiency. *Treatment:* Discontinue the drug and monitor serum calcium. Give fluids IV, with or without diuretics, for 2–3 days. Carefully monitor renal function and urinary output.

**Drug Interactions:** Use of gallium nitrate with nephrotoxic drugs (e.g., aminoglycosides, amphotericin B) may increase the incidence of renal insufficiency in clients with hypercalcemia due to cancer.

**Laboratory Test Interferences:** BUN and creatinine.

## Dosage
### • IV Infusion
*Serious hypercalcemia.*
**Adults:** 200 mg/m²/day for 5 consecutive days.
*Mild hypercalcemia.*
**Adults:** 100 mg/m²/day for 5 consecutive days.

## NURSING CONSIDERATIONS
### Administration/Storage
**IV** 1. Must give daily dose as an IV infusion over 24 hr.
2. Dilute the daily dose in 1 L of 0.9% NaCl injection or 5% dextrose injection; dilution is stable for 48 hr at room temperature and for 7 days if refrigerated.
3. If serum calcium levels are brought into the normal range in less than 5 days, treatment may be discontinued early.
4. Discard any unused portion; the product contains no preservative.
### Assessment
1. Determine that cancer-related hypercalcemia was previously unresponsive to saline hydration. In treating, first establish adequate hydration to increase renal excretion of calcium and correct for dehydration caused by hypercalcemia. Diuretic therapy should *not* be used prior to correction of hypovolemia.
2. Monitor CBC, serum calcium, phosphorus, and renal function studies. If hypocalcemia occurs, stop gallium infusion.
3. Monitor I&O. Hypercalcemia is frequently associated with impaired renal function; monitor serum creatinine and BUN closely and discontinue therapy if creatinine levels exceed 2.5 mg/dL.
4. A satisfactory urine output (2 L/day) should be established before therapy is initiated. Adequate hydration should be maintained throughout therapy; avoid overhydration with compromised CV function.
5. Report any visual or hearing disturbances as these may be drug related.
### Outcomes/Evaluate: Serum calcium levels within desired range (8.8–10.4 mg/dL)

# Ganciclovir sodium (DHPG)
(gan-**SYE**-kloh-veer)
**Pregnancy Category:** C
Cytovene, Vitrasert **(Rx)**
**Classification:** Antiviral

See also *Antiviral Agents.*
**Action/Kinetics:** Upon entry into viral cells infected by CMV, ganciclovir is converted to ganciclovir triphosphate by the CMV. Ganciclovir triphosphate inhibits viral DNA synthesis by competitive inhibition of viral DNA polymerases and direct incorporation into viral DNA; this results in eventual termination of viral DNA elongation. Ganciclovir is active against CMV, herpes simplex virus-1 and -2, Epstein-Barr virus, and varicella zoster virus. Use of the intraocular implant causes a significantly slower disease progression than did those treated with IV ganciclovir. **t½:** Approximately 2.9 hr. Believed to cross the blood-brain barrier. Most excreted unchanged through the urine. Renal impairment increases the t½ of the drug; make dosage adjustments based on $C_{CR}$.
**Uses: IV:** Immunocompromised clients with CMV retinitis, including AIDS clients. Diagnosis may be confirmed by culture of CMV from the blood, urine, or throat; note that a negative CMV culture does not rule out CMV retinitis. Prevention of CMV disease in transplant clients at risk; duration of treatment depends on duration and degree of immunosuppression. *Investigational:* Treatment of CMV infections (e.g., gastroenteritis, hepatitis, pneumonitis) in immunocompromised clients.

**PO:** Alternative to IV for maintenance treatment of CMV retinitis in immunocompromised (including AIDS) clients. Prevention of CMV disease in clients with advanced HIV infection at risk for developing CMV disease.

**Intraocular implant:** CMV retinitis in those with AIDS.

**Contraindications:** Hypersensitivity to acyclovir or ganciclovir. Lactation. Use when the absolute neutrophil count is less than 500/mm³ or the platelet count is less than 25,000/mm³.

**Special Concerns:** Safety and effectiveness of ganciclovir have not been established for nonimmunocompromised clients, treatment of other CMV infections such as pneumonitis or colitis, or congenital or neonatal CMV disease. Use with caution in impaired renal function, in elderly clients, or with preexisting cytopenias or with a history of cytopenic reactions to other drugs, chemicals, or irradiation. Use in children only if potential benefits outweigh potential risks, including carcinogenicity and reproductive toxicity. Not a cure for CMV retinitis and progression of the disease may continue in immunocompromised clients. Treatment with AZT and ganciclovir (e.g., in AIDS clients) will likely not be tolerated and lead to severe granulocytopenia.

**Side Effects:** *Hematologic:* Granulocytopenia, thrombocytopenia, neutropenia (may be irreversible), eosinophilia, leukopenia, anemia, hypochromic anemia, bone marrow depression, pancytopenia, *leukemia, lymphoma. CNS:* Ataxia, *coma,* neuropathy, confusion, abnormal dreams or thoughts, dizziness, headache, paresthesia, psychosis, nervousness, somnolence, tremor, agitation, amnesia, anxiety, depression, euphoria, hypertonia, hypesthesia, insomnia, manic reaction, *seizures,* trismus, emotional lability. *GI:* N&V, aphthous stomatitis, diarrhea, anorexia, dry mouth, *GI hemorrhage, pancreatitis,* abdominal pain, flatulence, dyspepsia, constipation, dysphagia, esophagitis, eructation, fecal incontinence, melena, mouth ulceration, tongue disorder, hepatitis, weight loss. *CV:* Hypertension or hypotension, arrhythmias, phlebitis,

deep thrombophlebitis, *cardiac arrest, intracranial hypertension, MI, stroke,* pericarditis, vasodilation, migraine. *Body as a whole:* Fever (most common), chills, edema, infections, malaise, *sepsis, multiple organ failure,* asthenia, enlarged abdomen, abscess, back pain, cellulitis, chest pain, facial edema, neck pain or rigidity. *Dermatologic:* Rash (most common), alopecia, pruritus, urticaria, sweating, acne, dry skin, fixed eruption, herpes simplex, maculopapular rash, skin discoloration, vesiculobullous rash, photosensivitiy, phototoxicity. *GU:* Hematuria, breast pain, kidney failure, abnormal kidney function, urinary frequency, UTI. *At injection site:* Catheter infection, catheter sepsis, inflammation or pain, abscess, edema, hemorrhage, phlebitis. *Musculoskeletal:* Arthralgia, bone pain, leg cramps, myalgia, myasthenia. *Ophthalmologic:* Abnormal vision, amblyopia, blindness, conjunctivitis, eye pain, glaucoma, retinitis, photophobia, cataracts, vitreous disorder. *Respiratory:* Dyspnea, increased cough, pneumonia. *Hepatic:* Cholestasis, cholangitis. *Miscellaneous:* Abnormal gait, decreased libido, deafness, *anaphylaxis,* taste perversion, tinnitus, acidosis, congenital anomaly, encephalopathy, impotence, transverse myelitis, infertility, splenomegaly, *Stevens-Johnson syndrome, unexplained death,* retinal detachment in CMV retinitis clients.

**OD  Overdose Management:** *Symptoms:* Neutropenia. Possibility of hypersalivation, anorexia, vomiting, bloody diarrhea, inactivity, cytopenia, testicular atrophy, increased BUN and liver function test results. *Treatment:* Hydration, hemodialysis.

**Drug Interactions**
*Adriamycin* / Additive cytotoxicity in rapidly dividing cells
*Amphotericin B* / Additive cytotoxicity in rapidly dividing cells; also, ↑ serum creatinine levels
*Cyclosporine* / ↑ Serum creatinine levels
*Dapsone* / Additive cytotoxicity in rapidly dividing cells

*Flucytosine* / Additive cytotoxicity in rapidly dividing cells

*Imipenem/Cilastatin combination* / Possibility of seizures

*Pentamidine* / Additive cytotoxicity in rapidly dividing cells

*Probenecid* / ↑ Effect of ganciclovir due to ↓ renal excretion

*Sulfamethoxazole/Trimethoprim combinations* / Additive cytotoxicity in rapidly dividing cells

*Vinblastine* / Additive cytotoxicity in rapidly dividing cells

*Vincristine* / Additive cytotoxicity in rapidly dividing cells

*AZT* / ↑ Risk of granulocytopenia and anemia

**Laboratory Test Interferences:** ↑ or ↓ Serum creatinine. ↑ BUN, alkaline phosphatase, CPK, LDH, AST, ALT. ↓ Blood glucose. Abnormal liver function test. Hypokalemia, hyponatremia.

## Dosage

- **IV Infusion, Capsules**
  *CMV retinitis.*

**Induction treatment:** 5 mg/kg over 1 hr q 12 hr for 14–21 days in clients with normal renal function. Do not use PO treatment for induction. **Maintenance, IV:** 5 mg/kg over 1 hr by IV infusion daily for 7 days or 6 mg/kg/day for 5 days each week. Dosage must be reduced in clients with renal impairment. **Maintenance, PO:** 1,000 mg t.i.d. with food. Or, 500 mg 6 times/day q 3 hr with food during waking hours.

*Prevention of CMV retinitis in those with advanced HIV infection and normal renal function.*
1,000 mg t.i.d. with food.

*Prophylaxis of CMV disease in transplant clients.*
**Initial dose, IV:** 5 mg/kg over 1 hr q 12 hr for 7–14 days. **Maintenance:** 5 mg/kg/day on 7 days each week (or 6 mg/kg/day on 5 days each week).

## NURSING CONSIDERATIONS

See also *Nursing Considerations* for *Antiviral Agents.*

**Administration/Storage**
1. Use capsules only in clients for whom the risk of a more rapid progression of the disease is offset by the benefit of avoiding daily IV infusions.

**IV** 2. Reconstitute by injecting 10 mL sterile water for injection followed by shaking. Discard if particulate matter or discoloration is noted. Because parabens is incompatible with ganciclovir, do not use bacteriostatic water for injection for reconstitution.

3. IV infusion concentrations greater than 10 mg/mL are not recommended. Further reconstitute ganciclovir with 100 mL of any of the following solutions: 5% dextrose, RL or Ringer's solution, 0.9% NaCl. Infuse over 1 hr. Doses greater than 6 mg/kg infused over 1 hr may result in increased toxicity.

4. Due to the high pH (9–11) of reconstituted ganciclovir, do not give IM or SC. Do not give by IV bolus or rapid IV injection.

5. To minimize phlebitis or pain at the injection site, give into veins with an adequate blood flow to allow rapid dilution and distribution.

6. Do not exceed 1.25 mg/kg/day in clients undergoing hemodialysis.

7. The reconstituted solution is stable for 12 hr at room temperature.

8. Follow guidelines for handling cytotoxic drugs during handling and disposal of drug. Avoid inhalation and contact with skin. Wear latex gloves and safety glasses when handling drug. Ideally, ganciclovir should be mixed by the pharmacist under a biologic hood.

**Assessment**
1. Document onset, duration of symptoms, and any previous treatments.

2. Determine CMV retinitis by indirect opthalmoscopy.

3. Assess orientation and mentation levels.

4. Monitor CBC and renal function studies; reduce dose with impaired renal function. Granulocytopenia and

thrombocytopenia are side effects of drug therapy; do not administer if neutrophil count drops below 500 cells/mm³ or the platelet count falls below 25,000/mm³. Concomitant therapy with AZT may increase neutropenia.

5. Monitor I&O. Ensure adequately hydrated before and during IV therapy.

6. May experience pain and/or phlebitis at infusion site because pH of *diluted* solution is high (pH 9–11). Follow administration guidelines carefully.

7. Review list of drug interactions as some may induce renal failure and have additive toxicity if given during ganciclovir therapy.

**Client/Family Teaching**

1. Drug therapy should not be interrupted unless deemed necessary by provider; a relapse may occur.

2. Take PO ganciclovir with food to increase bioavailability.

3. Drug is not a cure; is used to control symptoms.

4. Report any dizziness, confusion, and/or seizures immediately.

5. Use protection (sunglasses, clothing, hat, sunscreen) with sun exposure to prevent a photosensitivity reaction.

6. Report for scheduled labs; results may require adjustment of dose or discontinuation of therapy.

7. Have regular ophthalmologic examinations because retinitis may progress to blindness (retinal detachment). With intraocular implant identify side effects that require immediate reporting.

8. May impair fertility; determine if candidate for sperm/egg harvesting.

9. During and for 90 days following drug therapy, women of childbearing age should use safe contraception and men should practice barrier contraception.

10. Report any unusual behavior or altered thought processes.

**Outcomes/Evaluate**

• CMV prophylaxis in transplant and at-risk clients
• ↓ Progression of CMV retinitis

• Prevention of CMV retinitis in those with advanced HIV infection

# Gemcitabine hydrochloride

(jem-SIGHT-ah-been)
**Pregnancy Category:** D
Gemzar **(Rx)**
**Classification:** Antineoplastic, miscellaneous

See also *Antineoplastic Agents*.

**Action/Kinetics:** A nucleoside analog that kills cells undergoing DNA synthesis (S-phase) and by blocking the progression of cells through the G1/S-phase boundary. Metabolized within cells by nucleoside kinases to the active gemcitabine diphosphate and triphosphate nucleosides. The diphosphate inhibits ribonucleotide reductase, which is responsible for catalyzing reactions that generate the deoxynucleoside triphosphate for DNA synthesis. Inhibition of the reductase enzyme causes a decrease in the levels of deoxynucleotides. The triphosphate competes with triphosphate nucleosides for incorporation into DNA, resulting in inhibition of DNA synthesis. DNA polymerase is not able to remove the gemcitabine nucleoside and repair the growing DNA strands. The metabolite of gemcitabine nucleoside is excreted through the urine.

**Uses:** First-line treatment for locally advanced (nonresectable Stage II or Stage III) or metastatic (Stage IV) adenocarcinoma of the pancreas. The drug is indicated for those who have been treated previously with 5-fluorouracil.

**Contraindications:** Lactation.

**Special Concerns:** Use with caution in those with preexisting renal impairment or hepatic insufficiency. Safety and efficacy have not been determined in children.

**Side Effects:** *GI:* N&V, diarrhea, constipation, stomatitis. *CNS:* Somnolence, mild to severe paresthesias, insomnia. *CV:* Arrhythmia, hypertension, *MI, CVA. Hematologic:* Anemia, leukopenia, neutropenia, thrombocytopenia. *Respiratory:* Dyspnea, bronchospasm, cough, parenchymal lung toxicity (rare). *Dermatologic:* Alopecia, macular or finely granular maculopapular pruritic eruptions, pruritus. *Body as a whole:* Pain, fever, peripheral edema, flu syndrome (including fever), asthenia, chills, myalgia, sweating, malaise. *Miscellaneous:* **Hemorrhage, sepsis,** hemolytic uremic syndrome, infections, petechiae, rhinitis, **anaphylaxis (rare).**

**Laboratory Test Interferences:** ALT, AST, alkaline phosphatase, bilirubin, BUN, creatinine. Proteinuria, hematuria.

**OD Overdose Management:** *Symptoms:* Myelosuppression, paresthesias, severe rash. *Treatment:* Monitor with appropriate blood counts. Supportive therapy as needed.

**Dosage**
• **IV Only**

*Adenocarcinoma of the pancreas.*
**Adults:** 1,000 mg/m² given over 30 min once a week for up to 7 weeks (or until toxicity necessitates reducing or holding a dose). This is followed by a 1-week rest period. Subsequent cycles should consist of infusions once a week for 3 consecutive weeks out of 4. Those who complete the entire 7 weeks of initial therapy or a subsequent 3-week cycle at the 1,000-mg/m² dose may have the dose for subsequent cycles increased by 25% to 1,250 mg/m² provided that the absolute neutrophil count nadir exceeds 1,500 × 10⁶/L and the platlet nadir exceeds 100,000 × 10⁶/L and if nonhematologic toxicity has not been greater than World Health Organization Grade 1. If clients tolerate a dose of 1,250 mg/m² once weekly, the dose for the next cycle can be increased to 1,500 mg/m² provided the absolute neutrophil count and platelet nadirs are as defined above.

The dose should be reduced to 75% of the full dose if the absolute granulocyte count is 500–999 × 10⁶/L and the platelet count is 50,000–99,000 × 10⁶/L. The dose should be held if the absolute granulocyte count falls below 500 × 10⁶/L and the platelet count falls below 50,000 × 10⁶/L.

## NURSING CONSIDERATIONS

See also *Nursing Considerations* for *Antineoplastic Agents.*

**Administration/Storage**

**IV** 1. To reconstitute the drug, use 0.9% NaCl injection without preservatives. The maximum concentration upon reconstitution is 40 mg/mL; greater concentrations may cause incomplete dissolution.

2. Prolonging the infusion time beyond 60 min and more frequent administration than once weekly increases toxicity.

3. To reconstitute, add 5 mL of 0.9% NaCl injection to the 200-mg vial or 25 mL of 0.9% NaCl injection to the 1-g vial. Shake to dissolve. This results in a concentration of 40 mg/mL which may be further diluted, if needed, with 0.9% NaCl injection to concentrations as low as 0.1 mg/mL.

4. Do not refrigerate reconstituted gemcitabine as crystallization may occur. Store the diluted product at controlled room temperatures of 20°C–25°C (68°F–77°F). Reconstituted solutions are stable at these temperatures for 24 hr.

**Assessment**

1. Document disease stage, onset, duration of symptoms, organ(s) involved, and other agents trialed.

2. Obtain CBC, liver and renal function studies. Monitor CBC prior to each dose and liver and renal function tests periodically; causes thrombocytopenia and myelosuppression. Nadir: 1 week.

**Client/Family Teaching**

1. Anticipate IV therapy once weekly over 30 min for up to 7 weeks; then weekly for 3 out of every 4 weeks.

2. May experience fever and flu-like symptoms as well as a rash involving trunk and extremities.

---

3. Report any evidence of pain on voiding or hematuria.

4. Use reliable birth control during and for several months following therapy as drug can cause fetal harm.

**Outcomes/Evaluate:** Suppression of pancreatic malignant cell proliferation

# Gemfibrozil

(jem-**FIH**-broh-zill)

**Pregnancy Category:** B

Apo-Gemfibrozil ✹, Gemcor, Lopid, Novo-Gemfibrozil ✹, Nu-Gemfibrozil ✹ **(Rx)**

**Classification:** Antihyperlipidemic

**Action/Kinetics:** Gemfibrozil, which resembles clofibrate, decreases triglycerides, cholesterol, and VLDL and increases HDL; LDL levels either decrease or do not change. Also, decreases hepatic triglyceride production by inhibiting peripheral lipolysis and decreasing extraction of free fatty acids by the liver. Also, gemfibrozil decreases VLDL synthesis by inhibiting synthesis of VLDL carrier apolipoprotein B as well as inhibits peripheral lipolysis and decreases hepatic extraction of free fatty acids (thus decreasing hepatic triglyceride production). May be beneficial in inhibiting development of atherosclerosis. **Onset:** 2–5 days. **Peak plasma levels:** 1–2 hr; **t½:** 1.5 hr. Nearly 70% is excreted unchanged.

**Uses:** Hypertriglyceridemia (type IV and type V hyperlipidemia) unresponsive to dietary control or in clients who are at risk of pancreatitis and abdominal pain. Reduce risk of coronary heart disease in clients with type IIb hyperlipidemia who have not responded to diet, weight loss, exercise, and other drug therapy.

**Contraindications:** Gallbladder disease, primary biliary cirrhosis, hepatic or renal dysfunction.

**Special Concerns:** Use with caution during lactation. Safety and efficacy have not been established in children. The dose may have to be reduced in geriatric clients due to age-related decreases in renal function.

**Side Effects:** *GI:* Cholelithiasis, abdominal or epigastric pain, N&V, diarrhea, dyspepsia, constipation, acute appendicitis, colitis, pancreatitis, cholestatic jaundice, hepatoma. *CNS:* Dizziness, headache, fatigue, vertigo, somnolence, paresthesia, hypesthesia, depression, confusion, syncope, *seizures.* *CV:* Atrial fibrillation, extrasystole, peripheral vascular disease, *intracerebral hemorrhage.* *Hematopoietic:* Anemia, leukopenia, eosinophilia, thrombocytopenia, bone marrow hypoplasia. *Musculoskeletal:* Painful extremities, arthralgia, myalgia, myopathy, myasthenia, rhabdomyolysis, synovitis. *Allergic:* Urticaria, lupus-like syndrome, angioedema, *laryngeal edema,* vasculitis, *anaphylaxis.* *Dermatologic:* Eczema, dermatitis, pruritus, skin rashes, exfoliative dermatitis, alopecia. *Ophthalmic:* Blurred vision, retinal edema, cataracts. *Miscellaneous:* Increased chance of viral and bacterial infections, taste perversion, impotence, decreased male fertility, weight loss.

**Drug Interactions**

*Anticoagulants, oral* / ↑ Effect of anticoagulants; dosage adjustment necessary

*Lovastatin* / Possible rhabdomyolysis

*Simvastatin* / Possible rhabdomyolysis

**Laboratory Test Interferences:** ↑ AST, ALT, LDH, CPK, alkaline phosphatase, bilirubin. Hypokalemia. Positive antinuclear antibody. ↓ Hemoglobin, WBCs, hematocrit.

**Dosage**

• **Tablets**

**Adults:** 600 mg 30 min before the morning and evening meal (range: 900–1,500 mg/day). Dosage has not been established in children. Discontinue if significant improvement not observed within 3 months.

## NURSING CONSIDERATIONS

See also *Nursing Considerations* for *Clofibrate.*

**Assessment**

1. Document serum levels and note any previous therapy utilized. (Drug

usually reserved until triglycerides greater than 500 mg/dL.)

2. Assess compliance with therapeutic regimens and life-style changes including restriction of fat in diet, weight reduction, regular exercise, and avoidance of alcohol.

**Client/Family Teaching**

1. Take 30 min before meals.

2. Take as directed; continue to follow prescribed dietary guidelines and regular exercise program.

3. Use caution when driving or performing other dangerous tasks until drug effects realized; may experience dizziness or blurred vision.

4. Report any unusual bruising or bleeding. If also on anticoagulant therapy, a reduction in anticoagulant is indicated if gemfibrozil therapy is instituted.

5. Limit intake of alcohol.

6. Report any RUQ abdominal pain or change in color and consistency of stools.

7. Report any S&S associated with gallstones, such as abdominal pain and vomiting.

**Outcomes/Evaluate:** ↓ Serum cholesterol and triglyceride levels

---

# Gentamicin sulfate

(jen-tah-**MY**-sin)

**Pregnancy Category:** C

Alcomicin ✦, Cidomycin ✦, Diogent ✦, Garamycin, Garamycin Cream or Ointment, Garamycin Intrathecal, Garamycin IV Piggyback, Garamycin Ophthalmic Ointment, Garamycin Ophthalmic Solution, Garamycin Pediatric, Garatec ✦, Genoptic Ophthalmic Liquifilm, Genoptic S.O.P. Ophthalmic, Gentacidin Ophthalmic, Gentafair, Gentak Ophthalmic, Gentamicin, Gentamicin Ophthalmic, Gentamicin Sulfate IV Piggyback, Gentrasul Ophthalmic, G-myticin Cream or Ointment, Jenamicin, Minims Gentamcin ✦, Ocugram ✦, Pediatric Gentamicin Sulfate, PMS-Gentamicin Sulfate ✦, Schwinpharm Gentamicin ✦ **(Rx)**

**Classification:** Antibiotic, aminoglycoside

See also *Aminoglycosides.*

**Action/Kinetics: Therapeutic serum levels: IM,** 4–8 mcg/mL. **Toxic serum levels:** >12 mcg/mL (peak) and >2 mcg/mL (trough). Prolonged serum levels above 12 mcg/mL should be avoided. **t½:** 2 hr. Can be used with carbenicillin to treat serious *Pseudomonas* infections; do not mix these drugs in the same flask as carbenicillin will inactivate gentamicin.

**Uses: Systemic:** Serious infections caused by *Pseudomonas aeruginosa, Proteus, Klebsiella, Enterobacter, Serratia, Citrobacter,* and *Staphylococcus.* Infections include bacterial neonatal sepsis, bacterial septicemia, and serious infections of the skin, bone, soft tissue (including burns), urinary tract, GI tract (including peritonitis), and CNS (including meningitis). Should be considered as initial therapy in suspected or confirmed gram-negative infections. In combination with carbenicillin for treating life-threatening infections due to *P. aeruginosa.* In combination with penicillin for treating endocarditis caused by group D streptococci. In combination with penicillin for treating suspected bacterial sepsis or staphylococcal pneumonia in the neonate. Intrathecal administration is used in combination with systemic gentamicin for treating meningitis, ventriculitis, or other serious CNS infections due to *Pseudomonas. Investigational:* Pelvic inflammatory disease.

**Ophthalmic:** Ophthalmic infections due to *Staphylococcus, S. aureus, Streptococcus pneumoniae,* beta-hemolytic streptococci, *Corynebacterium* species, *Streptococcus pyogenes, Escherichia coli, Haemophilus influenzae, H. aegyptius, H. ducreyi, Klebsiella pneumoniae, Neisseria gonorrhoeae, Proteus* species, *Acinetobacter calcoaceticus, Enterobacter aerogenes, P. aeruginosa, Serratia marcescens, Moraxella lacunata.*

**Topical:** Prevention of infections following minor cuts, wounds, burns, and skin abrasions. Treat-

---

ment of primary or secondary skin infections. Treatment of infected skin cysts and other skin abscesses when preceded by incision and drainage to permit adequate contact between the drug and the infecting bacteria, infected stasis and other skin ulcers, infected superficial burns, paronychia, infected insect bites and stings, infected lacerations and abrasions and wounds from minor surgery.

**Contraindications:** Ophthalmic use to treat dendritic keratitis, vaccinia, varicella, mycobacterial infections of the eye, fungal diseases of the eye, use with steroids after uncomplicated removal of a corneal foreign body.

**Special Concerns:** Use with caution in premature infants and neonates. Ophthalmic ointments may retard corneal epithelial healing.

**Additional Side Effects:** Muscle twitching, numbness, *seizures,* increased BP, alopecia, purpura, pseudotumor cerebri. Photosensitivity when used topically. *After ophthalmic use:* Transient irritation, burning, stinging, itching, inflammation, angioneurotic edema, urticaria, vesicular and maculopapular dermatitis, mydriasis, conjunctival paresthesia, conjunctival hyperemia, nonspecific conjunctivitis, conjunctival epithelial defects, lid itching and swelling, bacterial/fungal corneal ulcers.

**Additional Drug Interactions:** With carbenicillin or ticarcillin, gentamicin may result in increased effect when used for *Pseudomonas* infections.

## Dosage

**• IM (usual), IV**
**Adults with normal renal function.**
   *Infections.*
1 mg/kg q 8 hr, up to 5 mg/kg/day in life-threatening infections; **children:** 2–2.5 mg/kg q 8 hr; **infants and neonates:** 2.5 mg/kg q 8 hr; **premature infants or neonates less than 1 week of age:** 2.5 mg/kg q 12 hr. Therapy may be required for 7–10 days.

   *Prevention of bacterial endocarditis, dental or respiratory tract procedures.*
**Adults:** 1.5 mg/kg gentamicin (not to exceed 80 mg) plus 1 g ampicillin, each IM or IV, 30–60 min before the procedure; one additional dose of each can be given 8 hr later (alternative: penicillin V, 1 g PO, 6 hr after initial dose).
   *Prophylaxis of bacterial endocarditis in GI or GU tract procedures or surgery.*
**Adults:** 1.5 mg/kg gentamicin (not to exceed 80 mg) plus 2 g ampicillin, each IM or IV, 30–60 min before procedure; dose should be repeated 8 hr later. **Children:** 2 mg/kg gentamicin plus penicillin G, 30,000 units/kg, or ampicillin, 50 mg/kg in same dosage interval as for adults. Pediatric dosage should not exceed single or 24-hr adult doses.
   *NOTE:* In clients allergic to penicillin, vancomycin, 1 g IV given slowly over 1 hr, may be substituted; the dose of vancomycin should be repeated 8–12 hr later. **Adults with impaired renal function:** To calculate interval (hr) between doses, multiply serum creatinine level (mg/100 mL) by 8.

**• IV**
   *Septicemia.*
**Initially:** 1–2 mg/kg infused over 30–60 min; **then,** maintenance doses may be administered.

**• Intrathecal**
   *Meningitis.*
**Use only the intrathecal preparation. Adults, usual:** 4–8 mg/day; **children and infants 3 months and older:** 1–2 mg/day
   *Pelvic inflammatory disease.*
**Initial:** 2 mg/kg IV; **then,** 1.5 mg/kg t.i.d. plus clindamycin, 500 mg IV q.i.d. Continue for at least 4 days and at least 48 hr after client improves. Continue clindamycin, 450 mg PO q.i.d. for 10–14 days.

**• Ophthalmic Solution (0.3%)**
   *Acute infections.*
**Initially:** 1–2 gtt in conjunctival sac q 15–30 min; **then,** as infection improves, reduce frequency.
   *Moderate infections.*

1–2 gtt in conjunctival sac 4–6 times/day.

*Trachoma.*

2 gtt in each eye b.i.d.–q.i.d.; treatment should be continued for up to 1–2 months.

• **Ophthalmic Ointment (0.3%)**

Depending on the severity of infection, ½-in. ribbon from q 3–4 hr to 2–3 times/day.

• **Topical        Cream/Ointment (0.1%)**

Apply 3–4 times/day to affected area. The area may be covered with a sterile bandage.

## NURSING CONSIDERATIONS

See also *Nursing Considerations* for *Aminoglycosides.*

**Administration/Storage**

1. When used intrathecally, the usual site is the lumbar area.

**IV** 2. For intermittent IV administration, dilute adult dose in 50–200 mL of sterile D5W or isotonic saline and administer over a 30–120-min period; use less volume for infants and children.

3. Do not mix with other drugs for parenteral use.

4. For parenteral use, the duration of treatment is 7–10 days; a longer course may be required for severe or complicated infections.

**Assessment**

1. Document type, duration, and onset of symptoms.

2. Obtain renal function studies and appropriate specimen for culture.

3. With eye disorders, note baseline ophthalmologic assessments.

4. Assess for tinnitus, vertigo, or hearing losses during therapy. Persistently increased gentamycin levels have been associated with 8th CN dysfunction.

**Client/Family Teaching**

1. Review the appropriate method and frequency for administration. Wash hands before and after treatment; prepare site and apply as directed.

2. With topical administration:

• Remove crusts of impetigo contagiosa before applying the cream or ointment to permit maximum contact between antibiotic and infection.

• Apply cream or ointment gently and cover with gauze dressing if desirable or as ordered.

• Avoid direct exposure to sunlight as photosensitivity reaction may occur.

• Avoid further contamination of infected skin.

3. Identify symptoms and wound changes that require medical attention; i.e., pain, redness, swelling, increased drainage or odor.

4. Report any evidence of visual impairment, vertigo, dizziness, hearing impairment, or worsening of symptoms.

5. Avoid vaccinia during treatment.

**Outcomes/Evaluate**

• Resolution of infection

• Therapeutic serum drug levels 4–8 mcg/mL; (peak 5–10 mcg/mL trough 1–2 mcg/mL)

# Glatiramer acetate

(glah-**TER**-ah-mer)

**Pregnancy Category:** B

Copaxone **(Rx)**

**Classification:** Drug for multiple sclerosis

**Action/Kinetics:** Thought to act by modifying immune processes responsible for pathology of multiple sclerosis. Some of drug enters lymphatic circulation reaching regional lymph nodes.

**Uses:** Reduce frequency of relapsing-remitting multiple sclerosis.

**Contraindications:** Hypersensitivity to glatiramer or mannitol.

**Special Concerns:** Use with caution during lactation. Safety and efficacy have not been determined in children less than 18 years of age. May interfere with useful immune function.

**Side Effects:** Side effects listed are those with incidence of 1% or more. *Immediate-post injection reaction:* Flushing, chest pain, palpitations, anxiety, dyspnea, laryngeal constriction, urticaria. *CNS:* Anxiety, hypertonia, tremor, vertigo, agitation, foot drop, nervousness, nystagmus, speech disorder, confusion, abnormal dreams, emotional lability, stupor, migraine. *GI:* Nausea, diarrhea, anorexia, vomiting, GI disorder, abdominal pain, gastroenteritis, bowel urgency, oral moniliasis, salivary gland enlargement, tooth caries, ulcerative stomatitis. *CV:* Vasodilation, palpitations, tachycardia, syncope, hypertension. *Body as a whole:* Infection, asthenia, pain, transient chest pain, flu syndrome, back pain, fever, neck pain, face edema, bacterial infection, chills, cyst, headache, injection site ecchymosis, accidental injury, neck rigidity, malaise, injection site edema or atrophy, abscess, peripheral edema, edema, weight gain. *Dermatologic:* Rash, pruritus, sweating, herpes simplex, erythema, urticaria, skin nodule, eczema, herpes zoster, pustular rash, skin atrophy and warts. *GU:* Urinary urgency, vaginal moniliasis, dysmenorrhea, amenorrhea, hematuria, impotence, menorrhagia, suspicious Pap smear, vaginal hemorrhage. *Hematologic:* Ecchymosis, lymphadenopathy. *Respiratory:* Dyspnea, allergic rhinitis, bronchitis, laryngismus, hyperventilation. *At injection site:* Pain, erythema, inflammation, pruritus, mass, induration, welt, hemorrhage, urticaria. *Miscellaneous:* Ear pain, eye disorder, arthralgia.

## Dosage

- **SC**

  *Multiple sclerosis.*

  **Adults:** 20 mg/day SC.

## NURSING CONSIDERATIONS

### Administration/Storage

1. SC sites include arms, abdomen, hips, and thighs.
2. Reconstitute with diluent provided (sterile water for injection). Gently swirl vial after diluent is added. Let stand at room temperature until solid material is dissolved.
3. Use reconstituted drug immediately as it contains no preservative.

Before reconstitution store at −20°C to −10°C (−4°F to −14°F).

### Assessment

1. Document age at onset, frequency of exacerbations, degree of physical disability, and other therapies trialed.
2. RR (relapsing–remitting) MS is characterized by recurrent attacks of neurologic dysfunction followed by complete or incomplete recovery; assess frequency.

### Client/Family Teaching

1. Use exactly as directed, do not stop without consulting provider.
2. Reconstitute with diluent provided and gently swirl vial. Let stand at room temperature until solid material is dissolved. Administer SC into arms, abdomen, hips or thighs, rotating sites.
3. Patient Information booklet is enclosed with drug for review of self–injection procedure.
4. Drug is used to slow accumulation of physical disablilty and to decrease frequency of clinical exacerbations with MS.
5. May experience pain, itching, swelling, and hardening of skin at injection site.
6. Chest tightness, flushing, SOB, and anxiety may occur within minutes of injection and last up to 30 min.
7. Practice reliable contraception.

**Outcomes/Evaluate:** ↓ Frequency and severity of MS exacerbations

---

# Glimepiride

(**GLYE**-meh-pye-ride)
**Pregnancy Category:** C
Amaryl **(Rx)**
**Classification:** Antidiabetic agent, sulfonylurea

---

See also *Hypoglycemic Agents.*
**Action/Kinetics:** Lowers blood glucose by stimulating the release of insulin from functioning pancreatic beta cells and by increasing the sensitivity of peripheral tissues to insulin. Completely absorbed from the GI tract within 1 hr. **Time to maximum effect:** 2–3 hr. Completely metabolized in the liver and metab-

olites are excreted through both the urine and feces.

**Uses:** As an adjunct to diet and exercise to lower blood glucose in non-insulin-dependent diabetes mellitus (Type II diabetes mellitus). In combination with insulin to decrease blood glucose in those whose hyperglycemia cannot be controlled by diet and exercise in combination with an oral hypoglycemic drug.

**Contraindications:** Diabetic ketoacidosis with or without coma. Use during lactation.

**Special Concerns:** The use of oral hypoglycemic drugs has been associated with increased CV mortality compared with treatment with diet alone or diet plus insulin. Safety and efficacy have not been determined in children.

**Side Effects:** The most common side effect is hypoglycemia. *GI:* N&V, GI pain, diarrhea, cholestatic jaundice (rare). *CNS:* Dizziness, headache. *Dermatologic:* Pruritus, erythema, urticaria, morbilliform or maculopapular eruptions. *Hematologic:* Leukopenia, agranulocytosis, thrombocytopenia, hemolytic anemia, aplastic anemia, pancytopenia. *Miscellaneous:* Hyponatremia, increased release of ADH, changes in accommodation and/or blurred vision.

**Drug Interactions:** See *Hypoglycemic Agents.*

**Dosage** ———
• **Tablets**

*Non-insulin-dependent diabetes mellitus (Type II diabetes).*

**Adults, initial:** 1–2 mg once daily, given with breakfast or the first main meal. The initial dose should be 1 mg in those sensitive to hypoglycemic drugs, in those with impaired renal or hepatic function, and in elderly, debilitated, or malnourished clients. The maximum initial dose is 2 mg or less daily. **Maintenance:** 1–4 mg once daily up to a maximum of 8 mg once daily. After a dose of 2 mg is reached, the dose should be increased in increments of 2 mg or

less at 1- to 2-week intervals (determined by the blood glucose response). **When combined with insulin therapy:** 8 mg once daily with the first main meal with low-dose insulin. The fasting glucose level for beginning combination therapy is greater than 150 mg/dL glucose in the plasma or serum.

*Type II diabetes—transfer from other hypoglycemic agents*
When transferring clients to glimipiride, no transition period is required. However, clients should be observed closely for 1 to 2 weeks for hypoglycemia when being transferred from longer half-life sulfonylureas (e.g., chlorpropamide) to glimepiride.

---

## NURSING CONSIDERATIONS

See also *Nursing Considerations* for *Hypoglycemic Agents.*
**Administration/Storage**
1. Dispense tablets in well-closed containers with safety caps.
2. Store tablets at 15°C–30°C (59°F–86°F).
**Assessment**
1. Note indications for therapy, if newly diagnosed or transferred therapy; onset and duration of disease.
2. List drugs currently prescribed and OTC to ensure none interact unfavorably.
3. Obtain baseline labs, including electrolytes, HbA1C, Ca, Mg, urinalysis, liver and renal function studies.
**Client/Family Teaching**
1. Review dose and frequency for administration.
2. Monitor finger sticks.
3. Continue regular exercise and dietary restrictions in addition to drug therapy.
4. Report as scheduled for teaching reinforcement, follow-up labs, and medication evaluation.
**Outcomes/Evaluate:** Blood sugar and HbA1C within desired range

# Glipizide
(**GLIP**-ih-zyd)

**Pregnancy Category:** C
Glucotrol, Glucotrol XL **(Rx)**
**Classification:** Sulfonylurea (anti-diabetic), second-generation

See also *Antidiabetic Agents.*
**Action/Kinetics:** Also has mild diuretic effects. **Onset:** 1–1.5 hr. **t½:** 2–4 hr. **Time to peak levels:** 1–3 hr. **Duration:** 10–16 hr. Metabolized in liver to inactive metabolites, which are excreted through the kidneys.
**Uses:** Adjunct to diet for control of hyperglycemia in clients with non-insulin-dependent diabetes.
**Additional Drug Interactions:** Cimetidine may ↑ effect of glipizide due to ↓ breakdown by liver.

**Dosage**
• **Tablets, Extended Release Tablets**
    *Diabetes.*
**Adults, initial:** 5 mg 30 min before breakfast; **then,** adjust dosage by 2.5–5 mg every few days, depending on the blood glucose response, until adequate control is achieved. **Maintenance:** 15–40 mg/day. Older clients should begin with 2.5 mg. The Extended Release Tablets are taken once daily (usually at breakfast) in doses of either 5 or 10 mg.

## NURSING CONSIDERATIONS

See also *Nursing Considerations* for *Antidiabetic Agents.*
**Administration/Storage**
1. Some clients are better controlled on once daily dosing while others are better controlled with divided dosing.
2. Divide maintenance doses greater than 15 mg/day; give before the morning and evening meals. Total daily doses of 30 mg or more may be given safely on twice daily dosing.
3. Assess client life-style to ensure that maximal changes in the areas of diet and exercise have been taken before increasing dosage. Once maximum dosage attained, if renal function is normal, consider adding Metformin to decrease production and absorption of gluocose if hyperglycemia is not controlled.

**Client/Family Teaching**
1. For greatest effect, take 30 min before meals.
2. Report any CNS side effects such as drowsiness or headache; differentiate from hypoglycemia.
3. May experience anorexia, constipation or diarrhea, vomiting, and gastralgia. If severe, record weight, I&O and report.
4. Skin reactions may occur and should be reported. Avoid sun exposure; when in the sun, use sunscreen and wear sunglasses and protective clothing.
5. Avoid alcohol in any form.
6. Practice barrier contraception.
7. Continue prescribed diabetic diet and regular exercise program. Monitor fingersticks; report loss of control.
**Outcomes/Evaluate:** BS and HbA1C levels within desired range

# Glucagon
(**GLOO**-kah-gon)
**Pregnancy Category:** B
**(Rx)**
**Classification:** Insulin antagonist

**Action/Kinetics:** Produced by the alpha islet cells of the pancreas, glucacon accelerates liver glycogenolysis by stimulating synthesis of cyclic AMP and increasing phosphorylase kinase activity. Increased blood glucose levels result from increased breakdown of glycogen to glucose and inhibition of glycogen synthetase. Glucagon stimulates hepatic gluconeogenesis by increasing the uptake of amino acids and converting them to glucose precursors. Also, lipolysis is increased, resulting in free fatty acids and glycerol for gluconeogenesis. Effective in overcoming hypoglycemia only if the liver has a glycogen reserve. **Onset, hypoglycemia:** 5–20 min. **Maximum effect:** 30 min. **Duration:** 1–2 hr. **t½:** 3–6 min. Metabolized in the liver, kidney, plasma membrane receptor sites, and plasma.
**Uses:** Used to terminate insulin-induced shock in diabetic or psychiatric clients. Client usually regains

consciousness 5–20 min after the parenteral administration of glucagon. The drug should only be used under medical supervision or in accordance with strict instructions received from the physician. Failure to respond may be an indication for IV administration of glucose—especially true in juvenile diabetics. As a diagnostic aid in radiologic examination of the GI tract when a hypotonic state is desirable. *Investigational:* Treatment of propranolol overdose and cardiovascular emergencies.

**Special Concerns:** Use with caution in clients with renal or hepatic disease, in those who are undernourished and emaciated, and in clients with a history of pheochromocytoma or insulinoma.

**Side Effects:** *GI:* N&V. *Allergy:* Respiratory distress, urticaria, hypotension. ***Stevens-Johnson syndrome when used as diagnostic aid.***

**OD** **Overdose Management:** *Symptoms:* N&V, hypokalemia. *Treatment:* Symptomatic.

**Drug Interactions**

*Anticoagulants, oral /* ↑ Effect of anticoagulants by ↑ hypoprothrombinemia

*Antidiabetic agents /* Hyperglycemic effect of glucagon antagonizes hypoglycemic effect of antidiabetics

*Corticosteroids, Epinephrine, Estrogens, Phenytoin /* Additive hyperglycemic effect of drugs listed

**Dosage** —————————

- **IM, IV, SC**
  *Hypoglycemia.*

**Children < 20 kg:** 0.5 mg; **Adults and children > 20 kg:** 1 mg; one to two additional doses may be given at 20-min intervals, if necessary.

*Insulin shock therapy.*

**IM, IV, SC:** 0.5–1 mg after 1 hr of coma; the client will usually awaken in 10–25 min. The dose may be repeated if there is no response.

*Diagnostic aid for GI tract.*

Dose dependent on desired onset of action and duration of effect necessary

for the examination. **IV:** 0.25–0.5 mg (onset: 1 min; duration: 9–17 min); 2 mg (onset: 1 min; duration 22–25 min). **IM:** 1 mg (onset: 8–10 min; duration: 12–27 min); 2 mg (onset: 4–7 min; duration: 21–32 min).

*For colon examination.*

**IM:** 2 mg 10 min prior to procedure.

*Treatment of toxicity of beta-adrenergic blocking agents.*

**Adults, IV, initial:** 2–3 mg given over 30 sec; may be repeated at the rate of 5 mg/hr until client is stabilized.

## NURSING CONSIDERATIONS
### Administration/Storage

1. Once client with hypoglycemia responds, give supplemental carbohydrates to prevent secondary hypoglycemia.

**IV** 2. Before reconstituting, store powder at room temperature.

3. Following reconstitution, use the solution immediately. If necessary, the solution may be stored at 5°C (41°F) for up to 2 days.

4. Reconstitute doses higher than 2 mg with sterile water for injection and use immediately.

5. With direct IV administration, inject at a rate not exceeding 1 mg/min.

6. Administer with dextrose solutions. A precipitate may form if saline solutions are used.

### Client/Family Teaching

1. Instruct family in the administration of glucagon SC or IM in the event of hypoglycemic reaction, loss of consciousness, or inability to swallow.

2. Following administration of glucagon, keep client on their side and administer a carbohydrate once they awaken.

3. Have rapidly available sugar, such as orange juice and Karo syrup in water (or life savers) to administer. If the shock was caused by a long-acting medication, administer slowly digestible carbohydrates, such as bread with honey.

4. Advise not to try to administer fluids by mouth if client has a reaction and is not fully conscious; they

could easily aspirate fluids into the lungs.

5. Record time of day and activity and report all hypoglycemic reactions so that insulin dosage can be adjusted.

**Outcomes/Evaluate**
- Reversal of S&S of hypoglycemia
- Termination of insulin-induced shock
- Inhibition of bowel peristalsis with small muscle relaxation during radiologic imaging of the GI tract

# Glyburide
(**GLYE**-byou-ryd)
**Pregnancy Category:** B
Albert Glyburide ✹, Apo-Glyburide ✹, Diabeta, Euglucon ✹, Gen-Glybe ✹, Glynase PresTab, Med-Glybe ✹, Micronase, Novo-Glyburide ✹, Nu-Glyburide ✹ **(Rx)**
**Classification:** Sulfonylurea (anti-diabetic), second-generation

See also *Antidiabetic Agents*.
**Action/Kinetics:** Has a mild diuretic effect. **Onset, nonmicronized:** 2–4 hr; **micronized:** 1 hr. **t½, nonmicronized:** 10 hr; **micronized:** Approximately 4 hr. **Time to peak levels:** 4 hr. **Duration, both forms:** 24 hr. Metabolized in liver to weakly active metabolites. Excreted in bile (50%) and through the kidneys (50%).

**Dosage**
- **Tablets, Nonmicronized (Dia-Beta/Micronase)**
  *Diabetes.*
**Adults, initial:** 2.5–5 mg/day given with breakfast (or the first main meal); **then,** increase by 2.5 mg at weekly intervals to achieve the desired response. **Maintenance:** 1.25–20 mg/day. Clients sensitive to sulfonylureas should start with 1.25 mg/day.
- **Tablets, Micronized (Glynase)**
  *Diabetes.*
**Adults, initial:** 1.5–3 mg/day given with breakfast (or the first main meal); **then,** increase by no more than 1.5 mg at weekly intervals to

achieve the desired response. **Maintenance:** 0.75–12 mg/day.

## NURSING CONSIDERATIONS

See also *Nursing Considerations* for *Antidiabetic Agents* and *Glipizide*.
**Administration/Storage**
1. For best results, administer prior to meals.
2. Do not exceed 20 mg/day of the nonmicronized product and 12 mg/day of the micronized product.
3. If daily dosage of the nonmicronized product exceeds 15 mg or the micronized product exceeds 6 mg, divide the dose and give before the morning and evening meals.
**Outcomes/Evaluate:** BS and HbA1C levels within desired range

# Gold sodium thiomalate (Sodium aurothiomalate)
(gold **SO**-dee-um thigh-oh-**MAH**-layt)
**Pregnancy Category:** C
Myochrysine ✹ **(Rx)**
**Classification:** Antirheumatic

**Action/Kinetics:** Exact mechanism not known. May inhibit lysosomal enzyme activity in macrophages and decrease macrophage phagocytic activity. Other mechanisms may include alteration of the immune response and alteration of biosynthesis of collagen. Gold salts suppress, but do not cure, arthritis and synovitis. Beneficial effects may not be seen for 3–12 months. Most experience transient side effects, although serious effects may be manifested in some. **Peak blood levels (IM):** 4–6 hr. **Steady-state plasma levels:** 1–5 mcg/mL. **t½:** increases with continued therapy. Gold may accumulate in tissues and persist for years. Significantly bound to plasma proteins. Eliminated slowly through both the urine (70%) and feces (30%). This preparation contains 50% gold.
**Uses:** Adjunct to the treatment of active, early rheumatoid arthritis in children and adults who have insufficient response to or are intolerant of full doses of one or more NSAIDs.

**Contraindications:** Hepatic disease, CV problems such as hypertension or CHF, severe diabetes, debilitated clients, renal disease, blood dyscrasias, agranulocytosis, hemorrhagic diathesis, clients receiving radiation treatments, colitis, lupus erythematosus, pregnancy, lactation, children under 6 years of age. Clients with eczema or urticaria.

**Side Effects:** *Skin:* Dermatitis (most common), pruritus, erythema, dermatoses, gray to blue pigmentation of tissues, alopecia, loss of nails. *GI:* Stomatitis (second most common), metallic taste, gastritis, colitis, gingivitis, glossitis, N&V, diarrhea (may be persistent), colic, anorexia, cramps, enterocolitis. *Hematologic:* Anemia, thrombocytopenia, granulocytopenia, leukopenia, eosinophilia, hemorrhagic diathesis. *Allergic:* Flushing, fainting, sweating, dizziness, **anaphylaxis,** syncope, bradycardia, angioneurotic edema, respiratory difficulties. *Other:* Interstitial pneumonitis, pulmonary fibrosis, nephrotic syndrome, glomerulitis (with hematuria), proteinuria, hepatitis, fever, headache, arthralgia, ophthalmologic problems including corneal ulcers, iritis, gold deposits, EEG abnormalities, peripheral neuritis. Corticosteroids may be used to treat symptoms such as stomatitis, dermatitis, GI, renal, hematologic, or pulmonary problems. Also, if symptoms are severe and do not respond to corticosteroids, a chelating agent such as dimercaprol may be used. Clients should be monitored carefully.

**OD  Overdose Management:** *Symptoms:* Hematuria, proteinuria, thrombocytopenia, granulocytopenia, N&V, diarrhea, fever, papulovesicular lesions, urticaria, exfoliative dermatitis, severe pruritus. *Treatment:* Discontinue use of the drug immediately. Give dimercaprol. Provide supportive treatment for hematologic or renal complications.

**Drug Interactions:** Concomitant use contraindicated with drugs known to cause blood dyscrasias (e.g., antimalarials, cytotoxic drugs, pyrazolone derivatives, immunosuppressive drugs).

**Laboratory Test Interferences:** Alters liver function tests. Urinary protein and RBCs, altered blood counts (indicative of toxic effect of drug).

## Dosage
* **IM**

   *Rheumatoid arthritis.*

**Adults:** w*eek 1:* 10 mg as a single injection; *week 2:* 25 mg as a single dose. Then, 25–50 mg/week until 0.8–1 g total has been given. Thereafter according to individual response. *Usual maintenance:* 25–50 mg every other week for up to 20 weeks. If condition remains stable, the dose can be given every third or fourth week indefinitely. **Pediatric, initial:** w*eek 1,* 10 mg; **then,** usual dose is 1 mg/kg, not to exceed 50 mg/injection using the same spacing of doses as for adults.

## NURSING CONSIDERATIONS
### Administration/Storage
1. Shake vial well to ensure uniformity of suspension before withdrawing medication. Do not use if contents have darkened (color should not exceed pale yellow).
2. Inject into gluteus maximus.
3. May reinstitute therapy following mild toxic symptoms but not after severe symptoms.
4. Geriatric clients manifest a lower tolerance to gold.

### Assessment
1. Document indications for therapy, previous treatments utilized, and the outcome.
2. Assess ROM; describe all areas of limitation and pain as well as active synovitis.
3. Monitor urinalysis, CBC, liver and renal function tests every 2 weeks.
4. Have client remain in a recumbent position for at least 20 min after injection to prevent falls resulting from transient vertigo or giddiness. Observe for flushing, dizziness,

G

sweating, and hypotension (nitritoid reaction).

5. Monitor I&O and electrolytes if prolonged diarrhea occurs.

**Client/Family Teaching**

1. Close medical supervision is required during gold therapy.

2. Do not become discouraged. Beneficial effects are slow to appear; therapy may be continued for up to 12 months in anticipation of relief.

3. Report any unusual bruising or bleeding, skin or mucous membrane lesions, or blood in urine or stools.

4. Rinse with dilute hydrogen peroxide for mild stomatitis; floss daily, use a soft bristle toothbrush, and rinse mouth frequently.

5. Avoid acidic or hot, spicy foods.

6. Practice reliable contraception during therapy.

7. Avoid direct sun exposure as a photosensitivity reaction may occur. Wear sunscreen, protective clothing, and a hat if exposure is necessary.

8. Continue anti-inflammatory doses of NSAIDs for several weeks into therapy.

**Outcomes/Evaluate:** ↓ Joint pain, swelling, and stiffness with ↑ ROM and mobility

---

# Gonadorelin acetate

(go-nad-oh-**RELL**-in)

**Pregnancy Category:** B

Factrel ✶(Hydrochloride salt), Lutrepulse, Relisorm ✶ **(Rx)**

**Classification:** Gonadotropin-releasing hormone.

**Action/Kinetics:** A synthetic hormone identical in amino acid sequence to the naturally occurring gonadotropin-releasing hormone. Thus, gonadorelin stimulates the synthesis and release of FSH and LH from the adenohypophysis. FSH and LH then stimulate the ovaries to synthesize estrogen and progesterone, which are necessary for development and release of an ovum. **t½, initial:** 2–10 min; **final:** 10–40 min. Metabolized to inactive peptide fragments, which are excreted in the urine.

**Uses:** Primary hypothalamic amenorrhea.

**Contraindications:** Sensitivity to gonadorelin acetate or gonadorelin HCl (used for determining gonadotropic function of the pituitary). Pituitary prolactinoma, causes of anovulation other than those of hypothalamic origin (e.g., ovarian cysts), hormone-dependent tumors.

**Special Concerns:** There is no indication for use of gonadorelin acetate during lactation. Safety and efficacy have not been determined in children less than 18 years of age.

**Side Effects:** *Ovarian hyperstimulation:* Ovarian enlargement, ascites with or without pain, pleural effusion. *Local, due to use of infusion pump:* Inflammation, infection, mild phlebitis, hematoma at site of catheter. ***Anaphylaxis: Bronchospasm,*** flushing, tachycardia, urticaria, induration at injection site. *Miscellaneous:* Multiple pregnancy.

**Drug Interactions:** Gonadorelin should not be used with ovarian stimulators.

---

**Dosage** ————————————

• **IV**

*Primary hypothalamic amenorrhea.*

5 mcg q 90 min (range: 1–20 mcg) delivered by Lutrepulse pump using the 0.8-mg solution at 50 mcL/pulse. The recommended treatment interval is 21 days. If there is no response after three treatment intervals, the dose should be increased cautiously and in stepwise fashion.

---

# NURSING CONSIDERATIONS

**Administration/Storage**

**IV** 1. The kit contains lyophilized powder for injection, diluent, catheter and tubing, alcohol swabs, IV cannula units, syringe and needle, elastic belt, batteries, Lutrepulse pump, pump manual, and package insert.

2. Reconstitute with 8 mL of diluent immediately before use and then transfer to the plastic reservoir.

3. The presterilized bag with the supplied infusion catheter set is

filled with the reconstituted solution for IV administration.

4. Administer IV using Lutrepulse pump, which can deliver 25 or 50 μL of solution over a period of 1 min and at a pulse frequency of 90 min. Depending on the concentration of the solution and the volume/pulse, the pump can deliver 2.5, 5, 10, or 20 mcg of gonadorelin.

5. The 8 mL of solution will last for approximately 7 consecutive days.

6. Change the cannula and peripheral IV site every 48 hr.

**Assessment**

1. Perform a thorough nursing history. Proper diagnosis is critical for treatment to be successful.

2. Determine that hypothalamic amenorrhea or hypogonadism is due to a deficiency in quantity or pulsing of endogenous gonadotropin-releasing hormone.

3. Note history of ovarian cysts or pituitary tumors; drug is contraindicated.

4. Obtain baseline ovarian ultrasound, pelvic exam, and mid-luteal phase serum progesterone level.

**Client/Family Teaching**

1. Demonstrate method for drug administration. Review detailed instructions regarding the proper use and care of the Lutrepulse infusion pump. Obtain phone number for 24 hr assistance.

2. Stress importance of using aseptic technique.

3. Assess infusion site for evidence of inflammation, phlebitis, erythema, infection, or hematoma.

4. Report symptoms of hyperstimulation of the ovaries; avoid having intercourse if symptoms evident as an ovarian cyst could rupture, resulting in hemoperitoneum.

5. Maintain careful recordkeeping in relation to menses, basal temperatures and graph recordings, and medication administration; report any side effects.

6. If ovulation occurs with the pump in place, the therapy should be continued for 2 more weeks to maintain the corpus luteum.

7. The clinical response to gonadorelin is monitored by ovarian ultrasound, mid-luteal phase serum progesterone levels, and regularly scheduled physical exams including a pelvic. The peripheral infusion site will be examined and changed every 48 hr. This therapy requires frequently scheduled visits and a relatively long-term commitment by the client.

**Outcomes/Evaluate:** Restoration of menstrual cycle with evidence of ovum production (response usually occurs within 2–3 weeks)

# Goserelin acetate
(GO-seh-rel-in)

**Pregnancy Category:** X (when used for endometriosis); D (when used for breast cancer)

Zoladex, Zoladex LA ✦ **(Rx)**

**Classification:** Antineoplastic, hormonal agent

See also *Antineoplastic Agents.*

**Action/Kinetics:** Goserelin acetate is a synthetic decapeptide analog of LHRH (or GnRH) which is a potent inhibitor of gonadotropin secretion from the pituitary gland. Initially, there is actually an increase in serum luteinizing hormone and FSH. This is followed by a long-term suppression of pituitary gonadotropins with serum levels of testosterone decreasing to those seen in surgically castrated males. When used for endometriosis, the drug controls the secretion of hormones required for the ovary to synthesize estrogen resulting in plasma estrogen levels seen in menopause. **Peak serum levels after SC implantation of 3.6 mg:** 12–15 days. **Mean peak serum levels:** Approximately 2.5 ng/mL. Available as an implant in a preloaded syringe. For the first 8 days of the treatment cycle, the rate of absorption is slower than for the remainder of the period. Rapidly cleared by a combination of hepatic metabolism and urinary excretion.

**Uses: Implant, 3.6 mg or 10.8 mg:** Palliative treatment of advanced prostatic carcinoma as an alternative to orchiectomy or estrogen administration when these are either unacceptable to the client or not indicated. **Implant, 3.6 mg only:** Endometriosis, including pain relief and reduction of endometriotic lesions. Palliative treatment of advanced breast cancer in premenopausal and postmenopausal women. For endometrial thinning prior to ablation for dysfunctional uterine bleeding.

**Contraindications:** Pregnancy, lactation, nondiagnosed vaginal bleeding, hypersensitivity to LHRH or LHRH agonist analogs. Use of the 10.8-mg implant in women.

**Special Concerns:** Safety and effectiveness have not been determined in clients less than 18 years of age. There may be transient worsening of symptoms during the first few weeks of therapy. Use with caution in males who are at particular risk of developing ureteral obstruction or spinal cord compression.

**Side Effects: In males.** *GU:* Sexual dysfunction, decreased erections, lower urinary tract symptoms, gynecomastia, renal insufficiency, urinary obstruction, UTI, bladder neoplasm, hematuria, impotence, urinary frequency, incontinence, urinary tract disorder, impaired urination. *CV:* CHF, **CVA, MI, heart failure, pulmonary embolus,** arrhythmia, hypertension, peripheral vascular disorder, chest pain, angina pectoris, cerebral ischemia, varicose veins. *CNS:* Lethargy, anorexia, dizziness, insomnia, asthenia, anxiety, depression, headache, paresthesia. *GI:* N&V, diarrhea, constipation, ulcer, hematemesis. *Respiratory:* Upper respiratory infection, COPD, increased cough, dyspnea, pneumonia. *Metabolic:* Gout, hypercalcemia, weight increase, diabetes mellitus. *Miscellaneous:* Pelvic or bone pain, anemia, chills, fever, breast pain, breast swelling or tenderness, abdominal or back pain, flu syndrome, sepsis, aggravation reaction, herpes simplex, pruritus, peripheral edema, injection site reaction, hot flashes, rash, sweating, complications of surgery.

**In females.** *GU:* Vaginitis, decreased or increased libido, pelvic symptoms, dyspareunia, dysmenorrhea, urinary frequency, UTI, vaginal bleeding (during the first 2 months) of varying duration and intensity. *CV:* **Hemorrhage,** hypertension, palpitations, tachycardia. *CNS:* Emotional lability, depression, headache, insomnia, dizziness, nervousness, anxiety, paresthesia, somnolence, abnormal thinking, malaise, fatigue, lethargy. *GI:* N&V, abdominal pain, increased appetite, anorexia, constipation, diarrhea, dry mouth, dyspepsia, flatulence. *Musculoskeletal:* Asthenia, back pain, myalgia, hypertonia, arthralgia, joint disorder, decrease of vertebral trabecular bone mineral density. *Dermatologic:* Sweating, acne, seborrhea, hirsutism, pruritus, alopecia, dry skin, ecchymosis, rash, skin discoloration. *Respiratory:* Pharyngitis, bronchitis, increased cough, epistaxis, rhinitis, sinusitis. *Miscellaneous:* Hot flashes, breast atrophy or enlargement, breast pain, tumor flare, pain, infection, application site reaction, flu syndrome, hair disorders, voice alterations, weight gain, allergic reaction, chest pain, fever, peripheral edema, hypercalcemia.

**Laboratory Test Interferences:** LDL and HDL cholesterol, triglycerides. Misleading results of pituitary-gonadotropic and gonadal function tests that are conducted during treatment.

## Dosage

- **SC Implant, 3.6 mg**

  *Prostatic carcinoma, endometriosis, advanced breast cancer, thinning prior to endometrial ablation for dysfunctional uterine bleeding.*

  3.6 mg q 28 days into the upper abdominal wall using sterile technique under the direction of a physician.

# VISUAL IDENTIFICATION GUIDE

Use this section to quickly verify the identity of a capsule, tablet, or other solid oral medication. More than 200 leading products are shown in actual size and color, organized alphabetically by generic name. Each product is labeled with its brand name, if applicable, as well as its strength and the name of its supplier.

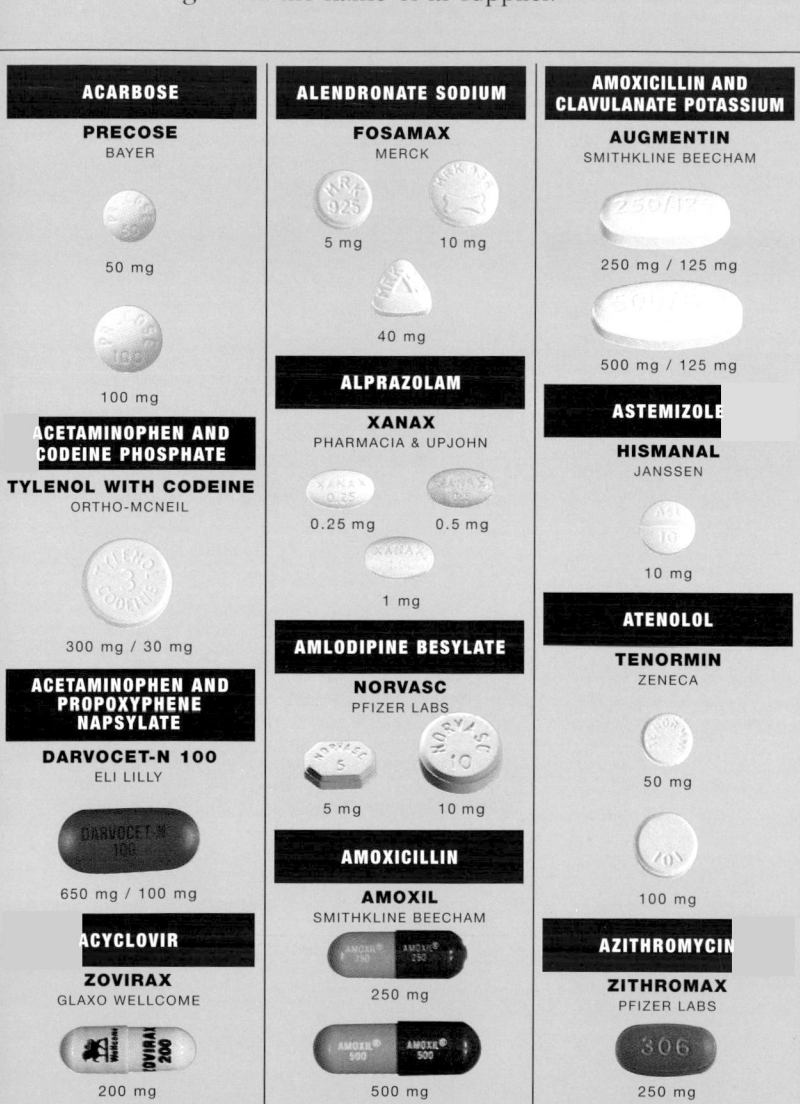

**ACARBOSE**

**PRECOSE**
BAYER

50 mg

100 mg

**ACETAMINOPHEN AND CODEINE PHOSPHATE**

**TYLENOL WITH CODEINE**
ORTHO-MCNEIL

300 mg / 30 mg

**ACETAMINOPHEN AND PROPOXYPHENE NAPSYLATE**

**DARVOCET-N 100**
ELI LILLY

650 mg / 100 mg

**ACYCLOVIR**

**ZOVIRAX**
GLAXO WELLCOME

200 mg

**ALENDRONATE SODIUM**

**FOSAMAX**
MERCK

5 mg

10 mg

40 mg

**ALPRAZOLAM**

**XANAX**
PHARMACIA & UPJOHN

0.25 mg

0.5 mg

1 mg

**AMLODIPINE BESYLATE**

**NORVASC**
PFIZER LABS

5 mg

10 mg

**AMOXICILLIN**

**AMOXIL**
SMITHKLINE BEECHAM

250 mg

500 mg

**AMOXICILLIN AND CLAVULANATE POTASSIUM**

**AUGMENTIN**
SMITHKLINE BEECHAM

250 mg / 125 mg

500 mg / 125 mg

**ASTEMIZOLE**

**HISMANAL**
JANSSEN

10 mg

**ATENOLOL**

**TENORMIN**
ZENECA

50 mg

100 mg

**AZITHROMYCIN**

**ZITHROMAX**
PFIZER LABS

250 mg

## BENAZEPRIL HCL

### LOTENSIN
NOVARTIS

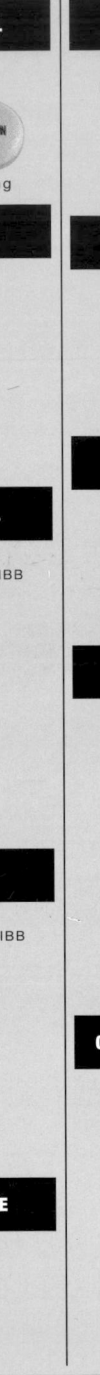

10 mg    20 mg

## BUMETANIDE

### BUMEX
ROCHE

0.5 mg

1 mg

## BUSPIRONE HCL

### BUSPAR
BRISTOL-MYERS SQUIBB

5 mg

10 mg

15 mg

## CAPTOPRIL

### CAPOTEN
BRISTOL-MYERS SQUIBB

12.5 mg

25 mg

50 mg

## CARBAMAZEPINE

### TEGRETOL
NOVARTIS

200 mg

## CEFADROXIL MONOHYDRATE

### DURICEF
BRISTOL-MYERS SQUIBB

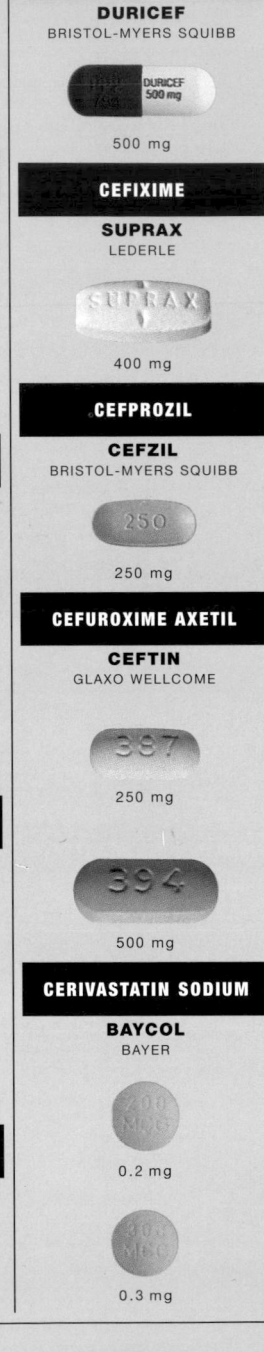

500 mg

## CEFIXIME

### SUPRAX
LEDERLE

400 mg

## CEFPROZIL

### CEFZIL
BRISTOL-MYERS SQUIBB

250 mg

## CEFUROXIME AXETIL

### CEFTIN
GLAXO WELLCOME

250 mg

500 mg

## CERIVASTATIN SODIUM

### BAYCOL
BAYER

0.2 mg

0.3 mg

## CIMETIDINE

### TAGAMET
SMITHKLINE BEECHAM

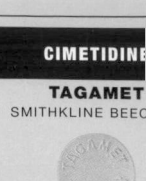

300 mg

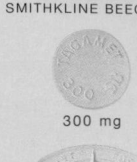

400 mg

## CIPROFLOXACIN HCL

### CIPRO
BAYER

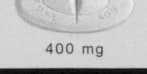

250 mg

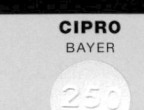

500 mg

## CLARITHROMYCIN

### BIAXIN
ABBOTT

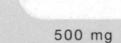

250 mg

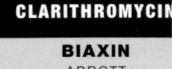

500 mg

## CLONAZEPAM

### KLONOPIN
ROCHE

0.5 mg    1 mg

## CLOPIDOGREL BISULFATE

### PLAVIX
SANOFI

75 mg

## CYCLOBENZAPRINE HCL

### FLEXERIL
MERCK

10 mg

## DIAZEPAM

### VALIUM
ROCHE

2 mg

5 mg

10 mg

## DICLOFENAC SODIUM

### VOLTAREN
NOVARTIS

50 mg          75 mg

## DICYCLOMINE HCL

### BENTYL
HOECHST MARION ROUSSEL

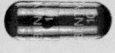 

10 mg          20 mg

## DIGOXIN

### LANOXIN
GLAXO WELLCOME

0.125 mg

0.25 mg

## DILTIAZEM HCL

### CARDIZEM CD
HOECHST MARION ROUSSEL

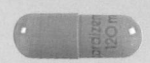

120 mg

180 mg

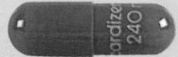

240 mg

## DIVALPROEX SODIUM

### DEPAKOTE
ABBOTT

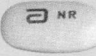

250 mg

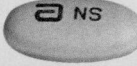

500 mg

## DOXAZOSIN MESYLATE

### CARDURA
ROERIG

 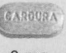

1 mg           2 mg

## ENALAPRIL MALEATE

### VASOTEC
MERCK

5 mg

10 mg

20 mg

## ERYTHROMYCIN BASE

### ERY-TAB
ABBOTT

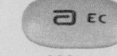

250 mg

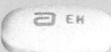

333 mg

### ERYTHROMYCIN
ABBOTT

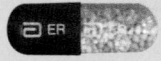

250 mg

### PCE
ABBOTT

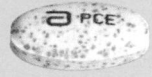

333 mg

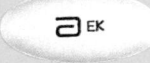

500 mg

## ERYTHROMYCIN STEARATE

### ERYTHROCIN STEARATE FILMTAB
ABBOTT

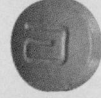

250 mg

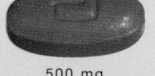

500 mg

## ESTROGENS, CONJUGATED

### PREMARIN
WYETH-AYERST

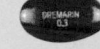 

0.3 mg         0.625 mg

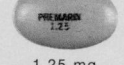

1.25 mg

## ESTROPIPATE

**OGEN**
PHARMACIA & UPJOHN

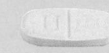
0.625 mg

1.25 mg

## ETODOLAC

**LODINE**
WYETH-AYERST

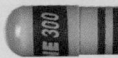
300 mg

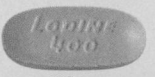
400 mg

## FAMOTIDINE

**PEPCID**
MERCK

20 mg

40 mg

## FEXOFENADINE HCL

**ALLEGRA**
HOECHST MARION ROUSSEL

60 mg

## FINASTERIDE

**PROSCAR**
MERCK

5 mg

## FIORINAL

**BUTALBITAL AND ASPIRIN AND CAFFEINE**
NOVARTIS

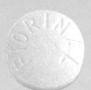
50 mg / 325 mg / 40 mg

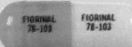
50 mg / 325 mg / 40 mg

## FLUOXETINE HCL

**PROZAC**
DISTA

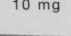
10 mg

20 mg

## FOSINOPRIL SODIUM

**MONOPRIL**
BRISTOL-MYERS SQUIBB

10 mg

20 mg

## FUROSEMIDE

**LASIX**
HOECHST MARION ROUSSEL

20 mg        40 mg

## GEMFIBROZIL

**LOPID**
PARKE-DAVIS

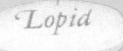
600 mg

## GLIMEPIRIDE

**AMARYL**
HOECHST MARION ROUSSEL

1 mg
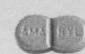
2 mg

4 mg

## GLIPIZIDE

**GLUCOTROL**
PRATT

5 mg

10 mg

## GLYBURIDE

**DIABETA**
HOECHST MARION ROUSSEL

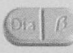
2.5 mg
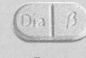
5 mg

## GLYBURIDE, MICRONIZED

**GLYNASE PRESTAB**
PHARMACIA & UPJOHN

3 mg

## GUANFACINE HCL

**TENEX**
A. H. ROBINS

1 mg

## HYDROCODONE BITARTRATE AND ACETAMINOPHEN

**VICODIN**
KNOLL

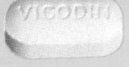
5 mg / 500 mg

## HYDROCODONE BITARTRATE AND IBUPROFEN

### VICOPROFEN
KNOLL

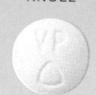

7.5 mg / 200 mg

## INDINAVIR SULFATE

### CRIXIVAN
MERCK

200 mg

400 mg

## IRBESARTAN

### AVAPRO
BRISTOL-MYERS SQUIBB

75 mg        150 mg

300 mg

## ISRADIPINE

### DYNACIRC
NOVARTIS

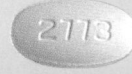

2.5 mg

5 mg

## KETOCONAZOLE

### NIZORAL
JANSSEN

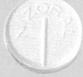

200 mg

## KETOROLAC TROMETHAMINE

### TORADOL
ROCHE

10 mg

## LEVOTHYROXINE SODIUM

### SYNTHROID
KNOLL

0.05 mg

0.1 mg

0.15 mg

## LISINOPRIL

### PRINIVIL
MERCK

10 mg        20 mg

### ZESTRIL
ZENECA

5 mg

10 mg

20 mg

## LORACARBEF

### LORABID
ELI LILLY

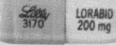

200 mg

## LORATADINE

### CLARITIN
SCHERING

10 mg

## LORAZEPAM

### ATIVAN
WYETH-AYERST

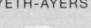

0.5 mg

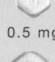

1 mg

## LOSARTAN POTASSIUM

### COZAAR
MERCK

25 mg

50 mg

## LOVASTATIN

### MEVACOR
MERCK

10 mg        20 mg

## MEDROXYPROGESTERONE ACETATE

### PROVERA
PHARMACIA & UPJOHN

2.5 mg        10 mg

## METFORMIN HCL

### GLUCOPHAGE
BRISTOL-MYERS SQUIBB

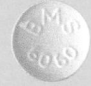

500 mg        850 mg

## METHYLPHENIDATE HCL

**RITALIN**
NOVARTIS

5 mg

10 mg

## METHYLPREDNISOLONE

**MEDROL**
PHARMACIA & UPJOHN

4 mg

## METOPROLOL TARTRATE

**LOPRESSOR**
NOVARTIS

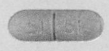

50 mg

100 mg

## MIBEFRADIL DIHYDROCHLORIDE

**POSICOR**
ROCHE

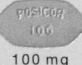

50 mg        100 mg

## MIRTAZAPINE

**REMERON**
ORGANON

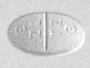 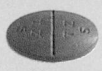

15 mg        30 mg

## MISOPROSTOL

**CYTOTEC**
G. D. SEARLE

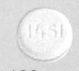 

100 mcg      200 mcg

## NABUMETONE

**RELAFEN**
SMITHKLINE BEECHAM

500 mg

## NAPROXEN

**NAPROSYN**
ROCHE

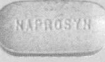

375 mg

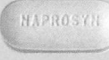

500 mg

## NAPROXEN SODIUM

**ANAPROX**
ROCHE

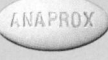

275 mg

**ANAPROX DS**
ROCHE

550 mg

## NEFAZODONE HCL

**SERZONE**
BRISTOL-MYERS SQUIBB

100 mg

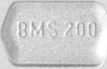

200 mg

## NEVIRAPINE

**VIRAMUNE**
ROXANE

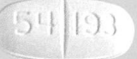

200 mg

## NIFEDIPINE

**PROCARDIA XL**
PRATT

30 mg        60 mg

90 mg

## NISOLDIPINE

**SULAR**
ZENECA

10 mg        20 mg

 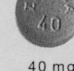

30 mg        40 mg

## NIZATIDINE

**AXID**
ELI LILLY

150 mg

## NORTRIPTYLINE HCL

**PAMELOR**
NOVARTIS

 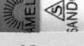

25 mg

50 mg

## OFLOXACIN

**FLOXIN**
ORTHO-MCNEIL

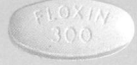

300 mg

## OMEPRAZOLE

**PRILOSEC**
ASTRA MERCK

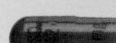

20 mg

## OXAPROZIN

**DAYPRO**
G. D. SEARLE

600 mg

## OXYCODONE AND ACETAMINOPHEN

**PERCOCET**
ENDO

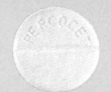

5 mg / 325 mg

## PAROXETINE HCL

**PAXIL**
SMITHKLINE BEECHAM

20 mg

## PENICILLIN V POTASSIUM

**PEN-VEE K**
WYETH-AYERST

250 mg

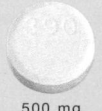

500 mg

## PENTOXIFYLLINE

**TRENTAL**
HOECHST MARION ROUSSEL

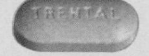

400 mg

## PHENYTOIN SODIUM, EXTENDED

**DILANTIN KAPSEALS**
PARKE-DAVIS

100 mg

## POTASSIUM CHLORIDE

**K-DUR**
KEY

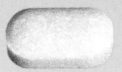

10 mEq

20 mEq

## MICRO-K 10 EXTENCAPS

A. H. ROBINS

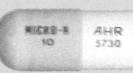

10 mEq

## PRAVASTATIN SODIUM

**PRAVACHOL**
BRISTOL-MYERS SQUIBB

20 mg

## PROPRANOLOL HCL

**INDERAL**
WYETH-AYERST

10 mg        20 mg

40 mg

## INDERAL LA

WYETH-AYERST

80 mg

## QUINAPRIL HCL

**ACCUPRIL**
PARKE-DAVIS

10 mg   20 mg

## RAMIPRIL

**ALTACE**
HOECHST MARION ROUSSEL

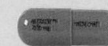

2.5 mg

5 mg

## RANITIDINE HCL

**ZANTAC**
GLAXO WELLCOME

150 mg

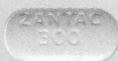

300 mg

## RITONAVIR

**NORVIR**
ABBOTT

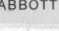

200 mg

## SAQUINAVIR MESYLATE

**INVIRASE**
ROCHE

200 mg

## SERTRALINE HCL

**ZOLOFT**
ROERIG

50 mg   100 mg

## SIBUTRAMINE HCL MONOHYDRATE

**MERIDIA**
KNOLL

5 mg

10 mg

15 mg

## SILDENAFIL CITRATE

**VIAGRA**
PFIZER

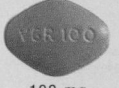

25 mg    50 mg

100 mg

## SIMVASTATIN

**ZOCOR**
MERCK

 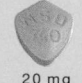

10 mg    20 mg

## SUCRALFATE

**CARAFATE**
HOECHST MARION ROUSSEL

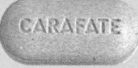

1 gm

## TAMOXIFEN

**NOLVADEX**
ZENECA

 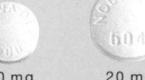

10 mg    20 mg

---

## TEMAZEPAM

**RESTORIL**
NOVARTIS

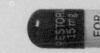

15 mg

30 mg

## TERAZOSIN

**HYTRIN**
ABBOTT

2 mg    5 mg

## THEOPHYLLINE

**THEO-DUR**
KEY

200 mg    300 mg

## TRIAMTERENE AND HYDROCHLOROTHIAZIDE

**MAXZIDE**
BERTEK

 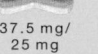

37.5 mg/    75 mg/
25 mg    50 mg

**DYAZIDE**
SMITHKLINE BEECHAM

37.5 mg / 25 mg

## TRIAZOLAM

**HALCION**
PHARMACIA & UPJOHN

0.125 mg    0.25 mg

## TRIMETHOPRIM AND SULFAMETHOXAZOLE

**BACTRIM DS**
ROCHE

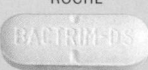

160 mg / 800 mg

---

## TROGLITAZONE

**REZULIN**
PARKE-DAVES

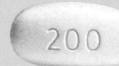

200 mg

300mg

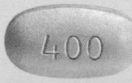

400 mg

## VERAPAMIL

**CALAN SR**
G. D. SEARLE

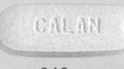

240 mg

## WARFARIN SODIUM

**COUMADIN**
DUPONT PHARMA

2 mg   2.5 mg   5 mg

## ZAFIRLUKAST

**ACCOLATE**
ZENECA

20 mg

## ZOLMITRIPTIN

**ZOMIG**
ZENECA

2.5 mg

5 mg

- **SC Implant, 10.8 mg**
  *Prostatic carcinoma.*
  10.8 mg q 12 weeks into the upper abdominal wall using sterile technique under the direction of a physician.

## NURSING CONSIDERATIONS

See also *Nursing Considerations* for *Antineoplastic Agents.*

**Administration/Storage**

1. Do not remove the sterile syringe containing the drug until immediately before use. Examine syringe for damage and to ensure drug is visible in the translucent chamber.
2. Administer drug under the supervision of a physician.
3. Clean the area with an alcohol swab; a topical (i.e., ethyl chloride) or a local anesthetic may be used prior to the injection.
4. To administer, stretch the skin with one hand and grip the needle with the fingers around the barrel of the syringe. Insert the needle into the SC fat; do not aspirate. If a large vessel is penetrated, blood will be seen immediately in the syringe; withdraw the needle and make the injection elsewhere with a new syringe.
5. The direction of the needle is changed so it parallels the abdominal wall. The needle is then pushed in until the barrel hub touches the skin and then withdrawn approximately 1 cm to create a space to inject the drug. The plunger is depressed to deliver the drug. The needle is then withdrawn and the area bandaged.
6. To confirm the drug has been delivered, ensure that the tip of the plunger is visible within the tip of the needle.
7. If there is need to remove goserelin surgically, it can be located by ultrasound.
8. Adhere to the 28-day and 12-week schedules as closely as possible.
9. Store at room temperatures not exceeding 25°C (77°F).
10. There is no evidence the drug accumulates with either hepatic and/or renal dysfunction.
11. Duration of treatment for endometriosis is 6 months.
12. Males with ureteral obstruction or spinal cord compression should have appropriate treatment prior to initiating goserelin therapy.

**Client/Family Teaching**

1. The most common side effects (especially hot flashes, decreased erections, and sexual dysfunction) are due to decreased testosterone levels.
2. There may be initial worsening of symptoms; results of transient increases of testosterone.
3. May experience an increase in bone pain and develop spinal cord compression or ureteral obstruction; these symptoms are usually only temporary but must be reported promptly so that appropriate treatment may be initiated.
4. Goserelin should not be used in women who are likely to become pregnant or who are pregnant. Drug may harm fetus and may impair fertility. Identify appropriate individuals for sperm or egg harvesting.
5. Advise clients with prostate cancer that if they decided against surgery (orchiectomy), for medication therapy, they must come in monthly for abdominal implants for the rest of their lives.
6. Identify appropriate resources and support groups.

**Outcomes/Evaluate**

- Symptom control; ↑ comfort
- ↓ Tumor size and spread
- ↓ Testosterone levels

# Granisetron hydrochloride

(gran-**ISS**-eh-tron)
**Pregnancy Category:** B
Kytril **(Rx)**
**Classification:** Antinauseant and antiemetic

**Action/Kinetics:** Selective 5-HT$_3$ (serotonin) receptor antagonist with little or no affinity for other 5-HT, beta-adrenergic, dopamine, or histamine receptors. During chemotherapy-induced vomiting, mucosal enterochromaffin cells release serotonin, which stimulates 5-HT$_3$ receptors. The stimulation of 5-HT$_3$ receptors by serotonin causes vagal discharge resulting in vomiting. Granisetron blocks serotonin stimulation and subsequent vomiting. In adult cancer clients undergoing chemotherapy, infusion of a single 40-mcg/kg dose over 5 min produced the following data. **Peak plasma level:** 63.8 ng/mL. **Plasma t½, terminal:** 8.95 hr. Metabolized in the liver with unchanged drug (12%) and metabolites excreted through both the urine and feces.

**Uses:** Prevention of N&V associated with initial and repeat cancer chemotherapy, including high-dose cisplatin. *Investigational:* Acute N&V following surgery.

**Contraindications:** Known hypersensitivity to the drug.

**Special Concerns:** Use with caution during lactation. Safety and efficacy in children less than 2 years of age have not been established.

**Side Effects: After IV use.** *CNS:* Headache, somnolence, agitation, anxiety, CNS stimulation, insomnia, extrapyramidal syndrome. *GI:* Diarrhea, constipation, taste disorder. *CV:* Hypertension, hypotension, arrhythmias (e.g., sinus bradycardia, atrial fibrillation, *AV block,* ventricular ectopy including nonsustained tachycardia, ECG abnormalities). *Allergic: Hypersensitivity reactions (anaphylaxis),* skin rashes. *Miscellaneous:* Asthenia, fever.

**After PO use.** *CNS:* Headache, dizziness, insomnia, anxiety, somnolence. *GI:* N&V, diarrhea, constipation, abdominal pain. *CV:* Hypertension, hypotension, angina, atrial fibrillation, syncope (rare). *Hypersensitivity:* Rarely, hypersensitivity reactions; *severe anaphylaxis,* shortness of breath, hypotension, urticaria. *Miscellaneous:* Fever, leukopenia, decreased appetite, anemia, alopecia, thrombocytopenia.

**Drug Interactions:** Because granisetron is metabolized by hepatic cytochrome P-450 drug-metabolizing enzymes, agents that induce or inhibit these enzymes may alter the clearance (and thus the half-life) of granisetron.

**Laboratory Test Interferences:** ↑ AST, ALT.

**Dosage** ————————
• **IV**
   *Antiemetic during cancer chemotherapy.*
**Adults and children over 2 years of age:** 10 mcg/kg infused over 5 min beginning 30 min before initiation of chemotherapy.
   *Antiemetic following surgery.*
1–3 mg.
• **Tablets**
   *Antiemetic.*
**Adults:** 1 mg b.i.d. with the first 1 mg-tablet given 1 hr before chemotherapy and the second 1-mg tablet given 12 hr after the first tablet only on days chemotherapy is given. Alternatively, 2 mg once daily taken 1 hr before chemotherapy.

## NURSING CONSIDERATIONS
### Administration/Storage
1. Give drug only on the day chemotherapy is given.
2. Dosage adjustment is not necessary for geriatric clients or with impaired renal or hepatic function.
**IV** 3. Prepare infusion at the time of administration by diluting in either NSS or D5W to a total volume of 20–50 mL; infuse over 5 min. Drug is stable for at least 24 hr when diluted in NSS or D5W and stored at room temperature under normal lighting.
4. Do not mix in solution with other drugs.
5. Do not freeze vial; protect from light.

### Assessment
1. Note indications for therapy; chemotherapy or postop N&V.
2. Anticipate administration 30 min before the start of emetogenic cancer chemotherapy.

**Outcomes/Evaluate:** Prevention of N&V

# Griseofulvin microsize

(griz-ee-oh-**FULL**-vin)
**Pregnancy Category:** C
Fulvicin-U/F, Grifulvin V, Grisactin 250, Grisactin 500, Grisovin-FP ✱ **(Rx)**

# Griseofulvin ultramicrosize

(griz-ee-oh-**FULL**-vin)
**Pregnancy Category:** C
Fulvicin-P/G, Grisactin Ultra, Gris-PEG **(Rx)**
**Classification:** Antibiotic, antifungal

See also *Anti-Infectives.*

**Action/Kinetics:** Derived from a species of *Penicillium.* Believed to interfere with cell division (metaphase) or DNA replication. When taken systemically, the drug is deposited in the newly formed skin and nails, which are then resistant to reinfection by the tinea. Absorbed from the duodenum. **Peak plasma concentration:** 0.5–2 mcg/mL after 4 hr. **t½:** 9–24 hr. Levels may be increased by giving the drug with a high-fat diet. GI absorption of the ultramicrosize products is about 1.5 times that of the microsize products; however, there is no evidence this causes any difference in the safety and effectiveness of the drug compared with the microsize form.

**Uses:** Tinea (ringworm) infections of skin (including athlete's foot), scalp, groin, and nails. Effective against tinea corporis, tinea pedis, tinea barbae, tinea unguium, tinea cruris, tinea capitis due to *Trichophyton* species, *Microsporum audouinii, M. canis, M. gypseum,* and *Epidermophyton floccosum.* It is the only PO drug effective against dermatophytid (tinea ringworm) infections. Not effective against *Candida.* Establish susceptibility of the infectious agent before treatment is begun.

**Contraindications:** Pregnancy. Porphyria or history thereof, hepatocellular failure, and hypersensitivity to drug. Exposure to artificial light or sunlight. Use for infections due to bacteria, candidiasis, actinomycosis, sporotrichosis, tinea versicolor, histoplasmosis, chromoblastomycosis, coccidioidomycosis, cryptococcosis, and North American blastomycosis.

**Special Concerns:** Cross sensitivity with penicillin is possible.

**Side Effects:** *Hypersensitivity:* Rashes, urticaria, ***angioneurotic edema,*** allergic reactions. *GI:* N&V, diarrhea, epigastric pain, ***GI bleeding.*** *CNS:* Dizziness, headache, confusion, mental fatigue, insomnia. *Miscellaneous:* Oral thrush, acute intermittent porphyria, paresthesias of extremities after long-term therapy, proteinuria, leukopenia, photosensitivity, worsening of lupus erythematosus, menstrual irregularities, hepatic toxicity, granulocytopenia.

**Drug Interactions**
*Alcohol, ethyl* / Tachycardia and flushing
*Anticoagulants, oral* / ↓ Effect of anticoagulants due to ↑ breakdown in liver
*Barbiturates* / ↓ Effect of griseofulvin due to ↓ absorption from GI tract
*Cyclosporine* / ↓ Plasma levels of cyclosporine → ↓ pharmacologic effect
*Oral contraceptives* / ↓ Effect of contraceptives → breakthrough bleeding, pregnancy, or amenorrhea
*Salicylates* / ↓ Serum salicylate levels

**Laboratory Test Interferences:** ↑ ALT, AST, alkaline phosphatase, BUN, and creatinine level values.

## Dosage

• **Capsules, Oral Suspension, Tablets**

*Tinea corporis, cruris, or capitis.*
**Adults:** 0.5 g griseofulvin microsize daily in a single dose or divided dose (or 330–375 mg ultramicrosize).

*Tinea pedis or unguium.*
**Adults:** 0.75–1 g/day of griseofulvin microsize (or 660–750 mg ultramicrosize). After response, decrease dose of microsize to 0.5 g/day. **Pediatric, 13.6–22.7 kg:** 125–250 mg

griseofulvin microsize daily (or 82.5–165 mg ultramicrosize); **pediatric, over 22.7 kg:** 250–500 mg microsize daily (or 165–330 mg ultramicrosize). *NOTE:* Dose has not been determined in children less than 2 years of age.

## NURSING CONSIDERATIONS

See also *General Nursing Considerations for All Anti-Infectives.*
**Administration/Storage**
1. Assure sufficient length of treatment; i.e., treatment for tinea capitis: 4 to 6 weeks; 2 to 4 weeks for tinea corporis; 4 to 8 weeks for tinea pedis; and 4 to 6 months (fingernails) and 6 to 18 months (toe nails) for tinea unguium.
2. With prolonged therapy, evaluate liver, renal, and hematologic function.
3. May not be the drug of choice with CAD and hyperlipidemia due to the high-fat consumption necessary to enhance absorption.
**Assessment**
1. Document location, size, and characteristics of skin infection.
2. Obtain baseline CBC, liver and renal function studies. Obtain cultures and scrapings as needed.
**Client/Family Teaching**
1. Eat high-fat food with drug (i.e., ice cream, bread and butter, gravy, fried chicken); fat enhances absorption of griseofulvin from the intestines.
2. Take all medication as prescribed to prevent any recurrence of infection. If the course of therapy is interrupted or not completed, therapy may have to be started all over again.
3. Practice appropriate hygiene to prevent reinfection.
4. Avoid exposure to intense natural and artificial light because photosensitivity reactions may occur. Wear protective clothing, sunglasses, and a sunscreen if exposure is necessary.
5. Report any fever, sore throat, and malaise, (all symptoms of leukopenia).
6. Use a nonhormonal form of birth control.
7. To be considered cured, repeated cultures and scrapings of affected sites must be negative.

8. Persistent N&V and diarrhea and any mental confusion should be immediately reported.
9. Avoid alcohol during therapy.
10. Anticipate long-term therapy, i.e., 2 weeks to 18 months depending on location of infection.
**Outcomes/Evaluate**
• Improvement in symptoms
• Negative cultures and scraping

# Guaifenesin (Glyceryl guaiacolate)
(gwye-FEN-eh-sin)
**Pregnancy Category:** C
Anti-Tuss, Balminil Expectorant ✹, Benylin-E ✹, Breonesin, Fenesin, Gee-Gee, Genatuss, GG-Cen, Glyate, Glycotuss, Glytuss, Guiatuss, Halotussin, Humibid L.A., Humibid Sprinkle, Hytuss, Hytuss-2X, Mytussin, Naldecon Senior EX, Robitussin, Scot-tussin, Sinumist-SR Capsulets, Uni-tussin **(OTC)**
**Classification:** Expectorant

**Action/Kinetics:** May increase the output of fluid of the respiratory tract by reducing the viscosity and surface tension of respiratory secretions, thereby facilitating their expectoration. Data on efficacy are lacking.
**Uses:** Dry, nonproductive cough due to colds and minor upper respiratory tract infections when there is mucus in the respiratory tract.
**Contraindications:** Chronic cough (e.g., due to smoking, asthma, or emphysema), cough accompanied by excess secretions. Use in children under age 12 for persistent or chronic cough due to asthma or cough accompanied by excessive mucus (unless prescribed by a provider).
**Special Concerns:** Persistent cough may indicate a serious infection; thus, the provider should be consulted if cough lasts for more than 1 week, is recurring, or is accompanied by high fever, rash, or persistent headache.
**Side Effects:** *GI:* N&V, GI upset. *CNS:* Dizziness, headache. *Dermatologic:* Rash, urticaria.

**OD    Overdose Management:** *Symptoms:* N&V. *Treatment:* Treat symptomatically.

**Drug Interactions:** Inhibition of platelet adhesiveness by guaifenesin may result in bleeding tendencies.

**Laboratory Test Interferences:** False + urinary 5-hydroxyindoleacetic acid. Color interference with determination of urinary vanillylmandelic acid.

**Dosage**

• **Capsules, Tablets, Oral Liquid, Syrup**
  *Expectorant.*

**Adults and children over 12 years:** 100–400 mg q 4 hr, not to exceed 2.4 g/day; **pediatric, 6–12 years:** 100–200 mg q 4 hr, not to exceed 1.2 g/day; **pediatric, 2–6 years:** 50–100 mg q 4 hr, not to exceed 600 mg/day. If less than 2 years of age, the dosage must be individualized by the provider.

• **Sustained-Release    Capsules, Sustained-Release Tablets**
  *Expectorant.*

**Adults and children over 12 years:** 600–1,200 mg q 12 hr, not to exceed 2.4 g/day; **pediatric, 6–12 years:** 600 mg q 12 hr, not to exceed 1.2 g/day; **pediatric, 2–6 years:** 300 mg q 12 hr, not to exceed 600 mg/day. *NOTE:* The liquid dosage forms may be more suitable for children less than 6 years of age.

## NURSING CONSIDERATIONS

**Assessment**

1. Document pulmonary assessment findings.
2. Note type, frequency, duration, and characteristics of cough and sputum production.

**Client/Family Teaching**

1. Take only as directed and do not exceed prescribed dose.
2. If symptoms persist more than 1 week, recur, or are accompanied by a persistent headache, fever, or rash, notify provider.
3. Report any evidence of increased bruising or bleeding .

4. Do not perform activities that require mental alertness; may cause drowsiness.
5. Increase fluids to 2.5 L/day to decrease secretion viscosity.
6. Avoid triggers: dust, chemicals, cigarette smoke, pollutants, and perfumes.

**Outcomes/Evaluate**

• Control of coughing episodes
• Mobilization of mucus

# Guanabenz acetate

(**GWON**-ah-benz)
**Pregnancy Category:** C
Wytensin **(Rx)**
**Classification:** Antihypertensive, centrally acting antiadrenergic

See also *Antihypertensive Agents.*

**Action/Kinetics:** Guanabenz stimulates alpha-2-adrenergic receptors in the CNS, resulting in a decrease in sympathetic impulses and in sympathetic tone. It also decreases the pulse rate, but postural hypotension has not been manifested. **Onset:** 60 min. **Peak effect:** 2–4 hr. **Peak plasma levels:** 2–5 hr. t½: 6 hr. **Duration:** 8–12 hr.

**Uses:** Hypertension, alone or as adjunct with thiazide diuretics.

**Contraindications:** Lactation, children under 12 years of age.

**Special Concerns:** Use with caution in severe coronary insufficiency, cerebrovascular disease, recent MI, hepatic or renal disease. Geriatric clients may be more sensitive to the hypotensive and sedative effects; dose reduction may be necessary due to age-related decreases in renal function. Sudden cessation may result in an increase in catecholamines and, rarely, "overshoot" hypertension.

**Side Effects:** *CNS:* Drowsiness and sedation (common), dizziness, weakness, headache, ataxia, depression, disturbances in sleep, excitement. *GI:* Dry mouth (common), N&V, diarrhea, constipation, abdominal discomfort, epigastric pain. *CV:* Palpitations, chest pain, arrhythmias,

AV dysfunction or block. *Dermatologic:* Rash, pruritus. *Miscellaneous:* Edema, blurred vision, muscle aches, dyspnea, nasal congestion, urinary frequency, gynecomastia, disturbances of sexual function, taste disorders, aches in extremities.

**OD** **Overdose Management:** *Symptoms:* Hypotension, sleepiness, irritability, miosis, lethargy, bradycardia. *Treatment:* Supportive treatment. VS and fluid balance should be monitored. Syrup of ipecac or gastric lavage followed by activated charcoal; administration of fluids, pressor agents, and atropine. Adequate airway should be maintained; artificial respiration may be required.

**Drug Interactions:** Use with CNS depressants may result in additive sedation.

**Dosage**
• **Tablets**
*Hypertension.*
**Adults, initial:** 4 mg b.i.d. alone or with a thiazide diuretic; **then,** increase by 4–8 mg/day q 1–2 weeks until control achieved. Maximum recommended dose: 32 mg b.i.d.

## NURSING CONSIDERATIONS

See also *Nursing Considerations* for *Antihypertensive Agents.*
**Administration/Storage:** The drug should be kept tightly closed and protected from light.
**Client/Family Teaching**
1. Do not drive or operate machinery until the drug's sedative effect assessed.
2. Report sleep disturbances; may indicate a depressive episode.
3. Avoid alcohol and other CNS depressants.
4. Continue prescribed dietary and exercise recommendations.
**Outcomes/Evaluate:** ↓ BP

# Guanadrel sulfate
(**GWON**-ah-drell)
**Pregnancy Category:** B
Hylorel **(Rx)**

**Classification:** Antihypertensive, peripherally acting antiadrenergic

See also *Antihypertensive Agents.*
**Action/Kinetics:** Similar to that of guanethidine. Inhibits vasoconstriction by blocking efferent, peripheral sympathetic pathways by depleting norepinephrine reserves and inhibiting norepinephrine release. Causes increased sensitivity to norepinephrine. **Onset:** 2 hr. **Peak plasma levels:** 1.5–2 hr. **Peak effect:** 4–6 hr. **t½:** Approximately 10 hr. **Duration:** 4–14 hr. Excreted through the urine as unchanged drug (40%) and metabolites.
**Uses:** Hypertension (usually step 2 therapy) in those not responding to a thiazide diuretic.
**Contraindications:** Pheochromocytoma, CHF, within 1 week of MAO drug use, within 2–3 days of elective surgery, lactation.
**Special Concerns:** Use with caution in bronchial asthma and peptic ulcer. Safety and efficacy not established in children. Geriatric clients may be more sensitive to the hypotensive effects.
**Side Effects:** *CNS:* Fainting, fatigue, headache, drowsiness, paresthesias, confusion, psychological problems, depression, syncope, sleep disorders, visual disturbances. *CV:* Chest pain, orthostatic hypotension, palpitations, peripheral edema. *Respiratory:* Exertional or resting SOB, coughing. *GI:* Increase in number of bowel movements, constipation, anorexia, indigestion, flatus, glossitis, N&V, dry mouth and throat, abdominal distress or pain. *GU:* Difficulty in ejaculation, impotence, nocturia, hematuria, urinary urgency or frequency. *Miscellaneous:* Leg cramps during both the day and night, excessive weight gain or loss, backache, neckache, joint pain or inflammation, aching limbs.
**OD** **Overdose Management:** *Symptoms:* Postural hypotension, syncope, dizziness, blurred vision. *Treatment:* Administration of a vasoconstrictor (e.g., phenylephrine) if hypotension persists. If used, monitor

carefully as client may be hypersensitive.

**Drug Interactions**

*Beta-adrenergic blocking agents* / Excessive hypotension, bradycardia

*Phenothiazines* / Reverses effect of guanadrel

*Phenylpropanolamine* / ↓ Effect of guanadrel

*Reserpine* / Excessive hypotension, bradycardia

*Sympathomimetics* / Hypotensive effect of guanadrel may be reversed; also, guanadrel may ↑ the effects of directly acting sympathomimetics

*Tricyclic antidepressants* / Reverses effect of guanadrel

*Vasodilators* / ↑ Risk of orthostatic hypotension

**Dosage** ───────────────

• **Tablets**

*Hypertension.*

**Individualized. Initial:** 5 mg b.i.d.; **then,** increase dosage to maintenance level of 20–75 mg/day in two to four divided doses. With a $C_{CR}$ of 30–60 mL/min, the initial dose should be 5 mg q 24 hr. If the $C_{CR}$ is less than 30 mL/min, the dosing interval should be increased to q 48 hr. Dose changes should be made carefully q 7 or more days for moderate renal insufficiency and q 14 or more days for severe insufficiency.

## NURSING CONSIDERATIONS

See also *Nursing Considerations* for *Antihypertensive Agents.*

**Administration/Storage**

1. Tolerance may occur with long-term therapy, necessitating a dosage increase.

2. While adjusting dosage, monitor both supine and standing BP.

**Client/Family Teaching**

1. May develop a dry mouth and become drowsy. Do not perform tasks that require mental alertness, such as driving, until drug effects realized.

2. Diarrhea may occur; if persistent, report as a severe electrolyte imbal-

ance may occur (particularly with the elderly).

**Outcomes/Evaluate:** Control of hypertension

─────────────────────────

# Guanethidine sulfate

(gwon-**ETH**-ih-deen)

**Pregnancy Category:** C

Apo-Guanethidine ✦, Ismelin Sulfate **(Rx)**

**Classification:** Antihypertensive, peripherally acting antiadrenergic

─────────────────────────

See also *Antihypertensive Agents.*

**Action/Kinetics:** Produces selective adrenergic blockade of efferent, peripheral sympathetic pathways by depleting norepinephrine reserve and inhibiting norepinephrine release. Induces a gradual, prolonged drop in both SBP and DBP, usually associated with bradycardia, decreased pulse pressure, a decrease in peripheral resistance, and small changes in CO. Is not a ganglionic blocking agent and does not produce central or parasympathetic blockade. With depleted catecholamines, guanethidine can directly depress the myocardium and can cause an increase in the sensitivity of tissues to catecholamines. Incompletely and variably absorbed from the GI tract (3%–30%) but is relatively constant for any given client. **Peak effect:** 6–8 hr. **Duration:** 24–48 hr. **Maximum effect:** 1–3 weeks. **Duration:** 7–10 days after discontinuation. **t½:** 4–8 days. From 25% to 50% excreted through the kidneys unchanged. Slowly excreted due to extensive tissue binding.

**Uses:** Moderate to severe hypertension—used alone or in combination. *NOTE:* The use of a thiazide diuretic may increase the effectiveness of guanethidine and reduce the incidence of edema. Also used for renal hypertension, including that secondary to pyelonephritis, renal artery stenosis, and renal amyloidosis.

**Contraindications:** Mild, labile hypertension; pheochromocytoma,

CHF not due to hypertension, use of MAO inhibitors, lactation.

**Special Concerns:** Administer with caution and at a reduced rate to clients with impaired renal function, coronary disease, CV disease especially when associated with encephalopathy, or severe cardiac failure or to those who have suffered a recent MI. Use with caution in hypertensive clients with renal disease and nitrogen retention or increasing BUN levels. Fever decreases dosage requirements. During prolonged therapy, cardiac, renal, and blood tests should be performed. Used with caution in peptic ulcer. Geriatric clients may be more sensitive to the hypotensive effects of guanethidine; also, it may be necessary to decrease the dose in these clients due to age-related decreases in renal function. Safety and efficacy have not been determined in children.

**Side Effects:** *CNS:* Dizziness, weakness, lassitude. Rarely, fatigue, psychic depression. *CV:* Syncope due to exertional or postural hypotension, bradycardia, fluid retention and edema with possible CHF. Less commonly, angina. *Respiratory:* Dyspnea, nasal congestion, asthma in susceptible individuals. *GI:* Persistent diarrhea (may be severe enough to cause discontinuation of use), increased frequency of bowel movements. N&V, dry mouth, and parotid tenderness are less common. *GU:* Inhibition of ejaculation, nocturia, urinary incontinence, priapism, impotence. *Hematologic:* Anemia, thrombocytopenia, leukopenia (rare). *Miscellaneous:* Dermatitis, scalp hair loss, blurred vision, myalgia, muscle tremors, chest paresthesia, weight gain, ptosis of the lids.

**OD** **Overdose Management:** *Symptoms:* Bradycardia, postural hypotension, diarrhea (may be severe). *Treatment:* If the client was previously normotensive, keep in a supine position (symptoms usually subside within 72 hr). If the client was previously hypertensive (especially with impaired cardiac reserve or other CV problems or renal disease),

intensive treatment may be needed. Vasopressors may be required. Severe diarrhea should be treated.

**Drug Interactions**

*Alcohol, ethyl* / Additive orthostatic hypotension

*Amphetamines* / ↓ Effect of guanethidine by ↓ uptake of the drug to its site of action

*Anesthetics, general* / Additive hypotension

*Antidepressants, tricyclic* / ↓ Effect of guanethidine by ↓ uptake of the drug to its site of action

*Antidiabetic drugs* / Additive effect ↓ in blood glucose

*Cocaine* / ↓ Effect of guanethidine by ↓ uptake of the drug at its site of action

*Digitalis* / Additive slowing of HR

*Ephedrine* / ↓ Effect of guanethidine by ↓ uptake of the drug at its site of action

*Epinephrine* / Guanethidine ↑ effect of epinephrine

*Haloperidol* / ↓ Effect of guanethidine by ↓ uptake of the drug at its site of action

*Levarterenol* / See *Norepinephrine*

*MAO inhibitors* / Reverse effect of guanethidine

*Metaraminol* / Guanethidine ↑ effect of metaraminol

*Methotrimeprazine* / Additive hypotensive effect

*Methoxamine* / Guanethidine ↑ effect of methoxamine

*Methylphenidate* / ↓ Effect of guanethidine

*Minoxidil* / Profound drop in BP

*Norepinephrine* / ↑ Effect of norepinephrine probably due to ↑ sensitivity of norepinephrine receptor and ↓ uptake of norepinephrine by the neuron

*Oral contraceptives* / ↓ Effect of guanethidine by ↓ uptake of the drug to its site of action

*Phenothiazines* / ↓ Effect of guanethidine by ↓ uptake of the drug to its site of action

*Phenylephrine* / ↑ Response to phenylephrine in guanethidine-treated clients

*Phenylpropanolamine* / ↓ Effect of guanethidine by ↓ uptake of the drug to its site of action

*Procainamide* / Additive hypotensive effect

*Procarbazine* / Additive hypotensive effect

*Propranolol* / Additive hypotensive effect

*Pseudoephedrine* / ↓ Effect of guanethidine by ↓ uptake of the drug at its site of action

*Quinidine* / Additive hypotensive effect

*Reserpine* / Excessive bradycardia, postural hypotension, and mental depression

*Sympathomimetics* / ↓ Effect of guanethidine; also, guanethidine potentiates the effects of directly acting sympathomimetics

*Thiazide diuretics* / Additive hypotensive effect

*Thioxanthenes* / ↓ Effect of guanethidine by ↓ uptake of the drug at its site of action

*Tricyclic antidepressants* / Inhibition of the effects of guanethidine

*Vasodilator drugs, peripheral* / Additive hypotensive effect

*Vasopressor drugs* / ↑ Effect of vasopressor agents probably due to ↑ sensitivity of norepinephrine receptor and ↓ uptake of vasopressor agent by the neuron

**Laboratory Test Interferences:** ↑ BUN, AST, and ALT. ↓ PT, serum glucose, and urine catecholamines. Alteration of electrolyte balance.

**Dosage** ———————————

• **Tablets**

  *Ambulatory clients.*
**Initial:** 10–12.5 mg/day; increase in 10–12.5-mg increments q 5–7 days; **maintenance:** 25–50 mg/day.

  *Hospitalized clients.*
**Initial:** 25–50 mg; increase by 25 or 50 mg/day or every other day; **maintenance:** approximately one-seventh of loading dose. **Pediatric, initial:** 0.2 mg/kg/day (6 mg/m²) given in one dose; **then,** dose may be

increased by 0.2 mg/kg/day q 7–10 days to maximum of 3 mg/kg/day.

## NURSING CONSIDERATIONS

See also *Nursing Considerations* for *Antihypertensive Agents.*

**Administration/Storage**

1. For severe hypertension, give the loading dose t.i.d. at 6-hr intervals with no nighttime dose.

2. Effects are cumulative; use small initial doses, increase gradually in small increments.

3. Often used with thiazide diuretics to reduce severity of sodium and water retention caused by guanethidine. When used together, reduce the dose of guanethidine.

4. When control is achieved, reduce the dose to the minimal dose required to maintain lowest possible BP.

5. Discontinue or decrease dosage at least 2 weeks before surgery; discontinue MAO inhibitors at least 1 week before starting guanethidine.

**Assessment**

1. Obtain baseline hepatic and renal function studies.

2. List drugs currently prescribed to ensure none interact unfavorably.

3. Assess VS; report bradycardia. An anticholinergic drug, i.e., atropine, may be indicated if severe.

4. Assess life-style and emotional state.

**Client/Family Teaching**

1. Limit alcohol intake; may precipitate orthostatic hypotension. Postural hypotension more prevalent in the morning; may be worsened by hot weather, alcohol, or exercise.

2. Avoid any sudden or prolonged standing or exercise.

3. Report any persistent nausea, vomiting, or diarrhea; severe electrolyte imbalances may occur.

4. Perform daily weights. Report any sudden increases in weight, ↑ SOB, reduction in urine volume or edema.

**Outcomes/Evaluate:** ↓ BP

---

# Guanfacine hydrochloride
(**GWON**-fah-seen)
**Pregnancy Category:** B
Tenex **(Rx)**
**Classification:** Antihypertensive, centrally acting

See also *Antihypertensive Agents.*

**Action/Kinetics:** Thought to act by central stimulation of alpha-2 receptors. Causes a decrease in peripheral sympathetic output and HR resulting in a decrease in BP. May also manifest a direct peripheral alpha-2 receptor stimulant action. **Onset:** 2 hr. **Peak plasma levels:** 1–4 hr. **Peak effect:** 6–12 hr. **t½:** 12–23 hr. **Duration:** 24 hr. Approximately 50% excreted through the kidneys unchanged.

**Uses:** Hypertension alone or with a thiazide diuretic. *Investigational:* Withdrawal from heroin use, to reduce the frequency of migraine headaches.

**Contraindications:** Hypersensitivity to guanfacine. Acute hypertension associated with toxemia. Children less than 12 years of age.

**Special Concerns:** Use with caution during lactation. Use with caution in clients with recent MI, cerebrovascular disease, chronic renal or hepatic failure, or severe coronary insufficiency. Geriatric clients may be more sensitive to the hypotensive and sedative effects. Safety and efficacy in children less than 12 years of age have not been determined.

**Side Effects:** *GI:* Dry mouth, constipation, nausea, abdominal pain, diarrhea, dyspepsia, dysphagia, taste perversion or alterations in taste. *CNS:* Sedation, weakness, dizziness, headache, fatigue, insomnia, amnesia, confusion, depression, vertigo, agitation, anxiety, malaise, nervousness, tremor. *CV:* Bradycardia, substernal pain, palpitations, syncope, chest pain, tachycarida, cardiac fibrillation, CHF, heart block, MI (rare), cardiovascular accident (rare). *Ophthalmic:* Visual disturbances, conjunctivitis, iritis, blurred vision. *Dermatologic:* Pruritus, dermatitis, purpura, sweating, skin rash with exfoliation, alopecia, rash. *GU:* Decreased libido, impotence, urinary incontinence or frequency, testicular disorder, nocturia, acute renal failure. *Musculoskeletal:* Leg cramps, hypokinesia, arthralgia, leg pain, myalgia. *Other:* Rhinitis, tinnitus, dyspnea, paresthesias, paresis, asthenia, edema, abnormal liver function tests.

**OD** **Overdose Management:** *Symptoms:* Drowsiness, bradycardia, lethargy, hypotension. *Treatment:* Gastric lavage. Supportive therapy, as needed. The drug is not dialyzable.

**Drug Interactions:** Additive sedative effects when used concomitantly with CNS depressants.

**Dosage** —————————————
• **Tablets**
  *Hypertension.*
  **Initial:** 1 mg/day alone or with other antihypertensives; if satisfactory results are not obtained in 3–4 weeks, dosage may be increased by 1 mg at 1–2-week intervals up to a maximum of 3 mg/day in one to two divided doses.
  *Heroin withdrawal.*
  0.03–1.5 mg/day.
  *Reduce frequency of migraine headaches.*
  1 mg/day for 12 weeks.

## NURSING CONSIDERATIONS

See also *Nursing Considerations* for *Antihypertensive Agents.*
**Administration/Storage**
1. Divide the daily dose if a decrease in BP is not maintained for over 24 hr; however, the incidence of side effects increases.
2. Adverse effects increase significantly when the daily dose exceeds 3 mg.
3. Initiate antihypertensive therapy in clients already taking a thiazide diuretic.
4. Abrupt cessation may result in increases in plasma and urinary catecholamines, symptoms of nervousness and anxiety, and BPs greater than those prior to therapy.

**Assessment**

1. Document indications for therapy, onset of symptoms, and any previous agents used and the outcome.

2. Determine the extent of CAD, and note any evidence of renal or liver dysfunction.

**Client/Family Teaching**

1. To minimize daytime drowsiness, take at bedtime. Do not perform activities that require mental alertness until drug effects realized.

2. Do not stop drug abruptly; may experience rebound effect.

3. May cause skin rash; report if persistent or severe.

4. Avoid OTC cough and cold remedies.

**Outcomes/Evaluate**

- ↓ BP
- ↓ S&S of heroin withdrawal
- ↓ Migraine headaches

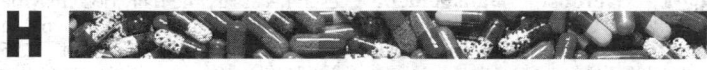

# Haloperidol
(hah-low-**PAIR**-ih-dohl)
**Pregnancy Category:** C
Apo-Haloperidol ✤, Haldol, Novo–Peridol ✤, Peridol ✤, PMS Haloperidol ✤ **(Rx)**

# Haloperidol decanoate
(hah-low-**PAIR**-ih-dohl)
**Pregnancy Category:** C (decanoate form)
Haldol Decanoate 50 and 100, Haldol LA ✤ **(Rx)**

# Haloperidol lactate
(hah-low-**PAIR**-ih-dohl)
**Pregnancy Category:** C
Haldol Lactate **(Rx)**
**Classification:** Antipsychotic, butyrophenone

**Action/Kinetics:** Precise mechanism not known. Haloperidol competitively blocks dopamine receptors in the tuberoinfundibular system to cause sedation. Also causes alpha-adrenergic blockade, decreases release of growth hormone, and increases prolactin release by the pituitary. Causes significant extrapyramidal effects, as well as a low incidence of sedation, anticholinergic effects, and orthostatic hypotension. Narrow margin between the therapeutically effective dose and that causing extrapyramidal symptoms. Also has antiemetic effects. **Peak plasma levels: PO,** 3–5 hr; **IM,** 20 min; **IM, decanoate:** approximately 6 days. **Therapeutic serum levels:** 3–10 ng/mL. **t½, PO:** 12–38 hr; **IM:** 13–36 hr; **IM, decanoate:** 3 weeks; **IV:** approximately 14 hr. **Plasma protein binding:** 90%. Metabolized in liver, slowly excreted in urine and bile.

**Uses:** Psychotic disorders including manic states, drug-induced psychoses, and schizophrenia. Aggressive and agitated clients, including chronic brain syndrome or mental retardation. Severe behavior problems in children (those with combative, explosive hyperexcitability not accounted for by immediate provocation). Short-term treatment of hyperactive children. Control of tics and vocal utterances associated with Gilles de la Tourette's syndrome in adults and children. The decanoate is used for prolonged therapy in chronic schizophrenia.

*Investigational:* Antiemetic for cancer chemotherapy, phencyclidine (PCP) psychosis, infantile autism. IV for acute psychiatric conditions.

**Contraindications:** Use with extreme caution, or not at all, in clients with parkinsonism. Lactation.

**Special Concerns:** PO dosage has not been determined in children less than 3 years of age; IM dosage is not recommended in children. Geriatric clients are more likely to exhibit orthostatic hypotension, anticholi-

---

nergic effects, sedation, and extrapyramidal side effects (such as parkinsonism and tardive dyskinesia).

**Side Effects:** Extrapyramidal symptoms, especially akathisia and dystonias, occur more frequently than with the phenothiazines. Overdosage is characterized by severe extrapyramidal reactions, hypotension, or sedation. The drug does not elicit photosensitivity reactions like those of the phenothiazines.

**OD** **Overdose Management:** *Symptoms:* CNS depression, hypertension or hypotension, extrapyramidal symptoms, agitation, restlessness, fever, hypothermia, hyperthermia, *seizures, cardiac arrhythmias,* changes in the ECG, autonomic reactions, *coma. Treatment:* Treat symptomatically. Antiparkinson drugs, diphenhydramine, or barbiturates can be used to treat extrapyramidal symptoms. Fluid replacement and vasoconstrictors (either norepinephrine or phenylephrine) can be used to treat hypotension. Ventricular arrhythmias can be treated with phenytoin. To treat seizures, use pentobarbital or diazepam. A saline cathartic can be used to hasten the excretion of sustained-release products.

**Drug Interactions**
*Amphetamine* / ↓ Effect of amphetamine by ↓ uptake of drug at its site of action
*Anticholinergics* / ↓ Effect of haloperidol
*Antidepressants, tricyclic* / ↑ Effect of antidepressants due to ↓ breakdown by liver
*Barbiturates* / ↓ Effect of haloperidol due to ↑ breakdown by liver
*Guanethidine* / ↓ Effect of guanethidine by ↓ uptake of drug at site of action
*Lithium* / ↑ Toxicity of haloperidol
*Methyldopa* / ↑ Toxicity of haloperidol
*Phenytoin* / ↓ Effect of haloperidol due to ↑ breakdown by liver
**Laboratory Test Interferences:** ↑ Alkaline phosphatase, bilirubin, serum transaminase; ↓ PT (clients on coumarin), serum cholesterol.

**Dosage** ⸻
• **Oral Solution, Tablets**
  *Psychoses.*
**Adults:** 0.5–2 mg b.i.d.–t.i.d. up to 3–5 mg b.i.d.–t.i.d. for severe symptoms; **maintenance:** reduce dosage to lowest effective level. Up to 100 mg/day may be required in some. **Geriatric or debilitated clients:** 0.5–2 mg b.i.d.–t.i.d. **Pediatric, 3–12 years or 15–40 kg:** 0.5 mg/day in two to three divided doses; if necessary the daily dose may be increased by 0.5-mg increments q 5–7 days for a total of 0.15 mg/kg/day for psychotic disorders and 0.075 mg/kg for nonpsychotic behavior disorders and Tourette's syndrome. Doses for children 3–6 years of age are 0.01–0.03 mg/kg/day PO for agitation and hyperkinesia and 0.5–4 mg/day for infantile autism.
• **IM, Lactate**
  *Acute psychoses.*
**Adults and adolescents, initial:** 2–5 mg; may be repeated if necessary q 4–8 hr to a total of 100 mg/day. Switch to **PO** therapy as soon as possible.
• **IM, Decanoate**
  *Chronic therapy.*
**Adults, initial dose:** 10–15 times the daily PO dose, not to exceed 100 mg initially, regardless of the previous oral antipsychotic dose; **then,** repeat q 4 weeks (decanoate is not to be given IV).

---

## NURSING CONSIDERATIONS

See also *Nursing Considerations* for *Antipsychotic Agents, Phenothiazines.*
**Administration/Storage**
1. Give the decanoate by deep IM injection using a 21-gauge needle. Do not exceed a volume of 3 mL/site.
2. Do not give decanoate IV.
**Assessment**
1. Document type, onset, and duration of symptoms.
2. Use with caution in the elderly; they tend to exhibit toxicity more

frequently; may also benefit from a periodic "drug holiday."

3. Document evidence of new onset of extrapyramidal symptoms; may be drug induced.

**Outcomes/Evaluate**

• Improved behavior patterns: ↓ agitation, ↓ hostility, ↓ psychosis, ↓ delusions

• Control of tics/vocal utterances

• ↓ Hyperactive behaviors

---

# Heparin calcium
(HEP-ah-rin)
**Pregnancy Category:** C
Calcilean ✽

# Heparin sodium injection
(HEP-ah-rin)
**Pregnancy Category:** C
Hepalean ✽, Hepalean-Lok ✽, Heparin Leo ✽ **(Rx)**

# Heparin sodium and sodium chloride
(HEP-ah-rin)
**Pregnancy Category:** C
Heparin Sodium and 0.45% Sodium Chloride, Heparin Sodium and 0.9% Sodium Chloride **(Rx)**

# Heparin sodium lock flush solution
(HEP-ah-rin)
**Pregnancy Category:** C
Heparin lock flush, Hep-Lock, Hep-Lock U/P **(Rx)**
**Classification:** Anticoagulant

See also *Anticoagulants*.

**Action/Kinetics:** Heparin potentiates the inhibitory action of antithrombin III on various coagulation factors including factors IIa, IXa, Xa, XIa, and XIIa. This occurs due to the formation of a complex with and causing a conformational change in the antithrombin III molecule. Inhibition of factor Xa results in interference with thrombin generation; thus, the action of thrombin in coagulation is inhibited. Heparin also increases the rate of formation of antithrombin III–thrombin complex causing inactivation of thrombin and preventing the conversion of fibrinogen to fibrin. By inhibiting the activation of fibrin-stabilizing factor by thrombin, heparin also prevents formation of a stable fibrin clot. Therapeutic doses of heparin prolong thrombin time, whole blood clotting time, activated clotting time, and PTT. Heparin also decreases the levels of triglycerides by releasing lipoprotein lipase from tissues; the resultant hydrolysis of triglycerides causes increased blood levels of free fatty acids. **Onset: IV,** immediate; **deep SC:** 20–60 min. **Peak plasma levels, after SC:** 2–4 hr. **t½:** 30–180 min in healthy persons. **t½** increases with dose, severe renal disease, and cirrhosis and in anephric clients and decreases with pulmonary embolism and liver impairment other than cirrhosis. *Metabolism:* Probably by reticuloendothelial system although up to 50% is excreted unchanged in the urine. Clotting time returns to normal within 2–6 hr.

**Uses:** Pulmonary embolism, peripheral arterial embolism, prophylaxis, and treatment of venous thrombosis and its extension. Atrial fibrillation with embolization. Diagnosis and treatment of disseminated intravascular coagulation. Low doses to prevent deep venous thrombosis and pulmonary embolism in pregnant clients with a history of thromboembolism, urology clients over 40 years of age, clients with stroke or heart failure, AMI or pulmonary infection, high-risk surgery clients, moderate and high-risk gynecologic clients with no malignancy, neurology clients with extracranial problems, and clients with severe musculoskeletal trauma. Prophylaxis of clotting in blood transfusions, extracorporeal circulation, dialysis procedures, blood samples for lab tests, and arterial and heart surgery. *Investigational:* Prophylaxis of post-MI, CVAs, and LV thrombi. By continuous infusion to treat myocardial ischemia in

---

unstable angina refractory to usual treatment. Adjunct to treat coronary occlusion with AMI. Prophylaxis of cerebral thrombosis in evolving stroke.

*Heparin lock flush solution:* Dilute solutions are used to maintain patency of indwelling catheters used for IV therapy or blood sampling. Not to be used therapeutically.

**Contraindications:** Active bleeding, blood dyscrasias (or other disorders characterized by bleeding tendencies such as hemophilia), purpura, thrombocytopenia, liver disease with hypoprothrombinemia, suspected intracranial hemorrhage, suppurative thrombophlebitis, inaccessible ulcerative lesions (especially of the GI tract), open wounds, extensive denudation of the skin, and increased capillary permeability (as in ascorbic acid deficiency). IM use.

Do not administer during surgery of the eye, brain, or spinal cord or during continuous tube drainage of the stomach or small intestine. Use is also contraindicated in subacute endocarditis, shock, advanced kidney disease, threatened abortion, severe hypertension, or hypersensitivity to drug. Premature neonates due to the possibility of a fatal "gasping syndrome."

**Special Concerns:** NaCl, 0.9%, is effective in maintaining patency of peripheral (noncentral) intermittent infusion devices and in reducing added medical costs. The following procedure has been recommended:

• Determine patency by aspirating lock.

• Flush with 2 mL NSS.

• Administer medication therapy. (Flush between drugs.)

• Flush with 2 mL NSS.

• Frequency of flushing to maintain patency when not actively in use varies from every 8 hr to every 24–48 hr.

• This does *NOT* apply to any central venous access devices.

**Side Effects:** *CV: Hemorrhage ranging from minor local ecchymoses to major hemorrhagic complications from any organ or tissue.* Higher incidence is seen in women over 60 years of age. Hemorrhagic reactions are more likely to occur in prophylactic administration during surgery than in the treatment of thromboembolic disease. White clot syndrome. *Hematologic:* Thrombocytopenia (both early and late). *Hypersensitivity:* Chills, fever, urticaria are the most common. Rarely, asthma, lacrimation, headache, N&V, rhinitis, *shock, anaphylaxis.* Allergic vasospastic reaction within 6–10 days after initiation of therapy (lasts 4–6 hr) including painful, ischemic, cyanotic limbs. Use a test dose of 1,000 units in clients with a history of asthma or allergic disease. *Miscellaneous:* Hyperkalemia, cutaneous necrosis, osteoporosis (after long-term high doses), delayed transient alopecia, priapism, suppressed aldosterone synthesis. Discontinuance of heparin has resulted in rebound hyperlipemia. *Following IM (usual), SC:* Local irritation, erythema, mild pain, ulceration, hematoma, and tissue sloughing.

**OD** **Overdose Management:** *Symptoms:* Nosebleeds, hematuria, tarry stools, petechiae, and easy bruising may be the first signs. *Treatment:* Drug withdrawal is usually sufficient to correct heparin overdosage. Protamine sulfate (1%) solution; each mg of protamine neutralizes about 100 USP heparin units.

**Drug Interactions**

*Alteplase, recombinant* / ↑ Risk of bleeding, especially at arterial puncture sites

*Anticoagulants, oral* / Additive ↑ PT

*Antihistamines* / ↓ Effect of heparin

*Aspirin* / Additive ↑ PT

*Cephalosporins* / ↑ Risk of bleeding due to additive effect

*Dextran* / Additive ↑ PT

*Digitalis* / ↓ Effect of heparin

*Dipyridamole* / Additive ↑ PT

*Hydroxychloroquine* / Additive ↑ PT

*Ibuprofen* / Additive ↑ PT

*Indomethacin* / Additive ↑ PT

*Insulin* / Heparin antagonizes effect of insulin
*Nicotine* / ↓ Effect of heparin
*Nitroglycerin* / ↓ Effect of heparin
*NSAIDs* / Additive ↑ PT
*Penicillins* / ↑ Risk of bleeding due to possible additive effects
*Salicylates* / ↑ Risk of bleeding
*Streptokinase* / Relative resistance to effects of heparin
*Tetracyclines* / ↓ Effect of heparin
*Ticlopidine* / Additive ↑ PT
**Laboratory Test Interferences:** ↑ AST and ALT.

## Dosage

*NOTE:* Adjusted for each client on the basis of laboratory tests.
• **Deep SC**
    *General heparin dosage.*
**Initial loading dose:** 10,000–20,000 units; **maintenance:** 8,000–10,000 units q 8 hr or 15,000–20,000 units q 12 hr. *Use concentrated solution.*
    *Prophylaxis of postoperative thromboembolism.*
5,000 units of concentrated solution 2 hr before surgery and 5,000 units q 8–12 hr thereafter for 7 days or until client is ambulatory.
• **Intermittent IV**
    *General heparin dosage.*
**Initial loading dose:** 10,000 units undiluted or in 50–100 mL saline; **then,** 5,000–10,000 units q 4–6 hr undiluted or in 50–100 mL saline.
• **Continuous IV Infusion**
    *General heparin dosage.*
**Initial loading dose:** 20,000–40,000 units/day in 1,000 mL saline (preceded initially by 5,000 units IV).
• **Special Uses**
    *Surgery of heart and blood vessels.*
**Initial,** 150–400 units/kg to clients undergoing total body perfusion for open heart surgery. *NOTE:* 300 units/kg may be used for procedures less than 60 min while 400 units/kg is used for procedures lasting more than 60 min. To prevent clotting in the tube system, add heparin to fluids in pump oxygenator.
    *Extracorporeal renal dialysis.*
See instructions on equipment.

*Blood transfusion.*
400–600 units/100 mL whole blood. 7,500 units should be added to 100 mL 0.9% sodium chloride injection; from this dilution, add 6–8 mL/100 mL whole blood.
    *Laboratory samples.*
70–150 units/10- to 20-mL sample to prevent coagulation.
    *Heparin lock sets.*
To prevent clot formation in a heparin lock set, inject 10–100 units/mL heparin solution through the injection hub in a sufficient quantity to fill the entire set to the needle tip.

## NURSING CONSIDERATIONS

See also *Nursing Considerations* for *Anticoagulants.*
**Administration/Storage**
1. Do *not* administer IM.
2. Administer by deep SC injection to minimize local irritation, hematoma, and tissue sloughing and to prolong action of drug.
• Z-track method: Use any fat roll, but abdominal fat rolls are preferred. Use a ½-in. or ⅝-in., 25- or 27-gauge needle. Grasp the skin layer of the fat roll and lift it up. Insert the needle at about a 45° angle to the skin's fat layer and then administer the medication. It is not necessary to aspirate to check if needle is in a blood vessel. Rapidly withdraw the needle while releasing the skin.
• "Bunch technique" method: Grasp tissue around the injection site, creating a tissue roll of about ½ in. in diameter. Insert needle into the tissue roll at a 90° angle to the skin surface and inject the medication. Again, it is not necessary to aspirate. Withdraw the needle rapidly when the skin is released.
• Do not administer within 2 in. of the umbilicus; due to increased vascularity of area.
3. Do not massage site.
4. Rotate sites of administration.
5. Slight discoloration does not affect potency.
**IV** 6. Hospitalize client for IV therapy.

---

7. May be diluted in dextrose, NSS, or Ringer's solution and administered over 4–24 hr with an infusion pump.

8. Protect solutions from freezing.

9. Have protamine sulfate, a heparin antagonist, available should excessive bleeding occur.

**Assessment**

1. Identify any bleeding incidents, i.e., bleeding tendencies, family history, or any other incidents of unexplained or active bleeding.

2. Note history of PUD; may be a potential site of bleeding.

3. Perform test dose (1,000 units SC) to clients with multiple allergies or asthma history.

4. Note any evidence of intracranial hemorrhage.

5. If receiving drugs that interact with anticoagulants, anticipate heparin dosage adjustment.

6. Monitor CBC, PT, PTT, and liver and renal function studies.

**Interventions:** for *Heparin Lock Flush Solution.*

1. Aspirate lock to determine patency. Maintain patency: inject 1 mL of flush solution into device diaphragm after each use (maintains catheter patency for up to 24 hr).

2. If administering a drug incompatible with heparin, flush with 0.9% NaCl injection or sterile water for injection before and immediately after incompatible drug administered. Inject another dose of heparin lock flush solution after the final flush.

3. Observe coagulation times carefully with underlying bleeding disorders; ↑ risk for hemorrhage.

4. The presence of heparin or NSS may cause interference with lab tests.

• To clear flush solution: aspirate and discard 1 mL of fluid from device before withdrawing blood sample.

• Inject 1 mL of flush solution into lock after blood samples are drawn.

• With excessively abnormal results, obtain a repeat sample from another site before initiating treatment.

5. Monitor for allergic reactions due to various biologic sources of heparin.

**Client/Family Teaching**

1. Review administration technique.

2. Report signs of active bleeding.

3. Report any excessive menstrual flow; may need to withhold or reduce dosage.

4. Alopecia is generally temporary.

5. Report alterations in GU function, urine color, or any injury.

6. Use an electric razor for shaving and a soft-bristle toothbrush to decrease gum irritation.

7. Arrange furniture to allow open space for unimpeded ambulation and to diminish chances of bumping into objects that may cause bruising and bleeding.

8. Use a night light to illuminate trips to the bathroom.

9. Avoid activities where excessive bumping, bruising or injury may occur.

10. Eat potassium-rich foods (e.g., baked potato, orange juice, bananas, beef, flounder, haddock, sweet potato, turkey, raw tomato).

11. Avoid eating large amounts of vitamin K foods, mostly yellow and dark green vegetables.

12. Report any increased bruising, bleeding of nose, mouth, gums, tarry stools, or GI upset.

13. Avoid alcohol, aspirin, and NSAIDs; increase anticoagulant response.

14. Alert all providers of therapy and wear or carry drug identification.

**Outcomes/Evaluate**

• Clot prophylaxis/treatment

• Indwelling catheter patency

# Histrelin acetate

(hiss-**TREL**-in)

**Pregnancy Category:** X

Supprelin, Synarel **(Rx)**

**Classification:** Gonadotropin-releasing hormone

**Action/Kinetics:** Histrelin contains a synthetic nonapeptide agonist of the naturally occurring GnRH. Initially the drug stimulates release of GnRH; however, chronic use desensitizes responsiveness of the pituitary gonadotropin, causing a reduction in ovarian and testicular steroidogenesis. Decreases in LH, FSH, and sex steroid levels are observed within 3 months of initiation of therapy.

**Uses:** To control the biochemical and clinical symptoms of central precocious puberty (either idiopathic or neurogenic) occurring before 8 years of age in girls or 9.5 years of age in boys.

**Contraindications:** Hypersensitivity to the product or any of its components. Lactation.

**Special Concerns:** Acute, serious hypersensitivity reactions may occur that require emergency medical treatment. Safety and efficacy in children less than 2 years of age have not been determined.

**Side Effects:** *Acute hypersensitivity reaction:* Angioedema, urticaria, ***CV collapse,*** hypotension, tachycardia, loss of consciousness, ***bronchospasm,*** dyspnea, flushing, pruritus. *CV:* Vasodilation (common), edema, palpitations, tachycardia, epistaxis, hypertension, migraine headache, pallor. *GI:* GI or abdominal pain, N&V, diarrhea, flatulence, decrease appetite, dyspepsia, GI cramps or distress, constipation, decreased appetite, thirst, gastritis. *CNS:* Headache (common), nervousness, dizziness, depression, changes in libido, mood changes, insomnia, anxiety, paresthesia, syncope, somnolence, cognitive changes, lethargy, impaired consciousness, tremor, hyperkinesia, convulsions (increased frequency), hot flashes or flushes, conduct disorder. *Endocrine:* Vaginal dryness, leukorrhea, metrorrhagia, breast pain, breast edema, decreased breast size, breast discharge, tenderness of female genitalia, anemia, goiter, hyperlipidemia, glycosuria. *Musculoskeletal:* Arthralgia, joint stiffness, muscle cramp or stiffness, myalgia, hypotonia, pain. *Respiratory:* Cough, upper respiratory infection, pharyngitis, respiratory congestion, asthma, breathing disorder, rhinorrhea, bronchitis, sinusitis, hyperventilation. *Dermatologic:* Commonly, redness, itching, and swelling at the injection site. Also, urticaria, sweating, keratoderma, pruritus, pain, dyschromia, alopecia, erythema. *Ophthalmologic:* Visual disturbances, abnormal pupillary function, polyopia, photophobia. *Otic:* Otalgia, hearing loss. *GU:* Vaginal bleeding (most often one episode within 1–3 weeks after starting therapy and lasting several days). Also, vaginitis, dysmenorrhea, and problems of the female genitalia including pruritus, irritation, odor, pain, infections, and hypertrophy. Dyspareunia, polyuria, dysuria, incontinence, urinary frequency, hematuria, nocturia. *Miscellaneous:* Pyrexia (common), weight gain, fatigue, viral infection, chills, various body pains, malaise, purpura.

**Dosage** ─────────────
- **SC**

  *Central precocious puberty.*
  10 mcg/kg given as a single, daily SC injection. Doses greater than 10 mcg/kg/day have not been evaluated.

## NURSING CONSIDERATIONS
### Administration/Storage
1. Reevaluate if prepubertal levels of sex hormones or a prepubertal gonadotropin response to GnRH administration are not achieved within the first 3 months of therapy.
2. Rotate injection site daily.
3. Contains no preservative; store vials at 2°C–8°C (36°F–46°F) and protect from light.
4. Use vials only once; discard any unused solution.
5. Remove vial from the packaging only at the time of use. Allow vial to reach room temperature before using.

### Assessment
1. Assess for histrelin-related hypersensitivity reactions.
2. Note results of physical and endocrinologic evaluation. This should include:
- Baseline height and weight
- Baseline hand and wrist X rays to determine bone age

- Sex steroid level (estradiol or testosterone)
- Adrenal steroid level (to R/O congenital hyperplasia)
- Beta-human chorionic gonadotropin level (to R/O chorionic gonadotropin-secreting tumor)
- GnRH stimulation test (to document activation of HPG [hypothalamic-pituitary-gonadal] axis)
- Pelvic ultrasound (adrenal, testicular) to R/O steroid-secreting tumor and to obtain baseline gonadal size
- CT of head (to R/O any undiagnosed intracranial tumor)

**Client/Family Teaching**

1. Review instructions provided with 7-day kit.
2. Drug contains no preservative; once vials entered, discard any unused solution.
3. Administer at room temperature.
4. Establish a daily administration schedule; rotate injection sites. If not administered daily, the pubertal process may be reactivated.
5. Compliance with therapy and scheduled clinical evaluations to assess progress and perform height measurements are important. Yearly bone growth determinations and serial GnRH testing document that gonadotropin responsiveness of the pituitary remains prepubertal during therapy.
6. Report any sudden swelling, dyspnea, dysphagia, rash, itching, and/or rapid heartbeat.
7. Hypogonadism may result if HPG axis reactivation fails after discontinuation of drug.
8. Drug should be discontinued when onset of puberty is desired; need F/U to assess menstrual cyclicity, reproductive function, and adult height attained.

**Outcomes/Evaluate:** Control of biochemical/physical manifestations of puberty

# Hyaluronidase

(hy-al-your-**ON**-ih-days)
**Pregnancy Category:** C
Wydase **(Rx)**

**Classification:** Enzyme, miscellaneous

**Action/Kinetics:** Hydrolyzes hyaluronic acid, a constituent of connective tissue, which promotes the diffusion of injected liquids. The purified enzyme has no effect on BP, respiration, temperature, and kidney function. It is antigenic and repeated use may induce the formation of antibodies that neutralize the effect. Local infection will not spread as long as it is not injected into the infected area. Effects last 24–48 hr.

**Uses:** Adjunct to promote absorption and dispersion of liquids and drugs, for hypodermoclysis, adjunct in urography to improve resorption of radiopaque agents, administration of local anesthetics. (Hyaluronidase can be added to primary drug solution or injected prior to administration of primary drug solution.)

**Contraindications:** Do not inject into acutely infected or cancerous areas.

**Special Concerns:** Use with caution during lactation.

**Side Effects:** Rarely, sensitivity reactions, including urticaria and **anaphylaxis.**

**OD** **Overdose Management:** *Symptoms:* Local edema or urticaria, chills, erythema, dizziness, N&V, tachycardia, hypotension. *Treatment:* Discontinue and begin supportive treatment immediately. Epinephrine, corticosteroids, and antihistamines may be required to treat symptoms.

**Dosage**
- **SC**
  *Drug and fluid dispersion.*
**Adults and older children, usual:** 150 units added to the injection solution.
  *SC urography.*
(When IV injection cannot be used.)
**With client in prone position:** 75 units **SC** over each scapula, followed by contrast medium in same site.
  *Hypodermoclysis.*
150 units, which facilitates absorption of 1,000 mL fluid (give at a rate no faster than would be used for IV

infusion); **pediatric, less than 3 years:** volume of single clysis should be limited to 200 mL; **premature infants, neonates:** volume should not exceed 25 mL/kg/day given at a rate no greater than 2 mL/min.

## NURSING CONSIDERATIONS
### Administration/Storage
1. Inject 0.02 mL intradermally as a preliminary skin test for sensitivity. A positive reaction occurs within 5 min when a wheal with pseudopods appears and persists for 20–30 min and is accompanied by localized itching. The appearance of erythema alone is not a positive reaction.
2. Methods for administering during clysis therapy:
• Inject under the skin before clysis started.
• After clysis is started, inject solution of hyaluronidase into tubing near the needle.
3. Control rate and volume of fluid for the older client so that it will not exceed those used for IV administration.
4. Do not inject hyaluronidase into a malignant area.
5. Check orders for dosage of hyaluronidase, type and amount of parenteral solution, rate of flow, and site of injection.
6. Incompatible with heparin and epinephrine.
7. Refrigerate the solution. The reconstituted sterile solution maintains potency for 2 weeks if stored below 30°C (86°F).

### Assessment
1. Document indications for therapy, presentation, and symptom onset.
2. Assess area receiving clysis for pale color, coldness, hardness, and pain; if evident, reduce flow rate.
3. Monitor PT/PTT, liver and renal function studies.
**Outcomes/Evaluate:** Enhanced absorption/dispersion of fluids

———COMBINATION DRUG———
# Hycodan Syrup and Tablets
(**HY**-koh-dan)
**(Rx) (C-III)**
**Pregnancy Category:** C
**Classification:** Antitussive

See also information on *Narcotic Analgesics* and *Cholinergic Blocking Agents.*
**Content:** Each tablet or 5 mL contains: *Antitussive, narcotic:* Hydrocodone bitartrate, 5 mg. *Anticholinergic:* Homatropine methylbromide, 1.5 mg.
**Uses:** Relief of symptoms of cough.
**Special Concerns:** May be habit-forming. Use with caution in children with croup, in geriatric or debilitated clients, impaired renal or hepatic function, hyperthyroidism, asthma, narrow-angle glaucoma, prostatic hypertrophy, urethral stricture, Addison's disease. Safety and effectiveness in children less than 6 years of age have not been determined.

### Dosage
• **Tablets, Syrup**
**Adults and children over 12 years:** 1 tablet or 5 mL q 4–6 hr as needed, not to exceed 6 tablets or 30 mL in 24 hr. Pediatric, 6–12 years: ½ tablet or 2.5 mL q 4–6 hr as needed, not to exceed 3 tablets or 15 mL in 24 hr.

## NURSING CONSIDERATIONS

See also *Nursing Considerations* for *Cholinergic Blocking Agents* and *Narcotic Analgesics.*
### Administration/Storage
1. The single maximum dose of medication for adults is 3 tablets or 15 mL of syrup after meals and at bedtime.
2. For children over 12 years of age, the maximum dosage is 2 tablets or 10 mL of syrup after meals and at bedtime.
3. For children 2–12 years of age,

the maximum dosage is 1 tablet or 5 mL of syrup after meals and at bedtime.

4. For children less than 2 years old, the maximum dosage is ¼ tablet or 1.25 mL of syrup after meals and at bedtime.

5. Doses should be taken at least 4 hr apart.

**Client/Family Teaching**

1. Drug may cause drowsiness and/or dizziness; avoid tasks that require mental alertness.

2. Report if symptoms persist, change, or intensify after 3–5 days of therapy.

3. May be habit-forming if used for prolonged periods.

4. Safely store and keep out of reach of children.

**Outcomes/Evaluate:** Relief of cough permitting uninterrupted periods of sleep

# Hydralazine hydrochloride
(hy-**DRAL**-ah-zeen)
**Pregnancy Category:** C
Apo-Hydralazine ✹, Apresoline, Novo-Hylazin ✹, Nu-Hydral ✹ **(Rx)**
**Classification:** Antihypertensive, direct action on vascular smooth muscle

See also *Antihypertensive Agents.*

**Action/Kinetics:** Exerts a direct vasodilating effect on vascular smooth muscle. Also alters cellular calcium metabolism that interferes with calcium movement within the vascular smooth muscle responsible for initiating or maintaining contraction. Preferentially dilates arterioles compared with veins; this minimizes postural hypotension and increases CO. Increases renin activity in the kidney, leading to an increase in angiotensin II, which then causes stimulation of aldosterone and thus sodium reabsorption. Because there is a reflex increase in cardiac function, hydralazine is commonly used with drugs that inhibit sympathetic activity (e.g., beta blockers, clonidine, methyldopa). Rapidly absorbed after PO use. Food increases bioavailability of the drug. **PO: Onset:** 45 min; **peak plasma level:** 1–2 hr; **duration:** 3–8 hr. **t½:** 3–7 hr. **IM: Onset:** 10–30 min; **peak plasma level:** 1 hr; **duration:** 2–4 hr. **IV: Onset:** 10–20 min; **maximum effect:** 10–80 min; **duration:** 2–4 hr. Metabolized in the liver and excreted through the kidney (2%–5% unchanged after PO use and 11%–14% unchanged after IV administration).

**Uses: PO:** In combination with other drugs for essential hypertension. **Parenteral:** Severe essential hypertension when PO use is not possible or when there is an urgent need to lower BP. Hydralazine is the drug of choice for eclampsia. *Investigational:* To reduce afterload in CHF, severe aortic insufficiency, and after valve replacement.

**Contraindications:** Coronary artery disease, angina pectoris, advanced renal disease (as in chronic renal hypertension), rheumatic heart disease (e.g., mitral valvular) and chronic glomerulonephritis.

**Special Concerns:** Use with caution in stroke clients and in those with pulmonary hypertension. Use with caution during lactation, in clients with advanced renal disease, and in clients with tartrazine sensitivity. Safety and efficacy have not been established in children. Geriatric clients may be more sensitive to the hypotensive and hypothermic effects of hydralazine; also, a decrease in dose may be necessary in these clients due to age-related decreases in renal function.

**Side Effects:** *CV:* Orthostatic hypotension, hypotension, *MI,* angina pectoris, palpitations, paradoxical pressor reaction, tachycardia. *CNS:* Headache, dizziness, psychoses, tremors, depression, anxiety, disorientation. *GI:* N&V, diarrhea, anorexia, constipation, paralytic ileus. *Allergic:* Rash, urticaria, fever, chills, arthralgia, pruritus, eosinophilia. Rarely, hepatitis, obstructive jaundice. *Hematologic:* Decrease in hemoglobin and RBCs, purpura, agranulocytosis, leukopenia. *Other:* Peripheral neuritis (paresthesias, numbness, tingling), dyspnea, impotence, nasal congestion, edema, muscle cramps, lacrimation, flushing, conjunctivitis, difficulty in urination, lupus-like syndrome, lymphadenopathy, splenomegaly. Side effects are less severe when dosage is increased slowly. *NOTE:* Hydralazine may cause symptoms resembling system lupus erythematosus (e.g., arthralgia, dermatoses, fever, splenomegaly, glomerulonephritis). Residual effects may persist for several years and long-term treatment with steroids may be necessary.

**OD** **Overdose Management:** *Symptoms:* Hypotension, tachycardia, skin flushing, headache. Also, myocardial ischemia, *cardiac arrhythmias, MI, and severe shock.* *Treatment:* If the CV status is stable, induce vomiting or perform gastric lavage followed by activated charcoal. Treat shock with volume expanders, without vasopressors; if a vasopressor is necessary, one should be used that is least likely to cause or aggravate tachycardia and cardiac arrhythmias. Renal function should be monitored.

**Drug Interactions**
*Beta-adrenergic blocking agents* / ↑ Effect of both drugs
*Indomethacin* / ↓ Effect of hydralazine
*Methotrimeprazine* / Additive hypotensive effect
*Procainamide* / Additive hypotensive effect
*Quinidine* / Additive hypotensive effect
*Sympathomimetics* / ↑ Risk of tachycardia and angina

**Dosage**
• **Tablets**
*Hypertension.*
**Adult, initial:** 10 mg q.i.d for 2–4 days; **then,** increase to 25 mg q.i.d. for rest of first week. For second and following weeks, increase to 50 mg q.i.d. **Maintenance:** individualized to lowest effective dose; maximum daily dose should not exceed 300 mg. **Pediatric, initial:** 0.75 mg/kg/

day (25 mg/m²/day) in two to four divided doses; dosage may be increased gradually up to 7.5 mg/kg/day (or 300 mg/day). Food increases the bioavailability of the drug.
• **IV, IM**
*Hypertensive crisis.*
**Adults, usual:** 20–40 mg, repeated as necessary. BP may fall within 5–10 min, with maximum response in 10–80 min. Usually switch to PO medication in 1–2 days. Dosage should be decreased in clients with renal damage. **Pediatric:** 0.1–0.2 mg/kg q 4–6 hr as needed.
*Eclampsia.*
5–10 mg q 20 min as an IV bolus. If no effect after 20 mg, another drug should be tried.

## NURSING CONSIDERATIONS

See also *Nursing Considerations* for *Antihypertensive Agents.*
**Administration/Storage**
1. To enhance bioavailability, give tablets with food.
**IV** 2. Make parenteral injections as quickly as possible after being drawn into the syringe. Administer undiluted at a rate of 10 mg over at least 1 min.
3. A metal filter will cause a change in color.
**Assessment**
1. Assess VS; BP (lying, sitting, and standing).
2. Note any hypersensitivity to the drug.
3. List other drugs prescribed that may interact unfavorably.
4. Note any coronary or renal disease.
5. Document pulmonary assessment noting lung sounds, presence of rales, dyspnea, JVD, or edema.
6. Explore life-style, dietary and exercise habits; identify areas for change.
**Interventions**
1. During parenteral administration, take the BP every 5 min until stable, then every 15 min during hypertensive crisis.

2. Monitor electrolytes and I&O; report any reduction in urine output or electrolyte abnormality.

3. The BP should be taken several times a day under standardized conditions, lying, sitting, and/or standing.

4. Clients with cardiac conditions may require closer monitoring during drug therapy.

5. Observe for the development of arthralgia, dermatoses, fever, anemia, or splenomegaly since these may require discontinuation of drug therapy.

**Client/Family Teaching**

1. Take with meals to avoid gastric irritation.

2. Headaches, palpitations, and mild postural hypotension may be experienced after the first dose; may persist for 7–10 days with continued treatment.

3. Record daily weights; report any rapid weight gain or edema.

4. Report evidence of a rheumatoid-like or influenza-like syndrome (fever, muscle, or joint aches); this requires discontinuing therapy.

5. Report tingling sensations or discomfort in the hands or feet, signs of peripheral neuropathies; may be reversed with other drugs, i.e., pyridoxine.

6. Avoid alcohol or other OTC agents that could lower BP or interact unfavorably.

7. Continue life-style modifications for BP management with diet, exercise, smoking cessation, limiting alcohol use, and reducing stress.

**Outcomes/Evaluate**
- ↓ BP
- Improvement in S&S of CHF

---

# Hydrochlorothiazide
(**hy**-droh-klor-oh-**THIGH**-ah-zyd)
**Pregnancy Category:** B
Apo-Hydro ✹, Diuchlor H ✹, Esidrex, Ezide, Hydro-DIURIL, Hydro-Par, Microzide, Neo-Codema ✹, Novo-Hydrazide ✹, Oretic, Urozide ✹ **(Rx)**
**Classification:** Diuretic, thiazide type

See also *Diuretics, Thiazide.*

**Action/Kinetics: Onset:** 2 hr. **Peak effect:** 4–6 hr. **Duration:** 6–12 hr. **t½:** 5.6–14.8 hr.

**Additional Use:** Microzide is available for once-daily, low-dose treatment for hypertension.

**Special Concerns:** Geriatric clients may be more sensitive to the usual adult dose.

**Additional Side Effects:** *CV:* Allergic myocarditis, hypotension. *Dermatologic:* Alopecia, exfoliative dermatitis, **toxic epidermal necrolysis,** erythema multiforme, **Stevens-Johnson syndrome.** *Miscellaneous: Anaphylactic reactions, respiratory distress including pneumonitis and pulmonary edema.*

**Dosage** ⸺
- **Oral Solution, Tablets**
  *Diuretic.*

**Adults, initial:** 25–200 mg/day for several days until dry weight is reached; **then,** 25–100 mg/day or intermittently. Some clients may require up to 200 mg/day.

  *Antihypertensive.*

**Adults, initial:** 25 mg/day as a single dose. The dose may be increased to 50 mg/day in one to two doses. Doses greater than 50 mg may cause significant reductions in serum potassium. **Pediatric, under 6 months:** 3.3 mg/kg/day in two doses; **up to 2 years of age:** 12.5–37.5 mg/day in two doses; **2–12 years of age:** 37.5–100 mg/day in two doses.

## NURSING CONSIDERATIONS

See also *Nursing Considerations* for *Diuretics, Thiazide.*

**Administration/Storage**

1. Divide daily doses in excess of 100 mg.

2. Give b.i.d. at 6–12-hr intervals.

3. When used with other antihypertensives, the dose of hydrochlorothiazide is usually not greater than 50 mg.

**Assessment:** Assess for glucose intolerance; monitor electrolytes and replace potassium as needed.

**Outcomes/Evaluate**
- ↓ BP
- ↑ Urine output; ↓ edema

---

————COMBINATION DRUG————
# Hydrocodone bitartrate and Acetaminophen
(**high**-droh-**KOH**-dohn, ah-**seat**-ah-**MIN**-oh-fen)
**Pregnancy Category:** C
Anexia 5/500, Anexia 7.5/650, Anexsia 10 mg Hydrocodone bitartrate, Anexsia 660 mg Acetaminophen, Lorcet 10/650, Lorcet Plus, Lortab 10/500 10 mg Hydrocodone bitartrate, Lortab 500 mg Acetaminophen **(Rx) (C-III)**
**Classification:** Analgesic

See also *Narcotic Analgesics* and *Acetaminophen.*

**Content:** Anexia 5/500: *Narcotic analgesic:* Hydrocodone bitartrate, 5 mg, and *Nonnarcotic analgesic:* Acetaminophen, 500 mg.

Anexia 10/650 and Lorcet 10/650: *Narcotic analgesic:* Hydrocodone bitartrate, 10 mg, and *Nonnarcotic analgesic:* Acetaminophen, 650 mg.
Anexia 7.5/650 and Lorcet Plus: *Narcotic analgesic:* Hydrocodone bitartrate, 7.5 mg, and *Nonnarcotic analgesic:* Acetaminophen, 650 mg.
Lortab 10/500: *Narcotic analgesic:* Hydrocodone bitartrate, 10 mg, and *Nonnarcotic analgesic:* Acetaminophen, 500 mg.

**Action/Kinetics:**    Hydrocodone produces its analgesic activity by an action on the CNS via opiate receptors. The analgesic action of acetaminophen is produced by both peripheral and central mechanisms.

**Uses:** Relief of moderate to moderately severe pain.

**Contraindications:** Hypersensitivity to acetaminophen or hydrocodone. Lactation.

**Special Concerns:** Use with caution, if at all, in clients with head injuries as the CSF pressure may be increased further. Use with caution in geriatric or debilitated clients; in those with impaired hepatic or renal function; in hypothyroidism, Addison's disease, prostatic hypertrophy, or urethral stricture; and in clients with

pulmonary disease. Use shortly before delivery may cause respiratory depression in the newborn. Safety and efficacy have not been determined in children.

**Side Effects:** *CNS:* Lightheadedness, dizziness, sedation, drowsiness, men-tal clouding, lethargy, impaired mental and physical performance, anxiety, fear, dysphoria, psychologic dependence, mood changes. *GI:* N&V. *Respiratory:* Respiratory depression (dose-related), irregular and periodic breathing. *GU:* Ureteral spasm, spasm of vesical sphincters, urinary retention.

**OD** **Overdose Management:** *Symptoms:* **Acetaminophen overdose may result in potentially fatal hepatic necrosis.** Also, renal tubular necrosis, hypoglycemic coma, and thrombocytopenia. Symptoms of hepatotoxic overdose include N&V, diaphoresis, and malaise. Symptoms of hydrocodone overdose include respiratory depression, somnolence progressing to stupor or **coma,** skeletal muscle flaccidity, cold and clammy skin, bradycardia, and hypotension. *Se-vere overdose may cause apnea, circulatory collapse, cardiac arrest, and death.* *Treatment (Acetaminophen):*
• Empty stomach promptly by lavage or induction of emesis with syrup of ipecac.
• Serum acetaminophen levels should be determined as early as possible but no sooner than 4 hr after ingestion.
• Determine liver function initially and at 24-hr intervals.
• The antidote, *N*-acetylcysteine, should be given within 16 hr of overdose for optimal results.

*Treatment (Hydrocodone):*
• Reestablish adequate respiratory exchange with a patent airway and assisted or controlled ventilation.
• Respiratory depression can be reversed by giving naloxone IV.
• Oxygen, IV fluids, vasopressors, and other supportive measures may be instituted as required.

---

**Drug Interactions**

*Anticholinergics* / ↑ Risk of paralytic ileus

*CNS depressants, including other narcotic analgesics, antianxiety agents, antipsychotics, alcohol* / Additive CNS depression

*MAO inhibitors* / ↑ Effect of either the narcotic or the antidepressant

*Tricyclic antidepressants* / ↑ Effect of either the narcotic or the antidepressant

**Dosage**
• **Tablets**
*Analgesia.*
1 tablet of Anexsia 7.5/650, Lorcet 10/650, or Lorcet Plus q 4–6 hr as needed for pain. The total 24-hr dose should not exceed 6 tablets. 1–2 tablets of Anexsia 5/500 q 4–6 hr as needed for pain. The total 24-hr dose should not exceed 8 tablets.

**NURSING CONSIDERATIONS**

See also *Nursing Considerations* for *Narcotic Analgesics* and *Acetaminophen.*

**Assessment**
1. Note onset, location, duration of symptoms, other agents prescribed, and the outcome. Determine if pain is acute or chronic; rate pain level.
2. Note history of hypothyroidism, prostatic hypertrophy, urethral stricture, Addison's, or pulmonary disease.
3. Monitor liver and renal function studies.
4. Coadministration of an NSAID may reduce the dosage required for pain relief.

**Client/Family Teaching**
1. Take only as prescribed.
2. Do not perform activities that require mental alertness; causes dizziness, lethargy, and impaired physical and mental performance.
3. Report any evidence of abnormal bleeding or bruising, respiratory difficulties, N&V, urinary difficulty, or excessive sedation.
4. Avoid alcohol and any other medications without approval.
5. Store drug appropriately, away from the bedside and safely out of the reach of children.

**Outcomes/Evaluate:** Desired pain control

————COMBINATION DRUG————
# Hydrocodone bitartrate and Ibuprofen
(high-droh-**KOH**-dohn/eye-byou-**PROH**-fen)
**Pregnancy Category:** C
Vicoprofen **(Rx) (C-III)**
**Classification:** Narcotic analgesic and nonsteroidal anti-inflammatory drug

See also *Hydrocodone bitartrate* and *Ibuprofen.*
**Content:** Each tablet contains *Narcotic:* Hydrocodone bitartrate, 7.5 mg and *NSAID:* Ibuprofen, 200 mg.
**Action/Kinetics: Peak plasma levels:** 1.7 hr for hydrocodone and 1.8 hr for ibuprofen. **t½ plasma, hydrocodone:** 4.5 hr; **ibuprofen:** 2.2 hr.
**Uses:** Short-term (less than 10 days) for management of acute pain.
**Additional Contraindications:** Use for osteoarthritis or rheumatoid arthritis. Use during labor and delivery or during lactation.
**Special Concerns:** Use with caution and at reduced doses in geriatric clients. Safety and efficacy have not been determined in children.

**Dosage**
• **Tablets**
*Analgesic.*
**Adults:** 1 tablet q 4–6 hr, as needed. Dosage should not exceed 5 tablets in a 24-hr period. Adjust dose and frequency of dosing to client needs.

**NURSING CONSIDERATIONS**

See also *Nursing Considerations* for *Hydrocodone bitartrate* and *Ibuprofen.*
**Assessment**
1. Document onset, location, and characteristics of pain; rate pain using a pain–rating scale.
2. Note any conditions that may preclude use of drug combination.
**Client/Family Teaching**
1. Take only as prescribed, do not exceed 5 tabs/day.

2. Drug is for short term use only, up to 10 days; may be habit forming.

3. Do not perform activities that require mental/physical alertness; may cause impairment.

4. Avoid alcohol and any other CNS depressants.

5. Report any S&S of GI bleeding, blurred vision, or other eye problems, skin rash, weight gain, or swelling of extremities.

**Outcomes/Evaluate:** Relief of pain

# Hydrocortisone (Cortisol)
(hy-droh-**KOR**-tih-zohn)

**Pregnancy Category:** C (topical and dental products)
**Parenteral:** Sterile Hydrocortisone Suspension. **Rectal:** Dermolate Anal-Itch, Cortenema ✤, Proctocort, ProctoCream.HC 2.5%, Rectocort ✤. **Retention Enema:** Cortenema, Hycort ✤, Rectocort ✤. **Roll-on Applicator:** Cortaid FastStick, Maximum Strength Cortaid Faststick, **Tablets:** Cortef, Hydrocortone. **Topical Cream:** Ala-Cort, Allercort, Alphaderm, Bactine, Cortate ✤, Cort-Dome, Cortifair, Dermacort, DermiCort, Dermolate Anti-Itch, Dermtex HC, Emo-Cort ✤, H₂Cort, Hi-Cor 1.0 and 2.5, Hydro-Tex, Hytone, Nutracort, Penecort, Prevex HC ✤, Synacort. **Topical Gel:** Extra Strength CortaGel, **Topical Liquid:** Scalpicin, T/Scalp, **Topical Lotion:** Acticort 100, Ala-Cort, Ala-Scalp, Allercort, Aquacort ✤, Cetacort, Cortate ✤, Cort-Dome, Delacort, Dermacort, Dermolate Scalp-Itch, Emo-Cort ✤, Gly-Cort, Hytone, LactiCare-HC, Lemoderm, Lexocort Forte, My Cort, Nutracort, Pentacort, Rederm, Sarna HC ✤, S-T Cort. **Topical Ointment:** Allercort, Cortoderm ✤, Cortril, Hytone, Lemoderm, Penecort. **Topical Solution:** Penecort, Emo-Cort Scalp Solution, Texacort Scalp Solution. **Topical Spray:** Cortaid, Dermolate Anti-Itch, Maximum Strength Coraid, Procort **(OTC) (Rx)**

# Hydrocortisone acetate
(hy-droh-**KOR**-tih-zohn)

**Pregnancy Category:** C (topical and dental products)
**Dental Paste:** Orabase-HCA. **Intrarectal Foam:** Cortifoam. **Ophthalmic/Otic:** Cortamed ✤. **Parenteral:** Hydrocortone Acetate. **Rectal:** Cort-Dome High Potency, Cortenema, Corticaine, Cortifoam. **Suppository:** Cortiment ✤, Rectocort ✤, **Topical Cream:** CaldeCORT Light, Carmol-HC, Cortaid, Cortef Feminine Itch, Corticaine, Corticreme ✤, FoilleCort, Gynecort, Gynecort Female Cream, Hyderm ✤, Lanacort, Lanacort 10, Lanacort 5, Maximum Strength Cortaid, Pharma-Cort, Rhulicort. **Topical Lotion:** Cortaid, Rhulicort. **Topical Ointment:** Anusol HC-1, Cortef Acetate, Dermaflex HC 1% ✤, Lanacort, Lanacort 5, Nov-Hydrocort., Maximum Strength Cortaid **(OTC) (Rx)**

# Hydrocortisone buteprate
(hy-droh-**KOR**-tih-zohn)

**Pregnancy Category:** C
**Topical Cream:** Pandel **(Rx)**

# Hydrocortisone butyrate
(hy-droh-**KOR**-tih-zohn)

**Pregnancy Category:** C (topical products)
**Topical Cream, Ointment, Solution:** Locoid **(Rx)**

# Hydrocortisone cypionate
(hy-droh-**KOR**-tih-zohn)

**Pregnancy Category:** C
**Oral Suspension:** Cortef **(Rx)**

# Hydrocortisone sodium phosphate
(hy-droh-**KOR**-tih-zohn)

**Pregnancy Category:** C
**Parenteral:** Hydrocortone Phosphate **(Rx)**

# Hydrocortisone sodium succinate
(hy-droh-**KOR**-tih-zohn)

**Pregnancy Category:** C

H

---

✤ = Available in Canada             ***bold italic*** = life threatening side effect

**Parenteral:** A-hydroCort, Solu-Cortef **(Rx)**

# Hydrocortisone valerate

(hy-droh-**KOR**-tih-zohn)
**Pregnancy Category:** C (topical products)
**Topical Cream/Ointment:** Westcort **(Rx)**
**Classification:** Corticosteroid, naturally occurring; glucocorticoid-type

See also *Corticosteroids.*
**Action/Kinetics:** Short-acting. **t½:** 80–118 min. Topical products are available without a prescription in strengths of 0.5% and 1%.

## Dosage
HYDROCORTISONE
• **Tablets**
20–240 mg/day, depending on disease.
• **IM Only**
One-third to one-half the PO dose q 12 hr.
• **Rectal**
100 mg in retention enema nightly for 21 days (up to 2 months of therapy may be needed; discontinue gradually if therapy exceeds 3 weeks).
• **Topical Ointment, Cream, Gel, Lotion, Solution, Spray**
Apply sparingly to affected area and rub in lightly t.i.d.–q.i.d.
HYDROCORTISONE ACETATE
• **Intralesional, Intra-articular, Soft Tissue**
5–50 mg, depending on condition.
• **Intrarectal Foam**
1 applicatorful (90 mg) 1–2 times/day for 2–3 weeks; **then** every second day.
• **Topical**
See *Hydrocortisone.*
HYDROCORTISONE BUTEPRATE
• **Topical Cream**
Apply a thin film to the affected area 1–2 times/day.
HYDROCORTISONE BUTYRATE
• **Topical Cream, Ointment, Solution**
Apply a thin film to the affected area b.i.d.–t.i.d.
HYDROCORTISONE CYPIONATE
• **Suspension**

20–240 mg/day, depending on the severity of the disease.
HYDROCORTISONE SODIUM PHOSPHATE
• **IV, IM, SC**
*General uses.*
**Initial:** 15–240 mg/day depending on use and on severity of the disease. Usually, one-half to one-third of the PO dose is given q 12 hr.
*Adrenal insufficiency, acute.*
**Adults, initial:** 100 mg IV; **then,** 100 mg q 8 hr in an IV fluid; **older children, initial:** 1–2 mg/kg by IV bolus; **then,** 150–250 mg/kg/day **IV** in divided doses; **infants, initial:** 1–2 mg/kg by IV bolus; **then,** 25–150 mg/kg/day in divided doses.
HYDROCORTISONE SODIUM SUCCINATE
• **IM, IV**
**Initial:** 100–500 mg; **then,** may be repeated at 2-, 4-, and 6-hr intervals depending on response and severity of condition.
HYDROCORTISONE VALERATE
• **Topical Cream**
See *Hydrocortisone.*

## NURSING CONSIDERATIONS

See also *Nursing Considerations* for *Corticosteroids.*
**Administration/Storage**
1. When using topical products, wash area prior to application to increase drug penetration.
2. Do not allow topical product to come in contact with the eyes.
3. Avoid prolonged use of topical products near the genital/rectal areas and eyes, on the face, and in creases of the skin.
4. For the buteprate and butyrate topical products, use an occlusive dressing only on advice of the provider if used to treat psoriasis or other deep-seated dermatoses.
5. Do not use buteprate products in the diaper area. With the butyrate products, do not use tight-fitting diapers or plastic pants.
6. No part of the intrarectal foam aerosol container should be inserted into the anus.
**IV** 7. Check label of parenteral hydrocortisone because IM and IV

preparations are not necessarily interchangeable.

8. Give reconstituted direct IV solution at a rate of 100 mg over 30 sec. Doses larger than 500 mg should be infused over 10 min. Drug may be further diluted in 50–100 mL of dextrose or saline solutions and administered as ordered within 24 hr.

**Assessment**

1. Document indications for therapy, type, location, onset, and duration of symptoms.
2. List other agents used and the outcome.
3. Assess CBC, chemistry profile, liver and renal function studies.

**Outcomes/Evaluate**

• Replacement of adrenocortical deficiency
• Restoration of skin integrity
• Relief of allergic manifestations

---

# Hydromorphone hydrochloride

(hy-droh-**MOR**-fohn)
**Pregnancy Category:** C
Dilaudid, Dilaudid-HP, Dilaudid-HP-Plus ✦, Dilaudid Sterile Powder ✦, Dilaudid-XP ✦, Hydromorph Contin ✦, PMS-Hydromorphone ✦ **(C-II) (Rx)**
**Classification:** Narcotic analgesic, morphine type

See also *Narcotic Analgesics.*
**Action/Kinetics:** Hydromorphone is 7–10 times more analgesic than morphine, with a shorter duration of action. It manifests less sedation, less vomiting, and less nausea than morphine, although it induces pronounced respiratory depression. **Onset:** 15–30 min. **Peak effect:** 30–60 min. **Duration:** 4–5 hr. **t½:** 2–3 hr. Give rectally for prolonged activity.

**Uses:** Analgesia for moderate to severe pain (e.g., surgery, cancer, biliary colic, burns, renal colic, MI, bone trauma). Dilaudid-HP is a concentrated solution intended for those tolerant to narcotics.

**Additional Contraindications:** Mi-

graine headaches. Use in children. Status asthmaticus, obstetrics, respiratory depression in absence of resuscitative equipment. Lactation.

**Special Concerns:** Do not confuse Dilaudid-HP with standard parenteral solutions of Dilaudid or with other narcotics as overdose and death can result. Use Dilaudid-HP with caution in clients with circulatory shock.

**Additional Side Effects:** Nystagmus.

**Dosage** ————————
• **Tablets, Liquid**
*Analgesia.*
**Adults:** 2 mg q 4–6 hr as necessary. For severe pain, 4 or more mg q 4–6 hr.
• **Suppositories**
*Analgesia.*
**Adults:** 3 mg q 6–8 hr.
• **SC, IM, IV**
*Analgesia.*
**Adults:** 1–2 mg q 4–6 hr. For severe pain, 3–4 mg q 4–6 hr.

## NURSING CONSIDERATIONS

See also *Nursing Considerations* for *Narcotic Analgesics.*
**Administration/Storage**
1. Refrigerate suppositories.
2. May be given as Dilaudid brand cough syrup. Be alert to an allergic response in those sensitive to yellow dye number 5.
**IV** 3. May be given by slow IV injection. Administer drug slowly to minimize hypotensive effects and respiratory depression. Dilute with 5 mL of sterile water or NSS and administer at a rate of 2 mg over 5 min.

**Assessment**
1. Document type, location, onset, and duration of symptoms. Use a scale to rate pain.
2. Assess for respiratory depression; more profound with hydromorphone than with other narcotic analgesics. Encourage to turn, cough, deep breathe or use incentive spi-

rometry every 2 hr to prevent atelectasis.

3. Drug may mask symptoms of acute pathology; assess abdomen carefully.

**Outcomes/Evaluate:** Relief of pain

# Hydroxychloroquine sulfate

(hy-drox-ee-**KLOR**-oh-kwin)
Plaquenil Sulfate **(Rx)**
**Classification:** 4-Aminoquinoline, antimalarial, and antirheumatic

See also *Antimalarial Drugs, 4-Aminoquinolines.*

**Action/Kinetics: Peak plasma levels:** 1–3 hr. Accumulates in the liver, spleen, kidney, heart, lung, and brain. About 50% of unchanged drug excreted in the urine. Enhance excretion by acidifying the urine and decrease by alkalizing the urine.

**Uses:** Prophylaxis and treatment of acute attacks of malaria due to *Plasmodium vivax, P. malariae, P. ovale,* and susceptible strains of *P. falciparum.* Acute or chronic rheumatoid arthritis (not a drug of choice; discontinue after 6 months if no beneficial effects noted). Discoid and SLE. Not used as a first line of therapy.

**Additional Contraindications:** Long-term therapy in children, ophthalmologic changes due to 4-aminoquinolines. Pregnancy.

**Special Concerns:** Use with caution in alcoholism or liver disease. Use in psoriasis may precipitate an acute attack.

**Additional Side Effects:** The appearances of skin eruptions or of misty vision and visual halos are indications for withdrawal. Clients on long-term therapy should be examined thoroughly at regular intervals for knee and ankle reflexes and hematopoietic studies.

**Drug Interactions**

*Digoxin* / Hydroxychloroquine ↑ serum digoxin levels
*Gold salts* / Dermatitis and ↑ risk of severe skin reactions
*Phenylbutazone* / Dermatitis and ↑ risk of severe skin reactions

**Dosage** ─────────

• **Tablets**

*Acute malarial attack.*

**Adults, initial:** 800 mg; **then,** 400 mg after 6–8 hr and 400 mg/day for next 2 days. **Children:** A total of 32 mg/kg given over a 3-day period as follows: **initial:** 12.9 mg/kg (not to exceed a single dose of 800 mg); **then,** 6.4 mg/kg (not to exceed a single dose of 400 mg) 6, 24, and 48 hr after the first dose.

*Suppression of malaria.*

**Adults:** 400 mg q 7 days. If therapy has not been initiated 14 days prior to exposure, an initial loading dose of 800 mg may be given in two divided doses 6 hr apart. **Children:** 6.4 mg/kg (not to exceed the adult dose) q 7 days. If therapy has not been initiated 14 days prior to exposure, an initial loading dose of 12.9 mg/kg may be given in two doses 6 hr apart.

*Rheumatoid arthritis.*

**Adults:** 400–600 mg/day taken with milk or meals; **maintenance** (usually after 4–12 weeks): 200–400 mg/day. Use in children is limited, but if use is warranted, a dose of 3–5 mg/kg/day, up to a maximum of 400 mg/day (given once or twice daily), may be used. (*NOTE:* Several months may be required for a beneficial effect to be seen in adults and children.)

*Lupus erythematosus.*

**Adults, usual:** 400 mg once or twice daily; **prolonged maintenance:** 200–400 mg/day.

## NURSING CONSIDERATIONS

See also *Nursing Considerations* for *Antimalarial Drugs, 4-Aminoquinolines,* and *General Nursing Considerations for All Anti-Infectives.*

**Administration/Storage**

1. Corticosteroids and salicylates may be used with hydroxychloroquine.

2. When a gradual decrease of steroid dose is indicated, reduce gradually (q 4–5 days). The dose of cortisone should be reduced by no more than 5–15 mg; hydrocortisone from

5–10 mg; predisone and predniso-lone from 1–2.5 mg; methylpredniso-lone and triamcinolone from 1–2 mg; and dexamethasone from 0.25–0.5 mg.

3. If the recommended maintenance dose is exceeded, the incidence of retinopathy increases.

**Assessment**

1. Document indications for thera-py, type and onset of symptoms, dates of exposure.

2. Record condition of skin; strength of ankle and knee reflexes; any joint swelling, discoloration, and warmth; ROM and pain level.

3. Determine history of liver disease or alcohol abuse.

4. Monitor CBC, liver/renal function studies, and ophthalmic exams q 3 mo.

**Client/Family Teaching**

1. Report any skin eruptions or muscular weakness.

2. Report any visual disturbances; obtain regular opthalmic exams; reti-nopathy is dose related.

3. Avoid excessive sun exposure; use sunscreen, hat, glasses, and pro-tective clothing.

4. When given for rheumatoid arthritis:

• GI irritation may be reduced by taking with meals or a glass of milk.

• Corticosteroids and salicylates or NSAIDs may be used concomitantly; continue anti-inflammatory dose for several weeks into therapy.

• Report all side effects. Anticipate excessive side effects; may necessitate dosage reduction. After 5–10 days of reduced dosage, provider may grad-ually increase drug to desired level.

• Reduce dosage when desired re-sponse attained so drug will again be effective in case of flare-up.

• Benefits may not occur until 6–12 months after therapy initiated.

5. When given for lupus erythemato-sus, administer with evening meal.

6. Initiate suppressive antimalarial therapy 2 weeks prior to exposure; continue for 6–8 weeks after leaving endemic area. If not started prior to exposure, double the initial loading dose and take in two doses 6 hr apart.

**Outcomes/Evaluate**

• Malarial prophylaxis

• Termination of acute malarial at-tack; suppression of symptoms

• ↓ Joint pain and swelling; ↑ mobility

# Hydroxyurea
(hy-**DROX**-ee-you-**ree**-ah)
**Pregnancy Category:** D
Hydrea (Abbreviation: HYD)
**Classification:** Antineoplastic, anti-metabolite

See also *Antineoplastic Agents*.

**Action/Kinetics:** Inhibits DNA syn-thesis but not synthesis of RNA or protein. As an antimetabolite, it in-terferes with the conversion of ribo-nucleotides to deoxyribonucleotides due to blockade of the ribonucleotide reductase system. May also inhibit incorporation of thymidine into DNA. Rapidly absorbed from GI tract. **Peak serum concentration:** 1–2 hr. **t½:** 3–4 hr. Crosses the blood-brain barrier. Degraded in liv-er; 80% excreted through the urine with 50% unchanged; also excreted as respiratory $CO_2$.

**Uses:** Chronic, resistant, myelocytic leukemia. Carcinoma of the ovary (recurrent, inoperable, or metastat-ic). Melanoma. With irradiation to treat primary squamous cell carcino-ma of the head and neck (but not the lip). *Investigational:* Sickle cell ane-mia, thrombocytopenia, HIV, psoria-sis.

**Contraindications:** Leukocyte count less than 2,500/mm³ or throm-bocyte count less than 100,000/mm³. Severe anemia.

**Special Concerns:** Use during pregnancy only if benefits clearly outweigh risks. Give with caution to clients with marked renal dysfunc-tion. Geriatric clients may be more sensitive to the effects of hydroxyurea necessitating a lower dose. Dosage has not been established in children.

**Additional Side Effects:** Erythrocyte abnormalities including megaloblastic erythropoiesis. Constipation, redness of the face, maculopapular rash.

**Laboratory Test Interferences:** ↑ Serum uric acid, BUN, and creatinine.

## Dosage

• **Capsules**

*Solid tumors, intermittent therapy or when used together with irradiation.*
**Dose individualized. Usual:** 80 mg/kg as a single dose every third day. Intermittent dosage offers advantage of reduced toxicity. If effective, maintain client on drug indefinitely unless toxic effects preclude such a regimen.

*Solid tumors, continuous therapy.*
20–30 mg/kg/day as a single dose.

*Resistant chronic myelocytic leukemia.*
20–30 mg/kg/day in a single dose or two divided daily doses.

*Concomitant therapy with irradiation for carinoma of the head and neck.*
80 mg/kg as a single dose every third day.

## NURSING CONSIDERATIONS

See also *Nursing Considerations* for *Antineoplastic Agents.*

**Administration/Storage**
1. Calculate dosage based on actual or ideal weight (whichever is less).
2. Continue therapy for at least 6 weeks before efficacy is assessed.
3. If unable to swallow a capsule, contents may be given in glass of water and drunk immediately; some material may not dissolve and may float on top of glass.
4. Start hydroxyurea at least 7 days before initiation of irradiation; continue through irradiation and indefinitely afterward as long as the client can tolerate the dose. The dosage of radiation is not usually adjusted with concomitant usage of hydroxyurea.
5. Do not store in excessive heat.

**Assessment**
1. Assess for exacerbation of postirradiation erythema.

2. Monitor uric acid, liver and renal function studies.
3. Obtain hematologic profiles weekly. Drug may cause severe granulocyte and platelet suppression. Nadir: 7 days; recovery: 14 days.

**Outcomes/Evaluate**
• Suppression of malignant process
• ↓ Tumor size and spread

# Hydroxyzine hydrochloride
(hy-**DROX**-ih-zeen)
Anxanil, Apo-Hydroxzine ✱, Atarax, Atarax 100, Atozine, E-Vista, Hyzine-50, Multipax ✱, Novo–Hydroxyzin ✱, Nu-Hydroxyzine ✱, PMS Hydroxyzine ✱, Quiess, Vistaquel 50, Vistaril, Vistazine 50 **(Rx)**

# Hydroxyzine pamoate
(hy-**DROX**-ih-zeen)
Vamate, Vistaril **(Rx)**
**Classification:** Nonbenzodiazepine antianxiety agent

**Action/Kinetics:** Manifests anticholinergic, antiemetic, antispasmodic, local anesthetic, antihistaminic, and skeletal relaxant effects. Has mild antiarrhythmic activity and mild analgesic effects. High sedative and antiemetic effects and moderate anticholinergic activity. **Onset:** 15–30 min. **t½:** 3 hr. **Duration:** 4–6 hr. Metabolized by the liver and excreted through the urine. The pamoate salt is believed to be converted to the hydrochloride in the stomach.

**Uses: PO:** Psychoneurosis and tension states, anxiety, and agitation. Anxiety observed in organic disease. Pruritus. Preanesthetic sedative; sedative following general anesthesia. **IM:** Acute hysteria or agitation, withdrawal symptoms (including delirium tremens) in the acute or chronic alcoholic, asthma. N&V (except that due to pregnancy). Pre- or postoperative and pre- or postpartum to allow decrease in dosage of narcotics.

**Contraindications:** Pregnancy (especially early) or lactation; treatment of morning sickness during pregnancy or as sole agent for treatment of psychoses or depression. Hypersensitivity to drug. IV, SC, or intra-arterially.

**Special Concerns:** Possible increased anticholinergic and sedative effects in geriatric clients.

**Side Effects:** Low incidence at recommended dosages. Drowsiness, dryness of mouth, involuntary motor activity, dizziness, urticaria, or skin reactions. Marked discomfort, induration, and even gangrene at site of IM injection.

**OD** **Overdose Management:** *Symptoms:* Oversedation. *Treatment:* Immediate induction of vomiting or performance of gastric lavage. General supportive care with monitoring of VS. Control hypotension with IV fluids and either norepinephrine or metaraminol (epinephrine should not be used).

**Drug Interactions:** Additive effects when used with other CNS depressants. See *Drug Interactions* for *Tranquilizers*.

**Laboratory Test Interferences:** Hydroxycorticosteroids.

**Dosage** ———————
• **Capsules, Oral Suspension, Syrup, Tablets. Hydroxyzine hydrochloride and hydroxyzine pamoate**
    *Antianxiety.*
**Adults:** 50–100 mg q.i.d.; **pediatric under 6 years:** 50 mg/day; **over 6 years:** 50–100 mg/day in divided doses.
    *Pruritus.*
**Adults:** 25 mg t.i.d.–q.i.d.; **children under 6 years:** 50 mg/day in divided doses; **children over 6 years:** 50–100 mg/day in divided doses.
    *Preoperative or post–general anesthetic sedative.*
**Adults:** 50–100 mg; **children:** 0.6 mg/kg.
• **IM. Hydroxyzine Hydrochloride**
    *Acute anxiety, including alcohol withdrawal.*
**Adults, initial:** 50–100 mg repeated q 4–6 hr as needed.

*N&V, pre- and postoperative, pre- and postpartum.*
**Adults:** 25–100 mg; **pediatric,** 1.1 mg/kg. Switch to **PO** as soon as possible.

## NURSING CONSIDERATIONS

See also *Nursing Considerations* for *Tranquilizers*.

**Administration/Storage**
1. Inject IM only. Make injection into the upper, outer quadrant of the buttocks or the midlateral muscles of the thigh. In children inject into the midlateral muscles of the thigh.
2. Shake suspension vigorously until it is completely resuspended.

**Assessment:** Document indications for therapy, type, onset, location, and duration of symptoms. Note any associated characteristics or contributing factors.

**Client/Family Teaching**
1. Frequent mouth rinsing, sucking hard candy, chewing sugarless gums, and increased fluid intake may relieve symptoms of dry mouth.
2. Wait and evaluate sedative effects of drug before performing tasks that require mental alertness.
3. Avoid alcohol or any other CNS depressants.
4. Drug is only for short-term management.

**Outcomes/Evaluate**
• ↓ Anxiety and agitation
• Relief of itching/allergic S&S
• Control of N&V

# Hylan G-F 20
(**HIGH**-lan)
Synvisc, **(Rx)**

See *Sodium hyaluronate*.

# Hyoscyamine sulfate
(high-oh-**SIGH**-ah-meen)
**Pregnancy Category:** C
Anaspaz, Cystospaz-M, Espasmotex, Levbid, Levsin, Levsinex, Levsin SL, Spasdel **(Rx)**
**Classification:** Cholinergic blocking agent

---

***bold italic*** = life threatening side effect

See also *Cholinergic Blocking Agents.*

**Action/Kinetics:** One of the belladonna alkaloids; acts by blocking the action of acetylcholine at the postganglionic nerve endings of the parasympathetic nervous system. $t\frac{1}{2}$: $3\frac{1}{2}$ hr for tablets, 7 hr for extended-release capsules, and 9 hr for extended-release tablets. Majority of the drug is excreted in the urine unchanged.

**Uses:** To control gastric secretion, visceral spasm, and hypermotilitiy in spastic colitis, spastic bladder, cystitis, pylorospasm, and associated abdominal cramps. Adjunctive therapy to treat irritable bowel syndrome and functional GI disorders. Adjunctive therapy in neurogenic bladder and neurogenic bowel disturbances. Treat infant colic (use elixir or solution). Use with morphine or other narcotics for symptomatic relief of biliary and renal colic. In Parkinsonism to reduce rigidity and tremors and to control sialorrhea and hyperhidrosis. To treat poisoning by anticholinesterase agents. To reduce GI motility to facilitate diagnostic procedures, such as endoscopy or hypersecretion in pancreatitis. To treat selected cases of partial heart block associated with vagal activity. Used as a preoperative medication to reduce salivary, tracheobronchial, and pharyngeal secretions.

**Special Concerns:** Heat prostration may occur if the drug is taken in the presence of high environmental temperatures. Use with caution during lactation.

**Side Effects:** See *Cholinergic Blocking Agents.*

**Dosage** ———————————
• **Extended-Release Capsules (0.375 mg) or Extended-Release Tablets (0.375 mg)**
**Adults and children over 12 years of age:** 0.375–0.750 mg q 12 hr, not to exceed 1.5 mg in 24 hr.
• **Tablets (0.125 mg)**
**Adults and children over 12 years of age:** 0.125–0.25 mg q 4 hr or as needed, not to exceed 1.5 mg in 24 hr.

• **Elixir (0.125 mg/5 mL)**
**Adults and children over 12 years of age:** 0.125 mg–0.25 mg (5–10 mL) q 4 hr, not to exceed 1.5 mg (60 mL) in 24 hr. **Children, 2 to 12 years of age:** 10 kg: 1.25 mL (0.031 mg) q 4 hr; 20 kg: 2.5 mL (0.062 mg) q 4 hr; 40 kg: 3.75 mL (0.093 mg) q 4 hr; 50 kg: 5 mL (0.125 mg) q 4 hr.
• **Drops (0.125 mg/mL)**
**Adults and children over 12 years of age:** 0.125–0.25 mg 5–10 mL q 4 hr, not to exceed 1.5 mg (12 mL) in 24 hr. **Children, 2 to 12 years of age:** 0.031–0.125 mg (0.251 mL) q 4 hr or as needed, not to exceed 0.75 mg (6 mL) in 24 hr. **Children, under 2 years of age:** 3.4 kg: 4 drops q 4 hr, not to exceed 24 drops in 24 hr; 5 kg: 5 drops q 4 hr, not to exceed 30 drops in 24 hr; 7 kg: 6 drops q 4 hr, not to exceed 36 drops in 24 hr; 10 kg: 8 drops q 4 hr, not to exceed 48 drops in 24 hr.
• **Injection (0.5 mg/mL)**
*GI disorders.*
**Adults:** 0.25–0.5 mg (0.5–1 mL). Some clients need only one dose while others require doses 2, 3, or 4 times a day at 4 hr intervals.
*Diagnostic procedures.*
**Adults:** 0.25–0.5 mg (0.5–1 mL) given IV 5 to 10 min prior to the procedure.
*Preanesthetic medication.*
**Adults and children over 2 years of age:** 0.005 mg/kg 30–60 min prior to the time of induction of anesthesia. May also be given at the time the preanesthetic sedative or narcotic is given.
*During surgery to reduce drug-induced bradycardia.*
**Adults and children over 2 years of age:** Increments of 0.125 mg (0.25 mL) IV repeated as needed.
*Reverse neuromuscular blockade.*
**Adults and children over 2 years of age:** 0.2 mg (0.4 mL) for every 1 mg neostigmine or equivalent dose of physostigmine or pyridostigmine.

## NURSING CONSIDERATIONS

See also *Nursing Considerations* for *Cholinergic Blocking Agents.*

## Administration/Storage
1. May take hyoscyamine SL tablets sublingually, PO, or chewed. May take hyoscyamine tablets PO or sublingually.
2. Depending on the use, give the injection SC, IM, or IV.
3. Visually inspect the injectable form for particulate matter/discoloration.

## Assessment
1. Document indications for therapy, type, onset, and duration of symptoms.
2. List other agents trialed and the outcome.
3. Determine any evidence of glaucoma, bladder neck or GI tract obstruction.

## Client/Family Teaching
1. Take as prescribed; report any loss of symptom control so provider can adjust dose and frequency of administration.
2. Do not perform activities that require mental alertness until drug effects realized; dizziness, drowsiness, and blurred vision may occur.
3. Diarrhea may be a symptom of intestinal obstruction, esp. with a colostomy or ileostomy; report promptly.
4. Avoid excessive temperatures and activity; drug may decrease perspiration, which may cause fever, heat prostration, or stoke.
5. Stop drug and report any mental confusion, impaired gait, disorientation, or hallucinations.

## Outcomes/Evaluate
- ↓ GI motility
- ↓ Secretion production
- Control of pain and spasm

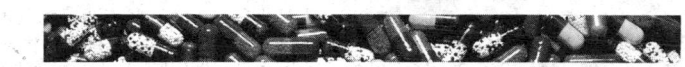

# Ibuprofen
(eye-byou-**PROH**-fen)

**Rx:** Actiprofen ✦, Alti-Ibuprofen ✦, Apo-Ibuprofen ✦, Children's Advil, Children's Motrin, IBU, Ibuprohm, Motrin, Novo-Profen ✦, Nu-Ibuprofen ✦, Saleto-400, -600, and -800. **OTC:** Advil Caplets and Tablets, Bayer Select Pain Relief Formula Caplets, Children's Advil Suspension, Children's Motrin Liquid Suspension, Children's Motrin Drops, Genpril Caplets and Tablets, Haltran, Ibuprin, Ibuprohm Caplets and Tablets, Junior Strength Motrin Caplets, Menadol, Midol IB, Motrin-IB Caplets and Tablets, Nuprin Caplets and Tablets, PediaCare Fever Drops, Saleto-200

**Classification:** Nonsteroidal anti-inflammatory drug (NSAID)

See also *Nonsteroidal Anti-Inflammatory Drugs.*

**Action/Kinetics: Time to peak levels:** 1–2 hr. **Onset:** 30 min for analgesia and approximately 1 week for anti-inflammatory effect. **Peak serum levels:** 1–2 hr. **t½:** 2 hr. **Duration:** 4–6 hr for analgesia and 1–2 weeks for anti-inflammatory effect. Food delays absorption rate but not total amount of drug absorbed.

**Uses:** Analgesic for mild to moderate pain. Primary dysmenorrhea, rheumatoid arthritis, osteoarthritis, antipyretic. *Investigational:* Resistant acne vulgaris (with tetracyclines); inflammation due to ultraviolet-B exposure (sunburn), juvenile rheumatoid arthritis. High doses to treat progressive lung deterioration in cystic fibrosis. OTC products are used for the relief of fever and minor aches and pains due to colds, flu, sore throats, headaches, and toothaches.

**Contraindications:** Use of ibuprofen is not recommended during pregnancy, especially during the last trimester.

**Special Concerns:** The dosage must be individually determined for children less than 12 years of age as safety and effectiveness have not been established.

**Additional Side Effects:** Dermatitis (maculopapular type), rash. Hypersensitivity reaction consisting of abdominal pain, fever, headache, *meningitis,* N&V, signs of liver damage; especially seen in clients with SLE.

**Additional Drug Interactions**

*Furosemide* / Ibuprofen ↓ diuretic effect of furosemide due to ↓ renal prostaglandin synthesis

*Lithium* / Ibuprofen ↑ plasma levels of lithium

*Thiazide diuretics* / Ibuprofen ↓ diuretic effect of furosemide due to ↓ renal prostaglandin synthesis

**Dosage** ────────────

- **Suspension, Chewable Tablets, Tablets**

*Rheumatoid arthritis, osteoarthritis.*
Either 300 mg q.i.d. or 400, 600, or 800 mg t.i.d.–q.i.d.; adjust dosage according to client response. Full therapeutic response may not be noted for 2 or more weeks.

*Juvenile arthritis.*
30–70 mg/kg/day in three to four divided doses (20 mg/kg/day may be adequate for mild cases).

*Mild to moderate pain.*
**Adults:** 400 mg q 4–6 hr, as needed.

*Antipyretic.*
**Pediatric, 2–12 years of age:** 5 mg/kg if baseline temperature is 102.5°F (39.1°C) or below or 10 mg/kg if baseline temperature is greater than 102.5°F (39.1°C). Maximum daily dose: 40 mg/kg.

*Primary dysmenorrhea.*
**Adults:** 400 mg q 4 hr, as needed.

- **Tablets for OTC Use**

*Mild to moderate pain, antipyretic, dysmenorrhea.*
200 mg q 4–6 hr; dose may be increased to 400 mg if pain or fever persist. Dose should not exceed 1,200 mg/day.

- **Suspension for OTC Use**

*Pain, fever.*
**Children, 2–11 years:** 7.5 mg/kg, up to q.i.d., to a maximum of 30 mg/kg/day.

## NURSING CONSIDERATIONS

See also *Nursing Considerations* for *Nonsteroidal Anti-Inflammatory Drugs.*

**Administration/Storage**

1. Do not use OTC ibuprofen as an antipyretic for more than 3 days.
2. Do not use as an analgesic for more than 10 days unless medically cleared.
3. Do not take more than 3.2 g/day of prescription products and no more than 1.2 g/day of OTC products.

**Assessment**

1. Document indications for therapy, onset, location, and type of symptoms.
2. Assess for evidence of lupus.
3. Obtain CBC, liver and renal function studies (X rays and eye exam) prior to initiating long-term drug therapy.

**Client/Family Teaching**

1. Take with a snack, milk, antacid, or meals to decrease GI upset. Report any N&V, diarrhea, or constipation.
2. Take the dosage prescribed for best results.
3. With history of CHF or compromised cardiac function, keep weight records, report edema; drug causes Na retention.
4. Report blurred vision; obtain periodic eye exams with long-term therapy.
5. Report as scheduled for follow-up evaluations: ROM, CBC, renal function, X rays, and stool for blood.

**Outcomes/Evaluate**

- ↓ Joint pain and ↑ mobility
- ↓ Fever, ↓ Inflammation
- ↓ Uterine cramping
- ↓ Lung deterioration with CF

---

# Ibutilide fumarate
(ih-**BYOU**-tih-lyd)
**Pregnancy Category:** C
Corvert **(Rx)**
**Classification:** Antiarrhythmic agent

---

**Action/Kinetics:** Class III antiarrhythmic agent. Delays repolarization by activation of a slow, inward current (mostly sodium), rather than by blocking outward potassium currents (the way other class III antiarrhythmics act). This results in prolongation in the duration of the atrial and ventricular action potential and refractoriness. Also a dose-related prolongation of the QT interval. High systemic plasma clearance that approximates liver blood flow; protein binding is less than 40%. **t½, terminal:** 6 hr. Over 80% is excreted in the urine (with 7% excreted unchanged) and approximately 20% is excreted through the feces.

**Uses:** For rapid conversion of atrial fibrillation or atrial flutter of recent onset to sinus rhythm. Determination of clients to receive ibutilide should be based on expected benefits of maintaining sinus rhythm and whether this outweighs both the risks of the drug and of maintenance therapy.

**Contraindications:** Use of certain class Ia antiarrhythmic drugs (e.g., disopyramide, quinidine, procainamide) and certain class III drugs (e.g., amiodarone and sotalol) concomitantly with ibutilide or within 4 hr of postinfusion.

**Special Concerns:** Ibutilide may cause potentially fatal arrhythmias, especially sustained polymorphic ventricular tachycardia, usually in association with QT prolongation (torsades de pointes). Effectiveness has not been determined in clients with arrhythmias of more than 90 days in duration. Breast feeding should be discouraged during therapy. Safety and efficacy have not been determined in children less than 18 years of age.

**Side Effects:** *CV: **Life-threatening arrhythmias, either sustained or nonsustained polymorphic ventricular tachycardia (torsades de pointes).*** Induction or worsening of ventricular arrhythmias. Nonsustained monomorphic ventricular extrasystoles, nonsustained monomorphic ventricular tachycardia, sinus tachycardia, SVT, hypotension, postural hypotension, bundle branch block, AV block, bradycardia, QT-segment prolongation, hypertension, palpitation, supraventricular extrasystoles, nodal arrhythmia, CHF, idioventricular rhythm, sustained monomorphic ventricular tachycardia. *Miscellaneous:* Headache, nausea, syncope, renal failure.

**OD Overdose Management:** *Symptoms:* Increased ventricular ectopy, monomorphic ventricular tachycardia, AV block, nonsustained polymorphic ventricular tachycardia. *Treatment:* Treat symptoms.

**Drug Interactions**
*Amiodarone* / ↑ Risk of prolonged refractoriness
*Antidepressants, tricyclic and tetracyclic* / ↑ Risk of proarrhythmias
*Digoxin* / Supraventricular arrhythmias, due to ibutilide, may mask the cardiotoxicity due to high digoxin levels
*Disopyramide* / ↑ Risk of prolonged refractoriness
*Histmne H₁ receptor antagonists* / ↑ Risk of proarrhythmias
*Quinidine* / ↑ Risk of prolonged refractoriness
*Phenothiazines* / ↑ Risk of proarrhythmias
*Procainamide* / ↑ Risk of prolonged refractoriness
*Sotalol* / ↑ Risk of prolonged refractoriness

**Dosage**
• **IV Infusion**
*Atrial fibrillation or atrial flutter of recent onset.*
**Clients weighing 60 kg or more, initial:** 1 mg (one vial) infused over 10 min. **Clients weighing less than 60 kg, initial:** 0.01 mg/kg infused over 10 min. If the arrhythmia does not terminate within 10 min after the end of the initial infusion (regardless of the body weight), a second 10-min infusion of equal strength may be given 10 min after completion of the first infusion.

**NURSING CONSIDERATIONS**
**Administration/Storage**
**IV** 1. Anticoagulate clients with

atrial fibrillation (>2–3 days duration) for at least 2 weeks.

2. May give undiluted or diluted in 50 mL of 0.9% NaCl injection or 5% dextrose injection before infusion. The contents of one vial (1 mg) mixed with 50 mL of diluent forms an admixture of approximately 0.017 mg/mL of ibutilide. Administer infusion over 10 min.

3. Either PVC or polyolefin bags are compatible with admixtures of ibutilide.

4. Admixtures with approved diluents are chemically and physically stable for 24 hr at room temperature and for 48 hr if refrigerated.

**Assessment**

1. Document onset of arrhythmia and any associated symptoms.

2. List drugs currently prescribed to ensure none interact unfavorably.

3. Monitor VS, I&O, and ECG.

4. Ibutilide must be given in a setting with continuous ECG monitoring and by those trained in the identification and treatment of acute ventricular arrhythmias, especially polymorphic ventricular tachycardia.

5. Document conversion to NSR (usually within 30–90 min). Drug infusion should cease: when arrhythmia is terminated or in the event of sustained or nonsustained ventricular tachycardia or marked prolongation of QT interval.

6. Observe for at least 4 hr following infusion or until QT interval has returned to baseline. Monitor longer if arrhythmic activity observed.

**Client/Family Teaching**

1. Explain the reasons for dosing and why new-onset atrial fibrillation should be terminated (to prevent embolus formation).

2. Review the benefits and possible adverse side effects.

3. Stress the importance of close medical follow-up to determine stability of rhythm.

**Outcomes/Evaluate:** Conversion of atrial fibrillation to stable sinus rhythm

# Idarubicin hydrochloride

(eye-dah-**ROOB**-ih-sin)
**Pregnancy Category:** D
Idamycin For Injection **(Rx)**
**Classification:** Antineoplastic agent

See also *Antineoplastic Agents.*

**Action/Kinetics:** An anthracycline that inhibits nucleic acid synthesis and interacts with the enzyme topoisomerase II. Rapidly taken up into cells due to significant lipid solubility. **t½ (terminal):** 22 hr when used alone and 20 hr when used with cytarabine. Metabolized in the liver to the active idarubicinol, which is excreted through both the bile and urine. Both idarubicin and idarubicinol are significantly bound (97% and 94%, respectively) to plasma proteins.

**Uses:** In combination with other drugs (often cytarabine) to treat AML in adults, including French-American-British classifications M1–M7. Comparison with daunorubicin indicates that idarubicin is more effective in inducing complete remissions in clients with AML.

**Contraindications:** Lactation. Pre-existing bone marrow suppression induced by previous drug therapy or radiotherapy (unless benefit outweighs risk). Administration by the IM or SC routes.

**Special Concerns:** Safety and effectiveness have not been demonstrated in children. Skin reactions may occur if the powder is not handled properly.

**Side Effects:** *GI:* N&V, mucositis, diarrhea, abdominal pain, abdominal cramps, **hemorrhage.** *Hematologic:* **Severe myelosuppression.** *Dermatologic:* Alopecia, generalized rash, urticaria, bullous erythrodermatous rash of the palms and soles, hives at injection site. *CNS:* Headache, **seizures,** altered mental status. *CV:* CHF, **serious arrhythmias including atrial fibrillation, chest pain, MI, cardiomyopathies,** decrease in LV ejection fraction. *NOTE:* Cardiac toxicity is more common in clients who have received anthracycline drugs previously or who have preexisting cardiac disease. *Miscellaneous:* Altered hepatic and renal function tests, infection (95% of clients), fever, pulmonary allergy, neurologic changes in peripheral nerves.

**OD** **Overdose Management:** *Symptoms:* Severe GI toxicity, myelosuppression. *Treatment:* Supportive treatment including antibiotics and platelet transfusions. Treat mucositis.

**Dosage**
• **IV**
*Induction therapy in adults with AML.*
12 mg/m²/day for 3 days by slow (10–15 min) IV injection in combination with cytarabine, 100 mg/m²/day given by continuous infusion for 7 days or as a 25-mg/m² IV bolus followed by 200 mg/m²/day for 5 days by continuous infusion. A second course may be given if there is evidence of leukemia after the first course. The drug should not be given if the bilirubin level is greater than 5 mg/dL.

## NURSING CONSIDERATIONS

See also *Nursing Considerations* for *Antineoplastic Agents.*
**Administration/Storage**
**IV** 1. Reconstitute the 5-, 10-, and 20-mg vials with 5, 10, and 20 mL, respectively, of 0.9% NaCl injection to give a final concentration of 1 mg/mL. Do not use diluents containing bacteriostatic agents.
2. To minimize aerosol formation during reconstitution; vial contents are under negative pressure. Avoid inhalation of any aerosol formed.
3. Give slowly into a freely flowing IV infusion over 10–15 min.
4. If extravasation suspected or evident, elevate extremity and apply intermittent ice packs (immediately for ½ hr, then 4 times/day at ½-hr intervals for 3 days) over the affected area.
5. Do not mix IV solution with any other drugs.

6. Reconstituted solutions are stable for 7 days if refrigerated and 3 days at room temperature. Discard unused solution.
7. If drug comes in contact with the skin, wash area thoroughly with soap and water. Use goggles, gloves, and protective gowns to prepare and administer.
**Assessment**
1. Document any preexisting cardiac disease.
2. Note any previous radiation therapy or treatment with anthracyclines.
3. Monitor CBC, platelets, and liver and renal function studies. Reduce dose with impaired hepatic or renal function; hold If bilirubin levels > 5 mg/dL.
**Client/Family Teaching**
1. Nausea and diarrhea are frequent side effects of drug therapy; take antiemetic 1 hr before drug therapy.
2. Hair loss may occur.
3. Report any evidence of SOB or chest pain as drug may cause myocardial toxicity.
4. Report any S&S of anemia, i.e., dyspnea, fatigue, or faintness. Severe myelosuppression may occur; report any hemorrhaging or infection.
5. Complaints of severe abdominal pain should be reported.
6. Use reliable contraception before, during, and for several months after therapy.
7. Avoid all OTC products without provider approval; avoid vaccinia during therapy.
8. Encourage a high fluid intake, and keep the urine slightly alkaline to prevent the formation of uric acid stones. Clients with gout may require colchicine or Indocin.
**Outcomes/Evaluate**
• Presence of leukemia cells (second course of therapy may be indicated after hematologic recovery)
• Complete remission; improved hematologic parameters

# Idoxuridine (IDU)

(eye-dox-**YOUR**-ih-deen)

**Pregnancy Category:** C
Herplex Liquifilm, Herplex-D ✽ **(Rx)**
**Classification:** Antiviral agent, ophthalmic

See also *Antiviral Agents.*

**Action/Kinetics:** Idoxuridine, which resembles thymidine, inhibits thymidylic phosphorylase and specific DNA polymerases required for incorporation of thymidine into viral DNA. Idoxuridine, instead of thymidine, is incorporated into viral DNA, resulting in faulty DNA and the inability of the virus to infect tissue or reproduce. May also be incorporated into mammalian cells. Does not penetrate the cornea well. Rapidly inactivated by nucleotidases or deaminases.

**Uses:** Herpes simplex keratitis, especially for initial epithelial infections characterized by the presence of thread-like extensions. *NOTE:* Idoxuridine will control infection but will not prevent scarring, loss of vision, or vascularization. Alternative form of therapy must be instituted if no improvement is noted after 7 days or if complete reepithelialization fails to occur after 21 days of therapy.

**Contraindications:** Hypersensitivity; deep ulcerations involving stromal layers of cornea. Lactation. Concomitant use of corticosteroids in herpes simplex keratitis (corticosteroids may accelerate the spread of the viral infection).

**Special Concerns:** Idoxuridine may be sensitizing, especially with dermal use. Safety and efficacy have not been determined in children.

**Side Effects:** Localized to eye. Temporary visual haze, irritation, pain, pruritus, inflammation, sensitivity to bright light, follicular conjunctivitis with preauricular adenopathy, mild edema of eyelids and cornea, allergic reactions (rare), photosensitivity, corneal clouding and stippling, small punctate defects. *NOTE:* Squamous cell carcinoma has been reported at the site of application.

**OD** **Overdose Management:** *Symptoms (frequent administration):* Defects on corneal epithelium. *Treatment:* If an excess amount of drug is instilled in the eye, flush with water or normal saline.

**Drug Interactions:** Concurrent use of boric acid may cause irritation.

## Dosage

• **Ophthalmic (0.1%) Solution.**
**Initially:** 1 gtt every hour during the day and q 2 hr during the night until definite improvement is noted (usually within 7 days). **Following improvement:** 1 gtt q 2 hr during the day and q 4 hr at night. Continue for 3–7 days after healing is complete. Alternate dosing schedule: 1 gtt q min for 5 min; repeat q 4 hr, day and night.

## NURSING CONSIDERATIONS

See also *General Nursing Considerations for All Anti-Infectives.*
**Administration/Storage**
1. For best results, keep the infected tissues saturated with idoxuridine.
2. Store solution at 2°C–8°C (36°F–46°F); protect from light.
3. Do not mix with other medications.
4. Store ointment at 2°C–15°C (36°F–59°F).
5. Do not use drug that was improperly stored because of loss of activity and increased toxic effects.
6. Topical corticosteroids may be used with idoxuridine in the treatment of herpes simplex with corneal edema, stromal lesions, or iritis.
7. To control secondary infections, antibiotics may be used with idoxuridine.
8. Atropine may be used concomitantly with idoxuridine, if appropriate.
9. Improvement usually observed within 7–8 days; if there is continuous improvement, therapy should be continued for 21 days.
10. Some strains of herpes simplex may be resistant to idoxuridine; if there is no decrease in fluorescein staining after 14 days of use, another

form of therapy should be undertaken.

**Client/Family Teaching**
1. Review method for instillation, frequency for administration, and proper storage. Use as scheduled ATC, even during the night.
2. Report any symptoms of vision loss. Hazy vision following instillation will be of short duration.
3. *Do not* apply boric acid to the eye during idoxuridine therapy; boric acid may cause irritation.
4. Avoid using eye makeup; sharing towels and washcloths during therapy; wash hands frequently.
5. Wear dark glasses if photophobia occurs.
6. If used concurrently with corticosteroids, the idoxuridine will be continued longer than the steroid, to prevent reinfection.
7. Report for scheduled ophthalmic exams to determine drug response and to assess application site.

**Outcomes/Evaluate**
• Control of ophthalmic infection
• Reepithelialization of eye lesions

# Ifosfamide

(eye-**FOS**-fah-myd)
**Pregnancy Category:** D
Ifex **(Rx)**
**Classification:** Antineoplastic, alkylating agent

See also *Antineoplastic Agents* and *Alkylating Agents*.

**Action/Kinetics:** Ifosfamide, a synthetic analog of cyclophosphamide, must be converted in the liver to active metabolites. The alkylated metabolites of ifosfamide then interact with DNA. **t½, elimination:** 7 hr. Excreted in the urine both as unchanged drug and metabolites.

**Uses:** As third-line therapy, in combination with other antineoplastic drugs, for germ cell testicular cancer. Ifosfamide should always be given with mesna to prevent ifosfamide-induced hemorrhagic cystitis. *Investigational:* Cancer of the breast, lung,

pancreas, ovary, and stomach. Also for sarcomas, acute leukemias (except AML), malignant lymphomas.

**Contraindications:** Severe bone marrow depression. Lactation.

**Special Concerns:** Use with caution in clients with compromised bone marrow reserve, impaired renal function, and during lactation. Safety and efficacy have not been established in children. May interfere with wound healing.

**Additional Side Effects:** *GU: Hemorrhagic cystitis,* hematuria, dysuria, urinary frequency. *CNS:* Confusion, depressive psychosis, somnolence, hallucinations. Less frequently: dizziness, disorientation, cranial nerve dysfunction, *seizures, coma. GI:* Salivation, stomatitis. *Miscellaneous:* Myelosuppression, alopecia, infection, liver dysfunction, phlebitis, fever of unknown origin, dermatitis, fatigue, hypertension, hypotension, polyneuropathy, pulmonary symptoms, *cardiotoxicity,* interference with normal wound healing.

**OD    Overdose Management:** *Symptoms:* See *Additional Side Effects. Treatment:* General supportive measures.

**Laboratory Test Interferences:** ↑ Liver enzymes, bilirubin.

**Dosage** ───────────────
• **IV**
*Testicular cancer.*
1.2 g/m²/day for 5 consecutive days. Treatment may be repeated q 3 weeks or if platelet counts are at least 100,000/mm³ and WBCs are at least 4,000/mm³.

## NURSING CONSIDERATIONS

See also *Nursing Considerations* for *Antineoplastic Agents*.
**Administration/Storage**
**IV** 1. To prevent bladder toxicity, give with at least 2 L/day of PO or IV fluid as well as with mesna.
2. Administer dosage slowly over 30 min.
3. Reconstitute by adding either sterile water for injection or bacterios-

tatic water for injection for a final concentration of 50 mg/mL. Solutions may be further diluted to achieve concentrations from 0.6 to 20 mg/mL by adding 5% dextrose injection, 0.9% NaCl injection, sterile water for injection, or RL injection. Infuse over 30 min.

4. Reconstituted solutions (50 mg/mL) are stable for 1 week at 30°C (86°F) or 3 weeks at 5°C (41°F).

5. Refrigerate dilutions of ifosfamide not prepared with bacteriostatic water for injection; use within 6 hr.

**Assessment**

1. Anticipate concomitant admisistration with mesna to minimize hemorrhagic cystitis.

2. Send urine for analysis prior to each dose of ifosfamide.

3. Monitor CBC; immunosuppression may activate latent infections such as herpes.

**Client/Family Teaching**

1. Hair loss and N&V are frequent side effects of drug therapy.

2. Hyperpigmentation of skin and mucous membranes may occur; report any injury or interference with normal wound healing.

3. Report confusion, hallucinations, or marked drowsiness.

4. Females should practice contraceptive measures during and for at least 4 months following treatments. Infertility may result if treatment lasts 6 months.

5. Consume 2 L/day of fluids. Report presence of frothy dark urine, jaundice, or light-colored stools; signs of hepatotoxicity requiring dosage adjustments.

6. Joint or flank pain may be caused by the increase in uric acid that results from the rapid cytolysis of tumor and RBCs.

7. Report symptoms of neurotoxicity (numbness, tingling). Elicit family support in making observations and evaluations and recording.

8. Do not take salicylates or alcohol.

9. Avoid crowds, vaccinations, and persons with known infections.

**Outcomes/Evaluate**

• ↓ Tumor size and spread

• Desired hematologic parameters

# Imiglucerase
(ihm-eh-**GLEW**-sir-ace)
**Pregnancy Category:** C
Cerezyme **(Rx)**
**Classification:** Drug for Gaucher's disease

**Action/Kinetics:** Produced by recombinant DNA technology. Is an analogue of the human enzyme β-glucocerebrosidase which is a lysosomal glycoprotein enzyme that catalyzes the hydrolysis of glucocerebroside to glucose and ceramide. Clients with Gaucher's disease have a deficiency of β-glucocerebrosidase resulting in an accumulation of glucocerebrosidase in tissue macrophages; leads to severe anemia, thrombocytopenia, hepatosplenomegaly, and skeletal complications. Imiglucerase replaces the enzyme normally found in the body. **t½:** 3.6–10.4 min following infusion.

**Uses:** Long-term replacement therapy for clients with confirmed Type 1 Gaucher's disease.

**Contraindications:** Hypersensitivity to the product.

**Special Concerns:** Be alert to the possible development of IgG antibodies reactive with imiglucerase. Use with caution during lactation.

**Side Effects:** *CNS:* Headache, dizziness. *GI:* Nausea, abdominal discomfort. *Hypersensitivity:* Pruritus, rash, allergic hypersensitivity reactions. *Miscellaneous:* Mild decrease in BP, decreased urinary frequency.

**Dosage** ————————
• **IV**
  *Gaucher's disease.*
**Initial:** Dose ranges from 2.5 U/kg 3 times/week to 60 U/kg once a week or q 4 weeks. The usual initial dose is 60 U/kg q 2 weeks. **Maintenance:** After client response has been established, a decrease in dosage may be attempted. Progressive decreases in dose can be made at intervals of 3–6 months with appropriate monitoring.

## NURSING CONSIDERATIONS

See also *Nursing Considerations* for *Alglucerase*.

**Administration/Storage**

**IV** 1. On the day of drug use and depending on the dose to be given, reconstitute the appropriate number of vials with 5.1 mL of sterile water for injection (final volume of 5.3 mL containing 40 U/mL). Withdraw 5 mL from each vial and pool volume to a final volume of 100–200 mL.

2. Give by IV infusion over 1–2 hr. Alternatively, may be given at a rate no greater than 1 U/kg/min, thus allowing for small dosage adjustments.

3. Store vials at 2°C–8°C (36°F–46°F).

4. Do not use vials with particulate matter or discoloration. Do not use after the expiration date on the vial.

5. Because the product contains no preservative, do not store the reconstituted drug for subsequent use.

**Assessment:** Imiglucerase is produced from recombinant DNA whereas alglucerase is derived from pooled human placenta tissue (which is in very short supply). The DNA technology reduces the risks of viral contamination and infection and may replace drugs of human origin.

**Client/Family Teaching:** May experience transient headache, nausea, abdominal discomfort, itching, rash, dizziness, decreased BP, and decreased urinary frequency with drug therapy.

**Outcomes/Evaluate:** Improved hematologic parameters (e.g., ↑ H&H, ↑ erythrocyte and platelet counts;)

———COMBINATION DRUG———

# Imipenem-Cilastatin sodium

(em-ee-**PEN**-em, sigh-lah-**STAT**-in)
**Pregnancy Category:** C
Primaxin I.M., Primaxin I.V. **(Rx)**
**Classification:** Antibiotic combined with inhibitor of dehydropeptidase I

See also *Anti-Infectives*.

**Content:** The Powder for IV injection and the Powder for IM injection contain: imipenem, 500 mg, and cilastatin sodium, 500 mg, or imipenem, 750 mg, and cilastatin sodium, 750 mg.

**Action/Kinetics:** Inhibits cell wall synthesis. Is bactericidal against a wide range of gram-positive and gram-negative organisms. Stable in the presence of beta-lactamases. Addition of cilastatin prevents the metabolism of imipenem in the kidneys by dehydropeptidase I, thus ensuring high levels of the imipenem in the urinary tract. **t½, after IV:** 1 hr for each component. **Peak plasma levels of imipenem, after 20 min IV infusion:** 14–24 mcg/mL for the 250-mg dose, 21–58 mcg/mL for the 500-mg dose, and 41–83 mcg/mL for the 1-g dose. **Peak plasma levels, after IM:** 10–12 mcg/mL within 2 hr. Compared with IV administration, imipenem is approximately 75% bioavailable after IM use with cilastatin being 95% bioavailable. **t½, imipenem:** 2–3 hr. About 70% of imipenem and cilastin is recovered in the urine within 10 hr of administration.

**Uses: IV:** To treat the following serious infections: lower respiratory tract, urinary tract, gynecologic, skin and skin structures, bone and joint, endocarditis, intra-abdominal, bacterial septicemia, and infections caused by more than one agent. Infections resistant to aminoglycosides, cephalosporins, or penicillins have responded to imipenem. Bacterial eradication may not be achieved in clients with cystic fibrosis, chronic pulmonary disease, and lower respiratory tract infections caused by *Pseudomonas aeruginosa*.

**IM:** This route of administration is not intended for severe or life-threatening infections (including endocarditis, or bacterial sepsis). Used for lower respiratory tract infections, intra-abdominal infections, skin and skin structure infections, gynecologic infections.

**Contraindications:** IM use in clients allergic to local anesthetics of the amide type and use in clients with heart block (due to the use of lidocaine HCl diluent) or severe shock. Use in clients with a $C_{CR}$ of less than or equal to 5 mL/min/1.73 m², unless hemodialysis is begun within 48 hr.

**Special Concerns:** Use with caution in pregnancy and lactation. Due to cross sensitivity, use with caution in clients with penicillin allergy. Safety and effectiveness have not been determined in children less than 12 years of age.

**Side Effects:** *GI: **Pseudomembranous colitis,*** nausea, diarrhea, vomiting, abdominal pain, heartburn, increased salivation, ***hemorrhagic colitis,*** gastroenteritis, glossitis, pharyngeal pain, tongue papillar hypertrophy, hepatitis, jaundice, staining of the teeth. *CNS:* Fever, confusion, ***seizures,*** dizziness, sleepiness, myoclonus, headache, vertigo, paresthesia, encephalopathy, tremor, psychic disturbances (including hallucinations). *CV:* Hypotension, tachycardia, palpitations. *Dermatologic:* Rash, urticaria, pruritus, flushing, cyanosis, facial edema, erythema multiforme, skin texture changes, hyperhidrosis, ***toxic epidermal necrolysis, Stevens-Johnson syndrome.*** *CV:* Hypotension, palpitations, tachycardia. *Respiratory:* Chest discomport, dyspnea, hyperventilation. *GU:* Pruritus vulvae, anuria/oliguria, acute renal failure, polyuria, urine discoloration. *Hematologic:* Pancytopenia, bone marrow depression, thrombocytopenia, neutropenia, leukopenia, hemolytic anemia. *Miscellaneous:* Candidiasis, superinfection, tinnitus, polyarthralgia, asthenia, muscle weakness, transient hearing loss in clients with existing hearing impairment, taste perversion, thoracic spine pain.

The following side effects may occur at the injection site: Thrombophlebitis, phlebitis, pain, erythema, vein induration, infused vein infection.

**Drug Interactions:** Use of ganciclovir with imipenem-cilastatin may result in generalized seizures.

**Laboratory Test Interferences:** ↑ AST, ALT, alkaline phosphatase, LDH, bilirubin, potassium, chloride, BUN, creatinine. Also, ↑ eosinophils, monocytes, lymphocytes, basophils. ↓ Serum sodium, neutrophils, hemoglobin, hematocrit. ↑ or ↓ WBCs, platelets. Positive Coombs' test and abnormal PT. Presence of protein, RBCs, WBCs, casts, bilirubin, or urobilinogen in the urine.

**Dosage** ─────────────

- **IV**

    *Fully susceptible gram-positive organisms, gram-negative organisms, anaerobes.*
    *Mild:* 250 mg q 6 hr; *moderate:* 500 mg q 6 hr or q 8 hr; *severe/life-threatening:* 500 mg q 6 hr.
    *Urinary tract infections due to fully susceptible organisms.*
    *Uncomplicated:* 250 mg q 6 hr; *complicated:* 500 mg q 6 hr.
    *Moderately susceptible organisms (especially some strains of* P. aeruginosa).
    *Mild:* 500 mg q 6 hr; *moderate,* 500 mg q 6 hr to 1 g q 6 hr; *severe/life-threatening,* 1 g q 6 or 8 hr.
    *Urinary tract infections due to moderately susceptible organisms.*
    *Uncomplicated:* 250 mg q 6 hr; *complicated:* 500 mg q 6 hr.
    The total daily dose should not exceed 50 mg/kg or 4 g, whichever is lower.

- **IM**

    *Lower respiratory tract, skin and skin structure, or gynecologic infections: mild to moderate.*
    500 or 750 mg q 12 hr depending on severity.
    *Intra-abdominal infections: mild to moderate.*
    750 mg q 12 hr. The total daily dose should not exceed 1.5 g.

**Pediatric, 3 months to 3 years, all uses:** 25 mg/kg q 6 hr, to a maximum of 2 g/day. **Pediatric, over 3 years, all uses:** 15 mg/kg q 6 hr.

## NURSING CONSIDERATIONS

See also *General Nursing Considerations for All Anti-Infectives.*

**Administration/Storage**

1. When used IM, give in a large muscle mass with a 21-gauge 2-in. needle.

2. For IM use, prepare with 1% lidocaine HCl solution without epinephrine. The 500-mg vial is prepared with 2 mL while the 750-mg vial is prepared with 3 mL of lidocaine HCl.

3. Continue IM use for at least 2 days after S&S of infection are absent. Safety and effectiveness have not been established for use for more than 14 days.

4. Reduce dosage with a $C_{CR}$ of 70 mL/min/1.73 m² or less. Check package insert for specific dosage information.

**IV** 5. Reconstitute for IV use by mixing with 100 mL of diluent.

6. Base initial dose on the type and severity of infection. Give doses between 250 and 500 mg by IV infusion over 20–30 min. Give doses of 1 g by IV infusion over 40–60 min. If nausea develops, decrease infusion rate.

7. The following solutions can be used as diluents: 0.9% NaCl, 5% or 10% dextrose injection, 5% dextrose and 0.9% NaCl, 5% dextrose injection with either 0.225% or 0.45% saline solution, 5% dextrose with 0.15% potassium chloride solution, mannitol (2.5%, 5%, or 10%).

8. Reconstituted IV solutions vary from colorless to yellow while reconstituted IM solutions vary from white to light tan in color. Variations in color do not affect the potency.

9. Do not mix with other antibiotics; however, the drug may be administered with other antibiotics, if necessary.

10. Most reconstituted IV solutions can be stored at room temperature for 4 hr and, if refrigerated, for 24 hr. The exception is imipenem-cilastatin reconstituted with 0.9% NaCl solution, which is stable at room temperature for 10 hr and, if refrigerated, for 48 hr. Use reconstituted IM solutions within 1 hr of preparation.

**Outcomes/Evaluate**

• Resolution of infection
• Symptomatic improvement

# Imipramine hydrochloride
(im-**IHP**-rah-meen)
**Pregnancy Category:** B
Apo-Imipramine ✦, Impril ✦, Janimine, Novo-Pramine ✦, PMS-Imipramine ✦, Tofranil **(Rx)**

# Imipramine pamoate
(im-**IHP**-rah-meen)
**Pregnancy Category:** B
Tofranil-PM **(Rx)**
**Classification:** Antidepressant, tricyclic

See also *Antidepressants, Tricyclic.*

**Action/Kinetics:** Moderate anticholinergic and sedative effects; high orthostatic hypotensive effects. Biotransformed into its active metabolite, desmethylimipramine (desipramine). **Effective plasma level of imipramine and desmethylimipramine:** 200–350 ng/mL. **t½:** 11–25 hr. **Time to reach steady state:** 2–5 days.

**Uses:** Symptoms of depression. Enuresis in children. Chronic, severe neurogenic pain. Bulimia nervosa.

**Additional Side Effects:** *High therapeutic dosage may increase frequency of seizures in epileptic clients and cause seizures in nonepileptic clients.* Elderly and adolescent clients may have low tolerance to the drug.

**Laboratory Test Interferences:** ↑ Metanephrine (Pisano test); ↓ Urinary 5-HIAA.

**Dosage** —————————

• **Tablets, Capsules**
  *Depression.*

**Hospitalized clients:** 50 mg b.i.d.–t.i.d. Can be increased by 25 mg every few days up to 200 mg/day. After 2 weeks, dosage may be increased gradually to maximum of 250–300 mg/day at bedtime. **Outpa-**

---

✦ = Available in Canada                    **bold italic** = life threatening side effect

**tients:** 75–150 mg/day. Maximum dose for outpatients is 200 mg. Decrease when feasible to maintenance dosage: 50–150 mg/day at bedtime.
**Adolescent and geriatric clients:** 30–40 mg/day up to maximum of 100 mg/day. **Pediatric:** 1.5 mg/kg/day in three divided doses; can be increased 1–1.5 mg/kg/day q 3–5 days to a maximum of 5 mg/kg/day.

*Childhood enuresis.*

**Age 5 years and over:** 25 mg/day 1 hr before bedtime. Dose can be increased to 50 mg/day up to 12 years of age and to 75 mg/day in children over 12 years of age. Dose should not exceed 2.5 mg/kg/day.

* **IM**
  *Antidepressant.*

**Adults:** Up to 100 mg/day in divided doses. IM route not recommended for use in children less than 12 years of age.

## NURSING CONSIDERATIONS

See also *Nursing Considerations* for *Antidepressants, Tricyclic.*
**Administration/Storage**
1. Dissolve crystals in the injectable form by immersing closed ampules into hot water for 1 min.
2. Total daily dose can be given once daily at bedtime.
3. Protect from direct sunlight and strong artificial light.
4. Use parenteral therapy only in clients unwilling or unable to take PO medication. Switch to PO medication as soon as possible.
5. Do not give IV.
6. When used for the treatment of enuresis, the drug can be given in doses of 25 mg in midafternoon and 25 mg at bedtime (this regimen may increase effectiveness).
7. When used as an enuretic in children, do not exceed 2.5 mg/kg/day.
**Client/Family Teaching**
1. Review appropriate times and methods for administration.
2. Report any increase in frequency of seizures in epileptics and any occurrence of seizures in nonepileptics.
3. Children may experience mild N&V, unusual tiredness, nervous-

ness, or insomnia; report if pronounced.
4. Do not perform activities that require mental alertness until drug effects realized; may cause sedation.
5. With enuresis, refer parents to regional centers with incontinence programs if bed-wetting persists.
**Outcomes/Evaluate**
* Improvement in S&S of depression
* Prevention of bed-wetting
* Control of severe neurogenic pain
* Therapeutic serum drug levels (200–350 ng/mL)

# Imiquimod
(ih-**MIH**-kwih-mod)
**Pregnancy Category:** B
Aldara **(Rx)**
**Classification:** Drug for genital and perianal warts

**Action/Kinetics:** May induce cytokines, including interferon-alpha and others, to modify immune response. Minimal percutaneous absorption.
**Uses:** External genital and perianal warts/condyloma acuminata in adults.
**Contraindications:** Due to lack of studies, not recommended for use in urethral, intravaginal, cervical, rectal, or intra-anal human papilloma viral disease.
**Special Concerns:** Safety and efficacy have not been determined in clients less than 18 years of age. Use with caution during lactation.
**Side Effects:** *Dermatologic:* Erythema, itching, erosion, burning, excoriation/flaking, edema, pain, induration, ulceration, scabbing, vesicles, soreness. *Systemic:* Fungal infection, fatigue, fever, flu-like symptoms, headache, diarrhea, myalgia.

**Dosage**
* **Cream**
  *Genital/perianal warts.*

**Adults:** Apply 3 times/week prior to normal sleeping hours; leave on skin for 6–10 hr. Following treatment, remove by washing the area with mild soap and water. Continue treatment until there is total clearance of warts (16 weeks or less).

## NURSING CONSIDERATIONS
### Administration/Storage
1. Wash hands before and after application.
2. Apply a thin layer to the wart area and rub in until cream is not visible.
3. Avoid using excessive amounts of cream; single-use packets contain sufficient cream to cover up to 20 cm².
4. Due to skin reactions, rest period of several days may be necessary. Treatment may resume once reactions subside.
5. May weaken condoms or vaginal diaphragms; do not use together.
6. For external use only. Avoid contact with eyes.
7. Do not occlude treatment area with bandages or other covers/wraps. However, non-occlusive dressings (e.g., cotton gauze or underwear) can be used to manage skin reactions.
8. Do not store at temperatures greater than 30°C (86°F). Avoid freezing.
**Assessment:** Describe clinical presentation noting number and size of warts/condyloma, location, and condition of pretreatment area; photographs may be useful in assessing response to therapy.
### Client/Family Teaching
1. Apply a thin layer of cream to completely cover each wart at bedtime, after bathing. Usually prescribed three times per week, once daily. Do not cover area with occlusive bandages or wraps.
2. Wash hands before and after treatment, avoid eye contact.
3. Drug is not cure for genital warts caused by HPV but helps clear and diminish wart area. New warts may occur during therapy.
4. Avoid sexual contact (genital, rectal, oral) while cream is on skin. Wash off before sexual activity; may also weaken condoms and dia-

phragms. Use extra protection and practice safe sex to avoid infecting and/or acquiring from partners.
5. May experience redness, peeling, burning, itching, and swelling in treatment area; report if severe skin reaction occurs as rest period may be needed before continuing therapy once subsided.
6. Wash application area with mild soap and water 6 to 10 hr after application.
7. Uncircumcised males treating warts under foreskin should retract foreskin and clean area daily.
**Outcomes/Evaluate:** Clearing of genital and perianal warts/condyloma

# Immune globulin IV (Human)
(im-MYOUN GLOH-byou-lin)
**Pregnancy Category:** C
Gamimune N 5% and 10%, Gammabulin Immuno ✚, Gammagard S/D, Gammar-P I.V., Iveegam, Polygam, Polygam S/D, Sandoglobulin, Venoglobulin-I, Venoglobulin-S Solvent Detergent Treated **(Rx)**
**Classification:** Immunoglobulin G antibody product. *NOTE:* The available products differ significantly with respect to the process by which they are made (e.g., donor pool and fractionation/purification) as well as isotonicity. Thus, information on each product should be carefully read before use. *NOTE:* Gammagard has been replaced by Gammagard S/D. Also, Gammagard S/D is a higher concentration than Gammagard; thus, the drug can be infused more quickly. Certain products have been treated by compounds that are capable of inactivating several blood-borne viruses.

**Action/Kinetics:** Derived from a human volunteer pool. Contains the various IgG antibodies normally occurring in humans. The products may also contain traces of IgA and IgM. Plasma in the manufacturing pool has been found nonreactive for hepatitis B antigen. Have been no documented cases of viral transmission. Antibodies present in the products will cause both opsonization and neutralization of microbes and toxins. Reconstituted products may contain sucrose, maltose, protein, and/or small amounts of sodium chloride. Immune globulin IV provides immediate antibody levels. The percentage of IgG in the products is over 90%. **t½:** Gamimune N and Sandoglobulin, 3 weeks; Venoglobulin-I, 29 days.

**Uses:** *All products:* Severe combined immunodeficiency and primary immunoglobulin deficiency syndromes, including congenital agammaglobulinemia, X-linked agammaglobulinemia with or without hyper IgM, combined immunodeficiency, and Wiskott-Aldrich syndrome. *Investigational:* Chronic fatigue syndrome, quinidine-induced thrombocytopenia.

*Gamimune N, Gammagard S/D, Polygam S/D, Sandoglobulin, Venoglobulin-I and Venoglobulin-S:* Acute and chronic idiopathic thrombocytopenic purpura in both children and adults.

*Gammagard S/D, Polygam S/D:* B-cell chronic lymphocytic leukemia in those with hypogammaglobulinemia or recurrent associated bacterial infections .

*Iveegam:* Kawasaki syndrome (given with aspirin within 10 days of onset of the disease).

*Gamimune N:* Prophylactic use to decrease infections and the incidence of graft-versus-host-disease in bone marrow clients and in HIV-infected children to prevent bacterial infections.

**Contraindications:** Clients with selective IgA deficiency who have antibodies to IgA (the products contain IgA). Sensitivity to human immune globulin.

**Special Concerns:** The various products are used for different conditions and at different doses; thus, check information carefully.

**Side Effects:** *CNS:* Headache, malaise, feeling of faintness. Aseptic meningitis syndrome, including symptoms of severe headache, nuchal rigidity, drowsiness, fever, photophobia, painful eye movements, N&V. *Allergic:* Hypersensitivity or **anaphylactic reactions.** *Body as a whole:* Fever, chills. *GI:* Headache, nausea, vomiting. *Miscellaneous:* Chest tightness, dyspnea; chest, back, or hip pain; mild erythema following infiltration; burning sensation in the head; tachycardia.

Agammaglobulinemic and hypogammaglobulinemic clients never having received immunoglobulin therapy or where the time from the last treatment is more than 8 weeks may manifest side effects if the infusion rate exceeds 1 mL/min. Symptoms include flushing of the face, hypotension, tightness in chest, chills, fever, dizziness, diaphoresis, and nausea.

**Dosage**

*NOTE:* Due to differences in products, dosage must be listed separately for each product.

**• IV Only for All Products**

GAMIMUNE N

*Immunodeficiency syndrome.*

100–200 mg/kg given once a month; if response is satisfactory, dose can be increased to 400 mg/kg or infusion may be repeated more frequently than once a month. Rate of infusion for all uses: 0.01–0.02 mL/kg/min for 30 min; if no discomfort is experienced, the rate can be increased up to 0.08 mL/kg/min.

*Idiopathic thrombocytopenic purpura.*

400 mg/kg for 5 consecutive days or 1,000 mg/kg/day for 1 day or 2 consecutive days. **Maintenance:** If platelet count falls to less than 30,000/mm³ or if bleeding occurs, 400 mg/kg may be given as a single infusion. If an adequate response is not seen, the dose can be increased to 800–1,000 mg/kg given as a single infusion. Maintenance infusions are given, as needed, to maintain platelet counts greater than 30,000/mm³.

*Bone marrow transplantation.*

500 mg/kg beginning on days 7 and 2 pretransplant or at the time conditioning therapy for transplantation is

initiated; then, give weekly throughout the 90-day post-transplant period.

*Pediatric HIV infection.*
400 mg/kg q 28 days.

GAMMAGARD S/D

*Immunodeficiency syndrome.*
200–400 mg/kg (minimum of 100 mg/kg/month).

*B-cell chronic lymphocytic leukemia.*
400 mg/kg q 3–4 weeks.

*Idiopathic thrombocytopenic purpura.*
1,000 mg/kg; additional doses depend on platelet count (up to three doses can be given on alternate days). Rate of infusion: 0.5 mL/kg/min initially; may be increased gradually, not to exceed 4 mL/kg/hr if there is no client distress.

GAMMAR-P I.V.

*Immunodeficiency syndrome.*
200–400 mg/kg q 3–4 weeks. An alternative is a loading dose of at least 200 mg/kg at more frequent intervals and then 200–600 mg/kg at 3-week intervals once a therapeutic plasma level has been reached. Rate of infusion: 0.01 mL/kg/min, increasing to 0.02 mL/kg/min after 15 to 30 min. Most clients will tolerate a gradual increase to 0.03–0.06 mL/kg/min.

IVEEGAM

*Immunodeficiency syndrome.*
200 mg/kg/month. If desired effect not achieved, the dose may be increased up to fourfold (i.e., up to 800 mg/kg/month) or the intervals between doses shortened. Rate of infusion for all uses: 1 mL/min to a maximum of 2 mL/min of the 5% solution. The product may be further diluted with saline or 5% dextrose.

*Kawasaki syndrome.*
400 mg/kg/day for 4 consecutive days or a single dose of 2,000 mg/kg given over a 10-hr period. Treatment should be initiated within 10 days of onset and should include aspirin, 100 mg/kg each day through the 14th day of illness; then, aspirin is given at a dose of 3–5 mg/kg/day for 5 weeks.

POLYGAM S/D

*Immunodeficiency syndrome.*
**Initial:** 200–400 mg/kg may be given; **then,** 100 mg/kg/month. Rate of administration for all uses: Initially, 0.5 mL/kg/hr. If there is no distress, the rate can be gradually increased, not to exceed 4 mL/kg/hr. Those who tolerate the 5% solution at a rate of 4 mL/kg/hr can receive the 10% solution starting at 0.5 mL/kg/hr.

*B-cell chronic lymphocytic leukemia.*
400 mg/kg q 3 to 4 weeks.

*Idiopathic thrombocytopenic purpura.*
1 g/kg. Depending on response, additional doses can be given—three separate doses on alternate days can be given, if needed.

SANDOGLOBULIN-I

*Immunodeficiency syndrome.*
200 mg/kg/month; increase to 300 mg/kg if client response satisfactory (i.e., IgG serum level of 300 mg/dL). Rate of administration for all uses: 3% solution at an initial rate of 0.5–1 mL/min; after 15–30 min can increase to 1.5–2.5 mL/min (subsequent infusions at a rate of 2–2.5 mL/min). If the 6% solution is used, the initial infusion rate should be 1–1.5 mL/min and increased after 15–30 min to a maximum of 2.5 mL/min.

*Idiopathic thrombocytopenic purpura.*
400 mg/kg for 2–5 consecutive days.

VENOGLOBULIN-I

*Immunodeficiency disease.*
200 mg/kg/month by IV infusion; can increase to 300–400 mg/kg if response is insufficient or can repeat infusion more frequently than once monthly. Rate of infusion for all uses: 0.01 to 0.02 mL/kg/min for the first 30 min; if no distress is noted, the rate may be increased to 0.04 mL/kg/min. Higher rates may be used if tolerated. The drug can be given sequentially into a primary IV line containing normal saline; it is not

compatible with 5% dextrose solution.

*Idiopathic thrombocytopenic purpura.*

**Induction:** Up to 2,000 mg/kg for 2 to 7 consecutive days; those who respond to induction therapy (platelet count of 30,000/mm³–50,000/mm³) may be discontinued after two to seven daily doses. **Maintenance:** Single infusion of 2,000 mg/kg q 2 weeks, as needed to maintain a platelet count of 30,000/mm³ in children and 20,000/mm³ in adults or to prevent bleeding episodes between infusions.

Venoglobulin-s

*Immunodeficiency disease.*

200 mg/kg/month; can increase to 300–400 mg/kg if response is insufficient or can repeat infusion more frequently than once monthly. Rate of infusion for all uses: Initially, 0.01–0.02 mL/kg/min or 1.2 mL/kg/hr for the first 30 min. If no discomfort is noted, the rate for the 5% solution may be increased to 0.04 mL/kg/min or 2.4 mL/kg/hr and the rate for the 10% solution may be increased to 0.05 mL/kg/min or 3 mL/kg/hr.

*Idiopathic thrombocytopenic purpura.*

**Induction:** 2,000 mg/kg over a maximum of 5 days. **Maintenance:** 1,000 mg/kg as needed to maintain platelet counts of 30,000/mm³ for children and 20,000/mm³ for adults or to prevent bleeding episodes between infusions.

# NURSING CONSIDERATIONS
## Administration/Storage
**IV** 1. Follow the administration guidelines explicitly and follow the manufacturer's directions carefully for reconstitution of either the 3% or 6% solution.

2. In agamma- or hypogammaglobulinemic clients, use the 3% solution. Initially, administer at a rate of 10–20 gtt/min (0.5–1 mL/min). After 15–30 min the rate may be increased to 30–50 gtt/min (1.5–2.5 mL/min). Subsequent infusions may be given at a rate of 40–50 gtt/min (2–2.5

mL/min). If the first bottle of the 3% solution is given in these clients with good tolerance, subsequent infusions may be given using the 6% solution.

3. Do not shake the solutions because excessive foaming will occur.

4. Infuse only if the solution is clear and at room temperature.

5. Give only IV ; the IM or SC routes have not been evaluated.

6. Give by a separate IV line without mixing with other IV fluids or medications.

7. A rapid decrease in serum IgG level in the first week postinfusion will be observed; this is expected and is due to the equilibration of IgG between the plasma and extravascular space.

8. Utilize an electronic infusion device for administration.

9. Have epinephrine readily available in the event of an acute anaphylactic reaction.

## Assessment
1. Document indications for therapy; for passive immunization note date and type of exposure; assess closely for anaphylaxis.

2. Administer within 2 weeks of exposure to hepatitis A, within 6 days after measles exposure, and within 7 days after hepatitis B exposure.

3. Any history of ITP warrants close hematologic monitoring. With ITP, monitor CBC closely and determine if pregnant; this warrants close observation and management.

4. Monitor VS; if hypotension occurs, decrease or interrupt infusion rate until hypotension subsides.

5. Administer in a closely monitored environment and away from persons with active infections if immunocompromised.

6. Monitor LFTs, hematologic parameters, IgG levels, and appropriate blood and urine chemistries.

## Client/Family Teaching
1. Immunoglobulin helps to prevent and/or reduce intensity of various infectious diseases. With thrombocytopenia, expect increased platelets and enhanced clotting.

2. Once-monthly therapy is needed to maintain appropriate IgG serum levels.

3. Drug may cause N&V, fever, chills, flushing, lightheadedness, and tightness in the chest; report immediately, may be dosage and rate related.

4. Close observation and frequent lab studies are essential with pregnant individuals to improve chances of a healthy baby and to ensure maternal safety.

5. Warm soaks to injection site and PO Tylenol may assist to relieve discomfort.

6. Drug is derived from human plasma (except for those engineered genetically); be aware of potential risks.

**Outcomes/Evaluate**
• IgG levels within normal range
• ↑ Antibody titer; passive immunity
• ↑ Platelets; ↓ hemorrhaging with ITP

# Indapamide
(in-**DAP**-ah-myd)
**Pregnancy Category:** B
Lozol **(Rx)**

# Indapamide Hemihydrate
(in-**DAP**-ah-myd)
**Pregnancy Category:** B
Gen-Indapamide ✿, Lozide ✿ **(Rx)**
**Classification:** Diuretic, thiazide type

See also *Diuretics, Thiazide*.
**Action/Kinetics: Onset:** 1–2 weeks after multiple doses. **Peak levels:** 2 hr. **Duration:** Up to 8 weeks with multiple doses. t½: 14 hr. Nearly 100% is absorbed from the GI tract. Excreted through the kidneys (70% with 7% unchanged) and the GI tract (23%).
**Uses:** Alone or in combination with other drugs for treatment of hypertension. Edema in CHF.
**Special Concerns:** Dosage has not been established in children. Geriatric clients may be more sensitive to the hypotensive and electrolyte effects.

**Dosage** ———
• **Tablets**
*Edema of CHF.*
**Adults:** 2.5 mg as a single dose in the morning. If necessary, may be increased to 5 mg/day after 1 week.
*Hypertension.*
**Adults:** 1.25 mg as a single dose in the morning. If the response is not satisfactory after 4 weeks, the dose may be increased to 2.5 mg taken once daily. If the response to 2.5 mg is not satisfactory after 4 weeks, the dose may be increased to 5 mg taken once daily (however, consideration should be given to adding another antihypertensive).

## NURSING CONSIDERATIONS

See also *Nursing Considerations* for *Diuretics, Thiazide* and *Antihypertensive Agents*.
**Administration/Storage**
1. May be combined with other antihypertensive agents if response inadequate. Initially, reduce the dose of other agents by 50%.
2. Doses greater than 5 mg/day do not increase effectiveness but may increase hypokalemia.
**Assessment:** Document indications for therapy, type, onset, and duration of symptoms. Note other agents trialed and the outcome.
**Outcomes/Evaluate**
• ↓ BP
• ↑ Urinary output with ↓ edema

# Indinavir sulfate
(in-**DIN**-ah-veer)
**Pregnancy Category:** C
Crixivan **(Rx)**
**Classification:** Antiviral drug, protease inhibitor

*See also* Anitiviral Drugs.
**Action/Kinetics:** Binds to active sites on the HIV protease enzyme resulting in inhibition of enzyme activity. Inhibition prevents cleavage of the viral polyproteins resulting in the formation of immature noninfectious viral particles. Varying degrees

of cross resistance have been noted between indinavir and other HIV-protease inhibitors. Rapidly absorbed in fasting clients; **time to peak plasma levels:** Approximately 0.8 hr. Administration with a meal high in calories, fat, and protein results in a significant decrease in the amount absorbed and in the peak plasma concentration. Approximately 60% bound to plasma proteins. **t½:** 1.8 hr. Metabolized in the liver with both parent drug and metabolites excreted through the feces (over 80%) and the urine.

**Uses:** Treatment of HIV infection in adults when antiretroviral therapy is indicated. May be used with other anti-HIV drugs.

**Contraindications:** Lactation. Do not take with astemizole, cisapride, midazolam, rifampin, terfenadine, and triazolam. Mild to moderate liver or kidney disease.

**Special Concerns:** Not a cure for HIV infections; clients may continue to develop opportunistic infections and other complications of HIV disease. Not been shown to reduce the risk of transmission of HIV through sexual contact or blood contamination. No data on the effect of indinavir therapy on clinical progression of HIV infection, including survival or the incidence of opportunistic infections. Hemophiliacs treated for HIV infections with protease inhibitors may manifest spontaneous bleeding episodes. Safety and efficacy have not been determined in children.

**Side Effects:** *GI:* N&V, diarrhea, abdominal pain, abdominal distention, acid regurgitation, anorexia, dry mouth, aphthous stomatitis, cheilitis, cholecystitis, cholestasis, constipation, dyspepsia, eructation, flatulence, gastritis, gingivitis, glossodynia, gingival hemorrhage, increased appetite, infectious gastroenteritis, jaundice, liver cirrhosis. *CNS:* Headache, insomnia, dizziness, somnolence, agitation, anxiety, bruxism, decreased mental acuity, depression, dream abnormality, dysesthesia, excitement, fasciculation, hypesthesia, nervousness, neuralgia, neurotic disorder, paresthesia, peripheral neuropathy, sleep disorder, tremor, vertigo. *CV:* CV disorder, palpitation. *Musculoskeletal:* Back pain, arthralgia, leg pain, myalgia, muscle cramps, muscle weakness, musculoskeletal pain, shoulder pain, stiffness. *Body as a whole:* Asthenia, fatigue, flank pain, malaise, chest pain, chills, fever, flu-like illness, fungal infection, malaise, pain, syncope. *Hematologic:* Anemia, lymphadenopathy, spleen disorder. *Respiratory:* Cough, dyspnea, halitosis, pharyngeal hyperemia, pharyngitis, pneumonia, rales, rhonchi, ***respiratory failure,*** sinus disorder, sinusitis, URI. *Dermatologic:* Body odor, contact dermatitis, dermatitis, dry skin, flushing, folliculitis, herpes simplex, herpes zoster, night sweats, pruritus, seborrhea, skin disorder, skin infection, sweating, urticaria. *GU:* Nephrolithiasis, dysuria, hematuria, hydronephrosis, nocturia, PMS, proteinuria, renal colic, urinary frequency, UTI, uterine abnormality, urine sediment abnormality, urolithiasis. *Ophthalmic:* Accommodation disorder, blurred vision, eye pain, eye swelling, orbital edema. *Miscellaneous:* Asymptomatic hyperbilirubinemia, food allergy, taste disorder.

**Drug Interactions**

*Astemizole* / ↓ Metabolism of astemizole → possibility of cardiac arrhythmias and prolonged sedation

*Cisapride* / ↓ Metabolism of cisapride → possibility of cardiac arrhythmias and prolonged sedation

*Clarithromycin* / ↑ Plasma levels of both indinavir and clarithromycin

*Fluconazole* / ↓ Plasma levels of indinavir

*Isoniazid* / ↑ Plasma levels of isoniazid

*Ketoconazole* / ↑ Plasma levels of indinavir

*Midazolam* / ↓ Metabolism of midazolam → possibility of cardiac arrhythmias and prolonged sedation

*Oral contraceptives* / ↑ Plasma levels of both estrogen and progestin components of the oral contraceptive product

*Quinidine* / ↑ Plasma levels of indinavir

*Rifabutin* / ↑ Plasma levels of rifabutin

*Rifampin* / ↓ Plasma levels of indinavir

*Stavudine* / ↑ Plasma levels of stavudine

*Terfenadine* / ↓ Metabolism of terfenadine → possibility of cardiac arrhythmias and prolonged sedation

*Triazolam* / ↓ Metabolism of triazolam → possibility of cardiac arrhythmias and prolonged sedation

*Trimethoprim/Sulfamethoxazole* / ↑ Plasma levels of trimethoprim (no change in levels of sulfamethoxazole

*AZT* / ↑ Plasma levels of both indinavir and AZT

**Laboratory Test Interferences:** ↑ Serum transaminases (ALT, AST), total serum bilirubin, serum amylase. ↓ Hemoglobin, platelet count, neutrophils. Hyperbilirubinemia.

**Dosage** ————————
• **Capsules**
*HIV infections.*
**Adults:** 800 mg (two 400-mg capsules) q 8 hr ATC. The dosage is the same whether the drug is used alone or in combination with other retroviral agents. Reduce the dose to 600 mg q 8 hr with mild to moderate hepatic insufficiency due to cirrhosis.

## NURSING CONSIDERATIONS

See also *Nursing Considerations* for *Antiviral Drugs*.
**Administration/Storage**
1. Capsules are sensitive to moisture. Store in the original container; the desiccant should remain in the bottle. Keep in a tightly closed container protected from moisture and at a room temperature of 15°C–30°C (59°F–86°F).
2. If indinavir and didanosine are given together, give at least 1 hr apart on an empty stomach.
3. If indinavir is taken with rifabutin, reduce the dose of rifabutin to one-half the standard dose.

4. When indinavir is taken with ketoconazole, reduce the dose of indinavir to 600 mg q 8 hr.
**Assessment**
1. Document symptom onset, confirmation of HIV, other agents trialed with the outcome.
2. Monitor CD4 cell count, viral load, and LFTs. Anticipate reduced dosage with impaired liver function; drug is hepatically metabolized.
3. Review list of drugs currently prescribed to ensure that none interact.
**Client/Family Teaching**
1. Take as prescribed at 8-hr intervals ATC with water 1 hr before or 2 hr after meals for optimal absorption. Alternatively, the drug may be taken with other liquids, such as skim milk, juice, coffee, or tea, or with a light meal (e.g., dry toast with jelly, juice, and coffee with skim milk and sugar; or corn flakes, skim milk, and sugar).
2. If a dose is missed by more than 2 hr, wait and take the next dose at the regularly scheduled time. If a dose is missed by less than 2 hr, take immediately.
3. Must adequately hydrate. To ensure adequate hydration, drink at least 1.5 L of liquids during a 24-hr period.
4. Report any symptoms of nephrolithiasis (e.g., flank pain with or without hematuria, including microscopic hematuria); therapy should be interrupted for 1–3 days.
5. Drug is not a cure for HIV; opportunistic infections may still occur.
6. Use reliable birth control and barrier protection; drug does not decrease the risk of transmitting disease through sexual contact or blood contamination.
**Outcomes/Evaluate:** Control of HIV infection progression

# Indomethacin
(in-doh-**METH**-ah-sin)
Apo-Indomethacin ✦, Indochron E-R, Indocid ✦, Indocid Ophthalmic Suspension ✦, Indocid SR ✦, Indocin, Indocin SR, Indocollyre ✦, Indotec ✦,

---

✦ = Available in Canada                    ***bold italic*** = life threatening side effect

Novo–Methacin ✿, Nu-Indo ✿, Pro-
Indo ✿, Rhodacine ✿ **(Rx)**

# Indomethacin sodium trihydrate

(in-doh-**METH**-ah-sin)
Indocin I.V. **(Rx)**
**Classification:** Nonsteroidal anti-
inflammatory drug, analgesic, antipyretic

See also *Nonsteroidal Anti-Inflammatory Drugs.*
**Action/Kinetics:** PO. **Onset:** 30
min for analgesia and up to 1 week
for anti-inflammatory effect. **Peak
plasma levels:** 1–2 hr (2–4 hr for
sustained-release). **Peak action for
gout:** 24–36 hr; swelling gradually
disappears in 3–5 days. **Peak activity
for antirheumatic effect:** About 4
weeks. **Duration:** 4–6 hr for analgesia and 1–2 weeks for anti-inflammatory effect. **Therapeutic plasma
levels:** 10–18 mcg/mL. **t½:** Approximately 5 hr (up to 6 hr for sustained-
release). **Plasma t½ following IV
in infants:** 12–20 hr, depending on
age and dose. Approximately 90%
plasma protein bound. Metabolized in
the liver and excreted in both the
urine and feces.
**Uses:** Not a simple analgesic; use
only for the conditions listed. Moderate to severe rheumatoid arthritis,
osteoarthritis, and ankylosing spondylitis (drug of choice). Acute gouty
arthritis and acute painful shoulder
(tendinitis, bursitis). *IV:* Pharmacologic closure of persistent patent ductus
arteriosus in premature infants. *Investigational:* Topically to treat cystoid
macular edema (0.5% and 1%
drops), sunburn, primary dysmenorrhea, prophylaxis of migraine, cluster
headache, polyhydramnios.
**Additional Contraindications:**
Pregnancy and lactation. PO indomethacin in children under 14 years
of age. GI lesions or history of recurrent GI lesions. *IV use:* GI or intracranial bleeding, thrombocytopenia, renal disease, defects of coagulation,
necrotizing enterocolitis. *Suppositories:* Recent rectal bleeding, history of
proctitis.

**Special Concerns:** Use in children
should be restricted to those unresponsive to or intolerant of other
anti-inflammatory agents; efficacy
has not been determined in children
less than 14 years of age. Geriatric clients are at greater risk of developing
CNS side effects, especially confusion. To be used with caution in clients with history of epilepsy, psychiatric illness, or parkinsonism and in
the elderly. Indomethacin should be
used with extreme caution in the
presence of existing, controlled
infections.
**Additional Side Effects:** Reactivation of latent infections may mask
signs of infection. More marked CNS
manifestations than for other drugs of
this group. Aggravation of depression or other psychiatric problems,
epilepsy, and parkinsonism.
**Additional Drug Interactions**
*Captopril* / Indomethacin ↓ effect of
captopril, probably due to inhibition of prostaglandin synthesis
*Diflunisal* / ↑ Plasma levels of indomethacin; also, possible fatal GI
hemorrhage
*Diuretics (loop, potassium-sparing,
thiazide)* / Indomethacin may
reduce the antihypertensive and
natriuretic action of diuretics
*Lisinopril* / Possible ↓ effect of lisinopril
*Prazosin* / Indomethacin ↓ antihypertensive effects of prazosin

## Dosage

- **Capsules, Oral Suspension**
  *Moderate to severe arthritis, osteo-
arthritis, ankylosing spondylitis.*
**Adults, initial:** 25 mg b.i.d.–t.i.d.;
may be increased by 25–50 mg at
weekly intervals, according to condition and, if tolerated, until satisfactory response is obtained. With persistent night pain or morning stiffness, a
maximum of 100 mg of the total daily dose can be given at bedtime.
**Maximum daily dosage:** 150–200
mg. In acute flares of chronic rheumatoid arthritis, the dose may need to be
increased by 25–50 mg/day until the
acute phase is under control.
  *Acute gouty arthritis.*

**Adults, initial:** 50 mg t.i.d. until pain is tolerable; **then,** reduce dosage rapidly until drug is withdrawn. Pain relief usually occurs within 2–4 hr, tenderness and heat subside in 24–36 hr, and swelling disappears in 3–4 days.

*Acute painful shoulder (bursitis/tendinitis).*
75–150 mg/day in three to four divided doses for 1–2 weeks.

• **Sustained-Release Capsules**
*Antirheumatic, anti-inflammatory.*
**Adults:** 75 mg, of which 25 mg is released immediately, 1–2 times/day.

• **Suppositories**
*Anti-inflammatory, antirheumatic, antigout.*
**Adults:** 50 mg up to q.i.d. **Pediatric:** 1.5–2.5 mg/kg/day in three to four divided doses (up to a maximum of 4 mg/kg or 250–300 mg/day, whichever is less).

• **IV Only**
*Patent ductus arteriosus.*
3 IV doses, depending on age of the infant, are given at 12–24-hr intervals. **Infants less than 2 days:** first dose, 0.2 mg/kg, followed by two doses of 0.1 mg/kg each; **infants 2–7 days:** three doses of 0.2 mg/kg each; **infants more than 7 days:** first dose, 0.2 mg/kg, followed by two doses of 0.25 mg/kg each. If patent ductus arteriosus reopens, a second course of one to three doses may be given. Surgery may be required if there is no response after two courses of therapy.

## NURSING CONSIDERATIONS

See also *Nursing Considerations* for *Nonsteroidal Anti-Inflammatory Drugs.*
**Administration/Storage**
1. Do not crush the sustained-release form; do not use for acute gouty arthritis.
2. With dysphagia, the capsule contents may be emptied into applesauce, food, or liquid to ensure that client receives the prescribed dose.
3. Suppositories (50 mg) may be used if unable to take PO medication. Store below 30°C (86°F).
4. Use the smallest effective dose, based on individual need. Adverse reactions are dose related.
**IV** 5. Store in amber-colored containers.
6. Prepare the IV solution with 1–2 mL of preservative-free NaCl or sterile water for injection. Prepare just prior to use.
7. Reconstitute to 0.1 mg/mL or 0.05 mg/mL immediately before use and infuse over 5–10 sec.
**Assessment**
1. Note indications for therapy, type, onset, and duration of symptoms; list other agents trialed and the outcome.
2. Assess and document characteristics of involved joint(s), including goniometric measurements and ROM.
**Client/Family Teaching**
1. Take with food or milk to decrease GI upset. Do not crush or break capsules; may sprinkle capsule contents on food if unable to swallow.
2. Use caution when operating potentially hazardous equipment; may cause lightheadedness and decreased alertness.
3. Withhold the drug and report if adverse side effects occur since many may be serious enough to stop therapy.
4. Record weights, especially if nausea or vomiting occur; report any abdominal pain or diarrhea.
5. Indomethacin masks infections; report any S&S of infection or fever.
6. Report for scheduled ophthalmologic exams and lab studies.
7. It will take from 2 to 4 weeks of therapy before significant improvement evident in arthritic conditions. Follow prescribed dosing regimen carefully and refrain from becoming discouraged.
**Outcomes/Evaluate**
• ↓ Pain and inflammation; ↑ joint mobility

• Closure of patent ductus arteriosus
• Therapeutic serum drug levels (10–18 mcg/mL)

# Insulin injection (crystalline zinc insulin, unmodified insulin, regular insulin)

(IN-sue-lin)
**Pork:** Iletin II ✱, Insulin-Toronto ✱, Regular Iletin II, Regular Purified Pork Insulin. **Beef/Pork:** Iletin ✱, Regular Iletin I. **Human:** Humulin-R ✱, Novolin R, Novolin R PenFill, Novolin R Prefilled, Velosulin Human BR **(OTC)**
**Classification:** Rapid-acting insulin

See also *Insulins*.

**Action/Kinetics:** Rarely administered as the sole agent due to its short duration of action. Injections of 100 units/mL are clear; cloudy, colored solutions should not be used. Regular insulin is the only preparation suitable for IV administration. Available only as 100 units/mL. **Onset, SC:** 30–60 min; **IV:** 10–30 min. **Peak, SC:** 2–4 hr; **IV:** 15–30 min. **Duration, SC:** 6–8 hr; **IV:** 30–60 min.

**Uses:** Suitable for treatment of diabetic coma, diabetic acidosis, or other emergency situations. Especially suitable for the client suffering from labile diabetes. During acute phase of diabetic acidosis or for the client in diabetic crisis, client is monitored by serum glucose and serum ketone levels.

**Dosage** —————
• **SC**
  *Diabetes.*
**Adults, individualized, usual, initial:** 5–10 units; **pediatric:** 2–4 units. Injection is given 15–30 min before meals and at bedtime.
  *Diabetic ketoacidosis.*
**Adults:** 0.1 unit/kg/hr given by continuous IV infusion.

# NURSING CONSIDERATIONS

See also *Nursing Considerations* for *Insulins*.
**Administration/Storage**
**IV** 1. When used IV, reduce the rate of insulin infusion when plasma glucose levels reach 250 mg/dL.
2. Due to the short half-life of regular insulin, do not give large single IV doses.
**Outcomes/Evaluate:** Glucose and HbA1C within desired range

# Insulin injection, concentrated

(IN-sue-lin)
**Pregnancy Category:** C
Regular (Concentrated) Iletin II U-500 **(Rx)**
**Classification:** Insulin, concentrated

See also *Insulins*.
**Action/Kinetics:** Concentrated insulin injection (500 U/mL). Depending on response, may be given SC or IM as a single or as two or three divided doses. Not suitable for IV administration because of possible allergic or anaphylactoid reactions.
**Uses:** Insulin resistance requiring more than 200 units insulin/day.
**Contraindications:** Allergy to pork or mixed pork/beef insulin (unless client has been desensitized).
**Special Concerns:** Use with caution during lactation.
**Additional Side Effects:** Deep secondary hypoglycemia 18–24 hr after administration.
**Drug Interactions:** Do not use together with PO hypoglycemic agents.

**Dosage** —————
• **SC, IM**
  **Individualized,** depending on severity of condition. Clients must be kept under close observation until dosage is established.

# NURSING CONSIDERATIONS

See also *Nursing Considerations* for *Insulins*.

## Administration/Storage

1. Administer only water clear solutions (concentrated insulin may appear straw-colored).

2. Use small-caliber syringe for accuracy of measurement.

3. Deep secondary hypoglycemia may occur 18–24 hr after administration; have 10%–20% dextrose solution available.

4. Keep insulin cool or refrigerated.

## Assessment

1. Observe closely for S&S of hyper- or hypoglycemia until dosage established.

2. Monitor BS frequently and HbA1C q 3 mo.

## Client/Family Teaching

1. Review technique for self-administration.

2. Be alert for signs of hypoglycemia, which may indicate that responsiveness to insulin has been regained and that a reduction in dosage is warranted.

**Outcomes/Evaluate:** Serum glucose levels and HbA1-C to within desired range

# Insulin lispro injection (rDNA origin)

(IN-sue-lin LYE-sproh)
**Pregnancy Category:** B
Humalog **(Rx)**
**Classification:** Insulin, rDNA origin

See also *Insulins.*

**Action/Kinetics:** Rapid-acting insulin derived from *Escherichia coli* that has been genetically altered by the addition of the gene for insulin lispro. Is a human insulin analog created when the amino acids at positions 28 and 29 on the insulin B-chain are reversed. Absorbed faster than regular human insulin. Compared with regular insulin, has a more rapid onset of glucose-lowering activity, an earlier peak for glucose lowering, and a shorter duration of glucose-lowering activity. However, is equipotent to human regular insulin (i.e., one unit of insulin lispro has the same glucose-lowering capacity as one unit of regular insulin). May lower the risk of nocturnal hypoglycemia in clients with type I diabetes. **Onset:** 15 min. **Peak effect:** 30–90 min. **t½:** 1 hr. **Duration:** 5 hr or less.

**Uses:** Diabetes mellitus.

**Contraindications:** Use during episodes of hypoglycemia. Hypersensitivity to insulin lispro.

**Special Concerns:** Since insulin lispro has a more rapid onset and shorter duration of action than regular insulin, clients with type I diabetes also require a longer acting insulin to maintain glucose control. Requirements may be decreased in impaired renal or hepatic function. Use with caution during lactation. Safety and efficacy have not been determined in children less than 12 years of age.

**Side Effects:** See *Insulins.*

**Drug Interactions:** See *Insulins.*

## Dosage

• **SC**

*Diabetes.*

Individualized, depending on severity of the condition.

## NURSING CONSIDERATIONS

See also *Nursing Considerations* for *Insulins.*

### Administration/Storage

1. When used as a mealtime insulin, give within 15 min before a meal as compared with human regular insulin, which is best given 30–60 min before a meal.

2. May be mixed with Humulin N, Humulin L, or Humulin U. A decrease in the rate of absorption (but not the total bioavailability) was seen when Humalog was mixed with Humulin N.

3. When Humalog is mixed with either Humulin U or Humulin N, give mixture within 15 min before a meal and immediately after mixing.

4. If Humalog is mixed with a longer acting insulin, Humalog should be drawn into the syringe first to

prevent clouding of the Humalog by the longer-acting insulin.

5. Do not give mixtures IV.

6. Store in the refrigerator at 2°C–8°C (36°F–46°F). Do not freeze. If refrigeration is not possible, can be stored unrefrigerated for up to 28 days, provided it is kept as cool as possible and away from direct heat and light.

**Assessment**

1. Document indications for therapy, disease onset, previous agents trialed, and the outcome.

2. Monitor CBC, HbA1C, urinalysis, and liver and renal function studies.

**Client/Family Teaching**

1. Review method for preparation, storage, and administration; rotate sites.

2. Drug has a more rapid onset of action and a shorter duration of action than regular insulin.

3. Take within 15 min of meals and immediately after mixing, with combined therapy.

4. Monitor fingersticks closely until response evident. Review S&S of hypoglycemia and appropriate management.

5. Clients with type I diabetes also require a longer-acting insulin preparation for adequate glucose control.

6. Report as scheduled for follow-up labs, reinforcement of teaching, and evaluation of response to medication.

**Outcomes/Evaluate:** BS and HbA1C within desired range

# Insulin zinc suspension (Lente)

(IN-sue-lin)

**Pork:** Iletin II ✿, Lente Iletin II, Lente L.
**Beef/Pork:** Iletin ✿, Lentin Iletin I.
**Human:** Humulin L, Novolin ge Lente ✿, Novolin L **(OTC)**
**Classification:** Intermediate-acting insulin

See also *Insulins.*

**Action/Kinetics:** Contains 70% crystalline and 30% amorphous insulin suspension. Considered intermediate-acting. Principal advantage is the absence of a sensitizing agent such as protamine. **Onset:** 1–2.5 hr. **Peak:** 7–15 hr. **Duration:** About 22 hr.
**Uses:** Allergy to other types of insulin and in clients disposed to thrombotic phenomena in which protamine may be a factor. Zinc insulin is not a replacement for regular insulin and is not suitable for emergency use.

**Dosage**

• **SC**

*Diabetes.*

**Adults, initial:** 7–26 units 30–60 min before breakfast. Dosage is then increased by daily or weekly increments of 2–10 units until satisfactory readjustment is established. A second smaller dose may be given prior to the evening meal or at bedtime. Clients on NPH can be transferred to insulin zinc suspension on a unit-for-unit basis. Clients being transferred from regular insulin should begin zinc insulin at two-thirds to three-fourths the regular insulin dosage. If the client is being transferred from protamine zinc insulin, the dose of zinc insulin should be about 50% of that required for protamine zinc insulin.

## NURSING CONSIDERATIONS

See *Nursing Considerations* for *Insulins.*
**Outcomes/Evaluate:** Normalization of BS and HbA1C levels

# Insulin zinc suspension, extended (Ultralente)

**Human:** Humulin-U ✿, Humulin U Ultralente., Novolin ge Ultralente ✿ **(OTC)**
**Classification:** Long-acting insulin

See also *Insulins.*

**Action/Kinetics:** Large crystals of insulin and a high content of zinc are responsible for the slow-acting properties of this preparation. Products containing both 40 units/mL and 100 units/mL are available. **Onset:** 4–8 hr. **Peak:** 10–30 hr. **Duration:** 36 hr or longer.

**Uses:** Mild to moderate hyperglycemia in stabilized diabetics. Not suitable for the treatment of diabetic coma or emergency situations.

**Dosage** ────────────────

• **SC**
 *Individualized.*
**Usual, initial:** 7–26 units as a single dose 30–60 min before breakfast.
**Do not administer IV.**

## NURSING CONSIDERATIONS

See *Nursing Considerations* for *Insulins.*
**Outcomes/Evaluate:** Normalization of BS and HbA1C levels

# Interferon alfa-2a recombinant (rl FN-A; IFLrA)
(in-ter-**FEER**-on **AL**-fah)
**Pregnancy Category:** C
Roferon-A **(Rx)**
**Classification:** Antineoplastic, miscellaneous agent

**Action/Kinetics:** Interferon alfa-2a is the product of recombinant DNA technology using strains of genetically engineered *Escherichia coli.* Activity is expressed as International Units, which are determined by comparing the antiviral activity of recombinant interferons with the activity of the international reference standard of human leukocyte interferon. Interferons bind to specific receptors on the cell surface, resulting in inhibition of virus replication in virus-infected cells, suppression of cell proliferation, increase in the phagocytic activity of macrophages, and enhancement of the toxic effects of leukocytes for target cells.
**Peak serum levels:** 3.8–7.3 hr. **t½:** 3.7–8.5 hr. Metabolized by the kidney.
**Uses:** Hairy cell leukemia in clients older than 18 years of age. Can be used in splenectomized and non-splenectomized clients. AIDS-related Kaposi's sarcoma in clients older than 18 years of age. Chronic myelogenous leukemia. Chronic hepatitis C. *Investigational:* The drug has been used for a large number of other conditions. Significant activity has been noted against the following neoplastic diseases: locally for superficial bladder tumors, carcinoid tumor, cutaneous T-cell lymphoma, essential thrombocythemia, low-grade non-Hodgkin's lymphoma. Limited activity has been noted in acute leukemias, cervical carcinoma, chronic lymphocytic leukemia, Hodgkin's disease, malignant gliomas, melanoma, multiple myeloma, mycosis fungoides/Sézary syndrome, nasopharyngeal carcinoma, osteosarcoma, ovarian carcinoma, renal carcinoma. Interferon alfa-2a also has significant activity against the following viral infections: chronic non-A, non-B hepatitis, condylomata acuminata, cutaneous warts, cytomegaloviruses, herpes keratoconjunctivitis; limited activity is seen against herpes simplex, HIV infection to slow progression, papillomaviruses, rhinoviruses, vaccinia virus, varicella zoster, and viral hepatitis B.
**Contraindications:** Lactation.
**Special Concerns:** Use with caution in clients with a history of unstable angina, uncontrolled CHF, COPD, diabetes mellitus prone to ketoacidosis, thrombophlebitis, pulmonary embolism, seizure disorders, severe renal and hepatic disease, compromised CNS function, and severe myelosuppression. Safety and efficacy in individuals less than 18 years of age have not been established.
**Side Effects:** *Flu-like symptoms:* Fever, headache, fatigue, arthralgia, myalgias, chills, weight loss, dizziness. *CV:* Hypotension, *arrhythmias,* syncope, hypertension, edema, palpitations, transient ischemic attacks, pulmonary edema, CHF, cardiac murmur, *MI, stroke, cardiomyopathy,* hot flashes, Raynaud's phenomenon, thrombophlebitis. *Respiratory:* Coughing, dyspnea, dryness or inflammation of oropharynx, chest pain or congestion, *bronchospasm,* pneumonia, tachypnea, rhinitis, rhinorrhea, sinus-

itis. *CNS:* Depression, confusion, dizziness, headache, paresthesia, anxiety, ataxia, aphasia, aphonia, dysarthria, amnesia, weakness, nervousness, emotional lability, impotence, numbness, lethargy, sleep disturbances, visual disturbances, vertigo, decreased mental · status, memory loss, disturbances of libido, involuntary movements, **suicidal ideation, seizures,** forgetfulness, neuropathy, tremor. *GI:* Anorexia, N&V, diarrhea, emesis, abdominal pain, hypermotility, abdominal fullness, abdominal pain, flatulence, constipation, gastric distress. *Hematologic:* Thrombocytopenia, neutropenia, leukopenia, decreased hemoglobin, severe anemia, severe cytopenias, coagulopathy, Coombs' positive hemolytic anemia, aplastic anemia. *Musculoskeletal:* Joint or bone pain, arthritis, polyarthritis, poor coordination, muscle contractions, gait disturbances. *Dermatologic:* Rash, pruritus, dry skin, ecchymosis, petechiae, skin flushing, alopecia, urticaria, diaphoresis, cyanosis, bruising. *Miscellaneous:* Generalized pain, back pain, inflammation at injection site, epistaxis, bleeding gums, weight loss, alteration of taste, altered hearing, edema, night sweats, earache, eye irritation, hypothyroidism, hypertriglyceridemia.

**Drug Interactions**
*Interleukin-2* / ↑ Risk of renal failure
*Theophylline* / ↓ Clearance of theophylline
**Laboratory Test Interferences:** ↑ AST, ALT, LDH, BUN, serum creatinine, alkaline phosphatase, bilirubin, uric acid, serum glucose, serum phosphorus. ↓ H&H. Hypocalcemia, proteinuria.

**Dosage** ─────
• **IM, SC**
*Hairy cell leukemia.*
**Induction:** 3 million IU/day for 16–24 weeks; **maintenance,** 3 million IU 3 times/week. Doses higher than 3 million IU are not recommended.
*AIDS-related Kaposi's sarcoma.*

**Induction:** 36 million IU/day for 10–12 weeks; or, 3 million IU/day on days 1–3; 9 million IU/day on days 4–6; and 18 million IU/day on days 7–9 followed by 36 million IU/day for the remainder of the 10 to 12-week induction period. **Maintenance:** 36 million IU 3 times/week. If severe side effects occur, the dose can be withheld or reduced by one-half.
*Chronic myelogenous leukemia.*
**Induction:** 9 million IU/day. The dose can be graded during the first week of therapy to improve short-term tolerance by giving 3 million IU/day for 3 days to 6 million IU/day for 3 days and then to the target dose of 9 million IU/day. **Maintenance:** Optimal dose and duration of therapy have not been determined. The regimen should be continued until the disease progresses.
*Chronic hepatitis C.*
3 million IU, SC or IM, 3 times/week for 12 months.

─────

**NURSING CONSIDERATIONS**
**Administration/Storage**
1. Discontinue treatment if hairy cell leukemia does not respond within 6 months.
2. If severe reactions occur, reduce dose of drug by one-half or withhold individual doses. Assess effect on bone marrow of previous radiation or chemotherapy.
3. Although optimal duration of treatment has not been established, clients have been treated for up to 20 consecutive months. Nadir: leukocytes, 20–40 days; platelets, 15–20 days.
4. Consider SC route with a platelet count less than 50,000/mm³.
5. Although not approved by the FDA, interferon alfa-2a has been given by continuous or intermittent IV infusion as well as ophthalmically and intravaginally.
6. The reconstituted solution is stable for 30 days when stored at 2°C–8°C (36°F–46°F) and for 24 hr when stored at room temperature. The undiluted drug is not stable in

syringes due to adhesion to syringe surfaces.

**Client/Family Teaching**

1. Review appropriate method for administration, care and safe storage of drug and equipment, and proper syringe disposal.

2. Most common side effects are flu-like symptoms, such as fever, fatigue, headache, chills, nausea, and loss of appetite; may be minimized by taking at bedtime.

3. Flu-like symptoms usually diminish in severity as treatment continues. Acetaminophen may be used for fever and headache.

4. Drink plenty of fluids (2–3 L/day) during therapy.

5. Hypotension may occur up to 2 days following drug therapy; sit before standing and rise slowly.

6. Do not change brands of interferon without approval; changes in dosage may occur with different brands.

7. Report for CBC, electrolytes, and liver function studies as scheduled.

8. Report any evidence of neurologic or psychologic disturbances.

9. Hair loss may occur.

10. Practice safe sex; use contraception.

11. Avoid alcohol and any other unprescribed CNS depressants.

**Outcomes/Evaluate**

- ↓ Tumor size and spread
- Inhibition of viral replication
- ↓ Lesions with Kaposi's sarcoma

---

# Interferon alfa-2b recombinant (rl FN-α2; α-2-interferon)

(in-ter-**FEER**-on **AL**-fah )

**Pregnancy Category:** C

Intron A **(Rx)**

**Classification:** Antineoplastic, miscellaneous agent

**Action/Kinetics:** A product of recombinant DNA technology using strains of genetically engineered *Escherichia coli*. The activity is expressed as International Units, which are determined by comparing the antiviral activity of the recombinant interferon with the activity of the international reference standard of human leukocyte interferon. Interferons bind to specific receptors on the cell surface, resulting in inhibition of virus replication in virus-infected cells, suppression of cell proliferation, increase in the phagocytic activity of macrophages, and enhancement of the toxic effects of leukocytes for target cells. **Peak serum levels after IM, SC:** 18–116 IU/mL after 3–12 hr. **t½, IM, SC:** 2–3 hr. **Peak serum levels after IV infusion:** 135–270 IU/mL at the end of the infusion. **t½, IV:** 2 hr. The main site of metabolism may be the kidney.

**Uses:** Hairy cell leukemia in clients older than 18 years of age (in both splenectomized and nonsplenectomized clients). Intralesional use for genital or venereal warts (*Condylomata acuminata*.) AIDS-related Kaposi's sarcoma in clients over 18 years of age. Chronic hepatitis C in clients at least 18 years of age with compensated liver disease and a history of blood or blood product exposure or who are HCV antibody positive. Chronic hepatitis B in clients over 18 years of age with compensated liver disease and HBV replication (clients must be serum HBsAg positive for at least 6 months and have HBV replication with elevated serum ALT). Adjunct therapy for malignant melanoma in those who are 18 years of age or older who are free of the disease but at a high risk for recurrence within 56 days of surgery. With an anthracycline drug for the initial treatment of clinically aggressive non-Hodgkin's lymphoma.

*Investigational:* The drug has been used for a large number of conditions. Significant activity has been noted against the following neoplastic diseases: locally for superficial bladder tumors, carcinoid tumor, chronic myelogenous leukemia, cutaneous T-cell lymphoma, essential thrombocythemia, low-grade non-Hodgkin's lymphoma, and chronic granulocytic leukemia. Limited activity has been noted in acute leukemias, cervical carcinoma, chronic lymphocytic leukemia, Hodgkin's disease, malignant gliomas, melanoma, multiple myeloma, nasopharyngeal carcinoma, osteosarcoma, ovarian carcinoma, renal carcinoma, and chronic granulomatous disease. Interferon alfa-2b has also been used to treat the following viral infections: Significant activity has been seen against cutaneous warts, CMVs, herpes keratoconjunctivitis, and herpes simplex. Limited activity has been noted against papillomaviruses, rhinoviruses, vaccinia virus, varicella zoster, and HIV (used with foscarnet/AZT). It has also been used to treat multiple sclerosis.

**Contraindications:** Lactation. To treat rapidly progressive visceral disease in AIDS-related Kaposi's sarcoma. Use in clients with decompensated liver disease, autoimmune hepatitis, history of autoimmune disease, or immunosuppressed transplant clients.

**Special Concerns:** Use with caution in clients with a history of unstable angina, uncontrolled CHF, COPD, diabetes mellitus prone to ketoacidosis, thrombophlebitis, pulmonary embolism, seizure disorders, severe renal and hepatic disease, compromised CNS function, and severe myelosuppression. Safety and efficacy in individuals less than 18 years of age have not been established.

**Side Effects:** *Flu-like symptoms:* Fever, headache, fatigue, myalgia, chills. *CV:* Hypotension, **arrhythmias,** tachycardia, syncope, hypertension, coagulation disorders, chest pain, palpitations, flushing, atrial fibrillation, bradycardia, **cardiac failure, cardiomyopathy,** extrasystoles, postural hypotension. *CNS:* Depression, confusion, somnolence, migraine, dizziness, ataxia, insomnia, irritability, paresthesia, anxiety, nervousness, emotional lability, amnesia, im-

paired concentration, weakness, tremor, syncope, abnormal coordination, hypoesthesia, hypesthesia, abnormal coordination, aggravated depression, aggressive reaction, hypertonia, hypokinesia, impaired consciousness, neuropathy, agitation, apathy, aphasia, dysphonia, extrapyramidal disorder, hot flashes, hyperesthesia, hyperkinesia, neurosis, paresis, paroniria, parosmia, personality disorder, **seizures, coma,** polyneuropathy, **suicide attempt.** *GI:* N&V, diarrhea, stomatitis, weight loss, anorexia, flatulence, thirst, dehydration, constipation, eructation, abdominal pain, loose stools, abdominal distention, dysphagia, esophagitis, gastric ulcer, **GI hemorrhage,** GI mucosal discoloration, gum hyperplasia, gingival bleeding, gingivitis, increased saliva, increased appetite, melena, oral leukoplakia, rectal bleeding after stool, **rectal hemorrhage,** ulcerative stomatitis, ascites, gallstones, gastroenteritis, halitosis. *Hematologic:* Thrombocytopenia, granulocytopenia, anemia, **hemolytic anemia,** leukopenia. *Musculoskeletal:* Arthralgia, leg cramps, asthenia, arthrosis, arthritis, muscle pain or weakness, back pain, bone pain, rigors, carpal tunnel syndrome. *Respiratory:* Pharyngitis, coughing, dyspnea, sinusitis, rhinitis, epistaxis, nasal congestion, dry mouth, **bronchospasm,** pleural pain, pneumonia, rhinorrhea, sneezing, wheezing, bronchitis, cyanosis, lung fibrosis. *EENT:* Alteration or loss of taste, tinnitus, hearing disorders, conjunctivitis, photophobia, vision disorders, eye pain, diplopia, dry eyes, earache, lacrimal gland disorder, periorbital edema, vertigo, speech disorder. *Dermatologic:* Rash, pruritus, alopecia, urticaria, dry skin, dermatitis, purpura, photosensitivity, acne, nail disorder, facial edema, moniliasis, reaction at injection site, abnormal hair texture, cold/clammy skin, cyanosis of the hand, epidermal necrolysis, dermatitis lichenoides, furunculosis, increased hair growth, erythema, melanosis, nonherpetic cold sores, peripheral ischemia, skin depigmentation or discoloration, vitiligo, folliculitis, lipoma, psoriasis. *GU:* Amenorrhea, hematuria, impotence, leukorrhea, menorrhagia, urinary frequency, nocturia, polyuria, uterine bleeding, increased BUN, incontinence, pelvic pain. *Endocrine:* Gynecomastia, thyroid disorder, aggravation of diabetes mellitus, virilism. *Hepatic:* Jaundice, upper right quadrant pain, **hepatic encephalopathy, hepatic failure.** *Other:* Pain, increased sweating, malaise, decreased libido, herpes simplex, lymphadenopathy, chest pain, abscess, cachexia, hypercalcemia, peripheral edema, stye, substernal chest pain, weakness, sepsis, dehydration, fungal infection, herpes zoster, viral infection, trichomoniasis.

**Drug Interactions**
*Aminophylline* / ↓ Clearance of aminophylline due to ↓ breakdown by the liver
*AZT* / ↑ Risk of neutropenia
**Laboratory Test Interferences:** ↑ AST, ALT, LDH, BUN, serum creatinine, alkaline phosphatase. ↓ H&H. Abnormal hepatic function tests, bilirubinemia.

**Dosage**
• **IM, SC**
*Hairy cell leukemia.*
2 million IU/m² 3 times/week. Higher doses are not recommended. May require 6 or more months of therapy for improvement. Do not use the 50-million-IU strength of the powder for injection for treating hairy cell leukemia.
*AIDS-related Kaposi's sarcoma*
30 million IU/m² 3 times/week SC or IM using only the 50-million-IU vial. Using this dose, clients should tolerate an average dose of 110 million IU/week at the end of 12 weeks of therapy and 75 million IU/week at the end of 24 weeks of therapy.
*Chronic hepatitis C.*
3 million IU 3 times/week for 16 weeks. At 16 weeks, extend treatment to 18 to 24 months at 3 million IU 3 times/week to improve the sustained response of normalization of ALT. Discontinue therapy if there is no response after 16 weeks.
*Chronic hepatitis B.*
30–35 million IU/week SC or IM, given as either 5 million IU/day or 10 million IU 3 times/week for 16 weeks. If serious side effects occur, the dose may be decreased by 50%.
• **IV**
*Malignant melanoma.*
20 million IU/m² IV on 5 consecutive days/week for 4 weeks. **Maintenance:** 10 million IU/m² SC 3 times/week for 48 weeks.
• **Intralesional**
*Condylomata acuminata (genital or venereal warts).*
1 million IU/lesion 3 times/week for 3 weeks. For this purpose, use only the vial containing 10 million units and reconstitute using no more than 1 mL diluent. To reduce side effects, give in the evening with acetaminophen. Maximum response usually occurs within 4–8 weeks. If results are unsatisfactory after 12–16 weeks, a second course may be started.

## NURSING CONSIDERATIONS

See also *Nursing Considerations* for *Interferon alfa-2a recombinant* and *Interferon alfa-n3.*
**Administration/Storage**
1. Prior to administration, the drug must be reconstituted with bacteriostatic water for injection, which is provided. The client may self-administer the dose at bedime.
2. If severe side effects occur, the dose can be reduced as much as 50% or therapy can be discontinued until side effects subside. For example, if the granulocyte count is less than 750/mm³ and the platelet count is less than 50,000/mm³, reduce the dose by 50%; if the granulocyte count is less than 500/mm³ and the platelet count is less than 30,000/mm³, interrupt drug therapy until counts return to normal or baseline levels. Nadir: 3–5 days.
3. Discontinue treatment for hairy

cell leukemia if no response within 6 months.

4. When used for venereal or genital warts, maximum response usually occurs 4–8 weeks after therapy is initiated. If results not satisfactory after 12–16 weeks, a second course of therapy may be undertaken.

5. Although the optimal duration of treatment has not been established, clients have been treated for up to 20 consecutive months.

6. If the platelet count is less than 50,000/mm³, give SC rather than IM.

7. Use a Tuberculin or similar syringe with a 25- to 30-gauge needle for intralesion administration. Do not give beneath the lesion too deeply or inject too superficially. As many as five lesions can be treated at one time.

8. The reconstituted solution is stable for 30 days when stored from 2°C–8°C (36°F–46°F) and for 48 hr when stored at 40°C (104°F) or less. The undiluted drug is not stable in syringes due to adhesion to syringe surfaces.

**IV** 9. Although not approved by the FDA, interferon alfa-2a has been given by continuous or intermittent IV infusion as well as ophthalmically and intravaginally.

10. For infusion solutions, after reconstitution, withdraw the appropriate dose and inject into a 100-mL bag of 0.9% NaCl injection. The final concentration should be 10 million IU/10 mL or more. Infuse over a 20-min period. Prepare solution immediately prior to use.

**Client/Family Teaching**

1. Flu-like symptoms may be minimized by administering the drug at bedtime. Use acetaminophen for fever and headache.

2. Consume 2–3 L/day of fluids.

3. Report for labs and bone marrow hairy cell determinations.

**Outcomes/Evaluate**

• Improved hematologic response with disease regression

• ↓ Size and number of genital/venereal warts

# Interferon alfa-n3
(in-ter-**FEER**-on **AL**-fah)
**Pregnancy Category:** C
Alferon N **(Rx)**
**Classification:** Antineoplastic

**Action/Kinetics:** Interferon alfa-n3 is made from pooled human leukocytes induced by incomplete infection with Sendai (avian) virus. The product is a sterile, aqueous formulation of purified, natural, human interferon alpha proteins. The drug binds to receptors on cell surfaces leading to a sequence of events including inhibition of virus replication and suppression of cell proliferation. Also, interferon alfa-n3 causes immunomodulation characterized by enhanced phagocytosis by macrophages, augmentation of the cytotoxicity of lymphocytes, and enhancement of human leukocyte antigen expression. Intralesional use of interferon alfa-n3 does not result in detectable plasma levels of the drug.

**Uses:** Intralesional treatment of refractory or recurring external condylomata acuminata (genital or venereal warts) in clients 18 years of age or older. *Investigational:* Alpha interferons are being tested for use in a large number of neoplastic diseases and viral infections.

**Contraindications:** Hypersensitivity to human interferon alpha; clients who are allergic to mouse immunoglobulin (IgG), egg protein, or neomycin (the production process involves a nutrient medium containing neomycin although it has not been detected in the final product). Lactation.

**Special Concerns:** Due to the manifestation of fever and flu-like symptoms with interferon alfa-n3 use, the drug should be used with caution in clients with debilitating diseases including unstable angina, uncontrolled CHF, COPD, diabetes mellitus with ketoacidosis, thrombophlebitis, pulmonary embolism, hemophilia, severe myelosuppression, or seizure disorders. Safety and effectiveness have not been determined in children less than 18 years of age.

**Side Effects:** *Flu-like symptoms:* Commonly, fever, headache, myalgias which decrease with repeated doses. Also, chills, fatigue, malaise. *CNS:* Dizziness, lightheadedness, insomnia, depression, nervousness, decreased ability to concentrate. *GI:* N&V, heartburn, diarrhea, tongue hyperesthesia, thirst, altered taste, increased salivation. *Musculoskeletal/Skin:* Arthralgia, back pain, hot sensation at bottom of feet, tingling of legs/feet, muscle cramps. *Respiratory:* Nose or sinus drainage, nose bleed, throat tightness, pharyngitis. *Miscellaneous:* Pruritus, swollen lymph nodes, heat intolerance, visual disturbances, sensitivity to allergens, papular rash on neck, hot flashes, herpes labialis, dysuria, photosensitivity, decreased WBC count.

*NOTE:* When used for treatment of cancer, the incidence of many of the preceding side effects was increased. Additional side effects were noted including: *GI:* Constipation, anorexia, stomatitis, dry mouth, mucositis, sore mouth. *Laboratory Test Values:* Abnormal hemoglobin, WBC count, alkaline phosphatase, total bilirubin, platelet count, AST, and GGT. *Miscellaneous:* Insomnia, blurred vision, ocular rotation pain, sore injection site, chest pains, low BP.

**Dosage** ————————————
- **Intralesional Injection**
  *Condylomata acuminata.*
  0.05 mL (250,000 IU)/wart twice a week for up to 8 weeks. The maximum recommended dose per treatment session is 0.5 mL (2.5 million IU). The safety and effectiveness of a second course of treatment have not been determined.

## NURSING CONSIDERATIONS

See also *Nursing Considerations* for *Interferon alfa-2a* and *alfa-2b Recombinant*.
**Administration/Storage**
1. Inject drug into the base of the wart using a 30-gauge needle.
2. For large warts, inject at several

points around the periphery of the wart using a total dose of 0.05 mL/wart.
3. Store drug at 2°C–8°C (36°F–46°F). Do not freeze or shake.
**Assessment**
1. Note any allergic reactions to egg protein or neomycin; may have increased sensitivity to drug.
2. Determine any preexisting debilitating diseases; note functional level.
3. For condylomata therapy, measure and document size and number of lesions.
**Client/Family Teaching**
1. Intralesional treatment should be continued for 8 weeks.
2. Genital warts may disappear both during and after treatment has been completed. When this occurs, unless new warts appear or warts become enlarged, there should be a 3-month waiting period after the first 8-week course of therapy.
3. Do not change brands of interferon without approval; manufacturing process, strength, and type of interferon may vary.
4. Fertile women should practice contraception.
5. Report early signs of hypersensitivity reactions (e.g., hives, chest tightness, generalized urticaria, hypotension, wheezing, anaphylaxis).
**Outcomes/Evaluate**
- ↓ Pain, number of genital warts
- Suppression of malignant cell proliferation

# Interferon alfacon-1
(in-ter-**FEER**-on **AL**-fah-kon)
**Pregnancy Category:** C
Infergen **(Rx)**
**Classification:** Drug for chronic hepatitis

See also *Interferon alfa-2a* and *Interferon-alfa 2b.*
**Action/Kinetics:** Prepared by recombinant technology. Has antiviral, antiproliferative, and immunomodulatory effects. Plasma levels are too small to measure.

---

**Uses:** Treatment of chronic hepatitis C infections in those over 18 years of age with compensated liver disease. *Investigational:* With G-CSF therapy to treat hairy-cell leukemia.

**Contraindications:** Hypersensitivity to alpha interferons or to products derived from *E. coli.* Use in autoimmune hepatitis or in decompensated hepatic disease.

**Special Concerns:** Use with caution in preexisting cardiac disease, in depression, in those with abnormally low peripheral blood cell counts, in those receiving myelosuppressive agents, and in autoimmune disorder. Use with caution during lactation. Safety and efficacy have not been determined in children less than 18 years of age.

**Side Effects:** *Flu-like symptoms:* Headache, fatigue, fever, myalgia, rigors, arthralgia, increased sweating. *Body as a whole:* Body pain, hot flushes, non-cardiac chest pain, malaise, asthenia, peripheral edema, access pain, allergic reactions, weight loss. *Hypersensitivity:* Urticaria, angioedema, bronchoconstriction, **anaphylaxis.** *CNS:* Insomnia, dizziness, paresthesia, amnesia, hypoesthesia, hypertonia, nervousness, depression, anxiety, emotional lability, abnormal thinking, agitation, decreased libido. *GI:* Abdominal pain, nausea, diarrhea, anorexia, dyspepsia, vomiting, constipation, flatulence, toothache, hemorrhoids, decreased saliva, tender liver. *CV:* Hypertension, palpitation. *Hematologic:* Granulocytopenia, thrombocytopenia, leukopenia, ecchymosis, lymphadenopathy, lymphocytosis. *Respiratory:* Pharyngitis, upper respiratory infection, cough, sinusitis, rhinitis, respiratory tract congestion, upper respiratory tract congestion, epistaxis, dyspnea, bronchitis. *Dermatologic:* Alopecia, pruritus, rash, erythema, dry skin. *Musculoskeletal:* Back, limb, neck, or skeletal pain. *GU:* Dysmenorrhea, vaginitis, menstrual disorder. *Ophthalmic:* Conjunctivitis, eye pain. *Otic:* Tinnitus, earache.

**Laboratory Test Alteration:** ↑ TSH, triglycerides. ↓ Hemoglobin, hematocrit. Abnormal thyroid tests.

**Dosage** ────────────
- **SC Injection**
  *Chronic hepatitis C infection.*

**Adults over 18 years of age:** 9 mcg SC as a single injection three times a week for 24 weeks. At least 48 hr should elapse between doses. Those who tolerate therapy but did not respond or relapsed following discontinuation may be subsequently treated with 15 mcg three times a week for 6 months.

## NURSING CONSIDERATIONS

See also *Nursing Considerations* for *Interferon alfa-2a* and *Interferon alfa-2b.*

### Administration/Storage
1. Do not give 15 mcg three times a week if client has not received or has not tolerated an initial course of therapy.
2. Reduce dose to 7.5 mcg following an intolerable adverse reaction. If adverse effects continue at reduced dosage, discontinue therapy or reduce dose further.
3. Store refrigerated but do not freeze. Avoid vigorous shaking.

### Assessment
1. Note any cardiac disease, hypertension, or severe psychiatric disorders as these preclude drug therapy.
2. Monitor CBC, TSH, HCV RNA, liver and renal function studies.

### Client/Family Teaching
1. Review dose and method of administration (SC); usually administered 3 times per week with 48 hr between doses.
2. May experience flu-like symptoms, including headache, fatigue, fever, muscle/joint pain, rigors, and increased sweating.
3. Stop drug and report any S&S of depression, suicide ideations or attempt.
4. Do not change brands of interferon without provider approval.

**Outcomes/Evaluate:** Improvement in LFTs

# Interferon beta-1a

(in-ter-**FEER**-on)
**Pregnancy Category:** C
Avonex (Interferon beta-1a)

# Interferon beta-1b (rIFN-B)

Betaseron (Interferon beta-1b) **(Rx)**
**Classification:** Drug for multiple sclerosis (MS)

**Action/Kinetics:** Interferon beta-1a is produced by mammalian cells into which the human interferon beta gene has been introduced. Interferon beta-1b is made by bacterial fermentation of a strain of *Escherichia coli* that is a genetically engineered plasmid containing the gene for human interferon beta$_{ser17}$. Interferon betas have antiviral, antiproliferative, and immunoregulatory effects. Mechanism for the beneficial effect in MS is unknown, although the effects are mediated through combination with specific cell receptors located on the cell membrane. The receptor-drug complex induces the expression of a number of interferon-induced gene products that are thought to be the mediators of the biologic effects of interferon beta-1a and beta-1b. t½ for interferon beta-1a: 10 hr. Kinetic information is not available for interferon beta-1b since serum levels are low or not detectable following SC administration to MS clients. Data from healthy volunteers indicate peak serum levels of beta-1b occur within 1–8 hr with a mean serum concentration of 40 IU/mL. Mean terminal half-lives ranged from 8 min to 4.3 hr.

**Uses: Interferon beta-1a:** Treatment of relapsing forms of MS to slow the appearance of physical disability and decrease the frequency of clinical exacerbations. **Interferon beta-1b:** Treatment of ambulatory clients with relapsing-remitting MS to reduce the frequency of clinical exacerbations. Remitting-relapsing MS is manifested by recurrent attacks of neurologic dysfunction fol-

lowed by complete or incomplete recovery. *Investigational:* Treatment of AIDS, AIDS-related Kaposi's sarcoma, metastatic renal cell carcinoma, herpes of the lips or genitals, malignant melanoma, cutaneous T-cell lymphoma, and acute non-A/non-B hepatitis.

**Contraindications:** Hypersensitivity to natural or recombinant interferon beta or human albumin. Use during lactation.

**Special Concerns:** The safety and efficacy for use in chronic progressive MS and in children less than 18 years of age have not been studied. Depression and attempted suicide and suicide have occurred. The drug has the potential to be an abortifacient. Use with caution in those with preexisting seizure disorder.

**Side Effects: Side effects common to interferon beta-1a and beta-1b.** *Body as a whole:* Headache, fever, flu-like symptoms, pain, asthenia, chills, reaction at injection site (including necrosis/inflammation), malaise. *GI:* Abdominal pain, diarrhea, dry mouth, *GI hemorrhage*, gingivitis, hepatomegaly, intestinal obstruction, periodontal abscess, proctitis. *CV:* Arrhythmia, hypotension, postural hypotension. *CNS:* Dizziness, speech disorder, convulsion, suicide attempt, abnormal gait, depersonalization, facial paralysis, hyperesthesia, neurosis, psychosis. *Respiratory:* Sinusitis, dyspnea, hemoptysis, hyperventilation. *Musculoskeletal:* Myalgia, arthritis. *Dermatologic:* Contact dermatitis, furunculosis, seborrhea, skin ulcer. *GU:* Epididymitis, gynecomastia, hematuria, kidney calculus, nocturia, vaginal hemorrhage, ovarian cyst. *Miscellaneous:* Abscess, ascites, cellulitis, hernia, hypothyroidism, *sepsis,* hiccoughs, thirst, leukorrhea.

**Interferon beta-1a.** *Body as a whole:* Infection. *GI:* Nausea, dyspepsia, anorexia, blood in stool, colitis, constipation, diverticulitis, gall bladder disorder, gastritis, gum hemorrhage, hepatoma, increased appetite, *intestinal perforation,* periodonitis, tongue disorder. *CV:* Syncope, vasodilation, arteritis, *heart arrest, hemorrhage, pulmonary embolus,* palpitation, pericarditis, peripheral ischemia, peripheral vascular disorder, spider angioma, telangiectasia. *CNS:* Sleep difficulty, muscle spasm, ataxia, amnesia, Bell's palsy, clumsiness, drug dependence, increased libido. *Respiratory:* URTI, emphysema, laryngitis, pharyngeal edema, pneumonia. *Musculoskeletal:* Arthralgia, bone pain, myasthenia, osteonecrosis, synovitis. *Dermatologic:* Urticaria, alopecia, nevus, herpes zoster, herpes simplex, basal cell carcinoma, blisters, cold clammy skin, erythema, genital pruritus, skin discoloration. *GU:* Vaginitis, breast fibroadenosis, breast mass, dysuria, fibrocystic change of the breast, fibroids, kidney pain, menopause, pelvic inflammatory disease, penis disorder, Peyronie's disease, polyuria, postmenopausal hemorrhage, prostatic disorder, pyelonephritis, testis disorder, urethral pain, urinary urgency, urinary retention, urinary incontinence. *Hematologic:* Anemia, ecchymosis at injection site, eosinophils greater than 10%, hematocrit less than 37%, increased coagulation time, ecchymosis, lymphadenopathy, petechia. *Metabolic:* Dehydration, hypoglycemia, hypomagnesemia, hypokalemia. *Ophthalmic:* Abnormal vision, conjunctivitis, eye pain, vitreous floaters. *Miscellaneous:* Otitis media, decreased hearing, facial edema, fibrosis at injection site, hypersensitivity at injection site, lipoma, neoplasm, photosensitivity, toothache, sinus headache, chest pain.

**Interferon beta-1b.** *Body as a whole:* Generalized edema, hypothermia, *anaphylaxis, shock,* adenoma, sarcoma. *GI:* Constipation, vomiting, GI disorder, aphthous stomatitis, cardiospasm, cheilitis, cholecystitis, cholelithiasis, duodenal ulcer, enteritis, esophagitis, fecal impaction or incontinence, flatulence, gastritis, glossitis, hematemesis, hepatic neoplasia, hepatitis, ileus, increased salivation, melena, nausea, oral leuko-

plakia, oral moniliasis, *pancreatitis, rectal hemorrhage,* salivary gland enlargement, stomach ulcer, peritonitis, tenesmus. *CV:* Migraine, palpitation, hypertension, tachycardia, peripheral vascular disorder, *hemorrhage,* angina pectoris, atrial fibrillation, cardiomegaly, *cardiac arrest, cerebral hemorrhage, heart failure, MI, pulmonary embolus, ventricular fibrillation* cerebral ischemia, endocarditis, pericardial effusion, spider angioma, subarachnoid hemorrhage, syncope, thrombophlebitis, thrombosis, varicose veins, vasospasm, venous pressure increase, ventricular extrasystoles. *CNS:* Mental symptoms, hypertonia, somnolence, hyperkinesia, acute/chronic brain syndrome, agitation, apathy, aphasia, ataxia, brain edema, *coma,* delirium, delusions, dementia, dystonia, encephalopathy, euphoria, hallucinations, hemiplegia, hypalgesia, incoordination, intracranial hypertension, decreased libido, manic reaction, meningitis, neuralgia, neuropathy, paralysis, paranoid reaction, decreased reflexes, stupor, subdural hematoma, torticollis, tremor. *Respiratory:* Laryngitis, apnea, asthma, atelectasis, lung carcinoma, hypoventilation, interstitial pneumonia, lung edema, pleural effusion, pneumothorax. *Musculoskeletal:* Myasthenia, arthrosis, bursitis, leg cramps, muscle atrophy, myopathy, myositis, ptosis, tenosynovitis. *Dermatologic:* Sweating, alopecia, erythema nodosum, exfoliative dermatitis, hirsutism, leukoderma, lichenoid dermatitis, maculopapular rash, photosensitivity, psoriasis, benign skin neoplasm, skin carcinoma, skin hypertrophy, skin necrosis, urticaria, vesiculobullous rash. *GU:* Dysmenorrhea, menstrual disorder, metrorrhagia, cystitis, breast pain, menorrhagia, urinary urgency, fibrocystic breast, breast neoplasm, urinary retention, anuria, balanitis, breast engorgement, cervicitis, impotence, kidney failure, tubular disorder, nephritis, oliguria, polyuria, salpingitis, urethritis, urinary incontinence, enlarged uterine fibroids, uterine neoplasm. *Hematolo-*

*gic:* Lymphocytes less than 1500/mm³, active neutrophil count less than 1500/mm³, WBCs less than 3000/mm³, lymphadenopathy, chronic lymphocytic leukemia, petechia, hemoglobin less than 9.4 g/dL, platelets less than 75,000/mm³, splenomegaly. *Metabolic:* Weight gain, weight loss, goiter, glucose less than 55 mg/dL or greater than 160 mg/dL, AST or ALT greater than 5 times baseline, total bilirubin greater than 2.5 times baseline, urine protein greater than 1+, alkaline phosphatase greater than 5 times baseline, BUN greater than 40 mg/dL, calcium greater than 11.5 mg/dL, cyanosis, edema, glycosuria, hypoglycemic reaction, hypoxia, ketosis. *Ophthalmic:* Conjunctivitis, abnormal vision, diplopia, nystagmus, oculogyric crisis, papilledema, blepharitis, blindness, dry eyes, iritis, keratoconjunctivitis, mydriasis, photophobia, retinitis, visual field defect. *Miscellaneous:* Pelvic pain, hydrocephalus, alcohol intolerance, otitis externa, otitis media, parosmia, taste loss, taste peversion.

**Laboratory Test Interferences:** ↑ ALT, total bilirubin, AST, BUN, urine protein. Hypoglycemia or hyperglycemia. Ketosis.

**Dosage** ───────────────
- **Interferon beta-1a: IM**
  *Relapsing forms of MS.*
  30 mcg IM once a week.
- **Inteferon beta-1b: SC**
  *Relapsing-remitting MS clients.*
  0.25 mg (8 mIU) every other day.

## NURSING CONSIDERATIONS
### Administration/Storage
1. Effectiveness beyond 2 years of use is not known.
2. To reconstitute and use interferon beta-1a, use the following process:
- Reconstitute with 1.1 mL of diluent and swirl gently to dissolve.
- Vials must be stored in a refrigerator at 2°C–8°C (36°F–46°F).
- Following reconstitution, use within 6 hr and store at the same temperatures as the unreconstituted drug.
3. To reconstitute and use interferon beta-1b, use the following process:
- Using a sterile syringe and needle, inject 1.2 mL of diluent provided (0.54% NaCl) into the vial. Swirl gently to dissolve the drug completely. (Do not shake.)
- Visually inspect reconstituted product; discard if it contains particulate matter or is discolored.
- Withdraw 1 mL of the reconstituted solution from the vial into a sterile syringe fitted with a 27-gauge needle and inject SC. Injection sites include the arms, abdomen, hips, and thighs.
- Since the reconstituted product contains no preservative, discard any unused portions after one use.
- Before and after reconstitution with diluent, store the drug at 2°C–8°C (36°F–46°F). Use the product within 3 hr of reconstitution.

### Assessment
1. Document age of diagnosis, frequency of exacerbations, other therapies prescribed and the outcome.
2. Note any hypersensitivity to human albumin or interferon beta.
3. Determine if pregnant; drug has abortifacient properties.
4. Monitor hematologic profile and hepatic enzyme levels q 3 mo.

### Client/Family Teaching
1. Review guidelines for drug reconstitution, proper dose, administration, and care and disposal of equipment.
2. Do not change dose or administration schedule without approval.
3. Flu-like symptoms are common; acetaminophen may provide some relief.
4. Report any evidence of mental changes, depression, or suicide ideations.
5. Practice reliable birth control; drug may harm fetus.
6. May cause photosensitivity reactions; wear protective clothing, sunscreen, sun glasses, and a hat.
7. Avoid alcohol in any form.

8. With diabetes, monitor FS and report any overt changes.

9. Identify support groups that may assist to cope with chronic diseases.

**Outcomes/Evaluate:** ↓ Frequency and severity of MS exacerbations

# Interferon gamma-1b

(in-ter-**FEER**-on **GAM**-uh)
**Pregnancy Category:** C
Actimmune **(Rx)**
**Classification:** Interferon

**Action/Kinetics:** Consists of a single-chain polypeptide of 140 amino acids. Produced by fermentation of a genetically engineered *Escherichia coli* bacterium containing the DNA that encodes for the human protein. Manifests potent phagocyte-activating effects including generation of toxic oxygen metabolites within phagocytes. Such metabolites result in the death of microorganisms such as *Staphylococcus aureus, Toxoplasma gondii, Leishmania donovani, Listeria monocytogenes,* and *Mycobacterium avium intracellulare.* Since interferon gamma regulates activity of immune cells, it is characterized as a lymphokine of the interleukin type. Interferon gamma interacts functionally with other interleukin molecules (e.g., interleukin-2) and all interleukins form part of a complex, lymphokine regulatory network. As an example, interferon gamma and interleukin-4 may interact reciprocally to regulate murine IgE levels; interferon gamma can suppress IgE levels and inhibit the production of collagen at the transcription level in humans. Slowly absorbed after SC injection. **t½, elimination:** SC, 5.9 hr. **Peak plasma levels:** 7 hr after SC.

**Uses:** Decrease the frequency and severity of serious infections associated with chronic granulomatous disease.

**Contraindications:** Hypersensitivity to interferon gamma or *E. coli*-derived products. Use during lactation.

**Special Concerns:** Safety and effectiveness have not been determined in children less than 1 year of age. Use with caution in clients with preexisting cardiac disease, including symptoms of ischemia, arrhythmia, or CHF, and in clients with myelosuppression, seizure disorders, or compromised CNS function.

**Side Effects:** The following side effects were noted in clients with chronic granulomatous disease receiving the drug SC. *GI:* Diarrhea, vomiting, nausea, abdominal pain, anorexia. *CNS:* Fever (over 50%), headache, fatigue, depression. *Miscellaneous:* Rash, chills, erythema or tenderness at injection site, pain at injection site, weight loss, myalgia, arthralgia, back pain.

When used in clients other than those with chronic granulomatous disease, in addition to the preceding, the following side effects were reported. *GI:* **GI bleeding,** pancreatitis, hepatic insufficiency. *CV:* Hypotension, heart block, **heart failure,** syncope, **tachyarrhythmia, MI.** *CNS:* Confusion, disorientation, symptoms of parkinsonism, gait disturbance, **seizures,** hallucinations, transient ischemic attacks. *Hematologic:* **Deep venous thrombosis, pulmonary embolism.** *Respiratory:* **Bronchospasm,** tachypnea, interstitial pneumonitis. *Metabolic:* Hyperglycemia, hyponatremia. *Miscellaneous:* Reversible renal insufficiency, worsening of dermatomyositis.

**Dosage**
- **SC**

  *Chronic granulomatous disease.*
  50 mcg/m² (1.5 million units/m²) for clients whose body surface is greater than 0.5 m². If the body surface is less than 0.5 m², the dose of interferon gamma should be 1.5 mcg/kg/dose. The drug is given 3 times/week (e.g., Monday, Wednesday, Friday).

## NURSING CONSIDERATIONS
### Administration/Storage
1. Preferred injection sites are the right and left deltoid and anterior thigh.

2. The product does not contain a preservative. Use the vial only for a

single dose and discard any unused portion.

3. Safety and effectiveness have not been determined for doses greater or less than 50 mcg/m².

4. If severe side effects occur, dose can be reduced by 50% or therapy can be discontinued until these subside.

5. May be administered using either sterilized glass or plastic disposable syringes.

6. Vials must be stored at 2°C–8°C (36°F–46°F) to assure optimal retention of activity. Do not freeze the vial.

7. Do not shake the vial; avoid vigorous agitation.

8. Discard vials stored at room temperature for more than 12 hr.

9. Do not store undiluted drug in syringes due to adhesion to syringe surfaces.

**IV** 10. Although not approved by the FDA, the drug has been given by continuous (10 days to 8 weeks) or intermittent (at 1, 6, or 24 hr) IV infusion as well as by IM injection.

**Assessment**

1. Determine age with onset of chronic granulomatous disease and what if any treatments in the past were used to reduce frequency and severity of infections.

2. Note history of CAD or CNS disorders; assess for symptoms.

3. Monitor urinalysis, CBC, liver and renal function studies q 3 mo.

**Client/Family Teaching**

1. Review appropriate method for administration, reconstitution, storage, and disposal of drug and equipment.

2. Keep drug in the refrigerator; do *not* shake container.

3. Take at bedtime with acetaminophen to minimize flu-like symptoms (fever and headaches).

4. Consume 2–3 L/day of fluids.

5. Avoid alcohol and any other CNS depressants.

6. Close medical supervision is imperative with this disease and genetically engineered drug therapy as dosage may require frequent adjustments. Report all concerns and any adverse effects.

**Outcomes/Evaluate:** Suppression of infective microorganisms associated with chronic granulomatous disease

# Ipecac syrup
(**IP**-eh-kak)
**Pregnancy Category:** C
PMS Ipecac Syrup ✸ **(OTC)**
**Classification:** Emetic

**Action/Kinetics:** Acts both locally on the gastric mucosa as an irritant and centrally to stimulate the CTZ. The central effect is caused by emetine and cephaeline, which are two alkaloids in the product. **Onset:** 20 min. **Duration:** 20–25 min. In contrast to apomorphine, a second dose may be given if necessary. **Ipecac syrup must not be confused with ipecac fluid extract, which is 14 times as potent.** Syrup of ipecac can be purchased without a prescription.

**Uses:** To empty the stomach promptly and completely after oral poisoning or drug overdose.

**Contraindications:** With corrosives or petroleum distillates, in individuals who are unconscious or semicomatose, severely inebriated, or in shock. Infants under 6 months of age.

**Special Concerns:** Use with caution during lactation. If used in children less than 12 months of age, there is an increased risk of aspiration of vomitus. Abuse may occur in anorexic or bulemic clients and its use in these groups has been associated with severe cardiomyopathies and death.

**Side Effects:** Diarrhea, drowsiness, coughing, or choking with emesis, mild CNS depression, GU upset (may last several hours) after emesis. Can be cardiotoxic if not vomited and allowed to be absorbed. Cardiotoxic effects include heart conduction disturbances, atrial fibrillation, or *fatal myocarditis*.

**OD** **Overdose Management:** *Symptoms:* If absorbed into the general circulation, symptoms may include cardiac conduction disturbances, bradycardia, atrial fibrillation, hypotension, or *fatal myocarditis.* *Treatment:* Activated charcoal to absorb ipecac syrup. Gastric lavage. Support the CV system with symptomatic treatment.

**Drug Interactions:** Activated charcoal adsorbs ipecac syrup, thus decreasing its effect.

**Dosage** ─────────
• **Syrup**
  *Emetic.*
**Adults and children over 12 years:** 15–30 mL followed by 240 mL of water; **infants up to 1 year:** 5–10 mL followed by one-half to one glass of water; **pediatric, 1–12 years:** 15 mL followed by one to two glasses of water.

## NURSING CONSIDERATIONS
**Administration/Storage**
1. Check label of medication closely so that the syrup and the fluid extract are not confused.
2. Dosage may be repeated in children over 1 year of age and adults once if vomiting does not occur within 30 min. Gastric lavage should be considered if vomiting does not occur within 15 min after the second dose.
3. Administer ipecac syrup with 200–300 mL of water.
4. There is controversy as to whether ipecac syrup should be given to children less than 1 year old. However, it appears to be both safe and effective.
**Assessment**
1. Estimate amount and time of ingestion and compare with plasma level of agent ingested.
2. Do not use if intoxicant is a convulsant (i.e., tricyclic antidepressants); may trigger seizures abruptly.
3. Do not use for petroleum-based or caustic substances such as kerosene, lye, Drano, or gasoline.
4. Assess respiratory status and level

of consciousness; do not use if there is no gag reflex or if semicomatose.
**Client/Family Teaching**
1. For use in the event of accidental poisoning.
2. Before administering ipecac syrup, contact regional poison control center or local hospital.
3. Store in a locked closet, out of the reach of children. Check expiration date periodically and always before use.
4. Review abuse potential, such as to induce vomiting after meals for weight reduction and its potential cardiac toxic effects. (Some states have banned OTC sales for this reason.)
**Outcomes/Evaluate:** Inducement of vomiting following drug overdose or poisoning

# Ipratropium bromide
(eye-prah-**TROH**-pee-um)
**Pregnancy Category:** B
Alti-Ipratropium Bromide ✲, Apo-Ipravent ✲, Atrovent, Novo-Ipramide ✲ **(Rx)**
**Classification:** Anticholinergic, quaternary ammonium compound

See also *Cholinergic Blocking Agents.*
**Action/Kinetics:** Chemically related to atropine. Antagonizes the action of acetylcholine. Prevents the increase in intracellular levels of cyclic guanosine monophosphate, which is caused by the interaction of acetylcholine with muscarinic receptors in bronchial smooth muscle; this leads to bronchodilation which is primarily a local, site-specific effect. Not easily absorbed into the systemic circulation; excreted through the feces. **$t\frac{1}{2}$, elimination:** 2 hr after inhalation.
**Uses: Aerosol or solution:** Bronchodilation in COPD, including chronic bronchitis and emphysema. **Nasal spray:** Symptomatic relief (using 0.06%) of rhinorrhea associated with allergic and nonallergic perennial rhinitis in clients over 12 years of age. Symptomatic relief (using 0.06%) of rhinorrhea associated with the common cold in those over 12 years of age. *NOTE:* The use of

ipratropium with sympathomimetic bronchodilators, methylxanthines, steroids, or cromolyn sodium (all of which are used in treating COPD) are without side effects.

**Contraindications:** Hypersensitivity to atropine, ipratropium, or derivatives. Hypersensitivity to soya lecithin or related food products, including soy bean or peanut (inhalation aerosol).

**Special Concerns:** Use with caution in clients with narrow-angle glaucoma, prostatic hypertrophy, or bladder neck obstruction and during lactation. Safety and efficacy have not been determined in children. Use of ipratropium as a single agent for the relief of bronchospasm in acute COPD has not been studied adequately.

**Side Effects:** *Inhalation aerosol. CNS:* Cough, nervousness, dizziness, headache, fatigue, insomnia, drowsiness, difficulty in coordination, tremor. *GI:* Dryness of oropharynx, GI distress, dry mouth, nausea, constipation. *CV:* Palpitations, tachycardia, flushing. *Dermatologic:* Itching, hives, alopecia. *Miscellaneous:* Irritation from aerosol, worsening of symptoms, rash, hoarseness, blurred vision, difficulty in accommodation, drying of secretions, urinary difficulty, paresthesias, mucosal ulcers.

*Inhalation solution. CNS:* Dizziness, insomnia, nervousness, tremor, headache. *GI:* Dry mouth, nausea, constipation. *CV:* Hypertension, aggravation of hypertension, tachycardia, palpitations. *Respiratory:* Worsening of COPD symptoms, coughing, dyspnea, bronchitis, bronchospasm, increased sputum, URI, pharyngitis, rhinitis, sinusitis. *Miscellaneous:* Urinary retention, UTIs, urticaria, pain, flu-like symptoms, back or chest pain, arthritis.

*Nasal spray. CNS:* Headache, dizziness. *GI:* Nausea, dry mouth, taste perversion. *CV:* Palpitation, tachycardia. *Respiratory:* URI, epistaxis, pharyngitis, nasal dryness, miscellaneous nasal symptoms, nasal irritation, blood-tinged mucus, dry throat, cough, nasal congestion, nasal burning, coughing. *Ophthalmic:* Ocular irritation, blurred vision, conjunctivitis. *Miscellaneous:* Hoarseness, thirst, tinnitis, urinary retention.

*All products. Allergic:* Skin rash; angioedema of the tongue, throat, lips, and face; urticaria, laryngospasm, **anaphylaxis**. *Anticholinergic reactions:* Precipitation or worsening of narrow angle glaucoma, prostatic disorders, tachycardia, urinary retention, constipation, and bowel obstruction.

**Dosage** ────────────
• **Respiratory Aerosol**
  *Treat bronchospasms.*
**Adults:** 2 inhalations (36 mcg) q.i.d. Additional inhalations may be required but should not exceed 12 inhalations/day.
• **Solution for Inhalation**
  *Treat bronchospasms.*
**Adults:** 500 mcg (1-unit-dose vial) administered t.i.d.–q.i.d. by oral nebulization with doses 6–8 hr apart.
• **Nasal Spray, 0.03%**
  *Perennial rhinitis.*
2 sprays (42 mcg) per nostril b.i.d.–t.i.d. for a total daily dose of 168–252 mcg/day.
• **Nasal Spray, 0.06%**
  *Rhinitis due to the common cold.*
2 sprays (84 mcg) per nostril t.i.d.–q.i.d. for a total daily dose of 504–672 mcg/day. The safety and efficacy for use for the common cold for more than 4 days have not been determined.

## NURSING CONSIDERATIONS

See also *Nursing Considerations* for *Cholinergic Blocking Agents.*
**Administration/Storage**
1. If also taking albuterol, ipratropium may be mixed in the nebulizer with albuterol if used within 1 hr.
2. Store the aerosol below 30°C (86°F); avoid excessive humidity.
3. Store the solution between 15°C and 30°C (59°F and 86°F); protect

from light. Store unused vials in the foil pouch.

4. Store the nasal spray tightly closed between 15°C and 30°C (59°F and 86°F). Avoid freezing.

**Assessment**

1. Document type, onset, characteristics of symptoms, any other agents used.

2. Perform full pulmonary assessment; review PFTs and X-ray reports.

3. Note any prostate enlargement or difficulty urinating.

**Client/Family Teaching**

1. Take as directed; shake well before using. Review administration technique.

2. If using more than one inhalation per dose, wait 3 min before administering the second inhalation.

3. Drug is not for use in terminating an acute attack; effects take up to 15 min. Have another prescribed agent readily available in this event.

4. Avoid contact with the eyes. A spacer may be useful with the inhaler and a mouthpiece with the nebulizer to help prevent solution (mist) contact with the eyes.

5. May experience a bitter taste and dry mouth; use frequent mouth rinses and hard candy to relieve.

6. Transient dizziness, insomnia, blurred vision, or excessive weakness may occur.

7. Stop smoking now to preserve current level of lung function and to prevent further damage; utilize smoking cessation program.

**Outcomes/Evaluate**

• Improved airway exchange and breathing patterns
• ↓ Wheezing, dyspnea
• Relief of rhinorrhea

# Irbesartan

(ihr-beh-**SAR**-tan)

**Pregnancy Category:** C (first trimester), D (second and third trimesters)

Avapro **(Rx)**

**Classification:** Antihypertensive, angiotensin II receptor antagonist

See also *Antihypertensive Drugs.*

**Action/Kinetics:** By binding to $AT_1$ angiotensin II receptor, blocks vasoconstrictor and aldosterone-secreting effects of angiotensin II. Rapid absorption after PO use. **Peak plasma levels:** 1.5–2 hr. Food does not affect bioavailability. **t½, terminal elimination:** 11–15 hr. Over 90% bound to plasma proteins. Metabolized in liver and both unchanged drug and metabolites excreted through urine and feces.

**Uses:** Treat hypertension alone or in combination with other antihypertensives.

**Special Concerns:** Safety and efficacy have not been determined in children.

**Side Effects:** *GI:* Diarrhea, dyspepsia, heartburn, abdominal pain, N&V, constipation, oral lesion, gastroenteritis, flatulence, abdominal distention. *CV:* Tachycardia, syncope, orthostatic hypotension, hypotension (especially in volume- or salt-depletion), flushing, hypertension, cardiac murmur, ***MI, cardio-respiratory arrest, heart failure, hypertensive crisis, CVA,*** angina pectoris, arrhythmias, conduction disorder, transient ischemic attack. *CNS:* Sleep disturbance, anxiety, nervousness, dizziness, numbness, somnolence, emotional disturbance, depression, paresthesia, tremor. *Musculoskeletal:* Extremity swelling, muscle cramp, arthritis, muscle ache, musculoskeletal pain, musculoskeletal chest pain, joint stiffness, bursitis, muscle weakness. *Respiratory:* Epistaxis, tracheobronchitis, congestion, pulmonary congestion, dyspnea, wheezing, upper respiratory infection, rhinitis, pharyngitis, sinus abnormality. *GU:* Abnormal urination, prostate disorder, urinary tract infection, sexual dysfunction, libido change. *Dermatologic:* Pruritus, dermatitis, ecchymosis, facial erythema, urticaria. *Ophthalmic:* Vision disturbance, conjunctivitis, eyelid abnormality. *Otic:* Hearing abnormality, ear infection, ear pain, ear abnormality. *Miscellaneous:* Gout, fever, fatigue, chills, facial edema, upper extremity edema, headache, influenza, rash, chest pain.

**Laboratory Test Interferences:** ↑ BUN (minor), serum creatinine.

**Dosage**
• **Tablets**

*Hypertension.*

150 mg once daily, up to 300 mg once daily. Lower initial dose of 75 mg is recommended for clients with depleted intravascular volume or salt. If BP is not controlled by irbesartan alone, hydrochlorothiazide may have an additive effect. Clients not adequately treated by 300 mg irbesartan are unlikely to get benefit from higher dose or b.i.d. dosing.

## NURSING CONSIDERATIONS

See also *Nursing Considerations* for *Antihypertensive Drugs.*

**Administration/Storage:** Adjustment of dose is not required in geriatric clients or in hepatic or renal impairment.

**Assessment**

1. Document indications for therapy, onset, duration, characteristics of symptoms, and other agents trialed.
2. Observe infants exposed to an angiotensin II inhibitor in utero for hypotension, oliguria, and hyperkalemia.

**Client/Family Teaching**

1. Take only as directed. May take with or without food.
2. Continue low-fat, low-cholesterol diet, regular exercise, tobacco cessation, salt restriction and life-style changes necessary to maintain lowered BP.
3. Practice reliable contraception. Stop drug and report if pregnancy suspected.

**Outcomes/Evaluate:** ↓ BP

# Irinotecan hydrochloride
(**eye**-rih-noh-**TEE**-kan)
**Pregnancy Category:** D
Camptosar **(Rx)**
**Classification:** Antineoplastic, hormone

See also *Antineoplastic Agents.*

**Action/Kinetics:** The cytotoxic effect is due to double-strand DNA damage produced during DNA synthesis when replication enzymes interact with the ternary complex formed by topoisomerase I, DNA, and either irinotecan or SN-38 (its active metabolite). Conversion of irinotecan to SN-38 occurs in the liver. **t½, terminal, irinotecan:** About 6 hr; **t½, terminal, SN-38:** About 10 hr. SN-38 is 95% bound to plasma proteins.

**Uses:** Metastatic carcinoma of the colon or rectum in those whose disease has recurred or progressed following 5-fluorouracil therapy.

**Contraindications:** Lactation.

**Special Concerns:** Clients who have previously received pelvic or abdominal irradiation are at an increased risk for severe myelosuppression when treated with irinotecan. Safety and efficacy have not been determined in children.

**Side Effects:** *GI:* Diarrhea, N&V, anorexia, abdominal cramping or pain, constipation, flatulence, stomatitis, dyspepsia. *Hematologic:* Leukopenia, anemia, neutropenia, serious **thrombocytopenia** (rare). *CNS:* Insomnia, dizziness. *Respiratory:* Dyspnea, increased coughing, rhinitis, **severe pulmonary events** (rare). *CV:* Vasodilation, flushing. *Body as a whole:* Asthenia, fever, pain, headache, back pain, chills, minor infections (usually UTI), edema, abdominal enlargement. *Dermatologic:* Alopecia, sweating, rashes. *Metabolic/nutritional:* Decreased body weight, dehydration.

**OD** **Overdose Management:** *Symptoms:* Extension of side effects. *Treatment:* Maximum supportive care to prevent dehydration due to diarrhea. Treat any infections.

**Drug Interactions**

*Antineoplastic agents* / ↑ Risk of myelosuppression and diarrhea

*Dexamethasone* / ↑ Risk of lymphocytopenia and hyperglycemia

---

*Prochlorperazine* / ↑ Risk of akathisia

**Laboratory Test Interferences:** AST, alkaline phosphatase.

## Dosage
• **IV Infusion**

*Metastatic carcinoma of the colon or rectum.*

**Initial:** 125 mg/m² given as an IV infusion over 90 min once weekly for 4 weeks. This is followed by a 2-week rest period. **Subsequent dosing:** Additional courses of treatment may be repeated q 6 weeks (4 weeks on therapy, 2 weeks off therapy). Doses can be adjusted to as high as 150 mg/m² or as low as 50 mg/m² in 25- to 50-mg/m² increments, depending on the client's tolerance. If intolerable toxicity does not occur, courses of treatment may be continued indefinitely. *NOTE:* Modifications of the dosage are based on the degree of neutropenia, neutropenic fever, diarrhea, and other toxicities. Consult the package insert for specific dosage modifications.

## NURSING CONSIDERATIONS

See also *Nursing Considerations* for *Antineoplastic Agents*.
### Administration/Storage
**IV** 1. Avoid extravasation. If extravasation occurs, flush site with sterile water and apply ice.
2. Since irinotecan causes vomiting, clients should receive antiemetic therapy. Antiemetic therapy includes dexamethasone, 10 mg, and a 5-HT₃ blocker such as granisetron or ondansetron. Give 30 min before administration of irinotecan.
3. Prepare the infusion solution by diluting in 5% dextrose injection (preferred) or 0.9% NaCl injection to a final concentration of 0.12–1.1 mg/mL; administer over 90 min.
4. Solutions diluted in 5% dextrose, stored in the refrigerator, and protected from light are stable for 48 hr. However, due to possible microbial contamination during dilution, use refrigerated admixtures within 24 hr or, if kept at room temperature, use within 6 hr. Do not refrigerate admixtures containing 0.9% NaCl. Freezing irinotecan or admixtures of irinotecan may cause drug precipitation.

### Assessment
1. Document indications for therapy; note any history of pelvic or abdominal irradiation and last 5-FU therapy.
2. List all drugs currently prescribed to ensure none exacerbate any side effects.
3. Drug is emetogenic; administer antiemetic 30 min prior to therapy.
4. May need IV atropine for those who experience early-onset abdominal cramps, diarrhea, or diaphoresis.
5. Assess infusion site carefully; flush site with sterile water and apply ice with extravasation.
6. Obtain CBC before each treatment. Hold if ANC below 500/mm³ or neutropenic fever occurs. Any significant reduction in WBC (less then 2,000/mm³), neutrophil count (less than 1,000/mm³), or platelet count (below 100,000 mm³) warrants a dose reduction.

### Client/Family Teaching
1. Diarrhea may occur within 24 hr of therapy; is cholinergic in nature and usually transient.
2. Report if temperature is over 101°F or diarrhea, vomiting, or dehydration develop.
3. With late-onset diarrhea (usually 10 days after therapy) take 4 mg of loperamide, followed by 2 mg q 2 h for 12 hr until diarrhea free.
4. Avoid laxatives unless approved.
5. Practice birth control during and for several months following therapy.
**Outcomes/Evaluate:** Inhibition of malignant cell proliferation

# Isoetharine hydrochloride
(eye-so-**ETH**-ah-reen)
**Pregnancy Category:** C
Arm-a-Med Isoetharine HCl, Beta-2, Bronkosol **(Rx)**

# Isoetharine mesylate
(eye-so-**ETH**-ah-reen)
**Pregnancy Category:** C

Bronkometer **(Rx)**
**Classification:** Adrenergic agent, bronchodilator

See also *Sympathomimetic Drugs.*

**Action/Kinetics:** Has a greater stimulating activity on beta-2 receptors of the bronchi than on beta-1 receptors of the heart. Causes relief of bronchospasms. **Inhalation: Onset,** 1–6 min; **peak effect:** 15–60 min; **duration:** 1–3 hr. Partially metabolized; excreted in urine.

**Uses:** Bronchial asthma, bronchospasms due to chronic bronchitis or emphysema, bronchiectasis, pulmonary obstructive disease.

**Special Concerns:** Dosage has not been established in children less than 12 years of age.

**Dosage** ─────────
• **Inhalation Solution**
*Hand nebulizer.*
**Adults:** 3–7 inhalations (use undiluted) of the 0.5% or 1% solution.
*Oxygen aerosolization or IPPB.*
**Adults:** Dose depends on strength of solution used (range: 0.062%–1%) and whether the solution is used undiluted or diluted according to the following: **1%:** 0.25–1 mL by IPPB or 0.25–0.5 mL by oxygen aerosolization diluted 1:3 with saline or other diluent. **0.2–0.5%:** 2 mL used undiluted; **0.2%:** 1.25–2.5 mL used undiluted; **0.167 or 0.17%:** 3 mL used undiluted; **0.125%:** 2–4 mL used undiluted; **0.1%:** 2.5-5 mL used undiluted; **0.08%:** 3 mL used undiluted; **0.062%:** 4 mL used undiluted.
• **Mesylate Metered Dose Inhaler**
**Adults:** 0.34 mg (1 inhalation) repeated after 1–2 min if needed; **then,** dose may be repeated q 4 hr.

## NURSING CONSIDERATIONS

See *Special Nursing Considerations for Adrenergic Bronchodilators* under *Sympathomimetic Drugs.*
**Administration/Storage**
1. One or 2 inhalations are usually sufficient; wait 1 min after initial dose to determine if another dose needed.

2. Usually does not need to be repeated more than q 4 hr.
3. Do not use if solution contains a precipitate or is brown.
**Assessment:** Document indications for therapy, pulmonary assessments, X rays and review PFTs; note any allergy to sulfites.
**Client/Family Teaching**
1. Review proper technique for administration.
2. Stop smoking; enroll in smoking cessation program.
**Outcomes/Evaluate:** Improved airway exchange; ↓ airway resistance

# Isoniazid (INH, Isonicotinic acid hydrazide)
(eye-so-**NYE**-ah-zid)
**Pregnancy Category:** C
Dom-Isoniazide ✿, Isotamine ✿, Laniazid, Laniazid C.T., Nydrazid Injection, PMS-Isoniazid ✿ **(Rx)**
**Classification:** Primary antitubercular agent

**General Statement:** Isoniazid is the most effective tuberculostatic agent. The metabolism of isoniazid is genetically determined and involves the level of a hepatic enzyme. Clients on isoniazid fall into two groups, depending on the manner in which they metabolize the drug. As a rule, 50% of whites and blacks inactivate the drug slowly, whereas the majority of American Indians, Eskimos, Japanese, and Chinese are rapid acetylators (inactivators).
1. **Slow acetylators:** These clients show earlier, favorable response but have more toxic reactions (e.g., neuropathies because of higher blood levels of drug).
2. **Rapid acetylators:** These clients have possible poor clinical response due to rapid inactivation, which is 5–6 times faster than slow acetylators. This group requires an increased daily dose of the drug. They are more likely to develop hepatitis.

---

✿ = Available in Canada                     ***bold italic*** = life threatening side effect

**Action/Kinetics:** Probably interferes with lipid and nucleic acid metabolism of growing bacteria, resulting in alteration of the bacterial wall. Is tuberculostatic. Readily absorbed after PO and parenteral (IM) administration and widely distributed in body tissues, including cerebrospinal, pleural, and ascitic fluids. **Peak plasma concentration: PO,** 1–2 hr. **t½, fast acetylators:** 0.5–6 hr; **t½, slow acetylators:** 2–5 hr. These values are increased in association with liver and kidney impairment. Metabolized in liver and excreted primarily in urine.

**Uses:** Tuberculosis caused by human, bovine, and BCG strains of *Mycobacterium tuberculosis*. The drug should not be used as the sole tuberculostatic agent. Prophylaxis of tuberculosis. *Investigational:* To improve severe tremor in clients with multiple sclerosis.

**Contraindications:** Severe hypersensitivity to isoniazid or in clients with previous isoniazid-associated hepatic injury or side effects.

**Special Concerns:** Severe and sometimes fatal hepatitis may occur even after several months of therapy; incidence is age-related and current alcohol use increases the risk. Increased risk of fatal hepatitis in minority women, especially Blacks and Hispanics; also increased risk postpartum. Extreme caution should be exercised in clients with convulsive disorders, in whom the drug should be administered only when the client is adequately controlled by anticonvulsant medication. Also, use with caution for the treatment of renal tuberculosis and, in the lowest dose possible, in clients with impaired renal function and in alcoholics.

**Side Effects:** *Neurologic:* Peripheral neuropathy characterized by symmetrical numbness and tingling of extremities (dose-related). Rarely, toxic encephalopathy, optic neuritis, optic atrophy, **seizures,** impaired memory, toxic psychosis. *GI:* N&V, epigastric distress, xerostomia. *Hypersensitivity:* Fever, skin rashes and eruptions, vasculitis, lymphadenopa-

thy. *Hepatic:* Liver dysfunction, jaundice, bilirubinemia, bilirubinuria, *serious and sometimes fatal hepatitis (especially in clients over 50 years of age).* Increases in serum AST and ALT. *Hematologic: Agranulocytosis,* eosinophilia, thrombocytopenia, *hemolytic, sideroblastic, or aplastic anemia. Metabolic/Endocrine:* Metabolic acidosis, pyridoxine deficiency, pellagra, hyperglycemia, gynecomastia. *Miscellaneous:* Tinnitus, urinary retention, rheumatic syndrome, lupus-like syndrome, arthralgia.

*NOTE:* Pyridoxine, 10–50 mg/day, may be given concomitantly with isoniazid to decrease CNS side effects. Ophthalmologic and liver function tests are recommended periodically.

**OD** **Overdose Management:** *Symptoms:* N&V, dizziness, blurred vision, slurred speech, visual hallucinations within 30–180 min. Severe overdosage may cause respiratory distress, *CNS depression (coma can occur), severe seizures,* metabolic acidosis, acetonuria, hyperglycemia. *Treatment:* Maintain respiration and undertake gastric lavage (within first 2–3 hr providing seizures are not present). To control seizures, give diazepam or a short-acting IV barbiturate followed by pyridoxine (1 mg IV/1 mg isoniazid ingested). Sodium bicarbonate, IV, to correct metabolic acidosis. Forced osmotic diuresis; monitor fluid I&O. For severe cases, hemodialysis or peritoneal dialysis should be considered.

**Drug Interactions**
*Aluminum salts* / ↓ Effect of isoniazid due to ↓ absorption from GI tract
*Anticoagulants, oral* / ↓ Anticoagulant effect
*Atropine* / ↑ Side effects of isoniazid
*Benzodiazepines* / ↑ Effect of benzodiazepines that undergo oxidative metabolism (e.g., diazepam, triazolam)
*Carbamazepine* / ↑ Risk of both carbamazepine and isoniazid toxicity

*Cycloserine* / ↑ Risk of cycloserine CNS side effects

*Disulfiram* / ↑ Risk of acute behavioral and coordination changes

*Enflurane* / Isoniazid may produce high levels of hydrazine, which increases defluorination of enflurane

*Ethanol* / ↑ Chance of isoniazid-induced hepatitis

*Halothane* / ↑ Risk of hepatotoxicity and hepatic encephalopathy

*Hydantoins (phenytoin)* / ↑ Effect of hydantoins due to ↓ breakdown in liver

*Ketoconazole* / ↓ Serum levels of ketoconazole → ↓ effect

*Meperidine* / ↑ Risk of hypotension or CNS depression

*PAS* / ↑ Effect of isoniazid by ↑ blood levels

*Rifampin* / Additive liver toxicity

**Laboratory Test Interferences:** Altered liver function tests. False + or ↑ potassium, AST, ALT, urine glucose (Benedict's test, Clinitest).

**Dosage**
- **Syrup, Tablets**
  *Active tuberculosis.*
  **Adults:** 5 mg/kg/day (up to 300 mg/day) as a single dose; **children and infants:** 10–20 mg/kg/day (up to 300 mg total) in a single dose.
  *Prophylaxis.*
  **Adults:** 300 mg/day in a single dose; **children and infants:** 10 mg/kg/day (up to 300 mg total) in a single dose.
- **IM**
  *Active tuberculosis.*
  **Adults:** 5 mg/kg (up to 300 mg) once daily. **Pediatric:** 10–20 mg/kg (up to 300 mg) once daily.
  *Prophylaxis.*
  **Adults/adolescents:** 300 mg/day.
  **Pediatric:** 10 mg/kg/day.
  *NOTE:* Pyridoxine, 6–50 mg/day, is recommended in the malnourished and those prone to neuropathy (e.g., alcoholics, diabetics).

## NURSING CONSIDERATIONS

See also *General Nursing Considerations for All Anti-Infectives.*

**Administration/Storage**
1. Store in dark, tightly closed containers.
2. Solutions for IM injection may crystallize at low temperature; warm to room temperature if precipitation is evident.
3. Anticipate a slight local irritation at the site of injection. Rotate and document injection sites.
4. Administer with pyridoxine, 10–50 mg/day, in malnourished, alcoholic, or diabetic clients to prevent symptoms of peripheral neuropathy.

**Assessment**
1. Document indications for therapy, type and onset of symptoms. List other therapies used and the outcome.
2. Obtain baseline labs, CXR, and AFB sputums; note date of PPD conversion. Monitor liver and renal function studies; reduce dose with renal dysfunction.
3. Perform pulmonary assessment; describe sputum characteristics.

**Client/Family Teaching**
1. Take on an empty stomach 1 hr before or 2 hr after meals.
2. Consume 2–3 L/day of fluids to ensure adequate hydration.
3. Pyridoxine is given to prevent neurotoxic drug effects (peripheral neuritis).
4. Avoid alcohol to prevent hepatic toxicity.
5. Withhold drug and report fatigue, weakness, malaise, and anorexia (S&S of hepatitis).
6. Report any visual disturbances; may precede optic neuritis.
7. With diabetes, monitor FS closely.
8. Take drugs as ordered; report for periodic lab and ophthalmic assessments.

**Outcomes/Evaluate**
- Negative sputum cultures for AFB
- ↓ Neurotoxic drug effects

• Symptomatic improvement (↓ fever, ↓ pulmonary secretions, ↑ appetite)

# Isophane insulin suspension (NPH)

(**EYE**-so-fayn **IN**-sue-lin)
**Pork:** Iletin II NPH ✿, NPH-N, NPH Iletin II. **Beef/Pork:** Iletin NPH ✿, NPH Iletin I. **Human:** Humulin N, Novolin ge NPH ✿, Novolin N, Novolin N PenFill, Novolin N Prefilled **(OTC)**
**Classification:** Intermediate-acting insulin

See also *Insulins*.
**Action/Kinetics:** Contains zinc insulin crystals modified by protamine, appearing as a cloudy or milky suspension. Not recommended for emergency use. Not suitable for IV administration or in the presence of ketosis. **Onset:** 1–1.5 hr. **Peak:** 4–12 hr. **Duration:** Up to 24 hr.

## Dosage
• **SC**
    *Diabetes.*
**Adult, individualized, usual, initial:** 7–26 units as a single dose 30–60 min before breakfast. A second smaller dose may be given, if needed, prior to the evening meal or at bedtime. If necessary, the daily dose may be increased in increments of 2–10 units at daily or weekly intervals until desired control is achieved.

Clients on insulin zinc may be transferred directly to isophane insulin on a unit-for-unit basis. If client is being transferred from regular insulin, the initial dose of isophane should be from two-thirds to three-fourths the dose of regular insulin.

## NURSING CONSIDERATIONS

See *Nursing Considerations* for *Insulins*.
**Outcomes/Evaluate**
• Normalization of BS and HbA1C levels
• Control of diabetes; ↓ organ damage

## ——COMBINATION DRUG——

# Isophane insulin suspension and insulin injection

(**EYE**-so-fayn **IN**-sue-lin)
**Human:** Humulin 30/70 ✿, Humulin 50/50, Humulin ge 50/50 ✿, Humulin 70/30, Novolin ge 30/70 ✿, Novolin 70/30, Novolin 70/30 PenFill, Novolin 70/30 Prefilled **(OTC)**
**Classification:** Mixture of insulins to achieve variable duration of action

See also *Insulins*.
**Content:** Contains from 10% to 50% insulin injection and from 50% to 70% isophane insulin. Except for Humulin 50/50 and Novolin ge 50/50, the larger number in the product refers to the percentage of isophane insulin suspension.
**Action/Kinetics:** This combination allows for a rapid onset (30–60 min) due to insulin injection and a long duration (24 hr) due to isophane insulin. **Peak effect:** 4–8 hr.

## Dosage
• **SC**
    *Diabetes.*
**Adults:** Individualized and given once daily 15–30 min before breakfast, or as directed. **Children:** Individualized according to client size.

## NURSING CONSIDERATIONS

See *Nursing Considerations* for *Insulins*.
**Outcomes/Evaluate:** Normalization of BS and HbA1C levels

# Isoproterenol

(eye-so-proh-**TER**-ih-nohl)
**Pregnancy Category:** C
Isuprel Glossets **(Rx)**

# Isoproterenol hydrochloride

(eye-so-proh-**TER**-ih-nohl)
**Pregnancy Category:** C
Dispos-a-Med Isoproterenol HCl, Isuprel, Isuprel Mistometer, Norisodrine Aerotrol **(Rx)**

# Isoproterenol sulfate

(eye-so-proh-**TER**-ih-nohl)

**Pregnancy Category:** C
Medihaler-Iso **(Rx)**
**Classification:** Sympathomimetic,
direct-acting

See also *Sympathomimetic Drugs.*

**Action/Kinetics:** Produces pronounced stimulation of both beta-1 and beta-2 receptors of the heart, bronchi, skeletal muscle vasculature, and the GI tract. Has both positive inotropic and chronotropic activity; systolic BP may increase while diastolic BP may decrease. Thus, mean arterial BP may not change or may be decreased. Causes less hyperglycemia than epinephrine, but produces bronchodilation and the same degree of CNS excitation. **Inhalation: Onset,** 2–5 min; **peak effect:** 3–5 min; **duration:** 30–120 min. **IV: Onset,** immediate; **duration:** less than 1 hr. **Sublingual: Onset,** 15–30 min; **duration:** 1–2 hr. Partially metabolized; excreted in urine.

**Uses:** Bronchodilator in asthma, chronic pulmonary emphysema, bronchiectasis, bronchitis, and other conditions involving bronchospasms (e.g., during surgery). Treat bronchospasms during anesthesia. Cardiac arrest, heart block, syncope due to complete heart block, Adams-Stokes syndrome. Certain cardiac arrhythmias including ventricular tachycardia, ventricular arrhythmias; syncope due to carotid sinus hypersensitivity. Hypoperfusion shock syndrome. Hypovolemic and septic shock as an adjunct to fluid and electrolyte replacement. Use in cardiac arrest until electric shock or pacemaker therapy are available.

**Contraindications:** Tachyarrhythmias, tachycardia, or heart block caused by digitalis intoxication, ventricular arrhythmias that require inotropic therapy, and angina pectoris.

**Special Concerns:** Use with caution in the presence of tuberculosis. Safety and effectiveness have not been determined in children less than 12 years of age. Use with caution during lactation.

**Additional Side Effects:** *CV: **Cardiac arrest,*** Adams-Stokes attack, hypotension, precordial pain or distress. *CNS:* Hyperactivity, hyperkinesia. *Respiratory:* Wheezing, bronchitis, increase in sputum, ***bronchial edema and inflammation, pulmonary edema, paradoxical airway resistance.*** Excessive inhalation causes refractory bronchial obstruction. *Miscellaneous:* Flushing, sweating, swelling of the parotid gland. Sublingual administration may cause buccal ulceration. Side effects of drug are less severe after inhalation.

**Drug Interactions**
*Bretylium* / Possibility of arrhythmias
*Guanethidine* / ↑ Pressor response of isoproterenol
*Halogenated hydrocarbon anesthetics* / Sensitization of the heart to catecholamines which may cause serious arrhythmias
*Oxytocic drugs* / Possibility of severe, persistent hypertension
*Tricyclic antidepressants* / Potentiation of pressor effect

**Dosage** ───────────
ISOPROTERENOL HYDROCHLORIDE
• **IV Infusion**
*Shock.*
5 mcg/min (1.25 mL/min of solution prepared by diluting 10 mL of 1:5,000 solution in 500 mL of D5W or 5 mL of 1:5,000 solution in 250 mL of D5W).
*Cardiac standstill and cardiac arrhythmias.*
**Adults:** 5 mcg/min (1.25 mL of either 1.25 mL/min of solution prepared by diluting 10 mL of 1:5,000 solution in 500 mL of D5W or 5 mL of 1:5,000 solution in 250 mL of D5W).
• **IV**
*Cardiac standstill and cardiac arrhythmias.*
1–3 mL (0.02–0.06 mg) of solution prepared by diluting 1 mL of 1:5,000 solution to 10 mL with sodium chloride or 5% dextrose solution. Dosage range: 0.01–0.2 mg.
*Bronchospasm during anesthesia.*

───────────
✦ = Available in Canada    **bold italic** = life threatening side effect

**Adults:** Dilute 1 mL of the 1:5,000 solution to 10 mL with sodium chloride injection or 5% dextrose solution and given an initial dose of 0.01–0.02 mg IV; repeat when necessary.

• **IM, SC**
  *Cardiac standstill and cardiac arrhythmias.*
**Adults:** 1 mL (0.2 mg) of 1:5,000 solution (range: 0.02–1 mg).
  **Intracardiac (in extreme emergencies):** 0.1 mL (0.02 mg) of 1:5,000 solution.

• **Hand Bulb Nebulizer**
  *Acute bronchial asthma.*
**Adults and children:** 5–15 deep inhalations of the 1:200 solution. In adults 3–7 inhalations of the 1:100 solution may be useful. If there is no relief after 5–10 min, the doses may be repeated one more time. Repeat treatment up to 5 times/day may be necessary if there are repeat attacks.
  *Bronchospasm in chronic obstructive lung disease.*
**Adults and children:** 5–15 deep inhalations of the 1:200 solution (in clients with severe attacks, 3–7 inhalations of the 1:100 solution may be useful). An interval of 3–4 hr should elapse between uses.

• **Metered-Dose Inhalation**
  *Acute bronchial asthma.*
**Adults, usual:** 1–2 inhalations beginning with 1 inhalation, and if no relief occurs within 2–5 min, a second inhalation may be used. **Maintenance:** 1–2 inhalations 4–6 times/day. No more than 2 inhalations at any one time or more than 6 inhalations in 1 hr should be taken.
  *Bronchospasm in chronic obstructive lung disease.*
**Adults and children:** 1–2 inhalations repeated at no less than 3–4 hr intervals (i.e., 4–6 times/day).

• **Nebulization by Compressed Air or Oxygen**
  *Bronchospasms in chronic obstructive lung disease.*
**Adults and children:** 0.5 mL of the 1:200 solution is diluted to 2–2.5 mL (for a concentration of 1:800–1:1,000). The solution is delivered over 15–20 min and may be repeated up to 5 times/day.

• **IPPB**
  *Bronchospasms in chronic obstructive lung disease.*
**Adults and children:** 0.5 mL of a 1:200 solution diluted to 2–2.5 mL with water or isotonic saline. The solution is delivered over 10–20 min and may be repeated up to 5 times/ day.

ISOPROTERENOL SULFATE
Dispensed from metered aerosol inhaler for bronchospasms. See preceding dosage for *Hydrochloride*.

## NURSING CONSIDERATIONS

See also *Special Nursing Considerations for Adrenergic Bronchodilators* under *Sympathomimetic Drugs.*
**Administration/Storage**
1. Administration to children, except where noted, is the same as that for adults, because a child's smaller ventilatory exchange capacity will permit a proportionally smaller aerosol intake. For acute bronchospasms in children, use 1:200 solution.
2. In children, no more than 0.25 mL of the 1:200 solution should be used for each 10–15 min of programmed treatment.
3. Elderly clients usually receive a lower dose.
4. Do not crush or chew sublingual tablets; place under the tongue and allow to disintegrate. Do not swallow saliva until absorption has taken place.
**IV** 5. Do not use the injection if it is pinkish to brownish in color. Protect from light and store at 15°C–30°C (59°F–86°F).
**Assessment**
1. Document indications for therapy, causative factors, type and onset of symptoms.
2. Perform pulmonary assessment; note PFTs and CXRs. Report respiratory problems that worsen after administration; refractory reactions may necessitate withdrawal of the drug.
3. Identify arrhythmias (especially

ventricular) and angina; may preclude drug therapy.

**Client/Family Teaching**
1. Review method for inhaler use; a spacer enhances instillation.
2. Rinse mouth and equipment with water; removes drug residue and minimizes dryness after inhalation.
3. Maintain fluid intake of 2–3 L/day; liquefies secretions.
4. Sputum and saliva may appear pink after inhalation therapy; do not become alarmed.
5. When also taking inhalant glucocorticoids, take isoproterenol first and wait 15 min before using the second inhaler.
6. Do not use more often than prescribed; excessive use can cause severe cardiac and respiratory problems.
7. Identify parotid gland; withhold drug and report if becomes enlarged.
8. Stop smoking now to preserve current level of lung function; enroll in smoking cessation program.

**Outcomes/Evaluate**
• Improved airway exchange
• ↓ Bronchoconstriction/bronchospasms
• Stable cardiac rhythm

# Isosorbide dinitrate chewable tablets
(eye-so-**SOR**-byd)
**Pregnancy Category:** C
Sorbitrate **(Rx)**

# Isosorbide dinitrate extended-release capsules
(eye-so-**SOR**-byd)
**Pregnancy Category:** C
Dilatrate-SR, Isordil Tembids **(Rx)**

# Isosorbide dinitrate extended-release tablets
(eye-so-**SOR**-byd)
**Pregnancy Category:** C

Cedocard-SR ✿, Coradur ✿, Isordil Tembids **(Rx)**

# Isosorbide dinitrate sublingual tablets
(eye-so-**SOR**-byd)
**Pregnancy Category:** C
Apo-ISDN ✿, Isordil, Sorbitrate **(Rx)**

# Isosorbide dinitrate tablets
(eye-so-**SOR**-byd)
**Pregnancy Category:** C
Apo-ISDN ✿, Isordil Titradose, Sorbitrate **(Rx)**
**Classification:** Coronary vasodilator, antianginal drug

See also *Antianginal Drugs, Nitrates/Nitrites.*

**Action/Kinetics: Sublingual, chewable. Onset:** 2–5 min; **duration:** 1–3 hr. **Oral Capsules/Tablets. Onset:** 20–40 min; **duration:** 4–6 hr. **Extended-release. Onset:** up to 4 hr; **duration:** 6–8 hr.

**Additional Use:** Diffuse esophageal spasm. Oral tablets are only for prophylaxis while sublingual and chewable forms may be used to terminate acute attacks of angina.

**Special Concerns:** Use with caution during lactation. Safety and efficacy have not been established in children.

**Additional Side Effects:** Vascular headaches occur especially frequently.

**Additional Drug Interactions**
*Acetylcholine* / Isosorbide antagonizes the effect of acetylcholine
*Norepinephrine* / Isosorbide antagonizes the effect of norepinephrine

**Dosage**
• **Tablets**
  *Antianginal.*
**Initial:** 5–20 mg q 6 hr; **maintenance:** 10–40 mg q 6 hr (usual: 20–40 mg q.i.d.).
• **Chewable Tablets**
  *Antianginal, acute attack.*

**Initial:** 5 mg q 2–3 hr. The dose can be titrated upward until angina is relieved or side effects occur.
*Prophylaxis.*
5–10 mg q 2–3 hr.
• **Extended-Release Capsules**
*Antianginal.*
**Initial:** 40 mg; **maintenance:** 40–80 mg q 8–12 hr.
• **Extended-Release Tablets**
*Antianginal.*
**Initial:** 40 mg; **maintenance:** 40–80 mg q 8–12 hr.
• **Sublingual**
*Acute attack.*
2.5–5 mg q 2–3 hr as required. The dose can be titrated upward until angina is relieved or side effects occur.
*Prophylaxis.*
5–10 mg q 2–3 hr.

## NURSING CONSIDERATIONS

See also *Nursing Considerations* for *Antianginal Drugs, Nitrates/Nitrites.*
**Client/Family Teaching**
1. Administer with meals to eliminate or reduce headaches; otherwise, take on an empty stomach to facilitate absorption.
2. Tolerance may develop. Short-acting products can be given b.i.d.–t.i.d. with the last dose no later than 7:00 p.m. while the extended-release products can be given once daily or twice daily at 8:00 a.m. and 2:00 p.m.
3. None of the products should be crushed or chewed, unless specifically ordered.
4. Review appropriate method for administration; do not chew sublingual tablets.
5. Chewable tablets should be held in the mouth for 1–2 min; allows absorption through buccal membranes.
6. Avoid alcohol or alcohol-containing products.
7. Acetaminophen may assist to relieve drug-induced headaches.
**Outcomes/Evaluate**
• ↓ Frequency and severity of anginal attacks
• ↑ Exercise tolerance

• Resolution of esophageal spasm

# Isosorbide mononitrate, oral

(eye-so-**SOR**-byd)
**Pregnancy Category:** C
Imdur, ISMO, Monoket **(Rx)**
**Classification:** Coronary vasodilator, antianginal drug

See also *Antianginal Drugs, Nitrates/Nitrites,* and *Isosorbide Dinitrate.*
**Action/Kinetics:** Isosorbide mononitrate is the major metabolite of isosorbide dinitrate. The mononitrate is not subject to first-pass metabolism. Bioavailability is nearly 100%. **Onset:** 30–60 min. **t½:** About 5 hr.
**Uses:** Prophylaxis of angina pectoris.
**Contraindications:** To abort acute anginal attacks. Use in acute MI or CHF.
**Special Concerns:** Use with caution in clients who may be volume depleted or who are already hypotensive. Use with caution during lactation. Safety and effectiveness have not been determined in children. The benefits have not been established in acute MI or CHF.
**Side Effects:** *CV:* Hypotension (may be accompanied by paradoxical bradycardia and increased angina pectoris). *CNS:* Headache, lightheadedness, dizziness. *GI:* N&V. *Miscellaneous:* Possibility of methemoglobinemia.
**OD** **Overdose Management:** *Symptoms:* Increased intracranial pressure manifested by throbbing headache, confusion, moderate fever. Also, vertigo, palpitations, visual disturbances, N&V, syncope, air hunger, dyspnea (followed by reduced ventilatory effort), diaphoresis, skin either flushed or cold and clammy, heart block, bradycardia, paralysis, ***coma, seizures, death.*** *Treatment:* Therapy should be directed toward an increase in central fluid volume. Vasoconstrictors should *not* be used.
**Drug Interactions**
*Ethanol* / Additive vasodilation

*Calcium channel blockers* / Severe orthostatic hypotension
*Organic nitrates* / Severe orthostatic hypotension

**Dosage** ⎯⎯⎯⎯⎯⎯⎯⎯⎯
IMDUR TABLETS
   *Prophylaxis of angina.*
**Initial:** 30 mg (given as one-half of the 60-mg tablet) or 60 mg once daily; **then,** dosage may be increased to 120 mg given as 2–60-mg tablets once daily. Rarely, 240 mg daily may be needed.
ISMO, MONOKET TABLETS
   *Prevention and treatment of angina.*
**Adults:** 20 mg b.i.d. with the doses 7 hr apart (it is preferable that first dose be given on awakening). An initial dose of 5 mg may be best for clients of small stature; the dose should then be increased to at least 10 mg by the second or third day of therapy.

## NURSING CONSIDERATIONS

See also *Nursing Considerations* for *Antianginal Drugs, Nitrates/Nitrites,* and *Isosorbide Dinitrate.*
**Administration/Storage**
1. The treatment regimen minimizes the development of refractory tolerance.
2. Give extended-release tablet in the morning on arising. Do not crush or chew; take with a half glass of water.
**Client/Family Teaching**
1. Consume 1–2 L/day of fluids to ensure adequate hydration.
2. Drug may cause marked hypotension.
3. Report if angina persists or recurs.
**Outcomes/Evaluate:** Angina prophylaxis

## Isotretinoin
(eye-so-**TRET**-ih-noyn)
**Pregnancy Category:** X
Accutane, Accutane Roche ✷,
Isotrex ✷ **(Rx)**

**Classification:** Vitamin A metabolite (antiacne, keratinization stabilizer)

**Action/Kinetics:** Reduces sebaceous gland size, decreases sebum secretion, and inhibits abnormal keratinization. Approximately 25% of the PO dosage form is bioavailable. **Peak plasma levels:** 3 hr. **Steady-state blood levels following 80 mg/day:** 160 ng/mL. Nearly 100% bound to plasma protein. **t½:** 10–20 hr. Metabolized in the liver to 4-oxo-isotretinoin, which is also active. Approximately equal amounts are excreted through the urine and in the feces.
**Uses:** Severe recalcitrant cystic acne unresponsive to other therapy. *Investigational:* Cutaneous disorders of keratinization, cutaneous T-cell lymphoma (mycosis fungoides), leukoplakia, prevention of secondary primary tumors in those treated for squamous-cell carcinoma of the head and neck.
**Contraindications:** Due to the possibility of fetal abnormalities or spontaneous abortion, women who are pregnant or intend to become pregnant should not use the drug. Certain conditions for use should be met in women with childbearing potential (see package insert). Use during lactation and in children.
**Special Concerns:** Intolerance to contact lenses may develop.
**Side Effects:** *Skin:* Cheilitis, skin fragility, pruritus, dry skin, desquamation of facial skin, drying of mucous membranes, brittle nails, photosensitivity, rash, hypo- or hyperpigmentation, urticaria, erythema nodosum, hirsutism, excess granulation of tissues as a result of healing, petechiae, peeling of palms and soles, skin infections, paronychia, thinning of hair, nail dystrophy, pyogenic granuloma, bruising. *CNS:* Headache, fatigue, pseudotumor cerebri (i.e., headaches, papilledema, disturbances in vision), depression. *Ocular:* Conjunctivitis, optic neuritis, corneal opacities, dry eyes, decrease in acuity of night vision, photophobia,

eyelid inflammation, cataracts, visual disturbances. *GI:* Dry mouth, N&V, abdominal pain, nonspecific GI symptoms, inflammatory bowel disease (including regional enteritis), anorexia, weight loss, inflammation and bleeding of gums. *Neuromuscular:* Arthralgia, muscle pain, bone and joint pain and stiffness, skeletal hyperostosis. *CV:* Flushing, palpitation, tachycardia. *GU:* White cells in urine, proteinuria, nonspecific urogenital findings, microscopic or gross hematuria, abnormal menses. *Other:* Epistaxis, dry nose and mouth, respiratory infections, disseminated herpes simplex, edema, transient chest pain, development of diabetes, hepatitis, hepatotoxicity, vasculitis, anemia, lymphadenopathy, flushing, palpitations.

**OD** **Overdose Management:** *Symptoms:* Abdominal pain, ataxia, cheilosis, dizziness, facial flushing, headache, vomiting. Symptoms are transient. *Treatment:* Symptoms are quickly resolved with drug cessation or decrease in dose.

**Drug Interactions**
*Alcohol* / Potentiation of ↑ in serum triglycerides
*Benzoyl peroxide* / ↑ Drying effects of isotretinoin
*Carbamazepine* / ↓ Carbamazepine plasma levels
*Minocycline* / ↑ Risk of development of pseudotumor cerebri or papilledema
*Tetracycline* / ↑ Risk of development of pseudotumor cerebri or papilledema
*Tretinoin* / ↑ Drying effects of isotretinoin
*Vitamin A* / ↑ Risk of toxicity
**Laboratory Test Interferences:** ↑ Plasma triglycerides, sedimentation rate, platelet counts, alkaline phosphatase, AST, ALT, GGTP, LDH, fasting blood glucose, uric acid in blood, cholesterol, CPK levels in clients who exercise vigorously. ↓ HDL, RBC parameters, WBC counts.

**Dosage**
• **Capsules**
*Recalcitrant cystic acne.*

**Adults, individualized, initial:** 0.5–1 mg/kg/day (range: 0.5–2 mg/kg/day) divided in two doses for 15–20 weeks. Adjust dose based on toxicity and clinical response; if cyst count decreases by 70% or more, drug may be discontinued. If necessary, a second course of therapy may be instituted after a rest period of 2 months. Doses of 0.05–0.5 mg/kg/day are effective but result in higher frequency of relapses.

*Keratinization disorders.*
Doses up to 4 mg/kg/day have been used.

*Prevent second tumors in squamous-cell carcinoma of the head and neck.*
50–100 mg/m².

## NURSING CONSIDERATIONS
### Administration/Storage
1. Do not crush capsules.
2. To enhance absorption, administer with meals.
3. Before using drug, have client complete consent form included with the package insert.
4. A rest period of 2 months is recommended if a second course of therapy is needed.

### Assessment
1. Document clinical presentation; photos may help.
2. Perform a pregnancy test on all sexually active women of childbearing age.
3. Determine other agents used and the outcome.
4. Monitor serum glucose levels, chemistry, CBC, urinalysis, and liver function studies, especially lipoprotein, cholesterol, and triglycerides.

### Client/Family Teaching
1. Avoid donating blood for 30 days after drug therapy has been discontinued.
2. A pregnancy test will be performed monthly because drug is teratogenic. Females of childbearing age should practice reliable birth control 1 month before, during, and 1 month following therapy; severe fetal damage may occur.
3. A 30-day prescription will be dispensed to ensure compliance.

4. Report if a persistent headache, N&V, or visual disturbances develop.

5. Clients who wear contact lenses may develop sensitivity to contacts during and after therapy. Excessively dry eyes may require an eye lubricant.

6. Condition may become worse before healing starts.

7. Avoid any OTC medications, especially vitamin A, without approval.

8. Eliminate or markedly reduce consumption of alcohol; may increase triglyceride levels.

9. Avoid prolonged sunlight exposure; may cause photosensitivity. Wear protective clothing, sunscreen, and sunglasses when exposed.

10. Lubricants may assist to diminish symptoms of dry, chapped skin and lips.

**Outcomes/Evaluate:** ↓ Severity/number of cystic acne lesions

---

# Isradipine
(iss-**RAD**-ih-peen)
**Pregnancy Category:** C
DynaCirc, DynaCirc CR **(Rx)**
**Classification:** Calcium channel blocking agent

---

See also *Calcium Channel Blocking Agents.*

**Action/Kinetics:** Binds to calcium channels resulting in the inhibition of calcium influx into cardiac and smooth muscle and subsequent arteriolar vasodilation. Reduced systemic resistance leads to a decrease in BP with a small increase in resting HR. In clients with normal ventricular function, the drug reduces afterload leading to some increase in CO. Well absorbed from the GI tract, although it undergoes significant first-pass metabolism. **Peak plasma levels:** 1 ng/mL after 1.5 hr. **Onset:** 2–3 hr. Food increases the time to peak effect by about 1 hr, although the total bioavailability does not change. **t½, initial:** 1.5–2 hr; **terminal,** 8 hr. Completely metabolized in the liver with 60%–65%

excreted through the kidneys and 25%–30% through the feces. Maximum effect may not be observed for 2–4 wks.

**Uses:** Alone or with thiazide diuretics in the management of essential hypertension. *Investigational:* Chronic stable angina.

**Contraindications:** Lactation.

**Special Concerns:** Safety and effectiveness have not been determined in children. Use with caution in clients with CHF, especially those taking a beta-adrenergic blocking agent. Bioavailability increases in those over 65 years of age, in impaired hepatic function, and in mild renal impairment.

**Side Effects:** *CV:* Palpitations, edema, flushing, tachycardia, SOB, hypotension, transient ischemic attack, *stroke,* atrial fibrillation, *ventricular fibrillation, MI,* CHF, angina. *CNS:* Headache, dizziness, fatigue, drowsiness, insomnia, lethargy, nervousness, depression, syncope, amnesia, psychosis, hallucinations, weakness, jitteriness, paresthesia. *GI:* Nausea, abdominal discomfort, diarrhea, vomiting, constipation, dry mouth. *Respiratory:* Dyspnea, cough. *Dermatologic:* Pruritus, urticaria. *Miscellaneous:* Chest pain, rash, pollakiuria, cramps of the legs and feet, nocturia, polyuria, hyperhidrosis, visual disturbances, numbness, throat discomfort, leukopenia, sexual difficulties.

**Drug Interactions:** Severe hypotension has been observed during fentanyl anesthesia with concomitant use of a beta-blocker and a calcium channel blocking agent.

**Laboratory Test Interferences:** ↑ Liver function tests.

**Dosage** ———————————
• **Capsules**
*Hypertension.*
**Adults, initial:** 2.5 mg b.i.d. alone or in combination with a thiazide diuretic. If BP is not decreased satisfactorily after 2–4 weeks, the dose may be increased in increments of 5

mg/day at 2 to 4-week intervals up to a maximum of 20 mg/day. Adverse effects increase, however, at doses above 10 mg/day.
- **Tablets, Controlled-Release**
  *Hypertension.*
  **Adults:** 5–10 mg once daily.

## NURSING CONSIDERATIONS

See *Nursing Considerations* for *Calcium Channel Blocking Agents*.
**Administration/Storage:** Store in a tight container protected from light.
**Client/Family Teaching**
1. Use caution, may cause dizziness and confusion; assess drug effects.
2. Report for scheduled lab tests: liver and renal function studies every 3–6 months.
**Outcomes/Evaluate:** ↓ BP; control of hypertension

# Itraconazole
(ih-trah-**KON**-ah-zohl)
**Pregnancy Category:** C
Sporanox **(Rx)**
**Classification:** Antifungal

**Action/Kinetics:** Believed to inhibit cytochrome P-450-dependent synthesis of ergosterol, a necessary component of fungal cell membranes. Absorption appears to increase when taken with a cola beverage. Concentrates in fatty tissues, omentum, liver, kidney, and skin. **t½, at steady-state:** 64 hr. Extensively metabolized by the liver; the major metabolite is hydroxyitraconazole, which also has antifungal activity. The drug and major metabolite are extensively bound (over 99%) to plasma proteins. Metabolites are excreted in both the urine and feces.
**Uses:** Treatment of blastomycosis (pulmonary and extrapulmonary) and histoplasmosis (including chronic cavitary pulmonary disease and disseminated, nonmeningeal histoplasmosis) in both immunocompromised and nonimmunocompromised clients. To treat aspergillus infections (pulmonary and extrapulmonary) in clients intolerant or refractory to amphotericin B. Ony-

chomycosis due to tinea unguium of the toenail with or without fingernail involvement. The drug is effective against *Blastomyces dermatitidis, Histoplasma capsulatum* and *H. duboisii, Aspergillus flavus* and *A. fumigatis,* and *Cryptococcus neoformans.* Oropharyngeal and esophageal candidiasis. In vitro activity has also been found for a number of other organisms, including *Sporothirx scheneckii, Trochophyton* species, *Candida albicans,* and *Candida* species. *Investigational:* (1) Superficial mycoses including dermatophytoses (tinea capitis, tinea corporis, tinea cruris, tinea pedis, and tinea manuum), pityriasis versicolor, candidiasis (vaginal, oral, chronic mucocutaneous), and sebopsoriasis. (2) Systemic mycoses including dimorphic infections (paracoccidioidomycosis, coccidioidomycosis), cryptococcal infections (meningitis, disseminated), and candidiasis. (3) Miscellaneous mycoses including fungal keratitis, alternariosis, leishmaniasis (cutaneous), subcutaneous mycoses (chromomycosis, sporotrichosis), and zygomycosis.
**Contraindications:** Concomitant use of astemizole, cisapride, triazolam, oral midazolam, or terfenadine. Hypersensitivity to the drug or its excipients. Lactation. Use for the treatment of onychomycosis in pregnant women or in women wishing to become pregnant.
**Special Concerns:** Safety and efficacy have not been determined in children although pediatric clients have been treated for systemic fungal infections.
**Side Effects:** *GI:* N&V, diarrhea, abdominal pain, anorexia, general GI disorders, flatulence, constipation, gastritis. *CNS:* Headache, dizziness, vertigo, insomnia, decreased libido, somnolence, depression. *CV:* Hypertension, orthostatic hypotension, vasculitis. *Dermatologic:* Rash (occurs more frequently in immunocompromised clients also taking immunosuppressant drugs), pruritus. *Allergic:* Rash, pruritus, urticaria,

angioedema, and rarely, **anaphylaxis and Stevens-Johnson syndrome.** *Miscellaneous:* Edema, fatigue, fever, malaise, abnormal hepatic function, hypokalemia, albuminuria, tinnitus, impotence, adrenal insufficiency, gynecomastia, breast pain in males, menstrual disorder, hepatitis (rare), neuropathy (rare).

**OD** **Overdose Management:** *Symptoms:* Extension of side effects. *Treatment:* Use supportive measures, including gastric lavage and sodium bicarbonate. Dialysis will not remove itraconazole.

**Drug Interactions**
*Astemizole* / ↑ Astemizole levels → serious CV toxicity including ventricular tachycardia, torsades de pointes, and death.
*Calcium blockers (especially amlodipine and nifedipine)* / Development of edema
*Cisapride* / Cisapride levels serious CV toxicity including ventricular tachycardia, torsades de pointes, and death.
*Cyclosporine and HMG-CoA reductase inhibitors* / Possible development of rhabdomyolysis. ↑ Cyclosporine levels (dose of cyclosporine should be ↓ by 50% if itraconazole doses are much greater than 100 mg/day)
*Digoxin* / ↑ Digoxin levels
*H₂ Antagonists* / ↓ Plasma levels of itraconazole
*Midazolam, oral* / ↑ Levels of oral midazolam → potentiation of sedative and hypnotic effects
*Isoniazid* / ↓ Plasma levels of itraconazole
*Phenytoin* / ↓ Plasma levels of itraconazole; also, metabolism of phenytoin may be altered
*Rifampin* / ↓ Plasma levels of itraconazole
*Quinidine* / Tinnitus and decreased hearing
*Sulfonylureas* / ↑ Risk of hypoglycemia
*Tacrolimus* / ↑ Levels of tacrolimus

*Terfenadine* / ↑ Terfenadine levels → serious CV toxicity including ventricular tachycardia, torsades de pointes, and death
*Triazolam* / Levels of triazolam potentiation of sedative and hypnotic effects
*Warfarin* / ↑ Anticoagulant effect of warfarin
**Laboratory Test Interferences:** Liver enzymes

**Dosage**
• **Capsules**
   *Blastomycosis or histoplasmosis.*
**Adults:** 200 mg once daily. If there is no improvement or the disease is progressive, the dose may be increased in 100-mg increments to a maximum of 400 mg/day. **Children, 3–16 years of age:** 100 mg/day (for systemic fungal infections).
   *Aspergilliosis.*
200–400 mg daily.
   *Life-threatening infections.*
**Adults:** A loading dose of 200 mg t.i.d. for the first 3 days should be given.
   *Onychomycosis.*
200 mg once a day for 12 consecutive weeks. Alternatively, for fingernail fungus, 200 mg b.i.d. for 1 week, followed by a 3-week rest and then a second 1-week pulse of 200 mg b.i.d.
   *Unlabeled uses.*
**Adults:** 50–400 mg/day for 1 day to more than 6 months, depending on the condition and the response.
• **Oral Solution**
   *Oropharyngeal candidiasis.*
200 mg/day for 1–2 weeks.
   *Esophageal candidiasis.*
100 mg/day for a minimum of 3 weeks.

**NURSING CONSIDERATIONS**
**Administration/Storage**
1. Take with food to ensure maximal absorption.
2. Give daily doses greater than 200 mg in two divided doses.
3. Continue treatment for a mini-

---

mum of 3 months until symptoms and lab tests indicate the active fungal infection has subsided. Recurrence of active infection may occur if there is an inadequate treatment period.

**Assessment**

1. Document indications for therapy, onset, duration of symptoms, and other agents prescribed, noting compliance and outcome. Drug is extremely expensive and should not generally be considered first-line therapy with typical fungal infections.

2. List drugs currently prescribed to prevent any unfavorable effects.

3. Monitor CBC, electrolytes, fungal cultures/scrapings, liver and renal function studies.

4. Drug is not intended for pregnant or nursing mothers.

5. The response rate of histoplasmosis in HIV-infected clients is similar to non-HIV-infected clients, although the clinical course of histoplasmosis in HIV-infected clients is more severe and usually requires maintenance therapy to prevent relapse.

6. Absorption may be decreased in HIV-infected clients with hypochlorhydria.

**Client/Family Teaching**

1. Take with food to enhance absorption and only as directed (usually for 3 months). Noncompliance or inadequate periods of treatment may lead to a recurrence of active infection.

2. Report any S&S that may suggest liver dysfunction; i.e., anorexia, unusual fatigue, N&V, diarrhea, yellow skin/eyes, dark urine, and pale stool.

3. Report symptoms that may indicate reactivation of histoplasmosis, such as weight loss, chest pain, SOB, fever, rales, and pain.

4. S&S of blastomycosis include SOB, rales, hemoptysis, chest pain, fever, cough, skin lesions, rashes, and weight loss; requires immediate attention.

**Outcomes/Evaluate:** Eradication of infecting organisms; symptom relief

# Ivermectin

(eye-ver-**MEK**-tin)
**Pregnancy Category:** C
Stromectol **(Rx)**
**Classification:** Anthelmintic

See also *Anthelmintics.*

**Action/Kinetics:** Binds selectively to glutamate-gated chloride channels that occur in invertebrate nerve and muscle cells. This leads to increase in permeability of cell membrane to chloride ions and hyperpolarization of nerve or muscle cell, resulting in paralysis and death of parasite. **Peak plasma levels:** About 4 hr. t½: About 19 hr. Metabolized in liver and excreted through feces.

**Uses:** Intestinal strongyloidiasis due to *Strongyloides stercoralis.* Onchocerciasis due to *Onchocerca volvulus.*

**Special Concerns:** Use during lactation only if benefits outweigh risks. Those with hyperreactive onchodermatitis (sowdah) may be more likely to have severe side effects. Control of extraintestinal strongyloidiasis is difficult in immunocompromised clients.

**Side Effects: When used to treat strongyloidiasis.** *GI:* Diarrhea, nausea, anorexia, constipation, vomiting, abdominal pain. *CNS:* Dizziness, somnolence, tremor, vertigo. *Dermatologic:* Pruritus, rash, urticaria. *Miscellaneous:* Asthenia, fatigue.

**When used to treat onchocerciasis.** *Mazzotti reaction:* Pruritus, edema, papular and pustular or frank urticarial rash, fever, inguinal lymph node enlargement and tenderness, axillary lymph node enlargement and tenderness, arthralgia, synovitis, cervical lymph node enlargement and tenderness. *Ophthalmic:* Limbitis, punctate opacity, abnormal sensation in the eyes, anterior uveitis, chorioretinitis, chorioiditis, conjunctivitis, eyelid edema, keratitis. *Miscellaneous:* Tachycardia, peripheral edema, facial edema, orthostatic hypotension, headache, myalgia, worsening of bronchial asthma.

**OD** **Overdose Management:** *Symptoms:* Asthenia, diarrhea, dizziness, edema, headache, nausea, rash, vomiting, abdominal pain, ataxia, dyspnea, paresthesia, seizure, urticaria. *Treatment:* Supportive therapy, including parenteral fluids and electrolytes, respiratory support, and pressor agents (if significant hypotension). Induce emesis or gastric lavage as soon as possible, followed by laxatives and other antipoison measures.

**Laboratory Test Interferences:** ↑ ALT, AST, hemoglobin. ↓ Leukocyte count. Eosinophilia.

**Dosage**

• **Tablets**

*Strongyloidiasis.*

Single oral dose to provide about 200 mcg/kg: **15–24 kg:** 0.5 tablet; **25–35 kg:** 1 tablet; **36–50 kg:** 1.5 tablets; **51–65 kg:** 2 tablets; **66–79 kg:** 2.5 tablets.

*Onchocerciasis.*

Single oral dose to provide about 150 mcg/kg: **15–25 kg:** 0.5 tablet; **26–44 kg:** 1 tablet; **45–64 kg:** 1.5 tablets; **65–84 kg:** 2 tablets.

## NURSING CONSIDERATIONS

See also *Nursing Considerations for Anthelmintics.*

**Administration/Storage**

1. For either use, take with water.
2. For strongyloidiasis, perform follow-up stool examinations to verify eradication of infection.
3. For onchocerciasis, consider retreatment at intervals as short as 3 months.

**Assessment:** Determine date of parasite exposure, characteristics of symptons, and lab confirmation of parasitic nematode.

**Client/Family Teaching**

1. Take as directed with a full glass of water.
2. Report if abdominal pain, chest discomfort, severe rash, joint inflammation, or vision alterations occur.
3. Must bring consecutive F/U stool specimens to lab to verify eradication of strongyloides parasite. With onchocerciasis, the adult parasite is not killed, thus retreatment is usually required.

**Outcomes/Evaluate:** Control/eradication of extraintestinal strongyloidiasis/onchocerciasis

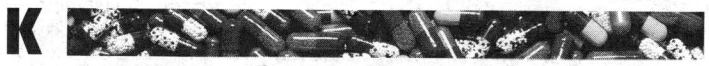

# Kanamycin sulfate

(kan-ah-**MY**-sin)

**Pregnancy Category:** D

Kantrex, Klebcil **(Rx)**

**Classification:** Aminoglycoside antibiotic and antitubercular agent (tertiary)

See also *Anti-Infectives* and *Aminoglycosides.*

**Action/Kinetics:** Activity resembles that of neomycin and streptomycin. **Peak therapeutic serum levels: IM,** 15–40 mcg/mL. t½: 2–3 hr. Toxic serum levels: >35 mcg/mL (peak) and >10 mcg/mL (trough).

**Uses: Parenteral:** As initial therapy for infections due to *Escherichia coli, Proteus, Enterobacter aerogenes, Klebsiella pneumoniae, Serratia marcescens,* and *Acinetobacter.* May be combined with a penicillin or cephalosporin before knowing results of susceptibility tests. *Investigational:* As part of a multiple-drug regimen for *Mycobacterium avium* complex in AIDS clients.

**PO:** As an adjunct to mechanical cleansing of large bowel for suppression of intestinal bacteria; hepatic coma.

**Special Concerns:** Use with caution in premature infants and neonates.

**Additional Side Effects:** Sprue-like syndrome with steatorrhea, malabsorption, and electrolyte imbalance.

**Additional Drug Interactions:** Procainamide ↑ muscle relaxation.

## Dosage

• **Capsules**

*Intestinal bacteria suppression.*

1 g every hour for 4 hr; **then,** 1 g q 6 hr for 36–72 hr.

*Hepatic coma.*

8–12 g/day in divided doses.

• **IM, IV**

**Adults and children:** 15 mg/kg/day in two to three equal doses. Maximum daily dose should not exceed 1.5 g regardless of route of administration.

For calculating dosage interval (in hr) in clients with impaired renal function, multiply serum creatinine (mg/100 mL) by 9.

• **IM**

*Tuberculosis.*

**Adults:** 15 mg/kg/day. Not recommended for use in children.

• **Intraperitoneal**

500 mg diluted in 20 mL sterile distilled water.

• **Inhalation**

250 mg in saline—nebulize b.i.d.–q.i.d.

*Irrigation of abscess cavities, pleural space, ventricular cavities.*

0.25% solution.

## NURSING CONSIDERATIONS

See also *General Nursing Considerations for All Anti-Infectives* and *Aminoglycosides.*

**Assessment:** Document indications for therapy, onset, duration, and characteristics of symptoms; reduce dose with renal dysfunction.

**Outcomes/Evaluate**

• Negative culture reports
• Desired bowel cleansing

---

# Ketoconazole

(kee-toe-**KON**-ah-zohl)

**Pregnancy Category:** C

Nizoral **(Rx)**., Nizoral AD **(OTC)**

**Classification:** Broad-spectrum antifungal

---

See also *Anti-Infectives.*

**Action/Kinetics:** Inhibits synthesis of sterols (e.g., ergosterol), damaging the cell membrane and resulting in loss of essential intracellular material. Also inhibits biosynthesis of triglycerides and phospholipids and inhibits oxidative and peroxidative enzyme activity. When used to treat *Candida albicans,* it inhibits transformation of blastospores into the invasive mycelial form. Use in Cushing's syndrome is due to its ability to inhibit adrenal steroidogenesis.

**Peak plasma levels:** 3.5 mcg/mL after 1–2 hr after a 200-mg dose. t½ [biphasic]: first, 2 hr; second, 8 hr. Requires acidity for dissolution. Metabolized in liver to inactive metabolites and most excreted through feces.

**Uses: PO:** Candidiasis, chronic mucocutaneous candidiasis, candiduria, histoplasmosis, chromomycosis, oral thrush, blastomycosis, coccidioidomycosis, paracoccidioidomycosis. Recalcitrant cutaneous dermatophyte infections not responding to other therapy. **Cream:** Tinea pedis. Tinea corporis and tinea cruris due to *Trichophyton rubrum, T. mentagrophytes,* and *Epidermophyton floccosum.* Tinea versicolor caused by *Microsporum furfur;* cutaneous candidiasis caused by *Candida* species; seborrheic dermatitis. **Shampoo:** To reduce scaling due to dandruff and tinea versicolor. *Investigational:* Onychomycosis due to *Candida* and *Trichophyton.* High doses to treat CNS fungal infections. Advanced prostate cancer, Cushing's syndrome.

**Contraindications:** Hypersensitivity, fungal meningitis. Topical product not for ophthalmic use. Use during lactation.

**Special Concerns:** Use tablets with caution in children less than 2 years of age. The safety and effectiveness of the shampoo and cream have not been determined in children. Use with caution during lactation.

**Side Effects:** *GI:* N&V, abdominal pain, diarrhea. *CNS:* Headache, dizziness, somnolence, fever, chills. *Hematologic:* Thrombocytopenia, leukopenia, **hemolytic anemia.** *Miscellaneous:* Hepatotoxicity, photophobia, pruritus, gynecomastia, impotence, bulging fontanelles, urticaria, decreased serum testosterone levels, anaphylaxis (rare). *Topical cream:* Stinging, irritation, pruritus. *Shampoo:* Increased hair loss, irritation, abnormal hair texture, itching, oiliness or dryness of the scalp and hair, scalp pustules.

**Drug Interactions**

*Antacids* / ↓ Absorption of ketoconazole due to ↑ pH induced by these drugs

*Anticoagulants* / ↓ Effect of anticoagulants

*Anticholinergics* / ↓ Absorption of ketoconazole due to ↑ pH induced by these drugs

*Astemizole* / ↑ Plasma levels of astemizole → serious CV effects

*Corticosteroids* / ↑ Risk of corticosteroid toxicity due to ↑ bioavailability

*Cyclosporine* / ↑ Levels of cyclosporine (may be used therapeutically to decrease the dose of cyclosporine)

*Histamine H₂ antagonists* / ↓ Absorption of ketoconazole due to ↑ pH induced by these drugs

*Isoniazid* / ↓ Bioavailability of ketoconazole

*Rifampin* / ↓ Serum levels of both drugs

*Terfenadine* / ↑ Plasma levels of terfenadine → serious CV effects

*Theophyllines* / ↓ Serum levels of theophylline

**Laboratory Test Interferences:** Transient ↑ serum liver enzymes. ↓ Serum testosterone.

**Dosage** ──────────

• **Tablets**

*Fungal infections.*

**Adults:** 200–400 mg once daily. **Pe-** diatric, over 2 years: 3.3–6.6 mg/kg once daily.

*CNS fungal infections.*

**Adults:** 800–1,200 mg/day.

*Advanced prostate cancer.*

400 mg q 8 hr.

*Cushing's syndrome.*

800–1,200 mg/day.

• **Topical Cream (2%)**

*Tinea corporis, tinea cruris, tinea versicolor, tinea pedis, cutaneous candidiasis.*

Cover the affected and immediate surrounding areas once daily (twice daily for more resistant cases). Duration of treatment is usually 2 weeks.

*Seborrheic dermatitis.*

Apply to affected area b.i.d. for 4 weeks or until symptoms clear.

• **Shampoo (1%, 2%)**

Use twice a week for 4 weeks with at least 3 days between each shampooing. **Then,** use as required to maintain control.

## NURSING CONSIDERATIONS

See also *General Nursing Considerations for All Anti-Infectives.*

**Administration/Storage**

1. Give a minimum of 2 hr before administration of drugs that increase gastric pH (such as antacids, anticholinergics, or H₂ blockers). If antacids needed, delay administration by 2 hr.

2. The minimum treatment for candidiasis (using tablets) is 1–2 weeks and for other systemic mycoses is 6 months.

**Client/Family Teaching**

1. Take tablets with food to decrease GI upset. Take 2 hr before drugs that alter gastric pH.

2. Apply shampoo to wet hair in sufficient quantities to cover the entire scalp for 1 min. Rinse with warm water; repeat, leaving shampoo on the scalp for 3 min. After the second washing, rinse thoroughly and dry hair with towel or warm air flow.

3. Report persistent fever, pain, or diarrhea.

4. With lack of stomach acid, dis-

**K**

---

*bold italic* = life threatening side effect

solve each tablet in 4 mL aqueous solution of 0.2 N HCl; use a straw to avoid contact with teeth. This is followed by drinking a glass of tap water.

5. Use caution when driving or when performing hazardous tasks; may cause headaches, dizziness, and drowsiness.

6. Avoid alcohol or alcohol-containing products.

7. Wear sunglasses, sunscreen, and protective clothing, avoid sun exposure to prevent photosensitivity reactions.

### Outcomes/Evaluate
• Eradication of fungal infections
• Control of dandruff with ↓ scaling

# Ketoprofen
(kee-toe-**PROH**-fen)
**Pregnancy Category: B**
**Rx:** Apo-Keto ✼, Apo-Keto-E ✼, Apo-Keto-SR ✼, Novo-Keto ✼, Novo-Keto-EC ✼, Nu-Ketoprofen ✼, Nu-Ketoprofen-E ✼, Orafen ✼, Orudis, Orudis-E ✼, Orudis-SR ✼, Oruvail, PMS-Ketoprofen ✼, PMS-Ketoprofen-E ✼, Rhodis ✼, Rhodis-EC ✼, Rhodis SR ✼, Rhovail ✼, **OTC:** Actron, Orudis KT.
**Classification:** Nonsteroidal anti-inflammatory drug

See also *Nonsteroidal Anti-Inflammatory Drugs.*

**Action/Kinetics:** Possesses anti-inflammatory, antipyretic, and analgesic properties. Known to inhibit both prostaglandin and leukotriene synthesis, to have antibradykinin activity, and to stabilize lysosomal membranes. **Onset:** 15–30 min. **Peak plasma levels:** 0.5–2 hr. **Duration:** 4–6 hr. **t½:** 2–4 hr. **t½, geriatrics:** Approximately 5 hr. Is 99% bound to plasma proteins. Food does not alter the bioavailability; however, the rate of absorption is reduced.

**Uses: Rx:** Acute or chronic rheumatoid arthritis and osteoarthritis (both capsules and sustained-release capsules). Primary dysmenorrhea. Analgesic for mild to moderate pain.

**OTC:** Temporary relief of aches and pains associated with the common cold, toothache, headache, muscle aches, backache, menstrual cramps, reduction of fever, and minor pain of arthritis.

*Investigational:* Juvenile rheumatoid arthritis, sunburn, prophylaxis of migraine, migraine due to menses.

**Contraindications:** Should not be used during late pregnancy. Use should be avoided during lactation and in children. Use of the extended-release product for acute pain.

**Special Concerns:** Safety and effectiveness have not been established in children. Geriatric clients may manifest increased and prolonged serum levels due to decreased protein binding and clearance. Use with caution in clients with a history of GI tract disorders, in fluid retention, hypertension, and heart failure.

**Additional Side Effects:** *GI:* Peptic ulcer, **GI bleeding,** dyspepsia, nausea, diarrhea, constipation, abdominal pain, flatulence, anorexia, vomiting, stomatitis. *CNS:* Headache. *CV:* Peripheral edema, fluid retention.

**Additional Drug Interactions**
*Acetylsalicylic acid* / ↑ Plasma ketoprofen levels due to ↓ plasma protein binding
*Hydrochlorothiazide* / ↓ Chloride and potassium excretion
*Methotrexate* / Concomitant use → toxic plasma levels of methotrexate
*Probenecid* / ↓ Plasma clearance of ketoprofen and ↓ plasma protein binding
*Warfarin* / Additive effect to cause bleeding

### Dosage
• **Rx: Extended Release Capsules, Capsules**
*Rheumatoid arthritis, osteoarthritis.*
**Adults, initial:** 75 mg t.i.d. or 50 mg q.i.d.; **maintenance:** 150–300 mg in three to four divided doses daily. Doses above 300 mg/day are not recommended. Alternatively, 200 mg once daily using the sustained-release formulation (Oruvail). Dosage should be decreased by one-half to one-third in clients with impaired renal function or in geriatric clients.

*Mild to moderate pain, dysmenorrhea.*

**Adults:** 25–50 mg q 6–8 hr as required, not to exceed 300 mg/day. Dosage should be reduced in smaller or geriatric clients and in those with liver or renal dysfunction. Doses greater than 75 mg do not provide any added therapeutic effect.

• **OTC: Tablets**

**Adults, over 16 years of age:** 12.5 mg with a full glass of liquid every 4 to 6 hr. If pain or fever persists after 1 hr follow with an additional 12.5 mg. Experience may determine that an initial dose of 25 mg gives a better effect. Dosage should not exceed 25 mg in a 4- to 6-hr period or 75 mg in a 24-hr period.

## NURSING CONSIDERATIONS

See also *Nursing Considerations* for *Nonsteroidal Anti-Inflammatory Drugs.*

**Administration/Storage:** Do not use the sustained-release form to treat pain in any client or for initial therapy in clients who are small, elderly, or who have renal or hepatic impairment.

**Assessment**

1. Document indications for therapy, type, onset, location, intensity, and symptom characteristics.

2. Note history of GI disorders, cardiac failure, hypertension, or fluid retention.

3. Determine if pregnant; note age. Not for children under 12 years of age.

4. Monitor bleeding and hematologic profiles, liver and renal function studies. In high doses, may prolong bleeding times by decreasing platelet aggregation. Reduce dose in the elderly and those with impaired renal function.

**Client/Family Teaching**

1. GI side effects may be minimized by taking with antacids, milk, or food.

2. Avoid alcohol.

3. Do not take any aspirin products unless specifically prescribed.

4. Report any new symptoms such as rash, headaches, black stools, disturbances in vision, petechiae, unexplained bruising, bleeding from the gums, or nose bleeds.

5. Report any evidence of liver dysfunction such as fatigue, upper right quadrant pain, clay-colored stools, or yellowing of the skin and sclera.

**Outcomes/Evaluate**

• ↓ Joint pain, inflammation; ↑ mobility

• ↓ Uterine cramping

# Ketorolac tromethamine

(kee-toh-**ROH**-lack)

**Pregnancy Category:** C

Acular, Acular PF, Toradol, Toradol IM **(Rx)**

**Classification:** Nonsteroidal anti-inflammatory drug

See also *Nonsteroidal Anti-Inflammatory Drugs.*

**Action/Kinetics:** Possesses anti-inflammatory, analgesic, and antipyretic effects. Completely absorbed following IM use. **Onset:** Within 30 min. **Maximum effect:** 1–2 hr after IV or IM dosing. **Duration:** 4–6 hr. **Peak plasma levels:** 2.2–3.0 mcg/mL 50 min after a dose of 30 mg. **t½, terminal:** 3.8–6.3 hr in young adults and 4.7–8.6 hr in geriatric clients. Over 99% is bound to plasma proteins. Metabolized in the liver with over 90% excreted in the urine and the remainder excreted in the feces.

**Uses: PO:** Short-term (up to 5 days) management of severe, acute pain that requires analgesia at the opiate level. Always initiate therapy with IV or IM followed by PO only as continuation treatment, if necessary. **IM/IV:** Ketorolac has been used with morphine and meperidine and shows an opioid-sharing effect. The combination can be used for breakthrough pain. **Ophthalmic:** Relieve itching caused by seasonal allergic conjunctivitis. Reduce occular pain and photo phobia following incisional refractive surgery.

**K**

**Contraindications:** Hypersensitivity to the drug, incomplete or partial syndrome of nasal polyps, angioedema, and bronchospasm due to aspirin or other NSAIDs. Use in clients with advanced renal impairment or in those at risk for renal failure due to volume depletion. Use in suspected or confirmed cardiovascular bleeding, hemorrhagic diathesis, or incomplete hemostasis and in those with a high risk of bleeding. Use as an obstetric preoperative medication or for obstetric analgesia. Routine use with other NSAIDs. Intrathecal or epidural administration. Use in labor and delivery. The ophthalmic solution should not be used in clients wearing soft contact lenses.

**Special Concerns:** Use with caution in impaired hepatic or renal function, during lactation, in geriatric clients, and in clients on high-dose salicylate regimens. The age, dosage, and duration of therapy should receive special consideration when using this drug. Safety and effectiveness have not been determined in children.

**Additional Side Effects:** *CV:* Vasodilation, pallor. *GI:* GI pain, peptic ulcers, nausea, dyspepsia, flatulence, GI fullness, stomatitis, excessive thirst, GI bleeding (higher risk in geriatric clients), *perforation. CNS:* Headache, nervousness, abnormal thinking, depression, euphoria. *Hypersensitivity:* **Bronchospasm, anaphylaxis.** *Miscellaneous:* Purpura, asthma, abnormal vision, abnormal liver function.

*Use of the ophthalmic solution:* Transient stinging and burning following instillation, ocular irritation, allergic reactions, superficial ocular infections, superficial keratitis.

**Drug Interactions:** Ketorolac may ↑ plasma levels of salicylates due to ↓ plasma protein binding.

**Dosage** ————————
• **IM**
*Analgesic, single dose.*
**Adults: less than 65 years of age:** One 60-mg dose. **Adults, over 65 years of age, in renal impair-**ment, or weight less than 50 kg: One 30-mg dose.
*Analgesic, multiple dose.*
**Adults, less than 65 years of age:** 30 mg q 6 hr, not to exceed 120 mg daily. **Adults, over 65 years of age, in renal impairment, or weight less than 50 kg:** 15 mg q 6 hr, not to exceed 60 mg daily.
• **IV**
*Analgesic, single dose.*
**Adults, less than 65 years of age:** One 30-mg dose. **Adults, over 65 years of age, in renal impairment, or weight less than 50 kg:** One 15-mg dose.
• **Tablets**
*Transition from IV/IM to PO.*
**Adults less than 65 years of age:** 20 mg as a first PO dose for clients who received 60 mg IM single dose, 30 mg IV single dose, or 30 mg multiple dose IV/IM; **then,** 10 mg q 4–6 hr, not to exceed 40 mg in a 24-hr period. **Adults, over 65 years of age, in renal impairment, or weight less than 50 kg:** 10 mg as a first PO dose for those who received a 30-mg IM single dose, a 15-mg IV single dose, or a 15-mg multiple dose IV/IM; **then,** 10 mg q 4–6 hr, not to exceed 40 mg in a 24-hr period.
• **Ophthalmic Solution**
*Seasonal allergic conjunctivitis.*
1 gtt (0.25 mg) q.i.d. Efficacy has not been determined beyond 1 week of use.
*Following cataract extraction.*
1 gtt to the affected eye(s) q.i.d. beginning 24 hr after surgery and continuing for 2 weeks postoperatively.

## NURSING CONSIDERATIONS

See also *Nursing Considerations* for *Nonsteroidal Anti-Inflammatory Drugs.*
**Administration/Storage**
1. Use as part of a regular analgesic schedule rather than on an as needed basis.
2. If given on p.r.n. basis, base the size of a repeat dose on the duration of pain relief from the previous

dose. If the pain returns within 3–5 hr, the next dose could be increased by up to 50% (as long as the total daily dose is not exceeded). If the pain does not return for 8–12 hr, the next dose could be decreased by as much as 50% or the dosing interval could be increased to q 8–12 hr.

3. Shortening the dosing intervals recommended will lead to an increased frequency and duration of side effects.

4. Correct hypovolemia before the drug is given.

**IV** 5. Do not mix IV/IM ketorolac in a small volume (i.e., a syringe) with morphine sulfate, meperidine HCl, promethazine HCl, or hydroxyzine HCl as ketorolac will precipitate from solution.

6. When used IM/IV, the IV bolus must be given over no less than 15 sec. Give IM slowly and deeply into the muscle.

7. Protect the injection from light.

**Assessment**

1. Document indications for therapy, type, location, intensity, duration, and onset of symptoms.

2. Note any previous experience with this drug or NSAIDs and the results.

3. Determine any liver or renal dysfunction; assess hydration.

**Client/Family Teaching**

1. Take only as directed; do not exceed prescribed dosage. Report if symptoms unrelieved.

2. Drug may cause drowsiness and dizziness.

3. Avoid alcohol and all OTC agents without approval.

**Outcomes/Evaluate**

• Effective pain control

• ↓ Ocular allergic manifestations

**L**

# Labetalol hydrochloride

(lah-**BET**-ah-lohl)

**Pregnancy Category:** C

Normodyne, Trandate **(Rx)**

**Classification:** Alpha- and beta-adrenergic blocking agent

See also *Beta-Adrenergic Blocking Agents* and *Antihypertensive Agents*.

**Action/Kinetics:** Decreases BP by blocking both alpha- and beta-adrenergic receptors. Standing BP is lowered more than supine. Significant reflex tachycardia and bradycardia do not occur although AV conduction may be prolonged. **Onset: PO,** 2–4 hr; **IV,** 5 min. **Peak plasma levels, PO:** 1–2 hr. **Peak effects, PO:** 2–4 hr. **Duration: PO,** 8–12 hr. **t½: PO,** 6–8 hr; **IV,** 5.5 hr. Significant first-pass effect; metabolized in liver. Food increases bioavailability of the drug.

**Uses: PO:** Alone or in combination with other drugs for hypertension.

**IV:** Hypertensive emergencies. *Investigational:* Pheochromocytoma, clonidine withdrawal hypertension.

**Contraindications:** Cardiogenic shock, cardiac failure, bronchial asthma, bradycardia, greater than first-degree heart block.

**Special Concerns:** Use with caution during lactation, in impaired renal and hepatic function, in chronic bronchitis and emphysema, and in diabetes (may prevent premonitory signs of acute hypoglycemia). Safety and efficacy in children have not been established.

**Side Effects:** See also *Beta-Adrenergic Blocking Agents.* **After PO Use.** *GI:* Diarrhea, cholestasis with or without jaundice. *CNS:* Fatigue, drowsiness, paresthesias, headache, syncope (rare). *GU:* Impotence, priapism, ejaculation failure, difficulty in micturition, Peyronie's disease, acute urinary bladder retention. *Respiratory:* Dyspnea, bronchospasm. *Musculo-*

*bold italic* = life threatening side effect

*skeletal:* Muscle cramps, asthenia, toxic myopathy. *Dermatologic:* Generalized maculopapular, lichenoid, or urticarial rashes; bullous lichen planus, psoriasis, facial erythema, reversible alopecia. *Ophthalmic:* Abnormal vision, dry eyes. *Miscellaneous:* SLE, positive antinuclear factor, antimitochondrial antibiodies, fever, edema, nasal stuffiness.

**After parenteral use.** *CV:* Ventricular arrhythmias. *CNS:* Numbness, somnolence, yawning. *Miscellaneous:* Pruritus, flushing, wheezing.

**After PO or parenteral use.** *GI:* N&V, dyspepsia, taste distortion. *CNS:* Dizziness, tingling of skin or scalp, vertigo. *Miscellaneous:* Postural hypotension, increased sweating.

**OD** **Overdose Management:** *Symptoms:* Excessive hypotension and bradycardia. *Treatment:* Induce vomiting or perform gastric lavage. Clients should be placed in a supine position with legs elevated. If required, the following treatment can be used:

• Epinephrine or a beta-2 agonist (aerosol) to treat bronchospasm.

• Atropine or epinephrine to treat bradycardia.

• Digitalis glycoside and a diuretic for cardiac failure; dopamine or dobutamine may also be used.

• Diazepam to treat seizures.

• Norepinephrine (or another vasopressor) to treat hypotension.

• Administration of glucagon (5–10 mg rapidly over 30 sec), followed by continuous infusion of 5 mg/hr, may be effective in treating severe hypotension and bradycardia.

**Drug Interactions**
*Beta-adrenergic bronchodilators /* Labetalol ↓ bronchodilator effect of these drugs
*Cimetidine /* ↑ Bioavailability of PO labetalol
*Glutethimide /* ↓ Effects of labetalol due to ↑ breakdown by liver
*Halothane /* ↑ Risk of severe myocardial depression → hypotension
*Nitroglycerin /* Additive hypotension

*Tricyclic antidepressants /* ↑ Risk of tremors
**Laboratory Test Interferences:** False + increase in urinary catecholamines. Transient ↑ serum transaminases, BUN, serum creatinine.

**Dosage**
• **Tablets**
  *Hypertension.*
**Individualize. Initial:** 100 mg b.i.d. alone or with a diuretic; **maintenance:** 200–400 mg b.i.d. up to 1,200–2,400 mg/day for severe cases.
• **IV**
  *Hypertension.*
**Individualize. Initial:** 20 mg slowly over 2 min; **then,** 40–80 mg q 10 min until desired effect occurs or a total of 300 mg has been given.
• **IV Infusion**
  *Hypertension.*
**Initial:** 2 mg/min; **then,** adjust rate according to response. **Usual dose range:** 50–300 mg.
  *Transfer from IV to PO therapy.*
**Initial:** 200 mg; **then,** 200–400 mg 6–12 hr later, depending on response. Thereafter, dosage based on response.

## NURSING CONSIDERATIONS

See also *Nursing Considerations* for *Beta-Adrenergic Blocking Agents* and *Antihypertensive Agents.*
**Administration/Storage**
1. When transferring to PO labetalol from other antihypertensive therapy, slowly reduce dosage of current therapy.
2. Full antihypertensive effect is usually seen within the first 1–3 hr after the initial dose or dose increment.
**IV** 3. To transfer from IV to PO therapy in hospitalized clients, begin when supine BP begins to increase.
4. Not compatible with 5% sodium bicarbonate injection.
5. May give IV undiluted (20 mg over 2 min) or reconstituted with dextrose or saline solutions (infuse at a rate of 2 mg/min). When given by IV infusion, use a device that allows precise control of flow rate.

**Assessment**

1. Assess effect of labetalol tablets on standing BP before discharge from the hospital. Obtain standing BP at different times during the day to assess full effects.

2. To reduce chance of orthostatic hypotension, clients should remain supine for 3 hr after receiving parenteral labetalol.

**Client/Family Teaching**

1. Use caution; may precipitate orthostatic hypotension and cause dizziness.

2. May cause increased sensitivity to cold; dress appropriately.

**Outcomes/Evaluate:** ↓ BP

# Lactulose
(**LAK**-tyou-lohs)

**Pregnancy Category:** B

Acilac ✦, Cephulac, Cholac, Chronulac, Comalose-R ✦, Constilac, Constulose, Duphalac, Duphalac Dry ✦, Gen-Lac ✦, Enulose, Evalose, Heptalac, Lactulax ✦, PMS Lactulose ✦ **(Rx)**

**Classification:** Ammonia detoxicant, laxative

**Action/Kinetics:** Lactulose, a disaccharide containing both lactose and galactose, causes a decrease in the blood concentration of ammonia in clients suffering from portal-systemic encephalopathy. Due to bacteria-induced degradation of lactulose in the colon, resulting in an acid medium. Ammonia will then migrate from the blood to the colon to form ammonium ion, which is trapped and cannot be absorbed. A laxative action due to increased osmotic pressure from lactic, formic, and acetic acids then expels the trapped ammonium. The decrease in blood ammonia concentration improves the mental state, EEG tracing, and diet protein tolerance of clients. The increased osmotic pressure also results in a laxative effect, which may take up to 24 hr. Partly absorbed from the GI tract. **Onset:** 24–48 hr.

**Uses:** Prevention and treatment of portal-systemic encephalopathy, including hepatic and prehepatic coma (Cephylac, Cholac, Enulose, Evalose, Heptalac are used). Chronic constipation (Chronulac, Constilac, Duphalac are used).

**Contraindications:** Clients on galactose-restricted diets.

**Special Concerns:** Safe use during lactation and in children has not been established. Infants who have been given lactulose have developed hyponatremia and dehydration. Use with caution in presence of diabetes mellitus.

**Side Effects:** *GI:* N&V, diarrhea, cramps, flatulence, gaseous distention, belching.

**Drug Interactions**

*Antacids* / May inhibit the drop in pH of the colon required for lactulose activity

*Neomycin* / May cause ↓ degradation of lactulose due to neomycin-induced ↑ in elimination of certain bacteria in the colon

**Dosage**

• **Syrup, Oral Solution**
*Encephalopathy.*

**Adults, initial:** 30–45 mL (20–30 g) t.i.d.–q.i.d.; adjust q 2–3 days to obtain two or three soft stools daily. Long-term therapy may be required in portal-systemic encephalopathy; **infants:** 2.5–10 mL/day (1.6–6.6 g/day) in divided doses; **older children and adolescents:** 40–90 mL/day (26.6–60 g/day) in divided doses.

*During acute episodes of constipation.*

30–45 mL (20–30 g) q 1–2 hr to induce rapid initial laxation.

*Chronic constipation.*

**Adults and children:** 15–30 mL/day (10–20 g/day) as a single dose after breakfast (up to 60 mL/day may be required).

## NURSING CONSIDERATIONS
**Administration/Storage**

1. To minimize sweet taste, dilute with water/juice or add to desserts.

2. When given by gastric tube, dilute well to prevent vomiting and possibility of aspiration pneumonia.

3. When administered by enema use a rectal balloon catheter to assist with retention.
4. Do not take with other laxatives.
5. Store below 30°C (86°F). Avoid freezing.

**Assessment:** Document mental status; monitor serum ammonia and potassium levels during therapy for encephalopathy. May also cause further potassium loss that will intensify disease symptoms.

**Client/Family Teaching**
1. Report any GI distress; may subside as therapy continues, otherwise dose may need to be reduced.
2. Medication contains carbohydrate; report flushed, dry skin, complaints of dry mouth and intense thirst, a fruity odor to the breath, abdominal pain, and low BP (S&S of hyperglycemia; more likely to occur with diabetes).
3. Keep skin clean and dry; reposition frequently because skin breakdown may occur rapidly.

**Outcomes/Evaluate**
• Improved level of consciousness
• ↓ Serum ammonia levels
• Relief of constipation

# Lamivudine (3TC)
(lah-**MIH**-vyou-deen)
**Pregnancy Category:** C
3TC ✹, Epivir **(Rx)**
**Classification:** Antiviral drug

See also *Antiviral Drugs*.
**Action/Kinetics:** Synthetic nucleoside analog effective against HIV. Converted to active 5'-triphosphate (L-TP) metabolite which inhibits HIV reverse transcription via viral DNA chain termination. L-TP also inhibits the RNA- and DNA-dependent DNA polymerase activities of reverse transcriptase. Rapidly absorbed after PO administration. Most eliminated unchanged through the urine.
**Uses:** In combination with AZT for the treatment of HIV infection, based on clinical or immunologic evidence of progression of the disease. There are no data on the effect of lamivudine and AZT on clinical

progression of HIV infection, such as the incidence of opportunistic infections or survival.
**Contraindications:** Lactation.
**Special Concerns:** Clients taking lamivudine and AZT may continue to develop opportunistic infections and other complications of HIV infection. Use with caution and at a reduced dose in those with impaired renal function. Data on the use of lamivudine and AZT in pediatric clients are lacking; however, use the combination with extreme caution in children with pancreatitis.
**Side Effects:** Side effects are for the combination of lamivudine plus AZT. *GI:* N&V, diarrhea, anorexia, or decreased appetite, abdominal pain, abdominal cramps, dyspepsia. *CNS:* Neuropathy, insomnia or other sleep disorders, dizziness, depressive disorders, paresthesias, peripheral neuropathies. *Respiratory:* Nasal signs and symptoms, cough. *Musculoskeletal:* Musculoskeletal pain, myalgia, arthralgia. *Body as a whole:* Headache, malaise, fatigue, fever or chills, skin rashes. *NOTE:* Pediatric clients have an increased risk to develop **pancreatitis.**
**Drug Interactions:** Use of lamivudine with trimethoprim-sulfamethoxazole resulted in a significant increase in lamivudine levels.

**Dosage**
• **Oral Solution, Tablets**
   *HIV infection.*
**Adults and adolescents, aged 12–16 years:** 150 mg b.i.d. in combination with AZT. For adults with low body weight (less than 50 kg), the recommended dose is 2 mg/kg b.i.d. in combination with AZT. **Children, 3 months to 12 years of age:** 4 mg/kg b.i.d. (up to a maximum of 150 mg b.i.d.) in combination with AZT. In clients over 16 years of age, the dose should be adjusted, as follows, in impaired renal function. Creatinine clearance ($C_{CR}$) less than 50 mL/min: 150 mg b.i.d., $C_{CR}$ 30–49 mL/min: 150 mg once daily. $C_{CR}$ 15–29 mL/min: 150 mg for the first dose followed by 100 mg once daily. $C_{CR}$

5–14 mL/min: 150 mg for the first dose followed by 50 mg once daily. $C_{CR}$ less than 5 mL/min: 50 mg for the first dose followed by 25 mg once daily.

## NURSING CONSIDERATIONS

See also *Nursing Considerations* for *Antiviral Drugs*.

**Administration/Storage**
1. Consult AZT prescribing information before using with lamivudine.
2. May be taken without regard to food.
3. Store PO solution at 2°C–25°C (36°F–77°F).

**Assessment**
1. Note disease confirmation, other agents trialed, and the outcome.
2. Monitor children for clinical symptoms of pancreatitis.
3. Monitor renal and hematologic parameters, including $CD_4$ and viral load. Adjust dose with impaired renal function.

**Client/Family Teaching**
1. Take exactly as prescribed with AZT twice a day.
2. Drug is not a cure; may continue to experience illnesses and opportunistic infections associated with HIV.
3. Use barrier protection with sexual partners to prevent HIV transmission.
4. With children, report symptoms of pancreatitis (i.e., abdominal pain, N&V, fever, loss of appetite, yellow skin discoloration).

**Outcomes/Evaluate:** Control of HIV disease progression with AZT

# Lamivudine/Zidovudine
((lah-**MIH**-vyou-deen, zye-**DOH**-vyou-deen))
**Pregnancy Category:** C
Combivir **(Rx)**
**Classification:** Antiviral drug combination

See also *Lamivudine, Zidovudine,* and *Antiviral Drugs*.

**Content:** Each Combivir tablet contains: *Antiviral:* Lamivudine, 150 mg and *Antiviral:* Zidovudine, 300 mg.
**Action/Kinetics:** Both drugs are reverse transcriptase inhibitors with activity against HIV. Combination results in synergistic antiretroviral effect. Each drug is rapidly absorbed.
**Uses:** Treatment of HIV infection.
**Contraindications:** Use in clients requiring dosage reduction, children less than 12 years of age, $C_{CR}$ less than 50 mL/min, body weight less than 50 kg, and in those experiencing dose-limiting side effects.
**Side Effects:** See individual drugs.

**Dosage**
• **Tablets**
  *HIV infection.*
**Adults and children over 12 years of age:** One combination tablet—150 mg lamivudine/300 mg zidovudine—b.i.d.

## NURSING CONSIDERATIONS

See also *Nursing Considerations* for *Lamivudine, Zidovudine* and *Antiviral Drugs*.

**Administration/Storage**
1. May be taken without regard to food.
2. Reduce dose in impaired renal function.

**Assessment**
1. Document disease onset, clinical characteristics, other agents trialed, and outcome.
2. Weigh client; not for use in those with low body weight or $C_{CR}$ less than 50 mL/min.
3. Monitor CBC, liver and renal function studies; report any dysfunction.
4. Assess for hepatomegaly and lactic acidosis (pH < 7.35 or serum lactate > 5-6 mEq/L).

**Client/Family Teaching**
1. Take as directed, with or without food, twice daily.
2. Report any severe fatigue, SOB, dizziness, or muscle pain; drug may cause neutropenia and anemia.
3. Drug is not a cure, may continue

to experience opportunistic infections.

4. Practice safe sex; drug does not prevent disease transmission.

**Outcomes/Evaluate:** Control of HIV; ↓ viral load

# Lamotrigine
(lah-**MAH**-trih-jeen)
**Pregnancy Category:** C
Lamictal **(Rx)**
**Classification:** Anticonvulsant

See also *Anticonvulsants.*

**Action/Kinetics:** Mechanism of anticonvulsant action not known. May act to inhibit voltage-sensitive sodium channels. This effect stabilizes neuronal membranes and modulates presynaptic transmitter release of excitatory amino acids such as glutamate and aspartate. Rapidly and completely absorbed after PO use. **Peak plasma levels:** 1.4–4.8 hr. t½, **after repeated doses: About 33 hr.** Metabolized by the liver with metabolites and unchanged drug excreted mainly through the urine (94%). Lamotrigine induces its own metabolism. Eliminated more rapidly in clients who have been taking antiepileptic drugs that induce liver enzymes. However, valproic acid decreases the clearance of lamotrigine.

**Uses:** Adjunct in the treatment of partial seizures in adults with epilepsy. *Investigational:* Adults with generalized clonic-tonic, absence, atypical absence, and myoclonic seizures. Infants and children with Lennox-Gastaut syndrome.

**Contraindications:** Use during lactation and in children less than 16 years of age.

**Special Concerns:** Use with caution in clients with diseases or conditions that could affect metabolism or elimination of the drug, such as in impaired renal, hepatic, or cardiac function.

**Side Effects:** Side effects listed are those with an incidence of 0.1% or greater. *CNS:* Dizziness, ataxia, somnolence, headache, incoordination, insomnia, tremor, depression, anxie-ty, irritability, decreased memory, speech disorder, confusion, disturbed concentration, sleep disorder, emotional lability, vertigo, mind racing, amnesia, nervousness, abnormal thinking, abnormal dreams, agitation, akathisia, aphasia, CNS depression, depersonalization, dyskinesia, dysphoria, euphoria, faintness, hallucinations, hostility, hyperkinesia, hypesthesia, myoclonus, panic attack, paranoid reaction, personality disorder, psychosis, stupor. *GI:* N&V, diarrhea, dyspepsia, constipation, tooth disorder, anorexia, dry mouth, abdominal pain, dysphagia, flatulence, gingivitis, gum hyperplasia, increased appetite, increased salivation, abnormal liver function tests, mouth ulceration, stomatitis, thirst. *CV:* Hot flashes, palpitations, flushing, migraine, syncope, tachycardia, vasodilation. *Musculoskeletal:* Arthralgia, joint disorder, myasthenia, dysarthria, muscle spasm, twitching. *Hematologic:* Anemia, ecchymosis, leukocytosis, leukopenia, lymphadenopathy, petechiae. *Respiratory:* Rhinitis, pharyngitis, increased cough, dyspnea, epistaxis, hyperventilation. *Dermatologic:* **Stevens-Johnson syndrome, toxic epidermal necrolysis,** pruritus, alopecia, acne, dry skin, eczema, erythema, hirsutism, maculopapular rash, sweating, urticaria. *Ophthalmologic:* Diplopia, blurred vision, nystagmus, abnormal vision, abnormal accommodation, conjunctivitis, oscillopsia, photophobia. *GU:* Dysmenorrhea, vaginitis, amenorrhea, female lactation, hematuria, polyuria, urinary frequency or incontinence, UTI, vaginal moniliasis. *Body as a whole: **Possibility of sudden unexplained death in epilepsy,*** flu syndrome, fever, infection, neck pain, malaise, **seizure exacerbation,** chills, halitosis, facial edema, weight gain or loss, peripheral edema, hyperglycemia. *Miscellaneous:* Ear pain, tinnitus, taste perversion.

**OD** **Overdose Management:** *Symptoms:* Possibility of dizziness, headache, somnolence, coma. *Treatment:* Hospitalization with general supportive care. If indicated, induce emesis or perform gastric lavage. Protect the airway.

**Drug Interactions**

*Acetaminophen* / ↓ Serum lamotrigine levels

*Carbamazepine* / Lamotrigine concentration is ↓ by about 40%

*Phenobarbital* / Lamotrigine concentration is ↓ by about 40%

*Phenytoin* / Lamotrigine concentration is ↓ by 45%–54%

*Primidone* / Lamotrigine concentration is ↓ by about 40%

*Valproic acid* / Lamotrigine concentration is ↑ twofold while valproic acid concentration is ↓ by 25%

**Dosage**
* **Tablets**

   *Treatment of partial seizures.*

**Adults and children over 16 years of age who are taking enzyme-inducing antiepileptic drugs, but not valproate:** 50 mg once a day for weeks 1 and 2, followed by 100 mg/day in two divided doses for weeks 3 and 4. **Maintenance dose:** 300–500 mg/day given in two divided doses. The dose should be increased by 100 mg/day every week until maintenance levels are reached. **Adults and children over 16 years of age who are taking enzyme-inducing antiepileptic drugs plus valproic acid:** 25 mg every other day for weeks 1 and 2, followed by 25 mg once daily for weeks 3 and 4. **Maintenance dose:** 100–150 mg/day in two divided doses. The dose should be increased by 25–50 mg/day every 1–2 weeks.

## NURSING CONSIDERATIONS

See also *Nursing Considerations* for *Anticonvulsants.*

**Administration/Storage**

1. Base dose on the therapeutic response since a therapeutic plasma level has not been determined.

2. If a change in seizure control or worsening of side effects is noted in clients receiving lamotrigine in combination with other antiepileptic drugs, a reevaluation of all the drugs in the regimen should be considered.

3. Discontinuing an enzyme-inducing antiepileptic drug should prolong the half-life of lamotrigine, whereas discontinuing valproic acid should shorten the half-life of lamotrigine.

4. If it is decided to discontinue lamotrigine therapy, a stepwise reduction of dose over 2 weeks (about 50% per week) is recommended unless safety concerns mandate a more rapid withdrawal.

**Assessment**

1. Document type, onset, and duration of symptoms, previous agents used, and the outcome.

2. If also prescribed other anticonvulsant agents (i.e., valproate, carbamazepine), monitor closely for adverse effects.

3. Monitor CBC, liver and renal function studies; reduce dose with liver or renal dysfunction.

**Client/Family Teaching:**

1. Do not stop abruptly; may cause increased seizure frequency. Drug should be gradually decreased over at least 2 weeks unless safety concerns require rapid withdrawal.

2. Do not perform activities that require mental alertness and/or coordination until drug effects realized; may cause dizziness, ataxia, somnolence, headache, and blurred vision.

3. Report loss of seizure control or if a rash occurs; provider may interrupt therapy.

4. Photosensitization may occur; wear protective clothing, sunscreen, and sunglasses until tolerance determined.

**Outcomes/Evaluate:** Control of seizures

# Lansoprazole
(lan-**SAHP**-rah-zohl)
**Pregnancy Category:** B
Prevacid **(Rx)**
**Classification:** GI drug, proton pump inhibitor

**Action/Kinetics:** Suppresses gastric acid secretion by inhibition of the $(H^+, K^+)$-ATPase system located at the secretory surface of the parietal cells in the stomach. Drug is a gastric acid (proton) pump inhibitor in that it blocks the final step of acid production. Both basal and stimulated gastric acid secretion are inhibited, regardless of the stimulus. May have antimicrobial activity against *Helicobacter pylori*. Absorption begins only after lansoprazole granules leave the stomach, but absorption is rapid. **Peak plasma levels:** 1.7 hr. **Mean plasma t½:** 1.5 hr. Over 97% bound to plasma proteins. Food does not appear to affect the rate of absorption, if given before meals. Metabolized in the liver with metabolites excreted through both the urine (33%) and feces (66%).

**Uses:** Short-term treatment (up to 4 weeks) for healing and symptomatic relief of active duodenal ulcer. With clarithromycin and amoxicillin as triple therapy to eradicate *Helicobacter pylori* infection in active or recurrent duodenal ulcers. Short-term treatment (up to 8 weeks) for healing and symptomatic relief of all grades of erosive esophagitis. Maintenance treatment of healed erosive esophagitis. Long-term treatment of pathologic hypersecretory conditions, including Zollinger-Ellison syndrome.

**Contraindications:** Lactation.

**Special Concerns:** Reduce dosage in impaired hepatic function. Symptomatic relief does not preclude the presence of gastric malignancy. Safety and efficacy have not been determined in children less than 18 years of age.

**Side Effects:** *GI:* Diarrhea, abdominal pain, nausea, melena, anorexia, bezoar, cardiospasm, cholelithiasis, constipation, dry mouth, thirst, dyspepsia, dysphagia, eructation, esophageal stenosis, esophageal ulcer, esophagitis, fecal discoloration, flatulence, gastric nodules, fundic gland polyps, gastroenteritis, *GI hemorrhage, rectal hemorrhage,* hematemesis, increased appetite, increased salivation, stomatitis, tenesmus, vomiting, ulcerative colitis. *CV:* Angina, hypertension or hypotension, *CVA, MI, shock,* palpitations, vasodilation. *CNS:* Headache, agitation, amnesia, anxiety, apathy, confusion, depression, syncope, dizziness, hallucinations, hemiplegia, aggravated hostility, decreased libido, nervousness, paresthesia, abnormal thinking. *GU:* Abnormal menses, breast enlargement, gynecomastia, breast tenderness, hematuria, albuminuria, glycosuria, impotence, kidney calculus. *Respiratory:* Asthma, bronchitis, increased cough, dyspnea, epistaxis, hemoptysis, hiccoughs, pneumonia, upper respiratory inflammation or infection. *Endocrine:* Diabetes mellitus, goiter, hypoglycemia or hyperglycemia. *Hematologic:* Anemia, eosinophilia, hemolysis. *Musculoskeletal:* Arthritis, arthralgia, musculoskeletal pain, myalgia. *Dermatologic:* Acne, alopecia, pruritus, rash, urticaria. *Ophthalmologic:* Amblyopia, eye pain, visual field defect. *Otic:* Deafness, otitis media, tinnitus. *Miscellaneous:* Gout, weight loss or gain, taste perversion, asthenia, candidiasis, chest pain, edema, fever, flu syndrome, halitosis, infection, malaise.

**Drug Interactions**

*Ampicillin* / ↓ Effect of ampicillin due to ↓ absorption

*Digoxin* / ↓ Effect of digoxin due to ↓ absorption

*Iron salts* / ↓ Effect of iron salts due to ↓ absorption

*Ketoconazole* / ↓ Effect of ketoconazole due to ↓ absorption

*Sucralfate* / Delayed absorption of lansoprazole

**Laboratory Test Interferences:** Abnormal liver function tests. ↑ AST, ALT, creatinine, alkaline phosphatase, globulins, GGTP, glucocorticoids, LDH, gastrin. ↑ or ↓ or abnormal WBC and platelets. Abnormal AG ratio, RBC. Bilirubinemia, hyperlipemia. ↑ or ↓ Electrolytes or cholesterol.

**Dosage** —————————————

• **Capsules, Delayed Release**
 *Duodenal ulcer.*

**Adults:** 15 mg daily before breakfast for 4 weeks.

*Maintenance of healed duodenal ulcer.*
**Adults:** 15 mg once daily.

*Duodenal ulcers associated with H. pylori.*
**Triple therapy:** Lansoprazole, 30 mg, plus clarithromycin, 500 mg, and amoxicilin, 1 g, b.i.d. for 14 days. **Double therapy:** Lansoprazole, 30 mg, plus amoxicillin, 1 g, t.i.d. for 14 days in those intolerant or resistant to clarithromycin.

*Erosive esophagitis.*
30 mg before eating for up to 8 weeks. If the client does not heal in 8 weeks, an additional 8 weeks of therapy may be given. If there is a recurrence, an additional 8-week course may be considered.

*Maintenance of healed erosive esophagitis.*
15 mg once daily for up to 12 months.

*Pathologic hypersecretory conditions.*
**Initial:** 60 mg once daily. Adjust the dose to client need. Dosage may be continued as long as necessary. Doses up to 90 or 120 mg (in divided doses) daily have been given.

## NURSING CONSIDERATIONS
### Administration/Storage
1. There is no significant effect on the amount or rate of absorption if lansoprazole is given before meals.
2. For those unable to swallow capsules, the delayed-release capsule may be opened and the contents sprinkled on a tablespoon of applesauce.
3. To give with a NG tube in place, open the capsule and mix intact granules with 40 mL of apple juice. Instill through the NG tube into the stomach, flushing with additional apple juice to clear the tube.
4. Adjust dosage in severe liver disease.
5. Store in a tight container protected from moisture. Store between 15°C and 30°C (59°F and 86°F).

### Assessment
1. Document indications for therapy, onset, duration of symptoms, and any other agents trialed.
2. Note findings of upper GI, barium swallow, or endoscopy.
3. Monitor CBC, electrolytes, triglycerides, liver and renal function studies; reduce dose with severe liver disease.
### Client/Family Teaching
1. Take exactly as prescribed; do not exceed dose or share medications.
2. Keep scheduled appointments. Drug is generally for short-term therapy and discontinued once condition is healed. Long-term effects are not known; users should be assessed for gastric malignancy.
### Outcomes/Evaluate
• Suppression of acid secretion
• Healing of ulcer/erosive esophagitis
• ↓ Pain; relief of heartburn

# Latanoprost
(lah-**TAH**-noh-prost)
**Pregnancy Category:** C
Xalatan **(Rx)**
**Classification:** Prostaglandin agonist

**Action/Kinetics:** A prostaglandin F$_2\alpha$ analog that decreases intraocular pressure by increasing the outflow of aqueous humor. Absorbed through the cornea where it is hydrolyzed by esterases to the active acid. **Peak levels in aqueous humor:** 2 hr. **Onset:** 3–4 hr. **Maximum effect:** 8–12 hr. The active acid is metabolized in the liver and excreted in the urine. **t½, elimination:** 17 min.
**Uses:** To reduce intraocular pressure in open-angle glaucoma and ocular hypertension in clients who are intolerant of other drugs to reduce intraocular pressure or who have been unresponsive to other drug therapy.
**Contraindications:** Use while wearing contact lenses.
**Special Concerns:** Latanoprost may gradually change eye color by

increasing the amount of brown pigment in the iris; the resultant color changes may be permanent. Use with caution during lactation. The drug product contains benzalkonium chloride, which may be absorbed by contact lenses. Safety and efficacy have not been determined in children.

**Side Effects:** *Ophthalmic:* Blurred vision, stinging, conjunctival hyperemia, foreign body sensation, itching, increased pigmentation of the iris, punctate epithelial keratopathy, dry eye, excessive tearing, eye pain, lid crusting, lid edema, lid erythema, lid discomfort or pain, photophobia, conjunctivitis, diplopia, discharge from the eye, retinal artery embolus, retinal detachment, vitreous hemorrhage from diabetic retinopathy (rare). *Systemic:* upper respiratory tract infection (e.g., cold, flu), pain in muscles/joints/back, chest pain/angina pectoris, rash, allergic skin reactions.

**Drug Interactions:** A precipitate may form if lanatoprost is used with eye drops containing thimerosal.

**Dosage** ⎯⎯⎯⎯⎯⎯⎯⎯⎯
• **Solution, 0.005%**
  *Elevated intraocular pressure.*
  1 gtt (1.5 mcg) in the affected eye(s) once daily in the evening. More frequent use may decrease the intraocular pressure lowering effect.

## NURSING CONSIDERATIONS
### Administration/Storage
1. At least 5 min should elapse between administration of lanatoprost and other topical ophthalmic drugs; esp. drops containing thimerosal.
2. Prior to administration, remove contact lenses. Reinsert 15 min following administration.
3 Protect from light. Refrigerate unopened bottles. Once opened, the container may be stored at room temperature (up to 25°C; 77°F) for 6 weeks.

### Client/Family Teaching
1. Wash hands before and after use. Avoid touching any part of the eye with the container tip to prevent contamination and eye infections. Contaminated solutions may cause eye damage and loss of vision.
2. Use only once daily, in the evening.
3. Remove contact lenses and do not reinsert for at least 15 min after administration.
4. Report any lid or eye reactions, especially conjunctivitis.
5. Iris color changes may occur due to an increase of brown pigment in the iris; this may be permanent.

**Outcomes/Evaluate:** ↓ Intraocular pressure

# Letrozole
(**LET**-roh-zohl)
**Pregnancy Category:** D
Femara **(Rx)**
**Classification:** Antineoplastic, hormone

⎯⎯⎯⎯⎯⎯⎯⎯⎯⎯⎯⎯⎯⎯⎯⎯

See also *Antineoplastic Agents.*

**Action/Kinetics:** A nonsteroidal competitive inhibitor of aromatase, resulting in inhibition of conversion of androgens to estrogens. It acts by competitively binding to heme of cytochrome P450 subunit of aromatase, leading to decreased biosynthesis of estrogen in all tissues. Does not cause increase in serum FSH and does not affect synthesis of adrenocorticosteroids, aldosterone, or thyroid hormones. **t½, elimination:** About 2 days. Steady state plasma levels after daily doses of 2.5 mg reached in 2 to 6 weeks. Inactive metabolites are excreted in urine.

**Uses:** Advanced breast cancer in postmenopausal women with disease progression following antiestrogen therapy.

**Special Concerns:** Use with caution during lactation and in those with severely impaired hepatic function. Safety and efficacy have not been determined in children.

**Side Effects:** *CNS:* Headache, somnolence, dizziness, vertigo, depression, anxiety. *GI:* N&V, constipation, diarrhea, abdominal pain, anorexia, dyspepsia. *Body as a whole:* Fatigue, viral infections, peripheral edema, asthenia, decreased weight. *Dermatologic:* Hot flashes, rash, pruritus, alopecia, increased sweating. *Respiratory:* Dyspnea, coughing, pleural effusion. *Miscellaneous:* Chest pain, hypertension, arthralgia, fracture.

**Laboratory Test Interferences:** ↑ AST, ALT, GGT. ↓ Lymphocyte counts. Hypercholesterolemia, hypercalcemia.

### Dosage

• **Tablets**

*Advanced breast cancer.*

**Adults and elderly:** 2.5 mg once/day. Continue until tumor progression is evident. Dosage adjustment is not needed in renal impairment if $C_{CR}$ is greater than or equal to 10 mL/min.

## NURSING CONSIDERATIONS

See also *Nursing Considerations* for *Antineoplastic Agents.*

**Assessment**

1. Note disease onset, clinical findings, previous antiestrogen therapy, and response.

2. Monitor liver and renal function studies.

**Client/Family Teaching**

1. Take as directed; may take without regard to meals.

2. Report any severe rash, diarrhea, pain, dyspnea, or chest pain.

**Outcomes/Evaluate:** ↓ Tumor mass; ↓ malignant cell proliferation

# Leucovorin calcium (citrovorum factor, folinic acid)

(loo-koh-**VOR**-in)

**Pregnancy Category:** C

Lederle Leucovorin Calcium ✤, Wellcovorin **(Rx)**

**Classification:** Folic acid derivative

**Action/Kinetics:** Derivative of folic acid; is a mixture of the diasterioisomers of the 5-formyl derivative of tetrahydrofolic acid. Does not require reduction by dihydrofolate reductase to be active in intracellular metabolism; thus, it is not affected by dihydrofolate inhibitors. Rapidly absorbed following PO administration. Quickly metabolized to 1,5-methyltetrahydrofolate, which is then metabolized by other pathways back to 5,10-methylene-tetrahydrofolate and then converted to 5-methyltetrahydrofolate using the cofactors $FADH_2$ and NADPH. Leucovorin can counteract the therapeutic and toxic effects of methotrexate (acts by inhibiting dihydrofolate reductase) but can enhance the effects of 5-fluorouracil (5-FU). Is rapidly absorbed. **Peak serum levels, PO:** Approximately 2.3 hr; **after IM:** 52 min; **after IV:** 10 min. **Onset, PO:** 20–30 min; **IM:** 10–20 min; **IV:** < 5 min. **Terminal t½:** 5.7 hr (PO), 6.2 hr (IM and IV). **Duration:** 3–6 hr. Excreted by the kidney.

**Uses: PO and Parenteral:** Prophylaxis and treatment of toxicity due to methotrexate and folic acid antagonists (e.g., pyrimethamine and trimethoprim). Leucovorin rescue following high doses of methotrexate for osteosarcoma. **Parenteral:** Megaloblastic anemias due to nutritional deficiency, sprue, pregnancy, and infancy when oral folic acid is not appropriate. Adjunct with 5-FU to prolong survival in the palliative treatment of metastatic colorectal carcinoma.

**Contraindications:** Pernicious anemia or megaloblastic anemia due to vitamin $B_{12}$ deficiency.

**Special Concerns:** It is recommended for megaloblastic anemia caused by pregnancy even though the drug is pregnancy category C. Use with caution during lactation. May increase the frequency of seizures in susceptible children. When leucovorin is used with 5-FU for advanced colorectal cancer, the dosage of 5-FU must be lower than usual as leucovorin enhances the toxicity of 5-FU. The benzyl alcohol in the parenteral form may caues a fatal gasping syndrome in premature infants.

L

**Side Effects: Leucovorin alone.**
Allergic reactions, including urticaria
and *anaphylaxis.*
**Leucovorin and 5-FU.** *GI:* N&V,
diarrhea, stomatitis, constipation,
anorexia. *Hematologic:* Leukopenia,
thrombocytopenia. *CNS:* Fatigue,
lethargy, malaise. *Miscellaneous:* Infection, alopecia, dermatitis.
**Drug Interactions**
*5-FU* / ↑ Toxicity of 5-FU
*Methotrexate* / High doses of leucovorin ↓ effect of intrathecally
administered methotrexate
*PAS* / ↓ Serum folate levels → folic
acid deficiency
*Phenobarbital* / ↓ Effect of phenobarbital → ↑ frequency of seizures,
especially in children
*Phenytoin* / ↓ Effect of phenytoin
due to ↑ rate of breakdown by
liver; also, phenytoin may ↓ plasma
folate levels
*Primidone* / ↓ Effect of primidone
→ ↑ frequency of seizures, especially in children
*Sulfasalazine* / ↓ Serum folate levels → folic acid deficiency

**Dosage**
• **IM, IV, Tablets**
*Advanced colorectal cancer.*
**Either** leucovorin, 200 mg/m² by
slow IV over a minimum of 3 min followed by 5-FU, 370 mg/m² IV **or**
leucovorin 20 mg/m² IV followed by
5-FU, 425 mg/m² IV. Treatment is
repeated daily for 5 days with the 5-
day treatment course repeated at 28-
day intervals for two courses and
then repeated at 4- to 5-week intervals
as long as the client has recovered
from the toxic effects.
*Leucovorin rescue after high-dose
methotrexate therapy.*
The dose of leucovorin is based on a
methotrexate dose of 12–15 mg/m²
given by IV infusion over 4 hr. The
dose of leucovorin is 15 mg (10
mg/m²) PO, IM, or IV q 6 hr for 10
doses starting 24 hr after the start of
the methotrexate infusion. Give leucovorin parenterally if there is nausea,
vomiting, or GI toxicity. If serum
methotrexate levels are greater than
0.2 µM at 72 hr and greater than 0.05

µM at 96 hr after administration, leucovorin should be continued at a
dose of 15 mg PO, IM, or IV q 6 hr
until methotrexate levels are less
than 0.05 µM. If serum methotrexate
levels are equal to or greater than 50
µM at 24 hr or equal to or greater than
5 µM at 48 hr after administration or
if there is a 100% or greater increase
in serum creatinine levels at 24 hr after methotrexate administration, the
dose of leucovorin should be 150
mg IV q 3 hr until methotrexate levels are less than 1 µM; **then,** give
leucovorin, 15 mg IV q 3 hr until
methotrexate levels are less than
0.05 µM. If significant clinical toxicity
is seen following methotrexate, leucovorin rescue should total 14 doses
over 84 hr in subsequent courses of
methotrexate therapy.
*Impaired methotrexate elimina-
tion or accidental overdose.*
Start leucovorin rescue as soon as
the overdose is discovered and within 24 hr of methotrexate administration when excretion is impaired.
Give leucovorin, 10 mg/m² PO, IM, or
IV q 6 hr until serum methotrexate
levels are less than $10^{-8}$ M. If the 24-
hr serum creatinine has increased
50% over baseline or if the 24- or 48-
hr methotrexate level is more than 5
$\times 10^{-6}$ M or greater than $9 \times 10^{-7}$ M,
respectively, the dose of leucovorin
should be increased to 100 mg/m²
IV q 3 hr until the methotrexate level is less than $10^{-8}$ M. Urinary alkalinization with sodium bicarbonate
solution (to maintain urine pH at 7 or
greater) and hydration with 3 L/day
should be undertaken at the same
time.
*Overdosage of folic acid antago-
nists.*
5–15 mg/day.
*Megaloblastic anemia due to folic
acid deficiency.*
**Adults and children:** Up to 1
mg/day.

## NURSING CONSIDERATIONS
**Administration/Storage**
1. The oral solution is stable for 14
days if refrigerated or for 7 days if
stored at room temperature.

L

**IV** 2. If used for methotrexate rescue, hydrate well and alkalinize urine to reduce nephrotoxicity.

3. Dilute with 5 mL bacteriostatic water for injection and use within 1 week. If sterile water for injection is added, use the solution immediately.

4. Give doses higher than 25 mg parenterally because PO absorption is saturated.

5. Do not use leucovorin calcium injection containing benzyl alcohol in doses greater than 10 mg/m$^2$.

6. Parenteral use is preferred if there is a possibility client may vomit or not absorb leucovorin.

7. In treating overdosage due to folic acid antagonists, give as soon as possible. As the time interval between the overdosage and administration of leucovorin increases, the effectiveness of leucovorin decreases.

8. Protect from light.

**Assessment**

1. Document indications for therapy: replacement or rescue. If for rescue therapy, administer promptly (first dose within 1 hr) following a high dose of folic acid antagonists; follow dosage exactly to be effective.

2. Note history of vitamin B$_{12}$ deficiency that has resulted in pernicious anemia or megaloblastic anemia. Leucovorin may obscure the diagnosis of pernicious anemia if previously undiagnosed.

3. Determine any history of seizure disorders and assess for a recurrence.

4. Monitor renal, B$_{12}$, folic acid, and hematologic values. Creatinine increases of 50% over pretreatment levels indicate severe renal toxicity.

5. Urine pH should be greater than 7.0; monitor q 6 hr during therapy. Urine alkalinization with NaHCO$_3$ or acetazolamide may be necessary to prevent nephrotoxic effects.

**Client/Family Teaching**

1. Report immediately any skin rash, itching, malaise, or difficulty breathing.

2. Parenteral therapy generally is used following chemotherapy because N&V may prevent oral absorption.

3. When high-dose therapy is used, be alert for mental confusion and impaired judgment. Safety measures and supervision help to ensure safety and protection.

4. Consume 3 L/day of fluids with rescue therapy.

**Outcomes/Evaluate**

• Symptomatic improvement (↓ fatigue, ↑ weight, improved orientation)

• ↑ Normoblasts (with megaloblastic anemias)

• Prevention/reversal of GI, renal, and bone marrow toxicity in methotrexate therapy or during overdosage of folic acid antagonists

# Leuprolide acetate

(loo-**PROH**-lyd)

**Pregnancy Category:** X

Lupron, Lupron Depot, Lupron Depot—3 Month, Lupron Depot—4 Month, Lupron Depot-Ped, Lupron for Pediatric Use **(Rx)**

**Classification:** Antineoplastic agent, hormonal

See also *Antineoplastic Agents.*

**Action/Kinetics:** Related to the naturally occurring GnRH. By desensitizing GnRH receptors, gonadotropin secretion is inhibited. Initially, however, LH and FSH levels increase, leading to increases of sex hormones. However, decreases in these hormones will be observed within 2–4 weeks. **Peak plasma levels:** 4 hr for various doses. t½: 3 hr.

**Uses:** Palliative treatment in advanced prostatic cancer when orchiectomy or estrogen treatment are not appropriate. Endometriosis (use depot form). Central precocious puberty (use depot-PED form). In combination with iron supplements for the presurgical treatment of anemia caused by uterine fibroid tumors (use depot form). *Investigational:* With flutamide for metastatic prostatic cancer.

---

**Contraindications:** Pregnancy, in women who may become pregnant while receiving the drug, and during lactation. Sensitivity to benzyl alcohol (found in leuprolide injection). Undiagnosed abnormal vaginal bleeding. Hypersensitivity to GnRH or GnRH agonist analogs. The 30-mg depot in women.

**Special Concerns:** Safety and efficacy have not been determined in children (except depot-PED). May cause increased bone pain and difficulty in urination during the first few weeks of therapy for prostatic cancer.

**Side Effects: Injection and Depot.** *GI:* N&V, anorexia, diarrhea, constipation, taste disorders/perversion, gingivitis, dysphagia, hepatic dysfunction. *CNS:* Pain, depression, emotional lability, insomnia, headache, dizziness, nervousness, paresthesias, anxiety, memory disorder, syncope, personality disorder, somnolence, spinal fracture/paralysis. *CV:* Peripheral edema, angina, ***cardiac arrhythmias, TIA/stroke,*** hypotension, vasodilation. *GU:* Hematuria, urinary frequency or urgency, dysuria, testicular pain, incontinence, cervix disorder, penile swelling, prostate pain. *Respiratory:* Dyspnea, hemoptysis, pneumonia, epistaxis, pulmonary infiltrates. *Endocrine:* Gynecomastia, breast tenderness, impotency, hot flashes, sweating, decreased testicular size, increased or decreased libido. *Musculoskeletal:* Myalgia, bone pain, pelvic fibrosis, ankylosing spondylosis. *Dermatologic:* Dermatitis, skin reactions, acne, seborrhea, hair growth, ecchymosis, hair loss, skin striae, erythema multiforme and other rashes, androgen-like effects. *Ophthalmic:* Ophthalmic disorder, abnormal vision. *Other:* Asthenia, diabetes, fever, chills, tinnitus, infection, body odor, hard nodule in throat, accelerated sexual maturation, hearing disorder, peripheral neuropathy.

**Injection.** *CV:* ***MI, pulmonary emboli.*** *GI:* ***GI bleeding,*** rectal polyps, peptic ulcer. *CNS:* Lethargy, mood swings, numbness, blackouts, fatigue. *Respiratory:* Cough, ***pulmonary fibrosis,*** pleural rub. *Dermatologic:* Carcinoma of the skin/ear, itching, dry skin, pigmentation, skin lesions. *GU:* Bladder spasms, urinary obstruction. *Miscellaneous:* Enlarged thyroid, inflammation, temporal bone swelling, blurred vision.

**Depot.** *CV:* Tachycardia, bradycardia, ***heart failure,*** varicose vein, palpitations. *GI:* Dysphagia, gingivitis. *CNS:* Delusions, confusion, hypesthesia. *GI:* Duodenal ulcer, dry mouth, thirst, appetite changes. *Respiratory:* Rhinitis, pharyngitis, pleural effusion. *Endocrine:* Lactation, menstrual disorder. *GU:* Penis disorder, testis disorder. *Ophthalmic:* Conjunctivitis, amblyopia, dry eyes. *Miscellaneous:* Nail disorder, flu syndrome, enlarged abdomen, lymphedema, dehydration, lymphadenopathy.

**Laboratory Test Interferences: Injection and Depot.** ↑ Calcium. ↓ WBC. Hypoproteinemia. **Injection:** ↑ BUN, creatinine. **Depot:** ↑ LDH, alkaline phosphatase, AST, uric acid, cholesterol, LDL, triglycerides, PT, PTT, glucose, WBC. ↓ Platelets, potassium. Hyperphosphatemia, abnormal LFTs. Misleading results from tests of pituitary gonadotropic and gonadal function up to 4–8 weeks after discontinuing depot therapy.

**Dosage**
- **Depot, Injection**

*Advanced prostatic cancer.*
Injection: 1 mg/day SC using the syringes provided. Depot (IM): 7.5 mg monthly, 22.5 mg q 3 months, or 30 mg q 4 months.

*Central precocious puberty.*
Injection: **Initial:** 50 mcg/kg/day SC as a single dose. Dose may increased by 10 mcg/kg/day, which is the maintenance dose. Depot-Ped: **Initial:** 0.3 mg/kg/4 weeks (minimum 7.5 mg) as a single IM dose.

*Endometriosis, uterine fibroids.*
3.75 mg IM once a month for at least 6 months for endometriosis and 3 months or less for uterine fibroids. If further treatment is contemplated, assess bone density prior to beginning therapy.

## NURSING CONSIDERATIONS

See also *Nursing Considerations* for *Antineoplastic Agents.*

**Administration/Storage**

1. Follow manufacturer's guidelines carefully to prepare the depot form. Reconstitute only with the diluent provided; after reconstitution, the preparation is stable for 24 hr. There is no preservative so discard if not used immediately.

2. When injecting depot form, do not use needles smaller than 22 gauge.

3. Give the injection using only the syringes provided.

4. Injection: Store below room temperature at 25°C (77°F) or less. Avoid freezing and protect from light. Store vial in carton until use.

5. Depot may be stored at room temperature.

**Assessment:** Document indications for therapy, onset of symptoms, other agents trialed, and the outcome.

**Client/Family Teaching**

1. Hot flashes may occur with drug therapy.

2. Record weight; report gains of more than 2 lb/day.

3. Immediately report any weakness, numbness, respiratory difficulty, or impaired urination.

4. Altered sexual effects (impotence, decreased testes size) may occur; identify appropriate resources for counseling and support.

5. Increased bone pain may be evident at the start of therapy; analgesics may be used for pain control.

**Outcomes/Evaluate**

• ↓ Tumor size and spread

• Improved symptoms with endometriosis

---

# Levamisole hydrochloride

(lee-**VAM**-ih-sohl)

**Pregnancy Category:** C

Ergamisol **(Rx)**

**Classification:** Antineoplastic, adjunct

---

**Action/Kinetics:** Used in combination with fluorouracil; considered to be an immunomodulator. Mechanism is to restore depressed immune function. As such, it stimulates formation of antibodies, stimulates T-cell activation and proliferation, potentiates monocyte and macrophage function (including phagocytosis and chemotaxis), and increases mobility adherence and chemotaxis of neutrophils. Rapidly absorbed from the GI tract. **Peak plasma levels:** 0.13 mcg/mL after 1.5–2 hr. **t½:** 3–4 hr. Metabolized by the liver and excreted mainly in the urine.

**Uses:** In combination with fluorouracil to treat clients with Dukes' stage C colon cancer following surgical resection.

**Contraindications:** Lactation.

**Special Concerns:** Safety and effectiveness have not been demonstrated in children. Agranulocytosis, caused by levamisole, may be accompanied by a flu-like syndrome, or it may be asymptomatic. Thus, hematologic monitoring is required.

**Side Effects:** *GI:* Commonly nausea and diarrhea; vomiting, stomatitis, anorexia, abdominal pain, constipation, flatulence, dyspepsia. *Hematologic:* Leukopenia, thrombocytopenia, anemia, granulocytopenia. *Dermatologic:* Commonly: dermatitis and pruritus; alopecia, skin discoloration. *CNS:* Dizziness, headache, inability to concentrate, weakness, memory loss, paresthesia, ataxia, somnolence, depression, insomnia, confusion, nervousness, anxiety, forgetfulness. *Musculoskeletal:* Arthralgia, myalgia. *Ophthalmologic:* Abnormal tearing, conjunctivitis, blurred vision. *Miscellaneous:* Fatigue, fever, rigors, chest pain, edema, taste perversion, altered sense of smell, infection, hyperbilirubinemia, epistaxis.

**Drug Interactions**

*Ethanol* / Disulfiram-like reaction when used with levamisole

*Phenytoin* / ↑ Phenytoin plasma levels

---

**Dosage**
• **Tablets**
**Adults, initial:** Levamisole, 50 mg q 8 hr for 3 days (starting 7–30 days after surgery) given together with fluorouracil, 450 mg/m²/day by IV push for 5 days (starting 21–34 days after surgery). **Maintenance:** Levamisole, 50 mg q 8 hr for 3 days q 2 weeks for 1 year; fluorouracil, 450 mg/m²/day by IV push once a week beginning 28 days after the beginning of the 5-day course and continuing for 1 year.

## NURSING CONSIDERATIONS
### Administration/Storage
1. Start levamisole no earlier than 7 and no later than 30 days after surgery; initiate fluorouracil therapy no earlier than 21 days and no later than 35 days after surgery. Before fluorouracil therapy is started, client should be out of the hospital, ambulatory, eating normally, have well-healed wounds, and have recovered from any postoperative complications.
2. If levamisole therapy has been started 7–20 days after surgery, start fluorouracil therapy at the same time as the second course of levamisole (i.e., 21–34 days after surgery).
### Assessment
1. Document indications for therapy, symptom onset, and any previous treatments.
2. Give concomitantly with IV fluorouracil.
3. Monitor CBC, electrolytes, and LFTs.
• Consider granulocyte colony-stimulating factors.
• If WBC is between 2,500 and 3,500/mm³ hold fluorouracil until WBC is 3,500/mm³.
• If WBC is less than 2,500/mm³, hold until 3,500/mm³ and then reinstitute fluorouracil at a dose reduced by 20%.
• If the WBC is less than 2,500/mm³ for more than 10 days even though fluorouracil has not been given, and despite Neupogen, the administration of levamisole should be discontinued.

• Administration of both levamisole and fluorouracil should be deferred until the platelet count is restored.
### Client/Family Teaching
1. Report immediately any malaise, confusion, fever, or chills (flu-like symptoms).
2. Avoid alcohol; may cause a disulfiram-like effect.
3. Female clients of childbearing age should practice safe contraception.
4. Report any stomatitis or diarrhea after fluorouracil administration; drug should be discontinued before the full five doses are given.
5. Need weekly lab studies for CBC prior to therapy and electrolyte and LFTs every 3 months for 1 year.
### Outcomes/Evaluate
• Control of tumor size and spread
• Restoration of immune function; inhibition of malignant cell proliferation

# Levarterenol bitartrate (Norepinephrine bitartrate)
(lee-var-**TER**-ih-nohl)
**Pregnancy Category:** C
Levophed **(Rx)**
**Classification:** Adrenergic agent, direct-acting

See also *Sympathomimetic Drugs.*
**Action/Kinetics:** Produces vasoconstriction (increase in BP) by stimulating alpha-adrenergic receptors. Also causes a moderate increase in contraction of heart by stimulating beta-1 receptors. Minimal hyperglycemic effect. **Onset:** immediate; **duration:** 1–2 min. Metabolized in liver and other tissues by the enzymes MAO and catechol-O-methyltransferase; however, the pharmacologic activity is terminated by uptake and metabolism in sympathetic nerve endings. Metabolites excreted in urine.
**Uses:** Hypotensive states caused by trauma, septicemia, blood transfusions, drug reactions, spinal anesthesia, poliomyelitis, central vasomotor depression, and MIs. Adjunct to

treatment of cardiac arrest and profound hypotension.

**Additional Contraindications:** Hypotension due to blood volume deficiency (except in emergencies), mesenteric or peripheral vascular thrombosis, in halothane or cyclopropane anesthesia (due to possibilities of fatal arrhythmias). Pregnancy (may cause fetal anoxia or hypoxia).

**Special Concerns:** Use with caution in clients taking MAO inhibitors or tricyclic antidepressants.

**Additional Side Effects:** Drug may cause bradycardia that can be abolished by atropine.

Dosage ─────────────
• **IV Infusion Only**
**Effect on BP determines dosage, initial:** 8–12 mcg/min or 2–3 mL of a 4-mcg/mL solution/min; **maintenance,** 2–4 mcg/min with the dose determined by client response.

## NURSING CONSIDERATIONS

See also *Nursing Considerations* for *Sympathomimetic Drugs.*
**Administration/Storage**
**IV** 1. Discard solutions that are brown or that have a precipitate.
2. Do not administer through the same tube as blood products.
3. Continue the infusion until BP is maintained without therapy. Avoid abrupt withdrawal of levarterenol.
4. Dilute in either D5W or 5% dextrose in saline.
5. For IV administration, use a large vein (preferably the antecubital or subclavian). Avoid veins with poor circulation.
6. Administer IV solutions with an electronic infusion device. Monitor the rate of flow constantly.
7. Have phentolamine available for use at the site of extravasation to dilate local blood vessels and to minimize local necrosis.
**Assessment**
1. Determine that client is adequately hydrated.
2. During administration, the client

should be in a closely monitored environment.
3. Monitor BP frequently by arterial line or *Dinemapp.* Assess I&O, ECG, VS, CVP, and PA wedge pressure readings.
4. Observe infusion site frequently for evidence of extravasation; ischemia and sloughing may occur. Check for blanching along the course of the vein; may indicate permeability of the vein wall, which could allow leakage to occur. If evident, change IV site and administer phentolamine to the site of the extravasation.
5. Withdraw drug gradually; may experience an initial rebound drop in BP. Extra fluids parenterally may diminish rebound hypotension and help stabilize BP during withdrawal of the drug.
**Outcomes/Evaluate**
• ↑ BP
• Improved tissue perfusion
• Urinary output > 30 mL/hr

# Levobunolol hydrochloride
(lee-voh-**BYOU**-no-lohl)
**Pregnancy Category:** C
AKBeta, Betagan ✤, Betagan Liquifilm, Novo-Levobunolol ✤, Ophtho-Bunolol ✤ **(Rx)**
**Classification:** Beta-adrenergic blocking agent

See also *Beta-Adrenergic Blocking Agents.*
**Action/Kinetics:** Acts on both beta-1- and beta-2-adrenergic receptors. May act by decreasing the formation of aqueous humor. **Onset:** <60 min. **Peak effect:** 2–6 hr. **Duration:** 24 hr.
**Uses:** To decrease intraocular pressure in chronic open-angle glaucoma or ocular hypertension.
**Special Concerns:** Safety and effectiveness have not been determined in children. Significant absorption in geriatric clients may result in myocardial depression. Also, use with

caution in angle-closure glaucoma (use with a miotic), in clients with muscle weaknesses, and in those with decreased pulmonary function.
**Additional Side Effects:** *Ophthalmic:* Stinging and burning (transient), decreased corneal sensitivity, blepharoconjunctivitis. *Dermatologic:* Urticaria, pruritus.

**Dosage**
• **Ophthalmic Solution (0.25%, 0.5%)**
**Adults, usual:** 1 gtt of 0.25% or 0.5% solution in affected eye(s) 1–2 times/day (depending on variations in diurnal intraocular pressure).

## NURSING CONSIDERATIONS

See also *Nursing Considerations* for *Beta-Adrenergic Blocking Agents.*
**Administration/Storage**
1. If other eye drops are to be administered, wait at least 5 min before instilling.
2. Apply gentle pressure to the inside corner of the eye for approximately 60 sec following instillation.
3. If intraocular pressure is not decreased sufficiently, pilocarpine, epinephrine, or systemic carbonic anhydrase inhibitors may be used.
4. Due to diurnal intraocular pressure variations, a satisfactory response to twice daily therapy is best determined by measuring intraocular pressure at different times during the day.
**Client/Family Teaching**
1. Do not close the eyes tightly or blink more frequently than usual after instillation of the drug.
2. Medication is used to lower pressures in the eye and to prevent vision loss.
3. Return for evaluation of intraocular pressure and drug's effectiveness.
**Outcomes/Evaluate:** ↓ Intraocular pressure

# Levocabastine hydrochloride
(**lee**-voh-kah-**BASS**-teen)
**Pregnancy Category:** C

Livostin Eye Drops ✿, Livostin Nasal Spray **(Rx)**
**Classification:** Ophthalmic antihistamine

**Action/Kinetics:** A histamine $H_1$ receptor antagonist for ophthalmic use. **Duration:** 2 hr. A small amount of the drug is absorbed into the systemic circulation.
**Uses:** Temporary relief of seasonal allergic conjunctivitis.
**Contraindications:** Use while soft contact lenses are being worn.
**Special Concerns:** The drug is only for ophthalmic use. Safety and efficacy have not been determined in children less than 12 years of age.
**Side Effects:** *Ophthalmologic:* Transient stinging and burning, visual disturbances, eye pain, eye dryness, red eyes, lacrimation, discharge from eyes, eyelid edema. *CNS:* Headache, fatigue, somnolence. *Miscellaneous:* Pharyngitis, cough, nausea, rash, erythema, dyspnea.

**Dosage**
• **Ophthalmic Suspension**
*Allergic conjunctivitis.*
1 gtt instilled in affected eye(s) q.i.d. for up to 2 weeks.

## NURSING CONSIDERATIONS
**Administration/Storage**
1. Shake suspension well before using. Do not use if it is discolored.
2. Do not permit dropper tip to touch the eyelids or surrounding areas; this prevents contamination to the dropper tip and suspension.
3. Keep the bottle tightly closed. Store at room temperature (15°C–30°C or 59°F–86°F) and do not freeze.
**Assessment**
1. Note other agents prescribed and the outcome.
2. Assess for evidence of infection or abnormal drainage from the eye.
3. Determine any changes in or loss of vision.
**Client/Family Teaching**
1. Thoroughly mix contents before instillation.
2. Soft contact lens *cannot* be worn during this therapy.

3. Some burning and stinging may be evident but should subside.

4. Report if symptoms do not improve or if they become worse after 2–4 days of therapy.

**Outcomes/Evaluate:** Relief of ocular itching with allergic conjunctivitis

# Levocarnitine
(lee-voh-**KAR**-nih-teen)
**Pregnancy Category:** B
Carnitor **(Rx)**
**Classification:** Metabolic agent for systemic carnitine deficiency

**Action/Kinetics:** Occurs naturally and is required in mammals for energy metabolism. Believed to facilitate the entry of long-chain fatty acids into cellular mitochondria, thus making available substrate for oxidation and subsequent production of energy. Primary systemic deficiency of carnitine is characterized by low plasma, RBC, and/or tissue levels of the substance. Secondary carnitine deficiency is the result of inborn errors of metabolism. **Maximum plasma levels:** 3.3 hr. **t½, distribution:** 0.585 hr; **t½, elimination:** 17.4 hr. About 76% of administered levocarnitine is excreted in the urine.

**Uses:** Along with supportive and other therapy for the treatment of primary systemic carnitine deficiency. Acute and chronic treatment of clients with an inborn error of metabolism that results in secondary carnitine deficiency.

**Contraindications:** Lactation.

**Side Effects:** *GI:* N&V, abdominal cramps, diarrhea, gastritis. *Miscellaneous:* Body odor, mild myasthenia in uremic clients.

## NURSING CONSIDERATIONS
**Administration/Storage**
1. Do not use PO solution parenterally.
2. To reduce taste fatigue, PO solution can be dissolved in drinks or other liquid foods. Consume slowly.
3. Space doses evenly throughout the day to maximize tolerance.

**IV** 4. Prior to use, visually inspect the parenteral product for particulate matter and discoloration.

**Assessment**
1. Document indications for therapy: primary systemic carnitine deficiency or secondary as a result of inborn errors of metabolism.
2. Note age at onset, duration and characteristics of symptoms, and clinical presentation. Document CV status and overall clinical condition.
3. Monitor CBC, blood chemistries, ECG, VS, and plasma carnitine concentrations.
4. Assess for evidence of hypoglycemia, cardiomyopathy, Reye-like encephalopathy, hypotonia, failure to thrive, or muscle weakness; especially during the first week of therapy and with dosage increases.

**Client/Family Teaching**
1. Take exactly as directed. Solution may be dissolved in fluids or liquid foods to prevent tiring of drug taste.
2. Consume solution slowly; increase dilution, and evenly space the doses throughout the day to minimize GI reactions and to maximize tolerance.
3. Transient nausea, vomiting, diarrhea, and abdominal cramps may occur.
4. A reduction in dosage may assist to minimze drug related body odor or GI intolerance; consult provider.
5. Report any unusual side effects or worsening of clinical condition promptly.

**Outcomes/Evaluate**
• Improved overall clinical condition.
• Carnitine levels between 35 and 69 μmol/L

# Levodopa
(lee-voh-**DOH**-pah)
Dopar, Larodopa, L-Dopa **(Rx)**
**Classification:** Antiparkinson agent

**Action/Kinetics:** Depletion of dopamine in the striatum of the brain is thought to cause the symptoms of Parkinson's disease. Levodopa, a dopamine precursor, is able to cross the blood-brain barrier to enter the CNS. It is decarboxylated to dopamine in the basal ganglia, thus replenishing depleted dopamine stores. **Peak plasma levels:** 0.5–2 hr (may be delayed if ingested with food). **t½, plasma:** 1–3 hr. Onset occurs in 2–3 weeks although some clients may require up to 6 months. Extensively metabolized both in the GI tract and the liver; metabolites are excreted in the urine.

**Uses:** Idiopathic, arteriosclerotic, or postencephalitic parkinsonism. Parkinsonism due to carbon monoxide or manganese intoxication. Levodopa only provides symptomatic relief and does not alter the course of the disease. When effective, it relieves rigidity, bradykinesia, tremors, dysphagia, seborrhea, sialorrhea, and postural instability. Used in combination with carbidopa. *Investigational:* Pain from herpes zoster; restless legs syndrome.

**Contraindications:** Concomitant use with MAO inhibitors. History of melanoma or in clients with undiagnosed skin lesions. Lactation. Hypersensitivity to drug, narrow-angle glaucoma, blood dyscrasias, hypertension, coronary sclerosis.

**Special Concerns:** Use with extreme caution in clients with history of MIs, convulsions, arrhythmias, bronchial asthma, emphysema, active peptic ulcer, psychosis or neurosis, wide-angle glaucoma, and renal, hepatic, or endocrine diseases. Use during pregnancy only if benefits clearly outweigh risks. Safety has not been established in children less than 12 years of age. Geriatric clients may require a lower dose as they have a reduced tolerance for the drug and its side effects (including cardiac effects). Clients may experience an "on-off" phenomenon in which they experience an improved clinical status followed by loss of therapeutic effect.

**Side Effects:** The side effects of levodopa are numerous and usually dose related. Some may abate with usage. *CNS:* Choreiform and/or dys-

tonic movements, paranoid ideation, psychotic episodes, *depression (with possibility of suicidal tendencies),* dementia, *seizures (rare),* dizziness, headache, faintness, confusion, insomnia, nightmares, hallucinations, delusions, agitation, anxiety, malaise, fatigue, euphoria. *GI:* N&V, anorexia, abdominal pain, dry mouth, sialorrhea, dysphagia, dysgeusia, hiccups, diarrhea, constipation, burning sensation of tongue, bitter taste, flatulence, weight gain or loss, GI bleeding (rare), duodenal ulcer (rare). *CV:* Cardiac irregularities, palpitations, orthostatic hypotension, hypertension, phlebitis, hot flashes. *Ophthalmologic:* Diplopia, dilated pupils, blurred vision, development of Horner's syndrome, oculogyric crisis. *Hematologic:* **Hemolytic anemia, agranulocytosis,** leukopenia. *Musculoskeletal:* Muscle twitching (early sign of overdose), tonic contraction of the muscles of mastication, increased hand tremor, ataxia. *Miscellaneous:* Blepharospasm (early sign of overdose), urinary retention, urinary incontinence, increased sweating, unusual breathing patterns, weakness, numbness, bruxism, alopecia, priapism, hoarseness, edema, dark sweat and/or urine, flushing, skin rash, sense of stimulation. Levodopa interacts with many other drugs (see what follows) and must be administered cautiously.

**OD** **Overdose Management:** *Symptoms:* Muscle twitching, blepharospasm. Also see *Side Effects. Treatment:* Immediate gastric lavage for acute overdose. Maintain airway and give IV fluids carefully. General supportive measures.

**Drug Interactions**
*Amphetamines* / Levodopa potentiates the effect of indirectly acting sympathomimetics
*Antacids* / ↑ Effect of levodopa due to ↑ absorption from GI tract
*Anticholinergic drugs* / Possible ↓ effect of levodopa due to ↑ breakdown of levodopa in stomach (due to delayed gastric emptying time)
*Antidepressants, tricyclic* / ↓ Effect of levodopa due to ↓ absorption

from GI tract; also, ↑ risk of hypertension

*Benzodiazepines* / ↓ Effect of levodopa

*Clonidine* / ↓ Effect of levodopa

*Digoxin* / ↓ Effect of digoxin

*Ephedrine* / Levodopa potentiates the effect of indirectly acting sympathomimetics

*Furazolidone* / ↑ Effect of levodopa due to ↓ breakdown by liver

*Guanethidine* / ↑ Hypotensive effect of guanethidine

*Hypoglycemic drugs* / Levodopa upsets diabetic control with hypoglycemic agents

*MAO inhibitors* / Concomitant administration may result in hypertension, lightheadedness, and flushing due to ↓ breakdown of dopamine and norepinephrine formed from levodopa

*Methionine* / ↓ Effect of levodopa

*Methyldopa* / Additive effects including hypotension

*Metoclopramide* / ↑ Bioavailability of levodopa; ↓ effect of metoclopramide

*Papaverine* / ↓ Effect of levodopa

*Phenothiazines* / ↓ Effect of levodopa due to ↓ uptake of dopamine into neurons

*Phenytoin* / Antagonizes the effect of levodopa

*Propranolol* / May antagonize the hypotensive and positive inotropic effect of levodopa

*Pyridoxine* / Reverses levodopa-induced improvement in Parkinson's disease

*Reserpine* / Inhibits response to levodopa by ↓ dopamine in the brain

*Thioxanthines* / ↓ Effect of levodopa in Parkinson clients

*Tricyclic antidepressants* / ↓ Absorption of levodopa → ↓ effect

**Laboratory Test Interferences:** ↑ BUN, AST, LDH, ALT, bilirubin, alkaline phosphatase, protein-bound iodine. ↓ H&H, WBCs. False + Coombs' test. Interference with tests for urinary glucose and ketones.

**Dosage** ────────────
- **Capsules, Tablets**
  *Parkinsonism.*

**Adults, initial:** 250 mg b.i.d.–q.i.d. taken with food; **then,** increase total daily dose by 100–750 mg/3–7 days until optimum dosage reached (should not exceed 8 g/day). Up to 6 months may be required to achieve a significant therapeutic effect.

## NURSING CONSIDERATIONS

See also *Nursing Considerations* for *Cholinergic Blocking Agents.*

**Administration/Storage**

1. If unable to swallow tablets or capsules, crush tablets or empty the capsule into a small amount of fruit juice at the time of administration.

2. Often administered together with an anticholinergic agent.

**Assessment**

1. Review medical history for any contraindications to therapy. Stop drug 24 hr before surgery and note when drug is to be restarted.

2. Assess and document baseline rigidity, tremors, motor function, and involuntary movements. Note mental status.

3. Note adverse side effects that may require ↓ drug dose or "drug holiday"

4. Monitor ECG, CBC, liver/renal function studies, and protein bound iodine tests.

**Client/Family Teaching**

1. Take with food to decrease GI upset.

2. Report headaches; may indicate drug-induced glaucoma. Twitching or eye spasms may indicate toxicity.

3. Dosage should not exceed 8 g/day; do not stop abruptly.

4. Avoid taking multivitamin preparations containing 10–25 mg of vitamin $B_6$ rapidly reverses the antiparkinson effect of levodopa.

5. Significant results may take up to 6 months to be realized; continue taking even though immediate results are not evident.

6. Drug may cause dizziness or drowsiness; review orthostatic effects. Do not perform tasks that require mental alertness until drug effects realized.

7. Sweat and urine may appear dark; this is not harmful.

8. Sustained erection may occur; report immediately.

9. Report any evidence of depression or psychosis or any other unusual mental or behavioral changes.

10. Report for all scheduled lab and medical visits so that the effectiveness of drug therapy can be evaluated and dosage adjusted as needed.

11. Identify appropriate support services.

**Outcomes/Evaluate:** Improvement in motor function, reflexes, gait, strength of grip, and amount of tremor

---

# Levofloxacin

(**lee**-voh-**FLOX**-ah-sin)

**Pregnancy Category:** C

Levaquin **(Rx)**

**Classification:** Fluoroquinolone antibiotic

See also Fluoroquinolones.

**Uses:** Acute maxillary sinusitis due to *Streptococcus pneumoniae, Haemophilus influenzae,* or *Moraxella catarrhalis.* Acute bacterial exacerbation of chronic bronchitis due to *Staphylococcus aureus, S. pneumoniae, H. influenzae, Haemophilus parainfluenzae,* or *M. catarrhalis.* Community acquired pneumonia due to *S. aureus, S. pneumoniae, H. influenzae, H. parainfluenzae, Klebsiella pneumoniae, M. catarrhalis, Chlamydia pneumoniae, Legionella pneumonophila,* or *Mycoplasma pneumoniae.* Uncomplicated mild to moderate infections of the skin and skin structures, including abscesses, cellulitis, furuncies, impetigo, pyoderma, and wound infections due to *S. aureus* or *Streptococcus pyogenes.* Mild to moderate complicated urinary tract infections due to *Enterococcus fae-*

*calis, Enterobacter cloacae, Escherichia coli, Klebsiella pneumoniae, Proteus mirabilis,* or *Pseudomonas aeruginosa.* Acute mild to moderate pyelonephritis due to E. coli.

**Contraindications:** Lactation.

**Special Concerns:** The dose must be reduced with impaired renal function. (See *Administration/Storage*.) Safety and efficacy have not been determined in those less than 18 years of age.

**Dosage** —————————————

• **Injection, Tablets**

   *Acute maxillary sinusitis.*
500 mg once daily for 10–14 days.

   *Acute bacterial exacerbation of chronic bronchitis.*
500 mg once daily for 7 days.

   *Community acquired pneumonia.*
500 mg once daily for 7–14 days.

   *Uncomplicated skin and skin structure infections.*
500 mg once daily for 7–10 days.

   *Complicated urinary tract infections.*
250 mg once daily for 10 days.

   *Acute pyelonephritis.*
250 mg once daily for 10 days.

---

## NURSING CONSIDERATIONS

See also *Nursing Considerations* for Fluoroquinolones, .

**Administration/Storage**

1. Reduce dose with impaired renal function when used for acute maxillary sinusitis, acute bacterial exacerbation of chronic bronchitis, community acquired pneumonia, and uncomplicated skin and skin structure infections. If $C_{CR}$ is between 20 and 49 mL/min, the initial dose is 500 mg and subsequent doses are 250 mg q 24 hr. If $C_{CR}$ is between 10 and 19 mL/min, the initial dose is 500 mg and subsequent doses are 250 mg q 48 hr. If the client is on hemodialysis or chronic ambulatory peritoneal dialysis, the initial dose is 500 mg and subsequent doses are 250 mg q 48 hr.

2. Oral doses are given at least 2 hr before or 2 hr after antacids containing magnesium or aluminum, as

well as sucralfate, iron products, and multivitamin preparations containing zinc.

3. Store tablets in a tight container at 15°C–30°C (59°F–85°F).

**IV** 4. The injectable form may be mixed with 0.9% NaCl injection, 5% dextrose injection, D5%/0.9% NaCl, 5% dextrose in RL, Plasma-Lyte 56/5% dextrose injection, D5%/0.45% NaCl, 0.15% potassium chloride injection, or M/6 sodium lactate injection.

5. Diluted solutions for IV use are stable for 72 hr up to a concentration of 5 mg/mL when stored in IV containers at 25°C or less (77°F or less). Such solutions are stable for 14 days when stored under refrigeration at 5°C (41°F). Diluted solutions that are frozen in glass bottles or plastic IV containers are stable for 6 months when stored at –20°C (–4°F).

6. Thaw frozen solutions at room temperature or in a refrigerator. Do not thaw in a microwave or by bath immersion. After initial thawing, do not refreeze.

**Client/Family Teaching**

1. Take only as directed; complete entire prescription.

2. Avoid multivitamins with zinc, iron products, sucralfate, and magnesium- or aluminum-containing antacids for 2 hr before and after dose.

3. Practice reliable birth control during therapy.

4. Use caution until drug effects realized; may experience dizziness, drowsiness or visual changes.

5. Notify provider if symptoms do not improve or worsen after 72 hr of therapy.

**Outcomes/Evaluate**

• Symptomatic improvement

• Resolution of infective organism

# Levomethadyl acetate hydrochloride

(lee-voh-**METH**-ah-dill)

**Pregnancy Category:** C

ORLAAM **(Rx)**

**Classification:** Narcotic analgesic only for use in opiate dependence

See also *Narcotic Analgesics.*

**Uses:** Treatment of opiate dependence. *NOTE:* This drug can be dispensed only by treatment programs approved by the FDA, DEA, and the designated state authority. The drug can be dispensed only in the oral form and according to treatment requirements stated in federal regulations. The drug has no approved uses outside of the treatment of opiate dependence.

**Special Concerns:** Usual dose must not be given on consecutive days due to the risk of fatal overdosage.

**Side Effects:** See *Narcotic Analgesics.* Induction with levomethadyl that is too rapid for the level of tolerance of the client may result in overdosage, including symptoms of both *respiratory and CV depression.*

**Dosage**

• **Oral Solution**

*Induction.*

**Initial:** 20–40 mg administered at 48–72-hr intervals; **then,** dose may be increased in increments of 5–10 mg until steady state is reached (usually within 1–2 weeks). Clients dependent on methadone may require higher initial doses of levomethadyl; the suggested initial 3-times/week dose for such clients is 1.2–1.3 times the daily methadone maintenance dose being replaced. This initial dose should not exceed 120 mg with subsequent doses given at 48- or 72-hr intervals, depending on the response. If additional opioids are required, supplemental amounts of methadone should be given rather than giving levomethadyl on 2 consecutive days.

*Maintenance.*

Most clients are stabilized on doses of 60–90 mg 3 times/week although the dose may range from 10 to 140 mg 3 times/week. The maximum *total* amount of levomethadyl recommended for any client is either 140,

**L**

140, 140 mg or 130, 130, 180 mg on a thrice-weekly schedule.

*Reinduction after an unplanned lapse in dosing: following a lapse of one levomethadyl dose.*

If the client comes to the clinic the day following a missed scheduled dose (e.g., misses Monday and arrives at clinic on Tuesday), the regular Monday dose is given, with the scheduled Wednesday dose given on Thursday and the Friday dose given on Saturday. The client's regular schedule can be resumed the following Monday. If the client misses one dose and comes to the clinic the day of the next scheduled dose (i.e., misses Monday, comes to clinic on Wednesday), the usual dose will be well tolerated in most cases although some clients will need a reduced dose.

*Reintroduction after a lapse of more than one levomethadyl dose.*

Restart the client at an initial dose of 50%–75% of the previous dose, followed by increases of 5–10 mg every dosing day (i.e., intervals of 48–72 hr) until the previous maintenance dose is reached.

*Transfer from levomethadyl to methadone.*

Transfer can be done directly, although the dose of methadone should be 80% of the levomethadyl dose being replaced. The first methadone dose should not be given sooner than 48 hr after the last levomethadyl dose. Increases or decreases of 5–10 mg may be made in the daily methadone dose to control symptoms of withdrawal or symptoms of excessive sedation.

*Detoxification from levomethadyl.*

Both gradual reduction (i.e., 5%–10% a week) and abrupt withdrawal have been used successfully.

## NURSING CONSIDERATIONS
### Administration/Storage

1. The drug is usually given 3 times/week—either on Monday, Wednesday, and Friday or on Tuesday, Thursday, and Saturday. If withdrawal is a problem with this interval, the preceding dose may be increased.

2. If the degree of tolerance is not known, may start on methadone to facilitate more rapid titration to an effective dose. Then can be converted to levomethadyl after a few weeks. The cross-over from methadone to levomethadyl should be accomplished in a single dose.

3. During maintenance therapy, if, e.g., those on a Monday, Wednesday, and Friday schedule complain of withdrawal symptoms on Sunday, the Friday dose may be increased in 5- to 10-mg increments up to 40% over the Monday/Wednesday dose up to a maximum of 140 mg.

4. Levomethadyl take-home doses are not permitted. If a situation arises where the client cannot come to the clinic for a regular dose of levomethadyl, they may be switched to receive one or more doses of methadone. These should be 80% of the client's Monday/Wednesday levomethadyl dose; the first dose of methadone should be taken no sooner than 48 hr after the last dose of levomethadyl. The number of take-home doses of methadone should be two less than the number of days expected absence and should not exceed the number of take-home doses allowed in the methadone regulations. Upon return to clinic, client should resume levomethadyl maintenance following the same dosage schedule prior to the temporary interruption. If more than 48 hr has elapsed since the last methadone dose, reintroduce on levomethadyl at a dose determined by the clinical evaluation.

### Assessment

1. Document that client is opiate dependent, length of dependence, type and method of specific drugs used.

2. Determine methadone usage as drug requirements may be higher.

3. Identify that client has been accepted/approved for drug through a federally approved treatment protocol.

4. In clients who have missed

scheduled doses, follow administration guidelines carefully.

**Client/Family Teaching**
1. Must comply with regularly scheduled doses of levomethadyl.
2. Although the program does not require daily dosing, it does require that the client physically come to clinic for scheduled medication administration (usually every other day).
3. Identify additional support groups/persons who may assist in their goal of freedom from addiction.
4. Determine other resources (child care, job retraining, food stamps, etc.) that would support them in their goal to live drug free.

**Outcomes/Evaluate:** Freedom from drug (opiate) dependence

# Levonorgestrel Implants
(**lee**-voh-nor-**JES**-trel)
**Pregnancy Category:** X
Norgestrel II, Norplant System **(Rx)**
**Classification:** Progestin, contraceptive system

See also *Progesterone and Progestins.*

**Action/Kinetics:** Levonorgestrel implants are marketed either in a set of six flexible Silastic capsules each containing 36 mg of levonorgestrel or two rods containing 150 mg of levonorgestrel; an insertion kit is provided to the provider to assist with implantation. Small amounts of the drug slowly diffuse through the wall of each capsule resulting in blood levels of levonorgestrel that are lower than those seen when levonorgestrel or norgestrel is taken as oral contraceptive. The dose released is initially 85 mcg/day, followed by a decrease to approximately 50 mcg/day after 9 months, to 35 mcg/day after 18 months, and then leveling off to 30 mcg/day thereafter. Blood levels of levonorgestrel vary over a wide range and cannot be used as the sole measure of the risk of pregnancy. If used properly, the risk of pregnancy is less than

1 for every 100 users. Levonorgestrel does not have any estrogenic effects. The implant system lasts up to 5 years and the contraceptive effect is rapidly reversed if the system is removed from the body.

**Uses:** Prevention of pregnancy (system lasts for up to 5 years). New capsules may be inserted after 5 years if continuing contraception is desired. A product (Norgestrel II) containing two rods of levonorgestrel instead of six rods is also available.

**Contraindications:** Active thrombophlebitis, thromboembolic disorders, undiagnosed abnormal genital bleeding, acute liver disease, benign or malignant liver tumors, known or suspected breast carcinoma, confirmed or suspected pregnancy.

**Special Concerns:** Menstrual bleeding irregularities are commonly observed. Women who have a family history of breast cancer or who have breast nodules should be monitored carefully. Use with caution in individuals in whom fluid retention might be dangerous and in those with a history of depression. Women being treated for hyperlipidemias should be monitored closely because an increase in LDL levels may occur. Capsules should not be inserted until 6 weeks after parturition in women who are breast-feeding.

**Side Effects:** *Menstrual irregularities:* Prolonged menses, spotting, irregular onset of menses, frequent menses, amenorrhea, scanty bleeding, cervicitis, vaginitis. *At implant site:* Pain or itching, infection, bruising following insertion or removal, hyperpigmentation (reversible upon removal). *GI:* Abdominal discomfort, nausea, change of appetite, weight gain. *CNS:* Headache, nervousness, dizziness. *Dermatologic:* Dermatitis, acne, hirsutism, scalp hair loss, excess hair growth. *Miscellaneous:* Breast discharge, breast pain, leukorrhea, musculoskeletal pain, fluid retention, possibility of ectopic pregnancy in long-term users, delayed follicular atresia.

**OD** **Overdose Management:**
*Symptoms:* Overdosage can result if more than six capsules are inserted. Symptoms include fluid retention and uterine bleeding irregularities. *Treatment:* All capsules should be removed.

**Drug Interactions**
*Carbamazepine* / ↓ Effectiveness → ↑ risk of pregnancy
*Phenytoin* / ↓ Effectiveness → ↑ risk of pregnancy

**Laboratory Test Interferences:** ↓ Sex hormone binding globulin levels, $T_4$ levels (slight). ↑ Uptake of $T_3$.

**Dosage**
• **Silastic Capsules**
Six levonorgestrel-containing (36 mg each) Silastic capsules implanted subdermally in the midportion of the upper arm (8–10 cm above the elbow crease). Capsules are distributed in a fan-like pattern 15° apart (total of 75°).

## NURSING CONSIDERATIONS

See also *Nursing Considerations* for *Progesterone and Progestins*.

**Administration/Storage**
1. To ensure effectiveness and to be sure the woman is not pregnant at the time of capsule implantation, implant capsules during the first 7 days of the cycle or immediately after an abortion.
2. Capsules should be inserted only by individuals instructed on the proper procedure for insertion. If capsules are placed too deeply, they may be more difficult to remove.
3. If all capsules cannot be removed at the first attempt, allow the site to heal before another attempt is made.
4. Expulsion is not common but may occur if the capsules are placed too shallow/too close to the incision or if infection occurs.
5. If infection occurs, treat and cure before replacing capsules.
6. After 5 years, remove capsules; if additional contraception desired, a new set of capsules can be inserted.

**Assessment**
1. A complete medical history, physical and gynecologic exam

should be performed prior to implantation or reimplantation and annually during use.
2. Ensure not pregnant at the time of implantation.
3. Determine if breast-feeding; do not insert until 6 weeks after delivery.
4. Note any history of thromboembolic disorders or depression.
5. Assess liver function and for evidence of hyperlipidemia.
6. Assess for family history of breast cancer. Document presence of breast nodules; these require careful monitoring.
7. Obtain baseline weight. Be aware that the effectiveness of levonorgestrel may be slightly decreased with weights exceeding 70.5 kg.

**Client/Family Teaching**
1. Review procedure for wound care postinsertion and identify symptoms of infection and rejection that should be reported. A small scar may be evident at the insertion site.
2. Expect some irregularity with the menstrual cycle such as longer periods, missed periods, and spotting in between during the first year of implantation.
3. Report for regularly scheduled F/U visits so that therapy can be carefully evaluated.
4. The capsules may be removed at any time for any reason; pregnancy can occur after the next menstrual cycle.
5. Additional protection must be used to prevent STDs.

**Outcomes/Evaluate:** Effective contraception

# Levothyroxine sodium $(T_4)$
(lee-voh-thigh-**ROX**-een)
**Pregnancy Category:** A
Eltroxin, Levo-T, Levothroid, Levoxyl, Synthroid, L-Thyroxine Sodium **(Rx)**
**Classification:** Thyroid preparation

See also *Thyroid Drugs*.
**Action/Kinetics:** Levothyroxine is the synthetic sodium salt of the levoisomer of $T_4$ (tetraiodothyronine). Levothyroxine, 0.05–0.6 mg

equals approximately 60 mg (1 grain) of thyroid. Absorption from the GI tract is incomplete and variable, especially when taken with food. Has a slower onset but a longer duration than sodium liothyronine. More active on a weight basis than thyroid. Is usually the drug of choice. Effect is predictable as thyroid content is standard. **Time to peak therapeutic effect:** 3–4 weeks. **t½:** 6–7 days in a euthyroid person, 9–10 days in a hypothyroid client, and 3–4 days in a hyperthyroid client. Is 99% protein bound. **Duration:** 1–3 weeks after withdrawal of chronic therapy. *NOTE:* All levothyroxine products are not bioequivalent; thus, changing brands is not recommended.

**Drug Interactions:** Concurrent use of aluminum hydroxide and levothyroxine may result in adsorption of levothyroxine to the aluminum and increased fecal elimination of levothyroxine.

**Dosage**
• **Tablets**
*Mild hypothyroidism.*
**Adults, initial:** 50 mcg once daily; **then,** increase by 25–50 mcg q 2–3 weeks until desired clinical response is attained; **maintenance, usual:** 75–125 mcg/day (although doses up to 200 mcg/day may be required in some clients).
*Severe hypothyroidism.*
**Adults, initial:** 12.5–25 mcg once daily; **then,** increase dose, as necessary, in increments of 25 mcg at 2- to 3-week intervals.
*Congenital hypothyroidism.*
**Pediatric, 12 years and older:** 2–3 mcg/kg once daily until the adult daily dose (usually 150 mcg) is reached. **6–12 years of age:** 4–5 mcg/kg/day or 100–150 mcg once daily. **1–5 years of age:** 5–6 mcg/kg/day or 75–100 mcg once daily. **6–12 months of age:** 6–8 mcg/kg/day or 50–75 mcg once daily. **Less than 6 months of age:** 8–10

mcg/kg/day or 25–50 mcg once daily.
• **IM, IV**
*Myxedematous coma.*
**Adults, initial:** 400 mcg by rapid IV injection, even in geriatric clients; **then,** 100–200 mcg/day, IV. **Maintenance:** 100–200 mcg/day, IV. Smaller daily doses should be given until client can tolerate PO medication.
*Hypothyroidism.*
**Adults:** 50–100 mcg once daily; **pediatric, IV, IM:** A dose of 75% of the usual PO pediatric dose should be given.

## NURSING CONSIDERATIONS

See also *Nursing Considerations* for *Thyroid Drugs.*
**Administration/Storage**
1. In infants and children who cannot swallow tablets, the correct dosage tablet may be crushed and suspended in a small amount of formula or water and given by dropper or spoon. The crushed tablet may also be sprinkled over cooked cereal or applesauce.
2. Transfer from liothyronine to levothyroxine: administer replacement drug for several days before discontinuing liothyronine. Transfer from levothyroxine to liothyronine: discontinue levothyroxine before starting low daily dose of liothyronine.
**IV** 3. Prepare solution for injection immediately before administration. Reconstitute by adding 5 mL of 0.9% NaCl injection or bacteriostatic NaCl injection and shake vial to ensure complete mixing.
4. Discard any unused portion of the IV medication.
5. Do not mix with other IV infusion solutions.
**Assessment**
1. Elderly clients are likely to have undetected cardiac problems. Obtain ECG prior to initiating therapy.
2. Monitor thyroid profile.
3. If pregnant, must continue taking thyroid preparations throughout the pregnancy.

L

4. Document height, weight, and psychomotor development in children.

5. List drugs currently consumed to ensure none interact unfavorably.

**Client/Family Teaching**

1. Do not switch brands; bioavailability may change.

2. Do not take with food unless specifically instructed; may interfere with absorption.

3. Report any persistent headaches, increased HR (hold if resting HR is greater than 100), chest pain, diarrhea, irritability, excitability, more than 5 lb/week weight loss, and excessive sweating.

4. Avoid iodine-rich foods.

5. Drug is not a cure for hypothyroidism; must be taken for lifetime to control symptoms.

**Outcomes/Evaluate**

• Promotion of normal metabolism
• ↑ Levels of $T_3$ and $T_4$, ↓ TSH

------COMBINATION DRUG------

# Librax
(**LIB**-rax)
**(Rx)**
**Classification:** Antianxiety agent

See also *Tranquilizers, Antimanic Drugs, and Hypnotics* and *Cholinergic Blocking Agents*.

**Content:** *Antianxiety agent:* Chlordiazepoxide, 5 mg. *Anticholinergic agent:* Clidinium bromide, 2.5 mg. See also information on individual components.

**Uses:** Possibly effective as an adjunct in the treatment of irritable colon, spastic colon, mucous colitis, and acute enterocolitis.

**Contraindications:** Pregnancy, glaucoma, prostatic hypertrophy.

**Dosage** ------
• **Capsules**
**Individualized. Adults, usual:** 1–2 capsules t.i.d.–q.i.d. before meals and at bedtime.

## NURSING CONSIDERATIONS

See *Nursing Considerations* for *Tranquilizers, Antimanic Drugs, and Hypnotics* and *Cholinergic Blocking Agents*.

**Outcomes/Evaluate**

• Restoration of normal bowel motility and relief of pain
• Symptomatic improvement

# Lidocaine hydrochloride
(**LYE**-doh-kayn)
**Pregnancy Category:** B
**IM:** LidoPen Auto-Injector, **(Rx). Direct IV or IV Admixtures:** Lidocaine HCl for Cardiac Arrhythmias, Xylocaine HCl IV for Cardiac Arrhythmias, Xylocard ✽ **(Rx). IV Infusion:** Lidocaine HCl in 5% Dextrose **(Rx)**
**Classification:** Antiarrhythmic, class IB

See also *Antiarrhythmic Agents*.
**Action/Kinetics:** Shortens the refractory period and suppresses the automaticity of ectopic foci without affecting conduction of impulses through cardiac tissue. Increases the electrical stimulation threshold of the ventricle during diastole. It does not affect BP, CO, or myocardial contractility. **IV: Onset,** 45–90 sec; **duration:** 10–20 min. **IM, Onset,** 5–15 min; **duration,** 60–90 min. **t½:** 1–2 hr. **Therapeutic serum levels:** 1.5–6 mcg/mL. **Time to steady-state plasma levels:** 3–4 hr (8–10 hr in clients with AMI). **Protein-binding:** 40%–80%. Ninety percent is rapidly metabolized in the liver to active metabolites. Since lidocaine has little effect on conduction at normal antiarrhythmic doses, use in acute situations (instead of procainamide) in instances in which heart block might occur.

**Uses: IV:** Treatment of acute ventricular arrhythmias such as those following MIs or occurring during surgery. The drug is ineffective against atrial arrhythmias. **IM:** Certain emergency situations (e.g., ECG equipment not available; mobile coronary care unit, under advice of a physician).

*Investigational:* IV in children who develop ventricular couplets or frequent premature ventricular beats.

**Contraindications:** Hypersensitivity to amide-type local anesthetics, Stokes-Adams syndrome, Wolff-

Parkinson-White syndrome, severe SA, AV, or intraventricular block (when no pacemaker is present).
**Special Concerns:** Use with caution during labor and delivery, during lactation, and in the presence of liver or severe kidney disease, CHF, marked hypoxia, digitalis toxicity with AV block, severe respiratory depression, or shock. In geriatric clients, the rate and dose for IV infusion should be decreased by one-half and slowly adjusted. Safety and efficacy have not been determined in children; the IM autoinjector product should not be used for children.
**Side Effects:** *Body as a whole:* Malignant hyperthermia characterized by tachycardia, tachypnea, labile BP, metabolic acidosis, temperature elevation. *CV: **Precipitation or aggravation of arrhythmias (following IV use),** hypotension, **bradycardia (with possible cardiac arrest), CV collapse.** CNS:* Dizziness, apprehension, euphoria, lightheadedness, nervousness, drowsiness, confusion, changes in mood, hallucinations, twitching, "doom anxiety," **convulsions,** unconsciousness. *Respiratory:* Difficulties in breathing or swallowing, **respiratory depression or arrest.** *Allergic:* Rash, cutaneous lesions, urticaria, edema, **anaphylaxis.** *Other:* Tinnitus, blurred or double vision, vomiting, numbness, sensation of heat or cold, twitching, tremors, soreness at IM injection site, fever, **venous thrombosis or phlebitis (extending from site of injection),** extravasation. During anesthesia, CV depression may be the first sign of lidocaine toxicity. During other usage, convulsions are the first sign of lidocaine toxicity.
**OD** **Overdose Management:** *Symptoms:* Symptoms are dependent on plasma levels. If plasma levels range from 4 to 6 mcg/mL, mild CNS effects are observed. Levels of 6 to 8 mcg/mL may result in significant CNS and CV depression while levels greater than 8 mcg/mL cause hypotension, decreased CO, respiratory depression, obtundation, **seizures,**

**and coma.** *Treatment:* Discontinue the drug and begin emergency resuscitative procedures. Seizures can be treated with diazepam, thiopental, or thiamylal. Succinylcholine, IV, may be used if the client is anesthetized. IV fluids, vasopressors, and CPR are used to correct circulatory depression.
**Drug Interactions**
*Aminoglycosides* / ↑ Neuromuscular blockade
*Beta-adrenergic blockers* / ↑ Lidocaine levels with possible toxicity
*Cimetidine* / ↓ Clearance of lidocaine → possible toxicity
*Phenytoin* / IV phenytoin → excessive cardiac depression
*Procainamide* / Additive cardiodepressant effects
*Succinylcholine* / ↑ Action of succinylcholine by ↓ plasma protein binding
*Tocainide* / ↑ Risk of side effects
*Tubocurarine* / ↑ Neuromuscular blockade
**Laboratory Test Interferences:** ↑ CPK following IM use.

**Dosage** ————————
• **IV Bolus**
  *Antiarrhythmic.*
**Adults:** 50–100 mg at rate of 25–50 mg/min. Bolus is used to establish rapid therapeutic plasma levels. Repeat if necessary after 5-min interval. Onset of action is 10 sec. **Maximum dose/hr:** 200–300 mg.
• **Infusion**
  *Antiarrhythmic.*
20–50 mcg/kg at a rate of 1–4 mg/min. No more than 200–300 mg/hr should be given. **Pediatric, loading dose:** 1 mg/kg IV or intratracheally q 5–10 min until desired effect reached (maximum total dose: 5 mg/kg).
• **IV Continuous Infusion**
  *Maintain therapeutic plasma levels following loading doses.*
**Adults:** Give at a rate of 1–4 mg/min (20–50 mcg/kg/min). Dose should be reduced in clients with heart failure, with liver disease, or who are taking drugs that interact with lido-

caine. **Pediatric:** 20–50 mcg/kg/min (usual is 30 mcg/kg/min).

• **IM**

*Antiarrhythmic.*

**Adults:** 4.5 mg/kg (approximately 300 mg for a 70-kg adult). Switch to IV lidocaine or oral antiarrhythmics as soon as possible although an additional IM dose may be given after 60–90 min.

## NURSING CONSIDERATIONS

See also *Nursing Considerations* for *Antiarrhythmic Agents.*

**Administration/Storage**

**IV** 1. *Do not add lidocaine to blood transfusion assembly.*

2. Do not use lidocaine solutions that contain epinephrine to treat arrhythmias. Make certain that vial states, "For Cardiac Arrhythmias." Check prefilled syringes closely to ensure appropriate dose has been obtained. (Lidocaine prefilled syringes come in both milligrams and grams.)

3. Use D5W to prepare solution; this is stable for 24 hr. Administer with an electronic infusion device.

4. Reduce IV bolus dosage in clients over 70 years of age, in those with CHF or liver disease, and in clients taking cimetidine or propranolol (i.e., where metabolism of lidocaine is reduced).

**Assessment**

1. Note any hypersensitivity to amide-type local anesthetics.

2. Elderly clients who have hepatic or renal disease or who weigh less than 45.5 kg will need to be watched especially closely for adverse side effects; adjust dosage as directed.

3. Document CNS status; report sudden changes in mental status, dizziness, visual disturbances, twitching, and tremors. These symptoms may precede convulsions. Note pulmonary findings; assess for respiratory depression, characterized by slow, shallow respirations. Monitor liver and renal function studies, electrolytes, and ECG; assess for hypotension and cardiac collapse.

4. View monitor strips for myocar-
dial depression, variations of rhythm, or aggravation of arrhythmia.

**Outcomes/Evaluate**

• Control of ventricular arrhythmias

• Therapeutic serum drug levels (1.5–6 mcg/mL)

# Lincomycin hydrochloride

(link-oh-**MY**-sin)

Lincocin **(Rx)**

**Classification:** Anti-infective

See also *Anti-Infectives.*

**Action/Kinetics:** Isolated from *Streptomyces lincolnensis.* Suppresses protein synthesis by microorganisms by binding to ribosomes (50S subunit), which is essential for transmittal of genetic information. Both bacteriostatic and bactericidal. Rapidly absorbed from the GI tract and is widely distributed. **Peak serum levels: PO,** 2.6 mcg/mL after 500 mg; **IM,** 9.5 mcg/mL after 600 mg; **IV,** 19 mcg/mL after 600 mg. **t½:** 4.4–6.4 hr. Do not use for trivial infections.

**Uses:** Not a first-choice drug but useful for clients allergic to penicillin. Spectrum resembles that of the erythromycins. Used for serious respiratory tract, skin, and soft tissue infections due to staphylococci, streptococci, or pneumococci and some gram-negative organisms. Septicemia. In conjunction with diphtheria antitoxin in the treatment of diphtheria.

**Contraindications:** Hypersensitivity to drugs. Use in infants up to 1 month of age.

**Special Concerns:** Safe use during pregnancy has not been established. Use with caution in clients with GI disease, liver or renal disease, or a history of allergy or asthma. Not for use in treating viral and minor bacterial infections.

**Side Effects:** *GI:* N&V, diarrhea, abdominal pain, tenesmus, flatulence, bloating, anorexia, weight loss, esophagitis. Nonspecific colitis, pseudomembranous colitis (may be severe). *Allergic:* Morbilliform rash (most common). Also, maculopapular rash, urticaria, pruritus, fever, hypotension. Rarely, polyarteritis, **anaphy-laxis,** erythema multiforme. *Hemato-logic:* Leukopenia, neutropenia, eosinophilia, thrombocytopenia, **agranulocytosis.** *Miscellaneous:* Superinfection.

*Following IV use:* Thrombophlebitis, erythema, pain, swelling. IV lincomycin may cause hypotension, syncope, and **cardiac arrest** (rare). *Following IM use:* Pain, induration, sterile abscesses. *Following topical use:* Erythema, irritation, dryness, peeling, itching, burning, oiliness. Also, sore throat, fatigue, urinary frequency, headache.

*NOTE:* The injection contains benzyl alcohol, which has been associated with a fatal gasping syndrome in infants.

**Drug Interactions**
*Antiperistaltic antidiarrheals (opiates, Lomotil)* / ↑ Diarrhea due to ↓ removal of toxins from colon
*Erythromycin* / Cross-interference → ↓ effect of both drugs
*Kaolin (e.g., Kaopectate)* / ↓ Effect due to ↓ absorption from GI tract
*Neuromuscular blocking agents* / ↑ Effect of blocking agents

**Laboratory Test Interferences:** ↓ Levels of AST, ALT, NPN, alkaline phosphatase, bilirubin, BSP retention, and ↓ platelet count.

**Dosage**
• **Capsules**
*Infections.*
**Adults:** 500 mg t.i.d.–q.i.d.; **children over 1 month of age:** 30–60 mg/kg/day in three to four divided doses, depending on severity of infection.
• **IM**
*Infections.*
**Adults:** 600 mg q 12–24 hr; **children over 1 month of age:** 10 mg/kg q 12–24 hr, depending on severity of infection.
• **IV**
*Infections.*
**Adults:** 0.6–1.0 g q 8–12 hr up to 8 g/day, depending on severity of infection; **children over 1 month of**

**age:** 10–20 mg/kg/day, depending on severity of infection.

*NOTE:* In impaired renal function, reduce dosage by 70%–75%.
• **Subconjunctival Injection**
0.75 mg/0.25 mL.

## NURSING CONSIDERATIONS

See also *General Nursing Considerations for All Anti-Infectives.*
**Administration/Storage**
1. Prepare drug for administration as directed on package insert.
2. Administer slowly IM to minimize pain.
**IV** 3. For IV use, carefully follow concentration and recommended rate for administration to prevent severe cardiopulmonary reactions.
4. Injection contains benzyl alcohol.
**Assessment**
1. Manage colitis by providing fluids, electrolytes, protein supplements, systemic corticosteroids, and vancomycin (may occur 2–9 days to several weeks after initiation of therapy).
2. Assess for transient flushing, sensations of warmth and cardiac disturbances, which may accompany IV infusions.
3. Monitor VS, CBC, and LFTs.
**Client/Family Teaching**
1. Take on an empty stomach between meals and not with a sugar substitute, to ensure optimum absorption. Report GI disturbances, including abdominal pain, diarrhea, anorexia, N&V, bloody or tarry stools, and excessive flatulence.
2. Do not use antiperistaltic agents if diarrhea occurs; may prolong or aggravate condition.
3. Avoid acne or topical mercury preparations containing a peeling agent in an area affected by medication because severe irritation can occur.
4. Do not take kaolin concomitantly because it will reduce absorption of lincomycin; if kaolin is required, administer 3 hr before.

**Outcomes/Evaluate**
* Negative culture reports
* Resolution of infection

# Liothyronine sodium ($T_3$)

(lye-oh-**THIGH**-roh-neen)
**Pregnancy Category:** A
Cytomel, Sodium-L-Triiodothyronine,
Triostat **(Rx)**
**Classification:** Thyroid preparation

See also *Thyroid Drugs.*
**Action/Kinetics:** Synthetic sodium salt of levoisomer of $T_3$. Has more predictable effects due to standard hormone content. From 15 to 37.5 mcg is equivalent to about 60 mg of desiccated thyroid. May be preferred when a rapid effect or rapidly reversible effect is required. Has a rapid onset, which may result in difficulty in controlling the dosage as well as the possibility of cardiac side effects and changes in metabolic demands. However, its short duration allows quick adjustment of dosage and helps control overdosage. **t½:** 24 hr for euthyroid clients, approximately 34 hr in hypothyroid clients, and approximately 14 hr in hyperthyroid clients. **Duration:** Up to 72 hr. Is 99% protein bound.
**Additional Contraindications:** Use of liothyronine is not recommended in children with cretinism because there is some question about whether the hormone crosses the blood-brain barrier.

**Dosage**
* **Tablets**
  *Mild hypothyroidism.*
**Adults, individualized, initial:** 25 mcg/day. Increase by 12.5–25 mcg q 1–2 weeks until satisfactory response has been obtained. **Usual maintenance:** 25–75 mcg/day (100 mcg may be required in some clients). Use lower initial dosage (5 mcg/day) for the elderly, children, and clients with CV disease. Increase only by 5-mcg increments.
  *Myxedema.*
**Adults, initial:** 5 mcg/day increased by 5–10 mcg/day q 1–2 weeks until 25 mcg/day is reached; **then,** increase q

1–2 weeks by 12.5–50 mcg. **Usual maintenance:** 50–100 mcg/day.
  *Simple (nontoxic) goiter.*
**Adults, initial:** 5 mcg/day; **then,** increase q 1–2 weeks by 5–10 mcg until 25 mcg/day is reached; **then,** dose can be increased by 12.5–25 mcg/week until the maintenance dose of 50–100 mcg/day is reached (usual is 75 mcg/day).
  *$T_3$ suppression test.*
75–100 mcg/day for 7 days followed by a repeat of the $I^{131}$ thyroid uptake test (a 50% or greater suppression of uptake indicates a normal thyroid-pituitary axis).
  *Congenital hypothyroidism.*
**Adults and children, initial:** 5 mcg/day; **then,** increase by 5 mcg/day q 3–4 days until the desired effect is achieved. Approximately 20 mcg/day may be sufficient for infants a few months of age while children 1 year of age may require 50 mcg/day. Children above 3 years may require the full adult dose.
* **IV Only**
  *Myxedema coma, precoma.*
**Adults, initial:** 25–50 mcg. Base subsequent doses on continuous monitoring of client's clinical status and response. Doses should be given at least 4 hr, and no more than 12 hr, apart. Total daily doses of 65 mcg in initial days of therapy are associated with a lower incidence of mortality. In cases of known CV disease, an initial dose of 10–20 mcg should be given.

# NURSING CONSIDERATIONS

See also *Nursing Considerations* for *Thyroid Drugs,* and *Levothyroxine.*
**Administration/Storage**
1. *Transfer from other thyroid preparations to liothyronine:* Discontinue old preparation before starting on low daily dose of liothyronine. *Transfer from liothyronine to another thyroid preparation:* Start therapy with replacement drug several days prior to complete withdrawal of sodium liothyronine.
2. If symptoms of hyperthyroidism noted, the drug can be withdrawn

for 2–3 days and can be reinstituted at a lower dose.

**IV** 3. A *Cytomel* injection kit is available for the emergency treatment of myxedema coma.

**Outcomes/Evaluate:** Thyroid hormone replacement

---

# Liotrix

(**LYE**-oh-trix)
**Pregnancy Category:** A
Thyrolar **(Rx)**
**Classification:** Thyroid preparation

---

See also *Thyroid Drugs.*

**General Statement:** Mixture of synthetic levothyroxine sodium ($T_4$) and liothyronine ($T_3$). The mixture contains the products in a 4:1 ratio by weight and in a 1:1 ratio by biologic activity. The two commercial preparations contain slightly different amounts of each component. Because of this discrepancy, a switch from one preparation to the other must be made cautiously. Liotrix has standard hormone content; thus, the effect is predictable.

**Dosage**
• **Tablets**
  *Hypothyroidism.*
**Adults and children, initial:** 50 mcg levothyroxine and 12.5 mcg liothyronine (Thyrolar); **then,** at monthly intervals, increments of like amounts can be made until the desired effect is achieved. **Usual maintenance:** 50–100 mcg of levothyroxine and 12.5–25 mcg liothyronine daily.
  *Congenital hypothyroidism.*
**Children, 0–6 months:** 8–10 mcg $T_4$/kg/day (25–50 mcg/day); **6–12 months:** 6–8 mcg $T_4$/kg/day (50–75 mcg/day); **1–5 years:** 5–6 mcg $T_4$/kg/day (75–100 mcg/day); **6–12 years:** 4–5 mcg $T_4$/kg/day (100–150 mcg/day); **over 12 years:** 2–3 mcg $T_4$/kg/day (over 150 mcg/day).

## NURSING CONSIDERATIONS

See also *Nursing Considerations* for *Thyroid Drugs* and individual agents.

**Administration/Storage**
1. The initial dose for geriatric clients should be ½ the usual adult dose; this can be doubled q 6–8 weeks until desired effect is attained.
2. In children, make dosing increments q 2 weeks until desired response attained.
3. Always do thyroid function tests before initiating dosage changes.
4. Administer as a single dose before breakfast.
5. Protect tablets from light, heat, and moisture.
6. Due to differences in the amounts of hormones between Euthroid and Thyrolar, do not switch brands once started on a particular brand.

**Outcomes/Evaluate:** Thyroid hormone replacement

---

# Lisinopril

(lie-**SIN**-oh-prill)
**Pregnancy Category:** C
Prinivil, Zestril **(Rx)**
**Classification:** Antihypertensive, ACE inhibitor

---

See also *Angiotensin-Converting Enzyme Inhibitors.*

**Action/Kinetics:** Both supine and standing BPs are reduced, although the drug is less effective in blacks than in Caucasians. Although food does not alter the bioavailability of lisinopril, only 25% of a PO dose is absorbed. **Onset:** 1 hr. **Peak serum levels:** 7 hr. **Duration:** 24 hr. **t½:** 12 hr. 100% of the drug is excreted unchanged in the urine.

**Uses:** Alone or in combination with a diuretic (usually a thiazide) to treat hypertension (step I therapy). In combination with digitalis and a diuretic for treating CHF not responding to other therapy. Use within 24 hr of acute MI to improve survival in hemodynamically stable clients (clients should receive the standard treatment, including thrombolytics, aspirin, and beta blockers).

**L**

---

**Special Concerns:** Use with caution during lactation. Safety and efficacy have not been established in children. Geriatric clients may manifest higher blood levels. Dosage should be reduced in clients with impaired renal function.

**Side Effects:** *CNS:* Dizziness, headache, fatigue, vertigo, insomnia, depression, sleepiness, paresthesias, malaise, nervousness, confusion. *GI:* Diarrhea, N&V, dyspepsia, anorexia, constipation, dysgeusia, dry mouth, abdominal pain, flatulence. *Respiratory:* Cough, dyspnea, bronchitis, upper respiratory symptoms, nasal congestion, sinusitis, pharyngeal pain, ***bronchospasm, asthma.*** *CV:* Hypotension, orthostatic hypotension, angina, tachycardia, palpitations, rhythm disturbances, ***stroke,*** chest pain, orthostatic effects, peripheral edema, ***MI, CVA.*** *Musculoskeletal:* Asthenia, muscle cramps, joint pain, shoulder and back pain, myalgia, arthralgia, arthritis. *Hepatic:* Hepatitis, cholestatic jaundice, pancreatitis. *Dermatologic:* Rash, pruritus, flushing, increased sweating, urticaria. *GU:* Impotence, oliguria, progressive azotemia, acute renal failure, UTI. *Miscellaneous: **Angioedema (may be fatal if laryngeal edema occurs),*** hyperkalemia, neutropenia, anemia, ***bone marrow depression,*** decreased libido, chest pain, fever, blurred vision, syncope, vasculitis of the legs, gout.

**OD** **Overdose Management:** *Symptoms:* Hypotension. *Treatment:* Supportive. To correct hypotension, IV normal saline is treatment of choice. Lisinopril may be removed by hemodialysis.

**Drug Interactions**
*Diuretics* / Excess ↓ BP
*Indomethacin* / Possible ↓ effect of lisinopril
*Potassium-sparing diuretics* / Significant ↑ serum potassium

**Laboratory Test Interferences:** ↑ Serum potassium, BUN, serum creatinine. ↓ H&H.

**Dosage**
• **Tablets**

*Essential hypertension, used alone.*
10 mg once daily. Adjust dosage depending on response (range: 20–40 mg/day given as a single dose). Doses greater than 80 mg/day do not give a greater effect.

*Essential hypertension in combination with a diuretic.*
**Initial:** 5 mg. The BP-lowering effects of the combination are additive. Dosage should be reduced in clients with renal impairment.

*CHF.*
**Initial:** 5 mg once daily (2.5 mg/day in clients with hyponatremia) in combination with diuretics and digitalis. **Dosage range:** 5–20 mg/day as a single dose.

*Acute MI.*
**First dose:** 5 mg; **then,** 5 mg after 24 hr, 10 mg after 48 hr, and then 10 mg daily. Continue dosing for 6 weeks. In clients with a systolic pressure less than 120 mm Hg when treatment is started or within 3 days after the infarct should be given 2.5 mg. If hypotension occurs (systolic BP less than 100 mm Hg), the dose may be temporarily reduced to 2.5 mg. If prolonged hypotension occurs, the drug should be withdrawn.

## NURSING CONSIDERATIONS

See also *Nursing Considerations* for *Angiotensin-Converting Enzyme Inhibitors* and *Antihypertensive Agents.*

**Administration/Storage**
1. When considering use of lisinopril in a client taking diuretics, discontinue the diuretic, if possible, 2–3 days before beginning lisinopril therapy. If the diuretic cannot be discontinued, the initial dose of lisinopril should be 5 mg; observe closely for at least 2 hr.
2. Maximum antihypertensive effects may not be observed for 2–4 weeks in some.
3. When starting treatment for CHF, give under medical supervision, especially if SBP less than 100 mm Hg.
4. With clients whose BP is controlled with lisinopril, 20 mg plus hydrochlorothiazide 25 mg, given separately should trial Prinzide 12.5

mg or Zestoretic 20–12.5 mg before Prinzide 25 mg or Zestoretic 20–25 mg is used.

5. The maximum recommended daily dose of lisinopril is 80 mg in a single daily dose. Clients usually do not require hydrochlorothiazide in doses exceeding 50 mg/day, especially if combined with other antihypertensives.

6. Use of potassium supplements, potassium-sparing diuretics, or potassium salt substitutes with Prinzide or Zestoretic may lead to increases in serum potassium.

7. Prinzide or Zestoretic is recommended for those with a $C_{CR}$ greater than 30 mL/min.

8. Anticipate reduced dosage with renal insufficiency—initial dose of 10 mg/day if $C_{CR}$ is greater than 30 mL/min, 5 mg/day if $C_{CR}$ is between 10 and 30 mL/min, and 2.5 mg/day in dialysis clients (i.e., $C_{CR}$ less than 10 mL/min).

**Client/Family Teaching**

1. Avoid symptoms of orthostatic hypotension (i.e., rise slowly from sitting or lying position and wait until symptoms subside).

2. Avoid all potassium supplements as well as foods high in potassium.

3. Review drug side effects; report for BP check and lab studies.

**Outcomes/Evaluate**

- ↓ BP
- Improved survival with acute MI

———COMBINATION DRUG———

# Lisinopril and Hydrochlorothiazide

(lie-**SIN**-oh-pril, hy-droh-kloh-roh-**THIGH**-ah-zyd)
**Pregnancy Category:** C
Prinzide, Zestoretic **(Rx)**
**Classification:** Antihypertensive

See also *Lisinopril* and *Hydrochlorothiazide*.
**Content:** Lisinopril is an ACE inhibitor and hydrochlorothiazide is a diuretic. Prinzide 12.5 and Zestoretic 20–12.5: Lisinopril, 20 mg, and hydrochlorothiazide, 12.5 mg. Prinzide

25 and Zestoretic 20–25: Lisinopril, 20 mg, and hydrochlorothiazide, 25 mg.
**Uses:** Hypertension in clients in whom combination therapy is appropriate. Not for initial therapy.

**Dosage**
- **Tablets**
  *Hypertension.*
**Individualized. Usual:** 1 or 2 tablets once daily of Prinzide 12.5, Prinzide 25, Zestoretic 20–12.5, or Zestoretic 20–25.

## NURSING CONSIDERATIONS

See also *Nursing Considerations* for *Antihypertensive Agents, Lisinopril,* and *Hydrochlorothiazide*.
**Administration/Storage**
1. With clients whose BP is controlled with lisinopril 20 mg plus hydrochlorothiazide 25 mg, given separately, trial Prinzide 12.5 or Zestoretic 20–12.5 before Prinzide 25 or Zestoretic 20–25 mg is used.
2. Maximum recommended daily dose of lisinopril is 80 mg in a single daily dose. Clients usually do not require hydrochlorothiazide in doses exceeding 50 mg/day, especially if combined with other antihypertensives.
3. Use of potassium supplements, potassium-sparing diuretics, or potassium salt substitutes with Prinzide or Zestoretic may lead to increases in serum potassium.
4. Prinzide or Zestoretic is recommended for those with a $C_{CR}$ greater than 30 mL/min.
**Client/Family Teaching**
1. Take BP and maintain written record for review.
2. Avoid symptoms of orthostatic hypotension (i.e., rise slowly from sitting or lying position and wait until symptoms subside).
3. Avoid all potassium supplements as well as foods high in potassium.
4. Report for BP check and labs.
**Outcomes/Evaluate:** Control of hypertension

L

# Lithium carbonate

(**LITH**-ee-um)
**Pregnancy Category:** D
Carbolith ✦, Duralith ✦, Eskalith,
Eskalith CR, Lithane, Lithizine ✦,
Lithobid, Lithonate, Lithotabs **(Rx)**

# Lithium citrate

(**LITH**-ee-um)
**Pregnancy Category:** D
PMS-Lithium ✦
**Classification:** Antipsychotic agent,
miscellaneous

**Action/Kinetics:** Mechanism for
the antimanic effect of lithium is unknown. Various hypotheses include:
(a) a decrease in catecholamine neurotransmitter levels caused by lithium's effect on $Na^+$-$K^+$ ATPase to improve transneuronal membrane
transport of sodium ion; (b) a decrease in cyclic AMP levels caused
by lithium which decreases sensitivity of hormonal-sensitive adenyl cyclase receptors; or (c) interference
by lithium with lipid inositol metabolism ultimately leading to insensi-
tivity of cells in the CNS to stimulation
by inositol.

Affects the distribution of calcium,
magnesium, and sodium ions and
affects glucose metabolism. **Peak
serum levels** (regular release): 1–4 hr;
(slow-release): 4–6 hr. **Onset:** 5–14
days. **Therapeutic serum levels:**
0.4–1.0 mEq/L (must be carefully
monitored because toxic effects may
occur at these levels and significant
toxic reactions occur at serum lithium
levels of 2 mEq/L). **t½ (plasma):** 24
hr (longer in presence of renal
impairment and in the elderly). Lithium and sodium are excreted by the
same mechanism in the proximal
tubule. Thus, to reduce the danger of
lithium intoxication, sodium intake
must remain at normal levels.

**Uses:** Control of manic and hypo-
manic episodes in manic-depressive
clients. Prophylaxis of bipolar
depression. *Investigational:* To reverse neutropenia induced by cancer chemotherapy and in children
with chronic neutropenia. Prophylaxis of cluster headaches and cyclic

migraine headaches. Treatment of
certain types of mental depression
(e.g., schizoaffective disorder, aug-
ment the antidepressant effect of tricyclic or MAO drugs in treating unipolar depression). Also for premenstrual tension, alcoholism
accompanied by depression, tardive
dyskinesia, bulimia, hyperthyroidism, excess ADH secretion. Lithium
succinate, in a topical form, has
been used for the treatment of genital herpes and seborrheic dermatitis.

**Contraindications:** Cardiovascular
or renal disease. Brain damage. Dehydration, sodium depletion, clients
receiving diuretics. Lactation.

**Special Concerns:** Safety and efficacy have not been established for
children less than 12 years of age.
Use with caution in geriatric clients
because lithium is more toxic to the
CNS in these clients; also, geriatric
clients are more likely to develop
lithium-induced goiter and clinical
hypothyroidism and are more likely to
manifest excessive thirst and larger
volumes of urine.

**Side Effects:** These are related to
the blood lithium level. *CNS:* Fainting,
drowsiness, slurred speech, confusion, dizziness, tiredness, lethargy,
ataxia, dysarthria, aphasia, vertigo,
stupor, restlessness, ***coma, seizures.***
Pseudotumor cerebri leading to papilledema and increased ICP. *GI:*
Anorexia, N&V, diarrhea, thirst, dry
mouth, bloated stomach. *Muscular:*
Tremors (especially of hand), muscle
weakness, fasciculations and/or
twitching, clonic movements of limbs,
increased deep tendon reflexes,
choreoathetoid movements, cogwheel rigidity. *Renal:* Nephrogenic
diabetes insipidus (polyuria, polydypsia), oliguria, albuminuria. *Endocrine:* Hypothyroidism, goiter, hyperparathyroidism. *CV:* Changes in
ECG, edema, hypotension, ***CV collapse,*** irregular pulse, tachycardia.
*Ophthalmologic:* Blurred vision,
downbeat nystagmus. *Dermatologic:*
Acneform eruptions, pruritic-macu-
lopapular rashes, drying and thinning of hair, alopecia, paresthesia,
cutaneous ulcers, lupus-like symp-

toms. *Miscellaneous:* Hoarseness; swelling of feet, lower legs, or neck; cold sensitivity; leukemia; leukocytosis; dyspnea on exertion.

**OD** **Overdose Management:** *Symptoms:* Symptoms dependent on serum lithium levels. Levels less than 2 mEq/L: N&V, diarrhea, muscle weakness, drowsiness, loss of coordination.

Levels of 2–3 mEq/L: Agitation, ataxia, blackouts, blurred vision, choreoathetoid movements, confusion, dysarthria, fasciculations, giddiness, hyperreflexia, hypertonia, manic-like behavior, myoclonic twitching or movement of entire limbs, slurred speech, tinnitus, urinary or fecal incontinence, vertigo.

Levels over 3 mEq/L: *Arrhythmias, coma,* hypotension, *peripheral vascular collapse, seizures (focal and generalized),* spasticity, stupor, twitching of muscle groups.

*Treatment:* Early symptoms are treated by decreasing the dose or stopping treatment for 24–48 hr:
• Use gastric lavage.
• Restore fluid and electrolyte balance (can use saline) and maintain kidney function.
• Increase lithium excretion by giving aminophylline, mannitol, or urea.
• Prevent infection. Maintain adequate respiration.
• Monitor thyroid function.
• Institute hemodialysis.

**Drug Interactions**
*Acetazolamide* / ↓ Lithium effect by ↑ renal excretion
*Aminophylline* / ↓ Lithium effect by ↑ renal excretion
*Bumetanide* / ↑ Lithium toxicity due to ↓ renal clearance
*Carbamazepine* / ↑ Risk of lithium toxicity
*Diazepam* / ↑ Risk of hypothermia
*Ethacrynic acid* / ↑ Lithium toxicity due to ↓ renal clearance
*Fluoxetine* / ↑ Serum levels of lithium
*Furosemide* / ↑ Lithium toxicity due to ↓ renal clearance

*Haloperidol* / ↑ Risk of neurologic toxicity
*Ibuprofen* / ↑ Chance of lithium toxicity due to ↓ renal clearance
*Indomethacin* / ↑ Chance of lithium toxicity due to ↓ renal clearance
*Iodide salts* / Additive effect to cause hypothyroidism
*Mannitol* / ↓ Lithium effect by ↑ renal excretion
*Mazindol* / ↑ Chance of lithium toxicity due to ↑ serum levels
*Methyldopa* / ↑ Chance of lithium toxicity due to ↑ serum levels
*Naproxen* / ↑ Chance of lithium toxicity due to ↑ serum levels
*Neuromuscular blocking agents* / Lithium ↑ effect of these agents → respiratory depression and apnea
*Phenothiazines* / ↓ Levels of phenothiazines and ↑ neurotoxicity
*Phenylbutazone* / ↑ Chance of lithium toxicity due to ↓ renal clearance
*Phenytoin* / ↑ Chance of lithium toxicity
*Piroxicam* / ↑ Chance of lithium toxicity due to ↓ renal clearance
*Probenecid* / ↑ Chance of lithium toxicity due to ↑ serum levels
*Sodium bicarbonate* / ↓ Lithium effect by ↑ renal excretion
*Sodium chloride* / Excretion of lithium is proportional to amount of sodium chloride ingested; if client is on salt-free diet, may develop lithium toxicity since less lithium excreted
*Spironolactone* / ↑ Chance of lithium toxicity due to ↑ serum levels
*Succinylcholine* / ↑ Muscle relaxation
*Sympathomimetics* / ↓ Pressor effect of sympathomimetics
*Tetracyclines* / ↑ Chance of lithium toxicity due to ↑ serum levels
*Theophyllines* / ↓ Effect of lithium due to ↑ renal excretion
*Thiazide diuretics, triamterene* / ↑ Chance of lithium toxicity due to ↓ renal clearance
*Tricyclic antidepressants* / ↑ Effect of tricyclic antidepressants
*Urea* / ↓ Lithium effect by ↑ renal excretion

**L**

***bold italic*** = life threatening side effect

**Laboratory Test Interferences:** False + urinary glucose test (Benedict's), ↑ serum glucose, creatinine kinase. False – or ↓ serum PBI, uric acid; ↑ TSH; ↓ $T_4$.

## Dosage

• **Capsules, Tablets, Extended-Release Tablets, Syrup**

*Acute mania.*

**Adults:** Individualized and according to lithium serum level (not to exceed 1.4 mEq/L) and clinical response. **Usual initial:** 300–600 mg t.i.d. or 600–900 mg b.i.d. of slow-release form; **elderly and debilitated clients:** 0.6–1.2 g/day in three doses. **Maintenance:** 300 mg t.i.d.–q.i.d.

Administration of drug is discontinued when lithium serum level exceeds 1.2 mEq/L and resumed 24 hr after it has fallen below that level.

*To reverse neutropenia.*
300–1,000 mg/day (to achieve serum levels of 0.5–1.0 mEq/L) for 7–10 days.

*Prophylaxis of cluster headaches.*
600–900 mg/day.

## NURSING CONSIDERATIONS

### Administration/Storage

1. To prevent toxic serum levels from occurring, determine blood levels 1–2 times/week during initiation of therapy, and monthly thereafter, on blood samples taken 8–12 hr after dosage.
2. Full beneficial effects of drug may not be noted for 6–10 days.

### Assessment

1. Conduct a drug history; determine if taking other medications likely to interact.
2. With arthritic conditions, document if taking any anti-inflammatory agents.
3. Monitor thyroid function studies; assess for decreased function.
4. Document mental status; monitor CV function, chemistry, urinalysis, weight, and ECG.

### Client/Family Teaching

1. Take with food or immediately after meals. Avoid any caffeinated beverages/foods because these may aggravate mania.
2. Report any episodes of persistent diarrhea; may indicate need for supplemental fluids or salt.
3. Maintain a constant level of salt intake to avoid fluctuations in lithium activity. Weight gain and edema may be related to sodium retention; report if excessive.
4. Drink 10–12 glasses of water each day; avoid dehydration (e.g., vigorous exercise, sunbathing, sauna) to prevent increased concentrations of lithium in urine.
5. Review the goals of therapy and drug side effects that require immediate reporting (diarrhea, vomiting with drowsiness, muscular weakness, lack of coordination).
6. Do not engage in physical activities that require alertness or physical coordination until drug effects are realized; may cause drowsiness.
7. Will take several weeks to realize a behavioral benefit from therapy.
8. Do not change brands of drug.
9. Lithium works well in the manic phase; concomitant antidepressant use may be necessary during depressive phases.
10. Transient acneiform eruptions, folliculitis, and altered sexual function in men have been reported.
11. Carry name and telephone number of persons to contact if needed or if family members note behavioral changes or physical changes contrary to expectations. Carry ID, noting diagnosis and prescribed meds.

### Outcomes/Evaluate

• Stabilization of mood swings
• ↓ Symptoms of mania ( ↓ hyperactivity, ↓ sleeplessness, and improved judgment)
• Therapeutic serum drug levels (0.4–1.0 mEq/L)

# Lodoxamide tromethamine

(loh-**DOX**-ah-myd)
**Pregnancy Category:** B
Alomide **(Rx)**
**Classification:** Antiallergic ophthalmic

**Action/Kinetics:** Mast cell stabilizer that inhibits type I immediate hypersensitivity reactions. Prevents the release of mast cell inflammatory mediators, including slow-reacting substances of anaphylaxis (peptidoleukotrienes), and inhibits eosinophil chemotaxis. The mechanism for the beneficial effect is not known with certainty but may be due to prevention of calcium influx into mast cells upon stimulation by antigens. **Elimination t½:** 8.5 hr. Excreted mainly through the urine.

**Uses:** To treat ocular disorders such as vernal keratoconjunctivitis, vernal conjunctivitis, and vernal keratitis.

**Contraindications:** Use in clients wearing soft contact lenses.

**Special Concerns:** Use with caution during lactation. The drug is for ophthalmic use only and should not be injected. Safety and efficacy have not been determined for use in children less than 2 years of age.

**Side Effects:** *Ophthalmologic:* Transient burning, stinging, or discomfort upon instillation. Ocular itching or pruritus, blurred vision, dry eye, tearing, discharge from eyes, hyperemia, crystalline deposits in eye, foreign body sensation, corneal erosion or ulcer, scales on lid or lash, eye pain, ocular edema or swelling, ocular warming sensation, ocular fatigue, chemosis, corneal abrasion, anterior chamber cells, keratopathy, keratitis, blepharitis, allergy, sticky sensation, epitheliopathy. *CNS:* Headache, dizziness, somnolence. *GI:* Nausea, stomach discomfort. *Miscellaneous:* Heat sensation, sneezing, dry nose, rash.

**Dosage**

- **Ophthalmic Solution**

  *Ocular disorders.*

  **Adults and children over 2 years of age:** 1–2 gtt in each affected eye q.i.d. for up to 3 months.

## NURSING CONSIDERATIONS

**Assessment:** Determine onset and symptoms; list other agents trialed.

**Client/Family Teaching**

1. Review appropriate method and frequency for administration. Some stinging and burning may be evident on instillation; report if symptoms persist after instillation.

2. Soft contact lenses *cannot* be worn during therapy.

**Outcomes/Evaluate:** ↓ Ocular inflammation

# Lomefloxacin hydrochloride

(**loh**-meh-**FLOX**-ah-sin)

**Pregnancy Category:** C

Maxaquin **(Rx)**

**Classification:** Antibacterial, fluoroquinolone derivative

See also *Fluoroquinolones.*

**Action/Kinetics: Mean peak plasma levels:** 4.2 mcg/mL after a 400-mg dose. The rate and extent of absorption are decreased if taken with food. **t½:** 8 hr. Metabolized in the liver with 65% excreted unchanged through the urine and 10% excreted unchanged in the feces.

**Uses:** Acute bacterial exacerbation of chronic bronchitis caused by *Haemophilus influenzae* or *Moraxella catarrhalis.* Uncomplicated UTIs due to *Escherichia coli, Klebsiella pneumoniae, Proteus mirabilis,* or *Staphylococcus saprophyticus.* Complicated UTIs due to *E. coli, K. pneumoniae, P. mirabilis, Pseudomonas aeruginosa, Citrobacter diversus,* or *Enterobacter cloacae.* Preoperatively to decrease the incidence of UTIs 3–5 days after surgery in clients undergoing transurethral procedures. Uncomplicated gonococcal infections. Prevent infection in preoperative transrectal prostate biopsy.

**Contraindications:** Use in minor urologic procedures for which prophylaxis is not indicated (e.g., simply cystoscopy, retrograde pyelography). Use for the empiric treatment of acute bacterial exacerbation of

L

chronic bronchitis due to *Streptococcus pneumoniae*. Lactation.

**Special Concerns:** Plasma clearance is reduced in the elderly. Safety and efficacy have not been determined in children less than 18 years of age. Serious hypersensitivity reactions that are occasionally fatal have occurred, even with the first dose. No dosage adjustment is needed for elderly clients with normal renal function. Not efficiently removed from the body by hemodialysis or peritoneal dialysis.

**Additional Side Effects:** *CNS:* Confusion, tremor, vertigo, nervousness, anxiety, hyperkinesia, anorexia, agitation, increased appetite, depersonalization, paranoia, **coma.** *GI:* GI inflammation or bleeding, dysphagia, tongue discoloration, bad taste in mouth. *GU:* Dysuria, hematuria, micturition disorder, anuria, strangury, leukorrhea, intermenstrual bleeding perineal pain, vaginal moniliasis, orchitis, epididymitis, proteinuria, albuminuria. *Hypersensitivity Reactions:* Urticaria, itching, pharyngeal or facial edema, **CV collapse,** tingling, loss of consciousness, dyspnea. *CV:* Hypotension, tachycardia, bradycardia, extrasystoles, cyanosis, **arrhythmia, cardiac failure,** angina pectoris, **MI, pulmonary embolism, cardiomyopathy,** phlebitis, cerebrovascular disorder. *Respiratory:* Dyspnea, respiratory infection, epistaxis, **bronchospasm,** cough, increased sputum, respiratory disorder, stridor. *Hematologic:* Eosinophilia, leukopenia, increase or decrease in platelets, increase in ESR, lymphocytopenia, decreased hemoglobin, anemia, bleeding, increased PT, increase in monocytes. *Dermatologic:* Urticaria, eczema, skin exfoliation, skin disorder. *Ophthalmologic:* Conjunctivitis, eye pain. *Otic:* Earache, tinnitus. *Musculoskeletal:* Back or chest pain, asthenia, leg cramps, arthralgia, myalgia. *Miscellaneous:* Increase or decrease in blood glucose, flushing, increased sweating, facial edema, influenza-like symptoms, decreased heat tolerance, purpura, lymphadenopathy, increased fibrinolysis, thirst, gout, hypoglycemia, phototoxicity.

**Laboratory Test Interferences:** ↑ ALT, AST, alkaline phosphatase, bilirubin, BUN, gamma-glutamyltransferase. ↑ or ↓ Potassium. Abnormalities of urine specific gravity or serum electrolytes.

## Dosage

• **Tablets**

*Acute bacterial exacerbation of chronic bronchitis. Cystitis.*

**Adults:** 400 mg once daily for 10 days.

*Complicated UTIs.*

**Adults:** 400 mg once daily for 14 days.

*Uncomplicated UTIs.*

400 mg once daily for 3 days.

*Prophylaxis of infection before surgery for transurethral procedures.* Single 400-mg dose 2–6 hr before surgery.

*Uncomplicated gonococcal infections.*

400 mg as a single dose (as an alternative to ciprofloxacin or ofloxacin).

## NURSING CONSIDERATIONS

See also *General Nursing Considerations for All Anti-Infectives* and *Fluoroquinolones.*

### Administration/Storage

1. May take without regard for meals.

2. Dosage modification is required for clients with $C_{CR}$ less than 40 mL/min/1.73 m² and more than 10 mL/min/1.73 m². Following an initial loading dose of 40 mg, give daily maintenance doses of 200 mg for the duration of treatment. Assess lomefloxacin levels to determine any need to alter dosing interval. Follow this same regimen for clients on hemodialysis.

### Assessment

1. Note indications for therapy, type and onset of symptoms.

2. Obtain cultures and renal function studies; modify dosage with renal dysfunction.

## Outcomes/Evaluate
- UTI prophylaxis
- Symptomatic relief
- Improved breathing patterns

# Lomustine
(loh-MUS-teen)
**Pregnancy Category:** D
CeeNu (Abbreviation: CCNU) **(Rx)**
**Classification:** Antineoplastic, alkylating agent

See also *Antineoplastic Agents* and *Alkylating Agents.*

**Action/Kinetics:** Alkylating agent that inhibits DNA and RNA synthesis through DNA alkylation. It also affects other cellular processes, including RNA, protein synthesis and the processing of ribosomal and nucleoplasmic messenger RNA; DNA base component structure; the rate of DNA synthesis and DNA polymerase activity. Is cell cycle nonspecific. Rapidly absorbed from the GI tract; crosses the blood-brain barrier resulting in concentrations higher than in plasma. **Peak plasma level:** 1–6 hr; **t½:** biphasic; **initial,** 6 hr; **postdistribution:** 1–2 days. From 15% to 20% of drug remains in body after 5 days. Fifty percent of drug excreted within 12 hr through the kidney, 75% within 4 days. Small amounts are excreted through the lungs and feces. Metabolites present in milk.

**Uses:** Used alone or in combination with other drugs. Primary and meta static brain tumors. Secondary therapy in Hodgkin's disease (in combination with other antineoplastics).

**Contraindications:** Use during lactation.

**Additional Side Effects:** High incidence of N&V 3–6 hr after administration and lasting for 24 hr. Renal and pulmonary toxicity. Dysarthria. *Delayed bone marrow suppression* may occur due to cumulative bone marrow toxicity. *Thrombocytopenia and leukopenia may lead to bleeding and overwhelming infections.* Secondary malignancies.

**Laboratory Test Interferences:** Elevated liver function tests (reversible).

**Dosage** ———————
- **Capsules**
**Adults and children, initial:** 130 mg/m² as a single dose q 6 weeks. If bone marrow function is reduced, decrease dose to 100 mg/m² q 6 weeks. Subsequent dosage based on blood counts of clients (platelet count above 100,000/mm³ and leukocyte count above 4,000/mm³). Undertake weekly blood tests and do not repeat therapy before 6 weeks.

## NURSING CONSIDERATIONS

See also *Nursing Considerations* for *Antineoplastic Agents.*
**Administration/Storage**
1. Store below 40°C (104°F).
2. Given alone or in combination with other drugs, surgery, or radiotherapy.
3. Causes platelet and leukocyte suppression. Nadir: 3–7 weeks.
**Client/Family Teaching**
1. Medication comes in capsules of three strengths and a combination of capsules will make up the correct dose; take all at one time.
2. May have N&V up to 36 hr after treatment; may be followed by 2–3 days of anorexia. Take antiemetics as prescribed. GI distress may be reduced by taking antiemetics before drug administration or by taking the drug after fasting.
3. Report feelings of depression caused by prolonged N&V so that various antiemetics can be tried and to ensure that psychological support is available as needed.
4. Any abnormal bruising or bleeding, sore throat or flu symptoms should be reported.
5. Avoid all OTC agents.
6. Intervals of 6 weeks are necessary between doses for optimum effect with minimal toxicity; hematologic profiles should be assessed weekly.

L

---

♣ = Available in Canada                    ***bold italic*** = life threatening side effect

**Outcomes/Evaluate:** Control/remission of metastatic processes

# Loperamide hydrochloride

(loh-**PER**-ah-myd)

**Pregnancy Category:** B

Alti-Loperamide ✦, Apo-Loperamide ✦, Imodium, Imodium A-D Caplets, Kaopectate II Caplets, Maalox Anti-Diarrheal Caplets, Novo-Loperamide ✦, Pepto Diarrhea Control, PMS-Loperamide Hydrochloride ✦ (Imodium is Rx, all others are OTC)

**Classification:** Antidiarrheal agent, systemic

**Action/Kinetics:** Slows intestinal motility by acting on the nerve endings and/or intramural ganglia embedded in the intestinal wall. The prolonged retention of the feces in the intestine results in reducing the volume of the stools, increasing viscosity, and decreasing fluid and electrolyte loss. Reported to be more effective than diphenoxylate. **Time to peak effect, capsules:** 5 hr; **PO solution:** 2.5 hr. **t½:** 9.1–14.4 hr. Twenty-five percent excreted unchanged in the feces.

**Uses: Rx:** Symptomatic relief of acute nonspecific diarrhea and of chronic diarrhea associated with inflammatory bowel disease. Decrease the volume of discharge from ileostomies.

**OTC:** Control symptoms of diarrhea, including traveler's diarrhea. *Investigational:* With trimethoprim-sulfamethoxazole to treat traveler's diarrhea.

**Contraindications:** Discontinue drug promptly if abdominal distention develops in clients with acute ulcerative colitis. In clients in whom constipation should be avoided. OTC if body temperature is over 101°F (38°C) and in presence of bloody diarrhea. Use in acute diarrhea associated with organisms that penetrate the intestinal mucosa, such as *E. coli, Salmonella,* and Shigella.

**Special Concerns:** Safe use in children under 2 years of age and during lactation has not been established.

Fluid and electrolyte depletion may occur in clients with diarrhea. Children less than 3 years of age are more sensitive to the narcotic effects of loperamide.

**Side Effects:** *GI:* Abdominal pain, distention, or discomfort. Constipation, dry mouth, N&V, epigastric distress. Toxic megacolon in clients with acute colitis. *CNS:* Drowsiness, dizziness, fatigue. *Other:* Allergic skin rashes.

**OD** **Overdose Management:** *Symptoms:* Constipation, CNS depression, GI irritation. *Treatment:* Give activated charcoal (it will reduce absorption up to ninefold). If vomiting has not occurred, perform gastric lavage followed by activated charcoal, 100 g, through a gastric tube. Give naloxone for respiratory depression.

**Dosage**

• **Rx Capsules, Liquid**

*Acute diarrhea.*

**Adults, initial:** 4 mg, followed by 2 mg after each unformed stool, up to maximum of 16 mg/day. **Pediatric:** D*ay 1 doses:* **8–12 years:** 2 mg t.i.d.; **6–8 years:** 2 mg b.i.d.; **2–5 years:** 1 mg t.i.d. using only the liquid. *After day 1:* 1 mg/10 kg after a loose stool (total daily dosage should not exceed day 1 recommended doses).

*Chronic diarrhea.*

**Adults:** 4–8 mg/day as a single or divided dose. Dosage not established for chronic diarrhea in children.

• **OTC Oral Solution, Tablets**

*Acute diarrhea.*

**Adults:** 4 mg after the first loose bowel movement followed by 2 mg after each subsequent bowel movement to a maximum of 8 mg/day for no more than 2 days. **Pediatric, 9–11 years:** 2 mg after the first loose bowel movement followed by 1 mg after each subsequent loose bowel movement, not to exceed 6 mg/day for no more than 2 days. **Pediatric, 6–8 years:** 1 mg after the first bowel movement followed by 1 mg after each subsequent loose bowel movement, not to exceed 4 mg/day for no more than 2 days.

## NURSING CONSIDERATIONS
### Administration/Storage
1. OTC products are not intended for use in children less than 6 years of age unless physician prescribed.
2. If no improvement within 10 days after using up to 16 mg/day for *chronic diarrhea,* symptoms are not likely to improve with further use. Seek medical intervention.
3. In *acute diarrhea,* discontinue after 48 hr and report if ineffective.
### Assessment
1. Note any allergy to piperidine derivatives.
2. Document indications for therapy, onset, frequency, and duration of symptoms. Identify any contributing causative factors.
### Client/Family Teaching
1. May cause a dry mouth; try ice, sugarless gum, and candy to alleviate.
2. Use caution while driving or performing tasks requiring alertness; may cause dizziness and drowsiness.
3. Record the number, frequency, and consistency of stools per day and the amount of medication consumed. Report if diarrhea lasts up to 5 days without relief.
4. Report if fever, nausea, abdominal pain, or abdominal distention occurs; may require dosage adjustment.
5. Dietary treatment of diarrhea is preferred, if possible, in children (avoid apple juices, high-fat and highly spiced foods).
### Outcomes/Evaluate: ↓ Diarrhea

## Loracarbef
(lor-ah-**KAR**-bef)
**Pregnancy Category:** B
Lorabid **(Rx)**
**Classification:** Beta-lactam antibiotic

See also *Anti-Infectives.*
**Action/Kinetics:** Related chemically to cephalosporins. Acts by inhibiting cell wall synthesis. Stable in the presence of certain bacterial beta-lactamases. **Average peak plasma levels:** 8 mcg/mL following a single 200-mg dose in a fasting subject after 90 min and 14 mcg/mL following a single 400-mg dose in a fasting subject after 90 min. Following doses of 7.5 mg/kg and 15 mg/kg of the oral suspension to children, average peak plasma levels were 13 and 19 mcg/mL, respectively, within 40–60 min. **Elimination t½:** 1 hr (increased to 5.6 hr in clients with a $C_{CR}$ from 10 to 50 mL/min/1.73 m² and to 32 hr in clients with a $C_{CR}$ of less than 10 mL/min/1.73 m²). Not metabolized in humans.
**Uses:** Secondary bacterial infections of acute bronchitis caused by *Streptococcus pneumoniae, Haemophilus influenzae,* or *Morazella catarrhalis* (including beta-lactamase-producing strains of both organisms). Acute bacterial exacerbations of chronic bronchitis caused by *S. pneumoniae, H. influenzae,* or *M. catarrhalis* (including beta-lactamase-producing strains of both organisms). Pneumonia caused by *S. pneumoniae* or *H. influenzae* (only non-beta-lactamase-producing strains). Otitis media caused by *S. pneumoniae, Streptococcus pyogenes, H. influenzae,* or *M. catarrhalis* (including beta-lactamase-producing strains of both organisms). Acute maxillary sinusitis caused by *S. pneumoniae, H. influenzae* (only non-beta-lactamase-producing strains), or *M. catarrhalis* (including beta-lactamase-producing strains). Pharyngitis and tonsillitis caused by *S. pyogenes.* Uncomplicated skin and skin structure infections caused by *Staphylococcus aureus* (including penicillinase-producing strains) or *S. pyogenes.* Uncomplicated UTIs caused by *Escherichia coli* or *Staphylococcus saprophyticus.* Uncomplicated pyelonephritis caused by *E. coli.*
**Contraindications:** Hypersensitivity to loracarbef or cephalosporin-class antibiotics.

**Special Concerns:** Use during labor and delivery only if clearly needed. Pseudomembranous colitis is possible with most antibacterial agents. Use with caution and at reduced dosage in clients with impaired renal function, in those with a history of colitis, in clients receiving concurrent treatment with potent diuretics, during lactation, and in clients with known penicillin allergies. Safety and efficacy in children less than 6 months of age have not been determined.

**Side Effects:** The incidence of certain side effects is different in the pediatric population compared with the adult population. *GI:* Diarrhea, N&V, abdominal pain, anorexia, pseudomembranous colitis. *Hypersensitivity:* Skin rashes, urticaria, pruritus, erythema multiforme. *CNS:* Headache, somnolence, nervousness, insomnia, dizziness. *Hematologic:* Transient thrombocytopenia, leukopenia, eosinophilia. *Miscellaneous:* Vasodilation, vaginitis, vaginal moniliasis, rhinitis.

**OD** **Overdose Management:** *Symptoms:* N&V, epigastric distress, diarrhea. *Treatment:* Hemodialysis may be effective in increasing the elimination of loracarbef from plasma from clients with chronic renal failure.

**Drug Interactions**
*Diuretics, potent* / ↑ Risk of renal dysfunction
*Probenecid* / ↓ Renal excretion resulting in ↑ plasma levels of loracarbef

**Dosage**
• **Capsules, Oral Suspension**
*Secondary bacterial infection of acute bronchitis.*
**Adults 13 years of age and older:** 200–400 mg q 12 hr for 7 days.
*Acute bacterial exacerbation of chronic bronchitis.*
**Adults 13 years of age and older:** 400 mg q 12 hr for 7 days.
*Pneumonia.*
**Adults 13 years of age and older:** 400 q 12 hr for 14 days.
*Pharyngitis, tonsillitis.*

**Adults 13 years of age and older:** 200 mg q 12 hr for 10 days. **Infants and children, 6 months–12 years:** 15 mg/kg/day in divided doses q 12 hr for 10 days.
*Sinusitis.*
**Adults 13 years of age and older:** 400 mg q 12 hr for 10 days.
*Acute otitis media.*
**Infants and children, 6 months–12 years:** 30 mg/kg/day in divided doses q 12 hr for 10 days. Use the suspension as it is more rapidly absorbed than the capsules, resulting in higher peak plasma levels when given at the same dose.
*Skin and skin structure infections (impetigo).*
**Infants and children, 6 months–12 years:** 15 mg/kg/day in divided doses q 12 hr for 7 days.

## NURSING CONSIDERATIONS

See also *General Nursing Considerations for All Anti-Infectives.*
**Administration/Storage**
1. The manufacturer provides a chart to assist with establishing the dosage regimen for pediatric clients.
2. Clients with $C_{CR}$ levels of 10–49 mL/min may be given one-half the recommended dose at the usual dosage interval. Clients with $C_{CR}$ less than 10 mL/min may be treated with the recommended dose given every 3–5 days. Clients on hemodialysis should receive another dose following dialysis.
3. Reconstitute the oral suspension by adding 30 mL water to the 50-mL bottle or 60 mL water to the 100-mL bottle. After mixing, the suspension may be kept at room temperature for 14 days without significant loss of potency. Keep tightly closed and discard any unused portion after 14 days.
**Assessment**
1. Note any sensitivity to cephalosporins and penicillin derivatives.
2. List drugs currently prescribed to ensure none interact unfavorably.
3. Obtain baseline cultures and renal function studies.

### Client/Family Teaching
1. Take at least 1 hr before or at least 2 hr after meals. Complete entire prescription.
2. Report persistent diarrhea, which may be secondary to pseudomembranous colitis and requires medical intervention.

### Outcomes/Evaluate
- Negative C&S reports
- Relief of ear/throat pain
- Improved breathing patterns
- Evidence of wound healing

# Loratidine
(loh-**RAH**-tih-deen)
**Pregnancy Category:** B
Claritin, Claritin Reditabs **(Rx)**
**Classification:** Antihistamine

See also *Antihistamines.*

**Action/Kinetics:** Metabolized in the liver to active metabolite descarboethoxyloratidine. Has low to no sedative and anticholinergic effects. Does not alter cardiac repolarization and has not been linked to development of torsades de pointes as seen with astemizole and terfenadine. **Onset:** 1–3 hr. **Maximum effect:** 8–12 hr. Food delays absorption. **t½, loratidine:** 8.4 hr; **t½, descarboethoxyloratidine:** 28 hr. **Duration:** 24 hr. Excreted through both the urine and feces.

**Uses:** Relief of nasal and nonnasal symptoms of seasonal allergic rhinitis, including runny nose, itchy and watery eyes, itchy palate, and sneezing. Treatment of chronic idiopathic urticaria.

**Special Concerns:** Use with caution, if at all, during lactation. Give a lower initial dose in liver impairment. Safety and efficacy have not been determined in children less than 2 years of age.

**Side Effects:** Most commonly, headache, somnolence, fatigue, and dry mouth. *GI:* Altered salivation, gastritis, dyspepsia, stomatitis, tooth ache, thirst, altered taste, flatulence. *CNS:* Hypoesthesia, hyperkinesia, migraine, anxiety, depression, agitation, paroniria, amnesia, impaired concentration. *Ophthalmologic:* Altered lacrimation, conjunctivitis, blurred vision, eye pain, blepharospasm. *Respiratory:* Upper respiratory infection, epistaxis, pharyngitis, dyspnea, coughing, rhinitis, sinusitis, sneezing, bronchitis, ***bronchospasm,*** hemoptysis, laryngitis. *Body as a whole:* Asthenia, increased sweating, flushing, malaise, rigors, fever, dry skin, aggravated allergy, pruritus, purpura. *Musculoskeletal:* Back/chest pain, leg cramps, arthralgia, myalgia. *GU:* Breast pain, menorrhagia, dysmenorrhea, vaginitis. *Miscellaneous:* Earache, dysphonia, dry hair, urinary discoloration.

### Dosage
- **Syrup, Tablets**
  *Allergic rhinitis, chronic idiopathic urticaria.*

**Adults and children 6 years and older:** 10 mg once daily on an empty stomach. *In clients with impaired liver function (GFR less than 30 mL/min):* 10 mg every other day.

## NURSING CONSIDERATIONS

See also *Nursing Considerations* for *Antihistamines.*

### Administration/Storage
1. Use the syrup or rapid-distintegrating tablets for children 6 to 11 years of age.
2. Use caution. The concentration of the syrup is 10 mg/10 mL.

### Assessment
1. Document indications for therapy, type, onset, and duration of symptoms. List other agents trialed and the outcome.
2. Monitor LFTs; note any dysfunction and reduce dose. Assess the elderly and clients with hepatic and renal impairment for increasing somnolence.
3. Document pulmonary findings; assess throat, nodes, and turbinates.
4. Perform a drug profile. Cautiously coadminister with drugs that inhibit hepatic metabolism (i.e., macrolide

---

antibiotics, cimetidine, ranitidine, ketoconazole, or theophylline).

**Client/Family Teaching**
1. Take on an empty stomach; food may delay absorption.
2. If using rapid-disintegrating tablets, place under the tongue. Disintegration occurs within seconds, after which the tablet contents may be swallowed with or without water.
3. Use rapid-disintegrating tablets within 6 months of opening the laminated foil pouch and immediately after opening the individual tablet blister.
4. Do not perform activities that require mental alertness until drug effects are realized; generally, does not cause drowsiness.
5. Identify triggers, i.e., foods, detergents, or materials that may have induced urticarial response.

**Outcomes/Evaluate**
• Relief of nasal congestion and seasonal allergic manifestations
• Control of skin eruption R/T antigenic offender

————COMBINATION DRUG————

# Loratidine and Pseudoephedrine sulfate

(loh-**RAH**-tih-deen, **soo**-doh-eh-**FED**-rin)

**Pregnancy Category:** B
Claritin-D, Claritin-D 24 Hour Extended Release Tablets, Claritin-D 24 hour, Chlor-Tripolon N.D. ✿, Claritin Extra ✿ **(Rx)**
**Classification:** Antihistamine/decongestant

See also *Loratidine* and *Pseudoephedrine Sulfate.*
**Content:** Each tablet of Claritin-D contains: *Antihistamine:* Loratidine, 5 mg. *Decongestant:* Pseudoephedrine sulfate, 120 mg. The product is formulated such that loratidine is released immediately and pseudoephedrine is released both immediately and over time.

Each tablet of Claritin-D 24 Hour Extended Release contains: *Antihistamine:* Loratidine, 10 mg. *Decongestant:* Pseudoephedrine sulfate, 240 mg. Tablet Extended Relaease 10

mg-240 mg.
**Uses:** To relieve symptoms of seasonal allergic rhinitis, including those with asthma.
**Contraindications:** Clients with narrow-angle glaucoma or urinary retention and in those receiving MAO inhibitors and within 14 days of such treatment. In clients with severe hypertension, severe CAD, hepatic insufficiency, and hypersensitivity to the components. In those who have difficulty swallowing due to possibility of upper GI tract obstruction.
**Special Concerns:** Use with caution in clients with hypertension, diabetes mellitus, ischemic heart disease, increased intraocular pressure, hyperthyroidism, renal impairment, or prostatic hypertrophy. The safety and efficacy in clients over 60 years of age and below 12 years of age have not been determined. Use with caution during lactation.
**Side Effects:** See individual components. The most common side effects for this product are: *CNS:* Headache, insomnia, somnolence, nervousness, dizziness, fatigue. *GI:* Dry mouth, dyspepsia, nausea. *Miscellaneous:* Pharyngitis, anorexia, thirst.

**Dosage**
• **Tablets**
  *Allergic rhinitis.*
**Adults and children over 12 years of age:** 1 tablet q 12 hr given on an empty stomach. Clients with a GFR less than 30 mL/min should receive 1 tablet daily.
• **Extended Release Tablets**
  *Allergic rhinitis.*
**Adults:** One 24 Hour Extended Release Tablet daily.

## NURSING CONSIDERATIONS

See also *Nursing Considerations* for *Antihistamines,* and individual agents.
**Administration/Storage:** Store away from heat, moisture, and direct light.
**Assessment:** Note any history of hypertension, CAD, and renal and hepatic dysfunction. Drug is contraindicated with glaucoma, MAO therapy

(or within 14 days of stopping), urinary retention, and seizures.

**Client/Family Teaching**
1. May take with food or milk to decrease GI upset.
2. Take in the morning upon first arising to prevent bedtime insomnia.
3. Drug may cause nervousness and dizziness; do not perform activities that require mental and physical alertness until drug effects realized.
4. Avoid alcohol, CNS depressants, and any OTC agents for sleep or pain.

**Outcomes/Evaluate:** Relief of nasal and sinus congestion

---

# Lorazepam
(lor-**AYZ**-eh-pam)
**Pregnancy Category:** D
Apo-Lorazepam ✤, Ativan, Lorazepam Intensol, Novo-Lorazem ✤, Nu-Loraz ✤, PMS-Lorazepam ✤, Pro-Lorazepam ✤ **(C-IV) (Rx)**
**Classification:** Antianxiety agent, benzodiazepine

---

See also *Tranquilizers, Antimanic Drugs, and Hypnotics.*
**Action/Kinetics:** Absorbed and eliminated faster than other benzodiazepines. **Peak plasma levels: PO,** 1–6 hr; **IM,** 1–1.5 hr. **t½:** 10–20 hr. Metabolized to inactive compounds, which are excreted through the kidneys.
**Uses: PO:** Anxiety, tension, anxiety with depression, insomnia, acute alcohol withdrawal symptoms. **Parenteral:** Amnesic agent, anticonvulsant, antitremor drug, adjunct to skeletal muscle relaxants, preanesthetic medication, adjunct prior to endoscopic procedures, treatment of status epilepticus, relief of acute alcohol withdrawal symptoms. *Investigational:* Antiemetic in cancer chemotherapy.
**Additional     Contraindications:** Narrow-angle glaucoma. Use cautiously in presence of renal and hepatic disease. Parenterally in children less than 18 years.

**Special Concerns:** PO dosage has not been established in children less than 12 years of age and IV dosage has not been established in children less than 18 years of age.
**Additional   Drug   Interactions:** With parenteral lorazepam, scopolamine → sedation, hallucinations, and behavioral abnormalities.

**Dosage**
- **Tablets, Concentrate**
  *Anxiety.*
  **Adults:** 1–3 mg b.i.d.–t.i.d.
  *Hypnotic.*
  **Adults:** 2–4 mg at bedtime. **Geriatric/debilitated clients, initial:** 0.5–2 mg/day in divided doses. Dose can be adjusted as required.
- **IM**
  *Preoperatively.*
  **Adults:** 0.05 mg/kg up to maximum of 4 mg 2 hr before surgery for maximum amnesic effect.
- **IV**
  *Preoperatively.*
  **Adults, initial:** 0.044 mg/kg or a total dose of 2 mg, whichever is less.
  *Amnesic effect.*
  **Adults:** 0.05 mg/kg up to a maximum of 4 mg administered 15–20 min prior to surgery.
  *Antiemetic in cancer chemotherapy.*
  **Initial:** 2 mg 30 min before beginning chemotherapy; **then,** 2 mg q 4 hr as needed.

---

## NURSING CONSIDERATIONS

See also *Nursing Considerations* for *Tranquilizers, Antimanic Drugs, and Hypnotics.*
**Administration/Storage**
1. If higher doses are required, increase the evening dose before the daytime doses.
**IV** 2. For IV use, dilute just before use with equal amounts of either sterile water for injection, NaCl injection, or 5% dextrose injection.
3. Do not exceed an IV rate of 2 mg/min.
4. Do not use if solution is discolored or contains a precipitate.

---

**Assessment**
1. Document indications for therapy, onset, duration of symptoms. Assess mental status; describe characteristics of anxiety.
2. List other agents used to treat this condition and the outcome.
**Client/Family Teaching**
1. Take only as directed; report loss of effectiveness.
2. Drug may cause dizziness and drowsiness; use with caution until drug effects realized.
3. Report immediately any increased depression or suicidal ideations.
4. Avoid alcohol and any other CNS depressants.
5. With long-term therapy, do not stop suddenly. Drug should be tapered by provider to prevent withdrawal symptoms.
**Outcomes/Evaluate**
• ↓ Levels of anxiety, tension, and depression
• Control of alcohol withdrawal
• Muscle relaxation/amnesia

# Losartan potassium

(loh-**SAR**-tan)
**Pregnancy Category:** C (first trimester), D (second and third trimesters)
Cozaar **(Rx)**
**Classification:** Antihypertensive, angiotensin II receptor antagonist

See also *Antihypertensive Agents.*
**Action/Kinetics:** Angiotensin II, a potent vasoconstrictor, is the primary vasoactive hormone of the renin-angiotensin system; it is involved in the pathophysiology of hypertension. Angiotensin II increases systemic vascular resistance, causes sodium and water retention, and leads to increased heart rate and vasoconstriction. Losartan competitively blocks the angiotensin $AT_1$ receptor located in vascular smooth muscle and the adrenal glands, which is involved in mediating the effects of angiotensin II. Thus, BP is reduced. No significant effects on heart rate, has minimal orthostatic effects, and does not affect potas-sium levels significantly. Also, losartan does act on the $AT_2$ receptor. Undergoes significant first-pass metabolism in the liver, where it is converted to an active carboxylic acid metabolite that is responsible for most of the angiotensin receptor blockade. Rapidly absorbed after PO administration, although food slows absorption. **Peak plasma levels of losartan and metabolite:** 1 hr and 3–4 hr, respectively. t½, **losartan:** 2 hr; t½, **metabolite:** 6–9 hr. The drug and metabolite are highly bound to plasma proteins. Maximum effects are usually seen within 1 week, although from 3 to 6 weeks may be required in some clients. Drug and metabolites are excreted through both the urine (35%) and feces (60%).
**Uses:** Treatment of hypertension, alone or in combination with other antihypertensive agents.
**Contraindications:** Lactation. Use after pregnancy is discouraged.
**Special Concerns:** When used alone, the effect to decease BP in blacks was less than in non-blacks. Dosage adjustments are not required in clients with renal impairment, unless they are volume depleted. In clients with severe CHF, there is a risk of oliguria and/or progressive azotemia with acute renal failure and/or death (which are rare). In those with unilateral or bilateral renal artery stenosis, there is a risk of increased serum creatinine or BUN. Lower doses are recommended in those with hepatic insufficiency. Safety and efficacy have not been determined in children less than 18 years of age.
**Side Effects:** *GI:* Diarrhea, dyspepsia, anorexia, constipation, dental pain, dry mouth, flatulence, gastritis, vomiting, taste perversion. *CV:* Angina pectoris, second-degree AV block, **CVA, MI, ventricular tachycardia, ventricular fibrillation,** hypotension, palpitation, sinus bradycardia, tachycardia, orthostatic effects. *CNS:* Dizziness, insomnia, anxiety, anxiety disorder, ataxia, confusion, depression, abnormal dreams, hypesthesia,

decreased libido, impaired memory, migraine, nervousness, paresthesia, peripheral neuropathy, panic disorder, sleep disorder, somnolence, tremor, vertigo. *Respiratory:* Upper respiratory infection, cough, nasal congestion, sinus disorder, sinusitis, dyspnea, bronchitis, pharyngeal discomfort, epistaxis, rhinitis, respiratory congestion. *Musculoskeletal:* Muscle cramps, myalgia, joint swelling, musculoskeletal pain, stiffness, arthralgia, arthritis, fibromyalgia, muscle weakness; pain in the back, legs, arms, hips, knees, shoulders. *Dermatologic:* Alopecia, dermatitis, dry skin, ecchymosis, erythema, flushing, photosensitivity, pruritus, rash, sweating, urticaria. *GU:* Impotence, nocturia, urinary frequency, UTI. *Ophthalmologic:* Blurred vision, burning/stinging in the eye, conjunctivitis, decrease in visual acuity. *Miscellaneous:* Gout, anemia, tinnitus, facial edema, fever, syncope.

**OD** **Overdose Management:** *Symptoms:* Hypotension, tachycardia, bradycardia (due to vagal stimulation). *Treatment:* Supportive treatment. Hemodialysis is not indicated.

**Drug Interactions:** Administration of losartan and phenobarbital resulted in a decreased plasma level (20%) of losartan.

**Laboratory Test Interferences:** Minor ↑ BUN, serum creatinine. Occasional ↑ liver enzymes and/or serum bilirubin. Small ↓ hemoglobin, hematocrit.

**Dosage**
• **Tablets**
  *Hypertension.*
**Adults:** 50 mg once daily. In those with possible depletion of intravascular volume (e.g., clients treated with a diuretic), use 25 mg once daily. If the antihypertensive effect (measured at trough) is inadequate, a twice-a-day regimen, using the same dose, may be tried; or an increase in dose may give a more satisfactory result. If BP is not controlled by losartan alone, a diuretic (e.g., hydrochlorothiazide) may be added.

## NURSING CONSIDERATIONS

See also *Nursing Considerations* for *Antihypertensive Agents.*

**Administration/Storage:** May be given with other antihypertensive drugs.

**Assessment**
1. Document indications for therapy, onset and duration of disease, previous agents used and the outcome.
2. Monitor CBC, liver and renal function studies. Correct any volume depletion prior to using to prevent sympathomimetic hypotension. Reduce starting dose with volume depletion or hepatic impairment. Observe for S&S of fluid or electrolyte imbalance.

**Client/Family Teaching**
1. Take only as directed at the same time(s) each day with or without food.
2. Regular exercise, proper low-salt diet, and life-style changes (i.e., no smoking, low alcohol, low-fat diet, low stress, adequate rest) may also contribute to enhanced BP control.
3. Do not change positions suddenly, dangle before rising, and rest until symptoms subside to prevent postural symptoms.
4. Avoid any OTC agents.
5. May cause photosensitivity reaction; use precautions.
6. Use effective contraception; report immediately if pregnancy is suspected because drug during second and third trimesters is associated with fetal injury and morbidity.

**Outcomes/Evaluate:** Desired level of BP control

————COMBINATION DRUG————

# Losartan potassium and Hydrochlorothiazide

(loh-**SAR**-tan, **hy**-droh-klor-oh-**THIGH**-ah-zyd)
**Pregnancy Category:** C (first trimester), D (second and third trimesters)

**Hyzaar (Rx)**
**Classification:** Antihypertensive

See also *Losartan potassium, Hydrochlorothiazide,* and *Diuretics, Thiazide.*

**Content:** Each tablet contains *Antihypertensive:* Losartan potassium, 50 mg, and *Diuretic:* Hydrochlorothiazide, 12.5 mg.

**Action/Kinetics:** Losartan undergoes significant first-pass metabolism in the liver, where it is converted to an active carboxylic acid metabolite that is responsible for most of the angiotensin receptor blockade. The drug is rapidly absorbed after PO administration, although food does slows absorption. **Peak plasma levels of losartan and metabolite:** 1 hr and 3–4 hr, respectively. **t½, losartan:** 2 hr; **t½, metabolite:** 6–9 hr. Losartan and its active metabolite are highly bound to plasma proteins. Maximum effects are usually seen within 1 week, although from 3 to 6 weeks may be required in some clients. The drug and metabolites are excreted through both the urine (35%) and feces (60%).

**Peak effects, hydrochlorothiazide:** 4 hr; **duration:** 6–12 hr. **Hydrochlorothiazide t½, plasma:** 5.6–14.8 hr. Most of an oral dose is excreted unchanged.

**Uses:** Treatment of hypertension. Not indicated for initial therapy. Use the combination of losartan potassium and hydrochlorothiazide when BP is not controlled adequately with losartan potassium alone. Also used for clients whose BP is inadequately controlled by 25 mg/day of hydrochlorothiazide or is controlled but experiences hypokalemia.

**Contraindications:** Use in pregnancy, especially during the second and third trimesters. In those with anuria or hypersensitivity to sulfonamide-derived drugs (e.g., hydrochlorothiazide). In severe renal impairment. Lactation.

**Special Concerns:** Use with caution in clients with impaired hepatic function or progressive liver disease. Hypersensitivity reactions to hydrochlorothiazide may occur in those with or without a history of allergy or bronchial asthma, although such reactions are more likely in these clients. Thiazides may worsen or activate systemic lupus erythematosus. Safety and efficacy have not been determined in children.

**Side Effects:** See individual drug entries.

**Drug Interactions:** See individual drug entries.

**Dosage**

• **Tablets**
*Hypertension.*
**Adults:** One tablet (losartan, 50 mg, and hydrochlorothiazide, 12.5 mg) daily. If BP is not controlled after approximately 3 weeks of therapy, the dose may be increased to 2 tablets daily. The total daily dose should not exceed 2 tablets.

## NURSING CONSIDERATIONS

See also *Nursing Considerations* for *Losartan potassium,* and *Antihypertensive Agents.*

**Administration/Storage:** May be administered with other antihypertensive drugs.

**Assessment**
1. Document duration of disease, previous agents used and the outcome.
2. Monitor CBC, liver and renal function studies. Not for use with liver dysfunction.
3. With renal impairment, determine that $C_{CR} > 30$ mL/min (if below 30 mL/min loop diuretics are preferable to thiazides).
4. Determine any sensitivity to sulfonamides, allergy, or bronchial asthma; may exhibit a hypersensitive reaction to hydrochlorothiazide.

**Client/Family Teaching**
1. Take only as directed at the same time(s) each day with or without food.
2. Regular exercise, proper low-salt diet, and life-style changes (i.e., no smoking, low alcohol, low-fat diet, low stress, adequate rest) contribute to enhanced BP control.

3. Do not change positions suddenly, dangle before rising, and rest until postural symptoms subside.
4. Avoid any OTC agents.
5. May cause photosensitivity.
6. Use effective contraception; report pregnancy as drug during second and third trimesters associated with fetal injury and morbidity.

**Outcomes/Evaluate:** Control of BP

# Lovastatin (Mevinolin)

(**LOW**-vah-**STAT**-in, me-**VIN**-oh-lin)
**Pregnancy Category:** X
Mevacor **(Rx)**
**Classification:** Antihyperlipidemic

**Action/Kinetics:** Isolated from a strain of *Aspergillus terreus*. It specifically inhibits HMG–coenzyme A reductase, an enzyme that is necessary to convert HMG–coenzyme A to mevalonate (an early step in the biosynthesis of cholesterol). Levels of VLDL, LDL, cholesterol, and plasma triglycerides are reduced, while the plasma concentration of HDL cholesterol is increased. Since the enzyme is not completely inhibited, mevalonate is available in amounts necessary to maintain homeostasis. Approximately 35% of a dose is absorbed. Extensive first-pass effect—less than 5% reaches the general circulation. Absorption is decreased by about one-third if the drug is given on an empty stomach rather than with food. **Onset:** within 2 weeks using multiple doses. **Time to peak plasma levels:** 2–4 hr. **Time to peak effect:** 4–6 weeks using multiple doses. **Duration:** 4–6 weeks after termination of therapy. Over 95% is bound to plasma proteins. Metabolized in the liver (its main site of action) to active metabolites. Over 80% of a PO dose is excreted in the feces, via the bile, and approximately 10% is excreted through the urine.

**Uses:** As an adjunct to diet in primary hypercholesterolemia (types IIa and IIb) in clients with a significant risk of CAD and who have not responded to diet or other measures. May also be useful in clients with combined hypercholesterolemia and hypertriglyceridemia. To slow the progression of coronary atherosclerosis in clients with CAD in order to lower total and LDL cholesterol levels. *Investigational:* Diabetic dyslipidemia, nephrotic hyperlipidemia, familial dysbetalipoproteinemia, and familial combined hyperlipidemia.

**Contraindications:** During pregnancy and lactation, active liver disease, persistent unexplained elevations of serum transaminases. Use in children less than 18 years of age.

**Special Concerns:** Use with caution in clients who have a history of liver disease or who are known heavy consumers of alcohol. Carefully monitor clients with impaired renal function.

**Side Effects:** *GI:* Flatus (most common), abdominal pain, cramps, diarrhea, constipation, dyspepsia, N&V, heartburn, anorexia, stomatitis, acid regurgitation, dry mouth. *CNS:* Headache, dizziness, tremor, vertigo, memory loss, paresthesia, anxiety, depression, insomnia. *Musculoskeletal:* Myalgia, muscle cramps, localized pain, arthralgia, myopathy, rhabdomyolysis with renal dysfunction secondary to myoglobinuria. *Hypersensitivity reaction:* Vasculitis, purpura, polymyalgia rheumatica, angioedema, lupus erythematosus-like syndrome, thrombocytopenia, *hemolytic anemia,* leukopenia, eosinophilia, positive ANA, arthritis, arthralgia, urticaria, asthenia, ESR increase, fever, chills, flushing, photosensitivity, malaise, dyspnea, *toxic epidermal necrolysis, anaphylaxis, erythema multiforme including Stevens-Johnson syndrome.* *Dermatologic:* Alopecia, pruritus, rash, skin changes, including nodules, discoloration, dryness, changes to hair and nails. *Hepatic:* Hepatitis (including chronic active hepatitis), cholestatic jaundice, fatty change in liver, cirrhosis, *fulminant hepatic necrosis,* hepatoma, pancreatitis. *GU:* Gynecomastia, loss

L

of libido, erectile dysfunction. *Ophthalmic:* Blurred vision, progression of cataracts, lens opacities, ophthalmoplegia. *Hematologic:* Anemia, leukopenia, transient asymptomatic eosinophilia, thrombocytopenia. *Miscellaneous:* Cardiac chest pain, dysgeusia, edema, alteration of taste, impairment of extraocular movement, facial paresis, peripheral neuropathy, peripheral nerve palsy.

**Drug Interactions**
*Cyclosporine* / ↑ Risk of rhabdomyolysis or severe myopathy
*Erythromycin* / ↑ Risk of rhabdomyolysis or severe myopathy
*Gemfibrozil* / ↑ Risk of rhabdomyolysis or severe myopathy
*Niacin* / ↑ Risk of rhabdomyolysis or severe myopathy
*Warfarin* / ↑ PT

**Laboratory Test Interferences:** ↑ AST, ALT, CPK, alkaline phosphatase, bilirubin. Thyroid function test abnormalities.

**Dosage** —————
• **Tablets**
**Adults/adolescents, initial:** 20 mg once daily with the evening meal. Dose range: 10–80 mg/day in single or two divided doses with meals. If serum cholesterol levels are greater than 300 mg/dL, initial dose should be 40 mg/day. Adjust dose at intervals of every 4 weeks, if necessary.

**NURSING CONSIDERATIONS**
**Administration/Storage**
1. Place client on standard cholesterol-lowering diet before starting lovastatin; continue during treatment.
2. Dosage modification is not necessary in clients with renal insufficiency.
3. For clients on immunosuppressive therapy, start with 10 mg/day; do not exceed 20 mg/day.
**Assessment**
1. Document serum cholesterol profile, other therapies used and the outcome.
2. Note hepatic disease and any heavy consumption of alcohol.
3. Determine if pregnant.

4. Request recent eye exam; slight changes have been noted in the lenses of some clients.
5. Assess LFTs q 4–6 weeks for the first 15 months of therapy. A threefold increase in serum transaminase or new-onset abnormal liver function is an indication to discontinue therapy.
6. Assess life-style, including diet (intake of fats, carbohydrates, and proteins), activity (regular exercise), alcohol consumption, and smoking history. Identify areas that may contribute to increased serum cholesterol levels.
**Client/Family Teaching**
1. Take with meals. Continue cholesterol-lowering diet and exercise program as prescribed.
2. Adhere to dietary restrictions, daily exercise, and weight loss in the overall management and control of hypercholesterolemia and hyperlipidemia.
3. Practice reliable birth control; drug is pregnancy category X.
4. Report malaise, muscle spasms, or fever. These may be mistaken for the flu, but could be serious side effects of drug therapy.
5. Any RUQ abdominal pain or change in color and consistency of stools should be reported.
6. Periodic LFTs and eye exams are mandatory; report any early visual disturbances.
**Outcomes/Evaluate:** ↓ Cholesterol/triglyceride levels

# Loxapine hydrochloride
(**LOX**-ah-peen)
**Pregnancy Category:** C
Loxapac ✿, Loxitane C, Loxitane IM **(Rx)**

# Loxapine succinate
(**LOX**-ah-peen)
**Pregnancy Category:** C
Loxapac ✿, Loxitane **(Rx)**
**Classification:** Antipsychotic, tricyclic

See also *Antipsychotic Agents, Phenothiazines.*
**Action/Kinetics:** Thought to act by blocking dopamine at postsynaptic

brain receptors. Causes significant extrapyramidal symptoms, moderate sedative effects, and a low incidence of anticholinergic effects, as well as orthostatic hypotension. **Onset:** 20–30 min. **Peak effects:** 1.5–3 hr. **Duration:** about 12 hr. **t½:** 3–4 hr. Partially metabolized in the liver; excreted in urine, and unchanged in feces.

**Uses:** Psychoses. *Investigational:* Anxiety neurosis with depression.

**Additional Contraindications:** History of convulsive disorders.

**Special Concerns:** Use with caution in clients with CV disease. Use during lactation only if benefits outweigh risks. Dosage has not been established in children less than 16 years of age. Geriatric clients may be more prone to developing orthostatic hypotension, anticholinergic, sedative, and extrapyramidal side effects.

**Additional Side Effects:** Tachycardia, hypertension, hypotension, lightheadedness, and syncope.

**Dosage** ───────────────

• **Capsules, Oral Solution**
  *Psychoses.*
**Adults, initial:** 10 mg (of the base) b.i.d. For severe cases, up to 50 mg/day may be required. Increase dosage rapidly over 7–10 days until symptoms are controlled. **Range:** 60–100 mg up to 250 mg/day. **Maintenance:** If possible reduce dosage to 15–25 mg b.i.d.–q.i.d.

• **IM**
  *Psychoses.*
**Adults:** 12.5–50 mg (of the base) q 4–6 hr; once adequate control has been established, switch to PO medication after control achieved (usually within 5 days).

## NURSING CONSIDERATIONS

See also *Nursing Considerations* for *Antipsychotic Agents, Phenothiazines.*

**Administration/Storage**
1. Measure the concentrate dosage *only* with the enclosed calibrated dropper.

2. Mix oral concentrate with orange or grapefruit juice immediately before administration to disguise unpleasant taste.

**Assessment**
1. Note indications for therapy, type, onset, and characteristics of symptoms.
2. List agents used previously and the outcome.
3. Document mental status and behavioral manifestations.

**Client/Family Teaching**
1. Drug may cause orthostatic effects.
2. Do not stop abruptly.
3. Caution, may cause photosensitivity.

**Outcomes/Evaluate:** ↓ Agitated/hyperactive behaviors

# Lymphocyte immune globulin, anti-thymocyte globulin (equine) sterile solution

(**LIM**-foh-sight im-**MYOUN GLOH**-byou- lin an-tih-**THIGH**-moh-sight **GLOH**-byou-lin, **EE**-kwine)
**Pregnancy Category:** C
Atgam **(Rx)**
**Classification:** Immunosuppressant

**Action/Kinetics:** Obtained from hyperimmune serum of horses immunized with human thymus lymphocytes. Reduces the number of circulating, thymus-dependent lymphocytes that form rosettes from sheep erythrocytes. Antilymphocytic effect may be due to alteration of the function of T-lymphocytes, which are responsible, in part, for cell-mediated immunity. **t½, serum:** 5.7 days when the drug is given with other immunosuppressants and measured as horse IgG.

**Uses:** Management of allograft rejection in renal transplant clients, given either at the time of rejection or as an adjunct with other immunosuppressants to delay onset of the first rejection episode. Treatment of moderate

L

to severe aplastic anemia in those who are unsuitable for bone marrow transplantation.

**Contraindications:** In those who have demonstrated a severe systemic reaction during prior administration of the drug or any other equine gamma globulin preparation.

**Special Concerns:** A systemic reaction, such as a generalized rash, tachycardia, dyspnea, hypotension, or anaphylaxis, precludes any further administration of the drug. Potency may vary from lot to lot. The possibility of transmission of infectious agents exists. Use with caution during lactation.

**Side Effects: General side effects.** *Whole body:* Fever, chills, systemic or localized infection, malaise, serum sickness, edema, sweating. *GI:* N&V, diarrhea, **GI bleeding or perforation,** sore mouth or throat, epigastric or stomach pain, abdominal pain. *CNS:* Headache, **seizures,** confusion, disorientation, dizziness, faintness, paresthesias. *CV:* Hypertension or hypotension, tachycardia, deep vein thrombosis, thrombophlebitis, CHF, vasculitis, renal artery thrombosis. *Hematologic:* Thrombocytopenia, leukopenia, eosinophilia, neutropenia, granulocytopenia, anemia, lymphadenopathy, aplasia, pancytopenia, hemolysis, hemolytic anemia. *Dermatologic:* Rashes. *Respiratory:* Dyspnea, apnea, cough, **pulmonary edema,** nosebleed. *Musculoskeletal:* Chest, back, or flank pain; arthralgia, myalgias, leg pains, abnormal involuntary movement or tremor, rigidity. *Miscellaneous:* Herpes simplex infection, swelling or redness at infusion site, swelling, **anaphylaxis, laryngospasm/edema,** hyperglycemia, **acute renal failure,** viral hepatitis, enlarged or ruptured kidney.

**When used for renal transplantation with other immunosuppressants.** *Whole body:* Fever, chills, weakness or faintness. *CNS:* Headache, dizziness, paresthesia, **seizures.** *GI:* Diarrhea, nausea and/or vomiting, stomatitis, hiccoughs, epigastric pain, malaise. *Hematologic:* Leukopenia, thrombocytopenia.

*Dermatologic:* Rash, pruritus, urticaria, wheal, flare. *CV:* Hypotension, peripheral thrombophlebitis, edema, hypertension, renal artery stenosis, tachycardia. *Musculoskeletal:* Arthralgia, chest or back pain (or both), myalgia. *Respiratory:* Dyspnea, laryngospasm, pulmonary edema. *Miscellaneous:* Clotted arteriovenous fistula, pain at infusion site, night sweats, **anaphylaxis,** herpes simplex reactivation, hyperglycemia, iliac vein obstruction, localized infection, lymphadenopathy, serum sickness, systemic infection, **toxic epidermal necrosis,** wound dehiscence.

**When used for aplastic anemia with support therapy.** *Whole body:* Fever, chills, diaphoresis, aches. *GI:* N&V, diarrhea. *CNS:* Headache, agitation, lethargy, listlessness, lightheadedness, **seizures,** encephalitis or postviral encephalopathy. *CV:* Chest pain, phlebitis, bradycardia, myocarditis, cardiac irregularity, hypotension, CHF, hypertension. *Hematologic:* Lymphadenopathy, postcervical lymphadenopathy, tender lymph nodes. *Respiratory:* Bilateral pleural effusion, respiratory distress. *Musculoskeletal:* Arthralgia, myalgia, joint stiffness, muscle aches. *Miscellaneous:* Periorbital edema, edema, hepatosplenomegaly, burning soles/palms, foot sole pain, proteinuria, **anaphylaxis.**

**Drug Interactions:** Previously masked reactions to Atgam may appear when the drug is given concomitantly with corticosteroids or other immunosuppressants.

**Laboratory Test Interferences:** ↑ SGOT, SGPT, alkaline phosphatase, serum creatinine.

## Dosage
- **IV Only**
  *Renal allograft recipients.*
**Adults:** 10–20 mg/kg daily. **Children:** 5–25 mg/kg daily. Usually used concomitantly with azathioprine and corticosteroids. When used to delay the onset of allograft rejection, a fixed dose of 15 mg/kg for

14 days is used; then, the dose is given every other day for 14 days for a total of 21 doses in 28 days. The first dose should be given within 24 hr before or after the transplant. When used to treat rejection, the recommended dose is 10–15 mg/kg daily for 14 days; additional alternate day therapy can be given for a total of 21 doses. The first dose can be delayed until after the diagnosis of the first rejection episode.

*Aplastic anemia.*
10–20 mg/kg daily for 8–14 days; additional alternate day therapy may be given for a total of 21 doses.

## NURSING CONSIDERATIONS
### Administration/Storage
**IV** 1. It is recommended that clients be skin tested with an intradermal injection of 0.1 mL of a 1:1,000 dilution (5 mg horse IgG) of Atgam in NaCl injection and a contralateral NaCl injection. Observe over 15–20 min for the first hour after intradermal injection. A local reaction of 10 mm or greater with a wheal or erythema (or both) with or without pseudopod formation and itching or a marked local swelling should be considered a positive test. *NOTE:* Anaphylaxis has still occurred following a negative skin test.
2. Dilution of Atgam with dextrose injection is not recommended, as low salt concentrations may cause precipitation.
3. The use of highly acidic infusion solutions is not recommended due to the possibility of physical instability over time.
4. The product can be transparent to slightly opalescent, colorless to faintly pink or brown. A slight granular or flaky deposit may form during storage.
5. In order to avoid excessive foaming and/or denaturation of protein, do not shake either diluted or undiluted Atgam.
6. When used for IV infusion, dilute in an inverted bottle of sterile vehicle so the undiluted drug does not come in contact with the air inside. Do not exceed a concentration of 4 mg/mL; gently rotate or swirl the diluted solution so it is thoroughly mixed. Allow the diluted drug to come to room temperature before administration.
7. Administer drug into a vascular shunt, arterial venous fistula, or a high-flow central vein through an in-line filter with a pore size of 0.2–1.0 micron. The in-line filter prevents administration of any insoluble material that may develop during product storage. Use of high-flow veins will minimize development of phlebitis and thrombosis.
8. Do not administer in less than 4 hr.
9. Diluted Atgam is stable for up to 24 hr at concentrations up to 4 mg/mL in 0.9% NaCl, D5%/0.25% NaCl, and D5%/0.45% NaCl. Store diluted solution in the refrigerator.

### Assessment
1. Document type of symptoms, date of transplant, and/or hematologic profile.
2. Administer concomitantly with corticosteroids, antihistamines, and antipyretics to help control drug-induced side effects.
3. With repeated treatments, exclude those exhibiting any evidence of a systemic reaction.
4. Monitor ECG, electrolytes, hematologic profile, liver and renal function studies.

### Interventions
1. Only those experienced with immunosuppressive therapy in treating aplastic anemia or renal transplant should use the drug.
2. Observe for evidence of concurrent infection, thrombocytopenia, or leukopenia.
3. Discontinue if any of the following occurs: (a) symptoms of anaphylaxis, (b) severe and unremitting thrombocytopenia or leukopenia in renal transplant clients.
4. Respiratory distress and pain in the chest, back, or flank may indicate anaphylactoid reaction. Stop drug immediately and report.

---

✦ = Available in Canada                    *bold italic* = life threatening side effect

5. Continuously observe for possible allergic reactions.

6. Clients with aplastic anemia may require platelet transfusions during therapy to maintain acceptable platelet levels .

**Outcomes/Evaluate**

• Interruption of cell-mediated renal allograft rejection

• ↓ Rejection and graft loss

• Hematologic remission

# M

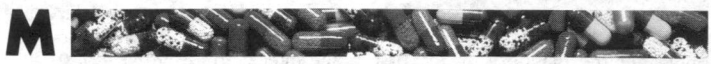

# Mafenide acetate

(**MAH**-fen-eyed)
**Pregnancy Category:** C
Sulfamylon **(Rx)**
**Classification:** Sulfonamide, topical

See also *Sulfonamides.*
**Action/Kinetics:** Active against many gram-positive and gram-negative organisms and in the presence of serum and pus. When applied topically, it diffuses through devascularized areas, is absorbed, and is rapidly metabolized.
**Uses:** Topical application to prevent infections in second- and third-degree burns.
**Contraindications:** Not to be used for already established infections.
**Special Concerns:** Use with caution during lactation and in those with acute renal failure. Use not recommended in infants less than 1 month of age.
**Side Effects:** *Allergic:* Rash, itching, swelling, hives, blisters, facial edema, erythema, eosinophilia. *Dermatologic:* Pain or burning (common) on application; excoriation of new skin, bleeding (rare). *Respiratory:* Hyperventilation or tachypnea, decrease in arterial $pCO_2$. *Metabolic:* Acidosis, increase in serum chloride. *Miscellaneous:* **Fatal hemolytic anemia with disseminated intravascular coagulation,** diarrhea.

**Dosage** ———————————
• **Cream**
1/16-in.-thick film applied over entire surface of burn with gloves once or twice daily until healing is progressing satisfactorily or until site is ready for grafting.

## NURSING CONSIDERATIONS

See also *General Nursing Considerations for All Anti-Infectives* and for *Sulfonamides.*
**Administration/Storage**
1. Continue until healing is progressing well or until the burn site is ready for grafting. Do not withdraw the drug if there is still the possibility of infections.
2. Avoid exposure to excessive heat.
**Client/Family Teaching**
1. Mafenide cream should be applied aseptically to a cleansed, debrided, burn site using a gloved hand.
2. Undertake daily bathing to assist in wound debridement.
3. Burns treated with mafenide are to be covered only with a thin dressing.
4. The drug causes pain on application; use analgesics as prescribed.
5. Report at once any unusual reactions including rashes, bruising, bleeding, swelling, or breathing difficulty.
**Outcomes/Evaluate:** Readiness for grafting at burn site; infection free

# Magnesium sulfate

(mag-**NEE**-see-um **SUL**-fayt)
**Pregnancy Category:** A
Epsom Salts **(OTC and Rx)**
**Classification:** Anticonvulsant, electrolyte, saline laxative

See also *Anticonvulsants* and *Laxatives.*
**Action/Kinetics:** Magnesium is an essential element for muscle contraction, certain enzyme systems, and nerve transmission. Extracellular

fluid levels: 1.5–2.5 mEq/L. Mg depresses the CNS and controls convulsions by blocking release of acetylcholine at the myoneural junction. Also, Mg decreases the sensitivity of the motor end plate to acetylcholine and decreases the excitability of the motor membrane. **Therapeutic serum levels:** 4–6 mEq/L (normal Mg levels: 1.5–3.0 mEq/L). **Onset: IM,** 1 hr; **IV,** immediate. **Duration: IM,** 3–4 hr; **IV,** 30 min. Excreted by the kidneys.

**Uses:** Seizures associated with toxemia of pregnancy, epilepsy, or when abnormally low levels of magnesium may be a contributing factor in convulsions, such as in hypothyroidism or glomerulonephritis. For eclampsia, IV use is restricted to control of life-threatening seizures. Acute nephritis in children to control hypertension, encephalopathy, and seizures. Replacement therapy in magnesium deficiency. Adjunct in TPN. Laxative. *Investigational:* Inhibit premature labor (not a first-line agent). IV use as an adjunct to treat acute exacerbations of moderate to severe asthma in clients who respond poorly to beta agonists. IV use to reduce early mortality in clients with acute MI (is given as soon as possible and continued for 24–48 hr).

**Contraindications:** In the presence of heart block or myocardial damage. In toxemia of pregnancy during the 2 hr prior to delivery.

**Special Concerns:** Use with caution in clients with renal disease because magnesium is removed from the body solely by the kidneys.

**Side Effects:** Magnesium intoxication. *CNS:* Depression. *CV:* Flushing, hypotension, *circulatory collapse, depression of the myocardium. Other:* Sweating, hypothermia, muscle paralysis, CNS depression, *respiratory paralysis.* Suppression of knee jerk reflex can be used to determine toxicity. *Respiratory failure may occur if given after knee jerk reflex disappears.* Hypocalcemia with signs of tetany

secondary to magnesium sulfate when used for eclampsia.

**OD** **Overdose Management:** *Symptoms:* Serum levels can predict symptoms of toxicity. Symptoms include *sharp decrease in BP and respiratory paralysis,* changes in ECG (increased PR interval, increased QRS complex, prolonged QT interval), *asystole, heart block.* At serum levels of 7–10 mEq/L there is hypotension, narcosis, and loss of deep tendon reflexes. *Levels of 12–15 mEq/L result in respiratory paralysis; greater than 15 mEq/L cause cardiac conduction problems. Levels greater than 25 mEq/L cause cardiac arrest.* Treatment:

• Use artificial ventilation immediately.

• Have 5–10 mEq of calcium (e.g., 10–20 mL of 10% calcium gluconate) readily available for IV injection to reverse heart block and respiratory depression.

• Hemodialysis and peritoneal dialysis are effective.

**Drug Interactions**
*CNS depressants (general anesthetics, sedative-hypnotics, narcotics)* / Additive CNS depression
*Digitalis* / Heart block when Mg intoxication is treated with calcium in digitalized clients
*Neuromuscular blocking agents* / Possible additive neuromuscular blockade

**Dosage**
• **IM**
   *Anticonvulsant.*
**Adults:** 1–5 g of a 25%–50% solution up to 6 times/day. **Pediatric:** 20–40 mg/kg using the 20% solution (may be repeated if necessary).
• **IV**
   *Anticonvulsant.*
**Adults:** 1–4 g using 10%–20% solution, not to exceed 1.5 mL/min of the 10% solution.
   *Hypomagnesemia, mild.*
**Adults:** 1 g as a 50% solution q 6 hr for 4 times (or total of 32.5 mEq/24 hr).

M

*Hypomagnesemia, severe.*
**Adults:** Up to 2 mEq/kg over 4 hr.
• **IV Infusion**
   *Anticonvulsant.*
**Adults:** 4–5 g in 250 mL 5% dextrose at a rate not to exceed 3 mL/min.
   *Hypomagnesemia, severe.*
**Adults:** 5 g (40 mEq) in 1,000 mL dextrose 5% or sodium chloride solution by **slow** infusion over period of 3 hr.
   *Hyperalimentation.*
**Adults:** 8–24 mEq/day; **infants:** 2–10 mEq/day.
• **Oral Solution**
   *Laxative.*
**Adults:** 10–15 g; **pediatric:** 5–10 g.

## NURSING CONSIDERATIONS

See also *Nursing Considerations* for *Anticonvulsants* and *Laxatives*.

**Administration/Storage**

1. When used as a laxative, dissolve in a glassful of ice water or other chilled fluid to lessen the disagreeable taste.

2. Dilutions for IM: deep injection of 50% concentrate is appropriate for adults. Use a 20% solution for children.

**IV** 3. For IV injections, administer undiluted only 1.5 mL of 10% solution per minute; discontinue when convulsions cease.

4. For IV infusion, dilute 4 g in 250 mL of D5W or NSS; do not exceed 3 mL/min.

**Assessment**

1. Document indications for therapy, onset and duration of symptoms.

2. Note any kidney disease.

3. Assess cardiac status and the ECG for evidence of any abnormality.

4. Obtain baseline magnesium levels and renal function.

5. With premature labor, continually assess fetal heart rate and intensity and timing of contractions.

**Interventions**

1. Before administering check if any of the following conditions exist:
• Absent patellar reflexes
• Respirations below 16/min
• Urine output < 100 mL in past 4 hr
• Early signs of hypermagnesemia:

flushing, sweating, hypotension, or hyperthermia
• Past history of heart block or myocardial damage; prolonged PR and widened QRS intervals

2. Adjust dose of CNS depressants.

3. Digitalis toxicity treated with calcium is extremely dangerous and may result in heart block.

4. With acute MI, administer immediately and continue for 24–48 hr.

5. Do not administer for 2 hr preceding delivery.

6. If mother received continuous IV Mg therapy 24 hr prior to delivery, assess newborn for neurologic and respiratory depression.

**Outcomes/Evaluate**
• Control of seizures
• Magnesium levels (1.8–3 mEq/L)
• Successful evacuation of stool

# Mannitol
(MAN-nih-tol)
**Pregnancy Category:** C
Osmitrol **(Rx)**
**Classification:** Diuretic, osmotic

**Action/Kinetics:** Increases the osmolarity of the glomerular filtrate, which decreases the reabsorption of water and increases excretion of sodium and chloride. It also increases the osmolarity of the plasma, which causes enhanced flow of water from tissues into the interstitial fluid and plasma. Thus, cerebral edema, increased ICP, and CSF volume and pressure are decreased. **Onset, IV:** 30–60 min for diuresis and within 15 min for reduction of cerebrospinal and intraocular pressures. **Peak:** 30–60 min. **Duration:** 6–8 hr diuresis and 4–8 hr for reduction of intraocular pressure. **t½:** 15–100 min. Over 90% excreted through the urine unchanged. A test dose is given in clients with impaired renal function or oliguria.
**Uses:** Diuretic to prevent or treat the oliguric phase of acute renal failure before irreversible renal failure occurs. Decrease ICP and cerebral edema by decreasing brain mass. Decrease elevated intraocular pressure when the pressure cannot be low-

ered by other means. To promote urinary excretion of toxic substances. As a urinary irrigant to prevent hemolysis and hemoglobin buildup during transurethral prostatic resection or other transurethral surgical procedures. *Investigational:* Prevent hemolysis during cardiopulmonary bypass surgery.

**Contraindications:** Anuria, pulmonary edema, severe dehydration, active intracranial bleeding except during craniotomy, progressive heart failure or pulmonary congestion after mannitol therapy, progressive renal damage following mannitol therapy.

**Special Concerns:** Use with caution during lactation. If blood is given simultaneously with mannitol, add at least 20 mEq of sodium chloride to each liter of mannitol solution to avoid pseudoagglutination. Sudden expansion of the extracellular volume that occurs after rapid IV mannitol may lead to fulminating CHF. Mannitol may obscure and intensify inadequate hydration or hypovolemia.

**Side Effects:** *Electrolyte:* Fluid and electrolyte imbalance, acidosis, loss of electrolytes, dehydration. *GI:* Nausea, vomiting, dry mouth, thirst, diarrhea. *CV:* Edema, hypotension or hypertension, increase in heart rate, angina-like chest pain, CHF, thrombophlebitis. *CNS:* Dizziness, headaches, blurred vision, *seizures.* *Miscellaneous:* Pulmonary congestion, marked diuresis, rhinitis, chills, fever, urticaria, pain in arms, skin necrosis.

**OD** **Overdose Management:** *Symptoms:* Increased electrolyte excretion, especially sodium, chloride, and potassium. Sodium depletion results in orthostatic tachycardia or hypotension and decreased CVP. Potassium loss can impair neuromuscular function and cause intestinal dilation and ileus. If urine flow is inadequate, pulmonary edema or water intoxication may occur. Other symptoms include hypotension, polyuria

that rapidly becomes oliguria, stupor, *seizures,* hyperosmolality, and hyponatremia. *Treatment:* Discontinue the infusion immediately and begin supportive measures to correct fluid and electrolyte imbalances. Hemodialysis is effective.

**Drug Interactions:** May cause deafness when used in combination with kanamycin.

**Laboratory Test Interferences:** ↑ or ↓ Inorganic phosphorus. ↑ Ethylene glycol values because mannitol also is oxidized to an aldehyde during test.

**Dosage** ———————————

• **IV Infusion Only**

*Test dose (oliguria or reduced renal function).*
Either 50 mL of a 25% solution, 75 mL of a 20% solution, or 100 mL of a 15% solution infused over 3–5 min. If urine flow is 30–50 mL/hr, therapeutic dose can be given. If urine flow does not increase, give a second test dose; if still no response, client must be reevaluated.

*Prevention of acute renal failure (oliguria).*
**Adults:** 50–100 g, as a 5%–25% solution, given at a rate to maintain urine flow of at least 30–50 mL/hr.

*Treatment of oliguria.*
**Adults:** 50–100 g of a 15%–25% solution.

*Reduction of intracranial pressure and brain mass.*
**Adults:** 1.5–2 g/kg as a 15%–25% solution, infused over 30–60 min.

*Reduction of intraocular pressure.*
**Adults:** 1.5–2 g/kg as a 20% solution (7.5–10 mL/kg) or as a 15% solution (10–13 mL/kg) given over 30–60 min. When used preoperatively, the dose should be given 1–1.5 hr before surgery to maintain the maximum effect.

*Antidote to remove toxic substances.*
**Adults:** Dose depends on the fluid requirement and urinary output. IV fluids and electrolytes are given to replace losses. If a beneficial effect is

**M**

not seen after 200 g mannitol, the infusion should be discontinued.

- **Irrigation Solution**
  *Urologic irrigation.*

**Adults:** Use as a 2.5% irrigating solution for the bladder (this concentration minimizes the hemolytic effect of water alone).

## NURSING CONSIDERATIONS

See also *Nursing Considerations* for *Diuretics, Thiazides.*

### Administration/Storage

**IV** 1. Use a filter if concentrated mannitol is used (15%, 20%, and 25%).

2. Concentrations greater than 15% may crystallize. To redissolve, warm the bottle in a hot water bath or autoclave; cool to body temperature before administering.

3. Do not add to other IV solutions or mix with other medications.

4. If blood is administered concurrently, add 20 mEq of NaCl to each liter of mannitol to prevent pseudoagglutination.

### Assessment

1. Document indications for therapy, type and onset of symptoms.

2. List other meds prescribed to ensure none alter therapeutic drug effects.

3. Assess and document neurologic findings.

4. When used to reduce ICP and brain mass, evaluate the circulatory and renal reserve, fluid and electrolyte balance, body weight, and total I&O before and after mannitol infusion.

5. Note any renal failure. Assess for S&S of electrolyte imbalances and dehydration and replace as needed. If renal failure or oliguria present, perform test dose.

6. Monitor VS and I&O. Slow infusion rate and report any S&S of pulmonary edema manifested by dyspnea, cyanosis, rales, and/or frothy sputum.

### Outcomes/Evaluate

- Desired diuresis with ↓ edema
- ↓ ICP, intraocular pressures

# Masoprocol
(mah-**SOH**-proh-kol)
**Pregnancy Category:** B
Actinex **(Rx)**
**Classification:** Dermatologic agent

**Action/Kinetics:** Mechanism of action is unknown. Less than 1%–2% is absorbed through the skin over a 4-day period following application.

**Uses:** Actinic (solar) keratoses.

**Contraindications:** Hypersensitivity to masoprocol or other ingredients in the formulation. Use with an occlusive dressing.

**Special Concerns:** Use with caution during lactation. Safety and efficacy have not been determined in children. The presence or absence of local skin reactions does not correlate with effectiveness of the drug.

**Side Effects:** *Dermatologic:* Commonly, erythema, flaking, itching, dryness, edema, burning, soreness, allergic contact dermatitis. Also, bleeding, crusting, eye irritation, oozing, rash, soreness, skin irritation, stinging, tightness, tingling, blistering, eczema, fissuring, leathery feeling to the skin, skin roughness, wrinkling, excoriation.

### Dosage

- **Cream**

Following washing and drying areas where actinic keratoses are located, the drug should be gently massaged into the area, until it is evenly distributed, morning and evening for 28 days.

## NURSING CONSIDERATIONS

**Administration/Storage:** For external use only.

### Assessment

1. Determine any sulfite sensitivity; may cause allergic-type reactions, esp. in asthmatics or atopic nonasthmatics.

2. Document symptoms and onset of skin disorder; list other treatments used and the outcome.

3. Assess carefully and describe characteristics (including location and size) of lesions to be treated.

**Client/Family Teaching**
1. Administer using the following guidelines:
• Wash hands.
• Wash and dry involved area thoroughly.
• Apply masoprocol evenly and gently and massage into actinic lesion.
• Wash hands immediately after application.
• Exercise special care if drug must be applied near the eyes, nose, or mouth. If drug comes in contact with the eyes, wash promptly with water.
• Apply each morning and evening for 28 days as directed.
• Do not cover treated areas with any type of occlusive dressing.
• Protect linens, fabrics, and clothing as cream may stain.
• Avoid all other skin products and makeup during therapy.
2. A local transient burning sensation may be felt immediately after applying.
3. Local skin reactions are frequent (bright-red skin, inflamed) and usually resolve within 2 weeks of discontinuing therapy.
4. Stop drug and report any evidence of severe reaction characterized by blistering or oozing lesions.
5. Avoid undue sun exposure, especially since solar keratoses may be sun induced.
**Outcomes/Evaluate:**  ↓  Number and size of actinic lesions

# Mazindol
(**MAYZ**-in-dohl)
**Pregnancy Category:** C
Mazanor, Sanorex **(C-IV) (Rx)**
**Classification:** Anorexiant

See also *Amphetamines and Derivatives.*
**Action/Kinetics:  Onset:** 30–60 min; **duration:** 8–15 hr. **t½:** Less than 24 hr. **Therapeutic blood levels:** 0.003–0.012 mcg/mL. Excreted in urine partially unchanged.

**Uses:** Short-term (8–12 weeks) treatment of exogenous obesity in conjunction with a weight reduction program including exercise, reduced caloric intake, and behavior modification.
**Additional Side Effects:** Testicular pain.

**Dosage** ───────────
• **Tablets**
**Adults, initial:** 1 mg once daily 1 hr before the first meal of the day; **then,** dose can be increased to 1 mg t.i.d. before meals or 2 mg once daily 1 hr before lunch.

## NURSING CONSIDERATIONS

See also *Nursing Considerations* for *Amphetamines and Derivatives.*
**Client/Family Teaching**
1. Review goals and time frame for achieving. Identify importance of diet, regular exercise, and reduced caloric intake in the overall management of obesity.
2. Take with meals if GI distress occurs.
3. Attend diet counseling and support groups.
**Outcomes/Evaluate:** Weight reduction

# Mebendazole
(meh-**BEN**-dah-zohl)
**Pregnancy Category:** C
Vermox **(Rx)**
**Classification:** Anthelmintic

See also *Anthelmintics.*
**Action/Kinetics:** Anthelmintic effect occurs by blocking the glucose uptake of the organisms, thereby reducing their energy until death results. It also inhibits the formation of microtubules in the helminth. **Peak plasma levels:** 2–4 hr. Poorly absorbed from the GI tract. Excreted in feces as unchanged drug or metabolites.
**Uses:** Whipworm, pinworm, roundworm, common and American hookworm infections; in single or

**M**

mixed infections. Mebendazole is not effective for hydatid disease.

**Contraindications:** Hypersensitivity to mebendazole.

**Special Concerns:** Use with caution in children under 2 years of age and during lactation.

**Side Effects:** *GI:* Transient abdominal pain and diarrhea. *Hematologic:* Reversible neutropenia. *Miscellaneous:* Fever.

**Drug Interactions:** Carbamazepine and hydantoin may ↓ effect due to ↓ plasma levels of mebendazole.

**Dosage** ────────────

• **Tablets, Chewable**
  *Whipworm, roundworm, and hookworm.*
**Adults and children:** 1 tablet morning and evening on 3 consecutive days.
  *Pinworms.*
1 tablet, one time. All treatments can be repeated after 3 weeks if the client is not cured.

## NURSING CONSIDERATIONS

See also *Nursing Considerations* for *Anthelmintics*.

**Client/Family Teaching**

1. Tablets may be chewed, swallowed, or crushed and mixed with food. Fasting or purging are not required.

2. Pinworms may be highly contagious:

• Carefully wash hands with soap and water before and after eating and toileting; clean nails and keep out of mouth.

• Advise school nurse of treatment.

• Do not share washcloths and towels. Wear tight underpants; change daily. Sleep alone; wear shoes during waking hours.

• Do not shake or share linens/clothing; wash in hot water.

• Clean toilet and seats with disinfectant daily; vacuum or wetmop bedroom floors daily.

3. Wash all fruits and vegetables. Thoroughly cook all meats and vegetables.

4. Immobilization followed by death of parasites is slow. Complete clearance from the GI tract may take up to 3 days after initiation of treatment.

**Outcomes/Evaluate**

• Three consecutive negative stool and/or perianal swabs

• Organism expulsion/destruction

# Mecamylamine hydrochloride

(mek-ah-**MILL**-ah-meen)

**Pregnancy Category:** C

Inversine **(Rx)**

**Classification:** Antihypertensive, ganglionic blocking agent

────────────

**Action/Kinetics: Onset (gradual):** ½–2 hr. **Duration:** 6–12 hr. May take 2–3 days to achieve full therapeutic potential. Less apt than other ganglionic blocking agents to induce tolerance. Excreted unchanged by the kidneys. The rate of excretion is influenced by urinary pH in that alkalinization of the urine decreases, and acidification increases, renal excretion.

**Uses:** Moderate to severe hypertension including uncomplicated malignant hypertension. Withdraw or substitute mecamylamine slowly because sudden withdrawal or switching to other antihypertensive agents may result in severe hypertensive rebound. Since mecamylamine reduces peristalsis, it is a useful addition to a thiazide-guanethidine regimen in clients who experience persistent diarrhea with guanethidine.

**Contraindications:** Mild, moderate, labile hypertension; coronary insufficiency, clients with recent MI, uremia, clients being treated with antibiotics and sulfonamides, glaucoma, organic pyloric stenosis, uncooperative clients. Lactation.

**Special Concerns:** Dosage has not been established in children. Geriatric clients may be more sensitive to the hypotensive effects of mecamylamine; also, a decrease in dose may be required in these clients due to age-related decreases in renal function. Use with caution in marked cerebral and coronary arteriosclerosis, after recent CVA, prostatic hypertrophy, urethral stricture, bladder neck obstruction. Abdominal distention, decreased bowel signs, and other symptoms of adynamic ileus are reasons for discontinuing the drug.

**Side Effects:** *GI:* N&V, constipation (may be preceded by small, frequent, liquid stools), dry mouth, glossitis, anorexia, ileus. *CNS:* Sedation, weakness, fatigue. Rarely, choreiform movements, mental aberrations, tremors, ***seizures***. *Respiratory:* Fibrosis, interstitial pulmonary edema. *CV:* Postural hypotension, orthostatic dizziness, syncope. *GU:* Urinary retention, decreased libido, impotence. *Miscellaneous:* Paresthesia, blurred vision, dilated pupils.

**OD** **Overdose Management:** *Symptoms:* Hypotension, ***peripheral vascular collapse,*** orthostatic hypotension, N&V, diarrhea, constipation, paralytic ileus, dizziness, anxiety, dry mouth, mydriasis, blurred vision, palpitations, increased intraocular pressure, urinary retention. *Treatment:* Vasopressors to treat hypotension.

**Dosage**
• **Tablets**
*Hypertension.*
**Adults, initial:** 2.5 mg b.i.d. Increase by increments of 2.5 mg q 2 or more days; **maintenance:** 25 mg/day in three divided doses.

## NURSING CONSIDERATIONS

See also *Nursing Considerations* for *Antihypertensive Agents.*
**Administration/Storage:** The morning dose may be small or omitted; larger doses are given at noon and in the evening.
**Client/Family Teaching**
1. For better control of hypertension, administer after meals.
2. Allow more time to prepare for the day's activities to permit the body time to adjust to postural drug effects.
3. If weak, dizzy, or faint after standing or exercising for a long time, lie down or sit down and lower head between knees.
4. Eat a diet high in fiber and consume foods and fluids that help prevent constipation.
**Outcomes/Evaluate:** ↓ BP

# Mechlorethamine hydrochloride (Nitrogen mustard)

(meh-klor-**ETH**-ah-meen)
**Pregnancy Category:** D
Mustargen **(Rx)**
**Classification:** Antineoplastic, alkylating agent

See also *Antineoplastic Agents* and *Alkylating Agents.*
**Action/Kinetics:** Cell-cycle nonspecific. Forms an unstable ethylenimmonium ion, which then alkylates or binds with various compounds, including nucleic acids. The cytotoxic activity is due to cross-linking of DNA and RNA strands and protein synthesis. When used for intracavitary tumors, exerts both an inflammatory reaction and sclerosis on serous membranes, which causes adherence of the drug to serosal surfaces. It reacts rapidly with tissues and within minutes after administration the active drug is no longer present. Metabolites are excreted through the urine.
**Uses:** **IV:** Bronchogenic carcinoma; chronic lymphocytic and chronic myelocytic leukemia; palliative treatment of stages III and IV of Hodgkin's disease, polycythemia vera, mycosis fungoides, lymphosarcoma. **Intracavity:** Intrapericardial, intraperitoneal, or intrapleural: Metastatic carcinoma resulting in effusion. *Investigational:* **Topical:** Cutaneous mycosis fungoides.
**Contraindications:** Use during lactation. During infectious disease.
**Special Concerns:** Extravasation into SC areas causes painful inflammation and induration. Use in children has been limited although the drug

has been used in MOPP (mechlorethamine, Oncovin, procarbazine, prednisone) therapy.

**Additional Side Effects:** High incidence of N&V. Amyloidosis, hyperuricemia, petechiae, SC hemorrhages, tinnitus, deafness, herpes zoster, or temporary amenorrhea. Extravasation into SC tissue causes painful inflammation.

**Drug Interactions:** Amphotericin B: Combination ↑ possibility of blood dyscrasias.

**Dosage** ————————————
• **IV**

**Adults, children:** a total dose of 0.4 mg/kg per course of therapy given as a single dose or in two to four divided doses of 0.1–0.2 mg/kg over 2–4 days. Depending on blood cell count, a second course may be given after 3 weeks.

• **Intrapleural, Intraperitoneal, Intrapericardial**

0.4 mg/kg (0.2 mg/kg has been used intrapericardially).

• **Topical Ointment, Solution**

Apply to entire skin surface once daily until 6–12 months after a complete response is obtained; **then,** use once to several times a week for up to 3 years.

## NURSING CONSIDERATIONS

See also *Nursing Considerations* for *Antineoplastic Agents.*

**Administration/Storage**

1. For intracavitary administration, may be further diluted in 100 mL of NSS; turn client every 60 sec for 5 min to the following positions: prone, supine, right side, left side, and knee-chest. Lack of effect often results from failure to move client often enough. Remaining fluid may be removed after 24–36 hr.

**IV** 2. Drug is highly irritating; avoid any contact with skin. Wear plastic or rubber gloves during preparation.

3. Best administered through tubing of a rapidly flowing IV saline infusion.

4. Prepare solution immediately before administration because it decomposes on standing.

5. Medication is available in a rubber-stoppered vial to which 10 mL of either sterile water for injection or NaCl injection is added to give a concentration of 1 mg/mL; administer over 3–5 min.

6. Insert the needle and keep it inserted until the medication is dissolved and the required dose withdrawn. Carefully discard the vial with the remaining solution so that no one will come in contact with it.

7. Use aqueous solution of equal parts 5% sodium thiosulfate and 5% sodium bicarbonate to clean glassware, tubings, and other articles after drug administration. Soak for 45 min.

8. Monitor IV closely because extravasation causes swelling, erythema, induration, and sloughing. In case of extravasation, remove IV, infuse area with isotonic sodium thiosulfate (4.14% solution of USP salt), and apply cold compresses. If sodium thiosulfate is not available, use isotonic NaCl solution or 1% lidocaine. Apply ice for 6–12 hr.

**Assessment**

1. Document indications for therapy and route of administration. Note any agents used previously.

2. Monitor I&O, uric acid, renal and hematologic function. Assess for dehydration, anemia, infection, and gout (allopurinol may lower uric acid levels). Drug causes granulocyte and platelet suppression. Nadir: 7–14 days; recovery 21 days.

**Interventions**

1. Administer phenothiazine and/or a sedative as ordered (30–45 min prior to medication and RTC as needed) to control severe N&V that usually occurs 1–3 hr after administration.

2. Administer in late afternoon or early evening, and follow with a sedative (sleeping pill) to control adverse symptoms and to induce sleep.

3. If drug comes in contact with the eye, irrigate with copious amounts of saline solution and consult opthalmologist. Irrigate skin with water for 15 min and then with 2%

sodium thiosulfate solution in the event of accidental contact.

**Client/Family Teaching**
1. Hair loss may occur.
2. Avoid vaccinia and exposure to infections or infected persons.
3. Drug may cause irreversible gonadal suppression.
4. Practice birth control during and for 4 months following therapy.

**Outcomes/Evaluate**
• ↓ Tumor size/spread
• Improved hematologic parameters
• Resolution of effusion

## Meclizine hydrochloride
(**MEK**-lih-zeen)
**Pregnancy Category:** B
Antivert, Antivert/25 and /50, Antivert/25 Chewable, Antrizine, Bonamine ✦, Bonine, Dizmiss, Dramamine II, Meni-D, Ru-Vert-M **(OTC and Rx)**
**Classification:** Antihistamine (piperidine-type), antiemetic, antimotion sickness

See also *Antihistamines* and *Antiemetics*.
**Action/Kinetics:** Mechanism for the antiemetic effect may be due to a central anticholinergic effect to decrease vestibular stimulation and depress labyrinthine activity. May also act on the CTZ to decrease vomiting. **Onset:** 30–60 min; **Duration:** 8–24 hr. **t½:** 6 hr.
**Uses:** Nausea and vomiting, dizziness of motion sickness, vertigo associated with diseases of the vestibular system.
**Special Concerns:** Safety for use during lactation and in children less than 12 years of age has not been determined. Pediatric and geriatric clients may be more sensitive to the anticholinergic effects of meclizine.
**Side Effects:** *CNS:* Drowsiness, excitation, nervousness, restlessness, insomnia, euphoria, vertigo, hallucinations (auditory or visual). *GI:* N&V, diarrhea, constipation, anorexia. *GU:* Urinary frequency or retention; diffi-

culty in urination. *CV:* Hypotension, tachycardia, palpitations. *Miscellaneous:* Dry nose and throat, blurred or double vision, tinnitus, rash, urticaria.

**Dosage**
• **Capsules, Tablets, Chewable Tablets**
*Motion sickness.*
**Adults:** 25–50 mg 1 hr before travel; may be repeated q 24 hr during travel.
*Vertigo.*
**Adults:** 25–100 mg/day in divided doses.

### NURSING CONSIDERATIONS

See also *Nursing Considerations* for *Antihistamines* and *Antiemetics*.
**Assessment**
1. Document onset, duration, and characteristics of symptoms.
2. Assess for other adverse symptoms; drug may mask signs of drug overdose or pathology such as increased ICP or intestinal obstruction.
**Client/Family Teaching**
1. Take only as directed and report if condition does not improve.
2. Antiemetics tend to cause drowsiness and dizziness. Do not drive or perform other hazardous tasks until drug response evident.
**Outcomes/Evaluate**
• Prevention of motion sickness
• Control of vertigo

## Meclofenamate sodium
(me-kloh-fen-**AM**-ayt)
Meclomen **(Rx)**
**Classification:** Nonsteroidal anti-inflammatory drug

See also *Nonsteroidal Anti-Inflammatory Drugs.*
**Action/Kinetics: Peak plasma levels:** 30–60 min. **t½:** 2–3.3 hr. Peak anti-inflammatory activity may not be observed for 2–3 weeks. Excreted through urine and feces.
**Uses:** Acute and chronic rheumatoid arthritis and osteoarthritis. Not indicated as the initial drug for rheuma-

toid arthritis due to GI side effects. Has been used in combination with gold salts or corticosteroids. Mild to moderate pain. Primary dysmenorrhea, excessive menstrual blood loss. *Investigational:* Sunburn, prophylaxis of migraine, migraine due to menses.

**Additional Contraindications:** Not recommended for use during pregnancy or lactation. Use in children less than 14 years of age.

**Special Concerns:** Safe use during lactation not established. Safety and efficacy not established in functional class IV rheumatoid arthritis.

**Additional Side Effects:** Severe diarrhea, nausea, headache, rash, dermatitis, abdominal pain, pyrosis, flatulence, malaise, fatigue, paresthesia, insomnia, depression, taste disturbances, nocturia, blood loss (through feces: 2 mL/day).

**Drug Interactions**
*Aspirin* / ↓ Plasma levels of meclofenamate
*Warfarin* / ↑ Effect of warfarin

**Laboratory Test Interferences:** ↑ Serum transaminase, alkaline phosphatase; rarely, ↑ serum creatinine or BUN.

**Dosage** ⎯⎯⎯⎯⎯⎯⎯
• **Capsules**
*Rheumatoid arthritis, osteoarthritis.*
**Adults, usual:** 200–400 mg/day in three to four equal doses. Initiate at lower dose and increase to maximum of 400 mg/day if necessary. After initial satisfactory response, lower dosage to decrease severity of side effects.
*Mild to moderate pain.*
**Adults:** 50 mg q 4–6 hr (100 mg may be required in some clients), not to exceed 400 mg/day.
*Excessive menstrual blood loss and primary dysmenorrhea.*
**Adults:** 100 mg t.i.d. for up to 6 days, starting at the onset of menses.

## NURSING CONSIDERATIONS

See also *Nursing Considerations* for *Nonsteroidal Anti-Inflammatory Drugs.*

**Administration/Storage**
1. Lower doses may be effective for chronic use.
2. Reduce dose or discontinue temporarily if diarrhea occurs.

**Client/Family Teaching**
1. May take with food or milk to diminish GI upset.
2. Report any changes in stool color or diarrhea.
3. Take as ordered and do not become discouraged; may take 2–3 weeks to see improvement in arthritic conditions.

**Outcomes/Evaluate**
• Improvement in joint pain and mobility with ↓ inflammation
• Relief of pain and dysmenorrhea

---

# Medroxyprogesterone acetate
(meh-**drox**-see-proh-**JESS**-ter-ohn)
**Pregnancy Category:** X
Alti-MPA ❋, Amen, Curretab, Cycrin, Depo-Provera, Depo-Provera C-150, Provera **(Rx)**
**Classification:** Progestational hormone, synthetic

---

See also *Progesterone and Progestins* and *Antineoplastic Agents.*

**Action/Kinetics:** Synthetic progestin devoid of estrogenic and androgenic activity. Prevents stimulation of endometrium by pituitary gonadotropins. Priming with estrogen is necessary before response is noted. Rapidly absorbed from GI tract. **Maximum levels:** 1–2 hr. **t½, after PO:** 2–3 hr for first 6 hr; then, 8–9 hr. **t½, long-acting forms IM:** About 10 weeks with maximum levels within 24 hr.

**Uses:** Secondary amenorrhea, abnormal uterine bleeding due to hormonal imbalance (no organic pathology). Adjunct in palliative treatment of inoperable, recurrent, or metastatic endometrial or renal carcinoma. Long-acting contraceptive (injectable form). *Investigational:* Polycystic ovary syndrome, precocious puberty. With estrogen to treat menopausal symptoms and hypermenorrhea. To stimulate respiration in obesity-hypoventilation syndrome (oral).

**Contraindications:** Clients with or a history of thrombophlebitis, thromboembolic disease, cerebral apoplexy. Liver dysfunction. Known or suspected malignancy of the breasts or genital organs. Missed abortion; as a diagnostic for pregnancy. Undiagnosed vaginal bleeding. Use during the first 4 months of pregnancy.

**Special Concerns:** The overall risk of breast, liver, ovarian, endometrial, and cervical cancer is not thought to increase with use of the injectable long-acting contraceptive preparation. Possibility of ectopic pregnancy. Use with caution in clients with a history of depression. Due to the possibility of fluid retention, use with caution in clients with epilepsy, migraine, asthma, or cardiac or renal dysfunction.

**Side Effects:** *GU:* Amenorrhea or infertility for up to 18 months. *CV:* Thrombophlebitis, ***pulmonary embolism.*** *GI:* Nausea (rare), jaundice. *CNS:* Nervousness, drowsiness, insomnia, fatigue, dizziness, headache (rare). *Dermatologic:* Pruritus, urticaria, rash, acne, hirsutism, alopecia, angioneurotic edema. *Miscellaneous:* ***Hyperpyrexia, anaphylaxis,*** decrease in glucose tolerance, weight gain, fluid retention.

**Drug Interactions:** Aminoglutethimide may ↑ metabolism of medroxyprogesterone → ↓ effect.

**Dosage** ——————
• **Tablets**
*Secondary amenorrhea.*
5–10 mg/day for 5–10 days, with therapy beginning at any time during the menstrual cycle. If endometrium has been estrogen primed: 10 mg medroxyprogesterone/day for 10 days beginning any time.
*Abnormal uterine bleeding with no pathology.*
5–10 mg/day for 5–10 days, with therapy beginning on day 16 or 21 of the menstrual cycle. If endometrium

has been estrogen primed: 10 mg/day for 10 days, beginning on day 16 of the menstrual cycle. Bleeding usually begins within 3–7 days.
• **IM**
*Endometrial or renal carcinoma.*
**Initial:** 400–1,000 mg/week; **then, if improvement noted,** 400 mg/month. Medroxyprogesterone is not intended to be the primary therapy.
*Long-acting contraceptive.*
150 mg of depot form q 3 months by deep IM injection given only during the first 5 days after the onset of a normal menstrual period, within 5 days postpartum if not breastfeeding, or 6 weeks postpartum if breastfeeding.

## NURSING CONSIDERATIONS

See also *Nursing Considerations* for *Antineoplastic Agents* and *Progesterone and Progestins.*
**Assessment**
1. Document type, onset, and duration of symptoms.
2. Note any thromboembolic disease.
3. Monitor calcium levels and LFTs. With severe hypercalcemia, have IV fluids, diuretics, corticosteroids, and phosphate supplements available; monitor closely once corrected.
**Client/Family Teaching**
1. With cancer therapy, the combined effect of the drug and osteolytic metastases may result in hypercalcemia. Report insomnia, lethargy, anorexia, and N&V. Increase fluid intake to minimize hypercalcemia.
2. Keep scheduled appointments for contraceptive evaluation. Additional barrier protection is necessary to prevent STDs and HIV transmission.
**Outcomes/Evaluate**
• Prevention of pregnancy
• Control of tumor size and spread
• Regular menses; normal hormone levels

# Mefenamic acid
(meh-fen-**NAM**-ick **AH**-sid)
**Pregnancy Category:** C

Ponstan ✹, Ponstel **(Rx)**
**Classification:** Nonsteroidal, anti-inflammatory drug

See also *Nonsteroidal Anti-Inflammatory Drugs.*
**Action/Kinetics:** Inhibits prostaglandin synthesis. Is an anti-inflammatory, antipyretic, and analgesic. **Peak plasma levels:** 2–4 hr; **t½:** 2–4 hr; **duration:** 4–6 hr. Slowly absorbed from the GI tract, metabolized by the liver, and excreted in the urine and feces.
**Uses:** Short-term relief (< 1 week) of mild to moderate pain (e.g., pain associated with tooth extraction and musculoskeletal disorders). Primary dysmenorrhea. *Investigational:* PMS, sunburn.
**Contraindications:** Ulceration or chronic inflammation of the GI tract, pregnancy or possibility thereof, children under 14, and hypersensitivity to the drug.
**Special Concerns:** Dosage has not been established in children less than 14 years of age. Use with caution in clients with impaired renal or hepatic function, asthma, or clients on anticoagulant therapy.
**Additional Side Effects:** *Autoimmune hemolytic anemia if used more than 12 months.* Diarrhea may be significant. Rash (maculopapular type).
**Drug Interactions**
*Anticoagulants* / ↑ Hypoprothrombinemia due to ↓ plasma protein binding
*Insulin* / ↑ Insulin requirement
*Lithium* / ↑ Plasma levels of lithium
**Laboratory Test Interferences:** False + test for urinary bile using diazo tablets.

**Dosage** ───────────
• **Capsules**
  *Analgesia, primary dysmenorrhea.*
**Adults and children over 14 years of age, initial:** 500 mg; **then,** 250 mg q 6 hr.

## NURSING CONSIDERATIONS

See also *Nursing Considerations* for *Nonsteroidal Anti-inflammatory Drugs.*
**Administration/Storage:** Do not use for more than a week at a time.
**Client/Family Teaching**
1. Take with food to minimize GI upset.
2. Use caution when driving or operating potentially hazardous machinery; drug may cause dizziness, lightheadedness, or confusion.
3. Report any unusual bleeding, rashes, itching, diarrhea, or increased sweating.
**Outcomes/Evaluate**
• Relief of pain
• Control of uterine cramping

# Mefloquine hydrochloride

(meh-**FLOH**-kwin)
**Pregnancy Category:** C
Lariam **(Rx)**
**Classification:** Antimalarial

**Action/Kinetics:** Related chemically to quinine and acts as a blood schizonticide. It may increase intravesicular pH in acid vesicles of parasite. Mefloquine is a mixture of enantiomeric molecules that results in differences in the rates of release, absorption, distribution, metabolism, elimination, and activity of the drug. It shows myocardial depressant activity with about 20% of the antifibrillatory activity of quinidine and 50% of the increase in the PR interval noted with quinine. **t½:** 13–24 days (average 3 weeks). Is 98% bound to plasma proteins and is concentrated in blood erythrocytes (i.e., the target cells in treatment of malaria).
**Uses:** Mild to moderate acute malaria caused by mefloquine-susceptible strains of *Plasmodium falciparum* (both chloroquine susceptible and resistant strains) or *P. vivax.* Data are not available regarding effectiveness in treating *P. ovale* or *P. malar-*

*iae.* Also, prophylaxis of *P. falciparum* and *P. vivax* infections, including prophylaxis of chloroquine-resistant strains of *P. falciparum.* *NOTE:* Clients with acute *P. vivax* malaria are at a high risk for relapse as mefloquine does not eliminate the exoerythrocytic (hepatic) parasites. Thus, these clients should also be treated with primaquine. *NOTE:* Strains of *P. falciparum* are reported to be resistant to mefloquine.

**Contraindications:** Hypersensitivity to mefloquine or related compounds.

**Special Concerns:** Use with caution during lactation and in those with psychiatric disturbances due to the possibility of emotional reactions. Safety and effectiveness have not been determined in children.

**Side Effects:** *NOTE:* At the doses used, it is difficult to distinguish side effects due to the drug from symptoms attributable to the disease itself. **When used for treatment of acute malaria.** *GI:* N&V, diarrhea, abdominal pain, loss of appetite. *CNS:* Dizziness, fever, headache, fatigue, emotional problems, *seizures.* *Miscellaneous:* Myalgia, chills, skin rash, tinnitus, bradycardia, hair loss, pruritus, asthenia. **When used for prophylaxis of malaria.** *CNS:* Dizziness, syncope, encephalopathy of unknown etiology. *Miscellaneous:* Vomiting, extrasystoles. **Postmarketing surveillance.** *CNS:* Vertigo, psychoses, confusion, anxiety, depression, *seizures,* hallucinations, insomnia, abnormal dreams, forgetfulness, motor and sensory neuropathy. *CV:* Hypertension, hypotension, tachycardia, palpitations. *Dermatologic:* Flushing, urticaria, Stevens-Johnson syndrome, erythema multiforme. *Miscellaneous:* Visual disturbances.

**OD** **Overdose Management:** *Symptoms:* Cardiotoxic effects, vomiting, diarrhea. *Treatment:* Induce vomiting and administer fluid therapy to treat vomiting and diarrhea.

**Drug Interactions**
*Beta-adrenergic blocking agents /* ECG abnormalities or cardiac arrest
*Chloroquine /* ↑ Risk of seizures
*Quinidine /* ↑ Risk of ECG abnormalities or cardiac arrest
*Quinine /* ↑ Risk of seizures, ECG abnormalities, or cardiac arrest; also, ↑ risk of convulsions
*Valproic acid /* Loss of seizure control and ↓ blood levels of valproic acid

**Laboratory Test Interferences: When used for prophylaxis:** Transient ↑ transaminases, leukocytosis, thrombocytopenia. When used for treatment of acute malaria: ↓ Hematocrit, transient ↑ transaminases, leukocytosis, thrombocytopenia.

**Dosage** ————
• **Tablets**
*Mild to moderate malaria caused by susceptible strains of* P. falciparum *or* P. vivax.
1,250 mg (5 tablets) as a single dose with at least 8 oz of water (not to be taken on an empty stomach).
*Prophylaxis of malaria.*
250 mg (1 tablet) once a week for 4 weeks; **then,** 1 tablet every other week. The CDC recommends a single dose taken weekly starting 1 week before travel, continued weekly during travel, and for 4 weeks after leaving malarious areas. **Pediatric, 15–19 kg:** ¼ **tablet (62.5 mg) weekly; 20–30 kg:** ½ **tablet (125 mg) weekly; 31–45 kg:** ¾ **tablet (187.5 mg) weekly; over 45 kg:** 1 tablet (250 mg) weekly. The CDC recommends a similar dosing schedule for children as for adults.

## NURSING CONSIDERATIONS

See also *General Nursing Considerations for All Anti-Infectives.*
**Administration/Storage:** Store tablets at 15°C–30°C (59°F–86°F).
**Assessment**
1. Note lab confirmation of causative organism.
2. Monitor liver function.

3. Note any psychiatric disturbances or severe emotional lability.

4. With life-threatening *P. falciparum* infection, initiate treatment with an IV antimalarial drug; follow with mefloquine, to complete therapy.

5. To reduce cardiotoxic effects, induce vomiting with overdose.

**Client/Family Teaching**

1. Do not take on an empty stomach; take with at least 8 oz of water.

2. Report any early evidence of visual disturbance; obtain periodic ophthalmic exams.

**Outcomes/Evaluate:** Acute malaria prophylaxis (with drug-sensitive malarial parasites)

# Megestrol acetate

(meh-**JESS**-trohl)
**Pregnancy Category:** D
Apo-Megestrol ✹, Linmegestrol ✹, Megace, Megace OS ✹, Nu-Megestrol ✹ **(Rx)**
**Classification:** Synthetic progestin

See also *Progesterone and Progestins* and *Antineoplastic Agents.*

**Action/Kinetics:** Antineoplastic activity is due to suppression of gonadotropins (antiluteinizing effect). Has appetite-enhancing properties (mechanism unknown). Contains tartrazine, which can cause allergic-type reactions, including asthma, often occurring in aspirin sensitivity.

**Uses: Tablets:** Palliative treatment of advanced endometrial or breast cancer. Should not be used instead of chemotherapy, radiation, or surgery.

**Oral suspension:** Treatment of anorexia, cachexia, or an unexplained, significant weight loss in clients with a diagnosis of AIDS.

**Contraindications:** Use as a diagnostic aid test for pregnancy, in known or suspected pregnancy, or for prophylaxis to avoid weight loss. Use during the first 4 months of pregnancy.

**Special Concerns:** Use with caution in clients with a history of thromboembolic disease. Use in HIV-infected women with endometrial or breast cancer has not been widely studied. Long-term use may increase the risk of respiratory infections and may cause secondary adrenal suppression. Safety and efficacy in children have not been determined.

**Side Effects:** *GI:* Diarrhea, flatulence, nausea, dyspepsia, vomiting, constipation, dry mouth, hepatomegaly, increased salivation, abdominal pain, oral moniliasis. *CV:* Hypertension, *cardiomyopathy,* palpitation. *CNS:* Insomnia, headache, paresthesia, confusion, *seizures,* depression, neuropathy, hypesthesia, abnormal thought process. *Respiratory:* Pneumonia, dyspnea, cough, pharyngitis, chest pain, lung disorder, increased risk of respiratory infection with chronic use. *Dermatologic:* Rash, alopecia, herpes, pruritus, vesiculobullous rash, sweating, skin disorder. *GU:* Impotence, decreased libido, urinary frequency, albuminuria, urinary incontinence, UTI, gynecomastia. *Body as a whole:* Asthenia, anemia, fever, pain, moniliasis, infection, sarcoma. *Miscellaneous:* Leukopenia, edema, peripheral edema, amblyopia.

**Laboratory Test Interferences:** Hyperglycemia, ↑ LDH.

**Dosage**
• **Oral Suspension**
*Appetite stimulant in AIDS clients.*
**Adults, initial:** 800 mg/day (20 mL/day). The dose should be adjusted to 400 mg/day (10 mL/day) after 1 month.
• **Tablets**
*Breast cancer.*
40 mg q.i.d.
*Endometrial cancer.*
40–320 mg/day in divided doses. To determine efficacy, treatment should be continued for at least 2 months.

## NURSING CONSIDERATIONS

See also *Nursing Considerations* for *Antineoplastic Agents, Progesterone and Progestins,* and *Medroxyprogesterone Acetate.*

**Administration/Storage:** The oral suspension is available in a lemon-lime flavor that contains 40 mg of micronized megestrol acetate/mL; shake well before using.

**Assessment**
1. Document indications for therapy, type and duration of symptoms.
2. Note any thromboembolic disease.
3. Determine if pregnant.
4. Note sensitivity to tartrazines.
5. With long-term therapy, assess for respiratory infections and adrenal suppression.

**Client/Family Teaching**
1. Take exactly as prescribed; do not skip or double up doses. May take with meals if GI upset occurs.
2. Report vaginal bleeding, edema, swelling or pain in leg veins, pain/weakness in thumb (CTS).
3. Females should practice birth control.

**Outcomes/Evaluate**
• ↓ Tumor size and spread
• Prevention of further weight loss

# Melphalan (L-PAM, L-Phenylalanine mustard, L-Sarcolysin)

(**MEL**-fah-lan)
**Pregnancy Category:** D
Alkeran (Abbreviation: MPL) **(Rx)**
**Classification:** Antineoplastic, alkylating agent

See also *Antineoplastic Agents* and *Alkylating Agents*.

**Action/Kinetics:** A bifunctional alkylating agent that forms an unstable ethylenimmonium ion that binds to or alkylates various intracellular substances including nucleic acids. It produces a cytotoxic effect by cross-linking of DNA and RNA strands as well as inhibition of protein synthesis. Absorption from GI tract is variable and incomplete. **t½ after PO:** 90 min. Inactivated in tissues and body fluids although it will remain active in the blood for approximately 6 hr. Within 24 hr, 10% is excreted unchanged in the urine.

**Uses:** Multiple myeloma. Epithelial carcinoma of ovary (nonresectable).

Use IV only when PO therapy is not appropriate. *Investigational:* Cancer of the breast and testes.

**Contraindications:** Lactation. Known resistance to drug.

**Special Concerns:** Safety and efficacy have not been determined in children less than 12 years of age. Use with extreme caution in those with compromised bone marrow function due to prior chemotherapy or radiation. Reduce IV dosage in impaired renal function.

**Additional Side Effects:** *Severe bone marrow depression (especially after IV use),* chromosomal aberrations (may be mutagenic), *leukemia (acute, nonlymphatic) in clients with multiple myeloma.* Also, hypersensitivity reactions including *anaphylaxis, pulmonary fibrosis,* interstitial pneumonia, vasculitis, *hemolytic anemia.*

**OD** **Overdose Management:** *Symptoms:* Severe N&V, decreased consciousness, *seizures,* muscle paralysis, cholinomimetic symptoms, diarrhea, severe mucositis, stomatitis, colitis, *hemorrhage of GI tract, bone marrow toxicity. Treatment:* General supportive treatment, blood transfusions, antibiotics. Monitor hematology for up to 6 weeks. Use of filgrastim or sargramostim may decrease the period of pancytopenia.

**Drug Interactions**
*Carmustine* / ↑ Risk of lung toxicity
*Cisplatin* / Cisplatin-induced renal dysfunction → ↓ melphalan excretion
*Cyclosporine* / ↑ Risk of nephrotoxicity
*Interferon alfa* / ↓ Levels of melphalan
*Nalidixic acid* / ↑ Risk of severe hemorrhagic necrotic enterocolitis in pediatric clients

**Laboratory Test Interferences:** ↑ Uric acid and urinary 5-HIAA levels.

**Dosage**
• **Tablets**
*Multiple myeloma.*
One of the following regimens may be used. (1) 6 mg given once daily for

2–3 weeks (adjust dose based on weekly blood counts). Drug is then discontinued for up to 4 weeks with blood count being monitored. When WBC and platelet counts are increasing, a maintenance dose of 2 mg/day can be started. (2) 10 mg/day for 7–10 days. Maximum leukocyte and platelet suppression occurs within 3–5 weeks with recovery within 4–8 weeks. When the WBC exceeds 4,000/mm³ and the platelet count is greater than 100,000/mm³, a maintenance dose of 2 mg/day can be started. Dose is then adjusted to 1–3 mg/day, depending on the hematologic response. Leukocytes should be kept in the range of 3,000–3,500 cells/mm³. (3) 0.15 mg/kg/day for 7 days followed by a rest period of at least 2 weeks (up to 5 weeks may be needed). During the rest period, the leukocyte count will decrease; when WBC and platelet counts are increasing, a maintenance dose of 0.05 mg/kg/day may be given. (4) 0.25 mg/kg/day for 4 consecutive days (or 0.2 mg/kg/day for 5 consecutive days) for a total dose of 1 mg/kg/course of therapy. The 4- to 5-day courses can be repeated q 4–6 weeks if the granulocyte and platelet counts have returned to normal.

*Epithelial ovarian cancer.*
0.2 mg/kg/day for 5 days repeated q 4–5 weeks (as long as blood counts return to normal).

• **IV**
*Multiple myeloma.*
**Adults, usual:** 16 mg/m² as a single infusion over 15–20 min. This dose should be given at 2-week intervals for a total of four doses. The dose should be reduced up to 50% in clients with a BUN less than or equal to 30 mg/dL.

## NURSING CONSIDERATIONS

See also *Nursing Considerations* for *Antineoplastic Agents.*
### Administration/Storage
**IV** 1. About one-third to one-half of clients with multiple myeloma show a favorable response to IV melphalan.

2. For IV use, reconstitute powder with 10 mL of the supplied diluent for a concentration of 5 mg/mL. After the diluent is added, shake vial vigorously until a clear solution is obtained. The dose to be given is then immediately diluted with 0.9% NaCl injection to a concentration of less than or equal to 0.45 mg/mL.
3. Complete IV administration within 60 min after reconstitution. After dilution with saline, about 1% label strength of melphalan hydrolyzes every 10 min.
4. Protect from light and dispense in glass.
5. A precipitate forms if the reconstituted IV product is stored at 5°C (41°F).
### Assessment
1. Document any previous radiation or chemotherapy treatments.
2. Monitor liver and renal function studies, uric acid, and CBC. Drug causes granulocyte and platelet suppression. Nadir: 14 days; recovery: 28–40 days.
3. Advise to use contraceptive measures during therapy and for several months after.
### Outcomes/Evaluate
• ↓ Malignant cell proliferation
• Improved hematologic parameters

# Menotropins
(men-oh-**TROH**-pinz)
**Pregnancy Category:** X
Humegon, Pergonal **(Rx)**
**Classification:** Ovarian stimulant

**Action/Kinetics:** Menotropins are a mixture of FSH and LH extracted from the urine of postmenopausal women. Causes growth and maturation of ovarian follicles. For ovulation to occur, HCG is administered the day following menotropins. **Time to peak effect, females:** 18 hr. In men, menotropins with HCG given for a minimum of 3 months induce spermatogenesis. Eliminated through the kidneys.
**Uses: Females:** In combination with HCG to induce ovulation in clients with anovulatory cycles not due to pri-

mary ovarian failure. **Males:** In combination with HCG to induce spermatogenesis in clients with primary or secondary hypogonadotrophic hypogonadism.

**Contraindications:** *Women:* Pregnancy. Primary ovarian failure as indicated by high levels of urinary gonadotropins, ovarian cysts, intracranial lesions, including pituitary tumors. Overt thyroid and adrenal dysfunction. Any cause of infertility other than anovulation. Abnormal bleeding of undetermined origin. Ovarian cysts or enlargement of the ovaries not due to polycystic ovarian syndrome. *Men:* Normal gonadotropin levels, primary testicular failure, disorders of fertility other than hypogonadotrophic hypogonadism. Thyroid or adrenal dysfunction. Absence of neoplastic disease should be established before treatment is initiated.

**Side Effects:** *Women. GU:* Ovarian overstimulation, hyperstimulation syndrome (maximal 7–10 days after discontinuation of drug), ovarian enlargement (20% of clients), adnexal torsion, ***ruptured ovarian cysts, ectopic pregnancy,*** multiple births (20%). *CV:* ***Hemoperitoneum, thromboembolism,*** tachycardia, pulmonary and vascular complications. *Hypersentivity:* Generalized urticaria, angioneurotic edema, facial edema, ***dysnpea indicating laryngeal edema.*** *CNS:* Headaches, malaise, dizziness. *GI:*N&V, abdominal pain, diarrhea, abdominal cramps, bloating. *At injection site:* Pain, rash, swelling, irritation. *Miscellaneous:* Fever, chills, musculoskeletal aches, joint pains, body rashes, dyspnea, tachypnea.

*Men.* Gynecomastia, breast pain, mastitis, nausea, abnormal lipoprotein fraction, abnormal AST and ALT.

**Dosage** ─────────────

• **IM**

*Induction of ovulation.*

**Individualized, initial:** 75 IU of FSH and 75 IU of LH for 7–12 days (maximum), followed by 10,000 USP units of HCG 1 day after last dose of menotropins. **Subsequent courses:** Same dosage schedule for two more courses, if ovulation has occurred. **Then,** dose may be increased to 150 IU of FSH and 150 IU of LH for 7–12 days, followed by HCG as in the preceding for two or more courses.

*Induction of spermatogenesis.* It may be necessary to give HCG alone, 5,000 IU 3 times/week, for 4–6 months prior to menotropins; **then,** 75 IU FSH and 75 IU LH **IM** 3 times/week and HCG 2,000 IU 2 times/week for at least 4 months. If no response after 4 months, double each dose of menotropins with the HCG dose unchanged.

───────────────────────

## NURSING CONSIDERATIONS

### Administration/Storage

1. Administer parenterally; menotropins are destroyed in the GI tract.

2. To prepare solution, dissolve the contents of one ampule in 1–2 mL sterile saline. Reconstituted solutions must be used immediately; discard any unused portions.

3. Store the lyophilized powder at room temperature or in the refrigerator (3°C–25°C, or 37°F–77°F).

### Assessment

1. Document indications for therapy and other therapy or drugs used.

2. Determine if tested for urinary gonadotropins (high levels) or evaluated for the presence of ovarian cysts; drug contraindicated.

3. Obtain CBC, electrolytes, urinary gonadotropin levels, thyroid and adrenal function studies; note neurovascular assessments (esp. peripheral pulses).

### Interventions

1. Obtain urinary estrogen excretion levels daily. If greater than 100 mcg or if daily estriol excretion exceeds 50 mcg, *withhold HCG* and report; these signal impending hyperstimulation syndrome.

2. If hospitalized for hyperstimulation, perform the following interventions:

• Place client on bed rest.

───────────────────────

• Monitor I&O; weigh daily.
• Monitor urine sp. gravity, serum and urine lytes.
• Assess for hemoconcentration. May need heparin to prevent hyper-coagulability.
• Increase fluid intake; replace electrolytes.
• Provide analgesics for comfort.
3. Monitor CBC; an occasional client will develop erythrocytosis.
4. Report any unexplained fever, ovarian enlargement, or complaints of abdominal pain.

**Client/Family Teaching**
1. Report any pain, coolness, or pale bluish color of an extremity (signs of arterial bloodclot).
2. Fever or the development of lower abdominal pain may be the result of overstimulation of the ovaries that has caused cysts to form, a loss of fluid into the peritoneum, or bleeding; report immediately. Need exam for this at least every other day during drug therapy and for 2 weeks thereafter; hospitalization is necessary if evident.
3. Collect a 24-hr urine daily to be analyzed for estrogen and deliver to lab facility.
4. Take basal body temperature and graph.
5. Signs that indicate ovulation include an increase in the basal body temperature, and an increase in the appearance and volume of cervical mucus.
6. Engage in daily intercourse from the day before chorionic gonadotropin is administered until ovulation occurs.
7. If symptoms indicate overstimulation of the ovaries, a significant ovarian enlargement may have occurred. Report and abstain from intercourse because of increased risk of ovarian cyst rupture.
8. Pregnancy usually occurs 4–6 weeks after completion of therapy. Multiple births may occur.

**Outcomes/Evaluate**
• Ovulation evidenced by ↑ estrogen levels and desired pregnancy
• Male spermatogenesis evidenced by ↑ testosterone levels

# Meperidine hydrochloride (Pethidine hydrochloride)

(meh-**PER**-ih-deen)
**Pregnancy Category:** C
Demerol Hydrochloride **(C-II) (Rx)**
**Classification:** Narcotic analgesic, synthetic

See also *Narcotic Analgesics*.
**Action/Kinetics:** Only one-tenth as potent an analgesic as morphine. Its analgesic effect is only one-half when given PO rather than parenterally. Has no antitussive effects and does not produce miosis. Produces moderate spasmogenic effects on smooth muscle. **Duration:** Less than that of most opiates; keep in mind when establishing a dosing schedule. Produces both psychologic and physical dependence; overdosage causes severe respiratory depression (see *Narcotic Overdose*). **Onset:** 10–45 min. **Peak effect:** 30–60 min. **Duration:** 2–4 hr. **t½:** 3–4 hr.
**Uses:** Analgesic for severe pain, hepatic and renal colic, obstetrics, preanesthetic medication, adjunct to anesthesia. Particularly useful for minor surgery, as in orthopedics, ophthalmology, rhinology, laryngology, and dentistry, and for diagnostic procedures such as cystoscopy, retrograde pyelography, and gastroscopy. Spasms of GI tract, uterus, urinary bladder. Anginal syndrome and distress of CHF.
**Additional       Contraindications:** Hypersensitivity to drug, convulsive states as in epilepsy, tetanus and strychnine poisoning, children under 6 months, diabetic acidosis, head injuries, shock, liver disease, respiratory depression, increased cranial pressure, and before labor during pregnancy.
**Special Concerns:** Use with caution during lactation and in older or debilitated clients. Use with extreme caution in clients with asthma. Atropine-like effects may aggravate glaucoma, especially when given

with other drugs which should be used with caution in glaucoma.

**Additional Side Effects:** Transient hallucinations, transient hypotension (high doses), visual disturbances. Meperidine may accumulate in clients with renal dysfunction, leading to an increased risk of CNS toxicity.

**OD** **Overdose Management:** *Symptoms:* Severe respiratory depression. See *Narcotic Analgesics.* *Treatment:* Naloxone 0.4 mg IV is effective in the treatment of acute overdosage. In PO overdose, gastric lavage and induced emesis are indicated. Treatment, however, is aimed at combating the progressive respiratory depression usually through artificial ventilation.

**Additional Drug Interactions**
*Antidepressants, tricyclic* / Additive anticholinergic side effects
*Hydantoins* / ↓ Effect of meperidine due to ↑ breakdown by liver
*MAO inhibitors* / ↑ Risk of severe symptoms including hyperpyrexia, restlessness, hyper- or hypotension, convulsions, or coma

**Dosage**
• **Tablets, Syrup, IM, SC**
  *Analgesic.*
**Adults:** 50–100 mg q 3–4 hr as needed; **pediatric:** 1.1–1.8 mg/kg, up to adult dosage, q 3–4 hr as needed.
  *Preoperatively.*
**Adults, IM, SC:** 50–100 mg 30–90 min before anesthesia; **pediatric, IM, SC:** 1–2 mg/kg 30–90 min before anesthesia.
  *Obstetrics.*
**Adults, IM, SC:** 50–100 mg q 1–3 hr.
• **IV**
  *Support of anesthesia.*
**IV infusion:** 1 mg/mL or **slow IV injection:** 10 mg/mL until client needs met.

## NURSING CONSIDERATIONS

See also *Nursing Considerations* for *Narcotic Analgesics.*
**Administration/Storage**
1. For repeated doses, IM administration is preferred over SC use.

2. More effective when given parenterally than when given PO.
3. Take the syrup with ½ glass of water to minimize anesthetic effect on mucous membranes.
4. If used concomitantly with phenothiazines or antianxiety agents, reduce the dose by 25%–50%.
**IV** 5. Meperidine for IV use is incompatible with the following drugs: aminophylline, barbiturates, heparin, iodide, methicillin, morphine sulfate, phenytoin, sodium bicarbonate, sulfadiazine, and sulfisoxazole.

**Assessment**
1. Document intensity, location, onset, duration, and level of pain (use a rating scale).
2. Note any head injury, seizure disorder, or conditions that compromise respirations.
3. Assess renal function; note any glaucoma.
**Client/Family Teaching**
1. Use pain rating scale to evaluate drug effectiveness.
2. Drug causes dizziness and drowsiness; do not engage in activities that require mental alertness.
3. Rise slowly, do not to change positions abruptly due to postural effect.
4. Store safely away from bedside; record dose and time of administration.
**Outcomes/Evaluate:** Desired level of analgesia

# Mephentermine sulfate
(meh-**FEN**-ter-meen)
**Pregnancy Category:** C
Wyamine Sulfate **(Rx)**
**Classification:** Adrenergic agent, indirectly acting; vasopressor

See also *Sympathomimetic Drugs.*
**Action/Kinetics:** Acts indirectly by releasing norepinephrine from its storage sites and directly by exerting a slight effect on alpha and beta-1 receptors and a moderate effect on beta-2 receptors mediating vasodilation. Causes increased CO; also elic-

its slight CNS effects. **IV: Onset,** immediate; **duration:** 15–30 min. **IM: Onset,** 5–15 min; **duration:** 1–2 hr. Metabolized in liver. Excreted in urine within 24 hr (rate increased in acidic urine).

**Uses:** Hypotension due to anesthesia, ganglionic blockade, or hemorrhage (only as emergency treatment until blood or blood substitutes can be given).

**Contraindications:** To treat hypotension caused by chlorpromazine. In combination with MAO inhibitors.

**Special Concerns:** Use with caution in CV disease and in chronically ill clients. Use with caution in treating shock secondary to hemorrhage. Safety and efficacy have not been demonstrated in children.

**Side Effects:** Anxiety, cardiac arrhythmias, increased BP (especially in those with heart disease).

**Additional Drug Interactions:** Mephentermine will potentiate hypotensive effects of phenothiazines.

**Dosage**

• **IV, IM**

*Hypotension during spinal anesthesia.*

**IV, Adults:** 30–45 mg; 30-mg doses may be repeated as required; or, **IV infusion, Adults and children:** 0.1% (1 mg/mL) mephentermine in D5W with the rate of infusion and duration dependent on client response. **IV, Pediatric:** 0.4 mg/kg (12 mg/m²) as a single dose.

*Prophylaxis of hypotension in spinal anesthesia.*

**IM, Adults:** 30–45 mg 10–20 min before anesthesia. **IM, Pediatric:** 0.4 mg/kg (12 mg/m²) as a single dose.

*Shock following hemorrhage.*

Not recommended, but IV infusion of 0.1% in D5W may maintain BP until blood volume is replaced.

## NURSING CONSIDERATIONS

See also *Nursing Considerations* for *Sympathomimetic Drugs.*
**Administration/Storage**

**IV** 1. For shock, the preferred method of administration is either injection of the undiluted parenteral solution containing 30 mg/mL or a continuous infusion of a 1-mg/mL solution in D5W directly into the vein.

2. Prepare the 0.1% solution by adding 10 or 20 mL of mephentermine (the 30-mg/mL strength) to either 250 or 500 mL of D5W, respectively.

**Assessment:** Determine cause of hypotensive episode; note any CV disease, hemorrhage, or chronic illness.

**Interventions:** Record BP q 5 min until stable; once stabilized, check q 15–30 min beyond the duration of the drug's action (IM 1–4 hr; IV 5–15 min).

**Outcomes/Evaluate:** Stabilization of BP

# Meprobamate
(meh-proh-**BAM**-ayt)

Apo-Meprobamate ✦, Equanil, Equanil Wyseals, Meditran ✦, Meprospan 200 and 400, Miltown 200, 400 and 600, Neuramate, Novo-Mepro ✦ **(C-IV) (Rx)**
**Classification:** Nonbenzodiazepine antianxiety agent

See also *Tranquilizers, Antimanic Drugs, and Hypnotics.*

**Action/Kinetics:** Also possesses muscle relaxant and anticonvulsant effects. Acts on the limbic system and the thalamus, as well as inhibits polysynaptic spinal reflexes. **Onset:** 1 hr. **Blood levels, chronic therapy:** 5–20 mcg/mL. **t½:** 6–24 hr. Extensively metabolized in liver and inactive metabolites and some unchanged drug (8%–19%) are excreted in the urine.

**Uses:** Short-term treatment (no more than 4 months) of anxiety.

**Contraindications:** Hypersensitivity to meprobamate or carisoprodol. Porphyria. Children less than 6 years of age.

**Special Concerns:** Use with caution in pregnancy, lactation, epilepsy, liver and kidney disease. Geriatric clients may be more sensitive to the depressant effects of meprobamate; also, due to age-related impaired renal function, the dose of meproba-mate may have to be reduced.

**Side Effects:** *CNS:* Ataxia, drowsi-ness, dizziness, weakness headache, paradoxical excitement, euphoria, slurred speech, vertigo. *GI:* N&V, di-arrhea. *Miscellaneous:* Visual distur-bances, allergic reactions including hematologic and dermatologic symptoms, paresthesias.

**OD** **Overdose Management:** *Symptoms:* Drowsiness, stupor, lethargy, ataxia, *shock, coma, respira-tory collapse, death.* Also, arrhyth-mias, tachycardia or bradycardia, re-duced venous return, *profound hy-potension, CV collapse.* Excessive oronasal secretions, *relaxation of pharyngeal wall leading to obstruction of airway.* *Treatment:* Induction of vomiting or gastric lavage if detected shortly after ingestion. It is imperative that gastric lavage be continued or gastroscopy be performed as incom-plete gastric emptying can cause re-lapse and death.

• Give fluids to treat hypotension. Avoid fluid overload.

• Institute artificial respiration.

• Use care in treating seizures due to combined CNS depressant effects.

• Use forced diuresis and vasopres-sors followed by hemodialysis or he-moperfusion if condition deterio-rates.

**Drug Interactions:** Additive de-pressant effects when used with CNS depressants, MAO inhibitors, and tri-cyclic antidepressants.

**Laboratory Test Interferences:** *With test methods:* ↑ 17-Hydroxycor-ticosteroids, 17-ketogenic steroids, and 17-ketosteroids. *Pharmacologic effects:* ↑ Alkaline phosphatase, bilirubin, serum transaminase, uri-nary estriol (calorimetric tests), por-phobilinogen. ↓ PT in clients on Coumarin.

**Dosage** ————————
• **Tablets**
*Anxiety.*
**Adults, initial:** 400 mg t.i.d.–q.i.d. (or 600 mg b.i.d.). May be increased,

if necessary, up to maximum of 2.4 g/day. **Pediatric, 6–12 years of age:** 100–200 mg b.i.d.–t.i.d. (the 600-mg tablet is not recommended for use in children).

---

## NURSING CONSIDERATIONS

See also *Nursing Considerations* for *Tranquilizers, Antimanic Drugs, and Hypnotics.*
**Administration/Storage:** Do not crush or chew tablets.
**Assessment**
1. Document onset and duration of symptoms; identify any causative factors.
2. Assess mental status and note be-havioral manifestations.
**Outcomes/Evaluate:** ↓ Symptoms of anxiety

---

# Mercaptopurine (6-Mercaptopurine)

(mer-kap-toe-**PYOUR**-een)
**Pregnancy Category:** D
Purinethol (Abbreviation: 6-MP) **(Rx)**
**Classification:** Antineoplastic, antimetabolite (purine analog)

**M**

See also *Antineoplastic Agents.*
**Action/Kinetics:** Cell-cycle specific for the S phase of cell division. Con-verted to thioinosinic acid by the en-zyme hypoxanthine-guanine phos-phoribosyltransferase. Thioinosinic acid then inhibits reactions involving inosinic acid. Also, both thioinosinic acid and 6-methylthioinosinate (also formed from mercaptopurine) inhib-it RNA synthesis. About 50% ab-sorbed from GI tract. **Plasma t½:** 47 min in adults and 21 min in children. Metabolites are excreted in urine with up to 39% excreted unchanged. Cross-resistance with thioguanine has been observed.
**Uses:** Acute lymphocytic or myelo-cytic leukemia. Lymphoblastic leukemia, especially in children. Acute myelogenous and myelo-monocytic leukemia. Effectiveness varies depending on use. The drug is not effective for leukemia of the

---

CNS, solid tumors, lymphomas, or chronic lymphatic leukemia. *Investigational:* Inflammatory bowel disease, chronic myelocytic leukemia, polycythemia vera, non-Hodgkin's lymphoma, psoriatic arthritis.

**Contraindications:** Use in resistance to mercaptopurine or thioguanine. To treat CNS leukemia, chronic lymphatic leukemia, lymphomas (including Hodgkin's disease), solid tumors. Lactation.

**Special Concerns:** Use with caution in clients with impaired renal function. Use during lactation only if benefits clearly outweigh risks. Severe bone marrow depression (anemia, leukopenia, thrombocytopenia) may occur. There is an increased risk of pancreatitis when used for inflammatory bowel disease.

**Additional Side Effects:** Hepatotoxicity, oral lesions, drug fever, hyperuricemia. Produces less GI toxicity than folic acid antagonists, and side effects are less frequent in children than in adults. Pancreatitis (when used for inflammatory bowel disease).

**OD** **Overdose Management:** *Symptoms:* Immediate symptoms include N&V, diarrhea, and anorexia while delayed symptoms include myelosuppression, gastroenteritis, and liver dysfunction. *Treatment:* Induction of emesis if detected soon after ingestion. Supportive measures.

**Drug Interactions**
*Allopurinol* / ↑ Effect of methotrexate due to ↓ breakdown by liver (reduce dose of methotrexate by 25%–33%)
*Trimethoprim–Sulfamethoxazole* / ↑ Risk of bone marrow suppression

**Dosage** ──────────
• **Tablets**
**Highly individualized:** 2.5 mg/kg/day. **Adults, usual:** 100–200 mg; **pediatric:** 50 mg. Dosage may be increased to 5 mg/kg/day after 4 weeks if beneficial effects are not noted. Dosage is increased until symptoms of toxicity appear. **Main-**

**tenance after remission:** 1.5–2.5 mg/kg/day.

## NURSING CONSIDERATIONS

See also *Nursing Considerations* for *Antineoplastic Agents.*
**Administration/Storage**
1. Since the maximum effect of mercaptopurine on the blood count may be delayed and the blood count may drop for several days after drug has been discontinued, discontinue therapy at first sign of abnormally large drop in leukocyte count. Nadir: 14 days.
2. Administer drug in one dose daily at any convenient time.
3. Discourage intake of alcoholic beverages.
**Assessment**
1. Document indications for therapy, onset of symptoms, and other treatments prescribed.
2. Obtain liver and renal function studies, uric acid, and hematologic profile. Drug causes granulocyte and platelet suppression. Nadir: 10–14 days; recovery: 21–28 days.
**Outcomes/Evaluate**
• Improved hematologic levels
• ↓ Malignant cell proliferation
• Symptoms of disease remission

## Meropenem
(**mer**-oh-**PEN**-em)
**Pregnancy Category:** B
Merrem IV **(Rx)**
**Classification:** Antibiotic, miscellaneous

See also *Anti-Infectives.*
**Action/Kinetics:** Broad-spectrum carbapenem antibiotic. Acts by inhibiting cell wall synthesis in gram-positive and gram-negative bacteria. **t½, elimination:** About 1 hr. Both unchanged drug (65% to 83%) and the inactive metabolite (20% to 32%) are excreted through the urine. Adjust dosage in impaired renal function.
**Uses:** Complicated appendicitis and peritonitis caused by *Escherichia coli, Klebsiella pneumoniae, Pseudomonas aeruginosa, Bacteroides fragilis, Bacteroides thetaiotaomi-*

*cron, Peptostreptococcus* species, and viridans group streptococci. Bacterial meningitis caused by *Streptococcus pneumoniae, Haemophilus influenzae* (β-lactamase- and non-β-lactamase-producing strains), and Neisseria meningitidis.

**Contraindications:** Hypersensitivity to meropenem or other drugs in the same class. Those who have had anaphylactic reactions to β-lactams.

**Special Concerns:** Use with caution during lactation. Safety and efficacy have not been determined for children less than 3 months of age.

**Side Effects:** *GI:* Diarrhea, N&V, constipation, abdominal pain, *GI hemorrhage,* pseudomembranous colitis, abdominal pain, melena, oral moniliasis, anorexia, cholestatic jaundice, jaundice, flatulence, ileus. *CNS:* Insomnia, agitation, headache, delirium, confusion, dizziness, nervousness, paresthesia, hallucinations, somnolence, anxiety, depression, *seizures. CV: Heart failure, cardiac arrest, MI, pulmonary embolus,* tachycardia, hypertension, bradycardia, hypotension, syncope. *Dermatologic:* Rash, pruritus, urticaria, sweating. *Body as a whole:* Pain, chest pain, *sepsis, shock, hepatic failure,* fever, abdominal enlargement, back pain. *GU:* Dysuria, kidney failure, presence of urine RBCs. *Respiratory:* Respiratory disorder, dyspnea. *At injection site:* Inflammation, phlebitis, thrombophlebitis, pain, edema. *Miscellaneous:* Anemia, peripheral edema, hypoxia, epistaxis, hemoperitoneum.

In children, the drug may cause diarrhea, rash, and vomiting when used for bacterial infections. Also, when used for meningitis in children, rash (diaper area moniliasis), diarrhea, oral moniliasis, and glossitis have been noted.

**Laboratory Test Alteration:** ↑ Eosinophils, ALT, AST, alkaline phosphatase, LDH, bilirubin, creatinine, BUN. ↓ Hemoglobin, hematocrit, WBCs. ↑ or ↓ platelets. Prolonged or shortened PT, PTT. Positive direct or indirect Coombs' test.

**Dosage** —————————————
• **IV**
  *Bacterial infections, meningitis.*
**Adults:** 1 g IV q 8 hr given over 15–30 min or as an IV bolus injection (5–20 mL) over 3–5 min. In clients with impaired renal function, the dose is reduced as follows: creatinine clearance 26–50 mL/min, 1 g q 12 hr; creatinine clearance 10–25 mL/min, one-half the recommended dose q 12 hr; creatinine clearance less than 10 mL/min, one-half the recommended dose q 24 hr. **Children, 3 months or older:** 20 or 40 mg/kg (depending on the type of infection) q 8 hr, up to a maximum of 2 g q 8 hr. For pediatric clients weighing 50 kg or more, administer 1 g q 8 hr for intra-abdominal infections and 2 g q 8 hr for meningitis given over 15–30 min or as an IV bolus injection (5–20 mL) over 3–5 min.

## NURSING CONSIDERATIONS

See also General *Nursing Considerations for* All *Anti-Infectives.*
**Administration/Storage**
**IV** 1. Do not mix with solutions containing other drugs.
2. Stability varies depending on the solution used to prepare the injection; consult package insert.
3. Store at controlled room temperature of 20°C–25°C (68°F–77°F).
**Assessment**
1. Document onset, duration, and characteristics of symptoms.
2. Note any drug or PCN sensitivity.
3. Monitor CBC, cultures, liver and renal function studies.
4. Determine any CNS disorders (i.e., brain lesions, history of seizures or bacterial meningitis); monitor closely.
5. Reduce dose with renal dysfunction and in the elderly.
**Outcomes/Evaluate:** Resolution of infection

**M**

# Mesalamine (5-aminosalicylic acid)

(mes-**AL**-ah-meen)

**Pregnancy Category:** B

Asacol, Mesasal, Novo-5 ASA ✳,
Pentasa, Quintasa ✳, Rowasa,
Salofalk ✳ **(Rx)**

**Classification:** Anti-inflammatory agent

**Action/Kinetics:** Chemically related to acetylsalicylic acid. Acts locally in the colon to inhibit cyclo-oxygenase and therefore prostaglandin synthesis, resulting in a reduction of inflammation of colitis. Following PR administration, between 10% and 30% is absorbed and is excreted through the urine as the N-acetyl-5-aminosalicylic acid metabolite; the remainder is excreted in the feces. PO tablets are coated with an acrylic-based resin that prevents release of mesalamine until it reaches the terminal ileum and beyond. Approximately 28% of the drug found in tablets is absorbed with the remaining drug available for action in the colon. Capsules are ethylcellulose coated, controlled release designed to release the drug throughout the GI tract; from 20% to 30% is absorbed. **t½, mesalamine:** 0.5–1.5 hr; **t½, N-acetyl mesalamine:** 5–10 hr. **Time to reach maximum plasma levels:** 4–12 hr for both mesalamine and metabolite. Excreted mainly through the kidneys.

**Uses: PO:** Maintaining remission and treatment of mild to moderate active ulcerative colitis. **Rectal:** Treatment of active mild to moderate distal ulcerative colitis, proctosigmoiditis, or proctitis.

**Contraindications:** Hypersensitivity to salicylates.

**Special Concerns:** Use with caution in clients with sulfasalazine sensitivity, in those with impaired renal function, and during lactation. Safety and efficacy have not been established in children. Pyloric stenosis may delay the drug in reaching the colon.

**Side Effects:** *Sulfite sensitivity:* Hives, wheezing, itching, *anaphylax-is. Intolerance syndrome:* Acute abdominal pain, cramping, bloody diarrhea, rash, fever, headache. *GI:* Abdominal pain or discomfort, flatulence, cramps, dyspepsia, nausea, diarrhea, hemorrhoids, rectal pain or burning, rectal urgency, constipation, bloating, worsening of colitis, eructation, pain following insertion of enema, vomiting (after PO use). *CNS:* Headache, dizziness, insomnia, fatigue, malaise, chills, fever, asthenia. *Respiratory:* Cold, sore throat; increased cough, pharyngitis, rhinitis following PO use. *Dermatologic:* Acne, pruritus, itching, rash. *Musculoskeletal:* Back pain, hypertonia, arthralgia, myalgia, leg and joint pain, arthritis. *Miscellaneous:* Flu-like symptoms, hair loss, anorexia, peripheral edema, urinary burning, sweating, pain, chest pain, conjunctivitis, dysmenorrhea, pancreatitis.

In addition to the preceding, PO use may result in the following side effects. *GI:* Anorexia, gastritis, gastroenteritis, cholecystitis, dry mouth, increased appetite, oral ulcers, tenesmus, perforated peptic ulcer, bloody diarrhea, duodenal ulcer, dysphagia, esophageal ulcer, fecal incontinence, GI bleeding, oral moniliasis, rectal bleeding, abnormal stool color and texture. *CNS:* Anxiety, depression, hyperesthesia, nervousness, confusion, peripheral neuropathy, somnolence, emotional lability, vertigo, paresthesia, migraine, tremor, transverse myelitis, Guillain-Barré syndrome. *Dermatologic:* Dry skin, psoriasis, pyoderma gangrenosum, urticaria, erythema nodosum, eczema, photosensitivity, lichen planus, nail disorder. *CV:* Pericarditis, myocarditis, vasodilation, palpitations, *fatal myocarditis,* chest pain, T-wave abnormalities. *GU:* Nephropathy, interstitial nephritis, urinary urgency, dysuria, hematuria, menorrhagia, epididymitis, amenorrhea, hypomenorrhea, metrorrhagia, nephrotic syndrome, urinary frequency, albuminuria, nephrotoxicity. *Hematologic:* **Agranulocytosis,** anemia, eosinophilia, leukopenia, thrombocytopenia, lymphadenopathy, thrombocythemia, ecchymosis. *Respiratory:* Worsening of asthma, sinusitis, interstitial pneumonitis, pulmonary infiltrates, fibrosing alveolitis. *Ophthalmologic:* Eye pain, blurred vision. *Miscellaneous:* Ear pain, tinnitus, taste perversion, neck pain, enlargement of abdomen, facial edema, gout, hypersensitivity pneumonitis, breast pain, Kawasaki-like syndrome.

**OD** **Overdose Management:** *Symptoms:* Salicylate toxicity manifested by tinnitus, vertigo, headache, confusion, drowsiness, sweating, hyperventilation, vomiting, and diarrhea. Severe toxicity results in disruption of electrolyte balance and blood pH, ***hyperthermia, and dehydration.*** *Treatment:* Therapy to treat salicylate toxicity, including emesis, gastric lavage, fluid and electrolyte replacement (if necessary), maintenance of adequate renal function.

**Laboratory Test Interferences:** ↑ AST, ALT, BUN, LDH, alkaline phosphatase, serum creatinine, amylase, lipase, GTTP.

## Dosage
- **Suppository**

One suppository (500 mg) b.i.d.
- **Rectal Suspension Enema**

4 g in 60 mL once daily for 3–6 weeks, usually given at bedtime. For maintenance, the drug can be given every other day or every third day at doses of 1–2 g.
- **Capsules, Extended-Release**

1 g (4 capsules) q.i.d. for a total daily dose of 4 g for up to 8 weeks.
- **Tablets, Enteric-Coated**

800 mg t.i.d. for a total dose of 2.4 g/day for 6 weeks.

## NURSING CONSIDERATIONS
### Administration/Storage
1. Take tablets whole, being careful not to break the outer coating.
2. Shake the bottle well to ensure suspension is homogeneous.
3. Have client lie on the left side with the lower leg extended and the upper right leg flexed forward. The knee-chest position may also be used for rectal administration.
4. Insert the applicator tip and squeeze bottle steadily to allow it to empty.
5. Retain the enema for approximately 8 hr.
6. For maximal effect, retain suppository rectally for 1–3 hr or more.
7. Beneficial effects using the suppository or enema may be seen within 3–21 days, with a full course of therapy lasting up to 6 weeks.

### Assessment
1. Determine any sulfite sensitivity.
2. Document character and frequency of stools. Assess abdomen; note bowel sounds; distension, pain/tenderness.
3. Monitor chemistries, liver and renal function studies, and abdominal films.

### Client/Family Teaching
1. Review technique for enema administration.
- Prior to use, shake bottle until all contents are thoroughly mixed. Remove cap, insert tip into rectum, and squeeze steadily to completely discharge contents.
- Lie on the left side with the lower leg extended and the upper right leg flexed forward. The knee-chest position may also be used for suppository administration.
- Retain the enema for 8 hr to ensure proper absorption of the drug in enema form; may best be accomplished by administering at bedtime, after bowel movement, and retaining throughout the sleep cycle.
- For maximal effect, retain suppository for 1–3 hr or more.
- Protect bed linens with towels or rubber pads.
2. Hold drug and report if severe abdominal pain, cramping, bloody diarrhea, rash, fever, or headache occurs.
3. Avoid smoking and cold foods; these increase bowel motility.
4. The therapy may last 3–6 weeks; follow as prescribed.

---

✦ = Available in Canada      ***bold italic*** = life threatening side effect

**Outcomes/Evaluate**
- Relief of pain and diarrhea
- Normalization of bowel patterns

# Mesna
(**MEZ**-nah)
**Pregnancy Category:** B
Mesnex, Uromitexan ✱ **(Rx)**
**Classification:** Antidote for use with
ifosfamide

**Action/Kinetics:** Ifosfamide is metabolized to products that cause hemorrhagic cystitis. In the kidney,
mesna reacts chemically with these
ifosfamide metabolites to cause their
detoxification. Following IV use,
mesna is rapidly oxidized to mesna
disulfide (dimesna), which is eliminated by the kidneys. **t½ in blood,
mesna:** 0.36 hr; **dimesna:** 1.17 hr. **t½,
terminal:** 7 hr.
**Uses:** Prophylactically to reduce the
incidence of hemorrhagic cystitis
caused by ifosfamide. *Investigational:*
Reduce incidence of hemorrhagic
cystitis caused by cyclophosphamide.
**Contraindications:** Hypersensitivity to thiol compounds. Lactation.
**Special Concerns:** This product
contains benzyl alcohol, which may
cause a fatal "gasping syndrome" in
infants.
**Side Effects:** Since mesna is used
with ifosfamide and other antineoplastic agents, it is difficult to identify those side effects due to mesna.
The following symptoms are believed possible. *GI:* Bad taste in
mouth (100%), soft stools, diarrhea,
limb pain, headache, fatigue, nausea, hypotension, and allergy.
**Laboratory Test Interferences:**
False + test for urinary ketones.

**Dosage**
- **IV Bolus**
  *Prophylaxis of ifosfamide-in-
  duced hemorrhagic cystitis.*
Dosage of mesna equal to 20% of
the ifosfamide dose given at the time
of ifosfamide and at 4 and 8 hr after
each dose of ifosfamide. Thus, the
total daily dose of mesna is 60% of the
ifosfamide dose (e.g., an ifosfamide

dose of 1.2 g/m² would mean doses
of mesna would be 240 mg/m² at
the time the ifosfamide dose was
given, 240 mg/m² after 4 hr, and 240
mg/m² after 8 hr). This dosage
should be given on each day that
ifosfamide is administered.

## NURSING CONSIDERATIONS
**Administration/Storage**
**IV** 1. If the dosage of ifosfamide is
increased or decreased, adjust mesna
dosage accordingly.
2. The drug can be reconstituted to a
final concentration of 20 mg mes-
na/mL fluid by adding 5% dextrose
injection, D5%/0.2% NaCl injection, D5%/0.33% NaCl injection,
D5%/0.45% NaCl, 0.9% NaCl injection, or RL injection.
3. Diluted solutions are stable for 24
hr at 25°C (77°F). However, when
mesna is exposed to oxygen, dimesna is formed; thus, use a new ampule
should be used for each administration.
4. Mesna is not compatible with cisplatin.
**Assessment**
1. Drug must be administered with
each dose of ifosfamide and at 4-
and 8-hr intervals following the initial
dose to be effective against drug-induced hemorrhagic cystitis.
2. Analyze morning urine specimen
each day before ifosfamide therapy.
3. Note age and any sensitivity to
benzyl alcohol.
**Client/Family Teaching**
1. May experience a bad taste in the
mouth during drug therapy; use
hard candy to mask taste.
2. N&V and diarrhea are frequent
side effects of drug therapy; report if
persistent or bothersome.
**Outcomes/Evaluate:** Prevention of
ifosfamide-induced    hemorrhagic
cystitis

# Mesoridazine besylate
(mez-oh-**RID**-ah-zeen)
Serentil **(Rx)**
**Classification:** Antipsychotic, piperidine-type phenothiazine

See also *Antipsychotic Agents, Phenothiazines.*

**Action/Kinetics:** Pronounced sedative and hypotensive effects, moderate anticholinergic effects, and a low incidence of extrapyramidal symptoms and antiemetic effects.

**Uses:** Schizophrenia, acute and chronic alcoholism, behavior problems in clients with mental deficiency and chronic brain syndrome, psychoneurosis.

**Special Concerns:** Use during pregnancy only if benefits clearly outweigh risks. Dosage has not been established in children less than 12 years of age. Geriatric, debilitated, and emaciated clients require a lower initial dose.

**Dosage** ─────────

• **Oral Solution, Tablets**
*Psychotic disorders.*
**Adults and adolescents:** 30–150 mg/day in two to three divided doses.

*Alcoholism.*
**Adults, initial:** 25 mg b.i.d.; **optimum total dose:** 50–200 mg/day.

• **IM**
*Psychotic disorders.*
**Adults and adolescents:** 25 mg (base); **then,** repeat the dose in 30–60 min as needed.

## NURSING CONSIDERATIONS

See also *Nursing Considerations* for *Antipsychotic Agents, Phenothiazines.*

**Administration/Storage**
1. Acidified tap or distilled water, orange juice, or grape juice may be used to dilute the concentrate prior to use.
2. Do not prepare or store bulk dilutions.

**Assessment**
1. Document onset, duration, and characteristics of symptoms; describe behavioral manifestations.
2. List other agents trialed and the outcome.
3. Observe for increased sedation, orthostatic and cholinergic effects.

Keep supine for at least 30 min after parenteral administration to minimize orthostatic effect.

**Outcomes/Evaluate:** Improved patterns of behavior with ↓ agitation, ↓ hyperactivity, and reality orientation

# Metaproterenol sulfate (Orciprenaline sulfate)
(met-ah-proh-**TER**-ih-nohl)
**Pregnancy Category:** C
Alupent, Arm-A-Med Metaproterenol Sulfate, Metaprel **(Rx)**
**Classification:** Adrenergic agent, direct-acting; bronchodilator

See also *Sympathomimetic Drugs.*
**Action/Kinetics:** Markedly stimulates beta-2 receptors, resulting in relaxation of smooth muscles of the bronchial tree, as well as peripheral vasodilation. Minimal effects on beta-1 receptors. Similar to isoproterenol but with a longer duration of action and fewer side effects. **Onset: Inhalation aerosol,** within 1 min; **peak effect:** 1 hr; **duration:** 1–5 hr. **Onset, hand bulb nebulizer or IPPB:** 5–30 min; **duration:** 4–6 hr after repeated doses. **PO: Onset,** 15–30 min; **peak effect:** 1 hr. **Duration:** 4 hr. Marked first-pass effect after PO use. Metabolized in the liver and excreted through the kidney.

**Uses:** Bronchodilator in asthma, bronchitis, emphysema, and other conditions associated with reversible bronchospasms. Treatment of acute asthmatic attacks in children over 6 years of age.

**Special Concerns:** Dosage of syrup or tablets not determined in children less than 6 years of age.

**Additional Side Effects:** *GI:* Diarrhea, bad taste or taste changes. *Respiratory:* Worsening of asthma, nasal congestion, hoarseness. *Miscellaneous:* Hypersensitivity reactions, rash, fatigue, backache, skin reactions.

**Drug Interactions:** Possible potentiation of adrenergic effects if used before or after other sympathomimetic bronchodilators.

## Dosage
- **Syrup, Tablets**
  *Bronchodilation.*

  **Adults and children over 27.2 kg or 9 years:** 20 mg t.i.d.–q.i.d.; **children under 27.2 kg or 6–9 years of age:** 10 mg t.i.d.–q.i.d.; **children less than 6 years of age:** 1.3–2.6 mg/kg/day of the syrup has been studied.

- **Inhalation. Hand Nebulizer**
  *Bronchodilation.*

  Usual dose is 10 inhalations (range: 5–15 inhalations) of undiluted 5% solution.

- **IPPB**
  *Bronchodilation.*

  0.3 mL (range: 0.2–0.3 mL) of 5% solution diluted to 2.5 mL saline or other diluent.

- **MDI**
  *Bronchodilation.*

  2–3 inhalations (1.30–2.25 mg) q 3–4 hr. Total daily dose should not exceed 12 inhalations (9 mg).

## NURSING CONSIDERATIONS

See also *Special Nursing Considerations for Adrenergic Bronchodilators* under *Sympathomimetic Drugs*.

**Administration/Storage**
Refrigerate unit dose vials at 2°C–8°C (35°F–46°F).

**Client/Family Teaching**
1. Review appropriate method for administration. Shake container before each use.
2. Report loss of effectiveness with prescribed dosage and frequency.
3. Store the inhalant solution at room temperature, but avoid excessive heat and light.
4. Do not use the solution if it is brown or shows a precipitate.
5. Do not use inhalant solutions more often than q 4 hr to relieve acute bronchospasms. In chronic bronchospastic disease, the dose can be given t.i.d.–q.i.d. A single dose of the nebulized drug may not completely abort an attack of acute asthma.

6. Stop smoking to preserve lung function.

**Outcomes/Evaluate**
- Improved airway exchange; ↑ oxygen saturation levels
- Relief of respiratory distress

# Metaraminol bitartrate
(met-ah-**RAM**-ih-nohl)
**Pregnancy Category:** C
Aramine **(Rx)**
**Classification:** Adrenergic agent, direct-acting; vasopressor

See also *Sympathomimetic Drugs.*
**Action/Kinetics:** Indirectly releases norepinephrine from storage sites and directly stimulates primarily alpha receptors and, to a slight extent, beta-1 receptors. Causes marked increases in BP due primarily to vasoconstriction and to a slight increase in CO. Reflex bradycardia is also manifested. Increases venous tone, causes pulmonary vasoconstriction, and increases pulmonary pressure, even if CO is decreased. CNS stimulation usually does not occur. **Onset: IV:** 1–2 min; **IM:** 10 min; **SC:** 5–20 min. **Duration, IV:** 20 min; **IM, SC:** About 60 min. Metabolized in the liver and excreted through the urine and feces. Urinary excretion of unchanged drug can be enhanced by acidifying the urine.

**Uses:** Hypotension associated with surgery, spinal anesthesia, hemorrhage, trauma, infections, tumors, and adverse drug reactions. Adjunct to the treatment of either septicemia or cardiogenic shock. *Investigational:* Injected intracavernosally to treat priapism due to phentolamine, papaverine, or other causes.

**Contraindications:** Use with cyclopropane or halothane anesthesia (unless clinical conditions mandate such use). As a substitute for blood or fluid replacement.

**Special Concerns:** Use with caution in cirrhosis, malaria, heart or thyroid disease, hypertension, or diabetes. Hypertension and ischemic ECG changes may occur when used to treat priapism. Use with caution during lactation. Use is not a substitute for the replacement of blood, plasma, fluids, and electrolytes.

**Additional Side Effects:** Rapidly induced hypertension may cause acute pulmonary edema, arrhythmias, and *cardiac arrest.* Due to its long duration of action, cumulative effects are possible with prolonged increases in BP.

**Drug Interactions**

*Digitalis glycosides* / ↑ Risk of ectopic arrhythmias

*Furazolidone* / Possible hypertensive crisis and intracranial hemorrhage

*Guanethidine* / Antihypertensive effects of guanethidine may be partially or totally reversed

*Halogenated hydrocarbons* / Sensitization of the heart to catecholamines; use of metaraminol may cause serious arrhythmias

*MAO Inhibitors* / Possible hypertensive crisis and intracranial hemorrhage

*Oxytocic drugs* / Possiblity of severe, persistent hypertension

*Tricyclic antidepressants* / ↓ Pressor effect of metaraminol

**Dosage** ⎯⎯⎯⎯⎯⎯⎯⎯⎯⎯
• **IM, SC**
    *Prophylaxis of hypotension.*
**Adults:** 2–10 mg given IM or SC; **pediatric:** 0.01 mg/kg (3 mg/m²) IM or SC.
• **IV Infusion**
    *Hypotension.*
**Adults:** 15–100 mg in 250–500 mL of 0.9% Nacl injection or 5% dextrose injection by IV infusion at a rate to maintain desired BP (up to 500 mg/500 mL has been used). **Pediatric:** 0.4 mg/kg (12 mg/m²) by IV infusion in a solution containing 1 mg/25 mL 0.9% Nacl injection or 5% dextrose injection.
• **Direct IV**
    *Severe shock.*
**Adults:** 0.5–5.0 mg by direct IV followed by IV infusion of 15–100 mg in 250–500 mL fluid. **Pediatric:** 0.01 mg/kg (0.3 mg/m²) by direct IV.

• **Endotracheal Tube**
If IV access is not possible, metaraminol may be given by an ET tube. Perform five quick insufflations; forcefully expel 5 mg diluted to 10 mL into the ET tube and follow with five quick insufflations.

## NURSING CONSIDERATIONS

See also *Nursing Considerations* for *Sympathomimetic Drugs.*

**Administration/Storage**

**IV** 1. Administer with an infusion device during IV therapy for accurate drug control and titration.

2. The following solutions may be used to dilute metaraminol: NaCl injection, 5% dextrose injection, Ringer's injection, RL injection, 5% dextran in saline, Normosol-R pH 7.4, and Normosol-M in 5% dextrose injection.

3. Storage at temperatures below –20°C (–4°F) should be avoided.

4. Use infusion solutions within 24 hr.

**Assessment**

1. Document type and onset of symptoms as well as any precipitating factors.

2. Take BP every 15 min. Monitor ECG, I&O, and VS. Ensure adequate hydration.

3. Assess IV site frequently; extravasation may result in tissue necrosis.

**Outcomes/Evaluate:** ↑ BP with hypotensive episode

# Metformin hydrochloride
(met-**FOR**-min)
**Pregnancy Category:** B
Apo-Metformin ✦, Gen-Metformin ✦, Glucophage, Novo-Metformin ✦, Nu-Metformin ✦ **(Rx)**
**Classification:** Oral antidiabetic

**Action/Kinetics:** Decreases hepatic glucose production, decreases intestinal absorption of glucose, and increases peripheral uptake and utilization of glucose. Does not cause hypoglycemia in either diabetic or nondiabetic clients, and it does not cause hyperinsulinemia. Insulin secretion remains unchanged, while

M

⎯⎯⎯⎯⎯⎯⎯⎯⎯⎯⎯⎯⎯⎯⎯⎯⎯⎯⎯⎯⎯⎯⎯⎯

fasting insulin levels and day-long plasma insulin response may decrease. In contrast to sulfonylureas, the body weight of clients treated with metformin remains stable or may decrease somewhat. Food decreases and slightly delays the absorption of metformin. Negligibly bound to plasma protein; steady-state plasma levels (less than 1 mcg/mL) are reached within 24–48 hr. Excreted unchanged in the urine; no biliary excretion. **t½, plasma elimination:** 6.2 hr. The plasma and blood half-lives are prolonged in decreased renal function.

**Uses:** Alone as an adjunct to diet to lower blood glucose in clients having non-insulin-dependent diabetes mellitus whose blood glucose cannot be managed satisfactorily via diet alone. Also, metformin may be used concomitantly with a sulfonylurea when diet and metformin or a sulfonylurea alone do not result in adequate control of blood glucose.

**Contraindications:** Renal disease or dysfunction (serum creatinine levels greater than 1.5 mg/dL in males and greater than 1.4 mg/dL in females) or abnormal creatinine clearance due to cardiovascular collapse, acute MI, or septicemia. In clients undergoing radiologic studies using iodinated contrast media, because use of such products may cause alteration of renal function, leading to acute renal failure and lactic acidosis. Acute or chronic metabolic acidosis, including diabetic ketoacidosis, with or without coma. Lactation.

**Special Concerns:** Cardiovascular collapse, acute CHF, acute MI, and other conditions characterized by hypoxia have been associated with lactic acidosis, which may also be caused by metformin. Use of oral hypoglycemic agents may increase the risk of cardiovascular mortality. Although hypoglycemia does not usually occur with metformin, it may result with deficient caloric intake, with strenuous exercise not supplemented by increased intake of calories, or when metformin is taken with sulfonylureas or alcohol. Because of age-related decreases in renal function, use with caution as age increases. Safety and efficacy have not been determined in children.

**Side Effects:** *Metabolic:* Lactic acidosis (fatal in approximately 50% of cases). *GI:* Diarrhea, N&V, abdominal bloating, flatulence, anorexia, unpleasant or metallic taste. *Hematologic:* Asymptomatic subnormal serum vitamin $B_{12}$ levels.

**OD** **Overdose Management:** *Symptoms:* Lactic acidosis.

**Drug Interactions**

*Alcohol* / Alcohol ↑ the effect of metformin on lactate metabolism

*Cimetidine* / Cimetidine ↑ (by 60%) peak metformin plasma and whole blood levels

*Furosemide* / Furosemide ↑ metformin plasma and blood levels; also, metformin ↓ the half-life of furosemide

*Iodinated contrast media* / ↑ Risk of acute renal failure and lactic acidosis

*Nifedipine* / Nifedipine ↑ the absorption of metformin, leading to ↑ plasma metformin levels

**Dosage** ———————————

• **Tablets**

*Non-insulin-dependent diabetes mellitus.*

**Adults, using 500-mg tablet:** Starting dose is one 500-mg tablet b.i.d. given with the morning and evening meals. Dosage increases may be made in increments of 500 mg every week, given in divided doses, up to a maximum of 2,500 mg/day. If a 2,500-mg daily dose is required, it may be better tolerated when given in divided doses t.i.d. with meals. **Adults, using 850-mg tablet:** Starting dose is 850 mg once daily given with the morning meal. Dosage increases may be made in increments of 850 mg every other week, given in divided doses, up to a maximum of 2,550 mg/day. **Usual maintenance dose:** 850 mg b.i.d. with the morning and evening meals. However, some clients may require 850 mg t.i.d. with meals.

## NURSING CONSIDERATIONS
### Administration/Storage
1. Individualize dosage based on tolerance and effectiveness.
2. Give with meals starting at a low dose with gradual escalation. This will reduce GI side effects and allow determination of the minimal dose necessary for adequate control of blood glucose.
3. No transition period is required when transferring clients from standard oral hypoglycemic drugs (other than chlorpropamide) to metformin. When transferring from chlorpropamide, exercise caution during the first 2 weeks because of chlorpropamide's long duration of action.
4. If the maximum dose of metformin for 4 weeks does not provide adequate control of blood glucose, gradual addition of an oral sulfonylurea (data are available for glyburide, chlorpropamide, tolbutamide, and glipizide) may be considered, while maintaining the maximum dose of metformin. The desired control of blood glucose may be attained by adjusting the dose of each drug.
5. If no response to 1–3 months of concomitant metformin and oral sulfonylurea therapy, consideration should be given to initiating insulin therapy and discontinuing the oral agents.
6. The initial and maintenance doses of metformin in geriatric and debilitated clients should be conservative because of the potential for decreased renal function. Do not titrate these clients to the maximum dose.

### Assessment
1. Document age at diabetes onset, previous therapies utilized, and the outcome.
2. Monitor CBC, BS, electrolytes, HbA1C, urinalysis, liver and renal function studies. Assess for liver or renal failure; may precipitate lactic acidosis (i.e., serum lactate levels greater than 5 mmol/L, decreased blood pH, increased anion gap).
3. Do not administer if procedures utilizing iodinated contrast agents ordered.
4. If anemia develops, exclude vitamin $B_{12}$ deficiency; may interfere with $B_{12}$ absorption.
5. If surgery is scheduled, withhold and do not administer until normal diet resumed.

### Client/Family Teaching
1. Take with food to diminish GI upset.
2. May cause a metallic taste; should subside.
3. Regular exercise, decreased caloric intake, and weight loss are the recommended primary treatment forms to reduce blood glucose levels; medication neither replaces nor excuses compliance with these modalities.
4. Inadequate caloric intake or strenuous exercise without caloric replacement may precipitate hypoglycemia.
5. Do regular blood sugar monitoring (fingersticks) and maintain record for provider review.
6. Avoid alcohol and any situations that may precipitate dehydration.
7. Consume plenty of fluids and report when illnesses with fever, vomiting, and diarrhea are persistent and severe.
8. Stop drug and immediately report any of the following symptoms: difficulty breathing, severe weakness, muscle pain, increased sleepiness, or sudden increased abdominal distress.

### Outcomes/Evaluate
• Control of BS; prevention of microvascular complications
• HbA1C within desired range (usually 6%–8%)

# Methadone hydrochloride
(**METH**-ah-dohn)
**Pregnancy Category:** C
Dolophine, Methadose **(C-II) (Rx)**
**Classification:** Narcotic analgesic, morphine type

---

See also *Narcotic Analgesics*.
**Action/Kinetics:** Produces only mild euphoria, which is the reason it is used as a heroin withdrawal substitute and for maintenance programs. Produces physical dependence; withdrawal symptoms develop more slowly and are less intense but more prolonged than those associated with morphine. Does not produce sedation or narcosis. Not effective for preoperative or obstetric anesthesia. Only one-half as potent PO as when given parenterally. **Onset:** 30–60 min. **Peak effects:** 30–60 min. **Duration:** 4–6 hr. **t½:** 15–30 hr. Both the duration and half-life increase with repeated use due to cumulative effects.
**Uses:** Severe pain. Drug withdrawal and maintenance of narcotic dependence.
**Additional Contraindications:** IV use, liver disease, during pregnancy, in children, or in obstetrics (due to long duration of action and chance of respiratory depression in the neonate).
**Special Concerns:** Use with caution during lactation.
**Additional Side Effects:** Marked constipation, excessive sweating, pulmonary edema, choreic movements.
**Drug Interactions:** Rifampin and phenytoin ↓ plasma methadone levels by ↑ breakdown by liver; thus, possible symptoms of narcotic withdrawal may develop.
**Laboratory Test Interferences:** ↑ Immunoglobulin G.

**Dosage**
• **Tablets, Oral Solution, Oral Concentrate**
    *Analgesia.*
**Adults, individualized:** 2.5–10 mg q 3–4 hr, although higher doses may be necessary for severe pain or due to development of tolerance.
    *Narcotic withdrawal.*
**Initial:** 15–20 mg/day PO (some may require 40 mg/day); **then,** depending on need of the client, slowly decrease dosage.

    *Maintenance following narcotic withdrawal.*
**Adults, individualized, initial:** 20–40 mg PO 4–8 hr after heroin is stopped; **then,** adjust dosage as required up to 120 mg/day.

## NURSING CONSIDERATIONS

See also *Nursing Considerations* for *Narcotic Analgesics*.
**Administration/Storage**
1. Dilute solution in at least 90 mL of water prior to administration.
2. If taking dispersible tablets, dilute in 120 mL of water, orange juice, citrus-flavored drink, or other acidic fruit drink. Allow at least 1 min for complete drug dispersion.
3. For repeated analgesic doses, IM administration is preferred over SC administration; Inspect sites for signs of irritation.
4. Duration of treatment for detoxification purposes is no longer than 21 days. Do not repeat treatment for 4 weeks.
**Client/Family Teaching**
1. If ambulatory and not suffering acute pain, side effects may be more pronounced.
2. Report if N&V develop because a lower dose of drug may relieve these symptoms.
3. To minimize drug's constipating effects, exercise regularly and increase intake of fluids, fruit, and bulk in the diet.
4. For clients on narcotic withdrawal therapy, store drug out of the reach of children.
5. Identify social service groups for assistance in child care, food and living arrangements, and expenses.
**Outcomes/Evaluate**
• Control of severe pain
• Detoxification and maintenance in narcotic-dependent individual

# Methamphetamine hydrochloride
(meth-am-**FET**-ah-meen)
**Pregnancy Category:** C
Desoxyn **(C-II) (Rx)**

**Classification:** Central nervous system stimulant, amphetamine-type

See also *Amphetamines and Derivatives.*

**Action/Kinetics: t½:** 4–5 hr, depending on urinary pH.

**Uses:** Attention-deficit disorders in children over 6 years of age. Obesity (use controversial and often not recommended).

**Contraindications:** Use for obesity. Attention-deficit disorders in children less than 6 years of age.

**Dosage** ─────────────

• **Tablets**

*Attention-deficit disorders in children 6 years and older.*

**Initial:** 5 mg 1–2 times/day; increase in increments of 5 mg/day at weekly intervals until optimum dose is reached (usually 20–25 mg/day).

• **Extended-Release Tablets**

*Attention-deficit disorders in children 6 years and older, maintenance.*

20–25 mg once daily.

*Obesity.*

Either one 5-mg tablet 30 min before each meal or 10–15 mg of the long-acting form in the morning. Duration of treatment should not exceed a few weeks.

## NURSING CONSIDERATIONS

See also *Nursing Considerations* for *Amphetamines and Derivatives.*

**Administration/Storage**

1. When used to facilitate verbalization during psychotherapeutic interview, give second dose only if the first dose has proven effective.

2. When used for attention-deficit disorders, the total daily dose can be given in two divided doses or once a day using the long-acting product. Do not use the long-acting product to initiate therapy. Evaluate client progress periodically to determine the need for continued treatment.

**Assessment**

1. Document indications for therapy, type, onset, and duration of symptoms. List other agents prescribed and the outcome.

2. Assess mental status and note behavioral manifestations.

**Outcomes/Evaluate:** ↑ Attention span and the ability to sit quietly and concentrate

# Methazolamide
(meth-ah-**ZOH**-lah-myd)

**Pregnancy Category:** C
Glauctabs, Neptazane **(Rx)**
**Classification:** Antiglaucoma drug

**Action/Kinetics:** Inhibition of carbonic anhdyrase decreases the secretion of aqueous humor resulting in a decrease in intraocular pressure. Has weak diuretic effects and, due to inhibition of carbonic anhydrase, produces an alkaline urine. Excretion of both urinary citrate and uric acid is decreased. Distributed to the plasma, CSF, aqueous humor of the eye, red blood cells, bile, and extracellular fluid. **Onset:** 2–4 hr. **Peak effect:** 6–8 hr. **Duration:** 10–18 hr. **t½, elimination:** 14 hr. About 25% excreted unchanged in the urine.

**Uses:** Treatment of chronic open-angle glaucoma, secondary glaucoma. Preoperatively in acute angle-closure glaucoma to lower IOP prior to surgery.

**Contraindications:** Use in marked kidney or liver disease or dysfunction, in adrenal gland failure, and in hyperchloremic acidosis. Long-term use in clients with angle-closure glaucoma, since organic closure of the angle may occur even if IOP is lowered. Lactation.

**Special Concerns:** Use with caution in those with pulmonary obstruction or emphysema as acidosis may be aggravated or precipitated. Use with caution in those with cirrhosis or hepatic insufficiency due to the possibility of hepatic coma. The safety and efficacy have not been determined for use in children.

**Side Effects:** *GI:* Taste alteration, N&V, diarrhea, melena. *CNS:* Paresthesias (especially a "tingling" feel-

**M**

ing in the extremities), fatigue, malaise, loss of appetite, drowsiness, confusion, **convulsions.** *Metabolic:* Metabolic acidosis, electrolyte imbalance. *GU:* Polyuria, hematuria, glycosuria. Rarely, crystalluria and renal calculi. *Dermatologic:* Urticaria, photosensitivity. *Miscellaneous:* Hearing dysfunction or tinnitus, transient myopia, hepatic insufficiency, flaccid paralysis.

*NOTE:* Side effects may be observed that are due to the sulfonamide. See *Sulfonamides.*

**Drug Interactions**

*Aspirin (high doses)* / Symptoms of anorexia, tachypnea, lethargy, coma, and death are possible
*Corticosteroids* / ↑ Risk of hypokalemia

**Dosage** ⎯⎯⎯⎯⎯⎯⎯⎯⎯⎯
• **Tablets**
*Glaucoma.*
50–100 mg b.i.d.–t.i.d.

**NURSING CONSIDERATIONS**

**Administration/Storage**

1. May be used with a miotic and osmotic agent.
2. Store at controlled room temperatures of 15°C–30°C (59°F–86°F).

**Assessment**

1. Document indications for therapy; note any sensitivity to sulfonamides.
2. List drugs currently prescribed to ensure none interact unfavorably.
3. Obtain baseline CBC, electrolytes, and LFTs.

**Client/Family Teaching**

1. Take as directed; do not exceed prescribed dosage.
2. Report for followup ocular evaluations and electrolyte determinations.
3. Report any unusual fever, bleeding, rash, or fatigue.

**Outcomes/Evaluate:** ↓ IOP

⎯⎯⎯⎯⎯⎯⎯⎯⎯⎯⎯⎯⎯⎯⎯⎯⎯⎯

# Methenamine hippurate

(meh-**THEEN**-ah-meen)
**Pregnancy Category:** C
Hip-Rex ✿, Hiprex, Urex **(Rx)**

# Methenamine mandelate

(meh-**THEEN**-ah-meen)
**Pregnancy Category:** C
Mandelamine ✿ **(Rx)**
**Classification:** Urinary tract anti-infective

⎯⎯⎯⎯⎯⎯⎯⎯⎯⎯⎯⎯⎯⎯⎯⎯⎯⎯

**Action/Kinetics:** Converted in an acid medium into ammonia and formaldehyde (the active principle), which denatures protein. Formaldehyde levels in the urine may be bacteriostatic or bactericidal, depending on the pH; it is most effective when the urine has a pH value of 5.5 or less, which is maintained by using the hippurate or mandelate salt. Readily absorbed from GI tract, but up to 60% may be hydrolyzed by gastric acid if tablets are not enteric-coated. To be effective, urinary formaldehyde concentration must be greater than 25 mcg/mL. **Peak levels of formaldehyde:** 2 hr if using hippurate and 3–8 hr if using mandelate (if urinary pH is 5.5 or less) **t½:** 3–6 hr. Seventy to 90% of drug and metabolites excreted in urine within 24 hr.

**Uses:** Acute, chronic, and recurrent UTIs by susceptible organisms, especially gram-negative organisms including *Escherichia coli.* As a prophylactic before urinary tract instrumentation. Never used as sole agent in the treatment of acute infections.

**Contraindications:** Renal insufficiency, severe liver damage, severe dehydration. Concurrent use of sulfonamides as an insoluble precipitate may form with formaldehyde.

**Special Concerns:** Use with caution in gout (methenamine may cause urate crystals to precipitate in the urine).

**Side Effects:** *GI:* N&V, diarrhea, anorexia, cramps, stomatitis. *GU:* Hematuria, albuminuria, crystalluria, dysuria, urinary frequency or urgency, bladder irritation. *Dermatologic:* Skin rashes, urticaria, pruritus, erythematous eruptions. *Other:* Headache, dyspnea, edema, lipoid pneumonitis.

**OD** **Overdose Management:** *Treatment:* Absorption following overdose may be minimized by inducing vomiting or by gastric lavage, followed by activated charcoal. Fluids should be forced.

**Drug Interactions**

*Acetazolamide* / ↓ Effect of methenamine due to inhibition of conversion to formaldehyde

*Sodium bicarbonate* / ↓ Effect of methenamine due to inhibition of conversion to formaldehyde

*Sulfonamides* / ↑ Chance of sulfonamide crystalluria due to acid urine produced by methenamine

*Thiazide diuretics* / ↓ Effect of methenamine due to ↑ alkalinity of urine produced by thiazides

**Laboratory Test Interferences:** False + urinary glucose with Benedict's solution. Drug interferes with determination of urinary catecholamines and estriol levels by acid hydrolysis technique (enzymatic techniques not affected). False + catecholamines, hydroxycorticosteroids, vanillylmandelic acid; false – 5-hydroxyindoleacetic acid.

**Dosage**
• **Tablets**
*Hippurate:* **Adults and children over 12 years:** 1 g b.i.d. in the morning and evening; **children, 6–12 years:** 0.5 g b.i.d.
• **Oral Suspension, Enteric-Coated Tablets**
*Mandelate:* **Adults:** 1 g q.i.d. after meals and at bedtime; **children 6–12 years:** 0.5 g q.i.d.; **children under 6 years:** 0.25 g/13.6 kg q.i.d.

**NURSING CONSIDERATIONS**

See also *General Nursing Considerations for All Anti-Infectives.*
**Assessment**
1. Document indications for therapy, onset and duration of symptoms.
2. Note any history of gout.
3. List other agents prescribed. Urine may become turbid and full of sediment when administered with sulfamethizole.
4. Obtain baseline C&S. Monitor urine for evidence of hematuria and/or albuminuria.

5. Maintain acidic urine when treating *Proteus* or *Pseudomonas* infections.
6. Oral methenamine mandelate suspensions have a vegetable oil base; particular care should thus be taken in the elderly or debilitated to prevent lipid pneumonia.

**Client/Family Teaching**
1. May take with food if GI upset occurs.
2. Maintain fluid intake of 1.5–2 L/day.
3. To maintain an acidic urine, alkalizing foods (e.g., milk products) or medication (e.g., acetazolamide, bicarbonate) should be avoided.
4. Foods (such as prunes, plums, and cranberry juice) may help maintain acid urine. Drugs such as ascorbic acid, methionine, ammonium chloride, or sodium diphosphate may additionally be required.
5. Use Labstix or Nitrazine paper to test that pH of urine is 5.5 or lower if ordered.
6. With high dosage, report any evidence of bladder irritation or painful and frequent micturition.
7. Report adverse drug effects such as N&V, skin rash, tinnitus, and muscle cramps as these may require termination of drug therapy.

**Outcomes/Evaluate**
• Resolution of UTI
• Negative urine C&S results

# Methicillin sodium
(meth-ih-**SILL**-in)
**Pregnancy Category:** B
Staphcillin **(Rx)**
**Classification:** Antibiotic, penicillin

See also *Anti-Infectives* and *Penicillins.*
**Action/Kinetics:** Semisynthetic, penicillinase-resistant salt suitable for soft tissue, penicillin G-resistant, and resistant staphylococcal infections. **Peak plasma levels: IM,** 10–20 mcg/mL after 30–60 min; **IV,** 15 min. t½: 30 min. Excreted chiefly in the urine.
**Additional Use:** Infections by penicillinase-producing staphylococci,

osteomyelitis, septicemia, enterocolitis, bacterial endocarditis.

**Special Concerns:** Use with caution in clients with renal failure. Safe use in neonates has not been established. Periodic renal function tests are indicated for long-term therapy.

## Dosage

- **IM, Continuous IV Infusion**
  *General infections.*
**Adults:** 4–12 g/day, depending on the infection, in divided doses q 4–6 hr. (*NOTE:* If C$_{CR}$ is less than 10 mL/min, the dose should not exceed 2 g q 12 hr.) **Pediatric:** 100–300 mg/kg/day in divided doses q 4–6 hr. **Infants over 7 days of age and weighing more than 2 kg:** 100 mg/kg/day in divided doses q 6 hr. **Infants more than 7 days of age and weighing less than 2 kg or less than 7 days of age and weighing more than 2 kg:** 75 mg/kg/day in divided doses q 8 hr. **Infants under 7 days of age and weighing less than 2 kg:** 50 mg/kg/day in divided doses q 12 hr.
  *Meningitis.*
**Infants over 7 days of age and weighing more than 2 kg:** 150–200 mg/kg/day. **Infants more than 7 days of age and weighing less than 2 kg or less than 7 days and weighing more than 2 kg:** 150 mg/kg/day. **Infants under 7 days of age and weighing less than 2 kg:** 100 mg/kg/day.

## NURSING CONSIDERATIONS

See also *General Nursing Considerations for All Anti-Infectives* and for *Penicillins.*

### Administration/Storage

1. Inject medication slowly; injections are particularly painful.
2. Inject deeply into gluteal muscle. Use caution to avoid sciatic nerve injury.
3. To prevent sterile abscesses at injection site, include 0.2–0.3 mL of air in syringe so irritating solution will not leak into tissue.
4. Sensitive to heat when dissolved. Therefore, solutions for IM administration must be used within 24 hr if

standing at room temperature or within 4 days if refrigerated. Solutions for IV use must be used within 8 hr.

**IV** 5. Do not use dextrose solutions for diluting methicillin; low acidity may destroy the antibiotic.
6. If used IV, thrombophlebitis can occur, especially in geriatric clients. Check for redness or edema at site of injection and for pain along the course of the vein; methicillin is a vesicant.
7. For IV administration, dilute 1 mL (500 mg) with 20–25 mL of sterile water for injection or NaCl injection USP and administer at a rate of 10 mL/min. May further dilute and administer IVPB over 30 min.
8. Do not mix methicillin with any other drug in the same syringe or IV solution.

### Assessment

1. Document indications for therapy, type and onset of symptoms.
2. Obtain blood cultures and CBC prior to start of therapy and weekly during therapy. Many strains of methicillin-resistant staphylococci have been identified.
3. Monitor CBC, electrolytes, liver and renal function studies.

### Client/Family Teaching

1. Drug contains sodium; calculate accordingly with strict sodium restrictions.
2. Report fever, nausea, and other signs of hepatotoxicity.
3. With any evidence of pallor, ecchymosis, hematuria, or bleeding tendencies, report as drug enhances anticoagulants.

### Outcomes/Evaluate

- Negative C&S reports
- Eradication of infection: ↓ fever, ↓ WBC, and ↓ symptoms

# Methimazole (Thiamazole)

(meth-**IM**-ah-zohl)
**Pregnancy Category:** D
Tapazole **(Rx)**
**Classification:** Antithyroid drug

See also *Antithyroid Drugs.*

**Action/Kinetics:** Onset is more rapid but effect is less consistent than that of propylthiouracil. Bioavailability may be affected by food. **t½:** 4–14 hr. **Onset:** 10–20 days. **Time to peak effect:** 2–10 weeks. **t½:** 6–13 hr. Crosses the placenta; high levels appear in breast milk. Metabolized in the liver and excreted through the kidneys (7% unchanged).

**Special Concerns:** Incidence of hepatic toxicity may be greater than for propylthiouracil.

**Dosage**
• **Tablets**
*Mild hyperthyroidism.*
**Adults, initial:** 15 mg/day.
*Moderately severe hyperthyroidism.*
**Adults, initial:** 30–40 mg/day.
*Severe hyperthyroidism.*
**Adults, initial:** 60 mg/day. For hyperthyroidism, the daily dose is usually given in three equal doses 8 hr apart. **Maintenance:** 5–15 mg/day as a single dose or divided into two doses. **Pediatric:** 0.4 mg/kg given once daily or divided into two doses; **maintenance:** 0.2 mg/kg. Alternatively, **initial:** 0.5–0.7 mg/kg/day (15–20 mg/m²/day in three divided doses); **maintenance:** ⅓–⅔ initial dose when client is euthyroid up to a maximum of 30 mg/day.
*Thyrotoxic crisis.*
**Adults,** 15–20 mg/4 hr during the first day as an adjunct to other treatments.

## NURSING CONSIDERATIONS

See also *Nursing Considerations* for *Antithyroid Drugs.*
**Assessment**
1. Document indications for therapy and type and onset of symptoms.
2. Monitor CBC, thyroid function, height, weight, and VS.
3. Assess for changes in extremity sensation; some clients may develop paresthesias.
**Client/Family Teaching**
1. May take with a snack to reduce

gastric irritation. Report if GI upset persists.
2. Take as prescribed at evenly spaced intervals and with evenly spaced doses throughout the day.
3. Report any unexpected symptoms immediately. The effects may not be evident for weeks; dosage may require adjustment.
4. Report any sore throats, fever, chills, and unexplained bleeding (S&S of agranulocytosis).
5. Report hair loss.
6. Drug is usually administered until client becomes euthyroid or for a year; then if more treatment is necessary, radiopharmaceuticals may be considered.
**Outcomes/Evaluate**
• Promotion of normal metabolism
• Serum thyroid function levels within desired range; ↓ T₄

# Methocarbamol
(meth-oh-**KAR**-bah-mohl)
Robaxin, Robaxin Injectable ✦, Robaxin-750 **(Rx)**
**Classification:** Centrally acting muscle relaxant

See also *Skeletal Muscle Relaxants, Centrally Acting.*
**Action/Kinetics:** Beneficial effect may be related to the sedative properties of the drug. Has no direct effect on the contractile mechanism of striated muscle, the motor endplate, or the nerve fiber and it does not directly relax tense skeletal muscles. Of limited usefulness. May be given IM or IV in polyethylene glycol 300 (50% solution). PO therapy should be initiated as soon as possible. **Onset:** 30 min. **Peak plasma levels:** 2 hr after 2 g. **t½:** 1–2 hr. Inactive metabolites are excreted in the urine.
**Uses:** Adjunct for the relief of acute, painful musculoskeletal conditions (e.g., sprains, strains). Adjunct in tetanus.
**Contraindications:** Hypersensitivity, when muscle spasticity is required to maintain upright position, seizure disorders, pregnancy, lacta-

tion, children under 12 years. Renal disease (parenteral dosage form only since it contains polyethylene glycol 300).

**Special Concerns:** Use with caution in epilepsy and during lactation. The injectable form should be used with caution in suspected or known epileptics.

**Side Effects:** *Following PO use.* *CNS:* Dizziness, drowsiness, lightheadedness, vertigo, lassitude, headache. *GI:* Nausea. *Miscellaneous:* Allergic symptoms including rash, urticaria, pruritus, conjunctivitis, nasal congestion, blurred vision, fever. *Following IV use (in addition to the preceding).* *CV:* Hypotension, bradycardia, syncope. *CNS:* Fainting, mild muscle incoordination. *Miscellaneous:* Metallic taste, GI upset, flushing, nystagmus, double vision, thrombophlebitis, sloughing or pain at injection site, *anaphylaxis.*

**OD** **Overdose Management:** *Symptoms:* CNS depression, including coma, is often seen when methocarbamol is used with alcohol or other CNS depressants. *Treatment:* Supportive, depending on the symptoms.

**Drug Interactions:** Central nervous system depressants (including alcohol) may ↑ the effect of methocarbamol.

**Laboratory Test Interferences:** Color interference in 5-HIAA and VMA.

**Dosage** ———————
• **Tablets**
  *Skeletal muscle disorders.*
**Adults, initial:** 1.5 g q.i.d. for the first 2–3 days (for severe conditions, 8 g/day may be given); **maintenance:** 1 g q.i.d., 0.75 g q 4 hr, or 1.5 g t.i.d.
• **IM, IV**
  *Skeletal muscle disorders.*
**Adults, usual initial:** 1 g; in severe cases, up to 2–3 g may be necessary. **IV administration should not exceed 3 days.**
  *Tetanus.*
**Adults:** 1–2 g IV, initially, into tube of previously inserted indwelling needle. An additional 1–2 g may be

added to the infusion for a total initial dose of 3 g. May be given q 6 hr (up to 24 g/day may be needed) until **PO** administration is feasible. **Pediatric, initial:** 15 mg/kg given into tube of previously inserted indwelling needle. Dose may be repeated q 6 hr.

## NURSING CONSIDERATIONS

See also *Nursing Considerations* for *Skeletal Muscle Relaxants.*

**Administration/Storage**
1. If drug is to be administered IM, inject no more than 5 mL into each gluteal region.
2. When administering IM to an adult, select a large muscle mass. When administering IM to a child, use the vastus lateralis. Document and rotate sites.
**IV** 3. If administered IV, do not exceed a rate of 3 mL/min.
4. For IV drip, one ampule may be added to no more than 250 mL of NaCl or 5% dextrose injection.
5. With IV, check frequently for infiltration. Extravasation of fluid may cause sloughing or thrombophlebitis.
6. Before removing IV, clamp off the tubing to prevent extravasation of the hypertonic solution, which may cause thrombophlebitis.

**Interventions**
1. Position in a recumbent position during IV administration; maintain this position for 10–15 min after injection to minimize the side effects of postural hypotension. Monitor VS.
2. Keep side rails up and supervise ambulation of elderly clients or those who have been immobilized prior to drug therapy.
3. Observe seizure precautions.

**Client/Family Teaching**
1. Drug causes drowsiness; do not operate dangerous machinery and equipment or drive a car.
2. Rise slowly from a recumbent position and dangle legs before standing up to minimize hypotensive effects.
3. Diplopia, blurred vision, and nystagmus may occur; should disappear

with continued use but report if persistent.

4. Report any urticaria, skin eruptions, rash, or pruritus; allergic responses and may necessitate drug withdrawal.

5. Nausea, anorexia, and a metallic taste may occur; report if severe or interfere with nutrition.

6. Avoid alcohol and any other CNS depressants.

7. Urine may turn black, brown, or green; will disappear once drug discontinued.

**Outcomes/Evaluate**
• Improvement in muscle spasticity, pain, and mobility
• Control of tetanus-induced neuromuscular manifestations

# Methotrexate, Methotrexate sodium

(meth-oh-**TREKS**-ayt)
**Pregnancy Category:** D (X for pregnant psoriatic or rheumatoid arthritis clients)
Amethopterin, Folex PFS, Rheumatrex Dose Pack (Abbreviation: MTX)
**(Rx)**
**Classification:** Antineoplastic, antimetabolite (folic acid analog)

See also *Antineoplastic Agents*.
**Action/Kinetics:** Cell-cycle specific for the S phase of cell division. Acts by inhibiting dihydrofolate reductase, which prevents reduction of dihydrofolate to tetrahydrofolate; this results in decreased synthesis of purines and consequently DNA. The most sensitive cells are bone marrow, fetal cells, dermal epithelium, urinary bladder, buccal mucosa, intestinal mucosa, and malignant cells. When used for rheumatoid arthritis it may affect immune function. Variable absorption from GI tract. **Peak serum levels, IM:** 30–60 min; **PO:** 1–2 hr. **t½:** initial, 1 hr; intermediate, 2–3 hr; final, 8–12 hr. May accumulate in the body. Excreted by kidney (55%–92% in 24 hr). Renal function tests are recommended before initiation of therapy; perform daily leukocyte counts during therapy.

**Uses:** Uterine choriocarcinoma (curative), chorioadenoma destruens, hydatidiform mole, acute lymphocytic and lymphoblastic leukemia, lymphosarcoma, and other disseminated neoplasms in children; meningeal leukemia, some beneficial effect in regional chemotherapy of head and neck tumors, breast tumors, and lung cancer. In combination for advanced stage non-Hodgkin's lymphoma. Advanced mycosis fungoides. High doses followed by leucovorin rescue in combination with other drugs for prolonging relapse-free survival in nonmetastatic osteosarcoma in individuals who have had surgical resection or amputation for the primary tumor. Severe, recalcitrant, disabling psoriasis. Rheumatoid arthritis (severe, active, classical, or definite) in clients who have had inadequate response to NSAIDs and at least one or more antirheumatic drugs (disease modifying). *Investigational:* Severe corticosteroid-dependent asthma to reduce corticosteroid dosage; adjunct to treat osteosarcoma. Psoriatic arthritis and Reiter's disease.

**Contraindications:** Psoriasis clients with kidney or liver disease; blood dyscrasias as hypoplasia, thrombocytopenia, anemia, or leukopenia. Alcoholism, alcoholic liver disease, or other chronic liver disease. Immunodeficiency syndromes. Pregnancy and lactation.

**Special Concerns:** Use with caution in impaired renal function and elderly clients. Use with extreme caution in the presence of active infection and in debilitated clients. Safety and efficacy have not been established for juvenile rheumatoid arthritis.

**Additional Side Effects:** *Severe bone marrow depression.* Hepatotoxicity, fibrosis, cirrhosis. *Hemorrhagic enteritis, intestinal ulceration or perforation,* acne, ecchymosis, hematemesis, melena, increased pigmentation, diabetes, leukoen-

*bold italic* = life threatening side effect

M

cephalopathy, chronic interstitial obstructive pulmonary disease, acute renal failure. Intrathecal use may result in chemical arachnoiditis, transient paresis, or **seizures.** Concomitant exposure to sunlight may aggravate psoriasis.

**OD** **Overdose Management:** *Symptoms:* See Antineoplastic Agents, Chapter 2. *Treatment:* Leucovorin, given as soon as possible, may decrease toxic effects. The dose used is 10 mg/m² PO or parenterally followed by 10 mg/m² PO q 6 hr for 72 hr. Charcoal hemoperfusion will reduce serum levels. In massive overdosage, hydration and urinary alkalinization are needed to prevent precipitation of methotrexate and metabolites in the renal tubules.

**Drug Interactions**

*Alcohol, ethyl* / Additive hepatotoxicity; combination can result in coma
*Aminoglycosides, oral* / ↓ Absorption of PO methotrexate
*Anticoagulants, oral* / Additive hypoprothrombinemia
*Chloramphenicol* / ↑ Effect of methotrexate by ↓ plasma protein binding
*Etretinate* / Possible hepatotoxicity if used together for psoriasis
*Folic acid–containing vitamin preparations* / ↓ Response to methotrexate
*Ibuprofen* / ↑ Effect of methotrexate by ↓ renal secretion
*NSAIDs* / Possible fatal interaction
*PABA* / ↑ Effect of methotrexate by ↓ plasma protein binding
*Phenylbutazone* / ↑ Effect of methotrexate by ↓ renal secretion
*Phenytoin* / ↑ Effect of methotrexate by ↓ plasma protein binding
*Probenecid* / ↑ Effect of methotrexate by ↓ renal clearance
*Procarbazine* / Possible ↑ nephrotoxicity
*Pyrimethamine* / ↑ Methotrexate toxicity
*Salicylates (aspirin)* / ↑ Effect of methotrexate by ↓ plasma protein binding; also, salicylates ↓ renal excretion of methotrexate

*Smallpox vaccination* / Methotrexate impairs immunologic response to smallpox vaccine
*Sulfonamides* / ↑ Effect of methotrexate by ↓ plasma protein binding
*Tetracyclines* / ↑ Effect of methotrexate by ↓ plasma protein binding
*Thiopurines* / ↑ Plasma levels of thiopurines

**Dosage**

• **Tablets (Methotrexate). IM, IV, IA, Intrathecal (Methotrexate Sodium)**
*Choriocarcinoma and similar trophoblastic diseases.*
**Dose individualized. PO, IM:** 15–30 mg/day for 5 days. May be repeated 3–5 times with 1-week rest period between courses.
*Acute lymphatic (lymphoblastic) leukemia.*
**Initial:** 3.3 mg/m² (with 60 mg/m² prednisone daily); **maintenance: PO, IM,** 30 mg/m² 2 times/week or **IV,** 2.5 mg/kg q 14 days.
*Meningeal leukemia.*
**Intrathecal:** 12 mg/m² q 2–5 days until cell count returns to normal.
*Lymphomas.*
**PO:** 10–25 mg/day for 4–8 days for several courses of treatment with 7- to 10-day rest periods between courses.
*Mycosis fungoides.*
**PO:** 2.5–10 mg/day for several weeks or months; **alternatively, IM:** 50 mg once weekly or 25 mg twice weekly.
*Lymphosarcoma.*
0.625–2.5 mg/kg/day in combination with other drugs.
*Osteosarcoma.*
Used in combination with other drugs, including doxorubicin, cisplatin, bleomycin, cyclophosphamide, and dactinomycin. **Usual IV starting dose for methotrexate:** 12 g/m²; dose may be increased to 15 g/m² to achieve a peak serum level of 10⁻³ mol/L at the end of the methotrexate infusion.
*Psoriasis.*
**Adults, usual: PO, IM, IV,** 10–25 mg/week, continued until beneficial

response observed. Weekly dose should not exceed 50 mg. **Alternate regimens: PO,** 2.5 mg q 12 hr for three doses or q 8 hr for four doses each week (not to exceed 30 mg/week); **or PO,** 2.5 mg daily for 5 days followed by 2 days of rest (dose should not exceed 6.25 mg/day). Once beneficial effects are noted, reduce dose to lowest possible level with longest rest periods between doses.

*Rheumatoid arthritis.*
**Initial:** Single PO doses of 7.5 mg/week or divided PO doses of 2.5 mg at 12-hr intervals for three doses given once a week; **then,** adjust dosage to achieve optimum response, not to exceed a total weekly dose of 20 mg. Once response has been reached, the dose should be reduced to the lowest possible effective dose.

## NURSING CONSIDERATIONS

See also *Nursing Considerations* for *Antineoplastic Agents.*
**Administration/Storage**
1. Use only sterile, preservative-free NaCl injection to reconstitute powder for intrathecal administration.
2. Prevent inhalation of medication particles and skin exposure.
3. When used for rheumatoid arthritis, improvement is thought to be maintained for up to 2 years with continuous therapy. When discontinued, the arthritis usually worsens within 3–6 weeks.
**IV** 4. Six hours prior to initiation of a methotrexate infusion, hydrate with 1 L/m$^2$ of IV fluid. Continue hydration at 125 mL/m$^2$/hr during the methotrexate infusion and for 2 days after the infusion has been completed.
5. Alkalinize the urine (see *Sodium Bicarbonate*) to a pH above 7 during methotrexate infusion.
6. Follow guidelines provided for leucovorin rescue schedule following high doses of methotrexate.
**Assessment**
1. Determine if receiving other or-

ganic acids, such as aspirin, phenylbutazone, probenecid, and/or sulfa drugs; these affect renal clearance of methotrexate and increase thrombocytopenia and GI side effects. Note any acute infections.
2. List drugs client currently prescribed to ensure none interact unfavorably with methotrexate.
3. Monitor CBC, uric acid, liver and renal function studies; report oliguria. Drug causes granulocyte and platelet suppression. Nadir: 10 days; recovery: 14 days.
4. Have calcium leucovorin—a potent antidote for folic acid antagonists—readily available in case of overdosage. Antidotes are ineffective if not administered within 4 hr of overdosage. Corticosteroids are sometimes given concomitantly with initial dose of methotrexate.
**Client/Family Teaching**
1. Take tablets at bedtime with an antacid to minimize GI upset.
2. Avoid salicylates and alcohol as liver toxicity and bleeding may result.
3. Report oral ulcerations, one of the first signs of toxicity.
4. Avoid vaccinations (especially for smallpox) because the impaired immunologic response may result in vaccinia.
5. Consume 2–3 L/day of fluids to prevent renal damage and facilitate drug excretion.
6. Test urine pH and report if less than 6.5; bicarbonate tablets may be prescribed to assist in alkalizing the urine.
7. Allopurinol may be prescribed to reduce uric acid levels.
8. Avoid sun exposure and use sunscreens, sunglasses, and appropriate clothing when necessary.
**Outcomes/Evaluate**
• Suppression of malignant cell proliferation with ↓ tumor size and spread
• Improvement in skin lesions with severe psoriasis
• ↓ Joint swelling/pain; ↑ mobility

**M**

---

# Methsuximide
(meth-**SUCKS**-ih-myd)
Celontin **(Rx)**
**Classification:** Anticonvulsant, succinimide type

See also *Anticonvulsants* and *Succinimides.*
**Action/Kinetics: Peak levels:** 1–4
hr. **t½:** 1–3 hr for methsuximide and
36–45 hr for the active metabolite.
**Therapeutic serum levels:** 10–40
mcg/mL.
**Uses:** Methsuximide is used for absence seizures refractory to other
drugs. May be given with other anticonvulsants when absence seizures
coexist with other types of epilepsy.
**Additional Side Effects:** Most common are ataxia, dizziness, and
drowsiness.
**Additional Drug Interactions:**
Methsuximide may ↑ the effect of
primidone.

**Dosage** ─────────────
• **Capsules**
*Absence seizures.*
**Adults and children, initial:** 300
mg/day for first week; **then,** if necessary, increase dosage by 300 mg/
day at weekly intervals until control
established. **Maximum daily dose:**
1.2 g in divided doses.

## NURSING CONSIDERATIONS

See also *Nursing Considerations* for
*Anticonvulsants* and *Succinimides.*
**Administration/Storage:** The 150-
mg dosage form can be used for
children.
**Assessment**
1. Document type and frequency of
seizures, noting characteristics, other
drugs prescribed, and the outcome.
2. Determine baseline level of consciousness and balance, as drug may
impair.
**Outcomes/Evaluate**
• Control of seizures
• Therapeutic drug levels (10–40
mcg/mL)

# Methyldopa
(meth-ill-**DOH**-pah)
**Pregnancy Category:** B (PO)
Aldomet, Apo-Methyldopa ✣,
Dopamet ✣, Medimet ✣,
Novo–Medopa ✣, Nu-Medopa ✣
**(Rx)**

# Methyldopate hydrochloride
(meth-ill-**DOH**-payt)
**Pregnancy Category:** B (PO), C (IV)
Aldomet Hydrochloride **(Rx)**
**Classification:** Antihypertensive, cen-
trally acting antiadrenergic

See also *Antihypertensive Agents.*
**Action/Kinetics:** The active
metabolite, alpha-methylnorepineph-
rine, lowers BP by stimulating central
inhibitory alpha-adrenergic receptors, false neurotransmission, and/or
reduction of plasma renin. Little
change in CO. **PO: Onset:** 7–12 hr.
**Duration:** 12–24 hr. All effects terminated within 48 hr. Absorption is
variable. **IV: Onset:** 4–6 hr. **Duration:** 10–16 hr. Seventy percent of
drug excreted in urine. **Full therapeutic effect:** 1–4 days. **t½:** 1.7 hr.
Metabolites excreted in the urine.
**Uses:** Moderate to severe hypertension. Particularly useful for clients
with impaired renal function, renal
hypertension, resistant cases of hypertension complicated by stroke,
CAD, or nitrogen retention, and for
hypertensive crisis (parenterally).
**Contraindications:** Sensitivity to
drug (including sulfites), labile and
mild hypertension, pregnancy, active hepatic disease, use with MAO inhibitors, or pheochromocytoma.
**Special Concerns:** Use with caution in clients with a history of liver or
kidney disease. A decrease in dose in
geriatric clients may prevent syncope.
**Side Effects:** *CNS:* Sedation (transient), weakness, headache, asthenia, dizziness, paresthesias, Parkinson-like symptoms, psychic disturbances, symptoms of CV impairment, choreoathetotic movements,
Bell's palsy, decreased mental acuity, verbal memory impairment. *CV:*
Bradycardia, orthostatic hypotension, hypersensitivity of carotid si-

# Methyldopa
(meth-ill-**DOH**-pah)

nus, worsening of angina, paradoxical hypertensive response (after IV), myocarditis, CHF, pericarditis, vasculitis. *GI:* N&V, abdominal distention, diarrhea or constipation, flatus, colitis, dry mouth, sore or "black tongue," pancreatitis, sialoadenitis. *Hematologic:* **Hemolytic anemia,** leukopenia, granulocytopenia, thrombocytopenia, **bone marrow depression.** *Endocrine:* Gynecomastia, amenorrhea, galactorrhea, lactation, hyperprolactinemia. *GU:* Impotence, failure to ejaculate, decreased libido. *Dermatologic:* Rash, **toxic epidermal necrolysis.** *Hepatic:* Jaundice, hepatitis, liver disorders, abnormal liver function tests. *Miscellaneous:* Edema, fever, lupus-like symptoms, nasal stuffiness, arthralgia, myalgia, **septic shock-like syndrome.**

**OD  Overdose  Management:**
*Symptoms:* CNS, GI, and CV effects including sedation, weakness, lightheadedness, dizziness, coma, bradycardia, acute hypotension, impairment of AV conduction, constipation, diarrhea, distention, flatus, N&V. *Treatment:* Induction of vomiting or gastric lavage if detected early. General supportive treatment with special attention to HR, CO, blood volume, urinary function, electrolyte imbalance, paralytic ileus, and CNS activity. In severe cases, hemodialysis is effective.

**Drug Interactions**
*Anesthetics, general* / Additive hypotension
*Antidepressants, tricyclic* / Tricyclic antidepressants may block hypotensive effect of methyldopa
*Haloperidol* / Methyldopa ↑ toxic effects of haloperidol
*Levodopa* / ↑ Effect of both drugs
*Lithium* / ↑ Possibility of lithium toxicity
*MAO inhibitors* / Metabolites of methyldopa, usually metabolized by MAO inhibitors, may → excessive sympathetic stimulation
*Methotrimeprazine* / Additive hypotensive effect

*Phenothiazines* / ↑ Risk of serious ↑ BP
*Propranolol* / Paradoxical hypertension
*Sympathomimetics* / Potentiation of hypertensive effect of sympathomimetics
*Thiazide diuretics* / Additive hypotensive effect
*Thioxanthenes* / Additive hypotensive effect
*Tolbutamide* / ↑ Hypoglycemia due to ↓ breakdown by liver
*Tricyclic antidepressants* / ↓ Effect of methyldopa
*Vasodilator drugs* / Additive hypotensive effect
*Verapamil* / ↑ Effect of methyldopa
**Laboratory Test Interferences:**
False + or ↑ : Alkaline phosphatase, bilirubin, BUN, BSP, cephalin flocculation, creatinine, AST, ALT, uric acid, Coombs' test, PT. Positive lupus erythematosus cell preparation and antinuclear antibodies.

**Dosage**
• **Methyldopa. Oral Suspension, Tablets**
   *Hypertension.*
**Initial:** 250 mg b.i.d.–t.i.d. for 2 days. Adjust dose q 2 days. If increased, start with evening dose. **Usual maintenance:** 0.5–3.0 g/day in two to four divided doses; **maximum:** 3 g/day. Transfer to and from other antihypertensive agents should occur gradually, with initial dose of methyldopa not exceeding 500 mg. *NOTE:* Do not use combination medication to initiate therapy. **Pediatric, initial:** 10 mg/kg/day in two to four divided doses, adjusting maintenance to a maximum of 65 mg/kg/day (or 3 g/day, whichever is less).
• **Methyldopate HCl. IV Infusion**
   *Hypertension.*
**Adults:** 250–500 mg q 6 hr; **maximum:** 1 g q 6 hr for hypertensive crisis.
   Switch to PO methyldopa, at same dosage level, when BP is brought under control. **Pediatric:** 20–40 mg/kg/day in divided doses q 6 hr;

**M**

**maximum:** 65 mg/kg/day (or 3 g/day, whichever is less).

## NURSING CONSIDERATIONS

See also *Nursing Considerations* for *Antihypertensive Agents.*

### Administration/Storage

1. Tolerance may occur following 2–3 months of therapy. Increasing the dose or adding a diuretic often restores effect on BP.

**IV** 2. If administered IV, mix with 100 mL of 5% dextrose or administer in D5W at a concentration of 10 mg/mL. Infuse over 30–60 min.

### Assessment

1. Document indications for therapy, onset of symptoms, other agents prescribed and the outcome.
2. Monitor CBC, LFTs, and Coombs' test. If blood transfusion required, ascertain that both direct and indirect Coombs' tests are done; if positive, consult with hematologist.
3. Assess for drug tolerance; may occur during the second or third month of therapy.
4. Note any jaundice; drug is contraindicated with active hepatic disease.

### Client/Family Teaching

1. To prevent dizziness and fainting, rise from bed slowly to a sitting position and dangle legs over the edge of the bed.
2. Sedation may occur when therapy is first started, but should disappear once the maintenance dose is established.
3. In rare cases, methyldopa may darken urine or turn it blue; this is not harmful.
4. Withhold drug and report any of the following symptoms: tiredness, fever, or yellowing of skin and sclera.
5. Continue to follow prescribed diet and exercise program in the overall goal of BP control.
6. Do not take any other medications or remedies unless appoved.
7. Always carry a card detailing current medication regimen.

**Outcomes/Evaluate:** ↓ BP

---COMBINATION DRUG---

# Methyldopa and Hydrochlorothiazide

(meth-ill-**DOH**-pah, hy-droh-klor-oh-**THIGH**-ah-zyd)

**Pregnancy Category:** C

Aldoril 15, Aldoril 25, Aldoril D30, Aldoril D50, Apo-Methazide ✹, Novo-Doparil ✹, PMS-Dopazide ✹ **(Rx)**

**Classification:** Antihypertensive

See also *Methyldopa* and *Hydrochlorothiazide.*

**Content:** *Antihypertensive:* Methyldopa, 250–500 mg. *Diuretic/antihypertensive:* Hydrochlorothiazide, 15–50 mg.

**Uses:** Hypertension (not for initial treatment).

**Contraindications:** Active hepatic disease.

**Special Concerns:** Use in pregnancy only if benefits outweigh risks.

### Dosage

- **Tablets**

**Adults:** 1 tablet b.i.d.–t.i.d. for first 48 hr; **then,** increase or decrease dose, depending on response, in intervals of not less than 2 days. Maximum daily dosage: methyldopa, 3.0 g; hydrochlorothiazide, 100–200 mg.

## NURSING CONSIDERATIONS

See also *Nursing Considerations* for *Antihypertensive Agents* and individual agents.

### Administration/Storage

1. If Aldoril is given together with antihypertensives other than thiazides, the initial dose of methyldopa should not be more than 500 mg/day in divided doses.
2. Additional methyldopa may be given separately if Aldoril alone does not control BP adequately.
3. If tolerance is observed after 2–3 months of therapy, the dose of either methyldopa and/or hydrochlorothiazide may be increased to restore control.

**Outcomes/Evaluate:** Control of hypertension

# Methylergonovine maleate

(meth-ill-er-**GON**-oh-veen)
**Pregnancy Category:** C
Methergine **(Rx)**
**Classification:** Oxytocic agent

**Action/Kinetics:** Synthetic drug related to ergonovine, a natural alkaloid obtained from ergot. Methylergonovine stimulates the rate, tone, and amplitude of uterine contractions. The uterus becomes more sensitive to the drug toward the end of pregnancy. **Onset** (uterine contractions): **PO,** 5–10 min; **IM,** 2–5 min; **IV,** immediate. **t½, IV:** 2–3 min (initial) and 20–30 min (final). **Duration, PO, IM:** 3 hr; **IV:** 45 min.

**Uses:** Management and prevention of postpartum and postabortal hemorrhage by producing firm uterine contractions and decreasing uterine bleeding. During the second stage of labor following delivery of the anterior shoulder, but only under full obstetric supervision. *Investigational:* Ergonovine has been used to diagnose Prinzmetal's angina (variant angina).

**Contraindications:** Pregnancy, toxemia, hypertension. Ergot hypersensitivity. To induce labor or threatened spontaneous abortions. Administration before delivery of the placenta.

**Special Concerns:** Use with caution in sepsis, obliterative vascular disease, impaired renal or hepatic function. Use with caution during lactation.

**Side Effects:** *CV:* Hypertension that may be associated with seizure or headache; hypotension, thrombophlebitis, palpitation. *GI:* N&V, diarrhea, foul taste. *CNS:* Dizziness, headache, tinnitus, hallucinations. *Miscellaneous:* Sweating, chest pain, dyspnea, hematuria, water intoxication, leg cramps, nasal congestion.

*NOTE: Use of methylergonovine during labor may result in uterine tetany with rupture, cervical and perineal lacerations, embolism of amniot-*ic fluid as well as hypoxia and intracranial hemorrhage in the infant.

**OD** **Overdose Management:** *Symptoms:* Initially, N&V, abdominal pain, increase in BP, tingling of extremities, numbness. Symptoms of severe overdose include hypotension, hypothermia, ***respiratory depression, seizures, coma.*** *Treatment:* Induce vomiting or perform gastric lavage. Administer a cathartic; institute diuresis. Maintain respiration, especially if seizures or coma occur. Treat seizures with anticonvulsant drugs. Warm extremities to control peripheral vasospasm.

**Drug Interactions:** Hypertension may occur if methylergonovine is used with vasoconstrictors.

## Dosage
- **IM, IV (Emergencies Only)**
0.2 mg q 2–4 hr following delivery of placenta, of the anterior shoulder, or during the puerperium.
- **Tablets**
0.2 mg t.i.d.–q.i.d. until danger of hemorrhage and uterine atony is over (usually within 2 days, but no more than 1 week).

## NURSING CONSIDERATIONS
### Administration/Storage
**IV** 1. Administer slowly over 1 min; check VS for evidence of shock or hypertension after IV administration. Have emergency drugs available.
2. Discard ampules that are discolored.
### Assessment
1. Document indications for therapy, onset and duration of symptoms.
2. Assess for S&S of ergotism (cold and numb fingers and toes, N&V, headache, muscle pain, chest pain, weakness).
3. Document fundal tone and nonphasic contractures; massage to check for relaxation or severe cramping.
4. Obtain baseline calcium and correct if low to improve drug effectiveness; monitor prolactin levels and

assess for decreased milk production.

**Client/Family Teaching**
1. Take only as directed; do not exceed dosage.
2. Avoid smoking; nicotine constricts blood vessels.
3. Report any S&S of ergotism (cold and numb fingers and toes, N&V, headache, muscle pain, chest pain, weakness).
4. Abdominal cramps may be experienced; report any severe cramping or increased bleeding.

**Outcomes/Evaluate:** Improved uterine tone; control of postpartum hemorrhage

# Methylphenidate hydrochloride

(meth-ill-**FEN**-ih-dayt)
**Pregnancy Category:** C
PMS-Methylphenidate ✱, Ritalin, Ritalin-SR **(C-II) (Rx)**
**Classification:** Central nervous system stimulant

**Action/Kinetics:** May act by blocking the reuptake mechanism of dopaminergic neurons. In children with attention-deficit disorders, methylphenidate causes decreases in motor restlessness with an increased attention span. In narcolepsy the drug acts on the cerebral cortex and subcortical structures (e.g., thalamus) to increase motor activity and mental alertness and decrease fatigue. **Peak blood levels, children:** 1.9 hr for tablets and 4.7 hr for extended-release tablets. **Duration:** 4–6 hr. **t½:** 1–3 hr. Metabolized by the liver and excreted by the kidney.

**Uses:** Attention-deficit disorders in children as part of overall treatment regimen. Narcolepsy. *Investigational:* Depression in elderly, cancer, and poststroke clients. Anesthesia-related hiccups.

**Contraindications:** Marked anxiety, tension and agitation, glaucoma. Severe depression, to prevent normal fatigue, diagnosis of Tourette's syndrome, motor tics. In children who manifest symptoms of primary

psychiatric disorders (psychoses) or acute stress.

**Special Concerns:** Use with caution during lactation. Safety and efficacy in children less than 6 years of age have not been established. Use with great caution in clients with history of hypertension or convulsive disease.

**Side Effects:** *CNS:* Nervousness, insomnia, headaches, dizziness, drowsiness, chorea, depressed mood (transient). Toxic psychoses, dyskinesia, Tourette's syndrome. Psychologic dependence. *CV:* Palpitations, tachycardia, angina, arrhythmias, hyper- or hypotension, cerebral arteritis or occlusion. *GI:* Nausea, anorexia, abdominal pain, weight loss (chronic use). *Allergic:* Skin rashes, fever, urticaria, arthralgia, exfoliative dermatitis, erythema multiforme with necrotizing vasculitis, erythema. *Hematologic:* Thrombocytopenic purpura, leukopenia, anemia. *Miscellaneous:* Hair loss, abnormal liver function.

In children, the following side effects are more common: anorexia, abdominal pain, weight loss (chronic use), tachycardia, insomnia.

**OD** **Overdose Management:** *Symptoms:* Characterized by CV symptoms (hypertension, cardiac arrhythmias, tachycardia), mental disturbances, agitation, headaches, vomiting, hyperreflexia, **hyperpyrexia, convulsions, and coma.** *Treatment:* Symptomatic. Excess CNS stimulation may be treated by keeping the client in quiet, dim surroundings to reduce external stimuli. Protect the client from self-injury. A short-acting barbiturate may be used. Emesis or gastric lavage should be undertaken if the client is conscious. Adequate circulatory and respiratory function must be maintained. Hyperpyrexia may be treated by cooling the client (e.g., cool bath, hypothermia blanket).

**Drug Interactions**
*Anticoagulants, oral* / ↑ Effect of anticoagulants due to ↓ breakdown by liver

*Anticonvulsants (phenobarbital, phenytoin, primidone)* / ↑ Effect of anticonvulsants due to ↓ breakdown by liver
*Guanethidine* / ↓ Effect of guanethidine by displacement from its site of action
*MAO inhibitors* / Possibility of hypertensive crisis, hyperthermia, convulsions, coma
*Tricyclic antidepressants* / ↑ Effect of antidepressants due to ↓ breakdown by liver

**Laboratory Test Interferences:** ↑ Urinary excretion of epinephrine.

**Dosage** ───────────

• **Tablets**
  *Narcolepsy.*
**Adults:** 5–20 mg b.i.d.–t.i.d. preferably 30–45 min before meals.
  *Attention-deficit disorders.*
**Pediatric, 6 years and older, initial:** 5 mg b.i.d. before breakfast and lunch; **then,** increase by 5–10 mg/week to a maximum of 60 mg/day.

• **Extended-Release Tablets**
  *Narcolepsy.*
**Adults:** 20 mg 1–3 times/day q 8 hr, preferably on an empty stomach.
  *Attention-deficit disorders.*
**Pediatric, 6 years and older:** 20 mg 1–3 times/day.

## NURSING CONSIDERATIONS

See also *Nursing Considerations* for *Pemoline.*

**Administration/Storage**
1. If receiving for attention-deficit disorders and no improvement is noticed in 1 month, or if stimulation occurs, discontinue the medication.
2. Discontinue periodically to assess client condition as drug therapy is not indefinite; discontinue at time of puberty.
3. Sustained-release tablets are effective for 8 hr and may be substituted for regular-release tablets if the 8-hr dosage of the sustained-release tablets is the same as the titrated 8-hr dosage of regular tablets.

**Assessment**
1. Document indications for therapy, type and onset of symptoms.

Note other drugs prescribed that may interact unfavorably.
2. Ensure psychologic evaluations show no evidence of psychotic disorder or severe stress.
3. Obtain baseline CBC, CNS evaluation, and ECG.

**Client/Family Teaching**
1. Take before breakfast and lunch to avoid interference with sleep.
2. Use caution when driving or operating hazardous machinery as drug may mask fatigue and/or cause physical incoordination, dizziness, or drowsiness.
3. Record weight 2 times/week and report any significant loss as weight loss may occur.
4. Report any overt changes in client mood or attention span.
5. Skin rashes, fever, or pain in the joints should be reported immediately.
6. Therapy may be interrupted every few months ("drug holiday") to determine if the drug is still necessary in those who do respond to therapy.
7. Avoid caffeine in any form.

**Outcomes/Evaluate**
• ↑ Ability to sit quietly/concentrate
• ↓ Daytime sleeping

# Methylprednisolone
(meth-ill-pred-**NISS**-oh-lohn)
**Pregnancy Category:** C
**Tablets:** Medrol, Meprolone **(Rx)**

# Methylprednisolone acetate
(meth-ill-pred-**NISS**-oh-lohn)
**Pregnancy Category:** C
**Cream:** Medrol Veriderm Cream ✿.
**Enema:** Medrol Enpak **(Rx). Parenteral:** depMedalone-40 and -80, Deposject 40 and 80, Depo-Medrol, D-Med 80, Duralone-40 and -80, Medralone-40 and -80, M-Prednisol-40 and -80 **(Rx)**

# Methylprednisolone sodium succinate
(meth-ill-pred-**NISS**-oh-lohn)

**M**

**Pregnancy Category:** C
**Parenteral:** A-methaPred, Solu-
Medrol **(Rx)**
**Classification:** Glucocorticoid

See also *Corticosteroids*.
**Action/Kinetics:** Low incidence of
increased appetite, peptic ulcer, psychic stimulation, and sodium and
water retention. May mask negative
nitrogen balance. **Onset:** Slow, 12–
24 hr. **t½, plasma:** 78–188 min. **Duration:** Long, up to 1 week. Rapid onset of sodium succinate by both IV
and IM routes. Long duration of action
of the acetate.
**Additional Use:** Severe hepatitis
due to alcoholism. Within 8 hr of severe spinal cord injury (to improve
neurologic function). Septic shock
(controversial).
**Special Concerns:** Use during
pregnancy only if benefits outweigh
risks.
**Additional Drug Interactions**
*Erythromycin* / ↑ Effect of methylprednisolone due to ↓ breakdown
by liver
*Troleandomycin* / ↑ Effect of
methylprednisolone due to ↓ breakdown by liver
**Laboratory Test Interferences:** ↓
Immunoglobulins A, G, M.

**Dosage** ————————————
METHYLPREDNISOLONE
• **Tablets**
*Rheumatoid arthritis.*
**Adults:** 6–16 mg/day. Decrease
gradually when condition is under
control. **Pediatric:** 6–10 mg/day.
*SLE.*
**Adults, acute:** 20–96 mg/day;
**maintenance:** 8–20 mg/day.
*Acute rheumatic fever.*
1 mg/kg body weight daily. Drug is al-
ways given in four equally divided
doses after meals and at bedtime.
METHYLPREDNISOLONE ACETATE
• **IM**
*Adrenogenital syndrome.*
40 mg q 2 weeks.
*Rheumatoid arthritis.*
40–120 mg/week.
*Dermatologic lesions, dermatitis.*

40–120 mg/week for 1–4 weeks; for
severe cases, a single dose of 80–120
mg should provide relief.
*Seborrheic dermatitis.*
80 mg/week.
*Asthma, rhinitis.*
80–120 mg.
• **Intra-articular, Soft Tissue and
Intralesional Injection**
4–80 mg, depending on site.
• **Retention Enema**
40 mg 3–7 times/week for 2 or more
weeks.
METHYLPREDNISOLONE SODIUM SUCCI-
NATE
• **IM, IV**
*Most conditions.*
**Adults, initial:** 10–40 mg, depending
on the disease; **then,** adjust dose
depending on response, with subsequent doses given either **IM, IV.**
*Severe conditions.*
**Adults:** 30 mg/kg infused IV over
10–20 min; may be repeated q 4–6 hr
for 2–3 days only. **Pediatric:** not
less than 0.5 mg/kg/day.

## NURSING CONSIDERATIONS

See also *Nursing Considerations* for
*Corticosteroids*.
**Administration/Storage**
1. Dosage must be highly individualized.
2. Methylprednisolone acetate is not
for IV use.
3. Use sodium succinate solutions
within 48 hr after preparation.
4. For alternate day therapy using
methylprednisolone, twice the usual
PO dose is given every other morning
(client receives beneficial effect
while minimizing side effects).
**Assessment**
1. Document indications for treatment and describe clinical presentation.
2. Monitor CBC, HbA1C, glucose,
and electrolytes.
**Outcomes/Evaluate**
• Relief of allergic manifestations
• ↓ Pain/inflammation; ↑ mobility
• ↓ Nerve fiber destruction in spinal
cord injury (SCI)

# Methysergide maleate

(meth-ih-**SIR**-jyd)
**Pregnancy Category:** X
Sansert **(Rx)**
**Classification:** Prophylactic for vascular headaches

**Action/Kinetics:** Semisynthetic ergot alkaloid derivative. May act by directly stimulating smooth muscle leading to vasoconstriction. Blocks the effects of serotonin, a powerful vasodilator believed to play a role in vascular headaches; it also inhibits the release of histamine from mast cells and prevents the release of serotonin from platelets. Has weak emetic and oxytocic activity. **Onset:** 1–2 days. **Peak plasma levels:** 60 ng/mL. **Duration:** 1–2 days. Excreted through the urine as unchanged drugs and metabolites.

**Uses:** Prophylaxis or reduction of the intensity and frequency of vascular headache (in clients having one or more per week or in cases where headaches are so severe preventive therapy is indicated).

**Contraindications:** Severe renal or hepatic disease, severe hypertension, CAD, peripheral vascular disease, tendency toward thromboembolic disease, cachexia (profound ill health or malnutrition), severe arteriosclerosis, pulmonary disease, phlebitis or cellulitis of lower limbs, collagen diseases or fibrotic processs, debilitated states, valvular heart disease, infectious disease, or peptic ulcer. Pregnancy, lactation, use in children.

**Special Concerns:** Geriatric clients may be more affected by peripheral vasoconstriction leading to the possibility of hypothermia.

**Side Effects:** The drug is associated with a high incidence of side effects. *Fibrosis:* ***Retroperitoneal fibrosis, cardiac fibrosis, pleuropulmonary fibrosis,*** Peyronie's-like disease. The fibrotic condition may result in vascular insufficiency in the lower legs. *CV:* Vasoconstriction of arteries leading to paresthesia, chest pain, abdominal pain, or extremities that are cold, numb, or painful. Tachycardia, postural hypotension. *CNS:* Dizziness, ataxia, drowsiness, vertigo, insomnia, euphoria, lightheadedness, and psychic reactions such as depersonalization, depression, and hallucinations. *GI:* N&V, diarrhea, heartburn, abdominal pain, increased gastric acid, constipation. *Hematologic:* Eosinophilia, neutropenia. *Other:* Peripheral edema, flushing of face, skin rashes, transient alopecia, myalgia, arthralgia, weakness, weight gain, telangiectasia.

**Drug Interactions:** Narcotic analgesics are inhibited by methysergide.

**Dosage**
• **Tablets**
**Adults:** Administer 4–8 mg/day in divided doses. Continuous administration should not exceed 6 months. May be readministered after a 3- to 4-week rest period.

## NURSING CONSIDERATIONS
### Administration/Storage
1. Administer with meals or milk to minimize GI irritation R/T increased hydrochloric acid production.
2. Discontinue gradually to avoid migraine headache rebound.
3. If drug is not effective after 3 weeks, it is not likely to be beneficial and should be discontinued.
### Assessment
1. Note frequency and severity of headaches and efforts made in the past to control or prevent them.
2. Obtain CBC, liver and renal function studies; assess for dysfunction.
3. Determine behavior prior to therapy. Review diet (tyramine foods, additives, preservatives, colorings), activity, substance use (including caffeine and nicotine), OTC medications, and stress levels; may have precipitated event.
### Client/Family Teaching
1. Take with meals or milk to minimize GI upset.
2. Report symptoms of nervousness,

**M**

---

weakness, insomnia, rashes, alopecia, or peripheral edema.

3. Report any unusual weight gain; check extremities for edema. If weight gain excessive, adjust caloric intake. Maintain a low-salt diet and see dietitian for assistance.

4. Keep a diary noting any events, foods, or activities that may relate to the onset of headaches.

5. Administration should not be continued on a regular basis for longer than 6 months without a 3- to 4-week rest.

6. General malaise, fatigue, weight loss, low-grade fever, or urinary tract problems may be symptoms of fibrosis (cardiac or pleuropulmonary); report any of these symptoms immediately.

7. Do not drive a car or engage in other hazardous tasks until drug effects are realized; may cause drowsiness.

8. If dizziness or lightheadedness occurs upon arising, rise slowly from a supine position and dangle the legs for a few minutes before standing erect. If feeling faint, lie down with the legs elevated.

9. Avoid alcohol, caffeine, nicotine, and cannabis, as these may precipitate vascular headaches.

10. Psychologic changes may occur, especially hallucinations; report if evident.

11. Must be discontinued gradually, as rebound headaches may occur.

**Outcomes/Evaluate:** ↓ Frequency and occurrence of severe vascular headaches

# Metipranolol hydrochloride

(met-ih-**PRAN**-oh-lohl)
**Pregnancy Category:** C
OptiPranolol **(Rx)**
**Classification:** Beta-adrenergic blocking agent

See also *Beta-Adrenergic Blocking Agents.*

**Action/Kinetics:** Blocks both beta-1- and beta-2-adrenergic receptors. Reduction in intraocular pressure may be related to a decrease in production of aqueous humor and a slight increase in the outflow of aqueous humor. A decrease from 20% to 26% in intraocular pressure may be seen if the intraocular pressure is greater than 24 mm Hg at baseline. May be absorbed and exert systemic effects. When used topically, has no local anesthetic effect and exerts no action on pupil size or accommodation. **Onset:** 30 min. **Maximum effect:** 1–2 hr. **Duration:** 12–24 hr.

**Uses:** To reduce IOP in clients with ocular hypertension and chronic open-angle glaucoma.

**Special Concerns:** Use with caution during lactation. Safety and effectiveness have not been determined in children.

**Side Effects:** *Ophthalmologic:* Local discomfort, dermatitis of the eyelid, blepharitis, conjunctivitis, browache, tearing, blurred vision, abnormal vision, photophobia, edema. Due to absorption, the following systemic side effects have been reported. *CV:* Hypertension, MI, atrial fibrillation, angina, bradycardia, palpitation. *CNS:* Headache, dizziness, anxiety, depression, somnolence, nervousness. *Respiratory:* Dyspnea, rhinitis, bronchitis, coughing. *Miscellaneous:* Allergic reaction, asthenia, nausea, epistaxis, arthritis, myalgia, rash.

**Dosage**
• **Ophthalmic Solution (0.3%)**
**Adults:** 1 gtt in the affected eye(s) b.i.d. Increasing the dose or more frequent administration does not increase the beneficial effect.

## NURSING CONSIDERATIONS

See also *Nursing Considerations* for *Beta-Adrenergic Blocking Agents.*
**Administration/Storage**
1. May be used concomitantly with other drugs to lower intraocular pressure.
2. Due to diurnal variation in response, measure intraocular pressure at different times during the day.

**Assessment**
1. Note ocular condition and record pretreatment pressures.
2. Document baseline ECG and VS.
**Client/Family Teaching**
1. Transient burning or stinging is common during administration; report if severe.
2. Take only as directed; report any persistent bothersome side effects or symptoms of intolerance.
3. Report for F/U visits to assess for systemic effects, measure intraocular pressures, and determine drug effectiveness.
**Outcomes/Evaluate:** ↓ IOP

# Metoclopramide
(meh-toe-kloh-**PRAH**-myd)
**Pregnancy Category:** B
Apo-Metoclop ✿, Maxeran ✿, Maxolon, Nu-Metoclopramide ✿, Octamide PFS, Reglan **(Rx)**
**Classification:** Gastrointestinal stimulant

**Action/Kinetics:** Dopamine antagonist that acts by increasing sensitivity to acetylcholine; this results in increased motility of the upper GI tract and relaxation of the pyloric sphincter and duodenal bulb. Gastric emptying time and GI transit time are shortened. No effect on gastric, biliary, or pancreatic secretions. Facilitates intubation of the small bowel and speeds transit of a barium meal. Produces sedation, induces release of prolactin, increases circulating aldosterone levels (is transient), and is an antiemetic. **Onset, IV:** 1–3 min; **IM,** 10–15 min; **PO,** 30–60 min. **Duration:** 1–2 hr. **t½:** 5–6 hr. Significant first-pass effect following PO use; unchanged drug and metabolites excreted in urine. Renal impairment decreases clearance of the drug.
**Uses: PO:** Acute and recurrent diabetic gastroparesis, gastroesophageal reflux. **Parenteral:** Facilitate small bowel intubation, stimulate gastric emptying, and increase intestinal transit of barium to aid in radiologic examination of stomach and small intestine. Prophylaxis of N&V in cancer chemotherapy and following surgery (when nasogastric suction is not desired). *Investigational:* To improve lactation. N&V due to various causes, including vomiting during pregnancy and labor, gastric ulcer, anorexia nervosa. Improve client response to ergotamine, analgesics, and sedatives when used to treat migraine (may increase absorption). Postoperative gastric bezoars. Atonic bladder. Esophageal variceal bleeding.
**Contraindications:** Gastrointestinal hemorrhage, obstruction, or perforation; epilepsy; clients taking drugs likely to cause extrapyramidal symptoms, such as phenothiazines. Pheochromocytoma.
**Special Concerns:** Use with caution during lactation and in hypertension. Extrapyramidal effects are more likely to occur in children and geriatric clients.
**Side Effects:** *CNS:* Restlessness, drowsiness, fatigue, lassitude, akathisia, anxiety, insomnia, confusion. Headaches, dizziness, extrapyramidal symptoms (especially acute dystonic reactions), Parkinson-like symptoms (including cogwheel rigidity, mask-like facies, bradykinesia, tremor), dystonia, myoclonus, *de-pression (with suicidal ideation),* tardive dyskinesia (including involuntary movements of the tongue, face, mouth, or jaw), seizures, hallucinations. *GI:* Nausea, bowel disturbances (usually diarrhea). *CV:* Hypertension (transient), hypotension, SVT, bradycardia. *Hematologic:* ***Agranulocytosis,*** leukopenia, neutropenia. Methemoglobinemia in premature and full-term infants at doses of 1–4 mg/kg/day IM, IV, or PO for 1–3 or more days. *Endocrine:* Galactorrhea, amenorrhea, gynecomastia, impotence (due to hyperprolactinemia), fluid retention (due to transient elevation of aldosterone). ***Neuroleptic malignant syndrome: Hyperthermia, altered consciousness, au-***

M

*tonomic dysfunction, muscle rigidity, death.* Miscellaneous: Incontinence, urinary frequency, porphyria, visual disturbances, flushing of the face and upper body, hepatotoxicity.

**OD  Overdose Management:** Symptoms: Agitation, irritability, hypertonia of muscles, drowsiness, disorientation, extrapyramidal symptoms. Treatment: Treat extrapyramidal effects by giving anticholinergic drugs, anti-Parkinson drugs, or antihistamines with anticholinergic effects. General supportive treatment. Reverse methemoglobinemia by giving methylene blue.

**Drug Interactions**
*Acetaminophen* / ↑ GI absorption of acetaminophen
*Anticholinergics* / ↓ Effect of metoclopramide
*Cimetidine* / ↓ Effect of cimetidine due to ↓ absorption from GI tract
*CNS depressants* / Additive sedative effects
*Cyclosporine* / ↓ Absorption of cyclosporine → ↑ immunosuppressive and toxic effects
*Digoxin* / ↓ Effect of digoxin due to ↓ absorption from GI tract
*Ethanol* / ↑ GI absorption of ethanol
*Levodopa* / ↑ GI absorption of levodopa and levodopa ↓ effects of metoclopramide on gastric emptying and lower esophageal pressure
*MAO inhibitors* / ↑ Release of catecholamines → toxicity
*Narcotic analgesics* / ↓ Effect of metoclopramide
*Succinylcholine* / ↑ Effect of succinylcholine due to inhibition of plasma cholinesterase
*Tetracyclines* / ↑ GI absorption of tetracyclines

**Dosage**
• **Tablets, Syrup, Concentrate**
*Diabetic gastroparesis.*
**Adults:** 10 mg 30 min before meals and at bedtime for 2–8 weeks (therapy should be reinstituted if symptoms recur).
*Gastroesophageal reflux.*
**Adults:** 10–15 mg q.i.d. 30 min before meals and at bedtime. If symptoms

occur only intermittently, single doses up to 20 mg prior to the provoking situation may be used.
*To enhance lactation.*
**Adults:** 30–45 mg/day.
• **IM, IV**
*Prophylaxis of vomiting due to chemotherapy.*
**Initial:** 1–2 mg/kg IV q 2 hr for two doses, with the first dose 30 min before chemotherapy; **then,** 10 mg or more q 3 hr for three doses. Inject slowly IV over 15 min.
*Prophylaxis of postoperative N&V.*
**Adults:** 10–20 mg IM near the end of surgery.
*Facilitate small bowel intubation.*
**Adults:** 10 mg given over 1–2 min; **pediatric, 6–14 years:** 2.5–5 mg; **pediatric, less than 6 years:** 0.1 mg/kg.
*Radiologic examinations to increase intestinal transit time.*
**Adults:** 10 mg as a single dose given IV over 1–2 min.

**NURSING CONSIDERATIONS**
**Administration/Storage**
1. After PO use, absorption of certain drugs from the GI tract may be affected (see *Drug Interactions*).
**IV** 2. Inject slowly IV over 1–2 min to prevent transient feelings of anxiety and restlessness.
3. Metoclopramide is physically and/or chemically incompatible with a number of drugs; check package insert if drug is to be admixed.
4. For IV use, dilute doses greater than 10 mg in 50 mL of D5W, D5%/0.45% NaCl, RL injection, Ringer's injection, or NaCl injection; infuse over 15 min.
**Assessment**
1. Document indications for therapy, type and onset of symptoms. List drugs prescribed, ensuring none interact unfavorably.
2. Assess abdomen for bowel sounds and distention; note any N&V.
**Client/Family Teaching**
1. Do not operate a car or hazardous machinery until drug effects realized; drug has a sedative effect.
2. Report any persistent side effects so

they can be properly evaluated and counteracted.

3. Avoid alcohol and any other CNS depressants.

4. Extrapyramidal effects (trembling hands, facial grimacing) should be reported; may be treated with IM diphenhydramine.

**Outcomes/Evaluate**

• Prevention of N&V

• Enhanced gastric motility

• Promotion of gastric emptying

• Prophylaxis of gastric bezoars

# Metolazone

(meh-**TOH**-lah-zohn)

**Pregnancy Category:** B

Mykrox, Zaroxolyn **(Rx)**

**Classification:** Diuretic, thiazide

See also *Diuretics, Thiazide*.

**Action/Kinetics: Onset:** 1 hr. **Peak blood levels, rapid availability tablets:** 2–4 hr; **t½, elimination:** About 14 hr. **Peak blood levels, slow availability tablets:** 8 hr. **Duration, rapid or slow availablity tablets:** 24 hr or more. Most excreted unchanged through the urine.

**Uses: Slow availability tablets:** Edema accompanying CHF; edema accompanying renal diseases, including nephrotic syndrome and conditions of reduced renal function. Alone or in combination with other drugs for the treatment of hypertension.

**Rapid availability tablets:** Treatment of newly diagnosed mild to moderate hypertension alone or in combination with other drugs. The rapid availability tablets are not to be used to produce diuresis.

*Investigational:* Alone or as an adjunct to treat calcium nephrolithiasis, premanagement of menstrual syndrome, and adjunct treatment of renal failure.

**Contraindications:** Anuria, prehepatic and hepatic coma, allergy or hypersensitivity to metolazone. Routine use during pregnancy. Lactation.

**Special Concerns:** Use with caution in those with severely impaired renal function. Safety and effectiveness have not been determined in children.

**Side Effects:** See *Diuretics, Thiazide*. The most commonly reported side effects are dizziness, headache, muscle cramps, malaise, lethargy, lassitude, joint pain/swelling, and chest pain.

**Additional Drug Interactions**

*Alcohol* / ↑ Hypotensive effect

*Barbiturates* / Hypotensive effect

*Narcotics* / Hypotensive effect

*NSAIDs* / ↓ Hypotensive effect of metolazone

*Salicylates* / Hypotensive effect of metolazone

**Dosage**

• **Slow Availability Tablets**

*Edema due to cardiac failure or renal disease.*

**Adults:** 5–20 mg once daily. For those who experience paroxysmal nocturnal dyspnea, a larger dose may be required to ensure prolonged diuresis and saluresis for a 24-hr period.

*Mild to moderate essential hypertension.*

**Adults:** 2.5–5 mg once daily.

• **Rapid Availability Tablets**

*Mild to moderate essential hypertension.*

**Adults, initial:** 0.5 mg once daily, usually in the morning. If inadequately controlled, the dose may be increased to 1 mg once a day. Increasing the dose higher than 1 mg does not increase the effect.

## NURSING CONSIDERATIONS

See also *Nursing Considerations* for *Diuretics, Thiazide*.

**Administration/Storage**

1. Formulations of slow availability tablets should not be interchanged with formulations of rapid availability tablets as they are not therapeutically equivalent.

2. The antihypertensive effect may

be observed from 3 to 4 days to 3 to 6 weeks.

3. If BP is not controlled with 1 mg of the rapid availability tablets, add another antihypertensive drug, with a different mechanism of action, to the therapy.

4. Store tablets at room temperature in a tight, light-resistant container.

**Assessment**

1. Document indications for therapy, noting onset, duration, and clinical characteristics.

2. Monitor BP, ECG, CBC, electrolytes, liver and renal function studies; assess for symptoms of electrolyte imbalance (i.e., ↓ Na, ↓ K, ↓ Mg and hypochloremic alkalosis).

**Client/Family Teaching**

1. Take exactly as directed.

2. May cause orthostatic hypotension and syncope; use caution.

3. Weigh self regularly; report increases of more than 3 lb/day.

**Outcomes/Evaluate:** ↓ Edema; ↓ BP

# Metoprolol succinate
(me-toe-**PROH**-lohl)
**Pregnancy Category:** C
Toprol XL **(Rx)**

# Metoprolol tartrate
(me-toe-**PROH**-lohl)
**Pregnancy Category:** B
Apo-Metoprolol ✦, Apo-Metoprolol (Type L) ✦, Betaloc ✦, Betaloc Durules ✦, Gen-Metoprolol ✦, Lopressor, Novo-Metoprol ✦, Nu-Metop ✦, PMS-Metoprolol-B ✦ **(Rx)**
**Classification:** Beta-adrenergic blocking agent

See also *Beta-Adrenergic Blocking Agents.*

**Action/Kinetics:** Exerts mainly beta-1-adrenergic blocking activity although beta-2 receptors are blocked at high doses. Has no membrane stabilizing or intrinsic sympathomimetic effects. Moderate lipid solubility. **Onset:** 15 min. **Peak plasma levels:** 90 min. **t½:** 3–7 hr. Effect of drug is cumulative. Food increases bioavailability. Exhibits significant first-pass effect. Metabolized in liver and excreted in urine.

**Uses: Metoprolol Succinate:** Alone or with other drugs to treat hypertension. Chronic management of angina pectoris.

**Metoprolol Tartrate:** Hypertension (either alone or with other antihypertensive agents, such as thiazide diuretics). Acute MI in hemodynamically stable clients. Angina pectoris. *Investigational:* IV to suppress atrial ectopy in COPD, aggressive behavior, prophylaxis of migraine, ventricular arrhythmias, enhancement of cognitive performance in geriatric clients, essential tremors.

**Additional Contraindications:** Myocardial infarction in clients with a HR of less than 45 beats/min, in second- or third-degree heart block, or if SBP is less than 100 mm Hg. Moderate to severe cardiac failure.

**Special Concerns:** Safety and effectiveness have not been established in children. Use with caution in impaired hepatic function and during lactation.

**Additional Drug Interactions**

*Cimetidine* / May ↑ plasma levels of metoprolol

*Contraceptives, oral* / May ↑ effects of metoprolol

*Methimazole* / May ↓ effects of metoprolol

*Phenobarbital* / ↓ Effect of metoprolol due to ↑ breakdown by liver

*Propylthiouracil* / May ↓ the effects of metoprolol

*Quinidine* / May ↑ effects of metoprolol

*Rifampin* / ↓ Effect of metoprolol due to ↑ breakdown by liver

**Laboratory Test Interferences:** ↑ Serum transaminase, LDH, alkaline phosphatase.

**Dosage**

• **Metoprolol Succinate Tablets**
  *Angina pectoris.*

**Individualized. Initial:** 100 mg/day in a single dose. Dose may be increased slowly, at weekly intervals, until optimum effect is reached or there is a pronounced slowing of

HR. Doses above 400 mg/day have not been studied.

*Hypertension.*
**Initial:** 50–100 mg/day in a single dose with or without a diuretic. Dosage may be increased in weekly intervals until maximum effect is reached. Doses above 400 mg/day have not been studied.

• **Metoprolol Tartrate Tablets**
*Hypertension.*
**Initial:** 100 mg/day in single or divided doses; **then,** dose may be increased weekly to maintenance level of 100–450 mg/day. A diuretic may also be used.

*Aggressive behavior.*
200–300 mg/day.

*Essential tremors.*
50–300 mg/day.

*Prophylaxis of migraine.*
50–100 mg b.i.d.

*Ventricular arrhythmias.*
200 mg/day.

• **Metoprolol Tartrate Injection (IV) and Tablets**
*Early treatment of MI.*
3 IV bolus injections of 5 mg each at approximately 2-min intervals. If clients tolerate the full IV dose, give 50 mg q 6 hr PO beginning 15 min after the last IV dose (or as soon as client's condition allows). This dose is continued for 48 hr followed by **late treatment:** 100 mg b.i.d. as soon as feasible; continue for 1–3 months (although data suggest treatment should be continued for 1–3 years). In clients who do not tolerate the full IV dose, begin with 25–50 mg q 6 hr PO beginning 15 min after the last IV dose or as soon as the condition allows.

## NURSING CONSIDERATIONS

See also *Nursing Considerations* for *Beta-Adrenergic Blocking Agents* and *Antihypertensive Agents.*
**Assessment**
1. Document indications for therapy; note any cardiac disease.
2. Monitor liver and renal function studies, ECG, and VS.

**Client/Family Teaching**
1. Take doses at the same time each day.
2. Continue with diet, regular exercise, and weight loss in the overall plan to control BP.
3. Report any symptoms of fluid overload such as sudden weight gain, edema, or dyspnea.
4. Dress appropriately; may cause an increased sensitivity to cold.
**Outcomes/Evaluate**
• ↓ BP; ↓ anginal attacks
• Prevention of myocardial reinfarction and associated mortality

# Metronidazole
(meh-troh-**NYE**-dah-zohl)
**Pregnancy Category:** B
Apo-Metronidazole ✦, Femazole, Flagyl, Flagyl ER, Flagyl I.V., Flagyl I.V. RTU, Metric 21, Metro-Cream Topical, MetroGel Topical, MetroGel-Vaginal, Metro I.V., Metryl, Metryl-500, Metryl I.V., NidaGel ✦, Novo–Nidazol ✦, PMS-Metronidazole ✦, Protostat, Satric, Satric 500, Trikacide ✦ **(Rx)**
**Classification:** Systemic trichomonacide, amebicide

See also *Anti-Infectives.*
**Action/Kinetics:** Effective against anaerobic bacteria and protozoa. Specifically inhibits growth of trichomonae and amoebae by binding to DNA, resulting in loss of helical structure, strand breakage, inhibition of nucleic acid synthesis, and cell death. Well absorbed from GI tract and widely distributed in body tissues. **Peak serum concentration: PO,** 6–40 mcg/mL, depending on the dose, after 1–2 hr. **t½: PO,** 6–12 hr average: 8 hr. Eliminated primarily in urine (20% unchanged), which may be red-brown in color following either PO or IV use. The mechanism for its effectiveness in reducing the inflammatory lesions of acne rosacea are not known.
**Uses: Systemic:** Amebiasis. Symptomatic and asymptomatic trichomoniasis; to treat asymptomatic partner. Amebic dysentery and amebic liver

**M**

abscess. To reduce postoperative anaerobic infection following colorectal surgery, elective hysterectomy, and emergency appendectomy. Anaerobic bacterial infections of the abdomen, female genital system, skin or skin structures, bones and joints, lower respiratory tract, and CNS. Also, septicemia, endocarditis, hepatic encephalopathy. PO for Crohn's disease and pseudomembranous colitis. *Investigational:* giardiasis, *Gardnerella vaginalis.*

**Topical:** Inflammatory papules, pustules, and erythema of rosacea. *Investigational:* Infected decubitus ulcers (use 1% solution prepared from oral tablets).

**Vaginal:** Bacterial vaginosis.

**Contraindications:** Blood dyscrasias; active organic disease of the CNS. Not recommended for trichomoniasis during the first trimester of pregnancy. During lactation. For topical use: hypersensitivity to parabens or other ingredients of the formulation. Consumption of alcohol during use.

**Special Concerns:** Safety and efficacy have not been established in children.

**Side Effects: Systemic Use.** *GI:* Nausea, dry mouth, metallic taste, vomiting, diarrhea, abdominal discomfort, constipation. *CNS:* Headache, dizziness, vertigo, incoordination, ataxia, confusion, irritability, depression, weakness, insomnia, syncope, seizures, peripheral neuropathy including paresthesias. *Hematologic:* Leukopenia, **bone marrow aplasia.** *GU:* Burning, dysuria, cystitis, polyuria, incontinence, dryness of vagina or vulva, dyspareunia, decreased libido. *Allergic:* Urticaria, pruritus, erythematous rash, flushing, nasal congestion, fever, joint pain. *Miscellaneous:* Furry tongue, glossitis, stomatitis (due to overgrowth of *Candida*) ECG abnormalities, thrombophlebitis.

**Topical Use:** Watery eyes if gel applied too closely to this area; transient redness; mild burning, dryness, and skin irritation.

**Vaginal Use:** Symptomatic candida vaginitis, N&V.

**OD Overdose Management:** *Symptoms:* Ataxia, N&V, peripheral neuropathy, *seizures* up to 5–7 days. *Treatment:* Supportive treatment.

**Drug Interactions**
*Barbiturates* / Possible therapeutic failure of metronidazole
*Cimetidine* / ↑ Serum levels of metronidazole due to ↓ clearance
*Disulfiram* / Concurrent use may cause confusion or acute psychosis
*Ethanol* / Possible disulfiram-like reaction, including flushing, palpitations, tachycardia, and N&V
*Hydantoins* / ↑ Effect of hydantoins due to ↓ clearance
*Lithium* / ↑ Lithium toxicity
*Warfarin* / ↑ Anticoagulant effect

**Dosage** _____

• **Capsules, Tablets**
  *Amebiasis: Acute amebic dysentery or amebic liver abscess.*
**Adult:** 500–750 mg t.i.d. for 5–10 days; **pediatric:** 35–50 mg/kg/day in three divided doses for 10 days.
  *Trichomoniasis, female.*
250 mg t.i.d. for 7 days, 2 g given on 1 day in single or divided doses, or 375 mg b.i.d. for 7 days. **Pediatric:** 5 mg/kg t.i.d. for 7 days. An interval of 4–6 weeks should elapse between courses of therapy. *NOTE:* Do not treat pregnant women during the first trimester. *Male:* Individualize dosage; usual, 250 mg t.i.d. for 7 days.
  *Giardiasis.*
250 mg t.i.d. for 7 days.
  *G. vaginalis.*
500 mg b.i.d. for 7 days.

• **Tablets, Extended-Release**
  *Bacterial vaginosis.*
One 750-mg tablet per day for 7 days.

• **IV**
  *Anaerobic bacterial infections.*
**Adults, initially:** 15 mg/kg infused over 1 hr; **then,** after 6 hr, 7.5 mg/kg q 6 hr for 7–10 days (daily dose should not exceed 4 g). Treatment may be necessary for 2–3 weeks, although PO therapy should be initiated as soon as possible.

*Prophylaxis of anaerobic infection during surgery.*
**Adults:** 15 mg/kg given over a 30- to 60-min period, with completion 1 hr prior to surgery and 7.5 mg/kg infused over 30–60 min 6 and 12 hr after the initial dose.
• **Topical (0.75%)**
*Rosacea.*
After washing, apply a thin film and rub in well in the morning and evening for 9 weeks.
• **Vaginal (0.75%)**
*Bacterial vaginosis.*
One applicatorful (5 g) in the morning and evening for 5 days. Metro-Gel Vaginal allows for once-daily dosing at bedtime.

## NURSING CONSIDERATIONS

See also *General Nursing Considerations for All Anti-Infectives.*
**Administration/Storage**
1. For topical use, therapeutic results should be seen within 3 weeks with continuing improvement through 9 weeks of therapy.
2. Cosmetics may be used after application of topical metronidazole.
**IV** 3. Do not give by IV bolus. Administer each single dose over 1 hr.
4. Do not use syringes with aluminum needles or hubs.
5. If a primary IV fluid setup is used, discontinue the primary solution during infusion of metronidazole.
6. The order of mixing to prepare the powder for injection is important:
• Reconstitute.
• Dilute in IV solutions in glass or plastic containers.
• Neutralize pH with sodium bicarbonate solution. Do not refrigerate neutralized solutions.
7. Premixed, ready to use Flagyl usually comes 5 mg/mL (500 mg metronidazole in 100 mL of solution) in plastic bags; administer over 1 hr.
8. IV metronidazole has a high sodium content.

**Assessment**
1. Document indications for therapy and symptom characteristics.
2. Monitor CBC and cultures.
**Client/Family Teaching**
1. Take with food or milk to reduce GI upset; may cause a metallic taste.
2. Report any symptoms of CNS toxicity, such as ataxia or tremor and any unusual bruising or bleeding.
3. Do not perform tasks that require mental alertness until drug effects are realized; dizziness may occur.
4. During treatment for trichomoniasis, partner should also have therapy since organisms may be located in the male urogenital tract and reinfect partner. Use a condom to prevent reinfections.
5. Do not engage in intercourse while using the vaginal gel.
6. Drug may turn urine brown; do not be alarmed.
7. No alcohol; a disulfiram-like reaction may occur. Symptoms include abdominal cramps, vomiting, flushing, and headache.
**Outcomes/Evaluate**
• Symptomatic improvement
• Negative culture reports

# Mexiletine hydrochloride
(mex-**ILL**-eh-teen)
**Pregnancy Category:** C
Mexitil **(Rx)**
**Classification:** Antiarrhythmic, class IB

See also *Antiarrhythmic Drugs.*
**Action/Kinetics:** Mexiletine is similar to lidocaine but is effective PO. The drug inhibits the flow of sodium into the cell, thereby reducing the rate of rise of the action potential. The drug decreases the effective refractory period in Purkinje fibers. BP and pulse rate are not affected following use, but there may be a small decrease in CO and an increase in peripheral vascular resistance. The drug also has both local anesthetic and anticonvulsant effects. **Onset:** 30–120 min. **Peak blood levels:** 2–3 hr. **Therapeutic plasma levels:** 0.5–2 mcg/mL. **Plasma t½:** 10–12

hr. Approximately 10% excreted unchanged in the urine; acidification of the urine enhances excretion, whereas alkalinization decreases excretion.

**Uses:** Documented life-threatening ventricular arrhythmias (such as ventricular tachycardia). *Investigational:* Prophylactically to decrease the incidence of ventricular tachycardia and other ventricular arrhythmias in the acute phase of MI. To reduce pain, dysesthesia, and paresthesia associated with diabetic neuropathy.

**Contraindications:** Cardiogenic shock, preexisting second- or third-degree AV block (if no pacemaker is present). Use with lesser arrhythmias. Lactation.

**Special Concerns:** There is the possibility of increased risk of death when used in clients with non-life-threatening cardiac arrhythmias. Use with caution in hypotension, severe CHF, or known seizure disorders. Dosage has not been established in children.

**Side Effects:** *CV: **Worsening of arrhythmias,*** palpitations, chest pain, increased ventricular arrhythmias (PVCs), CHF, angina or angina-like pain, hypotension, bradycardia, syncope, ***AV block or conduction disturbances,*** atrial arrhythmias, hypertension, ***cardiogenic shock,*** hot flashes, edema. *GI:* High incidence of N&V, heartburn. Also, diarrhea or constipation, changes in appetite, dry mouth, abdominal cramps or pain, abdominal discomfort, salivary changes, dysphagia, altered taste, pharyngitis, changes in oral mucous membranes, upper GI bleeding, peptic ulcer, esophageal ulceration. *CNS:* High incidence of lightheadedness, dizziness, tremor, coordination difficulties, and nervousness. Also, changes in sleep habits, headache, fatigue, weakness, tinnitus, paresthesias, numbness, depression, confusion, difficulty with speech, short-term memory loss, hallucinations, malaise, psychosis, ***seizures,*** loss of consciousness. *Hematologic:* Leukopenia, neutropenia, agranulocytosis, thrombocytopenia. *GU:* Decreased libido, impotence, urinary hesitancy or retention. *Dermatologic:* Rash, dry skin. Rarely, exfoliative dermatitis, and ***Stevens-Johnson syndrome.*** *Miscellaneous:* Blurred vision, visual disturbances, dyspnea, arthralgia, fever, diaphoresis, loss of hair, hiccoughs, laryngeal or pharyngeal changes, syndrome of SLE, myelofibrosis.

**OD** **Overdose Management:** *Symptoms:* CNS symptoms (dizziness, drowsiness, paresthesias, seizures) usually precede CV symptoms (hypotension, sinus bradycardia, intermittent left bundle branch block (LBBB), ***temporary asystole).*** ***Massive overdoses cause coma and respiratory arrest.*** *Treatment:* General supportive treatment. Give atropine to treat hypotension or bradycardia. Acidification of the urine may increase rate of excretion.

**Drug Interactions**

*Aluminum hydroxide* / ↓ Absorption of mexiletine

*Atropine* / ↓ Absorption of mexiletine

*Cimetidine* / ↑ or ↓ Plasma levels of mexiletine

*Magnesium hydroxide* / ↓ Absorption of mexiletine

*Metoclopramide* / ↑ Absorption of mexiletine

*Narcotics* / ↓ Absorption of mexiletine

*Phenobarbital* / ↓ Plasma levels of mexiletine

*Phenytoin* / ↑ Clearance → ↓ plasma levels of mexiletine

*Rifampin* / ↑ Clearance → ↓ plasma levels of mexiletine

*Theophylline* / ↑ Effect of theophylline due to ↑ serum levels

*Urinary acidifiers* / ↑ Rate of excretion of mexiletine

*Urinary alkalinizers* / ↓ Rate of excretion of mexiletine

**Laboratory Test Interferences:** ↑ AST. Positive ANA.

**Dosage** —————————————
• **Capsules**
  *Antiarrhythmic.*
**Adults, individualized, initial:** 200 mg q 8 hr if rapid control of arrhyth-

mia not required; dosage adjustment may be made in 50- or 100-mg increments q 2–3 days, if required. **Maintenance:** 200–300 mg q 8 hr, depending on response and tolerance of client. If adequate response is not achieved with 300 mg or less q 8 hr, 400 mg q 8 hr may be tried although the incidence of CNS side effects increases. If the drug is effective at doses of 300 mg or less q 8 hr, the same total daily dose may be given in divided doses q 12 hr (e.g., 450 mg q 12 hr). Maximum total daily dose: 1,200 mg.

*Rapid control of arrhythmias.*
**Initial loading dose:** 400 mg followed by a 200-mg dose in 8 hr.

*Diabetic neuropathy.*
**Initial:** 150 mg/day for 3 days; **then,** 300 mg/day for 3 days. **Maintenance:** 10 mg/kg/day.

## NURSING CONSIDERATIONS

See also *Nursing Considerations* for *Antiarrhythmic Drugs.*

**Administration/Storage**
1. Reduce dose with severe liver disease and marked right-sided CHF.
2. If transferring to mexiletine from other class I antiarrhythmics, initiate mexiletine at a dose of 200 mg and then titrate according to the response at the following times: 6–12 hr after the last dose of quinidine sulfate, 3–6 hr after the last dose of procainamide, 6–12 hr after the last dose of disopyramide, or 8–12 hr after the last dose of tocainide.
3. Hospitalize client when transferring to mexiletine if there is a chance that withdrawal of the previous antiarrhythmic may produce life-threatening arrhythmias.

**Assessment**
1. Document indications for therapy; list any other agents trialed and the outcome.
2. Note evidence of CHF; assess ECG for AV block.
3. Document pulmonary assessment findings; note $SaO_2$ or $PO_2$.
4. Monitor ECG, CXR, CBC, electrolytes, and liver and renal function studies.
5. Assess urinary pH; alkalinity decreases and acidity increases renal drug excretion.

**Client/Family Teaching**
1. Take with food or an antacid to ↓ GI upset.
2. Report any bruising, bleeding, fevers, or sore throat as well as any adverse CNS effects such as dizziness, tremor, impaired coordination, N&V.
3. Immediately report any increase in heart palpitations, irregularity, or rate less than 50 beats/min.
4. Do not perform tasks that require mental alertness until drug effects are realized.
5. Carry identification that lists drugs currently prescribed.

**Outcomes/Evaluate**
• Control of ventricular arrhythmias
• Therapeutic drug levels (0.5–2 mcg/mL)
• ↓ Symptoms of diabetic neuropathy

# Mezlocillin sodium
(mez-low-**SILL**-in)
**Pregnancy Category:** B
Mezlin **(Rx)**
**Classification:** Antibiotic, penicillin

See also *Anti-Infectives* and *Penicillins.*

**Action/Kinetics:** Mezlocillin is a broad-spectrum (gram-negative and gram-positive organisms, including aerobic and anaerobic strains) antibiotic used parenterally. **Therapeutic serum levels:** 35–45 mcg/mL. **t½: IV,** 55 min. Excreted mostly unchanged by the kidneys. Penetration to CSF is poor unless meninges are inflamed.

**Uses:** Septicemia and infections of the lower respiratory tract, urinary tract, abdomen, skin, and female genital tract caused by *Klebsiella, Proteus, Pseudomonas, Escherichia coli, Bacteroides, Peptococcus, Streptococcus faecalis* (enterococcus), *Peptostreptococcus,* and *Enterobac-*

*ter.* Also, *Neisseria gonorrhoeae* infections of the urinary tract and female genital system. Infections caused by *Streptococcus pneumoniae* and group A beta-hemolytic streptococcus.

**Additional Side Effects:** Bleeding abnormalities. Decreased hemoglobin or hematocrit values.

**Laboratory Test Interferences:** ↑ AST, ALT, serum alkaline phosphatase, serum bilirubin, serum creatinine, and/or BUN. ↓ Serum potassium.

**Dosage**

• **IV, IM**

*Serious infections.*

**Adults:** 200–300 mg/kg/day in four to six divided doses; **usual:** 3 g q 4 hr or 4 g q 6 hr. **Infants and children, 1 month–12 years:** 50 mg/kg q 4 hr given **IM** or **IV** over 30 min; **infants more than 2 kg and less than 1 week of age or less than 2 kg and less than 1 week of age:** 75 mg/kg q 12 hr; **infants less than 2 kg and more than 1 week of age:** 75 mg/kg q 8 hr; **infants more than 2 kg and more than 1 week of age:** 75 mg/kg q 6 hr.

*Life-threatening infections.*

**Adults:** Up to 350 mg/kg/day, not to exceed 24 g/day.

*Gonococcal urethritis.*

**Adults:** Single dose of 1–2 g with probenecid, 1 g.

*Prophylaxis of postoperative infection.*

**Adults:** 4 g 30–90 min prior to start of surgery; **then,** 4 g, IV, 6 and 12 hr later.

*Prophylaxis of infection in clients undergoing cesarean section.*

**First dose:** 4 g IV when cord is clamped; **second and third doses:** 4 g IV 4 and 8 hr after the first dose.

---

**NURSING CONSIDERATIONS**

See also *Nursing Considerations* for *Penicillins.*

**Administration/Storage**

1. IM doses should not exceed 2 g/ injection. Continue for at least 2 days after symptoms of infection have disappeared.

2. For group A beta-hemolytic streptococcus, continue therapy for at least 10 days.

**IV** 3. When given by IV infusion (including piggyback), discontinue administration of other drugs during mezlocillin infusion.

4. Drug is very irritating to veins. Direct IV administration should be slow to prevent phlebitis; 1 g over 3–5 min. May further dilute in 50–100 mL of dextrose or saline solution and administer over 30 min.

5. For pediatric IV administration, infuse over 30 min.

6. Vials and infusion bottles should be stored at temperatures below 30°C (86°F).

7. The powder and reconstituted solution may darken slightly, but potency is not affected.

**Assessment**

1. Note any sensitivity to penicillin or cephalosporins.

2. Monitor cultures, CBC, PT, PTT, electrolytes, and renal function studies. Reduce dose with impaired renal function.

**Client/Family Teaching**

1. Immediately report any evidence of increased bruising and/or bleeding.

2. Report symptoms of drug-induced anemia manifested by fatigue, pallor, weakness, vertigo, headache, dyspnea, and palpitations.

**Outcomes/Evaluate**

• Negative culture reports

• Therapeutic serum drug levels (35–45 mcg/mL)

---

# Mibefradil dihydrochloride

This drug was removed from the market 6/98.

See also *Antihypertensive Agents.*

**Action/Kinetics:** Blocks both T-type (low voltage) and L-type (high voltage) calcium channels, leading to reduction of peripheral vascular resistance and thus fall in BP. For angina, may reduce HR and total peripheral resistance causing decrease in cardiac workload and myocardial oxygen demand. Slows sinus and AV node conduction sometimes causing abnormally low HR. **Peak plasma levels:** 1–2 hr. Food has no effect on rate or extent of absorption. **t½, elimination:** 17–25 hr. Metabolized in liver and excreted in urine and feces.

**Uses:** Alone or in combination with other drugs for hypertension or chronic stable angina pectoris.

**Contraindications:** Sick sinus syndrome or second- or third-degree AV block without pacemaker. Coadministration of terfenadine, astemizole, or cisapride. Lactation. Safety and efficacy have not been determined in children.

**Special Concerns:** Use with caution in severe hepatic impairment, heart failure, compromised ventricular function, pretreatment HR below 50, or severe aortic stenosis. May cause dose-related changes in appearance of ECG T and U waves.

**Side Effects:** *CNS:* Dizziness, headache, lightheadedness, paresthesia, anxiety, depression, insomnia. *GI:* Dyspepsia, N&V, abdominal pain, constipation, diarrhea, flatulence, gastroenteritis, rectal hemorrhage. *CV:* Flushing, orthostatic complaints, postural hypotension, syncope, bradycardia, *cardiac failure,* nonspecific chest pain, hypotension. *Musculoskeletal:* Arthritis, back pain, chest pain, muscle cramps, pain of extremities, sprains and strains. *Respiratory:* Bronchitis, coughing, dyspnea, nasal congestion, pharyngitis, sinusitis, rhinitis. *Dermatologic:* Exfoliative dermatitis, rash. *Miscellaneous:* Leg edema, generalized weakness, trauma, increased sweating, ear buzzing, otitis, angioedema, urinary tract infection, conjunctivitis.

**Dosage**
• **Tablets**
*Hypertension, Chronic stable angina.*

**Adults:** 50 mg once daily, up to 100 mg once daily, depending on response. Full effect of a given dose on BP seen after 1 to 2 weeks.

## NURSING CONSIDERATIONS

See also *Nursing Considerations* for *Antihypertensive Agents.*
**Administration/Storage:** Swallow tablets whole; do not crush or chew.
**Assessment**
1. Document indications for therapy, onset of symptoms, and other agents/therapies trialed.
2. Monitor VS, ECG, liver, and renal function studies; note any dysfunction or HR below 50 bpm.
3. Assess for any heart failure, bradycardia, hepatic failure and altered cardiac conduction.
**Client/Family Teaching**
1. Take as directed; do not crush or chew tablets. May take with or without food.
2. Report if lightheadedness or fatigue occurs.
3. Avoid terfenadine, astemizole, and cisapride while taking this drug.
4. May experience headaches, runny nose, stomach upset, and swelling of legs; report if persistent.
5. Continue lifestyle changes (i.e.; regular exercise, low fat and low salt diet, smoking cessation, stress reduction and weight loss) as prescribed.
**Outcomes/Evaluate:** ↓ BP; control of angina

## Miconazole
(my-**KON**-ah-zohl)
**Pregnancy Category:** C
**Systemic:** Monistat I.V. **Topical:** Micatin, Monistat-Derm. **Vaginal:** Monistat 3, Monistat 7 (Rx and OTC)
**Classification:** Antifungal agent

See also *Anti-Infectives.*
**Action/Kinetics:** Miconazole may be fungistatic or fungicidal, depending on the concentration. It is a broad-spectrum fungicide that alters the permeability of the fungal mem-

**M**

brane by inhibiting synthesis of sterols; thus, essential intracellular materials are lost. The drug also inhibits biosynthesis of triglycerides and phospholipids and also inhibits oxidative and peroxidative enzyme activity. **Peak blood levels:** 1 mcg/mL. The drug is eliminated in three phases; **t½ of each phase:** 0.4, 2.1, and 24 hr. More than 90% of miconazole is bound to serum proteins. Excretion of the drug is unaltered in clients with renal insufficiency, including those on hemodialysis.

**Uses: Systemic.** Fungal infections caused by coccidioidomycosis, candidiasis, cryptococcosis, paracoccidioidomycosis, chronic mucocutaneous candidiasis, pseudoallescheriosis. When used for the treatment of either fungal meningitis or urinary bladder infection, IV infusion must be supplemented with intrathecal administration or bladder irrigation of the drug. **Topical, Vaginal:** Tinea pedis, tinea cruris, tinea corporis caused by *Trichophyton rubrum, T. mentagrophytes,* and *Epidermophyton floccosum* (both OTC and Rx). Moniliasis and tinea versicolor (Rx only).

**Contraindications:** Hypersensitivity. Use of topical products in or around the eyes.

**Special Concerns:** Safe use in children less than 1 year of age has not been established.

**Side Effects: Following systemic use.** *GI:* N&V, diarrhea, anorexia. *Hematologic:* Thrombocytopenia, aggregation of erythrocytes, rouleaux formation on blood smears. Transient decrease in hematocrit. *Dermatologic:* Pruritus, rash, flushing, phlebitis at injection site. *CV:* Transient tachycardia or arrhythmias following rapid injection of undiluted drug. *Miscellaneous:* Fever, chills, drowsiness, transient decrease in serum sodium values. Hyperlipemia due to the vehicle (polyethylene glycol 40 and castor oil). **Following topical use:** Vulvovaginal burning, pelvic cramps, hives, skin rash, headache, itching, irritation, maceration, and allergic contact dermatitis.

**Drug Interactions**
*Amphotericin B* / ↓ Activity of miconazole of each drug
*Coumarin anticoagulants* / Miconazole ↑ anticoagulant effect

**Dosage**
- **IV Infusion**
    *Candidiasis.*
  **Adults:** 600–1,800 mg/day for 1 to more than 20 weeks.
    *Coccidioidomycosis.*
  **Adults:** 1,800–3,600 mg for 3 to more than 20 weeks.
    *Cryptococcosis.*
  **Adults:** 1,200–2,400 mg/day for 3 to more than 12 weeks.
    *Paracoccidioidomycosis.*
  **Adults:** 200–1,200 mg/day for 2 to more than 16 weeks.
    *Pseudoallescheriosis.*
  **Adults:** 600–3,000 mg/day for 5 to more than 20 weeks. **Pediatric, less than 1 year of age:** 15–30 mg/kg/day; **1–12 years of age:** 20–40 mg/kg/day, not to exceed 15 mg/kg/dose.
- **Intrathecal**
  20 mg/dose of the undiluted solution as an adjunct to **IV** therapy.
- **Bladder Instillation**
  200 mg of diluted solution as adjunct in treatment of fungal infections of urinary bladder.
- **Topical, Aerosol Powder, Aerosol Solution, Cream, Lotion, Powder**
  Apply to cover affected areas in morning and evening (once daily for tinea versicolor) for 7 days.
- **Vaginal Cream or Suppository**
  Monistat 3: One suppository daily at bedtime for 7 days (100-mg suppositories) or 3 consecutive days (200-mg suppositories).
  Monistat 7: One applicator full of cream or one suppository at bedtime daily for 7 days. Course may be repeated after presence of other pathogens has been ruled out.

## NURSING CONSIDERATIONS

See also *General Nursing Considerations for All Anti-Infectives.*

## Administration/Storage

1. The lotion is preferred for intertriginous areas.

2. To reduce recurrence of symptoms, tinea cruris, tinea corporis, and candida should be treated for 2 weeks; tinea pedis should be treated for 1 month.

3. For intrathecal use, the drug is given as the undiluted solution (20 mg/dose) as an adjunct to IV treatment for fungal meningitis. Doses are alternated between lumbar, cervical, and cisternal punctures every 3–7 days; document sites.

4. The vaginal products should be refrigerated below 15°C–30°C (59°F–86°F).

**IV** 5. For IV infusion, dilute drug in at least 200 mL of either 0.9% NaCl or 5% dextrose solution and administered over a period of 30–60 min. Discard if solution darkens.

6. The IV dose may be divided over three infusions daily.

## Assessment

1. Determine any previous experience with this drug, any evidence of sensitivity, and response obtained.

2. Monitor cultures, CBC, electrolytes, and liver function studies.

3. Document clinical presentation, noting size, number, and extent of lesions.

## Client/Family Teaching

1. Review technique for administration; use only as directed.

2. Use sanitary pads to protect clothing and linens when using cream or suppositories.

3. When used for vaginal infections, refrain from intercourse or have sexual partner use a condom to prevent reinfection.

4. When used vaginally, continue miconazole treatment during menses.

5. Report if exposed to HIV and recurrent vaginal yeast infections occur.

6. Persistent N&V, diarrhea, dizziness, and pruritus should be reported.

## Outcomes/Evaluate

• Negative culture reports
• Resolution of vaginitis evidenced by ↓ in itching/burning; ↓ discharge
• ↓ Size and number of lesions

# Midazolam hydrochloride

(my-**DAYZ**-oh-lam)

**Pregnancy Category:** D

Versed **(C-IV) (Rx)**

**Classification:** Benzodiazepine sedative; adjunct to general anesthesia

See also *Tranquilizers, Antimanic Drugs, and Hypnotics.*

**Action/Kinetics:** Short-acting benzodiazepine with sedative–general anesthetic properties. Depresses the response of the respiratory system to carbon dioxide stimulation, which is more pronounced in clients with COPD. Possible mild to moderate decreases in CO, mean arterial BP, SV, and systemic vascular resistance. HR may rise somewhat in those with slow HRs (< 65/min) and decrease in others (especially those with HRs more than 85/min). **Onset, IM:** 15 min; **IV:** 2–2.5 min for induction (if combined with a preanesthetic narcotic, induction is about 1.5 min). If preanesthetic medication (morphine) is given, the **Peak plasma levels, IM:** 45 min. **Maximum effect:** 30–60 min. **Time to recovery:** Usually within 2 hr, although up to 6 hr may be required. About 97% bound to plasma protein. **t½, elimination:** 1.2–12.3 hr. Rapidly metabolized in the liver to inactive compounds; excreted through the urine.

**Uses: IV, IM:** Preoperative sedation, anxiolysis, and amnesia. **IV:** Sedation, anxiolysis, and amnesia prior to or during short diagnostic, therapeutic, or endoscopic procedures (either alone or with other CNS depressants). Induction of general anesthesia before administration of other anesthetics. Supplement to nitrous oxide and oxygen in balanced anesthesia. Sedation of intubated and mechanically ventilated clients as a component of anesthesia or

M

during treatment in a critical care setting. *Investigational:* Treat epileptic seizures. Alternative to terminate refractory status epilepticus.

**Contraindications:** Hypersensitivity to benzodiazepines. Acute narrow-angle glaucoma. Use in obstetrics. Use in coma, shock, or acute alcohol intoxication where VS are depressed. IA injection.

**Special Concerns:** Use with caution during lactation. Pediatric clients may require higher doses than adults. Hypotension may be more common in conscious sedated clients who have received a preanesthetic narcotic. Geriatric and debilitated clients require lower doses to induce anesthesia and they are more prone to side effects. Use IV with extreme caution in severe fluid or electrolyte disturbances.

**Side Effects:** Fluctuations in VS, including decreased respiratory rate and tidal volume, apnea, variations in BP and pulse rate are common. The following are general side effects regardless of the route of administration. *CV:* Hypotension, cardiac arrest. *CNS:* Oversedation, headache, drowsiness, grogginess, confusion, retrograde amnesia, euphoria, nervousness, agitation, anxiety, argumentativeness, restlessness, emergence delirium, increased time for emergence, dreaming during emergence, nightmares, insomnia, tonic-clonic movements, ataxia, muscle tremor, involuntary or athetoid movements, dizziness, dysphoria, dysphonia, slurred speech, paresthesia. *GI:* Hiccoughs, N&V, acid taste, retching, excessive salivation. *Ophthalmologic:* Double vision, blurred vision, nystagmus, pinpoint pupils, visual disturbances, cyclic eyelid movements, difficulty in focusing. *Dermatologic:* Hives, swelling or feeling of burning, warmth or cold feeling at injection site, hive-like wheal at injection site, pruritus, rash. *Miscellaneous:* Blocked ears, loss of balance, chills, weakness, faint feeling, lethargy, yawning, toothache, hematoma.

**More common following IM use:** Pain at injection site, headache, induration and redness, muscle stiffness.

**More common following IV use:** R*espiratory:* **Bronchospasm,** coughing, dyspnea, laryngospasm, hyperventilation, shallow respirations, tachypnea, airway obstruction, wheezing, respiratory depression and ***respiratory arrest*** when used for conscious sedation. *CV:* PVCs, bigeminy, bradycardia, tachycardia, vasovagal episode, nodal rhythm.*At injection site:* Tenderness, pain, redness, induration, phlebitis.

**Drug Interactions**

*Alcohol* / ↑ Risk of apnea, airway obstruction, desaturation or hypoventilation

*Anesthetics, inhalation* / ↓ Dose if midazolam used as an induction agent

*CNS Depressants* / ↑ Risk of apnea, airway obstruction, desaturation or hypoventilation

*Droperidol* / ↑ Hypnotic effect of midazolam when used as a premedication

*Fentanyl* / ↑ Hypnotic effect of midazolam when used as a premedication

*Indinavir* / Possible prolonged sedation and respiratory depression

*Meperidine* / See *Narcotics;* also, ↑ Risk of hypotension

*Narcotics* / ↑ Hypnotic effect of midazolam when used as premedications

*Propofol* / ↑ Effect of propofol

*Ritonavir* / Possible prolonged sedation and respiratory depression

*Thiopental* / ↓ Dose if midazolam used as an induction agent

**Dosage** ——————————

• **IM**

*Preoperative sedation, anxiolysis, amnesia.*

**Adults:** 0.07–0.08 mg/kg IM (average: 5 mg) 1 hr before surgery. **Children:** 0.1–0.15 mg/kg (up to 0.5 mg/kg may be needed for more anxious clients).

• **IV**

*Conscious sedation, anxiolysis, amnesia for endoscopic or CV proce-*

*dures in healthy adults less than 60 years of age.*

Using the 1 mg/mL (can be diluted with 0.9% sodium chloride or D5W) product, titrate slowly to the desired effect (usually slurred speech); initial dose should be no higher than 2.5 mg IV (may be as low as 1 mg IV) within a 2-min period, after which an additional 2 min should be waited to evaluate the sedative effect. If additional sedation is necessary, small increments should be given waiting an additional 2 min or more after each increment to evaluate the effect. Total doses greater than 5 mg are usually not required. **Children:** Dosage must be individualized by the physician.

*Conscious sedation for endoscopic or CV procedures in debilitated or chronically ill clients or clients aged 60 or over.*

Slowly titrate to the desired effect using no more than 1.5 mg initially IV (may be as little as 1 mg IV) given over a 2-min period after which an additional 2 min or more should be waited to evaluate the effect. If additional sedation is needed, no more than 1 mg should be given over 2 min; wait an additional 2 min or more after each increment in dose. Total doses greater than 3.5 mg are usually not needed.

*Induction of general anesthesia, before use of other general anesthetics, in unmedicated clients.*

**Adults, unmedicated clients up to 55 years of age, IV, initial:** 0.3–0.35 mg/kg given over 20–30 sec, waiting 2 min for effects to occur. If needed, increments of about 25% of the initial dose can be used to complete induction; or, induction can be completed using a volatile liquid anesthetic. Up to 0.6 mg/kg may be used but recovery will be prolonged. **Adults, unmedicated clients over 55 years of age who are good risk surgical clients, initial IV:** 0.15–0.3 mg/kg given over 20–30 sec. **Adults, unmedicated clients over 55 years of age with severe**

**systemic disease or debilitation, initial IV:** 0.15–0.25 mg/kg given over 20–30 sec. **Pediatric:** 0.05–0.2 mg/kg IV.

*Induction of general anesthesia, before use of other general anesthetics, in medicated clients.*

**Adults, premedicated clients up to 55 years of age, IV, initial:** 0.15–0.35 mg/kg. If less than 55 years of age, 0.25 mg/kg may be given over 20–30 sec, allowing 2 min for effect. **Adults, premedicated clients over 55 years of age who are good risk surgical clients, initial, IV:** 0.2 mg/kg. **Adults, premedicated clients over 55 years of age with severe systemic disease or debilitation, initial, IV:** 0.15 mg/kg may be sufficient.

*Maintenance of balanced anesthesia for short surgical procedures.*

**IV:** Incremental injections about 25% of the dose used for induction when signs indicate anesthesia is lightening.

*NOTE:* Narcotic preanesthetic medication may include fentanyl, 1.5–2 mcg/kg IV 5 min before induction; morphine, up to 0.15 mg/kg IM; meperidine, up to 1 mg/kg IM; or, Innovar, 0.02 mL/kg IM. Sedative preanesthetic medication may include secobarbital sodium, 200 mg PO or hydroxyzine pamoate, 100 mg PO. Except for fentanyl, all preanesthetic medications should be given 1 hr prior to midazolam. Doses should always be individualized.

## NURSING CONSIDERATIONS

See also *Nursing Considerations* for *Tranquilizers, Antimanic Drugs, and Hypnotics.*

**Administration/Storage**

1. When used for procedures via the mouth, use a topical anesthetic.
2. Give IM doses in a large muscle mass.

**IV** 3. When used for conscious sedation, do not give by rapid or single bolus IV.
4. When used for induction of general anesthesia, give the initial dose over 20–30 sec.

5. If preanesthetic medications with a depressant component are given (e.g., narcotic analgesics or CNS depressants), reduce the midazolam dosage by 50% compared with healthy, young unmedicated clients.

6. Give maintenance doses to all clients in increments of 25% of the dose first required to achieve the sedative endpoint.

7. Give a narcotic preanesthetic for bronchoscopic procedures.

8. Carefully monitor all IV doses with the immediate availability of oxygen, resuscitative equipment, and personnel who are skilled in maintaining a patent airway and for support of ventilation. Continue monitoring during the recovery period.

9. May be mixed in the same syringe with atropine, meperidine, morphine, or scopolamine

10. At a concentration of 0.5 mg/mL midazolam is compatible with D5W and 0.9% NaCl for up to 24 hr and with RL solution for up to 4 hr.

**Client/Family Teaching**

1. Drug may cause dizziness and drowsiness. Avoid alcohol, CNS depressants, and activities that require mental alertness for 24 hr following drug administration.

2. Repeat postprocedure instructions and obtain in writing as may not fully recall instructions; transient amnesia is normal and memory of procedure may be minimal.

**Outcomes/Evaluate:** Desired level of sedation and amnesia; ↓ anxiety

# Midodrine hydrochloride

(**MIH**-doh-dreen)
**Pregnancy Category:** C
Amatine ✹, ProAmatine **(Rx)**
**Classification:** Treat orthostatic hypotension

**Action/Kinetics:** Midodrine, a prodrug, is converted to an active metabolite—desglymidodrine—that is an alpha-1 agonist. Desglymidodrine produces an increase in vascular tone and elevation of BP by activating alpha-adrenergic receptors of the arteriolar and venous vascula-

ture. No effect on cardiac beta-adrenergic receptors. The active metabolite does not cross the blood-brain barrier; thus, there are no CNS effects. Standing systolic BP is increased by approximately 15–30 mm Hg at 1 hr after a 10-mg dose; duration: 2–3 hr. Rapidly absorbed from the GI tract. **Peak plasma levels, midodrine:** 30 min; **t½:** 25 min. **Peak plasma levels, desglymidodrine:** 1–2hr; **t½:** 3–4 hr. The bioavailability of the active metabolite is not affected by food. Desglymidodrine is eliminated in the urine.

**Uses:** Orthostatic hypotension in those whose lives are significantly impaired despite standard clinical care. *Investigational:* Management of urinary incontinence.

**Contraindications:** Use in severe organic heart disease, acute renal disease, urinary retention, pheochromocytoma, thyrotoxicosis, persistent and excessive supine hypertension.

**Special Concerns:** Use with caution in impaired renal or hepatic function, during lactation, in orthostatic hypotensive clients who are also diabetic, or in those with a history of visual problems or who are also taking fludrocortisone acetate. Safety and efficacy have not been determined in children.

**Side Effects:** *CNS:* Paresthesia, pain, headache, feeling of pressure or fullness in the head, confusion, abnormal thinking, nervousness, anxiety. Rarely, dizziness, insomnia, somnolence. *GI:* Dry mouth. Rarely, canker sore, nausea, GI distress, flatulence. *Dermatologic:* Piloerection, pruritus, rash, vasodilation, flushed face. Rarely, erythema multiforme, dry skin. *Miscellaneous:* Dysuria, supine hypertension. Rarely, visual field defect, skin hyperesthesia, impaired urination, asthenia, backache, pyrosis, leg cramps.

**OD** **Overdose Management:** *Symptoms:* Hypertension, piloerection, sensation of coldness, urinary retention. *Treatment:* Emesis and administration of an alpha-adrenergic blocking agent (e.g., phentolamine).

**Drug Interactions**

*Alpha-adrenergic agonists* / ↑ Pressor effects of midodrine

*Alpha-adrenergic antagonists* / Antagonism of the effects of midodrine

*Beta-adrenergic blockers* / ↑ Risk of bradycardia, AV block, or arrhythmias

*Cardiac glycosides* / ↑ Risk of bradycardia, AV block, or arrhythmias

*Fludrocortisone* / ↑ Intraocular pressure and glaucoma

*Psychopharmacologic drugs* / ↑ Risk of bradycardia, AV block, or arrhythmias

**Dosage** ————————————
• **Tablets**

*Orthostatic hypotension.*

10 mg t.i.d. given during the daytime hours when the client is upright and pursuing daily activities (e.g., shortly before or upon arising in the morning, midday, and late afternoon–not later than 6:00 p.m.). To control symptoms, dosing may be q 3 hr. Initial dose in impaired renal function: 2.5 mg t.i.d.

*Urinary incontinence.*

2.5–5 mg b.i.d.–t.i.d.

**NURSING CONSIDERATIONS**

**Assessment**

1. Document onset, duration, and characteristics of symptoms. Note other nonpharmacologic treatments (i.e., support stockings, increased salt in diet, fluid expansion, sleeping with head of bed raised) trialed and the outcome.

2. Orthostatic hypotension is defined as SBP reductions > 20 mm Hg or DBP of over 10 mm Hg reduction within 3 min of standing; assess carefully on several occasions.

3. Document any acute renal disease, urinary retention, pheochromocytoma, severe organic heart disease, or thyrotoxicosis, as these preclude drug therapy. Assess for liver and renal dysfunction.

**Client/Family Teaching**

1. Do not take after the evening meal or within 4 hr of bedtime.

2. Use OTC products containing phenylephrine or phenylpropanolamine (such as cold remedies and diet aids) cautiously; may increase supine BP.

3. May experience supine hypertension; check BP regularly while lying and sitting and keep a record for review.

4. Report blurred vision, pounding in ears, headache, cardiac awareness, increased dizziness, and syncope and stop medications.

**Outcomes/Evaluate:** Relief of symptomatic orthostatic hypotension: ↓ dizziness, ↓ lightheadedness, ↓ unsteadiness

# Miglitol

(**MIG**-lih-tohl)
**Pregnancy Category:** B
Glyset **(Rx)**
**Classification:** Antidiabetic, oral

See also *Antidiabetic Agents.*

**Action/Kinetics:** Acts by delaying digestion of ingested carbohydrates resulting in smaller rise in blood glucose levels after meals. Effect is due to reversible inhibition of membrane-bound intestinal glucoside hydrolase enzymes which hydrolyze oligosaccharides and disaccharides to glucose and other monosaccharides. Reduces levels of glycosylated hemoglobin in type II diabetes. Does not enhance insulin secretion or increase insulin sensitivity. Does not cause hypoglycemia when given in fasted state. Absorption is saturable at high doses (i.e., only 50% to 70% of 100 mg dose is absorbed while 25 mg dose is 100% absorbed). **Peak levels:** 2–3 hr. Drug is not metabolized and is eliminated unchanged in urine. Dose must be reduced in those with impaired renal function.

**Uses:** Alone as adjunct to diet to treat non-insulin-dependent diabetes. With sulfonylurea when diet plus either miglitol or a sulfonylurea alone do not result in adequate control (effects of sulfonylurea and miglitol are additive).

**Contraindications:** Lactation, diabetic ketoacidosis, inflammatory bowel disease, colonic ulceration, partial intestinal obstruction, those predisposed to intestinal obstruction, chronic intestinal diseases associated with marked disorders of digestion or absorption, conditions that may deteriorate due to increased gas formation in the intestine, hypersensitivity to drug.

**Special Concerns:** When given with sulfonylurea or insulin, miglitol causes further decrease in blood sugar and increased risk of hypoglycemia. Safety and efficacy have not been determined in children.

**Side Effects:** *GI:* Flatulence, diarrhea, abdominal pain, soft stools, abdominal discomfort. *Dermatologic:* Skin rash (transient).

**Drug Interactions**
*Amylase* / ↓ Effect of miglitol
*Charcoal* / Adsorbent effect ↓ effect of miglitol
*Digoxin* / May ↓ plasma levels of digoxin
*Pancreatin* / ↓ Effect of miglitol
*Propranolol* / Significant ↓ bioavailability of propranolol
*Ranitidine* / Significant ↓ bioavailability of ranitidine

**Dosage** —————————————
• **Tablets**
*Type II diabetes.*
Individualize dosage. **Initial:** 25 mg t.i.d. with first bite of each main meal (some may benefit from starting with 25 mg once daily to minimize GI side effects). After 4 to 8 weeks of 25 mg t.i.d. dose, increase dosage to 50 mg t.i.d. for about 3 months. Measure glycosylated hemoglobin; if not satisfactory, increase dose to 100 mg t.i.d. **Maintenance:** 50 mg t.i.d., up to 100 mg t.i.d. (maximum).

## NURSING CONSIDERATIONS

See also *Nursing Considerations* for *Antidiabetic Agents.*

**Assessment**
1. Document indications for therapy, other agents trialed, and outcome.
2. Determine any IBD, colonic ulceration, intestinal obstruction, or severe digestion/absorption problems.
3. Monitor BS, HbA1C, and renal function; avoid if creatinine > 2 mg/dL.

**Client/Family Teaching**
1. Take with first bite of each meal.
2. May experience abdominal pain and diarrhea which should diminish with continued treatment.
3. Any stress, fever, trauma, infection, or surgery may alter glucose control. Monitor finger sticks regularly.
4. Drug inhibits breakdown of table sugar; have glucose available for episodes of marked hypoglycemia.
5. Continue prescribed diet and regular exercise. Report for F/U as scheduled.

**Outcomes/Evaluate:** ↓ BS; HbA1C less than 8

# Milrinone lactate

(**MILL**-rih-nohn)
**Pregnancy Category:** C
Primacor **(Rx)**
**Classification:** Inotropic/vasodilator

**Action/Kinetics:** Selective inhibitor of peak III cyclic AMP phosphodiesterase isozyme in cardiac and vascular muscle, resulting in a direct inotropic effect and a direct arterial vasodilator activity. Also improves diastolic function as manifested by improvements in LV diastolic relaxation. In clients with depressed myocardial function, the drug produces a prompt increase in CO and a decrease in pulmonary wedge pressure and vascular resistance, without a significant increase in HR or myocardial oxygen consumption. Causes an inotropic effect in clients who are fully digitalized without causing signs of glycoside toxicity. Also, LV function has improved in clients with ischemic heart disease. **Therapeutic plasma levels:** 150–250 ng/mL. **t½:** 2.3 hr following doses of 12.5–125 mcg/kg to clients with CHF. Metabolized in the liver and excreted primarily through the urine.

**Uses:** Short-term treatment of CHF, usually in clients receiving digoxin and diuretics.

**Contraindications:** Hypersensitivity to the drug. Use in severe obstructive aortic or pulmonic valvular disease in lieu of surgical relief of the obstruction.

**Special Concerns:** Use with caution during lactation. Safety and efficacy have not been determined in children.

**Side Effects:** *CV: Ventricular and supraventricular arrhythmias, including ventricular ectopic activity, nonsustained ventricular tachycardia, sustained ventricular tachycardia, and ventricular fibrillation. Infrequently, life-threatening arrhythmias associated with preexisting arrhythmias,* metabolic abnormalities, abnormal digoxin levels, and catheter insertion. Also, hypotension, angina, chest pain. *Miscellaneous:* Mild to moderately severe headaches, hypokalemia, tremor, thrombocytopenia, bronchospasm (rare).

**OD** **Overdose Management:** *Symptoms:* Hypotension. *Treatment:* If hypotension occurs, reduce or temporarily discontinue administration of milrinone until the condition of the client stabilizes. General measures should be used for supporting circulation.

**Dosage**
• **IV Infusion**
**Adults, loading dose:** 50 mcg/kg administered slowly over 10 min. **Maintenance, minimum:** 0.59 mg/kg/24 hr (infused at a rate of 0.375 mcg/kg/min); **maintenance, standard:** 0.77 mg/kg/24 hr (infused at a rate of 0.5 mcg/kg/min); **maintenance, maximum:** 1.13 mg/kg/24 hr (infused at a rate of 0.75 mcg/kg/min).

## NURSING CONSIDERATIONS
**Administration/Storage**
**IV** 1. Give IV infusions at rates described in the package insert.
2. Adjust the infusion rate depending on the hemodynamic and clinical response.
3. Prepare dilutions using 0.45% or 0.9% NaCl injection or 5% dextrose injection.
4. Reduce infusion rate in renal impairment (see package insert for chart).
5. Do not give furosemide in IV lines containing milrinone as a precipitate will form.
6. Store at room temperatures of 15°C–30°C (59° F–86°F).

**Assessment**
1. Document indications for therapy, type and onset of symptoms. Identify other meds used and the outcome.
2. Monitor CBC, electrolytes, liver and renal function studies. Document ECG, CO, CVP, and PAWP; rule out acute MI.

**Interventions**
1. Monitor I&O, electrolyte levels, and renal function. Potassium loss due to excessive diuresis may result in arrhythmias in digitalized clients; correct hypokalemia.
2. Monitor VS; review parameters for interruption of infusion (e.g., SBP < 80; HR < 50).
3. Observe for increased supraventricular and ventricular arrhythmias.

**Outcomes/Evaluate**
• ↑ CO and ↓ PACWP
• Resolution of S&S of CHF
• Drug levels (150–250 ng/mL)

# Minocycline hydrochloride
(mih-no-**SYE**-kleen)
**Pregnancy Category:** D
Alti-Minocycline ✦, Apo-Minocycline ✦, Dynacin, Minocin, Novo-Minocycline ✦, Vectrin **(Rx)**
**Classification:** Antibiotic, tetracycline

See also *Anti-Infectives* and *Tetracyclines*.

**Action/Kinetics:** In fasting adults, 90% to 100% of an oral dose is absorbed. **Peak plasma levels:** 1–4 hr. Absorption is less affected by milk or food than for other tetracyclines. **t½, elimination:** 11–26 hr. Metabolized in the liver.

**Uses:** See also *Tetracyclines*. To eliminate meningococci from the nasopharynx of asymptomatic *Neisseria meningitidis* carriers in which the risk of meningococcal meningitis is high. *Note:* Due to adverse CNS effects, it is now recommended that rifampin be used in treating meningococcus carriers when the drug susceptibility is not known or when the organism is sulfa-resistant. Minocycline is indicated only when rifampin is contraindicated.

Granulomas of the skin caused by *Mycobacterium marinum*. In combination with gonococcal regimens for presumptive treatment of coexisting chlamydial infections. Uncomplicated gonogoccal urethritis in adult males. Treatment of uncomplicated urethral, endocervical, or rectal infections caused by *Chlamydia trachomatis* or *Ureaplasma urealyticum* in adults. Intrapleurally as a sclerosing agent to control pleural effusions assocated with metastatic tumors. Treatment of cholera and nocardiosis. Adjunctive treatment of inflammatory acne unresponsive to oral tetracycline HCl or oral erythromycin.

**Additional Side Effects:** Blue-gray pigmentation areas of cutaneous inflammation, vertigo, ataxia, drowsiness, **Stevens-Johnson syndrome** (rare).

**Dosage** ⎯⎯⎯⎯⎯⎯⎯⎯⎯
• **Capsules, Injection, Suspension, Tablets**
*Infections against which effective, including asymptomatic meningococcus carriers.*
**Adults, initial:** 200 mg; **then,** 100 mg q 12 hr. An alternative regimen is 100–200 mg initially followed by 50 mg q 6 hr. The length of treatment is

5 days for meningococcus carriers. **Children over 8 years of age, initial:** 4 mg/kg; **then,** 2 mg/kg q 12 hr.
*Mycobacterial infections.*
100 mg PO b.i.d. for 6–8 weeks.
*Uncomplicated gongococcal urethritis in adult males.*
100 mg b.i.d. for 5 days.
*Uncomplicated urethral, endocervical, or rectal infections due to* Chlamydia trachomatis *or* Ureaplasma urealyticum.
100 mg PO b.i.d. for at least 7 days.
*Nongonococcal urethritis caused by* C. trachomatis or Mycoplasma.
100/day PO in 1 or 2 divided doses for 1 to 3 weeks.
*Sclerosing agent to control pleural effusions associated with metastatic cancer.*
300 mg diluted with 40–50 mL of 0.9% NaCl injection and instilled into the pleural space through a thoracostomy tube.
*Cholera in conjunction with fluid and electrolyte replacement.*
**Initial:** 200 mg PO; **then,** 100 mg PO 12 hr for 48–72 hr.
*Adjunct to treat inflammatory acne unresponsive to PO tetracycline HCl or erythromycin.*
50 mg PO 1–3 times/day.

## NURSING CONSIDERATIONS

See also *Nursing Considerations* for *Anti-Infectives,* ,and *Tetracyclines*.
**Administration/Storage**
**IV** 1. Do not dissolve in solutions containing calcium; a precipitate will form.
2. After dissolving medication in the vial, further dilute to 500–1,000 mL with any of the following: dextrose injection, dextrose and NaCl injection, NaCl injection, Ringer's injection, RL injection.
3. Start administration of the final dilution immediately.
4. Discard reconstituted solutions after 24 hr at room temperature.
**Assessment**
1. Document indications for therapy, onset, duration, location, and characteristics of symptoms.
2. Monitor cultures and CBC; identi-

fy contacts when treating a contagious disease.

**Client/Family Teaching**
1. Take complete prescription as prescribed; may take with meals if GI upset occurs.
2. With STDs, partners should use condoms during therapy to prevent reinfections and have periodic cultures done.
3. Practice reliable birth control; may cause fetal harm.
4. Report any unusual bruising or bleeding, severe rash or diarrhea and lack of improvement after 72 hr of therapy.

**Outcomes/Evaluate:** Symptomatic improvement; resolution of infection

# Minoxidil, oral
(mih-**NOX**-ih-dil)
**Pregnancy Category:** C
Loniten **(Rx)**
**Classification:** Antihypertensive, depresses sympathetic nervous system

See also *Antihypertensive Agents.*

**Action/Kinetics:** Decreases elevated BP by decreasing peripheral resistance by a direct effect. Causes increase in renin secretion, increase in cardiac rate and output, and salt/water retention. Does not cause orthostatic hypotension. **Onset:** 30 min. **Peak plasma levels:** reached within 60 min; **plasma t½:** 4.2 hr. **Duration:** 24–48 hr. Ninety percent absorbed from GI tract; excretion: renal (90% metabolites). The time needed to reach the maximum effect is inversely related to the dose.

**Uses:** Severe hypertension not controllable by the use of a diuretic plus two other antihypertensive drugs. Usually taken with at least two other antihypertensive drugs (a diuretic and a drug to minimize tachycardia such as a beta-adrenergic blocking agent). Minoxidil can produce severe side effects; it should be reserved for resistant cases of hypertension. Close medical supervision required, including possible hospi-

talization during initial administration. Topically to promote hair growth in balding men.

**Contraindications:** Pheochromocytoma. Within 1 month after a MI. Dissecting aortic aneurysm.

**Special Concerns:** Safe use during lactation not established. Use with caution and at reduced dosage in impaired renal function. Geriatric clients may be more sensitive to the hypotensive and hypothermic effects of minoxidil; also, it may be necessary to decrease the dose in these clients due to age-related decreases in renal function. BP controlled too rapidly may cause syncope, stroke, MI, and ischemia of affected organs. Experience with use in children is limited.

**Side Effects:** *CV:* Edema, ***pericardial effusion that may progress to tamponade*** (acute compression of heart caused by fluid or blood in pericardium), CHF, angina pectoris, changes in direction of T waves, increased HR. In children, rebound hypertension following slow withdrawal. *GI:* N&V. *CNS:* Headache, fatigue. *Hypersensitivity:* Rashes, including bullous eruptions and ***Stevens-Johnson syndrome.*** *Hematologic:* Initially, decrease in hematocrit, hemoglobin, and erythrocyte count but all return to normal. Rarely, thrombocytopenia and leukopenia. *Other:* Hypertrichosis (enhanced hair growth, pigmentation and thickening of fine body hair 3–6 weeks after initiation of therapy), breast tenderness, darkening of skin.

**OD** **Overdose Management:** *Symptoms:* Excessive hypotension. *Treatment:* Give NSS IV (to maintain BP and urine output). Vasopressors, such as phenylephrine and dopamine, can be used but only in underperfusion of a vital organ.

**Drug Interactions:** Concomitant use with guanethidine may result in severe hypotension.

**Laboratory Test Interferences:** Nonspecific changes in ECG. ↑ Alka-

M

line phosphatase, serum creatinine, and BUN.

## Dosage

• **Tablets**

*Hypertension.*

**Adults and children over 12 years, Initial:** 5 mg/day. For optimum control, dose can be increased to 10, 20, and then 40 mg in single or divided doses/day. Daily dosage should not exceed 100 mg. **Children under 12 years: Initial,** 0.2 mg/kg/day. Effective dose range: 0.25–1.0 mg/kg/day. Dosage must be titrated to individual response. Daily dosage should not exceed 50 mg.

## NURSING CONSIDERATIONS

See also *Nursing Considerations* for *Antihypertensive Agents.*

**Administration/Storage**

1. Give once daily if the supine diastolic pressure has been reduced less than 30 mm Hg and twice daily (in two equal doses) if it has been reduced more than 30 mm Hg.

2. The interval between dosage adjustments should be at least 3 days as the full response is not obtained until then. However, if more rapid control is required, adjustments can be made q 6 hr but with careful monitoring.

**Assessment**

1. Anticipate BP decreases within 30 min.

2. List other agents trialed and the outcome. Note if diruetic prescribed.

3. Assess cardiopulmonary status.

4. Monitor CBC, glucose, electrolytes, and renal function studies.

**Client/Family Teaching**

1. Can be taken with fluids and without regard to meals.

2. Record weight daily; report any S&S of fluid overload (gain of 6 lb/week; edema of extremities, face, and abdomen; or dyspnea).

3. Report any symptoms of angina, fainting, dizziness, or dyspnea that occurs, especially when lying down.

4. Drug may cause elongation, thickening, and increased pigmentation of body hair, but a return to

pretreatment norm should occur once discontinued.

**Outcomes/Evaluate:** ↓ BP; control of hypertension

# Minoxidil, topical solution

(mih-**NOX**-ih-dill)
**Pregnancy Category:** C
Apo-Gain ✿, Gen-Minoxidil ✿, Minoxigaine ✿, Rogaine, Rogaine Extra Strength for Men **(Rx) (OTC)**
**Classification:** Hair growth stimulant

**Action/Kinetics:** Minoxidil topical solution stimulates vertex hair growth in clients with male pattern baldness. Mechanism may be related to dilation of arterioles and stimulation of resting hair follicles into active growth. Following topical administration, approximately 1.4% is absorbed into the systemic circulation. **Onset:** 4 months but is variable. **Duration:** New hair growth may be lost 3–4 months after withdrawal of therapy. Minoxidil and its inactive metabolites are excreted in the urine. Also, see *Minoxidil, oral.*

**Uses:** To treat male and female pattern baldness (alopecia androgenetica). Extra Strength (5%) is only for treatment of hereditary male pattern baldness. *Investigational:* Alopecia areata.

**Contraindications:** Lactation.

**Special Concerns:** Use with caution in clients with hypertension, coronary heart disease, or predisposition to heart failure. Safety and efficacy in clients under 18 years of age have not been determined. Increased systemic absorption may occur if the scalp is irritated or there are abrasions.

**Side Effects:** *Dermatologic:* Allergic contact dermatitis, irritant dermatitis, pruritus, dry skin, flaking of scalp, alopecia, hypertrichosis, erythema, worsening of hair loss. *Allergic:* Hives, facial swelling, allergic rhinitis. *CNS:* Dizziness, lightheadedness, headache, faintness, anxiety, depression, fatigue. *Respiratory:* Sinusitis, bronchitis, respiratory infection. *Mis-*

*cellaneous:* Conjunctivitis, decreased visual acuity, vertigo. *NOTE:* The incidence of side effects due to placebos is often similar to the incidence of side effects due to the drug itself.

**Drug Interactions**
*Corticosteroids, topical* / Enhance absorption of topical minoxidil
*Guanethidine* / Possible ↑ risk of orthostatic hypotension
*Petrolatum* / Enhances absorption of topical minoxidil
*Retinoids* / Enhance absorption of topical minoxidil

**Dosage**
• **Topical Solution: 2%, 5%**
*Stimulate hair growth.*
**Adults:** Apply 1 mL b.i.d. directly onto the scalp in the hair loss area. 5% solution not to be used on women.

**NURSING CONSIDERATIONS**
**Administration/Storage**
1. Only clients with normal, healthy scalps should use topical minoxidil. Dermatitis, scalp abrasions, scalp psoriasis, or severe sunburn may increase the absorption of topical minoxidil and lead to systemic side effects (See *Minoxidil, oral*).
2. Hair may be shampooed before treatment, but dry the hair and scalp prior to topical application.
3. The product comes with a metered spray attachment (for application to large areas of the scalp), extender spray attachment (for application to small scalp areas or under the hair), and a rub-on applicator tip (to spread the solution on the scalp). Follow the directions on the package insert carefully for each of these methods of application.
4. If the fingertips are used to apply the drug, wash the hands thoroughly after application.
5. At least 4 months of continuous therapy is necessary before evidence of hair growth can be expected. Further hair growth continues through 1 year of treatment.
6. The alcohol base in topical minoxidil will cause irritation and

burning of the eyes, abraded skin, or mucous membranes. If contact with any of these areas, wash the site with copious amounts of water.
7. Avoid inhaling the spray mist.

**Client/Family Teaching**
1. Review appropriate method and frequency for application; solution may dry and leave a residue on the hair, this is harmless.
2. More frequent than prescribed applications will not enhance hair growth but will increase systemic side effects. Review info booklet.
3. New hair growth will be soft and hard to see and is not permanent. Drug is a treatment, not a cure; cessation of therapy will lead to hair loss within a few months. Topical minoxidil must be used for an indefinite time period to sustain the effect.
4. Treatment has positive benefits for only approximately one-half the population. May take up to 4 months of continuous therapy before any response is noted.
5. Report any evidence of irritation or rash.
6. Do not apply any other topical products to the scalp without approval.
7. Consult provider before using if no family history of gradual hair loss, if hair loss is sudden or patchy, if hair loss is accompanied by other symptoms, or if the reasons for hair loss are not clear.

**Outcomes/Evaluate:** Stimulation of hair growth

# Mirtazapine
(mir-**TAZ**-ah-peen)
**Pregnancy Category:** C
Remeron **(Rx)**
**Classification:** Antidepressant, tetracyclic

See also *Antidepressants.*
**Action/Kinetics:** Enhances central noradrenergic and serotonergic activity, perhaps by antagonism at central presynaptic alpha-2 adrenergic inhibitory autoreceptors and het-

eroreceptors. Also a potent antagonist of 5-HT$_2$, 5-HT$_3$ and histamine H$_1$ receptors. Moderate antagonist of peripheral alpha-1 adrenergic receptors and muscarinic receptors. Rapidly and completely absorbed from the GI tract. **Peak plasma levels:** Within 2 hr. **t½:** 20–40 hr. Extensively metabolized in the liver and excreted in both the urine (75%) and feces (15%). Females exhibit significantly longer elimination half-lives than males.

**Uses:** Treatment of depression.

**Contraindications:** Use in combination with a MAO inhibitor or within 14 days of initiating or discontinuing therapy with a MAO inhibitor.

**Special Concerns:** Use with caution in those with impaired renal or hepatic disease, in geriatric clients, during lactation, in CV or cerebrovascular disease that can be exacerbated by hypotension (e.g., history of MI, angina, ischemic stroke), and in conditions that would predispose to hypotension (e.g., dehydration, hypovolemia, treatment with antihypertensive medications). The effect of mirtazapine for longer than 6 weeks has not been evaluated, although treatment is indicated for 6 months or longer. Safety and efficacy have not been determined in children.

**Side Effects:** Side effects with an incidence of 0.1% or greater are listed. *CNS:* Somnolence, dizziness, activation of mania or hypomania, suicidal ideation, sedation, drowsiness, abnormal dreams, abnormal thinking, tremor, confusion, hypesthesia, apathy, depression, hypokinesia, vertigo, twitching, agitation, anxiety, amnesia, hyperkinesia, paresthesia, ataxia, delirium, delusions, depersonalization, dyskinesia, extrapyramidal syndrome, increased libido, abnormal coordination, dysarthria, hallucinations, neurosis, dystonia, hostility, increased reflexes, emotional lability, euphoria, paranoid reaction. *GI:* N&V, anorexia, dry mouth, constipation, ulcer, eructation, glossitis, cholecystitis, gum hemorrhage, stomatitis, colitis, abnor-

mal liver function tests. *CV:* Hypertension, vasodilation, angina pectoris, **MI,** bradycardia, ventricular extrasystoles, syncope, migraine, hypotension. *Hematologic:* Agranulocytosis. *Body as a whole:* Asthenia, flu syndrome, back pain, malaise, abdominal pain, acute abdominal syndrome, chills, fever, facial edema, photosensitivity reaction, neck rigidity, neck pain, enlarged abdomen. *Respiratory:* Dyspnea, increased cough, sinusitis, epistaxis, bronchitis, asthma, pneumonia. *GU:* Urinary frequency, UTI, kidney calculus, cystitis, dysuria, urinary incontinence, urinary retention, vaginitis, hematuria, breast pain, amenorrhea, dysmenorrhea, leukorrhea, impotence. *Musculoskeletal:* Myalgia, myasthenia, arthralgia, arthritis, tenosynovitis. *Dermatologic:* Pruritus, rash, acne, exfoliative dermatitis, dry skin, herpes simplex, alopecia. *Metabolic/nutritional:* Increased appetite, weight gain, peripheral edema, edema, thirst, dehydration, weight loss. *Ophthalmic:* Eye pain, abnormal accommodation, conjunctivitis, keratoconjunctivitis, lacrimation disorder, glaucoma. *Miscellaneous:* Deafness, hyperacusis, ear pain.

**OD** **Overdose Management:** *Symptoms:* Disorientation, drowsiness, impaired memory, tachycardia. *Treatment:* General supportive measures. If the client is unconscious, establish and maintain an airway. Consider induction of emesis or gastric lavage and administration of activated charcoal. Monitor cardiac and vital signs.

**Drug Interactions**
*Alcohol* / Additive impairment of motor skills
*Diazepam* / Additive impairment of motor skills

**Laboratory Test Interferences:** ALT and nonfasting cholesterol and triglycerides.

**Dosage** ————————
• **Tablets**
*Treatment of depression.*

**Initial:** 15 mg/day given as a single dose, preferably in the evening before sleep. Those not responding to the 15-mg dose may respond to doses up to a maximum of 45 mg/day. Do not make dose changes at intervals of less than 1 to 2 weeks. Consider treatment for up to 6 months.

## NURSING CONSIDERATIONS

See also *Nursing Considerations* for *Antidepressants*.

**Assessment**

1. Document indications, onset, duration, and symptom characteristics.
2. Note precipitating events that may relate to depression, i.e., death, divorce, illness, or job loss.
3. List drugs currently and previously prescribed to ensure no MAO inhibitor use within past 2 weeks.
4. Monitor ECG, CBC, LFTs, cholesterol, and triglyceride levels.

**Client/Family Teaching**

1. Take as directed; do not exceed prescribed dosing schedule.
2. Report any S&S of infection or flu (fever, sore throat, stomatitis, etc.); drug may cause agranulocytosis.
3. Do not engage in activities that require mental alertness until drug effects realized; dizziness and drowsiness may occur.
4. Avoid alcohol and OTC agents; may potentiate drug's cognitive and motor skill impairment.
5. Report as scheduled for follow-up labs and evaluation of clinical response to drug therapy.

**Outcomes/Evaluate:** Improved sleeping and eating patterns; less anxiety, ↓ agitation; improved mood, ↑ interest in social activities

## Misoprostol

(my-soh-**PROST**-ohl)
**Pregnancy Category:** X
Cytotec **(Rx)**
**Classification:** Prostaglandin

**Action/Kinetics:** Synthetic prostaglandin $E_1$ analog that inhibits gastric acid secretion, protects the gastric mucosa by increasing bicarbonate and mucous production, and decreases pepsin levels during basal conditions. May also stimulate uterine contractions that may endanger pregnancy. Rapidly converted to the active misoprostol acid. **Time for peak levels of misoprostol acid:** 12 min. **t½, misoprostol acid:** 20–40 min. Misoprostol acid is less than 90% bound to plasma protein. *NOTE:* Misoprostol does not prevent development of duodenal ulcers in clients on NSAIDs.

**Uses:** Prevention of aspirin and other nonsteroidal anti-inflammatory-induced gastric ulcers in clients with a high risk of gastric ulcer complications (e.g., geriatric clients with debilitating disease) or in those with a history of ulcer. *Investigational:* Treat duodenal ulcers including those unresponsive to histamine $H_2$ antagonists. With cyclosporine and prednisone to decrease the incidence of acute graft rejection in renal transplant clients (the drug improves renal function).

**Contraindications:** Allergy to prostaglandins, pregnancy, during lactation (may cause diarrhea in nursing infants).

**Special Concerns:** Use with caution in clients with renal impairment and in clients older than 64 years of age. Safety and efficacy have not been established in children less than 18 years of age. Misoprostol may cause miscarriage with potentially serious bleeding.

**Side Effects:** *GI:* Diarrhea, abdominal pain, nausea, dyspepsia, flatulence, vomiting, constipation. *Gynecologic:* Spotting, cramps, dysmenorrhea, hypermenorrhea, menstrual disorders, postmenopausal vaginal bleeding. *Miscellaneous:* Headache.

**OD Overdose Management:** *Symptoms:* Abdominal pain, diarrhea, dyspnea, sedation, tremor, fever, palpitations, bradycardia, hypotension, *seizures. Treatment:* Use supportive therapy.

**M**

---

✦ = Available in Canada          ***bold italic*** = life threatening side effect

## Dosage
• **Tablets**

**Adults:** 200 mcg q.i.d. with food. Dose can be reduced to 100 mcg if the larger dose cannot be tolerated. In renal impairment, the 200-mcg dose can be reduced if necessary.

## NURSING CONSIDERATIONS

### Administration/Storage
1. Reduce diarrhea by giving after meals and at bedtime; avoid magnesium-containing antacids. Diarrhea is usually self-limiting.
2. Maximum plasma levels are decreased if drug is taken with food.
3. Take for the duration of NSAID therapy.
4. Drug may increase gastric bicarbonate and mucous production.

### Assessment
1. Obtain a negative pregnancy test on females of childbearing age.
2. Document any ulcer disease; assess GI symptoms and clinical presentation.

### Client/Family Teaching
1. Do not share medications.
2. Avoid foods/spices that may aggravate condition: caffeine, alcohol, and black pepper.
3. Take misoprostol exactly as prescribed for the duration of aspirin or NSAID therapy.
4. May experience abdominal discomfort and/or diarrhea; take misoprostol after meals and at bedtime to minimize these side effects.
5. Report persistent diarrhea or increased menstrual bleeding.
6. All women of childbearing age must practice effective contraceptive measures; drug has abortifacient properties.

**Outcomes/Evaluate:** Prevention of drug-induced gastric ulcers

# Mitomycin
(my-toe-**MY**-sin)
Mutamycin (Abbreviation: MTC) **(Rx)**
**Classification:** Antineoplastic, antibiotic

See also *Antineoplastic Agents.*

**Action/Kinetics:** Antibiotic produced by *Streptomyces caespitosus* that inhibits DNA synthesis. At high doses both RNA and protein synthesis are inhibited. Most active during late $G_1$ and early S stages. Not recommended as a single agent for primary treatment or in place of surgery and/or radiotherapy. **t½, initial:** 5–15 min; **final:** 50 min. Metabolized in liver; 10% excreted unchanged in urine, more when dose is increased.

**Uses:** Palliative treatment and adjunct to surgical or radiologic treatment of disseminated adenocarcinoma of the stomach and pancreas. Used in combination with other agents. *Investigational:* Superficial bladder cancer; cancer of the breast, head and neck, lung, cervix; colorectal cancer; biliary cancer; chronic myelocytic leukemia. Ophthalmic solution used as an adjunct to surgical excision to treat primary or recurrent pterygia.

**Contraindications:** Pregnancy and lactation. Thrombocytopenia, coagulation disorders, increase in bleeding tendency due to other causes. In clients with a serum creatinine level greater than 1.7 mg/dL.

**Special Concerns:** Use with extreme caution in presence of impaired renal function.

**Additional Side Effects:** *Severe bone marrow depression, especially leukopenia and thrombocytopenia.* Pulmonary toxicity including dyspnea with nonproductive cough. *Microangiopathic hemolytic anemia with renal failure and hypertension (hemolytic uremic syndrome),* especially when used long-term in combination with fluorouracil. Cellulitis. Extravasation causes severe necrosis of surrounding tissue. *Respiratory distress syndrome in adults, especially when used with other chemotherapy.*

**Drug Interactions:** Severe bronchospasm and SOB when used with vinca alkaloids.

## Dosage
• **IV Only**
10–20 mg/m² as a single dose via in-

fusion q 6–8 wk. Subsequent courses of treatment are based on hematologic response and should not be repeated until leukocyte count is at least 4,000/mm³ and platelet count is at least 100,000/mm³.

## NURSING CONSIDERATIONS

See also *Nursing Considerations* for *Antineoplastic Agents.*

**Administration/Storage**

**IV** 1. Drug is toxic; avoid extravasation. Observe infusion site closely for evidence of erythema or complaints of discomfort. Apply ice and use thiosulfate for infiltrate.

2. Reconstitute 5-, 20-, or 40-mg vial with 10, 40, or 80 mL sterile water for injection, respectively, as indicated on label and administer over 5–10 min. Medication will dissolve if allowed to remain at room temperature.

3. Drug at concentration of 0.5 mg/mL is stable for 14 days under refrigeration or for 7 days at room temperature.

4. Diluted to a concentration of 20–40 mcg/mL, the drug is stable for 3 hr in D5W, for 12 hr in isotonic saline, and for 24 hr in sodium lactate injection.

5. Mitomycin (5–15 mg) and heparin (1,000–10,000 units) in 30 mL of isotonic saline is stable for 48 hr at room temperature.

**Assessment**

1. Document pulmonary function. Obtain CXR; pulmonary infiltrates and fibrosis can occur with cumulative doses. Observe closely for early evidence of pulmonary complications, such as dyspnea, nonproductive cough, and abnormal lung sounds and ABGs.

2. Obtain baseline CBC, PT, PTT, and renal function; do not initiate if serum creatinine level is greater than 1.7 mg/dL. Drug may cause platelet and granulocyte suppression. Nadir: 28 days; recovery: 40–55 days.

**Outcomes/Evaluate:**  ↓ Tumor size/spread

# Mitotane (O,P'-DDD)

(**MY**-toe-tayn)

**Pregnancy Category:** C

Lysodren **(Rx)**

**Classification:** Antineoplastic, antihormone

See also *Antineoplastic Agents.*

**Action/Kinetics:** Directly suppresses activity of adrenal cortex and changes the peripheral metabolism of corticosteroids, resulting in a decrease in 17-hydroxycorticosteroids. About 40% absorbed from GI tract; detectable in serum for 6–9 weeks after administration. Mostly stored in adipose tissue. **t½:** After therapy terminated, 18–159 days. Unchanged drug is excreted in the feces while metabolites are excreted in the urine. Steroid replacement therapy may have to be instituted (i.e., increased) to correct adrenal insufficiency. Therapy is continued as long as drug seems effective. Beneficial results may not become apparent until after 3 months of therapy.

**Uses:** Inoperable carcinoma (both functional and nonfunctional) of the adrenal cortex. *Investigational:* Cushing's syndrome.

**Contraindications:** Hypersensitivity to drug. Discontinue temporarily after shock or severe trauma. Lactation.

**Special Concerns:** Use with caution in the presence of liver disease other than metastatic lesions. Longterm usage may cause brain damage and functional impairment. Use during lactation only if benefits outweigh risks.

**Side Effects:** *CNS:* Continuous doses may result in brain damage and impairment of function. Depression, lethargy, somnolence, dizziness, vertigo. *GI:* N&V, anorexia, diarrhea. *CV:* Hypertension, orthostatic hypotension, flushing. *Dermatologic:* Transient skin rashes. *Ophthalmic:* Visual blurring, diplopia, lens opacity, toxic retinopathy. *GU:* Hematuria, hemorrhagic cystitis, albuminuria.

**M**

---

*Miscellaneous:* Adrenal insufficiency, generalized aching, hyperpyrexia. **Additional Side Effects:** Adrenal insufficiency. *CNS:* Depression, sedation, vertigo, lethargy. *Ophthalmic:* Blurring, diplopia, retinopathy, opacity of lens. *Renal:* Hemorrhagic cystitis, hematuria, proteinuria. *CV:* Flushing, orthostatic hypotension, hypertension. *Miscellaneous:* Hyperpyrexia, skin rashes, aching of body.

**Drug Interactions**

*Corticosteroids* / ↑ Metabolism of corticosteroids resulting in need for higher doses

*Warfarin* / Mitotane may ↑ rate of metabolism of warfarin, requiring an increase of dosage

**Laboratory Test Interferences:** ↓ PBI and urinary 17-hydroxycorticosteroids.

**Dosage**
- **Tablets**
  *Carcinoma of the adrenal cortex.*
  **Adults, initial:** 2–6 g/day in three to four equally divided doses (maximum tolerated dose may range from 2 to 16 g/day). Adjust dosage upward or downward according to severity of side effects or lack thereof. **Pediatric, initial:** 1–2 g/day in divided doses; **then,** dose can be increased gradually to 5–7 g/day.
  *Cushing's syndrome.*
  **Initial:** 3–6 g/day in three to four divided doses; **then,** 0.5 mg 2 times/week to 2 g/day.

## NURSING CONSIDERATIONS

See also *Nursing Considerations* for *Antineoplastic Agents.*

**Administration/Storage**

1. Initiate in hospital until stable dosage schedule is achieved.

2. Continue treatment for 3 months. If no beneficial effects are noted after 3 months at the maximum tolerated dose, a clinical failure can be concluded.

3. To counteract shock or trauma, be prepared to administer steroid medications in high doses; depressed adrenals may not produce sufficient steroids.

**Assessment**

1. Note any sensitivity to mitotane; document any episodes of shock or severe trauma that would necessitate discontinuation of drug therapy.

2. Assess for evidence of brain damage by performing behavioral and neurologic assessments.

**Client/Family Teaching**

1. Report any symptoms of adrenal insufficiency, such as weakness, increased fatigue, lethargy, and GI effects (including weight loss, N&V, and anorexia).

2. Always wear identification in case of trauma or shock; carry list of drugs currently prescribed.

3. Avoid tasks that require mental alertness until drug effects are realized.

4. Desired effects may not be evident for 3 months. If none noted after 3 months at the maximum tolerated dosage, drug will be stopped and a clinical failure concluded.

5. Avoid situations that may cause injury or exposure to infections.

**Outcomes/Evaluate**
- ↓ Tumor size and spread
- Desired cortisol levels

# Mitoxantrone hydrochloride

(my-toe-**ZAN**-trohn)
**Pregnancy Category:** D
Novantrone **(Rx)**
**Classification:** Antineoplastic agent, antibiotic

See also *Antineoplastic Agents.*

**Action/Kinetics:** Most active in the late S phase of cell division but is not cell-cycle specific. Appears to bind to DNA by intercalation between base pairs and a nonintercalative electrostatic interaction, causing an inhibition of DNA and RNA synthesis. Distribution to tissues such as the brain, spinal cord, spinal fluid, and eyes is low. **t½:** Approximately 6 days. Highly bound to plasma proteins. Excreted through both the feces (via the bile) and the urine (up to 65% unchanged).

**Uses:** In combination with other drugs, for the initial treatment of acute nonlymphocytic leukemias, including monocytic, promyelocytic, myelocytic, and acute erythroid leukemias. In combination with steroids to treat pain from advanced hormone-refractory prostate cancer. *Investigational:* Alone or in combination with other drugs to treat breast and liver cancer; non-Hodgkin's lymphomas.

**Contraindications:** Preexisting myelosuppression (unless benefits outweigh risks). Lactation. Intrathecal use.

**Special Concerns:** Safety and efficacy have not been established in children. May be mutagenic.

**Side Effects:** *Hematologic:* Severe myelosuppression, ecchymosis, petechiae. *GI:* N&V, diarrhea, stomatitis, mucositis, abdominal pain, GI bleeding. *CNS:* Headache, seizures. *CV:* CHF, decreases in LV ejection fraction, arrhythmias, tachycardia, chest pain, hypotension. *Respiratory:* Cough, dyspnea. *Miscellaneous:* Conjunctivitis, urticaria, rashes, renal failure, hyperuricemia, alopecia, fever, phlebitis (at infusion site), tissue necrosis (as a result of extravasation), jaundice. In addition, there is an increased risk of pneumonia, urinary tract and fungal infections, and sepsis.

**OD** **Overdose Management:** *Symptoms:* Severe leukopenia with infection. *Treatment:* Antibiotic therapy. Monitor hematology.

**Laboratory Test Interferences:** Transient ↑ AST and ALT.

**Dosage** —————————
• **IV Infusion**
*Initial therapy for acute nonlymphocytic leukemia, induction.*
Mitoxantrone, 12 mg/m²/day on days 1–3 combined with cytosine arabinoside, 100 mg/m² as a continuous 24-hr infusion on days 1–7. If the response is incomplete, a second induction course may be given using the same daily dosage, but giving mitoxantrone for 2 days and cytosine arabinoside for 5 days. *Consolidation therapy, approximately 6 weeks after final induction therapy:* mitoxantrone, 12 mg/m²/day on days 1 and 2 combined with cytosine arabinoside, 100 mg/m² as a continuous 24-hr infusion on days 1–5. A second consolidation course of therapy may be given 4 weeks after the first.

---

## NURSING CONSIDERATIONS

See also *Nursing Considerations* for *Antineoplastic Agents.*
### Administration/Storage
**IV** 1. Do not mix in the same infusion with other drugs.
2. Must be diluted prior to use with at least 50 mL of either 5% dextrose injection or 0.9% NaCl injection.
3. Give diluted solution into a freely running IV infusion of either 5% dextrose injection or 0.9% NaCl over at least 3 min.
4. Avoid extravasation at the injection site. Do not allow contact with the eyes, mucous membranes, or skin.
5. Do not freeze.
6. Closely follow hospital procedures for the handling and disposal of antineoplastic drugs.
### Assessment
1. Note any cardiac disease; perform baseline ECG and assess for symptoms of cardiotoxicity.
2. Anticipate N&V, mucositis, and stomatitis; initiate appropriate protocol. Assess need for allopurinol therapy.
3. Monitor VS, CBC, uric acid, liver and renal function studies. Drug may cause granulocyte and platelet suppression. Nadir: 10–14 days; recovery: 21 days.
### Client/Family Teaching
1. Drug may temporarily discolor urine and/or sclera greenish blue for 24 hr after therapy.
2. Report any persistent diarrhea, N&V, abnormal bruising and bleeding, severe dyspnea, or evidence of infection.

**M**

---

3. Consume 2–3 L/day of fluids to prevent hyperuricemia.

4. Avoid vaccinia and crowds, especially during flu season.

5. Practice reliable contraception.

**Outcomes/Evaluate:** Improved hematologic parameters; suppression of malignant cell proliferation

---

# Mivacurium chloride
(mih-vah-**KYOUR**-ee-um)
**Pregnancy Category:** C
Mivacron **(Rx)**
**Classification:** Neuromuscular blocking agent

See also *Neuromuscular Blocking Agents.*

**Action/Kinetics:** Competitively inhibits the action of acetylcholine on the motor end plate, resulting in a block of neuromuscular transmission. Time to maximum neuromuscular blockade is similar to atracurium (2.3–4.9 min in adults depending on the dose and 1.6–2.8 min in children depending on the dose). **Clinically effective neuromuscular block, adults:** 15–20 min after 0.15 mg/kg; **children:** 6–15 min after 0.2 mg/kg. Spontaneous recovery may be 95% complete in 25–30 min after an initial dose of 0.15 mg/kg in adults during opioid/nitrous oxide/oxygen anesthesia. Repeated administration or continuous infusion (for up to 2.5 hr) does not cause tachyphylaxis or cumulative neuromuscular blockade. Higher doses may cause transient decreases in mean arterial BP (especially seen in obese clients) and increases in HR in some clients within 1–3 min following the dose (can be minimized by giving the drug over 30–60 sec). The product is actually a mixture of isomers with varying elimination half-lives. Inactivated by plasma cholinesterase with metabolites excreted in the urine and bile.

**Uses:** Adjunct to general anesthesia to facilitate tracheal intubation and to provide relaxation of skeletal muscle during surgery or mechanical ventilation.

**Contraindications:** Sensitivity to mivacurium or other similar agents. Use of multidose vials in clients with allergy to benzyl alcohol.

**Special Concerns:** Use with caution during lactation. Use with caution in clients with significant CV disease and in those with any history of a greater sensitivity to the release of histamine or related mediators such as asthma. Volatile anesthetics may decrease the dosing requirement and prolong the duration of action. The duration of action of mivacurium may be prolonged in clients with decreased plasma cholinesterase. Reduced clearance of one or more isomers is observed in clients with end-stage kidney or liver disease. Geriatric clients show a longer duration of neuromuscular blockade. Acid-base or serum electrolyte abnormalities may potentiate or antagonize the action of neuromuscular blocking agents. Antagonism of neuromuscular blockade may be delayed in the presence of debilitation, carcinomatosis, and concomitant use of certain broad-spectrum antibiotics, anesthetic agents, and other drugs that enhance neuromuscular blockade. In children 2–12 years of age, mivacurium has a faster onset, shorter duration, and a faster recovery following reversal than adults. The drug has not been studied in children less than 2 years of age.

**Side Effects:** *Neuromuscular:* Prolonged neuromuscular blockade, muscle spasms. *CV:* Flushing of face, neck, or chest; hypotension, tachycardia, bradycardia, cardiac arrhythmias, phlebitis. *Respiratory:* **Bronchospasm,** wheezing, hypoxemia. *Dermatologic:* Rash, urticaria, erythema, reaction at injection site. *CNS:* Dizziness.

**OD** **Overdose Management:** *Symptoms:* Neuromuscular blockade beyond the time needed for surgery and anesthesia. Increased risk of hemodynamic side effects such as hypotension. *Treatment:*

• Primary treatment is maintenance of a patent airway and controlled ventilation until there is recovery of normal neuromuscular function.

• Neostigmine (0.03–0.064 mg/kg) or edrophonium (0.5 mg/kg) can be given once there is evidence of recovery from neuromuscular blockade.

• A peripheral nerve stimulator can be used to assess recovery and antagonism of neuromuscular block.

**Drug Interactions**

See *Neuromuscular Blocking Agents.*

Also, there is enhanced neuromuscular blockade when magnesium is given to pregnant women for toxemia.

**Dosage**
• **IV Only**
*Facilitation of tracheal intubation.*

**Adults:** 0.15 mg/kg given over 5–15 sec. Maintenance doses of 0.1 mg/kg provide about 15 min of additional clinically effective blockade.

**Children, 2–12 years:** The dosage requirements on a mg/kg basis are higher in children and onset and recovery occur more rapidly. **Initial:** 0.2 mg/kg given over 5–15 sec.

*Facilitation of tracheal intubation using continuous IV infusion.*

Continuous IV infusion may be used to maintain neuromuscular block.

**Adults:** On evidence of spontaneous recovery from an initial dose, an initial infusion rate of 9–10 mcg/kg/min is recommended. If continuous infusion is started at the same time as the administration of an initial dose, a lower initial infusion rate (such as 4 mcg/kg/min) should be used. In either case, the initial infusion rate should be adjusted according to the response to peripheral nerve stimulation and to clinical criteria. An average infusion rate of 6–7 mcg/kg/min will maintain neuromuscular block within the range of 89%–99% for extended periods of time in adults receiving opioid/nitrous oxide/oxygen anesthesia.

**Children:** Require higher infusion rates. During opioid/nitrous oxide/

oxygen anesthesia, the infusion rate needed to maintain 89%–99% blockade averages 14 mcg/kg/min (range: 5–31 mcg/kg/min).

*Tracheal intubation in clients with renal or hepatic impairment.*

0.15 mg/kg. Infusion rates should be decreased by as much as 50% in these clients depending on the degree of renal or hepatic impairment.

*Use in clients with reduced cholinesterase activity.*

Initial doses greater than 0.03 mg/kg are not recommended.

*Use in clients who are cachectic, are debilitated, or have carcinomatosis or neuromuscular disease.*

A test dose of 0.015–0.02 mg/kg is recommended.

*Use with isoflurane or enflurane anesthesia.*

An initial dose of 0.15 mg/kg may be used for intubation prior to administration of the isoflurane or enflurane. If mivacurium is given after establishment of anesthesia, the initial dose should be reduced by as much as 25% and the infusion rate should be decreased by as much as 35%–40%. When used with halothane, no adjustment of the initial dose is necessary but the infusion rate should be decreased by as much as 20%.

*Use in burn clients.*

A test dose of not more than 0.015–0.02 mg/kg is recommended, followed by additional dosing guided by the use of a neuromuscular block monitor.

*Use in obese clients weighing equal to or greater than 30% more than their ideal body weight (IBW).*

The initial dose is calculated using the IBW according to the following formulas:

Men: IBW in kg = $(106 + [6 \times$ height in inches above 5 ft])/2.2

Women: IBW in kg = $(100 + [5 \times$ height in inches above 5 ft])/2.2

*Use in clients with clinically significant CV disease or in those with any history of a greater sensitivity to the release of histamine or related mediators (asthma).*

**M**

An initial dose less than or equal to 0.15 mg/kg given over 60 sec.

## NURSING CONSIDERATIONS

See also *Nursing Considerations* for *Neuromuscular Blocking Agents*.

### Administration/Storage

**IV** 1. Give only in carefully adjusted dosage under the supervision of trained clinicians who know the action of the drug as well as possible complications from its use. Have resuscitative equipment readily available.

2. For adults and children, the amount of infusion solution required per hour depends on the clinical requirements, the concentration of mivacurium in the infusion solution, and the weight of the client. Consult tables provided by the manufacturer to determine the infusion rates using either the premixed infusion of 0.5 mg/mL or the injection containing 2 mg/mL.

3. Dosage adjustment may be necessary in the presence of significant liver, kidney, or CV disease; in obese clients weighing more than 30% of their ideal body weight for height; asthma; those with reduced plasma cholinesterase activity; and the use of inhalation general anesthetics.

4. Do not introduce additives into mivacurium premixed infusion in flexible plastic containers.

5. Ensure the premixed infusion is clear and the container undamaged. Is for single-client use only; discard any unused portion.

6. Vials (2 mg/mL) may be diluted to 0.5 mg/mL with 5% dextrose injection, 5% dextrose/0.9% NaCl, 0.9% NaCl, RL injection, or 5% dextrose/RL and then given by Y-site injection and titrated to desired response. The dilution is stable when stored in PVC bags at 5°C–25°C (41°F–77°F). Use the dilution within 24 hr; it is for single-client use only; discard any unused portion.

7. Injection is compatible with sufentanil citrate injection, alfentanil hydrochloride injection, fentanyl citrate injection, midazolam hydrochloride injection, and droperidol injection. However, it may not be compatible with alkaline solutions having a pH greater than 8.5 (e.g., barbiturate solutions).

8. The injection and premixed infusion are stored at 15°C–25°C (59°F–77°F). Avoid exposure to direct ultraviolet light; do not freeze or expose to excessive heat.

### Assessment

1. Note indications for therapy. Review conditions and drugs that antagonize and enhance neuromuscular blockade and assess for their presence.

2. Note any CV disease or asthma.

3. Monitor ABGs, electrolytes, liver and renal function studies; reduce dose with dysfunction.

4. Multidose vials contain benzyl alcohol; assess for intolerance.

5. Clients homozygous for the atypical plasma cholinesterase gene are quite sensitive to drugs' blocking effects.

6. Burn clients may show resistance depending on the time elapsed since the burn and the size of the burn; however, clients with burns may have decreased plasma cholinesterase, which offsets the resistance.

### Interventions

1. Administer in a carefully monitored environment by persons specially trained in the use of neuromuscular blocking agents.

2. To avoid distress, ensure client unconscious or sedated before administering mivacurium.

3. Use a peripheral nerve stimulator to measure neuromuscular function (assess response), adjust dosage, and confirm recovery (5-sec head lift and grip strength).

4. Geriatric clients show a longer duration of neuromuscular blockade.

5. Monitor VS. Mivacurium will not counteract the bradycardia produced by many anesthetic agents or by vagal stimulation.

6. Advise that transient flushing, wheezing, and tachycardia may be experienced.

## Outcomes/Evaluate
- Skeletal muscle relaxation
- Suppression of twitch response

# Moexipril hydrochloride
(moh-**EX**-ih-prill)
**Pregnancy Category:** C (first trimester), D (second and third trimesters)
Univasc **(Rx)**
**Classification:** Angiotensin-converting enzyme inhibitor

See also *Angiotensin-Converting Enzyme Inhibitors.*
**Action/Kinetics:** Converted in the liver to the active moexiprilat. **Onset:** 1 hr. **Duration:** 24 hr. Food decreases absorption of the drug. **t½, moexiprilat:** 2–9 hr. About 50% is bound to plasma protein. Active metabolite is excreted through both the urine and feces.
**Uses:** Treatment of hypertension alone or in combination with thiazide diuretics.
**Contraindications:** In those with a history of angioedema as a result of previous treatment with ACE inhibitors. Lactation.
**Special Concerns:** Use with caution in clients with impaired renal function or renal artery stenosis, hyperkalemia, CHF, severe hepatic impairment, and volume depletion. Those who are salt or volume depleted are at a greater risk of developing hypotension. Safety and efficacy have not been determined in children.
**Side Effects:** *GI:* Abdominal pain, N&V, diarrhea, dysgeusia, constipation, dry mouth, dyspepsia, pancreatitis, hepatitis, changes in appetite, weight changes. *CNS:* Insomnia, sleep disturbances, headache, dizziness, fatigue, drowsiness/sleepiness, malaise, nervousness, anxiety, mood changes. *CV:* Chest pain, hypotension, palpitations, angina pectoris, **CVA, MI,** orthostatic hypotension, rhythm disturbances, peripheral edema. *Respiratory:* Cough, bronchospasm, dyspnea, URI, sinusitis.

*GU:* Oliguria, urinary frequency, renal insufficiency. *Dermatologic:* Flushing, rash, diaphoresis, photosensitivity, pruritus, urticaria, pemphigus. *Musculoskeletal:* Myalgia, arthralgia. *Miscellaneous:* Angioedema, neutropenia, syncope, anemia, tinnitus, flu syndrome, pharyngitis, pain, rhinitis.
**Drug Interactions**
*Diuretics* / Excessive hypotension
*Lithium* / Moexipril ↑ serum levels of lithium → lithium toxicity
*Potassium-sparing diuretics* / ↑ Hyperkalemic effect of moexipril
*Potassium supplements* / ↑ Hyperkalemic effect of moexipril

**Dosage**
- **Tablets**
  *Hypertension.*
**Initial, adults not receiving diuretics:** 7.5 mg 1 hr before meals once daily. Dose is adjusted depending on response. **Maintenance:** 7.5–30 mg daily in one or two divided doses 1 hr before meals. **Initial, adults receiving diuretics:** Discontinue diuretic 2–3 days before beginning moexipril at a dose of 7.5 mg. If BP is not controlled, diuretic therapy can be resumed. If diuretic cannot be discontinued, give moexipril in an initial dose of 3.75 mg once daily 1 hr before meals. In those with impaired renal function, start with 3.75 mg once daily if creatinine clearance is less than 40 mL/min/1.73 m². The dose may be increased to a maximum of 15 mg/day.

## NURSING CONSIDERATIONS

See also *Nursing Considerations* for *Angiotensin-Converting Enzyme Inhibitors.*
**Assessment**
1. Document indications for therapy, onset of disease, other agents trialed and the outcome.
2. Assess for dehydration, CHF, or hyperkalemia.
3. Monitor ECG, electrolytes, liver and renal function studies; reduce dose with renal impairment.

---

✦ = Available in Canada                    ***bold italic*** = life threatening side effect

### Client/Family Teaching

1. Take on an empty stomach 1 hr before meals.
2. Rise slowly from a sitting or lying position; report any symptoms of persistent dizziness, lightheadedness, or fainting.
3. Seek help if angioedema (respiratory difficulty or swelling of lips, eyes, tongue, face, or extremities) or neutropenia (fever, sore throat) occurs.
4. Use reliable contraception;stop drug and report if pregnancy is suspected, as drug is harmful to fetus.
5. Do not take potassium supplements or use potassium-containing salt substitutes; drug may increase potassium levels.

**Outcomes/Evaluate:** ↓ BP

# Monoctanoin
(mahn-**OCK**-tah-noyn)
**Pregnancy Category:** C
Moctanin **(Rx)**
**Classification:** Solubilizer for gallstones

**Action/Kinetics:** A semisynthetic esterified glycerol that causes complete dissolution of gallstones in approximately one-third of treated clients, with an additional one-third manifesting a decrease in the size of stones. The decreased size may allow the stone to pass spontaneously.

**Uses:** To solubilize cholesterol gallstones located in the biliary tract, especially when other treatments have failed or cannot be undertaken. Most effective if the stones are radiolucent.

**Contraindications:** Biliary tract infection, recent duodenal ulcer or jejunitis, clinical jaundice, impaired hepatic function, acute pancreatitis, porto-systemic shunting, or any active life-threatening problems that would be complicated by perfusion into the biliary tract.

**Special Concerns:** Use with caution during lactation. Safety and effectiveness in children have not been established.

**Side Effects:** *GI:* Irritation of GI and biliary tracts, ascending cholangitis, erythema in antral and duodenal mucosa, ulceration or irritation of the mucosa of the common bile duct, increased fistula drainage, duodenal erosion, abdominal pain or discomfort, N&V, diarrhea, indigestion, anorexia, burning epigastrium, bile shock. *CNS:* Fever, fatigue, lethargy, depression, headache. *Other:* Leukopenia, pruritus, chills, diaphoresis, hypokalemia, intolerance, allergic symptoms.

**Laboratory Test Interferences:** ↑ Serum amylase.

### Dosage

• **Infusion via Catheter Inserted into Common Bile Duct**
    *Cholesterol gallstones.*
Perfuse at rate not to exceed 3–5 mL/hr at a pressure of 10 cm water (to minimize irritation) for 7–21 days.

## NURSING CONSIDERATIONS
### Administration/Storage

1. Do not administer drug IM or IV.
2. For maximum effects, maintain drug at a temperature of 37°C (98.6°F).
3. To reduce viscosity and enhance the bathing effect on stones, add the 13 mL of sterile water for injection to each 120-mL vial.
4. Perfusion pressure should never exceed 15 cm water (use overflow manometer or peristaltic pump).
5. Continue the perfusion for approximately 9–10 days after which conduct X-ray or endoscopy studies. If tests do not show a reduction in size or dissolution of stones, discontinue the drug.
6. If abdominal pain, nausea, vomiting, or diarrhea occurs, stop the perfusion for 1 hr, aspirate the duct, and restart the infusion. If symptoms persist, stop the perfusion for 1 hr, aspirate the duct, and restart the infusion at a reduced rate of 3 mL/hr. If symptoms still persist, temporarily discontinue the ˙perfusion during meals.
7. Irritation of the GI and biliary tracts may occur. These usually disappear within 2–7 days after the termination of therapy.

8. Intended only for direct biliary duct infusion.

9. If stored below 15°C (59°F), the preparation may be a semisolid. To reliquify, heat to 21°C–27°C (70°F–80°F) and then store at a room temperature of 15°C–30°C (59°F–86°F).

**Assessment**

1. Note any history of biliary tract infection or recent duodenal ulcer.

2. Assess for hepatic or renal dysfunction.

**Interventions**

1. Report any complaints of GI irritation.

2. Test stools for blood.

3. Report any evidence of fever, lethargy, depression, pruritus, diaphoresis, and hypokalemia.

4. Maintain patent tubes and asepsis with dressing and site care.

**Outcomes/Evaluate:** Dissolution/↓ size of gallstones with freedom from complication of prolonged bile duct infusion

# Moricizine hydrochloride
(mor-**IS**-ih-zeen)
**Pregnancy Category:** B
Ethmozine **(Rx)**
**Classification:** Antiarrhythmic, class I

See also *Antiarrhythmic Agents*.

**Action/Kinetics:** Causes a stabilizing effect on the myocardial membranes as well as local anesthetic activity. Shortens phase II and III repolarization leading to a decreased duration of the action potential and an effective refractory period. Also, there is a decrease in the maximum rate of phase O depolarization and a prolongation of AV conduction in clients with ventricular tachycardia. Whether the client is at rest or is exercising, has minimal effects on cardiac index, stroke index volume, systemic or pulmonary vascular resistance or ejection fraction, and pulmonary capillary wedge pressure. There is a small increase in resting BP and HR. The time, course, and intensity of antiarrhythmic and electrophysiologic effects are not re-

lated to plasma levels of the drug. **Onset:** 2 hr. **Peak plasma levels:** 30–120 min. **t½:** 1.5–3.5 hr (reduced after multiple dosing). **Duration:** 10–24 hr. 95% is protein bound. Significant first-pass effect. Metabolized almost completely by the liver with metabolites excreted through both the urine and feces; the drug induces its own metabolism. Food delays the rate of absorption resulting in lower peak plasma levels; however, the total amount absorbed is not changed.

**Uses:** Documented life-threatening ventricular arrhythmias (e.g., sustained ventricular tachycardia) where benefits of the drug are determined to outweigh the risks. *Investigational:* Ventricular premature contractions, couplets, and nonsustained ventricular tachycardia.

**Contraindications:** Preexisting second- or third-degree block, right bundle branch block when associated with bifascicular block (unless the client has a pacemaker), cardiogenic shock. Use during lactation.

**Special Concerns:** There is the possibility of increased risk of death when used in clients with non-life-threatening cardiac arrhythmias. Safety and effectiveness in children less than 18 years of age have not been determined. Geriatric clients have a higher rate of side effects. Increased survival rates following use of antiarrhythmic drugs have not been proven in clients with ventricular arrhythmias. Use with caution in clients with sick sinus syndrome due to the possibility of sinus bradycardia, sinus pause, or sinus arrest. Use with caution in clients with CHF.

**Side Effects:** *CV: Proarrhythmias, including new rhythm disturbances or worsening of existing arrhythmias;* ECG abnormalities, including conduction defects, sinus pause, junctional rhythm, AV block; palpitations, *sustained ventricular tachycardia,* cardiac chest pain, CHF, *cardiac death,* hypotension, hypertension, atrial fibrillation, atrial flutter, syn-

M

cope, bradycardia, **cardiac arrest, MI, pulmonary embolism,** vasodilation, thrombophlebitis, **cerebrovascular events.** *CNS:* Dizziness (common), anxiety, headache, fatigue, nervousness, paresthesias, sleep disorders, tremor, anxiety, hypoesthesias, depression, euphoria, somnolence, agitation, confusion, **seizures,** hallucinations, loss of memory, vertigo, coma. *GI:* Nausea, dry mouth, abdominal pain, vomiting, diarrhea, dyspepsia, anorexia, ileus, flatulence, dysphagia, bitter taste. *Musculoskeletal:* Asthenia, abnormal gait, akathisia, ataxia, abnormal coordination, dyskinesia, pain. *GU:* Urinary retention, dysuria, urinary incontinence, urinary frequency, impotence, kidney pain, decreased libido. *Respiratory:* Dyspnea, apnea, asthma, hyperventilation, pharyngitis, cough, sinusitis. *Opthalmologic:* Nystagmus, diplopia, blurred vision, eye pain, periorbital edema. *Dermatologic:* Rash, pruritus, dry skin, urticaria. *Miscellaneous:* Sweating, drug fever, hypothermia, temperature intolerance, swelling of the lips and tongue, speech disorder, tinnitus, jaundice.

**OD** **Overdose Management:** *Symptoms:* Vomiting, hypotension, lethargy, worsening of CHF, **MI, conduction disturbances, arrhythmias (e.g., junctional bradycardia, ventricular tachycardia, ventricular fibrillation, asystole), sinus arrest, respiratory failure.** *Treatment:* In acute overdose, induce vomiting, taking care to prevent aspiration. Client should be hospitalized and closely monitored for cardiac, respiratory, and CNS changes. Provide life support, including an intracardiac pacing catheter, if necessary.

**Drug Interactions**
*Cimetidine* / ↑ Plasma levels of moricizine due to ↓ excretion
*Digoxin* / Additive prolongation of the PR interval (but no significant increase in the rate of second- or third-degree AV block)
*Propranolol* / Additive prolongation of the PR interval

*Theophylline* / ↓ Plasma levels of theophylline due to ↑ rate of clearance
**Laboratory Test Interferences:** ↑ Bilirubin and liver transaminases.

**Dosage** ─────────
• **Tablets**
  *Antiarrhythmic.*
**Adults:** 600–900 mg/day in equally divided doses q 8 hr. If needed, the dose can be increased in increments of 150 mg/day at 3-day intervals until the desired effect is obtained. In clients with hepatic or renal impairment, the initial dose should be 600 mg or less with close monitoring and dosage adjustment.

## NURSING CONSIDERATIONS

See also *Nursing Considerations* for *Antiarrhythmic Agents.*
**Administration/Storage**
1. When transferring clients from other antiarrhythmics to moricizine, withdraw the previous drug for one to two plasma half-lives before starting moricizine. For example, when transferring from quinidine or disopyramide, moricizine can be started 6–12 hr after the last dose; when transferring from procainamide, moricizine can be initiated 3–6 hr after the last dose; when transferring from mexiletine, propafenone, or tocainide, moricizine can be started 8–12 hr after the last dose; and, when transferring from flecainide, moricizine can be started 12–24 hr after the last dose.
2. If clients are well controlled on an 8-hr regimen, they might be given the same total daily dose q 12 hr to increase compliance.
**Assessment**
1. Document cardiac history, note preexisting conditions and ECG abnormalities.
2. Monitor ECG, electrolytes, CXR, PFTs, liver and renal function studies; correct any electrolyte disturbance and reduce dose with liver or renal dysfunction.
3. Monitor cardiac rhythm closely to observe for drug-induced rhythm disturbances.

4. Clients should be hospitalized for initial dosing. Antiarrhythmic response may be determined by ECG, exercise testing, or programmed electrical stimulation testing.
5. Assess pacing parameters with pacemakers.
6. Monitor VS and report any persistent temperature elevations.
**Client/Family Teaching**
1. Take before meals; food delays rate of absorption.
2. Drug may cause dizziness. Use care when rising from a lying or sitting position.
3. Advise family member or significant other to learn CPR.
**Outcomes/Evaluate:** Termination of life-threatening ventricular arrhythmias

## Morphine hydrochloride
(**MOR**-feen)
**Pregnancy Category:** C
Morphitec-1, -5, -10, -20 ✿, M.O.S. ✿, M.O.S.-S.R. ✿ **(Rx)**

## Morphine sulfate
(**MOR**-feen **SUL**-fayt)
**Pregnancy Category:** C
Astramorph PF, Duramorph, Infumorph, Kadian, M-Eslon ✿, Morphine HP ✿, M.O.S.-Sulfate ✿, MS Contin, MS-IR, MSIR Capsules, Oramorph SR, RMS, RMS Rectal Suppositories, Roxanol, Roxanol 100, Roxanol Rescudose, Roxanol UD, Statex ✿ **(C-II) (Rx)**
**Classification:** Narcotic analgesic, morphine type

See also *Narcotic Analgesics.*
**Action/Kinetics:** Morphine is the prototype for opiate analgesics. **Onset:** approximately 15–60 min, based on epidural or intrathecal use. **Peak effect:** 30–60 min. **Duration:** 3–7 hr. **t½:** 1.5–2 hr. Oral morphine is only one-third to one-sixth as effective as parenteral products.
**Uses:** Intrathecally, epidurally, PO (including sustained-release products), or by continuous IV infusion for acute or chronic pain. In low doses, morphine is more effective against dull, continuous pain than against intermittent, sharp pain. Large doses, however, will dull almost any kind of pain. Preoperative medication. To facilitate induction of anesthesia and reduce dose of anesthetic. *Investigational:* Acute LV failure (for dyspneic seizures) and pulmonary edema. Morphine should not be used with papaverine for analgesia in biliary spasms but may be used with papaverine in acute vascular occlusions.
**Additional    Contraindications:** Epidural or intrathecal morphine if infection is present at injection site, in clients on anticoagulant therapy, bleeding diathesis, if client has received parenteral corticosteroids within the past 2 weeks.
**Special Concerns:** May increase the length of labor. Clients with known seizure disorders may be at greater risk for morphine-induced seizure activity.

## Dosage
• **Capsules, Tablets, Oral Solution, Soluble Tablets, Syrup**
*Analgesia.*
10–30 mg q 4 hr.
• **Sustained-Release Tablets**
*Analgesia.*
30 mg q 8–12 hr, depending on client needs and response. Kadian is indicated for once-daily dosing at doses of 20, 50, or 100 mg where analgesia is indicated for just a few days.
• **IM, SC**
*Analgesia.*
**Adults:** 5–20 mg/70 kg q 4 hr as needed; **pediatric:** 100–200 mcg/kg up to a maximum of 15 mg.
• **IV Infusion**
*Analgesia.*
**Adults:** 2.5–15 mg/70 kg in 4–5 mL of water for injection (should be administered slowly over 4–5 min).
• **IV Infusion, Continuous**
*Analgesia.*
**Adults:** 0.1–1 mg/mL in D5W by a controlled-infusion pump.
• **Rectal Suppositories**
**Adults:** 10–20 mg q 4 hr.

- **Intrathecal**
**Adults:** 0.2–1 mg as a single daily injection.
- **Epidural**
**Initial:** 5 mg/day in the lumbar region; if analgesia is not manifested in 1 hr, increasing doses of 1–2 mg can be given, not to exceed 10 mg/day. For continuous infusion, 2–4 mg/day with additional doses of 1–2 mg if analgesia is not satisfactory.

## NURSING CONSIDERATIONS

See also *Nursing Considerations* for *Narcotic Analgesics*.
### Administration/Storage
1. May be administered with food to diminish GI upset. Do not crush or chew controlled-release tablets.
2. Immediate-release capsules may be swallowed intact or the contents of the capsule may be sprinkled on food or stirred in juice to avoid the bitter taste. The contents of the capsule may also be delivered through a nasogastric or a gastric tube.
3. For intrathecal use, do not give more than 2 mL of the 5-mg/10-mL preparation or 1 mL of the 10-mg/10-mL product.
4. Give intrathecally only in the lumbar region; repeated injections are not recommended.
5. To reduce the chance of side effects with intrathecal administration, a constant IV infusion of naloxone (0.6 mg/hr for 24 hr after intrathecal injection) is recommended.
6. In certain circumstances (e.g., tolerance, severe pain), the physician may prescribe doses higher than those listed under *Dosage*. Dose may be lower in geriatric clients or those with respiratory disease.
**IV** 7. For IV use, dilute 2–10 mg with at least 5 mL sterile water or NSS and administer over 4–5 min. For continous infusions, reconstitute to a concentration of 0.1–1 mg/mL and administer as prescribed to control symptoms.
8. Rapid IV administration increases the risk of adverse effects; have a narcotic antagonist (e.g., naloxone) available.

### Assessment
1. Document location and characteristics of pain. Rate utilizing a pain-rating scale.
2. List other agents prescribed and the outcome.
3. Note any seizure disorder.
### Client/Family Teaching
1. Drug may cause dizziness and drowsiness; avoid activities that require mental alertness.
2. Practice cough and deep-breathing exercises or incentive spirometry to minimize the development of atelectasis.
3. Avoid alcohol and any other CNS depressants.
4. Record use for breakthrough pain when SR therapy prescribed, to ensure adequate dosage.
### Outcomes/Evaluate
- Relief of pain
- Control of respirations during mechanical ventilation

# Mupirocin
(myou-**PEER**-oh-sin)
**Pregnancy Category:** B
Bactroban **(Rx)**

# Mupirocin Calcium
**Pregnancy Category:** B
Bactroban Nasal **(Rx)**
**Classification:** Anti-infective, topical

**Action/Kinetics:** Binds to bacterial isoleucyl transfer RNA synthetase, which results in inhibition of protein synthesis by the organism. Not absorbed into the systemic circulation. Serum present in exudative wounds decreases the antibacterial activity. Metabolized to the inactive monic acid in the skin which is removed by normal skin desquamation. No cross resistance with other antibiotics such as chloramphenicol, erythromycin, gentamicin, lincomycin, methicillin, neomycin, novobiocin, penicillin, streptomycin, or tetracyclines.
**Uses: Topical:** To treat impetigo due to *Staphylococcus aureus, Streptococcus pyogenes,* and beta-hemolytic streptococcus. **Nasal:** Eradication of nasal colonization with

methicillin-resistant *S. aureus* in adult clients and health care workers.
**Contraindications:** Ophthalmic use. Lactation. Use if absorption of large quantities of polyethylene glycol is possible (i.e., large, open wounds). Use with other nasal products.
**Special Concerns:** Superinfection may result from chronic use. Safety and efficacy have not been established in children for mupirocin nasal.
**Side Effects: Topical use:** Superinfection, rash, burning, stinging, pain, nausea, tenderness, erythema, swelling, dry skin, contact dermatitis, and increased exudate.

**Nasal use:** Headache, rhinitis, respiratory disorder (including upper respiratory tract congestion), pharyngitis, taste perversion, burning, stinging, cough, pruritus, blepharitis, diarrhea, dry mouth, ear pain, epistaxis, nausea, rash.

**Dosage** —
• **Topical Ointment**
A small amount of ointment is applied to the affected area t.i.d. If no response is seen after 3–5 days, the client should be reevaluated.
• **Nasal Ointment**
Divide about one-half of the ointment from the single-use tube between the nostrils and apply in the morning and evening for 5 days.

**NURSING CONSIDERATIONS**
**Administration/Storage**
1. A gauze dressing may be used if desired.
2. After application in the nose, close the nostrils by pressing them together for about 1 min.
3. Store the topical ointment between 15°C–30°C (59°F–86°F); store the nasal ointment below 25°C (77°F).
**Assessment:** Document type, onset, duration, and characteristics of symptoms.
**Client/Family Teaching**
1. Review technique for administering

topical and/or nasal medications; use aseptic measures and hand washing before and after therapy to prevent contamination.
2. Report any symptoms of chemical irritation or hypersensitivity such as increased rash, itching, pain at site, or lack of healing.
3. Do not use other nasal products during nasal therapy.
4. Report if no improvement in skin infection is noted after 3–5 days of therapy.
5. Notify school nurse to ensure appropriate screening is performed when treating school-aged children with impetigo.
**Outcomes/Evaluate:** Healing of skin lesions; symptomatic improvement

# Muromonab-CD3
(myour-oh-**MON**-ab)
**Pregnancy Category:** C
Orthoclone OKT 3 **(Rx)**
**Classification:** Immunosuppressive agent

**Action/Kinetics:** Muromonab-CD3 is a murine monoclonal antibody that is a purified $IgG_{2a}$ immunoglobulin. Acts to prevent rejection of transplanted kidney tissue by blocking the action of T cells, which play a significant role in acute rejection. Specifically, the CD3 molecule in the membrane of T cells is blocked; this molecule is necessary for signal transduction. Does not cause myelosuppression. Antibodies to muromonab-CD3 have been observed after approximately 20 days. **Average serum levels after 3 days:** 0.9 mcg/mL. **Time to steady-state trough levels:** 3 days. **Duration:** 1 week for return of circulating CD3 positive T cells to pretreatment levels.
**Uses:** To reverse acute allograft rejection in kidney transplant clients; used in combination with azathioprine, cyclosporine, corticosteroids. Treatment of steroid-resistant acute

allograft rejection in cardiac and hepatic transplant clients.

**Contraindications:** Hypersensitivity to drug (or any product of murine origin), clients with anti-mouse titers greater than or equal to 1:1,000. Clients with fluid overload or uncompensated CHF as confirmed by chest X ray or more than a 3% weight gain within the week prior to treatment. History of seizures or predisposition to seizures. Use during pregnancy and lactation.

**Special Concerns:** Should not be used in pregnancy as it is an IgG antibody with potential hazard to the fetus. Although used in children, safety and effectiveness have not been assessed. Following the first two to three doses, a cytokine release syndrome due to the release of cytokines by activated lymphocytes or monocytes may occur. Clients at greatest risk for cytokine release syndrome are those with unstable angina, recent MI, symptomatic ischemic heart disease, heart failure, pulmonary edema, COPD, intravascular volume overload or depletion, cerebrovascular disease, advanced symptomatic vascular disease or neuropathy, history of seizures, or septic shock.

**Side Effects:** *Cytokine release syndrome (CRS):* Flu-like symptoms, such as pyrexia, chills, dyspnea, N&V, chest pain, diarrhea, tremor, wheezing, headache, tachycardia, rigor, and hypertension. *Rarely, severe, life-threatening shock-like syndrome including serious CV and CNS effects.*

*Within the first 45 days of therapy for renal transplants: Infections (which may be life-threatening) due to CMV, HSV, Staphylococcus epidermidis, Pneumocystis carinii, Legionella, Cryptococcus, Serratia, and other gram-negative bacteria.*

*Within the first 45 days of therapy for liver transplants: CMV, fungal infections, HSV, Legionella, and other severe, life-threatening gram-positive, gram-negative, and viral infections.*

*Within the first 45 days of therapy for heart transplants:* Most common-ly herpes simplex, fungal, and cytomegaloviral infections. *Hypersensitivity reactions: Cardiovascular collapse, cardiorespiratory arrest, shock,* loss of consciousness, hypotension, tachycardia, tingling, angioedema, *airway obstruction, bronchospasm,* dyspnea, urticaria, pruritus. *Neuro-psychiatric: Seizures,* encephalopathy, cerebral edema, *aseptic meningitis,* headaches. *CV: Cardiac arrest, shock, heart failure, CV collapse, MI,* hypotension, angina, tachycardia, bradycardia, hemodynamic instability, hypertension, LV dysfunction, arrhythmias, chest pain or tightness. *Respiratory: Respiratory arrest, ARDS, respiratory failure, cardiogenic or noncardiogenic pulmonary edema, apnea,* dyspnea, *bronchospasm,* wheezing, SOB, hypoxemia, tachypnea, hyperventilation, abnormal chest sounds, pneumonia, pneumonitis. *Dermatologic:* Rash, urticaria, pruritus, erythema, flushing, diaphoresis, *Stevens-Johnson syndrome. GI:* Nausea, vomiting, diarrhea, abdominal pain, *bowel infarction, GI hemorrhage. Hematologic:* Pancytopenia, *aplastic anemia,* neutropenia, leukopenia, thrombocytopenia, lymphopenia, leukocytosis, lymphadenopathy, *arterial and venous thrombosis of allografts and other vascular beds (heart, lung, brain, bowel), disturbances of coagulation. Musculoskeletal:* Arthralgia, arthritis, myalgia, stiffness, aches and pain. *Hepatic:* Hepatomegaly, splenomegaly, hepatitis (usually secondary to viral infection or lymphoma). *GU:* Anuria, oliguria, delayed graft function, abnormal urinary cytology (including exfoliation of damaged lymphocytes, collecting ducts, and cellular casts). *Ophthalmic:* Blindness, blurred vision, diplopia, photophobia, conjunctivitis. *Otic:* Hearing loss, otitis media, tinnitus, vertigo, nasal and ear stuffiness. *Body as a whole:* Fever, chills, rigors, flu-like syndrome, fatigue, malaise, generalized weakness, anorexia. *Miscellaneous:* Palsy of cranial nerve VI, *increased risk of developing neoplasms.*

**OD** **Overdose Management:**
*Symptoms:* Hyperthermia, myalgia, severe chills, diarrhea, vomiting, edema, oliguria, pulmonary edema, acute renal failure. *Treatment:* Observe client carefully and provide symptomatic and supportive treatment.

**Drug Interactions**
*Azathioprine, corticosteroids, cyclosporine* / Psychosis, infections, malignancies, seizures, encephalopathy, and thrombosis when taken with muromonab-CD3
*Indomethacin* / Encephalopathy and other CNS effects

**Laboratory Test Interferences:** ↑ AST, ALT. Transient and reversible ↑ in BUN and serum creatinine.

**Dosage**
• **IV Bolus**
*Reverse acute allograft rejection in kidney transplants.*
**Adults:** 5 mg/day for 10–14 days, beginning treatment once acute renal rejection is diagnosed.
*Cardiac/hepatic allograft rejection, steroid-resistant.*
5 mg/day for 10–14 days with treatment beginning after determination that corticosteroids will not reverse the rejection.

**NURSING CONSIDERATIONS**
**Administration/Storage**
**IV** 1. Give methylprednisolone sodium succinate, 8 mg/kg IV, 1–4 hr before dose to decrease incidence of first-dose reactions. Acetaminophen and antihistamines, given together, may reduce early reactions.
2. Initiate treatment as soon as acute renal rejection is diagnosed.
3. Give the dose in less than 1 min.
4. Do not give the drug by IV infusion or with any other drug solutions.
5. If the body temperature is 37.8°C (100°F), do not initiate drug therapy.
6. Draw the solution (which is a protein) into a syringe through a 0.2- or 0.22-μm filter; discard the filter and attach a 20-gauge needle.
7. Do not add or infuse other drugs

through the same IV line. If the same IV line is used for sequential infusion of different drugs, flush the line with saline before and after infusion of muromonab-CD3.
8. The appearance of a few translucent particles of protein does not affect the potency of the preparation.
9. Use the ampule immediately after opening, as there is no bacteriostatic agent in the product. Discard any unused drug.
10. Decrease the dose of other immunosuppressant drugs as follows during muromonab-CD3 use: prednisone, 0.5 mg/kg/day; azathioprine, 25 mg/day. Cyclosporine should be discontinued. Maintenance doses of these drugs can be resumed approximately 3 days prior to termination of muromonab-CD3 therapy.
11. Store at 2°C–8°C (36°F–46°F) and do not freeze or shake.

**Assessment**
1. Determine any past use and assess closely for evidence of antibodies. Drug is usually only given for one course of therapy.
2. Note any sensitivity to murine derivatives.
3. Monitor CBC and T-cell assays with $CD_3$ antigen daily.

**Interventions**
1. Anticipate pretreatment administration of an antihistamine, antipyretic, and methylprednisolone sodium succinate and hydrocortisone sodium succinate posttreatment to minimize intensity of side effects.
2. Monitor I&O and weights; assess for a positive fluid balance and report rapid weight gain.
3. Obtain CXR, assess lung sounds, and report any evidence of congestion.
4. Take the temperature q 4 hr. If the temperature goes above 37.7°C (100°F), withhold the drug until the temperature drops.
5. Monitor for a decrease in urine volume and creatinine clearance;

these are signs of transplant rejection.

6. Administer acetaminophen for flu-like symptoms and febrile reaction.

7. Symptoms of aseptic meningitis are usually evident within 3 days. Fever, headache, nuchal rigidity, and photophobia characterize this condition.

**Client/Family Teaching**

1. Chills, fever, SOB, and malaise are first-dose symptoms that will diminish on consecutive treatment days.

2. Report any dyspnea, edema, weight gain, chest pain, N&V, or infection immediately.

3. Perform frequent, careful oral care to minimize occurrence of oral inflammation.

4. Avoid vaccinia and crowds.

5. Continue to practice birth control for 12 weeks following therapy.

**Outcomes/Evaluate**

• Reversal of kidney transplant rejection and improved organ function

• Absence of graft rejection

# Mycophenolate mofetil
(**my**-koh-**FEN**-oh-layt)
**Pregnancy Category:** C
CellCept **(Rx)**
**Classification:** Immunosuppressant

**Action/Kinetics:** Rapidly absorbed after PO administration and hydrolyzed to the active mycophenolic acid (MPA). MPA has potent cytostatic effects on lymphocytes. Inhibits proliferative responses of T- and B-lymphocytes to both mitogenic and allospecific stimulation. MPA also suppresses antibody formation of B-lymphocytes. MPA and additional metabolites are excreted in the urine. **t½:** 17.9 hr.

**Uses:** Prophylaxis of organ rejection in those receiving allogeneic renal transplants. Mycophenolate should be used concomitantly with cyclosporine and corticosteroids.

**Contraindications:** Hypersensitivity to mycophenolate or MPA. Lactation.

**Special Concerns:** Clients receiving immunosuppressant drugs are at a higher risk of developing lymphomas and other malignancies, especially of the skin. Higher blood levels are seen in those with severe impaired renal function. Use with caution in active serious digestive system disease. Safety and efficacy have not been determined in children.

**Side Effects:** *Hematologic:* Severe neutropenia, anemia, leukopenia, thrombocytopenia, hypochromic anemia, leukocytosis. *GI:* **GI tract hemorrhage/perforations,** GI tract ulceration, diarrhea, constipation, nausea, dyspepsia, vomiting, oral moniliasis, anorexia, esophagitis, flatulence, gastritis, gastroenteritis, GI moniliasis, gingivitis, gum hyperplasia, hepatitis, ileus, infection, mouth ulceration, rectal disorder. *CNS:* Tremor, insomnia, dizziness, anxiety, depression, hypertonia, paresthesia, somnolence. *GU:* Urinary tract infection, hematuria, kidney tubular necrosis, urinary tract disorder, albuminuria, dysuria, hydronephrosis, impotence, pain, pyelonephritis, urinary frequency. *CV:* Hypertension, angina pectoris, atrial fibrillation, cardiovascular disorder, hypotension, palpitation, peripheral vascular disorder, postural hypotension, tachycardia, thrombosis, vasodilation. *Respiratory:* Infection, dyspnea, increased cough, pharyngitis, bronchitis, pneumonia, asthma, lung disorder, lung edema, pleural effusion, rhinitis, sinusitis. *Dermatologic:* Acne, rash, alopecia, fungal dermatitis, hirsutism, pruritus, benign skin neoplasm, skin disorder, skin hypertrophy, skin ulcer, sweating. *Metabolic/Endocrine:* Peripheral edema, dehydration, hypercholesterolemia, hypophosphatemia, edema, hypokalemia, hyperkalemia, hyperglycemia, diabetes mellitus, parathyroid disorder. *Musculoskeletal:* Arthralgia, joint disorder, leg cramps, myalgia, myasthenia. *Ophthalmologic:* Amblyopia, cataract, conjunctivitis. *Body as a whole:* Pain,

abdominal pain, fever, chills, headache, infection, malaise, *sepsis,* asthenia, chest pain, back pain. *Miscellaneous:* Increased incidence of lymphoma/lymphoproliferative disease, nonmelanoma skin carcinoma, and other malignancies. Increased incidence of opportunistic infections, including herpes simplex, CMV, herpes zoster, *Candida, Aspergillus/Mucor* invasive disease, and *Pneumocystis carinii.* Enlarged abdomen, accidental injury, cyst, facial edema, flu syndrome, *hemorrhage,* hernia, weight gain, pelvic pain, ecchymosis, polycythemia.
**OD    Overdose    Management:**
*Symptoms:* Nausea, vomiting, diarrhea, hematologic abnormalities, especially neutropenia. *Treatment:* Reduce dose of the drug. Removal of MPA by bile acid sequestrants (e.g., cholestyramine).

**Drug Interactions**
*Acyclovir* / ↑ Plasma levels of both drugs due to competition for renal tubular excretion
*Antacids containing aluminum/magnesium* / ↓ Absorption of mycophenolate
*Cholestyramine* / ↓ Absorption of mycophenolate
*Ganciclovir* / ↑ Plasma levels of both drugs due to competition for renal tubular excretion
*Phenytoin* / ↓ Plasma protein binding of phenytoin
*Probenecid* / Significant ↑ plasma levels of MPA
*Salicylates* / ↑ Free fraction of MPA
*Theophylline* / ↓ Plasma protein binding of theophylline
**Laboratory Test Interferences:** ↑ Alkaline phosphatase, creatinine, gamma glutamyl transpeptidase, LDH, AST, ALT. Also, hypercalcemia, hyperlipemia, hyperuricemia, hypervolemia, hypocalcemia, hypoglycemia, hypoproteinemia, acidosis.

**Dosage**
• **Capsules**

*Prevent rejection following allogeneic renal transplantation.*
**Adults:** 1 g b.i.d. in combination with corticosteroids and cyclosporine.

---

**NURSING CONSIDERATIONS**
**Administration/Storage**
1. Start mycophenolate therapy within 72 hr following transplantation.
2. Give on an empty stomach.
3. Avoid doses of 1 g b.i.d. in chronic renal impairment (i.e., GFR less than 25 mL/min/1.73 m²) outside the immediate posttreatment period.
4. Mycophenolate is teratogenic; do not open or crush capsules. Avoid inhalation or direct contact with the skin or mucous membranes; wash the area thoroughly with soap and water if contact occurs. Rinse the eyes with plain water.
**Assessment**
1. Note date of transplant, other agents used and the outcome.
2. Document a negative pregnancy test 1 week prior to initiating therapy in all women of childbearing age.
3. Monitor hematologic profiles and observe closely for the development of severe neutropenia (day 31 to day 180) posttransplant with this therapy.
**Client/Family Teaching**
1. Take exactly as directed on an empty stomach twice a day; taken with cyclosporine and steroids.
2. With increased immunosuppression the susceptibility to infection and the risk of lymphoproliferative disease and other malignancies may be increased.
3. Women of childbearing age should practice two reliable forms of contraception simultaneously before, during, and for 6 weeks following therapy.
4. Report for all scheduled lab studies to evaluate response to therapy and to identify any potential problems early. (If ANC is less than 1.3 × 10³, then drug therapy must be inter-

**M**

rupted or decreased.) Obtain CBC weekly during first month, twice monthly for the second and third months, and then monthly thereafter for the first year.

**Outcomes/Evaluate:** Prevention of transplant rejection; improved organ function

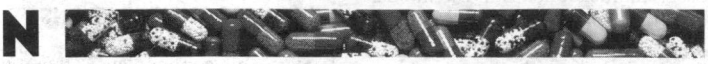

# Nabumetone
(nah-**BYOU**-meh-tohn)
**Pregnancy Category:** B
Relafen **(Rx)**
**Classification:** Nonsteroidal anti-inflammatory agent

See also *Nonsteroidal Anti-Inflammatory Drugs.*
**Action/Kinetics: Time to peak plasma levels:** 2.5–4 hr. **t½ of active metabolite:** 22.5–30 hr.
**Uses:** Acute and chronic treatment of osteoarthritis and rheumatoid arthritis. Has also been used to treat mild to moderate pain including postextraction dental pain, postsurgical episiotomy pain, and soft tissue athletic injuries.
**Contraindications:** Lactation.
**Special Concerns:** Safety and efficacy have not been determined in children.

**Dosage** ————————
• **Tablets**
*Osteoarthritis, rheumatoid arthritis.*
**Adults, initial:** 1,000 mg as a single dose; **maintenance:** 1,500–2,000 mg/day. Doses greater than 2,000 mg/day have not been studied.

## NURSING CONSIDERATIONS

See also *Nursing Considerations for Nonsteroidal Anti-Inflammatory Drugs.*
**Administration/Storage**
1. May be taken with or without food.
2. The total daily dose may be given either once or in two divided doses.
3. Use the lowest effective dose for chronic treatment.
**Assessment**
1. Document type, onset, and characteristics of symptoms. List any other drugs used and the outcome.
2. Note any swelling, pain, inflammation, trauma, or decreased ROM.
3. Monitor CBC, liver and renal function studies with chronic therapy.
**Client/Family Teaching**
1. Take as directed; may take with food to decrease GI upset.
2. Review side effects that require immediate reporting: persistent headaches, altered vision, rash, swelling of extremities, blood in stools.
3. Do not perform tasks that require mental alertness until drug effects realized.
4. Avoid alcohol and alcohol-containing products and aspirin-containing products.
**Outcomes/Evaluate**
• Relief of pain
• Improved mobility; ↑ ROM

# Nadolol
(**NAY**-doh-lohl)
**Pregnancy Category:** C
Alti-Nadolol ✤, Apo-Nadol ✤, Corgard, Novo-Nadolol ✤ **(Rx)**
**Classification:** Beta-adrenergic blocking agent

See also *Beta-Adrenergic Blocking Agents.*
**Action/Kinetics:** Manifests both beta-1- and beta-2-adrenergic blocking activity. Has no membrane stabilizing or intrinsic sympathomimetic activity. Low lipid solubility. **Peak serum concentration:** 3–4 hr. **t½:** 20–24 hr (permits once-daily dosage). **Duration:** 17–24 hr. Absorption variable, averaging 30%; steady plasma level achieved after 6–9 days of administration. Excreted unchanged by the kidney.

**Uses:** Hypertension, either alone or with other drugs (e.g., thiazide diuretic). Angina pectoris. *Investigational:* Prophylaxis of migraine, ventricular arrhythmias, aggressive behavior, essential tremor, tremors associated with lithium or parkinsonism, antipsychotic-induced akathisia, rebleeding of esophageal varices, situational anxiety, reduce intraocular pressure.

**Contraindications:** Bronchial asthma or bronchospasm, including severe COPD.

**Special Concerns:** Dosage has not been established in children.

**Dosage** ———————
• **Tablets**
*Hypertension.*
**Initial:** 40 mg/day; **then,** may be increased in 40- to 80-mg increments until optimum response obtained. **Maintenance:** 40–80 mg/day although up to 240–320 mg/day may be needed.
*Angina.*
**Initial:** 40 mg/day; **then,** increase dose in 40- to 80-mg increments q 3–7 days until optimum response obtained. **Maintenance:** 40–80 mg/day, although up to 160–240 mg/day may be needed.
*Aggressive behavior.*
40–160 mg/day.
*Antipsychotic-induced akathisia.*
40–80 mg/day.
*Essential tremor.*
120–240 mg/day.
*Lithium-induced tremors.*
20–40 mg/day.
*Tremors associated with parkinsonism.*
80–320 mg/day.
*Prophylaxis of migraine.*
40–80 mg/day.
*Rebleeding from esophageal varices.*
40–160 mg/day.
*Situational anxiety.*
20 mg.
*Ventricular arrhythmias.*
10–640 mg/day.

*Reduction of intraocular pressure.*
10–20 mg b.i.d.
*NOTE:* Dosage for all uses should be decreased in clients with renal failure.

## NURSING CONSIDERATIONS

See also *Nursing Considerations* for *Beta-Adrenergic Blocking Agents* and *Antihypertensive Agents.*
**Client/Family Teaching**
1. Report any rapid weight gain, increased SOB, or swelling of extremities.
2. Do not perform tasks that require mental alertness until drug effects realized; may cause dizziness.
3. May cause increased sensitivity to cold; dress appropriately.
**Outcomes/Evaluate**
• ↓ BP, ↓ HR
• ↓ Frequency/intensity of angina attacks

# Nafarelin acetate
(**NAF**-ah-rel-in)
**Pregnancy Category:** X
Synarel **(Rx)**
**Classification:** Gonadotropin-releasing hormone

**Action/Kinetics:** Produced through biotechnology; differs by only one amino acid from naturally occurring GnRH. Stimulates the release of LH and FSH from the adenohypophysis. Causes estrogen and progesterone synthesis in the ovary, resulting in the maturation and subsequent release of an ovum. With repeated use of the drug, however, the pituitary becomes desensitized and no longer produces endogenous LH and FSH; thus endogenous estrogen is not produced, leading to a regression of endometrial tissue, cessation of menstruation, and a menopausal-like state. Broken down by the enzyme peptidase. **Peak serum levels:** 10–40 min. t½: 3 hr; 80% is bound to plasma proteins.
**Uses:** Endometriosis (including reduction of endometriotic lesions) in

clients aged 18 or older; use restricted to no more than 6 months. Central precocious puberty in children of both sexes.

**Contraindications:** Hypersensitivity to GnRH or analogs. Abnormal vaginal bleeding of unknown origin. Pregnancy or possibility of becoming pregnant. Lactation.

**Special Concerns:** Use of nafarelin in pregnancy is not recommended; pregnancy should be ruled out before initiating therapy. Safety and effectiveness in children have not been established.

**Side Effects:** *Due to hypoestrogenic effects:* Hot flashes (common), decreased libido, vaginal dryness, headaches, emotional lability, insomnia. *Due to androgenic effects:* Acne, myalgia, reduced breast size, edema, seborrhea, weight gain, increased libido, hirsutism. *Musculoskeletal:* Decrease in vertebral trabecular bone density and total vertebral bone mass. *Miscellaneous:* Nasal irritation, depression, weight loss.

**Laboratory Test Interferences:** ↑ Cholesterol and triglyceride levels, plasma phosphorus, eosinophils. ↓ Serum calcium, WBCs.

**Dosage** ——————————
- **Nasal Spray**
  *Endometriosis.*
200 mcg into one nostril in the morning and 200 mcg into the other nostril at night (400 mcg b.i.d. may be required by some women).
  *Central precocious puberty.*
400 mcg (2 sprays) into each nostril in the morning (i.e., 4 sprays) and in the evening (total of 8 sprays/day). If adequate suppression is not achieved, 3 sprays (600 mcg) into alternating nostrils t.i.d. (i.e., a total of 9 sprays/day).

**NURSING CONSIDERATIONS**
**Administration/Storage**
1. Initiate therapy between days 2 and 4 of the menstrual cycle.
2. Use for longer than 6 months is not recommended due to the lack of safety data.

3. Store at room temperature in an upright position protected from light.
**Assessment**
1. Perform a complete history, noting any history of osteoporosis, alcohol, tobacco, or corticosteroid use; major risk factors for bone mineral loss that would preclude repeated courses with this drug.
2. Note description of menstrual cycles and any abnormal vaginal bleeding of unknown origin; drug is contraindicated. Document abdominal/vaginal assessments and ultrasound findings.
3. Determine if pregnant; drug is teratogenic.
**Client/Family Teaching**
1. Begin treatment between the second and fourth day of the menstrual cycle. Keep accurate records of menstrual patterns and cycles.
2. Use the spray upon arising and just before bedtime, alternating nostrils to decrease mucosal irritation.
3. Menses should cease while on therapy; report if regular menses continues.
4. Breakthrough bleeding may occur if successive doses are missed.
5. Use a nonhormonal form of contraception; drug may cause fetal harm.
6. If a topical nasal decongestant is required during treatment, use at least 30 min after nafarelin to prevent interference with drug absorption.
7. Drug may cause hypoestrogenic and androgenic side effects; report if evident as a change in drug dosage or therapy may be indicated.
**Outcomes/Evaluate**
- Restoration of pituitary-gonadal function in 4–8 weeks
- ↓ Number/size of endometriotic lesions

# Nafcillin sodium
(naf-**SILL**-in)
**Pregnancy Category:** B
Nafcil, Nallpen, Unipen **(Rx)**
**Classification:** Antibiotic, penicillin

See also *Anti-Infectives* and *Penicillins*.

**Action/Kinetics:** Penicillinase-resistant and acid stable. Parenteral therapy is recommended initially for severe infections. **Peak plasma levels: PO,** 7 mcg/mL after 30–60 min; **IM,** 14–20 mcg/mL after 30–60 min. **t½:** 60 min. Significantly bound to plasma proteins.

**Uses:** Infections by penicillinase-producing staphylococci and resistant staphylococcal infections; also certain pneumococci and streptococci. As initial therapy if staphylococcal infection is suspected (i.e., until results of culture have been obtained).

**Additional Side Effects:** Sterile abscesses and thrombophlebitis occur frequently, especially in the elderly.

**Dosage**
• **IV**
**Adults:** 0.5–1 g q 4 hr.
• **IM**
**Adults:** 0.5 g q 4–6 hr. **Children and infants:** 25 mg/kg b.i.d. **Neonates:** 10 mg/kg b.i.d. Or, for neonates weighing less than 2,000 g and less than 7 days of age, a dose of 25 mg/kg b.i.d. can be given; for neonates weighing less than 2,000 g but older than 7 days, a dose of 75 mg/kg/day divided q 6 hr.
• **Capsules**
*Mild to moderate infections.*
**Adults:** 250–500 mg q 4–6 hr.
*Severe infections.*
**Adults:** Up to 1 g q 4–6 hr.
*Pneumonia/scarlet fever.*
**Children:** 25 mg/kg/day in four divided doses.
*Staphylococcal infections.*
**Children:** 50 mg/kg/day in four divided doses. **Neonates:** 10 mg/kg t.i.d.–q.i.d.
*Streptococcal pharyngitis.*
**Children:** 250 mg t.i.d.
*NOTE:* IV administration is not recommended for neonates or infants.

## NURSING CONSIDERATIONS

See also *Nursing Considerations* for *Penicillins*.

**Administration/Storage**

1. Reconstitute for PO use by adding powder to bottle of diluent. Replace cap tightly and shake thoroughly until all powder is in solution. Check carefully for undissolved powder at the bottom of bottle. Store in refrigerator and discard unused portion after 1 week.

2. Serum levels after PO administration are low and unpredictable.

3. Administer IM by deep intragluteal injection.

**IV** 4. Do not administer IV to newborn infants.

5. Reserve IV use for therapy of 24–48 hr duration due to the possibility of thrombophlebitis, especially in geriatric clients. Reduce rate of flow and report any pain, redness, or edema at site of IV administration.

6. Reconstitute for parenteral use by adding required amount of sterile water. Shake vigorously. Date, time, and initial bottle. Refrigerate after reconstitution and discard unused portion after 48 hr.

7. For direct IV administration, dissolve powder in 15–30 mL of sterile water for injection or NSS and inject over 5- to 10-min period into the tubing of flowing IV infusion. For IV drip, dissolve the required amount in 100–150 mL of NSS and administer by IV drip over a period of 30–90 min.

**Client/Family Teaching**

1. Take capsules 1 hr before or 2 hr after meals with a full glass of water. Report any GI distress.

2. Report any unusual side effects or worsening of condition.

**Outcomes/Evaluate:** Negative culture reports with ↓ WBC, ↓ temperature and symptomatic improvement

# Naftifine hydrochloride
(**NAF**-tih-feen)
**Pregnancy Category:** B

Naftin **(Rx)**
**Classification:** Antifungal agent

See also *Anti-Infectives.*
**Action/Kinetics:** Synthetic antifungal agent with a broad spectrum of activity. Thought to inhibit squalene 2,3-epoxidase, which is responsible for synthesis of sterols. The decreased levels of sterols (especially ergosterol) and the accumulation of squalene in cells result in fungicidal activity. Although used topically, approximately 6% of the drug is absorbed. Naftifine and its metabolites are excreted via the feces and urine. **t½:** 2–3 days.
**Uses:** To treat tinea cruris, tinea pedis, and tinea corporis caused by *Candida albicans, Epidermophyton floccosum, Microsporum canis, M. audouinii, M. gypseum, Trichophyton rubrum, T. mentagrophytes,* and *T. tonsurans.*
**Contraindications:** Ophthalmic use.
**Special Concerns:** Consideration should be given to discontinuing nursing while using naftifine and for several days after the last application. Safety and efficacy in children have not been determined.
**Side Effects:** *Topical cream:* Burning, stinging, dryness, itching, local irritation, erythema. *Topical gel:* Burning, stinging, itching, rash, tenderness, erythema.

**Dosage** ————————————
• **Topical Cream (1%), Topical Gel (1%)**
Massage into affected area and surrounding skin once daily if using the cream and twice daily (morning and evening) if using the gel.

## NURSING CONSIDERATIONS

See also *General Nursing Considerations for All Anti-Infectives.*
**Client/Family Teaching**
1. Wash hands before and after use.
2. Avoid contact with eyes, nose, mouth, or other mucous membranes; for external use only.
3. Occlusive dressings, diapers, or wrappings should not be used; do not cover area.

4. Report any excessive itching or burning.
5. Beneficial effects are usually observed within 1 week; treatment should be continued for 1–2 weeks after symptoms diminish. If no beneficial effects after 4 weeks of treatment, seek reevaluation.
**Outcomes/Evaluate:** Negative culture results for pathogenic fungi; clinical improvement

# Nalbuphine hydrochloride
(**NAL**-byou-feen)
Nubain **(Rx)**
**Classification:** Narcotic agonist/antagonist

See also *Narcotic Analgesics.*
**Action/Kinetics:** Synthetic compound resembling oxymorphone and naloxone. Potent analgesic with both narcotic agonist and antagonist actions. Analgesic potency is approximately equal to that of morphine, while its antagonistic potency is approximately one-fourth that of nalorphine. **Onset: IV,** 2–3 min; **SC or IM,** <15 min. **Peak effect: 30–60 min. Duration: 3–6 hr;** t½: 5 hr.
**Uses:** Moderate to severe pain. Preoperative analgesia, anesthesia adjunct, obstetric analgesia.
**Contraindications:** Hypersensitivity to drug. Children under 18 years.
**Special Concerns:** Safe use during pregnancy (except for delivery) and lactation not established. Use with caution in presence of head injuries and asthma, MI (if client is nauseous or vomiting), biliary tract surgery (may induce spasms of sphincter of Oddi), renal insufficiency. Clients dependent on narcotics may experience withdrawal symptoms following use of nalbuphine.
**Additional Side Effects:** Even though nalbuphine is an agonist-antagonist, it may cause dependence and may precipitate withdrawal symptoms in an individual physically dependent on narcotics. *CNS:* Sedation is common. Crying, feelings of unreality, and other psychologic

reactions. *GI:* Cramps, dry mouth, bitter taste, dyspepsia. *Skin:* Itching, burning, urticaria, sweaty, clammy skin. *Other:* Blurred vision, difficulty with speech, urinary frequency.

**Drug Interactions:** Concomitant use with CNS depressants, other narcotics, phenothiazines, may result in additive depressant effects.

**Dosage**

- **SC, IM, IV**
  *Analgesia.*
  **Adults:** 10 mg/70 kg q 3–6 hr as needed (single dose should not exceed 20 mg q 3–6 hr; total daily dose should not exceed 160 mg).

## NURSING CONSIDERATIONS

See also *Nursing Considerations* for *Narcotic Analgesics.*

**Administration/Storage**
**IV** May be administered IV, undiluted. Administer each 10 mg or less over a 3- to 5-min period.

**Assessment**
1. Note any narcotic dependence; may precipitate withdrawal symptoms with narcotic addiction.
2. Document sulfite sensitivity.
3. Determine onset, location, duration, and intensity of pain. Use a pain-rating scale to assess pain.
4. Note any history of head injuries, asthma, or cardiac dysfunction.

**Outcomes/Evaluate:** Desired level of pain control

# Nalidixic acid
(nah-lih-**DICKS**-ick **AH**-sid)
**Pregnancy Category:** B
NegGram **(Rx)**
**Classification:** Urinary germicide

**Action/Kinetics:** Thought to inhibit the DNA synthesis, probably by interfering with DNA polymerization. Is either bacteriostatic or bactericidal. Rapidly absorbed from the GI tract. **Peak plasma concentration:** 20–40 mcg/mL after 1–2 hr; **peak urine levels:** 150–200 mcg/mL after 3–4 hr. **t½, plasma:** 1.5 hr (increased to 21 hr in anuric cli-

ents); **t½, urine:** 6 hr. Metabolized in the liver to hydroxynalidixic acid (comparable activity to nalidixic acid) and inactive compounds which are rapidly excreted. Extensively protein bound.

Sensitivity determinations are recommended before and periodically during prolonged administration of nalidixic acid. Renal and liver function tests are advisable if course of therapy exceeds 2 weeks.

**Uses:** Acute and chronic UTIs caused by susceptible gram-negative organisms, including *Escherichia coli, Proteus, Enterobacter,* and Klebsiella.

**Contraindications:** To be used with caution in clients with liver disease, severely impaired kidney function, epilepsy, and severe cerebral arteriosclerosis. Lactation. Use not recommended for infants less than 3 months of age.

**Special Concerns:** Use with care in prepubertal children.

**Side Effects:** *GI:* N&V, diarrhea, abdominal pain. *CNS:* Drowsiness, headache, dizziness, weakness, vertigo, toxic psychoses, intracranial hypertension, *seizures (rare)*. Also, increased intracranial pressure with bulging anterior fontanel, papilledema, and headache; sixth cranial nerve palsy in children and infants. *Allergic:* Photosensitivity (e.g., erythema, painful bullae on exposed skin), skin rashes, arthralgia (joint swelling and stiffness), pruritus, urticaria, angioedema, eosinophilia, anaphylaxis (rare). *Hematologic:* Leukopenia, thrombocytopenia, *hemolytic anemia* (especially in clients with G6PD deficiency). *Ophthalmic:* Reversible subjective visual disturbances, including overbrightness of lights, difficulty in focusing, changes in color perception, double vision, decreased visual acuity. *Other:* Metabolic acidosis, cholestatic jaundice, cholestasis, paresthesia.

**OD** **Overdose Management:** *Symptoms:* Toxic psychoses, convulsions, increased intracranial pres-

N

sure, nausea, vomiting, lethargy, metabolic acidosis. *Treatment:* Gastric lavage if the overdose is identified early. If absorption has occurred, fluid administration is increased with supportive measures. In severe cases, use of anticonvulsants may be necessary.

**Drug Interactions**
*Antacids, oral* / ↓ Effect of nalidixic acid due to ↓ absorption from GI tract
*Anticoagulants, oral* / ↑ Effect of anticoagulants due to ↓ plasma protein binding
*Nitrofurantoin* / ↓ Effect of nalidixic acid

**Laboratory Test Interferences:** False + for urinary glucose with Benedict's solution, Fehling's solution, or Clinitest Reagent tablets. Falsely elevated 17-ketosteroids.

**Dosage**
• **Oral Suspension, Tablets**
**Adults: initially,** 1 g q.i.d. for 1–2 weeks; **maintenance,** if necessary, 0.5 g q 6 hr. Maximum daily dose: 4 g. **Children, 3 months to 12 years, initial:** 55 mg/kg/day in four equally divided doses; **maintenance:** 33 mg/kg/day.

**NURSING CONSIDERATIONS**

See also *General Nursing Considerations for All Anti-Infectives.*
**Administration/Storage:** Underdosage (less than 4 g/day) initially may lead to emergence of bacterial resistance.
**Assessment**
1. Obtain CBC, urine culture, liver and renal function studies; note any dysfunction.
2. Assess for any adverse CNS effects (seizures, psychosis, severe headaches, or ↑ ICP); withhold drug and report.
**Client/Family Teaching**
1. Take 1 hr before meals, on an empty stomach. If GI upset occurs, may be taken with food. Drink at least 2–3 L/day of water.
2. Do not perform tasks that require mental alertness; may cause drowsi-ness, confusion, blurred vision, and dizziness.
3. Avoid prolonged exposure to sunlight or ultraviolet light; wear protective clothing and sunscreen if exposed. Photosensitivity may remain for 3 months following therapy.
**Outcomes/Evaluate:** Negative urine cultures; symptomatic improvement (↓ dysuria, ↓ frequency)

# Nalmefene hydrochloride
(NAL-meh-feen)
**Pregnancy Category:** B
Revex **(Rx)**
**Classification:** Narcotic antagonist

See also *Narcotic Antagonists.*
**Action/Kinetics:** Prevents or reverses respiratory depression, sedation, and hypotension due to opioids, including propoxyphene, nalbuphine, pentazocine, and butorphanol. Has a significantly longer duration of action than naloxone. Does not produce respiratory depression, psychotomimetic effects, or pupillary constriction (i.e., it has no intrinsic activity). Also, tolerance, physical dependence, or abuse potential have not been noted. **Onset, after IV:** 2 min. **Duration:** Up to 8 hr. t½: 10.8 hr. Metabolized by the liver and excreted in the urine.
**Uses:** For complete or partial reversal of the effects of opioid drugs postoperatively. Management of known or suspected overdose of opiates.
**Special Concerns:** Nalmefene will precipitate acute withdrawal symptoms in those who have some degree of tolerance and dependence on opioids. Use with caution in high CV risk clients or in those who have received potentially cardiotoxic drugs. Reversal of buprenorphine-induced respiratory depression may be incomplete; therefore artificial respiration may be necessary. Use with caution during lactation. Safety and effectiveness have not been determined in children.
**Side Effects:** *CV:* Tachycardia, hypertension, hypotension, vasodilation, bradycardia, arrhythmia. *GI:*

N&V, diarrhea, dry mouth. *CNS:* Dizziness, somnolence, depression, agitation, nervousness, tremor, confusion, withdrawal syndrome, myoclonus. *Body as a whole:* Fever, headache, chills, postoperative pain. *Miscellaneous:* Pharyngitis, pruritus, urinary retention.

**Laboratory Test Interferences:** ↑ AST.

**Dosage** ————————
• **IV**

*Reversal of postoperative depression due to opiates.*

**Adults:** Titrate in 0.25-mcg/kg incremental doses at 2–5-min intervals until the desired degree of reversal is achieved (i.e., adequate ventilation and alertness without significant pain or discomfort). In cases where the client is known to be at an increased CV risk, the incremental dose should be 0.1 mcg/kg (the drug may be diluted 1:1 with saline or sterile water). A total dose greater than 1 mcg/kg does not provide additional effects.

*Management of known or suspected overdose of opiates.*

**Adults, initial:** 0.5 mg/70 kg; **then,** 1 mg/70 kg 2–5 min later, if needed. Doses greater than 1.5 mg/70 kg do not increase the beneficial effect. If there is a reasonable suspicion of dependence on opiates, a challenge dose of nalmefene of 0.1 mg/70 kg should be given first; if there is no evidence of withdrawal in 2 min, the recommended dose can be given.

## NURSING CONSIDERATIONS

See also *Nursing Considerations* for *Narcotic Antagonists.*

**Administration/Storage**

1. Should IV access be lost or not readily obtainable, nalmefene can be given by the SC or IM route at doses of 1 mg. This dose is effective in 5–15 min.

**IV** 2. Treatment should follow, not precede, establishment of a patent airway, ventilatory assistance,

administration of oxygen, and circulatory access.

3. Nalmefene is supplied in two concentrations—ampules containing 1 mL (blue label) at a concentration suitable for postoperative use (100 mcg) and ampules containing 2 mL (green label) suitable for management of overdose (1 mg/mL), i.e., **10 times as concentrated.** Follow specific guidelines, depending on the use.

**Assessment**

1. Document type and amount of agent used and when administered/ingested.

2. Note any opioid dependence; may induce acute withdrawal symptoms.

3. Identify high CV risk or those who have received cardiotoxic drugs as this increases the risk for cardiac complications.

4. Observe carefully for recurrent respiratory depression. Compared to naloxone (1.1 hr) the half-life of nalmefene is much longer (10.8 hr). Overdose with long-acting opiates (e.g., methadone, LAAM) may cause recurrence of respiratory depression.

5. With renal failure, if more than one dose is required, administer incremental doses slowly (over 60 sec) to prevent the occurrence of dizziness and hypertension.

6. Client may experience N&V, fever, headaches, chills, pain, dizziness, and tachycardia.

**Outcomes/Evaluate:** Reversal of opioid-induced drug effects; ↓ risk of renarcotization

## Naloxone hydrochloride

(nal-**OX**-ohn)
**Pregnancy Category:** B
Narcan **(Rx)**
**Classification:** Narcotic antagonist

See also *Narcotic Antagonists.*

**Action/Kinetics:** Combines competitively with opiate receptors and blocks or reverses the action of narcotic analgesics. Since the duration of action of naloxone is shorter than that of the narcotic analgesics, the respiratory depression may return when the narcotic antagonist has worn off. **Onset: IV,** 2 min; **SC, IM:** **<5 min. Time to peak effect: 5–15 min. Duration:** Dependent on dose and route of administration but may be as short as 45 min. **t½:** 60–100 min. Metabolized in the liver to inactive products; eliminated through the kidneys.

**Uses:** Respiratory depression induced by natural and synthetic narcotics, including butorphanol, methadone, nalbuphine, pentazocine, and propoxyphene. Drug of choice when nature of depressant drug is not known. Diagnosis of acute opiate overdosage. Not effective when respiratory depression is induced by hypnotics, sedatives, or anesthetics and other nonnarcotic CNS depressants. Adjunct to increase BP in septic shock. *Investigational:* Treatment of Alzheimer's dementia, alcoholic coma, and schizophrenia.

**Contraindications:** Sensitivity to drug. Narcotic addicts (drug may cause severe withdrawal symptoms). Not recommended for use in neonates.

**Special Concerns:** Safe use during lactation and in children is not established.

**Side Effects:** N&V, sweating, hypertension, tremors, sweating due to reversal of narcotic depression. If used postoperatively, excessive doses may cause ***ventricular tachycardia and fibrillation,*** hypo- or hypertension, pulmonary edema, and ***seizures (infrequent).***

**Dosage**
- **IV, IM, SC**

*Narcotic overdose.*

**Initial:** 0.4–2 mg IV; if necessary, additional IV doses may be repeated at 2- to 3-min intervals. If no response after 10 mg, reevaluate diagnosis. **Pediatric, initial:** 0.01 mg/kg IV; **then,** 0.1 mg/kg IV, if needed. The SC or IM route may be used if an IV route is not available.

*To reverse postoperative narcotic depression.*

**Adults: IV, initial,** 0.1- to 0.2-mg increments at 2- to 3-min intervals; **then,** repeat at 1- to 2-hr intervals if necessary. Supplemental IM dosage increases the duration of reversal. **Children: Initial,** 0.005–0.01 mg IV at 2- to 3-min intervals until desired response is obtained.

*Reverse narcotic-induced depression in neonates.*

**Initial:** 0.01 mg/kg IV, IM, or SC. May be repeated using adult administration guidelines.

---

## NURSING CONSIDERATIONS

See also *Nursing Considerations* for *Narcotic Antagonists.*

### Administration/Storage

**IV** 1. May administer undiluted at a rate of 0.4 mg over 15 sec with narcotic overdosage. May reconstitute 2 mg in 500 mL of NSS or 5% dextrose to provide a concentration of 4 mcg/mL or 0.004 mg/mL. The rate of administration varies with client response.

2. Do not mix with preparations containing bisulfite, metabisulfite, long-chain or high molecular weight anions, or solutions with an alkaline pH.

3. When mixed with other solutions, use within 24 hr.

### Assessment

1. Identify any evidence of narcotic addiction. Note agent and drug half-life.

2. Document cardiopulmonary and neurologic assessments.

### Interventions

1. The duration of the narcotic may exceed naloxone (the antagonist). Therefore, more than one dose may be necessary to counteract the effects of the narcotic.

2. Monitor VS at 5-min intervals, then every 30 min once stabilized.

3. Titrate to avoid interfering with pain control or readminister narcotic at a lower dosage to maintain pain control.

**Outcomes/Evaluate:** Reversal of narcotic-induced respiratory depression

# Naltrexone

(nal-**TREX**-ohn)
**Pregnancy Category:** C
ReVia **(Rx)**
**Classification:** Narcotic antagonist

See also *Narcotic Antagonists.*

**Action/Kinetics:** Competitively binds to opiate receptors, thereby reversing or preventing the effects of narcotics. **Peak plasma levels:** 1 hr. **Duration:** 24–72 hr. Metabolized in the liver; a major metabolite—6-beta-naltrexol—is active. **Peak serum levels, after 50 mg: naltrexone,** 8.6 ng/mL; **6-beta-naltrexol,** 99.3 ng/mL. **t½: naltrexone,** approximately 4 hr; **6-beta-naltrexol,** 13 hr. Naltrexone and its metabolites are excreted in the urine.

**Uses:** To prevent narcotic use in former narcotic addicts. Adjunct to the psychosocial treatment for alcoholism. *Investigational:* To treat eating disorders and postconcussional syndrome not responding to other approaches.

**Contraindications:** Clients taking narcotic analgesics, those dependent on narcotics, those in acute withdrawal from narcotics. Liver failure, acute hepatitis.

**Special Concerns:** Use with caution during lactation. Safety during lactation and in children under 18 years of age has not been established.

**Side Effects:** *CNS:* Headache, anxiety, nervousness, sleep disorders, dizziness, change in energy level, depression, confusion, restlessness, disorientation, hallucinations, nightmares, bad dreams, paranoia, fatigue, drowsiness. *GI:* N&V, diarrhea, constipation, anorexia, abdominal pain or cramps, flatulence, ulcers, increased appetite, weight gain or loss, increased thirst, xerostomia, hemorrhoids. *CV:* Phlebitis, edema, increased BP, changes in ECG, palpitations, epistaxis, tachycardia. *GU:* Delayed ejaculation, increased urinary frequency or urinary

discomfort, increased or decreased interest in sex. *Respiratory:* Cough, sore throat, nasal congestion, rhinorrhea, sneezing, excess secretions, hoarseness, SOB, heaving breathing, sinus trouble. *Dermatologic:* Rash, oily skin, itching, pruritus, acne, cold sores, alopecia, athlete's foot. *Musculoskeletal:* Joint/muscle pain, muscle twitches, tremors, pain in legs, knees, or shoulders. *Ophthalmologic:* Blurred vision, aching or strained eyes, burning eyes, light-sensitive eyes, swollen eyes. *Other:* Hepatotoxicity, tinnitus, painful or clogged ears, chills, swollen glands, inguinal pain, cold feet, "hot" spells, "pounding" head, fever, yawning, side pains.

A severe narcotic withdrawal syndrome may be precipitated if naltrexone is administered to a dependent individual. The syndrome may begin within 5 min and may last for up to 2 days.

**Dosage** ———
- **Tablets**

  *To produce blockade of opiate actions.*
  **Initial:** 25 mg followed by an additional 25 mg in 1 hr if no withdrawal symptoms occur. **Maintenance:** 50 mg/day.
  *Alternate dosing schedule for blockade of opiate actions.*
  The weekly dose of 350 mg may be given as: (a) 50 mg/day on weekdays and 100 mg on Saturday; (b) 100 mg/48 hr; (c) 100 mg every Monday and Wednesday and 150 mg on Friday; or, (d) 150 mg q 72 hr.
  *Alcoholism.*
  50 mg once daily for up to 12 weeks. Treatment for longer than 12 weeks has not been studied.

## NURSING CONSIDERATIONS

See also *Nursing Considerations* for *Narcotic Antagonists.*
**Administration/Storage**
1. *Never* initiate therapy until determined that client is not dependent

**N**

on narcotics (i.e., a naloxone challenge test should be completed).

2. Client should be opiate free for at least 7–10 days before beginning therapy.

3. When initiating therapy, begin with 25 mg and observe for 1 hr for any signs of narcotic withdrawal.

4. The blockade produced by naltrexone may be overcome by taking large doses of narcotics; such doses may be fatal.

5. Clients taking naltrexone may not respond to preparations containing narcotics for use in coughs, diarrhea, or pain.

**Assessment**

1. Determine if addicted to opiates and when the last dose was ingested; must be opiate free for 7–10 days before initiating therapy. Check urinalysis to confirm absence of opiates; note if naloxone challenge test performed.

2. Monitor ECG and VS. Report if respirations severely lowered or difficulty breathing evident.

3. Obtain LFTs; monitor monthly during the first 6 months of therapy.

**Client/Family Teaching**

1. May take with food or milk to diminish GI upset.

2. Headaches, restlessness, and irritability may be caused by naltrexone.

3. Report loss of appetite, unusual fatigue, yellowing of skin or sclera, or itching. Abdominal pain or difficulty with bowel function may warrant a dosage reduction.

4. Remain drug free; identify individuals, agencies, and support groups that may assist in remaining drug free.

5. Attend support groups and behavioral therapy sessions.

**Outcomes/Evaluate:** Maintenance of narcotic-free state in detoxified addicts

# Naproxen
(nah-PROX-en)
**Pregnancy Category:** B
Apo-Naproxen ✷, EC-Naprosyn, Naprosyn, Napron X, Naxen ✷,

Novo–Naprox ✷, Nu-Naprox ✷, PMS-Naproxen ✷ **(Rx)**

# Naproxen sodium
(nah-PROX-en)
**Pregnancy Category:** B
Anaprox, Anaprox DS, Apo-Napro-Na ✷, Apo-Napro-Na DS ✷, Naprelan, Novo–Naprox Sodium ✷, Novo-Naprox Sodium DS ✷, Synflex ✷, Synflex DS ✷ **(Rx)**, Aleve **(OTC)**
**Classification:** Nonsteroidal, anti-inflammatory analgesic

See also *Nonsteroidal Anti-Inflammatory Drugs.*

**Action/Kinetics: Peak serum levels of naproxen:** 2–4 hr; **for sodium salt:** 1–2 hr. **t½ for naproxen:** 12–15 hr; **for sodium salt:** 12–13 hr. **Onset, immediate release for analgesia:** 1–2 hr. **Duration, analgesia:** Approximately 7 hr. **Onset, 24 hr (both immediate and delayed release):** 30 min; **duration:** 24 hr. The onset of anti-inflammatory effects may take up to 2 weeks and may last 2–4 weeks. More than 90% bound to plasma protein. Food delays the rate but not the amount of drug absorbed.

**Uses: Rx.** Mild to moderate pain. Musculoskeletal and soft tissue inflammation including rheumatoid arthritis, osteoarthritis, bursitis, tendinitis, ankylosing spondylitis. Primary dysmenorrhea, acute gout. Juvenile rheumatoid arthritis (naproxen only). *NOTE:* The delayed-release or enteric-coated products are not recommended for initial treatment of pain because, compared to other naproxen products, absorption is delayed. *Investigational:* Antipyretic in cancer clients, sunburn, acute migraine (sodium salt only), prophylaxis of migraine, migraine due to menses, PMS (sodium salt only). **OTC.** Relief of minor aches and pains due to the common cold, headache, toothache, muscular aches, backache, minor arthritis pain, pain due to menstrual cramps. Decrease fever.

**Contraindications:** Use of naproxen and naproxen sodium simultaneously. Lactation. Use of delayed-release product for initial treatment of acute pain.

**Special Concerns:** Safety and effectiveness of naproxen have not been determined in children less than 2 years of age; the safety and effectiveness of naproxen sodium have not been established in children. Geriatric clients may manifest increased total plasma levels of naproxen.

**Drug Interactions**

*Methotrexate* / Possibility of a fatal interaction

*Probenecid* / ↓ Plasma clearance of naproxen

**Laboratory Test Interferences:** Naproxen may increase urinary 17-ketosteroid values. Both forms may interfere with urinary assays for 5-HIAA.

**Dosage** ⎯⎯⎯⎯⎯⎯⎯⎯⎯⎯

Naproxen

• **Oral Suspension, Tablets**

*Rheumatoid arthritis, osteoarthritis, ankylosing spondylitis, pain, dysmenorrhea, acute tendinitis, bursitis.*

**Adults, individualized, usual:** 250–500 mg b.i.d. May increase to 1.5 g for short periods of time. Improvement should be observed within 2 weeks; if no improvement is seen, an additional 2-week course of therapy should be considered.

*Acute gout.*

**Adults, initial:** 750 mg; **then,** 250 mg naproxen q 8 hr until symptoms subside.

*Juvenile rheumatoid arthritis.*

Naproxen only, 10 mg/kg/day in two divided doses. If the suspension is used, the following dosage can be used: **13 kg:** 2.5 mL b.i.d.; **25 kg:** 5 mL b.i.d.; **38 kg:** 7.5 mL b.i.d.

• **Delayed Release Tablets**

*Rheumatoid arthritis, osteoarthritis, ankylosing spondylitis, pain, dysmenorrhea, acute tendinitis, bursitis.*

375–500 mg b.i.d.

Naproxen sodium

• **Tablets (Rx)**

*Rheumatoid arthritis, osteoarthritis, ankylosing spondylitis, pain, dysmenorrhea, acute tendinitis, bursitis.*

**Adults:** 275–550 mg b.i.d. in the morning and evening. May be increased to 1.65 g for short periods of time.

*Acute gout.*

**Adults, initial:** 825 mg; **then,** 275 mg q 8 hr until symptoms subside.

*Mild to moderate pain, primary dysmenorrhea, acute bursitis and tendinitis.*

**Adults, initial:** 550 mg; **then,** 275 mg q 6–8 hr as needed. Total daily dose should not exceed 1,375 mg.

• **Controlled Release Tablets**

*Rheumatoid arthritis, osteoarthritis, ankylosing spondylitis, pain, dysmenorrhea, acute tendinitis, bursitis.*

**Adults:** 750 mg or 1,000 mg once daily, not to exceed 1,000 mg/day.

*Acute gout.*

**Adults:** 1,000 mg once daily. For short periods of time, 1,500 mg may be given.

• **Tablets (OTC)**

**Adults:** 200 mg q 8–12 hr with a full glass of liquid. For some clients, 400 mg initially followed by 200 mg 12 hr later will provide better relief. Dose should not exceed 600 mg in a 24-hr period. Geriatric clients should not take more than 200 mg q 12 hr. Not for use in children less than 12 years of age unless directed by a physician.

## NURSING CONSIDERATIONS

See also *Nursing Considerations* for *Nonsteroidal Anti-Inflammatory Drugs.*

**Administration/Storage**

1. It is recommended that the medication be taken in the morning and in the evening. The doses do not have to be equal.

2. Do not give to children.

3. Naproxen suspension can be used to treat children with rheumatoid arthritis.

4. Delayed-release naproxen is not

recommended for treatment of acute pain.

5. Do not use the OTC product for more than 10 days for pain or 3 days for fever unless prescribed.

**Assessment**

1. Note any hypersensitivity to any NSAIDs.

2. Document indications for therapy, onset and characteristics of symptoms. With pain, rate using a pain-rating scale and determine if another product should be used initially.

3. Note any joint swelling, pain, trauma, inflammation, or decreased ROM.

4. Determine any GI bleeding or ulcers; use GI protectant if needed. Enteric coated product (EC-Naprosyn) reduces GI side effects.

5. Monitor CBC, liver and renal function studies with chronic therapy.

**Client/Family Teaching**

1. Take with food to ↓ GI upset; in the morning and evening for optimal effects.

2. Report any persistent abdominal pain or dark-colored stools immediately.

**Outcomes/Evaluate**

• Improved joint pain and mobility
• Relief of headaches
• ↓ Uterine cramping

# Natamycin

(nah-tah-**MY**-sin)
**Pregnancy Category:** C
Natacyn **(Rx)**
**Classification:** Antifungal (ophthalmic)

See also *Anti-Infectives.*

**Action/Kinetics:** Antifungal antibiotic derived from *Streptomyces natalensis*. Binds to the fungal cell membrane, resulting in alteration of permeability and loss of essential intracellular materials. Is fungicidal. After topical administration, therapeutic levels are reached in the corneal stroma but not in the intraocular fluid. Not absorbed systemically.

**Uses:** For ophthalmic use only. Drug of choice for *Fusarium sola-*

*nae* keratitis. For treatment of fungal blepharitis, conjunctivitis, and keratitis caused by susceptible organisms. It is active against a variety of yeasts and filamentous fungi including *Candida, Aspergillus, Cephalosporium, Fusarium,* and *Penicillium.* Before initiating therapy, determine the susceptibility of the infectious organism to drug in smears and cultures of corneal scrapings. Effectiveness of natamycin for use as single agent in fungal endophthalmitis not established.

**Contraindications:** Hypersensitivity to drug.

**Special Concerns:** Use with caution during lactation. Effectiveness as a single agent to treat fungal endophthalmitis has not been established. Safety and effectiveness have not been determined in children.

**Side Effects:** Eye irritation, occasional allergies.

**Dosage** —————
• **Ophthalmic Suspension (5%)**
*Fungal keratitis.*
**Initially,** 1 gtt in conjunctival sac q 1–2 hr; can be reduced usually, after 3–4 days to 1 gtt 6–8 times/day. Continue therapy for 14–21 days, during which dosage can be reduced gradually at 4 to 7-day intervals.
*Fungal blepharitis/conjunctivitis.*
1 gtt 4–6 times/day.

# NURSING CONSIDERATIONS

See also *General Nursing Considerations for All Anti-Infectives.*

**Administration/Storage**

1. Store at room temperature or in refrigerator avoiding exposure to light and excessive heat. Do not freeze.

2. Shake well before using.

3. Avoid contamination of dropper.

4. Discontinue if toxicity suspected.

5. Review therapy if no improvement noted after 7–10 days.

**Assessment:** Note indications for therapy; document clinical presentation.

**Client/Family Teaching**

1. Continue for 14–21 days even

though condition may appear controlled.

2. Report any increased itching, pain, burning, or stinging.

3. To prevent reinfection, do not share eye makeup, washcloths, towels, or eye medications.

**Outcomes/Evaluate:** Ophthalmic and symptomatic improvement

---

# Nedocromil sodium
(neh-**DAH**-kroh-mill)
**Pregnancy Category:** B
Tilade **(Rx)**
**Classification:** Antiasthmatic

**Action/Kinetics:** Inhibits the release of various mediators, such as histamine, leukotriene $C_4$, and prostaglandin $D_2$, from a variety of cell types associated with asthma. Has no intrinsic bronchodilator, antihistamine, or glucocorticoid activity; also, systemic bioavailability is low. **t½:** 3.3 hr. About 89% bound to plasma protein; excreted unchanged.

**Uses:** Maintenance therapy in adults and children (age six and older) with mild to moderate bronchial asthma.

**Contraindications:** Use for the reversal of acute bronchospasms, especially status asthmaticus.

**Special Concerns:** Use with caution during lactation. Safety and efficacy have not been established in children less than 12 years of age. Nedocromil has not been shown to be able to substitute for the total dose of corticosteroids.

**Side Effects:** *Respiratory:* Coughing, pharyngitis, rhinitis, upper respiratory tract infection, increased sputum, bronchitis, dyspnea, ***bronchospasm.*** *GI tract:* N&V, dyspepsia, abdominal pain, dry mouth, diarrhea. *CNS:* Dizziness, dysphonia. *Skin:* Rash, sensation of warmth. *Body as a whole:* Headache, chest pain, fatigue, arthritis. *Miscellaneous:* Viral infection, unpleasant taste.

**Laboratory Test Interferences:** ↑ ALT.

**Dosage**
• **Metered Dose Inhaler**
*Bronchial asthma.*
**Adults and children over 12 years of age:** Two inhalations q.i.d. at regular intervals in order to provide 14 mg/day. If the client is under good control on q.i.d. dosing (i.e., requiring inhaled or oral beta agonist no more than twice a week or no worsening of symptoms occur with respiratory infections), a lower dose can be tried. In such instances, the dose should first be reduced to 10.5 mg/day (i.e., used t.i.d.); then, after several weeks with good control, the dose can be reduced to 7 mg/day (i.e., used b.i.d.).

---

## NURSING CONSIDERATIONS
**Administration/Storage**

1. Each actuation releases 1.75 mg.

2. Must be used regularly, even during symptom-free period, in order to achieve beneficial effects.

3. Clients must be taught the proper method of use of the drug. An illustrated pamphlet is included in each pack of nedocromil.

4. Add nedocromil to existing treatment (e.g., bronchodilators). When clinical response is seen and if asthma is under good control, a gradual decrease in the concomitant medication can be tried.

5. Store between 2°C–30°C (36°F–86°F) and do not freeze.

**Assessment**

1. Document symptoms, noting type, onset, and duration. List other agents trialed and the outcome.

2. Assess respiratory status thoroughly; not for use with status asthmaticus or for reversal of acute bronchospasm.

3. Monitor peak flow and vital capacity measurements.

4. Document systemic and inhaled steroid therapy accurately. When a reduction is in progress, nedocromil cannot substitute for total steroid dose/requirements.

5. Review drug usage and time be-

**N**

tween prescriptions to ensure proper use.

**Client/Family Teaching**

1. Review correct procedure for administration; use the step-by-step instructions provided with the drug.

2. Beneficial *preventative* effects will not be obtained if not correctly administered by topical lung application. Drug is an inhaled anti-inflammatory that reduces lung inflammation.

3. Do not stop therapy during symptom-free periods; drug must be taken at regular intervals. Continue to use with other prescribed therapies.

4. Report any persistent headaches, unpleasant taste in mouth that interferes with nutrition, severe nausea, or chest pain.

5. Report any coughing or bronchospasm following use of nedocromil; drug should be discontinued, lungs assessed, and alternative therapy substituted.

**Outcomes/Evaluate:** ↓ Severity/frequency of asthmatic episodes

# Nefazodone hydrochloride

(nih-**FAY**-zoh-dohn)

**Pregnancy Category:** C

Serzone **(Rx)**

**Classification:** Antidepressant

**Action/Kinetics:** Exact antidepressant mechanism not known. Inhibits neuronal uptake of serotonin and norepinephrine and antagonizes central 5-HT$_2$ receptors and alpha-1-adrenergic receptors (which may cause postural hypotension). Produces none to slight anticholinergic effects, moderate sedation, and slight orthostatic hypotension. **Peak plasma levels:** 1 hr. **t½:** 2–4 hr. **Time to reach steady state:** 4–5 days. Extensively metabolized by the liver with less than 1% excreted unchanged in the urine. Food delays the absorption of nefazodone and decreases the bioavailability by approximately 20%.

**Uses:** Treatment of depression.

**Contraindications:** Use with terfenadine or astemizole; in combination with an MAO inhibitor or within 14 days of discontinuing MAO inhibitor therapy. Clients hypersensitive to nefazodone or other phenylpiperazine antidepressants.

**Special Concerns:** Use with caution in clients with a recent history of MI, unstable heart disease and taking digoxin, or a history of mania. Use with caution during lactation. Safety and efficacy have not been determined in individuals below 18 years of age. There is a possibility of a suicide attempt in depression that may persist until significant remission occurs.

**Side Effects:** *CNS:* Dizziness, insomnia, agitation, somnolence, lightheadedness, activation of mania or hypomania, confusion, memory impairment, paresthesia, abnormal dreams, decreased concentration, ataxia, incoordination, psychomotor retardation, tremor, hypertonia, decreased libido, vertigo, twitching, depersonalization, hallucinations, *suicide thoughts/attempt*, apathy, euphoria, hostility, abnormal gait, abnormal thinking, derealization, paranoid reaction, dysarthria, myoclonus, *neuroleptic malignant syndrome (rare)*. *CV:* Postural hypotension, hypotension, sinus bradycardia, tachycardia, hypertension, syncope, ventricular extrasystoles, angina pectoris, *CVA (rare)*. *GI:* Nausea, dry mouth, constipation, dyspepsia, diarrhea, increased appetite, vomiting, eructation, periodontal abscess, gingivitis, colitis, gastritis, mouth ulceration, stomatitis, esophagitis, peptic ulcer, rectal hemorrhage. *Dermatologic:* Pruritus, dry skin, acne, alopecia, urticaria, maculopapular rash, vesiculobullous rash, eczema. *Musculoskeletal:* Asthenia, arthralgia, arthritis, tenosynovitis, muscle stiffness, bursitis. *Respiratory:* Pharyngitis, increased cough, dyspnea, bronchitis, asthma, pneumonia, laryngitis, voice alteration, epistaxis, hiccups. *Hematologic:* Ecchymosis, anemia, leukopenia, lymphadenopathy. *Ophthalmologic:*

Blurred vision, abnormal vision, visual field defect, dry eye, eye pain, abnormal accommodation, diplopia, conjunctivitis, mydriasis, keratoconjunctivitis, photophobia, night blindness. *Body as a whole:* Headache, infection, flu syndrome, chills, fever, neck rigidity, allergic reaction, malaise, photosensitivity, facial edema, hangover effect, enlarged abdomen, hernia, pelvic pain, halitosis, cellulitis, weight loss, gout, dehydration. *GU:* Urinary frequency, UTI, urinary retention, vaginitis, breast pain, cystitis, urinary urgency, metrorrhagia, amenorrhea, polyuria, vaginal hemorrhage, breast enlargement, menorrhagia, urinary incontinence, abnormal ejaculation, hematuria, nocturia, kidney calculus. *Miscellaneous:* Peripheral edema, thirst, abnormal LFTs, ear pain, hyperacusis, deafness, taste loss.

**OD** **Overdose Management:** *Symptoms:* N&V, somnolence, increased incidence of severity of any of the reported side effects. *Treatment:* Symptomatic and supportive in the cases of hypotension or excessive sedation. Gastric lavage may be used.

**Drug Interactions**
*Alprazolam* / ↑ Plasma levels of alprazolam
*Astemizole* / ↑ Plasma levels of astemizole resulting in QT prolongation and possible serious CV events, including death due to ventricular tachycardia of the torsades de pointes type
*Digoxin* / ↑ Plasma levels of digoxin
*MAO inhibitors* / Serious and possibly fatal reactions including symptoms of hyperthermia, rigidity, myoclonus, autonomic instability with possible rigid fluctuations of VS, and mental status changes that may include extreme agitation progressing to delirium and coma
*Propranolol* / ↓ Plasma levels of propranolol
*Terfenadine* / ↑ Plasma levels of terfenadine resulting in QT prolongation and possible serious CV events, including death due to ventricular tachycardia of the torsades de pointes type
*Triazolam* / ↑ Plasma levels of triazolam
**Laboratory Test Interferences:** ↑ AST, ALT, LDH. ↓ Hematocrit. Hypercholesterolemia, hypoglycemia.

**Dosage** ─────────────
• **Tablets**
  *Antidepressant.*
**Adults, initial:** 200 mg/day given in two divided doses. Increase dose in increments of 100–200 mg/day at intervals of no less than 1 week. The effective dose range is 300–600 mg/day. The initial dose for elderly or debilitated clients is 100 mg/day given in two divided doses.

─────────────

## NURSING CONSIDERATIONS
### Administration/Storage
1. Several weeks may be required for the full beneficial effect to be observed.
2. Although long-term use has not been studied, it is usually recommended that the drug be given for a period of 6 months or longer.
3. At least 14 days should elapse between discontinuation of an MAO inhibitor and initiation of therapy with nefazodone; also, at least 7 days should elapse after stopping nefazodone and before starting an MAO inhibitor.

### Assessment
1. Document indications for therapy, onset and duration of symptoms, and any underlying or precipitating factors.
2. List drugs currently prescribed to ensure none interact unfavorably.
3. Determine any CAD, recent MI, or conditions requiring digoxin administration.
4. Monitor CBC, ECG, liver and renal function studies.

### Client/Family Teaching
1. Take before meals; food may inhibit absorption.
2. Do not perform activities that re-

quire mental alertness or coordination until drug effects realized; may cause dizziness, drowsiness, confusion, incoordination, decreased concentration and response time.

3. Avoid alcohol and any other CNS depressants. No OTC agents without approval.

4. May take several weeks (2–4) before any effects are realized; do not become discouraged.

5. Report any unusual sensations or side effects, increased depression, or suicidal thoughts/behavior.

6. Use reliable birth control during therapy.

**Outcomes/Evaluate:** Symptomatic improvement; ↓ depression, as evidenced by improved sleeping and eating patterns, ↓ fatigue, and ↑ social involvement and activity

# Nelfinavir mesylate

(nel-**FIN**-ah-veer)
**Pregnancy Category:** B
Viracept **(Rx)**
**Classification:** Antiviral, protease inhibitor

See also *Antiviral Drugs.*

**Action/Kinetics:** HIV-1 protease inhibitor, resulting in prevention of cleavage of gagpol polyprotein resulting in production of immature, non-infectious viruses. Activity is increased when used with didanosine, lamivudine, stavudine, zalcitabine, or zidovudine. **Peak plasma levels:** 2–4 hr. **Steady-state plasma levels:** 3–4 mcg/mL. Food increases plasma levels 2–3 fold. **t½, terminal:** 3.5–5 hr. Metabolites (one of which is as active as parent compound) and unchanged drug excreted mainly in feces.

**Uses:** Treat HIV infection when antiretroviral therapy is required.

**Contraindications:** Administration with astemizole, cisapride, midazolam, rifampin, terfenadine, or triazolam.

**Special Concerns:** Use with caution with hepatic impairment. Safety and efficacy have not been deter-

mined in children less than 2 years of age.

**Side Effects:** Side effects were determined when used in combination with other antiviral drugs. *GI:* N&V, diarrhea, flatulence, abdominal pain, anorexia, dyspepsia, epigastric pain, GI bleeding, hepatitis, mouth ulcers, pancreatitis. *CNS:* Anxiety, depression, dizziness, emotional lability, hyperkinesia, insomnia, migraine, paresthesia, *seizures,* sleep disorder, somnolence, *suicide ideation. Hematologic:* Anemia, leukopenia, thrombocytopenia. *Respiratory:* Dyspnea, rhinitis, sinusitis, pharyngitis. *GU:* Kidney calculus, sexual dysfunction, urine abnormality. *Ophthalmic:* Eye disorder, acute iritis. *Musculoskeletal:* Arthralgia, arthritis, cramps, myalgia, myasthenia, myopathy. *Dermatologic:* Dermatitis, folliculitis, fungal dermatitis, maculopapular rash, pruritus, urticaria, sweating. *Miscellaneous:* Asthenia, dehydration, allergic reaction, back pain, fever, headache, malaise, pain, accidental injury.

**OD** **Overdose Management:** *Symptoms:* See side effects. *Treatment:* Emesis or gastric lavage, followed by activated charcoal.

**Drug Interactions**

*Anticonvulsants /* Possible ↓ plasma levels of nelfinavir

*Astemizole /* Potential for serious and life-threatening cardiac arrhythmias

*Indinavir /* Significant ↑ in nelfinavir levels

*Oral contraceptives /* ↓ Effect of oral contraceptives; use alternative contraceptive measures

*Rifabutin /* ↑ Levels of rifabutin; reduce dose of rifabutin by one-half

*Rifampin /* Significant ↓ in nelfinavir levels; do not coadminister

*Terfenadine /* Potential for serious and life-threatening cardiac arrhythmias

**Laboratory Test Interferences:** ↑ ALT, AST, creatine phosphokinase, alkaline phosphatase, amylase, lactic dehydrogenase, GGT. Hyperlipidemia, hyperuricemia, hypoglycemia. Abnormal liver function tests.

## Dosage
• **Powder, Tablets**
*HIV.*
**Adults:** 750 mg (i.e., 3-250 mg tablets) t.i.d. in combination with nucleoside analogs. **Children, 2 to 13 years:** 20-30 mg/kg/dose t.i.d.

## NURSING CONSIDERATIONS

See also *Nursing Considerations* for *Antiviral Drugs*.
**Assessment**
1. Document onset of disease, clinical characteristics, and other agents trialed.
2. List drugs prescribed/consumed to ensure none interact unfavorably.
3. Monitor CBC, $CD_4$ counts, viral load, liver and renal function.
**Client/Family Teaching**
1. Take as prescribed with snack or light meal to enhance absorption.
2. Do not reconstitute powder with water in its original container. Mix powder with small amount of water, milk, formula, soy formula, soy milk or dietary supplement. Once mixed, consume entire amount for full dose. Do not mix with acidic foods or juice (e.g., orange or apple juice, apple sauce) due to their bitter taste.
3. Report any evidence of increased bruising or bleeding.
4. Drug is to be administered in combination with nucleoside analogs as prescribed.
5. Drug is not cure but helps to manage symptoms.
6. If diarrhea is bothersome, report as loperamide may be prescribed.
7. Drug does not prevent transmission of disease; continue to practice safe sex.
**Outcomes/Evaluate:** Control of HIV symptoms; ↓ viral load

# Neomycin sulfate
(nee-oh-**MY**-sin)
**Pregnancy Category:** D
Mycifradin Sulfate, Myciguent, Neobiotic **(Rx)**
**Classification:** Antibiotic, aminoglycoside

See also *Anti-Infectives* and *Aminoglycosides*.
**Action/Kinetics: Peak plasma levels: PO,** 1–4 hr; **Therapeutic serum level:** 5–10 mcg/mL. **t½:** 2–3 hr.
**Uses: PO:** Hepatic coma, sterilization of gut prior to surgery, inhibition of ammonia-forming bacteria in GI tract in hepatic encephalopathy. Therapy of intestinal infections due to pathogenic strains of *Escherichia coli,* primarily in children. *Investigational:* Hypercholesterolemia.
   **Topical:** Prophylaxis or treatment of infection in burns, minor cuts, wounds, and skin abrasions. As an aid to healing and for treating superficial skin infections.
**Additional Contraindications:** Intestinal obstruction (PO). Topical products should not be used in or around the eyes.
**Special Concerns:** Safe use during pregnancy has not been determined. Due to the possibility of toxicity, some experts do not recommend the parenteral use of neomycin for any purpose. Use with caution in clients with extensive burns, trophic ulceration, or other conditions where significant systemic absorption is possible.
**Side Effects:** Chronic use of topical neomycin to inflamed skin of those with contact dermatitis and chronic dermatosis increases the chance of hypersensitivity. Ototoxicity, nephrotoxicity. Sprue-like syndrome with steatorrhea, malabsorption, and electrolyte imbalance. Skin rashes after topical or parenteral administration. Chronic use in allergic contact dermatitis and chronic dermatoses increases the risk of sensitization.
**Additional Drug Interactions**
*Digoxin* / ↓ Effect of digoxin due to ↓ absorption from GI tract
*Penicillin V* / ↓ Effect of penicillin due to ↓ absorption from GI tract
*Procainamide* / ↑ Muscle relaxation produced by neomycin

**N**

---

## Dosage

- **Oral Solution**

*Preoperatively in colorectal surgery.*

1 g each of neomycin and erythromycin base for a total of three doses: the first two doses 1 hr apart the afternoon before surgery and the third dose at bedtime the night before surgery.

*Hepatic coma, adjunct.*

**Adults,** 4–12 g/day in divided doses for 5–6 days; **children:** 50–100 mg/kg/day in divided doses for 5–6 days.

- **Topical Cream, Ointment**

Neomycin alone or in combination with other antibiotics (bacitracin or gramicidin) and/or an anti-inflammatory agent (corticosteroid). Apply ointment (0.5%) or cream (0.5%) 1–3 times/day to affected area. If necessary, a bandage may be used to cover the area.

## NURSING CONSIDERATIONS

See also *Nursing Considerations* for *Aminoglycosides*.

### Administration/Storage

1. Carefully follow recommended procedure to prepare the GI tract for surgery.
2. Have available neostigmine to counteract renal failure, respiratory depression and arrest (side effects that may occur when neomycin is administered intraperitoneally).
3. When used topically, clean the affected area and apply a small amount equal to the surface area of a fingertip.

### Assessment

1. Document indications for therapy. Note clinical presentation and symptom characteristics.
2. Describe abdominal assessment findings.
3. Review lab data.

### Interventions

1. Monitor I&O and serum electrolyte levels. Encourage fluid intake of 2–3 L/day.
2. Expect slight laxative effect produced by PO neomycin. Withhold

and report in case of suspected intestinal obstruction.

3. Anticipate low-residue diet for preoperative disinfection and a laxative immediately preceding PO administration of neomycin sulfate.
4. Clean the affected area before applying topical ointment or solution.

### Outcomes/Evaluate

- Improved level of consciousness
- Healing of skin wounds
- Bowel sterilization before intestinal surgery

# Neostigmine bromide
(nee-oh-**STIG**-meen)
**Pregnancy Category:** C
Prostigmin Bromide **(Rx)**

# Neostigmine methylsulfate
(nee-oh-**STIG**-meen)
**Pregnancy Category:** C
Prostigmin Injection, PMS-Neostigmine Methylsulfate ✤ **(Rx)**
**Classification:** Indirectly acting cholinergic-acetylcholinesterase inhibitor

**Action/Kinetics:** Acetylcholinesterase inhibitor that causes an increase in the concentration of acetylcholine at the myoneural junction, thus facilitating transmission of impulses across the myoneural junction. In myasthenia gravis, muscle strength is increased. May also act on the autonomic ganglia of the CNS. Prevents or relieves postoperative distention by increasing gastric motility and tone and prevents or relieves urinary retention by increasing the tone of the detrusor muscle of the bladder. Shorter acting than ambenonium chloride and pyridostigmine. Atropine is often given concomitantly to control side effects. **Onset: PO,** 45–75 min; **IM,** 20–30 min; **IV,** 4–8 min. **Time to peak effect, parenteral:** 20–30 min. **Duration:** All routes, 2.5–4 hr. t½, **PO:** 42–60 min; **IM:** 51–90 min; **IV:** 47–60 min. Eliminated through the urine (about 40% unchanged).

**Uses:** Diagnosis and treatment of myasthenia gravis. Prophylaxis and treatment of postoperative distention or urinary retention. Antidote for tubocurarine and other nondepolarizing drugs.

**Contraindications:** Hypersensitivity, mechanical obstruction of GI or urinary tract, peritonitis, history of bromide sensitivity. Vesical neck obstruction of urinary bladder. Lactation.

**Special Concerns:** Safety and effectiveness in children have not been established. Use with caution in clients with bronchial asthma, bradycardia, vagotonia, epilepsy, hyperthyroidism, peptic ulcer, cardiac arrhythmias, or recent coronary occlusion. May cause uterine irritability and premature labor if given IV to pregnant women near term. In geriatric clients, the duration of action may be increased.

**Side Effects:** *GI:* N&V, diarrhea, abdominal cramps, involuntary defecation, salivation, dysphagia, flatulence, increased gastric and intestinal secretions. *CV:* Bradycardia, tachycardia, hypotension, ECG changes, nodal rhythm, *cardiac arrest,* syncope, *AV block,* substantial pain, thrombophlebitis after IV use. *CNS:* Headache, *seizures,* malaise, weakness, dysarthria, dizziness, drowsiness, loss of consciousness. *Respiratory:* Increased oral, pharyngeal, and bronchial secretions; *bronchospasms, skeletal muscle paralysis, laryngospasm, central respiratory paralysis, respiratory depression or arrest,* dyspnea. *Ophthalmologic:* Miosis, double vision, lacrimation, accommodation difficulties, hyperemia of conjunctiva, visual changes. *Musculoskeletal:* Muscle fasciculations or weakness, muscle cramps or spasms, arthralgia. *Other:* Skin rashes, urinary frequency and incontinence, sweating, flushing, allergic reactions, anaphylaxis, urticaria. These effects can usually be reversed by parenteral administration of 0.6 mg of atropine sulfate, which should be readily available.

Cholinergic crisis, due to overdosage, must be distinguished from myasthenic crisis (worsening of the disease), since cholinergic crisis involves removal of drug therapy, while myasthenic crisis involves an increase in anticholinesterase therapy.

**OD** **Overdose Management:** *Symptoms:* Abdominal cramps, vomiting, diarrhea, epigastric distress, excessive salivation, cold sweating, pallor, blurred vision, urinary urgency, fasciculation and *paralysis of voluntary muscles (including the tongue),* miosis, increased BP (may be accompanied by bradycardia), sensation of internal trembling, panic, severe anxiety. *Treatment:* Discontinue medication temporarily. Give atropine, 0.5–1 mg IV (up to 5–10 or more mg may be needed to get the HR to 80 beats/min). Supportive treatment including artificial respiration and oxygen.

**Drug Interactions**

*Aminoglycosides* / ↑ Neuromuscular blockade

*Atropine* / Atropine suppresses symptoms of excess GI stimulation caused by cholinergic drugs

*Corticosteroids* / ↓ Effect of neostigmine

*Magnesium salts* / Antagonize the effects of anticholinesterases

*Mecamylamine* / Intense hypotensive response

*Organophosphate-type insecticides/pesticides* / Added systemic effects with cholinesterase inhibitors

*Succinylcholine* / ↑ Neuromuscular blocking effects

**Dosage** —————————————

NEOSTIGMINE BROMIDE

• **Tablets**

*Treat myasthenia gravis.*

**Adults:** 15 mg q 3–4 hr; adjust dose and frequency as needed. **Usual maintenance:** 150 mg/day with dosing intervals determined by client response. **Pediatric,** 2 mg/kg (60 mg/m$^2$) daily in six to eight divided doses.

NEOSTIGMINE METHYLSULFATE

---

♣ = Available in Canada                    ***bold italic*** = life threatening side effect

- **IM, IV, SC**
  *Diagnosis of myasthenia gravis.*
  **Adults, IM, SC:** 1.5 mg given with 0.6 mg atropine; **pediatric, IM:** 0.04 mg/kg (1 mg/m²); or, **IV:** 0.02 mg/kg (0.5 mg/m²).
  *Treat myasthenia gravis.*
  **Adults, IM, SC:** 0.5 mg. **Pediatric, IM, SC:** 0.01–0.04 mg/kg q 2–3 hr.
  *Antidote for tubocurarine.*
  **Adults, IV:** 0.5–2 mg slowly with 0.6–1.2 mg atropine sulfate. Can repeat if necessary up to total dose of 5 mg. **Pediatric, IV:** 0.04 mg/kg with 0.02 mg/kg atropine sulfate.
  *Prevention of postoperative GI distention or urinary retention.*
  **Adults, IM, SC:** 0.25 mg (1 mL of the 1:4,000 solution) immediately after surgery repeated q 4–6 hr for 2–3 days.
  *Treatment of postoperative GI distention.*
  **Adults, IM, SC:** 0.5 mg (1 mL of the 1:2,000 solution) as required.
  *Treatment of urinary retention.*
  **Adults, IM, SC:** 0.5 mg (1 mL of the 1:2,000 solution). If urination does not occur within 1 hr after 0.5 mg, the client should be catheterized. After the bladder is emptied, 0.5 mg is given q 3 hr for at least five injections.

## NURSING CONSIDERATIONS
### Administration/Storage
1. Determine interval doses individually to achieve optimum effects.
2. If greater fatigue occurs at certain times of the day, a larger part of the daily dose can be administered at these times.
3. Do not give if high concentrations of halothane or cyclopropane are present.
**IV** 4. May administer IV form undiluted at a rate of 0.5 mg/min.

### Assessment
1. Note any bromide sensitivity or hypersensitivity to drugs in this category.
2. Identify drugs client is taking to determine if any interact unfavorably.

### Interventions
1. Report symptoms of generalized cholinergic stimulation (evidence of a toxic reaction).
2. Assess for stability and vision. If difficulty with coordination or vision caution to avoid use of heavy machinery until the effects of the medication wear off.
3. Monitor VS for the first hour after drug administration. Report if the pulse is less than 80 as the drug should be withheld. If hypotension occurs, have the client remain recumbent until BP stabilizes.
4. When used as an antidote for nondepolarizing drugs, provide ventilatory assistance.
5. If taking for myasthenia gravis, any onset of weakness 1 hr after administration usually indicates overdosage of drug. Weakness 3 hr or more after administration usually indicates underdosage and/or resistance. Document as well as any associated difficulty with respirations or increase in muscle weakness.

### Client/Family Teaching
1. With myasthenia, maintain a written record of periods of muscle strength or weakness so that dosage can be evaluated and adjusted accordingly; space activities to avoid excessive fatigue.
2. Take the dose exactly as prescribed; taking it late may result in myasthenic crisis whereas taking it early may result in cholinergic crisis.
3. Increasing weakness should be reported immediately; drug tolerance can develop.
4. Wear and/or carry identification indicating therapy with neostigmine and why.

### Outcomes/Evaluate
- ↑ Muscle strength and function with myasthenia gravis
- Relief of postoperative ileus or urinary retention
- Reversal of respiratory depression R/T nondepolarizing drugs

# Nevirapine
((neh-**VYE**-rah-peen))
**Pregnancy Category:** C

Viramune **(Rx)**
**Classification:** Antiviral

See also *Antiviral Drugs.*
**Action/Kinetics:** By binding tightly to reverse transcriptase, nevirapine prevents viral RNA from being converted into DNA. In combination with a nucleoside analogue, it reduces the amount of virus circulating in the body and increases CD4+ cell counts. Readily absorbed, with peak plasma levels occurring 4 hr after a 200-mg dose. Extensively metabolized in the liver. Excreted through both the urine (about 90%) and the feces (about 10%). Induces its own metabolism such that following chronic use the half-life decreases from about 45 hr following a single dose to 25 to 30 hr following multiple dosing with 200 or 400 mg daily.
**Uses:** In combination with nucleoside analogues (e.g., AZT, lamivudine, didanosine, zalcitabine) for the treatment of HIV-1 infections in adults who have experienced clinical and immunologic deterioration. Always use in combination with at least one other antiretroviral agent, as resistant viruses emerge rapidly when nevirapine is used alone. The use of nevirapine with protease inhibitors (e.g., saquinavir, indinavir, ritonavir) is not recommended.
**Contraindications:** Lactation.
**Special Concerns:** The duration of benefit from therapy may be limited. Nevirapine is not a cure for HIV infections; clients may continue to experience illnesses associated with HIV infections, including opportunistic infections. Nevirapine has not been shown to reduce the risk of transmitting HIV to others through sexual contact or blood contamination. Use with caution in impaired renal or hepatic function. Safety and efficacy have not been determined in children.
**Side Effects:** *GI:* Nausea, abnormal LFTs, diarrhea, abdominal pain, ulcerative stomatitis, hepatitis. *CNS:* Headache, fatigue, paresthesia. *He-*
*matologic:* Decreased hemoglobin, decreased platelets, decreased neutrophils. *Miscellaneous:* **Rash (may be severe and life-threatening),** fever, peripheral neuropathy, myalgia.
**Drug Interactions**
*Oral contraceptives* / ↓ Plasma levels of oral contraceptives → ↓ effect
*Protease inhibitors* / ↓ Plasma levels of protease inhibitors
*Rifabutin* / ↓ Nevirapine trough concentrations
*Rifampin* / Nevirapine trough concentrations
**Laboratory Test Interferences:** ALT, AST, GGT, total bilirubin.

**Dosage**
• **Tablets**
*HIV-1 infections.*
**Initial:** 200 mg/day for 14 days.
**Maintenance:** 200 mg b.i.d. (e.g., 7:00 a.m. and 7:00 p.m.) in combination with a nucleoside analogue antiretroviral agent.

## NURSING CONSIDERATIONS

See also *Nursing Considerations* for *Antiviral Drugs,* and *Anti-Infectives.*
**Administration/Storage**
1. Clients who interrupt nevirapine dosing for more than 7 days should restart therapy using one 200-mg tablet for the first 14 days, followed by 200 mg b.i.d. (7 a.m. and 7 p.m.).
2. Can be taken with or without food.
3. If a dose is skipped, take the next dose as soon as possible; do not double the dose.
4. Store tablets in a tightly closed bottle at 15°C–30°C (59°F–86°F).
**Assessment**
1. Document disease onset, symptom characteristics, other agents trialed and the outcome.
2. List drugs currently prescribed to ensure none interact unfavorably.
3. Monitor CBC, CD4 counts, viral load, liver and renal function studies.
**Client/Family Teaching**
1. Drug is not a cure but helps control disease symptoms.
2. Take exactly as directed; do not

double up with missed doses. Should be taken with another antiretroviral agent to prevent emergence of resistant viruses.

3. A rash may occur in the first few weeks of therapy. Notify provider and do not increase dosage until rash subsides.

4. Any severe rash or rash accompanied by flu-like symptoms warrants immediate notification.

5. Drug does not prevent transmission through sexual contact or blood contamination. Practice barrier contraception or nonhormonal form of birth control.

**Outcomes/Evaluate:**   Improved CD4 cell counts; ↓ Viral load

---

# Niacin (Nicotinic acid)

(**NYE**-ah-sin, nih-koh-**TIN**-ick **AH**-sid)

**Pregnancy Category:** C

Nia-Bid, Niaspan, Nico-400, Nicobid, Nicolar, Nicotinex, Slo-Niacin, Span-Niacin, Tega-Span (Rx and OTC)

# Niacinamide

(nye-ah-**SIN**-ah-myd)

**Pregnancy Category:** C

Papulex ✤ (Rx: Injection; OTC: Tablets)

**Classification:** Vitamin B complex

---

**Action/Kinetics:** Niacin (nicotinic acid) and niacinamide are water-soluble, heat-resistant vitamins prepared synthetically. Niacin (after conversion to the active niacinamide) is a component of the coenzymes nicotinamide-adenine dinucleotide and nicotinamide-adenine dinucleotide phosphate, which are essential for oxidation-reduction reactions involved in lipid metabolism, glycogenolysis, and tissue respiration. Deficiency of niacin results in pellagra, the most common symptoms of which are dermatitis, diarrhea, and dementia. In high doses niacin also produces vasodilation. Reduces serum cholesterol and triglycerides in types II, III, IV, and V hyperlipoproteinemia (mechanism unknown). **Peak serum levels:** 45 min; **t½:** 45 min.

**Uses:** Prophylaxis and treatment of pellagra; niacin deficiency. Treat hyperlipidemia in clients not responding to either diet or weight loss. Reduce the risk of recurrent nonfatal MI and promote regression of atherosclerosis when combined with bile-binding resins.

**Contraindications:** Severe hypotension, hemorrhage, arterial bleeding, liver dysfunction, peptic ulcer. Use of the extended-release tablets and capsules in children.

**Special Concerns:** Extended-release niacin may be hepatotoxic. Use with caution in diabetics, gall bladder disease, and clients with gout.

**Side Effects:** *GI:* N&V, diarrhea, peptic ulcer activation, abdominal pain. *Dermatologic:* Flushing, warm feeling, skin rash, pruritus, dry skin, itching and tingling feeling, keratosis nigricans. *Other:* Hypotension, headache, macular cystoid edema, amblyopia. *NOTE:* Megadoses are accompanied by serious toxicity including the symptoms listed in the preceding as well as liver damage, hyperglycemia, hyperuricemia, arrhythmias, tachycardia, and dermatoses.

**Drug Interactions**

*Chenodiol* / ↓ Effect of chenodiol

*Probenecid* / Niacin may ↓ uricosuric effect of probenecid

*Sulfinpyrazone* / Niacin ↓ uricosuric effect of sulfinpyrazone

*Sympathetic blocking agents* / Additive vasodilating effects → postural hypotension

---

**Dosage**

NIACIN

• **Extended-Release Capsules, Tablets, Extended-Release Tablets, Capsules, Elixir**

   *Vitamin.*

**Adults:** Up to 500 mg/day; **pediatric:** Up to 300 mg/day.

   *Antihyperlipidemic.*

**Adults, initial:** 1 g t.i.d.; **then:** increase dose in increments of 500 mg/day q 2–4 weeks as needed. **Maintenance:** 1–2 g t.i.d. (up to a maximum of 8 g/day).

- **IM, IV**
  *Pellagra.*
  **Adults, IM:** 50–100 mg 5 or more times/day. **IV, slow:** 25–100 mg 2 or more times/day. **Pediatric, IV slow:** Up to 300 mg/day.
  NIACINAMIDE
- **Tablets**
  *Vitamin.*
  **Adults:** Up to 500 mg/day. **Pediatric:** Up to 300 mg/day. Capsules not recommended for use in children.

## NURSING CONSIDERATIONS
### Administration/Storage
**IV** May administer IV form diluted (to 2 mg/mL solution concentration) at a rate not exceeding 2 mg/min.
### Assessment
1. Obtain baseline glucose, HbA1-C, and plasma lipid levels; monitor periodically throughout therapy.
2. Note any history of PUD or liver or gallbladder dysfunction.
3. Assess diet, exercise, and any lifestyle changes necessary to decrease coronary risk factors.
4. The extended-release capsules and tablets are not useful in lowering triglycerides. When using the regular strength tablets for hyperlipidemia, start low and go slow to enhance client tolerance.
### Client/Family Teaching
1. Take nicotinic acid PO only with cold water (no hot beverages). Can be taken with meals if GI upset occurs.
2. May experience a warm flushing in the face and ears within 2 hr after taking. One aspirin may be taken to reduce effect. Alcohol may increase these effects.
3. Lie down if feeling weak and dizzy after taking niacin (until this feeling passes) and inform provider.
4. Identify foods sources high in niacin (dairy products, meats, tuna, and eggs); assess levels of consumption.
5. With diabetes, do not take niacin unless specifically ordered and then the blood glucose levels must be closely monitored for hyperglyce-

mia; also monitor for ketonuria and glucosuria. Antidiabetic agents may require a dosage increase.
6. Report any skin color changes or yellowing of the sclera.
7. Clients predisposed to gout may experience flank, joint, or stomach pains, which should be reported immediately.
8. If blurred vision or skin lesions occur, remain out of direct sunlight.
9. No unsupervised excessive vitamin ingestion; high doses may impair liver function.
### Outcomes/Evaluate
- ↓ Serum cholesterol and triglyceride levels
- Relief of symptoms of pellagra and niacin deficiency

# Nicardipine hydrochloride
(nye-**KAR**-dih-peen)
**Pregnancy Category:** C
Cardene, Cardene IV, Cardene SR
**(Rx)**
**Classification:** Calcium channel blocking agent (antianginal, antihypertensive)

See also *Calcium Channel Blocking Agents.*
**Action/Kinetics:** Moderately increases CO and significantly decreases peripheral vascular resistance. **Onset of action:** 20 min. **Maximum plasma levels:** 30–120 min. Significant first-pass metabolism. Food (especially fats) will decrease the amount of drug absorbed from the GI tract. Steady-state plasma levels are reached after 2–3 days of therapy. **Therapeutic serum levels:** 0.028–0.050 mcg/mL. **$t\frac{1}{2}$, at steady state:** 8.6 hr. **Maximum BP-lowering effects, immediate release:** 1–2 hr; **maximum BP-lowering effects, sustained release:** 2–6 hr. **Duration:** 8 hr. Highly bound to plasma protein (> 95%) and metabolized by the liver with excretion through both the urine and feces.

**Uses: Immediate release:** Chronic stable angina (effort-associated angina) alone or in combination with beta-adrenergic blocking agents.

**Immediate and sustained released:** Hypertension alone or in combination with other antihypertensive drugs.

**IV:** Short-term treatment of hypertension when PO therapy is not desired or possible.

*Investigational:* CHF.

**Contraindications:** Clients with advanced aortic stenosis due to the effect on reducing afterload. During lactation.

**Special Concerns:** Safety and efficacy in children less than 18 years of age have not been established. Use with caution in clients with CHF, especially in combination with a beta blocker due to the possibility of a negative inotropic effect. Use with caution in clients with impaired liver function, reduced hepatic blood flow, or impaired renal function. Initial increase in frequency, duration, or severity of angina.

**Side Effects:** *CV:* Pedal edema, flushing, increased angina, palpitations, tachycardia, other edema, abnormal ECG, hypotension, postural hypotension, syncope, *MI, AV block,* ventricular extrasystoles, peripheral vascular disease. *CNS:* Dizziness, headache, somnolence, malaise, nervousness, insomnia, abnormal dreams, vertigo, depression, confusion, amnesia, anxiety, weakness, psychoses, hallucinations, paranoia. *GI:* N&V, dyspepsia, dry mouth, constipation, sore throat. *Neuromuscular:* Asthenia, myalgia, paresthesia, hyperkinesia, arthralgia. *Miscellaneous:* Rash, dyspnea, SOB, nocturia, polyuria, allergic reactions, abnormal liver chemistries, hot flashes, impotence, rhinitis, sinusitis, nasal congestion, chest congestion, tinnitus, equilibrium disturbances, abnormal or blurred vision, infection, atypical chest pain.

**OD Overdose Management:** *Symptoms:* Marked hypotension, bradycardia, palpitations, flushing, drowsiness, confusion, and slurred speech following PO overdose. Lethal overdose may cause systemic hypotension, bradycardia (following initial tachycardia), and progressive AV block. *Treatment:*
• Treatment is supportive. Monitor cardiac and respiratory function.
• If client is seen soon after ingestion, emetics or gastric lavage should be considered, followed by cathartics.
• *Hypotension:* IV calcium, dopamine, isoproterenol, metaraminol, or norepinephrine. Also, provide IV fluids. Place client in Trendelenburg position.
• *Ventricular tachycardia:* IV procainamide or lidocaine; cardioversion may be necessary. Also, provide slow-drip IV fluids.
• *Bradycardia, asystole, AV block:* IV atropine sulfate (0.6–1 mg), calcium gluconate (10% solution), isoproterenol, norepinephrine; also, cardiac pacing may be indicated. Provide slow-drip IV fluids.

**Drug Interactions**
*Cimetidine* / ↑ Bioavailability of nicardipine → ↑ plasma levels
*Cyclosporine* / ↑ Plasma levels of cyclosporine possibly leading to renal toxicity
*Ranitidine* / ↑ Bioavailability of nicardipine

**Dosage** ————
• **Capsules, Immediate Release**
*Angina, hypertension.*
**Initial, usual:** 20 mg t.i.d. (range: 20–40 mg t.i.d.). Wait 3 days before increasing dose to ensure steady-state plasma levels.
• **Capsules, Sustained Release**
*Hypertension.*
**Initial:** 30 mg b.i.d. (range: 30–60 mg b.i.d.).
*NOTE:* In renal impairment, the initial dose should be 20 mg t.i.d. In hepatic impairment, the initial dose should be 20 mg b.i.d.
• **IV**
*Hypertension.*
**Individualize dose. Initial:** 5 mg/hr; the infusion rate may be increased to a maximum of 15 mg/hr (by 2.5-mg/hr increments q 15 min). For a more rapid reduction in BP,

initiate at 5 mg/hr but increase the rate q 5 min in 2.5-mg/hr increments until a maximum of 15 mg/hr is reached. **Maintenance:** 3 mg/hr. The IV infusion rate to produce an average plasma level similar to a particular PO dose is as follows: 20 mg q 8 hr is equivalent to 0.5 mg/hr; 30 mg q 8 hr is equivalent to 1.2 mg/hr; and 40 mg q 8 hr is equivalent to 2.2 mg/hr.

## NURSING CONSIDERATIONS

See also *Nursing Considerations* for *Calcium Channel Blocking Agents.*

**Administration/Storage**

1. When used for treating angina, may be administered safely along with sublingual nitroglycerin, prophylactic nitrates, or beta blockers.

2. When used to treat hypertension, may be administered safely along with diuretics or beta blockers.

3. During initial therapy and when dosage is increased, clients may experience an increase in the frequency, duration, or severity of angina.

4. If transfer to PO antihypertensives other than nicardipine is planned, initiate therapy after discontinuing the infusion. If PO nicardipine is to be used at a dosage regimen of three times daily, give the first dose 1 hr prior to discontinuing IV infusion.

**IV** 5. Ampules must be diluted before infusion. Acceptable diluents are 5% dextrose, D5%/0.45% NaCl, D5% with 40 mEq potassium, 0.45% NaCl, and 0.9% NaCl. Nicardipine is incompatible with 5% sodium bicarbonate and RL solution.

6. The infusion concentration should be 0.1 mg/mL. The diluted product is stable at room temperature for 24 hr.

7. Store ampules at room temperature; freezing does not affect the product. Protect ampules from light and elevated temperatures.

**Assessment**

1. Document indications for therapy. List other agents prescribed and the outcome.

2. Note any history of CHF and if beta blockers prescribed; warrants close monitoring.

3. Monitor ECG, liver and renal function studies; note any dysfunction.

4. Monitor VS. When the immediate-release product is used for hypertension, the maximum lowering of BP occurs 1–2 hr after dosing. Evaluate BP at trough (8 hr after dosing). When the sustained-release product is used, maximum lowering of BP occurs 2–6 hr after dosing.

5. Monitor BP frequently during and following IV infusion. Avoid too rapid or excessive decrease in BP and discontinue infusion if significant hypotension or tachycardia.

**Client/Family Teaching**

1. Take at the same time each day.

2. Report any persistent and/or bothersome side effects such as dizziness, flushing, or increased incidents of angina or evidence of weight gain or edema.

3. Maintain proper intake of fluids to avoid constipation. Avoid caffeine and alcohol.

4. Male clients may experience impotence.

5. Anginal attacks may persist up to 30 min following drug ingestion due to reflex tachycardia; use nitrates as prescribed.

6. Report any change in psychologic state—depression, anxiety, sleep problems, or decreased mental acuity. Particularly important when working with elderly clients since there may be a tendency to misdiagnose the problem as senility.

**Outcomes/Evaluate**

• Control of hypertension
• ↓ Frequency/intensity of anginal attacks
• Therapeutic drug levels (0.028–0.050 mcg/mL)

# Nicotine polacrilex (Nicotine Resin Complex)

(**NIK**-oh-teen)
**Pregnancy Category:** X
Nicorette, Nicorette DS, Nicorette Plus ✱ (OTC)
**Classification:** Smoking deterrent

**Action/Kinetics:** Following chewing, nicotine is released from an ion exchange resin in the gum product, providing blood nicotine levels approximating those produced by smoking cigarettes. The amount of nicotine released depends on the rate and duration of chewing. Following repeated administration q 30 min, nicotine blood levels reach 25–50 ng/mL. If the gum is swallowed, only a minimum amount of nicotine is released. Metabolized mainly by the liver, with about 10%–20% excreted unchanged in the urine.

**Uses:** Adjunct with behavioral modification in smokers wishing to give up the smoking habit. Is considered only as an initial aid, with the ultimate goal being abstention from all forms of nicotine. Most likely to benefit are individuals with the following characteristics:

a. smoke brands of cigarettes containing more than 0.9 mg nicotine;

b. smoke more than 15 cigarettes daily;

c. inhale cigarette smoke deeply and frequently;

d. smoke most frequently during the morning;

e. smoke the first cigarette of the day within 30 min of arising;

f. indicate cigarettes smoked in the morning are the most difficult to give up;

g. smoke even if the individual is ill and confined to bed;

h. find it necessary to smoke in places where smoking is not allowed. *NOTE:* Nicotine may be effective in improving the course of difficult-to-treat ulcerative colitis.

**Contraindications:** Pregnancy, lactation, nonsmokers, serious arrhythmias, angina, vasospastic disease, active temporomandibular joint disease. Use in individuals less than 18 years of age.

**Special Concerns:** Safety and effectiveness in children and adolescents who smoke have not been determined. Use with caution in hypertension, PUD, oral or pharyngeal inflammation, gastritis, stomatitis, hyperthyroidism, insulin-dependent diabetes, and pheochromocytoma.

**Side Effects:** *CNS:* Dizziness, irritability, headache. *GI:* N&V, indigestion, GI upset, salivation, eructation. *Other:* Sore mouth or throat, hiccoughs, sore jaw muscles.

**OD** **Overdose Management:** *Symptoms: GI:* N&V, diarrhea, salivation, abdominal pain. *CNS:* Headache, dizziness, confusion, weakness, fainting, *seizures. Respiratory:* Labored breathing, *respiratory paralysis (cause of death).* Other: Cold sweat, disturbed hearing and vision, hypotension, and rapid, weak pulse. *Treatment:* Syrup of ipecac if vomiting has not occurred, saline laxative, gastric lavage followed by activated charcoal (if client is unconscious), maintenance of respiration, maintenance of CV function.

**Drug Interactions**

*Caffeine* / Possibly ↓ blood levels of caffeine due to ↑ rate of breakdown by liver

*Catecholamines* / ↑ Levels of catecholamines

*Cortisol* / ↑ Levels of cortisol

*Furosemide* / Possible ↓ diuretic effect of furosemide

*Glutethimide* / Possible ↓ absorption of glutethimide

*Imipramine* / Possibly ↓ blood levels of imipramine due to ↑ rate of breakdown by liver

*Pentazocine* / Possibly ↓ blood levels of pentazocine due to ↑ rate of breakdown by liver

*Theophylline* / Possibly ↓ blood levels of theophylline due to ↑ rate of breakdown by liver

**Dosage** ——————
• **Gum**

**Initial:** One piece of gum chewed whenever the urge to smoke occurs; best results are obtained when the gum is chewed on a fixed schedule, at intervals of 1 to 2 hr, with at least 9 pieces chewed per day. **maintenance:** 9–12 pieces of gum daily during the first month, not to exceed 30 pieces daily of the 2-mg strength and 20 pieces daily of the 4-mg strength.

## NURSING CONSIDERATIONS
### Administration/Storage
1. Available as a 2-mg (Nicorette) and 4-mg (Nicorette DS) gum. Those who smoke more than 25 cigarettes/day should be started on the 4-mg dose.
2. Evaluate monthly; if client has not smoked for 3 months, slowly withdraw the gum. Should not be used for longer than 6 months.
3. Suggested procedures for gradual withdrawal of the gum include:
• Decreasing the total number of pieces/day by one or more pieces q 4–7 days.
• Decreasing the chewing time with each piece from the normal 30 min to 10–15 min for 4–7 days; then gradually decreasing the number of pieces used per day.
• Increasing the chewing time for more than 30 min and reducing the number of pieces used per day.
• Substituting one or more pieces of sugarless gum for an equal number of pieces of nicotine gum; then, increasing the number of pieces of sugarless gum substituted for nicotine gum q 4–7 days.
• Replacing the 4-mg gum with the 2-mg gum and applying any of the first four procedures listed in the preceding.
### Assessment
1. Document nicotine profile: type and brand (cigarettes, chewing tobacco, or cigars), amount used per day, when used, and what increases usage.
2. Note any temporomandibular

joint syndrome or cardiac arrhythmia; precludes gum therapy.
### Client/Family Teaching
1. Must want to stop smoking and should do so immediately.
2. Use gum only as directed. When client has the urge to smoke, chew one piece slowly for about 30 min. If a slight tingling becomes evident, stop chewing until sensation subsides.
3. Acidic beverages, such as coffee, juices, soft drinks, and wine, interfere with buccal absorption of nicotine from the gum; thus, avoid eating and drinking 15 min before and during chewing as effects may be diminished.
4. Gum will not stick to dentures or appliances.
5. Identify individuals and local support groups that can help with smoking cessation and provide emotional and psychologic support throughout the endeavor. Participate in a formal smoking cessation program.

**Outcomes/Evaluate:** Control of nicotine withdrawal symptoms with smoking cessation

# Nicotine transdermal system
(**NIK**-oh-teen)
**Pregnancy Category:** D
Habitrol, Prostep **(Rx)**, Nicoderm CQ Step 1, Step 2, or Step 3, Nicotrol **(OTC)**
**Classification:** Smoking deterrent

**Action/Kinetics:** Nicotine transdermal system is a multilayered film that provides systemic delivery of varying amounts of nicotine over a 24-hr period after applying to the skin. Nicotine's reinforcing activity is due to stimulation of the cortex (via the locus ceruleus), producing increased alertness and cognitive performance and a "reward" effect due to an action in the limbic system. At low doses the stimulatory effects predominate, whereas at high doses the reward effects predominate. The nicotine

N

transdermal system produces an initial (first day of use) increase in BP, an increase in HR (3%–7%), and a decrease in SV after 10 days. Metabolized in the liver to a large number of metabolites, all of which are less active than nicotine. **t½, following removal of the system from the skin:** 3–4 hr.

**Uses:** As an aid to stopping smoking for the relief of nicotine withdrawal symptoms. Should be used in conjunction with a comprehensive behavioral smoking cessation program.

**Contraindications:** Hypersensitivity or allergy to nicotine or any components of the therapeutic system. Use in children and during pregnancy, labor, and delivery. Lactation. Use in those with heart disease, hypertension, a recent MI, severe or worsening angina pectoris, and those taking certain antidepressants or antiasthmatic drugs. Use in severe renal impairment.

**Special Concerns:** Pregnant smokers should be encouraged to try to stop smoking using educational and behavioral interventions before using the nicotine transdermal system. The product should only be used during pregnancy if the potential benefit outweighs the potential risk of nicotine to the fetus. The use of nicotine transdermal systems for longer than 3 months has not been studied. Clients with coronary heart disease (history of MI and/or angina pectoris), serious cardiac arrhythmias, or vasospastic diseases (e.g., Buerger's disease, Prinzmetal's variant angina) should be screened carefully before using the transdermal system. Use with caution in clients with hyperthyroidism, pheochromocytoma, insulin-dependent diabetes (nicotine causes the release of catecholamines), in active peptic ulcers, in accelerated hypertension, and during lactation.

**Side Effects:** *NOTE:* The incidence of side effects is complicated by the fact that clients manifest effects of nicotine withdrawal or by concurrent smoking.

*Dermatologic:* Erythema, pruritus, or burning at the site of application; cutaneous hypersensitivity, sweating, rash at application site. *Body as a whole:* Allergy, back pain. *GI:* Diarrhea, dyspepsia, dry mouth, abdominal pain, constipation, N&V. *Musculoskeletal:* Arthralgia, myalgia. *CNS:* Abnormal dreams, somnolence, dizziness, impaired concentration, headache, insomnia. *CV:* Tachycardia, hypertension. *Respiratory:* Increased cough, pharyngitis, sinusitis. *GU:* Dysmenorrhea.

**OD** **Overdose Management:** *Symptoms:* Pallor, cold sweat, N&V, abdominal pain, salivation, diarrhea, headache, dizziness, disturbed hearing and vision, mental confusion, weakness, tremor. Large overdoses may cause prostration, hypotension, *respiratory failure, seizures, and death. Treatment:* Remove the transdermal system immediately. The surface of the skin may be flushed with water and dried; soap should not be used as it may increase the absorption of nicotine. Diazepam or barbiturates may be used to treat seizures and atropine can be given for excessive bronchial secretions or diarrhea. Respiratory support for respiratory failure and fluid support for hypotension and CV collapse. If transdermal systems are ingested PO, activated charcoal should be given to prevent seizures. If the client is unconscious, the charcoal should be administered by an NGT. A saline cathartic or sorbitol added to the first dose of activated charcoal may hasten GI passage of the system. Doses of activated charcoal should be repeated as long as the system remains in the GI tract as nicotine will continue to be released for many hours.

**Dosage** ————————
• **Transdermal System**
HABITROL (RX)
**Healthy clients, initial:** 21 mg/day for 4–8 weeks; **then,** 14 mg/day for 2–4 weeks and 7 mg/day for 2–4 weeks. **Light smokers, those who weigh less than 100 lb or who**

**have CV disease:** 14 mg/day for 4–8 weeks; **then,** 7 mg/day for 2–4 weeks.

PROSTEP (RX)

**Clients weighing 100 lb or more:** 22 mg/day for 4–8 weeks; **then,** 11 mg/day for 2–4 weeks. **Clients weighing less than 100 lb:** 11 mg/day for 4–8 weeks.

NICODERM CQ (OTC)

**Light smokers (10 or less cigarettes/day):** One 14-mg/24-hr patch for 16 or 24 hr/day for 6 weeks; **then,** one 7-mg/24-hr patch for 16 or 24 hr/day for 2 weeks. **Heavy smokers (> 10 cigarettes/day):** One 21-mg/24-hr patch for 16 or 24 hr/day for 6 weeks; **then,** one 14-mg/24-hr patch for 16 or 24 hr/day for 2 weeks, followed by one 7-mg/24-hr patch for 16 or 24 hr for 2 weeks.

NICOTROL (OTC)

**Those who smoke > 10 cigarettes/day:** 15 mg/day for 6 weeks. The patch is to be worn for 16 hr and removed at bedtime.

## NURSING CONSIDERATIONS
**Administration/Storage**

1. There will be differences in the duration and length of therapy, depending on the product prescribed.

2. Apply the transdermal system promptly after its removal from the protective pouch to prevent loss of nicotine due to evaporation. Only use systems where the pouch is intact.

3. Apply system once daily to a nonhairy, clean, and dry site on the trunk or upper, outer arm. After 16 or 24 hr (depending on the regimen established), remove the system. When indicated, apply a new system to an alternate skin site. Do not reuse skin sites for at least a week.

4. When a used system is removed, fold it over and place in the protective pouch that contained the new system. Dispose of the used system to ensure access is prevented by children or pets.

5. The goal of therapy with nicotine transdermal systems is complete abstinence. If the client has not stopped smoking by the fourth week of therapy, discontinue treatment.

6. Assess the need for adjustment of the dose during the first 2 weeks of therapy.

7. Nicotine will continue to be absorbed from the skin for several hours after removal of the system.

8. Do not store systems above 30°C (86°F) because they are sensitive to heat.

**Assessment**

1. Document nicotine profile: type and brand (cigarettes, chewing tobacco, or cigars), amount used per day, when used, and what increases usage.

2. Determine any CAD, liver or renal dysfunction.

3. List meds currently prescribed. Cessation of smoking, with or without nicotine replacement, may alter the response to certain drugs.

4. Document any skin disorders; nicotine transdermal systems may be irritating with skin disorders such as atopic or eczematous dermatitis.

**Client/Family Teaching**

1. Use extreme caution during application; avoid contact with active systems. If contact occurs, wash area with water only. The eyes should not be touched. These systems can be a dermal irritant and cause contact dermatitis.

2. Any persistent skin irritations such as erythema, edema, or pruritus at the application site as well as any generalized skin reactions such as hives, urticaria, or a generalized rash should be reported and the system removed.

3. Follow manufacturer's guidelines for proper system application. Review information sheet that comes with the product which contains instructions on how to use and dispose of the transdermal systems properly.

4. Stop smoking completely. If smoking continues, may experience

**N**

adverse side effects due to higher nicotine levels in the body.

5. Participate in a formal smoking cessation program. The success or failure of smoking cessation depends on the quality, intensity, and frequency of supportive care.

6. Nicotine in any form can be toxic and addictive; nicotine transdermal systems may lead to dependence. To minimize this risk, withdraw use of the transdermal system gradually after 4–8 weeks of use.

7. Symptoms of nicotine withdrawal include craving, nervousness, restlessness, irritability, mood lability, anxiety, drowsiness, sleep disturbances, impaired concentration, increased appetite, headache, myalgia, constipation, fatigue, and weight gain; report if evident as dosage may require adjustment.

8. Change site of application daily; do not reuse for 1 week.

9. With Nicotrol, remove patch at bedtime and apply upon arising.

10. Keep all products used and unused away from children and pets; sufficient nicotine is still present in used systems to cause toxicity.

11. If therapy is unsuccessful after 4 weeks, discontinue and identify reasons for failure so that a later attempt may be more successful.

**Outcomes/Evaluate:** Smoking cessation; control of nicotine withdrawal symptoms

# Nifedipine
(nye-**FED**-ih-peen)
**Pregnancy Category:** C
Adalat, Adalat CC, Adalat P.A. 10 and 20 ✶, Adalat XL ✶, Apo-Nifed ✶, Apo-Nifed PA ✶, Gen-Nifedipine ✶, Novo-Nifedin ✶, Nu-Nifed ✶, Procardia, Procardia XL, Taro-Nifedipine ✶ **(Rx)**
**Classification:** Calcium channel blocking agent (antianginal, antihypertensive)

See also *Calcium Channel Blocking Agents*.

**Action/Kinetics:** Variable effects on AV node effective and functional refractory periods. CO is moderately increased while peripheral vascular resistance is significantly decreased. **Onset:** 20 min. **Peak plasma levels:** 30 min (up to 4 hr for extended-release). **t½:** 2–5 hr. **Therapeutic serum levels:** 0.025–0.1 mcg/mL. **Duration:** 4–8 hr (12 hr for extended-release). Low-fat meals may slow the rate but not the extent of absorption. Metabolized in the liver to inactive metabolites.

**Uses:** Vasospastic (Prinzmetal's or variant) angina. Chronic stable angina without vasospasm, including angina due to increased effort (especially in clients who cannot take beta blockers or nitrates or who remain symptomatic following clinical doses of these drugs). Essential hypertension (sustained-release only). *Investigational:* PO, sublingually, or chewed in hypertensive emergencies. Also prophylaxis of migraine headaches, primary pulmonary hypertension, severe pregnancy-associated hypertension, esophageal diseases, Raynaud's phenomenon, CHF, asthma, premature labor, biliary and renal colic, and cardiomyopathy. To prevent strokes and to decrease the risk of CHF in geriatric hypertensives.

**Contraindications:** Hypersensitivity. Lactation.

**Special Concerns:** Use with caution in impaired hepatic or renal function and in elderly clients. Initial increase in frequency, duration, or severity of angina (may also be seen in clients being withdrawn from beta blockers and who begin taking nifedipine).

**Side Effects:** *CV:* Peripheral and pulmonary edema, MI, hypotension, palpitations, syncope, CHF (especially if used with a beta blocker), decreased platelet aggregation, arrhythmias, tachycardia. Increased frequency, length, and duration of angina when beginning nifedipine therapy. *GI:* Nausea, diarrhea, constipation, flatulence, abdominal cramps, dysgeusia, vomiting, dry mouth, eructation, gastroesophageal reflux, melena. *CNS:* Dizziness, lightheadedness, giddiness, nervousness, sleep disturbances, headache, weakness, depression, migraine, psychoses, hallucinations, disturbances in equilibrium, somnolence, insomnia, abnormal dreams, malaise, anxiety. *Dermatologic:* Rash, dermatitis, urticaria, pruritus, photosensitivity, erythema multiforme, ***Stevens-Johnson syndrome.*** *Respiratory:* Dyspnea, cough, wheezing, SOB, respiratory infection, throat, nasal, or chest congestion. *Musculoskeletal:* Muscle cramps or inflammation, joint pain or stiffness, arthritis, ataxia, myoclonic dystonia, hypertonia, asthenia. *Hematologic:* Thrombocytopenia, leukopenia, purpura, anemia. *Other:* Fever, chills, sweating, blurred vision, sexual difficulties, flushing, transient blindness, hyperglycemia, hypokalemia, gingival hyperplasia, allergic hepatitis, hepatitis, tinnitus, gynecomastia, polyuria, nocturia, erythromelalgia, weight gain, epistaxis, facial and periorbital edema, hypoesthesia, gout, abnormal lacrimation, breast pain, dysuria, hematuria.

**Additional Drug Interactions**

*Anticoagulants, oral* / Possibility of ↑ PT

*Cimetidine* / ↑ Bioavailability of nifedipine

*Digoxin* / ↑ Effect of digoxin by ↓ excretion by kidney

*Magnesium sulfate* / ↑ Neuromuscular blockade and hypotension

*Quinidine* / Possible ↓ effect of quinidine due to ↓ plasma levels; ↑ risk of hypotension, bradycardia, AV block, pulmonary edema, and ventricular tachycardia

*Ranitidine* / ↑ Bioavailability of nifedipine

*Theophylline* / Possible ↑ effect of theophylline

**Laboratory Test Interferences:** ↑ Alkaline phosphatase, CPK, LDH, AST, ALT. Positive Coombs' test.

**Dosage**
- **Capsules**

**Individualized. Initial:** 10 mg t.i.d. (range: 10–20 mg t.i.d.); **maintenance:** 10–30 mg t.i.d.–q.i.d. Clients with coronary artery spasm may respond better to 20–30 mg t.i.d.–q.i.d. Doses greater than 120 mg/day are rarely needed while doses greater than 180 mg/day are not recommended.

- **Sustained-Release Tablets**

**Initial:** 30 or 60 mg once daily for Procardia XL and 30 mg once daily for Adalat CC. Titrate over a 7- to 14-day period. Dosage can be increased as required and as tolerated, to a maximum of 120 mg/day for Procardia XL and 90 mg/day for Adalat CC.

*Investigational, hypertensive emergencies.*

10–20 mg given PO, sublingually (by puncturing capsule and squeezing contents under the tongue), or chewed (capsule is punctured several times and then chewed).

## NURSING CONSIDERATIONS

See also *Nursing Considerations* for *Calcium Channel Blocking Agents.*

**Administration/Storage**

1. Do not exceed a single dose (other than sustained-released) of 30 mg.

2. Before increasing the dose, carefully monitor BP.

3. Use only the sustained-release tablets to treat hypertension.

4. Sublingual nitroglycerin and long-acting nitrates may be used concomitantly with nifedipine.

5. Concomitant therapy with beta-adrenergic blocking agents may be used. In these cases, note any potential drug interactions.

6. Clients withdrawn from beta blockers may manifest symptoms of increased angina which cannot be prevented by nifedipine; in fact, nifedipine may increase the severity of angina in this situation.

7. Clients with angina may be switched to the sustained-release product at the nearest equivalent total daily dose. However, use doses greater than 90 mg/day with caution.

8. Protect capsules from light and

**N**

---

moisture and store at room temperature in the original container.

9. During initial therapy and when dosage is increased, clients may experience an increase in the frequency, duration, or severity of angina.

10. Food may decrease the rate but not the extent of absorption. Thus, the drug can be taken without regard to meals.

**Assessment**

1. Document any sensitivity to other CCBs.

2. Note any pulmonary edema, ECG abnormalities, or palpitations. Document cardiopulmonary assessment findings.

**Interventions**

1. During titration period, note evidence of hypotensive response and increased HR that result from peripheral vasodilation; these may precipitate angina.

2. Although beta-blocking drugs may be used concomitantly with chronic stable angina, the combined effects of the drugs cannot be predicted (especially in clients with compromised LV function or cardiac conduction abnormalities). Pronounced hypotension, heart block, and CHF may occur.

3. If therapy with a beta blocker is to be discontinued, gradually decrease dosage to prevent withdrawal syndrome.

**Client/Family Teaching**

1. May take with or without food. Sustained-release tablets should not be chewed or divided.

2. There is no cause for concern if an empty tablet appears in the stool.

3. Maintain a fluid intake of 2–3 L/day to avoid constipation.

4. Do not use OTC agents unless approved; avoid alcohol and caffeine.

5. Report any symptoms of persistent headache, flushing, nausea, palpitations, weight gain, dizziness, or lightheadedness.

6. Perform daily weights and note any extremity swelling. Peripheral edema may result from arterial vasodilatation that is precipitated by nifedipine or swelling may indicate increasing ventricular dysfunction and should be reported.

7. If also receiving beta-adrenergic blocking agents, report any evidence of hypotension, exacerbation of angina, or evidence of heart failure.

8. Once beta-blocking agents have been discontinued, increased anginal pain may occur; report if evident.

**Outcomes/Evaluate**

• ↓ Frequency and intensity of anginal episodes; ↓ BP

• Improved peripheral circulation

• Prevention of strokes and ↓ risk of CHF in geriatric hypertensives

---

# Nilutamide

((nye-**LOO**-tah-myd))

**Pregnancy Category:** C

Anadron ✦, Nilandron **(Rx)**

**Classification:** Antineoplastic, hormone

---

See also *Antineoplastic Agents*.

**Action/Kinetics:** Antiandrogen activity with no estrogen, progesterone, mineralocorticoid, or glucocorticoid effects. Binds to the androgen receptor, thus preventing the normal androgenic response. Rapidly and completely absorbed from the GI tract. Extensively metabolized with at least one metabolite showing significant activity. Metabolites excreted through the urine. **t½, elimination:** Approximately 41–49 hr.

**Uses:** In combination with surgical castration for the treatment of metastatic prostate cancer (stage $D_2$).

**Contraindications:** Severe hepatic impairment, severe respiratory insufficiency, hypersensitivity to nilutamide.

**Special Concerns:** Many clients experience a delay in adaptation to the dark ranging from seconds to a few minutes. Safety and efficacy have not been determined in children.

**Side Effects:** *GI:* Nausea, constipation, dry mouth, diarrhea, hepatitis, GI disorder, **GI hemorrhage,** melena. *CNS:* Dizziness, paresthesia, nervousness. *CV:* Hypertension, **heart failure,** angina, syncope. *Respiratory:* Interstitial pneumonitis, dyspnea, lung disorder, increased cough, rhinitis. *Metabolic/nutritional:* Edema, weight loss, intolerance to alcohol. *Ophthalmic:* Cataract, photophobia, impaired adaptation to dark, abnormal vision. *Miscellaneous:* Leukopenia, hot flushes, UTI, malaise, pruritus, arthritis, aplastic anemia (rare).

**Drug Interactions**
*Phenytoin* / ↓ Metabolism of phenytoin → delayed elimination and ↑ risk of toxicity
*Theophylline* / Metabolism of theophylline delayed elimination and risk of toxicity
*Vitamin K antagonists* / Metabolism of vitamin K antagonists delayed elimination and risk of toxicity
**Laboratory Test Interferences:** AST, ALT, alkaline phosphatase, haptoglobin, BUN, creatinine. Hyperglycemia.

**Dosage**
• **Tablets**
*Metastatic prostate cancer.*
300 mg (six 50-mg tablets) once daily for 30 days followed by 150 mg (three 50-mg tablets) once daily.

## NURSING CONSIDERATIONS

See also *Nursing Considerations* for *Antineoplastic Agents.*
**Administration/Storage**
1. To ensure maximum beneficial effects, initiate treatment on the same day as or the day after surgical castration.
2. Can be taken with or without food.
3. Protect from light and store at room temperature at 15°C–30°C (59°F–86°F).
**Assessment**
1. Note duration of symptoms, previous therapy, and the outcome.
2. Drug should be given on the day of or the day following surgery for prostate cancer.
3. Obtain baseline CBC, LFTs, and

CXR. Assess cardiopulmonary status closely; drug may cause interstitial pneumonitis.
**Client/Family Teaching**
1. Review guidelines concerning the dosage and dosing frequency.
2. Wear tinted glasses to prevent delay in adaptation to the dark. Use caution driving through tunnels or at night.
3. Immediately report any symptoms of dyspnea, cough, or chest pain.
**Outcomes/Evaluate:** Control of malignant cell proliferation with prostatic cancer

# Nimodipine
(nye-**MOH**-dih-peen)
**Pregnancy Category:** C
Nimotop, Nimotop I.V. ✦ **(Rx)**
**Classification:** Calcium channel blocking agent

See also *Calcium Channel Blocking Agents.*
**Action/Kinetics:** Has a greater effect on cerebral arteries than arteries elsewhere in the body (probably due to its highly lipophilic properties). Mechanism to reduce neurologic deficits following subarachnoid hemorrhage not known. **Peak plasma levels:** 1 hr. **t½:** 1–2 hr. Significantly bound (over 95%) to plasma protein. Undergoes first-pass metabolism in the liver; metabolites excreted through the urine.
**Uses:** Improvement of neurologic deficits due to spasm following subarachnoid hemorrhage from ruptured congenital intracranial aneurysms; clients should have Hunt and Hess grades of I–III. *Investigational:* Migraine headaches and cluster headaches.
**Contraindications:** Lactation.
**Special Concerns:** Safety and efficacy have not been established in children. Use with caution in clients with impaired hepatic function and reduced hepatic blood flow. The half-life may be increased in geriatric clients.

N

**Side Effects:** *CV:* Hypotension, peripheral edema, CHF, ECG abnormalities, tachycardia, bradycardia, palpitations, rebound vasospasm, hypertension, hematoma, **DIC, DVT.** *GI:* Nausea, dyspepsia, diarrhea, abdominal discomfort, cramps, **GI hemorrhage,** vomiting. *CNS:* Headache, depression, lightheadedness, dizziness. *Hepatic:* Abnormal liver function test, hepatitis, jaundice. *Hematologic:* Thrombocytopenia, anemia, purpura, ecchymosis. *Dermatologic:* Rash, dermatitis, pruritus, urticaria. *Miscellaneous:* Dyspnea, muscle pain or cramps, acne, itching, flushing, diaphoresis, wheezing, hyponatremia.

**Laboratory Test Interferences:** ↑ Nonfasting serum glucose, LDH, alkaline phosphatase, ALT. ↓ Platelet count.

**Dosage** ⎯⎯⎯⎯⎯⎯⎯⎯⎯⎯
• **Capsules**
**Adults:** 60 mg q 4 hr beginning within 96 hr after subarachnoid hemorrhage and continuing for 21 consecutive days. The dosage should be reduced to 30 mg q 4 hr in clients with hepatic impairment.

## NURSING CONSIDERATIONS

See also *Nursing Considerations* for *Calcium Channel Blocking Agents.*
**Administration/Storage:** If unable to swallow the capsule (e.g., unconscious or at time of surgery), make a hole in both ends of the capsule (soft gelatin) with an 18-gauge needle and withdraw the contents into a syringe. The medication can be administered into the client's NG tube and washed down with 30 mL of NSS.
**Assessment**
1. Obtain baseline labs; note any hepatic dysfunction and reduce dose if evident.
2. Determine if pregnant.
3. Perform baseline neurologic scores and thoroughly document deficits. Monitor VS, I&O, and weights.
4. Initiate therapy within 96 hr of subarachnoid hemorrhage.
**Client/Family Teaching**
1. Take the drug on time; sleep must be interrupted to give the medication q 4 hr ATC for 21 days.
2. Report any side effects such as nausea, lightheadedness, dizziness, muscle cramps, or muscle pain.
3. SOB, the need to take deep breaths on occasion, wheezing, or other evidence of adverse effects should be reported.
**Outcomes/Evaluate**
• ↓ Neurologic deficits due to venospasm following subarachnoid hemorrhage
• Termination of migraine and cluster headaches

# Nisoldipine
(**NYE**-sohl-dih-peen)
**Pregnancy Category:** C
Sular **(Rx)**
**Classification:** Calcium channel blocking drug

**Action/Kinetics:** Inhibits the transmembrane influx of calcium into vascular smooth muscle and cardiac muscle, resulting in dilation of arterioles. Has greater potency on vascular smooth muscle than on cardiac muscle. Chronic use results in a sustained decrease in vascular resistance and small increases in SI and LV ejection fraction. Weak diuretic effect and no clinically important chronotropic effects. Well absorbed following PO use; however, absolute bioavailability is low due to presystemic metabolism in the gut wall. Foods high in fat result in a significant increase in peak plasma levels. **Maximum plasma levels:** 6–12 hr. **t½, terminal:** 7–12 hr. Almost completely bound to plasma proteins. Metabolized in the liver and excreted through the urine.
**Uses:** Treatment of hypertension alone or in combination with other antihypertensive drugs.
**Contraindications:** Nisoldipine should not be taken with grapefruit juice as it interferes with metabolism, resulting in a significant increase in plasma levels of the drug. Use in those with known hypersensitivity to dihydropyridine calcium channel blockers. Lactation.

**Special Concerns:** Geriatric clients may show a two- to threefold higher plasma concentration; therefore caution should be used in dosing. Use with caution and at lower doses in those with hepatic insufficiency. Use with caution in clients with CHF or compromised ventricular function, especially in combination with a beta blocker.

**Side Effects:** *CV:* Increased angina and/or MI in clients with CAD. Initially, excessive hypotension, especially in those taking other antihypertensive drugs. Vasodilation, palpitation, atrial fibrillation, *CVA, MI,* CHF, first-degree AV block, hypertension, hypotension, jugular venous distension, migraine, postural hypotension, ventricular extrasystoles, SVT, syncope, systolic ejection murmur, T-wave abnormalities on ECG, venous insufficiency. *Body as a whole:* Peripheral edema, cellulitis, chills, facial edema, fever, flu syndrome, malaise. *GI:* Anorexia, nausea, colitis, diarrhea, dry mouth, dyspepsia, dysphagia, flatulence, gastritis, *GI hemorrhage,* gingival hyperplasia, glossitis, hepatomegaly, increased appetite, melena, mouth ulceration. *CNS:* Headache, dizziness, abnormal dreams, abnormal thinking and confusion, amnesia, anxiety, ataxia, cerebral ischemia, decreased libido, depression, hypesthesia, hypertonia, insomnia, nervousness, paresthesia, somnolence, tremor, vertigo. *Musculoskeletal:* Arthralgia, arthritis, leg cramps, myalgia, myasthenia, myositis, tenosynovitis. *Hematologic:* Anemia, ecchymoses, leukopenia, petechiae. *Respiratory:* Pharyngitis, sinusitis, asthma, dyspnea, end-inspiratory wheeze and fine rales, epistaxis, increased cough, laryngitis, pleural effusion, rhinitis. *Dermatologic:* Acne, alopecia, dry skin, exfoliative dermatitis, fungal dermatitis, herpes simplex, herpes zoster, maculopapular rash, pruritus, pustular rash, skin discoloration, skin ulcer, sweating, urticaria. *GU:* Dysuria, hematuria, impotence, nocturia, urinary frequency, vaginal hemorrhage, vaginitis. *Metabolic:* Gout, hypokalemia, weight gain or loss. *Ophthalmic:* Abnormal vision, amblyopia, blepharitis, conjunctivitis, glaucoma, itchy eyes, keratoconjunctivitis, retinal detachment, temporary unilateral loss of vision, vitreous floater, watery eyes. *Miscellaneous:* Diabetes mellitus, thyroiditis, chest pain, ear pain, otitis media, tinnitus, taste disturbance.

**OD** **Overdose Management:** *Symptoms:* Pronounced hypotension. *Treatment:* Active CV support, including monitoring of CV and respiratory function, elevation of extremities, judicious use of calcium infusion, pressor agents, and fluids. Dialysis is not likely to be beneficial, although plasmapheresis may be helpful.

**Drug Interactions:** Cimetidine significantly ↑ the plasma levels of nisoldipine.

**Laboratory Test Interferences:** ↑ Serum creatine kinase, NPN, BUN, serum creatinine. Abnormal LFTs.

**Dosage**
- **Tablets, Extended-Release**
  *Hypertension.*

Dose must be adjusted to the needs of each person. **Initial:** 20 mg once daily; **then,** increase by 10 mg/week or longer intervals to reach adequate BP control. **Usual maintenance:** 20–40 mg once daily. Doses beyond 60 mg once daily are not recommended. **Initial dose, clients over 65 years and those with impaired renal function:** 10 mg once daily.

## NURSING CONSIDERATIONS

See also *Nursing Considerations* for *Calcium Channel Blocking Agents.*
**Administration/Storage**
1. Swallow tablets whole; do not chew, divide, or crush.
2. Do not give tablets with grapefruit juice or a high-fat meal.
3. Closely monitor dosage adjustments in clients over 65 years of age

---

✦ = Available in Canada                    **bold italic** = life threatening side effect

and those with impaired liver function.

**Assessment**

1. Document indications for therapy, onset and duration of symptoms, other agents trialed, and the outcome.

2. Anticipate reduced dosage in the elderly and those with impaired liver function.

3. Obtain baseline ECG and note any history or evidence of CHF or compromised LV function.

4. List other drugs currently prescribed to ensure none interact unfavorably.

**Client/Family Teaching**

1. Take as directed; avoid consumption with high-fat foods or grapefruit juices.

2. Headaches, peripheral edema, and dizziness may occur; report if persistent.

3. Report as scheduled for BP evaluation during titration period. Maintain record of BP.

**Outcomes/Evaluate:** Desired reduction in BP

# Nitrofurantoin

(nye-troh-fyour-**AN**-toyn)
**Pregnancy Category:** B
Apo-Nitrofurantoin ✿, Furadantin **(Rx)**

# Nitrofurantoin macrocrystals

(nye-troh-fyour-**AN**-toyn)
**Pregnancy Category:** B
Macrobid, Macrodantin, Nephronex ✿, Novo-Furan ✿ **(Rx)**
**Classification:** Urinary germicide

See also *Anti-Infectives*.

**Action/Kinetics:** Interferes with bacterial carbohydrate metabolism by inhibiting acetyl coenzyme A; also interferes with bacterial cell wall synthesis. Bacteriostatic at low concentrations and bactericidal at high concentrations. Tablets are readily absorbed from the GI tract; bioavailability is increased by food. $t\frac{1}{2}$: 20 min (60 min in anephric clients). **Urine levels:** 50–250 mcg/

mL. If the $C_{CR}$ is less than 40 mL/min, urine antibacterial levels are inadequate, with the subsequent higher blood levels increasing the possibility of toxicity. Antibacterial activity is best in an acid urine. From 30% to 50% excreted unchanged in the urine. Nitrofurantoin macrocrystals (Macrodantin) are available; this preparation maintains effectiveness while decreasing GI distress.

**Uses:** UTIs due to susceptible strains of *Escherichia coli, Staphylococcus aureus* (not for treatment of pyelonephritis or perinephric abscesses), enterococci, and certain strains of *Enterobacter* and *Klebsiella*.

**Contraindications:** Anuria, oliguria, and clients with impaired renal function ($C_{CR}$ below 40 mL/min); pregnant women, especially near term; infants less than 1 month of age; and nursing mothers.

**Special Concerns:** To be used with extreme caution in clients with anemia, diabetes, electrolyte imbalance, avitaminosis B, or a debilitating disease. Safety during lactation has not been established.

**Side Effects:** Nitrofurantoin is a potentially toxic drug with many side effects. *GI:* N&V, anorexia, diarrhea, abdominal pain, parotitis, pancreatitis. *CNS:* Headache, dizziness, vertigo, drowsiness, nystagmus, confusion, depression, euphoria, psychotic reactions (rare). *Hematologic:* Leukopenia, thrombocytopenia, eosinophilia, megaloblastic anemia, **agranulocytosis,** granulocytopenia, **hemolytic anemia (especially in clients with G6PD deficiency).** *Allergic:* Drug fever, skin rashes, pruritus, urticaria, angioedema, exfoliative dermatitis, erythema multiforme *(rarely, Stevens-Johnson syndrome),* **anaphylaxis,** arthralgia, myalgia, chills, sialadenitis, asthma symptoms in susceptible clients; maculopapular, erythematous, or eczematous eruption. *Pulmonary:* Sudden onset of dyspnea, cough, chest pain, fever and chills; pulmonary infiltration with consolidation or pleural effusion on x-ray, elevated sedimentation rate, eosinophilia. *After subacute or chronic use:* dyspnea, nonproductive cough, malaise, interstitial pneumonitis. Permanent impairment of pulmonary function with chronic therapy. A lupus-like syndrome associated with pulmonary reactions. *Hepatic:* Hepatitis, cholestatic jaundice, chronic active hepatitis, hepatic necrosis (rare). *CV:* Benign intracranial hypertension, changes in ECG, collapse, cyanosis. *Miscellaneous:* Peripheral neuropathy, asthenia, alopecia, superinfections of the GU tract, muscle pain.

**OD** **Overdose Management:** *Symptoms:* Vomiting (most common). *Treatment:* Induce emesis. High fluid intake to promote urinary excretion. The drug is dialyzable.

**Drug Interactions**
*Acetazolamide* / ↓ Effect of nitrofurantoin due to ↑ alkalinity of urine produced by acetazolamide
*Antacids, oral* / ↓ Effect of nitrofurantoin due to ↓ absorption from GI tract
*Anticholinergic drugs* / ↑ Effect of nitrofurantoin due to ↑ absorption from stomach
*Magnesium trisilicate* / ↓ Absorption of nitrofurantoin from GI tract
*Nalidixic acid* / Nitrofurantoin ↓ effect of nalidixic acid
*Probenecid* / High doses ↓ secretion of nitrofurantoin → toxicity
*Sodium bicarbonate* / ↓ Effect of nitrofurantoin due to ↑ alkalinity of urine produced by sodium bicarbonate

**Laboratory Test Interferences:** ↑ AST, ALT, serum phosphorus. ↓ Hemoglobin.

**Dosage** ——————
• **Capsules, Oral Suspension**
  *UTIs.*
**Adults:** 50–100 mg q.i.d., not to exceed 600 mg/day. For cystitis, Macrobid is given in doses of 100 mg b.i.d. for 7 days. **Pediatric, 1 month of age and over:** 5–7 mg/kg/day in four equal doses.
  *Prophylaxis of UTIs.*

**Adults:** 50–100 mg at bedtime. **Pediatric, 1 month of age and over:** 1 mg/kg/day at bedtime or in two divided doses daily.

## NURSING CONSIDERATIONS

See also *General Nursing Considerations for All Anti-Infectives.*
**Administration/Storage**
1. Administer PO medication with meals or milk to promote absorption and reduce gastric irritation.
2. Preferably, administer capsules containing crystals, instead of tablets, because crystals cause less GI intolerance.
3. Store PO medications in amber-colored bottles.
4. Continue dosage for a minimum of 3 days after obtaining a negative urine culture.
**Assessment**
1. Monitor CBC, urine C&S, liver and renal functions; also CXR and PFTs with chronic therapy.
2. Observe for acute or delayed-onset anaphylactic reaction.
3. Drug may alter certain lab determinations.
4. Monitor for recurrent UTI symptoms and report because urinary superinfections may occur.
5. Blacks and ethnic groups of Mediterranean and Near Eastern origin should be assessed for symptoms of anemia.
**Client/Family Teaching**
1. Take with food to minimize GI upset and enhance absorption; complete full course of therapy.
2. Increase fluid intake, drink at least 2 quarts of water a day. Acidic foods (prunes, cranberry juice, plums) enhance drug action whereas alkaline foods (milk products) minimize drug action.
3. Acid urine enhances antibacterial activity. Drug may turn urine a dark yellow or brown color.
4. Report any persistent or bothersome side effects. Symptoms of respiratory dysfunction require immediate intervention.

**N**

---

5. Immediately report any numbness and tingling in the extremities or flu-like symptoms. These are indications for drug withdrawal because the condition may worsen and become irreversible.

6. Report persistent N&V and diarrhea as these may be symptoms of a GI superinfection.

**Outcomes/Evaluate**
• Negative urine culture results
• Resolution of infection; symptomatic improvement ($\downarrow$ dysuria, $\downarrow$ frequency)

# Nitroglycerin IV
(nye-troh-**GLIH**-sir-in)
**Pregnancy Category:** C
Nitro-Bid IV, Nitroglycerin in 5% Dextrose, Tridil **(Rx)**
**Classification:** Antianginal agent (coronary vasodilator)

See also *Antianginal Drugs, Nitrates/ Nitrites.*
**Action/Kinetics: Onset:** 1–2 min; **duration:** 3–5 min (dose-dependent).

**Uses:** Hypertension associated with surgery (e.g., associated with ET intubation, skin incision, sternotomy, anesthesia, cardiac bypass, immediate postsurgical period). CHF associated with acute MI. Angina unresponsive to usual doses of organic nitrate or beta-adrenergic blocking agents. Cardiac-load reducing agent. Produce controlled hypotension during surgical procedures.

**Special Concerns:** Dosage has not been established in children.

## Dosage
• **IV Infusion Only**
**Initial:** 5 mcg/min delivered by precise infusion pump. May be increased by 5 mcg/min q 3–5 min until response is seen. If no response seen at 20 mcg/min, dose can be increased by 10–20 mcg/min until response noted. Monitor titration continuously until client reaches desired level of response.

## NURSING CONSIDERATIONS

See also *Nursing Considerations* for *Antianginal Drugs, Nitrates/Nitrites.*
**Administration/Storage**
**IV** 1. Dilute with 5% dextrose USP or 0.9% NaCl injection. Not for direct IV use; must first be diluted.

2. Use only a glass IV bottle and administration set provided by the manufacturer; nitroglycerin is readily adsorbed onto many plastics. Avoid adding unnecessary plastic to IV system.

3. Aspirate medication into a syringe and then inject immediately into a glass bottle (or polyolefin bottle) to minimize contact with plastic.

4. Do not administer with any other medications in the IV system.

5. Do not interrupt IV nitroglycerin for administration of a bolus of any other medication.

6. To provide correct dosage, remove 15 mL of solution from the IV tubing if concentration of solution is changed.

7. Administer IV solution with an electronic infusion device (volumetric) and in a closely monitored environment.

**Assessment**
1. Document indications and goals of therapy.

2. Assess and rate pain, noting location, onset, duration, and any precipitating factors.

**Interventions**
1. Obtain written parameters for BP and pulse; monitor throughout therapy.

2. Monitor VS and ECG. Note any evidence of hypotension, nausea, sweating, and/or vomiting. Monitor CVP and/or PA pressure as ordered; document presence of tachycardia or bradycardia:
• Elevate the legs to restore BP.
• Reduce the rate of flow or administer additional IV fluids.

3. Assess for thrombophlebitis at the IV site; remove if reddened.

4. After the initial positive response to therapy, dosage increments will be smaller and made at longer intervals.

5. Sinus tachycardia may occur in a client with angina pectoris who is receiving a maintenance dose of nitroglycerin (HR of 80 beats/min or less reduces myocardial demand).

6. Check that topical, PO, or sublingual doses are adjusted or held if client is on concomitant therapy with IV nitroglycerin.

7. Wean from IV nitroglycerin by gradually decreasing doses to avoid posttherapy or CV distress. Usually initiated when the client is receiving the peak effect from PO or topical vasodilators; monitor for hypertension and angina.

8. Administer nonnarcotic analgesic (usually acetaminophen) because headache is a common side effect of drug therapy.

**Outcomes/Evaluate**
- Resolution/control of angina
- ↓ BP; ↑ activity tolerance
- Improvement in S&S of CHF (↑ output, ↓ rales, ↓ CVP)

# Nitroglycerin sublingual
(nye-troh-**GLIH**-sir-in)
**Pregnancy Category:** C
Nitrostat **(Rx)**
**Classification:** Antianginal agent (coronary vasodilator)

See also *Antianginal Drugs, Nitrates/ Nitrites*.
**Action/Kinetics: Sublingual. Onset:** 1–3 min; **duration:** 30–60 min.
**Uses:** Agents of choice for prophylaxis and treatment of angina pectoris.
**Special Concerns:** Dosage has not been established in children.

**Dosage**
- **Sublingual Tablets**
150–600 mcg under the tongue or in the buccal pouch at first sign of attack; may be repeated in 5 min if necessary (no more than 3 tablets should be taken within 15 min). For prophylaxis, tablets may be taken 5–10 min prior to activities that may precipitate an attack.

**NURSING CONSIDERATIONS**

See also *Nursing Considerations* for *Antianginal Drugs, Nitrates/Nitrites*.
**Administration/Storage**
1. Place sublingual tablets under the tongue and allow to dissolve; they should not be swallowed.
2. Store in the original container at room temperature protected from moisture. Discard unused tablets if 6 months has elapsed since the original container was opened.
**Client/Family Teaching**
1. Date sublingual container upon opening (usually only good for 6 months).
2. Let tablet dissolve under the tongue; may sting when it comes in contact with the mucosa.
3. Take *before* stressful activity, i.e., exercise, sex.
4. Report immediately if pain is not controlled.
**Outcomes/Evaluate**
- Angina prophylaxis
- Termination of anginal attack

# Nitroglycerin sustained-release capsules
(nye-troh-**GLIH**-sir-in)
**Pregnancy Category:** C
Nitroglyn **(Rx)**

# Nitroglycerin sustained-release tablets
(nye-troh-**GLIH**-sir-in)
**Pregnancy Category:** C
Nitrogard-SR ✦, Nitrong, Nitrong SR ✦ **(Rx)**
**Classification:** Antianginal agent (coronary vasodilator)

See also *Antianginal Drugs, Nitrates/Nitrites*.
**Action/Kinetics: Sustained-release.**
**Onset:** 20–45 min; **duration:** 3–8 hr.
**Uses:** To prevent anginal attacks. "Possibly effective" for the prophylaxis or treatment of anginal attacks.
**Special Concerns:** Dosage has not been established in children.

---

✦ = Available in Canada                                      *bold italic* = life threatening side effect

**Dosage**
- **Sustained-Release Capsules**
2.5, 6.5, or 9 mg q 8–12 hr.
- **Sustained-Release Tablets**
1.3, 2.6, or 6.5 mg q 8–12 hr.

## NURSING CONSIDERATIONS

See also *Nursing Considerations* for *Antianginal Drugs, Nitrates/Nitrites.*
**Administration/Storage**
1. Do not chew sustained-release tablets and capsules; not intended for sublingual use.
2. Give the smallest effective dose 2–4 times/day.
3. Tolerance may develop.
**Outcomes/Evaluate:** Angina prophylaxis

# Nitroglycerin topical ointment

(nye-troh-**GLIH**-sir-in)
**Pregnancy Category:** C
Nitro-Bid, Nitrol, Nitrol TSAR Kit ✹,
Nitrong ✹ **(Rx)**
**Classification:** Antianginal agent (coronary vasodilator)

See also *Antianginal Drugs, Nitrates/Nitrites.*
**Action/Kinetics: Onset:** 30–60 min; **duration:** 2–12 hr (depending on amount used per unit of surface area).
**Uses:** Prophylaxis and treatment of angina pectoris due to CAD.
**Special Concerns:** Dosage has not been established in children.

**Dosage**
- **Topical Ointment (2%)**
1–2 in. (15–30 mg) q 8 hr; up to 4–5 in. (60–75 mg) q 4 hr may be necessary. One inch equals approximately 15 mg nitroglycerin. Determine optimum dosage by starting with ½ in. q 8 hr and increasing by ½ in. with each successive dose until headache occurs; then, decrease to largest dose that does not cause headache. When ending treatment, reduce both the dose and frequency of administration over 4–6 weeks to prevent sudden withdrawal reactions.

## NURSING CONSIDERATIONS

See also *Nursing Considerations* for *Antianginal Drugs, Nitrates/Nitrites.*
**Client/Family Teaching**
1. Squeeze ointment carefully onto dose-measuring application papers, which are packaged with the medicine. Use applicator to spread ointment or fold paper in half and rub back and forth.
2. Use the paper to spread the ointment onto a nonhairy area of skin. Application to the chest may be psychologically helpful, but ointment may be applied to other nonhairy areas.
3. Rotate sites to prevent irritation. Keep a record of areas used to avoid unnecessary repetitive use of sites.
4. Apply ointment in a thin, even layer covering an area of skin 5–6 in. in diameter. Remember to remove last dose.
5. Tape the application paper over the area, or cover the area with a piece of plastic wrap-type material. A clear plastic cover causes less leakage of ointment, decreases skin irritation, increases the amount absorbed, and prevents clothing stains. Date, time, and initial tape at site.
6. Once the dose is established, use the same type of covering to ensure that the same amount of drug is absorbed during each application.
7. Clean around tube opening and tightly cap tube after use.
8. To prevent systemic absorption protect skin from contact with the ointment. Wash hands thoroughly after application to prevent headache.
9. Remove at bedtime or as directed to prevent tolerance or loss of drug effect. Remember to reapply upon awakening the next morning.
**Outcomes/Evaluate:** Termination and prevention of acute anginal episodes

# Nitroglycerin transdermal system

(nye-troh-**GLIH**-sir-in)
**Pregnancy Category:** C

Deponit 0.2 mg/hr and 0.4 mg/hr, Minitran 0.1 mg/hr, 0.2 mg/hr, 0.4 mg/hr, and 0.6 mg/hr, Nitrek 0.2 mg/hr, 0.4 mg/hr, and 0.6 mg/hr, Nitrodisc 0.2 mg/hr, 0.3 mg/hr, and 0.4 mg/hr, Nitro-Dur 0.1 mg/hr, 0.2 mg/hr, 0.3 mg/hr, 0.4 mg/hr, 0.6 mg/hr, and 0.8 mg/hr, Transderm-Nitro 0.1 mg/hr, 0.2 mg/hr, 0.4 mg/hr, and 0.6 mg/hr **(Rx)**
**Classification:** Antianginal agent (coronary vasodilator)

See also *Antianginal Drugs, Nitrates/Nitrites*.
**Action/Kinetics:   Onset:** 30–60 min; **duration:** 8–24 hr. The amount released each hour is indicated in the name.
**Uses:** Prophylaxis of angina pectoris due to CAD. *NOTE:* There is some evidence that nitroglycerin patches stop preterm labor.
**Special Concerns:** Dosage has not been established in children.

**Dosage**
• **Topical Patch**
**Initial:** 0.2–0.4 mg/hr (initially the smallest available dose in the dosage series) applied each day to skin site free of hair and free of excessive movement (e.g., chest, upper arm).
**Maintenance:** Additional systems or strengths may be added depending on the clinical response.

## NURSING CONSIDERATIONS

See also *Nursing Considerations* for *Antianginal Drugs, Nitrates/Nitrites*.
**Administration/Storage**
1. Follow instructions for specific products on package insert.
2. When terminating therapy, gradually reduce the dose and frequency of application over 4–6 weeks.
3. Tolerance is a significant factor affecting efficacy if the system is used continuously for more than 12 hr/day. Thus, a dosage regimen would include a daily period where the patch is on for 12–14 hr and a period of 10–12 hr when the patch is off (i.e., while asleep).
4. Remove patch before defibrillating as patch may explode.

5. The various products differ in the mechanism for the delivery system; the most important factor is the amount of drug released per hour. A wide range of client variability will be noted. Variables in the rate of absorption include the skin, physical exercise, and elevated ambient temperature.
6. It is important to note that there is a wide variety between clients in the actual amount of nitroglycerin absorbed each day. Physical exercise and increased ambient temperatures may increase the amount absorbed.
**Client/Family Teaching**
1. Apply only as directed. Make sure skin is completely dry before applying.
2. Remove old pad and rotate sites of application each day to avoid skin irritation. Do not apply to distal areas of extremities.
3. Date patch as a reminder that drug has been administered.
4. Once applied, do not disturb or open patch. Do not stop therapy abruptly.
5. Remove at bedtime or as directed to prevent a diminished response (tolerance) to the drug. Remember to reapply a new system upon awakening the next morning.
6. Bathing or swimming should not interfere with therapy.
**Outcomes/Evaluate:**   Control/prevention of anginal episodes

# Nitroglycerin translingual spray
(nye-troh-**GLIH**-sir-in)
**Pregnancy Category:** C
Nitrolingual **(Rx)**
**Classification:** Antianginal agent (coronary vasodilator)

See also *Antianginal Drugs, Nitrates/Nitrites*.
**Action/Kinetics:   Onset:** 2 min; **duration:** 30–60 min.
**Uses:** Coronary artery disease to relieve an acute attack or used prophylactically   10–15   min   before

beginning activities that can cause an acute anginal attack.
**Special Concerns:** Dosage has not been established in children.

## Dosage
* **Spray**
  *Termination of acute attack.*
  One to two metered doses (400–800 mcg) on or under the tongue q 5 min as needed; no more than three metered doses should be administered within a 15-min period.
  *Prophylaxis.*
  One to two metered doses 5–10 min before beginning activities that might precipitate an acute attack.

## NURSING CONSIDERATIONS

See also *Nursing Considerations* for *Antianginal Drugs, Nitrates/Nitrites.*
**Client/Family Teaching**
1. Do *not* inhale the spray. Spray under the tongue.
2. Seek immediate medical attention if chest pain persists.
**Outcomes/Evaluate:** Control/prevention of acute anginal episodes

# Nitroprusside sodium
(nye-troh-**PRUS**-eyed)
**Pregnancy Category:** C
Nitropress **(Rx)**
**Classification:** Antihypertensive, direct action on vascular smooth muscle

**Action/Kinetics:** Direct action on vascular smooth muscle, leading to peripheral vasodilation of arteries and veins. Acts on excitation-contraction coupling of vascular smooth muscle by interfering with both influx and intracellular activation of calcium. No effect on smooth muscle of the duodenum or uterus and is more active on veins than on arteries. May also improve CHF by decreasing systemic resistance, preload and afterload reduction, and improved CO. **Onset** (drug must be given by IV infusion): 0.5–1 min; **peak effect:** 1–2 min; **t½:** 2 min; **duration:** Up to 10 min after infusion stopped. Nitroprusside reacts with hemoglobin to produce cyanmethemoglobin and

cyanide ion. Caution must be exercised as nitroprusside injection can result in toxic levels of cyanide. However, when used briefly or at low infusion rates, the cyanide produced reacts with thiosulfate to produce thiocyanate, which is excreted in the urine.
**Uses:** Hypertensive crisis to reduce BP immediately. To produce controlled hypotension during anesthesia to reduce bleeding. Acute CHF. *Investigational:* In combination with dopamine for acute MI. Left ventricular failure with coadministration of oxygen, morphine, and a loop diuretic.
**Contraindications:** Compensatory hypertension where the primary hemodynamic lesion is aortic coarctation or AV shunting. Use to produce controlled hypotension during surgery in clients with known inadequate cerebral circulation or in moribund clients. Clients with congenital optic atrophy or tobacco amblyopia (both of which are rare). Acute CHF associated with decreased peripheral vascular resistance (e.g., high-output heart failure that may be seen in endotoxic sepsis). Lactation.
**Special Concerns:** Use with caution in hypothyroidism, liver or kidney impairment, during lactation, and in the presence of increased ICP. Geriatric clients may be more sensitive to the hypotensive effects of nitroprusside; also, a decrease in dose may be necessary in these clients due to age-related decreases in renal function.
**Side Effects:** Excessive hypotension. *Large doses may lead to cyanide toxicity. Following rapid BP reduction:* Dizziness, nausea, restlessness, headache, sweating, muscle twitching, palpitations, abdominal pain, apprehension, retching, retrosternal discomfort. *Other side effects:* Bradycardia, tachycardia, ECG changes, venous streaking, rash, methemoglobinemia, decreased platelet aggregation, flushing, hypothyroidism, ileus, irritation at injection site, hypothyroidism. *Symptoms of thiocyanate toxicity:* Blurred vision, tinnitus, confusion, hyperreflexia,

seizures. *CNS symptoms (transitory):* Restlessness, agitation, increased ICP, and muscle twitching. Vomiting or skin rash.

**OD** **Overdose Management:** *Symptoms:* Excessive hypotension, cyanide toxicity, thiocyanate toxicity. *Treatment:*
• Measure cyanide levels and blood gases to determine venous hyperoxemia or acidosis.
• To treat cyanide toxicity, discontinue nitroprusside and give sodium nitrite, 4–6 mg/kg (about 0.2 mL/kg) over 2–4 min (to convert hemoglobin into methemoglobin); follow by sodium thiosulfate, 150–200 mg/kg (about 50 mL of the 25% solution). This regimen can be given again, at half the original doses, after 2 hr.

**Drug Interactions:** Concomitant use of other antihypertensives, volatile liquid anesthetics, or certain depressants ↑ response to nitroprusside.

**Dosage** ―――――――
• **IV Infusion Only**
*Hypertensive crisis.*
**Adults:** average, 3 mcg/kg/min. **Range:** 0.3–10 mcg/kg/min. Smaller dose is required for clients receiving other antihypertensives. **Pediatric:** 1.4 mcg/kg/min adjusted slowly depending on the response.

Monitor BP and use as guide to regulate rate of administration to maintain desired antihypertensive effect. Rate of administration should not exceed 10 mcg/kg/min.

## NURSING CONSIDERATIONS

See also *Nursing Considerations* for *Antihypertensive Agents.*
**Administration/Storage**
**IV** 1. Dissolve contents of the vial (50 mg) in 2–3 mL of D5W. This stock solution must be diluted further in 250–1,000 mL D5W.
2. If properly protected from light, the reconstituted solution is stable for 24 hr.
3. Discard solutions that are any color but light brown.

4. Do not add any other drug or preservative to solution.
5. Protect dilute solutions during administration by wrapping bag and tubing with opaque material such as aluminum foil or foil-lined bags; change setup every 24 hr. Explain that covering the IV bag protects the medication from light and maintains drug stability. Administer IV solution with an electronic infusion device in a monitored environment.
6. Cyanide toxicity is possible if more than 500 mcg/kg nitroprusside is given faster than 2 mcg/kg/min. To reduce this possibility, sodium thiosulfate can be co-infused with nitroprusside at rates of 5–10 times that of nitroprusside.
7. Protect drug from heat, light, and moisture. Store at 15°C–30°C (59°F–86°F).

**Assessment**
1. Document symptom characteristics and other therapies trialed.
2. Note any hypothyroidism or $B_{12}$ deficiency.
3. Monitor CBC, electrolytes, ABGs, PAWP, and liver and renal function studies.

**Interventions**
1. Monitor VS, I&O, and ECG. Monitor BP closely and titrate infusion.
2. Observe for symptoms of thiocyanate toxicity. Evaluate thiocyanate levels q 24–48 hr; levels should be less than 100 mcg thiocyanate/mL or 3 μmol cyanide/mL. Metabolic acidosis may precede cyanide toxicity.

**Outcomes/Evaluate**
• ↓ BP
• Improvement in S&S of refractory CHF

―――――――――――――

# Nizatidine
(nye-**ZAY**-tih-deen)
**Pregnancy Category:** C
Axid **(Rx)**, Axid AR **(OTC)**
**Classification:** Histamine $H_2$ receptor antagonist

―――――――――――――

See also *Histamine H₂ Antagonists.*
**Action/Kinetics:** Decreases gastric acid secretion by blocking the effect

of histamine on histamine $H_2$ receptors. Does not affect the P-450 and P-448 drug metabolizing enzymes.**Onset:** 30 min. **Peak plasma levels:** 0.5–3 hr after a PO dose. **Time to peak effect:** 0.5–3 hr. **Duration, nocturnal:** Up to 12 hr; **basal:** Up to 8 hr. **t½:** 1–2 hr. Approximately 60% of a PO dose is excreted unchanged in the urine. Clients with moderate to severe renal impairment manifest a significant prolongation of t½ with decreased clearance.

**Uses:** Treatment of acute duodenal ulcer and maintenance following healing of a duodenal ulcer. GERD, including erosive and ulcerative esophagitis. Short-term treatment of benign gastric ulcer. OTC use to prevent meal-induced heartburn.

**Contraindications:** Hypersensitivity to $H_2$ receptor antagonists. Cirrhosis of the liver, impaired renal or hepatic function. Lactation.

**Special Concerns:** Safety and efficacy have not been determined in children.

**Side Effects:** *CNS:* Headache, fatigue, somnolence, insomnia, dizziness, abnormal dreams, anxiety, nervousness, confusion (rare). *GI:* N&V, diarrhea, pancreatitis, constipation, abdominal discomfort, flatulence, dyspepsia, anorexia, dry mouth. *Dermatologic:* Exfoliative dermatitis, erythroderma, pruritus, urticaria, erythema multiforme. *CV:* Asymptomatic ventricular tachycardia; *rarely, cardiac arrhythmias or arrest following rapid IV use. Respiratory:* Rhinitis, pharyngitis, sinusitis, cough. *Body as a whole:* Asthenia, back pain, chest pain, infection, fever, myalgia. *Miscellaneous:* Impotence, loss of libido, thrombocytopenia, sweating, gynecomastia, hyperuricemia, eosinophilia, gout, and cholestatic or hepatocellular effects (resulting in increased AST, ALT, or alkaline phosphatase).

**Drug Interactions**
*Antacids containing Al and Mg hydroxides* / ↓ Nizatidine absorption by about 10%
*Aspirin, high doses* / ↑ Salicylate serum levels

*Simethicone* / ↓ Nizatidine absorption by about 10%

**Laboratory Test Interferences:** False + test for urobilinogen.

## Dosage
AXID
- **Capsules**
  *Active duodenal ulcer.*

**Adults:** Either 300 mg once daily at bedtime or 150 mg b.i.d. The dose should be 150 mg/day if the $C_{CR}$ is 20–50 mL/min and 150 mg every other day if $C_{CR}$ is less than 20 mL/min.

  *Prophylaxis following healing of duodenal ulcer.*

**Adults:** 150 mg/day at bedtime. The dose should be 150 mg every other day if $C_{CR}$ is 20–50 mL/min and 150 mg every 3 days if $C_{CR}$ is less than 20 mL/min.

  *Treatment of benign gastric ulcer.*

**Adults:** 150 mg b.i.d. or 300 mg at bedtime

  *Gastroesophageal reflux disease, including erosive and ulcerative esophagitis.*

**Adults:** 150 mg b.i.d.
AXID AR
- **Tablets**
  *Heartburn.*
1 tablet b.i.d.

## NURSING CONSIDERATIONS

See also *Nursing Considerations* for *Histamine $H_2$ Antagonists.*

**Administration/Storage**
1. Maintain treatment for active duodenal ulcer for up to 8 weeks.
2. Gastric malignancy may be present even though a clinical response to nizatidine has occurred.
3. Doses of 150 and 300 mg can be mixed with commercial juices (apple juice, *Gatorade, Ocean Spray,* and others); such preparations are stable for 48 hr when refrigerated. However, a 10% loss in potency is seen if mixed with *V8* or *Cran-Grape* juices.

**Assessment**
1. Document type, onset, location, duration, and characteristics of symptoms.
2. Note any allergies to $H_2$ receptor antagonists.

3. Monitor hepatic and renal function studies; reduce dosage with renal insufficiency.

4. Note *H. pylori* results and diagnostic findings, i.e., radiographic and/or endoscopic.

**Client/Family Teaching**

1. Take at bedtime due to potential sedative effects.

2. Use caution when performing tasks that require mental alertness until drug effects realized.

3. Continue to take as ordered even if symptoms subside.

4. Report any side effects, such as rashes, flaking of skin, or extreme sleepiness.

5. Avoid alcohol, caffeine, spicy foods, and aspirin-containing products.

6. **Do not smoke,** as this interferes with drug's effects.

**Outcomes/Evaluate:** Improvement in ulcer pain and irritation; ↓ GERD symptoms

# Norfloxacin

(nor-**FLOX**-ah-sin)
**Pregnancy Category:** C
Chibroxin Ophthalmic Solution, Noroxin, Noroxin Ophthalmic Solution ✦ (Rx)
**Classification:** Fluoroquinolone anti-infective

See also *Anti-Infectives* and *Fluoroquinolones.*

**Action/Kinetics:** Active against gram-positive and gram-negative organisms by inhibiting bacterial DNA synthesis. Not effective against obligate anaerobes. **Peak plasma levels:** 1.4–1.6 mcg/mL after 1–2 hr following a dose of 400 mg and 2.5 mcg/mL 1–2 hr after a dose of 800 mg. **t½:** 3–4.5 hr. Food decreases the absorption of norfloxacin. Approximately 30% excreted unchanged in the urine and 30% through the feces.

**Uses: Systemic:** Uncomplicated UTIs caused by *Escherichia coli, Klebsiella pneumoniae, Enterobacter cloacae, Proteus mirabilis, P. vulgaris, Pseudomonas aeruginosa, Citrobacter freundii, Staphylococcus aureus, S. epidermidis, Enterococcus faecalis, Enterobacter aerogenes, S. saprophyticus,* and *S. agalactiae.* Complicated UTIs caused by *Enterococcus faecalis, E. coli, K. pneumoniae, P. mirabilis, P. aeruginosa,* or *Serratia marcescens.* Urethral gonorrhea and endocervical gonococcal infections due to penicillinase- or non-penicillinase-producing *Neisseria gonorrhoeae.* Prostatitis due to *E. coli.*

**Ophthalmic:** Superficial ocular infections involving the cornea or conjunctiva due to *Staphylococcus, S. aureus, Streptococcus pneumoniae, E. coli, Haemophilus aegyptius, H. influenzae, Klebsiella pneumoniae, Neisseria gonorrhoeae, Proteus* species, *Enterobacter aerogenes, Serratia marcescens, Pseudomonas aeruginosa,* and *Vibrio* species.

**Contraindications:** Hypersensitivity to nalidixic acid, cinoxacin, or norfloxacin. Lactation, infants, and children. Ophthalmic use for dendritic keratitis, vaccinia, varicella, mycobacterial infections of the eye, fungal disease of the eye, and use with steroid combinations after uncomplicated removal of a corneal foreign body.

**Special Concerns:** Use with caution in clients with a history of seizures and in impaired renal function. Geriatric clients eliminate norfloxacin more slowly.

**Side Effects:** See also *Side Effects* for *Fluoroquinolones.*

*GI:* Nausea, vomiting, diarrhea, abdominal pain or discomfort, dry/painful mouth, dyspepsia, flatulence, constipation, pseudomembranous colitis, stomatitis. *CNS:* Headache, dizziness, fatigue, malaise, drowsiness, depression, insomnia, confusion, psychoses. *Hematologic:* Decreased hematocrit, eosinophilia, leukopenia, neutropenia, either increased or decreased platelets. *Dermatologic:* Photosensitivity, rash, pruritus, exfoliative dermatitis, *toxic epidermal necrolysis,* erythema, erythema multiforme, *Stevens-Johnson syndrome.* Other: Paresthesia, hypersensitivity, fever, visual disturbances, hearing loss, crystalluria, cylindruria, candiduria, myoclonus (rare), hepatitis, pancreatitis, arthralgia.

*Following ophthalmic use:* Conjunctival hyperemia, photophobia, chemosis, bitter taste in mouth.

**Additional Drug Interactions:** Nitrofurantoin ↓ antibacterial effect of norfloxacin.

**Laboratory Test Interferences:** ↑ AST, ALT, alkaline phosphatase, BUN, serum creatinine, and LDH.

**Dosage**

• **Tablets**

*Uncomplicated UTIs due to* E. coli, K. pneumoniae, or P. mirabilis.
400 mg q 12 hr for 3 days.

*Uncomplicated UTIs due to other organisms.*
400 mg q 12 hr for 7–10 days.

*Complicated UTIs.*
400 mg q 12 hr for 10–21 days. Maximum dose for UTIs should not exceed 800 mg/day.

*Uncomplicated gonorrhea.*
800 mg as a single dose.

*Impaired renal function, with $C_{CR}$ equal to or less than 30 mL/min/1.73 m².*
400 mg/day for 7–10 days.

*Prostatis due to* E. coli.
400 mg q 12 hr for 28 days.

• **Ophthalmic Solution**

*Acute infections.*
**Initially,** 1–2 gtt q 15–30 min; **then,** reduce frequency as infection is controlled.

*Moderate infections.*
1–2 gtt 4–6 times/day.

## NURSING CONSIDERATIONS

See also *Nursing Considerations* for *Fluoroquinolones.*

**Assessment**

1. Document indications for therapy and type, location, onset, and duration of symptoms.

2. Note any seizure disorder or impaired renal function; reduce dose with impaired function.

3. Obtain baseline CBC and cultures.

4. Determine if pregnant.

**Client/Family Teaching**

1. Take 1 hr before or 2 hr after meals, with a glass of water; food decreases the absorption of norfloxacin.

2. Take at evenly spaced intervals, generally every 12 hr.

3. Antacids should not be taken with or for 2 hr after a dose of norfloxacin.

4. To prevent crystalluria consume 2–3 L/day of fluids.

5. Use caution if operating equipment or driving a motor vehicle; may cause dizziness.

6. Advise females of childbearing age to practice contraception during drug therapy.

7. Avoid prolonged sun exposure; wear sunglasses, protective clothing, and a sunscreen to prevent photosensitivity reactions.

**Outcomes/Evaluate**

• Negative culture reports

• Symptomatic improvement (with UTI: ↓ dysuria, hematuria, and frequency; with ophthalmic use: ↓ itching, burning, and discharge).

# Nortriptyline hydrochloride

(nor-**TRIP**-tih-leen)
**Pregnancy Category:** C
Aventyl, Pamelor **(Rx)**
**Classification:** Antidepressant, tricyclic

See also *Antidepressants, Tricyclic.*

**Action/Kinetics:** Manifests moderate anticholinergic and sedative effects but slight orthostatic hypotensive effects. **Effective plasma levels:** 50–150 ng/mL. **t½:** 18–44 hr. **Time to reach steady state:** 4–19 days.

**Uses:** Treatment of symptoms of depression. Chronic, severe neurogenic pain. Dermatologic disorders including chronic urticaria, angioedema, and nocturnal pruritus in atopic eczema.

**Contraindications:** Use in children.

**Special Concerns:** Safety and efficacy have not been determined in children.

**Laboratory Test Interferences:** ↓ Urinary 5-HIAA.

**Dosage** ⸺
- **Capsules, Oral Solution**
  *Depression.*
  **Adults:** 25 mg t.i.d.–q.i.d. Dose individualized; begin at a low dosage and increase as needed. **Doses above 150 mg/day are not recommended. Elderly clients:** 30–50 mg/day in divided doses.
  *Dermatologic disorders.*
  75 mg/day.

## NURSING CONSIDERATIONS

See also *Nursing Considerations* for *Antidepressants, Tricyclic.*
**Administration/Storage:** Store at controlled room temperatures.
**Assessment:** Document indications for therapy, type, onset, and characteristics of symptoms. Identify any causative factors.
**Client/Family Teaching:** Take after meals and at bedtime to minimize GI upset.
**Outcomes/Evaluate**
- Control of symptoms of depression ( ↓ fatigue, improved sleeping and eating patterns, effective coping)
- ↓ Nocturnal pruritus
- Relief of chronic neurogenic pain

# Nystatin
(nye-**STAT**-in)
**Pregnancy Category:** C (A for vaginal use)
**Tablets:** Mycostatin, Nilstat. **Oral Suspension:** Mycostatin, Nadostine ✹, Nilstat, Nystex, PMS Nystatin ✹. **Troches:** Mycostatin Pastilles. **Vaginal Tablets:** Mycostatin, Nadostine ✹. **Topical:** Mycostatin, Nadostine ✹, Nilstat, Nyaderm ✹, Nystex, Nystop, **Topical Powder:** Nystop **(Rx)**
**Classification:** Antibiotic, antifungal

See also *Anti-Infectives.*
**Action/Kinetics:** Derived from *Streptomyces noursei*; is both fungistatic and fungicidal against all species of *Candida.* Binds to fungal cell membranes (sterols), resulting in altered cellular permeability and leakage of potassium and other essential intracellular components. Poorly absorbed from the GI tract; unabsorbed nystatin is excreted in the feces.
**Uses:** *Candida* infections of the skin, mucous membranes, GI tract, vagina, and mouth (thrush). The drug is too toxic for systemic infections although it can be given PO for intestinal moniliasis infections, as it is not absorbed from the GI tract.
**Contraindications:** Use for systemic mycoses. Use of topical products in or around the eyes.
**Special Concerns:** Occlusive dressings should not be used when treating candidiasis. Lozenges should not be used in children less than 5 years of age.
**Side Effects:** Nystatin has few toxic effects. *GI:* Epigastric distress, N&V, diarrhea. *Other:* Rarely, irritation.

**Dosage** ⸺
- **Capsule, Lozenge, Oral Suspension, Tablets**
  *Intestinal candidiasis.*
  **Tablets,** 500,000–1,000,000 units t.i.d.; continue treatment for 48 hr after cure to prevent relapse.
  *Oral candidiasis.*
  **Oral Suspension, adults and children:** 400,000–600,000 units q.i.d. (½ dose in each side of mouth, held as long as possible before swallowing); **infants:** 200,000 units q.i.d. (same procedure as with adults); **premature or low birth weight infants:** 100,000 units q.i.d. **Lozenge, adults and children:** 200,000–400,000 units 4–5 times/day, up to 14 days. *NOTE:* Lozenges should not be chewed or swallowed.
- **Vaginal Tablets**
  100,000 units (1 tablet) inserted in vagina once each day for 2 weeks.
- **Topical Cream, Ointment, Powder (100,000 units/g each)**
  Apply to affected areas b.i.d.–t.i.d., or as indicated, until healing is complete.

**N**

---

✹ = Available in Canada                    ***bold italic*** = life threatening side effect

## NURSING CONSIDERATIONS

See also *General Nursing Considerations for All Anti-Infectives.*

### Administration/Storage

1. A powder for extemporaneous compounding of the oral suspension is available. To reconstitute, add ⅛ tsp of the powder (about 500,000 units) to approximately ½–1 cup water and stir well. This product is administered immediately after mixing.

2. Protect drug from heat, light, moisture, and air.

3. The suspension can be stored for 7 days at room temperature or for 10 days in the refrigerator without loss of potency.

4. For *Candida* infections of the feet, the powder can be freely dusted on the feet as well as in socks and shoes.

5. The cream is generally used in *Candida* infections involving intertriginous areas; however, moist lesions should be treated with powder.

6. Refrigerate vaginal tablets.

**Assessment:** Document onset, location, duration, and clinical presentation of symptoms.

### Client/Family Teaching

1. Review the appropriate method and technique for administration. Use as directed for the amount of time designated to ensure desired results.

2. Do not mix oral suspension in foods because the medication will be inactivated.

3. Drop 1 mL of oral suspension in each side of mouth or apply with a swab to treat oral moniliasis. Swish around and keep in the mouth as long as possible before swallowing.

4. For pediatric use, 250,000 units of cherry flavor nystatin has been frozen in the form of popsicles.

5. Do not use mouthwash with oral candidiasis as this may alter normal flora and promote infections.

6. Vaginal tablets may be administered PO for candidiasis. These should be sucked on as a lozenge and not chewed or swallowed.

7. Insert vaginal tablets high in vagina with applicator.

8. Continue using vaginal tablets even when menstruating; treatment should be continued for 2 weeks. Avoid tampons.

9. Continue vaginal tablets in the gravid client for 3–6 weeks before term to reduce incidence of thrush in the newborn.

10. Discontinue and report if vaginal tablets cause irritation, redness, or swelling.

11. Drug may stain; sanitary pads may help protect clothing and linens.

12. Apply cream or ointment to mycotic lesions with a swab or wear gloves to avoid direct contact with hands as contact dermatitis may ensue.

13. To prevent reinfection, avoid intercourse during therapy or use condoms. Advise partner to seek treatment if symptomatic.

### Outcomes/Evaluate

- Negative culture results
- Improvement in skin and mucous membrane irritation with less discomfort and itching

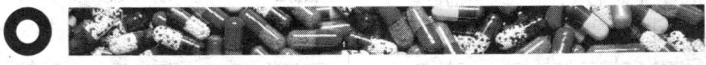

## Octreotide acetate

(ock-**TREE**-oh-tyd)

**Pregnancy Category:** B

Sandostatin **(Rx)**

**Classification:** Antineoplastic

**Action/Kinetics:** Similar to the natural hormone somatostatin. It suppresses secretions of serotonin and GI peptides including gastrin, insulin, glucagon, secretin, motilin, vasoactive intestinal peptide, and pancreatic polypeptide. The drug stimulates fluid and electrolyte absorption from the GI tract and inhibits growth hormone. It may alter the absorption of dietary fats in some clients. Rapidly absorbed from injection sites. **Peak levels:** 5.5 ng/mL after approximately 25 min. **t½:** 1.7 hr. **Duration:** Up to 12 hr. About one-third of a dose is excreted unchanged in the urine.

**Uses:** Metastatic carcinoid tumors; vasoactive intestinal tumors (VIPomas). The drug inhibits severe diarrhea in both situations and causes improvement in hypokalemia in VIPomas. Acromegaly. *Investigational:* GI fistula, variceal bleeding, pancreatic fistula, irritable bowel syndrome, and dumping syndrome. Also, treatment of diarrhea due to AIDS, short bowel syndrome, diabetes, pancreatic cholera syndrome, chemotherapy or radiation therapy in cancer patients, and idiopathic secretory diarrhea. Other potential uses include enteric fistula, pancreatitis, pancreatic surgery, glucagonoma, insulinoma, Zollinger-Ellison syndrome, intestinal obstruction, local radiotherapy, chronic pain management, antineoplastic therapy, to decrease insulin requirements in diabetes mellitus, in thyrotropin- and TSH-secreting tumors.

**Special Concerns:** Use with caution in diabetics, in clients with gallbladder disease, in clients with severe renal failure requiring dialysis, and during lactation.

**Side Effects:** *GI:* Nausea, diarrhea or loose stools, abdominal pain or distention, malabsorption of fat, vomiting; less commonly, constipation, pancreatitis, anorexia, flatulence, abdominal distention, abnormal stools, hepatitis, jaundice, appendicitis, GI bleeding, hemorrhoids. *CNS:* Headache, dizziness, lightheadedness, fatigue; less commonly, anxiety, seizures, depression, vertigo, decrease in libido, syncope, tremor, Bell's palsy, paranoia, pituitary apoplexy. *CV:* Sinus bradycardia in acromegalics, hypertension, thrombophlebitis, SOB, CHF, ischemia, palpitations, orthostatic hypotension, conduction abnormalities, hypertensive reaction, tachycardia,

arrhythmias, chest pain. *Endocrine:* Hyperglycemia or hypoglycemia in acromegalics, biochemical hypothyroidism in acromegalics. Galactorrhea, hypoadrenalism, diabetes insipidus, gynecomastia, amenorrhea, polymenorrhea, vaginitis. *Musculoskeletal:* Backache, joint pain, arthritis, joint effusion, muscle pain, Raynaud's phenomenon. *Dermatologic:* Pain, wheal, or erythema at injection site; flushing, edema, pruritus, hair loss, rash, cellulitis, petechiae, urticaria. *GU:* Pollakiuria, UTI, nephrolithiasis, hematuria. *Hematologic:* Hematoma at injection site, bruise, iron deficiency anemia, epistaxis. *Other:* Gallbladder abnormalities, especially stones or biliary sludge; flu symptoms, malabsorption of fat, blurred vision, otitis, allergic reaction, visual disturbances, ***anaphylactoid reactions, including anaphylactic shock.***

**OD Overdose Management:** *Symptoms:* Hyperglycemia and hypoglycemia manifested by dizziness, drowsiness, loss of sensory or motor function, incoordination, disturbed consciousness, and visual blurring. *Treatment:* Withdraw drug temporarily and treat symptomatically.

**Drug Interactions:** Octreotide may interfere with drugs such as diazoxide, insulin, beta-adrenergic blocking agents, or sulfonylureas. Close monitoring is necessary.

**Laboratory Test Interferences:** ↑ Liver enzymes, CK.

**Dosage** ———————
• **SC (Recommended), IV Bolus (Emergencies)**
  *Metastatic carcinoid tumors.*
**Initial, SC:** 50 mcg 1–2 times/day. **Then,** 100–600 mcg/day in two to four divided doses for the first 2 weeks; **maintenance, usual:** 450 mcg/day (range: 50–1,500 mcg/day).
  *VIPomas.*
**Initial, SC:** 200–300 mcg/day in two to four divided doses during the initial 2 weeks of therapy (range: 150–750 mcg/day). Doses may then

---

🍁 = Available in Canada                    ***bold italic*** = life threatening side effect be adjusted but the daily dose usually does not exceed 450 mcg.

*Acromegaly.*
**Initial:** 50 mcg t.i.d.; **then,** 100–500 mcg t.i.d. The goal is to achieve growth hormone levels less than 5 ng/mL or IGF-1 levels less than 1.9 U/mL in males and less than 2.2 U/mL in females.

*GI fistula.*
50–200 mcg q 8 hr.

*Variceal bleeding.*
25–50 mcg/hr via continuous IV infusion for 18 hr to 5 days.

*AIDS-related diarrhea.*
100–500 mcg SC t.i.d.

*Idiopathic secretory diarrhea, short-bowel syndrome.*
Either 25 mcg/hr by IV infusion or 50 mcg SC b.i.d.

*Diabetes, pancreatic cholera syndrome, diarrhea due to chemotherapy or radiation therapy in cancer clients.*
50–100 mcg SC t.i.d. for 3 days.

*Pancreatic fistula.*
50–200 mcg q 8 hr.

*Irritable bowel syndrome.*
100 mcg as a single dose to 125 mcg SC b.i.d.

*Dumping syndrome.*
50–150 mcg/day.

## NURSING CONSIDERATIONS
### Administration/Storage
1. Experience is lacking for doses greater than 750 mcg/day.
2. Avoid multiple injections at the same site within a short period of time. Preferred sites for injection are the abdomen, hip, and thigh.
3. GI side effects can be minimized by giving the drug between meals and at bedtime.
**IV** 4. Inspect ampules for particulate matter and discoloration; if present, do not use.
5. Reactions at the site of injection can be minimized by letting the solution warm to room temperature before administering the injection and by giving the injection slowly.
6. Store ampules for long periods at 2°C–8°C (36°F–46°F) although they may be stored at room temperature the day they will be used.

7. Octreotide is not compatible with TPN solutions due to the formation of glycosyl octreotide conjugate, which may decrease its efficacy.
8. Octreotide is stable in sterile isotonic saline solutions or sterile solutions of D5W for 24 hr. The drug may be diluted in volumes of 50–200 mL and infused IV over 15–30 min or given by IV push over 3 min. In carcinoid crisis, the drug may be given by rapid IV bolus.

### Assessment
1. Document indications for therapy, type, onset, and duration of symptoms. List other agents trialed and the outcome.
2. Monitor thyroid function studies; drug may cause biochemical hypothyroidism, necessitating replacement therapy.
3. Monitor serum electrolyte and glucose levels. The drug alters serum glucose levels and may require an adjustment of antidiabetic drug dosage.
4. Drug may alter fat absorption and gallbladder function, assess client carefully and monitor the appropriate lab values (e.g., quantitative 72-hr fecal fat and serum carotene [fat malabsorption]) and ultrasonography studies during long-term therapy.
5. Monitor I&O. Perform abdominal assessments routinely, noting character and frequency of stools and any abnormal findings.

### Client/Family Teaching
1. Drug is usually administered SC. There may be pain at the site of injection; rotate sites. Review guidelines for administration, dose, frequency, and site rotation.
2. Dosage of drug is highly individualized; take only as prescribed. Usually two injections a day are necessary when treating endocrine tumors.
3. More frequent side effects with this drug include N&V, dizziness, headache, diarrhea, abdominal cramps, flatulence, steatorrhea with bulky bowel movements, and weakness; report if persistent.
4. Keep the medication refrigerated.
5. Clients with diabetes should

monitor blood sugars frequently and report significant variations.

**Outcomes/Evaluate**

- Relief of severe diarrhea and control of secondary electrolyte imbalance with metastatic disease
- ↓ Tumor growth

# Ofloxacin
(oh-**FLOX**-ah-zeen)
**Pregnancy Category:** C
Floxin, Floxin I.V., Floxin Otic, Ocuflox **(Rx)**
**Classification:** Antibacterial, fluoroquinolone

See also *Anti-Infectives.*

**Action/Kinetics:** Effective against a wide range of gram-positive and gram-negative aerobic and anaerobic bacteria. Penicillinase has no effect on the activity of ofloxacin. Widely distributed to body fluids. **Maximum serum levels:** 1–2 hr. t½, **first phase:** 5–7 hr; **second phase:** 20–25 hr. **Peak serum levels at steady state, after PO doses:** 1.5 mcg/mL after 200-mg doses, 2.4 mcg/mL after 300-mg doses, and 2.9 mcg/mL after 400-mg doses. **Peak serum levels after IV doses:** 2.7 mcg/mL after 200-mg dose and 4 mcg/mL after 400-mg dose. Between 70% and 80% is excreted unchanged in the urine.

**Uses: Systemic:** Pneumonia or acute bacterial exacerbations of chronic bronchitis or community-acquired pneumonia due to *Haemophilus influenzae* or *Streptococcus pneumoniae.* Not a drug of first choice in the treatment of presumed or confirmed pneumococcal pneumonia. Not effective for syphilis.

Acute, uncomplicated urethral and cervical gonorrhea due to *Neisseria gonorrhoeae;* nongonococcal urethritis, and cervicitis due to *Chlamydia trachomatis.* Mixed infections of the urethra and cervix due to *N. gonorrhoeae* and *C. trachomatis.*

Mild to moderate skin and skin structure infections due to *Staphylo-coccus aureus, Streptococcus pyogenes,* or *Proteus mirabilis.*

Uncomplicated cystitis due to *Citrobacter diversus, Enterobacter aerogenes, E. coli, Klebsiella pneumoniae, Proteus mirabilis,* or *Pseudomonas aeruginosa.* Complicated UTIs due to *Escherichia coli, K. pneumoniae, P. mirabilis, C. diversus,* or *P. aeruginosa.* Prostatitis due to *E. coli.* Monotherapy for pelvic inflammatory disease.

IV therapy is indicated when the client is unable to take PO medication.

**Ophthalmic:** Treatment of conjunctivitis caused by *S. aureus, Staphylococcus epidermidis, S. pneumoniae, Enterobacter cloacae, H. influenzae, P. mirabilis,* and *P. aeruginosa.* Corneal ulcers caused by susceptible organisms.

**Otic:** Otitis externa in clients one year of age and older. Acute otitis media from age one to twelve with tympanostomy tubes. Chronic suppurative otitis media in those twelve years and older who have perforated tympanic membranes.

**Contraindications:** Hypersensitivity to quinolone antibacterial agents. Use during lactation. Use for syphilis (ineffective). Ophthalmic use in dendritic keratitis, vaccinia, varicella, mycobacterial infections of the eye, fungal diseases of the eye, and with steroid combinations after uncomplicated removal of a corneal foreign body.

**Special Concerns:** Safety and effectiveness of the systemic forms have not been established in children, adolescents under the age of 18 years, pregnant women, and lactating women. Safety and effectiveness of the ophthalmic form have not been established in children less than 1 year of age. Use with caution in clients with known or suspected CNS disorders such as severe cerebral atherosclerosis, epilepsy, or factors that predispose to seizures. The effectiveness of the IV dosage form in treating severe infections has not been determined.

---

**Side Effects:** See also *Side Effects* for *Fluroquinolones.*

*GI:* Nausea, diarrhea, vomiting, abdominal pain or discomfort, dry or painful mouth, dyspepsia, flatulence, constipation, pseudomembranous colitis, dysgeusia, decreased appetite. *CNS:* Headache, dizziness, fatigue, malaise, somnolence, depression, insomnia, seizures, sleep disorders, nervousness, anxiety, cognitive change, dream abnormality, euphoria, hallucinations, vertigo. *CV:* Chest pain, edema, hypertension, palpitations, vasodilation. *Hypersensitivity reactions:* Dyspnea, **anaphylaxis.** *GU:* External genital pruritus in women, vaginitis, vaginal discharge; burning, irritation, pain, and rash of the female genitalia; glucosuria, proteinuria, hematuria, pyuria, dysmenorrhea, menorrhagia, metrorrhagia, urinary frequency or pain. *Respiratory:* Cough, rhinorrhea. *Dermatologic:* Diaphoresis, vasculitis, photosensitivity, rash, pruritus. *Hematologic:* Leukocytosis, lymphocytopenia, eosinophilia. *Musculoskeletal:* Asthenia, extremity pain, arthralgia, myalgia, possibility of osteochondrosis. *Miscellaneous:* Chills, malaise, syncope, hyperglycemia or hypoglycemia, whole body pain, thirst, weight loss, photophobia, trunk pain, paresthesia, visual disturbances, hypersensitivity, hearing loss, fever.

*After ophthalmic use:* Transient ocular burning or discomfort, stinging, redness, itching, photophobia, tearing, and dryness.

**Laboratory Test Interferences:** ↑ ALT, AST.

**Dosage** ——————————
• **Tablets, IV**
*Pneumonia, exacerbation of chronic bronchitis.*
400 mg q 12 hr for 10 days.
*Acute uncomplicated gonorrhea.*
One 400-mg dose. The Centers for Disease Control also recommend adding doxycycline.
*Cervicitis/urethritis due to* C. trachomatis or N. gonorrhoeae.
300 mg q 12 hr for 7 days.

*Mild to moderate skin and skin structure infections.*
400 mg q 12 hr for 10 days.
*Cystitis due to* E. coli *or* K. pneumoniae.
200 mg q 12 hr for 3 days.
*Cystitis due to other organisms.*
200 mg q 12 hr for 7 days.
*Complicated UTIs.*
200 mg q 12 hr for 10 days.
*Prostatitis.*
300 mg q 12 hr for 6 weeks.
*Chlamydia.*
300 mg PO b.i.d. for 7 days.
*Epididymitis.*
300 mg PO b.i.d. for 10 days.
*Pelvic inflammatory disease, outpatient.*
400 mg PO b.i.d. for 14 days.
*NOTE:* The dose should be adjusted in clients with a $C_{CR}$ of 50 mL/min or less. If the $C_{CR}$ is 10–50 mL/min, the dosage interval should be q 24 hr, and if $C_{CR}$ is less than 10 mL/min, the dose should be half the recommended dose given q 24 hr.
• **Ophthalmic Solution (0.3%)**
*Conjunctivitis.*
**Initial:** 1–2 gtt in the affected eye(s) q 2–4 hr for the first 2 days; **then,** 1–2 gtt q.i.d. for five additional days.
• **Otic Solution (0.3%)**
*Otitis externa, otitis media.*
Apply b.i.d.

## NURSING CONSIDERATIONS

See also *Nursing Considerations* for *Fluoroquinolones* and *Anti-Infectives.*
**Administration/Storage**
1. Do not take with food.
2. Store in tightly closed containers at a temperature below 30°C (86°F).
3. Do not inject the ophthalmic solution subconjunctivally and do not introduce directly into the anterior chamber of the eye.
**IV** 4. For IV use, give slowly over at least 60 min; do not give by rapid or bolus IV infusion.
5. The IV product must be diluted prior to use to a final concentration of 4 mg/mL. The following solutions may be used for dilution: 0.9% NaCl; 5% dextrose; D5%/0.9% NaCl; D5%/RL; 5% sodium bicarbonate;

Plasma-Lyte 56 in 5% dextrose; D5%/0.45% NaCl and 0.15% KCl; sodium lactate (M/6); water for injection. Infuse slowly, over 1 hr.

6. Ofloxacin in premixed bottles or flexible containers does not have to be diluted further as it is already pre-mixed in 5% dextrose. Store the pre-mixed product at 25°C or less (77°F). Protect from excessive heat, freezing, and light.

**Assessment**

1. Note any sensitivity to quinolone derivatives.

2. Document indications for therapy, type, onset, and symptom characteristics.

3. Monitor CBC, cultures, liver and renal function studies; reduce dose with altered renal function. Review other prescribed agents; probenecid may block tubular excretion.

4. Assess for any CNS disorders. Report any CNS effects such as tremors, restlessness, confusion, and hallucinations; therapy may need to be discontinued.

**Client/Family Teaching**

1. Do not take with food. Take PO medication 1 hr before or 3 hr after meals.

2. Avoid vitamins, iron or mineral combinations, aluminum- or magnesium-based antacids 2 hr before and 2 hr after ingestion of ofloxacin.

3. Do not perform activities that require mental alertness until drug effects are realized; may cause drowsiness and lightheadedness.

4. Exercise care to avoid contamination of the ophthalmic applicator tip with material from the eye, fingers, or other sources.

5. After ophthalmic use, may experience burning, stinging, itching, or tearing but this should subside.

6. Drink 2–3 L/day of fluids to assist in drug elimination.

7. Most common side effects include N&V and diarrhea; report if persistent.

8. Avoid direct sunlight, as a photosensitivity reaction may occur. If exposed, wear sunglasses, protective clothing, and sunscreen.

9. Clients with diabetes should monitor their blood sugars closely during drug therapy as extreme variations may occur.

**Outcomes/Evaluate:** Negative culture reports; symptomatic improvement

# Olanzapine
((oh-**LAN**-zah-peen))
**Pregnancy Category:** C
Zyprexa **(Rx)**
**Classification:** Antipsychotic agent, miscellaneous

**Action/Kinetics:** A thienbenzodiazepine antipsychotic believed to act by antagonizing dopamine $D_{1-4}$ and serotonin ($5HT_2$) receptors. Also binds to muscarinic, histamine $H_1$, and alpha-1 adrenergic receptors, which can explain many of the side effects. Well absorbed from the GI tract. **Peak plasma levels:** 6 hr after PO dosing. Undergoes significant first-pass metabolism with about 40% metabolized before it reaches the systemic circulation. Food does not affect the rate or extent of absorption. Significantly bound to plasma proteins. Unchanged drug and metabolites are excreted through both the urine and feces.

**Uses:** Management of psychotic disorders.

**Contraindications:** Lactation.

**Special Concerns:** Use with caution in geriatric clients, as the drug may be excreted more slowly in this population. Use with caution in impaired hepatic function. Use care in giving olanzapine to those where there is a chance of increased core body temperature (e.g., strenuous exercise, exposure to extreme heat, concomitant anticholinergic drug administration, dehydration). Due to anticholinergic side effects, use with caution in clients with significant prostatic hypertrophy, narrow-angle glaucoma, or a history of paralytic ileus. Safety and efficacy have not been determined in children less than 18 years of age.

**Side Effects:** *Neuroleptic malignant syndrome:* Hyperpyrexia, muscle rigidity, altered mental status, irregular pulse or BP, tachycardia, diaphoresis, cardiac dysrhythmia, rhabdomyolysis, *acute renal failure, death. GI:* Dysphagia, constipation, dry mouth, increased appetite, increased salivation, N&V, thirst, aphthous stomatitis, eructation, esophagitis, rectal incontinence, flatulence, gastritis, gastroenteritis, gingivitis, glossitis, hepatitis, melena, mouth ulceration, oral moniliasis, periodontal abscess, *rectal hemorrhage,* tongue edema. *CNS:* Tardive dyskinesia, seizures, somnolence, agitation, insomnia, nervousness, hostility, dizziness, anxiety, personality disorder, akathisia, hypertonia, tremor, amnesia, impaired articulation, euphoria, stuttering, *suicide,* abnormal gait, alcohol misuse, antisocial reaction, ataxia, CNS stimulation, coma, delirium, depersonalization, hypesthesia, hypotonia, incoordination, decreased libido, obsessive-compulsive symptoms, phobias, somatization, stimulant misuse, stupor, vertigo, withdrawal syndrome. *CV:* Tachycardia, orthostatic/postural hypotension, hypotension, *CVA, hemorrhage, heart arrest* , migraine, palpitation, vasodilation, ventricular extrasystoles. *Body as a whole:* Headache, fever, abdominal pain, chest pain, neck rigidity, intentional injury, flu syndrome, chills, facial edema, hangover effect, malaise, moniliasis, neck pain, pelvic pain, photosensitivity. *Respiratory:* Rhinitis, increased cough, pharyngitis, dyspnea, apnea, asthma, epistaxis, hemoptysis, hyperventilation, voice alteration. *GU:* Premenstrual syndrome, hematuria, metrorrhagia, urinary incontinence, UTI, abnormal ejaculation, amenorrhea, breast pain, cystitis, decreased or increased menstruation, dysuria, female lactation, impotence, menorrhagia, polyuria, pyuria, urinary retention, urinary frequency, impaired urination, enlarged uterine fibroids. *Hematologic:* Leukocytosis, lymphadenopathy, thrombocytopenia. *Metabolic/nutritional:* Weight gain or loss, peripheral edema, lower extremity edema, dehydration, hyperglycemia, hyperkalemia, hyperuricemia, hypoglycemia, hypokalemia, hyponatremia, ketosis, water intoxication. *Musculoskeletal:* Joint pain, extremity pain, twitching, arthritis, back and hip pain, bursitis, leg cramps, myasthenia, rheumatoid arthritis. *Dermatologic:* Vesiculobullous rash, alopecia, contact dermatitis, dry skin, eczema, hirsutism, seborrhea, skin ulcer, urticaria. *Ophthalmic:* Amblyopia, blepharitis, corneal lesion, cataract, diplopia, dry eyes, eye hemorrhage, eye inflammation, eye pain, ocular muscle abnormality. *Otic:* Deafness, ear pain, tinnitus. *Miscellaneous:* Diabetes mellitus, goiter, cyanosis, taste perversion.

**OD Overdose Management:** *Symptoms:* Drowsiness, slurred speech. Possible obtundation, seizures, dystonic reaction of the head and neck. CV symptoms, arrhythmias. *Treatment:* Establish and maintain an airway and ensure adequate oxygenation and ventilation. Gastric lavage followed by activated charcoal and a laxative can be considered, although dystonic reaction may cause aspiration with induced emesis. CV monitoring should begin immediately with continuous ECG monitoring to detect possible arrhythmias. Hypotension and circulatory collapse are treated with IV fluids or sympathomimetic agents. *Do not use epinephrine, dopamine, or other sympathomimetic with beta-agonist activity, as beta stimulation may worsen hypotension.*

**Drug Interactions**
*Antihypertensive agents* / ↑ Effect of antihypertensive agents
*Carbamazepine* / ↑ Clearance of olanzepine due to ↑ rate of metabolism
*CNS depressants* / ↑ Effect of CNS depressants
*Levodopa and Dopamine agonists* / Olanzapine may antagonize the effects of levodopa and dopamine agonists

**Laboratory Test Interferences:** ALT, AST, GGT, alkaline phosphatase, serum prolactin, eosinophils, CPK. Hyperprolactinemia.

## Dosage

• **Tablets**

*Psychoses.*

**Adults, initial:** 5–10 mg once daily without regard to meals. Goal is 10 mg daily; increments to reach 10 mg can be in 5-mg amounts but at an interval of 1 week. Doses higher than 10 mg daily are recommended only after clinical assessment and should not be greater than 20 mg/day. The recommended initial dose is 5 mg in those who are debilitated, who have a predisposition to hypotensive reactions, who may have factors that cause a slower metabolism of olanzapine (e.g., non-smoking female clients over 65 years of age), or who may be more sensitive to the drug. It is recommended that clients who respond to the drug be continued on it at the lowest possible dose to maintain remission with periodic evaluation to determine continued need for the drug.

## NURSING CONSIDERATIONS

**Administration/Storage:** Protect from light and store at a controlled room temperature of 20°C–25°C (68°F–77°F).

**Assessment**

1. Document onset, duration, and characteristics of symptoms; note presenting behavioral manifestations. List other agents trialed and the outcome.

2. Monitor ECG, CBC, liver and renal function studies.

**Client/Family Teaching**

1. Take only as directed; do not share medications; do not exceed prescribed dosage.

2. Avoid activities or situations where overheating may occur, e.g., strenuous exercise.

3. Do not drive or perform activities that require mental alertness until drug effects realized.

4. Caution about orthostatic effects when changing positions suddenly, especially from a lying to a standing position.

5. Report any suicidal ideations, abnormal bleeding, sudden muscle pain or weakness, and irregular heart beat.

6. Avoid alcohol and any other CNS depressants or OTC agents.

7. Practice reliable birth control.

8. Report as scheduled for medication renewals, therapy sessions, and evaluation of drug effectiveness.

**Outcomes/Evaluate:** Improved patterns of behavior with ↓ agitation, ↓ hostility and psychosis, and fewer delusions

# Olopatadine hydrochloride

(oh-loh-pah-**TIH**-deen)

**Pregnancy Category:** C

Patanol **(Rx)**

**Classification:** Antihistamine, ophthalmic

See also *Antihistamines.*

**Action/Kinetics:** Selective histamine H-1 receptor antagonist. Little is absorbed into the systemic circulation.

**Uses:** Prevention of itching in allergic conjunctivitis.

**Contraindications:** Not to be injected. Not to be instilled while the client is wearing contact lenses.

**Special Concerns:** Use with caution during lactation. Safety and efficacy have not been determined for children less than 3 years of age.

**Side Effects:** *Ophthalmic:* Burning or stinging, dry eye, foreign body sensation, hyperemia, keratitis, lid edema, pruritus. Nose/throat: Pharyngitis, rhinitis, sinusitis. *Miscellaneous:* Headache, asthenia, cold syndrome, taste perversion.

## Dosage

• **Solution (0.1%)**

*Allergic conjunctivitis.*

---

**Adults and children over 3 years of age:** 1–2 drops in each affected eye b.i.d. at an interval of 6–8 hr.

## NURSING CONSIDERATIONS

See also *Nursing Considerations* for *Antihistamines, .*

**Administration/Storage:** Store at 4°C–30°C (39°F–86°F).

**Assessment:** Document indications for therapy; note onset, duration, location, occurrence, and characteristics of symptoms. Identify triggers.

**Client/Family Teaching**

1. Wash hands before and after administration; do not let the dropper tip touch the eyelids or surrounding areas to prevent contamination of the dropper and solution.
2. Burning and stinging as well as swelling, redness, and foreign body sensation may occur; report if persistent.
3. Remove contact lens before instilling eye drops.
4. Review potential triggers and how to avoid and reduce contact to prevent increased irritation.

**Outcomes/Evaluate:** Relief of allergic ocular manifestations.

# Olsalazine sodium
(ohl-**SAL**-ah-zeen)
**Pregnancy Category:** C
Dipentum **(Rx)**
**Classification:** Anti-inflammatory drug

**Action/Kinetics:** A salicylate that is converted by bacteria in the colon to 5-PAS (5-para-aminosalicylate), which exerts an anti-inflammatory effect for the treatment of ulcerative colitis. 5-PAS is slowly absorbed resulting in a high concentration of drug in the colon. The anti-inflammatory activity is likely due to inhibition of synthesis of prostaglandins in the colon. After PO use the drug is only slightly absorbed (2.4%) into systemic circulation where it has a short half-life (< 1 hr) and is more than 99% bound to plasma proteins.

**Uses:** To maintain remission of ulcerative colitis in clients who cannot take sulfasalazine.

**Contraindications:** Hypersensitivity to salicylates.

**Special Concerns:** Use with caution during lactation. Safety and efficacy have not been established in children. May cause worsening of symptoms of colitis.

**Side Effects:** *GI:* Diarrhea (common), pain or cramps, nausea, dyspepsia, bloating, anorexia, vomiting, stomatitis. *CNS:* Headache, drowsiness, lethargy, fatigue, dizziness, vertigo. *Miscellaneous:* Arthralgia, rash, itching, upper respiratory tract infection. *NOTE:* The following symptoms have been reported on withdrawal of therapy: diarrhea, nausea, abdominal pain, rash, itching, headache, heartburn, insomnia, anorexia, dizziness, lightheadedness, rectal bleeding, depression.

**OD** **Overdose Management:** *Symptoms:* Diarrhea, decreased motor activity. *Treatment:* Treat symptoms.

**Dosage**
• **Capsules**
**Adults:** Total of 1 g/day in two divided doses.

## NURSING CONSIDERATIONS
**Assessment**

1. Note any sensitivity to salicylates and/or an intolerance to sulfasalazine.
2. Document indications for therapy, type, onset, and duration of symptoms.
3. With renal disease, monitor urinalysis, BUN, and creatinine. With chronic therapy monitor CBC and renal function studies.
4. Review radiographic/endoscopic findings.

**Client/Family Teaching**

1. Drug should be taken with food and in evenly divided doses.
2. Report any persistent diarrhea.

**Outcomes/Evaluate:** Symptom remission with ulcerative colitis

# Omeprazole
(oh-**MEH**-prah-zohl)
**Pregnancy Category:** C
Losec ✦, Prilosec **(Rx)**

**Classification:** Agent to suppress gastric acid secretion

**Action/Kinetics:** Thought to be a gastric pump inhibitor in that it blocks the final step of acid production by inhibiting the H+–K+ ATPase system at the secretory surface of the gastric parietal cell. Both basal and stimulated acid secretions are inhibited. Serum gastrin levels are increased during the first 1 or 2 weeks of therapy and are maintained at such levels during the course of therapy. Because omeprazole is acid-labile, the product contains an enteric-coated granule formulation; however, absorption is rapid. **Peak plasma levels:** 0.5–3.5 hr. **Onset:** Within 1 hr. **t½:** 0.5–1 hr. **Duration:** Up to 72 hr (due to prolonged binding of the drug to the parietal H+–K+; ATPase enzyme). Significantly bound (95%) to plasma protein. Metabolized in the liver and inactive metabolites are excreted through the urine. Consider dosage adjustment in Asians.

**Uses:** Short-term (4- to 8-week) treatment of active duodenal ulcer, active benign gastric ulcer, erosive esophagitis (all grades), and heartburn and other symptoms associated with GERD. In combination with clarithromycin for eradication of *Helicobacter pylori* and active duodenal ulcer. Long-term maintenance therapy for healed erosive esophagitis. Long-term treatment of pathologic hypersecretory conditions such as Zollinger-Ellison syndrome, multiple endocrine adenomas, and systemic mastocytosis. *Investigational:* In combination with amoxicillin for eradication of *H. pylori.*

**Contraindications:** Lactation. Use as maintenance therapy for duodenal ulcer disease.

**Special Concerns:** Bioavailability may be increased in geriatric clients. Use with caution during lactation. Symptomatic effects with omeprazole do not preclude gastric malignancy. Safety and effectiveness have not been determined in children.

**Side Effects:** *CNS:* Headache, dizziness. Possibly, anxiety disorders, abnormal dreams, vertigo, insomnia, nervousness, apathy, paresthesia, somnolence, depression, aggression, hallucinations, hemifacial dysesthesia, tremors, confusion. *GI:* Diarrhea, N&V, abdominal pain, abdominal swelling, constipation, flatulence, anorexia, fecal discoloration, esophageal candidiasis, mucosal atrophy of the tongue, dry mouth, irritable colon, gastric fundic gland polyps, gastroduodenal carcinoids. *Hepatic:* **Pancreatitis.** Overt liver disease, including hepatocellular, cholestatic, or mixed hepatitis; *liver necrosis, hepatic failure,* hepatic encephalopathy. *CV:* Angina, chest pain, tachycardia, bradycardia, palpitation, peripheral edema, elevated BP. *Respiratory:* Upper respiratory infection, pharyngeal pain, bronchospasms, cough, epistaxis. *Dermatologic:* Rash, severe generalized skin reaction including *toxic epidermal necrolysis, Stevens-Johnson syndrome;* erythema multiforme, skin inflammation, urticaria, pruritus, alopecia, dry skin, hyperhidrosis. *GU:* UTI, acute interstitial nephritis, urinary frequency, hematuria, proteinuria, glycosuria, testicular pain, microscopic pyuria, gynecomastia. *Hematologic:* Pancytopenia, thrombocytopenia, anemia, leukocytosis, neutropenia, hemolytic anemia, *agranulocytosis.* *Musculoskeletal:* Asthenia, back pain, myalgia, joint pain, muscle cramps, muscle weakness, leg pain. *Miscellaneous:* Rash, angioedema, fever, pain, gout, fatigue, malaise, weight gain, tinnitus, alteration in taste.

When used with clarithromycin the following *additional* side effects were noted: Tongue discoloration, rhinitis, pharyngitis, and flu syndrome.

*NOTE:* Data are lacking on the effect of long-term hypochlorhydria and hypergastrinemia on the risk of developing tumors.

**OD** **Overdose Management:** *Symptoms:* Confusion, drowsiness, blurred vision, tachycardia, nausea, diaphoresis, flushing, headache, dry mouth. *Treatment:* Symptomatic and supportive. Omeprazole is not readily dialyzable.

**Drug Interactions**

*Ampicillin (esters)* / Possible ↓ absorption of ampicillin esters due to ↑ ↑ pH of stomach

*Diazepam* / ↑ Plasma levels of diazepam due to ↓ rate of metabolism by the liver

*Iron salts* / Possible ↓ absorption of iron salts due to ↑ pH of stomach

*Ketoconazole* / Possible ↓ absorption of ketoconazole due to ↑ pH of stomach

*Phenytoin* / ↑ Plasma levels of phenytoin due to ↓ rate of metabolism of the liver

*Warfarin* / Prolonged rate of elimination of warfarin due to ↓ rate of metabolism by the liver

**Laboratory Test Interferences:** ↑ AST, ALT, gamma-glutamyl transpeptidase, alkaline phosphatase, bilirubin, serum creatinine. Glycosuria, hyponatremia, hypoglycemia.

**Dosage** —————————

• **Capsules, Eneric-Coated**

*Active duodenal ulcer.*

**Adults,** 20 mg/day for 4–8 weeks.

*Erosive esophagitis, heartburn, symptoms associated with GERD.*

**Adults:** 20 mg/day for 4–8 weeks.

**Maintenance of healing erosive esophagitis:** 20 mg daily.

*Treatment of H. pylori, reduction of risk of duodenal ulcer recurrence.*

**Days 1–14:** Omeprazole, 40 mg daily in the morning, plus clarithromycin, 500 mg t.i.d. Days 15–28: Omeprazole, 20 mg daily.

*Pathologic hypersecretory conditions.*

Adults, initial: 60 mg/day; then, dose individualized although doses up to 120 mg t.i.d. have been used. Daily doses greater than 80 mg should be divided.

*Gastric ulcers.*

Adults: 40 mg once daily for 4–8 weeks.

## NURSING CONSIDERATIONS

**Administration/Storage:** Capsules should be stored in a tight container protected from light and moisture. Store between 15°C and 30°C (59°F and 86°F).

**Assessment**

1. Document indications for therapy, type, onset, and duration of symptoms.

2. Determine if pregnant.

3. Record abdominal assessments, radiographic/ endoscopic findings and note *H. pylori* results.

4. Monitor CBC and LFTs; note any hepatic dysfunction.

**Client/Family Teaching**

1. Antacids can be administered with omeprazole.

2. The capsule should be taken before eating and is to be swallowed whole; it should not be opened, chewed, or crushed.

3. Review the list of side effects associated with drug therapy; report any persistent symptoms, especially diarrhea.

4. Report any changes in urinary elimination or pain and discomfort associated with voiding.

5. Avoid alcohol and all OTC agents without approval.

6. Drug inhibits total gastric acid secretion and is for short-term use only. Side effects of prolonged therapy and suppression of acid secretion alter bacterial colonization and lead to hypochlorhydria and hypergastrinemia which may cause an increased risk for the development of gastric tumors.

**Outcomes/Evaluate:** Promotion of ulcer healing; relief of pain; ↓ gastric acid production

# Ondansetron hydrochloride

(on-**DAN**-sih-tron)

**Pregnancy Category:** B

Zofran **(Rx)**

**Classification:** Antiemetic

**Action/Kinetics:** It is believed that cytotoxic chemotherapy results in the release of serotonin from ente-

rochromoffin cells of the small intestine. The released serotonin may stimulate the vagal afferent nerves through the 5-HT$_3$ receptors, thus stimulating the vomiting reflex. Ondansetron, a 5-HT$_3$ antagonist, blocks this effect of serotonin. Whether the drug acts centrally and/or peripherally to antagonize the effect of serotonin is not known. **Time to peak plasma levels, after PO:** 1.7–2.1 hr. **t½, after IV use:** 3.5–4.7 hr; **after PO use:** 3.1–6.2 hr, depending on the age. A decrease in clearance and increase in half-life are observed in clients over 75 years of age, although no dosage adjustment is recommended. Clients less than 15 years of age show a shortened plasma half-life after IV use (2.4 hr). ignificantly metabolized with 5% of a dose excreted unchanged in the urine.
**Uses: Parenteral:** Prevent N&V resulting from initial and repeated courses of cancer chemotherapy, including high-dose cisplatin. Prophylaxis and treatment of selected cases of postoperative N&V, especially situations where there is multiple retching and long periods of N&V. **Oral:** Prevention of N&V due to initial and repeated courses of cancer chemotherapy. Prevenion of N&V associated with radiotherapy in clients receiving either total body irradiation, single high-dose fraction, or daily fractions to the abdomen. Prevention of postoperative N&V.
**Special Concerns:** Use with caution during lactation. Safety and effectiveness in children 3 years of age and younger are not known.
**Side Effects:** *GI:* Diarrhea (most common), constipation, xerostomia, abdominal pain. *CNS:* Headache, dizziness, drowsiness, sedation, malaise, fatigue, anxiety, agitation, extrapyramidal syndrome, ***clonic-tonic seizures.*** *CV:* Tachycardia, chest pain, hypotension, ECG alterations, angina, bradycardia, syncope, vascular occlusive events. *Dermatologic:* Pain, redness, and burning at injection site; cold sensation, pruritus, paresthe-

sia. *Hypersensitivity (rare):* ***Anaphylaxis, bronchospasm, shock,*** SOB, hypotension, angioedema, urticaria. *Miscellaneous:* Rash, ***bronchospasm,*** transient blurred vision, hypokalemia, weakness, fever, musculoskeletal pain, shivers, dysuria, postoperative carbon dioxide-related pain, akathisia, acute dystonic reactions, gynecologic disorder, urinary retention, wound problem.
**Laboratory Test Alteration:** ↑ AST, ALT.

**Dosage**
• **IM, IV**
*Prevention of N&V due to chemotherapy.*
**Adults and children, 4–18 years:** Three doses of 0.15 mg/kg each. The first dose is infused over 15 min starting 30 min before the start of chemotherapy; the second and third doses are given 4 hr and 8 hr, respectively, after the first dose. Alternatively, a single 32-mg dose may be given over 15 min beginning 30 min before the start of chemotherapy.
*N&V postoperatively.*
**Adults:** 4 mg over 2–5 min immediately before induction of anesthesia or postoperatively as needed. **Children, 2 to 12 years weighing 40 kg or less:** 0.1 mg/kg over 2–5 min. **Children, 2 to 12 years weighing over 40 kg:** 4 mg over 2–5 min.
• **Tablets**
*In clients receiving moderately emetogenic chemotherapy agents.*
**Adults and children over 12 years of age:** 8 mg 30 min before treatment followed by a second 8-mg dose 8 hr after the first dose; **then,** 8 mg b.i.d. for 1–2 days after chemotherapy. **Children, 4–12 years:** 4 mg t.i.d. The first dose is given 30 min before chemotherapy with subsequent doses 4 and 8 hr after the first dose. **Then,** 4 mg q 8 hr for 1–2 days after completion of chemotherapy.
*Prevention of N&V due to total body irradiation.*

8 mg 1–2 hr before each fraction of radiotherapy administered each day.

*Prevention of N&V in single high-dose fraction radiotherapy to the abdomen.*

8 mg 1–2 hr before radiotherapy with subsequent doses 8 hr after the first dose for 1–2 days after completion of radiotherapy.

*Prevention of N&V due to daily fractionated radiotherapy to the abdomen.*

8 mg 1–2 hr before radiotherapy, with subsequent doses 8 hr after the first dose for each day radiotherapy is given.

*Prevention of postoperative N&V.*

**Adults:** 16 mg given as a single dose 1 hr before induction of anesthesia.

## NURSING CONSIDERATIONS

See also *Nursing Considerations* for *Antiemetics*.

### Administration/Storage

1. With impaired hepatic function, do not exceed 8 mg PO or 8 mg IV daily infused over 15 min beginning 30 min prior to the start of chemotherapy.

2. Tablets may be used to prepare a liquid product with cherry syrup, Syrpalta, Ora Sweet, or Ora Sweet Sugar Free. The concentration is 4 mg/5mL and is stable for 42 days at 4°C (39°F).

3. Suppositories can be made by adding pulverized tablets to a melted fatty acid base, mixing thoroughly, and pouring into suppository molds. They are stable for 30 or more days if stored in light-resistant containers under refrigeration.

**IV** 4. Dilute the 2-mg/mL injection in 50 mL of 5% dextrose injection or 0.9% NaCl injection before administration; infuse over 15 min.

5. The diluted drug is stable at room temperature, with normal lighting, for 48 hr after dilution with 0.9% NaCl; 5% dextrose injection, D5%/0.9% NaCl, D5%/0.45% NaCl, and 3% NaCl injection.

### Assessment

1. Document indications for therapy, onset and duration of symptoms, other agents prescribed, and the outcome.

2. Monitor LFTs; note any liver dysfunction and adjust dosage.

### Client/Family Teaching

1. Take the medications exactly as prescribed in order to ensure desired results.

2. Report any rash, diarrhea, constipation, or altered respirations (bronchospasms).

### Outcomes/Evaluate

- Prevention/control of chemotherapy-induced N&V
- Prophylaxis/relief of postoperative N&V

---

# Oprelvekin (Interleukin 11)

(oh-**PREL**-veh-kin)

**Pregnancy Category:** C

Neumega **(Rx)**

**Classification:** Recombinant human interleukin

**Action/Kinetics:** Produced by DNA recombinant technology. Interleukin 11 is a thrombopoietic growth factor that directly stimulates proliferation of hematopoietic stem cells and megakaryocyte progenitor cells and induces megakaryocyte maturation. This results in increased platelet production. **Peak serum levels:** 3.2 hr. **t½, terminal:** 6.9 hr. Metabolized and excreted through urine.

**Uses:** Prevention of thrombocytopenia following myelosuppressive chemotherapy in clients with nonmyeloid malignancies who are at high risk of severe thrombocytopenia. **Contraindications:** Use following myeloablative chemotherapy. Lactation.

**Special Concerns:** Use with caution in CHF or those who may be susceptible to developing CHF, and in those with history of heart failure who are well compensated and receiving appropriate medical therapy. Use with caution in those with history of atrial arrhythmia, in preexisting papilledema or with tumors involving CNS. Safety and efficacy have not been determined in children.

**Side Effects:** *Body as a whole:* Edema, neutropenic fever, headache, fever, rash, conjunctival infection, asthenia, chills, pain, infection, flu-like symptoms. *GI:* N&V, mucositis, diarrhea, oral moniliasis, abdominal pain, constipation, dyspepsia. *CV:* Tachycardia, vasodilation, palpitations, syncope, atrial fibrillation or flutter, thrombocytosis, **thrombotic events.** *CNS:* Dizziness, insomnia, nervousness. *Respiratory:* Dyspnea, rhinitis, increased cough, pharyngitis, pleural effusion. *Miscellaneous:* Anorexia, ecchymosis, myalgia, bone pain, alopecia, mild visual blurring (transient).

In cancer clients: Also, amblyopia, dehydration, exfoliative dermatitis, eye hemorrhage, paresthesia, skin discoloration.

**Laboratory Test Alteration:** ↓ Hemoglobin, serum albumin, transferrin, gamma globulins (all due to expansion of plasma volume).

**OD Overdose Management:** *Symptoms:* Increased incidence of cardiovascular events if doses greater than 50 mcg/kg are given. *Treatment:* Discontinue drug and observe for signs of toxicity.

**Dosage**
• **SC Injection**
*Prevent thrombocytopenia.*
**Adults:** 50 mcg/kg once daily SC either in the abdomen, thigh, or hip. Dose of 75–100 mcg/kg in children will produce plasma levels consistent with a 50 mcg/kg dose in adults.

## NURSING CONSIDERATIONS
**Administration/Storage**
1. Initiate dosing 6 to 24 hr after completion of chemotherapy. Continue dosing until post-nadir platelet count is 50,000 cells/mcL or more. Duration of dosing is usually 10 to 21 days. Dosing beyond 21 days is not recommended.
2. Discontinue treatment 2 or more

days before starting next planned cycle of chemotherapy.
3. Reconstitute with 1 mL of sterile water for injection without preservative. Direct water at side of vial and swirl gently. Avoid excessive or vigorous shaking.
4. Reconstituted solution contains 5 mg/mL. Use within 3 hr as there is no preservative. Store vial either in refrigerator or at room temperature. Do not shake or freeze reconstituted solution.
5. Do not re-enter or reuse single-use vial. Discard any unused portion.
6. Store lyophilized drug and diluent at 2°C–8°C (36°F–46°F).
**Assessment**
1. Document indications for therapy, onset, duration, and clinical manifestations.
2. Monitor CBC and platelet counts.
3. List chemotherapy agent and platelet nadir; initiate therapy 6-24 hr after chemotherapy completed. Stop oprelvekin at least 2 days before next round of chemotherapy.
**Client/Family Teaching**
1. Review administration and dosage guidelines. Use only as directed, SC, into abdomen, thigh, or hip; rotate sites.
2. Report any unusual side effects or any evidence of increased bruising or bleeding.
3. Drug is used to prevent chemotherapy induced low platelets by stimulating bone marrow to increase platelet production.
**Outcomes/Evaluate:** Thrombocytopenia prophylaxis; ↑ platelet production

# Oxacillin sodium
(ox-ah-**SILL**-in)
**Pregnancy Category:** B
Bactocill, Prostaphlin **(Rx)**
**Classification:** Antibiotic, penicillin

See also *Anti-Infectives* and *Penicillins.*
**Action/Kinetics:** Penicillinase-resistant, acid-stable drug used for

resistant staphylococcal infections.
**Peak plasma levels: PO,** 1.6–10
mcg after 30–60 min; **IM,** 5–11
mcg/mL after 30 min. **t½:** 30 min.
**Uses:** Infections caused by penicillinase-producing staphylococci; also certain pneumococci and streptococci.

**Dosage** ——————————
• **Capsules, Oral Solution**
  *Mild to moderate infections of the upper respiratory tract, skin, soft tissue.*
**Adults and children (over 20 kg):**
500 mg q 4–6 hr for at least 5 days.
**Children less than 20 kg:** 50 mg/kg/day in equally divided doses q 6 hr for at least 5 days.
  *Septicemia, deep-seated infections.*
Parenteral therapy (see below) followed by PO therapy. **Adults:** 1 g q 4–6 hr; **children:** 100 mg/kg/day in equally divided doses q 4–6 hr.
• **IM, IV**
  *General infections.*
**Adults and children over 40 kg:**
250–500 mg q 4–6 hr. **Children less than 40 kg:** 50 mg/kg/day in equally divided doses q 6 hr.
  *Severe infections of the lower respiratory tract or disseminated infections.*
**Adults and children over 40 kg:**
Up to 1 g q 4–6 hr. **Children less than 40 kg:** Up to 100 mg/kg/day.
**Neonates and premature infants, less than 2,000 g:** 50 mg/kg/day divided q 12 hr if less than 7 days of age and 100 mg/kg/day divided q 8 hr if more than 7 days of age.
**Neonates and premature infants, more than 2,000 g:** 75 mg/kg/day divided q 8 hr if less than 7 days of age and 150 mg/kg/day divided q 6 hr if more than 7 days of age. Maximum daily dose: **Adults,** 12 g; **children,** 100–300 mg/kg.

## NURSING CONSIDERATIONS

See also *Nursing Considerations* for *Penicillins.*
**Administration/Storage**
1. Administer IM by deep intragluteal injection, rotate injection sites,
and observe for pain and swelling at IM injection site.
**IV** 2. Reconstitution: Add sterile water for injection or NaCl injection in amount indicated on vial. Shake until solution is clear. For parenteral use, reconstituted solution may be kept for 3 days at room temperature or 1 week in refrigerator. Discard outdated solutions.
3. IV administration (two methods):
• For rapid, direct administration, add an equal amount of sterile water or isotonic saline to reconstituted dosage (usually 250- to 500-mg vial with 5 mL of solution) and administer over a period of 10 min.
• For IV infusion, add reconstituted solution to either dextrose, saline, or invert sugar solution for a concentration of 0.5–40 mg/mL and administer over a 6-hr period, during which time drug remains potent.
• Observe for pain, redness, and edema at the site of IV injection and along the course of the vein.
4. Treatment of osteomyelitis may require several months of intensive PO therapy.
**Outcomes/Evaluate:** Improvement in S&S of infection; negative culture reports

# Oxamniquine
(ox-**AM**-nih-kwin)
**Pregnancy Category:** C
Vansil **(Rx)**
**Classification:** Anthelmintic, antischistosomal

**Action/Kinetics:** Causes *Schistosoma mansoni* (trematode parasite) to shift from the mesenteric veins to the liver, where they are destroyed. More effective against male than against female schistosomes, but females cease laying eggs following treatment; thus, the infection eventually subsides due to decreased reproduction. **Peak plasma concentration:** 1–1.5 hr. **t½:** 1–2.5 hr. Well absorbed after PO administration. Inactive metabolites are excreted in urine.
**Uses:** All stages of acute and chronic *S. mansoni* infections (transmitted

by snails), including involvement of the liver and spleen. *Investigational:* With praziquantel to treat neurocysticercosis (single dose only).

**Special Concerns:** Use with caution during lactation.

**Side Effects:** Well tolerated. *CNS:* Transient drowsiness and dizziness, headaches, EEG abnormalities. *Convulsions (mostly in epileptics);* therefore, closely monitor clients with history of convulsive disorders. *GI:* N&V, abdominal pain, anorexia. *Dermatologic:* Urticaria, mild to moderate increases in liver enzymes but with no evidence of hepatotoxicity.

**Dosage** ─────
• **Capsules**
**Adults:** 12–15 mg/kg as single PO dose. **Adults, 30–40 kg:** 500 mg; **41–60 kg:** 750 mg; **61–80 kg:** 1,000 mg; **81–100 kg:** 1,250 mg. **Children (under 30 kg):** 10 mg/kg followed in 2–8 hr with a second 10-mg/kg dose.

## NURSING CONSIDERATIONS

See also *Nursing Considerations* for *Anthelmintics.*
**Client/Family Teaching**
1. Administer after food to minimize GI distress.
2. Do not drive a car or operate hazardous machinery because drug may cause dizziness and/or drowsiness.
3. Report any evidence of seizures or CNS symptoms.
4. May discolor urine orange/red; report so that hematuria may be ruled out.
5. Cough, pulmonary infiltrates, elevated liver enzymes, hives, and itching have been associated with death of parasites and not drug toxicity. These symptoms may occur several days to 1 month following treatment.
**Outcomes/Evaluate:** Eradication of *S. mansoni* parasitic infection

---

# Oxaprozin
(ox-ah-**PROH**-zin)
**Pregnancy Category:** C
Daypro **(Rx)**
**Classification:** Nonsteroidal anti-inflammatory drug

See also *Nonsteroidal Anti-Inflammatory Drugs.*
**Uses:** Acute and chronic use to manage rheumatoid arthritis and osteoarthritis.

**Dosage** ─────
• **Tablets**
*Rheumatoid arthritis.*
**Adults:** 1,200 mg once daily. Lower and higher doses may be required in certain clients.
*Osteoarthritis.*
**Adults:** 1,200 mg once daily. For clients with a lower body weight or with a milder disease, 600 mg/day may be appropriate.
The maximum daily use for either rheumatoid arthritis or osteoarthritis is 1,800 mg (or 26 mg/kg, whichever is lower) given in divided doses.

## NURSING CONSIDERATIONS

See also *Nursing Considerations* for *Nonsteroidal Anti-Inflammatory Drugs.*
**Administration/Storage:** Regardless of the use, individualize and use the lowest effective dose to minimize side effects.
**Assessment**
1. Document indications for therapy, type, onset, and symptom characteristics. List other agents used and the outcome.
2. Assess involved joint(s) and determine baseline ROM, the extent of any inflammation and rate pain level.
3. Monitor CBC, liver and renal function studies (q 6–12 months).
**Outcomes/Evaluate:** Relief of joint pain and inflammation with improved mobility

---

# Oxazepam
(ox-**AY**-zeh-pam)
**Pregnancy Category:** D
Apo-Oxazepam ✸, Novo-Oxapam ✸, Oxpam ✸, PMS-Oxazepam ✸, Serax, Zapex ✸ **(C-IV) (Rx)**

**Classification:** Antianxiety agent, benzodiazepine

See also *Tranquilizers, Antimanic Drugs, and Hypnotics.*
**Action/Kinetics:** Absorbed more slowly than most benzodiazepines. **Peak plasma levels:** 2–4 hr. **t½:** 5–20 hr. Broken down in the liver to inactive metabolites, which are excreted through both the urine and feces. Reputed to cause less drowsiness than chlordiazepoxide.
**Uses:** Anxiety, tension, anxiety with depression. Adjunct in acute alcohol withdrawal.
**Special Concerns:** Dosage has not been established in children less than 12 years of age; use is not recommended in children less than 6 years of age.
**Additional Side Effects:** Paradoxical reactions characterized by sleep disorders and hyperexcitability during first weeks of therapy. Hypotension has occurred with parenteral administration.

**Dosage** ——————
• **Capsules, Tablets**
    *Anxiety, mild to moderate.*
**Adults:** 10–30 mg t.i.d.–q.i.d.
    *Anxiety, tension, irritability, agitation.*
**Geriatric and debilitated clients:** 10 mg t.i.d.; can be increased to 15 mg t.i.d.–q.i.d.
    *Alcohol withdrawal.*
**Adults:** 15–30 mg t.i.d.–q.i.d.

**NURSING CONSIDERATIONS**

See also *Nursing Considerations* for *Tranquilizers, Antimanic Drugs, and Hypnotics.*
**Client/Family Teaching**
1. Review goals of therapy, dosage, and frequency of administration.
2. Drug may cause dizziness and drowsiness; use caution until drug effects realized.
3. Report any persistant insomnia or hyperactivity.
4. Do not stop abruptly with long-term therapy.
**Outcomes/Evaluate**
• ↓ Symptoms of anxiety and tension

• Control of alcohol withdrawal symptoms

---

# Oxiconazole nitrate
(ox-ee-**KON**-ah-zohl)
**Pregnancy Category:** B
Oxistat **(Rx)**
**Classification:** Antifungal agent, topical

---

See also *Anti-Infectives.*
**Action/Kinetics:** Acts by inhibiting ergosterol synthesis, which is required for cytoplasmic membrane integrity of fungi. Active against a broad range of organisms including many strains of *Trichophyton rubrum* and *T. mentagrophytes*. Systemic absorption is low.
**Uses:** Topical treatment of tinea pedis (athlete's foot), tinea cruris (jock itch), tinea versicolor, and tinea corporis (ringworm) due to *T. rubrum, T. mentagrophytes*, and *Epidermophyton floccosum*.
**Contraindications:** Ophthalmic or vaginal use.
**Special Concerns:** Use with caution during lactation.
**Side Effects:** *Dermatologic:* Pruritus, burning, stinging, irritation, erythema, fissuring, maceration, contact dermatitis, scaling, tingling, pain, dyshidrotic eczema, folliculitis, papules, rash, nodules.

**Dosage** ——————
• **Cream (1%), Lotion (1%)**
**Adults and childen:** Apply 1% cream or lotion to cover affected areas once daily in the evening. To prevent recurrence, continue treatment for 2 weeks for tinea corporis and tinea cruris and for 1 month for tinea pedis.

---

**NURSING CONSIDERATIONS**
**Assessment**
1. Assess and describe area of involvement, noting presentation, onset, duration, and characteristics of symptoms.
2. The diagnosis should be reviewed if no clinical response after the designated treatment period (tinea corporis and tinea cruris require 2

weeks of therapy; tinea pedis requires 1 month of therapy to prevent recurrence.

**Client/Family Teaching**
1. Wash hands before and after application; use only as directed.
2. Report any itching and/or burning; treatment should be discontinued if sensitivity or chemical irritation appear.
3. Follow prescribed therapy; some infections may require 2 weeks to a month of daily treatments to ensure there is no recurrence.
4. Drug is for external use only; avoid eye contact.

**Outcomes/Evaluate:** Resolution of fungal infection; symptomatic improvement

# Oxybutynin chloride

(ox-ee-**BYOU**-tih-nin)
**Pregnancy Category:** B
Apo-Oxybutynin ✦, Ditropan, Nu-Oxybutyn ✦ **(Rx)**
**Classification:** Antispasmodic

**Action/Kinetics:** Causes increased vesicle capacity, decreases frequency of uninhibited contractions of the detrusor muscle, and delays initial urgency to void by exerting a direct antispasmodic effect. Has no effect at either the neuromuscular junction or autonomic ganglia. Has 4–10 times the antispasmodic effect of atropine but only one-fifth the anticholinergic activity. **Onset:** 30–60 min; **Time to peak effect:** 3–6 hr; **duration:** 6–10 hr. Eliminated through the urine.

**Uses:** Neurogenic bladder disease characterized by urinary retention, urinary overflow, incontinence, nocturia, urinary frequency or urgency, reflex neurogenic bladder.

**Contraindications:** Glaucoma (angle closure), GI obstruction, paralytic ileus, intestinal atony (in elderly or debilitated), megacolon, toxic megacolon complicating ulcerative colitis, severe colitis, myasthenia gravis, obstructive uropathy, unstable CV status in acute hemorrhage.

**Special Concerns:** *Use with caution when increased cholinergic effect is undesirable and in the elderly.* Safe use in children less than 5 years of age has not been determined. Use with caution in geriatric clients; during lactation; in clients with autonomic neuropathy, renal, or hepatic disease; and in clients with hiatal hernia with reflex esophagitis. Heat stroke and fever (due to decreased sweating) may occur if given at high environmental temperatures.

**Side Effects:** *GI:* N&V, constipation, bloated feeling, decreased GI motility. *CNS:* Drowsiness, insomnia, weakness, dizziness, restlessness, hallucinations. *EENT:* Dry mouth, decreased lacrimation, mydriasis, amblyopia, cycloplegia. *CV:* Tachycardia, palpitations, vasodilation. *Miscellaneous:* Decreased sweating, urinary hesitancy and retention, impotence, suppression of lactation, ***severe allergic reactions,*** drug idiosyncrasies, urticaria, and other dermal manifestations. *NOTE:* The drug may aggravate symptoms of prostatic hypertrophy, hypertension, coronary heart disease, CHF, hyperthyroidism, cardiac arrhythmias, and tachycardia.

**OD** **Overdose Management:** *Symptoms:* Intense CNS disturbances (restlessness, psychoses), circulatory changes (flushing, hypotension) and failure, respiratory failure, paralysis, coma. *Treatment:* Stomach lavage, physostigmine (0.5–2 mg IV; repeat as necessary up to maximum of 5 mg). Supportive therapy, if necessary. Counteract excitement with sodium thiopental (2%) or chloral hydrate (100–200 mL of 2% solution) rectally. Artificial respiration may be necessary if respiratory muscles become paralyzed.

**Drug Interactions:** See *Cholinergic Blocking Agents.*

**Dosage** —
• **Syrup, Tablets**
**Adults:** 5 mg b.i.d.–t.i.d. Maximum dose: 5 mg q.i.d. **Children, over 5**

---

✦ = Available in Canada                    ***bold italic*** = life threatening side effect

**years:** 5 mg b.i.d. Maximum dose: 5 mg t.i.d.

## NURSING CONSIDERATIONS

See also *Nursing Considerations* for *Cholinergic Blocking Agents.*
**Administration/Storage:** Dispense in tight, light-resistant containers and store at 15°C–30°C (59°F–86°F).
**Assessment**
1. Document type, onset, frequency, and duration of symptoms.
2. Review conditions that may be aggravated by oxybutynin and determine if present (renal, hepatic disease, hiatal hernia, reflux esophagitis).
**Client/Family Teaching**
1. Take only as directed.
2. Use caution driving a car or in operating dangerous machinery; drug may cause drowsiness and blurred vision.
3. Withhold medication and report if diarrhea occurs (especially with an ileostomy or colostomy); may be an early symptom of intestinal obstruction.
4. Consume 2–3 L/day of fluids to ensure adequate hydration and to relieve symptoms of dry mouth.
5. Vegetables, fruit, fiber, and fluids should be consumed in adequate quantities to prevent constipation.
6. Wear sunglasses, sunscreen, and protective clothing during exposure; drug may cause a photosensitivity reaction.
7. Avoid overexposure to heat and acknowledge the body's need for increased fluids in hot weather because sweating is inhibited by the drug and heat stroke may occur.
8. Report any loss of effect as dosage may require adjustment.
9. With neurogenic bladder, return as scheduled for cystometry and to evaluate response to therapy and need for continuation of medication.
**Outcomes/Evaluate**
• Relief of spasms and associated GU pain
• Normal urinary elimination patterns
• Positive cystometry findings

————COMBINATION DRUG————

# Oxycodone and acetaminophen

(ox-ee-**KOH**-dohn, ah-**SEAT**-ah-**MIN**-oh-fen)
**Pregnancy Category:** C
Endocet, Oxycocet ✹, Percocet ✹, Percocet-Demi ✹, Roxicet **(C-II) (Rx)**
**Classification:** Analgesic

See also *Acetaminophen* and *Narcotic Analgesics.*
**Content: Endocet and Roxicet Tablets:** *Narcotic analgesic:* Oxycodone hydrochloride, 5 mg. *Analgesic:* Acetaminophen, 325 mg. **Roxicet Oral Solution:** *Narcotic analgesic:* Oxycodone hydrochloride, 5 mg/5 mL. *Analgesic:* Acetaminophen, 325 mg/5 mL.
**Uses:** Relief of moderate to moderately severe pain.
**Contraindications:** Hypersensitivity to either oxycodone or acetaminophen.
**Special Concerns:** Can produce drug dependence and has abuse potential. The respiratory depressant effects of oxycodone can be exaggerated in clients with head injury, other intracranial lesions, or a preexisting increase in intracranial pressure. Use with caution in clients who are elderly, are debilitated, have severely impaired hepatic or renal function, are hyperthyroid, have Addison's disease, have prostatic hypertrophy, or have urethral stricture. Use for acute abdominal conditions may obscure the diagnosis or clinical course. Use with caution during lactation. Safety and efficacy in children have not been established.
**Side Effects:** Commonly, dizziness, lightheadedness, N&V, and sedation; these effects are more common in ambulatory clients than nonambulatory clients. Other side effects include euphoria, dysphoria, constipation, skin rash, and pruritus. See also individual components.
**Drug Interactions**
*Anticholinergic drugs* / Production of paralytic ileus

*Antidepressants, tricyclic /* ↑ Effect of either the tricyclic antidepressant or oxycodone

*CNS depressants (including other narcotic analgesics, phenothiazines, antianxiety drugs, sedative-hypnotics, anesthetics, alcohol) /* Additive CNS depression

*MAO inhibitors /* ↑ Effect of either the MAO inhibitor or oxycodone

**Dosage** ⎯⎯⎯⎯⎯⎯⎯⎯⎯⎯
• **Oral Solution, Tablets**
  *Analgesic.*
**Adults:** 5 mL of the oral solution q 6 hr or 1 tablet q 6 hr as needed for pain.

## NURSING CONSIDERATIONS

See also *Nursing Considerations* for *Acetaminophen* and *Narcotic Analgesics.*

**Assessment**
1. Document indications for therapy, type, onset, and duration of symptoms. Use a pain-rating scale to rate pain level.
2. List other agents prescribed and the outcome.
3. Note CNS assessment findings and level of consciousness.

**Client/Family Teaching**
1. Take only as directed; may take with food to decrease GI upset.
2. Drug may cause dizziness and drowsiness; do not perform activities that require mental or physical alertness and do not change positions abruptly.
3. May cause constipation, N&V, dry mouth, and physical dependence; review interventions to offset side effects.
4. Avoid alcohol and any other CNS depressants without provider approval. (*NOTE:* Oral solution contains small amounts of alcohol.)

**Outcomes/Evaluate:** Desired pain control

# Oxycodone hydrochloride
(ox-ee-**KOH**-dohn)

**Pregnancy Category:** C
OxyContin, Roxicodone, Roxicodone Intensol, Supeudol ✸ (C-II) (Rx)

# Oxycodone terephthalate
(ox-ee-**KOH**-dohn teh-ref-**THAL**-ayt)

**Pregnancy Category:** C
(C-II) (Rx)
**Classification:** Narcotic analgesic, morphine type

See also *Narcotic Analgesics.*
**Action/Kinetics:** Semisynthetic opiate causing mild sedation and little or no antitussive effect. Most effective in relieving acute pain. **Onset:** 15–30 min. **Peak effect:** 60 min. **Duration:** 4–6 hr. t½: 3.2 hr for immediate-release product and 4.5 hr for extended-release. Dependence liability is moderate. Oxycodone terephthalate is only available in combination with aspirin (e.g., Percodan) or acetaminophen.

**Uses:** Moderate to severe pain. The extended-release product (OxyContin) is indicated for moderate to severe pain, including that due to cancer, injuries, arthritis, lower back problems, and other musculoskeletal conditions that require treatment for more than a few days.

**Additional Contraindications:** Use in children.

**Special Concerns:** OxyContin 80 mg controlled release is indicated only for opiate-tolerant clients.

**Additional Drug Interactions:** Clients with gastric distress, such as colitis or gastric or duodenal ulcer, and clients who have glaucoma should not receive Percodan, which also contains aspirin.

**Dosage** ⎯⎯⎯⎯⎯⎯⎯⎯⎯⎯
• **Capsule, Oral Solution, Concentrated Solution, Tablet, Extended Release Tablet**
  *Analgesia.*
**Adults:** 5 mg q 6 hr.
• **Extended Release Tablet**
  *Analgesia.*

**Adults, opioid-naive:** 10 mg q 12 hr. **Adults, with prior narcotic therapy:** 10–30 mg b.i.d.

## NURSING CONSIDERATIONS

See also *Nursing Considerations* for *Narcotic Analgesics*.

**Assessment:** Document onset, location, and duration of pain and characteristics of symptoms. Use a pain-rating scale to rate pain levels.

**Client/Family Teaching**
1. Take medication with food to minimize GI upset.
2. Swallow extended-release tablets whole. Ingesting broken, crushed, or chewed extended-release tablets may lead to rapid release and absorption and the possibility of toxic effects.
3. Use caution and do not perform activities that require mental alertness.
4. Avoid alcohol in any form.

**Outcomes/Evaluate:** Relief of pain

---

# Oxymorphone hydrochloride

(ox-ee-**MOR**-fohn)
**Pregnancy Category:** C
Numorphan **(C-I) (Rx)**
**Classification:** Narcotic analgesic, morphine type

See also *Narcotic Analgesics*.

**Action/Kinetics:** On a weight basis, is said to be 2–10 times more potent as an analgesic than morphine although potency depends on the route of administration. It produces mild depression of the cough reflex and significant respiratory depression and emesis. **Onset:** 5–10 min. **Peak effect:** 30–60 min. **Duration:** 3–6 hr.

**Uses:** Moderate to severe pain. **Parenteral:** Preoperative analgesia, to support anesthesia, obstetrics, relief of anxiety in clients with dyspnea associated with acute LV failure and pulmonary edema.

**Dosage**
• **SC, IM**
*Analgesia.*

**Adults, initial:** 1–1.5 mg q 4–6 hr; dose can be increased carefully until analgesic response obtained.
*Analgesia during labor.*
**Adults:** 0.5–1.0 mg IM.
• **IV**
*Analgesia.*
**Adults, initial:** 0.5 mg.
• **Suppositories**
*Analgesia.*
**Adults:** 5 mg q 4–6 hr. **Not recommended for children under 12 years of age.**

## NURSING CONSIDERATIONS

See also *Nursing Considerations* for *Narcotic Analgesics*.

**Administration/Storage**
1. Store suppositories in the refrigerator.
**IV** 2. If the drug is to be administered IV, dilute the dosage in 5 mL of sterile water or NSS and administer over 2–3 min.

**Assessment:** Document indications for therapy, noting onset, location, and duration of pain; rate pain on rating scale to evaluate drug's effectiveness.

**Client/Family Teaching**
1. C&DB several times each hour while awake to prevent atelectasis; incentive spirometry may be useful.
2. Drug may aggravate gallbladder conditions; report any abdominal complaints.
3. Use safety precautions; drug causes drowsiness and dizziness.

**Outcomes/Evaluate:** Relief of pain; control of anxiety

---

# Oxytocin, parenteral

(ox-eh-**TOE**-sin)
**Pregnancy Category:** X
Pitocin, Toesen ✿ **(Rx)**
**Classification:** Oxytocic agent

**Action/Kinetics:** Synthetic compound identical to the natural hormone isolated from the posterior pituitary. Has uterine stimulant, vasopressor, and weak antidiuretic properties. May act on uterine myofibril activity to increase the number of contracting myofibrils. Uterine sensitivity to oxytocin, as well as amplitude and duration of uterine contractions, increases gradually during gestation and just before parturition increases rapidly. Facilitates ejection of milk from the breasts by stimulating smooth muscle. **Onset, IV:** immediate; **IM,** 3–5 min; **Peak effects:** 40 min. **Steady-state plasma levels:** Reached within 40 min. **t½:** 1–6 min (decreased in late pregnancy and lactation). **Duration, IV:** 20 min after infusion is stopped; **IM:** 2–3 hr. Eliminated through the urine, liver, and functional mammary gland.

**Uses:** *Antepartum:* Induction or stimulation of labor at term. To overcome true primary or secondary uterine inertia. Induction of labor with oxytocin is indicated only under certain *specific* conditions and is not usual because serious toxic effects can occur.

Oxytocin is indicated:
1. For uterine inertia.
2. For induction of labor in cases of erythroblastosis fetalis, maternal diabetes mellitus, preeclampsia, and eclampsia.
3. For induction of labor after premature rupture of membranes in last month of pregnancy when labor fails to develop spontaneously within 12 hr.
4. For routine control of postpartum hemorrhage and uterine atony.
5. To hasten uterine involution.
6. To complete inevitable abortions after the 20th week of pregnancy.
7. Intranasally for initial letdown of milk.

*Investigational:* Breast engorgement, oxytocin challenge test for determining antepartum fetal HR.

**Contraindications:** Hypersensitivity to drug. Significant cephalopelvic disproportion; unfavorable fetal positions or presentations that are undeliverable without conversion prior to delivery. In obstetric emergencies where the benefit-to-risk ratio for either the mother or fetus favors surgical intervention. Fetal distress where delivery is not imminent, pro-longed use in uterine inertia or severe toxemia, hypertonic or hyperactive uterine patterns, when adequate uterine activity does not achieve satisfactory progress. Induction of augmentation of labor where vaginal delivery is contraindicated, including invasive cervical cancer, cord presentation or prolapse, total placenta previa and vasa previa, active herpes genitalis.

Also, predisposition to thromboplastin and amniotic fluid embolism (dead fetus, abruptio placentae), history of previous traumatic deliveries, or women with four or more deliveries. Oxytocin should never be given IV undiluted or in high concentrations. Oxytocin citrate is contraindicated in severe toxemia, CV or renal disease. Intranasal oxytocin is contraindicated during pregnancy.

**Side Effects:** *Mother:* Tetanic uterine contractions, *anaphylaxis,* cardiac arrhythmia, *fatal afibrinogenemia,* N&V, PVCs, increased blood loss, pelvic hematoma, hypertension, tachycardia, and ECG changes. Also, rarely, anxiety, dyspnea, precordial pain, edema, cyanosis or reddening of the skin, and CV spasm. Water intoxication from prolonged IV infusion, *death due to hypertensive episodes, subarachnoid hemorrhage, postpartum hemorrhage, or uterine rupture.* Excessive dosage may cause uterine hypertonicity, spasm, tetanic contraction, or uterine rupture.

*Fetus:* **Death,** PVCs, bradycardia, tachycardia, arrhythmias, hypoxia, *intracranial hemorrhage due to overstimulation of the uterus during labor leads to uterine tetany with marked impairment of uteroplacental blood flow.*

*NOTE:* Hypersensitivity reactions occur rarely. When they do, they occur most often with natural oxytocin administered IM or in concentrated IV doses and least frequently after IV infusion or diluted doses. Accidental swallowing of buccal tablets is not harmful.

---

**OD**    **Overdose Management:**
*Symptoms: Hyperstimulation of the uterus resulting in hypertonic or tetanic contractions. Or, a resting tone of 15–20 cm water between contractions can result in uterine rupture, cervical and vaginal lacerations, tumultuous labor, uteroplacental hypoperfusion, postpartum hemorrhage, and a variable deceleration of fetal heart rate, fetal hypoxia, hypercapnia, or death. Water intoxication with seizures can occur if large doses (40–50 mL/min) of the drug are infused for long periods of time.* Treatment: Discontinue the drug and restrict fluid intake. Start diuresis and give a hypertonic saline solution IV. Correct electrolyte imbalance and control seizures with a barbiturate. If the client is comatose, provide special nursing care.

**Drug Interactions**
*Cyclopropane /* Hypotension; also, maternal sinus bradycardia with abnormal AV rhythms
*Sympathomimetic amines /* Severe hypertension and possible stroke

**Dosage**
• **IV Infusion, IM**
*Induction or stimulation of labor.*
Dilute 10 units (1 mL) to 1,000 mL isotonic saline or 5% dextrose for IV infusion. **Initial:** 0.001–0.002 unit/min (0.1–0.2 mL/min); dose can be gradually increased at 15- to 30-min intervals by 0.001 unit/min (0.1 mL/min) to maximum of 0.02 unit/min (2 mL/min).
*Reduction of postpartum bleeding.*
Dilute 10–40 units (1–4 mL) to 1,000 mL with isotonic saline or 5% dextrose for IV infusion. Administer at a rate to control uterine atony, usually at a rate of 0.02–0.1 unit/min.
*Incomplete or therapeutic abortion.*
10 units at a rate of 0.02–0.04 unit/min by IV infusion or 10 units IM after placental delivery.

# NURSING CONSIDERATIONS
**Administration/Storage**
**IV** 1. Use Y-tubing system, with one bottle containing IV solution and oxytocin, and the other containing only the IV solution. This allows for the discontinuation of the drug while maintaining the patency of the vein when it is decided to change to the drug-free infusion bottle. Give parenteral oxytocin infusions only with an electronic infusion device.
2. Oxytocin is rapidly broken down by sodium bisulfite. Have magnesium sulfate immediately available to relax the uterus in case of tetanic uterine contractions.
3. The provider should be immediately available during drug administration.

**Assessment**
1. Note any sensitivity to the drug.
2. Document indications for therapy and onset of symptoms.
3. Determine fetal maturity, pelvic adequacy, and fetal presentation prior to initiating drug.
4. Check for dilation, assess resting uterine tone and time the duration and frequency, noting characteristics of uterine contractions. Note maternal and fetal HRs and intrauterine pressure.
5. Carefully review history for any contraindications prior to administering oxytocin.

**For induction and stimulation of labor and/or oxytocin challenge test:**
**Interventions**
1. Before initiating therapy, inform client of the rationale for using oxytocic agents and reassure that the procedure is not unusual. Explain that the medication will induce contractions that may feel like menstrual cramps initially but can be very painful; analgesics can be used when necessary.
2. Remain with the client during the induction period and throughout the stimulation of labor.
3. Record VS and check I&O q 15 min.
4. Note resting uterine tone and assess the uterine contractions for frequency, duration, and strength of the contractions.
5. Monitor the fetal HR and rhythm at least every 10 min. Document and

immediately report any alterations from the normal pattern.

6. Prevent uterine rupture and fetal damage by clamping off IV oxytocin, starting medication-free IV fluids, turning client on her left side to prevent fetal anoxia, providing oxygen, and reporting when the following events occur:

• If the contractions occur more frequently than every 2 min and last longer than 60–90 sec with no period of uterine relaxation in between.

• If the contractions are excessively strong and/or exceed 50–65 mm Hg.

• If resting uterine tone is 15–20 mm Hg or more.

• If the fetal HR indicates bradycardia, tachycardia, or irregularities of rhythm.

7. Assess for water intoxication following prolonged administration of oxytocin. Monitor I&O and serum electrolytes closely.

8. Observe for lethargy, confusion, and stupor. Note if the client has developed neuromuscular hyperexcitability with increased reflexes and muscular twitching. These symptoms should be reported immediately since convulsions and coma may occur if left untreated. Magnesium sulfate should be readily available for IV administration.

• **During the fourth stage of labor when oxytocin is administered for prevention or control of hemorrhage:**

1. Describe the location, size, and firmness of the uterus. Report if the uterus is displaced or boggy and follow designated hospital protocol.

2. In clients with spinal anesthesia, visually inspect for any evidence of bleeding. Sensation is diminished and hemorrhage may occur insidiously.

3. Note the amount and color of the lochia. Report any bright red lochia, excessive bleeding, or the passage of clots.

4. Monitor the client's VS until they remain stable.

5. Closely monitor I&O. Observe client for S&S of water intoxication; document and report immediately.

**Outcomes/Evaluate**

• Induction of labor with effective uterine contractions

• ↑ Uterine tone with ↓ postpartum bleeding

# Paclitaxel
(**PACK**-lih-**tax**-el)
**Pregnancy Category:** D
Taxol (**Rx**)
**Classification:** Antineoplastic, miscellaneous

See also *Antineoplastic Agents*.
**Action/Kinetics:** Naturally occurring antineoplastic agent that promotes the assembly of microtubules from tubulin dimers and stabilizes microtubules by preventing depolymerization. The stabilization results in the inhibition of the normal dynamic reorganization of the microtubule network that is required for vital interphase and mitotic cellular functions. Also induces abnormal "bundles" of microtubules throughout the cell cycle and multiple esters of microtubules during mitosis. Following IV administration, there is a biphasic decline in plasma levels. The initial rapid decline is due to distribution to the peripheral compartment and significant elimination, whereas the second phase is due, in part, to a slow efflux of the drug from the peripheral compartment. Metabolized by the liver with small amounts of unchanged drug excreted in the urine.

**Uses:** Metastatic carcinoma of the ovary after failure of first-line or subsequent chemotherapy. Breast cancer after combination chemotherapy has failed or there has been relapse

*bold italic* = life threatening side effect

within 6 months of adjuvant chemotherapy (prior therapy must have included an anthracycline unless contraindicated). Second-line treatment of AIDS-related Kaposi's sarcoma. *Investigational:* Alone or in combination with other chemotherapeutic drugs for advanced head and neck cancer, previously untreated extensive-stage small-cell lung cancer, adenocarcinoma of the upper GI tract, hormone-refractory prostate cancer, advanced non-small-cell lung cancer, and leukemias.

**Contraindications:** Hypersensitivity to paclitaxel, in those with a hypersensitivity to products containing polyoxymethylated castor oil (Cremophor EL), clients with a baseline neutropenia below 1,500 cells/mm³, and those with AIDS-related Kaposi's sarcoma with baseline neutrophil counts below 1,000 cells/mm³. Lactation.

**Special Concerns:** Use with caution in clients with impaired hepatic function. Safety and efficacy have not been determined in children.

**Side Effects:** *Hypersensitivity reactions:* Severe symptoms usually occur during the first hour of therapy and occur during both the first or second course of therapy despite premedication. Severe symptoms include *dyspnea, angioedema,* hypotension, or generalized urticaria all of which require immediate cessation of the drug and aggressive treatment therapy. Symptoms not requiring treatment include milder dyspnea, flushing, skin reactions, hypotension, or tachycardia. *Hematologic:* Neutropenia and leukopenia (common), thrombocytopenia, anemia, infections, bleeding, packed cell transfusions, platelet transfusions. *CV:* Bradycardia and hypotension (including during the infusion), hypertension, *severe CV events (including asymptomatic ventricular tachycardia, bigeminy, syncope, complete AV block),* abnormal ECG (including nonspecific repolarization abnormalities, sinus tachycardia, premature beats). *Musculoskeletal:* Peripheral neuropathy (including mild paresthesia), myalgia, arthralgia. *GI:* N&V, diarrhea, mucositis. *Miscellaneous:* Alopecia, fever associated with severe neutropenia; infections of the urinary tract and upper respiratory tract as well as **sepsis due to neutropenia.**

**OD Overdose Management:** *Symptoms:* **Bone marrow suppression,** peripheral neurotoxicity, mucositis. Accidental inhalation may cause dyspnea, chest pain, burning eyes, sore throat, and nausea. *Treatment:* Treat symptomatically.

**Drug Interactions**

*Cisplatin* / More profound myelosuppression when paclitaxel was given after cisplatin than when paclitaxel was given before cisplatin, due to a ⅓ decrease in paclitaxel clearance

*Doxorubicin* / ↑ Levels of doxorubicin and doxorubicinol

*Ketoconazole* / Inhibition of metabolism of paclitaxel by ketoconazole

**Laboratory Test Interferences:** ↑ Bilirubin, alkaline phosphatase, ALT, AST.

**Dosage** ──────────────
• **IV Infusion**
    *Metastatic carcinoma of the ovary.*
**Adults:** 135 mg/m² given IV over 3 hr q 3 weeks after failure of first-line or subsequent chemotherapy.
    *Metastatic breast cancer.*
**Adults:** 175 mg/m² given IV over 3 hr q 3 weeks after failure of chemotherapy for metastatic disease or relapse after 6 months of adjuvant chemotherapy.
    *AIDS-related Kaposi's sarcoma.*
135 mg/m² given IV over 3 hr q 3 weeks or 100 mg/m² given IV over 3 hr q 2 weeks.

## NURSING CONSIDERATIONS

See also *Nursing Considerations* for *Antineoplastic Agents.*

**Administration/Storage**

**IV** 1. The undiluted concentrate of paclitaxel should not come in contact with plasticized polyvinylchloride equipment or devices used to prepare solutions for infusion.

2. Premedicate before use to prevent severe hypersensitivity reac-

tions. Premedication may consist of oral dexamethasone, 20 mg, given 12 and 6 hr before paclitaxel; diphenhydramine (or equivalent), 50 mg IV, 30–60 min before paclitaxel; and cimetidine, 300 mg IV, or ranitidine, 50 mg IV, 30–60 min before paclitaxel.

3. In those with advanced HIV disease, reduce the dose of dexamethasone to 10 mg PO; initiate or repeat treatment only if neutrophil count is 1,000 cells/mm³ or greater; begin concomitant hematopoietic growth factor as needed.

4. Dilute paclitaxel concentrate prior to infusion in 0.9% NSS, 5% dextrose injection, D5%/0.9% NaCl, or D5%/RL to a final concentration of 0.3–1.2 mg/mL. Diluted solutions are stable for up to 24 hr at room temperature.

5. Administer diluted solution through an in-line filter with a microporous membrane not greater than 0.22 μm.

6. The dilutions may show haziness, which is due to the formulation vehicle. No significant loss of potency has been noted following simulated delivery of the solution through IV tubing containing an in-line (0.22-μm) filter.

7. To minimize client exposure to the plasticizer DHEP which may be leached from PVC infusion bags or sets, store diluted paclitaxel solutions in bottles (glass, polypropylene) or plastic bags (polypropylene, polyolefin) and administered through polyethylene-lined administration sets.

8. Unopened vials of the concentrate are stable when stored under refrigeration, protected from light, in the original package.

9. Do not undertake repeat courses until the neutrophil count is at least 1,500 cells/mm³ and the platelet count is at least 100,000 cells/mm³. The dose should be reduced by 20% for subsequent courses in those who experience a neutrophil count below 500 cells/mm³ for 1 week or more or if there is severe peripheral neuropathy during therapy.

10. Use gloves when handling the drug. If the solution comes in contact with the skin, wash the skin immediately and thoroughly with soap and water. If the drug comes in contact with mucous membranes, thoroughly flush the membranes with water.

11. *Treatment of Hypersensitivity Reactions:* Stop the infusion and treat with bronchodilators (such as albuterol or theophylline), epinephrine, antihistamines, and corticosteroids.

**Assessment**

1. Document tumor location, previous therapy (include agents, dosage, and duration), especially radiation because this may enhance myelosuppressive drug effects. Determine if client has received this drug and the response.

2. Administer pretreatment medications, usually corticosteroids, diphenhydramine, and $H_2$ antagonists. After pretreatment medication, if symptoms of severe hypersensitivity reaction (dyspnea, hypotension, angioedema, or generalized urticaria) appear, interrupt infusion and report. Hypersensitivity reactions usually occur during the first hour and despite premedication.

3. Document any severe hypersensitivity reaction so that client is *NOT* rechallenged with paclitaxel.

4. Monitor VS, I&O, CBC, liver and renal function studies; ensure that neutrophil count is 1,500 cells/mm³ before drug administration (with AIDS-related Kaposi's sarcoma with baseline neutrophil counts > 1,000 cells/mm³) and that platelet count is at least 100,000 cells/mm³. Neutrophil nadir: 11 days; platelet nadir 8–9 days.

**Client/Family Teaching**

1. Anticipate hair loss.

2. Joint pain and discomfort may be experienced 2–3 days after therapy but should resolve in several days.

3. Report any fever, chills, sore throat, infection, abnormal bruising or bleeding, or CNS symptoms, especially peripheral neuropathy.

**P**

4. Avoid alcohol, aspirin, and NSAIDs.

5. Use reliable contraception during and for 4 months following therapy.

**Outcomes/Evaluate:** ↓ Tumor size and spread

# Pamidronate disodium

(pah-**MIH**-droh-nayt)
**Pregnancy Category:** C
Aredia **(Rx)**
**Classification:** Bone growth regulator, antihypercalcemic

**Action/Kinetics:** Inhibits both normal and abnormal bone resorption without inhibiting bone formation and mineralization. Precise mechanism is not known, but the drug may inhibit dissolution of hydroxyapatite crystal or have an effect on bone reabsorbing cells. Causes decreased serum phosphate levels probably due to a decreased release of phosphate from bone and increased renal excretion as parathyroid levels return to normal. Urinary calcium/creatinine and urinary hydroxyproline/creatinine ratios decrease and usually return to normal or below normal after treatment. **t½:** Biphasic, 1.6 hr (alpha) and 27.3 hr (beta). Approximately 50% of an IV infused dose is excreted unchanged in the urine within 72 hr.

**Uses:** In conjunction with hydration to treat moderate to severe hypercalcemia associated with malignancy (with or without bone metastases). Moderate to severe Paget's disease. In conjunction with antimyeloma chemotherapy to treat osteolytic bone lesions of multiple myeloma or osteolytic bone metastases of breast cancer. *Investigational:* Postmenopausal osteoporosis; hyperparathyroidism; prophylaxis of glucocorticoid-induced osteoporosis; reduce bone pain in clients with prostatic carcinoma; treat immobilization-induced hypercalcemia.

**Contraindications:** Hypersensitivity to biphosphonates.

**Special Concerns:** Use with caution during lactation. Safety and effectiveness have not been determined in children. Pamidronate has not been tested in clients who have creatinine levels greater than 5 mg/dL.

**Side Effects:** *Metabolic/Electrolytes:* Hypocalcemia, hypokalemia, hypomagnesemia, hypophosphatemia, hypomagnesemia. *Body as a whole:* Slight increase in body temperature, fluid overload, generalized pain, back pain, fatigue, fever, moniliasis. *GI:* N&V, constipation, abdominal pain, anorexia, **GI hemorrhage,** ulcerative stomatitis. *CNS:* Somnolence, insomnia, dizziness, headache, paresthesia, abnormal vision, slight possibility of **seizures.** *CV:* Hypertension, atrial fibrillation, syncope, tachycardia. *Respiratory:* Rales, rhinitis, upper respiratory tract infection. *GU:* UTI. *Musculoskeletal:* Bone pain. *At site of administration:* Redness, swelling or induration, pain on palpation. *Miscellaneous:* Anemia, hypothyroidism, sweating.

## Dosage
• **IV Infusion**

*Moderate hypercalcemia (corrected serum calcium of about 12–13.5 mg/dL) of malignancy.*
**Initial therapy:** 60–90 mg. The 60-mg dose is given as an initial single dose over at least 4 hr; the 90-mg dose must be given as an initial single dose over 24 hr.

*Severe hypercalcemia (corrected serum calcium greater than 13.5 mg/dL) of malignancy.*
**Initial therapy:** 90 mg as a single initial dose given over 24 hr. If retreatment is necessary, use the same dose as for initial therapy; at least 7 days should elapse before retreatment.

*Moderate to severe Paget's disease.*
30 mg/day given as a 4-hr infusion on 3 consecutive days (total dose: 90 mg). If retreatment is necessary, the same dosage schedule is used.

*Osteolytic bone lesions of multiple myeloma.*
90 mg given as a 4-hr infusion every month. Those with marked Bence-Jones proteinuria and dehydration

should receive adequate hydration before infusion of pamidronate.

*Osteolytic bone metastases.*
90 mg given as a 2-hr infusion q 3 to 4 weeks.

## NURSING CONSIDERATIONS
### Administration/Storage
**IV** 1. If hypercalcemia recurs, retreatment can be instituted provided a minimum of 7 days has elapsed to allow full response to the initial dose.

2. Reconstitute drug by adding 10 mL sterile water for injection, which results in a concentration of 30, 60, or 90 mg/10 mL with a pH of 6–7.4.

3. For hypercalcemia of malignancy, dilute in 1,000 mL of sterile 0.45% or 0.9% NaCl or 5% dextrose injection. This solution is stable for 24 hr at room temperature.

4. For treating Paget's disease or osteolytic bone lesions of multiple myeloma, dilute the recommended dose in 500 mL of sterile 0.45% or 0.9% NaCl or 5% dextrose injection.

5. If reconstituted with sterile water for injection, the drug may be stored in the refrigerator for up to 24 hr at 2°C–8°C (36°F–46°F).

6. Do not mix with calcium-containing infusion solutions such as Ringer's solution.

7. Give as a single IV solution and in a separate line.

### Assessment
1. Note indications for therapy, i.e., hypercalcemia of malignancy, symptomatic Paget's disease, postmenopausal osteoporosis, bone pain.

2. Document any biphosphonate hypersensitivity.

3. Note any evidence of cardiac disease.

4. Obtain baseline ECG, serum calcium, magnesium, potassium, phosphorus, CBC, and renal function studies.

### Interventions
1. Monitor VS and I&O. Ensure adequate administration of fluids to correct hypovolemia and correct any volume deficits before administering diuretics.

2. During drug administration, vigorous saline hydration should be undertaken for moderate to severe hypercalcemia to restore the urine output to about 2 L/day. For less severe hypercalcemia, more conservative approaches can be taken including saline hydration with or without loop diuretics. Overhydration should be avoided, especially with heart failure. Weigh daily and observe for edema.

3. Assess for seizure activity; incorporate seizure precautions.

### Client/Family Teaching
1. Review dietary sources of calcium (dark green vegetables, yogurt, cheese, milk, etc.) that should be avoided.

2. May experience transient mild temperature elevations for up to 48 hr following therapy.

3. Maintain adequate hydration; keep a log of I&O.

4. Report any increase in N&V, bone pain, thirst, or lethargy R/T hypercalcemia.

### Outcomes/Evaluate
• Desired calcium levels
• ↓ Bone pain/instability

# Pancrelipase
# (Lipancreatin)
(pan-kree-**LY**-payz)
**Pregnancy Category:** C
Cotazym, Cotazym-S, Creon 5, 10, or 20, Creon 8, 10, or 25 ✹, Digess 8000 ✹, Ilozyme, Ku-Zyme HP, Pancrease, Pancrease MT 4, 10, 16, or 20, Protilase, Viokase, Ultrase MT12, 20, or 24, Viokase ✹, Zymase **(Rx)**
**Classification:** Digestant

**Action/Kinetics:** Enzyme concentrate from hog pancreas, which contains lipase, amylase, and protease, enzymes that replace or supplement naturally occurring enzymes. More active at neutral or slightly alkaline pH. Has 12 times the lipolytic activity and 4 times both the proteolytic and amylolytic activity of pancreatin.

---

✹ = Available in Canada · · · **bold italic** = life threatening side effect

Certain products have an enteric coating that protects the enzymes from deactivation in the stomach.

**Uses:** Pancreatic deficiency diseases such as chronic pancreatitis, cystic fibrosis of the pancreas, pancreatectomy, ductal obstructions caused by cancer of the pancreas or common bile duct, steatorrhea of malabsorption syndrome or postgastrectomy or postgastrointestinal surgery. Presumptive test for pancreatic function, especially in insufficiency due to chronic pancreatitis.

**Contraindications:** Hog protein sensitivity. Acute pancreatitis, acute exacerbation of chronic pancreatic disease.

**Special Concerns:** Safety for use during lactation and in children less than 6 months of age not established. Methacrylic acid copolymer, which is found in the enteric coating of certain products, may cause fibrosing colonopathy.

**Side Effects:** *GI:* Nausea, diarrhea, abdominal cramps following high doses. *Other:* Inhalation of the powder is irritating to the skin and mucous membranes and may result in an asthma attack. High doses cause hyperuricemia and hyperuricosuria.

**OD Overdose Management:** *Symptoms:* Diarrhea, intestinal upset.

**Drug Interactions**
*Calcium carbonate* / ↓ Effect of pancreatic enzymes
*Iron* / Response to oral iron may ↓ if given with pancreatic enzymes
*Magnesium hydroxide* / ↓ Effect of pancreatic enzymes

**Dosage**
• **Capsules; Enteric-Coated Microspheres, Microtablets, Spheres, Pellets; Powder; Tablets**
*Pancreatic insufficiency.*
**Adults and children over 12 years of age:** 4,000–48,000 units of lipase with each meal and with snacks. **Children, 7–12 years:** 4,000–12,000 units of lipase with each meal and snacks; **1–6 years:** 4,000–8,000 units of lipase with each meal and 4,000 units lipase with snacks. **6–12 months:** 2,000 units lipase with each meal. Dosage has not been established in children less than 6 months of age. Severe deficiencies may require up to 64,000–88,000 units of lipase with meals (or the frequency of administration can be increased if side effects are not manifested).

*Pancreatectomy or obstruction of pancreatic ducts.*
**Adults:** 8,000–16,000 units of lipase at 2 hr intervals or as directed by a physician.
*Cystic fibrosis.*
Use 0.7 g of the powder with meals.

## NURSING CONSIDERATIONS
### Administration/Storage
1. When administering to young children, the contents of the capsule can be sprinkled on food.
2. After several weeks of use, adjust the dosage according to the therapeutic response.
3. Store unopened preparations in tight containers at a temperature not to exceed 25°C (77°F).
4. Do not crush or chew enteric-coated products (i.e., microspheres, microtablets). If unable to swallow, the capsule may be opened and shaken on a small amount of soft, cold food (e.g., applesauce, gelatin) that does not require chewing. This should be swallowed immediately without chewing (the enzymes may irritate the mucosa). Follow with a glass of juice or water to ensure complete swallowing of the product. Enteric-coated products that come in contact with foods with a pH greater than 5.5 will dissolve.
5. Generally, 300 mg of pancrelipase is required to digest every 17 g of dietary fat.
6. Products are not bioequivalent and thus should not be interchanged without approval.
### Assessment
1. Obtain a thorough nursing history and document indications for therapy.
2. Determine any sensitivity or allergy to pork, since hog protein is the main constituent of pancrelipase.
### Client/Family Teaching
1. Review the appropriate dietary

recommendations (usually low fat, high calorie, high protein); utilize a dietitian for dietary counseling and assistance in meal planning. It takes 300 mg of pancrelipase to digest 17 g of dietary fat.

2. Take just before or with meals and snacks and with plenty of liquids to prevent oral mucosal irritation. Omit if dose missed.

3. Report any nausea, cramping, or diarrhea. The dosage needs to be adjusted to control steatorrhea.

**Outcomes/Evaluate**
• Improved digestion/nutritional status with deficiency states
• Control of diarrhea, ↓ steatorrhea

---

# Pancuronium bromide

(pan-kyou-**ROH**-nee-um)
**Pregnancy Category:** C
Gen-Pancuronium ✦, Pavulon **(Rx)**
**Classification:** Neuromuscular blocking agent, nondepolarizing

See also *Neuromuscular Blocking Agents.*

**Action/Kinetics:** Five times as potent as d-tubocurarine. Anticholinesterase agents will reverse effects. Possesses vagolytic activity although it is not likely to cause histamine release. **Onset:** Within 45 sec. **Time to peak effect:** 3–4.5 min (depending on the dose). **Duration:** 35–45 min (increased with multiple doses). t½, **elimination:** 89–161 min. Forty percent is excreted through the urine either unchanged or as metabolites; 10% is excreted through the bile. In clients with renal failure, the t½ is doubled. Significantly bound to plasma protein.

**Uses:** Adjunct to anesthesia to produce relaxation of skeletal muscle. Facilitate ET intubation. Facilitate management of clients undergoing mechanical ventilation.

**Special Concerns:** Children up to 1 month of age may be more sensitive to the effects of atracurium. Clients with myasthenia gravis or Eaton-Lambert syndrome may have profound effects from small doses.

**Additional Side Effects:** *Respiratory:* **Apnea, respiratory insufficiency.** *CV:* Increased HR and MAP. *Miscellaneous:* Salivation, skin rashes, *hypersensitivity reactions (e.g., bronchospasm,* flushing, hypotension, redness, tachycardia).

**Additional Drug Interactions**
*Azathioprine* / Reverses effects of pancuronium
*Bacitracin* / Additive muscle relaxation
*Enflurane* / ↑ Muscle relaxation
*Isoflurane* / ↑ Muscle relaxation
*Metocurine* / ↑ Muscle relaxation but duration is not prolonged
*Quinine* / ↑ Effect of pancuronium
*Sodium colistimethate* / ↑ Muscle relaxation
*Succinylcholine* / ↑ Intensity and duration of action of pancuronium
*Tetracyclines* / Additive muscle relaxation
*Theophyllines* / ↓ Effects of pancuronium; also, possible cardiac arrhythmias
*Tricyclic antidepressants with halothane* / Administration of pancuronium may cause severe arrhythmias
*Tubocurarine* / ↑ Muscle relaxation but duration is not prolonged

**Dosage** ⸺
• **IV Only**
  *Muscle relaxation during anesthesia.*
**Adults and children over 1 month of age, initial:** 0.04–0.1 mg/kg. Additional doses of 0.01 mg/kg may be administered as required (usually q 20–60 min). **Neonates:** A test dose of 0.02 mg/kg should be administered first to determine responsiveness.
  *ET intubation.*
0.06–0.1 mg/kg as a bolus dose. Can undertake intubation in 2 to 3 min.

## NURSING CONSIDERATIONS

See also *Nursing Considerations* for *Neuromuscular Blocking Agents.*
**Administration/Storage**
**IV** 1. Additional doses significantly increase the duration of skeletal muscle relaxation.

---

2. May be mixed with 5% dextrose, D5%/NSS, RL, and 0.9% NSS. When mixed with any of these solutions, the drug is stable with no change in pH or potency for 2 days in glass or plastic containers.

3. Administer in a continuously monitored environment.

4. Have appropriate anticholinesterase agents available to reverse drug effects. These include pyridostigmine bromide, neostigmine, or edrophonium and are usually administered with atropine or glycopyrrolate.

**Interventions**

1. Provide ventilatory support.

2. Monitor and record VS, ECG, and I&O. Drug can cause vagal stimulation resulting in bradycardia, hypotension, and cardiac arrhythmias.

3. A peripheral nerve stimulator should be used to evaluate neuromuscular response and recovery.

4. Consciousness is not affected by pancuronium. Explain all procedures and provide emotional support. Do not conduct any discussions that should not be overheard.

5. With short-term therapy, reassure clients that they will be able to talk and move once the drug effects are reversed.

6. Muscle fasciculations may cause client to be sore or injured after recovery. Administer prescribed nondepolarizing agent and reassure that the soreness is likely caused by the unsynchronized contractions of adjacent muscle fibers just before the onset of paralysis.

7. Position for comfort and so that the body is in proper alignment. Turn and perform mouth care and eye care frequently (protect eyes; blink reflex is suppressed).

8. Assess airway at frequent intervals. Have a suction machine at the bedside.

9. Check to be certain that the ventilator alarms are set and on at all times. *Never* leave client unmonitored.

10. Determine client need and administer medications for anxiety, pain, and/or sedation regularly.

**Outcomes/Evaluate**

• Desired level of paralysis; suppression of twitch response

• Facilitation of ET intubation; tolerance of mechanical ventilation

# Papaverine

(pah-**PAV**-er-een)
**Pregnancy Category:** C
Pavabid Plateau Caps, Pavagen TD
**(Rx)**
**Classification:** Peripheral vasodilator

**Action/Kinetics:** Direct spasmolytic effect on smooth muscle, possibly by inhibiting cyclic nucleotide phosphodiesterase, thus increasing levels of cyclic AMP. This effect is seen in the vascular system, bronchial muscle, and in the GI, biliary, and urinary tracts. Large doses produce CNS sedation and sleepiness. May also directly relax cerebral vessels as it increases cerebral blood flow and decreases cerebral vascular resistance. Depresses cardiac conduction and irritability and prolongs the myocardial refractory period. Localized in fat tissues and liver. Steady plasma concentration maintained when drug is given q 6 hr. **Peak plasma levels:** 1–2 hr. **t½:** 30–120 min. Sustained-release products may be poorly and erratically absorbed. Metabolized in the liver and inactive metabolites excreted in the urine.

**Uses:** Relief of cerebral and peripheral ischemia associated with arterial spasm and myocardial ischemia complicated by arrhythmias.

**Contraindications:** Complete AV block; administer with extreme caution in presence of coronary insufficiency and glaucoma.

**Special Concerns:** Safe use during lactation or for children not established. Use with caution in glaucoma.

**Side Effects:** *CV:* Flushing of face, hypertension, increase in HR and depth of respiration. Large doses can depress AV and intraventricular conduction, causing serious arrhythmias. *GI:* Nausea, anorexia, abdominal distress, constipation or diarrhea, dry mouth and throat. *CNS:* Headache, drowsiness, sedation, vertigo. *Miscellaneous:* Sweating, malaise, pruritus, skin rashes, chronic hepatitis, hepatic hypersensitivity, jaundice, eosinophilia, altered LFTs.

**OD** **Overdose Management:** *NOTE:* Both acute and chronic poisoning may result from use of papaverine. Symptoms are extensions of side effects.

*Symptoms (Acute Poisoning):* Nystagmus, diplopia, drowsiness, weakness, lassitude, incoordination, coma, cyanosis, ***respiratory depression.*** *Treatment (Acute Poisoning):* Delay absorption by giving tap water, milk, or activated charcoal followed by gastric lavage or induction of vomiting and then a cathartic. BP should be maintained and measures taken to treat respiratory depression and coma. Hemodialysis is effective.

*Symptoms (Chronic Poisoning):* Ataxia, blurred vision, drowsiness, anxiety, headache, GI upset, depression, urticaria, erythematous macular eruptions, blood dyscrasias, hypotension. *Treatment (Chronic Poisoning):* Discontinue medication. Monitor and treat blood dyscrasias. Provide symptomatic treatment. Treat hypotension by IV fluids, elevation of legs, and a vasopressor with inotropic effects.

**Drug Interactions**
*Diazoxide IV* / Additive hypotensive effect
*Levodopa* / Papaverine ↓ effect of levodopa by blocking dopamine receptors
**Laboratory Test Interferences:** ↑ AST, ALT, and bilirubin.

**Dosage**
• **Capsules, Timed-Release**
*Ischemia.*
150 mg q 12 hr. May be increased to 150 mg q 8 hr or 300 mg q 12 hr in difficult cases.

## NURSING CONSIDERATIONS
**Assessment**
1. Document indications for therapy, type, onset, and duration of symptoms.

2. Determine any cardiac dysfunction; monitor VS, ECG, and LFTs.
3. Document mental status; assess all extremities for color, warmth, and pulses.
**Client/Family Teaching**
1. Take with meals or milk to minimize GI upset.
2. Do not perform activities that require mental alertness until drug effects are realized; may cause dizziness or drowsiness.
3. Avoid tobacco products as nicotine may cause vasospasm.
**Outcomes/Evaluate:** ↓ Pain symptoms R/T ischemia

# Paregoric (Camphorated opium tincture)
(pair-eh-**GOR**-ick)
**Pregnancy Category:** C
**(C-III) (Rx)**
**Classification:** Antidiarrheal agent, systemic

See also *Narcotic Analgesics.*
**Action/Kinetics:** The active principle of the mixture is opium (0.04% morphine). The preparation also contains benzoic acid, camphor, and anise oil. Morphine increases the muscular tone of the intestinal tract, decreases digestive secretions, and inhibits normal peristalsis. The slowed passage of the feces through the intestines promotes desiccation, which is a function of the time the feces spend in the intestine. **t½:** 2–3 hr.
**Duration:** 4–5 hr.
**Uses:** Acute diarrhea.
**Contraindications:** See *Morphine Sulfate.* Do not use in clients with diarrhea caused by poisoning until toxic substance has been eliminated. Treatment of pseudomembranous colitis due to lincomycin, penicillins, and cephalosporins. Rubbing paregoric on the gums of a teething child is no longer recommended.
**Special Concerns:** Many physicians do not recommend use of paregoric in treating neonatal opioid dependence.

---

**Side Effects:** See *Narcotic Analgesics.*
**Drug Interactions:** See *Narcotic Analgesics.*

### Dosage
• **Liquid**
**Adult:** 5–10 mL 1–4 times/day (5 mL contains 2 mg of morphine). **Pediatric:** 0.25–0.5 mL/kg 1–4 times/day.

## NURSING CONSIDERATIONS

See also *Nursing Considerations* for *Narcotic Analgesics.*
**Administration/Storage**
1. Administer with water to ensure that it reaches the stomach; mixture will have a milky appearance.
2. Store medication in a light-resistant container.
3. Carefully distinguish between paregoric and tincture of opium. Tincture of opium contains 25 times more morphine than paregoric.
4. Paregoric preparations are subject to the Controlled Substances Act and must be charted accordingly.
5. Have naloxone available to treat any overdosage.
**Assessment**
1. Document onset, duration, and condition requiring paregoric, level of effectiveness, other agents prescribed and the outcome.
2. Note any hepatic dysfunction or drug dependence.
**Client/Family Teaching**
1. Adhere to prescribed regimen.
2. Report if the diarrhea persists.
3. Stop medication once diarrhea has abated. Continued use may result in constipation.
**Outcomes/Evaluate:** Relief of diarrhea

---

## Paromomycin sulfate
(pair-oh-moh-**MY**-sin)
Humatin **(Rx)**
**Classification:** Antibiotic, aminoglycoside

See also *Aminoglycosides.*
**Action/Kinetics:** Obtained from *Streptomyces rimosus forma paromomycina.* Spectrum of activity resembles that of neomycin and kanamycin. Poorly absorbed from the GI tract and is ineffective against systemic infections when given PO.
**Uses:** Inhibition of ammonia-forming bacteria in GI tract in hepatic encephalopathy, intestinal amebiasis, preoperative suppression of intestinal flora. Hepatic coma. *Investigational:* Anthelmintic, to treat *Dientamoeba fragilis, Diphyllobothrium latum, Taenia saginata, T. solium, Dipylidium caninum,* and *Hymenolepis nana.*
**Contraindications:**    Intestinal obstruction.
**Special Concerns:** Use during pregnancy only if benefits outweigh risks. To be used with caution in the presence of GI ulceration because of possible systemic absorption.
**Additional Side Effects:** Diarrhea or loose stools. Heartburn, emesis, and pruritus ani. Superinfections, especially by monilia.
**Drug Interactions:** Penicillin is inhibited by paromomycin.

### Dosage
• **Capsules**
*Hepatic coma.*
**Adults:** 4 g/day in divided doses for 5–6 days.
*Intestinal amebiasis.*
**Adults and children:** 25–35 mg/kg/day administered in three doses with meals for 5–10 days.
*D. fragilis infections.*
25–30 mg/kg/day in three divided doses for 1 week.
*H. nana infections.*
45 mg/kg/day for 5–7 days.
*D. latum, T. saginata, T. solium, D. caninum infections.*
**Adults:** 1 g/ q 15 min for a total of four doses; **pediatric:** 11 mg/kg/15 min for four doses.

## NURSING CONSIDERATIONS

See also *Nursing Considerations* for *Aminoglycosides.*
**Administration/Storage:** Do not administer parenterally and or concurrently with penicillin.
**Client/Family Teaching**
1. Take before or after meals.

2. Report any persistent diarrhea, dehydration, and general weakness.
**Outcomes/Evaluate:** Suppression of intestinal flora

# Paroxetine hydrochloride
(pah-**ROX**-eh-teen)
**Pregnancy Category:** B
Paxil **(Rx)**
**Classification:** Antidepressant

**Action/Kinetics:** Inhibits neuronal reuptake of serotonin in the CNS resulting in potentiation of serotonergic activity in the CNS. It appears to have weak effects on neuronal uptake of norepinephrine and dopamine. Has no anticholinergic effects, does not cause orthostatic hypotension, produces a slight sedative effect. Completely absorbed from the GI tract. **Time to peak plasma levels:** 5.2 hr. **Peak plasma levels:** 61.7 ng/mL. t½: 21 hr. **Time to reach steady state:** About 10 days. Plasma levels are increased in impaired renal and hepatic function as well as in geriatric clients. Extensively metabolized in the liver to inactive metabolites. Approximately two-thirds of the drug is excreted through the urine and one-third is excreted in the feces.

**Uses:** Treatment of major depressive episodes, panic disorder with or without agoraphobia (as defined in DSM-IV), and obsessive-compulsive disorders (as defined in DSM-III-R). *Investigational:* Headaches, diabetic neuropathy, premature ejaculation.

**Contraindications:** Use in clients taking MAO inhibitors. Use of alcohol.

**Special Concerns:** Use with caution and initially at reduced dosage in elderly clients as well as in those with impaired hepatic or renal function, with a history of mania, with a history of seizures, in clients with diseases or conditions that could affect metabolism or hemodynamic responses, and during lactation. Concurrent administration of paroxetine with lithium or digoxin should be undertaken with caution. Safety and efficacy have not been determined in children.

**Side Effects:** The side effects listed were observed with a frequency up to 1 in 1,000 clients.

*CNS:* Headache, somnolence, insomnia, agitation, *seizures,* tremor, anxiety, activation of mania or hypomania, dizziness, nervousness, paresthesia, drugged feeling, myoclonus, CNS stimulation, confusion, amnesia, impaired concentration, depression, emotional lability, vertigo, abnormal thinking, akinesia, alcohol abuse, ataxia, *convulsions, possibility of a suicide attempt* depersonalization, hallucinations, hyperkinesia, hypertonia, incoordination, lack of emotion, manic reaction, paranoid reaction. *GI:* Nausea, abdominal pain, diarrhea, dry mouth, vomiting, constipation, decreased appetite, flatulence, oropharynx disorder ("lump" in throat, tightness in throat), dyspepsia, increased appetite, bruxism, dysphagia, eructation, gastritis, glossitis, increased salivation, mouth ulceration, *rectal hemorrhage,* abnormal LFTs. *Hematologic:* Anemia, leukopenia, lymphadenopathy, purpura. *CV:* Palpitation, vasodilation, postural hypotension, hypertension, syncope, tachycardia, bradycardia, conduction abnormalities, abnormal ECG, hypotension, migraine, peripheral vascular disorder. *Dermatologic:* Sweating, rash, pruritus, acne, alopecia, dry skin, ecchymosis, eczema, furunculosis, urticaria. *Metabolic/Nutritional:* Edema, weight gain, weight loss, hyperglycemia, peripheral edema, thirst. *Respiratory:* Respiratory disorder (cold symptoms or upper respiratory infection), pharyngitis, yawn, increased cough, rhinitis, asthma, bronchitis, dyspnea, epistaxis, hyperventilation, pneumonia, respiratory flu, sinusitis. *GU:* Abnormal ejaculation (usually delay), erectile difficulties, sexual dysfunction, impotence, urinary frequency, urinary difficulty or hesitancy, decreased libido, anorgasmia in women, difficulty in reaching cli-

**P**

---

max/orgasm in women, abortion, amenorrhea, breast pain, cystitis, dysmenorrhea, dysuria, menorrhagia, nocturia, polyuria, urethritis, urinary incontinence, urinary retention, vaginitis. *Musculoskeletal:* Asthenia, back pain, myopathy, myalgia, myasthenia, neck pain, arthralgia, arthritis. *Ophthalmologic:* Blurred vision, abnormality of accommodation, eye pain, mydriasis. *Otic:* Ear pain, otitis media, tinnitus. *Miscellaneous:* Fever, chest pain, trauma, taste perversion or loss, chills, malaise, allergic reaction, **carcinoma,** face edema, moniliasis, anorexia.

*NOTE:* Over 4- to 6-week period, there was evidence of adaptation to side effects such as nausea and dizziness but less adaptation to dry mouth, somnolence, and asthenia.

**OD** **Overdose Management:** *Symptoms:* N&V, drowsiness, sinus tachycardia, dilated pupils. *Treatment:*
• Establish and maintain an airway.
• Ensure adequate oxygenation and ventilation.
• Induction of emesis, lavage, or both; following evacuation, 20–30 g activated charcoal may be given q 4–6 hr during the first 24–48 hr after ingestion.
• An ECG should be taken and cardiac function monitored if there is any evidence of abnormality.
• Provide supportive care with monitoring of VS.

**Drug Interactions**
*Antiarrhythmics, Type IC* / Possible ↑ effect due to ↓ breakdown by the liver
*Cimetidine* / ↑ Effect of paroxetine due to ↓ breakdown by the liver
*Digoxin* / Possible ↓ plasma levels
*MAO inhibitors* / Possibility of serious, and sometimes fatal, reactions including hyperthermia, rigidity, myoclonus, autonomic instability with possible rapid fluctuations in VS, and mental status changes including extreme agitation progressing to delirium and coma
*Phenobarbital* / Possible ↓ effect of paroxetine due to ↑ breakdown by the liver

*Phenytoin* / Possible ↓ effect of paroxetine due to ↑ breakdown by the liver; also, paroxetine ↓ levels of phenytoin
*Procyclidine* / ↓ Dose of procyclidine as significant anticholinergic effects are seen
*Theophylline* / ↑ Theophylline levels
*Tryptophan* / Possibility of headache, nausea, sweating, and dizziness when taken together
*Warfarin* / Possibility of ↑ bleeding tendencies

**Dosage**
• **Tablets**
*Depression.*
**Adults:** 20 mg/day, usually given as a single dose in the morning. Some clients not responding to the 20-mg dose may benefit from increasing the dose in 10-mg/day increments, up to a maximum of 50 mg/day. Dose changes should be made at intervals of at least 1 week.
*Panic disorders.*
**Adults, initial:** 10 mg/day usually given in the morning; **then,** increase by 10-mg increments each week until a dose of 40 mg/day is reached. Maximum daily dose: 60 mg.
*Obsessive-compulsive disorders.*
**Adults, initial:** 20 mg/kg; **then,** increase by 10-mg increments a day in intervals of at least 1 week until a dose of 40 mg/kg is reached. Maximum daily dose: 60 mg.
*Headaches.*
10–50 mg/day.
*Diabetic neuropathy.*
10–60 mg/day.
*Premature ejaculation in men.*
20 mg/day.
*NOTE:* Geriatric or debilitated clients, those with severe hepatic or renal impairment, **initial:** 10 mg/day, up to a maximum of 40 mg/day for all uses.

## NURSING CONSIDERATIONS
### Administration/Storage
1. Even though beneficial effects may be seen in 1–4 weeks, continue therapy as prescribed.
2. Effectiveness is maintained for up

to 1 year with daily doses averaging 30 mg.

**Assessment**

1. Document type, onset, and duration of symptoms, any previous treatment, and the outcome.

2. Note clinical presentation and behavioral manifestations.

3. Document any mania, altered metabolic or hemodynamic states, or seizures.

4. List drugs currently prescribed to ensure no unfavorable interactions. Do not use in combination with a MAO or within 14 days of discontinuing treatment with a MAO.

5. Monitor weight, VS, ECG, electrolytes, CBC, liver and renal function studies; note any dysfunction.

6. During management of overdose, always entertain the possibility of multiple drug involvement.

**Client/Family Teaching**

1. Take only as directed. Prescriptions will be for small quantities to ensure compliance and discourage overdose.

2. Do not engage in tasks that require mental alertness until drug effects realized.

3. Avoid alcohol and OTC products.

4. Report excessive weight loss and adjust diet.

5. Notify provider if pregnancy is suspected or planned.

6. Report any thoughts of suicide or increased suicide ideations. Advise family not to leave severely depressed individuals alone; possibility of a suicide attempt is inherent in depression and may persist until significant remission is observed.

7. Participate in therapy sessions designed to assist with underlying problems.

**Outcomes/Evaluate**

• ↓ Depression

• Improved eating/sleeping patterns; ↑ social involvement/activity

• ↓ Panic attacks; ↓ obsessive repetitive behaviors

---

*COMBINATION DRUG*

# Pediazole

(**PEE**-dee-ah-zohl)
**Pregnancy Category:** C
**(Rx)**
**Classification:** Antibacterial

---

See also *Erythromycins* and *Sulfonamides.*

**Content:** This product is available as granules that, when reconstituted, provide an oral suspension.

*Antibacterial, antibiotic:* Erythromycin ethylsuccinate, 200 mg/5 mL erythromycin activity. *Antibacterial, sulfonamide:* Sulfisoxazole, 600 mg/5 mL. See also information on individual components.

**Uses:** Acute otitis media in children caused by Haemophilus influenzae.

**Contraindications:** Pregnancy at term and in children less than 2 months of age. Use with caution during other times of pregnancy.

**Dosage**

• **Oral Suspension**

**Usual:** Equivalent of 50 mg/kg/day of erythromycin and 150 mg/kg/day of sulfisoxazole, up to a maximum of 6 g/day. **Over 45 kg:** 10 mL q 6 hr; **24 kg:** 7.5 mL q 6 hr; **16 kg:** 5 mL q 6 hr; **8 kg:** 2.5 mL q 6 hr; **less than 8 kg:** Calculate dose according to body weight.

## NURSING CONSIDERATIONS

See also *General Nursing Considerations for All Anti-Infectives*; *Erythromycins;* and *Sulfonamides.*

**Administration/Storage**

1. Refrigerate the reconstituted suspension and use within 14 days.

2. Continue therapy for 10 days.

**Client/Family Teaching**

1. Review the appropriate method, dosage, and frequency for administration.

2. May take without regard to meals.

3. Keep medication refrigerated; shake well before using.

**P**

---

4. Return as scheduled for F/U to ensure desired response to therapy.
**Outcomes/Evaluate:** Resolution of infection; symptomatic improvement

# Pegademase bovine
(peg-**AD**-eh-mace **BOH**-veen)
**Pregnancy Category:** C
Adagen **(Rx)**
**Classification:** Enzyme

**Action/Kinetics:** Derived from bovine intestine and is the conjugate of numerous strands of monomethoxypolyethylene glycol, which is attached covalently to the enzyme ADA. In deficiency clients, adenosine, 2'-deoxyadenosine, and their metabolites are toxic to lymphocytes. Replacement with pegademase bovine improves immune function and decreases the frequency of opportunistic infections. The time required to correct the metabolic abnormalities may range from a few weeks to 6 months. Adequate dosage may be evaluated by measuring ADA levels and by monitoring the level of dATP in erythrocytes. **Peak plasma levels, after IM:** 2–3 days. **t½:** 3 to more than 6 days. After initiation of therapy, the trough level should be between 15 and 35 μmol/hr/mL before a maintenance injection is given.

**Uses:** Enzyme replacement for the treatment of SCID in which there is a deficiency of ADA. Pegademase bovine may be used in infants from birth and in children of any age at the time of diagnosis of deficiency. The drug is ineffective in clients with immunodeficiency due to other causes.

**Contraindications:** Severe thrombocytopenia. IV use.

**Special Concerns:** Use with caution during lactation. There is no evidence to support the safety and effectiveness of pegademase bovine either before or as support therapy for bone marrow transplantation. Use with caution in mild to moderate thrombocytopenia.

**Side Effects:** Data are limited but pain at the injection site and headache have been reported.

**Drug Interactions:** Since vidarabine is a substrate for ADA, use of vidarabine with pegademase bovine may alter the activities of both drugs.

**Dosage**
- **IM**

**Individualized.** Dose is given q 7 days. *First dose:* 10 units/kg. *Second dose:* 15 units/kg. *Third dose:* 20 units/kg. *Maintenance doses:* 20 units/kg/week. If necessary, the weekly dose may be increased by 5 units/kg but the maximum single dose should not exceed 30 units/kg.

## NURSING CONSIDERATIONS
### Administration/Storage
1. Do not mix with any other drug prior to administration.
2. Store in the refrigerator between 2°C and 8°C (36°F–46°F). Do not store frozen or at room temperature. Do not use if there is any chance the vial has been frozen.
3. For IM use only.
### Assessment
1. Document onset of SCID with ADA deficiency. Record baseline level of ADA activity in plasma and erythrocyte dATP. Antibodies to pegademase bovine may develop and should be suspected if the preinjection level of ADA is less than 10 μmol/hr/mL and if other causes for the decrease have been ruled out (e.g., improper storage of vials, improper handling of plasma samples).
2. Note if failed bone marrow transplant or if not suitable for transplant; usual cure for ADA deficiency.
3. Protect from opportunistic infections until immune response/function has returned.
4. Assess for thrombocytopenia. Monitor plasma ADA activity and RBC dATP levels to determine drug response and adequate dosing levels.
### Client/Family Teaching
1. Report any early S&S of infection immediately.

2. After initial therapy, ADA activity should be measured every 1–2 weeks during the first 8–12 weeks of therapy. Between 3 and 9 months, activity should be measured twice a month and then monthly until after 18–24 months of therapy. ADA activity can then be monitored every 2–4 months.

3. Lab studies of dATP, once it has decreased to acceptable levels, should be measured 2–4 times during the remainder of the first year of therapy and 2–3 times yearly thereafter provided that therapy has not been interrupted; report as scheduled.

**Outcomes/Evaluate**
- Plasma ADA activity in the range of 15–35 µmol/hr/mL
- ↓ Erythrocyte dATP to less than or equal to 0.005–0.015 µmol/mL packed erythrocytes or less than or equal to 1% of the total erythrocyte adenine nucleotide (ATP + dATP) content, with a normal ATP level (preinjection sample)

# Pegaspargase (PEG-L-asparaginase)

(peg-**ASS**-pair-gays)
**Pregnancy Category:** C
Oncaspar **(Rx)**
**Classification:** Antineoplastic, miscellaneous

See also *Antineoplastic Agents.*
**Action/Kinetics:** Pegaspargase is a modification of the enzyme L-asparaginase. L-asparaginase, derived from *Escherichia coli,* is modified by conjugating covalently units of monomethoxypolyethylene glycol (PEG), thus forming the active PEG-L-asparaginase. Leukemic cells are not able to synthesize asparagine due to a lack of the enzyme asparaginase synthetase and are thus dependent on exogenous asparaginase for survival. Rapid depletion of asparagine, due to administration of asparaginase, kills leukemic cells. Normal cells, which can synthesize

their own asparagine, are less affected.

**Uses:** Clients with acute lymphoblastic leukemia who have developed hypersensitivity to the native forms of L-asparaginase. Pegaspargase is used in combination with other antineoplastic drugs including vincristine, methotrexate, cytarabine, daunorubicin, and doxorubicin. Use of pegaspargase as a single agent should only be undertaken when therapy with multiple drugs is determined to be inappropriate for the client.

**Contraindications:** Pancreatitis or history thereof. Clients who have had significant hemorrhagic events associated with prior L-asparaginase therapy. Previous allergic reactions, such as generalized urticaria, bronchospasm, laryngeal edema, hypotension, or other side effects to pegaspargase that are not acceptable. Lactation.

**Special Concerns:** Clients taking pegaspargase are at a higher risk for bleeding problems, especially with simultaneous use of other drugs that have anticoagulant properties (e.g., aspirin, NSAIDs). Safety and efficacy have not been determined in clients from 1 to 21 years of age with known previous hypersensitivity to L-asparaginase.

**Side Effects:** Most commonly hypersensitivity reactions, chemical hepatotoxicity, and coagulopathies. *Allergic reactions:* ***Hypersensitivity reactions*** (acute or delayed), including ***life-threatening anaphylaxis,*** may occur during therapy, especially in clients with known hypersensitivity to other forms of L-asparaginase. Also, skin rashes, erythema, edema, pain, fever, chills, urticaria, dyspnea, ***bronchospasm,*** increased ALT, N&V, malaise, arthralgia, induration, hives, tenderness, swelling, lip edema. *GI:* Pancreatitis (may be severe), abdominal pain, anorexia, diarrhea, constipation, flatulence, GI pain, indigestion, mucositis, mouth tenderness, severe colitis. *Coagulation disorders:* Decreased anticoagulant effect, **DIC,** decreased fibrinogen, increased thromboplastin, increased coagulation time, prolonged PTs, prolonged PTTs, **clinical hemorrhage (may be fatal),** decreased antithrombin III, superficial and deep venous thrombosis, sagittal sinus thrombosis, venous catheter thrombosis, atrial thrombosis, decreased platelet count, purpura, ecchymosis, easy bruisability. *Hepatic:* Jaundice, abnormal liver function test, liver fatty deposits, hepatomegaly, ascites, **liver failure.** *CV:* Hypotension (may be severe), tachycardia, thrombosis, chest pain, hypertension, subacute bacterial endocarditis, edema. *Hematologic:* **Hemolytic anemia,** leukopenia, pancytopenia, thrombocytopenia, **agranulocytosis,** anemia. *CNS:* **Convulsions, status epilepticus,** temporal lobe seizures, headache, paresthesia, mild to severe confusion, disorientation, dizziness, emotional lability, somnolence, **coma,** mental status changes, Parkinson-like syndrome. *Respiratory:* Dyspnea, **bronchospasm,** increased cough, epistaxis, upper respiratory infection. *Dermatologic:* Injection site hypersensitivity, rash, petechial rash, erythema simplex, pruritus, itching, alopecia, fever blister, hand whiteness, fungal changes, nail whiteness and ridging. *GU:* Hematuria, increased urinary frequency, abnormal kidney function, severe hemorrhagic cystitis, **renal failure,** uric acid nephropathy. *Musculoskeletal:* Arthralgia, myalgia, bone pain, joint disorder, diffuse and local musculoskeletal pain, joint stiffness, cramps. *Miscellaneous:* Pain in the extremities, injection site reaction (including pain, swelling, or redness), night sweats, peripheral edema, increased or decreased appetite, excessive thirst, weight loss, face edema, lesional edema, **septic shock, sepsis,** infection, malaise, fatigue, metabolic acidosis.

**Drug Interactions:** Depletion of serum proteins by pegaspargase may ↑ the toxicity of other drugs which are protein bound. ↑ Predisposition to bleeding when used with warfarin, heparin, dipyridamole, aspirin, or NSAIDs. May ↓ the effect of methotrexate.

**Laboratory Test Interferences:** ↑ AST, amylase, lipase, gamma-glutamyltranspeptidase, BUN, creatinine. Bilirubinemia, hyperglycemia, hyperuricemia, hypoglycemia, hypoproteinemia, hyperammonemia, hyponatremia, hypoalbuminemia, proteinuria.

**Dosage** ———————————
- **IM (Preferred), IV**
  *As a component of selected multidrug regimens.*
  **Adults:** 2,500 IU/m$^2$ q 14 days. This dose is also used if the drug is given as a sole agent. **Children with a BSA greater than 0.6 m$^2$:** 2,500 IU/m$^2$ q 14 days. **Children with a BSA less than 0.6 m$^2$:** 82.5 IU/kg q 14 days.

## NURSING CONSIDERATIONS

See also *Nursing Considerations* for *Antineoplastic Agents.*

**Administration/Storage**

1. The preferred route of administration is IM due to a lower risk of hepatotoxicity, coagulopathy, and GI and renal disorders.

2. Do not give if there is any indication it has been frozen; freezing destroys pegaspargase activity.

3. When given IM, do not exceed 2 mL to a single injection site; if more than 2 mL is necessary, use multiple injection sites.

4. When remission is obtained, appropriate maintenance therapy may be instituted.

5. Do not shake; avoid excessive agitation. Do not use if cloudy, if a precipitate is present, or if it's been stored at room temperature for more than 48 hr.

6. Store at 2°C–8°C (36°F–46°F).

7. Use only one dose per vial; do not reenter the vial. Discard any unused portions.

**IV** 8. When used IV, administer over a 1- to 2-hr period in 100 mL of NSS or D5W, through an infusion tube of a solution that is already running.

**Assessment**

1. Document previous therapy and outcome. Use the National Cancer Institute Common Toxic Criteria to grade the severity of any hypersensitivity reaction.

2. Anticipate concomitant administration with other antineoplastic agents.

3. Monitor continuously for anaphylaxis during the first hour of therapy.

4. Assess for early S&S of infection due to immunosuppressive drug effects.

5. IM administration may decrease many of the drug-associated adverse systemic effects.

6. Monitor liver and renal function studies, uric acid, hematologic and coagulation profiles.

**Client/Family Teaching**

1. Report any increased bruising or bleeding, any early S&S of infection.

2. Avoid agents that may increase bleeding tendency (e.g., aspirin or NSAIDs).

3. Any persistent N&V, yellow skin discoloration, or severe abdominal pain should be evaluated immediately.

4. Report any altered mental status or evidence of seizure activity.

5. Drug lowers resistance to infections; avoid situations that may put one at risk (i.e., crowds, persons with infectious diseases, vaccinia).

**Outcomes/Evaluate:** Improved hematologic parameters; remission of acute lymphoblastic leukemia

---

# Pemoline

(**PEM**-oh-leen)

**Pregnancy Category:** B

Cylert, Cylert Chewable **(C-IV) (Rx)**

**Classification:** CNS stimulant

**Action/Kinetics:** Believed to act by dopaminergic mechanisms. Causes a decrease in hyperactivity and a prolonged attention span in children. **Peak serum levels:** 2–4 hr. **Duration:** Up to 8 hr. **t½:** 12 hr. **Steady state:** 2–3 days; beneficial effects may not be noted for 3–4 weeks.

Approximately 50% is bound to plasma protein. Metabolized by the liver, and approximately 50% is excreted unchanged by the kidneys.

**Uses:** Attention-deficit disorders. Due to possible life-threatening hepatic failure, not usually first-line therapy. *Investigational:* Narcolepsy.

**Contraindications:** Hypersensitivity to drug. Tourette's syndrome. Children under 6 years of age.

**Special Concerns:** Safe use during lactation has not been established. Use with caution in impaired renal or kidney function. Chronic use in children may cause growth suppression.

**Side Effects:** *CNS:* Insomnia (most common). Dyskinesia of the face, tongue, lips, and extremities; precipitation of Tourette's syndrome. Mild depression, headache, nystagmus, dizziness, hallucinations, irritability, *seizures.* Exacerbation of behavior disturbances and thought disorders in psychotic children. *GI:* Transient weight loss, gastric upset, nausea. *Miscellaneous:* Skin rash, *hepatic failure.*.

**OD** **Overdose Management:** *Symptoms:* Symptoms of CNS stimulation and sympathomimetic effects including agitation, confusion, delirium, euphoria, headache, muscle twitching, mydriasis, vomiting, hallucinations, flushing, sweating, tachycardia, hyperreflexia, tremors, *hyperpyrexia,* hypertension, *seizures (may be followed by coma). Treatment:* Reduce external stimuli. If symptoms are not severe, induce vomiting or undertake gastric lavage. Chlorpromazine can be used to decrease the CNS stimulation and sympathomimetic effects.

**Laboratory Test Interferences:** ↑ AST, ALT, serum LDH.

**Dosage**

- **Tablets, Chewable Tablets**
  *Attention-deficit disorders.*

**Children, 6 years and older, initial:** 37.5 mg/day as a single dose in the morning; increase at 1-week intervals by 18.75 mg until desired response is attained up to maximum of 112.5 mg/day. **Usual maintenance:** 56.25–75 mg/day.

*Narcolepsy.*
**Adults:** 50–200 mg/day in two divided doses.

## NURSING CONSIDERATIONS
### Administration/Storage
1. Administer as a single dose in the morning.
2. Interrupt treatment once or twice annually to determine whether behavioral symptoms still necessitate drug therapy.
### Assessment
1. Document indications for therapy, type, onset, and duration of symptoms; describe clinical presentation.
2. List other agents prescribed and the outcome.
### Client/Family Teaching
1. Administer early in the morning to minimize insomnia.
2. Do not perform activities that require mental alertness until drug effects are realized.
3. Avoid excessive consumption of caffeine-containing products.
4. Advise school health department of medication regimen.
5. Measure height every month, and weigh child twice a week. Graph all measurements and bring to each visit. Report any weight loss or failure to grow.
6. Continue therapy; behavioral changes take 3–4 weeks to occur.
7. Instruct when to interrupt drug administration, and to observe and record behavior without the medication, to determine whether therapy should be resumed.
8. Stress importance of bringing the child in periodically for LFTs to assess for toxicity.
9. Identify signs of overdosage, such as agitation, restlessness, hallucinations, and tachycardia; withhold drug, protect the child, and report immediately.
### Outcomes/Evaluate:
Improved attention span; ↓ hyperactivity with ability to sit quietly and concentrate

# Penbutolol sulfate
(pen-**BYOU**-toe-lohl)
**Pregnancy Category:** C
Levatol **(Rx)**
**Classification:** Beta-adrenergic blocking agent

See also *Beta-Adrenergic Blocking Agents.*
**Action/Kinetics:** Has both beta-1- and beta-2-receptor blocking activity. It has no membrane-stabilizing activity but does possess minimal intrinsic sympathomimetic activity. High lipid solubility. **t½:** 5 hr. 80%–98% protein bound. Metabolized in the liver and excreted through the urine.
**Uses:** Mild to moderate arterial hypertension.
**Contraindications:** Bronchial asthma or bronchospasms, including severe COPD.
**Special Concerns:** Dosage has not been established in children. Geriatric clients may manifest increased or decreased sensitivity to the usual adult dose.

### Dosage
• **Tablets**
*Hypertension.*
**Initial:** 20 mg/day either alone or with other antihypertensive agents. **Maintenance:** Same as initial dose. Doses greater than 40 mg/day do not result in a greater antihypertensive effect.

## NURSING CONSIDERATIONS

See also *Nursing Considerations* for *Antihypertensive Agents.*
**Administration/Storage:** Doses of 10 mg/day are effective but full effects are not evident for 4–6 weeks. The full effect of a 20- to 40-mg dose may not be observed for 2 weeks.
**Client/Family Teaching**
1. May cause postural hypotension; to avoid, rise slowly from a sitting or lying position.
2. Take only as prescribed; full effects may not be realized for a month or more.
3. May cause an increased sensitivity to cold; dress appropriately.

**Outcomes/Evaluate:** ↓ BP

# Penciclovir
(pen-**SIGH**-kloh-veer)
**Pregnancy Category:** B
Denavir **(Rx)**
**Classification:** Antiviral drug

See also Antiviral Drugs.
**Action/Kinetics:** Active against herpes simplex virus (HSVs), including HSV-1 and HSV-2. In infected cells, viral thymidine kinase phosphorylates penciclovir to a monophosphate form which then is converted to penciclovir triphosphate by cellular kinases. Penciclovir triphosphate inhibits HSV polymerase competitively with deoxyguanosine triphosphate which inhibits herpes viral DNA synthesis and replication. Not absorbed through the skin.
**Uses:** Treatment of recurrent herpes labialis (cold sores) in adults.
**Contraindications:** Lactation. Application of the drug to mucous membranes.
**Special Concerns:** Use with caution if applied around the eyes due to the possibility of irritation. The effect of the drug in immunocompromised clients has not been determined. Safety and efficacy have not been determined in children.
**Side Effects:** *Dermatologic:* Reaction at the site of application, hypesthesia, local anesthesia, erythematous rash, mild erythema. *Miscellaneous:* Headache, taste perversion.

**Dosage** ─────────────
• **Cream (10 mg/g)**
*Cold sores.*
Apply q 2 hr while awake for 4 days.

## NURSING CONSIDERATIONS

See also *Nursing Considerations* for *Antiviral Drugs.*
**Administration/Storage**
1. Start treatment as soon as possible during the prodrome or when lesions appear.
2. Use only on the lips and face.

**Assessment:** Document onset, location, description, and extent of lesions. Note frequency of occurrence and any triggers or prodrome.
**Client/Family Teaching**
1. Apply q 2 hr while awake for 4 days at the first symptoms of a cold sore.
2. Avoid contact with mucous membranes; apply to lips and face only.
3. Use sunscreens and lip balms with a sunscreen when sun exposed to prevent recurrence and to diminish intensity of outbreaks.
4. Report if lesions do not improve or if a foul odor or purulent drainage appears.
**Outcomes/Evaluate:** ↓ Intensity/pain; clearing of herpes labialis lesions

# Penicillamine
(pen-ih-**SILL**-ah-meen)
Cuprimine, Depen **(Rx)**
**Classification:** Antirheumatic, heavy metal antagonist, to treat cystinuria

**Action/Kinetics:** A chelating agent for mercury, lead, iron, and copper; forms soluble complexes, thus decreasing toxic levels of the metal (e.g., copper in Wilson's disease). Anti-inflammatory activity may be due to its ability to inhibit T-lymphocyte function and therefore decrease cell-mediated immune response. It may also protect lymphocytes from hydrogen peroxide generated at the site of inflammation by inhibiting release of lysosomal enzymes and oxygen radicals. Beneficial effects may not be seen for 2 to 3 months when used for rheumatoid arthritis. In cystinuria, is able to reduce excess cystine excretion, probably by disulfide interchange between penicillamine and cystine. This results in penicillamine-cysteine disulfide, which is a complex that is more soluble than cystine and is thus readily excreted. Well absorbed from the GI tract and excreted in urine. Food decreases the absorption of penicillamine over 50%. **Peak plasma lev-**

P

**els:** 1–3 hr. About 80% is bound to plasma albumin. **t½:** Approximately 2 hr. Metabolites are excreted through the urine.

**Uses:** Wilson's disease, cystinuria, and rheumatoid arthritis—severe active disease unresponsive to conventional therapy. Heavy metal antagonist. *Investigational:* Primary biliary cirrhosis. Scleroderma.

**Contraindications:** Pregnancy, lactation, penicillinase-related aplastic anemia or agranulocytosis, hypersensitivity to drug. Clients allergic to penicillin may cross-react with penicillamine. Renal insufficiency or history thereof.

**Special Concerns:** The use of penicillamine for juvenile rheumatoid arthritis has not been established. Clients older than 65 years may be at greater risk of developing hematologic side effects.

**Side Effects:** This drug manifests a large number of potentially serious side effects. Clients should be carefully monitored. *GI:* Altered taste perception (common), N&V, diarrhea, anorexia, GI pain, stomatitis, oral ulcerations, reactivation of peptic ulcer, glossitis, cheilosis, colitis, gingivostomatitis (rare). *CNS:* Tinnitus, myasthenia gravis, peripheral sensory and motor neuropathies (with or without muscle weakness), reversible optic neuritis, polyradiculopathy (rare). *Hematologic:* Thrombocytopenia, leukopenia, *agranulocytosis, aplastic anemia,* eosinophilia, monocytosis, red cell aplasia, thrombocytopenia, *hemolytic anemia,* leukocytosis, thrombocytosis. *Renal:* Proteinuria, hematuria, nephrotic syndrome, *Goodpasture's syndrome* (a severe and ultimately fatal glomerulonephritis). *Allergic:* Rashes (common), lupus-like syndrome, drug fever, pruritus, pemphigoid-type symptoms (e.g., bullous lesions), drug fever, arthralgia, lymphadenopathy, dermatoses, urticaria, thyroiditis, hypoglycemia, migratory polyarthralgia, polymyositis, allergic alveolitis. *Respiratory:* Obliterative bronchiolitis, pulmonary fibrosis, pneumonitis, bronchial asthma, interstitial pneumonitis. *Dermatologic:* Increased skin friability, excessive skin wrinkling, development of small white papules at venipuncture and surgical sites, alopecia or falling hair, lichen planus, dermatomyositis, nail disorders, *toxic epidermal necrolysis,* cutaneous macular atrophy. *Hepatic:* Pancreatitis, hepatic dysfunction, intrahepatic cholestasis, toxic hepatitis (rare). *Other:* Thrombophlebitis, hyperpyrexia, polymyositis, mammary hyperplasia, renal vasculitis (may be fatal), hot flashes, lupus erythematosus–like syndrome.

**Drug Interactions**

*Antacids* / ↓ Effect of penicillamine due to ↓ absorption from GI tract

*Antimalarial drugs* / ↑ Risk of blood dyscrasias and adverse renal effects

*Cytotoxic drugs* / ↑ Risk of blood dyscrasias and adverse renal effects

*Digoxin* / Penicillamine ↓ effect of digoxin

*Gold therapy* / ↑ Risk of blood dyscrasias and adverse renal effects

*Iron salts* / ↓ Effect of penicillamine due to ↓ absorption from GI tract

**Laboratory Test Interferences:** ↑ Serum alkaline phosphatase, LDH. Positive thymol turbidity test and cephalin flocculation test.

**Dosage**

- **Capsules, Tablets**

    *Rheumatoid arthritis.*

**Adults, individualized, initial:** 125–250 mg/day. Dosage may be increased at 1- to 3-month intervals by 125- to 250-mg increments until adequate response is attained. **Maximum:** 500–750 mg/day. Up to 500 mg/day can be given as a single dose; higher dosages should be divided. **Maintenance, individualized. Range:** 500–750 mg/day. If the client is in remission for 6 or more months, a gradual stepwise decrease in dose of 125 or 250 mg/day at about 3-month intervals can be attempted.

    *Wilson's disease.*

Dosage is usually calculated on the basis of the urinary excretion of copper. One gram of penicillamine promotes excretion of 2 mg of copper. **Adults and adolescents, usual, initial:** 250 mg q.i.d. Dosage may have to be increased to 2 g/day. A further increase does not produce additional excretion. **Pediatric, 6 months—young children:** 250 mg as a single dose given in fruit juice.

*Antidote for heavy metals.*
**Adults:** 0.5–1.5 g/day for 1–2 months; **pediatric:** 30–40 mg/kg/day (600–750 mg/m²/day) for 1–6 months.

*Cystinuria.*
Individualized and based on excretion rate of cystine (100–200 mg/day in clients with no history of stones, below 100 mg with clients with history of stones or pain). Initiate at low dosage (250 mg/day) and increase gradually to minimum effective dosage. **Adult, usual:** 2 g/day (range: 1–4 g/day); **pediatric:** 7.5 mg/kg q.i.d. If divided in fewer than four doses, give larger dose at night.

*Primary biliary cirrhosis.*
**Adults:** 600–900 mg/day.

## NURSING CONSIDERATIONS
### Administration/Storage
1. If unable to tolerate dosage for cystinuria, the bedtime dosage should be larger and should be continued.
2. Administer the contents of the capsule in 15–30 mL of chilled juice or pureed fruit if unable to swallow capsules or tablets.
3. When treating rheumatoid arthritis, discontinue if doses up to 1.5 g/day for 2–3 months do not produce improvement.
4. Alternative dosage forms may be prepared if needed. An elixir containing 50 mg/mL may be prepared by dissolving the contents of 48 capsules in 100 mL of water. This is then filtered, and 100 mL of cherry syrup and 30 mL of alcohol stirred in. The volume is then brought up to 240 mL with water. The preparation is shaken well and stored in the refrigerator. Suppositores (750 mg) may be prepared by melting 51 g of cocoa butter and dissolving the contents of 150 capsules in the cocoa butter; the mixture is poured into a prelubricated suppository mold and then frozen and stored in a refrigerator.

### Assessment
1. Determine indications for therapy, presenting symptoms, other therapies prescribed and the outcome.
2. Note if taking any medication with which penicillamine will interact unfavorably. Also, it impedes absorption of many drugs.
3. Assess hearing to detect evidence of hearing loss.
4. Document CNS assessment and neurologic status.
5. With arthritis, assess joints for pain, stiffness, soreness, swelling, and ↓ ROM.
6. Test for pregnancy; drug can cause fetal damage.
7. Monitor CBC, LFTs, and urinalysis.

### Interventions
1. Note complaints of N&V or diarrhea. Check for any alterations in taste; monitor weight and I&O.
2. Inspect mucosal surfaces at regular intervals. If ulcers appear and are severe or persistent, may need to reduce drug dose as it may interfere with wound healing.
3. Routinely monitor CBC. If WBC falls below 3,500/mm³ or the platelet count falls below 100,000/mm³, withhold drug and report. If counts are low for three successive lab tests, a temporary interruption of therapy is indicated.
4. Monitor LFTs; report jaundice or other signs of hepatic dysfunction.
5. White papules appearing at the site of venipuncture or at surgical sites may indicate sensitivity to penicillamine or the presence of infection.
6. If to undergo surgery, anticipate dosage reduction to 250 mg/day until wound healing is complete.
7. Penicillamine increases the body's need for pyridoxine. Give pyridoxine (25 mg/day) daily.

**P**

---

8. A positive ANA test indicates client may develop a lupus-like syndrome in the future. The drug need not be discontinued.

9. If cystinuria occurs, encourage a high fluid intake throughout the day and at bedtime.

10. For Wilson's disease, avoid multivitamin preparations containing copper.

**Client/Family Teaching**

1. Give on an empty stomach 1 hr before or 2 hr after meals. Also wait 1 hr after ingestion of any other food, milk, or drug.

2. Take temperature nightly during the first few months of therapy. A fever may indicate a hypersensitivity reaction.

3. Report any evidence of fever, sore throat, chills, bruising, or bleeding; early symptoms of granulocytopenia.

4. If stomatitis occurs, report immediately and stop drug. Practice regular oral hygiene such as brushing teeth with a soft toothbrush, flossing daily, and using mouth rinses free of alcohol.

5. A loss of taste perception or a metallic taste may develop; relates to zinc chelation and may last for 2 months or more.

6. If to receive an oral iron preparation, at least 2 hr should elapse between ingestion of penicillamine and the dose of therapeutic iron. Iron decreases the cupruretic effects of penicillamine.

7. Skin tends to become friable and susceptible to injury; avoid activities that could injure the skin. Advise elderly clients to avoid excessive pressure on the shoulders, elbows, knees, toes, and buttocks.

8. Report cloudy urine or urine that is smoky brown (signs of proteinuria and hematuria).

9. Practice reliable birth control; report missed menstrual period or other symptoms of pregnancy.

10. With Wilson's disease:

• Eat a diet low in copper. Exclude foods such as chocolate, nuts, shellfish, mushrooms, liver, molasses, broccoli, and copper-enriched cereals.

• Use distilled or demineralized water if the drinking water contains more than 0.1 mg/L copper.

• Unless taking iron supplements, take sulfurated potash or Carbo-Resin with meals to minimize the absorption of copper.

• It may take 1–3 months for neurologic improvements to occur. Therefore, continue the therapy even if no improvements seem evident.

• Check any vitamin preparations being used to ensure that they do not contain copper.

11. If cystinuria occurs, advise the following:

• Drink large amounts of fluid to prevent the formation of renal calculi. Drink 500 mL of fluid at bedtime and another pint during the night, when the urine tends to be the most concentrated and most acidic. The greater the fluid intake, the lower the required dose of penicillamine.

• Measure specific gravity and determine pH. The urine specific gravity should be maintained at less than 1.010 and the pH maintained at 7.5–8.0.

• Obtain yearly X ray of the kidneys to detect the presence of renal calculi.

• Eat a diet low in methionine, a major precursor of cystine. Exclude foods high in cystine such as rich meat, soups and broths, milk, eggs, cheeses, and peas.

• If client is pregnant or is a child, a diet low in methionine is also low in calcium; consider calcium supplementation.

12. With rheumatoid arthritis, continue using other therapies and medications to achieve relief from symptoms because penicillamine may take 4–6 months to have a therapeutic effect. As improvement begins, analgesic drugs and NSAIDs may be slowly discontinued.

**Outcomes/Evaluate**

• ↑ Urinary excretion of copper

• ↓ Cystine excretion and prevention of renal calculi in cystinuria

• ↓ Joint pain, swelling, inflammation, and stiffness with ↑ mobility

———*COMBINATION DRUG*———
# Penicillin G benzathine and Procaine combined
(pen-ih-**SILL**-in, **BEN**-zah-theen, **PROH**-kain)
**Pregnancy Category:** B
Bicillin C-R, Bicillin C-R 900/300 **(Rx)**
**Classification:** Antibiotic, penicillin

See also *Anti-Infectives* and *Penicillins*.

**Content:** The injection contains the following: *300,000 units/dose:* 150,000 units each of penicillin G benzathine and penicillin G procaine. *600,000 units/dose:* 300,000 units each of penicillin G benzathine and penicillin G procaine. *1,200,000 units/dose:* 600,000 units each of penicillin G benzathine and penicillin G procaine. *2,400,000 units/dose:* 1,200,000 units each of penicillin G benzathine and penicillin G procaine. *Injection, 900/300 per dose:* 900,000 units of penicillin G benzathine and 300,000 units of penicillin G procaine.

**Uses:** Streptococcal infections (A, C, G, H, L, and M) without bacteremia, of the upper respiratory tract, skin, and soft tissues. Scarlet fever, erysipelas, pneumococcal infections, and otitis media.

**Contraindications:** Use to treat syphilis, gonorrhea, yaws, bejel, and pinta.

**Dosage** ———
• **IM Only**
*Streptococcal infections.*
**Adults and children over 27 kg:** 2,400,000 units, given at a single session using multiple injection sites or, alternatively, in divided doses on days 1 and 3; **children 13.5–27 kg:** 900,000–1,200,000 units; **infants and children under 13.5 kg:** 600,000 units.
*Pneumococcal infections, except meningitis.*
**Adults:** 1,200,000 units; **pediatric:** 600,000 units. Give q 2–3 days until temperature is normal for 48 hr.

## NURSING CONSIDERATIONS
See also *Nursing Considerations* for *Penicillins*.
**Administration/Storage**
1. For adults, administer by deep IM injection in the upper outer quadrant of the buttock. For infants and children, use the midlateral aspect of the thigh.
2. Rotate injection sites for repeated doses.
**Outcomes/Evaluate:** Resolution of infection

# Penicillin G benzathine, parenteral
(pen-ih-**SILL**-in, **BEN**-zah-theen)
**Pregnancy Category:** B
Bicillin 1200 L-A ✿, Bicillin L-A, Megacillin Suspension ✿, Permapen **(Rx)**
**Classification:** Antibiotic, penicillin

See also *Anti-Infectives* and *Penicillins*.
**Action/Kinetics:** Penicillin G is neither penicillinase resistant nor acid stable. The product is a long-acting (repository) form of penicillin in an aqueous vehicle; it is administered as a sterile suspension. **Peak plasma levels: IM** 0.03–0.05 unit/mL.
**Uses:** Most gram-positive (streptococci, staphylococci, pneumococci) and some gram-negative (gonococci, meningococci) organisms. Syphilis. Prophylaxis of glomerulonephritis and rheumatic fever. Surgical infections, secondary infections following tooth extraction, tonsillectomy.

**Dosage** ———
• **Parenteral Suspension (IM Only)**
*Upper respiratory tract infections, erysipeloid, yaws.*
**Adults:** 1,200,000 units as a single dose; **older children:** 900,000 units as a single dose; **children under 27 kg:** 300,000–600,000 units as a single dose; **neonates:** 50,000 units/kg as a single dose.
*Early syphilis.*

**P**

**Adults:** 2,400,000 units as a single dose.

*Late syphilis.*
**Adults:** 2,400,000 units q 7 days for 3 weeks.

*Neurosyphilis.*
**Adults:** Penicillin G, 12,000,000–24,000,000 units IV/day for 10–14 days followed by penicillin G benzathine, 2,400,000 units IM q week for 3 weeks.

*Congenital syphilis, older children.*
50,000 units/kg IM (up to adult dose of 2,400,000 units).

*Prophylaxis of rheumatic fever.*
**Adults and children over 27.3 kg:** 1,200,000 units/ q 4 weeks; **children and infants less than 27.3 kg:** 50,000 units/kg as a single dose.

## NURSING CONSIDERATIONS

See also *Nursing Considerations* for *Penicillins.*

**Administration/Storage**
1. Shake multiple-dose vial vigorously before withdrawing the desired dose because medication tends to clump on standing. Check that all medication is dissolved and that no residue is present at bottom of bottle.
2. Use a 20-gauge needle and do not allow medication to remain in the syringe and needle for long periods of time before administration because the needle may become plugged and the syringe "frozen."
3. Inject slowly and steadily into the muscle and *do not massage* injection site.
4. For adults, use the upper outer quadrant of the buttock; for infants and small children, the midlateral aspect of the thigh should be used. Do not administer in the gluteal region in children less than 2 years of age.
5. *Do not administer IV.* Before injection of medication, aspirate needle to ascertain that needle is not in a vein.
6. Rotate and chart site of injections.
7. Divide between two injection sites if dose is large or available muscle mass is small.

**Client/Family Teaching**
1. Must return for repository penicillin injections.
2. Obtain sexual counseling. Sexual partner should also undergo treatment.

**Outcomes/Evaluate**
• Prophylaxis of poststreptococcal rheumatic fever
• Resolution of infection

# Penicillin G potassium for injection
(pen-ih-**SILL**-in)
**Pregnancy Category:** B
Pfizerpen **(Rx)**

# Penicillin G (Aqueous) sodium for injection
(pen-ih-**SILL**-in )
**Pregnancy Category:** B
**(Rx)**
**Classification:** Antibiotic, penicillin

See also *Anti-Infectives* and *Penicillins.*

**Action/Kinetics:** The low cost still makes penicillin G the first choice for treatment of many infections. Rapid onset makes it especially suitable for fulminating infections. Is neither penicillinase resistant nor acid stable. **Peak plasma levels: IM or SC,** 6–20 units/mL after 15–30 min **t½:** 30 min.

**Uses:** Streptococci of groups A, C, G, H, L, and M are sensitive to penicillin G. High serum levels are effective against streptococci of the D group.

**Additional Side Effects:** Rapid IV administration may cause hyperkalemia and cardiac arrhythmias. Renal damage occurs rarely.

**Dosage**
• **Penicillin G Potassium and Sodium Injections (IM, Continuous IV Infusion)**
*Streptococcal infections.*
**Adults:** 300,000–30 million units/day, depending on the use. **Pediatric:** 100,000–250,000 units/kg/day (given in divided doses q 4 hr). **Infants over 7 days of age weighing**

**more than 2 kg:** 100,000 units/kg/day (given in divided doses q 6 hr). **Infants over 7 days of age weighing less than 2 kg:** 75,000 units/day (given in divided doses q 8 hr). **Infants less than 7 days of age weighing more than 2 kg:** 50,000 units/kg/day (given in divided doses q 8 hr). **Infants less than 7 days of age weighing less than 2 kg:** 50,000 units/kg/day (given in divided doses q 12 hr).

*Meningitis.*
**Infants over 7 days of age weighing more than 2 kg:** 200,000 units/kg. **Infants over 7 days of age weighing less than 2 kg:** 150,000 units/kg. **Infants less than 7 days of age weighing more than 2 kg:** 150,000 units/kg. **Infants less than 7 days of age weighing less than 2 kg:** 100,000 units/kg/day for 14 days.

*Gram-negative bacillary bacteremia.*
20 million or more units daily.

*Anthrax.*
A minimum of 5 million units/day (up to 12–20 million units have been used).

*Clostridial infections.*
20 million units/day used with an antitoxin.

*Actinomycosis, cervicofacial.*
1–6 million units/day; *thoracic and abdominal disease:* **initial,** 12–20 million units/day IV for 6 weeks followed by penicillin V, PO, 500 mg q.i.d. for 2–3 months.

*Rat-bite fever, Haverhill fever.*
12–20 million units/day for 3–4 weeks.

*Endocarditis due to* Listeria.
15–20 million units/day for 4 weeks (in adults).

*Endocarditis due to* Erysipelothrix rhusiopathiae.
12–20 million units/day for 4–6 weeks.

*Meningitis due to* Listeria.
15–20 million units/day for 2 weeks (in adults).

*Pasteurella infections causing bacteremia and meningitis.*
4–6 million units/day for 2 weeks.

*Severe fusospirochetal infections of the oropharynx, lower respiratory tract, and genital area.*
5–10 million units/day.

*Pneumococcal infections causing empyema.*
5–24 million units/day in divided doses q 4–6 hr.

*Pneumococcal infections causing meningitis.*
20–24 million units/day for 14 days.

*Pneumococcal infections causing endocarditis, pericarditis, peritonitis, suppurative arthritis, osteomyelitis, mastoiditis.*
12–20 million units/day for 2–4 weeks.

*Adjunct with antitoxic to prevent diphtheria.*
2–3 million units/day in divided doses for 10–12 days.

*Meningococcal meningitis.*
20–30 million units/day by continuous IV drip for 14 days (or until there is no fever for 7 days) or 200,000–300,000 units/kg/day q 2–4 hr in divided doses for a total of 24 doses.

*Neurosyphilis.*
12–24 million units/day for 10–14 days (can be followed by benzathine penicillin G, 2.4 million units IM weekly for 3 weeks).

*Congenital syphilis in newborns.*
50,000 units/kg/day (IV) in divided doses q 8–12 hr for 10–14 days; *in infants after newborn period:* 50,000 units/kg q 4–6 hr for 10–14 days.

*Gonococcal infections in infants.*
100,000 units/kg/day in two equal doses.

• **Oral Solution, Tablets**
*General use.*
**Adults:** 200,000–500,000 units q 6–8 hr; **pediatric under 12 years of age:** 25,000–90,000 units/kg/day in three to six divided doses. *NOTE:* 250 mg Penicillin G potassium, PO, is equivalent to 400,000 units.

*Upper respiratory tract infections due to streptococci.*
200,000–250,000 units q 6–8 hr for 10 days (for severe infections, use

400,000–500,000 units q 8 hr for 10 days or 800,000 units q 12 hr).

*Infections of the respiratory tract due to pneumococci.*
400,000–500,000 units q 6 hr until client has no fever for 48 hr.

*Infections of the skin and skin structures due to staphylococci.*
200,000–500,000 units q 6–8 hr until cured.

*Infections of the oropharynx due to fusospirochetes.*
400,000–500,000 units q 6–8 hr.

*Prophylaxis of rheumatic fever and/or chorea.*
200,000–250,000 units b.i.d. chronically.

## NURSING CONSIDERATIONS

See also *Nursing Considerations* for *Penicillins.*

### Administration/Storage
1. Take PO products at least 1 hr before or 2 hr after meals.
2. IM administration is preferred; discomfort is minimized by using solutions of up to 100,000 units/mL.
3. Use 1%–2% lidocaine solution as diluent for IM (if ordered) to lessen pain at injection site. Do not use procaine as diluent for aqueous penicillin.
4. Electrolyte contents: Penicillin G Sodium (1 mg =1,600 units) contains 2 mEq sodium/1 million units; Penicillin G Potassium (1 mg =1,600 units) contains 1.7 mEq potassium and 0.3 mEq sodium/1 million units.
**IV** 5. Use sterile water, isotonic saline USP, or 5% D5W and mix with recommended volume for desired strength.
6. For intermittent IV administration (q 6 hr) reconstitute with 100 mL of dextrose or saline solution and infuse over 1 hr.
7. Loosen powder by shaking bottle before adding diluent.
8. Hold vial horizontally and rotate slowly while directing the stream of the diluent against the wall of the vial.
9. Shake vigorously after addition of diluent.
10. Solutions may be stored at room temperature for 24 hr or in refrigerator for 1 week. Discard remaining solution.
11. The following drugs should *not* be mixed with penicillin during IV administration: aminophylline, amphotericin B, ascorbic acid, chlorpheniramine, chlorpromazine, gentamicin, heparin, hydroxyzine, lincomycin, metaraminol, novobiocin, oxytetracycline, phenylephrine, phenytoin, polymyxin B, prochlorperazine, promazine, promethazine, sodium bicarbonate, sodium salts of barbiturates, sulfadiazine, tetracycline, tromethamine, vancomycin, vitamin B complex.

### Assessment
1. Document indications for therapy, type, onset, and duration of symptoms.
2. Order drug by specifying sodium or potassium salt.
3. Monitor I&O. Dehydration decreases drug excretion and may raise blood level of penicillin G to dangerously high levels causing kidney damage. GI disturbances may lead to dehydration.
4. Very high doses (>20 million units) may cause seizures or platelet dysfunction, especially with impaired renal function.
5. Obtain baseline CBC, liver and renal function studies and cultures.

### Outcomes/Evaluate
• Symptomatic improvement; negative culture reports
• Prophylaxis of rheumatic fever or chorea

# Penicillin G Procaine Suspension, Sterile
(pen-ih-**SILL**-in, **PROH**-caine)
**Pregnancy Category:** B
Ayercillin ✜, Crysticillin 300 A.S. and 600 A.S., Wycillin **(Rx)**
**Classification:** Antibiotic, penicillin

See also *Anti-Infectives* and *Penicillins.*

**Action/Kinetics:** Long-acting (repository) form in aqueous or oily vehicle. Destroyed by penicillinase. Because of slow onset, a soluble penicillin is often administered concomitantly for fulminating infections.

**Uses:** Penicillin-sensitive staphylococci, pneumococci, streptococci, and bacterial endocarditis (for *Streptococcus viridans* and *S. bovis* infections). Gonorrhea, all stages of syphilis. *Prophylaxis:* Rheumatic fever, pre- and postsurgery. Diphtheria, anthrax, fusospirochetosis (Vincent's infection), erysipeloid, rat-bite fever.

**Dosage**

• **IM Only**

*Pneumococccal, staphylococcal, streptococcal infections; erysipeloid, rat-bite fever, anthrax, fusospirochetosis.*

**Adults, usual:** 600,000–1,200,000 units/day for 10–14 days. **Newborns, usual:** 50,000 units/kg/day in a single dose.

*Bacterial endocarditis.*

**Adults:** 1,200,000 units penicillin G procaine q.i.d. for 2–4 weeks with streptomycin, 500 mg b.i.d. for the first 14 days.

*Diphtheria carrier state.*

300,000 units/day for 10 days.

*Diphtheria, adjunct with antitoxin.*

300,000–600,000 units/day.

*Gonococcal infections.*

4.8 million units divided into at least two doses and given with 1 g PO probenecid (given 30 min before the injections).

*Neurosyphilis.*

2.4 million units/day for 10 days (given at two sites) with probenecid 500 mg PO q.i.d.; **then,** benzathine penicillin G, 2.4 million units/week for 3 weeks.

*Congenital syphilis in infants, symptomatic and asymptomatic.*

50,000 units/kg/day for 10–14 days.

*Syphilis: primary, secondary, latent with negative spinal fluid.*

**Adults and children over 12 years:** 600,000 units/day for 8 days (total of 4.8 million units).

## NURSING CONSIDERATIONS

See also *Nursing Considerations* for *Penicillins.*

**Administration/Storage**

1. Note on package whether medication is to be refrigerated, since some brands require this to maintain stability.

2. Shake multiple-dose vial thoroughly to ensure uniform suspension before injection. If the medication is clumped at the bottom of the vial, shake until clump dissolves.

3. Use a 20-gauge needle and aspirate immediately after withdrawing medication from the vial; otherwise needle may become clogged and syringe may "freeze."

4. Administer into two sites if dose is large or available muscle mass is small.

5. Aspirate to check that the needle is not in a vein.

6. Inject deep into muscle at a slow rate.

7. Do not massage after injection.

8. Rotate and chart injection sites.

9. For IM use only.

**Assessment:** Document indications for therapy, onset of symptoms, any other treatments prescribed, and pretreatment cultures.

**Client/Family Teaching**

1. Report a wheal or other skin reactions at injection site that may indicate reaction to procaine as well as to penicillin.

2. Obtain sexual counseling; have sexual partner also undergo treatment.

3. With a history of rheumatic fever or congenital heart disease, must use antibiotic prophylaxis prior to any invasive medical or dental procedure.

**Outcomes/Evaluate:** Resolution of infection; infection prophylaxis

# Penicillin V potassium (Phenoxymethyl-penicillin potassium)

(pen-ih-**SILL**-in)

**Pregnancy Category:** B

Apo-Pen-VK ✽, Beepen-VK, Betapen-VK, Ledercillin VK, Nadopen-V

---

✹, Novo-Pen-VK ✹, Nu-Pen-VK ✹, Penicillin VK, Pen-V, Pen-Vee K, PVF K ✹, Robicillin VK, V-Cillin K, Veetids 125, 250, and 500 **(Rx)**
**Classification:** Antibiotic, penicillin

See also *Anti-Infectives* and *Penicillins*.

**Action/Kinetics:** Related closely to penicillin G. Products are not penicillinase resistant but are acid stable and resist inactivation by gastric secretions. Well absorbed from the GI tract and not affected by foods. **Peak plasma levels:** Penicillin V, **PO:** 2.7 mcg/mL after 30–60 min; penicillin V potassium, **PO:** 1–9 mcg/mL after 30–60 min. **t½:** 30 min. Periodic blood counts and renal function tests are indicated during long-term usage.

**Uses:** Penicillin-sensitive staphylococci, pneumococci, streptococci, gonococci. Vincent's infection of the oropharynx. Lyme disease. *Prophylaxis:* Rheumatic fever, chorea, bacterial endocarditis, pre- and postsurgery. Should *not* be used as prophylaxis for GU instrumentation or surgery, sigmoidoscopy, or childbirth or during the acute stage of severe pneumonia, bacteremia, arthritis, empyema, pericarditis, and meningitis. Penicillin G, IV, should be used for treating neurologic complications due to Lyme disease.

**Special Concerns:** More and more strains of staphylococci are resistant to penicillin V, necessitating culture and sensitivity studies.

**Additional Drug Interactions**
*Contraceptives, oral* / ↓ Effectiveness of oral contraceptives
*Neomycin, oral* / ↓ Absorption of penicillin V

**Dosage** ⎯⎯⎯⎯⎯⎯⎯⎯
• **Oral Solution, Tablets**
*Streptococcal infections.*
**Adults and children over 12 years:** 125–250 mg q 6–8 hr for 10 days. **Children, usual:** 25–50 mg/kg/day in divided doses q 6–8 hr.
*Pneumococcal or staphylococcal infections, fusospirochetosis of oropharynx.*

**Adults and children over 12 years:** 250–500 mg q 6–8 hr.
*Prophylaxis of rheumatic fever/chorea.*
125–250 mg b.i.d.
*Prophylaxis of bacterial endocarditis.*
**Adults and children over 27 kg:** 2 g 30–60 min prior to procedure; **then,** 1 g q 6 hr. **Pediatric:** 1 g 30–60 min prior to procedure; **then,** 500 mg/ q 6 hr.
*Anaerobic infections.*
250 mg q.i.d. See also *Penicillin G, Procaine, Aqueous, Sterile.*
*Prophylaxis of septicemia caused by* Staphylococcus pneumoniae in children with sickle cell anemia.
125 mg b.i.d.
*Streptococcal pharyngitis in children.*
250 mg b.i.d. for 10 days.
*Streptococcal otitis media and sinusitis.*
250–500 mg q 6 hr for 14 days.
*Lyme disease.*
250–500 mg q.i.d. for 10–20 days (for children less than 2 years of age, 50 mg/kg/day in four divided doses for 10–20 days).
*NOTE:* 250 mg penicillin V is equivalent to 400,000 units.

## NURSING CONSIDERATIONS

See also *Nursing Considerations* for *Penicillins.*
**Administration/Storage**
1. Administer without regard to meals. Blood levels may be slightly higher when administered on an empty stomach.
2. Do not administer at the same time as neomycin because malabsorption of penicillin V may occur.
**Client/Family Teaching**
1. Clients with a history of rheumatic fever or congenital heart disease need to use and understand the importance of antibiotic prophylaxis prior to any invasive medical or dental procedure.
2. Report if throat and/or ear symptoms do not improve after 48 hr of therapy; may need to reevaluate and alter therapy.

3. With oral administration, if a reaction is going to occur, you usually see it after the second dose. Seek medical intervention immediately if respiratory distress or skin wheals appear.

4. Use an additional nonhormonal form of birth control if taking oral contraceptives because their effectiveness may be diminished.

**Outcomes/Evaluate**
• Symptomatic improvement
• Negative lab C&S reports
• Endocarditis/rheumatic fever prophylaxis

# Pentamidine isethionate
(pen-**TAM**-ih-deen)
**Pregnancy Category:** C
NebuPent, Pentacarinate ✦, Pentam (Rx)
**Classification:** Antibiotic, miscellaneous (antiprotozoal)

**Action/Kinetics:** Inhibits synthesis of DNA, RNA, phospholipids, and proteins, thereby interfering with cell metabolism. It may interfere also with folate transformation. About one-third of the dose may be excreted unchanged in the urine. Plasma levels following inhalation are significantly lower than after a comparable IV dose.

**Uses: Parenteral:** Pneumonia caused by *Pneumocystis carinii*. **Inhalation:** Prophylaxis of *P. carinii* in high-risk HIV-infected clients defined by one or both of the following: (a) a history of one or more cases of pneumonia caused by *P. carinii* and/or (b) a peripheral CD4+ lymphocyte count less than 200/mm³. *Investigational:* Trypanosomiasis, visceral leishmaniasis.

**Contraindications:** Clients manifesting anaphylaxis to inhaled or parenteral pentamidine.

**Special Concerns:** Use with caution in clients with hepatic or kidney disease, hypertension or hypotension, hyperglycemia or hypoglycemia, hypocalcemia, leukopenia, thrombocytopenia, anemia, ven-

tricular tachycardia, pancreatitis, Stevens-Johnson syndrome.

**Side Effects: Parenteral.** C*V:* Hypotension, ***ventricular tachycardia,*** phlebitis. *GI:* Nausea, anorexia, bad taste in mouth. *Hematologic:* Leukopenia, thrombocytopenia, anemia. *Electrolytes/glucose:* Hypoglycemia, hypocalcemia, hyperkalemia. *CNS:* Dizziness without hypotension, confusion, hallucinations. *Miscellaneous:* Acute renal failure, ***Stevens-Johnson syndrome,*** elevated serum creatinine, elevated LFTs, pain or induration at IM injection site, sterile abscess at injection site, rash, neuralgia.

**Inhalation.** Most frequent include the following. *GI:* Decreased appetite, N&V, metallic taste, diarrhea, abdominal pain. *CNS:* Fatigue, dizziness, headache. *Respiratory:* SOB, cough, pharyngitis, chest pain, chest congestion, ***bronchospasm,*** pneumothorax. *Miscellaneous:* Rash, night sweats, chills, myalgia, headache, anemia, edema.

**Dosage**
• **IV, Deep IM**
**Adults and children:** 4 mg/kg/day for 14 days. Dosage should be reduced in renal disease.
• **Aerosol**
*Prevention of* P. carinii pneumonia.
300 mg q 4 weeks given via the Respirgard II nebulizer.

## NURSING CONSIDERATIONS

See also *General Nursing Considerations for All Anti-Infectives.*
**Administration/Storage**
1. For use in the nebulizer, reconstitute by dissolving vial contents in 6 mL sterile water for injection. Do not use saline solution because it causes the drug to precipitate.
2. Deliver the dose using the nebulizer until the chamber is empty (30–45 min). The suggested flow rate is 5–7 L/min from a 40- to 50-psi (pounds per square inch) air or oxygen source.

P

3. When used for nebulization, do not mix with any other drug.

4. The solution for nebulization is stable at room temperature for 48 hr if protected from light.

5. To prepare IM solution, dissolve one vial in 3 mL of sterile water for injection.

**IV** 6. To prepare IV solution, dissolve one vial in 3–5 mL of sterile water for injection or 5% dextrose injection. The drug is then further diluted in 50–250 mL of 5% dextrose solution. This solution then can be infused slowly over 60 min.

7. IV solutions in concentrations of 1 and 2.5 mg/mL in 5% dextrose injection are stable for 48 hr at room temperature.

**Assessment**

1. Document indications for therapy and assess extent of infection.

2. Determine history of kidney disease, hypertension, and past blood disorders. Monitor cultures, CBC, electrolytes, blood sugar, calcium, $CD_4$ counts, liver and renal function.

3. Note results of tuberculosis screening tests.

4. Auscultate lung sounds; document CXR and respiratory assessment findings.

**Interventions**

1. Observe for symptoms of hypoglycemia, hypocalcemia, and/or hyperkalemia.

2. During IV therapy monitor BP frequently (q 15 min during therapy and q 2 hr following therapy until stable).

3. Monitor VS and I&O.

4. Obtain apical pulse; auscultate for any evidence of arrhythmia.

5. During administration of aerosolized pentamidine, appropriate precautions should be followed to protect the health care worker. Do not administer if pregnant; remove contact lenses. Wear:

• Eye protection with side shields

• Disposable gowns

• Respiratory protective equipment such as an organic dust-mist respirator unless client is under hood stalls or in a ventilated booth

• Gloves

• Administer with the Respirgard II nebulizer

• Document worker exposure(s) and report any persistent or unusual symptoms, especially chronic URIs

6. Follow appropriate institutional guidelines and Occupational Safety and Health Association (OSHA) standards for administration of drug.

7. Incorporate Universal Precautions to protect immunocompromised clients.

**Client/Family Teaching**

1. Report any bruising, hematuria, blood in stools, or other evidence of bleeding.

2. Avoid aspirin-containing compounds, alcohol, IM injections, or rectal thermometers.

3. Use a soft toothbrush, electric razor, and night light to prevent injury and falls.

4. Be alert for S&S of hypoglycemia (which may be severe); report after consuming juice with sugar.

5. Report early signs of Stevens-Johnson syndrome (characterized by high fever, severe headaches, stomatitis, conjunctivitis, rhinitis, urethritis, and balanitis).

6. Increase intake of fluids to 2–3 L/day.

7. Rise from a prone position slowly and dangle legs before standing as drug may cause dizziness and postural hypotension.

8. During inhalation, a metallic taste may be experienced.

**Outcomes/Evaluate**

• (Parenterally) Improvement in symptoms of *P. carinii* pneumonia

• (Inhalation) *P. carinii* pneumonia prophylaxis

———COMBINATION DRUG———

# Pentazocine hydrochloride with Naloxone hydrochloride

(pen-**TAZ**-oh-seen, nah-**LOX**-ohn)

**Pregnancy Category:** C

Talwin NX **(C-IV) (Rx)**

# Pentazocine lactate

(pen-**TAZ**-oh-seen)

**Pregnancy Category:** C
Talwin **(C-IV) (Rx)**
**Classification:** Narcotic agonist/antagonist

See also *Narcotic Analgesics.*

**General Statement:** To reduce the possibility of abuse, the PO dosage form of pentazocine has been combined with naloxone (Talwin NX), which will prevent the effects of IV administered pentazocine but will not affect the efficacy of pentazocine when taken PO. If pentazocine with naloxone is used IV, fatal reactions may occur, which include vascular occlusion, pulmonary emboli, ulceration, and abscesses, and withdrawal in narcotic-dependent individuals.

**Content:** Each tablet of pentazocine HCl with naloxone HCl contains: pentazocine HCl, 50 mg, and naloxone HCl, 0.5 mg.

**Action/Kinetics:** Manifests both narcotic agonist and antagonist properties. Agonist effects are due to combination with kappa and sigma opioid receptors; antagonistic effect is due to an action on mu opioid receptors. The drug also elevates systemic and pulmonary arterial pressure, systemic vascular resistance, and LV end-diastolic pressure, which results in an increased cardiac workload. One-third as potent as morphine as an analgesic. **Onset: IM,** 15–20 min; **PO,** 15–30 min; **IV,** 2–3 min. **Peak effect: IM,** 15–60 min; **PO,** 60–180 min. **Duration, all routes:** 3 hr. However, onset, duration, and degree of relief depend on both dose and severity of pain. **t½:** 2–3 hr. Extensive first-pass metabolism in the liver.

**Uses: PO:** Moderate to severe pain. **Parenteral:** Preoperative or preanesthetic medication, obstetrics, supplement to surgical anesthesia. Moderate to severe pain.

**Additional Contraindications:** Increased ICP or head injury. Not recommended for use in children under 12 years of age. Avoid using methadone or other narcotics for pentazocine withdrawal.

**Special Concerns:** Use with caution in impaired renal or hepatic function, as well as after MI, when N&V are present. Use with caution in women delivering premature infants and in clients with respiratory depression. Safety and efficacy in children less than 12 years of age have not been determined.

**Additional Side Effects:** *CNS:* Syncope, dysphoria, nightmares, hallucinations, disorientation, paresthesias, confusion, **seizures.** *Miscellaneous;* Decreased WBCs, edema of the face, chills. Both psychologic and physical dependence are possible, although the addiction liability is thought to be no greater than for codeine. Multiple parenteral doses may cause severe sclerosis of the skin, SC tissues, and underlying muscle.

**Dosage** —————————————
PENTAZOCINE HYDROCHLORIDE WITH NALOXONE
• **Tablets**
*Analgesia.*
**Adults:** 50 mg q 3–4 hr, up to 100 mg. Daily dose should not exceed 600 mg.
PENTAZOCINE LACTATE
• **IM, IV, SC**
*Analgesia.*
**Adults:** 30 mg q 3–4 hr; doses exceeding 30 mg IV or 60 mg IM not recommended. Total daily dosage should not exceed 360 mg.
*Obstetric analgesia.*
**Adults:** 30 mg IM given once; or, 20 mg IV q 2–3 hr for two or three doses.

## NURSING CONSIDERATIONS

See also *Nursing Considerations* for *Narcotic Analgesics.*
**Administration/Storage**
1. Do not mix soluble barbiturates in the same syringe with pentazocine as a precipitate will form.
**IV** 2. IV pentazocine may be administered undiluted. However, if the drug is to be diluted, place 5 mg of drug into 5 mL of sterile water for

injection. Administer each 5 mg or less over a 1-min period.

**Assessment**

1. Document indications for therapy, other agents used and the outcome.

2. Note characteristics of pain; rate using a pain-rating scale.

3. Note any evidence of head injury or increased ICP; document mental status; determine any history of hepatic, renal, or cardiac dysfunction.

**Client/Family Teaching**

1. Drug may cause dizziness and drowsiness.

2. Avoid alcohol and any other CNS depressants.

**Outcomes/Evaluate:** Relief of pain

---

# Pentobarbital

(pen-toe-**BAR**-bih-tal)
**Pregnancy Category:** D
Nembutal **(C-II) (Rx)**

# Pentobarbital sodium

(pen-toe-**BAR**-bih-tal)
**Pregnancy Category:** D
Nembutal Sodium, Nova-Rectal ✦,
Novo-Pentobarb ✦ **(C-II) (Rx)**
**Classification:** Sedative-hypnotic, barbiturate type

---

See also *Barbiturates*.
**Action/Kinetics:** Short-acting. t½: 19–34 hr. Is 60%–70% protein bound.

**Uses: PO:** Sedative. Short-term treatment of insomnia (no more than 2 weeks). Preanesthetic. **Rectal:** Sedation, short-term treatment of insomnia (no more than 2 weeks). **Parenteral:** Short-term treatment of insomnia (no more than 2 weeks). Preanesthetic. Anticonvulsant in anesthetic doses for emergency treatment of acute convulsive states (e.g., status epilepticus, eclampsia, meningitis, tetanus, and toxic reactions to strychnine or local anesthetics). *Investigational:* Parenterally to induce coma to protect the brain from ischemia and increased ICP following stroke and head trauma.

**Special Concerns:** Dosage should be reduced in geriatric and debilitat-

ed clients and in those with impaired hepatic or renal function.

**Dosage**

• **Capsules**
  *Sedation.*
**Adults:** 20 mg t.i.d.–q.i.d. **Pediatric:** 2–6 mg/kg/day, depending on age, weight, and degree of sedation desired.

  *Preoperative sedation.*
**Adults:** 100 mg. **Pediatric:** 2–6 mg/kg/day (maximum of 100 mg), depending on age, weight, and degree of sedation desired.

  *Hypnotic.*
**Adults:** 100 mg at bedtime.

• **Suppositories, Rectal**
  *Hypnotic.*
**Adults:** 120–200 mg at bedtime; **infants, 2–12 months (4.5–9 kg):** 30 mg; **1–4 years (9–18.2 kg):** 30 or 60 mg; **5–12 years (18.2–36.4 kg):** 60 mg; **12–14 years (36.4–50 kg):** 60 or 120 mg.

• **IM**
  *Hypnotic/preoperative sedation.*
**Adults:** 150–200 mg; **pediatric:** 2–6 mg/kg (not to exceed 100 mg).

  *Anticonvulsant.*
**Pediatric, initially:** 50 mg; **then,** after 1 min, additional small doses may be given, if needed, until the desired effect is achieved.

• **IV**
  *Sedative/hypnotic.*
**Adults:** 100 mg followed in 1 min by additional small doses, if required, up to a total of 500 mg.

  *Anticonvulsant.*
**Adults, initial:** 100 mg; **then,** after 1 min, additional small doses may be given, if needed, up to a total of 500 mg. **Pediatric, initially:** 50 mg; **then,** after 1 min, additional small doses may be given, if needed, until the desired effect is achieved.

## NURSING CONSIDERATIONS

See also *Nursing Considerations* for *Barbiturates*.
**Administration/Storage**

1. Parental pentobarbital is incompatible with most other drugs; therefore, do not mix other drugs in the same syringe. Do not use solution if

it is discolored or contains a precipitate.

2. Administer no more than 5 mL at one site IM because of possible tissue irritation (pain, necrosis, gangrene).

3. The parenteral product is not for SC use.

4. Suppositories are not to be divided.

**IV** 5. The IV dose is given in fractions because pentobarbital is a potent CNS depressant that may cause adverse respiratory and circulatory responses. Adults generally receive 100 mg initially; children and debilitated clients, 50 mg. Subsequent fractions are administered after 1-min observation periods. Overdose or too rapid administration may cause spasms of the larynx and/or pharynx.

6. Do not exceed an IV rate of 50 mg/min.

7. Pentobarbital solutions are highly alkaline.

8. Assess IV site for patency. Interrupt infusion and report any complaint of pain at injection site or in the limb.

**Assessment**

1. Document indications for therapy, onset and type of symptoms, and any other agents prescribed.

2. With insomnia, assist to identify type and any causative factors; review sleep patterns.

3. Obtain baseline liver and renal function studies; anticipate reduced dose with impairment as well as with the debilitated and elderly.

4. Observe for signs of respiratory depression; usually the first sign of drug overdose.

5. During treatment of cerebral edema (barbiturate coma), monitor and document ICP readings, and neurologic status.

6. Initiate appropriate safety measures once the medication has been administered. This is particularly important when working with confused or elderly clients.

7. Administer analgesics as needed since sedatives and hypnotics do not control pain.

**Client/Family Teaching**

1. Drug may cause drowsiness and morning-after "hangover."

2. Avoid alcohol or any other CNS depressants.

3. With insomnia, drug is for short-term use only; with long-term use one can experience rebound insomnia.

**Outcomes/Evaluate**

- Improved sleeping patterns
- Desired level of sedation
- Control of seizures

# Pentosan polysulfate sodium

(**PEN**-toh-san)
**Pregnancy Category:** B
Elmiron **(Rx)**
**Classification:** Urinary analgesic

**Action/Kinetics:** Mechanism for urinary analgesic activity is not known. It appears to adhere to the bladder wall mucosal membrane and may act as a buffer to control cell permeability, thus preventing irritating solutes in the urine from reaching the cells. Also has a weak anticoagulant effect. Less than 3% of an administered dose is absorbed from the GI tract. **t½:** 4.8 hr. Metabolized by the liver and spleen.

**Uses:** Relief of bladder pain or discomfort associated with interstitial cystitis.

**Contraindications:** Hypersensitivity to pentosan polysulfate sodium or related compounds.

**Special Concerns:** Use with caution during lactation, in those with hepatic insufficiency or spleen disorders, and in those who have a history of heparin-induced thrombocytopenia. Safety and efficacy have not been determined in children less than 16 years of age.

**Side Effects:** *GI:* Diarrhea, N&V, abdominal pain, dyspepsia, anorexia, colitis, constipation, esophagitis, flatulence, gastritis, mouth ulcer. *CNS:* Headache, severe emotional lability or depression, hyperkinesia, dizziness,

P

insomnia. *CV:* Bleeding complications, including ecchymosis, epistaxis, gum hemorrhage. *Hematologic:* Anemia, leukopenia, thrombocytopenia. *Respiratory:* Dyspnea, pharyngitis, rhinitis. *Dermatologic:* Alopecia, rash, pruritus, urticaria, increased sweating. *Ophthalmic:* Amblyopia, conjunctivitis, optic neuritis, retinal hemorrhage. *Miscellaneous:* Hepatic toxicity, liver function abnormalities, allergic reactions, tinnitus, photosensitivity.

**Laboratory Test Interferences:** ↑ PTT, PT.

**Dosage**
- **Capsules**
  *Interstitial cystitis.*
  100 mg t.i.d.

## NURSING CONSIDERATIONS

**Administration/Storage:** Store at controlled room temperatures of 15°C–30°C (59°F–86°F).

**Assessment**
1. Document onset, duration, frequency of occurrence, and characteristics of symptoms. Note other agents trialed and the outcome.
2. Determine any spleen disorder, liver dysfunction, or intolerance to heparin.
3. Obtain baseline CBC and urine for C&S.

**Client/Family Teaching**
1. Advise to take each capsule as directed with a full glass of water 1 hr before or 2 hr after a meal.
2. Report any unusual bruising or bleeding; drug has a mild anticoagulant effect.
3. Notify provider if pain persists or worsens.

**Outcomes/Evaluate:** Relief of bladder pain/discomfort with interstitial cystitis

# Pentostatin (2'-deoxycoformycin; DCF)

(**PEN**-toh-**stah**-tin)
**Pregnancy Category:** D
Nipent **(Rx)**

**Classification:** Antineoplastic antibiotic

See also *Antineoplastic Agents.*

**Action/Kinetics:** Isolated from *Streptomyces antibioticus;* inhibits the enzyme ADA. Inhibition of ADA, especially in the presence of adenosine or deoxyadenosine, results in cellular toxicity (T cells, B cells) due to elevated intracellular levels of dATP; this blocks the synthesis of DNA through inhibition of ribonucleotide reductase. Also inhibits RNA synthesis and causes increased DNA damage. **t½, distribution:** 11 min; **terminal:** 5.7 hr. Approximately 90% is excreted in the urine as unchanged pentostatin or metabolites.

**Uses:** Hairy cell leukemia in adults who are refractory to alpha-interferon; such individuals have progressive disease after a minimum of 3 months of alpha-interferon therapy or no response after a minimum of 6 months of alpha-interferon therapy.

**Contraindications:** In combination with fludarabine phosphate. Lactation.

**Special Concerns:** Treat clients with infection only if the potential benefit outweighs the risk; infection should be treated before pentostatin therapy is initiated or resumed. Safety and effectiveness have not been determined in children.

**Side Effects:** *Hematologic:* Leukopenia, anemia, thrombocytopenia, ecchymosis, lymphadenopathy, petechia, abnormal erythrocytes, leukocytosis, pancytopenia, purpura, splenomegaly, eosinophilia, hematologic disorder, hemolysis, lymphoma-like reaction. *GI:* N&V, anorexia, abdominal pain, diarrhea, constipation, flatulence, stomatitis, colitis, dysphagia, dyspepsia, eructation, gastritis, ***GI hemorrhage,*** gum hemorrhage, intestinal obstruction, leukoplakia, melena, periodontal abscess, proctitis, abnormal stools, esophagitis, gingivitis, mouth disorder. *Hepatic:* Hepatitis, hepatomegaly, ***hepatic failure.*** *CNS:* Headache, anxiety, abnormal thinking, confusion, depression, dizziness, insomnia, nervousness, paresthesia, somnolence, agitation, amnesia, ataxia, abnormal dreams, depersonalization, emotional lability, hyperesthesia, hypesthesia, hypertonia, incoordination, decreased libido, neuropathy, stupor, tremor, vertigo, *coma, seizures. CV:* Arrhythmia, abnormal ECG, *hemorrhage,* thrombophlebitis, aortic stenosis, arterial anomaly, cardiomegaly, CHF, *cardiac arrest,* flushing, hypertension, *MI,* palpitation, varicose vein, *shock. Dermatologic:* Rash, skin disorder, eczema, dry skin, herpes simplex, herpes zoster, maculopapular rash, pruritus, seborrhea, skin discoloration, sweating, vesiculobullous rash, acne, alopecia, exfoliative dermatitis, contact dermatitis, fungal dermatitis, benign skin neoplasm, psoriasis, SC nodule, skin hypertrophy, urticaria. *GU:* GU disorder, dysuria, hematuria, fibrocystic breasts, gynecomastia, hydronephrosis, oliguria, polyuria, pyuria, toxic nephropathy, urinary frequency, urinary retention, urinary urgency, UTI, impaired urination, urolithiasis, vaginitis. *Musculoskeletal:* Myalgia, arthralgia, asthenia, facial paralysis, abnormal gait, arthritis, bone pain, osteomyelitis, neck rigidity, pathologic fracture. *Respiratory:* Cough, upper respiratory infection, lung disorder, bronchitis, dyspnea, epistaxis, lung edema, pneumonia, pharyngitis, rhinitis, sinusitis, asthma, atelectasis, hemoptysis, hyperventilation, hypoventilation, increased sputum, laryngitis, larynx edema, lung fibrosis, pleural effusion, pneumothorax, *pulmonary embolus. Body as a whole:* Fever, infection, fatigue, weight loss or gain, peripheral edema, pain, allergic reaction, chills, sepsis, chest pain, back pain, flu syndrome, malaise, neoplasm, abscess, enlarged abdomen, ascites, acidosis, dehydration, diabetes mellitus, gout, abnormal healing, cellulitis, facial edema, cyst, fibrosis, granuloma, hernia, hemorrhage or inflammation of the injection site, moniliasis, pelvic pain, photosensitivity, *anaphylaxis,* mucous

membrane disorder, immune system disorder, neck pain. *Ophthalmic:* Abnormal vision, conjunctivitis, eye pain, blepharitis, cataract, diplopia, exophthalmos, lacrimation disorder, optic neuritis, retinal detachment. *Miscellaneous:* Ear pain, deafness, otitis media, parosmia, taste perversion, tinnitus.

**OD** **Overdose Management:** *Symptoms: Severe renal, hepatic, pulmonary, and CNS toxicity; death can result.* *Treatment:*    General    supportive measures.

**Drug Interactions**
*Fludarabine* / Use with pentostatin may cause ↑ risk of fatal pulmonary toxicity
*Vidarabine* / ↑ Effect of vidarabine, including side effects
**Laboratory Test Interferences:** ↑ Liver function test, BUN, creatinine, LDH, CPK, gamma globulins. Albuminuria, glycosuria, hyponatremia, hypocholesterolemia.

**Dosage**
- **IV Bolus, IV Infusion**
  *Alpha-interferon-refractory hairy cell leukemia.*
  4 mg/m² every other week.

## NURSING CONSIDERATIONS

See also *Nursing Considerations* for *Antineoplastic Agents.*
**Administration/Storage**
**IV** 1. The optimum duration of treatment has not been determined; if major toxicity has not occurred, continue treatment until a complete response has been achieved. This should be followed by two additional doses and then treatment should be stopped. If, after 12 months, there is only a partial response, discontinue treatment.
2. Withhold if there is severe rash, CNS toxicity, infection, or elevated serum creatinine.
3. Temporarily withhold if the absolute neutrophil count falls below 200 cells/mm³ during treatment in a client who had an initial neutrophil count greater than 500 cells/mm³. Continue

treatment when the count returns to pretreatment levels.

4. Store vials in the refrigerator at 2°C–8°C (36°F–46°F). Reconstituted vials or reconstituted vials further diluted may be stored at room temperature and ambient light for up to 8 hr.

5. To reconstitute, 5 mL of sterile water for injection is added to the vial; the vial is mixed thoroughly to obtain complete dissolution for a concentration of 2 mg/mL.

6. May be given by IV bolus or diluted in 25–50 mL of 5% dextrose injection or 0.9% NaCl injection and administered over 30 min. Dilution of the entire contents of the reconstituted vial with 25 or 50 mL provides a concentration of diluted pentostatin of 0.33 or 0.18 mg/mL, respectively. Such a dilution does not interact with polyvinylchloride infusion containers or administration sets.

**Assessment**

1. Note any previous experience with alpha-interferon and the response.

2. Obtain baseline hematologic parameters, liver and renal function studies.

3. Question client initially and note any symptoms of infection.

**Client/Family Teaching**

1. Report the development of rashes as these may require discontinuation of drug therapy.

2. Practice effective birth control.

3. Avoid direct sun exposure; use protection when necessary.

4. Report for scheduled lab studies to evaluate hematologic parameters. Periodic bone marrow aspirates and biopsies may be necessary.

**Outcomes/Evaluate:** Improved hematologic parameters (↑ hemoglobin, granulocyte, and platelet counts) with hairy cell leukemia

# Pentoxifylline

(pen-tox-**EYE**-fih-leen)
**Pregnancy Category:** C
Trental **(Rx)**
**Classification:** Agent affecting blood viscosity

**Action/Kinetics:** Pentoxifylline and its active metabolites decrease the viscosity of blood and improve erythrocyte flexibility. This results in increased blood flow to the microcirculation and an increase in tissue oxygen levels. Although not known with certainty, the mechanism may include (1) decreased synthesis of thromboxane $A_2$, thus decreasing platelet aggregation, (2) increased blood fibrinolytic activity (decreasing fibrinogen levels), and (3) decreased RBC aggregation and local hyperviscosity by increasing cellular ATP. **Peak plasma levels:** 2–4 hr. Significant first-pass effect. **t½:** pentoxifylline, 0.4–0.8 hr; metabolites, 1–1.6 hr. Excreted in the urine.

**Uses:** Intermittent claudication; not intended to replace surgery. *Investigational:* To improve circulation in clients with cerebrovascular insufficiency, transient ischemic attacks, sickle cell thalassemia, diabetic angiopathies and neuropathies, high-altitude sickness, strokes, acute and chronic hearing disorders, circulation disorders of the eye, severe recurrent aphthous stomatitis, leg ulcers, asthenozoospermia, and Raynaud's phenomenon.

**Contraindications:** Intolerance to pentoxifylline, caffeine, theophylline, or theobromine. Recent cerebral or retinal hemorrhage.

**Special Concerns:** Use with caution in impaired renal function and during lactation. Safety and efficacy in children less than 18 years of age not established. Geriatric clients may be at greater risk for manifesting side effects.

**Side Effects:** *CV:* Angina, chest pain, hypotension, edema. *GI:* Abdominal pain, flatus/bloating, dyspepsia, salivation, bad taste in mouth, N&V, anorexia, constipation, dry mouth and thirst, cholecystitis. *CNS:* Dizziness, headache, tremor, malaise, anxiety, confusion, depression, *seizures. Ophthalmologic:* Blurred vision, conjunctivitis, scotomata. *Dermatologic:* Pruritus, rash, urticaria, brittle fingernails, angioedema. *Respiratory:* Dyspnea, laryngitis, nasal congestion, epistaxis. *Miscellaneous:* Flu-like symptoms, leukopenia, sore throat, swollen neck glands, change in weight, earache, malaise.

**OD Overdose Management:** *Symptoms:* Agitation, fever, flushing, hypotension, nervousness, *seizures,* somnolence, tremors, loss of consciousness. *Treatment:* Gastric lavage followed by activated charcoal. Monitor BP and ECG. Support respiration, control seizures, and treat arrhythmias.

**Drug Interactions**
*Antihypertensives* / Small ↓ in BP; dose of antihypertensive may need to be ↑
*Theophylline* / ↑ Theophylline levels → ↑ risk of toxicitiy
*Warfarin* / Prolonged PT

**Dosage**
* **Extended-Release Tablets**
  *Intermittent claudication.*
  **Adults:** 400 mg t.i.d. with meals. Treatment should be continued for at least 8 weeks. If side effects occur, dosage can be reduced to 400 mg b.i.d.
  *Severe idiopathic recurrent aphthous stomatitis.*
  400 mg t.i.d. for 1 month.

## NURSING CONSIDERATIONS
**Assessment**
1. Note any history of sensitivity to caffeine, theophylline, or theobromine.
2. Document indications for therapy and type, onset, and duration of symptoms. List other agents trialed and any studies performed (i.e., Dopplers) to rule out blockage.
3. Determine if pregnant.
4. Monitor CBC and renal function studies.

**Client/Family Teaching**
1. Take the medication with meals to minimize GI upset.
2. Report any angina and palpitations if evident.
3. Continue the treatment for at least 8 weeks, even though effectiveness may not yet be apparent.
4. Do not perform activities that require mental alertness until drug effects are realized as dizziness and blurred vision may occur.
5. Avoid nicotine-containing products; nicotine constricts blood vessels.
6. Walk every day to the point of pain but not through it, rest and then resume walking. Wear cotton socks and comfortable, well-fitting shoes.
7. Report for lab studies to evaluate drug effectiveness.

**Outcomes/Evaluate:** ↓ Pain and cramping in lower extremities during activity

————*COMBINATION DRUG*————
# Percocet
(**PER**-koh-set)
**Pregnancy Category:** C
**(C-II) (Rx)**
**Classification:** Analgesic

See also *Acetaminophen* and *Narcotic Analgesics.*

**Content:** Each tablet contains: *Nonnarcotic analgesic:* Acetaminophen, 325 mg. *Narcotic analgesic:* Oxycodone HCl, 5 mg. Also see information on individual components.

**Uses:** Moderate to moderately severe pain.

**Special Concerns:** Use with caution during lactation. Safety and effectiveness have not been determined in children. Dependence to oxycodone can occur.

**Dosage**
* **Tablets**
**Adults, usual:** 1 tablet q 6 hr as required for pain.

## NURSING CONSIDERATIONS

See also *Nursing Considerations* for *Narcotic Analgesics* and *Acetaminophen.*

**Administration/Storage:** Adjust dosage depending on the response of the client, tolerance, and the severity of the pain.

**Assessment:** Document location, onset, duration, and characteristics of pain. Use a pain-rating scale to rate pain.

**Client/Family Teaching**

1. May cause dizziness and drowsiness.
2. Drug is for short-term use; chronic pain conditions require alternative pharmacologic agents.
3. Avoid alcohol and any other CNS depressants.

**Outcomes/Evaluate:** Relief of pain

# Pergolide mesylate

(**PER**-go-lyd)
**Pregnancy Category:** B
Permax **(Rx)**
**Classification:** Antiparkinson agent

See also *Antiparkinson Agents*.

**Action/Kinetics:** Potent dopamine receptor (both $D_1$ and $D_2$) agonist. Believed to act by directly stimulating postsynaptic dopamine receptors in the nigrostriatal system, thus relieving symptoms of parkinsonism. Also inhibits prolactin secretion; causes a transient rise in serum levels of growth hormone and a decrease in serum levels of LH. About 90% of the drug is bound to plasma proteins. Metabolized in the liver and excreted through the urine.

**Uses:** Adjunctive treatment to levodopa/carbidopa in Parkinson's disease.

**Special Concerns:** Use with caution during lactation and in clients prone to cardiac dysrhythmias, preexisting dyskinesia, and preexisting states of confusion or hallucinations. Safety and efficacy have not been determined in children.

**Side Effects:** The most common side effects are listed. *CV:* Postural hypotension, palpitation, vasodilation, syncope, hypotension, hypertension, *arrhythmias, MI. GI:* Nausea (common), vomiting, diarrhea, constipation, dyspepsia, anorexia, dry mouth. *CNS:* Dyskinesia (common), dizziness, dystonia, hallucinations, confusion, insomnia, somnolence,

anxiety, tremor, depression, abnormal dreams, psychosis, personality disorder, extrapyramidal syndrome, akathisia, paresthesia, incoordination, akinesia, neuralgia, hypertonia, speech disorders. *Musculoskeletal:* Arthralgia, bursitis, twitching, myalgia. *Respiratory:* Rhinitis, dyspnea, hiccup, epistaxis. *Dermatologic:* Sweating, rash. *Ophthalmologic:* Abnormal vision, double vision, eye disorders. *GU:* UTI, urinary frequency, hematuria. *Whole body:* Pain in chest, abdomen, neck, or back; headache, asthenia, flu syndrome, chills, facial edema, infection. *Miscellaneous:* Taste alteration, peripheral edema, anemia, weight gain.

**OD** **Overdose Management:** *Symptoms:* Might include agitation, hypotension, vomiting, hallucinations, involuntary movements, palpitations, tingling of arms and legs. *Treatment:* Activated charcoal (usually recommended instead of or in addition to gastric lavage or induction of vomiting). Maintain BP. An antiarrhythmic drug may be helpful. A phenothiazine or butyrophenone may help any CNS stimulation. Support ventilation.

**Drug Interactions**

*Butyrophenones /* ↓ Effect of pergolide due to dopamine antagonist effect

*Metoclopramide /* ↓ Effect of pergolide due to dopamine antagonist effect

*Phenothiazines /* ↓ Effect of pergolide due to dopamine antagonist effect

*Thioxanthines /* ↓ Effect of pergolide due to dopamine antagonist effect

**Dosage**
• **Tablets**
  *Parkinsonism.*

**Adults, initial:** 0.05 mg/day for the first 2 days; **then,** increase dose gradually by 0.1 or 0.15 mg/day every third day over the next 12 days. The dosage may then be increased by 0.25 mg/day every third day until the therapeutic dosage level is reached. The mean therapeutic daily dosage is 3 mg used concurrently with levodopa/carbidopa (expressed as levodopa) at a dose of 650 mg/day. The effectiveness of doses of pergolide greater than 5 mg/day has not been evaluated.

## NURSING CONSIDERATIONS

See also *Nursing Considerations* for *Antiparkinson Agents*.

### Administration/Storage
1. Usually given in divided doses 3 times/day.
2. When determining the therapeutic dose for pergolide, the dosage of concurrent levodopa/carbidopa may be decreased cautiously.

### Assessment
1. Note any sensitivity to ergot derivatives.
2. Document any cardiac arrhythmias.
3. Describe location of tremor, rigidity, motor fluctuations and movements.

### Client/Family Teaching
1. Pergolide is to be taken concurrently with prescribed dose of levodopa/carbidopa. Do not exceed prescribed dosage.
2. Do not perform tasks that require mental alertness until drug effects realized; may cause drowsiness or dizziness.
3. Rise slowly from a sitting or lying position to minimize hypotensive effects of pergolide. Activities may need to be curtailed until side effects subside.
4. Report for all scheduled lab and medical appointments so that drug therapy may be evaluated and adjusted as needed.

### Outcomes/Evaluate: Improved levodopa/carbidopa response evidenced by ↓ muscle weakness, ↓ rigidity, ↓ salivation, and improved mobility

# Perphenazine
(per-**FEN**-ah-zeen)
Apo-Perphenazine ✹, Phenazine ✹, PMS-Perphenazine ✹, Trilafon **(Rx)**

**Classification:** Antipsychotic, antiemetic, piperazine-type phenothiazine

See also *Antipsychotic Agents, Phenothiazines*.

**Action/Kinetics:** Resembles chlorpromazine. High incidence of extrapyramidal effects; strong antiemetic effects; moderate anticholinergic effects; and a low incidence of orthostatic hypotension and sedation. **Onset, IM:** 10 min. **Maximum effect, IM:** 1–2 hr. **Duration, IM:** 6 hr (up to 24 hr).

**Uses:** Psychotic disorders. To treat severe N&V.

**Special Concerns:** Use during pregnancy only if benefits clearly outweigh risks. Dosage has not been established in children less than 12 years of age. Geriatric, emaciated, or debilitated clients usually require a lower initial dose.

### Dosage
- **Oral Solution, Syrup, Tablets**
  *Psychoses.*
**Nonhospitalized clients:** 4–8 mg t.i.d. or 8–16 mg repeat-action tablets b.i.d. **Hospitalized clients:** 8–16 mg b.i.d.–q.i.d. or 8–32 mg repeat-action tablets b.i.d. Total daily dosage should not exceed 64 mg.
  *Severe N&V.*
**Adults:** 8–16 mg/day in divided doses (24 mg/day may be required in some clients).
- **IM**
  *Psychotic disorders.*
**Adults and adolescents, nonhospitalized:** 5 mg q 6 hr, not to exceed 15 mg/day. **Hospitalized clients: initial,** 5–10 mg; total daily dose should not exceed 30 mg.
  *Severe N&V.*
**Adults and adolescents:** 5 mg (initially, 10 mg in severe cases) q 6 hr, not to exceed 15 mg in ambulatory clients or 30 mg in hospitalized clients.
- **IV**
  *Severe N&V.*
**Adults:** Up to 5 mg diluted to 0.5 mg/mL with 0.9% sodium chloride

---

✹ = Available in Canada        ***bold italic*** = life threatening side effect

injection. Should be given in divided doses of not more than 1 mg q 1–3 hr. Can also be given as an infusion at a rate not to exceed 1 mg/min. Use should be restricted to hospitalized recumbent adults. Maximum single dose should not exceed 5 mg.

## NURSING CONSIDERATIONS

See also *Nursing Considerations* for *Antipsychotic Agents, Phenothiazines.*

### Administration/Storage

1. Dilute each 5.0 mL of oral concentrate with 60 mL of water, milk, carbonated beverage, or orange juice.
2. Do not mix with tea, coffee, cola, grape juice, or apple juice as it will precipitate.
3. When rapid action is required, administer IM using 5 mg. Inject deep into the muscle, and repeat at 6-hr intervals as needed. Place client in a recumbent position and retain in that position for at least 1 hr after IM administration.
4. Protect from light and store solutions in an amber-colored container.
**IV** 5. For IV use dilute with NSS to a concentration of 0.5 mg/mL and administer 1 mg over at least 1 min.

### Assessment

1. Document indications for therapy, describe behavioral manifestations, and note onset of symptoms.
2. List other agents prescribed, duration of therapy, and the outcome.
3. Obtain baseline CBC, ECG, and LFTs.

### Interventions

1. Monitor VS closely;may cause hypotension, tachycardia, and/or bradycardia.
2. Supervise activity until drug effects realized.
3. Observe for tardive dyskinesia and other extrapyramidal symptoms; this would require a dosage reduction or discontinuation of therapy.

### Client/Family Teaching

1. Drug may cause drowsiness and dizziness.
2. Report any rash, fever, or urinary retention.
3. May discolor urine pinkish brown.
4. Report symptoms of tardive dyskinesia and extrapyramidal symptoms.
5. Wear protective clothes and sunscreen when sun exposure necessary; may discolor skin a bluish color.
6. Drug impairs body temperature regulation; dress appropriately and avoid temperature extremes.
7. Avoid alcohol and CNS depressants.

### Outcomes/Evaluate

• ↓ Agitation/excitability or withdrawn behaviors
• Control of severe N&V

# Phenazopyridine hydrochloride (Phenylazodiamino-pyridine HCl)

(fen-**AY**-zoh-**PEER**-ih-deen)

**Pregnancy Category:** B

Azo-Standard, Baridium, Phenazo ✳, Prodium, Pyridiate, Pyridiate No. 2, Pyridium, Pyronium ✳, Urogesic **(OTC) (Rx)**

**Classification:** Urinary analgesic

**Action/Kinetics:** An azo dye with local analgesic and anesthetic effects on the urinary tract. Sixty-five percent excreted unchanged or as metabolites within 24 hr.

**Uses:** Relief of pain, urgency or frequency, and burning in chronic UTIs or irritation, including cystitis, urethritis and pyelitis, trauma, surgery, or urinary tract instrumentation. May also be used as an adjunct to antibacterial therapy. The underlying cause of the irritation must be determined.

**Contraindications:** Renal insufficiency. Use in children less than 12 years of age. Chronic use to treat undiagnosed pain of the urinary tract.

**Side Effects:** *GI:* Nausea. *Hematologic:* Methemoglobinemia, **hemolytic anemia** (especially in clients with G6PD deficiency). *Dermatologic:* Yellowish tinge of the skin or sclerae may indicate accumulation of drug due to renal insufficiency, pruritus, rash. *Miscellaneous:* Renal and hepatic toxicity, headache, anaphylactoid reaction, staining of contact lenses.

**OD** **Overdose Management:** *Symptoms:* Methemoglobinemia following massive overdoses. Hemolysis due to G6PD deficiency. *Treatment:* Methylene blue, 1–2 mg/kg IV or 100–200 mg PO of ascorbic acid to treat methemoglobinemia.

**Laboratory Test Interferences:** Ehrlich's test for urine urobilinogen, phenolsulfonphthalein excretion test for kidney function, urine bilirubin, Clinistix or Tes-Tape, colorimetric laboratory test procedures (e.g., urine ketone tests, urine protein tests, urine steroid determinations).

**Dosage**
• **Tablets**
**Adults:** 200 mg t.i.d. with or after meals for not more than 2 days when used together with an antibacterial agent for UTI. **Pediatric, 6–12 years:** 4 mg/kg t.i.d. with food for 2 days.

## NURSING CONSIDERATIONS
**Assessment**
1. Document indications for therapy, type, onset, and characteristics of symptoms.
2. Assess for any liver/renal dysfunction.
**Client/Family Teaching**
1. Take with or after meals to prevent GI upset.
2. Use for only 2 days when taken together with an antibacterial agent for UTIs; continue antibiotic for entire prescription.
3. Consume 2–3 L/day of fluids.
4. With diabetes, check finger sticks regularly.
5. May cause staining of contact lenses.
6. Drug turns urine orange-red; may stain fabrics. Wear a sanitary napkin to avoid staining garments. A 0.25% sodium dithionate or sodium hydro-

sulfite solution, available from a pharmacy, will remove these stains.
7. Report any itching or yellowing of skin.

**Outcomes/Evaluate:** Relief of pain and discomfort with UTI

# Phendimetrazine tartrate
(fen-dye-**ME**-trah-zeen)
**Pregnancy Category:** C
Adipost, Bontrol PDM and Slow-Release, Dital, Dyrexan-OD, Melfiat-105 Unicelles, Plegine, Prelu-2, Rexigen Forte **(C-III) (Rx)**
**Classification:** Anorexiant

See also *Amphetamines and Derivatives.*
**Action/Kinetics: Duration, tablets:** 4 hr. **t½:** 5.5 hr (average).
**Uses:** Short-term (8–12 weeks) treatment of exogenous obesity in conjunction with a weight reduction program including exercise, reduced caloric intake, and behavior modification.

**Dosage**
• **Capsules, Tablets**
**Adults:** 35 mg 2–3 times/day 1 hr before meals. **Maximum daily dose:** 70 mg t.i.d.
• **Extended-Release Capsules, Extended-Release Tablets**
**Adults:** 105 mg/day 30–60 min before the morning meal.

## NURSING CONSIDERATIONS

See Nursing Considerations for *Amphetamines* and *Derivatives.*
**Assessment:** List indications for therapy, noting pretreatment weight, ECG, and labs. Identify other methods trialed and the outcome.
**Client/Family Teaching**
1. Must combine therapy with exercise and reduced caloric intake in the overall management of obesity.
2. This agent is for short-term therapy only. Attend formal behavioral modification programs.
**Outcomes/Evaluate:** Control of appetite; weight loss

P

---

# Phenelzine sulfate

(FEN-ell-zeen)
**Pregnancy Category:** C
Nardil **(Rx)**
**Classification:** Antidepressant, mono-amine oxidase inhibitor

**Action/Kinetics:** MAO inhibitor that prevents the enzyme from metabolizing biogenic amines. Antidepressant effect of phenelzine believed to be due to accumulation of biogenic amines in presynaptic granules, increasing the concentration of neurotransmitter released upon nerve stimulation. **Onset:** Few days to several months. Beneficial effects at doses of 60 mg/day may not be seen for at least 4 weeks. Clinical effects of the drug may be observed for up to 2 weeks after termination of therapy.

**Uses:** Depression characterized as atypical, nonendogenous, or neurotic; most often used in those clients who have mixed anxiety and depression and phobic or hypochondriacal symptoms. Not usually first-line therapy; reserve for those who have failed to respond to drugs more commonly used. *Investigational:* Alone or as an adjunct to treat bulimia nervosa, agoraphobia with panic attcks, globus hystericus syndrome, and chronic headache. Also for orthostatic hypotension, refractory migraine headaches, narcolepsy, obsessive-compulsive disorder, panic attacks, posttraumatic stress disorder, and social phobia.

**Contraindications:** Pheochromocytoma, CHF, history of liver disease, abnormal LFTs. Use with other sympathomimetic drugs due to the possibility of hypertensive crisis. Phenelzine is also contraindicated with the use of many other drugs (see *Drug Interactions*). Use in children under the age of 16 years.

**Special Concerns:** Use with caution in combination with antihypertensive drugs, including thiazide diuretics and β-blockers, due to the possibility of severe hypotensive effects. The safe use during pregnancy or lactation has not been determined. Use with caution in geriatric clients.

**Side Effects:** *CNS:* Dizziness, headache, drowsiness, sleep disturbances (insomnia, hypersomnia), fatigue, weakness, tremors, twitching, myoclonic movements, hyperreflexia, jitteriness, palilalia, euphoria, nystagmus, paresthesias, ataxia, *shock-like coma,* toxic delirium, manic reaction, *convulsions,* acute anxiety reaction, precipitation of schizophrenia. *GI:* Constipation, dry mouth, GI disturbances, reversible jaundice. Rarely, *fatal necrotizing hepatocellular damage. CV:* Postural hypotension, edema. *GU:* Anorgasmia, ejaculatory disturbances, urinary retention. *Metabolic:* Weight gain, hypernatremia, hypermetabolic syndrome. *Dermatologic:* Skin rash, sweating. *Ophthalmic:* Blurred vision, glaucoma. *Miscellaneous:* Leukopenia, edema of the glottis, fever associated with increased muscle tone.

**Laboratory Test Alteration:** ↑ Serum transaminases.

**OD** **Overdose Management:** *Symptoms:* Drowsiness, dizziness, fainting, irritability, hyperactivity, agitation, severe headache, hallucinations, trismus, opisthotonus, rigidity, convulsions, coma, rapid and irregular pulse, hypertension, hypotension, cardiovascular collapse, precordial pain, respiratory depression, respiratory failure, hyperpyrexia, diaphoresis, cold and clammy skin, death. Symptoms of overdose may be absent or minimal during the initial 12-hr period after ingestion but then slowly increase, reaching a maximum effect within 24 to 48 hr. *Treatment:* If detected early, induction of emesis or gastric lavage followed by a charcoal slurry. Use of IV diazepam for CNS symptoms. For hypotension and CV collapse, IV fluids and, if necessary, BP titration with an IV infusion of a dilute pressor drug. Respirations should be supported by use of supplemental oxygen and mechanical ventilation. Fluid and electrolyte balance must be maintained. Phenothiazine derivatives and CNS stimulants should **not** be used.

**Drug Interactions**

*Alcohol* / Possibility of excitation, seizures, delirium, hyperpyrexia, circulatory collapse, coma, death

*Anesthetics, general* / ↑ Hypotensive effect; use together with caution. Phenelzine should be discontinued at least 10 days before elective surgery

*Anticholinergic drugs, atropine* / MAO inhibitors ↑ effect of anticholinergic drugs

*Antidepressants, tricyclic* / Comcomitant use may result in excitation, sweating, tachycardia, tachypnea, hyperpyrexia, disseminated intravascular coagulation, delirium, tremors, convulsions, death. At least 7-10 days should elapse between discontinuing a MAO inhibitor and initiating a new drug. However, such combinations have been used together successfully

*Antihypertensive drugs* / Exaggerated hypotensive effects

*Beta-adrenergic blocking drugs* / Exaggerated hypotensive effects

*Buspirone* / Elevated BP

*Fluoxetine* / Possibility of hyperthermia, rigidity, myoclonic movements, death. At least 10 days should elapse between discontinuation of phenelzine and initiation of fluoxetine; and, at least 5 weeks should elapse between discontinuing fluoxetine and beginning phenelzine

*Narcotics* / Possibility of excitation, seizures, delirium, hyperpyrexia, circulatory collapse, coma, death

*Phenothiazines* / ↑ Effect of phenothizines due to ↓ breakdown by the liver; also, ↑ chance of severe extrapyramidal effects and hypertensive crisis

*Succinylcholine* / ↑ Effect of succinylcholine due to ↓ breakdown in the plasma by pseudocholinesterase

*Sympathomimetic drugs—amphetamine, cocaine, dopa, ephedrine, epinephrine, metaraminol, methyldopa, methylphenidate, norepinephrine, phenylephrine, phenylpropanolamine. Many OTC cold products, hay fever medications, and nasal decongestants contain one or more of these drugs* / All peripheral, metabolic, cardiac, and central effects are potentiated for up to 2 weeks after termination of MAO inhibitor therapy. Symptoms include acute hypertensive crisis with possible intracranial hemorrhage, hyperthermia, coma, and possibly death

*Thiazide diuretics* / Exaggerated hypotensive effects

*Tryptophan* / Possibility of behavioral and neurologic effects, including disorientation, confusion, amnesia, delirium, agitation, hypomania, ataxia, myoclonus, hyperreflexia, shivering, ocular oscillation, and Babinski signs

*Tyramine-rich foods—beer, broad beans, certain cheeses (Brie, cheddar, Camembert, Stilton), Chianti wine, chicken livers, caffeine, cola beverages, figs, licorice, liver, pickled or kippered herring, dry sausage (Genoa salami, hard salami, pepperoni, Lebanon bologna), tea, cream, yogurt, yeast extract, and chocolate* / Possible precipitation of hypertensive crisis, including severe headache, hyperension, intracranial hemorrhage, death

**Dosage**
- **Tablets**
  *Treatment of depression.*
  **Adults, initial:** 15 mg t.i.d.; **then,** increase the dose to 60 mg/day at a fairly rapid pace (some may require 90 mg/day). **Maintenance:** After the maximum beneficial effect has been observed, the dose should be reduced slowly over several weeks to a range of 15 mg/day or every other day to as high as 45 mg/day or every other day. **Geriatric, initial:** 0.8–1 mg/kg daily in divided doses; **then,** increase s needed to a maximum of 60 mg/day.

## NURSING CONSIDERATIONS
### Assessment

1. Document indications for therapy, onset and duration of symptoms, previous agents trialed and the outcome. Note clinical presentation and failure with other classes of antidepressants. Assess for prior use of MAO inhibitors. These drugs have a narrow safety margin and require close supervision and restriction of foods and drugs and use with other medical conditions.

2. List drugs currently prescribed and those used within the past two weeks (especially sympathomimetic drugs) to ensure none interact unfavorably.

3. Obtain pregnancy test; drugs cross placental barrier and may be teratogenic.

4. Monitor VS, ECG, electrolytes, liver and renal function studies.

5. Assess diet for foods that affect MAO inhibitors (especially tyramine-rich foods).

### Interventions

1. Monitor VS every 4 to 8 hr when initiating therapy and at regular intervals thereafter to detect any hypertension or arrhythmias.

2. Observe for any early symptoms of CHF, such as rales, SOB, or the presence of peripheral edema.

3. Obtain weight prior to initiating therapy and biweekly therafter. May experience weight loss, nausea, anorexia, and/or diarrhea.

4. Monitor closely during initiation of therapy for indications of suicidal ideations. Suicide attempts are more frequent when client emerges from the deepest phases of depression.

5. Report increased agitation, anxiety, mania, or any marked changes in behavior.

6. Do not administer in the evening because of the risk of insomnia.

7. Monitor I&O and note any evidence of urinary retention or bladder distension. Retention is more common among the elderly, males and those who are immobilized.

8. Increase fluids to 3 L/day and the intake of fuits, fruit juices, and fiber to avoid constipation.

9. Reports of red-green vision warrant further evaluation as this may indicate ophthalmic damage.

10. If client has been taking elevated doses of MAO inhibitors over a long period of time, any drug withdrawal should be accomplished by gradually reducing the dosage of drug to a maintenance level before discontinuing the drug entirely.

### Client/Family Teaching

1. Take as directed and with meals to decrease GI irritation.

2. Avoid taking other drugs while on this therapy and for two week after therapy has been discontinued unless specifically ordered. This includes OTC preparations for coughs, colds, congestion, or allergic reactions.

3. Review list of tyramine-containing foods to avoid (i.e., beer, Chianti wine, chicken livers, caffeine, cola beverages, certain cheeses such as Brie, cheddar, Camembert, and Stilton; figs, licorice, liver, pickled or kippered herring, dried fish, bananas, raisins, tenderizers, game meats, avocados, dry sausage such as Genoa salami, hard salami, pepperoni, and Lebanon bologna; tea, sour cream, yogurt, yeast extract, and chocolate.

4. Several weeks of therapy are required before significant changes may occur. Continue taking if there is improvement since this is necessary to maintain proper blood levels of the drugs as well as the feelings of symptomatic improvement. Report any S&S of suicidal behavior.

5. With diabetes monitor fingersticks closely and report any major variations; may potentiate the effect of insulin and sulfonylureas.

6. Report any visual changes, stiff neck, photophobia, unusual soreness or sweating, or changes in pupil size immediately as these may signal a hypertensive crisis.

7. Practice reliable birth control during and for several weeks before and after therapy.

8. Frequent mouth rinses, sugarless gum or hard candy, and increased

fluid intake may diminish dry mouth side effects.

9. If feeling faint lie down immediately. Rise slowly from a supine position and dangle legs before standing to minimize orthostatic hypotension.

10. Maintain activity in moderation. MAO inhibitors suppress anginal pain which may indicate myocardial ischemia.

11. Record weight regularly. If weight gain becomes significant, i.e., more than 5 lb/week for more than 2 weeks, a reducing diet or a change in drug therapy or dosage may be warranted. Increased SOB and edema may signal CHF.

12. Therapy requires regular F/U care since the dose will be gradually increased until the desired response is obtained. (Generally if there is no response observed by the third week of therapy, it is not likely client will respond to increased dosages.)

**Outcomes/Evaluate**
• Improvement in mood, energy, and interest levels
• ↓ Somatic complaints; normal sleep patterns
• Improved sense of self and abilty to problem solve

————COMBINATION DRUG————

# Phenergan with Codeine syrup

(FEN-er-gan, KOH-deen)
**Pregnancy Category:** C
**(C-V) (Rx)**
**Classification:** Antihistamine, antitussive

See also *Antihistamines* and *Codeine*.
**Content:** *Antihistamine:* Promethazine HCl, 6.25 mg/5 mL. *Antitussive, narcotic:* Codeine phosphate, 10 mg/5 mL.
**Uses:** Relief of coughs and other upper respiratory tract problems associated with the common cold or with allergy.
**Contraindications:** Clients with lower respiratory tract symptoms, including asthma. Use in children less than 2 years of age.

**Special Concerns:** Use with caution during lactation.

**Dosage** ————
• **Syrup**
**Adults:** 5 mL q 4–6 hr, not to exceed 30 mL/day; **pediatric, 6–12 years:** 2.5–5 mL q 4–6 hr, not to exceed 30 mL/day; **pediatric, 2–6 years:** 1.25–2.5 mL q 4–6 hr. The maximum daily dose of medication for children between 2 and 6 years of age depends on body weight. The amount of drug administered should not exceed:9 mL for 18 kg of body weight, or8 mL for 16 kg of body weight, or7 mL for 14 kg of body weight, or6 mL for 12 kg of body weight.

## NURSING CONSIDERATIONS

See also *Nursing Considerations* for *Antihistamines* and *Narcotics*.
**Assessment:** Determine duration and characteristics of cough; assess for allergy symptoms. Note ENT and pulmonary assessment findings.
**Client/Family Teaching**
1. Report if symptoms persist or intensify.
2. Consume 2–3 L/day of fluids and include additional roughage in the diet to avoid constipation.
3. Drug may be habit-forming and is not for long-term indiscriminate use.
**Outcomes/Evaluate:** ↓ Cough/congestion

————COMBINATION DRUG————

# Phenergan with Dextromethorphan syrup

(FEN-er-gan, dex-froh-meth-OR-fan)
**(Rx)**
**Pregnancy Category:** C
**Classification:** Antihistamine, antitussive

See also *Antihistamines* and *Dextromethorphan*.
**Content:** *Antihistamine:* Promethazine HCl, 6.25 mg/5 mL. *Nonnarcotic antitussive:* Dextromethorphan HCl, 15 mg/5 mL.

**Uses:** To treat symptoms of cough and upper respiratory problems observed with the common cold and allergies.

**Contraindications:** Use in children less than 2 years of age.

**Special Concerns:** Use with caution during lactation.

**Dosage** —————
• **Syrup**
**Adults:** 5 mL q 4–6 hr, not to exceed 30 mL/day. **Pediatric, 6–12 hr:** 2.5–5 mL q 4–6 hr, not to exceed 20 mL/day; **2–6 years:** 1.25–2.5 mL q 4–6 hr, not to exceed 10 mL/day.

## NURSING CONSIDERATIONS

See also *Nursing Considerations* for *Antihistamines* and *Dextromethorphan*.

**Assessment**
1. Determine onset, duration, and characteristics of symptoms.
2. List other agents used and the outcome.
3. Auscultate lungs and document pulmonary findings.

**Outcomes/Evaluate:** Control of cough; relief of congestion

————*COMBINATION DRUG*————

# Phenergan VC with Codeine syrup
(**FEN**-er-gan, **KOH**-deen)
**Pregnancy Category:** C
**(C-V) (Rx)**

# Phenergan VC syrup
(**FEN**-er-gan)
**Pregnancy Category:** C
**(Rx)**
**Classification:** Anthistamine, decongestant, antitussive

See also *Antihistamines, Phenylephrine,* and *Codeine.*

**Content:** Phenergan VC contains the following: *Antihistamine:* Promethazine HCl, 6.25 mg/5 mL. *Decongestant:* Phenylephrine HCl, 5 mg/5 mL. Phenergan VC with Codeine contains the preceding plus: *Narcotic antitussive:* Codeine phosphate, 10 mg/5 mL.

**Uses:** Phenergan VC: Nasal congestion accompanying allergy or the common cold. Phenergan VC with Codeine: Cough and nasal congestion accompanying allergy or the common cold.

**Contraindications:** Use for lower respiratory tract symptoms, including asthma. Use in children less than 2 years of age.

**Special Concerns:** Use with caution during lactation.

**Dosage** —————
• **Phenergan VC Syrup, Phenergan VC with Codeine Syrup**
**Adults:** 5 mL q 4–6 hr, not to exceed 30 mL/day. **Pediatric, 6–12 years:** 2.5–5 mL q 4–6 hr, not to exceed 30 mL/day; **2–6 years:** 1.25–2.5 mL q 4–6 hr. The maximum daily dose of medication for children between 2 and 6 years of age depends on body weight. The amount of drug administered should not exceed:9 mL for 18 kg of body weight, or8 mL for 16 kg of body weight, or7 mL for 14 kg of body weight, or6 mL for 12 kg of body weight

## NURSING CONSIDERATIONS

See also *Nursing Considerations* for *Antihistamines, Phenylephrine,* and *Codeine.*

**Assessment:** Note onset, duration, and characteristics of symptoms. Document ENT and pulmonary assessment findings.

**Client/Family Teaching**
1. May cause dizziness and drowsiness.
2. Avoid alcohol and CNS depressants.
3. Drug is not for long-term use; report if symptoms do not subside or get worse after 5 days.

**Outcomes/Evaluate:** Control of cough/congestion with less night time awakenings

# Phenobarbital
(fee-no-**BAR**-bih-tal)
**Pregnancy Category:** D
Barbilixir ✷, Solfoton **(C-IV) (Rx)**

# Phenobarbital sodium

(fee-no-**BAR**-bih-tal)
**Pregnancy Category:** D
Luminal Sodium **(C-IV) (Rx)**
**Classification:** Sedative, anticonvulsant, barbiturate type

See also *Barbiturates*.
**Action/Kinetics:** Long-acting. **t½:** 53–140 hr. **Onset:** 30 to more than 60 min. **Duration:** 10–16 hr. **Anticonvulsant therapeutic serum levels:** 15–40 mcg/mL. **Time for peak effect, after IV:** up to 15 min. Distributed more slowly than other barbiturates due to lower lipid solubility. Is 50%–60% protein bound. Twenty-five percent eliminated unchanged in the urine.

**Uses: PO:** Sedative, hypnotic (short-term), anticonvulsant (partial and generalized tonic-clonic or cortical focal seizures); emergency control of acute seizure disorders such as status epilepticus, meningitis, tetanus, eclampsia, toxicity of local anesthetics. **Parenteral:** Sedative, hypnotic (short-term), preanesthetic, anticonvulsant, emergency control of acute seizure disorders.

**Special Concerns:** The dose should be reduced in geriatric and debilitated clients as well as those with impaired hepatic or renal function.
**Additional Side Effects:** Chronic use may result in headache, fever, and megaloblastic anemia.

## Dosage

PHENOBARBITAL, PHENOBARBITAL SODIUM
• **Capsules, Elixir, Tablets**
*Sedation.*
**Adults:** 30–120 mg/day in two to three divided doses. **Pediatric:** 2 mg/kg (60 mg/m²) t.i.d.
*Hypnotic.*
**Adults:** 100–200 mg at bedtime. **Pediatric:** Dose should be determined by provider, based on age and weight.
*Anticonvulsant.*
**Adults:** 60–100 mg/day in single or divided doses. **Pediatric:** 3–6 mg/kg/day in single or divided doses.

• **IM, IV**
*Sedation.*
**Adults:** 30–120 mg/day in two to three divided doses.
*Preoperative sedation.*
**Adults:** 100–200 mg IM only, 60–90 min before surgery. **Pediatric:** 1–3 mg/kg IM or IV 60–90 min prior to surgery.
*Hypnotic.*
**Adults:** 100–320 mg IM or IV.
*Acute convulsions.*
**Adults:** 200–320 mg IM or IV; may be repeated in 6 hr if needed. **Pediatric:** 4–6 mg/kg/day for 7–10 days to achieve a blood level of 10–15 mcg/mL (or 15 mg/kg/day, IV or IM).
*Status epilepticus.*
**Adults:** 15–20 mg/kg IV (given over 10–15 min); may be repeated if needed. **Pediatric:** 15–20 mg/kg given over a 10- to 15-min period.

# NURSING CONSIDERATIONS

See also *Nursing Considerations* for *Barbiturates*.
**Administration/Storage**
1. When used for seizures, give the major fraction of the dose according to when seizures are likely to occur (i.e., on arising for daytime seizures and at bedtime when seizures occur at night).
2. When used as an anticonvulsant in infants and children, a loading dose of 15–20 mg/kg achieves blood levels of about 20 mcg/mL shortly after administration. In order to achieve therapeutic blood levels of 10–20 mcg/mL, higher doses per kilogram may be necessary compared with adults.
3. When used IM, inject into a large muscle (e.g., gluteus maximus, vastus lateralis). Injection into or near peripheral nerves may cause permanent neurological deficit.
4. In most cases, when used for epilepsy, drug must be taken regularly to avoid seizures, even when no seizures are imminent.
5. When used for seizures, give the lowest dose possible to avoid adding

P

---

to the depression that may follow seizures.

**IV** 6. Reserve IV use for conditions when other routes are not feasible. There is the possibility of overdose, including respiratory depression, even with slow injection of fractional doses.

7. Freshly prepare the aqueous solution for injection.

8. Some ready-dissolved solutions for injection are available; the vehicle is propylene glycol, water, and alcohol.

9. For IV administration, inject slowly at a rate of 50 mg/min.

10. Avoid extravasation as tissue damage and necrosis may result.

**Assessment**

1. Document indications for therapy, type, onset, and duration of symptoms.

2. List other agents prescribed and the outcome.

3. Assess liver and renal function studies. Reduce dose with impairment and in debilitated or in elderly clients.

**Client/Family Teaching**

1. Take only as directed and do not stop abruptly.

2. Drug may initially cause drowsiness; assess drug effects before performing tasks that require mental alertness.

3. Phenobarbital may require an increase in vitamin D consumption; consume foods high in vitamin D.

4. Drug decreases the effect of oral contraceptives; practice other nonhormonal forms of birth control.

5. Avoid alcohol and OTC agents without approval.

**Outcomes/Evaluate**

• Sedation; control of seizures

• Therapeutic anticonvulsant drug levels (10–40 mcg/mL)

# Phensuximide
(fen-**SUCKS**-ih-myd)
Milontin **(Rx)**
**Classification:** Anticonvulsant, succinimide type

See also *Anticonvulsants* and *Succinimides*.

**Action/Kinetics:** Less effective and less toxic than other succinimides. May color the urine pink, red, or red-brown. **t½:** 5–12 hr. **Peak effect:** 1–4 hr. Excreted through the bile and urine.

**Uses:** Absence seizures.

**Special Concerns:** Use with caution in clients with intermittent porphyria.

**Additional Side Effects:** Kidney damage, hematuria, urinary frequency.

**Dosage**
• **Capsules**
  *Absence seizures.*
**Adults and children, initial:** 0.5 g b.i.d.; **then,** dose can be increased by 0.5 g/day at 1-week intervals until seizures are controlled or the daily dosage reaches 3 g. May be used with other anticonvulsants in the presence of multiple types of epilepsy.

## NURSING CONSIDERATIONS

See also *Nursing Considerations* for *Anticonvulsants* and *Succinimides*.

**Client/Family Teaching**

1. May discolor urine a pink-brown. Report changes in elimination such as pain, frequency, or blood.

2. Report any loss of seizure control.

**Outcomes/Evaluate:** Control of seizures

# Phentolamine mesylate
(fen-**TOLL**-ah-meen)
**Pregnancy Category:** C
Regitine, Rogitine ✸ **(Rx)**
**Classification:** Alpha-adrenergic blocking agent

**Action/Kinetics:** Phentolamine competitively blocks both presynaptic (alpha-2) and postsynaptic (alpha-1) adrenergic receptors producing vasodilation and a decrease in peripheral resistance. The drug has little effect on BP. In CHF, phentolamine reduces afterload and pulmonary arterial pressure as well as increases

CO. **Onset** (parenteral): Immediate. **Duration:** Short. Poorly absorbed from the GI tract. About 10% excreted unchanged in the urine after parenteral use.

**Uses:** Prophylaxis or treatment of hypertension in pheochromocytoma as a result of stress or manipulation prior to or during surgery. Dermal necrosis and sloughing following IV use or extravasation of norepinephrine. To test for pheochromocytoma (not the method of choice). *Investigational:* Hypertensive crisis secondary to MAO inhibitor/sympathomimetic amine interactions, as well as rebound hypertension due to withdrawal of clonidine, propranolol, or other antihypertensive drugs. In combination with papaverine as an intracavernous injection for impotence.

**Contraindications:** Coronary artery disease including angina, MI, or coronary insufficiency.

**Special Concerns:** Use during pregnancy and lactation only if benefits clearly outweigh risks. Geriatric clients may have a greater risk of developing hypothermia. Use with great caution in the presence of gastritis, ulcers, and clients with a history thereof. Use of cardiac glycosides should be deferred until cardiac rhythm returns to normal.

**Side Effects:** *CV:* Acute and prolonged hypotension, tachycardia, and arrhythmias, especially after parenteral administration. Orthostatic hypotension, flushing. *GI:* N&V, diarrhea. *Other:* Dizziness, weakness, nasal stuffiness.

**OD** **Overdose Management:** *Symptoms: **Hypotension, shock.*** *Treatment:* Maintain BP by giving IV norepinephrine (DO NOT USE EPINEPHRINE).

**Drug Interactions**
*Ephedrine* / Phentolamine antagonizes vasoconstrictor and hypertensive effect
*Epinephrine* / Phentolamine antagonizes vasoconstrictor and hypertensive effect

*Norepinephrine* / Suitable antagonist to treat overdosage induced by phentolamine
*Propranolol* / Concomitant use during surgery for pheochromocytoma is indicated

**Dosage**
• **IV, IM**
*Prevent hypertension in pheochromocytoma, preoperative.*
**Adults, IV:** 5 mg 1–2 hr before surgery; dose may be repeated if needed. **Pediatric, IV, IM:** 1 mg (or 0.1 mg/kg) 1–2 hr before surgery; dose may be repeated if needed.
*Prevent or control hypertension during surgery.*
**Adults, IV:** 5 mg. **IV infusion:** 0.5–1 mg/min. **Pediatric, IV:** 0.1 mg/kg (3 mg/m$^2$). May be repeated, if necessary. During surgery 5 mg for adults and 1 mg for children may be given to prevent or control symptoms of epinephrine intoxication (e.g., paroxysms of hypertension, respiratory depression, seizures, tachycardia).
*Dermal necrosis/sloughing following IV or extravasation of norepinephrine.*
*Prevention:* 10 mg/1,000 mL norepinephrine solution; *treatment:* 5–10 mg/10 mL saline injected into area of extravasation within 12 hr. **Pediatric:** 0.1–0.2 mg/kg to a maximum of 10 mg.
*CHF.*
**Adults, IV infusion:** 0.17–0.4 mg/min.
*Diagnosis of pheochromocytoma.*
**Adults, rapid IV, initial:** 2.5 mg (if response is negative, a 5-mg test should be undertaken before concluding the test is negative); **children, rapid IV:** 1 mg. **Adults, IM:** 5 mg; **children, IM:** 3 mg.
• **Intracavernosal**
*Impotence.*
**Adults:** Papaverine, 30 mg, and 0.5–1 mg phentolamine; adjust dose according to response.

**NURSING CONSIDERATIONS**
**Administration/Storage**
**IV** 1. For IV administration, reconsti-

tute 5 mg with 1 mL sterile water or 0.9% NaCl and inject over 1 min.

2. Drug may also be further diluted: 5–10 mg in 500 mL of D5W and titrated to desired response.

3. When the IV administration of norepinephrine or dopamine results in infiltration, administer solutions of phentolamine SC at the site and within 12 hr for beneficial effects. Use 5–10 mg of phentolamine in 10–15 mL of 0.9% NaCl.

**Assessment:** Note any history of CAD, gastritis, or PUD; obtain VS and ECG.

**Interventions**

1. Monitor VS frequently during parenteral administration until stabilized.

2. To avoid postural hypotension, keep supine for at least 30 min after injection. Then dangle legs over the side of the bed and rise slowly to avoid orthostatic hypotension.

3. With S&S of drug overdose, place in Trendelenburg position. Have levarterenol available to minimize hypotension. *Do not use epinephrine.*

For the diagnosis of pheochromocytoma:

1. The test should not be undertaken on normotensive clients.

2. Sedatives, analgesics, and other nonessential medication should be withheld for 24 hr (and preferably 72 hr) prior to the test.

3. When testing for pheochromocytoma, keep in a supine position, preferably in a dark, quiet room.

4. If the IV test is used, BP should be measured immediately after the injection, at 30-sec intervals for the first 3 min and at 60-sec intervals for the next 7 min. If the IM test is used, BP should be measured every 5 min for 30–45 min.

5. The test is most reliable with sustained hypertension and least reliable with paroxysmal hypertension.

6. A positive response is a drop of more than 35 mm Hg systolic and 25 mm Hg diastolic pressure. Maximal decreases in BP usually occur within 2 min after injection and return to

preinjection pressure within 15–30 min. A negative response is indicated when the BP is unchanged, elevated, or reduced less than 35 mm Hg systolic and 25 mm Hg diastolic pressure.

**Outcomes/Evaluate**
- ↓ BP
- Prevention of tissue necrosis
- Positive test for pheochromocytoma

---

# Phenylephrine hydrochloride

(fen-ill-**EF**-rin)

**Pregnancy Category:** C

**Nasal:** Alconefrin 12, 25, and 50, Children's Nostril, Doktors, Duration, Neo-Synephrine Solution, Nostril, Rhinall, Vicks Sinex. **Ophthalmic:** AK-Dilate, Dionephrine ✿, Mydfrin 2.5%, Neo-Synephrine, Neo-Synephrine Viscous, Phenoptic, Prefrin Liquifilm, Relief. **Parenteral:** Neo-Synephrine. (Rx: Parenteral and Ophthalmic Solutions 2.5% or greater; OTC: Nasal products and ophthalmic solutions 0.12% or less)

**Classification:** Alpha-adrenergic agent (sympathomimetic)

---

See also *Sympathomimetic Drugs* and *Nasal Decongestants*.

**Action/Kinetics:** Stimulates alpha-adrenergic receptors, producing pronounced vasoconstriction and hence an increase in both SBP and DBP; reflex bradycardia results from increased vagal activity. Also acts on alpha receptors producing vasoconstriction in the skin, mucous membranes, and the mucosa as well as mydriasis by contracting the dilator muscle of the pupil. Resembles epinephrine, but it has more prolonged action and few cardiac effects. **IV: Onset,** immediate; **duration,** 15–20 min. **IM, SC: Onset,** 10–15 min; **duration:** 0.5–2 hr for IM and 50–60 min for SC. *Nasal decongestion (topical):* **Onset:** 15–20 min; **duration,** 30 min–4 hr. *Ophthalmic:* **Time to peak effect for mydriasis,** 15–60 min for 2.5% solution and 10–90 min for 10% solution. **Duration:** 0.5–1.5 hr for 0.12%, 3 hr for 2.5%, and 5–7 hr with 10% (when used for mydriasis). Excreted in urine.

**Uses: Systemic:** Vascular failure in shock, shock-like states, drug-induced hypotension or hypersensitivity. To maintain BP during spinal and inhalation anesthesia; to prolong spinal anesthesia. As a vasoconstrictor in regional analgesia. Paroxysmal SVT. **Nasal:** Nasal congestion due to allergies, sinusitis, common cold, or hay fever. **Ophthalmologic: 0.12%:** Temporary relief of redness of the eye associated with colds, hay fever, wind, dust, sun, smog, smoke, contact lens. **2.5% and 10%:** Decongestant and vasoconstrictor, treatment of uveitis with posterior synechiae, open-angle glaucoma, refraction without cycloplegia, ophthalmoscopic examination, funduscopy, prior to surgery.

**Contraindications:** Severe hypertension, ventricular tachycardia.

**Special Concerns:** Use with extreme caution in geriatric clients, severe arteriosclerosis, bradycardia, partial heart block, myocardial disease, hyperthyroidism and during pregnancy and lactation. Nasal and ophthalmic use of phenylephrine may be systemically absorbed. Use of the 2.5% or 10% ophthalmic solutions in children may cause hypertension and irregular heart beat. In geriatric clients, chronic use of the 2.5% or 10% ophthalmic solutions may cause rebound miosis and a decreased mydriatic effect.

**Side Effects:** *CV:* Reflex bradycardia, arrhythmias (rare). *CNS:* Headache, excitability, restlessness. *Ophthalmologic:* Rebound miosis and decreased mydriatic response in geriatric clients, blurred vision.

**OD** **Overdose Management:** *Symptoms:* Ventricular extrasystoles, short paroxysms of ventricular tachycardia, sensation of fullness in the head, tingling of extremities. *Treatment:* Administer an alpha-adrenergic blocking agent (e.g., phentolamine).

**Additional Drug Interactions**
*Anesthetics, halogenated hydrocarbon* / May sensitize myocardium → serious arrhythmias
*Bretylium* / ↑ Effect of phenylephrine → possible arrhythmias

**Dosage**
- **IM, IV, SC**
  *Vasopressor, mild to moderate hypotension.*
  **Adults:** 2–5 mg (range: 1–10 mg), not to exceed an initial dose of 5 mg IM or SC repeated no more often than q 10–15 min; or, 0.2 mg (range: 0.1–0.5 mg), not to exceed an initial dose of 0.5 mg IV repeated no more often than q 10–15 min. **Pediatric:** 0.1 mg/kg (3 mg/m²) IM or SC repeated in 1–2 hr if needed.
  *Vasopressor, severe hypotension and shock.*
  **Adults:** 10 mg by continuous IV infusion using 250–500 mL 5% dextrose injection or 0.9% sodium chloride injection given at a rate of 0.1–0.18 mg/min initial; **then,** give at a rate of 0.04–0.06 mg/min.
  *Prophylaxis of hypotension during spinal anesthesia.*
  **Adults:** 2–3 mg IM or SC 3–4 min before anesthetic given; subsequent doses should not exceed the previous dose by more than 0.1–0.2 mg. No more than 0.5 mg should be given in a single dose. **Pediatric:** 0.044–0.088 mg/kg IM or SC.
  *Hypotensive emergencies during spinal anesthesia.*
  **Adults, initial:** 0.2 mg IV; dose can be increased by no more than 0.2 mg for each subsequent dose not to exceed 0.5 mg/dose.
  *Prolongation of spinal anesthesia.*
  2–5 mg added to the anesthetic solution increases the duration of action up to 50% without increasing side effects or complications.
  *Vasoconstrictor for regional anesthesia.*
  Add 1 mg to every 20 mL of local anesthetic solution. If more than 2 mg phenylephrine is used, pressor reactions can be expected.

P

---

*Paroxysmal SVT.*
**Initial:** 0.5 mg (maximum) given by rapid IV injection (over 20–30 seconds). Subsequent doses are determined by BP and should not exceed the previous dose by more than 0.1–0.2 mg and should never be more than 1 mg.

• **Nasal Solution, Nasal Spray**
**Adults and children over 12 years of age:** 2–3 gtt of the 0.25% or 0.5% solution into each nostril q 3–4 hr as needed. In resistant cases, the 1% solution can be used but no more often than q 4 hr. **Children, 6–12 years of age:** 2–3 gtt of the 0.25% solution q 3–4 hr as needed. **Infants, greater than 6 months of age:** 1–2 gtt of the 0.16% solution into each nostril q 3–4 hr.

• **Ophthalmic Solution, 0.12%, 2.5%, 10%**
*Vasoconstriction, pupillary dilation.*
1 gtt of the 2.5% or 10% solution on the upper limbus a few minutes following 1 gtt of topical anesthetic (prevents stinging and dilution of solution by lacrimation). An additional drop may be needed after 1 hr.
*Uveitis.*
1 gtt of the 2.5% or 10% solution with atropine. To free recently formed posterior synechiae, 1 gtt of the 2.5% or 10% solution to the upper surface of the cornea. Treatment should be continued the following day, if needed. In the interim, hot compresses should be applied for 5–10 min t.i.d. using 1 gtt of 1% or 2% atropine sulfate before and after each series of compresses.
*Glaucoma.*
1 gtt of 10% solution on the upper surface of the cornea as needed. Both the 2.5% and 10% solutions may be used with miotics in clients with open-angle glaucoma.
*Surgery.*
2.5% or 10% solution 30–60 min before surgery for wide dilation of the pupil.
*Refraction.*
**Adults:** 1 gtt of a cycloplegic (homatropine HBr, atropine sulfate, cyclopentolate, tropicamide HCl, or a combination of homatropine and cocaine HCl) in each eye followed in 5 min with 1 gtt of 2.5% phenylephrine solution and in 10 min with another drop of cycloplegic. The eyes are ready for refraction in 50–60 min.
**Children:** 1 gtt of atropine sulfate, 1%, in each eye followed in 10–15 min with 1 gtt of phenylephrine solution, 2.5%, and in 5–10 min with a second drop of atropine sulfate, 1%. The eyes are ready for refraction in 1–2 hr.
*Ophthalmoscopic examination.*
1 gtt of 2.5% solution in each eye. The eyes are ready for examination in 15– 30 min and the effect lasts for 1–3 hr.
*Minor eye irritations.*
1–2 gtt of the 0.12% solution in the eye(s) up to q.i.d. as needed.

## NURSING CONSIDERATIONS

See also *Nursing Considerations* for *Sympathomimetic Drugs* and *Nasal Decongestants.*
**Administration/Storage**
1. Store drug in a brown bottle and away from light.
2. Anticipate that before administering the 10% ophthalmic solution, instillation of a drop of local anesthetic will be necessary.
3. When the drug is used as a nasal decongestant, instruct clients to blow their noses before administration.
**IV** 4. For IV administration, dilute each 1 mg with 9 mL of sterile water and administer over 1 min. Further dilution of 10 mg in 500 mL of dextrose, Ringer's, or saline solution may be titrated to client response.
5. When drug is used parenterally, monitor infusion site closely to avoid extravasation. If evident, local SC administration of phentolamine should be performed to prevent tissue necrosis.
6. Prolonged exposure to air or strong light may result in oxidation and discoloration. Solution should not be used if it changes color, becomes cloudy, or contains a precipitate.

**Assessment**

1. Document indications for therapy, type and onset of symptoms; note goals of therapy.

2. During IV administration monitor cardiac rhythm and BP continuously until stabilized, noting any evidence of bradycardia or arrhythmias.

**Client/Family Teaching**

1. Ophthalmic instillations and nasal decongestants may produce systemic sympathomimetic effects; chronic excessive use may cause rebound congestion.

2. Wear sunglasses in bright light. Report symptoms of photosensitivity and blurred vision if they persist after 12 hr. Blurred vision should decrease with repeated use.

3. With ophthalmic solution, report if there is no relief of symptoms within 2 days.

4. When using for nasal decongestion, report if no relief of symptoms within 3 days. Rebound nasal congestion may occur with longer therapy.

**Outcomes/Evaluate**

- ↑ BP
- Termination of paroxysmal SVT
- Relief of nasal congestion
- ↓ Conjunctivitis/allergic manifestations
- Dilatation of pupils

# Phenylpropanolamine hydrochloride

(fen-ill-**proh**-pah-**NOHL**-ah-meen)
Acutrim 16 Hour, Acutrim Late Day, Acutrim II Maximum Strength, Control, Dexatrim, Dexatrim Maximum Strength and Maximum Strength Caplets, Dexatrim Maximum Strength Pre-Meal Caplets, Efed II Yellow, Maigret-50, Phenyldrine, Propagest, Unitrol (OTC except Maigret-50 and Rhindecon)
**Classification:** Sympathomimetic decongestant, appetite suppressant

See also *Stimulants,* and *Sympathomimetic Drugs.*

**Action/Kinetics:** Thought to stimulate both alpha and beta receptors as well as to act indirectly through release of norepinephrine from storage sites. Increases in BP are due mainly to increased CO rather than to vasoconstriction; has minimal CNS effects. Acts on alpha-adrenergic receptors to produce a decongestant effect in the nasal mucosa. **Onset, decongestant:** 15–30 min; **peak plasma levels:** 1–2 hr; **duration, capsules and tablets:** 3 hr; **extended-release tablets:** 12–16 hr. **Peak plasma levels:** 100 ng. **t½:** 3–4 hr. Eighty percent to 90% excreted in the urine unchanged.

**Uses:** Nasal congestion due to colds, hay fever, allergies. Short-term (8–12 weeks) treatment of exogenous obesity in conjunction with a weight reduction program including reduced caloric intake, exercise, and behavior modification. *Investigational:* Mild to moderate stress incontinence in women.

**Contraindications:** Arteriosclerosis, depression, glaucoma, hypertension, diabetes, kidney disease, hyperthyroidism, during or within 14 days of use of MAO inhibitors, hypersensitivity to sympathomimetics. Not recommended as an anorexiant for children less than 12 years of age. Sustained-release forms during lactation and in children less than 12 years of age.

**Special Concerns:** Safety and efficacy during pregnancy and lactation and for children not established. Children less than 6 years of age may be at greater risk for developing psychiatric disorders when using phenylpropanolamine. The anorexiant dose must be individualized for children 12–18 years of age.

**Side Effects:** *CNS:* Dizziness, headache, insomnia, restlessness, bizarre behavior. Serious effects due to abuse include: agitation, tremor, increased motor activity, hallucinations, *seizures, stroke, and death. CV:* Palpitations, *hypertension (may be severe and lead to crisis),* tachycardia. *Miscellaneous:* Dry mouth, dysuria, renal failure, nausea, nasal dryness.

---

✦ = Available in Canada          *bold italic* = life threatening side effect

**Additional Drug Interactions**
*Bromocriptine* / Worsening of side effects of bromocriptine; possibility of ventricular tachycardia and cardiac dysfunction
*Caffeine* / ↑ Serum caffeine levels, ↑ risk of pharmacologic and toxic effects
*Indomethacin* / Possibility of severe hypertensive episode

**Dosage**
• **Capsules, Tablets**
*Decongestant.*
**Adults:** 25 mg q 4 hr or 50 mg q 6–8 hr (not to exceed 150 mg/day); **Children, 2–6 years:** 6.25 mg q 4 hr, not to exceed 37.5 mg in 24 hr; **6–12 years:** 12.5 mg q 4 hr, not to exceed 75 mg in 24 hr.
*Anorexiant.*
**Adults:** 25 mg t.i.d. 30 min before meals, not to exceed 75 mg in 24 hr.
• **Extended-Release Capsules, Extended-Release Tablets**
*Decongestant.*
**Adults:** 75 mg q 12 hr.
*Anorexiant.*
**Adults:** 75 mg once daily in the morning.

## NURSING CONSIDERATIONS

See also *Nursing Considerations* for *Stimulants* and *Sympathomimetic Drugs.*
**Client/Family Teaching**
1. Continue regular exercise, reduced caloric intake, and behavioral modification programs in the overall management of obesity.
2. Men should report difficulties in voiding; they may experience drug-induced urinary retention.
3. Drug may cause dizziness and tremors.
4. Avoid any caffeine-containing products or foods.
**Outcomes/Evaluate**
• ↓ Nasal congestion
• ↓ Appetite; weight loss

# Phenytoin (Diphenylhydantoin)
(FEN-ih-toyn, dye-fen-ill-hy-DAN-toyn)

**Pregnancy Category:** C
Dilantin Infatab, Dilantin-125, Novo-Phenytoin ✶ **(Rx)**

# Phenytoin sodium, extended
(FEN-ih-toyn)
**Pregnancy Category:** C
Dilantin Kapseals **(Rx)**

# Phenytoin sodium, parenteral
(FEN-ih-toyn)
**Pregnancy Category:** C
Dilantin Sodium **(Rx)**

# Phenytoin sodium prompt
(FEN-ih-toyn)
**Pregnancy Category:** C
Diphenylan Sodium **(Rx)**
**Classification:** Anticonvulsant, hydantoin type; antiarrhythmic (type I)

See also *Anticonvulsants* and *Antiarrhythmic Agents.*
**Action/Kinetics:** Acts in the motor cortex of the brain to reduce the spread of electrical discharges from the rapidly firing epileptic foci in this area. This is accomplished by stabilizing hyperexcitable cells possibly by affecting sodium efflux. Also, phenytoin decreases activity of centers in the brain stem responsible for the tonic phase of grand mal seizures. Has few sedative effects.

Monitor serum levels because the serum concentrations of phenytoin increase disproportionately as the dosage is increased. Phenytoin extended is designed for once-a-day dosage. It has a slow dissolution rate—no more than 35% in 30 min, 30%–70% in 60 min, and less than 85% in 120 min. Absorption is variable following PO dosage. **Peak serum levels: PO,** 4–8 hr. Since the rate and extent of absorption depend on the particular preparation, the same product should be used for a particular client. **Peak serum levels (following IM):** 24 hr (wide variation). **Therapeutic serum levels:** 5–20 mcg/mL. **t½:** 8–60 hr (average: 20–30 hr). **Steady state:** 7–10 days after initiation. Biotransformed in the liver. Both inactive metabolites and unchanged drug are excreted in the urine.

As an antiarrhythmic, phenytoin increases the electrical stimulation threshold of heart muscle, although it is less effective than quinidine, procainamide, or lidocaine. **Onset:** 30–60 min. **Duration:** 24 hr or more. **t½:** 22–36 hr. **Therapeutic serum level:** 10–20 mcg/mL.

**Uses:** Chronic epilepsy, especially of the tonic-clonic, psychomotor type. Not effective against absence seizures and may even increase the frequency of seizures in this disorder. Parenteral phenytoin is sometimes used to treat status epilepticus and to control seizures during neurosurgery.

PO for certain PVCs and IV for PVCs and tachycardia. Particularly useful for arrhythmias produced by digitalis overdosage.

*Investigational:* Paroxysmal choreoathetosis; to treat blistering and erosions in clients with recessive dystrophic epidermolysis bullosa; episodic dyscontrol; trigeminal neuralgia; as a muscle relaxant in neuromyotonia, myotonia congenita, or myotonic muscular dystrophy; to treat cardiac symptoms in overdosage of tricyclic antidepressants. Severe preeclampsia.

**Contraindications:** Hypersensitivity to hydantoins, exfoliative dermatitis, sinus bradycardia, second- and third-degree AV block, clients with Adams-Stokes syndrome, SA block. Lactation.

**Special Concerns:** Use with caution in acute, intermittent porphyria. Administer with extreme caution to clients with a history of asthma or other allergies, impaired renal or hepatic function, and heart disease (hypotension, severe myocardial insufficiency). Abrupt withdrawal may cause status epilepticus. Combined drug therapy is required if petit mal seizures are also present.

**Side Effects:** *CNS:* Most commonly, drowsiness, ataxia, dysarthria, confusion, insomnia, nervousness, irritability, depression, tremor, numbness, headache, psychoses, *increased seizures.* Choreoathetosis following IV use. *GI:* Gingival hyperplasia, N&V, either diarrhea or constipation. *Dermatologic:* Various dermatoses including a measles-like rash (common), scarlatiniform, maculopapular, and urticarial rashes. Rarely, drug-induced lupus erythematosus, *Stevens-Johnson syndrome,* exfoliative or purpuric dermatitis, and *toxic epidermal necrolysis.* Alopecia, hirsutism. Skin reactions may necessitate withdrawal of therapy. *Hematopoietic:* Leukopenia, granulocytopenia, thrombocytopenia, pancytopenia, *agranulocytosis,* macrocytosis, megaloblastic anemia, leukocytosis, monocytosis, eosinophilia, simple anemia, *aplastic anemia, hemolytic anemia. Hepatic:* Liver damage, toxic hepatitis, hypersensitivity reactions involving the liver including hepatocellular degeneration and *fatal hepatocellular necrosis. Ophthalmic:* Diplopia, nystagmus, conjunctivitis. *Miscellaneous:* Hyperglycemia, chest pain, edema, fever, photophobia, weight gain, *pulmonary fibrosis,* lymph node hyperplasia, gynecomastia, periarteritis nodosa, depression of IgA, soft tissue injury at injection site, coarsening of facial features, Peyronie's disease, enlarged lips.

*Rapid parenteral administration may cause serious CV effects, including hypotension, arrhythmias, CV collapse, and heart block, as well as CNS depression.*

Many clients have a partial deficiency in the ability of the liver to degrade phenytoin, and as a result, toxicity may develop after a small PO dose. Liver and kidney function tests and hematopoietic studies are indicated prior to and periodically during drug therapy.

**OD** **Overdose Management:** *Symptoms:* Initially, ataxia, dysarthria, and nystagmus followed by unresponsive pupils, hypotension, and *coma.* Plasma levels greater than 40 mcg/mL result in significant decreases in mental capacity. *Treatment:* Treat symptoms. Hemodialysis may be effective. In children, total-exchange transfusion has been used.

## Drug Interactions

*Acetaminophen* / ↓ Effect of acetaminophen due to ↑ breakdown by liver; however, hepatotoxicity may be ↑

*Alcohol, ethyl* / In alcoholics, ↓ effect of phenytoin due to ↑ breakdown by liver

*Allopurinol* / ↑ Effect of phenytoin due to ↓ breakdown in liver

*Amiodarone* / ↑ Effect of phenytoin or amiodarone due to ↓ breakdown by liver

*Antacids* / ↓ Effect of phenytoin due to ↓ GI absorption

*Anticoagulants, oral* / ↑ Effect of phenytoin due to ↓ breakdown by liver. Also, possible ↑ anticoagulant effect due to ↓ plasma protein binding

*Antidepressants, tricyclic* / May ↑ incidence of epileptic seizures or ↑ effect of phenytoin by ↓ plasma protein binding

*Barbiturates* / Effect of phenytoin may be ↑, ↓, or not changed; possible ↑ effect of barbiturates

*Benzodiazepines* / ↑ Effect of phenytoin due to ↓ breakdown by liver

*Carbamazepine* / ↓ Effect of phenytoin or carbamazepine due to ↑ breakdown by liver

*Charcoal* / ↓ Effect of phenytoin due to ↓ absorption from GI tract

*Chloramphenicol* / ↑ Effect of phenytoin due to ↓ breakdown by liver

*Chlorpheniramine* / ↑ Effect of phenytoin

*Cimetidine* / ↑ Effect of phenytoin due to ↓ breakdown by liver

*Clonazepam* / ↓ Plasma levels of clonazepam or phenytoin; or, ↑ risk of phenytoin toxicity

*Contraceptives, oral* / Estrogen-induced fluid retention may precipitate seizures; also, ↓ effect of contraceptives due to ↑ breakdown by liver

*Corticosteroids* / Effect of corticosteroids ↓ due to ↑ breakdown by liver; also, corticosteroids may mask hypersensitivity reactions due to phenytoin

*Cyclosporine* / ↓ Effect of cyclosporine due to ↑ breakdown by liver

*Diazoxide* / ↓ Effect of phenytoin due to ↑ breakdown by liver

*Dicumarol* / Phenytoin ↓ effect of dicumarol due to ↑ breakdown by liver

*Digitalis glycosides* / ↓ Effect of digitalis glycosides due to ↑ breakdown by liver

*Disopyrimide* / ↓ Effect of disopyramide due to ↑ breakdown by liver

*Disulfiram* / ↑ Effect of phenytoin due to ↓ breakdown by liver

*Dopamine* / IV phenytoin results in hypotension and bradycardia; also, ↓ effect of dopamine

*Doxycycline* / ↓ Effect of doxycycline due to ↑ breakdown by liver

*Estrogens* / See *Contraceptives, oral*

*Fluconazole* / ↑ Effect of phenytoin due to ↓ breakdown by liver

*Folic acid* / ↓ Effect of phenytoin

*Furosemide* / ↓ Effect of furosemide due to ↓ absorption

*Haloperidol* / ↓ Effect of haloperidol due to ↑ breakdown by liver

*Ibuprofen* / ↑ Effect of phenytoin

*Isoniazid* / ↑ Effect of phenytoin due to ↓ breakdown by liver

*Levodopa* / Phenytoin ↓ effect of levodopa

*Levonorgestrel* / ↓ Effect of norgestrel

*Lithium* / ↑ Risk of lithium toxicity

*Loxapine* / ↓ Effect of phenytoin

*Mebendazole* / ↓ Effect of mebendazole

*Meperidine* / ↓ Effect of meperidine due to ↑ breakdown by liver; toxic effects of meperidine may ↑ due to accumulation of active metabolite (normeperidine)

*Methadone* / ↓ Effect of methadone due to ↑ breakdown by liver

*Metronidazole* / ↑ Effect of phenytoin due to ↓ breakdown by liver

*Metyrapone* / ↓ Effect of metyrapone due to ↑ breakdown by liver

*Mexiletine* / ↓ Effect of mexiletine due to ↑ breakdown by liver

*Miconazole* / ↑ Effect of phenytoin due to ↓ breakdown by liver

*Nitrofurantoin* / ↓ Effect of phenytoin

*Omeprazole* / ↑ Effect of phenytoin due to ↓ breakdown by liver

*Phenacemide* / ↑ Effect of phenytoin due to ↓ breakdown by liver

*Phenothiazines* / ↑ Effect of phenytoin due to ↓ breakdown by liver

*Phenylbutazone* / ↑ Effect of phenytoin due to ↓ breakdown by liver and ↓ plasma protein binding

*Primidone* / Possible ↑ effect of primidone

*Pyridoxine* / ↓ Effect of phenytoin

*Quinidine* / ↓ Effect of quinidine due to ↑ breakdown by liver

*Rifampin* / ↓ Effect of phenytoin due to ↑ breakdown by liver

*Salicylates* / ↑ Effect of phenytoin by ↓ plasma protein binding

*Sucralfate* / ↓ Effect of phenytoin due to ↓ absorption from GI tract

*Sulfonamides* / ↑ Effect of phenytoin due to ↓ breakdown in liver

*Sulfonylureas* / ↓ Effect of sulfonylureas

*Theophylline* / ↓ Effect of both drugs due to ↑ breakdown by liver

*Trimethoprim* / ↑ Effect of phenytoin due to ↓ breakdown by liver

*Valproic acid* / ↑ Effect of phenytoin due to ↓ breakdown by liver and ↓ plasma protein binding; phenytoin may also ↓ effect of valproic acid due to ↑ breakdown by liver

**Laboratory Test Interferences:** Alters LFTs, ↑ blood glucose values, and ↓ PBI values. ↑ Gamma globulins. Phenytoin ↓ immunoglobulins A and G. False + Coombs' test.

## Dosage

• **Oral Suspension, Chewable Tablets**

*Seizures.*

**Adults, initial:** 100 mg (125 mg of the suspension) t.i.d.; adjust dosage at 7- to 10-day intervals until seizures are controlled; **usual, maintenance:** 300–400 mg/day, although 600 mg/day (625 mg of the suspension) may be required in some. **Pediatric, initial:** 5 mg/kg/day in two to three divided doses; **maintenance,** 4–8 mg/kg (up to maximum of 300 mg/day). Children over 6 years may require up to 300 mg/day. **Geriatric:** 3 mg/kg initially in divided doses; **then,** adjust dosage according to serum levels and response. Once dosage level has been established, the extended capsules may be used for once-a-day dosage.

• **Capsules, Extended-Release Capsules**

*Seizures.*

**Adults, initial:** 100 mg t.i.d.; adjust dose at 7- to 10-day intervals until control is achieved. An initial loading dose of 12–15 mg/kg divided into two to three doses over 6 hr followed by 100 mg t.i.d. on subsequent days may be preferred if seizures are frequent. **Pediatric:** See dose for Oral Suspension and Chewable Tablets.

*Arrhythmias.*

**Adults:** 200–400 mg/day.

• **IV**

*Status epilepticus.*

**Adults, loading dose:** 10–15 mg/kg at a rate not to exceed 50 mg/min; **then,** 100 mg PO or IV q 6–8 hr. **Pediatric, loading dose:** 15–20 mg/kg in divided doses of 5–10 mg/kg given at a rate of 1–3 mg/kg/min.

*Arrhythmias.*

**Adults:** 100 mg q 5 min up to maximum of 1 g.

• **IM**

Dose should be 50% greater than the PO dose.

*Neurosurgery.*

100–200 mg q 4 hr during and after surgery (during first 24 hr, no more than 1,000 mg should be administered; after first day, give maintenance dosage).

## NURSING CONSIDERATIONS

See also *Nursing Considerations* for *Anticonvulsants* and *Antiarrhythmic Agents.*

**P**

---

**Administration/Storage**

1. Full effectiveness of PO administered hydantoins is delayed and may take 6–9 days to be fully established. A similar period of time will elapse before effects disappear completely.

2. When hydantoins are substituted for or added to another anticonvulsant medication, their dosage is gradually increased, while dosage of the other drug is decreased proportionally.

3. Avoid IM, SC, or perivascular injections. Pain, inflammation, and necrosis may be caused by the highly alkaline solutions.

4. If receiving tube feedings of Isocal or Osmolite, the PO absorption of phenytoin may be decreased. Do not administer together.

5. Due to potential differences in bioavailability between PO products, do not interchange brands. Also, when switching from extended to prompt products, dosage adjustments may be required.

**IV** 6. Use of IV infusion is not recommended, as the drug is poorly soluble and may form a precipitate. Inject slowly and directly into a large vein through a large-gauge needle or IV catheter.

7. For parenteral preparations:
• Use only a clear solution.
• Dilute with special diluent supplied by manufacturer.
• Shake the vials until the solution is clear. It may take about 10 min for the drug to dissolve.
• To hasten the process, warm the vial in warm water after adding the diluent.
• The drug is incompatible with acid solutions.

8. *Do not* add phenytoin to an already running IV solution.

9. If IV infusion is used, a rate of 50 mg/min should not be exceeded in adults or 1–3 mg/kg/min in neonates.

10. Following IV administration, administer NSS through the same needle or IV catheter to avoid local irritation of the vein due to alkalinity of the solution. Do not use dextrose solutions.

11. For treatment of status epilepticus, inject the IV slowly at a rate not to exceed 50 mg/min. If necessary, repeat the dose 30 min after the initial administration.

**Assessment**

1. Document indications for therapy, onset and duration of symptoms.

2. Note history and nature of seizures, addressing location, frequency, duration, causes, and characteristics.

3. Determine if hypersensitive to hydantoins or has exfoliative dermatitis. Consider fosphenytoin in those unable to tolerate phenytoin.

4. Do not breast-feed baby following delivery.

5. Monitor ECG hematologic, liver, and renal function studies.

**Interventions**

1. During IV administration, monitor for hypotension.

2. Monitor serum drug levels:
• Seven to 10 days may be required to achieve recommended serum levels. Drug is highly protein bound; may order free and bound drug levels to better assess response. The drug is metabolized much more slowly by elderly clients; thus most may be managed with once a day dosing.
• If receiving drugs that interact with hydantoins or with impaired liver function, obtain level more frequently. Dilantin induces hepatic microsomal enzymes for drug metabolism.

3. Oral form has variable absorption; do not administer with tube feedings. Administer separately, flush, and clamp tube for 20 min to ensure absorption.

**Client/Family Teaching**

1. May take with food to minimize GI upset. Do not take within 2–3 hr of antacid ingestion.

2. Use care when performing tasks that require mental alertness. Drug may cause drowsiness, dizziness, and blurred vision.

3. Do not substitute products or exchange brands because bioavailability of phenytoin may vary. Seizure control may be lost or toxic blood levels may develop if a substitution is made.

4. Prompt-release forms of the medication cannot be substituted for another unless the dosage is also adjusted.
• If taking phenytoin extended, do not substitute chewable tablets for capsules. The strengths of the medications are not equal.
• If taking phenytoin extended, check bottle carefully. Chewable tablets are never in the extended form.
• With extended, take only a single dose daily; take only as directed and only in the brand prescribed.
5. If a dose is missed, take as soon as it is remembered. Then resume the usual schedule. Do not double up to make up for the missed dose. If the doses of drug are scheduled throughout the day, and one of the doses is missed, take the drug as soon as it is realized unless it's within 4 hr of the next dose. In that case, omit unless otherwise instructed.
6. Do not take any other agents. Hydantoins interact with many other medications and may require adjustment of the anticonvulsant dose.
7. Avoid alcohol in any form and CNS depressants.
8. With diabetes, monitor blood sugar and report changes; may have to to adjust insulin dosage and/or diet.
9. Hydantoin may cause the urine to appear pink, red, or brown; do not be alarmed.
10. To minimize bleeding from the gums and prevent gingival hyperplasia, practice good oral hygiene. Brush teeth with a soft toothbrush, massage the gums, and floss every day. Advise dentist of therapy.
11. Hydantoin has an androgenic effect on the hair follicle. Acne may develop; practice good skin care.
12. Report any excessive hair growth on the face and trunk and any discolorations or skin rash; may require dermatologist referral.
13. Complaints of weakness, ease of fatigue, headaches, or feeling faint may be signs of folic acid deficiency or megaloblastic anemia. Dietitian evaluation of food intake may be indicated as well as hematologic evaluations.
14. Report for lab studies as ordered, including a CBC, drug levels, and renal and liver function studies.
15. Drug may alter thyroid function results. If thyroid studies are conducted, for ensured accuracy, they should be repeated 10 days after therapy has been discontinued.
16. Do not stop abruptly. Report all bothersome side effects because these may be dose-related.
17. Practice reliable birth control; drug may interfere with oral contraceptives.

**Outcomes/Evaluate**
• Control of seizures
• Termination of ventricular arrhythmias; restoration of stable cardiac rhythm
• Therapeutic drug levels (5–20 mcg/mL)

# Phosphorated carbohydrate solution
(FOS-for-**ay**-ted **kar**-boh-**HIGH**-drayt)
Emecheck, Emetrol, Nausea Relief, Nausetrol **(OTC)**
**Classification:** Antiemetic

See also *Antiemetics*.
**Action/Kinetics:** A hyperosmolar carbohydrate solution containing fructose, dextrose, and orthophosphoric acid with controlled hydrogen ion concentration. It relieves N&V due to a direct action on the wall of the GI tract that decreases smooth muscle contraction and delays gastric emptying time; the effect is directly related to the amount used. There is some question as to the effectiveness of this product.
**Uses:** Symptomatic relief of N&V.
**Contraindications:** Diabetic clients due to the presence of carbohydrates. Individuals with hereditary fructose intolerance.

**Special Concerns:** Since nausea may be a symptom of a serious condition, a physician should be consulted if symptoms are not relieved or recur often.

**Side Effects:** *GI:* Abdominal pain and diarrhea due to large doses of fructose.

**Dosage** ————————

• **Oral Solution, Liquid**

*N&V due to psychogenic factors, functional vomiting.*

**Adults:** 15–30 mL at 15-min intervals until vomiting ceases; if the first dose is rejected, the same dosage should be given in 5 min. Should not be taken for more than five doses (1 hr). **Infants and children:** 5–10 mL at 15-min intervals in the same manner as adults.

*Regurgitation in infants.*

5 or 10 mL, 10–15 min before each feeding; in refractory cases, 10 or 15 mL, 30 min before feeding.

*Morning sickness.*

15–30 mL on arising; repeat q 3 hr or when nausea threatens.

*N&V due to drug therapy or inhalation anesthesia, motion sickness.*

**Adults and older children:** 15 mL; **young children:** 5 mL.

## NURSING CONSIDERATIONS

See also *Nursing Considerations* for *Antiemetics.*

**Assessment**

1. Document indications for therapy, onset and duration of symptoms, other agents utilized and the outcome.

2. Note any diabetes or hereditary fructose intolerance.

**Client/Family Teaching**

1. Do not dilute and do not take PO fluids immediately before a dose or for at least 15 min after a dose.

2. Report if symptoms persist, recur often, or become worse.

3. Increase fluid intake to prevent the development of dehydration.

**Outcomes/Evaluate:** Relief of N&V

# Physostigmine salicylate

(fye-zoh-**STIG**-meen)

**Pregnancy Category:** C
Antilirium **(Rx)**

# Physostigmine sulfate

(fye-zoh-**STIG**-meen)
**Pregnancy Category:** C
Eserine Sulfate **(Rx)**
**Classification:** Indirectly acting cholinergic-acetylcholinesterase inhibitor

See also *Neostigmine* and *Ophthalmic Cholinergic Agents.*

**Action/Kinetics:** Reversible acetylcholinesterase inhibitor causing an increased concentration of acetylcholine at nerve endings, which can antagonize anticholinergic drugs. Produces miosis, increased accommodation, and a decrease in intraocular pressure with decreased resistance to outflow of aqueous humor. When used for chronic open-angle glaucoma, ciliary muscle contraction may open the intertrabecular spaces, facilitating aqueous humor outflow. **Onset, IV:** 3–5 min. **Duration, IV:** 1–2 hr. **t½:** 1–2 hr. No dosage alteration is necessary in clients with renal impairment. **Onset, miosis:** 20–30 min; **duration, miosis:** 12–36 hr. **Reduction of IOP, peak:** 2–6 hr; **duration:** 12–36 hr.

**Uses:** Overdosage due to cholinergic blocking drugs (e.g., atropine) and tricyclic antidepressant overdosage. Reduce intraocular pressure in open-angle glaucoma. Friedreich's and other inherited ataxias (FDA has granted orphan status for this use). *Investigational:* Angle-closure glaucoma during or after iridectomy, secondary glaucoma if no inflammation present. Treat delirium tremens (DTs) and Alzheimer's disease. May also antagonize the CNS depressant effect of diazepam.

**Contraindications:** Active uveal inflammation, any inflammatory disease of the iris or ciliary body, glaucoma associated with iridocyclitis. Asthma, gangrene, diabetes, CV disease, GI or GU tract obstruction, any vagotonic state, in those receiving choline esters or depolarizing neuromuscular blocking drugs.

**Special Concerns:** Use with caution during lactation, in clients with chronic angle-closure glaucoma, or in clients with narrow angles. Safety and efficacy have not been established for ophthalmic use in children. Systemic use in children should be reserved for life-threatening situations only. Benzyl alcohol, found in the parenteral product, may cause a fatal "gasping syndrome" in premature infants. The parenteral form also contains sulfites that may cause allergic reactions.

**Additional Side Effects:** If IV administration is too rapid, bradycardia, hypersalivation, breathing difficulties, and *seizures* may occur. Conjunctivitis when used for glaucoma.

**OD** **Overdose Management:** *Symptoms:* Cholinergic crisis. *Treatment:* IV atropine sulfate: **Adults:** 0.4–0.6 mg; **infants and children up to 12 years of age:** 0.01 mg/kg q 2 hr as needed (maximum single dose should not exceed 0.4 mg). A short-acting barbiturate may be used for seizures not relieved by atropine.

**Drug Interactions**
*Anticholinesterases, systemic* /
Additive effects → toxicity
*Succinylcholine* / ↑ Risk of respiratory and CV collapse

**Dosage** —————————
• **IM, IV**
*Anticholinergic drug overdose.*
**Adults, IM, IV:** 0.5–2 mg at a rate of 1 mg/min; may be repeated if necessary. **Pediatric, IV:** 0.02 mg/kg IM or by slow IV injection (0.5 mg given over a period of at least 1 min). Dose may be repeated at 5–10 min if needed to a maximum of 2 mg if no toxic effects are manifested.
*Postanesthesia.*
0.5–1 mg given IM or by slow IV (less than 1 mg/min). May be repeated at 10- to 30-min intervals to attain desired response.
• **Ophthalmic Ointment**
*Glaucoma.*

**Adults and children:** 1 cm of the 0.25% sulfate ointment applied to the lower fornix up to t.i.d.

## NURSING CONSIDERATIONS

See also *Nursing Considerations* for *Neostigmine, Cholinergic Blocking Agents,* and *Ophthalmic Cholinergic Agents.*

**Administration/Storage**
1. The ophthalmic ointment may be used at night for prolonged effect of the medication.
2. Store the ophthalmic ointment tightly closed and protected from heat.
**IV** 3. May administer IV undiluted: 1 mg/min; 0.5 mg/min for children. Product contains benzyl alcohol.
**Assessment:** Determine type of overdosage (drug or plant ingestion), amount and time ingested.
**Interventions**
1. During IV administration, monitor ECG and VS; report any bradycardia, hypersalivation, respiratory difficulty, or seizure activity.
2. Have client void prior to administering. If incontinence occurs, may be caused by too high a dose.
**Client/Family Teaching**
1. During ophthalmic instillation, wipe away any excess medication from around the eyes.
2. Wash hands before and after administration to prevent contamination and systemic absorption.
3. Some stinging and burning of the eyes may occur. This should disappear with continued use. If painful spasms occur, apply cold compresses. If itching, pain, or tearing persists, do not continue using until medically cleared.
4. Night vision may be impaired.
5. N&V may occur; report if the symptoms persist or are severe.
**Outcomes/Evaluate**
• Reversal of toxic CNS symptoms R/T drug overdosage or plant toxins
• ↓ Intraocular pressures

**P**

# Phytonadione (Vitamin K₁)

(fye-toe-nah-**DYE**-ohn)

**Pregnancy Category:** C

Aqua-Mephyton, Mephyton **(Rx)**

**Classification:** Fat-soluble vitamin

**Action/Kinetics:** Vitamin K is essential for the hepatic synthesis of factors II, VII, IX, and X, all of which are essential for blood clotting. Vitamin K deficiency causes an increase in bleeding tendency, demonstrated by ecchymoses, epistaxis, hematuria, GI bleeding, and postoperative and intracranial hemorrhage. Similar to natural vitamin K, it has a more rapid and more prolonged effect than menadiol sodium diphosphate and is generally more effective. GI absorption occurs only via intestinal lymphatics and requires the presence of bile salts. Vitamin K is not effective in reversing the anticoagulant effect of heparin. Frequent determinations of PT are indicated during therapy. **IM: Onset,** 1–2 hr. *Control of bleeding:* Parenteral, 3–6 hr. *Normal PT:* 12–14 hr. **PO: Onset,** 6–12 hr.

**Uses:** Primary and drug-induced hypoprothrombinemia, especially that caused by anticoagulants of the coumarin and phenindione type. Vitamin K cannot reverse the anticoagulant activity of heparin.

Parenteral use for vitamin K malabsorption syndromes. Adjunct during whole blood transfusions. Preoperatively to prevent the danger of hemorrhages in surgical clients who may require anticoagulant therapy.

Certain forms of liver disease. Hemorrhagic states associated with obstructive jaundice, celiac disease, ulcerative colitis, sprue, biliary fistula, cystic fibrosis of the pancreas, regional enteritis, resection of intestine. Prophylaxis of hemorrhagic disease of the newborn.

**Contraindications:** Severe liver disease.

**Special Concerns:** Use with caution in clients with sulfite sensitivity. Use with caution during lactation as phytonadione is excreted in breast milk. Safety and efficacy have not been determined in children. Benzyl alcohol, contained in some preparations, may cause toxicity in newborns.

**Side Effects:** May be transient flushing of the face, sweating, a sense of constriction of the chest, and weakness. Cramp-like pain, weak and rapid pulse, convulsive movements, chills and fever, hypotension, cyanosis, or hemoglobinuria has been reported occasionally. *Shock and cardiac and respiratory failure* may be observed. *Allergic:* Rash, urticaria, *anaphylaxis.* *After PO use:* N&V, stomach upset, headache. *After parenteral use:* Flushing, alteration of taste, sweating, hypotension, dizziness, rapid and weak pulse, dyspnea, cyanosis, delayed skin reactions. Pain, swelling, and tenderness at injection site. *IV administration may cause severe reactions (e.g., shock, cardiac or respiratory arrest, anaphylaxis) leading to death.* These effects may occur when receiving vitamin K for the first time. *Newborns: Fatal kernicterus,* hemolysis, jaundice, hyperbilirubinemia (especially in premature infants).

**Drug Interactions**

*Antibiotics* / May inhibit the body's production of vitamin K and may lead to bleeding. Vitamin K supplements should be given

*Anticoagulants, oral* / Vitamin K antagonizes anticoagulant effect

*Cholestyramine* / ↓ Effect of phytonadione due to ↓ absorption from GI tract

*Colestipol* / ↓ Effect of phytonadione due to ↓ absorption from GI tract

*Hemolytics* / ↑ Potential for toxicity

*Mineral oil* / ↓ Effect of phytonadione due to ↓ absorption from GI tract

*Quinidine, Quinine* / ↑ Requirement for vitamin K

*Salicylates* / High doses of salicylates → ↑ requirements for vitamin K

*Sulfonamides* / ↑ Requirements for vitamin K

*Sucralfate /* ↓ Effect of phytonadione due to ↓ absorption from GI tract

## Dosage

- **Tablets**

*Hypoprothrombinemia, drug-induced.*

**Adults:** 2.5–10 mg (up to 25 mg); dose may be repeated after 12–48 hr if needed.

*Vitamin supplement, prothrombogenic, drug-induced hypoprothrombinemia.*

**Pediatric:** 5–10 mg.

- **IM, SC**

*Vitamin supplement, prothrombogenic, drug-induced hypoprothrombinemia.*

**Adults:** 2.5–10 mg (up to 25 mg) which may be repeated after 6–8 hr if needed. **Infants:** 1–2 mg; **children:** 5–10 mg.

*Prophylaxis of hypoprothrombinemia during prolonged TPN.*

**Adults, IM:** 5–10 mg once weekly; **pediatric:** 2–5 mg IM once weekly.

*Infants receiving milk substitutes or who are breastfed.*

1 mg/month if vitamin K in diet is less than 0.1 mg/L.

*Prevention of hemorrhagic disease in the newborn.*

0.5–1 mg IM within 1 hr after delivery. The dose may be repeated in 2–3 weeks if the mother took anticoagulant, anticonvulsant, antituberculosis, or recent antibiotic therapy during pregnancy. Alternatively, 1–5 mg given to the mother 12–24 hr before delivery.

*Treatment of hemorrhagic disease in the newborn.*

1 mg SC or IM (higher doses may be needed if the mother has been taking oral anticoagulants).

## NURSING CONSIDERATIONS

### Administration/Storage

1. Mix suspension (injection) only with water or D5W.
2. Mix colloidal injection with D5W, isotonic NaCl, or D5/NSS.
3. Protect vitamin K from light.
4. Store injectable emulsion or colloidal solutions in cool, 5°C–15°C (41°F–59°F), dark place.
5. Do not freeze.
6. Heparin may be used to reverse effects from overdosage.

### Assessment

1. Document sensitivity to sulfites.
2. Note drugs prescribed to ensure none interact.
3. Monitor PT/PTT, liver and hematologic values.
4. Determine history or lab evidence of advanced liver disease. This results in loss of protein synthesis and is not responsive to vitamin K.

### Interventions

1. Note any frank bleeding. Test stools, urine, and GI drainage for occult blood.
2. Observe hospitalized clients with poor nutrition (receiving TPN), uremia, recent surgery, and multiple antibiotic therapy for vitamin K deficiency.
3. Administer slowly. Rapid parenteral administration can produce dyspnea, chest and back pain, and even death.
4. With decreased bile secretion, administer bile salts to ensure absorption of PO phytonadione.
5. If receiving bile acid–binding resins such as colestipol or cholestyramine, monitor PT and assess carefully for malabsorption of vitamin K.

### Client/Family Teaching

1. Take only as directed.
2. Dietary sources high in vitamin K include dairy products, meats, and green leafy vegetables. The dietary requirement is low since it is also synthesized by colonized bacteria in the intestine.
3. Report any evidence of unusual bruising or bleeding.
4. Use a soft toothbrush, electric razor, and a night light at night; wear shoes and avoid IM shots and flossing to prevent injury with bleeding.
5. Avoid alcohol, aspirin, and ibuprofen compounds (NSAIDs) as well as any other OTC preparations.

**Outcomes/Evaluate**
- Prevention/control of bleeding
- Prophylaxis of hypoprothrombinemia during prolonged TPN
- Prevention of hemorrhagic disease in the newborn

# Pilocarpine hydrochloride
(pie-low-**CAR**-peen)
**Pregnancy Category:** C
Adsorbocarpine, Akarpine, Diocarpine ✺, Isopto Carpine, Miocarpine ✺, Pilocar, Pilopine HS, Piloptic-½ -1, -2, -3, -4, and -6, Pilopto-Carpine, Pilostat, Salagen **(Rx)**

# Pilocarpine nitrate
(pie-low-**CAR**-peen)
**Pregnancy Category:** C
Minims Pilocarpine ✺, Pilagan **(Rx)**

# Pilocarpine ocular therapeutic system
(pie-low-**CAR**-peen)
**Pregnancy Category:** C
Ocusert Pilo-20 and -40 **(Rx)**
**Classification:** Direct-acting cholinergic agent (miotic)

See also *Ophthalmic Cholinergic Agents.*
**Action/Kinetics:** *Hydrochloride or Nitrate Solution:* **Onset:** 45–60 min; **peak effect:** 75 min; **duration:** 4–14 hr. *Hydrochloride Gel:* **Onset:** 60 min; **peak effect:** 3–12 hr; **duration:** 18–24 hr. *Nitrate:* The ocular therapeutic system is placed in the cul-de-sac of the eye for release of pilocarpine. The drug is released from the ocular therapeutic system three times faster during the first few hours and then decreases (within 6 hr) to a rate of 20 or 40 mcg/hr for 1 week. *Ocular system:* **onset:** 60 min. **peak effect:** 1.5–2 hr; **duration:** 7 days. When used to treat dry mouth due to radiotherapy in head and neck cancer clients, pilocarpine stimulates residual functioning salivary gland tissue to increase saliva production.
**Uses: HCl:** Chronic simple glaucoma (especially open-angle). Chronic angle-closure glaucoma, including

after iridectomy. Acute angle-closure glaucoma (alone or with other miotics, epinephrine, beta-adrenergic blocking agents, carbonic anhydrase inhibitors, or hyperosmotic agents). To reverse mydriasis (i.e., after cycloplegic and mydriatic drugs). Pre- and postoperative intraocular tension. The nitrate product is also used for emergency miosis. Salagen (Pilocarpine HCl) has been approved for treatment of radiation-induced dry mouth in head and neck cancer clients. **Nitrate:** Glaucoma. Emergency relief of mydriasis in acutely glaucomatous clients. Reversal of mydriasis caused by cycloplegic agents. **Ocular Therapeutic System:** Glaucoma alone or with other ophthalmic medications. *Investigational:* Hydrochloride used to treat xerostomia in clients with malfunctioning salivary glands.
**Contraindications:** Lactation.
**Special Concerns:** Use with caution during lactation, in those with narrow angles (angle closure may result), or in those with known or suspected cholelithiasis or biliary tract disease. Use with caution in clients with controlled asthma, chronic bronchitis, or COPD. Safety and efficacy have not been established in children.
**Additional Side Effects:** The following side effects have been attributed to the pilocarpine ocular system. *Opthalmic:* Conjunctival irritation, including mild erythema with or without a slight increase in mucous secretion upon initial use.

    **Oral use (tablets).** *Dermatologic:* Sweating, flushing, rash, pruritus. *GI:* N&V, dyspepsia, diarrhea, abdominal pain, taste perversion, anorexia, increased appetite, esophagitis, tongue disorder. *CV:* Hypertension, tachycardia, bradycardia, ECG abnormality, palpitations, syncope. *CNS:* Dizziness, asthenia, headache, tremor, anxiety, confusion, depression, abnormal dreams, hyperkinesia, hypesthesia, nervousness, paresthesias, speech disorder, twitching. *Respiratory:* Sinusitis, rhinitis, pharyngitis, epistaxis, increased sputum, stridor, yawning. *Ophthalmic:* Lacrimation, amblyopia, conjunctivitis, abnormal vision, eye pain, glaucoma. *GU:* Urinary frequency, dysuria, metrorrhagia, urinary impairment. *Body as a whole:* Chills, edema, body odor, hypothermia, mucous membrane abnormality. *Miscellaneous:* Dysphagia, voice alteration, myalgias, seborrhea.

**OD** **Overdose Management:** *Treatment:* Titrate with atropine (0.5–1 mg SC or IM) and supportive measures to maintain circulation and respiration. If there is severe cardiovascular depression or bronchoconstriction, epinephrine (0.3–1 mg SC or IV) may be used.

## Dosage

PILOCARPINE HYDROCHLORIDE
* **Ophthalmic Gel, 4%**
    *Glaucoma.*

**Adults and adolescents:** ½-in. ribbon in the lower conjunctival sac of the affected eye(s) once daily at bedtime.

PILOCARPINE HYDROCHLORIDE
* **Ophthalmic Solution,** ¼%, ½%, 1%, 2%, 3%, 4%, 5%, 6%, 8%
Doses listed are all for adults and adolescents.

*Chronic glaucoma.*
1 gtt of a 0.5%–4% solution q.i.d.
*Acute angle-closure glaucoma.*
1 gtt of a 1% or 2% solution q 5–10 min for three to six doses; then, 1 gtt q 1–3 hr until pressure is decreased.
*Miotic, to counteract sympathomimetics.*
1 gtt of a 1% solution.
*Miosis, prior to surgery.*
1 gtt of a 2% solution q 4–6 hr for one or two doses before surgery.
*Miosis before iridectomy.*
1 gtt of a 2% solution for four doses immediately before surgery.

PILOCARPINE NITRATE
* **Ophthalmic Solution, 1%, 2%, 4%**
Doses listed are all for adults and adolescents.

*Chronic glaucoma.*

1–2 gtt of a 1%–4% solution b.i.d.–q.i.d.
*Emergency miosis.*
1–2 gtt of a 2% or 4% solution.
*Reversal of mydriasis.*
Dose and strength determined by the cycloplegic used.
* **Ocular System**
Insert and remove as directed by physician or package insert. Ocusert Pilo-20 is approximately equal to the 0.5% or 1% drops, while Ocusert Pilo-40 is approximately equal to the 2% or 3% solution.
* **Tablets (Salagen)**
*Treat radiation-induced dry mouth in head and neck cancer clients.*
**Initial: 5 mg t.i.d.; then,** up to 10 mg t.i.d., if needed.

## NURSING CONSIDERATIONS

See also *Nursing Considerations* for *Ophthalmic Cholinergic Agents.*
**Administration/Storage**
1. Concentrations greater than 4% of pilocarpine HCl may be more effective in clients with dark pigmented eyes; however, the incidence of side effects increases.
2. Myopia may be observed during the first several hours of therapy with the ocular therapeutic system. Thus, insert the system at bedtime so by morning the myopia is stable.
3. For acute, narrow-angle glaucoma, give pilocarpine in the unaffected eye to prevent angle-closure glaucoma.
4. Store the solution, protected from light, at 8°C–30°C (46°F–86°F). Refrigerate the gel at 2°C–8°C (36°F–46°F) until dispensed. Do not freeze gel; discard any unused portion after 8 weeks. Refrigerate the ocular therapeutic system at 2°C–8°C (36°F–46° F).
**Assessment:** Clients with acute infectious conjunctivitis or keratitis should be carefully evaluated before use of the pilocarpine ocular system.
**Client/Family Teaching**
1. Review how to insert and how to check the conjunctival sac for pres-

P

ence of the ocular system. Follow these general guidelines for insertion:

• Wash hands.
• Do not permit drug to touch any surface.
• Rinse insert with cool water.
• Pull down lower eyelid.
• Place according to manufacturer's directions.
• System may be moved under closed eyelids to upper eyelid for sleep. Use caution and report any pain as corneal abrasion or irritation may be present.
• Insert at bedtime to diminish side effects; check for presence of ocular system at bedtime and also upon awakening each day. If retention is a problem, the system can be placed in the superior cul-de-sac. The unit can be moved from the lower to upper conjunctival cul-de-sac by gentle digital massage through the eyelid. For best retention, move the unit to the upper conjunctival cul-de-sac before sleep.
• Report if eye irritation, redness, or mucus production persist with the ocular system.
2. If other glaucoma medication (i.e., drops) is used with the gel at bedtime, instill the drops at least 5 min before the gel.
3. Report for periodic tonometric readings to evaluate effectiveness of the drug.
4. Use only as directed. Refrigerate gel and ocular system.

**Outcomes/Evaluate**
• ↓ Intraocular pressures; pupillary constriction
• ↑ Saliva production; relief of radiation-induced dry mouth S&S

# Pindolol
(**PIN**-doh-lohl)
**Pregnancy Category:** B
Alti-Pindolol ✴, Apo-Pindol ✴, Gen-Pindolol ✴, Novo–Pindol ✴, Nu-Pindol ✴, Visken **(Rx)**
**Classification:** Beta-adrenergic blocking agent

See also *Beta-Adrenergic Blocking Agents.*

**Action/Kinetics:** Manifests both beta-1 and beta-2 adrenergic blocking activity. Also has significant intrinsic sympathomimetic effects and minimal membrane-stabilizing activity. Moderate lipid solubility. **t½:** 3–4 hr; however, geriatric clients have a variable half-life ranging from 7 to 15 hr, even with normal renal function. Metabolized by the liver, and the metabolites and unchanged (35%–40%) drug are excreted through the kidneys.
**Uses:** Hypertension (alone or in combination with other antihypertensive agents as thiazide diuretics). *Investigational:* Ventricular arrhythmias and tachycardias, antipsychotic-induced akathisia, situational anxiety.
**Contraindications:** Bronchial asthma or bronchospasm, including severe COPD.
**Special Concerns:** Dosage has not been established in children.
**Laboratory Test Interferences:** ↑ AST and ALT. Rarely, ↑ LDH, uric acid, alkaline phosphatase.

**Dosage**
• **Tablets**
*Hypertension.*
**Initial:** 5 mg b.i.d. (alone or with other antihypertensive drugs). If no response in 3–4 weeks, increase by 10 mg/day q 3–4 weeks to a maximum of 60 mg/day.
*Antipsychotic-induced akathisia.*
5 mg/day.

## NURSING CONSIDERATIONS

See also *Nursing Considerations* for *Beta-Adrenergic Blocking Agents* and *Antihypertensive Agents.*
**Assessment**
1. Document indications for therapy, onset and duration of symptoms, and any other agents trialed.
2. Assess diet, sodium consumption, weight, exercise regimens, and lifestyle.
3. Document VS and cardiopulmonary assessments.
**Outcomes/Evaluate:** ↓ BP; ↓ restlessness

# Pipecuronium bromide

(pih-peh-kyour-**OHN**-ee-um)
**Pregnancy Category:** C
Arduan **(Rx)**
**Classification:** Neuromuscular blocking agent, nondepolarizing

See also *Neuromuscular Blocking Agents.*

**Action/Kinetics:** Competes for cholinergic receptors at the motor end plate and is antagonized by acetylcholinesterase inhibitors. Has no effect on consciousness, pain threshold, or cerebration; thus, use must be accompanied by adequate anesthesia. **Maximum time for blockade:** 5 min following single doses of 70–85 mcg/kg. **Time to recovery to 25% of control:** 30–175 min under balanced anesthesia following single doses of 70 mcg/kg. **t½, distribution:** 6.22 min (4.33 min in renal transplant clients); **t½, elimination:** 1.7 hr (4 hr in renal transplant clients). Increased plasma levels are seen in clients with impaired renal function. Metabolized in the liver; metabolites and unchanged drug eliminated in the urine.

**Uses:** Adjunct to general anesthesia to provide relaxation of skeletal muscle during surgery. Skeletal muscle relaxation for ET intubation. Recommended for procedures lasting 90 or more minutes.

**Contraindications:** Due to the long duration of action, do not use in myasthenia gravis or Eaton-Lambert syndrome, as low doses can lead to a profound effect. Clients undergoing cesarean section. Use of pipecuronium before succinylcholine in order to reduce side effects of succinylcholine. In those requiring prolonged mechanical ventilation in the ICU or prior to or following other nondepolarizing neuromuscular blocking agents.

**Special Concerns:** Although the drug is used in infants and children, no information is available on maintenance dosing. Also, children 1–14 years of age under balanced or halo-

thane anesthesia may be less sensitive to the drug than adults. Use with caution in clients with impaired renal function. The drug should be administered only if there are adequate facilities for intubation, artificial respiration, oxygen therapy, and administration of an antagonist. Obesity may prolong the duration of action. Conditions resulting in an increased volume of distribution (e.g., old age, edematous states, slower circulation time in CV disease) may cause a delay in the time of onset.

**Side Effects:** *Neuromuscular: Prolongation of blockade including skeletal muscle paralysis resulting in respiratory insufficiency or apnea.* Muscle atrophy, difficult intubation. *CV:* Hypotension, bradycardia, hypertension, CVA, thrombosis, myocardial ischemia, atrial fibrillation, ventricular extrasystole. *CNS:* Hypesthesia, CNS depression. *Respiratory:* Dyspnea, respiratory depression, laryngismus, atelectasis. *Metabolic:* Hypoglycemia, hyperkalemia, increased creatinine. *Miscellaneous:* Rash, urticaria, anuria.

**OD** **Overdose Management:** *Symptoms: Skeletal muscle paralysis including depressed respiration.* Treatment: Artificial respiration until effects of drug have worn off. Antagonize neuromuscular blockade by administration of neostigmine, 0.04 mg/kg. Do not use edrophonium.

**Drug Interactions**

*Aminoglycosides /* ↑ Intensity and duration of neuromuscular blockade

*Bacitracin /* ↑ Intensity and duration of neuromuscular blockade

*Colistin/Sodium colistimethate /* ↑ Intensity and duration of neuromuscular blockade

*Enflurane /* ↑ Duration of action of pipecuronium

*Halothane /* ↑ Duration of action of pipecuronium

*Isoflurane /* ↑ Duration of action of pipecuronium

*Magnesium salts /* ↑ Intensity of neuromuscular blockade when used for toxemia of pregnancy

P

*Polymyxin B* / ↑ Intensity and duration of neuromuscular blockade
*Quinidine* / ↑ Risk of recurrent paralysis
*Tetracyclines* / ↑ Intensity and duration of neuromuscular blockade

## Dosage
- **IV Only**
  *Adjunct to general anesthesia.*

**Adults:** Initial dose may be based on the creatinine clearance and the ideal body weight (see information provided by manufacturer). Dose is individualized. The dose range is 50–100 mcg/kg.

*ET intubation using balanced anesthesia.*
70–85 mcg/kg with halothane, isoflurane, or enflurane in clients with normal renal function who are not obese; duration of muscle relaxation is 1–2 hr using this dosage range.

*Use following recovery from succinylcholine.*
50 mcg/kg in clients with normal renal function who are not obese; duration of muscle relaxation using this dose is 45 min. *Maintenance.*
**Adults:** 10–15 mcg/kg given at 25% recovery of control $T_1$ will provide muscle relaxation for an average of 50 min using balanced anesthesia; lower doses should be used in clients receiving inhalation anesthetics. **Pediatric:** The duration of action in infants following a dose of 40 mcg/kg ranged from 10 to 44 min while the duration in children following a dose of 57 mcg/kg ranged from 18 to 52 min.

## NURSING CONSIDERATIONS

See also *Nursing Considerations* for *Neuromuscular Blocking Agents.*
### Administration/Storage
**IV** 1. Administer only under the supervision of individuals experienced with the use of neuromuscular blocking agents.
2. Reconstitute using 0.9% NaCl, D5/NSS, D5W, RL, sterile water for injection, and bacteriostatic water for injection.
3. If used in newborns, do not reconstitute with bacteriostatic water

for injection because it contains benzyl alcohol.
4. When reconstituted with bacteriostatic water for injection, store the solution at room temperature or in the refrigerator; use within 5 days.
5. When reconstituted with sterile water or other IV solutions, refrigerate and use within 24 hr.
6. Do not dilute with or administer from large volumes of IV solutions.
7. Store at 2°C–30°C (35°F–86°F) and protect from light.
### Assessment
1. Document indications for therapy and anticipated duration of use.
2. Determine height and weight; note if obese; correlate drug dose for *ideal* body weight.
3. Assess for myasthenia gravis or Eaton-Lambert syndrome.
4. List drugs prescribed because many interact unfavorably with pipecuronium.
5. Determine if diarrhea is present and the duration; may alter desired neuromuscular blockade.
6. Monitor ECG, VS, electrolytes, and renal function studies.
### Interventions
1. The twitch response should be used to evaluate neuromuscular response and recovery and to minimize overdosage potential. Use a peripheral nerve stimulator to assess the height of the twitch wave.
2. Allow more time for pipecuronium to achieve maximum effect in older clients with slowed circulation, CV diseases, and/or edematous states. *Do not* increase drug dose because this will produce a longer duration of action.
3. Monitor VS and observe postrecovery for adequate clinical evidence of antagonism:
- 5-sec head lift
- Adequate pronation
- Effective airway and ventilatory patterns
4. Monitor ECG. Drug can cause vagal stimulation resulting in bradycardia, hypotension, and cardiac arrhythmias.
5. Muscle fasciculations may cause client to be sore or injured after

recovery. Administer prescribed nondepolarizing agent and reassure that the soreness is likely caused by the unsynchronized contractions of adjacent muscle fibers just before the onset of paralysis.

6. Document length of time client is receiving the drug. It should be used only on a short-term basis and in a continuously monitored environment.

7. Remember client is fully conscious and aware of surroundings and conversations.

8. Drug does not affect pain or anxiety; administer analgesics and anti-anxiety agents as needed.

9. Prolonged use, as in an ICU setting, may lead to skeletal muscle weakness and symptoms consistent with muscle disuse atrophy. This may complicate ventilator weaning and some clients may require extensive physical therapy.

**Outcomes/Evaluate**
• Skeletal muscle relaxation
• Suppression of twitch response

# Piperacillin sodium
(pie-PER-ah-sill-in)
**Pregnancy Category:** B
Pipracil **(Rx)**
**Classification:** Antibiotic, penicillin

See also *Penicillins*.
**Action/Kinetics:** Semisynthetic, broad-spectrum penicillin for parenteral use. It is not penicillinase resistant. Penetrates CSF in the presence of inflamed meninges. **Peak serum level:** 244 mcg/mL. **t½:** 36–72 min. Excreted unchanged in urine and bile.

**Uses:** Intra-abdominal infections, gynecologic infections, septicemia, skin and skin structure infections, bone and joint infections, UTIs, lower respiratory tract infections, gonococcal infections, streptococcal infections. Mixed infections prior to the identification of the causative organisms. Prophylaxis in surgery including GI, biliary, hysterectomy, cesarean section. Aminoglycosides

have been used with piperacillin sodium, especially in clients with impaired host defenses.
**Additional Side Effects:** Rarely, prolonged muscle relaxation.
**Laboratory Test Interferences:** Positive Coombs' test; ↑ (especially in infants) AST, ALT, LDH, bilirubin.

## Dosage
• **IM, IV**
*Serious infections.*
**IV:** 3–4 g q 4–6 hr (12–18 g/day) as a 20- to 30-min infusion.
*Complicated UTIs.*
**IV:** 8–16 g/day (125–200 mg/kg/day) in divided doses q 6–8 hr.
*Uncomplicated UTIs and most community-acquired pneumonias.*
**IM, IV:** 6–8 g/day (100–125 mg/kg/day) in divided doses q 6–12 hr.
*Uncomplicated gonorrhea infections.*
2 g **IM** with 1 g probenecid **PO** 30 min before injection (both given as single dose).
*Prophylaxis in surgery.*
**First dose: IV,** 2 g prior to surgery; **second dose:** 2 g either during surgery (abdominal) or 4–6 hr after surgery (hysterectomy, cesarean); **third dose:** 2 g at an interval depending on use. Dosage should be decreased in renal impairment.
Dosages have not been established in infants and children under 12 years of age although the following doses have been suggested: **Neonates,** 100 mg/kg q 12 hr; **children,** 200–300 mg/kg/day (up to a maximum of 24 g/day) divided q 4–6 hr.
*For cystic fibrosis.*
350–500 mg/kg/day divided q 4–6 hr.

## NURSING CONSIDERATIONS

See also *Nursing Considerations* for *Penicillins* and *Zosyn*.
**Administration/Storage**
1. For IM administration, use upper, outer quadrant of gluteus or well-developed deltoid muscle. Do not use lower or mid-third of upper arm.

2. Do not administer more than 2 g IM at any one site.

**IV** 3. For IV administration reconstitute each gram with at least 5 mL diluent, such as sterile or bacteriostatic water for injection, NaCl for injection, or bacteriostatic NaCl for injection. Shake until dissolved.

4. Inject IV slowly over a period of 3–5 min to avoid vein irritation.

5. Administer by intermittent IV infusion in at least 50 mL of dextrose or saline solutions over a period of 20–30 min.

6. After reconstitution, store at room temperature for 24 hr, refrigerate for 1 week, or freeze for 1 month.

**Assessment**
1. Document indications for therapy, onset and characteristics of symptoms.

2. Monitor cultures, electrolytes, hematologic, liver, and renal function studies.

3. Assess for diarrhea or other evidence of superinfection.

**Outcomes/Evaluate**
• Infection prophylaxis with surgery
• Symptomatic improvement
• Negative C&S reports

————COMBINATION DRUG————

# Piperacillin sodium and Tazobactam sodium

(pie-**PER**-ah-**sill**-in, tay-zoh-**BAC**-tam)
**Pregnancy Category:** B
Tazocin ✹, Zosyn **(Rx)**
**Classification:** Antibiotic, penicillin

See also *Piperacillin sodium* and *Penicillins*.

**Content:** The powder for injection contains: piperacillin sodium, 2 g, with tazobactam, 0.25 g; piperacillin sodium, 3 g, with tazobactam sodium, 0.372 g; or, piperacillin sodium, 4 g, with tazobactam sodium, 0. 5 g.

**Action/Kinetics:** This product is a combination of piperacillin sodium and tazobactam sodium, a beta-lactamase inhibitor. Tazobactam inhibits beta-lactamases, thus ensuring activity of piperacillin against beta-lacta-

mase-producing microorganisms. Thus, tazobactam broadens the antibiotic spectrum of piperacillin to those bacteria normally resistant to it. **Peak plasma levels:** Attained immediately after completion of an IV infusion. **t½, piperacillin and tazobactam:** 0.7–1.2 hr. Both drugs are eliminated through the kidney with piperacillin excreted unchanged and tazobactam excreted both unchanged and as inactive metabolites. The t½ of both drugs is increased in clients with renal impairment and in hepatic cirrhosis (dose adjustment not required).

**Uses:** (1) Appendicitis complicated by rupture or abscess and peritonitis caused by piperacillin-resistant, beta-lactamase-producing strains of *Escherichia coli, Bacteroides fragilis, B. ovatus, B. thetaiotaomicron,* and *B. vulgatus.* (2) Uncomplicated and complicated skin and skin structure infections (including cellulitis, cutaneous abscesses, and ischemic/diabetic foot infections) caused by piperacillin-resistant, beta-lactamase-producing strains of *Staphylococcus aureus.* (3) Postpartum endometritis or pelvic inflammatory disease caused by piperacillin-resistant, beta-lactamase-producing strains of *E. coli.* (4) Community-acquired pneumonia of moderate severity caused by piperacillin-resistant, beta-lactamase-producing strains of *Haemophilus influenzae.* (5) Moderate to severe nosocomial pneumonia caused by piperacillin-resistant, beta-lactamase-producing strains of *S. aureus.* (6) Infections caused by piperacillin-susceptible organisms for which piperacillin is effective may also be treated with this combination. The treatment of mixed infections caused by piperacillin-susceptible organisms and piperacillin-resistant, beta-lactamase-producing organisms susceptible to this combination do not require addition of another antibiotic.

**Contraindications:** Hypersensitivity to penicillins, cephalosporins, or beta-lactamase inhibitors.

**Special Concerns:** Use with caution during lactation. Safety and efficacy have not been determined in children less than 12 years of age.

**Side Effects:** See Penicillins. The highest incidence of side effects include the following. GI: Diarrhea, constipation, N&V, dyspepsia, stool changes, abdominal pain. CNS: Headache, insomnia, fever, agitation, dizziness, anxiety. Dermatologic: Rash, including maculopapular, bullous, urticarial, and eczematoid; pruritus. Hematologic: Thrombocytopenia, eosinophilia, leukopenia, neutropenia. Miscellaneous: Pain, moniliasis, hypertension, chest pain, edema, rhinitis, dyspnea.

**Drug Interactions**
*Heparin* / Possible ↑ effect of heparin
*Oral anticoagulants* / Possible ↑ effect of oral anticoagulants
*Tobramycin* / ↓ Area under the curve, renal clearance, and urinary recovery of tobramycin
*Vecuronium* / Prolongation of the neuromuscular blockade of vecuronium

**Laboratory Test Interferences:** ↓ H&H. Transient ↑ AST, ALT, alkaline phosphatase, and bilirubin. ↑ Serum creatinine, BUN. Prolonged PT and PTT. Positive direct Coombs' test. Proteinuria, hematuria, pyuria, abnormalities in electrolytes (↑ and ↓ sodium, potassium, calcium), hyperglycemia, ↓ total protein or albumin.

**Dosage** ─────────────
• **IV Infusion**
  *Susceptible infections.*
**Adults:** 12 g/day piperacillin and 1.5 g/day tazobactam, given as 3.375 g (i.e., 3 g piperacillin and 0.375 g tazobactam) q 6 hr for 7–10 days. In clients with renal insufficiency, the IV dose is adjusted depending on the extent of impaired function. If $C_{CR}$ is 20–40 mL/min, the dose is 8 g/day piperacillin and 1 g/day tazobactam in divided doses of 2.25 g q 6 hr. If the $C_{CR}$ is less than 20 mL/min, the dose is 6 g/day piperacillin and 0.75

g/day tazobactam in divided doses of 2.25 g q 8 hr.
  *Moderate to severe nosocomial pneumonia due to piperacillin-resistant, beta-lacatamase-producing* S. aureus.
**Adults:** 3.375 g q 4 hr with an aminoglycoside.

## NURSING CONSIDERATIONS

See also *Nursing Considerations* for *Piperacillin sodium* and *Penicillins*.
**Administration/Storage**
**IV** 1. For IV administration or by infusion, reconstitute the powder for injection with 5 mL suitable diluent/g piperacillin. IV diluents that can be used include 0.9% NaCl for injection, sterile water for injection, dextran 6% in saline, dextrose 5%, potassium chloride 40 mEq, bacteriostatic saline/parabens, bacteriostatic water/parabens, bacteriostatic saline/benzyl alcohol, bacteriostatic water/benzyl alcohol. *LR is not compatible.*
2. After the diluent is added, shake the vial well until the powder is dissolved. It may be further diluted to the desired final volume with the diluent.
3. If intermittent IV infusion is used, the 5 mL diluent/g piperacillin is further diluted to a volume of at least 50 mL. Give the infusion over a period of 30 min. During the infusion, discontinue the primary infusion solution.
4. If concomitant therapy with aminoglycosides is indicated, give piperacillin/tazobactam and the aminoglycoside separately, as penicillin can inactivate the aminoglycoside if they are mixed.
5. Use single-dose vials immediately after reconstitution. Discard any unused drug after 24 hr if stored at room temperature or after 48 hr if stored in the refrigerator at 2°C–8°C (36°F–46°F).
6. After reconstitution, is stable in glass and plastic syringes, IV bags, and tubing. Is stable in IV bags for up to 24 hr at room temperature and up to 1 week in the refrigerator. Is stable

P

in an ambulatory IV infusion pump for 24 hr at room temperature.

**Assessment**

1. Document indications for therapy, type, location, and onset of symptoms.

2. Determine any sensitivity to penicillins, cephalosporins, beta-lactamase inhibitors, or other allergens.

3. List other drugs prescribed to ensure none interact unfavorably. Use of heparin and oral anticoagulants may require dosage adjustments.

4. Monitor electrolytes, urinalysis, hematologic and coagulation profile, liver and renal function studies. Reduce dosage with renal impairment.

**Outcomes/Evaluate:** Resolution of infection

# Piperazine citrate
(pie-**PER**-ah-zeen)
**(Rx)**
**Classification:** Anthelmintic

See also *Anthelmintics.*

**Action/Kinetics:** Acts to paralyze the muscles of parasites; this dislodges the parasites and promotes their elimination by peristalsis. Has little effect on larvae in tissues. Readily absorbed from the GI tract, is partially metabolized by the liver, and the remainder is excreted in urine. Rate of elimination differs among clients although it is excreted nearly unchanged in the urine within 24 hr.

**Uses:** Pinworm (oxyuriasis) and roundworm (ascariasis) infestations. Particularly recommended for pediatric use.

**Contraindications:** Impaired liver or kidney function, seizure disorders, hypersensitivity. Lactation.

**Special Concerns:** Safe use during pregnancy has not been established. Due to neurotoxicity, prolonged, repeated, or excessive use in children should be avoided.

**Side Effects:** Piperazine has low toxicity. *GI:* N&V, diarrhea, cramps. *CNS:* Tremors, headache, vertigo, decreased reflexes, paresthesias, *seizures,* ataxia, chorea, memory decrement. *Ophthalmologic:* Nystagmus,

blurred vision, cataracts, strabismus. *Allergic:* Urticaria, fever, skin reactions, purpura, lacrimation, rhinorrhea, arthralgia, **bronchospasm,** cough. *Miscellaneous:* Muscle weakness.

**Drug Interactions:** Concomitant administration of piperazine and phenothiazines may result in an increase in extrapyramidal effects (including violent convulsions) caused by phenothiazines.

**Laboratory Test Interferences:** False – or ↓ uric acid values.

**Dosage**

• **Syrup, Tablets**
  *Pinworms.*
**Adults and children:** 65 mg/kg/day as a single dose for 7 days up to a maximum daily dose of 2.5 g.
  *Roundworms.*
**Adults:** One dose of 3.5 g/day for 2 consecutive days; **pediatric:** One dose of 75 mg/kg/day for 2 consecutive days, not to exceed 3.5 g/day. For severe infections, repeat therapy after 1 week.

## NURSING CONSIDERATIONS

See also *Nursing Considerations* for *Anthelmintics.*

**Assessment**

1. Note any evidence of impaired hepatic or renal function.

2. Document any seizure disorder or chronic neurologic disease.

3. Determine previous treatments and length of therapy; excessive therapy should be avoided in children due to neurotoxic effects.

4. Use cautiously with severe malnutrition or anemia.

**Client/Family Teaching**

1. Take on an empty stomach before breakfast or in two divided doses.

2. Report any adverse drug effects immediately.

3. Strict hygiene is required to prevent reinfection.

4. Keep pleasant-tasting medication out of reach of children.

5. Drug causes paralysis of ascariasis parasite and they are expelled live by peristalsis. Flush toilet 2–3 times to

ensure that contents are completely removed.

**Outcomes/Evaluate**
• Eradication of infecting parasite
• Negative stool exams and peri-anal swabs

# Pirbuterol acetate
(peer-**BYOU**-ter-ohl)
**Pregnancy Category:** C
Maxair Autohaler **(Rx)**
**Classification:** Sympathomimetic, bronchodilator

See also *Sympathomimetic Drugs.*
**Action/Kinetics:** Causes bronchodilation by stimulating beta-2-adrenergic receptors. Has minimal effects on beta-1 receptors. Also inhibits histamine release from mast cells, causes vasodilation, and increases ciliary motility. **Onset, inhalation:** Approximately 5 min. **Time to peak effect:** 30–60 min. **Duration:** 5 hr.
**Uses:** Alone or with theophylline or steroids, for prophylaxis and treatment of bronchospasm in asthma and other conditions with reversible bronchospasms, including bronchitis, emphysema, bronchiectasis, obstructive pulmonary disease. May be used with or without theophylline or steroids.
**Contraindications:** Cardiac arrhythmias due to tachycardia; tachycardia caused by digitalis toxicity.
**Special Concerns:** Safety and efficacy have not been determined in children less than 12 years of age.
**Additional Side Effects:** *CV:* PVCs, hypotension. *CNS:* Hyperactivity, hyperkinesia, anxiety, confusion, depression, fatigue, syncope. *GI:* Diarrhea, dry mouth, anorexia, loss of appetite, bad taste or taste change, abdominal pain, abdominal cramps, stomatitis, glossitis. *Dermatologic:* Rash, edema, pruritus, alopecia. *Miscellaneous:* Flushing, numbness in extremities, weight gain.

**Dosage**
• **Inhalation Aerosol**

**Adults and children over 12 years:** 0.2–0.4 mg (1–2 inhalations) q 4–6 hr, not to exceed 12 inhalations (2.4 mg) daily.

## NURSING CONSIDERATIONS

See also *Nursing Considerations* for *Sympathomimetic Drugs* and *Adrenergic Bronchodilators.*
**Assessment:** Document indications for therapy, noting onset, duration, and characteristics of symptoms. Perform cardiopulmonary assessment and note CXR and PFTs.
**Client/Family Teaching**
1. Review methods, frequency, and indication for administration. Use a chamber (spacer) to enhance dispersion.
2. Seek medical intervention if condition or peak flows deteriorate or if inhaler is ineffective in relieving symptoms at prescribed dosage.
**Outcomes/Evaluate:** Improved airway exchange; ↓ airway resistance

# Piroxicam
(peer-**OX**-ih-kam)
Alti-Piroxicam ✦, Apo-Piroxicam ✦, Dom-Piroxicam ✦, Feldene, Gen-Piroxicam ✦, Novo-Pirocam ✦, Nu-Pirox ✦, PMS-Piroxicam ✦, Pro-Piroxicam ✦, Rho-Piroxicam ✦ **(Rx)**
**Classification:** Nonsteroidal anti-inflammatory drug

See also *Nonsteroidal Anti-Inflammatory Drugs.*
**Action/Kinetics:** May inhibit prostaglandin synthesis. Effect is comparable to that of aspirin, but with fewer GI side effects and less tinnitus. May be used with gold, corticosteroids, and antacids. **Peak plasma levels:** 1.5–2 mcg/mL after 3–5 hr (single dose). **Steady-state plasma levels** (after 7–12 days): 3–8 mcg/mL. **t½:** 50 hr. **Analgesia, onset:** 1 hr; **duration:** 2–3 days. **Anti-inflammatory activity, onset:** 7–12 days; **duration:** 2–3 weeks. Metabolites and unchanged drug excreted in urine and feces.
**Uses:** Acute and chronic treatment of rheumatoid arthritis and osteoarthri-

**P**

tis. *Investigational:* Juvenile rheumatoid arthritis, primary dysmenorrhea, sunburn.

**Contraindications:** Safe use during pregnancy has not been determined. Lactation.

**Special Concerns:** Safety and efficacy have not been established in children. Increased plasma levels and elimination half-life may be observed in geriatric clients (especially women).

**Laboratory Test Interferences:** Reversible ↑ BUN.

### Dosage

- **Capsules**

  *Anti-inflammatory, antirheumatic.*

  **Adults:** 20 mg/day in one or more divided doses. Effect of therapy should not be assessed for 2 weeks.

## NURSING CONSIDERATIONS

See also *Nursing Considerations* for *Nonsteroidal Anti-Inflammatory Drugs*.

**Administration/Storage**

1. Steady-state plasma levels may not be reached for 2 weeks.

2. Clients over 70 years of age generally require one-half the usual adult dose of medication.

3. Not recommended for children under 14 years of age.

**Assessment**

1. Document indications for therapy, type of symptoms, other agents prescribed, and the outcome.

2. Assess involved joints and note ROM, erythema, swelling, pain, and warmth.

**Client/Family Teaching**

1. Take with food or milk to decrease GI upset. A stomach protectant (i.e., Cytotec) may be prescribed for those with a history of ulcer disease.

2. Take at anti-inflammatory dose to prevent further joint destruction during acute exacerbations.

3. Therapeutic effects of the medication cannot be evaluated fully for at least 2 weeks after beginning treatment.

4. Aspirin decreases the effectiveness of piroxicam and may increase the occurrence of side effects. Avoid aspirin, ethanol, and any other OTC products unless directed.

5. Report any increased abdominal pain, abnormal bruising or bleeding, malaise, or changes in the color of the stool immediately.

6. Drug side effects may not be evident for 7–10 days.

7. Report as scheduled for lab studies.

**Outcomes/Evaluate:** ↓ Joint pain and inflammation with improved mobility

---

# Plicamycin (Mithramycin)

(plye-kah-**MY**-sin, mith-rah-**MY**-sin)

**Pregnancy Category:** X
Mithracin (Abbreviation: MTH) **(Rx)**
**Classification:** Antineoplastic antibiotic

---

See also *Antineoplastic Agents*.

**Action/Kinetics:** Antibiotic produced by *Streptomyces plicatus, S. argillaceus,* and *S. tanashiensis.* Complexes with DNA in the presence of magnesium (or other divalent cations), resulting in inhibition of cellular and enzymatic RNA synthesis. Decreases blood calcium by blocking the hypercalcemic effect of vitamin D, acting on osteoclasts, and preventing the action of parathyroid hormone. Cleared rapidly from the blood and is concentrated in the Kupffer cells of the liver, renal tubular cells, and along formed bone surfaces. Crosses the blood-brain barrier. Excreted through the urine.

**Uses:** Malignant testicular tumors usually associated with metastases and when radiation or surgery is not an alternative. Hypercalcemia and hypercalciuria associated with advanced malignancy and not responsive to other therapy.

**Additional    Contraindications:** Thrombocytopenia, thrombocytopathy, coagulation disorders, and increased tendency to hemorrhage. Impaired bone marrow function. Pregnancy (category: X). Lactation.

Do not use for children under 15 years of age.

**Special Concerns:** Use with caution in impaired liver or kidney function.

**Additional Side Effects:** Severe thrombocytopenia, *__hemorrhagic tendencies.__* Facial flushing. Hepatic and renal toxicity. Extravasation may cause irritation or cellulitis. Electrolyte imbalance including hypocalcemia, hypokalemia, and hypophosphatemia.

**OD Overdose Management:** *Symptoms:* Hematologic toxicity. *Treatment:* Monitor hematologic status, especially clotting factors. Also, closely monitor serum electrolytes and hepatic and renal functions.

**Laboratory Test Interferences:** ↓ Serum calcium, potassium, and phosphorus. ↑ Serum BUN, creatinine, AST, ALT, alkaline phosphatase, bilirubin, isocitric dehydrogenase, ornithine carbamyltransferase, LDH. ↑ BSP retention.

**Dosage** ───────────────
• **IV Only**
  *Testicular tumor.*
**Dose individualized. Usual:** 25–30 (maximum) mcg/kg (given over a period of 4–6 hr) daily for 8–10 (maximum) days. Alternatively, 25–50 mcg/kg on alternate days for an average of eight doses.
  *Hypercalcemia, hypercalciuria.*
**Dose individualized:** 15–25 mcg/kg (given over a period of 4–6 hr) daily for 3–4 days. Additional courses of therapy may be warranted at weekly intervals if initial course is unsuccessful.

## NURSING CONSIDERATIONS

See also *Nursing Considerations* for *Antineoplastic Agents*.

**Administration/Storage**

**IV** 1. Store vials of medication in refrigerator at temperatures below 10°C (36°F). Discard unused portion of drug.

2. Reconstitute fresh for each day of therapy.

3. Drug is unstable in acid solution (pH 5 and below) and in reconstituted solutions (pH 7) and thus deteriorates rapidly.

4. Add 4.9 mL of sterile water to the 2.5-mg vial of plicamycin (or as recommended on the package insert) and shake to dissolve the drug. Final concentration 500 mcg/mL.

5. Add the calculated dosage of drug to the IV solution ordered (recommended 1 L of D5W) and adjust the rate of flow as ordered (recommended infusion time is 4–6 hr/L).

6. Closely check peripheral IV for extravasation. Stop IV if extravasation occurs; apply moderate heat to disperse drug and to reduce pain and tissue damage. Restart IV at another site.

7. Use only for hospitalized clients.

**Assessment**

1. Document indications for therapy and any other treatments prescribed.

2. Monitor CBC, calcium, potassium, phosphorus, hepatic and renal function studies; correct electrolytes and minerals throughout therapy.

3. Assess for evidence of abnormal bleeding such as epistaxis, hemoptysis, hematemesis, purpura, or ecchymoses. Drug may cause granulocyte and platelet suppression. Nadir: 10–14 days; recovery: 21 days.

**Interventions**

1. Administer antiemetic drugs before or during mithramycin therapy.

2. Monitor I&O. Correct dehydration; administer 2–3 L/day of fluids during therapy.

3. Rapid IV drug flow precipitates more severe GI side effects; administer slowly over 4–6 hr.

4. Monitor electrolytes; calcium and phosphate may rebound after therapy.

5. Remind clients to practice reliable birth control during and for several months following therapy.

**Outcomes/Evaluate**
• ↓ Tumor size/spread
• ↓ Serum calcium levels

P

───────────────────────────────

# Podofilox

(poh-**DAHF**-ih-lox)
**Pregnancy Category:** C
Condyline ✢, Condylox, Wartec ✢
**(Rx)**
**Classification:** Keratolytic

**Action/Kinetics:** An antimitotic agent that causes necrosis of visible wart tissue when applied topically. Small amounts are absorbed into the system 1–2 hr after application. **t½:** 1–4.5 hr. The drug does not accumulate following multiple treatments.

**Uses:** Topical treatment of external genital warts and perianal warts (gel only). *Investigational:* Systemically for treatment of cancer.

**Contraindications:** Use of solution or gel for mucous membrane warts or solution for perianal warts. Lactation.

**Special Concerns:** It is essential that genital warts be distinguished from squamous cell carcinoma prior to initiation of treatment. Safety and effectiveness have not been demonstrated in children. Avoid contact with the eyes.

**Side Effects: Solution.** D*ermatologic:* Commonly, burning, pain, inflammation, erosion, and itching. Also, tenderness, chafing, scarring, vesicle formation, dryness and peeling, tingling, bleeding, ulceration, malodor, crusting edema, foreskin irretraction. *Miscellaneous:* Pain with intercourse, insomnia, dizziness, hematuria, vomiting.

**Gel.** *Dermatologic:* Commonly, burning, pain, inflammation, erosion, itching, and bleeding. Also, stinging, erythema, desquamation, scabbing, discoloration, tenderness, dryness, crusting, fissures, soreness, ulceration, swelling/edema, tingling, rash, blisters.

**Systemic Use.** *GI:* N&V, diarrhea, oral ulcers. *Hematologic:* Bone marrow depression, leukocytosis, pancytosis. *CNS:* Altered mental status, lethargy, **coma, seizures.** *Miscellaneous:* Peripheral neuropathy, fever, tachypnea, ***respiratory failure,*** hematuria, renal failure.

**OD** **Overdose Management:**
*Symptoms:* N&V, diarrhea, fever, altered mental status, hematologic toxicity, peripheral neuropathy, lethargy, tachypnea, ***respiratory failure,*** hematuria, leukocytosis, pancytosis, renal failure, ***seizures, coma.*** *Treatment:* Wash the skin free of any remaining drug. General supportive therapy to treat symptoms.

**Dosage**
* **Topical Solution, Topical Gel**
  *External genital warts, perianal warts (gel only).*
**Adults, initial:** Apply b.i.d. in the morning and evening (i.e., q 12 hr) for 3 consecutive days; **then,** withhold use for 4 consecutive days. The 1-week cycle of treatment may be repeated up to 4 times until there is no visible sign of wart tissue. Alternative treatment should be considered if the response is incomplete after four treatments.

## NURSING CONSIDERATIONS
### Administration/Storage
1. Treatment should be limited to less than 10 cm² of wart tissue and to 0.5 mL or less of the solution or 0.5 g of the gel daily. Higher amounts do not increase efficacy but may increase the incidence of side effects.
2. Do not freeze the solution or gel; avoid exposure to excessive heat.
### Assessment
1. Note histologic confirmation of differentiation of lesion from squamous cell carcinoma.
2. Document the number and size of condyloma, location, and condition of pretreatment area(s).
### Client/Family Teaching
1. Wash hands before and after application. Apply the solution with the cotton-tipped applicator supplied and the gel with either the applicator or a finger. Apply only the minimum amount of solution required to cover the lesion.
2. Allow the solution or gel to dry before allowing the return of opposing skin surfaces to their normal positions.

3. After each treatment, dispose of the used applicator properly.

4. Adhere to the exact dosing instructions (on for 3 days, off for 4 days) to prevent adverse side effects.

5. Avoid contact with the eyes. If contact does occur, immediately flush the eye with large amounts of water and report.

**Outcomes/Evaluate:** Absence/ ↓ number and size of condylomas

# Polymyxin B sulfate, parenteral

(pol-ee-**MIX**-in)
**Pregnancy Category:** C
Aerosporin **(Rx)**

# Polymyxin B sulfate, sterile ophthalmic

(pol-ee-**MIX**-in)
**Pregnancy Category:** C
**(Rx)**
**Classification:** Antibiotic, polymyxin

See also *Anti-Infectives.*

**Action/Kinetics:** Derived from the spore-forming soil bacterium *Bacillus polymyxa.* Bactericidal against most gram-negative organisms; rapidly inactivated by alkali, strong acid, and certain metal ions. Increases the permeability of the plasma cell membrane of the bacterium (i.e., similar to detergents), causing leakage of essential metabolites and ultimately inactivation. **Peak serum levels: IM,** 2 hr. **t½:** 4.3–6 hr. Longer in presence of renal impairment. Sixty percent of drug excreted in urine. Virtually unabsorbed from the GI tract except in newborn infants. Remains in plasma after parenteral administration.

**Uses: Systemic:** Acute infections of the urinary tract and meninges, septicemia caused by *Pseudomonas aeruginosa.* Meningeal infections caused by *Haemophilus influenzae,* UTIs caused by *Escherichia coli,* bacteremia caused by *Enterobacter aerogenes* or *Klebsiella pneumoniae.*

Combined with neomycin for irrigation of the urinary bladder to prevent bacteriuria and bacteremia from indwelling catheters.

**Ophthalmic:** Conjunctival and corneal infections (e.g., conjunctivitis, keratitis, keratoconjunctivitis, corneal ulcers, blepharitis, blepharoconjunctivitis, acute meibomianitis, dacryocystitis) due to *E. coli, H. influenzae, H. parainfluenzae, K. pneumoniae, E. aerogenes,* and *P. aeruginosa.* Used alone or in combination for ear infections.

**Contraindications:** Hypersensitivity. A potentially toxic drug to be reserved for the treatment of severe, resistant infections in hospitalized clients. Not indicated for clients with severely impaired renal function or nitrogen retention. Ophthalmic use in dendritic keratitis, vaccinia, varicella, mycobacterial infections of the eye, fungal diseases of the eye, use with steroid combinations after uncomplicated removal of a foreign body from the cornea. Ophthalmic use in deep-seated ophthalmic infections or in those likely to become systemic infections.

**Special Concerns:** Safe use during pregnancy has not been established.

**Side Effects:** *Nephrotoxic:* Albuminuria, cylindruria, azotemia, hematuria, proteinuria, leukocyturia, electrolyte loss. *Neurologic:* Dizziness, flushing of face, mental confusion, irritability, nystagmus, muscle weakness, drowsiness, paresthesias, blurred vision, slurred speech, ataxia, ***coma, seizures. Neuromuscular blockade may lead to respiratory paralysis.*** *GI:* N&V, diarrhea, abdominal cramps. *Miscellaneous:* Fever, urticaria, skin exanthemata, eosinophilia, ***anaphylaxis.***

*Following intrathecal use:* Meningeal irritation with fever, stiff neck, headache, increase in leukocytes and protein in the CSF. Nerve-root irritation may result in neuritic pain and urine retention. *Following IM use:* Irritation, severe pain. *Following IV use:* Thrombophlebitis. *Following ophthalmic use:* Burning,

P

---

stinging, irritation, inflammation, angioneurotic edema, itching, urticaria, vesicular and maculopapular dermatitis.

**Drug Interactions**
*Aminoglycoside antibiotics* / Additive nephrotoxic effects
*Cephalosporins* / ↑ Risk of renal toxicity
*Phenothiazines* / ↑ Risk of respiratory depression
*Skeletal muscle relaxants (surgical)* / Additive muscle relaxation

**Laboratory Test Interferences:** False + or ↑ levels of urea nitrogen and creatinine. Casts and RBCs in urine.

**Dosage** ─────────────
• **IV**
*Infections.*
**Adults and children:** 15,000 25,000 units/kg/day (maximum) in divided doses q 12 hr. **Infants,** up to 40,000 units/kg/day.
• **IM**
**Not usually recommended due to pain at injection site.**
*Infections.*
**Adults and children:** 25,000–30,000 units/kg/day in divided doses q 4–6 hr. **Infants,** up to 40,000 units/kg/day.
    Both IV and IM doses should be reduced in renal impairment.
• **Intrathecal**
*Meningitis.*
**Adults and children over 2 years:** 50,000 units/day for 3–4 days; **then,** 50,000 units every other day until 2 weeks after cultures are negative; **children under 2 years,** 20,000 units/day for 3–4 days or 25,000 units once every other day; dosage of 25,000 units should be continued every other day for 2 weeks after cultures are negative.
• **Ophthalmic Solution**
1–2 gtt 2–6 times/day, depending on the infection. Treatment may be necessary for 1–2 months or longer.

## NURSING CONSIDERATIONS

See also *General Nursing Considerations for All Anti-Infectives.*

**Administration/Storage**
1. When used in the eye(s), tilt the head back and place the medication in the conjunctival sac. Light finger pressure should be applied on the lacrimal sac for 1 min.
2. To avoid contamination, do not allow the tip of the container to touch any surface.
3. Store and dilute as directed on package insert.
4. Lessen pain on IM injection by reducing drug concentration as much as possible. It is preferable to give drug more frequently in more dilute doses. If ordered, procaine hydrochloride (2 mL of a 0.5%–1.0% solution per 5 units of dry powder) may be used for mixing the drug for IM injection.
**IV** 5. For IV administration, reconstitute 500,000 units with 300–500 mL of D5W and infuse over 60–90 min.
6. *Never use preparations containing procaine hydrochloride for IV or intrathecal use.*

**Assessment**
1. Note indications: type, onset, and duration of symptoms.
2. Determine kidney function and urinary output; note edema. Assess respiratory function; note any prior problems.
3. Obtain specimens for C&S.

**Interventions**
1. Note any muscle weakness and early signs of muscle paralysis related to neuromuscular blockade. Assess for evidence of respiratory paralysis; withhold drug and report.
2. Monitor I&O; reduce dose with impaired renal function; observe for nephrotoxicity, characterized by albuminuria, urinary casts, nitrogen retention, and hematuria.
3. Use safety precautions; supervise ambulatory or bedridden clients with neurologic disturbances.
4. Anticipate a prolonged regimen of topical application of solution because drug is not toxic when used in wet dressings, and provider may wish to prevent emergence of resistant strains.

**Client/Family Teaching**
1. Avoid hazardous tasks until drug

effects realized; may cause dizziness, vertigo, and ataxia.

2. Consume at least 2 L/day of fluids.

3. Report any neurologic disturbances, i.e., dizziness, blurred vision, irritability, circumoral and peripheral numbness and tingling, weakness, and ataxia. These usually disappear within 24–48 hr after drug discontinued and are associated with high drug levels.

**Outcomes/Evaluate:** Negative cultures; resolution of infection; symptomatic improvement

# Porfimer sodium

(**POOR**-fih-mer)
**Pregnancy Category:** C
Photofrin **(Rx)**
**Classification:** Antineoplastic, miscellaneous

**Action/Kinetics:** A photosensitizing drug used in the photodynamic therapy (PDT) of tumors. The effects are both light and oxygen dependent. Following IV injection, porfimer is retained for a prolonged period of time in tumors, skin, and organs of the reticuloendothelial system (including liver and spleen). Drug administration is followed by illumination with 630 nm of light, which causes a photochemical (not a thermal) effect. Cellular damage is the result of propagation of radical reactions, including formation of superoxide and hydroxyl radicals. Tumor death may also occur through ischemic necrosis secondary to vascular occlusion that is likely mediated through release of thromboxane A$_2$. **t½, elimination:** 250 hr. **Mean plasma levels after 48 hr:** 2.6 mcg/mL. About 90% bound to serum proteins.

**Uses:** Completely obstructing esophageal cancer or those with partially obstructing esophageal cancer who cannot be treated satisfactorily with Nd:YAG laser therapy. Treatment of non-small cell lung cancer.

**Contraindications:** Known allergies to porphyrins. Use of PDT in existing tracheoesophageal or bronchoesophageal fistulas or tumors eroding into a major blood vessel. Lactation.

**Special Concerns:** Those treated with porfimer sodium will be photosensitive and must observe precautions to avoid exposure of the skin and eyes to direct sunlight or bright indoor lighting. Safety and efficacy have not been determined in children.

**Side Effects:** Side effects listed are those possible from porfimer PDT. Over 95% of clients experienced one or more side effects. Location of the tumor was predictive for three side effects: esophageal edema if the tumor was in the upper one-third of the esophagus, atrial fibrillation if in the middle third, and anemia if in the lower third. Clients with large tumors (greater than 10 cm) were more likely to manifest anemia. Some GI, CV, and respiratory side effects may be due to mediastinal inflammation.

*GI:* Constipation, N&V, abdominal pain, dysphagia, esophageal edema, esophageal tumor bleeding, hematemesis, dyspepsia, esophageal stricture, diarrhea, eructation, esophagitis, melena, esophageal perforation, gastric ulcer, ileus, jaundice, peritonitis. *Respiratory:* Pleural effusion, dyspnea, pneumonia, pharyngitis, respiratory insufficiency, coughing, tracheoesophageal fistula, bronchitis, ***bronchospasm, laryngotracheal edema, pulmonary hemorrhage, respiratory failure,*** pneumonitis, pulmonary edema, stridor. *CNS:* Insomnia, anorexia, confusion, anxiety. *CV:* Atrial fibrillation, cardiac failure, tachycardia, hypertension, hypotension, angina pectoris, bradycardia, ***MI,*** sick sinus syndrome, SVT. *Body as a whole:* Fever, pain, chest pain, back pain, peripheral edema, asthenia, substernal chest pain, generalized edema, surgical complications. *Ophthalmic:* Abnormal vision, diplopia, eye pain, photophobia, photosensitivity reaction. *Miscellaneous:* Anemia (due to tumor bleeding), moniliasis, UTI, *sepsis.*

**OD** **Overdose Management:** *Symptoms:* Photosensitivity. Increased symptoms and damage to normal tissue following an overdose of light. *Treatment:* Treat photosensitivity by protecting eyes and skin from direct sunlight or bright indoor light for 30 days. Clients should then be tested for residual photosensitivity. Porfimer is not dialyzable.

**Drug Interactions**
*Allopurinol* / ↓ Effect of porfimer
*Beta-carotene* / ↓ PDT activity
*Calcium channel blockers* / ↓ Effect of porfimer
*Ethanol* / ↓ PDT activity
*Glucocorticoids* / ↓ PDT activity
*Griseofulvin* / ↑ Photosensitivity reaction
*Mannitol* / ↓ PDT activity
*Phenothiazines* / ↑ Photosensitivity reaction
*Sulfonamides* / ↑ Photosensitivity reaction
*Tetracyclines* / ↑ Photosensitivity reaction
*Thiazide diuretics* / ↑ Photosensitivity reaction

**Dosage** ⎯⎯⎯⎯⎯⎯⎯⎯
• **IV Injection**
*Esophageal cancer.*
The first stage is IV injection of porfimer, 2 mg/kg, given over 3–5 min. Illumination with laser light (300 J/cm of tumor length at a wavelength of 630 nm) 40–50 hr later is the second stage of therapy. A second laser light application may be given 96–120 hr after the porfimer injection, which is preceded by gentle debridement of residual tumor. This regimen may be repeated 30 days after the initial therapy; up to three courses of treatment (each separated by a minimum of 30 days) may be given.

**NURSING CONSIDERATIONS**
**Administration/Storage**
**IV** 1. Vials of porfimer sodium are freeze-dried cake or powder for injection. Reconstitute each vial with 31.8 mL of either 5% dextrose injec-

tion or 0.9% NaCl injection. The final concentration is 2.5 mg/mL with a pH of 7–8. Shake well until the drug is dissolved. The reconstituted product is an opaque solution; detection of particulate matter by visual inspection is difficult.
2. Protect reconstituted drug from bright light and administer immediately.
3. Do not mix with other drugs in the same solution.
4. Take care to avoid extravasation at the injection site. If extravasation occurs, protect the area from light.
5. The laser light is delivered to the tumor by cylindrical *Optiguide* fiberoptic diffusers that are passed through the operating channel of an endoscope.
6. Wipe any spills with a damp cloth. Avoid skin and eye contact due to the potential for photosensitivity reactions when exposed to light. Use of rubber gloves and eye protection is recommended.
7. Dispose of contaminated materials using a polyethylene bag in a manner consistent with local regulations.
8. Store the unreconstituted drug at 20°C–25°C (68°F–77°F).

**Assessment**
1. Document indications for therapy, symptom onset, any other treatments/procedures trialed.
2. Evaluate before each course of treatment for evidence of tracheoesophageal or bronchoesophageal fistula.
3. Note size and location of the tumor to help anticipate and prepare for potential side effects. For example, if tumor is in the upper third of the esophagus, esophageal edema may develop; if in the middle third may see atrial fibrillation; and if in the lower third may see anemia. With tumors that are larger than 10 cm, anemia may occur.

**Client/Family Teaching**
1. Review the method of therapy and stages, e.g., IV injection of drug followed in 2–4 days by illumination with laser light. This laser therapy may be repeated in another 2–4 days after residual tumor debride-

ment and then repeated for up to three courses of therapy.

2. Avoid any exposure to sunlight or to bright lighting for 30 days as drug renders one photosensitive. Skin must be covered and protected.

**Outcomes/Evaluate:** Control of malignant cell proliferation

---

# Potassium Salts Potassium acetate, parenteral

**Pregnancy Category:** C
**(Rx)**

# Potassium acetate, Potassium bicarbonate, and Potassium citrate (Trikates)

**Oral Solution:** Tri-K **(Rx)**

# Potassium bicarbonate

K + Care ET **(Rx)**

# Potassium bicarbonate and Citric acid

**Effervescent Tablets:** K+ Care ET, Klor-Con/EF **(Rx)**

# Potassium bicarbonate and Potassium chloride

**Effervescent Granules:** Neo-K ✱ **(Rx)**.
**Effervescent Tablets:** Klorvess, K-Lyte/Cl, K-Lyte/Cl 50, Potassium-Sandoz ✱ **(Rx)**

# Potassium bicarbonate and Potassium citrate

**Effervescent Tablets:** Effer-K, Effervescent Potassium, K-Lyte **(Rx)**

# Potassium chloride

**Extended-Release Capsules:** K-Lease, K-Norm, Micro-K Extencaps, Micro-K 10 Extencaps **(Rx)**. **Injection:** Potassium Chloride for Injection Concentrate **(Rx)**. **Oral Solution:** Cena-K 10% and 20%, K-10 ✱, Kaochlor-10 and -20 ✱, Kaochlor 10%, Kaochlor S-F 10%, Kaon-Cl 20% Liquid, Kay Ciel, KCl 5% ✱, Klorvess 10% Liquid, Potasalan, Rum-K **(Rx)**.

**Powder for Oral Solution:** Gen-K, Kay Ciel, K+ Care, K-Lor, Klor-Con Powder, Klor-Con/25 Powder, K-Lyte/Cl Powder, Micro-K LS **(Rx)**. ,
**Extended-Release Tablets:** Apo-K ✱, K+ 10, Kalium Durules ✱, Kaon-Cl, Kaon-Cl-10, K-Dur 10 and 20, K-Long ✱, Klor-Con 8 and 10, Klotrix, K-Tab, Novolente-K ✱, Slow-K, Slo-Pot 600 ✱, Slow-K ✱, Ten-K **(Rx)**

# Potassium chloride, Potassium bicarbonate, and Potassium citrate

**Effervescent Granules:** Klorvess Effervescent Granules **(Rx)**

# Potassium gluconate

**Elixir:** Kaon, Kaylixir, K-G Elixir, Potassium-Rougier ✱, Royonate ✱ **(Rx)**.
**Tablets:** Kaon ✱ **(Rx)**

# Potassium gluconate and Potassium chloride

**Oral Solution and Powder for Oral Solution:** Kolyum **(Rx)**

# Potassium gluconate and Potassium citrate

**Oral Solution:** Twin-K **(Rx)**
**Classification:** Electrolyte

---

**General Statement:** Potassium is the major cation of the body's intracellular fluid. It is essential for the maintenance of important physiologic processes, including cardiac, smooth, and skeletal muscle function, acid-base balance, gastric secretions, renal function, protein and carbohydrate metabolism. Symptoms of hypokalemia include weakness, cardiac arrhythmias, fatigue, ileus, hyporeflexia or areflexia, tetany, polydipsia, and, in severe cases, flaccid paralysis and inability to concentrate urine. Loss of potassium is usually accompanied by a loss of chloride resulting in hypochloremic metabolic alkalosis.

The usual adult daily requirement of potassium is 40–80 mg. In adults, the normal extracellular concentration of potassium ranges from 3.5 to

**P**

---

5 mEq/L with the intracellular levels being 150–160 mEq/L. Extracellular concentrations of up to 5.6 mEq/L are normal in children.

Both hypokalemia and hyperkalemia, if uncorrected, can be fatal; thus, potassium must always be administered cautiously.

Potassium is readily and rapidly absorbed from the GI tract. Though a number of salts can be used to supply the potassium cation, potassium chloride is the agent of choice since hypochloremia frequently accompanies potassium deficiency. Dietary measures can often prevent and even correct potassium deficiencies. Potassium-rich foods include most meats (beef, chicken, ham, turkey, veal), fish, beans, broccoli, brussels sprouts, lentils, spinach, potatoes, milk, bananas, dates, prunes, raisins, avocados, watermelon, cantaloupe, apricots, and molasses.

From 80% to 90% of potassium intake is excreted by the kidney and is partially reabsorbed from the glomerular filtrate.

**Uses: PO:** Treat hypokalemia due to digitalis intoxication, diabetic acidosis, diarrhea and vomiting, familial periodic paralysis, certain cases of uremia, hyperadrenalism, starvation and debilitation, and corticosteroid or diuretic therapy. Also, hypokalemia with or without metabolic acidosis and following surgical conditions accompanied by nitrogen loss, vomiting and diarrhea, suction drainage, and increased urinary excretion of potassium. Prophylaxis of potassium depletion when dietary intake is not adequate in the following conditions: clients on digitalis and diuretics for CHF, hepatic cirrhosis with ascites, excess aldosterone with normal renal function, significant cardiac arrhythmias, potassium-losing nephropathy, and certain states accompanied by diarrhea. *Investigational:* Mild hypertension.

*NOTE:* Potassium chloride should be used when hypokalemia is associated with alkalosis; potassium bicarbonate, citrate, acetate, or gluconate should be used when hypokale-

mia is associated with acidosis.

**IV:** Prophylaxis and treatment of moderate to severe potassium loss when PO therapy is not feasible. Potassium acetate is used as an additive for preparing specific IV formulas when client needs cannot be met by usual nutrient or electrolyte preparations. Potassium acetate is also used in the following conditions: marked loss of GI secretions due to vomiting, diarrhea, GI intubation, or fistulas; prolonged parenteral use of potassium-free fluids (e.g., dextrose or NSS); diabetic acidosis, especially during treatment with insulin and dextrose infusions; prolonged diuresis; metabolic alkalosis; hyperadrenocorticism; primary aldosteronism; overdose of adrenocortical steroids, testosterone, or corticotropin; attacks of hereditary or familial periodic paralysis; during the healing phase of burns or scalds; and cardiac arrhythmias, especially due to digitalis glycosides.

**Contraindications:** Severe renal function impairment with azotemia or oliguria, postoperatively before urine flow has been reestablished. Crush syndrome, Addison's disease, hyperkalemia from any cause, anuria, heat cramps, acute dehydration, severe hemolytic reactions, adynamia episodica hereditaria, clients receiving potassium-sparing diuretics or aldosterone-inhibiting drugs. Solid dosage forms in clients in whom there is a reason for delay or arrest in passage of tablets through the GI tract.

**Special Concerns:** Safety during lactation and in children has not been established. Geriatric clients are at greater risk of developing hyperkalemia due to age-related changes in renal function. Administer with caution in the presence of cardiac and renal disease. Potassium loss is often accompanied by an obligatory loss of chloride resulting in hypochloremic metabolic alkalosis; thus, the underlying cause of the potassium loss should be treated.

**Side Effects: Hypokalemia.** *CNS:* Dizziness, mental confusion. *CV:* Arrhythmias; weak, irregular pulse;

hypotension, **heart block,** ECG abnormalities, **cardiac arrest.** *GI:* Abdominal distention, anorexia, N&V, *Neuromuscular:* Weakness, paresthesia of extremities, flaccid paralysis, areflexia, muscle or **respiratory paralysis,** weakness and heaviness of legs. *Other:* Malaise.

**Hyperkalemia.** *CV:* Bradycardia, then tachycardia, **cardiac arrest.** *GI:* N&V, diarrhea, abdominal cramps, GI bleeding or obstruction. Ulceration or perforation of the small bowel from enteric-coated potassium chloride tablets. *GU:* Oliguria, anuria. *Neuromuscular:* Weakness, tingling, paralysis. *Other:* Skin rashes, hyperkalemia.

**Effects due to solution or IV technique used.** Fever, infection at injection site, venous thrombosis, phlebitis extending from injection site, extravasation, venospasm, hypervolemia, hyperkalemia.

**OD** **Overdose Management:** *Symptoms:* Mild (5.5–6.5 mEq/L) to moderate (6.5–8 mEq/L) hyperkalemia (may be asymptomatic except for ECG changes). ECG changes include progression in height and peak of T waves, lowering of the R wave, decreased amplitude and eventually disappearance of P waves, prolonged PR interval and QRS complex, shortening of the QT interval, **ventricular fibrillation, death. Muscle weakness that may progress to flaccid quadriplegia and respiratory failure,** although dangerous cardiac arrhythmias usually occur before onset of complete paralysis. *Treatment (plasma potassium levels greater than 6.5 mEq/L):* All measures must be monitored by ECG. Measures consist of actions taken to shift potassium ions from plasma into cells by:

• **Sodium bicarbonate:** IV infusion of 50–100 mEq over period of 5 min. May be repeated after 10–15 minutes if ECG abnormalities persist.

• **Glucose and insulin:** IV infusion of 3 g glucose to 1 unit regular insulin to shift potassium into cells.

• **Calcium gluconate—or other calcium salt** (only for clients not on digitalis or other cardiotonic glycosides): IV infusion of 0.5–1 g (5–10 mL of a 10% solution) over period of 2 min. Dosage may be repeated after 1–2 min if ECG remains abnormal. When ECG is approximately normal, the excess potassium should be removed from the body by administration of polystyrene sulfonate, hemodialysis or peritoneal dialysis (clients with renal insufficiency), or other means.

• **Sodium polystyrene sulfonate, hemodialysis, peritoneal dialysis:** To remove potassium from the body.

**Drug Interactions**

*ACE inhibitors* / May cause potassium retention → hyperkalemia
*Digitalis glycosides* / Cardiac arrhythmias
*Potassium-sparing diuretics* / Severe hyperkalemia with possibility of cardiac arrhythmias or arrest

**Dosage**

Highly individualized. Oral administration is preferred because the slow absorption from the GI tract prevents sudden, large increases in plasma potassium levels. Dosage is usually expressed as mEq/L of potassium. The bicarbonate, chloride, citrate, and gluconate salts are usually administered PO. The chloride, acetate, and phosphate may be administered by **slow IV** infusion.

• **IV Infusion**
*Serum K less than 2.0 mEq/L.*
400 mEq/day at a rate not to exceed 40 mEq/hr. A maximum concentration of 80 mEq/L should be used.
*Serum K more than 2.5 mEq/L.*
200 mEq/day at a rate not to exceed 20 mEq/hr. A maximum concentration of 40 mEq/L should be used.
**Pediatric:** Up to 3 mEq potassium/kg (or 40 mEq/m²) daily. The volume administered should be adjusted depending on the body size.

P

---

- **Effervescent Granules, Effervescent Tablets, Elixir, Extended-Release Capsules, Extended Release Granules, Extended-Release Tablets, Oral Solution, Powder for Oral Solution, Tablets**

*Prophylaxis of hypokalemia.*
16–24 mEq/day.
*Potassium depletion.*
40–100 mEq/day.

*NOTE:* Usual dietary intake of potassium is 40–250 mEq/day.

For clients with accompanying metabolic acidosis, an alkalizing potassium salt (potassium bicarbonate, potassium citrate, or potassium acetate) should be selected.

## NURSING CONSIDERATIONS
### Administration/Storage

1. Give PO doses 2–4 times/day. Hypokalemia should be corrected slowly over a period of 3–7 days to minimize the development of hyperkalemia.

2. With esophageal compression, administer dilute liquid solutions of potassium rather than tablets.

**IV** 3. All parenteral products must be diluted with a suitable large volume of parenteral solution, mixed well, and given by slow IV infusion. The usual concentration of potassium chloride is 40 mEq/L of IV fluid (up to a maximum of 80 mEq/L).

4. "Layering" of potassium should be avoided by properly agitating the prepared IV solution. Potassium should never be added to an IV bottle that is hanging.

5. Potassium should not be administered IV undiluted. Usual method is to administer by slow IV infusion in dextrose solution at a concentration of 40–80 mEq/L and at a rate not to exceed 10–20 mEq/hr.

6. Ensure uniform distribution of potassium by inverting container during addition of potassium solution and then by agitating container. Squeezing the plastic container will not prevent potassium chloride from settling to the bottom.

7. Check site of administration frequently for pain and redness because drug is extremely irritating.

8. In critical clients, potassium chloride may be given slow IV in a solution of saline (unless contraindicated) since dextrose may lower serum potassium levels by producing an intracellular shift.

9. Administer all concentrated potassium infusions and riders with an infusion control device.

10. Have sodium polystyrene sulfonate (Kayexalate) available for oral or rectal administration in the event of hyperkalemia.

### Assessment

1. Note indications for therapy; document baseline serum electrolytes and ECG.

2. Note any impaired renal function. Assess for adequate urinary flow before administering potassium. Impaired function can lead to hyperkalemia.

### Interventions

1. If abdominal pain, distention, or GI bleeding develops, withhold and report.

2. Note any complaints of weakness, fatigue, or the presence of cardiac arrhythmias. These may be symptoms of hypokalemia indicating a low *intracellular* potassium level, although the level may appear to be within normal limits.

3. Monitor I&O. Withhold drug and report if client develops oliguria, anuria, or azoturia.

4. Observe for symptoms of adrenal insufficiency or extensive tissue breakdown.

5. Report complaints of weakness or heaviness of the legs, the presence of a gray pallor, cold skin, listlessness, mental confusion, flaccid paralysis, hypotension, or cardiac arrhythmias (S&S of hyperkalemia). Stop medication as the client may go into CV collapse.

6. Monitor serum potassium levels during parenteral therapy; normal level is 3.5–5.0 mEq/L.

### Client/Family Teaching

1. Dilute or dissolve PO liquids, effervescent tablets, or soluble powders in 3–8 oz of cold water, fruit or vegetable juice, or other suitable liq-

uid and drink slowly. Chill to increase palatability.

2. If GI upset occurs, products can be taken after meals or with food with a full glass of water.

3. Swallow enteric-coated tablets and extended-release capsules and tablets; do not dissolve them in the mouth.

4. Salt substitutes should not be used concomitantly with potassium preparations.

5. If receiving potassium-sparing diuretics, such as spironolactone or triamterene, do not take potassium supplements or eat foods high in potassium.

6. Identify high-potassium sources in the diet: spinach, collards, brussel sprouts, beet greens, tomato juice, celery. Once parenteral potassium is discontinued, ingest potassium-rich foods such as citrus juices, bananas, apricots, raisins, and nuts. The daily adult requirement is usually 40–80 mg. Utilize a dietitian to assist with meal planning.

**Outcomes/Evaluate:** Correction of potassium deficiency; potassium levels within desired range

---

# Pramipexole
(prah-mih-**PEX**-ohl)
**Pregnancy Category:** C
Mirapex **(Rx)**
**Classification:** Antiparkinson drug

**Action/Kinetics:** Thought to act by stimulating dopamine (especially $D_3$) receptors in striatum. Rapidly absorbed. **Peak levels:** 2 hr. Food increases time for maximum levels to occur. **t½, terminal:** About 8 hr (12 hr in geriatric clients). Excreted mainly unchanged in urine. Clearance decreases with age.

**Uses:** Idiopathic Parkinson's disease.

**Contraindications:** Lactation.

**Special Concerns:** Safety and efficacy have not been determined in children.

**Side Effects:** *CNS:* Hallucinations (especially in elderly), dizziness,

somnolence, insomnia, confusion, amnesia, hypesthesia, dystonia, akathisia, abnormal thinking, decreased libido, myoclonus. *CV:* Orthostatic hypotension. *Body as a whole:* Asthenia, general edema, malaise, fever. *GI:* Nausea, constipation, anorexia, dysphagia. *Miscellaneous:* Vision abnormalities, impotence, peripheral edema, decreased weight.

**Drug Interactions**

*Butyrophenones* / Possible ↓ effect of pramipexole

*Cimetidine* / ↑ Levodopa levels and half-life

*CNS Depressants* / Additive CNS depression

*Levodopa* / ↑ Levodopa levels; also, may cause or worsen pre-existing dyskinesia

*Metoclopramide* / Possible ↓ effect of pramipexole

*Phenothiazines* / Possible ↓ effect of pramipexole

*Thioxanthines* / Possible ↓ effect of pramipexole

**Dosage** ————
• **Tablets**
  *Parkinsonism.*

**Initial:** Start with 0.125 mg t.i.d.; **then,** increase dose by 0.125 mg t.i.d. weekly for seven weeks (i.e., dose at week seven is 1.5 mg t.i.d.). **Maintenance:** 1.5–4.5 mg/day in equally divided doses t.i.d. with or without comcomitant levodopa (about 800 mg/day).

Impaired renal function, $C_{CR}$, over 60 mL/min: Start with 0.125 mg t.i.d., up to maximum of 1.5 mg t.i.d. $C_{CR}$, 25–59 mL/min: Start with 0.125 mg b.i.d., up to maximum of 1.5 mg b.i.d. $C_{CR}$, 15–24 mL/min: Start with 0.125 mg once daily, up to maximum of 1.5 mg once daily.

## NURSING CONSIDERATIONS
**Administration/Storage**

1. Take with food to decrease nausea.

2. Consider decrease in levodopa dose if taken with pramipexole.

3. Discontinue pramipexole over 1 week period.

---

**Assessment**
1. Document disease onset, extent of motor function, reflexes, gait, strength of grip, and amount of tremor.
2. With tremor, assess for muscle weakness, muscle rigidity, difficulty walking, or changing directions.
3. Monitor LFTs, VS, ECG, and renal function studies.

**Client/Family Teaching**
1 Take only as prescribed; may take with food to decrease nausea.
2. Rise slowly from sitting or lying position to prevent postural effects.
3. Do not drive or perform activities that require mental/motor alertness until stabilized on drug. May cause dizziness, fainting, blackouts, hypotension, and sedative effects.
4. Practice reliable contraception.
5. Report any vision problems; obtain regular eye exams.
6. May cause hallucinations; report if evident.
7. Do not stop abruptly; must do so over one week period.

**Outcomes/Evaluate:** Control of Parkinsonian symptoms (e.g., improvement in motor function, reflexes, gait, strength of grip, and amount of tremor)

---

# Pravastatin sodium
(prah-vah-**STAH**-tin)
**Pregnancy Category:** X
Pravachol **(Rx)**
**Classification:** Antihyperlipidemic agent

**Action/Kinetics:** Competitively inhibits HMG-CoA reductase, the enzyme catalyzing the conversion of HMG-CoA to mevalonate in the biosynthesis of cholesterol. This results in an increased number of LDL receptors on cell surfaces and enhanced receptor-mediated catabolism and clearance of circulating LDL. Also inhibits LDL production by inhibiting hepatic synthesis of VLDL, the precursor of LDL. Elevated levels of total cholesterol, dLDL cholesterol, and apolipoprotein B (a membrane transport complex for LDL) promote development of atherosclerosis and

are lowered by pravastatin. Drug increases survival in heart transplant recipients. Rapidly absorbed from the GI tract. **Peak plasma levels:** 1–1.5 hr. Significant first-pass extraction and metabolism in the liver, which is the site of action of the drug; thus, plasma levels may not correlate well with lipid-lowering effectiveness. **t½, elimination:** 77 hr. Metabolized in the liver; approximately 20% of a PO dose is excreted through the urine and 70% in the feces.

**Uses:** Adjunct to diet for reducing elevated total and LDL cholesterol levels in clients with primary hypercholesterolemia (type IIa and IIb) when the response to a diet with restricted saturated fat and cholesterol has not been effective. Reduce the risk of heart attack and slow progression of coronary atherosclerosis in those with hypercholesterolemia and heart disease. *Investigational:* To lower cholesterol levels in those with heterozygous familial hypercholesterolemia, familial combined hyperlipidemia, diabetic dyslipidemia in non-insulin-dependent diabetics, hypercholesterolemia secondary to nephrotic syndrome, homozygous familial hypercholesterolemia in those not completely devoid of LDL receptors but who have a decreased level of LDL receptor activity.

**Contraindications:** To treat hypercholesterolemia due to hyperalphaproteinemia. Active liver disease; unexplained, persistent elevations in liver function tests. Use during pregnancy and lactation and in children less than 18 years of age.

**Special Concerns:** Use with caution in clients with a history of liver disease, renal insufficiency, or heavy alcohol use.

**Side Effects:** *Musculoskeletal:* Rhabdomyolysis with renal dysfunction secondary to myoglobinuria, myalgia, myopathy, arthralgias, localized pain. *CNS:* CNS vascular lesions characterized by *perivascular hemorrhage,* edema, and mononuclear cell infiltration of perivascular spaces; headache, dizziness, psychic disturbances. Dizziness, vertigo, memory loss, anxiety, insomnia, depression. *GI:* N&V, diarrhea, abdominal pain, cramps, constipation, flatulence, heartburn, anorexia. *Hepatic:* Hepatitis (including chronic active hepatitis), fatty change in liver, cirrhosis, *fulminant hepatic necrosis, hepatoma,* pancreatitis, cholestatic jaundice. *GU:* Gynecomastia, erectile dysfunction, loss of libido. *Ophthalmic:* Progression of cataracts, lens opacities, ophthalmoplegia. *Hypersensitivity reaction:* Vasculitis, purpura, polymyalgia rheumatica, *angioedema,* lupus erythematosus–like syndrome, thrombocytopenia, *hemolytic anemia,* leukopenia, positive ANA, arthritis, arthralgia, urticaria, asthenia, ESR increase, fever, chills, photosensitivity, malaise, dyspnea, *toxic epidermal necrolysis, Stevens-Johnson syndrome. Dermatologic:* Alopecia, pruritus, skin nodules, discoloration of skin, dryness of skin and mucous membranes, changes in hair and nails. *Neurologic:* Dysfunction of certain cranial nerves resulting in alteration of taste, impairment of extraocular movement, and facial paresis; paresthesia, peripheral neuropathy, tremor, vertigo, memory loss peripheral nerve palsy. *Respiratory:* Common cold, rhinitis, cough. *Hematologic:* Anemia, transient asymptomatic eosinophilia, thrombocytopenia, leukopenia. *Miscellaneous:* Rash, pruritus, cardiac chest pain, fatigue, influenza.

**Drug Interactions**
*Bile acid sequestrants* / ↓ Bioavailability of pravastatin
*Clofibrate* / ↑ Risk of myopathy
*Cyclosporine* / ↑ Risk of myopathy or rhabdomyolysis
*Erythromycin* / ↑ Risk of myopathy or rhabdomyolysis
*Gemfibrozil* / ↑ Risk of myopathy or rhabdomyolysis
*Niacin* / ↑ Risk of myopathy or rhabdomyolysis
*Warfarin* / ↑ Anticoagulant effect of warfarin

**Laboratory Test Interferences:** ↑ CPK, AST, ALT, alkaline phosphatase, bilirubin. Abnormalities in thyroid function tests.

**Dosage**
• **Tablets**
**Initial:** 10–20 mg once daily at bedtime (geriatric clients should take 10 mg once daily at bedtime). **Maintenance dose:** 10–40 mg once daily at bedtime (maximum dose for geriatric clients is 20 mg/day).

## NURSING CONSIDERATIONS

See also *Nursing Considerations* for *Antihyperlipidemic Agents.*
**Administration/Storage**
1. Place on a standard cholesterol-lowering diet for 3–6 months before beginning pravastatin and continue during therapy.
2. Drug may be taken without regard to meals.
3. The maximum effect is seen within 4 weeks during which time periodic lipid determinations should be undertaken.
**Assessment**
1. Determine that secondary causes for hypercholesterolemia are ruled out. Secondary causes include hypothyroidism, poorly controlled diabetes mellitus, dysproteinemias, obstructive liver disease, nephrotic syndrome, alcoholism, and other drug therapy.
2. Determine if pregnant.
3. Assess for liver disease or alcohol abuse.
4. Document any other risk factors for CAD.
5. Monitor cholesterol profile, CBC, liver and renal function studies.
**Interventions**
1. Obtain LFTs prior to pravastatin therapy q 6 weeks during the first 3 months of therapy, q 2–3 months during the remainder of the first year, then at 6-month intervals.
2. Pravastatin should be discontinued if markedly elevated CPK levels occur or myopathy is diagnosed.
3. Pravastatin should be discontin-

P

---

ued temporarily in clients experiencing an acute or serious condition (e.g., sepsis, hypotension, major surgery, trauma, uncontrolled epilepsy, or severe metabolic, endocrine, or electrolyte disorders) predisposing to the development of renal failure secondary to rhabdomyolysis.

**Client/Family Teaching**
1. Review the prescribed dietary recommendations (restricted cholesterol and saturated fats); continue diet during drug therapy.
2. Continue a regular exercise program and strive to attain recommended weight loss.
3. Report any unexplained muscle pain, tenderness, or weakness, especially if accompanied by malaise or fever.
4. Practice reliable birth control; report if pregnancy is suspected as drug therapy hazardous to a developing fetus.

**Outcomes/Evaluate:** ↓ Serum cholesterol and LDL levels; heart attack prophylaxis in those with atherosclerosis and hypercholesterolemia

# Praziquantel
(pray-zih-**KWON**-tell)
**Pregnancy Category:** B
Biltricide **(Rx)**
**Classification:** Anthelmintic

See also *Anthelmintics.*

**Action/Kinetics:** Causes increased cell permeability in the helminth, resulting in a loss of intracellular calcium with massive contractions, and paralysis of musculature with breakdown of the integrity of the organism. Also causes vacuolization and disintegration of phagocytes to the parasite, resulting in death. **Maximum serum levels:** 1–3 hr. **t½:** 0.8–1.5 hr. Levels in the CSF are approximately 14%–20% of the total amount of the drug in the plasma. Significant first-pass effect. Excreted primarily in the urine.

**Uses:** Schistosomal infections due to *Schistosoma japonicum, S. mansoni, S. mekongi,* and *S. hematobium.* Liver flukes (*Clonorchis sinensis,*

*Opisthorchis viverrini*). *Investigational:* Neurocysticercosis, other tissue flukes, and intestinal cestodes. Low doses of oxamniquine and praziquantel as a single-dose treatment of schistosomiasis.

**Contraindications:** Ocular cysticercosis. Lactation.

**Special Concerns:** Safety in children less than 4 years of age not established.

**Side Effects:** *GI:* Nausea, abdominal discomfort. *CNS:* Malaise, headache, dizziness, drowsiness. *Miscellaneous:* Fever, urticaria (rare). *NOTE:* These side effects may also be due to the helminth infection itself.

**OD** **Overdose Management:** *Symptoms:* Extension of side effects. *Treatment:* Administer a fast-acting laxative.

**Drug Interactions:** Hydantoins may decrease serum praziquantel levels, resulting in ineffective treatment.

**Dosage**
• **Tablets**
*Schistosomiasis.*
Three doses of 20 mg/kg as a 1-day treatment with an interval between doses not less than 4 hr or more than 6 hr.
*Chonorchiasis and opisthorchiasis.*
Three doses of 25 mg/kg as a 1-day treatment with an interval between doses not less than 4 hr or more than 6 hr..

## NURSING CONSIDERATIONS

See also *Nursing Considerations* for *Anthelmintics.*

**Assessment**
1. Document indications for therapy, onset, characteristics, duration of symptoms, and source of infestation.
2. Determine if the schistosomiasis or fluke infection is accompanied by cerebral cysticercosis; if so, hospitalize for treatment.
3. Note any liver dysfunction as reduced dosage may be indicated.
4. List drugs currently prescribed to ensure none interact unfavorably or deactivate drug (i.e., hydantoins).

**Client/Family Teaching**
1. Swallow tablets unchewed with liquid during meals. Keeping the tablets in the mouth may cause gagging or vomiting; the tablets should not be chewed as their bitter taste can cause retching and vomiting.
2. Use caution while driving or performing tasks requiring alertness; may cause dizziness and drowsiness.
3. Do not nurse a baby on treatment day and for 3 days following treatment.

**Outcomes/Evaluate:** Eradication of parasitic infestation; negative cultures

# Prazosin hydrochloride
(**PRAY**-zoh-sin)
**Pregnancy Category:** C
Alti-Prazosin ✦, Apo-Prazo ✦, Minipress, Novo-Prazin ✦, Nu-Prazo ✦, Rho-Prazosin ✦ **(Rx)**
**Classification:** Antihypertensive, alpha-1-adrenergic blocking agent

See also *Alpha-1-Adrenergic Blocking Agents* and *Antihypertensive Agents*.

**Action/Kinetics:** Produces selective blockade of postsynaptic alpha-1-adrenergic receptors. Dilates arterioles and veins, thereby decreasing total peripheral resistance and decreasing DBP more than SBP. CO, HR, and renal blood flow are not affected. Can be used to initiate antihypertensive therapy; most effective when used with other agents (e.g., diuretics, beta-adrenergic blocking agents). **Onset:** 2 hr. Absorption not affected by food. **Maximum effect:** 2–3 hr; **duration:** 6–12 hr. t½: 2–3 hr. Full therapeutic effect: 4–6 weeks. Metabolized extensively; excreted primarily in feces.

**Uses:** Mild to moderate hypertension alone or in combination with other antihypertensive drugs. *Investigational:* CHF refractory to other treatment. Raynaud's disease, benign prostatic hypertrophy.

**Special Concerns:** Safe use in children has not been established. Use with caution during lactation. Geriatric clients may be more sensitive to the hypotensive and hypothermic effects of prazosin; also, it may be necessary to decrease the dose in these clients due to age-related decreases in renal function.

**Side Effects: First-dose effect:** *Marked hypotension* and syncope 30–90 min after administration of initial dose (usually 2 or more mg), increase of dosage, or addition of other antihypertensive agent. *CNS:* Dizziness, drowsiness, headache, fatigue, paresthesias, depression, vertigo, nervousness, hallucinations. *CV:* Palpitations, syncope, tachycardia, orthostatic hypotension, aggravation of angina. *GI:* N&V, diarrhea or constipation, dry mouth, abdominal pain, pancreatitis. *GU:* Urinary frequency or incontinence, impotence, priapism. *Respiratory:* Dyspnea, nasal congestion, epistaxis. *Dermatologic:* Pruritus, rash, sweating, alopecia, lichen planus. *Miscellaneous:* Asthenia, edema, symptoms of lupus erythematosus, blurred vision, tinnitus, arthralgia, myalgia, reddening of sclera, eye pain, conjunctivitis, edema, fever.

**OD Overdose Management:** *Symptoms:* Hypotension, *shock.* *Treatment:* Keep client supine to restore BP and HR. If shock is manifested, use volume expanders and vasopressors; maintain renal function.

**Drug Interactions**
*Antihypertensives (other)* / ↑ Antihypertensive effect
*Beta-adrenergic blocking agents* / Enhanced acute postural hypotension following the first dose of prazosin
*Clonidine* / ↓ Antihypertensive effect of clonidine
*Diuretics* / ↑ Antihypertensive effect
*Indomethacin* / ↓ Effect of prazosin
*Nifedipine* / ↑ Hypotensive effect
*Propranolol* / Especially pronounced additive hypotensive effect

*Verapamil* / ↑ Hypotensive effect; ↑ sensitivity to prazosin-induced postural hypotension
**Laboratory Test Interferences:** ↑ Urinary metabolites of norepinephrine, VMA.

**Dosage**
• **Capsules**
  *Hypertension.*
**Individualized: Initial,** 1 mg b.i.d.–t.i.d.; **maintenance:** if necessary, increase gradually to 6–15 mg/day in two to three divided doses. Daily dose should not exceed 20 mg, although some clients have benefitted from doses of 40 mg daily. If used with diuretics or other antihypertensives, reduce dose to 1–2 mg t.i.d. **Pediatric, less than 7 years of age, initial:** 0.25 mg b.i.d.–t.i.d. adjusted according to response. **Pediatric, 7–12 years of age, initial:** 0.5 mg b.i.d.–t.i.d. adjusted according to response.

## NURSING CONSIDERATIONS

See also *Nursing Considerations* for *Antihypertensive Agents* and *Alpha-1-Adrenergic Blocking Agents*.
**Administration/Storage:** Reduce the dose to 1 or 2 mg t.i.d. if a diuretic or other antihypertensive agent is added to the regimen and then retitrate client.
**Client/Family Teaching**
1. Take the first dose at bedtime. Also, take the first dose of each increment at bedtime to reduce the incidence of syncope.
2. Do not drive or operate machinery for 24 hr after the first dose; may cause dizziness and drowsiness.
3. Food may delay absorption and minimize side effects of the drug.
4. Avoid rapid postural changes that may precipitate weakness, dizziness, and syncope. Lie down or sit down and put head below knees to avoid fainting if a rapid heartbeat is felt.
5. Avoid dangerous situations that may lead to fainting.
6. Report any bothersome side effects because reduction in dosage may be indicated. Use sips of water

and sugarless gum or candies for dry mouth effects.
7. Do not stop medication unless directed.
8. Avoid cold, cough, and allergy medications. The sympathomimetic component of such medications will interfere with the action of prazosin.
9. Comply with prescribed drug regimen; full drug effect may not be evident for 4–6 weeks.
**Outcomes/Evaluate:** ↓ BP; ↓ symptoms of refractory CHF

# Prednisolone
(pred-**NISS**-oh-lohn)
**Pregnancy Category:** C
**Syrup:** Prelone. **Tablets:** Delta-Cortef **(Rx)**

# Prednisolone acetate
(pred-**NISS**-oh-lohn)
**Pregnancy Category:** C
**Parenteral:** Articulose-50, Key-Pred 25 and 50, Predalone 50, **Ophthalmic Suspension:**, Diopred ✿, Econopred Ophthalmic, Econopred Plus, Ophtho-Tate ✿, Pred Forte Ophthalmic, Pred Mild Ophthalmic **(Rx)**

# Prednisolone acetate and Prednisolone sodium phosphate
(pred-**NISS**-oh-lohn)
**Pregnancy Category:** C
**(Rx)**

# Prednisolone sodium phosphate
(pred-**NISS**-oh-lohn)
**Pregnancy Category:** C
**Oral Solution:** Pediapred **(Rx)**. **Ophthalmic Solution:** AK-Pred Ophthalmic, Inflamase Forte Ophthalmic, Inflamase Mild Ophthalmic, Inflamase Forte Ophthalmic **(Rx)**. **Parenteral:** Hydeltrasol, Key-Pred-SP **(Rx)**

# Prednisolone tebutate
(pred-**NISS**-oh-lohn)
**Pregnancy Category:** C
Hydeltra-T.B.A., Prednisol TPA **(Rx)**
**Classification:** Corticosteroid, synthetic

See also *Corticosteroids*.

**Action/Kinetics:** Intermediate-acting. Is five times more potent than hydrocortisone and cortisone. Minimal side effects except for GI distress. Moderate mineralocorticoid activity. **Plasma t½:** over 200 min.

**Contraindications:** Lactation.

**Special Concerns:** Use during pregnancy only if benefits outweigh risks. Use with particular caution in diabetes.

**Dosage**

PREDNISOLONE

• **Tablets, Syrup**

*Most uses.*

5–60 mg/day, depending on disease being treated.

*Multiple sclerosis (exacerbation).*

200 mg/day for 1 week; **then,** 80 mg on alternate days for 1 month.

*Pleurisy of tuberculosis.*

0.75 mg/kg/day (then taper) given concurrently with antituberculosis therapy.

PREDNISOLONE ACETATE

• **IM**

4–60 mg/day. **Not for IV use.**

*Multiple sclerosis (exacerbation).*

See *Prednisolone*.

• **Intralesional, Intra-articular, Soft Tissue Injection**

4–100 mg (larger doses for large joints).

• **Ophthalmic Suspension (0.12%, 0.125%, 1%)**

1–2 gtt in the conjunctival sac q hr during the day and q 2 hr during the night; **then,** after response obtained, decrease dose to 1 gtt/ q 4 hr and then later 1 gtt t.i.d.–q.i.d.

PREDNISOLONE ACETATE AND PREDNISOLONE SODIUM PHOSPHATE

• **IM Only**

20–80 mg acetate and 5–20 mg sodium phosphate every few days for 3–4 weeks.

• **Intra-articular, Intrasynovial**

20–40 mg prednisolone acetate and 5–10 mg prednisolone sodium phosphate.

PREDNISOLONE SODIUM PHOSPHATE

• **PO Solution**

*Most uses.*

5–60 mg/day in single or divided doses.

*Adrenocortical insufficiency.*

**Pediatric:** 0.14 mg/kg (4 mg/m²) daily in three to four divided doses.

*Other pediatric uses.*

0.5–2 mg/kg (15–60 mg/m²) daily in three to four divided doses.

• **IM, IV**

4–60 mg/day.

*Multiple sclerosis (exacerbation).*

See *Prednisolone*.

• **Intralesional, Intra-articular, Soft Tissue Injection**

2–30 mg, depending on site and severity of disease.

• **Ophthalmic Solution (0.125%, 1%)**

See *Prednisolone acetate*.

PREDNISOLONE TEBUTATE

• **Intra-articular, Intralesional, Soft Tissue Injection**

4–30 mg, depending on site and severity of disease. Doses higher than 40 mg are not recommended.

**NURSING CONSIDERATIONS**

See also *Nursing Considerations* for *Corticosteroids*.

**Administration/Storage**

1. Before administering, check spelling and dose carefully; is frequently confused with prednisone.

2. Check to see if provider wants PO form administered with an antacid.

3. Prednisolone sodium phosphate oral solution produces a 20% higher peak plasma level than is seen with tablets.

**IV** 4. The IV form (sodium phosphate) may be administered at a rate not to exceed 10 mg/min.

**Assessment**

1. Document indications for therapy, type and onset of symptoms. Note any previous experiences with this drug and the outcome.

2. Monitor VS, CBC, electrolytes, blood sugar, weight, and mental status.

P

**Outcomes/Evaluate**
• Replacement therapy during adrenocortical hypofunction
• Symptomatic relief of allergic, immune, and inflammatory manifestations

# Prednisone
(**PRED**-nih-sohn)
**Pregnancy Category:** C
**Oral Solution:** Prednisone Intensol Concentrate **(Rx). Syrup:** Liquid Pred **(Rx). Tablets:** Alti-Prednisone ✱, Apo-Prednisone ✱, Deltasone, Jaa Prednisone ✱, Meticorten, Novo-Prednisone ✱, Orasone 1, 5, 10, 20, and 50, Panasol-S, Sterapred DS, Winpred ✱ **(Rx)**
**Classification:** Corticosteroid, synthetic

See also *Corticosteroids*.
**Action/Kinetics:** Three to five times as potent as cortisone or hydrocortisone. May cause moderate fluid retention. Metabolized in the liver to prednisolone, the active form.
**Special Concerns:** Use during pregnancy only if benefits outweigh risks. Dose must be highly individualized.

**Dosage**
• **Oral Concentrate, Syrup, Tablets**
  *Acute, severe conditions.*
**Initial:** 5–60 mg/day in four equally divided doses after meals and at bedtime. Decrease gradually by 5–10 mg q 4–5 days to establish minimum maintenance dosage (5–10 mg) or discontinue altogether until symptoms recur.
  *Replacement.*
**Pediatric:** 0.1–0.15 mg/kg/day.
  *COPD.*
30–60 mg/day for 1–2 weeks; then taper.
  *Ophthalmopathy due to Graves' disease.*
60 mg/day; **then,** taper to 20 mg/day.
  *Duchenne's muscular dystrophy.*
0.75–1.5 mg/kg/day (used to improve strength).

## NURSING CONSIDERATIONS

See also *Nursing Considerations* for *Corticosteroids*.
**Assessment**
1. Document indications for therapy, type, onset, and duration of symptoms. List other agents prescribed and the outcome.
2. Monitor CBC, electrolytes, blood sugar, weights, and mental status.
**Client/Family Teaching**
1. Take with food to decrease GI upset.
2. With long-term therapy, do not stop abruptly.
3. Report any S&S of adrenal insufficiency or loss of effectiveness.
4. Avoid ethanol and all OTC agents.
**Outcomes/Evaluate:** Relief of allergic, immune, and inflammatory manifestations

# Primaquine phosphate
(**PRIM**-ah-kwin)
**(Rx)**
**Classification:** 8-Aminoquinoline, antimalarial

**Action/Kinetics:** Mechanism of action not known, but the drug binds to and may alter the properties of DNA leading to decreased protein synthesis. Both the gametocyte and exoerythrocyte forms are inhibited. Some gametocytes are destroyed while others cannot undergo maturation division in the gut of the mosquito. Well absorbed from GI tract. **Peak plasma levels:** 1–3 hr. **Poorly distributed in body tissues. t½ elimination:** 4 hr. Rapidly metabolized.
**Uses:** Only for the radical cure of *Plasmodium vivax* malaria, the prophylaxis of relapse in *P. vivax* malaria, or following the termination of chloroquine phosphate suppressive therapy in areas where *P. vivax* is endemic.
**Contraindications:** Concomitant use with quinacrine. In clients with rheumatoid arthritis or lupus erythematosus who are acutely ill or who have a tendency to develop granulocytopenia. Concomitant use

with other bone marrow depressants or hemolytic drugs.

**Special Concerns:** Use during pregnancy only when benefits outweigh risks.

**Side Effects:** *GI:* Abdominal cramps, epigastric distress, N&V. *Hematologic:* Leukopenia. Methemoglobinemia in NADH methemoglobin reductase deficient individuals. Blacks and members of certain Mediterranean ethnic groups (Sardinians, Sephardic Jews, Greeks, Iranians) manifest a high incidence of G6PD deficiency and as a result have a low tolerance for primaquine. These individuals manifest **marked hemolytic anemia** following primaquine administration. *Miscellaneous:* Headache, pruritus, interference with visual accommodation, **cardiac arrhythmias,** hypertension.

**OD** **Overdose Management:** *Symptoms:* Abdominal cramps, vomiting, burning and epigastric distress, cyanosis, methemoglobinemia, anemia, moderate leukocytosis or leukopenia, CNS and CV disturbances. Granulocytopenia and **acute hemolytic anemia** in sensitive clients. *Treatment:* Treat symptoms.

**Drug Interactions**

*Bone marrow depressants, hemolytic drugs* / Additive side effects

*Quinacrine* / Quinacrine interferes with metabolic degradation of primaquine and thus enhances its toxic side reactions. **Do not give primaquine** to clients who are receiving or have received quinacrine within the past 3 months.

**Dosage** ———————
• **Tablets**

*Acute attack of vivax malaria, clients with parasitized RBCs.*

15 mg (base) daily for 14 days together with chloroquine phosphate (to destroy erythrocytic parasites).

*Suppression of malaria.*

**Adults:** 26.3 mg (15 mg base) daily for 14 days or 78.9 mg once a week for 8 weeks; **children:** 0.5 mg/kg/day (0.3 mg/kg base) for 14 days.

## NURSING CONSIDERATIONS

See also *General Nursing Considerations for All Anti-Infectives* and *Antimalarial Drugs, 4-Aminoquinolines.*

**Administration/Storage**

1. Store in tightly closed containers.
2. For suppression therapy, initiate during the last 2 weeks of or after suppressive therapy with chloroquine or a similar drug.

**Assessment**

1. Note any history of rheumatoid arthritis or lupus.
2. List other medications currently prescribed to ensure no unfavorable interactions.
3. Determine if pregnant. Do not give during first trimester and preferably not until after delivery.
4. Ensure that baseline hematologic profile and cultures have been performed. Monitor for indications to withdraw drug: dark urine that indicates hemolysis and a marked fall in hemoglobin, platelets, or erythrocyte count.
5. Assess dark-skinned clients closely. Because of a possible inborn deficiency of G6PD, these clients are particularly susceptible to hemolytic anemia while on primaquine.

**Client/Family Teaching**

1. Take immediately before or after meals or with antacids to minimize gastric irritation.
2. For suppressive therapy, take drug on same day each week.
3. Monitor color of urine and report any darkening or brown discoloration.
4. Must complete a full course of therapy for effective results.
5. Review symptoms of overdose (GI, CNS, and CV disturbances); report if evident.

**Outcomes/Evaluate:** Termination of acute malarial attacks/suppression of malarial symptoms; negative cultures

# Primidone
(**PRIH**-mih-dohn)

---

Apo-Primidone ✤, Mysoline, Sertan ✤ (Rx)

**Classification:** Anticonvulsant, miscellaneous

**Action/Kinetics:** Closely related to the barbiturates; however, the anticonvulsant mechanism is unknown. Produces a greater sedative effect than barbiturates when used for seizure treatment. Side effects usually subside with use. **Peak plasma levels:** 3 hr. Primidone is converted in the liver to two active metabolites, phenobarbital and phenylethylmalonamide (PEMA). **Peak plasma levels (PEMA):** 7–8 hr. **t½ (primidone):** 5–15 hr; **t½ (PEMA):** 10–18 hr; **t½ (phenobarbital):** 53–140 hr. The appearance of phenobarbital in the plasma may be delayed several days after initiation of therapy. **Therapeutic plasma levels, primadone:** 5–12 mcg/mL; **phenobarbital,** 15–40 mcg/mL. Primidone and metabolites are excreted through the kidneys, although 40% of primidone is excreted unchanged.

**Uses:** Alone or with other anticonvulsants to treat psychomotor seizures, focal seizures, or tonic-clonic seizures (including those refractory to barbiturate-hydantoin regimens). *Investigational:* Benign familial tremor.

**Contraindications:** Porphyria. Hypersensitivity to phenobarbital. Lactation.

**Special Concerns:** Safe use during pregnancy has not been determined. Use during lactation may result in drowsiness in the neonate. Children and geriatric clients may react to primidone with restlessness and excitement. Due to differences in bioavailability, brand interchange is not recommended.

**Side Effects:** *CNS:* Drowsiness, ataxia, vertigo, fatigue, hyperirritability, emotional disturbances, personality disturbances with mood changes and paranoia. *GI:* N&V, anorexia, painful gums. *Hematologic:* Megaloblastic anemia, thrombocytopenia. *Ophthalmologic:* Diplopia, nystagmus. *Miscellaneous:* Impotence, morbilliform and maculopapular skin rashes. Occasionally has caused hyperexcitability, especially in children. *Postpartum hemorrhage and hemorrhagic disease of the newborn.* Symptoms of SLE.

**Drug Interactions**
See also *Barbiturates.*
*Acetazolamide* / ↓ Effect of primidone due to ↓ levels
*Carbamazepine* / ↓ Plasma levels of primidone and phenobarbital and ↑ plasma levels of carbamazepine
*Hydantoins* / ↑ Plasma levels of primidone, phenobarbital, and PEMA
*Isoniazid* / ↑ Effect of primidone due to ↓ breakdown by liver
*Nicotinamide* / ↑ Effect of primidone due to ↓ rate of clearance from body
*Succinimides* / ↓ Plasma levels of primidone and phenobarbital

**Dosage**
• **Oral Suspension, Tablets**
*Seizures, in clients on no other anticonvulsant medication.*
**Adults and children over 8 years, initial:** Days 1–3, 100–125 mg at bedtime; days 4–6, 100–125 mg b.i.d.; days 7–9, 100–125 mg t.i.d.; **maintenance:** 250 mg t.i.d.–q.i.d. (may be increased to 250 mg 5–6 times/day; not to exceed 500 mg q.i.d.). **Children under 8 years, initial:** days 1–3, 50 mg at bedtime; days 4–6, 50 mg b.i.d.; days 7–9, 100 mg b.i.d.; **maintenance:** 125 mg b.i.d.–250 mg t.i.d. (10–25 mg/kg in divided doses).
*Seizures, in clients receiving other anticonvulsants.*
**Initial:** 100–125 mg at bedtime; **then,** increase to maintenance levels as other drug is slowly withdrawn (transition should take at least 2 weeks).
*Benign familial tremor.*
750 mg/day.

## NURSING CONSIDERATIONS

See also *Nursing Considerations* for *Anticonvulsants.*
**Assessment**
1. Document age of seizure onset,

frequency of occurrence, characteristics, and cause if known.

2. List other agents prescribed and the outcome.

3. Monitor CBC, liver and renal function studies.

**Client/Family Teaching**

1. May be taken with food if GI upset occurs.

2. Review the following conditions that should be reported:

- Hyperexcitability in children
- Excessive loss of hair
- Edema of eyelids and legs
- Visual disturbances
- Mental status changes
- Impotence
- Loss of seizure control

3. With pregnancy, vitamin K may be prescribed during the last month of pregnancy. This is to prevent postpartum hemorrhage in the mother and hemorrhagic disease of the newborn.

**Outcomes/Evaluate**

- Control of refractory seizures
- Therapeutic drug levels (5–12 mcg/mL)

# Probenecid
(proh-**BEN**-ih-sid)
**Pregnancy Category:** B
Benemid, Benuryl ✮ **(Rx)**
**Classification:** Antigout agent, uricosuric agent

**Action/Kinetics:** A uricosuric agent that increases the excretion of uric acid by inhibiting the tubular reabsorption of uric acid; this results in a decreased serum level of uric acid. Also inhibits the renal secretion of penicillins and cephalosporins; this effect is often taken advantage of in the treatment of infections because concomitant administration of probenecid will increase plasma levels of antibiotics. **Peak plasma levels:** 2–4 hr. **Time to peak effect, uricosuric:** 0.5 hr; **for suppression of penicillin excretion:** 2 hr. **Therapeutic plasma levels for inhibition of antibiotic secretion:** 40–60 mcg/mL; **therapeutic plasma levels for**

**uricosuric effect:** 100–200 mcg/mL. **t½:** approximately 5–8 hr. **Duration for inhibition of penicillin excretion:** 8 hr. Metabolized in the liver to active metabolites; excreted in urine (5%–10% unchanged). Excretion is increased in alkaline urine.

**Uses:** Hyperuricemia in chronic gout and gouty arthritis. Adjunct in therapy with penicillins or cephalosporins to elevate and prolong plasma antibiotic levels.

**Contraindications:** Hypersensitivity to drug, blood dyscrasias, uric acid, and kidney stones. Use for hyperuricemia in neoplastic disease or its treatment. Use in children less than 2 years of age. Concomitant use of salicylates or use with penicillin in renal impairment.

**Special Concerns:** Use with caution in renal disease, porphyria, G6PD deficiency, history of allergy to sulfa drugs, and peptic ulcer.

**Side Effects:** *CNS:* Headaches, dizziness. *GI:* Anorexia, N&V, diarrhea, constipation, and abdominal discomfort. *Allergic:* Skin rash, dermatitis, pruritus, drug fever, and rarely **anaphylaxis.** *GU:* Nephrotic syndrome, uric acid stones with or without hematuria, urinary frequency, renal colic or costovertebral pain. *Miscellaneous:* Flushing, **hemolytic anemia (possibly related to G6PD deficiency),** anemia, sore gums, **hepatic necrosis, aplastic anemia,.**

Initially, the drug may increase frequency of acute gout attacks due to mobilization of uric acid.

**Drug Interactions**

*Acyclovir* / Probenecid ↓ renal excretion of acyclovir

*Allopurinol* / Additive effects to ↓ uric acid serum levels

*AZT* / ↑ Bioavailability of AZT; possible malaise, myalgia, fever

*Benzodiazepines* / More rapid onset and longer duration of the effects of benzodiazepines

*Cephalosporins* / ↑ Effect of cephalosporins due to ↓ excretion by kidney

*Ciprofloxacin* / 50% ↑ in systemic levels of ciprofloxacin

*Clofibrate* / ↑ Levels of clofibric acid (active) → ↑ effects

*Dapsone* / ↑ Effect of dapsone

*Dyphylline* / ↑ Effect of dyphylline due to ↓ excretion by kidney

*Methotrexate* / ↑ Effect and toxicity of methotrexate due to ↓ excretion by kidney

*NSAIDs* / ↑ Effect of NSAIDs due to ↓ excretion by kidney

*Pantothenic acid* / ↑ Effects of pantothenic acid

*Penicillamine* / ↓ Effect of penicillamine

*Penicillins* / ↑ Effect of penicillins due to ↓ excretion by kidney

*Pyrazinamide* / Probenecid inhibits hyperuricemia produced by pyrazinamide

*Rifampin* / ↑ Effect of rifampin due to ↓ excretion by kidney

*Salicylates* / Salicylates inhibit uricosuric activity of probenecid

*Sulfinpyrazone* / ↑ Effect of sulfinpyrazone due to ↓ excretion by kidney

*Sulfonamides* / ↑ Effect of sulfonamides due to ↓ plasma protein binding

*Sulfonylureas, oral* / ↑ Action of sulfonylureas → hypoglycemia

*Thiopental* / ↑ Effect of thiopental

## Dosage

• **Tablets**

*Gout.*

**Adults, initial:** 250 mg b.i.d. for 1 week. **Maintenance:** 500 mg b.i.d. Dosage may have to be increased further (by 500 mg/day q 4 weeks to maximum of 2 g) until urate excretion is less than 700 mg in 24 hr. Colbenemid, a combination tablet containing colchicine (0.5 mg) and probenecid (500 mg), is available.

*Adjunct to penicillin or cephalosporin therapy.*

**Adults:** 500 mg q.i.d. Dosage is decreased for elderly clients with renal damage. **Pediatric, 2–14 years, initial:** 25 mg/kg (or 700 mg/m²); **maintenance,** 10 mg/kg q.i.d. (or 300 mg/m² q.i.d.). **For children 50 kg or more:** give adult dosage.

*Gonorrhea, uncomplicated.*

**Adults:** 1 g (as a single dose) 30 min before 4.8 million units of penicillin G procaine aqueous; **pediatric, less than 45 kg:** 25 mg/kg (up to a maximum of 1 g) with appropriate antibiotic therapy.

*Neurosyphilis.*

**Adults:** 0.5 g q.i.d. with penicillin G procaine aqueous, 2.4 million units/day IM, both for 10–14 days.

*Pelvic inflammatory disease.*

**Adults:** 1 g (as a single dose) plus cefoxitin, 2 g IM given concurrently.

## NURSING CONSIDERATIONS

### Administration/Storage

1. Do not start therapy until an acute gouty attack has subsided. If an acute attack is precipitated during therapy, continue the drug.

2. To prevent kidney stones, take at least 6 to 8 full (8-oz) glasses of water.

3. Maintain an alkaline urine by taking sodium bicarbonate, 3–7.5 g/day, or potassium citrate, 7.5 g/day.

### Assessment

1. Document indications for therapy, type and onset of symptoms.

2. Determine any PUD, G6PD deficiency, uricemia R/T neoplastic disease, kidney stones, or blood dyscrasia.

3. Assess involved joints, noting pain, inflammation, heat, swelling, deformity, and ROM.

4. Monitor CBC, uric acid, liver and renal function studies. Note urate excretion levels.

5. Hypersensitivity reactions may occur more frequently with intermittent therapy.

6. Assess for toxic plasma antibiotic levels if excretion is inhibited by probenecid. Make appropriate dosage adjustments.

### Client/Family Teaching

1. Take with food or milk to minimize gastric irritation. Report gastric intolerance so dosage may be corrected without loss of therapeutic effect.

2. Take a liberal amount of fluid (2.5–3 L/day) to prevent the formation of sodium urate stones. Avoid cranberry juice or vitamin C prepara-

tions, which acidify urine. Sodium bicarbonate may be used to maintain an alkaline urine to prevent urates from crystallizing and forming kidney stones.

3. Acute gout attacks may initially be more frequent due to mobilization of uric acid. Report any increase in the number of acute attacks at the initiation of therapy since colchicine may need to be added. Continue to take during acute attacks along with colchicine unless otherwise specified.

4. Report any unexplained fever, fatigue, skin rash, persistent GI upset, flushing, increased sweating, headaches, or dizziness.

5. Do not take salicylates or use caffeine or alcohol during uricosuric therapy. Acetaminophen preparations may be used for analgesic purposes.

6. Monitor FS closely; drug may increase hypoglycemic effects of PO antidiabetic agents.

**Outcomes/Evaluate**
- ↓ Uric acid levels; ↓ gout attacks
- ↓ Joint pain and swelling
- Elevated/prolonged plasma antibiotic (penicillin or cephalosporin) levels

# Procainamide hydrochloride

(proh-**KAYN**-ah-myd)
**Pregnancy Category:** C
Apo-Procainamide ✦, Procan SR ✦, Procanbid, Pronestyl, Pronestyl-SR
**(Rx)**
**Classification:** Antiarrhythmic, class IA

See also *Antiarrhythmic Agents*.
**Action/Kinetics:** Produces a direct cardiac effect to prolong the refractory period of the atria and to a lesser extent the bundle of His-Purkinje system and ventricles. Large doses may cause AV block. Some anticholinergic and local anesthetic effects.
**Onset: PO,** 30 min; **IV,** 1–5 min.
**Time to peak effect, PO:** 90–120 min; **IM,** 15–60 min; **IV,** immediate.
**Duration:** 3 hr. **t½:** 2.5–4.7 hr. **Therapeutic serum level:** 4–8 mcg/mL. **Protein binding:** 15%. From 40% to 70% excreted unchanged. Metabolized in the liver (16%–21% by slow acetylators and 24%–33% by fast acetylators) to the active N-acetylprocainamide (NAPA); has antiarrhythmic properties with a longer half-life than procainamide.
**Uses:** Documented ventricular arrhythmias (e.g., sustained ventricular tachycardia) that may be life threatening in clients where benefits of treatment clearly outweigh risks. Antiarrhythmic drugs have not been shown to improve survival in clients with ventricular arrhythmias.
**Contraindications:** Hypersensitivity to drug, complete AV heart block, lupus erythematosus, torsades de pointes, asymptomatic ventricular premature contractions. Lactation.
**Special Concerns:** There is an increased risk of death in those with non-life-threatening arrhythmias. Although used in children, safety and efficacy have not been established. Use with extreme caution in clients for whom a sudden drop in BP could be detrimental, in CHF, acute ischemic heart disease, or cardiomyopathy. Also, use with caution in clients with liver or kidney dysfunction, preexisting bone marrow failure or cytopenia of any type, development of first-degree heart block while on procainamide, myasthenia gravis, and those with bronchial asthma or other respiratory disorders. May cause more hypotension in geriatric clients; also, in this population, the dose may have to be decreased due to age-related decreases in renal function.
**Side Effects:** *Body as a whole:* Lupus erythematosus–like syndrome especially in those on maintenance therapy and who are slow acetylators. Symptoms include arthralgia, pleural or abdominal pain, arthritis, pleural effusion, pericarditis, fever, chills, myalgia, skin lesions, hematologic

P

---

changes. *CV:* Following IV use: Hypotension, *ventricular asystole or fibrillation, partial or complete heart block.* Rarely, second-degree heart block after PO use. *GI:* N&V, diarrhea, anorexia, bitter taste, abdominal pain. *Hematologic:* Thrombocytopenia, *agranulocytosis,* neutropenia. *Rarely, hemolytic anemia. Dermatologic:* Urticaria, pruritus, angioneurotic edema, flushing, maculopapular rash. *CNS:* Depression, dizziness, weakness, giddiness, psychoses, hallucinations. *Other:* Granulomatous hepatitis, weakness, fever, chills.

**OD Overdose Management:** *Symptoms:* Plasma levels of 10–15 mcg/mL are associated with toxic symptoms. Progressive widening of the QRS complex, prolonged QT or PR intervals, lowering of R and T waves, increased AV block, increased ventricular extrasystoles, *ventricular tachycardia or fibrillation. IV overdose may result in hypotension, CNS depression, tremor, respiratory depression. Treatment:*

• Induce emesis or perform gastric lavage followed by administration of activated charcoal.

• To treat hypotension, give IV fluids and/or a vasopressor (dopamine, phenylephrine, or norepinephrine).

• Infusion of ⅙ molar sodium lactate IV reduces the cardiotoxic effects.

• Hemodialysis (but not peritoneal dialysis) is effective in reducing serum levels.

• Renal clearance can be enhanced by acidification of the urine and with high flow rates.

• A ventricular pacing electrode can be inserted as a precaution in the event AV block develops.

**Drug Interactions**
*Acetazolamide* / ↑ Effect of procainamide due to ↓ excretion by kidney
*Anticholinergic agents, atropine* / Additive anticholinergic effects
*Antihypertensive agents* / Additive hypotensive effect
*Cholinergic agents* / Anticholinergic activity of procainamide antagonizes effect of cholinergic drugs

*Cimetidine* / ↑ Effect of procainamide due to ↑ bioavailability
*Disopyramide* / ↑ Risk of enhanced prolongation of conduction or depression of contractility and hypotension
*Ethanol* / Effect of procainamide may be altered, but because the main metabolite is active as an antiarrhythmic, specific outcome not clear
*Kanamycin* / Procainamide ↑ muscle relaxation produced by kanamycin
*Lidocaine* / Additive cardiodepressant effects
*Magnesium salts* / Procainamide ↑ muscle relaxation produced by magnesium salts
*Neomycin* / Procainamide ↑ muscle relaxation produced by neomycin
*Propranolol* / ↑ Serum procainamide levels
*Quinidine* / ↑ Risk of enhanced prolongation of conduction or depression of contractility and hypotension
*Ranitidine* / ↑ Effect of procainamide due to ↑ bioavailability
*Sodium bicarbonate* / ↑ Effect of procainamide due to ↓ excretion by the kidney
*Succinylcholine* / Procainamide ↑ muscle relaxation produced by succinylcholine
*Trimethoprim* / ↑ Effect of procainamide due to ↑ serum levels
**Laboratory Test Interferences:** May affect LFTs. False + ↑ in serum alkaline phosphatase. Positive ANA test. High levels of lidocaine and meprobamate may inhibit fluorescence of procainamide and NAPA.

**Dosage**
• **Capsules,    Extended-Release Tablets, Tablets**
**Adults, initial:** 50 mg/kg/day in divided doses q 3 hr. **Usual, 40–50 kg:** 250 mg q 3 hr of standard formulation or 500 mg q 6 hr of sustained-release; **60–70 kg:** 375 mg q 3 hr of standard formulation or 750 mg q 6 hr of sustained-release; **80–90 kg:** 500 mg q 3 hr of standard formulation or 1 g q 6 hr of sustained-release; **over**

**100 kg:** 625 mg q 3 hr of standard formulation or 1.25 g q 6 hr of sustained-release. **Pediatric:** 15–50 mg/kg/day divided q 3–6 hr (up to a maximum of 4 g/day).
• **Procanbid    Extended-Release Tablets**
   *Life-threatening arrhythmias.*
500 or 1,000 mg b.i.d.
• **IM**
   *Ventricular arrhythmias.*
**Adults, initial:** 50 mg/kg/day divided into fractional doses of ⅛–¼ given q 3–6 hr until PO therapy is possible. **Pediatric:** 20–30 mg/kg/day divided q 4–6 hr (up to a maximum of 4 g/day).
   *Arrhythmias associated with surgery or anesthesia.*
**Adults:** 100–500 mg.
• **IV**
**Initial loading infusion:** 20 mg/min (for up to 25–30 min). **Maintenance infusion:** 2–6 mg/min. **Pediatric, initial loading dose:** 3–5 mg/kg/dose over 5 min (maximum of 100 mg); **maintenance:** 20–80 mcg/kg/min continuous infusion (maximum of 2 g/day).

## NURSING CONSIDERATIONS

See also *Nursing Considerations* for *Antiarrhythmic Agents*.
**Administration/Storage**
1. Extended-release tablets are not recommended for use in children or for initiating treatment.
2. IM therapy may be used as an alternative to PO in clients with less threatening arrhythmias but who are nauseated or vomiting, who cannot take anything PO (e.g., preoperatively), or who have malabsorptive problems.
3. If more than three IM injections are required, assess the age, renal function, and blood levels of procainamide and NAPA; adjust dosage accordingly.
**IV** 4. Reserve IV use for emergency situations.
5. For IV initial therapy, dilute the drug with 5% dextrose solution; give a maximum of 1 g slowly to minimize

side effects by one of the following methods:
• Direct injection into a vein or into tubing of an established infusion line at a rate not to exceed 50 mg/min. Dilute either the 100- or 500-mg/mL vials prior to injection to facilitate control of the dosage rate. Doses of 100 mg may be given q 5 min until arrhythmia is suppressed or until 500 mg has been given (then wait 10 or more min before resuming administration).
• Loading infusion containing 20 mg/mL (1 g diluted with 50 mL of 5% dextrose injection) given at a constant rate of 1 mL/min for 25–30 min to deliver 500–600 mg.
6. For IV maintenance infusion, the dose is usually 2–6 mg/min. Administer with an electronic infusion device for safety and accuracy.
7. Discard solutions that are darker than light amber or otherwise colored. Solutions that have turned slightly yellow on standing may be used. Consult with pharmacist if unsure.
**Assessment**
1. Document indications for therapy, type, onset, and duration of symptoms. List other agents prescribed and the outcome.
2. Assess cardiopulmonary status and note findings.
3. Monitor ECG, CBC, electrolytes, ANA titers, liver and renal function studies.
**Interventions**
1. Place in a supine position during IV infusion and monitor BP. Discontinue if SBP falls 15 mm Hg or more during administration or if increased SA or AV block is noted.
2. Assess for symptoms of SLE, manifested by polyarthralgia, arthritis, pleuritic pain, fever, myalgia, and skin lesions.
**Client/Family Teaching**
1. Take with a full glass of water to lessen GI symptoms. Take either 1 hr before or 2 hr after meals.
2. If GI symptoms are severe and persistent may take with meals or

---

✦ = Available in Canada                    ***bold italic*** = life threatening side effect

with a snack to ensure compliance with drug therapy.

3. Sustained-release preparations should be swallowed whole. They should not be crushed, broken, or chewed. The wax matrix of sustained-release tablets may be evident in the stool and is considered normal.

4. Report any sore throat, fever, rash, chills, bruising, or diarrhea.

5. Do not take any OTC drugs.

**Outcomes/Evaluate**

• Termination of arrhythmias with restoration of stable cardiac rhythm

• Therapeutic drug levels (4–8 mcg/mL)

# Procarbazine hydrochloride (MIH, N-Methylhydrazine)

(pro-**KAR**-bah-zeen)
**Pregnancy Category:** D
Matulane, Natulan ✶ (Abbreviation: PCB) **(Rx)**
**Classification:** Antineoplastic, miscellaneous

See also *Antineoplastic Agents.*

**Action/Kinetics:** May inhibit synthesis of protein, RNA, and DNA and inhibit transmethylation of methyl groups of methionine into t-RNA. Absences of t-RNA could result in cessation of protein synthesis and subsequently DNA and RNA synthesis. Also, hydrogen peroxide formed during auto-oxidation of the drug may attack protein sulfhydryl groups found in residual protein that is tightly bound to DNA. Well absorbed from GI tract. Drug equilibrates between plasma and CSF (peak CSF levels occur within 30–90 min and peak plasma levels occur within 60 min). **t½, after IV:** 10 min. Metabolized in the liver and kidneys to cytotoxic products. About 70% eliminated in urine, mostly as metabolites, after 24 hr.

**Uses:** As an adjunct in the treatment of Hodgkin's disease (stage III and stage IV) as part of MOPP (nitrogen mustard, vincristine, procarbazine,

prednisone) or ChlVPP (chlorambucil, vinblastine, procarbazine, prednisone) therapies. *Investigational:* Non-Hodgkin's lymphomas, malignant melanoma, primary brain tumors, lung cancer, multiple myeloma, polycythemia vera.

**Contraindications:** Inadequate bone marrow reserve as shown by bone marrow aspiration (i.e., in clients with leukopenia, thrombocytopenia, or anemia). Lactation. Hypersensitivity to drug.

**Special Concerns:** Use with caution in impaired kidney or liver function. Due to the possibility of tremors, convulsions, and coma, close monitoring is necessary when used in children.

**Side Effects:** *GI:* N&V, anorexia, stomatitis, dry mouth, dysphagia, abdominal pain, hematemesis, melena, diarrhea, constipation. *CNS:* Paresthesias, neuropathies, headache, dizziness, depression, apprehension, nervousness, insomnia, nightmares, hallucinations, falling, weakness, fatigue, lethargy, drowsiness, unsteadiness, ataxia, foot drop, decreased reflexes, tremors, confusion, *coma, convulsions.* *CV:* Hypotension, tachycardia, syncope. *Respiratory:* Pleural effusion, pneumonitis, cough. *Hematologic:* Leukopenia, anemia, thrombocytopenia, pancytopenia, eosinophilia, *hemolytic anemia,* petechiae, purpura, epistaxis, hemoptysis. *GU:* Hematuria, urinary frequency, nocturia. *Dermatologic:* Dermatitis, pruritus, rash, urticaria, herpes, hyperpigmentation, flushing, alopecia. *Ophthalmic:* Retinal hemorrhage, nystagmus, photophobia, diplopia, inability to focus, papilledema. *Hepatic:* Jaundice, hepatic dysfunction. *Miscellaneous:* Gynecomastia in prepubertal and early pubertal boys, pain, myalgia and arthralgia, pyrexia, diaphoresis, chills, intercurrent infections, edema, hoarseness, generalized allergic reactions, hearing loss, slurred speech, second nonlymphoid malignancies (including acute myelocytic leukemia, malignant myelosclerosis) and azoospermia in those treated with procarbazine combined with other chemotherapy or radiation.

**OD Overdose Management:**
*Symptoms:* N&V, diarrhea, enteritis, hypotension, tremors, seizures, coma, hematologic and hepatic toxicity. *Treatment:* Induce vomiting or undertake gastric lavage. IV fluids. Frequent blood counts and LFTs should be performed.

**Drug Interactions**
*Alcohol* / Antabuse-like reaction
*Antihistamines* / Additive CNS depression
*Antihypertensive drugs* / Additive CNS depression
*Barbiturates* / Additive CNS depression
*Chemotherapy* / Depressed bone marrow activity
*Digoxin* / ↓ Digoxin plasma levels if combination therapy used
*Guanethidine* / Excitation and hypertension
*Hypoglycemic agents, oral* / ↑ Hypoglycemic effect
*Insulin* / ↑ Hypoglycemic effect
*Levodopa* / Flushing and hypertension within 1 hr of levodopa administration
*MAO inhibitors* / Possibility of hypertensive crisis
*Methyldopa* / Excitation and hypertension
*Narcotics* / Significant CNS depression → possible deep coma and death
*Phenothiazines* / Additive CNS depression; also, possibility of hypertensive crisis
*Reserpine* / Excitation and hypertension
*Sympathomimetics, indirectly acting* / Possibility of hypertensive crisis
*Tricyclic antidepressants* / Possible toxic and fatal reactions, including excitability, fluctuations in BP, seizures, and coma
*Tyramine-containing foods* / Possibility of hypertensive crisis

**Dosage**
• **Capsules**

*When used alone.*
**Adults:** 2–4 mg/kg/day for first week; **then,** 4–6 mg/kg/day until leukocyte count falls below 4,000/mm³ or platelet count falls below 100,000/mm³. If toxic symptoms appear, discontinue drug and resume treatment at rate of 1–2 mg/kg/day; **maintenance:** 1–2 mg/kg/day. **Children, highly individualized:** 50 mg/m²/day for first week; then 100 mg/m² (to nearest 50 mg) until maximum response obtained or until leukopenia or thrombocytopenia occurs. When maximum response is reached, maintain the dose at 50 mg/m²/day.

*When used in combination with other antineoplastic drugs (e.g., MOPP or ChIVPP therapies).*
100 mg/m² for 14 days.

## NURSING CONSIDERATIONS

See also *Nursing Considerations* for *Antineoplastic Agents.*
**Assessment**
1. Document indications for therapy and other agents prescribed.
2. Document cardiopulmonary and neurologic assessments.
3. Monitor CBC, uric acid, liver and renal function studies. May cause granulocyte and platelet suppression. Nadir: 14 days; recovery: 21–28 days.
**Client/Family Teaching**
1. Consult provider before taking any other medication because procarbazine has MAO inhibitory activity. The use of sympathomimetic drugs and foods with a high tyramine content (yeasts, yogurt, caffeine, chocolate, aged cheese, liver, smoked or pickled fish, fermented sausage, etc.) is contraindicated during therapy and for 2 weeks after discontinuing therapy; ingestion of these products may precipitate a hypertensive crisis.
2. Do not drive or perform tasks that require mental alertness until drug effects are realized.
3. Consume adequate fluids (2–3 L/day) to prevent dehydration.

4. Drug increases effect of insulin and oral hypoglycemic agents; hypoglycemic symptoms should be reported because adjustment of antidiabetic medication may be necessary.

5. Avoid exposure to sun or to ultraviolet rays because a photosensitive skin reaction may occur. Wear sunscreen, sunglasses, and protective clothing if exposure is necessary.

6. Avoid alcohol because a disulfiram-type reaction may occur.

7. Contraception should be practiced by both men and women.

8. Report persistent constipation (especially if diet, increased fluids, and bulk are ineffective), as laxatives may be prescribed.

**Outcomes/Evaluate:** Suppression of malignant cell proliferation

---

# Prochlorperazine
(proh-klor-**PAIR**-ah-zeen)
Compazine, Stemetil Suppositories ✶
**(Rx)**

# Prochlorperazine edisylate
(proh-klor-**PAIR**-ah-zeen)
Compazine Edisylate **(Rx)**

# Prochlorperazine maleate
(proh-klor-**PAIR**-ah-zeen)
Compazine Maleate **(Rx)**
**Classification:** Antipsychotic, antiemetic, piperazine-type phenothiazine

---

See also *Antipsychotic Agents, Phenothiazines.*

**Action/Kinetics:** Prochlorperazine causes a high incidence of extrapyramidal and antiemetic effects, moderate sedative effects, and a low incidence of anticholinergic effects and orthostatic hypotension. It also possesses significant antiemetic effects.

**Uses:** Psychoneuroses. Postoperative N&V, radiation sickness, vomiting due to toxins. Generally not used for clients who weigh less than 44 kg or who are under 2 years of age. Severe N&V.

**Special Concerns:** Safe use during pregnancy has not been established. Dosage has not been established in children less than 2 years of age or 9.1 kg body weight. Geriatric, emaciated, and debilitated clients usually require a lower initial dose.

## Dosage
• **Edisylate Syrup, Maleate Extended-Release Capsules, Tablets**
*Psychotic disorders.*
**Adults and adolescents:** 5–10 mg (base) t.i.d.–q.i.d. (dose can be increased gradually q 2–3 days as needed and tolerated). For extended-release capsules, up to 100–150 mg/day can be given. **Pediatric, 2–12 years:** 2.5 mg (base) b.i.d.–t.i.d.
*N&V.*
**Adults and adolescents:** 5–10 mg (base) t.i.d.–q.i.d. (up to 40 mg/day). For extended-release capsules, the dose is 15–30 mg once daily in the morning (or 10 mg q 12 hr, up to 40 mg/day). **Pediatric, 18–39 kg:** 2.5 mg (base) t.i.d. (or 5 mg b.i.d.), not to exceed 15 mg/day; **14–17 kg:** 2.5 mg (base) b.i.d.–t.i.d., not to exceed 10 mg/day; **9–13 kg:** 2.5 mg (base) 1–2 times/day, not to exceed 7.5 mg/day. The total daily dose for children should not exceed 10 mg the first day; on subsequent days, the total daily dose should not exceed 20 mg for children 2–5 years of age or 25 mg for children 6–12 years of age.
*Anxiety.*
**Adults and adolescents:** 5 mg (base) t.i.d.–q.i.d. up to 20 mg/day for no longer than 12 weeks.
• **IM, Edisylate Injection**
*Psychotic disorders, for immediate control of severely disturbed clients.*
**Adults and adolescents:** 10–20 mg (base); dose can be repeated q 2–4 hr as needed (usually up to three or four doses). **Maintenance:** 10–20 mg (base) q 4–6 hr. **Pediatric:** 0.132 mg/kg.
*Anxiety.*
**Adults and adolescents:** 5–10 mg (base); dose can be repeated q 2–4 hr as needed.

*N&V.*

**Adults and adolescents:** 5–10 mg with the dose repeated q 3–4 hr as needed. **Pediatric, 2–12 years:** 0.132 mg/kg.

*N&V during surgery.*

**Adults and adolescents:** 5–10 mg (base) 1–2 hr before induction of anesthesia; to control symptoms during or after surgery, the dose can be repeated once after 30 min.

• **IV, Edisylate Injection**
*N&V.*

**Adults and adolescents:** 2.5–10 mg as a slow injection or infusion (rate should not exceed 5 mg/min up to 40 mg/day).

*N&V during surgery.*

**Adults and adolescents:** 5–10 mg (base) given as a slow injection or infusion 15–30 min before induction of anesthesia; to control symptoms during or after surgery the dose can be repeated once. The rate of infusion should not exceed 5 mg/mL/min.

• **Rectal Suppositories**
**Pediatric, 2–12 years:** 2.5 mg b.i.d.–t.i.d. with no more than 10 mg given on the first day. No more than 20 mg/day for children 2–5 years of age and 25 mg/day for children 6–12 years of age.

## NURSING CONSIDERATIONS

See also *Nursing Considerations* for *Antipsychotic Agents, Phenothiazines.*

**Administration/Storage**

1. Store all forms of the drug in tight-closing amber-colored bottles; store suppositories below 37°C (98.6°F).
2. Add desired dosage of concentrate to 60 mL of beverage (e.g., tomato or fruit juice, milk, soup) or semisolid food just before administration to disguise the taste.
3. Drug should not be administered SC due to local irritation.
4. Drug should not be mixed with other agents in a syringe.
5. Prochlorperazine should not be diluted with any material containing the preservative parabens.

6. When given IM to children for N&V, the duration of action may be 12 hr.
7. Parenteral prescribing limits are 20 mg/day for children 2–5 years of age and 25 mg/day for children 6–12 years of age.

**Assessment**

1. Document indications for therapy, onset of symptoms, and presenting behaviors.
2. Assess mental status and note behavioral manifestations.
3. Monitor CBC, LFTs, and ECG.

**Interventions**

1. Monitor I&O and VS.
2. Auscultate bowel sounds and assess function.
3. Incorporate safety precautions during the treatment of an overdose.
4. If client was taking spansules, continue treatment until all signs of overdosage are no longer evident. Saline laxatives may be used to hasten the evacuation of pellets that have not yet released their medication.

**Client/Family Teaching**

1. Do not exceed the prescribed dose of drug.
2. If child shows signs of restlessness and excitement, withhold the drug and report.
3. Do not drive or operate machinery until drug effects are realized; drowsiness or dizziness may occur.
4. Report symptoms of extrapyramidal effects and tardive dyskinesia.
5. Use protection when in the sun to prevent photosensitivity reaction.
6. Rise and change positions slowly to prevent orthostatic effects.

**Outcomes/Evaluate**

• Control of N&V
• Reduction in agitation, excitability, or withdrawn behaviors

# Progesterone gel
(pro-**JES**-ter-ohn)
Crinone 4%, Crinone 8% **(Rx)**
**Classification:** Progesterone product

See also *Progesterone and Progestins.*

**Action/Kinetics: t½, absorption:** 25–50 hr. **t½, elimination:** 5–20 min. Extensively bound to plasma proteins. Metabolized in liver; excreted through urine and feces.

**Uses:** Progesterone supplementation or replacement as part of assisted reproductive technology treatment for infertile women with progesterone deficiency. Secondary amenorrhea.

**Contraindications:** Undiagnosed vaginal bleeding, liver disease or dysfunction, known or suspected malignancy of breast or genital organs, missed abortion, active thrombophlebitis or thromboembolic disease (or history of such). Concurrent use with other local intravaginal therapy.

**Special Concerns:** Safety and efficacy have not been determined in children.

**Side Effects:** See Progesterone and Progestins.

**Dosage** ————————
• **Vaginal gel: Crinone 8%**
*Assisted reproductive technology.*
90 mg once daily for women who require progesterone supplementation. Administer 90 mg b.i.d. in women with partial or complete ovarian failure who require progesterone replacement. If pregnancy occurs, treatment may be continued until placental autonomy has been achieved (up to 10–12 weeks).
• **Vaginal gel: Crinone 4%**
*Secondary amenorrhea.*
45 mg every other day up to total of 6 doses. For women who fail to respond, Crinone 8% (90 mg) may be given every other day up to total of 6 doses.

## NURSING CONSIDERATIONS

See also *Nursing Considerations* for *Progesterone and Progestins.*
**Administration/Storage**
1. Dosage increase from 4% gel can only be accomplished by using 8% gel. Increasing volume of gel does not increase amount of progesterone absorbed.
2. If other local intravaginal therapy

is to be used, there should be at least 6-hr period before or after Crinone administration.
3. Store at controlled room temperature below 25°C (77°F).
**Assessment**
1. Document indications for therapy, and physical and GYN exams.
2. Assess for liver disease, breast or genital malignancy, undiagnosed vaginal bleeding, or history of thromboembolic disease; these preclude drug therapy.
**Client/Family Teaching**
1. Review product information sheet on how to use product; use only as directed.
2. Do not use with other intravaginal products; if concurrent therapy prescribed, wait for 6 hr.
3. May experience breast enlargement, constipation, headaches, sleepiness, and perineal pain.
4. Report any overt symptoms or depression.
**Outcomes/Evaluate:** Progesterone replacement/supplementation

# Promazine hydrochloride
(**PROH**-mah-zeen)
Prozine-50, Sparine **(Rx)**
**Classification:** Antipsychotic, dimethylaminopropyl-type phenothiazine

See also *Antipsychotic Agents, Phenothiazines.*
**Action/Kinetics:** The use of promazine is accompanied by significant anticholinergic, sedative, and hypotensive effects; moderate antiemetic effect; and weak extrapyramidal effects. This drug is ineffective in reducing destructive behavior in acutely agitated psychotic clients.
**Uses:** Psychotic disorders.
**Special Concerns:** Safe use during pregnancy has not been established. Dosage has not been established in children less than 12 years of age. Geriatric, emaciated, and debilitated clients may require a lower initial dosage.

**Dosage** ————————
• **Tablets**

*Psychotic disorders.*
**Adults:** 10–200 mg q 4–6 hr; adjust dose as needed and tolerated. Total daily dose should not exceed 1,000 mg. **Pediatric, 12 years and older:** 10–25 mg q 4–6 hr; adjust dose as needed and tolerated.

• **IM**
*Psychotic disorders, severe and moderate agitation.*
**Adults, initial:** 50–150 mg; adjust dose if necessary after 30 min. **Maintenance:** 10–200 mg q 4–6 hr as needed and tolerated. Switch to PO therapy as soon as possible. **Pediatric over 12 years:** 10–25 mg q 4–6 hr for chronic psychotic disorders (maximum dose: 1 g/day).

IM doses may be given IV continuously.

## NURSING CONSIDERATIONS

See also *Nursing Considerations* for *Antipsychotic Agents, Phenothiazines.*
**Administration/Storage**
1. Dilute concentrate as directed on bottle. Taste can be disguised when given with citrus fruit juice, milk, or flavored drinks.
2. IM injections should be given in the gluteal region.
**IV** 3. IV doses should be diluted to 25 mg/mL with 0.9% NaCl injection and given slowly.
**Assessment:** Document indications for therapy, onset of symptoms, and presenting behaviors. Note other agents trialed and the outcome.
**Outcomes/Evaluate:** Improved behavior patterns with a reduction in agitation, excitability, or withdrawn behaviors

# Promethazine hydrochloride
(proh-**METH**-ah-zeen)
**Parenteral:** Anergan 50, Phenergan,
**Suppositories:** Phenergan, **Syrup:** Phenergan Fortis, Phenergan Plain,
**Tablets:** Histanil ✹, Phenergan, PMS Promethazine ✹ **(Rx)**
**Classification:** Antihistamine, phenothiazine-type

See also *Antihistamines* and *Antiemetics.*
**Action/Kinetics:** Antiemetic effects are likely due to inhibition of the CTZ. Effective in vertigo by its central anticholinergic effect which inhibits the vestibular apparatus and the integrative vomiting center as well as the CTZ. May cause severe drowsiness. **Onset, PO, IM, PR:** 20 min; **IV:** 3–5 min. **Duration, antihistaminic:** 6–12 hr; **sedative:** 2–8 hr. Slowly eliminated through urine and feces.
**Uses:** PO and PR for prophylaxis and treatment of motion sickness. Prophylaxis of N&V due to anesthesia or surgery (also postoperatively). Pre- or postoperative sedative, obstetric sedative. Hypersensitivity reactions, including perennial and seasonal allergic rhinitis, vasomotor rhinitis, allergic conjunctivitis, urticaria, angioedema, allergic reactions to blood or plasma, dermographism. Adjunct in the treatment of anaphylaxis or anaphylactoid reactions. Adjunct to analgesics for postoperative pain. IV with meperidine or other narcotics in special surgical procedures as bronchoscopy, ophthalmic surgery, or in poor-risk clients.
**Contraindications:** Lactation. Comatose clients, CNS depression due to drugs, previous phenothiazine idiosyncrasy, acutely ill or dehydrated children (due to greater susceptibility to dystonias). Children up to 2 years of age. SC or intra-arterial use due to tissue necrosis and gangrene.
**Special Concerns:** Safe use during pregnancy has not been established. Use in children may cause paradoxical hyperexcitability and nightmares. Geriatric clients are more likely to experience confusion, dizziness, hypotension, and sedation.
**Additional Side Effects:** Leukopenia and ***agranulocytosis (especially if used with cytotoxic agents).***

**Dosage**
• **Suppositories, Syrup, Tablets**
*Hypersensitivity reactions.*

**P**

---

**Adults:** 12.5 mg q.i.d. before meals and at bedtime (or 25 mg at bedtime if needed). **Pediatric over 2 years:** 0.125 mg/kg (3.75 mg/m²) q 4–6 hr; 0.5 mg/kg (15 mg/m²) at bedtime if needed; or, 6.25–12. mg t.i.d. (or 25 mg at bedtime if needed).

*Antiemetic.*
**Adults:** 25 mg (usual); 12.5–25 mg q 4–6 hr as needed. **Pediatric, over 2 years:** 0.25–0.5 mg/kg (7.5–15 mg/m²) q 4–6 hr as needed (or 12.5–25 mg q 4–6 hr).

*Sedation.*
**Adults:** 25–50 mg at bedtime; **pediatric, over 2 years:** 0.5–1 mg/kg (15–30 mg/m²) or 12.5–25 mg at bedtime.

*Motion sickness.*
**Adults:** 25 mg b.i.d. **Pediatric, over 2 years:** 12.5–25 mg b.i.d.

*Analgesia adjunct.*
**Adults:** 50 mg with an equal amount of meperidine and an appropriate dose of an atropine-like agent. **Pediatric, over 2 years:** 1.2 mg/kg with an equal amount of meperidine and an atropine-like agent.

- **IM, IV**
*Hypersensitivity reactions.*
**Adults:** 25 mg repeated in 2 hr if needed; **pediatric, 2–12 years:** 12.5 mg or less, not to exceed half the adult dose. Resume PO therapy as soon as possible.

*Antiemetic.*
**Adults:** 12.5–25 mg q 4 hr if needed. If used postoperatively, reduce doses of concomitant hypnotics, analgesics, or barbiturates. **Pediatric, 2–12 years:** Do not exceed half the adult dose. Do not use when the cause of vomiting is unknown.

*Sedation.*
**Adults:** 25–50 mg at bedtime. May be combined with hypnotics for pre- and postoperative sedation. **Pediatric, 2–12 years:** Do not exceed half the adult dose.

*Sedation during labor.*
**Adults:** 50 mg during early stages of labor, not to exceed 100 mg/24 hr.

*Analgesia adjunct.*
**Adults:** 25–50 mg in combination with reduced doses of analgesics

and hypnotics; give atropine-like drugs as needed. **Pediatric, 2–12 years:** 1.2 mg/kg in combination with an equal dose of analgesic or barbiturate and an appropriate dose of an atropine-like drug.

## NURSING CONSIDERATIONS

See also *Nursing Considerations* for *Antihistamines,* and *Antiemetics.*

**Administration/Storage:** Decrease dosage in dehydrated clients or those with oliguria.

**Assessment:** Document indications for therapy, type and onset of symptoms. Note age; older clients may manifest more adverse side effects.

**Client/Family Teaching**
1. Take only as directed and do not exceed dose, as arrhythmias may occur. May take with food or milk to decrease GI upset.
2. When used to prevent motion sickness, take 30–60 min before travel. On successive travel days, take on rising and again before the evening meal.
3. Avoid activities that require mental alertness until drug effects realized.
4. Do not consume alcohol or any OTC agents.
5. Drug may alter skin testing; stop 72 hr before testing.

**Outcomes/Evaluate**
- Prevention of vertigo
- Control of N&V
- Promotion of sleep
- Control of allergic manifestations

# Propafenone hydrochloride
(proh-pah-**FEN**-ohn)
**Pregnancy Category:** C
Rythmol **(Rx)**
**Classification:** Antiarrhythmic, class IC

**Action/Kinetics:** Manifests local anesthetic effects and a direct stabilizing action on the myocardium. Reduces upstroke velocity (Phase O) of the monophasic action potential, reduces the fast inward current carried by sodium ions in the Purkinje fibers, increases diastolic excitability threshold, and prolongs the effective refractory period. Also, spontaneous activity is decreased. Slows AV conduction and causes first-degree heart block. Has slight beta-adrenergic blocking activity. **Peak plasma levels:** 3.5 hr. **Therapeutic plasma levels:** 0.5–3 mcg/mL. Significant first-pass effect. Most metabolize rapidly (**t½:** 2–10 hr) to two active metabolites: 5-hydroxypropafenone and N-depropylpropafenone. However, approximately 10% (as well as those taking quinidine) metabolize the drug more slowly (**t½:** 10–32 hr). Because the 5-hydroxy metabolite is not formed in slow metabolizers and because steady-state levels are reached after 4–5 days in all clients, the recommended dosing regimen is the same for all clients.

**Uses:** Documented life-threatening ventricular arrhythmias such as sustained ventricular tachycardia where the benefits outweigh the risks. Do not use in less severe ventricular arrhythmias even if the client is symptomatic. Antiarrhythmic drugs have not been shown to improve survival in clients with ventricular arrhythmias. *Investigational:* SVTs including atrial fibrillation or flutter and arrhythmias associated with Wolff-Parkinson-White syndrome.

**Contraindications:** Uncontrolled CHF, cardiogenic shock, sick sinus node syndrome or AV block in the absence of an artificial pacemaker, bradycardia, marked hypotension, bronchospastic disorders, electrolyte disorders, hypersensitivity to the drug. MI more than 6 days but less than 2 years previously. Lactation.

**Special Concerns:** With use of procainamide there is an increased risk of death in those with non-life-threatening arrhythmias. Use with caution during labor and delivery. The safety and effectiveness have not been determined in children. Use with caution in clients with impaired hepatic or renal function. Geriatric clients may require lower dosage.

**Side Effects:** *CV: New or worsened arrhythmias.* First-degree AV block, intraventricular conduction delay, palpitations, PVCs, proarrhythmia, bradycardia, atrial fibrillation, angina, syncope, CHF, *ventricular tachycardia, second-degree AV block,* increased QRS duration, chest pain, hypotension, bundle branch block. Less commonly, atrial flutter, AV dissociation, flushing, hot flashes, sick sinus syndrome, sinus pause or arrest, SVT, *cardiac arrest. CNS:* Dizziness, headache, anxiety, drowsiness, fatigue, loss of balance, ataxia, insomnia. Less commonly, abnormal speech, abnormal dreams, abnormal vision, confusion, depression, memory loss, *apnea,* psychosis/mania, vertigo, *seizures, coma,* numbness, paresthesias. *GI:* Unusual taste, constipation, nausea and/or vomiting, dry mouth, anorexia, flatulence, abdominal pain, cramps, diarrhea, dyspepsia. Less commonly, gastroenteritis and liver abnormalities (cholestasis, hepatitis, elevated enzymes, hepatitis). *Hematologic: Agranulocytosis,* increased bleeding time, anemia, granulocytopenia, bruising, leukopenia, purpura, anemia, thrombocytopenia. *Miscellaneous:* Blurred vision, dyspnea, weakness, rash, edema, tremors, diaphoresis, joint pain, possible decrease in spermatogenesis. Less commonly, tinnitus, unusual smell sensation, alopecia, eye irritation, hyponatremia, inappropriate ADH secretion, impotence, increased glucose, kidney failure, lupus erythematosus, muscle cramps or weakness, nephrotic syndrome, pain, pruritus.

**OD Overdose Management:** *Symptoms:* Bradycardia, hypotension, IA and intraventricular conduction disturbances, somnolence. *Rarely, high-grade ventricular arrhythmias and seizures. Treatment:* To control BP and cardiac rhythm, defibrillation and infusion of dopamine or isoproterenol. If seizures occur, diazepam, IV, can be given. External cardiac massage and mechanical respiratory assistance may be required.

**Drug Interactions**

*Beta-adrenergic blockers* / ↑ Plasma levels of beta blockers metabolized by the liver

*Cimetidine* / ↓ Plasma levels of propafenone

*Cyclosporine* / ↑ Blood trough levels of cyclosporine; ↓ renal function

*Digoxin* / ↑ Plasma levels of digoxin necessitating a ↓ in the dose of digoxin

*Local anesthetics* / May ↑ risk of CNS side effects

*Quinidine* / ↑ Serum levels of propafenone in rapid metabolizers → possible ↑ effect

*Rifampin* / ↓ Effect of propafenone due to ↑ clearance

*Warfarin* / May ↑ plasma levels of warfarin necessitating ↓ dose of warfarin

**Laboratory Test Interferences:** ↑ ANA titers.

## Dosage

• **Tablets**

**Adults, initial:** 150 mg q 8 hr; dose may be increased at a minimum of q 3–4 days to 225 mg q 8 hr and, if necessary, to 300 mg q 8 hr.

## NURSING CONSIDERATIONS

See also *Nursing Considerations* for *Antiarrhythmic Agents.*

**Administration/Storage**

1. Always undertake initiation of therapy in a hospital setting.

2. The effectiveness and safety of doses exceeding 900 mg/day have not been determined.

3. There is no evidence that the use of propafenone affects the survival or incidence of sudden death with recent MI or SVT.

**Assessment**

1. Assess ECG and baseline arrhythmias; note any cardiac problems.

2. Monitor CBC, electrolytes, liver and renal function studies. Determine any renal or hepatic disease.

**Interventions**

1. May induce new or more severe arrhythmias; dose should be titrated in

each client on the basis of response and tolerance.

2. Report any significant widening of the QRS complex or any evidence of second- or third-degree AV block.

3. Dose should be increased more gradually in elderly clients as well as those with previous myocardial damage.

4. Monitor VS. Weigh client and place on strict I&O.

5. Evaluate hematologic studies to determine presence of anemia, agranulocytosis, leukopenia, thrombocytopenia, or altered prothrombin and coagulation times.

6. Client may complain of an unusual taste in the mouth which may interfere with eating and nutritional status.

**Client/Family Teaching**

1. Drink adequate quantities of fluid (2–3 L/day) and add bulk to the diet to avoid constipation.

2. Report any incidence of increased or unusual bruising or bleeding or S&S of hepatic dysfunction such as yellow sclera, dark-yellow urine, or yellow pigmentation of the skin.

3. Report any evidence of urinary tract problems or decreased urinary output.

4. Record BP and pulse readings.

**Outcomes/Evaluate**

• Termination of life-threatening ventricular tachycardia

• Therapeutic drug levels (0.5–3 mcg/mL)

# Propantheline bromide

(proh-**PAN**-thih-leen)

**Pregnancy Category:** C

Norpanth, Pro-Banthine, Propanthel

✱ **(Rx)**

**Classification:** Anticholinergic, antispasmodic (quaternary ammonium compound)

See also *Cholinergic Blocking Agents.*

**Action/Kinetics: Duration:** 6 hr. Metabolized in the liver and excreted through the urine.

**Uses:** Adjunct in peptic ulcer therapy. Spastic and inflammatory disease of GI and urinary tracts. Control of sali-

vation and enuresis. Duodenography. Second-line therapy for urinary incontinence.
**Special Concerns:** Safety and effectiveness for use in children with peptic ulcer have not been established.

**Dosage** ————————
• **Tablets**
  *GI problems.*
  **Adults:** 15 mg 30 min before meals and 30 mg at bedtime. Reduce dose to 7.5 mg t.i.d. for mild symptoms, geriatric clients, or clients of small stature. **Pediatric:** 0.375 mg/kg (10 mg/m²) q.i.d. with dose being adjusted as needed.
  *Urinary incontinence.*
  **Adults:** 7.5–30 mg 3–5 times/day; in some, doses as high as 15–60 mg q.i.d. may be needed.

## NURSING CONSIDERATIONS

See also *Nursing Considerations* for *Cholinergic Blocking Agents.*
**Assessment**
1. Document indications for therapy, type, onset, and duration of symptoms.
2. With ulcer disease or persistent GI complaints, determine *H. pylori* results.
3. A liquid diet is recommended during initiation of therapy with edematous duodenal ulcer.
**Client/Family Teaching**
1. Drug may cause drowsiness or dizziness. Do not drive or operate equipment until drug effects realized.
2. May impair visual acuity; dark glasses may be necessary. Report if symptoms are persistent.
3. Increase dietary intake of fluids and fiber to minimize the constipating effects of drug therapy.
4. Report any symptoms of urinary retention and persistent constipation.
**Outcomes/Evaluate**
• Relief of GI pain R/T PUD
• Control of urinary incontinence

# Propoxyphene hydrochloride
(proh-**POX**-ih-feen) C
**Pregnancy Category:** C
642 Tablets ♣, Darvon, Dolene, Doloxene, Doraphen, Doxaphene, Novo-Propoxyn ♣, Profene, Progesic, Pro Pox, Propoxycon **(C-IV) (Rx)**

# Propoxyphene napsylate
(proh-**POX**-ih-feen)
**Pregnancy Category:** C
Darvon-N **(C-IV) (Rx)**
**Classification:** Analgesic, narcotic, miscellaneous

**Action/Kinetics:** Resembles narcotics with respect to its mechanism and analgesic effect; it is one-half to one-third as potent as codeine. Is devoid of antitussive, anti-inflammatory, or antipyretic activity. When taken in excessive doses for long periods, psychologic dependence and occasionally physical dependence and tolerance will be manifested. **Peak plasma levels:** *hydrochloride:* 2–2.5 hr; *napsylate:* 3–4 hr. **Analgesic onset:** 30–60 min. **Peak analgesic effect:** 2–2.5 hr. **Duration:** 4–6 hr. **Therapeutic serum levels:** 0.05–0.12 mcg/mL. **t½, propoxyphene:** 6–12 hr; **norpropoxyphene:** 30–36 hr. Extensive first-pass effect; metabolites are excreted in the urine.
**Uses:** Relief of mild to moderate pain. Napsylate has been used experimentally to suppress the withdrawal syndrome from narcotics.
**Contraindications:** Hypersensitivity to drug. Use in children.
**Special Concerns:** Safe use during pregnancy has not been established. Use with caution during lactation.
**Side Effects:** *GI:* N&V, constipation, abdominal pain. *CNS:* Sedation, dizziness, lightheadedness, headache, weakness, euphoria, dysphoria. *Other:* Skin rashes, visual disturbances. Propoxyphene can produce psychologic dependence, as well as physical dependence and tolerance.

P

**OD  Overdose  Management:**
*Symptoms:* Stupor, respiratory depression, **apnea,** hypotension, pulmonary edema, **circulatory collapse, cardiac arrhythmias,** conduction abnormalities, **coma, seizures,** respiratory-metabolic acidosis. *Treatment:* Maintain an adequate airway, artificial respiration, and naloxone, 0.4–2 mg IV (repeat at 2- to 3-min intervals) to combat respiratory depression. Gastric lavage or administration of activated charcoal may be helpful. Correct acidosis and electrolyte imbalance. Acidosis due to lactic acid may require IV sodium bicarbonate.

**Drug Interactions**
*Alcohol, antianxiety drugs, antipsychotic agents, narcotics, sedative-hypnotics* / Concomitant use may lead to drowsiness, lethargy, stupor, respiratory, depression, and coma
*Carbamazepine* / ↑ Effect of carbamazepine due to ↓ breakdown by liver
*CNS depressants* / Additive CNS depression
*Orphenadrine* / Concomitant use may lead to confusion, anxiety, and tremors
*Phenobarbital* / ↑ Effect of phenobarbital due to ↓ breakdown by liver
*Skeletal muscle relaxants* / Additive respiratory depression
*Warfarin* / ↑ Hypoprothrombinemic effects of warfarin

**Dosage**
- **Capsules (Hydrochloride)**
  *Analgesia.*
**Adults:** 65 mg q 4 hr, not to exceed 390 mg/day.
- **Tablets (Napsylate)**
  *Analgesia.*
**Adults:** 100 mg q 4 hr, not to exceed 600 mg/day. Dose of propoxyphene should be reduced in clients with renal or hepatic impairment.

**NURSING CONSIDERATIONS**

See also *Nursing Considerations* for *Narcotic Analgesics.*
**Assessment**
1. Document indications for therapy; note onset, duration, location, and characteristics of pain. Use a pain-rating scale to assess pain. Note other agents prescribed, and the outcome.
2. Note any opiate or alcohol dependency.
3. Monitor liver and renal function studies; reduce dose with renal and liver dysfunction.
4. Determine if client smokes; smoking reduces drug effect by increasing metabolism.
5. Use with caution in the elderly and review drug profile to ensure other prescribed agents do not cause additive CNS effects.

**Client/Family Teaching**
1. May take with food to decrease GI upset.
2. Avoid activities that require mental alertness; drug may cause dizziness and drowsiness.
3. Do not consume alcohol or any OTC agents.

**Outcomes/Evaluate:** Relief of pain

————COMBINATION DRUG————

# Propranolol and Hydrochlorothiazide
(proh-**PRAN**-oh-lohl, hy-droh-**klor**-oh-**THIGH**-ah-zyd)
**Pregnancy Category:** C
Inderide 40/25, Inderide 80/25, Inderide LA 80/50, Inderide LA 120/50, Inderide LA 160/50 **(Rx)**
**Classification:** Antihypertensive

See also *Propranolol* and *Hydrochlorothiazide.*
**Content:** *Antihypertensive/diuretic:* Hydrochlorothiazide, 25 mg (Inderide) or 50 mg (Inderide LA).
*Beta-adrenergic blocking agent:* Propranolol HCl, 40 or 80 mg (Inderide) or 80, 120, or 160 mg (Inderide LA).
Also see information on individual components.
**Uses:** Hypertension (not indicated for initial therapy).
**Special Concerns:** Use with caution during lactation. Safety and effectiveness have not been established in children. The risk of hypothermia is increased in geriatric clients.

## Dosage

• **Inderide Tablets**
**Individualized:** 1–2 tablets b.i.d., up to 320 mg propranolol HCl daily.
• **Inderide LA Capsules**
1 capsule once daily.

## NURSING CONSIDERATIONS

See also *Nursing Considerations* for *Antihypertensive Agents* and individual agents.

**Administration/Storage**

1. Because of side effects from hydrochlorothiazide, do not use Inderide if propranolol must be given in excess of 320 mg/day.

2. If another antihypertensive agent is required, initial dosage should be one-half the usual dose to prevent an excessive drop in BP.

3. Inderide LA is not a milligram-to-milligram substitute for Inderide because the LA produces lower blood levels.

**Outcomes/Evaluate:** ↓ BP; control of hypertension

# Propranolol hydrochloride

(proh-**PRAN**-oh-lohl)
**Pregnancy Category:** C
Apo-Propranolol ✱, Detensol ✱, Dom-Propranolol ✱, Inderal, Inderal 10, 20, 40, 60, 80, and 90, Inderal I.A, Novo-Pranol ✱, Nu-Propranolol ✱, PMS Propranolol ✱, Propranolol Intensol **(Rx)**
**Classification:** Beta-adrenergic blocking agent; antiarrhythmic (type II)

See also *Beta-Adrenergic Blocking Agents*.

**Action/Kinetics:** Manifests both beta-1- and beta-2-adrenergic blocking activity. Antiarrhythmic action is due to both beta-adrenergic receptor blockade and a direct membrane-stabilizing action on the cardiac cell. Has no intrinsic sympathomimetic activity and has high lipid solubility.
**Onset, PO:** 30 min; **IV:** immediate.
**Maximum effect:** 1–1.5 hr. **Dura-**

**tion:** 3–5 hr. **t½:** 2–3 hr (8–11 hr for long-acting). **Therapeutic serum level, antiarrhythmic:** 0.05–0.1 mcg/mL. Completely metabolized by liver and excreted in urine. Although food increases bioavailability, absorption may be decreased.
**Uses:** Hypertension (alone or in combination with other antihypertensive agents). Angina pectoris, hypertrophic subaortic stenosis, prophylaxis of MI, pheochromocytoma, prophylaxis of migraine, essential tremor. Cardiac arrhythmias including ventricular tachycardias and arrhythmias, tachycardias due to digitalis intoxication, supraventricular arrhythmias, PVCs, resistant tachyarrhythmias due to anesthesia/catecholamines.

*Investigational:* Schizophrenia, tremors due to parkinsonism, aggressive behavior, antipsychotic-induced akathisia, rebleeding due to esophageal varices, situational anxiety, acute panic attacks, gastric bleeding in portal hypertension, vaginal contraceptive, anxiety, alcohol withdrawal syndrome, winter depression.

**Contraindications:** Bronchial asthma, bronchospasms including severe COPD.

**Special Concerns:** It is dangerous to use propranolol for pheochromocytoma unless an alpha-adrenergic blocking agent is already in use.

**Additional Side Effects:** Psoriasis-like eruptions, skin necrosis, SLE (rare).

**Additional Drug Interactions**

*Haloperidol* / Severe hypotension
*Hydralazine* / ↑ Effect of both agents
*Methimazole* / May ↑ effects of propranolol
*Phenobarbital* / ↓ Effect of propranolol due to ↑ breakdown by liver
*Propylthiouracil* / May ↑ the effects of propranolol
*Rifampin* / ↓ Effect of propranolol due to ↑ breakdown by liver
*Smoking* / ↓ Serum levels and ↑ clearance of propranolol

---

**Laboratory Test Interferences:** ↑ Blood urea, serum transaminase, alkaline phosphatase, LDH. Interference with glaucoma screening test.

## Dosage

• **Tablets, Sustained-Release Capsules, Oral Solution, Concentrate**

*Hypertension.*

**Initial:** 40 mg b.i.d. or 80 mg of sustained-release/day; **then,** increase dose to maintenance level of 120–240 mg/day given in two to three divided doses or 120–160 mg of sustained-release medication once daily. Maximum daily dose should not exceed 640 mg. **Pediatric, initial:** 0.5 mg/kg b.i.d.; dose may be increased at 3- to 5-day intervals to a maximum of 1 mg/kg b.i.d. The dosage range should be calculated by weight and not by body surface area.

*Angina.*

**Initial:** 80–320 mg b.i.d., t.i.d., or q.i.d.; or, 80 mg of sustained-release once daily; **then,** increase dose gradually to maintenance level of 160 mg/day of sustained-release capsule. The maximum daily dose should not exceed 320 mg.

*Arrhythmias.*

10–30 mg t.i.d.–q.i.d. given after meals and at bedtime.

*Hypertrophic subaortic stenosis.*

20–40 mg t.i.d.–q.i.d. before meals and at bedtime or 80–160 mg of sustained-release medication given once daily.

*MI prophylaxis.*

180–240 mg/day given in three to four divided doses. Total daily dose should not exceed 240 mg.

*Pheochromocytoma, preoperatively.*

60 mg/day for 3 days before surgery, given concomitantly with an alpha-adrenergic blocking agent.

*Inoperable tumors.*

30 mg/day in divided doses.

*Migraine.*

**Initial:** 80 mg sustained-release medication given once daily; **then,** increase dose gradually to maintenance of 160–240 mg/day in divided doses. If a satisfactory response has not been observed after 4–6 weeks, the drug should be discontinued and withdrawn gradually.

*Essential tremor.*

**Initial:** 40 mg b.i.d.; **then,** 120 mg/day up to a maximum of 320 mg/day.

*Aggressive behavior.*

80–300 mg/day.

*Antipsychotic-induced akathisia.*

20–80 mg/day.

*Tremors associated with Parkinson's disease.*

160 mg/day.

*Rebleeding from esophageal varices.*

20–180 mg b.i.d.

*Schizophrenia.*

300–5,000 mg/day.

*Acute panic symptoms.*

40–320 mg/day.

*Anxiety.*

80–320 mg/day.

*Intermittent explosive disorder.*

50–1,600 mg/day.

*Nonvariceal gastric bleeding in portal hypertension.*

24–480 mg/day.

• **IV**

*Life-threatening arrhythmias or those occurring under anesthesia.*

1–3 mg not to exceed 1 mg/min; a second dose may be given after 2 min, with subsequent doses q 4 hr. Clients should begin PO therapy as soon as possible. Although use in pediatrics is not recommended, investigational doses of 0.01–0.1 mg/kg/dose, up to a maximum of 1 mg/dose (by slow push), have been used for arrhythmias.

## NURSING CONSIDERATIONS

See also *Nursing Considerations* for *Beta-Adrenergic Blocking Agents* and *Antihypertensive Agents*.

**Administration/Storage**

1. Do not administer for a minimum of 2 weeks in client who has discontinued MAO inhibitor drugs.

**IV** 2. If signs of serious myocardial depression occur, slowly infuse isoproterenol (Isuprel) IV.

3. For IV use, dilute 1 mg in 10 mL of D5W and administer IV over at least

1 min. May be further reconstituted in 50 mL of dextrose or saline solution and infused IVPB over 10–15 min.

4. After IV administration, have available emergency drugs and equipment to combat hypotension or circulatory collapse.

**Assessment**

1. Document indications for therapy, type, onset, duration of symptoms, and other agents prescribed.

2. Note ECG, VS, and cardiopulmonary assessment. Assess for pulmonary disease, bronchospasms, or depression.

3. Report rash, fever, and/or purpura; may be symptoms of a hypersensitivity reaction.

4. Monitor VS, I&O. Observe for S&S of CHF (e.g., SOB, rales, edema, and weight gain).

**Client/Family Teaching**

1. Drug may cause drowsiness; assess drug response before performing activities that require mental alertness.

2. Do not smoke; smoking decreases serum levels of the drug and interferes with drug clearance.

3. Drug may mask most symptoms of hypoglycemia; monitor finger sticks carefully.

4. Check BP and HR weekly; report any significant changes.

5. Do not stop abruptly; may precipitate hypertension, myocardial ischemia, or cardiac arrhythmias.

6. Dress appropriately; drug may cause increased sensitivity to cold.

7. Avoid alcohol and any OTC agents containing alpha-adrenergic stimulants or sympathomimetics.

8. Report any persistent side effects, e.g., skin rashes, abnormal bleeding, unusual crying, or feelings of depression.

**Outcomes/Evaluate**

- ↓ BP, ↓ HR
- ↓ Frequency/intensity of angina; prevention of myocardial reinfarction
- Migraine prophylaxis
- Control of tachyarrhythmias
- Desired behavioral changes

- Relief/control of chronic pain
- Therapeutic drug levels as an antiarrhythmic (0.05–0.1 mcg/mL)

# Propylthiouracil
(proh-pill-thigh-oh-**YOUR**-ah-sill)
**Pregnancy Category:** D
Propyl-Thyracil ✦ (Rx)
**Classification:** Antithyroid preparation

See also *Antithyroid Drugs.*

**Action/Kinetics:** May be preferred for treatment of thyroid storm, as it inhibits peripheral conversion of thyroxine to triiodothyronine. Rapidly absorbed from the GI tract. **Duration:** 2–3 hr. **t½:** 1–2 hr. **Onset:** 10–20 days. **Time to peak effect:** 2–10 weeks. Eighty percent is protein bound. Metabolized by the liver and excreted through the kidneys.

**Special Concerns:** Incidence of vasculitis is increased.

**Drug Interactions:** Propylthiouracil may produce hypoprothrombinemia, adding to the effect of anticoagulants.

**Dosage**
- **Tablets**

    *Hyperthyroidism.*

**Adults, initial:** 300 mg/day (up to 900 mg/day may be required in some clients with severe hyperthyroidism) given as one to four divided doses; **maintenance, usual:** 100–150 mg/day. **Pediatric, 6–10 years, initial:** 50–150 mg/day in one to four divided doses; **over 10 years, initial:** 150–300 mg/day in one to four divided doses. Maintenance for all pediatric use is based on response. **Alternative dose for children, initial:** 5–7 mg/kg/day (150–200 mg/m²/day) in divided doses q 8 hr; **maintenance:** ⅓–⅔ the initial dose when the client is euthyroid.

    *Thyrotoxic crisis.*

**Adults:** 200–400 mg q 4 hr during the first day as an adjunct to other treatments.

    *Neonatal thyrotoxicosis.*

10 mg/kg daily in divided doses.

---

✦ = Available in Canada    *bold italic* = life threatening side effect

## NURSING CONSIDERATIONS

See also *Nursing Considerations* for *Antithyroid Drugs*.

### Client/Family Teaching

1. Take only as directed. May take with meals to decrease GI upset.
2. Avoid dietary sources of iodine (shellfish, kelp, iodized salt).
3. Report any fever, sore throat, enlarged cervical lymph nodes, or rash immediately.
4. Alert provider of unusual bruising or bleeding; report for labs.
5. Report S&S of hypothyroidism (cold intolerance, increased fatigue, mental depression).

### Outcomes/Evaluate

• Normal metabolism; control of symptoms (↑ weight, ↓ sweating, ↓ HR)
• Suppression of thyroid hormones (↓ T$_3$, T$_4$) after 3 weeks of therapy

---

# Protamine sulfate

(**PROH**-tah-meen)
**Pregnancy Category:** C
**(Rx)**
**Classification:** Heparin antagonist

**Action/Kinetics:** Protamine sulfate is a strongly basic polypeptide that complexes with strongly acidic heparin to form an inactive stable salt. The complex has no anticoagulant activity. Heparin is neutralized within 5 min after IV protamine. **Duration:** 2 hr (but depends on body temperature). The t½ of protamine is shorter than heparin; thus, repeated doses may be required. Upon metabolism, the complex may liberate heparin (heparin rebound).

**Uses:** Only for treatment of heparin overdose.

**Contraindications:** Previous intolerance to protamine. Not suitable for treating spontaneous hemorrhage, postpartum hemorrhage, menorrhagia, or uterine bleeding. Administration of over 50 mg over a short period.

**Special Concerns:** Use with caution during lactation. Safety and efficacy have not been determined in children. Rapid administration may cause severe hypotension and anaphylaxis.

**Side Effects:** *CV:* Sudden fall in BP, bradycardia, transitory flushing, warm feeling, *acute pulmonary hypertension, circulatory collapse (possibly irreversible) with myocardial failure* and decreased CO. Pulmonary edema in clients on cardiopulmonary bypass undergoing CV surgery. *Anaphylaxis:* Severe respiratory distress, capillary leak, and noncardiogenic pulmonary edema. *GI:* N&V. *CNS:* Lassitude. *Other:* Dyspnea, back pain in conscious clients undergoing cardiac catheterization, hypersensitivity reactions.

**OD Overdose Management:** *Symptoms:* Bleeding. Rapid administration may cause dyspnea, bradycardia, flushing, warm feeling, severe hypotension, hypertension. In assessing overdose, there may be the possibility of multiple drug overdoses leading to drug interactions and unusual pharmacokinetics. *Treatment:* Replace blood loss with blood transfusions or fresh frozen plasma. Fluids, epinephrine, dobutamine, or dopamine to treat hypotension.

### Dosage

• **Slow IV**

No more than 50 mg of protamine sulfate should be given in any 10-min period. One milligram of protamine sulfate can neutralize about 90 USP units of heparin derived from lung tissue or about 115 USP units of heparin derived from intestinal mucosa. *NOTE:* The dose of protamine sulfate depends on the amount of time that has elapsed since IV heparin administration. For example, if 30 min has elapsed, one-half the usual dose of protamine sulfate may be sufficient because heparin is cleared rapidly from the circulation.

---

## NURSING CONSIDERATIONS

### Administration/Storage

**IV** 1. Incompatible with several penicillins and with cephalosporins.
2. To minimize side effects, give slowly over 10 min. May also be

diluted in 50 mL of 5% dextrose or saline solution and administered at a rate of 50 mg over 10–15 min. Do not store diluted solutions.

3. Refrigerate at 2°C–8°C (36°F–46°F).

**Assessment:**

1. Determine amount, time of overdose and source to ensure appropriate antidote dosing.

2. Request type and crossmatch; assess need for fresh frozen plasma or whole blood.

3. Coagulation studies should be performed 5–15 min after protamine has been administered; repeat in 2–8 hr to assess for heparin rebound (increased bleeding, lowered BP, and/or shock).

4. Monitor VS, I&O and assess for sudden variations; i.e.,sudden fall in BP, bradycardia, dyspnea, transitory flushing, or sensations of warmth.

**Outcomes/Evaluate:** Stable H&H; control of heparin-induced hemorrhage

# Pseudoephedrine hydrochloride

(soo-doh-eh-**FED**-rin)
**Pregnancy Category:** B
Allermed, Balminil Decongestant Syrup ✱, Cenafed, Children's Congestion Relief, Children's Sudafed Liquid, Congestion Relief, Decofed Syrup, DeFed-60, Dorcol Children's Decongestant Liquid, Efidac/24, Eltor 120 ✱, Genaphed, Halofed, PediaCare Infants' Oral Decongestant Drops, PMS-Pseudoephedrine ✱, Pseudo, Pseudo-Gest, Seudotabs, Sinustop Pro, Sudafed, Sudafed 12 Hour **(OTC)**

# Pseudoephedrine sulfate

(soo-doh-eh-**FED**-rin)
**Pregnancy Category:** B
Afrin Extended-Release Tablets, Drixoral Day ✱, Drixoral N.D. ✱, Drixoral Non-Drowsy Formula **(OTC)**
**Classification:** Direct- and indirect-acting sympathomimetic, nasal decongestant

See also *Sympathomimetic Drugs.*

**Action/Kinetics:** Produces direct stimulation of both alpha-(pronounced) and beta-adrenergic receptors, as well as indirect stimulation through release of norepinephrine from storage sites. Results in decongestant effect on the nasal mucosa. Systemic administration eliminates possible damage to the nasal mucosa. **Onset:** 15–30 min. **Time to peak effect:** 30–60 min. **Duration:** 3–4 hr. **Extended-release: duration,** 8–12 hr. Urinary excretion slowed by alkalinization, causing reabsorption of drug.

**Uses:** Nasal congestion associated with sinus conditions, otitis, allergies. Relief of eustachian tube congestion.

**Additional    Contraindications:** Lactation. Use of sustained-release products in children less than 12 years of age.

**Special Concerns:** Use with caution in newborn and premature infants due to a higher risk of side effects. Geriatric clients may be more prone to age-related prostatic hypertrophy.

**Dosage**
HYDROCHLORIDE

• **Oral Solution, Syrup, Tablets**
   *Decongestant.*

**Adults:** 60 mg q 4–6 hr, not to exceed 240 mg in 24 hr. **Pediatric, 6–12 years:** 30 mg using the oral solution or syrup q 4–6 hr, not to exceed 120 mg in 24 hr, **2–6 years:** 15 mg using the oral solution or syrup q 4–6 hr, not to exceed 60 mg in 24 hr. For children less than 2 years of age, the dose must be individualized.

• **Extended-Release    Capsules, Tablets**
   *Decongestant.*

**Adults and children over 12 years:** 120 mg q 12 hr or 240 mg q 24 hr. Use is not recommended for children less than 12 years of age.
SULFATE

• **Extended-Release Tablets**
   *Decongestant.*

**Adults and children over 12 years:** 120 mg q 12 hr. Use is not recommended for children less than 12 years of age.

## NURSING CONSIDERATIONS

See also *Nursing Considerations* for *Sympathomimetic Drugs*.

**Client/Family Teaching**
1. Avoid taking at bedtime as may cause stimulation that can produce insomnia.
2. With hypertension, report headaches, dizziness, or increased BP readings.
3. Extended-release products should not be crushed or chewed.
4. Report if symptoms do not improve after 3–5 days.

**Outcomes/Evaluate:** Relief of nasal, sinus, or eustachian tube congestion

# Psyllium hydrophilic muciloid

(**SILL**-ee-um hi-droh-**FILL**-ik)
Effer-syllium, Fiberall Natural Flavor, Fiberall Orange Flavor, Fiberall Wafers, Fibrepur ✿, Hydrocil Instant, Konsyl, Konsyl-D, Metamucil, Metamucil Lemon-Lime Flavor, Metamucil Orange Flavor, Metamucil Sugar Free, Metamucil Sugar Free Orange Flavor, Modane Bulk, Natural Vegetable, Novo–Mucilax ✿, Perdiem Fiber, Prodiem Plain ✿, Reguloid Natural, Reguloid Orange, Reguloid Sugar Free Orange, Reguloid Sugar Free Regular, Serutan, Siblin, Syllact, V-Lax **(OTC)**
**Classification:** Laxative, bulk-forming

See also *Laxatives*.
**Action/Kinetics:** Obtained from the fruit of various species of plantago. The powder forms a gelatinous mass with water, which adds bulk to the stools and stimulates peristalsis. Also has a demulcent effect on an inflamed intestinal mucosa. Products may also contain dextrose, sodium bicarbonate, monobasic potassium phosphate, citric acid, and benzyl benzoate. Laxative effects usually occur in 12–24 hr. The full effect may take 2–3 days. Dependence may occur.

**Uses:** Prophylaxis of constipation in clients who should not strain during defecation. Short-term treatment of constipation; useful in geriatric clients with diminished colonic motor response and during pregnancy and postpartum to reestablish normal bowel function. To soften feces during fecal impaction.

**Contraindications:** Severe abdominal pain or intestinal obstruction.

**Side Effects:** Obstruction of the esophagus, stomach, small intestine, and rectum.

**Drug Interactions:** Do not use concomitantly with salicylates, nitrofurantoin, or cardiac glycosides (e.g., digitalis).

**Dosage**
Dose depends on the product. General information on adult dosage follows.
• **Granules/Flakes**
**Adults:** 1–2 teaspoons 1–3 times/day spread on food or with a glass of water.
• **Powder**
**Adults:** 1 rounded teaspoon in 8 oz of liquid 1–3 times/day.
• **Effervescent Powder**
**Adults:** 1 packet in water 1–3 times/day.
• **Chewable Pieces**
**Adults:** 2 pieces followed by a glass of water 1–3 times/day.

## NURSING CONSIDERATIONS

See Nursing Considerations for *Laxatives*.
**Administration/Storage**
1. The powder may be noxious and irritating when removing from the packets or canister. Open in a well-ventilated area and avoid inhaling particulate matter.
2. Mix powder with liquid just prior to administering; otherwise, the mixture may become thick and difficult to drink.

**Outcomes/Evaluate:** Prophylaxis/relief of constipation

# Pyrantel pamoate

(pie-**RAN**-tell)
Antiminth, Combantrin ✹, Pin-Rid,
Pin-X, Reese's Pinworm **(OTC)**
**Classification:** Anthelmintic

See also *Anthelmintics*.

**Action/Kinetics:** Has neuromuscular blocking effect which paralyzes the helminth, allowing it to be expelled through the feces. Also inhibits cholinesterases. Poorly absorbed from GI tract. **Peak plasma levels:** 0.05–0.13 mcg/mL after 1–3 hr. Partially metabolized in liver. Fifty percent is excreted unchanged in feces and less than 15% excreted unchanged in urine.

**Uses:** Pinworm (enterobiasis) and roundworm (ascariasis) infestations. Multiple helminth infections, as it is also effective against roundworm and hookworm.

**Contraindications:** Pregnancy. Hepatic disease.

**Special Concerns:** Use with caution in presence of liver dysfunction. Safe use in children less than 2 years of age has not been established.

**Side Effects:** *GI* (most frequent): Anorexia, N&V, abdominal cramps, diarrhea. *Hepatic:* Transient elevation of AST. *CNS:* Headache, dizziness, drowsiness, insomnia. *Miscellaneous:* Skin rashes.

**Drug Interactions:** Use with piperazine for ascariasis results in antagonism of the effect of both drugs.

**Dosage** ————————————
• **Liquid Oral Suspension, Tablets**
**Adults and children:** One dose of 11 mg/kg (maximum). **Maximum total dose:** 1.0 g.

## NURSING CONSIDERATIONS

See also *Nursing Considerations* for *Anthelmintics*.
**Client/Family Teaching**
1. Drug may be taken without regard to food intake. Can be taken with milk or fruit juices.
2. Drug may cause dizziness or drowsiness; do not engage in activities that require mental alertness.
3. Purging is not required.
4. When treating pinworms, review client/family precautions R/T transmission. (See *Anthelmintics*.)
**Outcomes/Evaluate:** Resolution of infection; negative stool and perianal swabs

# Pyridostigmine bromide

(peer-id-oh-**STIG**-meen)
**Pregnancy Category:** C
Mestinon, Mestinon-SR ✹, Regonol
**(Rx)**
**Classification:** Indirectly acting cholinergic-acetylcholinesterase inhibitor

For all information, see also *Neostigmine*.

**Action/Kinetics:** Has a slower onset, longer duration of action, and fewer side effects than neostigmine. **Onset, PO:** 30–45 min for syrup and tablets and 30–60 min for extended-release tablets; **IM:** 15 min; **IV:** 2–5 min. **Duration, PO:** 3–6 hr for syrup and tablets and 6–12 hr for extended-release tablets; **IM, IV:** 2–4 hr. Poorly absorbed from the GI tract; excreted in urine up to 72 hr after administration.

**Uses:** Myasthenia gravis. Antidote for nondepolarizing muscle relaxants (e.g., tubocurarine).

**Additional Contraindications:** Sensitivity to bromides.

**Special Concerns:** Safe use during pregnancy and during lactation has not been established. May cause uterine irritability and premature labor if given IV to pregnant women near term. In geriatric clients, the duration of action may be increased.

**Additional Side Effects:** Skin rash. Thrombophlebitis after IV use.

**OD Overdose Management:** *Symptoms:* Abdominal cramps, vomiting, diarrhea, epigastric distress, excessive salivation, cold sweating, pallor, blurred vision, urinary urgency, fasciculation and *paralysis of voluntary muscles* (including the tongue),

---

*bold italic* = life threatening side effect

P

miosis, increased BP (may be accompanied by bradycardia), sensation of internal trembling, panic, severe anxiety. *Treatment:* Discontinue medication temporarily. Give atropine, 0.5–1 mg IV (up to 5–10 mg or more may be needed to get HR to 80 beats/min). Supportive treatment including artificial respiration and oxygen.

## Dosage

- **Syrup, Tablets**
  *Myasthenia gravis.*
**Adults:** 60–120 mg q 3–4 hr with dosage adjusted to client response. **Maintenance:** 600 mg/day (range: 60 mg–1.5 g). **Pediatric:** 7 mg/kg (200 mg/m²) daily in five to six divided doses.

- **Sustained-Release Tablets**
  *Myasthenia gravis.*
**Adults:** 180–540 mg 1–2 times/day with at least 6 hr between doses. Sustained-release tablets not recommended for use in children.

- **IM, IV**
  *Myasthenia gravis.*
**Adults, IM, IV:** 2 mg (about ⅟₃₀ the adult dose) q 2–3 hr.
  *Neonates of myasthenic mothers.*
**IM:** 0.05–0.15 mg/kg q 4–6 hr.
  *Antidote for nondepolarizing drugs.*
**Adults, IV:** 10–20 mg with 0.6–1.2 mg atropine sulfate given IV.

## NURSING CONSIDERATIONS

See also *Nursing Considerations* for *Neostigmine.*

### Administration/Storage
1. During dosage adjustment, administer in a closely monitored environment.
**IV** 2. Parenteral dosage is ⅟₃₀ of the PO dose. May give undiluted at a rate of 0.5 mg IV over 1 min for myasthenia and at a rate of 5 mg IV over 1 min (with atropine) for reversal of nondepolarizing drug effects.

### Assessment
1. Monitor VS and observe for toxic reactions demonstrated by generalized cholinergic stimulation.
2. Assess for muscular weakness;

may signal impending myasthenic crisis and cholinergic overdose.
3. Determine the best individualized administration schedule according to client's routines and life-style.

### Client/Family Teaching
1. Myasthenia is an autoimmune disease with an unclear etiology. Medications correct acetycholine and cholinesterase imbalance at myoneural junction, which facilitates muscle contraction.
2. Do not crush and do not take extended-release tablets more often than q 6 hr; may be taken with conventional tablets, if prescribed.
3. With rest, muscle weakness and fatigue are temporarily resolved.
4. Rest and report symptoms of toxic reaction and myasthenic crisis.
5. Take medication as prescribed, since too early administration may result in cholinergic crisis whereas too late administration may result in myasthenic crisis.
6. Drug resistance may develop; close medical supervision and prompt reporting of all side effects is paramount.
7. Identify local support groups that may assist client to understand and cope with this disorder.

### Outcomes/Evaluate
- Improvement in muscle strength/function
- Reversal of nondepolarizing drugs

# Pyridoxine hydrochloride (Vitamin B₆)
(peer-ih-**DOX**-een)
**Pregnancy Category:** A
Nestrex (Rx: Injection; OTC: Tablets)
**Classification:** Vitamin B complex

**Action/Kinetics:** A water-soluble, heat-resistant vitamin that is destroyed by light. Acts as a coenzyme in the metabolism of protein, carbohydrates, and fat. As the amount of protein increases in the diet, the pyridoxine requirement increases. However, pyridoxine deficiency alone is rare. **t½:** 2–3 weeks. Metabolized in the liver and excreted through the urine.

**Uses:** Pyridoxine deficiency including poor diet, drug-induced (e.g., oral contraceptives, isoniazid), and inborn errors of metabolism. *Investigational:* Hydrazine poisoning, PMS, high urine oxalate levels, N&V due to pregnancy.

**Special Concerns:** Safety and effectiveness have not been established in children.

**Side Effects:** *CNS:* Unstable gait; decreased sensation to touch, temperature, and vibration; paresthesia, sleepiness; numbness of feet; awkwardness of hands; perioral numbness. *NOTE:* Abuse and dependence have been noted in adults administered 200 mg/day.

**OD Overdose Management:** *Symptoms:* Ataxia, severe sensory neuropathy. *Treatment:* Discontinue pyridoxine; allow up to 6 months for CNS sensation to return.

**Drug Interactions**

*Chloramphenicol* / ↑ Pyridoxine requirements
*Contraceptives, oral* / ↑ Pyridoxine requirements
*Cycloserine* / ↑ Pyridoxine requirements
*Ethionamide* / ↑ Pyridoxine requirements
*Hydralazine* / ↑ Pyridoxine requirements
*Immunosuppressants* / ↑ Pyridoxine requirements
*Isoniazid* / ↑ Pyridoxine requirements
*Levodopa* / Daily doses exceeding 5 mg pyridoxine antagonize the therapeutic effect of levodopa
*Penicillamine* / ↑ Pyridoxine requirements
*Phenobarbital* / Pyridoxine ↓ serum levels of phenobarbital
*Phenytoin* / Pyridoxine ↓ serum levels of phenytoin

**Dosage**

• **Capsules, Enteric-Coated Tablets, Extended-Release Tablets, Tablets**

*Dietary supplement.*

**Adults:** 10–20 mg/day for 2 weeks; **then,** 2–5 mg/day as part of a multivitamin preparation for several weeks. **Pediatric,** 2.5–10 mg/day for 3 weeks; **then,** 2–5 mg/day as part of a multivitamin preparation for several weeks.

*Pyridoxine dependency syndrome.*

**Adults and children, initial:** 30–600 mg/day; **maintenance,** 30 mg/day for life. **Infants, maintenance:** 2–10 mg/day for life.

*Drug-induced deficiency.*

**Adults, prophylaxis:** 10–50 mg/day for penicillamine or 100–300 mg/day for cycloserine, hydralazine, or isoniazid. **Adults, treatment:** 50–200 mg/day for 3 weeks followed by 25–100 mg/day to prevent relapse. **Adults, alcoholism:** 50 mg/day for 2–4 weeks; if anemia responds, continue pyridoxine indefinitely.

*Hereditary sideroblastic anemia.*

**Adults:** 200–600 mg/day for 1–2 months; **then,** 30–50 mg/day for life.

• **IM, IV**

*Pyridoxine dependency syndrome.*

**Adults:** 30–600 mg/day. **Pediatric:** 10–100 mg initially.

*Drug-induced deficiency.*

**Adults:** 50–200 mg/day for 3 weeks followed by 25–100 mg/day as needed.

*Cycloserine poisoning.*

**Adults:** 300 mg/day.

*Isoniazid poisoning.*

**Adults:** 1 g for each gram of isoniazid taken.

## NURSING CONSIDERATIONS

### Administration/Storage

1. If receiving levodopa, avoid preparations of vitamins containing $B_6$ because vitamin $B_6$ decreases the availability of levodopa to the brain.

**IV** 2. May be administered direct IV or placed in infusion solutions.

### Assessment

1. Document indications for therapy.

P

---

2. Take a complete drug history. If taking cycloserine, isoniazid, or oral contraceptives, report, as these drugs increase pyridoxine requirements.

**Client/Family Teaching**

1. Foods high in vitamin B$_6$ include potatoes, lima beans, broccoli, bananas, chicken breast, liver, whole-grain cereals. Well-balanced diets are the best source of vitamins; see a dietitian as needed.

2. If prescribed levodopa, avoid vitamin supplements containing vitamin B$_6$. More than 5 mg of the vitamin antagonizes the effect of levodopa. At the same time, concomitant administration of carbidopa will prevent the effect of vitamin B$_6$ on levodopa.

3. If taking phenobarbital and/or phenytoin, obtain serum drug levels routinely, as pyridoxine alters serum concentrations.

4. Pyridoxine may inhibit lactation.

5. Identify reasons for drug therapy, e.g., to prevent toxicity (peripheral neuropathy) with long term isoniazid or contraceptive therapy, to replace vitamin B$_6$ with inborn errors of metabolism or with poor nutrition.

**Outcomes/Evaluate**

• Relief of symptoms of pyridoxine deficiency

• Prophylaxis of drug-induced deficiency; ↓ toxic drug side effects

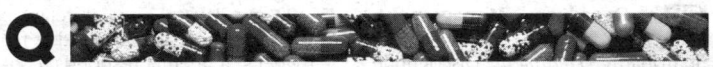

# Quetiapine fumarate

(kweh-**TYE**-ah-peen)
**Pregnancy Category:** C
Seroquel **(Rx)**
**Classification:** Antipsychotic drug

**Action/Kinetics:** Mechanism unknown but may act as an antagonist at dopamine D$_2$ and serotonin 5HT$_2$ receptors. Side effects may be due to antagonism of other receptors (e.g., histamine H$_1$, dopamine D$_1$, adrenergic alpha-1 and alpha-2, serotonin 5HT$_{1A}$). Rapidly absorbed. **Peak plasma levels:** 1.5 hr. Metabolized by liver and excreted through urine and feces. **t½, terminal:** About 6 hr.

**Uses:** Management of psychoses.

**Contraindications:** Lactation.

**Special Concerns:** Use with caution in liver disease, in those at risk for aspiration pneumonia, and in those with history of seizures or conditions that lower seizure threshold (e.g., Alzheimer's). Safety and efficacy have not been determined in children.

**Side Effects:** Side effects with incidence of 1% or more are listed. *Body as a whole:* Asthenia, rash, fever, weight gain, back pain, flu syndrome. *CNS:* Headache, somnolence, dizziness, hypertonia, dysarthria. *GI:* Constipation, dry mouth, dyspepsia, anorexia, abdominal pain. *CV:* Orthostatic hypotension, syncope, tachycardia, palpitation. *Respiratory:* Pharyngitis, rhinitis, increased cough, dyspnea. *Miscellaneous:* Peripheral edema, sweating, leukopenia, ear pain. *Note: **Neuroleptic malignant syndrome** and **seizures,** although rare, may occur.*

**Laboratory Test Alteration:** ↑ ALT during initial therapy, AST, total cholesterol, triglycerides.

**OD** **Overdose Management:** *Symptoms:* Drowsiness, sedation, tachycardia, hypotension, dystonic reaction of the head and neck, seizures, obtundation. *Treatment:* Cardiovascular monitoring for arrhythmias. If antiarrhythmic therapy is used, disopyramide, procainamide, and quinidine increase risk of prolongation of QT. Treat hypotension and circulatory shock with IV fluids or sympathomimetic drugs (do not use epinephrine or dopamine as they may worsen hypotension). Use anticholinergic drugs to treat severe extrapyramidal symptoms.

**Drug Interactions**

*Barbiturates* / ↓ Effect of quetiapine due to ↑ breakdown by liver

*Carbamazepine* / ↓ Effect of quetiapine due to ↑ breakdown by liver

*Dopamine agonists* /Quetiapine antagonizes effect

*Glucocorticoids* / ↓ Effect of quetiapine due to ↑ breakdown by liver

*Levodopa* / Quetiapine antagonizes effect

*Phenytoin* / ↓ Effect of quetiapine due to ↑ breakdown by liver

*Rifampin* / ↓ Effect of quetiapine due to ↑ breakdown by liver

*Thioridazine* / ↑ Clearance of quetiapine

**Dosage** ⎯⎯⎯⎯⎯⎯⎯⎯
• **Tablets**
*Psychoses.*
**Initial:** 25 mg b.i.d., with increases of 25 to 50 mg b.i.d. or t.i.d. on second and third day, as tolerated. Target dose range, by fourth day, is 300 to 400 mg daily. Further dosage adjustments can occur at intervals of two or more days. The antipsychotic dose range is 150 to 750 mg/day.

⎯⎯⎯⎯⎯⎯⎯⎯⎯⎯⎯⎯⎯⎯⎯

## NURSING CONSIDERATIONS

**Administration/Storage**
1. Total daily dose is divided and given two or three times a day.
2. Slower rate of dose titration and lower target dose is considered for elderly, in hepatic impairment, debilitated clients, and in those predisposed to hypotension.
3. Titration is not required when restarting clients who have had an interval of less than one week off quetiapine. Initial titration schedule is followed if clients have been off drug for more than one week.

**Assessment**
1. Determine clinical presentation and behavioral manifestations requiring therapy.
2. Note any predisposition to hypotensive reactions if debilitated or if hepatic impairment present.
3. Document ophthalmic exam initially, and at 6 mo intervals, to assess for cataract formation.

4. Assess for history of cardiovascular disease; note VS, ECG, and LFTs.

**Client/Family Teaching**
1. May take with or without food.
2. Do not perform activities that require mental alertness until after titration period and until drug effects realized; may impair judgement and motor skills, and cause sleepiness.
3. Avoid alcohol and any OTC agents without approval.
4. Use reliable contraception; report if pregnancy suspected. Do not breastfeed.
5. Report any evidence of extrapyramidal symptoms; tardive dyskinesia (involuntary movements).
6. Avoid situations where overheating or dehydration may occur.

**Outcomes/Evaluate:** Control of manifestations of psychotic disorders

# Quinapril hydrochloride
(**KWIN**-ah-prill)
**Pregnancy Category:** D
Accupril **(Rx)**
**Classification:** Angiotensin-converting enzyme inhibitor

⎯⎯⎯⎯⎯⎯⎯⎯⎯⎯⎯⎯⎯⎯⎯

See also *Angiotensin-Converting Enzyme Inhibitors*.

**Action/Kinetics: Onset:** 1 hr. **Time to peak serum levels:** 1 hr. **Peak decrease in BP:** 2–4 hr. Metabolized to quinaprilat, the active metabolite. **t½, quinaprilat:** 2 hr. **Duration:** 24 hr. Significantly bound to plasma proteins. Metabolized with approximately 60% excreted through the urine and 37% excreted in the feces. Also appears to improve endothelial function, an early marker of coronary atherosclerosis.

**Uses:** Alone or in combination with a thiazide diuretic for the treatment of hypertension. Adjunct with a diuretic or digitalis to treat CHF in those not responding adequately to diuretics or digitalis.

**Special Concerns:** Use with caution during lactation. Safety and effectiveness have not been determined in children. Geriatric clients may be more sensitive to the effects of quinapril and manifest higher peak quinaprilat blood levels.

**Side Effects:** *CV:* Vasodilation, tachycardia, **heart failure,** palpitations, **MI, CVA, hypertensive crisis,** angina pectoris, orthostatic hypotension, **cardiac rhythm disturbances, cardiogenic shock.** *GI:* Dry mouth or throat, constipation, N&V, abdominal pain, **GI hemorrhage.** *CNS:* Somnolence, vertigo, nervousness, depression, headache, dizziness, fatigue. *Hematologic:* **Agranulocytosis,** bone marrow depression, thrombocytopenia. *Dermatologic:* **Angioedema of the lips, tongue, glottis, and larynx;** sweating, pruritus, exfoliative dermatitis, photosensitivity, dermatopolymyositis. *Body as a whole:* Malaise, back pain. *GU:* Oliguria and/or progressive azotemia and rarely **acute renal failure and/or death in severe heart failure.** Worsening renal failure. *Respiratory:* Pharyngitis, cough, asthma, bronchospasm. *Miscellaneous:* Oligohydramnios in fetuses exposed to the drug in utero. Abnormal liver function tests, pancreatitis, syncope, hyperkalemia, amblyopia, viral infections.

**OD Overdose Management:** *Symptoms:* Commonly, hypotension. *Treatment:* IV infusion of normal saline to restore blood pressure.

**Drug Interactions**
*Potassium-containing salt substitutes* / ↑ Risk of hyperkalemia
*Potassium-sparing diuretics* / ↑ Risk of hyperkalemia
*Potassium supplements* / ↑ Risk of hyperkalemia
*Tetracyclines* / ↓ Absorption of tetracycline due to high magnesium content of quinapril tablets

**Dosage**
• **Tablets**
*Hypertension.*
**Initial:** 10 mg/day; **then,** adjust dosage based on BP response at peak (2–6 hr) and trough (predose) blood levels. The dose should be adjusted at 2-week intervals. **Maintenance:** 20, 40, or 80 mg daily as a single dose or in two equally divided doses. With im-

paired renal function, the initial dose should be 10 mg if the $C_{CR}$ is greater than 60 mL/min, 5 mg if the $C_{CR}$ is between 30 and 60 mL/min, and 2.5 mg if the $C_{CR}$ is between 10 and 30 mL/min. If the initial dose is well tolerated, the drug may be given the following day as a b.i.d. regimen.
*CHF.*
**Initial:** 5 mg b.i.d. If this dose is well tolerated, titrate clients at weekly intervals until an effective dose, usually 20–40 mg daily in two equally divided doses, is attained. Undesirable hypotension, orthostasis, or azotemia may prevent this dosage level from being reached.

---

## NURSING CONSIDERATIONS

See also *Angiotensin-Converting Enzyme Inhibitors* and *Antihypertensive Agents.*
**Administration/Storage**
1. If taking a diuretic, discontinue the diuretic 2–3 days prior to beginning quinapril. If the BP is not controlled, reinstitute the diuretic. If the diuretic cannot be discontinued, the initial dose should be 1.25 mg.
2. If the antihypertensive effect decreases at the end of the dosing interval with once-daily therapy, consider either twice-daily administration or increasing the dose.
3. The antihypertensive effect may not be observed for 1–2 weeks.
**Assessment**
1. Observe infants exposed to quinapril in utero for the development of hypotension, oliguria, and hyperkalemia.
2. If angioedema occurs, stop drug, assess airway, and observe until swelling resolved. Antihistamines may be useful in relieving symptoms.
3. Monitor VS, I&O, weights, electrolytes, CBC, and renal function studies. Agranulocytosis and bone marrow depression seen more often with renal impairment, especially if collagen vascular disease (e.g., SLE, scleroderma) present.
4. Clients with unilateral or bilateral renal artery stenosis may manifest

increased BUN and serum creatinine if given quinapril. Assess renal function closely the first few weeks of therapy.

**Client/Family Teaching**
1. Take as directed.
2. Report any unusual bruising or bleeding.
3. Any increased SOB, palpitations, swelling, or persistent nonproductive cough should be evaluated.

**Outcomes/Evaluate:** ↓ BP

# Quinidine bisulfate
(**KWIN**-ih-deen)
**Pregnancy Category:** D
Biquin Durules ✦ **(Rx)**

# Quinidine gluconate
(**KWIN**-ih-deen)
**Pregnancy Category:** C
Quinaglute Dura-Tabs, Quinalan, Quinate ✦ **(Rx)**

# Quinidine polygalacturonate
(**KWIN**-ih-deen)
**Pregnancy Category:** C
Cardioquin **(Rx)**

# Quinidine sulfate
(**KWIN**-ih-deen)
**Pregnancy Category:** C
Apo-Quinidine ✦, Quinidex Extentabs, Quinora **(Rx)**
**Classification:** Antiarrhythmic, class IA

See also *Antiarrhythmic Agents.*

**Action/Kinetics:** Reduces the excitability of the heart and depresses conduction velocity and contractility. Prolongs the refractory period and increases conduction time. It also decreases CO and possesses anticholinergic, antimalarial, antipyretic, and oxytocic properties. **PO: Onset:** 0.5–3 hr. **Maximum effects, after IM:** 30–90 min. **t½:** 6–7 hr. **Time to peak levels, PO:** 3–5 hr for gluconate salt, 1–1.5 hr for sulfate salt, and 6 hr for polygalacturonate salt; **IM:** 1 hr. **Therapeutic serum levels:** 2–6 mcg/mL. **Protein bind-**

**ing:** 60%–80%. **Duration:** 6–8 hr for tablets/capsules and 12 hr for extended-release tablets. Metabolized by liver. Urine pH affects rate of urinary excretion (10%–50% excreted unchanged).

**Uses:** Premature atrial, AV junctional, and ventricular contractions. Treatment and control of atrial flutter, established atrial fibrillation, paroxysmal atrial tachycardia, paroxysmal AV junctional rhythm, paroxysmal and chronic atrial fibrillation, paroxysmal ventricular tachycardia not associated with complete heart block, maintenance therapy after electrical conversion of atrial flutter or fibrillation. The parenteral route is indicated when PO therapy is not feasible or immediate effects are required. *Investigational:* Gluconate salt for life-threatening *Plasmodium falciparum* malaria.

**Contraindications:** Hypersensitivity to drug or other cinchona drugs. Myasthenia gravis, history of thrombocytopenic purpura associated with quinidine use, digitalis intoxication evidenced by arrhythmias or AV conduction disorders. Also, complete heart block, left bundle branch block, or other intraventricular conduction defects manifested by marked QRS widening or bizarre complexes. Complete AV block with an AV nodal or idioventricular pacemaker, aberrant ectopic impulses and abnormal rhythms due to escape mechanisms. History of drug-induced torsades de pointes or long QT syndrome.

**Special Concerns:** Safety in children and during lactation has not been established. Quinidine should be used with extreme caution in clients in whom a sudden change in BP might be detrimental or in those suffering from extensive myocardial damage, subacute endocarditis, bradycardia, coronary occlusion, disturbances in impulse conduction, chronic valvular disease, considerable cardiac enlargement, frank CHF, and renal or hepatic disease.

Cautious use is also recommended in clients with acute infections, hyperthyroidism, muscular weakness, respiratory distress, and bronchial asthma. The dose in geriatric clients may have to be reduced due to age-related changes in renal function.

**Side Effects:** *CV:* Widening of QRS complex, hypotension, *cardiac asystole,* ectopic ventricular beats, *ventricular tachycardia or fibrillation, torsades de pointes,* paradoxical tachycardia, *arterial embolism,* ventricular extrasystoles (one or more every 6 beats), prolonged QT interval, *complete AV block, ventricular flutter. GI:* N&V, abdominal pain, anorexia, diarrhea, urge to defecate as well as urinate, esophagitis (rare). *CNS:* Syncope, headache, confusion, excitement, vertigo, apprehension, delirium, dementia, ataxia, depression. *Dermatologic:* Rash, urticaria, exfoliative dermatitis, photosensitivity, flushing with intense pruritus, eczema, psoriasis, pigmentation abnormalities. *Allergic:* Acute asthma, angioneurotic edema, *respiratory arrest,* dyspnea, fever, *vascular collapse,* purpura, vasculitis, hepatic dysfunction (including granulomatous hepatitis), *hepatic toxicity. Hematologic:* Hypoprothrombinemia, *acute hemolytic anemia,* thrombocytopenic purpura, *agranulocytosis,* thrombocytopenia, leukocytosis, neutropenia, shift to left in WBC differential. *Ophthalmologic:* Blurred vision, mydriasis, alterations in color perception, decreased field of vision, double vision, photophobia, optic neuritis, night blindness, scotomata. *Other:* Liver toxicity including hepatitis, lupus nephritis, tinnitus, decreased hearing acuity, arthritis, myalgia, increase in serum skeletal muscle CPK, lupus erythematosus.

**OD** **Overdose Management:** *Symptoms: CNS:* Lethargy, confusion, *coma, seizures, respiratory depression or arrest,* headache, paresthesia, vertigo. CNS symptoms may be seen after onset of CV toxicity. *GI:* Vomiting, diarrhea, abdominal pain, hypokalemia, nausea. *CV:* Sinus tachycardia, *ventricular tachycardia or fibrillation, torsades de pointes, depressed automaticity and conduction* (including bundle branch block, sinus bradycardia, SA block, prolongation of QRS and QTc, sinus arrest, AV block, ST depression, T inversion), syncope, *heart failure.* Hypotension due to decreased conduction and CO and vasodilation. *Miscellaneous:* Cinchonism, visual and auditory disturbances, hypokalemia, tinnitus, acidosis. *Treatment:*
* Perform gastric lavage, induce vomiting, and administer activated charcoal if ingestion is recent.
* Monitor ECG, blood gases, serum electrolytes, and BP.
* Institute cardiac pacing, if necessary.
* Acidify the urine.
* Use artificial respiration and other supportive measures.
* Infusions of ⅙ molar sodium lactate IV may decrease the cardiotoxic effects.
* Treat hypotension with metaraminol or norepinephrine after fluid volume replacement.
* Use phenytoin or lidocaine to treat tachydysrhythmias.
* Hemodialysis is effective but not often required.

**Drug Interactions**
*Acetazolamide, Antacids* / ↑ Effect of quinidine due to ↓ renal excretion
*Amiodarone* / ↑ Quinidine levels with possible fatal cardiac dysrhythmias
*Anticholinergic agents, Atropine* / Additive effect on blockade of vagus nerve action
*Anticoagulants, oral* / Additive hypoprothrombinemia with possible hemorrhage
*Barbiturates* / ↓ Effect of quinidine due to ↑ breakdown by liver
*Cholinergic agents* / Quinidine antagonizes effect of cholinergic drugs
*Cimetidine* / ↑ Effect of quinidine due to ↓ breakdown by liver
*Digoxin, Digitoxin* / ↑ Symptoms of digoxin or digitoxin toxicity

*Disopyramide* / Either ↑ disopyramide levels or ↓ quinidine levels
*Guanethidine* / Additive hypotensive effect
*Methyldopa* / Additive hypotensive effect
*Metoprolol* / ↑ Effect of propranolol in fast metabolizers
*Neuromuscular blocking agents* / ↑ Respiratory depression
*Nifedipine* / ↓ Effect of quinidine
*Phenobarbital, Phenytoin* / ↓ Effect of quinidine by ↑ rate of metabolism in liver
*Potassium* / ↑ Effect of quinidine
*Procainamide* / ↑ Effects of procainamide with possible toxicity
*Propafenone* / ↑ Serum propafenone levels in rapid metabolizers
*Propranolol* / ↑ Effect of propranolol in fast metabolizers
*Reserpine* / Additive cardiac depressant effects
*Rifampin* / ↓ Effect of quinidine due to ↑ breakdown by liver
*Skeletal muscle relaxants* / ↑ Skeletal muscle relaxation
*Sodium bicarbonate* / ↑ Effect of quinidine due to ↓ renal excretion
*Sucralfate* / ↓ Serum levels of quinidine → ↓ effect
*Thiazide diuretics* / ↑ Effect of quinidine due to ↓ renal excretion
*Tricyclic antidepressants* / ↑ Effect of antidepressant due to ↓ clearance
*Verapamil* / ↓ Clearance of verapamil → ↑ hypotension, bradycardia, AV block, ventricular tachycardia, and pulmonary edema
**Laboratory Test Interferences:** False + or ↑ PSP, 17-ketosteroids, PT.

## Dosage
• **Quinidine Bisulfate Controlled-Release Tablets**
   *Antiarrhythmic.*
**Initial:** Test dose of 200 mg in the morning (to ascertain hypersensitivity). In the evening, administer 500 mg. **Then,** beginning the next day, 500–750 mg/12 hr. **Maintenance:** 0.5–1.25 g morning and evening.
• **Quinidine Polygalacturonate**

**Tablets, Quinidine Sulfate Tablets**
   *Premature atrial and ventricular contractions.*
**Adults:** 200–300 mg t.i.d.–q.i.d.
   *Paroxysmal SVTs.*
**Adults:** 400–600 mg q 2–3 hr until the paroxysm is terminated.
   *Conversion of atrial flutter.*
**Adults:** 200 mg q 2–3 hr for five to eight doses; daily doses can be increased until rhythm is restored or toxic effects occur.
   *Conversion of atrial flutter, maintenance therapy.*
**Adults:** 200–300 mg t.i.d.–q.i.d. Large doses or more frequent administration may be required in some clients.
• **Quinidine Gluconate Sustained-Release Tablets, Quinidine Sulfate Sustained-Release Tablets**
   *All uses.*
**Adults:** 300–600 mg q 8–12 hr.
• **Quinidine Gluconate Injection (IM or IV)**
   *Acute tachycardia.*
**Adults, initial:** 600 mg IM; **then,** 400 mg IM repeated as often as q 2 hr.
   *Arrhythmias.*
**Adults:** 330 mg IM or less IV (as much as 500–750 mg may be required).
   P. falciparum *malaria.*
Two regimens may be used. (1) *Loading dose:* 15 mg/kg in 250 mL NSS given over 4 hr; **then,** 24 hr after beginning the loading dose, institute 7.5 mg/kg infused over 4 hr and given q 8 hr for 7 days or until PO therapy can be started. (2) *Loading dose:* 10 mg/kg in 250 mL NSS infused over 1–2 hr followed immediately by 0.02 mg/kg/min for up to 72 hr or until parasitemia decreases to less than 1% or PO therapy can be started.

## NURSING CONSIDERATIONS

See also *Nursing Considerations* for *Antiarrhythmic Agents.*
**Administration/Storage**
1. A preliminary test dose may be given. **Adults:** 200 mg quinidine sulfate or quinidine gluconate adminis-

tered PO or IM. **Children:** Test dose of 2 mg of quinidine sulfate per kilogram of body weight.

2. The sustained-release forms are not interchangeable.

**IV** 3. Prepare IV solution by diluting 10 mL of quinidine gluconate injection (800 mg) with 50 mL of 5% glucose solution; give at a rate of 1 mL/min.

4. Use only colorless clear solution for injection. Light may cause quinidine to crystallize, which turns solution brownish.

**Assessment**

1. Note any allergic reactions to antiarrhythmic drugs or tartrazine, which is found in some formulations. Perform a test dose by administering one regular PO tablet; observe for hypersensitivity reactions and check for intolerance.

2. Document indications for therapy, type, onset, and symptom characteristics.

3. Obtain CXR; monitor electrolytes, CBC, liver and renal function studies.

4. Assess VS and ECG; note heart and lung sounds.

**Interventions**

1. Report any increased AV block, cardiac irritability, or rhythm suppression during IV administration.

2. Monitor I&O, VS; observe for hypotension. Drug induces urinary alkalization.

3. Report any neurologic deficits/sensory impairment (i.e., numbness, confusion, pyschosis, depression, or involuntary movements).

4. Report any persistent diarrhea. Among the elderly, there is a higher risk of toxicity, reduced CO, and unpredictable effects from drug.

5. Clients with long-standing atrial fibrillation or CHF with atrial fibrillation run a risk of embolization from mural thrombi when converting to sinus rhythm.

**Client/Family Teaching**

1. Take with food to minimize GI effects.

2. Avoid activities that require mental alertness until drug effects realized; may cause dizziness or blurred vision.

3. Add fruit and grain to diet. A high intake of fruits and vegetables (alkaline-ash foods) may prolong drug half-life.

4. Report any of the following symptoms:
- Severe skin rash, hives or itching
- Severe headache
- Unexplained fever
- Ringing in the ears, buzzing, or hearing loss
- Unusual bruising or bleeding
- Blurred vision
- Irregular heart beat, palpitations, or faintness
- Continued diarrhea

5. Wear dark glasses if photophobic.

6. Report for labs, ECG, PFTs, and ophthalmic exams.

**Outcomes/Evaluate**
- Restoration of stable cardiac rhythm
- Therapeutic drug levels (2–6 mcg/mL)

---

# Quinine sulfate
(**KWYE**-nine)
**Pregnancy Category:** X
Formula Q, Legatrim, M-KYA, Quinamm **(Rx)**
**Classification:** Antimalarial

**Action/Kinetics:** Natural alkaloid having antimalarial properties, antipyretic, analgesic, and oxytocic properties. Use of quinine in treating malaria is important due to emergence of resistant forms of vivax and falciparum; no resistant forms of the parasite have been found for quinine. Antimalarial mechanism not known precisely; quinine does affect DNA replication and may raise intracellular pH. Eradicates the erythrocytic stages of plasmodia. Increases the refractory period of skeletal muscle, decreases the excitability of the motor end-plate region, and affects the distribution of calcium within the muscle fiber, thus making it useful for nocturnal leg cramps. Is oxytocic and may cause congenital malformations. Rapidly and completely absorbed from the upper small intestine; widely distributed in body tissues. **Peak plasma levels:**

1–3 hr; **plasma levels following chronic use:** 7 mcg/mL. **t½:** 4–5 hr. Highly bound to protein (70%–85%); about 5% excreted unchanged in urine. Small amounts found in saliva, bile, feces, and gastric juice. Acidifying the urine increases the rate of excretion.

Pharmacokinetics of quinine are affected by malaria, with a decrease in volume of distribution and systemic clearance. Protein binding, which is normally 70% to 85%, increases to more than 90% in clients with cerebral malaria, in pregnancy, and in children.

**Uses:** Alone or in combination with pyrimethamine and a sulfonamide or a tetracycline for resistant forms of *Plasmodium falciparum.* As alternative therapy for chloroquine, sensitive stains of *P. falciparum, P. malariae, P. ovale,* and *P. vivax.* Mefloquine and clindamycin may also be used with quinine, depending on where the malaria was acquired. *Investigational:* Prevention and treatment of nocturnal recumbency leg cramps.

**Contraindications:** Clients with tinnitus, G6PD deficiency, optic neuritis, history of blackwater fever, and thrombocytopenia purpura associated with previous use of quinine.

**Special Concerns:** Use with caution in clients with cardiac arrhythmias and during lactation. Hemolysis, with a potential for hemolytic anemia, may occur in clients with G6PD deficiency.

**Side Effects:** Use of quinine may result in a syndrome referred to as *cinchonism.* Mild cinchonism is characterized by tinnitus, headache, nausea, slight visual disturbances. Larger doses, however, may cause severe CNS, CV, GI, or dermatologic effects.

*Allergic:* Flushing, cutaneous rashes (papular, scarlatinal, urticarial), fever, facial edema, pruritus, dyspnea, tinnitus, sweating, asthmatic symptoms, visual impairment, gastric upset. *GI:* N&V, epigastric pain, hepatitis. *Ophthalmologic:* Blurred vision with scotomata, photophobia, diplopia, night blindness, decreased visual fields, impaired color vision and perception, amblyopia, mydriasis, optic atrophy. *CNS:* Headache, confusion, restlessness, vertigo, syncope, fever, apprehension, excitement, delirium, hypothermia, dizziness, ***convulsions.*** *Otic:* Tinnitus, deafness. *Hematologic:* Acute hemolysis, hemolytic anemia, thrombocytopenic purpura, agranulocytosis, hypoprothrombinemia. *CV:* Symptoms of angina, ventricular tachycardia, conduction disturbances, vasculitis. *Miscellaneous:* Sweating, hypoglycemia, lichenoid photosensitivity.

**OD** **Overdose Management:** *Symptoms:* Dizziness, intestinal cramping, skin rash, tinnitus. With higher doses, symptoms include apprehension, confusion, fever, headache, vomiting, and seizures. *Treatment:*
• Induce vomiting or undertake gastric lavage.
• Maintain BP and renal function.
• If necessary, provide artificial respiration.
• Sedatives, oxygen, and other supportive measures may be required.
• Give IV fluids to maintain fluid and electrolyte balance.
• Treat angioedema or asthma with epinephrine, corticosteroids, and antihistamines.
• Urinary acidification will hasten excretion; however, in the presence of hemoglobinuria, acidification of the urine will increase renal blockade.

**Drug Interactions**
*Acetazolamide* / ↑ Blood levels (and therefore potential for toxicity) of quinine due to ↓ rate of elimination
*Aluminum-containing antacids* / Absorption of quinine ↓ or delayed
*Anticoagulants, oral* / Additive hypoprothrombinemia due to ↓ synthesis of vitamin K–dependent clotting factors
*Cimetidine* / ↑ Effect of quinine due to ↓ rate of excretion
*Digoxin* / ↑ Serum levels of digoxin

Q

*Heparin* / Effect ↓ by quinine
*Mefloquine* / ↑ Risk of ECG abnormalities or cardiac arrest; also, ↑ risk of convulsions. Do not use together; delay mefloquine administration at least 12 hr after the last dose of quinine.
*Neuromuscular blocking agents (depolarizing and nondepolarizing)* / ↑ Respiratory depression and apnea
*Rifabutin, Rifampin* / ↑ Hepatic clearance of quinine; can persist for several days following discontinuation of the rifampin
*Sodium bicarbonate* / ↑ Blood levels (and therefore potential for toxicity) of quinine due to ↓ rate of elimination

**Dosage** —————————
• **Capsules, Tablets**
  *Chloroquine-resistant malaria.*
  **Adults:** 650 mg q 8 hr for at least 3 days (7 days in Southeast Asia) along with pyrimethamine, 25 mg b.i.d. for the first 3 days and sulfadiazine, 2 g/day for the first 5 days. There are two alternative regimens: (1) quinine, 650 mg q 8 hr for at least 3 days (7 days in Southeast Asia) along with a tetracycline, 250 mg q 6 hr for 10 days or (2) quinine, 650 mg q 8 hr for 3 days with sulfadoxine, 1.5 g and pyrimethamine, 75 mg as a single dose.
  *Chloroquine-sensitive malaria.*
  **Adults:** 600 mg q 8 hr for 5–7 days.
  **Pediatric:** 10 mg/kg q 8 hr for 5–7 days.
  *Nocturnal leg cramps.*
  **Adults:** 260–300 mg at bedtime.

## NURSING CONSIDERATIONS

See also *General Nursing Considerations for All Anti-Infectives.*

**Administration/Storage**
1. Dispense in a light-resistant and child-resistant container; store at controlled room temperatures of 15°C–30°C (59°F–86°F).
**IV** 2. The parenteral form is available from the Centers for Disease Control if client unable to take PO.

**Assessment**
1. Document indications for therapy, onset and duration of symptoms, dates of travel, and any other agents trialed.
2. Note any history or evidence of cardiac arrhythmias or disease.
3. Assess leg cramps to determine that they only occur at night when recumbent.
4. Obtain baseline CBC and ophthalmic exam and monitor throughout drug therapy.

**Client/Family Teaching**
1. Do not take with antacids. To minimize GI irritation, take with food or after meals.
2. Do not drive a car or operate machinery until drug effects realized; may cause dizziness or blurred vision.
3. Use sunglasses to protect from photophobia.
4. If also taking cimetidine or digoxin, may require dosage adjustment; report side effects.
5. Females should use birth control; drug may harm fetus.
6. Report new ringing in the ears, blurring of vision, and headache, which may be followed by digestive disturbances, impairment of hearing and sight, confusion, and delirium. This may indicate intolerance or overdosage and requires immediate medical intervention.

**Outcomes/Evaluate:**   Termination of acute malarial attack/control of malaria symptoms

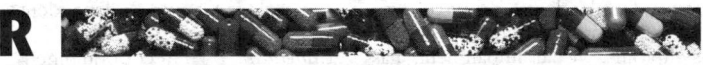

# Raloxifene hydrochloride
(ral-**OX**-ih-feen)

**Pregnancy Category:** X
Evista **(Rx)**

**Classification:** Estrogen receptor modulator

**Action/Kinetics:** Selective estrogen receptor modulator that reduces bone resorption and decreases overall bone turnover. Considered an estrogen antagonist that acts by combining with estrogen receptors. Has not been associated with endometrial proliferation, breast enlargement, breast pain, or increased risk of breast cancer. Also decreases total and LDL cholesterol levels. Absorbed rapidly after PO; significant first-pass effect. Excreted primarily in feces with small amounts excreted in urine.

**Uses:** Prevention of osteoporosis in postmenopausal women. Not effective in reducing hot flashes or flushes associated with estrogen deficiency.

**Contraindications:** In women who are or who might become pregnant, active or history of venous thromboembolic events (e.g., DVT, pulmonary embolism, retinal vein thrombosis). Use in premenopausal women, during lactation, or in pediatric clients. Concurrent use with systemic estrogen or hormone replacement therapy.

**Special Concerns:** Use with caution with highly protein-bound drugs, including clofibrate, diazepam, diazoxide, ibuprofen, indomethacin, and naproxen. Effect on bone mass density beyond 2 years of treatment is not known.

**Side Effects:** *CV:* Hot flashes, migraine. *Body as a whole:* Infection, flu syndrome, chest pain, fever, weight gain, peripheral edema. *CNS:* Depression, insomnia. *GI:* Nausea, dyspepsia, vomiting, flatulence, GI disorder, gastroenteritis. *GU:* Vaginitis, urinary tract infection, cystitis, leukorrhea, endometrial disorder. *Respiratory:* Sinusitis, pharyngitis, increased cough, pneumonia, laryngitis. *Musculoskeletal:* Arthralgia, myalgia, leg cramps, arthritis. *Dermatologic:* Rash, sweating.

**Laboratory Test Alteration:** ↑ Apolipoprotein A1, steroid-binding globulin, thyroxine-binding globulin, corticosteroid-binding globulin. ↓ Total cholesterol, LDL cholesterol, fibrinogen, apolipoprotien B, lipoprotein.

**Drug Interactions**
*Cholestryamine* / ↓ Absorption of raloxifene
*Warfarin* / ↓ Prothrombin time

**Dosage** ——————————
• **Tablets**
  *Prevention of osteoporosis in postmenopausal women.*
  **Adults:** 60 mg once daily.

**NURSING CONSIDERATIONS**

**Administration/Storage**
1. May be taken without regard for meals.
2. Take supplemental calcium and vitamin D if daily dietary intake is inadequate.

**Assessment**
1. Document indications for therapy; note date menopause passed.
2. Assess for history or evidence of CHF, active cancer or blood clots in legs, lungs or eyes.
3. Monitor LFTs; assess for any dysfunction.

**Client/Family Teaching**
1. Take exactly as directed once daily with or without food; if dietary calcium and vitamin D intake is inadequate, consume supplemental.
2. Drug is used by women after menopause to prevent bones from becoming weak and thin.
3. Avoid prolonged immobilization and restrictions of movement as with travel due to increased risk of venous thromboembolic events. Stop 3 days prior to and during prolonged immobilization such as with surgery or prolonged bedrest.
4. Drug is not effective in reducing hot flashes or flushes associated with low estrogen as it does not stimulate breast or uterus.
5. Regular weight bearing exercises as well as tobacco and alcohol cessation/modification should be practiced.

R

———————————————————————

6. Report any pain in calves or swelling in legs, sudden chest pain, SOB, or coughing up blood, as well as any vision changes.

**Outcomes/Evaluate:** Postmenopausal osteoporosis prophylaxis

# Ramipril
(**RAM**-ih-prill)
**Pregnancy Category:** D
Altace **(Rx)**
**Classification:** Angiotensin-converting enzyme inhibitor

See also *Angiotensin-Converting Enzyme Inhibitors.*

**Action/Kinetics: Onset:** 1–2 hr. **Time to peak serum levels:** 1 hr (1–2 hr for ramiprilat, the active metabolite). Ramiprilat has approximately six times the ACE inhibitory activity than ramipril. **t½:** 1–2 hr (13–17 hr for ramiprilat); prolonged in impaired renal function. **Duration:** 24 hr. Metabolized in the liver with 60% excreted through the urine and 40% in the feces. Food decreases the rate, but not the extent, of absorption of ramipril.

**Uses:** Alone or in combination with other antihypertensive agents (especially thiazide diuretics) for the treatment of hypertension. Treatment of CHF following MI to decrease risk of CV death and decrease the risk of failure-related hospitalization and progression to severe or resistant heart failure.

**Contraindications:** Use during lactation.

**Special Concerns:** Geriatric clients may manifest higher peak blood levels of ramiprilat.

**Side Effects:** *CV:* Hypotension, chest pain, palpitations, angina pectoris, *MI, arrhythmias. GI:* N&V, abdominal pain, diarrhea, dysgeusia, anorexia, constipation, dry mouth, dyspepsia, enzyme changes suggesting pancreatitis, dysphagia, gastroenteritis, increased salivation. *CNS:* Headache, dizziness, fatigue, insomnia, sleep disturbances, somnolence, depression, nervousness, malaise, vertigo, anxiety, amnesia, *convul-*

*sions,* tremor. *Respiratory:* Cough, dyspnea, upper respiratory tract infection, asthma, *bronchospasm. Hematologic:* Leukopenia, eosinophilia. Rarely, decreases in hemoglobin or hematocrit. *Dermatologic:* Diaphoresis, photosensitivity, pruritus, rash, dermatitis, purpura. *Body as a whole:* Paresthesias, angioedema, asthenia, syncope, fever, muscle cramps, myalgia, arthralgia, arthritis, neuralgia, neuropathy, influenza, edema. *Miscellaneous:* Impotence, tinnitus, hearing loss, vision disturbances, epistaxis, weight gain, proteinuria.

**Laboratory Test Interferences:** ↓ H&H.

**Dosage** —————————————
• **Capsules**
  *Hypertension.*
**Initial:** 2.5 mg once daily in clients not taking a diuretic; **maintenance:** 2.5–20 mg/day as a single dose or two equally divided doses. *Clients taking diuretics or who have a $C_{CR}$ less than 40 mL/min/1.73 m²:* initially 1.25 mg/day; dose may then be increased to a maximum of 5 mg/day.
  *CHF following MI.*
**Initial:** 2.5 mg b.i.d. Clients intolerant of this dose may be started on 1.25 mg b.i.d. The target maintenance dose is 5 mg b.i.d.

## NURSING CONSIDERATIONS

See also *Nursing Considerations* for *Angiotensin-Converting Enzyme Inhibitors* and *Antihypertensive Agents.*

**Administration/Storage**

1. For ease in swallowing, the contents of the capsule can be mixed with water, apple juice, or apple sauce.

2. If the antihypertensive effect decreases at the end of the dosing interval with once-daily dosing, consider either twice-daily administration or an increase in dose.

3. If taking a diuretic, discontinue the diuretic 2–3 days prior to beginning ramipril. If BP is not controlled, reinstitute the diuretic. If the diuretic

cannot be discontinued, consider an initial dose of ramipril of 1.25 mg.

**Client/Family Teaching**
1. Use caution; drug may cause dizziness and postural effects with sudden changes in position.
2. Report any persistent, dry, nonproductive cough, increased SOB, edema, or unusual bruising or bleeding.
3. Do not take any OTC agents without approval.

**Outcomes/Evaluate**
- ↓ BP
- Resolution of S&S of CHF

# Ranitidine bismuth citrate

((rah-**NIH**-tih-deen **BIS**-muth))
**Pregnancy Category:** C, when used with clarithromycin
Tritec **(Rx)**
**Classification:** Histamine H₂ antagonist/treatment for H. pylori

See also *Histamine H₂ Antagonists,* and *Ranitidine. NOTE:* Since clarithromycin is used with ranitidine bismuth citrate, information on clarithromycin must also be consulted.

**Action/Kinetics:** A complex of ranitidine, bismuth, and citrate which is freely soluble in water; solubility decreases as pH is decreased. An admixture of ranitidine and bismuth citrate is almost completely insoluble in water. It is believed the greater solubility of the complex facilitates penetration of the drug into the mucous layer that protects the epithelial cells in the GI mucosa. **Peak levels of ranitidine from complex:** 0.5–5 hr. **t½, elimination, ranitidine from ranitidine bismuth citrate:** 2.8–3.1 hr. Ranitidine is eliminated through the kidneys. **t½, terminal, bismuth:** 11–28 days. Bismuth is excreted primarily in the feces.

**Uses:** In combination with clarithromycin for treatment of active duodenal ulcers associated with *Helicobacter pylori* infections. *NOTE:* Ranitidine bismuth citrate should not be prescribed alone for the treatment of active duodenal ulcer.

**Contraindications:** Hypersensitivity to the complex or any of its ingredients. Hangover. Use in those with a history of acute porphyria or in those with a creatinine clearance less than 25 mL/min.

**Special Concerns:** Use with caution during lactation. Safety and efficacy of ranitidine bismuth citrate plus clarithromycin in pediatric clients have not been determined.

**Side Effects:** See also side effects for *Ranitidine. GI:* N&V, diarrhea, constipation, abdominal discomfort, gastric pain. *CNS:* Headache, dizziness, sleep disorder, tremors (rare). *Hypersensitivity:* Rash, anaphylaxis (rare). *Miscellaneous:* Pruritus, gynecologic problems, taste disturbance, chest symptoms, transient changes in liver enzymes.

**Drug Interactions**
*Antacids* / Possible ↓ plasma levels of ranitidine and bismuth
*Clarithromycin* / ↑ Plasma levels of ranitidine and bismuth

**Laboratory Test Interferences:** False + test for urine protein using Multistix. ↑ ALT, AST.

**Dosage**
- **Tablets**
  *Eradication of* H. pylori *infection. Ranitidine bismuth citrate:* 400 mg b.i.d. for 4 weeks. *Clarithromycin:* 500 mg t.i.d. for the first 2 weeks of therapy.

## NURSING CONSIDERATIONS

See also *Nursing Considerations* for *Histamine H₂ Antagonists,* and *Ranitidine.*

**Administration/Storage**
1. Bismuth may cause a temporary and harmless darkening of the tongue or stool; do not confuse with melena.
2. Both ranitidine bismuth citrate and clarithromycin can be taken with or without food.
3. Protect drug from light and store at 2°C–30°C (36°F–86°F).

**R**

**Assessment**
1. Document indications for therapy, onset and duration of symptoms, other agents trialed and the outcome.
2. Note serum *H. pylori* or endoscopic confirmation of disease.
3. Obtain baseline CBC, liver and renal function studies.
4. Determine any experience with these agents. Not for use with acute porphyria, a hangover, or $C_{CR}$ < 25 mL/min.

**Client/Family Teaching**
1. Take exactly as directed; do not skip doses or try and double up on missed doses. Take missed dose when remembered.
2. The cause for the ulcer is the bacteria *H. pylori;* this medication helps kill this bacteria. Must be taken with clarithromycin in order to be effective against *H. pylori*.
3. May experience diarrhea, headache, nausea, vomiting, and itchy skin; report if persistent and use only acetaminophen for headaches.
4. Use sugarless candies or rinse mouth frequently to diminish bad taste.
5. Stools and tongue may appear black in color; do not be alarmed.
6. Do not smoke; smoking slows ulcer healing and may cause a recurrence.
7. Avoid any other medications (prescription or OTC) without approval.

**Outcomes/Evaluate:** Healing of ulcer; ↓ pain and discomfort

# Ranitidine hydrochloride
(rah-**NIH**-tih-deen)
**Pregnancy Category:** B
Alti-Ranitidine HCl ✤, Apo-Ranitidine ✤, Novo-Ranidine ✤, Nu-Ranit ✤, Zantac, Zantac-C ✤, Zantac Efferdose, Zantac GELdose Capsules **(Rx)**, Zantac 75 **(OTC)**
**Classification:** $H_2$ receptor antagonist

See also *Histamine $H_2$ Antagonists.*
**Action/Kinetics:** Competitively inhibits gastric acid secretion by blocking the effect of histamine on histamine $H_2$ receptors. Both daytime and nocturnal basal gastric acid secretion, as well as food- and pentagastrin-stimulated gastric acid are inhibited. Weak inhibitor of cytochrome P-450 (drug-metabolizing enzymes); thus, drug interactions involving inhibition of hepatic metabolism are not expected to occur. Food increases the bioavailability. **Peak effect: PO,** 1–3 hr; **IM, IV,** 15 min. **t½:** 2.5–3 hr. **Duration, nocturnal:** 13 hr; **basal:** 4 hr. **Serum level to inhibit 50% stimulated gastric acid secretion:** 36–94 ng/mL. From 30% to 35% of a PO dose and from 68% to 79% of an IV dose excreted unchanged in urine.

**Uses:** Short-term (4–8 weeks) and maintenance treatment of duodenal ulcer. Pathologic hypersecretory conditions such as Zollinger-Ellison syndrome and systemic mastocytosis. Short-term treatment of active, benign gastric ulcers. Maintenance of healing of gastric ulcers. Gastroesophageal reflux disease, including erosive esophagitis. Maintenance of healing of erosive esophagitis. *Investigational:* Prophylaxis of pulmonary aspiration of acid during anesthesia, prevent gastric damage from NSAIDs, prevent stress ulcers, prevent acute upper GI bleeding, as part of multidrug regimen to eradicate Helicobacter pylori.

**Contraindications:** Cirrhosis of the liver, impaired renal or hepatic function.

**Special Concerns:** Use with caution during lactation and in clients with decreased hepatic or renal function. Safety and efficacy not established in children.

**Side Effects:** *GI:* Constipation, N&V, diarrhea, abdominal pain, pancreatitis (rare). *CNS:* Headache, dizziness, malaise, insomnia, vertigo, confusion, anxiety, agitation, depression, fatigue, somnolence, hallucinations. *CV:* Bradycardia or tachycardia, premature ventricular beats following rapid IV use (especially in clients predisposed to cardiac rhythm disturbances), *cardiac arrest*. *Hematologic:* Thrombocytopenia, granulocytopenia, leukopenia, pancytopenia (sometimes with marrow hypoplasia), *agranulocytosis, autoimmune hemolytic or aplastic anemia.* *Hepatic:* Hepatotoxicity, jaundice, hepatitis, increase in ALT. *Dermatologic:* Erythema multiforme, rash, alopecia. *Allergic:* **Bronchospasm, anaphylaxis,** angioneurotic edema (rare), rashes, fever, eosinophilia. *Other:* Arthralgia, gynecomastia, impotence, loss of libido, blurred vision, pain at injection site, local burning or itching following IV use.

**Drug Interactions**

*Antacids* / Antacids may ↓ the absorption of ranitidine

*Diazepam* / ↓ Effect of diazepam due to ↓ absorption from GI tract

*Glipizide* / Ranitidine ↑ effect of glipizide

*Procainamide* / Ranitidine ↓ excretion of procainamide → possible ↑ effect

*Theophylline* / Possible ↑ pharmacologic and toxicologic effects of theophylline

*Warfarin* / Ranitidine may ↑ hypoprothrombinemic effects of warfarin

**Laboratory Test Interferences:** False + test for urine protein using Multistix.

**Dosage**

• **Capsules (Soft Gelatin), Effervescent Tablets and Granules, Syrup, Tablets**

*Duodenal ulcer, short-term.*

**Adults:** 150 mg b.i.d. or 300 mg at bedtime to heal ulcer, although 100 mg b.i.d. will inhibit acid secretion and may be as effective as the higher dose. **Maintenance:** 150 mg at bedtime.

*Pathologic hypersecretory conditions.*

**Adults:** 150 mg b.i.d. (up to 6 g/day has been used in severe cases).

*Benign gastric ulcer.*

**Adults:** 150 mg b.i.d. for active ulcer. **Maintenance:** 150 mg at bedtime

*Gastroesophageal reflux disease.*

**Adults:** 150 mg b.i.d.

*Erosive esophagitis.*

**Adults:** 150 mg q.i.d.

*Maintenance of healing of erosive esophagitis.*

**Adults:** 150 mg b.i.d.

• **IM, IV**

*Treatment and maintenance for duodenal ulcer, hypersecretory conditions, gastroesophageal reflux.*

**Adults, IM:** 50 mg q 6–8 hr. **Intermittent IV injection or infusion:** 50 mg q 6–8 hr, not to exceed 400 mg/day. **Continuous IV infusion:** 6.25 mg/hr.

*Zollinger-Ellison clients.*

**Continuous IV infusion:** Dilute ranitidine in 5% dextrose injection to a concentration no greater than 2.5 mg/mL with an initial infusion rate of 1 mg/kg/hr. If after 4 hr the client shows a gastric acid output of greater than 10 mEq/hr or if symptoms appear, the dose should be increased by 0.5-mg/kg/hr increments and the acid output measured. Doses up to 2.5 mg/kg/hr may be necessary.

## NURSING CONSIDERATIONS

See also *Nursing Considerations* for *Histamine H$_2$ Antagonists.*

**Administration/Storage**

1. If the C$_{CR}$ is less than 50 mL/min, give 150 mg PO q 24 hr or 50 mg parenterally q 18–24 hr.

2. Give antacids concomitantly for gastric pain although they may interfere with ranitidine absorption.

3. Dissolve Efferdose tablets and granules in 6–8 oz of water before taking.

4. About one-half of clients may heal completely within 2 weeks; thus, endoscopy may show no need for further treatment.

5. No dilution is required for IM use.

6. Store the syrup between 4°C and 25°C (39°F and 77°F).

**IV** 7. For IV injection, dilute 50 mg with 0.9% NaCl injection to a total volume of 20 mL. Give the diluted solution over 5 min or more. For intermittent IV, dilute 50 mg in 100 mL 5% dextrose injection and give over 15–20 min.

---

8. The premixed injection does not require dilution; give only by slow IV drip over 15–20 min. Do not introduce additives into the solution. If used with a primary IV fluid system, discontinue the primary solution during drug infusion.

9. For continuous IV infusion, add ranitidine injection to 5% dextrose injection

10. The drug is stable for 48 hr at room temperature when mixed with 0.9% NaCl, 5% or 10% dextrose injection, RL injection, or 5% sodium bicarbonate injection.

**Assessment**

1. Document indications for therapy, onset and duration of symptoms, other agents used and anticipated treatment period.

2. Assess stomach pain, noting characteristics, frequency of occurrence and things that alter it.

3. Obtain CBC and assess for infections.

4. Determine if test for *H. pylori*, UGI, or endoscopy performed.

5. Assess for renal or liver disease.

6. Determine if pregnant.

7. Skin tests using allergens may elicit false negative results; stop drug 24–72 hr prior to testing.

**Client/Family Teaching**

1. Take with or immediately following meals. Wait 1 hr before taking an antacid.

2. Do not drive or operate machinery until drug effects are realized; dizziness or drowsiness may occur.

3. Avoid alcohol, aspirin-containing products, and beverages that contain caffeine (tea, cola, coffee); these increase stomach acid.

4. Avoid things that may aggravate symptoms, i.e., ETOH, aspirin, NSAIDs, caffeine, and black pepper.

5. Do not smoke; smoking interferes with healing and drug's effectiveness.

6. Report any evidence of diarrhea and maintain adequate hydration.

7. Report any confusion or disorientation.

8. Symptoms of breast tenderness will usually disappear after several weeks; report if persistent and evaluate need to stop drug.

9. Report as scheduled to determine extent of healing and expected length of therapy.

**Outcomes/Evaluate**

• ↓ Gastric acid production
• ↓ Abdominal pain/discomfort
• Endoscopic/radiographic evidence of duodenal ulcer healing

# Remifentanil hydrochloride

((rem-ih-**FEN**-tah-nil))
**Pregnancy Category:** C
Ultiva **(Rx)**
**Classification:** Narcotic analgesic

See also *Narcotic Analgesics.*

**Action/Kinetics:** Narcotic analgesic that binds with mu-opioid receptors. Rapid onset and peak effect with a short duration of action. Depresses respiration in a dose-dependent manner and causes muscle rigidity. Rapidly metabolized by nonspecific blood and tissue esterases; not metabolized appreciably by the liver or lung. **t½, elimination:** 3–10 min. **Recovery:** Within 5–10 min.

**Uses:** As an analgesic during the induction and maintenance of general anesthesia and for continuation as an analgesic in the immediate postoperative period. It is also an analgesic component of monitored anesthesia care.

**Contraindications:** Epidural or intrathecal use due to the presence of glycine in the formulation. Hypersensitivity to fentanyl analogues. Use as the sole agent in general anesthesia because LOC cannot be ensured and due to a high incidence of apnea, muscle rigidity, and tachycardia.

**Special Concerns:** Use with caution in obese clients and during lactation. Respiratory depression and other narcotic effects may be seen in newborns whose mothers are given remifentanil shortly before delivery. Geriatric clients are twice as sensitive as younger clients to the effects of the drug. Not studied in children less than 2 years of age.

**Side Effects:** *GI:* N&V, constipation, abdominal discomfort, xerostomia, gastroesophageal reflux, dysphagia, diarrhea, heartburn, ileus. *CNS:* Shivering, fever, dizziness, headache, agitation, chills, warm sensation, anxiety, involuntary movement, prolonged emergence from anesthesia, tremors, disorientation, dysphoria, nightmares, hallucinations, paresthesia, nystagmus, twitch, sleep disorder, seizures, amnesia. *CV:* Hypotension, bradycardia, tachycardia, hypertension, atrial and ventricular arrhythmias, heart block, ECG change consistent with myocardial ischemia, syncope. *Musculoskeletal:* Muscle rigidity, muscle stiffness, musculoskeletal chest pain, delayed recovery from neuromuscular block. *Respiratory:* Respiratory depression, apnea, hypoxia, cough, dyspnea, bronchospasm, laryngospasm, rhonchi, stridor, nasal congestion, pharyngitis, pleural effusion, hiccoughs, pulmonary edema, rales, bronchitis, rhinorrhea. *Dermatologic:* Pruritus, rash, urticaria, erythema, sweating, flushing, pain at IV site. *GU:* Urine retention, oliguria, dysuria, urine incontinence. *Hematologic:* Anemia, lymphopenia, leukocytosis, thrombocytopenia. *Metabolic:* Abnormal liver function, hyperglycemia, electrolyte disorders. *Miscellaneous:* Decreased body temperature, ***anaphylactic reaction,*** visual disturbances, postoperative pain.

**OD** **Overdose Management:** *Symptoms:* Apnea, chest-wall rigidity, seizures, hypoxemia, hypotension, bradycardia. *Treatment:* Discontinue administration, maintain a patent airway, initiate assisted or controlled ventilation with oxygen, and maintain adequate CV function. A neuromuscular blocking agent or a mu-opiate receptor antagonist may be used to treat muscle rigidity. IV fluids, vasopressors, and other supportive measures are indicated to treat hypotension. Bradycardia or hypotension may also be treated with atropine or glycopyrrolate. IV nalox-

one is used to treat respiratory depression or muscle rigidity. Reversal of the opioid effects may lead to acute pain and sympathetic hyperactivity.

**Drug Interactions:** Remifentanil is synergistic with other anesthetics. Doses of thiopental, propofol, isoflurane, and midazolam have been reduced by up to 75% with the coadministration of remifentanil.

**Laboratory Test Interferences:** CPK-MB levels.

**Dosage** _____

• **Continuous IV Infusion Only**
  *Induction of anesthesia through intubation.*
0.5–1 mcg/kg/min given with a hypnotic or volatile agent. If endotracheal intubation is to occur less than 8 min after the start of the infusion of remifentanil, the initial dose of 1 mcg/kg may be given over 30 to 60 sec.
  *Maintenance of nitrous oxide (66%) anesthesia.*
The dose of remifentanil is 0.4 mcg/kg/min (range of 0.1–2 mcg/kg/min). A supplemental IV bolus dose of 1 mcg/kg may be given.
  *Maintenance of isoflurane (0.4 to 1.5 MAC) or propofol (100–200 mcg/kg/min) anesthesia.*
The dose of remifentanil is 0.25 mcg/kg/min (range of 0.05–2 mcg/kg/min). A supplemental IV bolus dose of 1 mcg/kg may be given.
  *Continuation as an analgesic into the immediate postoperative period.*
The dose of remifentanil is 0.1 mcg/kg/min (range of 0.025–0.2 mcg/kg/min). The infusion rate may be adjusted every 5 min in 0.025-mcg/kg/min increments to balance the client's level of analgesia and respiratory rate.
  *Analgesic component of monitored anesthesia care.*
**Single IV dose:** 1 mcg/kg administered over 30 to 60 sec and given 90 sec before the local anesthetic. If remifentanil is given with midazolam (2 mg), the dose should be 0.5

**R**

---

mcg/kg. **Continuous IV infusion:** 0.1 mcg/kg beginning 5 min before the local anesthetic. After the local anesthetic, the dose of remifentanil is 0.05 mcg/kg/min (range 0.025–0.2 mcg/kg/min) at 5-min intervals in order to balance the level of analgesia and respiratory rate. If remifentanil is given with midazolam (2 mg), the dose should be 0.025 mcg/kg/min (range 0.025–0.2 mcg/kg/min).

## NURSING CONSIDERATIONS

See also *Nursing Considerations* for *Narcotic Analgesics.*
**Administration/Storage**
**IV** 1. Individualize need for preanesthetic drugs and the choice of anesthetic.
2. Decrease the starting dose by 50% in clients over 65 years of age. Cautiously titrate to the desired effect.
3. Use the adult dose for pediatric clients 2 years of age and older.
4. Base the starting dose in obese clients (i.e., greater than 30% over their ideal body weight) on ideal body weight.
5. Give continuous infusions only by an infusion device. The injection site should be close to the venous cannula.
6. Due to the rapid onset and short duration, administration during anesthesia can be titrated upward in 25% to 100% increments or downward in 25% to 50% decrements every 2 to 5 min to attain the desired level of opiate effect. In response to light anesthesia or transient periods of intense surgical stress, supplemental bolus doses of 1 mcg/kg may be given every 2 to 5 min.
7. Administer under close supervision of an anesthesia practitioner into the immediate postoperative period. Infusion rates greater than 0.2 mcg/kg/min are associated with respiratory depression.
8. When remifentanil infusion is discontinued, clear the IV tubing to prevent inadvertent administration at a later time.
9. Due to its duration, no opioid

activity will be present within 5–10 min of discontinuation.
10. Stable for 24 hr at room temperature after reconstitution and further dilution to concentrations of 20–250 mcg/mL. Dilution may be with sterile water for injection, 5% dextrose injection, 5% dextrose and 0.9% NaCl injection, 0.9% NaCl injection, or 0.45% NaCl injection.
11. Compatible with propofal when coadministered into a running IV administration set.
12. Store at 2°C–25°C (36°F–77°F).
**Assessment**
1. Document indications and expected duration of therapy.
2. Determine if pain is acute or chronic in nature; describe distinguishing characteristics and use a pain-rating scale to rate pain level.
3. Monitor liver and renal function studies.
4. Observe for progressive respiratory depression.
**Client/Family Teaching**
1. Do not perform activites that require mental alertness for 24 hr; drug causes dizziness, drowsiness, and impaired physical and mental performance.
2. Avoid alcohol and any other CNS depressants for 24 hr after procedure.
**Outcomes/Evaluate:** Pain control and analgesia

# Repaglinide
(re-**PAY**-glin-eyed)
**Pregnancy Category:** C
Prandin **(Rx)**
**Classification:** Oral antidiabetic

See also *Antidiabetic Agents, Hypoglycemic Agents.*

**Action/Kinetics:** Lowers blood glucose by stimulating release of insulin from pancreas. Action depends on functioning beta cells in pancreatic islets. Drug closes ATP-dependent potassium channels in beta-cell membrane due to binding at sites. Blockade of potassium channel depolarizes beta cell which leads to opening of calcium channels. This causes calcium influx which induces insulin secretion. Rapidly and completely absorbed from GI tract. **Peak plasma levels:** 1 hr. Completely metabolized in liver with most excreted in feces.

**Uses:** Adjunct to diet and exercise in type 2 diabetes mellitus. In combination with metformin to lower blood glucose where hyperglycemia can not be controlled by exercise, diet, or either drug alone.

**Contraindications:** Lactation. Diabetic ketoacidosis, with or without coma. Type 1 diabetes.

**Special Concerns:** Use with caution in impaired hepatic function. Safety and efficacy have not been determined in children.

**Side Effects:** *CV:* Chest pain, angina, ischemia. *GI:* Nausea, diarrhea, constipation, vomiting, dyspepsia. *Respiratory:* URI, sinusitis, rhinitis, bronchitis. *Musculoskeletal:* Arthralgia, back pain. *Miscellaneous:* Hypoglycemia, headache, paresthesia, chest pain, urinary tract infection, tooth disorder, allergy.

**OD** **Overdose Management:** *Symptoms:* Hypoglycemia. *Treatment:* Oral glucose. Also adjust drug dosage or meal patterns.

**Drug Interactions:** See *Antidiabetic Agents, Hypoglycemic Agents.*

**Dosage** ————
- **Tablets**

  *Type 2 diabetes mellitus.*
  Individualize dosage. **Initial:** In those not previously treated or whose HbA1-C is less than 8%, give 0.5 mg. For those previously treated or whose HbA1-C is 8% or more, give 1 or 2 mg before each meal. **Dose range:** 0.5–4 mg taken with meals. **Maximum daily dose:** 16 mg.

## NURSING CONSIDERATIONS

See also *Nursing Considerations* for *Antidiabetic Agents, Hypoglycemic Agents.*

**Administration/Storage**
1. May be dosed after meals 2, 3, or 4 times daily, depending on client's meal patterns.
2. Usually taken within 15 min of meal but time may vary from immediately preceding meal to as long as 30 min before meal.
3. When used to replace another oral hypoglycemic, it may be started the day after final dose of other drug is given.
4. If necessary to combine with metformin, starting dose and dose adjustments of repaglinide are the same as if repaglinide was used alone.

**Assessment**
1. Document onset, duration, and characteristics of disease; note other agents/methods trialed and outcome.
2. Monitor VS, HbA1-C, and LFTs.

**Client/Family Teaching**
1. Take as prescribed.
2. Continue regular exercise, diabetic diet, and lifestyle modifications in order to control BS and prevent organ damage.
3. Record finger sticks for provider review; report any unusual or intolerable side effects.

**Outcomes/Evaluate:** HbA1-C within desired range; control of BS

# Respiratory Syncytial Virus Immune Globulin Intravenous (Human) (RSV-IGIV)

**Pregnancy Category:** C
RespiGam **(Rx)**
**Classification:** Immunosuppressant

**Action/Kinetics:** Is an IgG containing neutralizing antibody to RSV. The immunoglobulin is obtained and purified from pooled adult human plasma that has been selected for high titers of neutralizing antibody against RSV. Each milliliter contains 50 mg of immunoglobulin, primarily IgG with trace amounts of IgA and IgM.

R

**Uses:** Prevention of serious lower respiratory tract infection caused by RSV in children less than 24 months old with bronchopulmonary dysplasia or a history of premature birth (less than 35 weeks gestation).

**Contraindications:** History of a severe prior reaction associated with administration of RSV-IGIV or other human immunoglobulin products. Clients with selective IgA deficiency who have the potential for developing antibodies to IgA and which could cause anaphylaxis or allergic reactions to blood products that contain IgA.

**Special Concerns:** Safety and efficacy have not been determined in children with congenital heart disease. Give close attention to the infusion rate as side effects may be related to the rate of administration. Since RSV-IGIV is made from human plasma, there is the possibility for transmission of blood-borne pathogenic organisms, although the risk is considered to be low due to screening of donors and viral inactivation and removal steps in the manufacturing process.

**Side Effects:** Infusion of RSV-IGIV may cause fluid overload, especially in children with bronchopulmonary dysplasia. Aseptic meningitis syndrome has been reported within several hours to 2 days following RSV-IGIV treatment. Symptoms include severe headache, drowsiness, fever, photophobia, painful eye movements, muscle rigidity, nausea, and vomiting. The CSF shows pleocytosis, predominately granulocytic, as well as elevated protein levels.

*Allergic:* Hypotension, ***anaphylaxis, angioneurotic edema,*** respiratory distress. *CNS:* Fever, pyrexia, sleepiness. *Respiratory:* Respiratory distress, wheezing, rales, tachypnea, cough. *GI:* Vomiting, diarrhea, gagging, gastroenteritis. *CV:* Tachycardia, increased pulse rate, hypertension, hypotension, heart murmur. *Dermatologic:* Rash, pallor, cyanosis, eczema, cold and clammy skin. *Miscellaneous:* Hypoxia, hypoxemia, inflammation at injection site, edema, rhinorrhea, conjunctival hemorrhage.

Reactions similar to other immunoglobulins may occur as follows. *Body as a whole:* Dizziness, flushing, ***immediate allergic, anaphylactic, or hypersensitivity reactions.*** *CV:* Blood pressure changes, palpitations, chest tightness. *Miscellaneous:* Anxiety, dyspnea, abdominal cramps, pruritus, myalgia, arthralgia.

**OD** **Overdose Management:** *Symptoms:* Symptoms due to fluid volume overload. *Treatment:* Administration of diuretics and modification of the infusion rate.

**Drug Interactions:** Antibodies found in immunoglobulin products may interfere with the immune response to live virus vaccines, including those for mumps, rubella, and measles. Also, the antibody response to diphtheria, tetanus, pertussis, and *Haemophilus influenzae b* may be lower in RSV-IGIV recipients.

## Dosage
- **IV Injection**
  *Prevention of RSV infections.*
  1.5 mL/kg/hr for 15 min. If the clinical condition of the client allows, the rate can be increased to 3 mL/kg/hr for the next 15-min period and, finally, increased to a maximum rate of 6 mL/kg/hr from 30 min to the end of the infusion. *Do not exceed these rates of infusion.*

## NURSING CONSIDERATIONS
### Administration/Storage
**IV** 1. Enter the single-use vial only once. Initiate infusion within 6 hr and complete within 12 hr of removal from the vial.

2. Do not use if the solution is turbid.

3. Give separately from other drugs or medications.

4. Give through an IV line (preferably a separate line) using a constant infusion pump. Administration may be "piggy-backed" into an existing line if that line contains one of the following dextrose solutions (with or without NaCl): 2.5%, 5%, 10%, or 20% dextrose in water. If a preexisting

line must be used, do not dilute RSV-IGIV more than 1:2 with one of the above solutions. Do not predilute RSV-IGIV before infusion.

5. Although use of filters is not necessary, an in-line filter with a pore size greater than 15 μm may be used.

6. Store the injection at 2°C–8°C (35.6°F–46.4°F). Do not freeze or shake (to prevent foaming).

**Assessment**

1. Document indications for therapy, any previous experiences with this drug and the outcome.

2. Note any IgA deficiency.

3. Assess VS, I&O, and cardiopulmonary status prior to infusion, before each rate increase, and thereafter at 30-min intervals until 30 min following infusion completion. Observe for fluid overload (increased HR, increased respiratory rate, rales, retractions), especially in infants with bronchopulmonary dysplasia. A loop diuretic (e.g., furosemide or bumetanide) should be available for management of fluid overload.

**Client/Family Teaching**

1. The first dose of RSV-IGIV should be given prior to the beginning of the RSV season and monthly throughout the RSV season (in the Northern Hemisphere, this is from November through April) in order to maintain protection.

2. Drug is derived from human plasma; review potential risks related to blood-borne pathogenic agents.

3. Report any severe headaches, painful eye movements, drowsiness, fever, N&V, or muscle rigidity (symptoms of aseptic meningitis); must be evaluated to rule out other causes of meningitis.

4. If virus vaccines are given during or within 10 months after RSV-IGIV infusion, reimmunization is recommended.

**Outcomes/Evaluate:** RSV prophylaxis; ↓ severity of RSV illness

# Reteplase recombinant
(**REE**-teh-place)

**Pregnancy Category:** C
Retavase **(Rx)**
**Classification:** Inhibitor of platelet aggregation

**Action/Kinetics:** Plasminogen activator that catalyzes the cleavage of endogenous plasminogen to generate plasmin. Plasmin, in turn, degrades the matrix of the thrombus, causing a thrombolytic effect. **t½:** 13 to 16 min. Cleared primarily by the liver and kidney.

**Uses:** In adults for the management of acute MI for improvement of ventricular function, reduction of the incidence of CHF, and reduction of mortality.

**Contraindications:** Active internal bleeding; history of CVA; recent intracranial or intraspinal surgery or trauma; intracranial neoplasm, arteriovenous malformation, or aneurysm; known bleeding diathesis; severe uncontrolled hypertension.

**Special Concerns:** Use with caution during lactation. Safety and efficacy have not been determined in children.

**Side Effects:** *Bleeding disorders:* From internal bleeding sites, including intracranial, retroperitoneal, GI, GU, or respiratory. *Hemorrhage may occur.* From superficial bleeding sites, including venous cutdowns, arterial punctures, sites of recent surgery. *CV: Cholesterol embolism,* coronary thrombolysis resulting in arrhythmias associated with perfusion (no different from those seen in the ordinary course of acute MI), cardiogenic shock, sinus bradycardia, accelerated idioventricular rhythm, ventricular premature depolarizations, SVT, ventricular tachycardia, *ventricular fibrillation,* AV block, pulmonary edema, *heart failure, cardiac arrest, recurrent ischemia, myocardial rupture, cardiac tamponade, venous thrombosis or embolism, electromechanical dissociation, mitral regurgitation, pericardial effusion, pericarditis.* *Hypersensitivity:* Serious allergic reactions. *NOTE:* Many of the CV side effects listed are frequent

R

sequelae of MI and may or may not be attributable to reteplase recombinant.

**Drug Interactions:** Use with abciximab, aspirin, dipyridamole, heparin, or vitamin K antagonists may increase the risk of bleeding.

**Laboratory Test Interferences:** Plasminogen, fibrinogen. Degradation of fibrinogen in blood samples removed for analysis.

## Dosage

• **IV only**

*Acute MI.*

**Adults:** 10 + 10 unit double-bolus. Each bolus is given over 2 min, with the second bolus given 30 min after initiation of the first bolus injection.

## NURSING CONSIDERATIONS

See also *Nursing Considerations* for *Alteplase*.

### Administration/Storage

**IV** 1. Initiate treatment as soon as possible after symptom onset.

2. Have available antiarrhythmic therapy for bradycardia and/or ventricular irritability.

3. Give each bolus injection by an IV line in which no other medication is being simultaneously infused or injected. Do not add any other medication to the solution containing reteplase recombinant.

4. Reconstitution is performed using the diluent, syringe, needle, and dispensing pin provided with the drug. Reconstitution is undertaken as follows:

• Remove the flip-cap from one vial of sterile water for injection (preservative free), and, with the syringe provided, withdraw 10 mL of the sterile water.

• Open the package containing the dispensing pin. Remove the needle from the syringe and discard. Remove the protective cap from the spike end of the dispensing pin and connect the syringe to the dispensing pin. Remove the protective flip-cap from one vial of reteplase.

• Remove the protective cap from the spike end of the dispensing pin, and insert the spike into the vial of reteplase. Transfer the 10 mL of sterile water through the dispensing pin into the vial.

• With the dispensing pin and syringe still attached to the vial, gently swirl the vial is to dissolve the reteplase recombinant. **Do not shake.**

• Withdraw the 10 mL of reconstituted reteplase recombinant back into the syringe (a small amount will remain due to overfill).

• Detach the syringe from the dispensing pin, and attach the sterile 20-gauge needle provided. The solution is ready to administer.

5. Since reteplase contains no antibacterial preservatives, reconstitute just prior to use. When reconstituted as directed, the solution may be used within 4 hr when stored at 2°C–30°C (36°F–86°F).

6. Keep the kit sealed until use and store at 2°C–25°C (36°F–77°F).

### Assessment

1. Document indications for therapy, noting onset, duration, and characteristics of chest pain.

2. List drugs currently prescribed to ensure none interact unfavorably.

3. Note evidence of CVA, internal bleeding, trauma, neurosurgery, or bleeding disorders.

4. Obtain CBC, type and cross, coagulation times, cardiac panel, and liver and renal function studies.

5. Note cardiopulmonary assessments and ECG.

### Interventions

1. During administration, continuously monitor cardiac rhythm. Have medications available for management of bradycardia and ventricular irritability.

2. Record VS every 15 min during infusion and for 2 hr following.

3. Administer first dose over 2 min and the second dose 30 min later if no serious bleeding is observed. In the event of any uncontrolled bleeding, terminate the heparin infusion and withhold the second dose.

4. Observe all puncture sites and areas for evidence of bleeding. Arterial sticks require 30 min of manual pressure followed by application of a pressure dressing.

5. Assess for reperfusion reactions such as:
• Arrhythmias usually of short duration, which may include bradycardia or ventricular tachycardia
• Reduction of chest pain
• Return of elevated ST segment and smaller Q waves
6. Maintain bedrest and observe for S&S of abnormal bleeding (hematuria, hematemesis, melena, CVA, cardiac tamponade).

**Client/Family Teaching**
1. Review goals of therapy and inherent risks of drug therapy during acute coronary artery occlusion.
2. To be effective, therapy should be instituted as soon as possible after symptom onset.
3. Encourage family members to learn CPR.

**Outcomes/Evaluate:**    Improved ventricular function; ↓ incidence of CHF, and ↓ mortality with AMI

---

# Rh<sub>o</sub> (D) Immune Globulin IV (Human)
(roh (dee) im-**MYOUN GLOH**-byou-lin)
**Pregnancy Category:** C
HypRho-D Full Dose ✦, WinRho SD
**(Rx)**
**Classification:** Immunosuppressant

**Action/Kinetics:** Sterile, freeze-dried gamma globulin (IgG) fraction containing antibodies to Rh<sub>o</sub> (D) derived from human plasma. The manufacturing process is effective in inactivating lipid-enveloped viruses, including hepatitis B and C and HIV. Contains approximately 2 mcg IgA/1,500 international units (300 mcg). It suppresses the immune response of nonsensitized Rh<sub>o</sub> (D) antigen-negative individuals following Rh<sub>o</sub> (D) antigen-positive red blood cell exposure. Mechanism is unknown. Suppression of Rh isoimmunization decreases the possibility of hemolytic disease in an Rh<sub>o</sub> (D) antigen-positive fetus in present and future pregnancies. **Peak levels, after IV:** 2

hr; **after IM:** 5–10 days. **t½, after IV:** 24 days; **after IM:** 30 days.
**Uses:** Suppression of Rh isoimmunization in non-sensitized Rh<sub>o</sub> (D) antigen-negative women within 72 hr after spontaneous or induced abortions, amniocentesis, chorionic vilus sampling, ruptured tubal pregnancy, abdominal trauma, transplacental hemorrhage, or in the normal course of pregnancy unless the blood type of the fetus or father is known to be Rh<sub>o</sub> (D) antigen-negative. Suppression of Rh isoimmunization in Rh<sub>o</sub> (D) antigen-negative female children and female adults in their childbearing years transfused with Rh<sub>o</sub> (D) antigen-positive RBCs or blood components containing Rh<sub>o</sub> (D) antigen-positive RBCs. Treatment of non-splenectomized Rh<sub>o</sub> (D) antigen-positive children with chronic or acute immune thrombocytopenic purpura (ITP), adults with chronic ITP, or children and adults with ITP secondary to HIV infection in clinical situations requiring an increase in platelet count to prevent excessive hemorrhage.
**Contraindications:** History of anaphylactic or severe systemic reaction to human globulin (i.e., due to the presence of trace amounts of IgA). Administration to Rh<sub>o</sub> (D) antigen-negative or splenectomized individuals, as efficacy has not been shown. Use in Rh<sub>o</sub> (D) antigen-negative clients who are Rh immunized (Rh antibody-positive), as evidenced by standard manual Rh antibody screening tests. Use in infants.
**Special Concerns:** Use with extreme caution in those with a hemoglobin level less than 8 g/dL due to the possibility of increasing the severity of anemia.
**Side Effects: When used for Rh isoimmunization suppression.** Side effects are infrequent but include discomfort and slight swelling at the injection site and a slight elevation in temperature. There is the possibility of ***anaphylaxis.***
     **When used for ITP.** Most com-

monly, headaches, chills, and fever. Decreased hemoglobin.

## Dosage

- **IM, IV.**

  *Pregnancy.*

  1,500 IU (300 mcg) at 28 weeks gestation. If given early in the pregnancy, administer at 12-week intervals in order to maintain an adequate level of passively acquired anti-Rh (antibodies). Give 600 IU (120 mcg) to the mother as soon as possible after delivery of a confirmed Rh₀ (D) antigen-positive baby and within 72 hr after delivery. If the Rh status of the baby is not known at 72 hr, give the drug to the mother. If more than 72 hr have elapsed, do not withhold the drug but give as soon as possible up to 28 days after delivery.

  *Other obstetric conditions.*

  600 IU (120 mcg) immediately after abortion, amniocentesis (after 24 weeks gestation), or any other manipulation late in pregnancy (after 34 weeks gestation) associated with an increased risk of Rh isoimmunization. Give 1,500 IU (300 mcg) immediately after amniocentesis before 34 weeks gestation or after chorionic vilus sampling. Repeat this dose q 12 weeks during pregnancy. Give as soon as possible in the event of threatened abortion.

  *Incompatible blood transfusions or massive fetal hemorrhage.*

  **IV:** 3,000 IU (600 mcg) q 8 hr until the total dose is given. **IM:** 6,000 IU (1,200 mcg) q 12 hr until the total dose is given.

- **IV only**

  *ITP.*

  **Initial:** 250 IU (50 mcg)/kg (125–200 IU/kg if the hemoglobin level is less than 10 g/dL). Give the initial dose as a single dose or two divided doses on separate days. If subsequent therapy is required, give 125–300 IU (25–60 mcg)/kg by IV only.

## NURSING CONSIDERATIONS

### Administration/Storage

1. For IM use, reconstitute aseptically with 1.25 mL of 0.9% NaCl injection using the same method as for IV use. Administer into the deltoid muscle of the upper arm or the anterolateral aspects of the upper thigh. Do not use the gluteal region routinely due to the risk of sciatic nerve injury. If the gluteal area is used, give only in the upper, outer quadrant.

2. If hemoglobin level is less than 10 g/dL, give a reduced dose of the drug (125–200 IU/kg) in order to reduce the risk of increasing the severity of anemia.

**IV** 3. The drug must be given IV for treating ITP, as the SC or IM routes are not effective.

4. For IV use, reconstitute aseptically with 2.5 mL of 0.9% NaCl injection. Introduce the diluent slowly onto the inside wall of the vial and wet the pellet by gentle swirling until dissolved. Do not shake. Administer into a suitable vein over 3 to 5 min.

5. Use only 0.9% NaCl injection to reconstitute the product.

6. Store vials of unreconstituted drug at 2°C–8°C (35°F–46°F). If the reconstituted drug is not used immediately, it may be stored at room temperature for no more than 4 hr. Discard any unused portion. Do not freeze either the unreconstituted or the reconstituted product.

### Assessment

1. Document indications and condition requiring therapy.

2. Determine Rh factor to ensure client is not antibody positive. Obtain blood sample for type and cross from mother and the neonate's cord. The neonate should be Rh₀(D) positive and the mother must be Rh₀(D) negative and (Dᵘ) negative. A large fetomaternal hemorrhage late in pregnancy or following delivery may cause a weak mixed field positive (Dᵘ) test result. Assess for a large fetomaternal hemorrhage and adjust the dose of Rh₀ (D) immune globulin accordingly. Give drug if there is any doubt about the blood type of the mother.

3. Reduce dose if hemoglobin is < 10 or there is evidence of a large fetomaternal hemorrhage.

4. When used to treat ITP, monitor clinical response by assessing platelet counts, red cell counts, hemoglobin, and reticulocyte levels.

**Client/Family Teaching:** When an Rh-negative mother carries an Rh-positive fetus, the fetal RBCs cross the placenta and enter the mother's circulation, evoking maternal antibody production against the Rh factor. When these antibodies cross to the fetal circulation, they destroy fetal RBCs, hence the need for monitoring and administration with all subsequent pregnancies. The medication prevents sensitization of an Rh-negative mother by an Rh-positive fetus, ultimately preventing hemolytic disease of the newborn.

**Outcomes/Evaluate**
• Suppression of Rh isoimmunization
• Prevention of hemolytic disease of the newborn
• ↑ Platelets

---

# Ribavirin

(rye-bah-**VYE**-rin)
**Pregnancy Category:** X
Virazole **(Rx)**
**Classification:** Antiviral agent

See also *Antiviral Drugs.*

**Action/Kinetics:** Has antiviral activity against respiratory syncytial virus (RSV), influenza virus, and HSV. Precise mechanism not known; may act as a competitive inhibitor of cellular enzymes that act on guanosine and xanthosine. Ribavirin is distributed to the plasma, respiratory tract, and RBCs and is rapidly taken up by cells. **t½ from plasma:** 9.5 hr; **from RBCs:** 40 days. Eliminated through both the urine and feces.

**Uses:** Hospitalized pediatric clients (including infants) with severe lower respiratory tract infections (viral pneumonia including bronchiolitis) due to RSV. Underlying conditions, such as prematurity or cardiopulmonary disease, may increase the severity of the RSV infection. Ribavirin is intended to be used along

with standard treatment (including fluid management) for such clients with severe lower respiratory tract infections. *Investigational:* Ribavirin aerosol has been used against influenza A and B. Oral ribavirin has been used against herpes genitalis, acute and chronic hepatitis, measles, and Lassa fever.

**Contraindications:** Use in adults. Infants requiring artificial respiration (the drug may precipitate in the equipment and interfere with appropriate ventilation of the client). Children with mild RSV lower respiratory tract infections who require a shorter hospital stay than required for a full course of ribavirin therapy. Pregnancy or women who may become pregnant during drug therapy (the drug may cause fetal harm and is known to be teratogenic). Lactation.

**Special Concerns:** Deterioration of respiratory function in infants with COPD or asthma.

**Side Effects:** *Pulmonary:* Worsening of respiratory status, pneumothorax, apnea, bacterial pneumonia, dependence on ventilator, ***bronchospasm,*** pulmonary edema, hypoventilation, cyanosis, dyspnea, atelectasis. *CV:* Hypotension, ***cardiac arrest,*** manifestations of digitalis toxicity, bradycardia, bigeminy, tachycardia. *Hematologic:* Anemia (with IV or PO ribavirin), reticulocytosis. *Other:* Conjunctivitis and rash (with the aerosol).

*NOTE:* The following symptoms have been noted in health care workers: headache, conjunctivitis, rhinitis, nausea, rash, dizziness, pharyngitis, lacrimation, bronchospasm, chest pain. Also, damage to contact lenses after prolonged close exposure to the aerosolized product.

**Dosage**
• **Aerosol Only, to an Infant Oxygen Hood Using the Small Particle Aerosol Generator-2 (SPAG-2)**
The concentration administered is 20 mg/mL and the average aerosol

---

concentration for a 12-hr period is 190 mcg/L of air. Treatment is continued for 12–18 hr a day for 3 (minimum)–7 days (maximum). See *Administration/Storage*.

## NURSING CONSIDERATIONS
### Administration/Storage
1. Treatment is most effective if initiated within the first 3 days of the RSV, which causes lower respiratory tract infections.
2. Administer ribavirin aerosol using only the SPAG-2 aerosol generator.
3. Do *not* institute therapy in clients requiring artificial respiration.
4. Do not give any other aerosolized medications if using ribavirin aerosol.
5. Solubilize with sterile water (USP) for injection or inhalation in the 100-mL vial. Transfer the solution to the SPAG-2 reservoir utilizing a sterilized 500-mL wide-mouth Erlenmeyer flask and further dilute to a final volume of 300 mL with sterile water.
6. Replace solutions in the SPAG-2 reservoir daily. Also, if the liquid level is low, discard before new drug solution is added.
7. The dose and administration schedule for infants who require mechanical ventilation are the same as for those who do not.
8. For nonmechanically ventilated infants, the aerosol is delivered to an infant oxygen hood from the SPAG-2 aerosol generator. If a hood cannot be used, the aerosol is given by face mask or oxygen tent. However, due to the larger size of a tent, the delivery dynamics may be altered.
9. Store reconstituted solutions at room temperature for 24 hr.
10. Women of childbearing age are not to administer the drug. *Post* this advisement so they do not come in contact with the drug.
### Interventions
1. Health care workers administering drug should use goggles and respirator to protect mucous membranes; remove contact lens, and monitor exposure times. Review side effects related to drug administration.
2. It is essential that constant monitoring be undertaken for both the fluid and respiratory status of the client.
3. Assess frequently for evidence of respiratory distress; stop therapy and report if distress occurs. Do not leave child unattended and unstimulated in the tent for long periods.
4. Monitor and record VS and I&O.
5. Anticipate limited use in infants and adults with COPD or asthma.
6. With prolonged therapy assess for anemia; monitor CBC values.
**Outcomes/Evaluate:** Improved airway exchange; resolution of RSV pneumonia

## Rifabutin
(**rif**-ah-**BYOU**-tin)
**Pregnancy Category:** B
Mycobutin **(Rx)**
**Classification:** Antitubercular drug

**Action/Kinetics:** Inhibits DNA-dependent RNA polymerase in susceptible strains of *Escherichia coli* and *Bacillus subtilis*. Rapidly absorbed from the GI tract. **Peak plasma levels after a single dose:** 3.3 hr. **Mean terminal t½:** 45 hr. About 85% is bound to plasma proteins. High-fat meals slow the rate, but not the extent, of absorption. About 30% of a dose is excreted in the feces and 53% in the urine, primarily as metabolites. The 25-O-desacetyl metabolite is equal in activity to rifabutin.
**Uses:** Prevention of disseminated *Mycobacterium avium* complex (MAC) disease in clients with advanced HIV infection.
**Contraindications:** Hypersensitivity to rifabutin or other rifamycins (e.g., rifampin). Use in clients with active tuberculosis. Lactation.
**Special Concerns:** Safety and efficacy have not been determined in children, although the drug has been used in HIV-positive children.
**Side Effects:** *GI:* Anorexia, abdominal pain, diarrhea, dyspepsia, eructation, flatulence, N&V, taste perversion. *Respiratory:* Chest pain, chest

pressure or pain with dyspnea. *CNS:* Insomnia, **seizures,** paresthesia, aphasia, confusion. *Musculoskeletal:* Asthenia, myalgia, arthralgia, myositis. *Body as a whole:* Fever, headache, generalized pain, flu-like syndrome. *Dermatologic:* Rash, skin discoloration. *Hematologic:* Neutropenia, leukopenia, anemia, eosinophilia, thrombocytopenia. *Miscellaneous:* Discolored urine, nonspecific T wave changes on ECG, hepatitis, hemolysis, uveitis.

**OD** **Overdose Management:** *Symptoms:* Worsening of side effects. *Treatment:* Gastric lavage followed by instillation into the stomach of an activated charcoal slurry.

**Drug Interactions:** Rifabutin has liver enzyme-inducing properties and may be expected to have similar interactions as does rifampin. However, rifabutin is a less potent enzyme inducer than rifampin.

*AZT* / ↓ Steady-state plasma levels of AZT after repeated rifabutin dosing

*Oral contraceptives* / Rifabutin may ↓ the effectiveness of oral contraceptives

**Laboratory Test Interferences:** ↑ AST, ALT, alkaline phosphatase.

**Dosage** ⎯⎯⎯⎯⎯⎯⎯⎯⎯⎯
• **Capsules**
*Prophylaxis of MAC disease in clients with advanced HIV infection.*
**Adults:** 300 mg/day.

## NURSING CONSIDERATIONS

See also *General Nursing Considerations for All Anti-Infectives.*
**Administration/Storage**
1. Give doses of 150 mg b.i.d. with food if N&V or other GI upset occurs.
2. Urine, feces, saliva, sputum, perspiration, tears, and skin may be colored brown-orange. Soft contact lenses may be permanently stained.
**Assessment**
1. Document indications for therapy, noting type, onset, and characteristics of symptoms.
2. Monitor CBC for neutropenia.

3. Ensure that CXR, PPD, and sputum AFB cultures have been performed to rule out active tuberculosis. Clients who develop active tuberculosis during therapy must be covered with appropriate antituberculosis medications.
**Client/Family Teaching**
1. If N&V or other GI upset occurs, may take doses of 150 mg b.i.d. with food.
2. Urine, feces, saliva, sputum, perspiration, tears, skin, and mucous membranes may be colored brown-orange. Soft contact lenses may be permanently stained.
3. Any S&S of muscle or eye pain, irritation, or inflammation should be reported.
4. Report any persistent vomiting or abnormal bruising or bleeding.
5. Practice nonhormonal form of birth control.
**Outcomes/Evaluate:** Prevention of disseminated *Mycobacterium avium* complex (MAC) with advanced HIV

# Rifampin
(rih-**FAM**-pin)
**Pregnancy Category:** C
Rifadin, Rimactane, Rofact ✦ **(Rx)**
**Classification:** Primary antitubercular agent

**Action/Kinetics:** Semisynthetic antibiotic derived from *Streptomyces mediterranei.* Suppresses RNA synthesis by binding to the beta subunit of DNA dependent RNA polymerase. This prevents attachment of the enzyme to DNA and blockade of RNA transcription. Both bacteriostatic and bactericidal; most active against rapidly replicating organisms. Well absorbed from the GI tract; widely distributed in body tissues. **Peak plasma concentration:** 4–32 mcg/mL after 2–4 hr. **t½:** 1.5–5 hr (higher in clients with hepatic impairment). In normal clients t½ decreases with usage. Metabolized in liver; 60% is excreted in feces.
**Uses:** All types of tuberculosis. Must be used in conjunction with at least

**R**

one other tuberculostatic drug (such as isoniazid, ethambutol, pyrazinamide) but is the drug of choice for retreatment. Also for treatment of asymptomatic meningococcal carriers to eliminate *Neisseria meningitidis. Investigational:* Used in combination for infections due to *Staphylococcus aureus* and *S. epidermidis* (endocarditis, osteomyelitis, prostatitis); Legionnaire's disease; in combination with dapsone for leprosy; prophylaxis of meningitis due to *Haemophilus influenzae* and gram-negative bacteremia in infants.

**Contraindications:** Hypersensitivity; not recommended for intermittent therapy.

**Special Concerns:** Safe use during lactation has not been established. Safety and effectiveness not determined in children less than 5 years of age. Use with extreme caution in clients with hepatic dysfunction.

**Side Effects:** *GI:* N&V, diarrhea, anorexia, gas, pseudomembranous colitis, pancreatitis, sore mouth and tongue, cramps, heartburn, flatulence. *CNS:* Headache, drowsiness, fatigue, ataxia, dizziness, confusion, generalized numbness, fever, difficulty in concentrating. *Hepatic:* Jaundice, hepatitis. Increases in AST, ALT, bilirubin, alkaline phosphatase. *Hematologic:* Thrombocytopenia, eosinophilia, hemolysis, leukopenia, **hemolytic anemia.** *Allergic:* Flu-like symptoms, dyspnea, wheezing, SOB, purpura, pruritus, urticaria, skin rashes, sore mouth and tongue, conjunctivitis. *Renal:* Hematuria, hemoglobinuria, renal insufficiency, acute renal failure. *Miscellaneous:* Visual disturbances, muscle weakness or pain, arthralgia, decreased BP, osteomalacia, menstrual disturbances, edema of face and extremities, adrenocortical insufficiency, increases in BUN and serum uric acid. *NOTE:* Body fluids and feces may be red-orange.

**OD** **Overdose Management:** *Symptoms:* Shortly after ingestion, N&V, and lethargy will occur. Followed by severe hepatic involvement (liver enlargement with tenderness, increased direct and total bilirubin, change in hepatic enzymes) with unconsciousness. Also, brownish red or orange discoloration of urine, saliva, tears, sweat, skin, and feces. *Treatment:* Gastric lavage followed by activated charcoal slurry introduced into the stomach. Antiemetics to control N&V. Forced diuresis to enhance excretion. If hepatic function is seriously impaired, bile drainage may be required. Extracorporeal hemodialysis may be necessary.

**Drug Interactions**
*Acetaminophen* / ↓ Effect of acetaminophen due to ↑ breakdown by liver
*Aminophylline* / ↓ Effect of aminophylline due to ↑ breakdown by liver
*Anticoagulants, oral* / ↓ Effect of anticoagulants due to ↑ breakdown by liver
*Antidiabetics, oral* / ↓ Effect of oral antidiabetic due to ↑ breakdown by liver
*Barbiturates* / ↓ Effect of barbiturates due to ↑ breakdown by liver
*Benzodiazepines* / ↓ Effect of benzodiazepines due to ↑ breakdown by liver
*Beta-adrenergic blocking agents* / ↓ Effect of beta-blocking agents due to ↑ breakdown by liver
*Chloramphenicol* / ↓ Effect of chloramphenicol due to ↑ breakdown by liver
*Clofibrate* / ↓ Effect of clofibrate due to ↑ breakdown by liver
*Contraceptives, oral* / ↓ Effect of oral contraceptives due to ↑ breakdown by liver
*Corticosteroids* / ↓ Effect of corticosteroids due to ↑ breakdown by liver
*Cyclosporine* / ↓ Effect of cyclosporine due to ↑ breakdown by liver
*Digitoxin* / ↓ Effect of digitoxin due to ↑ breakdown by liver
*Digoxin* / ↓ Serum levels of digoxin
*Disopyramide* / ↓ Effect of disopyramide due to ↑ breakdown by liver
*Estrogens* / ↓ Effect of estrogens due to ↑ breakdown by liver
*Halothane* / ↑ Risk of hepatotoxicity and hepatic encephalopathy

*Hydantoins* / ↓ Effect of hydantoins due to ↑ breakdown by liver

*Isoniazid* / ↑ Risk of hepatotoxicity

*Ketoconazole* / ↓ Effect of either ketoconazole or rifampin

*Methadone* / ↓ Effect of methadone due to ↑ breakdown by liver

*Mexiletine* / ↓ Effect of mexiletine due to ↑ breakdown by liver

*Quinidine* / ↓ Effect of quinidine due to ↑ breakdown by liver

*Sulfones* / ↓ Effect of sulfones due to ↑ breakdown by liver

*Theophylline* / ↓ Effect of theophylline due to ↑ breakdown by liver

*Tocainide* / ↓ Effect of tocainide due to ↑ breakdown by liver

*Verapamil* / ↓ Effect of verapamil due to ↑ breakdown by liver

**Laboratory Test Interferences:** ↑ AST, ALT, alkaline phosphatase, BUN, bilirubin, uric acid, BSP retention values. False + Coombs' test.

## Dosage

• **Capsules, IV**

*Pulmonary tuberculosis.*

**Adults:** Single dose of 600 mg/day; **children over 5 years:** 10–20 mg/kg/day, not to exceed 600 mg/day.

*Meningococcal carriers.*

**Adults:** 600 mg b.i.d. for 2 days; **children:** 10–20 mg/kg q 12 hr for four doses. Dosage should not exceed 600 mg/day.

## NURSING CONSIDERATIONS

See also *General Nursing Considerations for All Anti-Infectives.*

**Administration/Storage**

1. Administer capsules once daily 1 hr before or 2 hr after meals to ensure maximum absorption.

2. A PO suspension (10 mg/mL) may be prepared as follows: The contents of either four 300-mg rifampin capsules or eight 150-mg capsules are emptied into a 4-oz amber glass bottle. Add 20 mL of simple syrup; shake vigorously; then add 100 mL of simple syrup and shake again. The suspension is stable for 4 weeks when stored at room temperature or in the refrigerator.

3. Check to be sure that there is a desiccant in the bottle containing capsules of rifampin because these are relatively moisture sensitive.

4. If administered concomitantly with PAS, give drugs 8–12 hr apart because the acid interferes with the absorption of rifampin.

5. When used for tuberculosis, continue therapy for 6–9 months.

**IV** 6. Reconstitute 600-mg vial using 10 mL of sterile water for injection. Gently swirl vial to dissolve. The resultant solution contains 60 mg/mL rifampin; it is stable at room temperature for 24 hr.

7. Add the volume of reconstituted solution needed to 500 mL of D5W and infuse over 3 hr, or it may be added to 100 mL D5W and infused over 30 min. Sterile saline may be used when dextrose is contraindicated; however, the stability of rifampin is slightly less.

8. The diluted solution must be used within 4 hr or drug may precipitate from solution.

9. Injectable solution appears dark reddish brown.

**Assessment**

1. Note indications for therapy, type, onset, and duration of symptoms.

2. List any previous therapy.

3. Monitor CBC, liver and renal function studies, and cultures; note impaired liver or renal function and blood dyscrasias.

4. Document any GI disturbances or auditory nerve impairment.

5. Obtain baseline CXR; auscultate and document lung sounds and characteristics of sputum. Note PPD skin test results.

**Client/Family Teaching**

1. Take drug on an empty stomach 1 hr before or 2 hr after meals; report if GI upset occurs.

2. Must take daily for months to effectively treat tuberculosis. Do not stop taking or skip doses of medication.

3. Avoid alcohol; increases risk of liver toxicity.

R

---

4. Headache, drowsiness, confusion, fever, and muscle and joint aches may occur during the first few weeks of therapy; report if symptoms persist or increase in intensity.

5. Rifampin may impart a red-orange color to urine, feces, saliva, sputum, and tears; contact lenses may become *permanently* discolored.

6. Practice alternative birth control since oral contraceptives may not be effective; drug has teratogenic properties.

**Outcomes/Evaluate**
- Adjunct in treating tuberculosis
- Prophylaxis of meningitis due to *H. influenzae* and gram-negative bacteremia in infants

———COMBINATION DRUG———

# Rifampin and Isoniazid
(rih-**FAM**-pin/**eye**-soh-**NYE**-ah-zid)
**Pregnancy Category:** C
Rifamate, Rimactane/INH Dual Pack
**(Rx)**
**Classification:** Antitubercular drug combination

See also *Rifampin* and *Isoniazid*.
**Content:** Each capsule contains the following antituberculosis drugs: rifampin, 300 mg, and isoniazid, 150 mg.
**Uses:** Pulmonary tuberculosis following completion of initial therapy. Concomitant treatment with pyridoxine is recommended in malnourished clients, in those predisposed to neuropathy (e.g., alcoholics, diabetics), and in adolescents.
**Contraindications:** To treat meningococcal infections or asymptomatic carriers of *Neisseria meningitidis* to eliminate meningococci from the nasopharynx. In those who have previous isoniazid-induced hepatic injury or who have had severe side effects to isoniazid.
**Special Concerns:** Use with caution in impaired liver function, as rifampin and isoniazid can cause liver dysfunction and fatal hepatitis, respectively. Use with caution, if at all, during lactation.
**Side Effects:** See individual entries for Rifampin and Isoniazid.

**Dosage** ————
- **Capsules**
  *Pulmonary tuberculosis.*
  **Adults:** Two capsules once daily.

## NURSING CONSIDERATIONS

See also *Nursing Considerations* for *Rifampin* and *Isoniazid*.
**Assessment**
1. Document symptom onset, source of contact, other agents prescribed.
2. Note previous experience with this drug. Renal hypersensitivity has been reported when therapy was resumed after interruption.
3. Note any alcohol abuse, liver or renal dysfunction.
4. Monitor CBC, CXR, and liver and renal function studies.
**Client/Family Teaching**
1. Take exactly as prescribed (should be taken either 1 hr before or 2 hr after a meal); do not skip doses or share medications.
2. Body secretions (urine, feces, tears, sputum, sweat) and skin may become discolored orange-red. Soft contact lenses may become permanently stained.
3. Report any numbness or tingling in hands and feet (S&S of peripheral neuropathy or toxicity). Coadministration of pyridoxine may help prevent CNS toxic effects.
4. Symptoms of fatigue, weakness, malaise, N&V, and anorexia (symptoms of hepatitis) should be reported immediately.
5. Oral contraceptives may not work; drug is teratogenic.
6. Therapy will be continued until bacterial conversion and maximal improvement is noted.
**Outcomes/Evaluate:** Successful treatment and resolution of tubercle bacilli

———COMBINATION DRUG———

# Rifampin, Isoniazid, and Pyrazinamide
(rih-**FAM**-pin/**eye**-soh-**NYE**-ah-zid/pie-rah-**ZIN**-ah-myd)
**Pregnancy Category:** C
Rifater **(Rx)**
**Classification:** Antitubercular drug combination

See also *Rifampin* and *Isoniazid.*
**Content:** Each tablet contains the following antituberculosis drugs: rifampin, 120 mg; isoniazid, 50 mg; and pyrazinamide, 300 mg.
**Uses:** Initial phase of the short-course (2-month) treatment of pulmonary tuberculosis. Either streptomycin or ethambutol may be added unless the likelihood of resistance to isoniazid or rifampin is low. Concomitant treatment with pyridoxine is recommended in malnourished client's, in those predisposed to neuropathy (e.g., alcoholics, diabetics), and in adolescents. The 2-month treatment with Rifater is followed by a 4-month course of therapy with rifampin and isoniazid (Rifamate).
**Contraindications:** Hypersensitivity to any of the components. Severe hepatic damage, acute gout. Lactation.
**Special Concerns:** Use with caution in impaired liver function, as rifampin and isoniazid can cause liver dysfunction and fatal hepatitis, respectively. Use with caution in diabetes mellitus. Safety and efficacy have not been determined in children less than 15 years of age.
**Side Effects:** For side effects caused by isoniazid or rifampin, consult those drug entries. The side effects due to pyrazinamide follow. *Hepatic:* Hepatotoxicity, porphyria. *GI:* N&V, anorexia. *Hematologic:* Thrombocytopenia, sideroblastic anemia with erythroid hyperplasia, vacuolation of erythrocytes, and increased serum concentration. *Hypersensitivity:* Rashes, urticaria, pruritus. *Miscellaneous:* Hyperuricemia, gout, mild arthralgia and myalgia, fever, acne, photosensitivity, dysuria, interstitial nephritis.

**Dosage**
• **Tablets**
*Short-course treatment of pulmonary tuberculosis.*
**Clients weighing less than 44 kg:** 4 tablets/day given at the same time.
**Clients weighing 45–54 kg:** 5 tablets/day given at the same time. **Cli-**ents weighing more than 55 kg:** 6 tablets/day given at the same time.

## NURSING CONSIDERATIONS

See also *Nursing Considerations* for *Rifampin* and *Isoniazid.*
**Administration/Storage**
1. Intended for use during the first 2 months of therapy.
2. Protect tablets from excessive humidity and store at room temperature.
**Assessment**
1. Document symptom onset, source of contact, other agents prescribed.
2. Monitor CBC, CXR, serum uric acid, and liver function studies.
3. Note any alcohol abuse, liver or renal dysfunction.
4. Assess those with preexisting liver disease or those at risk for drug-related hepatitis (e.g., alcoholics) closely. The drug should be withdrawn if signs of hepatocellular damage or hyperuricemia accompanied by an acute gouty arthritis occur. However, if hyperuricemia accompanied by an acute gouty arthritis occurs without liver dysfunction, can transfer to a regimen that does not contain pyrazinamide.
**Client/Family Teaching**
1. Take tablets either 1 hr before or 2 hr after a meal with a full glass of water and 1 hr before antacids.
2. Therapy is short-term (2 months) and will be followed by a 4-month course of rifamate.
3. Avoid tyramine- (cheese, red wine) and histamine- (skipjack, tuna, other tropical fish) containing foods.
4. Drug contains rifampin, which may cause a red-orange discoloration to body secretions (sweat, sputum, urine, feces, tears) and skin. Soft contact lenses may become permanently stained.
5. Report any numbness or tingling in hands and feet; suggestive of peripheral neuropathy or toxicity. Coadministration of pyridoxine may help prevent CNS toxic effects.

**R**

***bold italic*** = life threatening side effect

6. Symptoms of fatigue, weakness, malaise, N&V, and anorexia (symptoms of hepatitis) should be reported.
7. Avoid alcohol or any alcohol-containing products.

**Outcomes/Evaluate:** Treatment of pulmonary tuberculosis/resolution of tubercle bacilli infection.

# Riluzole

((**RIL**-you-zohl))
**Pregnancy Category:** C
Rilutek **(Rx)**
**Classification:** Drug for amyotrophic lateral sclerosis

**Action/Kinetics:** Mechanism not known. Possible effects include (a) inhibition of glutamate release, (b) inactivation of voltage-dependent sodium channels, and (c) interference with intracellular events that follow transmitter binding at excitatory amino acid receptors. Well absorbed following PO use; high-fat meals decrease absorption. **t½, elimination, after repeated doses:** 12 hr. About 96% is bound to plasma proteins. Extensively metabolized, mainly in the liver, and excreted in the urine.

**Uses:** Treatment of clients with ALS; the drug extends both survival and time to tracheostomy.

**Contraindications:** Lactation.

**Special Concerns:** Hepatic and renal impairment will decrease excretion and lead to higher plasma levels; thus, use with caution in these clients. Use with caution in the elderly, as age-related changes in renal and hepatic function may cause a decreased clearance. It has been noted that clearance of riluzole in Japanese clients is 50% lower compared with Caucasians; clearance may also be lower in women. Safety and efficacy have not been determined in children.

**Side Effects:** Side effects listed occurred at a frequency of 0.1% or more. *GI:* N&V, diarrhea, anorexia, abdominal pain, dyspepsia, flatulence, dry mouth, stomatitis, tooth disorder, oral moniliasis, dysphagia, constipation, increased appetite, intestinal obstruction, fecal impaction, *GI hemorrhage,* GI ulceration, gastritis, fecal incontinence, jaundice, hepatitis, glossitis, gum hemorrhage, pancreatitis, tenesmus, esophageal stenosis. *Body as a whole:* Asthenia, malaise, weight loss or gain, peripheral edema, flu syndrome, hostility, abscess, *sepsis,* photosensitivity reaction, cellulitis, facial edema, hernia, peritonitis, reaction at injection site, chills, *attempted suicide,* enlarged abdomen, neoplasm. *CNS:* Dizziness (more common in women), vertigo, somnolence, circumoral paresthesia, headache, aggravation reaction, hypertonia, depression, insomnia, agitation, tremor, hallucination, personality disorders, abnormal thinking, coma, paranoid reaction, manic reaction, ataxia, extrapyramidal syndrome, hypokinesis, emotional lability, delusions, apathy, hypesthesia, incoordination, confusion, *convulsion,* amnesia, increased libido, stupor subdural hematoma, abnormal gait, delirium, depersonalization, facial paralysis, hemiplegia, decreased libido. *CV:* Hypertension, tachycardia, phlebitis, palpitation, postural hypotension, *heart arrest, heart failure,* syncope, hypotension, migraine, peripheral vascular disease, angina pectoris, *MI,* ventricular extrasystoles, *cerebral hemorrhage,* atrial fibrillation, bundle branch block, CHF, pericarditis, lower extremity embolus, *myocardial ischemia, shock.* Hematologic: Neutropenia, anemia, leukocytosis, leukopenia, ecchymosis. *Respiratory:* Decreased lung function, pneumonia, rhinitis, increased cough, sinusitis, apnea, bronchitis, dyspnea, respiratory disorder, increased sputum, hiccup, pleural disorder, asthma, epistaxis, hemoptysis, yawn, hyperventilation, lung edema, hypoventilation, *lung carcinoma,* hypoxia, laryngitis, pleural effusion, pneumothorax, respiratory moniliasis, stridor. *Musculoskeletal:* Arthralgia, back pain, leg cramps, dysarthria, myoclonus, arthrosis, myasthenia, *bone neoplasm.* GU: Urinary retention, urinary urgency,

R

urine abnormality, urinary incontinence, kidney calculus, hematuria, impotence, *prostate carcinoma,* kidney pain, metrorrhagia, priapism. *Dermatologic:* Pruritus, eczema, alopecia, exfoliative dermatitis, skin ulceration, urticaria, psoriasis, seborrhea, skin disorder, fungal dermatitis. *Metabolic:* Gout, respiratory acidosis, edema, thirst, hypokalemia, hyponatremia. *Miscellaneous:* Accidental or intentional injury, *death,* diabetes mellitus, thyroid neoplasia, amblyopia, ophthalmitis.

**Drug Interactions**
*Amitriptyline* / ↓ Elimination of riluzole → higher plasma levels
*Caffeine* / ↓ Elimination of riluzole → higher plasma levels
*Charcoal-broiled foods* / ↑ Elimination of riluzole → lower plasma levels
*Omeprazole* / ↑ Elimination of riluzole → lower plasma levels
*Quinolones* / ↓ Elimination of riluzole → higher plasma levels
*Rifampin* / ↑ Elimination of riluzole → lower plasma levels
*Smoking (cigarettes)* / ↑ Elimination of riluzole → lower plasma levels
*Theophyllines* / ↓ Elimination of riluzole → higher plasma levels

**Laboratory Test Interferences:** ↑ Gamma glutamyl transferase, alkaline phosphatase, gamma globulins. Abnormal liver function tests, + direct Coombs' test.

**Dosage** ————————
• **Tablets**
*Treatment of ALS.*
50 mg q 12 hr. Higher daily doses will not increase the beneficial effect but will increase the incidence of side effects.

## NURSING CONSIDERATIONS
### Administration/Storage
1. Take 1 hr before or 2 hr after a meal to avoid decreased bioavailability. Take at the same time each day. If a dose is missed, take the next tablet as originally planned.
2. Protect from bright light.

**Assessment**
1. Document symptom onset, presentation, ethnic background, and familial associations.
2. Assess renal and liver function tests. Elevations of several liver functions, especially bilirubin, should preclude the use of riluzole.
3. Monitor serum aminotransferases (including SGPT). SGPT levels should be measured every month during the first 3 months of therapy, every 3 months for the remainder of the first year, and then periodically.

**Client/Family Teaching**
1. Take 1 hr before or 2 hr after meals to maintain drug bioavailability.
2. Take as prescribed at the same time each day. Do not double up if dose is missed or forgotten.
3. Report any febrile illnesses.
4. Drug may cause dizziness, drowsiness, or vertigo. Do not perform activities that require mental alertness until drug effects realized.
5. Severe dry mouth symptoms may require use of salagen.
6. Avoid alcohol, as alcohol may potentiate liver toxicity.

**Outcomes/Evaluate:** Extension of survival or time to tracheostomy with ALS

# Rimantadine hydrochloride
(rih-**MAN**-tih-deen)
**Pregnancy Category:** C
Flumadine **(Rx)**
**Classification:** Antiviral agent

See also *Antiviral Drugs* and *Amantadine.*

**Action/Kinetics:** May act early in the viral replication cycle, possibly by inhibiting the uncoating of the virus. A virus protein specified by the virion $M_2$ gene may play an important role in the inhibition of the influenza A virus by rimantadine. Has little or no activity against influenza B virus. Plasma trough levels following 100 mg b.i.d. for 10 days range from 118 to 468 ng/mL;

R

however, levels are higher in clients over the age of 70 years. Metabolized in the liver, and both unchanged drug (25%) and metabolites excreted through the urine.

**Uses:** In adults for prophylaxis and treatment of illness caused by strains of influenza A virus. In children for prophylaxis against influenza A virus.

**Contraindications:** Hypersensitivity to amantadine, rimantadine, or other drugs in the adamantine class. Use during lactation.

**Special Concerns:** Use with caution in clients with renal or hepatic insufficiency. An increased incidence of seizures is possible in clients with a history of epilepsy who have received amantadine. Influenza A virus strains resistant to rimantadine can emerge during treatment and be transmitted, causing symptoms of influenza. Safety and efficacy of rimantadine in the treatment of symptomatic influenza infections in children have not been established. Safety and efficacy for prophylaxis of infections have not been determined in children less than 1 year of age. The incidence of side effects in geriatric clients is higher than in other clients.

**Side Effects:** GI and CNS side effects are the most common. *GI:* N&V, anorexia, dry mouth, abdominal pain, diarrhea, dyspepsia, constipation, dysphagia, stomatitis. *CNS:* Insomnia, dizziness, headache, nervousness, fatigue, asthenia, impairment of concentration, ataxia, somnolence, agitation, depression, gait abnormality, euphoria, hyperkinesia, tremor, hallucinations, confusion, *convulsions,* agitation, diaphoresis, hypesthesia. *Respiratory:* Dyspnea, *bronchospasm,* cough. *CV:* Pallor, palpitation, hypertension, *cerebrovascular disorder, cardiac failure,* pedal edema, heart block, tachycardia, syncope. *Miscellaneous:* Tinnitus, taste loss or change, parosmia, eye pain, rash, nonpuerperal lactation, increased lacrimation, increased frequency of micturition, fever, rigors.

**OD** **Overdose Management:** *Symptoms:* Extensions of side effects including the possibility of agitation, hallucinations, *cardiac arrhythmias, and death. Treatment:* Supportive therapy. IV physostigmine at doses of 1–2 mg IV in adults and 0.5 mg in children, not to exceed 2 mg/hr, has been reported to be beneficial in treating overdose for amantadine (a related drug).

**Drug Interactions**
*Acetaminophen* / ↓ Peak concentration and area under the curve for rimantadine
*Aspirin* / ↓ Peak plasma levels and area under the curve for rimantadine
*Cimetidine* / ↓ Clearance of rimantadine

**Dosage** ———————————
• **Syrup, Tablets**
    *Prophylaxis.*
**Adults and children over 10 years of age:** 100 mg b.i.d. In clients with severe hepatic dysfunction ($C_{CR} < 10$ mL/min) and in elderly nursing home clients, the dose should be reduced to 100 mg/day. **Children, less than 10 years of age:** 5 mg/kg once daily, not to exceed a total dose of 150 mg/day.
    *Treatment.*
**Adults:** 100 mg b.i.d. In clients with severe hepatic dysfunction and in elderly nursing home clients, reduce the dose to 100 mg/day.

---

## NURSING CONSIDERATIONS

See also *Nursing Considerations* for *Amantadine.*

**Administration/Storage:** For treatment of influenza A virus infections, initiate therapy as soon as possible, preferably within 48 hr after onset of S&S. Continue treatment for approximately 7 days from the initial onset of symptoms.

**Assessment**
1. Document indications for therapy, noting onset and duration of symptoms or exposure.
2. Determine if immunized.
3. List other drugs prescribed to ensure none interact unfavorably.

4. Assess liver and renal function studies to determine any dysfunction; reduce dosage with severe hepatic dysfunction and with elderly nursing home clients.

5. Note any epilepsy; assess for loss of seizure control.

**Client/Family Teaching**

1. Take only as directed; do not share meds.

2. Initiate as soon as symptoms appear and continue for 7 days.

3. Drug may cause dizziness.

4. Early annual vaccination is the method of choice for influenza prophylaxis. The 2- to 4-week time frame required to develop an antibody response can be managed with rimantadine.

**Outcomes/Evaluate:** Prevention/management of influenza A virus

---

# Risperidone
(ris-**PAIR**-ih-dohn)
**Pregnancy Category:** C
Risperdal **(Rx)**
**Classification:** Antipsychotic

---

**Action/Kinetics:** Mechanism may be due to a combination of antagonism of dopamine ($D_2$) and serotonin (5-$HT_2$) receptors. Also has high affinity for the alpha-1, alpha-2, and histamine-1 receptors. Metabolized significantly in the liver to the active metabolite 9-hydroxyrisperidone, which has equal receptor-binding activity as risperidone. Thus, the effect is likely due to both the parent compound and the metabolite. Food does not affect either the rate or extent of absorption. The ability to convert risperidone to 9-hydroxyrisperidone is subject to genetic variation. A low percentage of Asians have the ability to metabolize the drug. **Peak plasma levels, risperidone:** 1 hr; **peak plasma levels, 9-hydroxyrisperidone:** 3 hr for extensive metabolizers and 17 hr for poor metabolizers. **t½, risperidone and 9-methylrisperidone:** 3 and 21 hr, respectively, for extensive metabolizers and 20 and 30 hr,

respectively, for poor metabolizers. The clearance of the drug is decreased in geriatric clients and in clients with hepatic and renal impairment.

**Uses:** Treatment of psychotic disorders.

**Contraindications:** Lactation.

**Special Concerns:** Use with caution in clients with known CV disease (including history of MI or ischemia, heart failure, conduction abnormalities), cerebrovascular disease, and conditions that predispose the client to hypotension (e.g., dehydration, hypovolemia, use of antihypertensive drugs). Use with caution in clients who will be exposed to extreme heat or when taken with other CNS drugs or alcohol. The effectiveness of risperidone for more than 6–8 weeks has not been studied. Safety and effectiveness have not been established for children.

**Side Effects:** *Neuroleptic malignant syndrome:* Hyperpyrexia, muscle rigidity, altered mental status, autonomic instability (i.e., irregular pulse or BP, tachycardia, diaphoresis, cardiac dysrhythmia), elevated CPK, rhabdomyolysis, *acute renal failure, death. CNS:* Tardive dyskinesia (especially in geriatric clients), somnolence, insomnia, agitation, anxiety, aggressive reaction, extrapyramidal symptoms, headache, dizziness, increased dream activity, decreased sexual desire, nervousness, impaired concentration, depression, apathy, catatonia, euphoria, increased libido, amnesia, increased duration of sleep, dysarthria, vertigo, stupor, paresthesia, confusion. *GI:* Constipation, nausea, dyspepsia, vomiting, abdominal pain, increased or decreased salivation, toothache, anorexia, flatulence, diarrhea, increased appetite, stomatitis, melena, dysphagia, hemorrhoids, gastritis. *CV:* Prolongation of the QT interval that might lead to *torsades de pointes,*. Orthostatic hypotension, tachycardia, palpitation, hypertension or hypotension, *AV block, MI. Respiratory:*

---

Rhinitis, coughing, upper respiratory infection, sinusitis, pharyngitis, dyspnea. *Body as a whole:* Arthralgia, back pain, chest pain, fever, fatigue, rigors, malaise, edema, flu-like symptoms, increase or decrease in weight. *Hematologic:* Purpura, anemia, hypochromic anemia. *GU:* Polyuria, polydipsia, urinary incontinence, hematuria, dysuria, menorrhagia, orgastic dysfunction, dry vagina, erectile dysfunction, nonpuerperal lactation, amenorrhea, female breast pain, leukorrhea, mastitis, dysmenorrhea, female perineal pain, intermenstrual bleeding, *vaginal hemorrhage,* failure to ejaculate. *Dermatologic:* Rash, dry skin, seborrhea, increased pigmentation, increased or decreased sweating, acne, alopecia, hyperkeratosis, pruritus, skin exfoliation. *Ophthalmic:* Abnormal vision, abnormal accommodation, xerophthalmia. *Miscellaneous:* Increased prolactin, photosensitivity, diabetes mellitus, thirst, myalgia, epistaxis.

**OD** **Overdose Management:** *Symptoms:* Exaggeration of known effects, especially drowsiness, sedation, tachycardia, hypotension, and extrapyramidal symptoms. *Treatment:* Establish and secure airway, and ensure adequate oxygenation and ventilation. Follow gastric lavage with activated charcoal and a laxative. Monitor CV system, including continuous ECG readings. Provide general supportive measures. Hypotension and circulatory collapse can be treated with IV fluids or sympathomimetic drugs; however, do not use epinephrine and dopamine, as beta stimulation may worsen hypotension due to risperidone-induced alpha blockade. Anticholinergic drugs can be given for severe extrapyramidal symptoms.

**Drug Interactions**
*Carbamazepine* / ↑ Clearance of risperidone following chronic use of carbamazepine
*Clozapine* / ↓ Clearance of risperidone following chronic use of clozapine

*Levodopa* / Risperidone antagonizes the effects of levodopa and dopamine agonists
**Laboratory Test Interferences:** ↑ CPK, serum prolactin, AST, ALT. Hyponatremia.

**Dosage**
• **Oral Solution, Tablets**
 *Antipsychotic.*
**Adults, initial:** 1 mg b.i.d. Once daily dosing can also be used. Can be increased by 1 mg b.i.d. on the second and third days, as tolerated, to reach a dose of 3 mg b.i.d. by the third day. Further increases in dose should occur at intervals of about 1 week. **Maximal effect:** 4–6 mg/day. Doses greater than 6 mg/day were not shown to be more effective and were associated with greater incidence of side effects. Safety of doses greater than 16 mg/day have not been studied. The initial dose is 0.5 mg b.i.d. for clients who are elderly or debilitated, those with severe renal or hepatic impairment, and those predisposed to hypotension or in whom hypotension would pose a risk. Dosage increases in these clients should be in increments of 0.5 mg b.i.d. Dosage increases above 1.5 mg b.i.d. should occur at intervals of about 1 week.

## NURSING CONSIDERATIONS

See also *Nursing Considerations* for *Antipsychotic Drugs.*
**Administration/Storage**
1. Use a lower starting dose in geriatric clients and those with impaired renal or hepatic function. The PO solution may ease administration to geriatric clients and those in an acute-care setting.
2. When restarting clients who have had an interval of risperidone, follow the initial 3-day dose titration schedule.
3. If switching from other antipsychotic drugs to risperidone, immediate discontinuation of the previous antipsychotic drug is recommended when starting risperidone therapy. When switching from a depot antipsychotic injection, initiate risperidone

in place of the next scheduled injection.

**Assessment**

1. Document indications for therapy; note onset and duration as well as presenting behavioral manifestations and mental status.

2. Perform appropriate baseline assessments. Electrolyte imbalance, bradycardia, and concomitant administration with drugs that prolong the QT interval may increase the risk of torsades de pointes.

3. Reduce dose with severe liver, cardiac, or renal dysfunction.

4. Note any history of drug dependency.

5. Observe for altered mental status, muscle rigidity, dyskinetic movements, or overt changes in VS.

6. The antiemetic effect of risperidone may mask the S&S of overdose with certain drugs or conditions such as intestinal obstruction, Reye's syndrome, and brain tumor.

**Client/Family Teaching**

1. Take only as directed; do not share meds or stop abruptly.

2. Drug may impair judgment, motor skills, and thinking and cause blurred vision; determine drug effects before engaging in activities that require mental alertness.

3. Rise slowly from a lying to a sitting position and dangle legs before standing, as drug may cause orthostatic hypotension.

4. May alter temperature regulation; avoid exposure to extreme heat.

5. Wear protective clothing, sunscreen, hat, and sunglasses when sun exposure is necessary; may cause a photosensitivity reaction.

6. Report any abnormal bruising or bleeding or yellow skin discoloration.

7. Practice birth control. Report if pregnancy is suspected or desired.

8. Avoid alcohol and any other OTC agents or CNS depressants.

9. Risperidone elevates serum prolactin levels. Explore the potential relationship of prolactin and human breast cancer development; report

any evidence or history of breast cancer.

10. Any suicide ideations or bizarre behavior should be reported immediately. Due to the possibility of suicide attempts with schizophrenia, advise that close supervision of high-risk clients is necessary and that prescriptions will be written for the smallest quantity of tablets. Stress importance of close F/U.

**Outcomes/Evaluate:** Improved behavior patterns with ↓ agitation, ↓ hyperactivity, and reality orientation

# Ritodrine hydrochloride
(**RYE**-toe-dreen)
**Pregnancy Category:** B
Ritodrine HCl in 5% Dextrose, Yutopar
**(Rx)**
**Classification:** Uterine relaxant

**Action/Kinetics:** Stimulates beta-2 receptors of smooth muscle of the uterus, which results in inhibition of uterine contractility. May also directly inhibit the actin-myosin interaction. Beta-adrenergic blocking agents inhibit the drug. Increased blood levels of insulin, glucose, and free fatty acids and decreased levels of potassium have been observed during IV infusion. **Onset, IV:** 5 min. **Peak plasma concentration, IV:** After a 9-mg infusion over 60 min, 32–50 ng/mL; **PO:** after a dose of 10 mg, 5–15 ng/mL. **Time to peak serum levels:** 20–60 min. $t\frac{1}{2}$, **after IV:** 15–17 hr. Ninety percent of drug excreted within 24 hr through the urine.

**Uses:** Management of preterm labor in selected clients after week 20 of gestation. When indicated, initiate therapy as early as possible after diagnosis. However, decision to use ritodrine should include determination of fetal maturity.

**Contraindications:** Before week 20 of pregnancy and when continuation of pregnancy is hazardous to mother (e.g., eclampsia, severe preeclampsia, intrauterine fetal death, antepartum hemorrhage, pulmonary

R

hypertension, chorioamnionitis, and maternal hyperthyroidism, cardiac disease or uncontrolled diabetes mellitus). Also, medical conditions (e.g., uncontrolled hypertension, pheochromocytoma, bronchial asthma, hypovolemia, cardiac arrhythmias due to tachycardia or digitalis toxicity) that would be aggravated by beta-adrenergic agonists. Use in diabetics.

**Special Concerns:** Maternal pulmonary edema has been noted in women treated with ritodrine. The use in advanced labor (i.e., greater than 4 cm cervical dilation or effacement greater than 80%) has not been established.

**Side Effects:** All effects are related to the stimulation of beta receptors by the drug. **IV.** C*V:* Increase in maternal and fetal HR, increase in maternal systolic and marked decrease in diastolic BP (widening of pulse pressure), persistent tachycardia (may indicate pulmonary edema), palpitations, *arrhythmias including ventricular tachycardia,* chest pain or tightness, angina, heart murmur, *myocardial ischemia.* Sinus bradycardia following drug withdrawal. *GI:* N&V, bloating, ileus, epigastric distress, diarrhea or constipation. *CNS:* Headache, migraine headache, tremors, malaise, nervousness, jitteriness, restlessness, anxiety, emotional changes, drowsiness, weakness. *Metabolic:* Transient increases in insulin and blood glucose, increases in cyclic AMP and free fatty acids, decrease in potassium, glycosuria, lactic acidosis. *Respiratory:* Dyspnea, *maternal pulmonary edema,* hyperventilation. *Hematologic:* Leukopenia or agranulocytosis after 2–3 weeks of IV therapy (leukocyte count returned to normal after cessation of drug). *Other:* Erythema, *anaphylactic shock,* rash, intrauterine growth retardation, hemolytic icterus, sweating, chills, impaired liver function. *NOTE:* Neonatal effects are infrequent but may include hypoglycemia and ileus; also, hypocalcemia and hypotension in neonates whose mothers were treated with other betamimetic drugs.

**OD** **Overdose Management:** *Symptoms:* Excessive beta-adrenergic stimulation, including tachycardia (in both the mother and fetus), palpitations, *cardiac arrhythmias,* hypotension, dyspnea, tremor, dyspnea, nervousness, N&V. *Treatment:* Supportive measures. A beta-adrenergic blocking agent can be used as an antidote. The drug is dialyzable.

**Drug Interactions**
*Anesthetics, general* / Additive hypotension or cardiac arrhythmias
*Atropine* / ↑ Systemic hypertension
*Beta-adrenergic blocking agents* / Inhibition of the effect of ritodrine
*Corticosteroids* / ↑ Risk of pulmonary edema
*Diazoxide* / Additive hypotension or cardiac arrhythmias
*Magnesium sulfate* / Additive hypotension or cardiac arrhythmias
*Meperidine* / Additive hypotension or cardiac arrhythmias
*Sympathomimetics* / Additive or potentiated effects of sympathomimetics

**Laboratory Test Interferences:** ↑ Plasma glucose and insulin; ↓ plasma potassium.

**Dosage** ————————
- **IV**
  *Preterm labor.*
**Initial:** 0.05 mg/min (10 gtt/min using microdrip chamber); **then,** depending on response, increase by 0.05 mg/min (10 microdrops/min) q 10 min until desired response occurs. **Effective dose range:** 0.15–0.35 mg/min (30–70 gtt/min). Continue infusion antepartum for a minimum of 12 hr after contractions cease.

## NURSING CONSIDERATIONS
### Administration/Storage
**IV** 1. Reconstitute with dextrose solution (150 mg in 500 mL). Final dilution will contain 0.3 mg/mL ritodrine. Avoid solutions containing NaCl, as their use increases the risk of pulmonary edema.
2. To minimize hypotension, admin-

ister IV dose while in the left lateral position.

3. Use a Y set-up, infusion pump, and microdrip tubing (60 microdrops/mL) for drug administration.

4. Do not use discolored solutions or those containing precipitate. Use diluted solution within 48 hr.

5. If other drugs must be given by the IV route, the use of piggyback or another IV site allows continued independent control of the infusion rate of ritodrine.

**Assessment**

1. Note characteristics, onset, and duration of contractions.

2. Assess for any preeclampsia, hypertension, or diabetes.

3. Determine that ultrasound and amniocentesis have been performed to establish fetal maturity. Establish gestational age prior to initiating drug therapy. Ritodrine should not be used before week 20.

**Interventions**

1. Avoid concomitant administration of beta-adrenergic blocking drugs; these inhibit action of ritodrine.

2. Assess response to IV therapy by evaluating strength and frequency of uterine contractions and by monitoring fetal HR; report increased fetal HR.

3. Monitor and record VS.

• Maintain BP by positioning in a left lateral position and evaluating level of hydration.

• Report any increase in SBP, decrease in DBP, and tachycardia.

4. Monitor I&O; auscultate lung sounds to assess fluid status.

5. Prevent circulatory overload. Closely monitor IV flow rate and infused volume.

6. Assess for any respiratory dysfunction (i.e., rales, dyspnea, frothy sputum) that may precede pulmonary edema, especially when also receiving corticosteroids.

7. Assess for S&S of electrolyte imbalance, esp. hypokalemia, hyperglycemia, and acidosis with diabetes.

8. Assess postpartum client who has received both ritodrine and general anesthetic for potentiation of hypotensive effects.

9. Neonates of mothers who have received ritodrine should be assessed for hyper- or hypoglycemia, hypocalcemia, hypotension, and ileus. Have emergency medication and equipment to support neonate.

**Client/Family Teaching**

1. Medication is administered to stop labor and requires close medical supervision to ensure appropriate dosage.

2. Report any chest pain, tightness, palpitations, dizziness, weakness, tremors, or difficulty breathing immediately.

3. Once infusion has been completed, ambulation may be resumed in 3–4 days if symptoms do not recur.

4. If contractions resume, membranes rupture, or spotting and/or bleeding occur, lie down immediately and notify provider.

**Outcomes/Evaluate:** Inhibition of uterine contractions; suppression of labor

# Ritonavir
(rih-**TOH**-nah-veer)
**Pregnancy Category:** B
Norvir **(Rx)**
**Classification:** Antiviral drug, protease inhibitor

See also *Anitiviral Drugs.*

**Action/Kinetics:** Ritonavir is a peptidomimetic inhibitor of both the HIV-1 and HIV-2 proteases. Inhibition of HIV protease results in the enzyme incapable of processing the "gag-pool" polyprotein precursor that leads to production of noninfectious immature HIV particles. **Peak concentrations after 600 mg of the solution:** 2 hr after fasting and 4 hr after nonfasting. **t½:** 3–5 hr. The drug is metabolized by the cytochrome P450 system. Metabolites and unchanged drug are excreted through both the feces and urine.

**Uses:** Alone or in combination with nucleoside analogues (ddC or AZT)

R

for the treatment of HIV infection. Use of ritonavir may result in a reduction in both mortality and AIDS-defining clinical events. Clinical benefit has not been determined for periods longer than 6 months.

**Special Concerns:** Ritonavir is not considered a cure for HIV infection; clients may continue to manifest illnesses associated with advanced HIV infection, including opportunistic infections. Also, therapy with ritonavir has not been shown to decrease the risk of transmitting HIV to others through sexual contact or blood contamination. Use with caution in those with impaired hepatic function and during lactation. Hemophiliacs treated with protease inhibitors may manifest spontaneous bleeding episodes. Safety and efficacy have not been determined in children less than 12 years of age.

**Side Effects:** Side effects listed are those with a frequency of 2% or greater. *GI:* N&V, diarrhea, taste perversion, anorexia, flatulence, constipation, abdominal pain, dyspepsia, local throat irritation. *Nervous:* Circumoral paresthesia, peripheral paresthesia, dizziness, insomnia, paresthesia, somnolence, abnormal thinking. *Body as a whole:* Asthenia, headache, malaise, fever. *Dermatologic:* Sweating, rash. *Miscellaneous:* Vasodilation, hyperlipidemia, myalgia, pharyngitis.

**OD** **Overdose Management:** *Symptoms:* Extension of side effects. *Treatment:* General supportive measures, including monitoring of VS and observing the clinical status. Elimination of unabsorbed drug may be assisted by emesis or gastric lavage, with attention given to maintaining a patent airway. Activated charcoal may also help in removing any unabsorbed drug. Dialysis is not likely to be of benefit in removing the drug from the body.

**Drug Interactions:** Ritonavir is expected to produce large increases in the plasma levels of a number of drugs, including amiodarone, astemizole, bepridil, bupropion, cisapride, clozapine, encainide, erythromycin, flecainide, meperidine, methylphenidate, pentoxifylline, phenothiazines, piroxicam, propafenone, propoxyphene, quinidine, rifabutin, tefenadine, and warfarin. This may lead to an increased risk of arrhythmias, hematologic complications, seizures, or other serious adverse effects.

Ritonavir may produce a decrease in the plasma levels of the following drugs: atovaquone, clofibrate, daunorubicin, diphenoxylate, metoclopramide, and sedative/hypnotics.

Coadministration of ritonavir with the following drugs may cause extreme sedation and respiratory depression and thus should not be combined: alprazolam, clorazepate, diazepam, estazolam, flurazepam, midazolam, triazolam, and zolpidem.

**Laboratory Test Interferences:** ↑ Triglycerides, AST, ALT, GGT, CPK, uric acid.

**Dosage** ————————————
- **Capsules, Oral Solution**
  *Treatment of HIV infection.*
600 mg b.i.d. If nausea is experienced upon initiation of therapy, dose escalation may be tried as follows: 300 mg b.i.d. for 1 day, 400 mg b.i.d. for 2 days, 500 mg b.i.d. for 1 day, and then 600 mg b.i.d. thereafter.

## NURSING CONSIDERATIONS

See also *Nursing Considerations* for *Antiviral Drugs.*
**Administration/Storage**
1. Clients prescribed combination regimens with nucleoside analogues may improve GI tolerance by starting therapy with ritonavir alone and then adding the nucleoside before completing 2 weeks of ritonavir monotherapy.
2. Store capsules in the refrigerator at 2°C–8°C (36°F–46°F) and protect from light. Keep PO solution under the same conditions until dispensed. Refrigeration of the solution is recommended after dispensing; however, this is not necessary if the solution is stored in the original container, used

within 30 days, and kept below 25°C (77°F).

**Assessment**

1. Document symptom onset, serum confirmation of diagnosis, and other agents trialed with the outcome.

2. Obtain baseline CBC, T-lymphocytes ($CD_4$), and liver function tests and monitor throughout therapy. Document impaired liver function, as drug is hepatically metabolized.

3. List other agents prescribed to ensure none interact unfavorably, as drug is metabolized via P450 system.

**Client/Family Teaching**

1. Ritonavir should be taken with food, if possible. Taste may be improved by mixing with chocolate milk, Ensure, or Advera within 1 hr of dosing.

2. Take each day as prescribed. Do not alter dosage or discontinue without approval. If a dose is missed, the next dose should be taken as soon as possible; if a dose is skipped, do not double the next dose.

3. Use reliable birth control and barrier protection; drug does not reduce the risk of transmitting disease through sexual contact or blood contamination.

4. Drug is not a cure for HIV; illnesses associated with advanced HIV infection may still occur, including opportunistic infections.

**Outcomes/Evaluate:** Inhibition of disease progression and death with HIV infection

---

# Rituximab

(rih-**TUK**-sih-mab)
**Pregnancy Category:** C
Rituxan **(Rx)**
**Classification:** Antineoplastic agent, monoclonal antibody

---

See also *Antineoplastic Agents.*

**Action/Kinetics:** Genetically engineered chimeric murine/human monoclonal antibody which binds specifically to CD20 antigen found on surface of normal and malignant B lymphocytes causing cell lysis. Cell lysis may result due to complement-dependent cytotoxicity and antibody-dependent cellular cytotoxicity. CD20 regulates early steps in activation process for cell cycle initiation and differentiation and possibly functions as calcium ion channel. Causes significant decreases in both IgM and IgG serum levels from months 5 to 11. **Mean serum t½:** 59.8 hr after first infusion and 174 hr after 4th infusion.

**Uses:** Treat relapsed or refractory low-grade or follicular, CD20 positive, B-cell non-Hodgkin's lymphoma.

**Contraindications:** Use in known Type I hypersensitivity or anaphylactic reactions to murine proteins or any component of product. Lactation.

**Special Concerns:** Use with caution in preexisting cardiac conditions, including arrhythmias and angina. Infusion-related symptoms may occur from 30 to 120 min at beginning of first infusion and with less frequency with subsequent infusions. Safety of immunization with any vaccine, especially live viral vaccines, has not been studied. Safety and efficacy have not been determined in children.

**Side Effects: Infusion-related events:** Fever, chills, and rigors are most common. Also, nausea, urticaria, fatigue, headache, pruritus, bronchospasm, hypotension, angioedema, dyspnea, rhinitis, vomiting, flushing, and pain at disease sites. **Retreatment events:** Asthenia, throat irritation, flushing, tachycardia, anorexia, leukopenia, thrombocytopenia, anemia, peripheral edema, dizziness, depression, respiratory symptoms, night sweats, pruritus.

**General side effects.** *CV:* Arrhythmias, including ventricular tachycardia and supraventricular tachycardias; trigeminy, angina, hypotension, hypertension, tachycardia, postural hypotension, bradycardia. *Hematologic:* Thrombocytopenia (up to 30 days following last dose), severe anemia, neutropenia, leukopenia, coagulation disorder. *Body as a whole:* Asthenia, arthralgia, pain, chills, malaise. *GI:* Abdominal pain, N&V, diarrhea, dyspepsia, taste perversion. *CNS:* Headache, paresthesia, anxiety, agitation, insomnia, hypesthesia, nervousness. *Respiratory:* **Bronchospasm**, increased cough, rhinitis, dyspnea, bronchiolitis obliterans, hypoxia, asthma, sinusitis, respiratory disorder, bronchitis. *Dermatologic:* Pruritus, rash, urticaria, flushing. *Miscellaneous:* Angioedema, lacrimation disorder, back pain, peripheral edema, chest pain, anorexia, abdominal enlargement, conjunctivitis, tumor pain, pain at injection site, hypertonia.

**Laboratory Test Alteration:** ↑ LDH. Hyperglycemia, hypocalcemia.

**Dosage**
• **IV infusion**
 *Non-Hodgkin's lymphoma.*
375 mg/m² as IV infusion once a week for four doses (days 1, 8, 15, 22). *Do not administer as IV push or bolus.*

## NURSING CONSIDERATIONS

See also *Nursing Considerations* for *Antineoplastic Agents,* .

**Administration/Storage**

**IV** 1. To prepare for administration, withdraw (using aseptic techniques) necessary amount of rituximab and dilute to final concentration of 1 to 4 mg/mL into infusion bag containing either 0.9% NaCl or D5/W. Discard any unused portion left in vial.

2. Solutions for infusion are stable at 2°C–8°C (36°F–46°F) for 24 hr and at room temperature for additional 12 hr.

3. Due to the potential of hypersensitivity reactions, consider premedication with acetaminophen and diphenhydramine.

4. Due to the possibility of transient hypotension during infusion, consider withholding antihypertensive medication 12 hr prior to rituximab.

5. For first infusion, give at initial rate of 50 mg/hr. If hypersensitivity or infusion-related events do not occur, escalate infusion rate in 50 mg/hr increments every 30 min to maximum of 400 mg/hr. If hypersensitivity or infusion-related events occur, temporarily slow or interrupt infusion; infusion can continue at one-half previous rate until symptoms improve. Subsequent infusions can be given at initial rate of 100 mg/hr, and increased by 100 mg/hr increments at 30 min intervals to maximum of 400 mg/hr (as long as tolerated).

6. Protect vials from direct sunlight.

**Assessment**

1. Note any cardiac disease and assess for arrhythmias.

2. Therapy usually consists of once weekly infusions for four doses.

3. Infusion related reaction consisting of fever and chills/rigors may occur with first infusion.

4. Interrupt infusion if severe reaction occurs; may resume infusion at 50% initial rate once symptoms resolved.

**Outcomes/Evaluate:** Control of malignant cell proliferation

# Rocuronium bromide

(roh-kyou-ROH-nee-um)
**Pregnancy Category:** B
Zemuron **(Rx)**
**Classification:** Neuromuscular blocking agent

See also *Neuromuscular Blocking Agents.*

**Action/Kinetics:** A nondepolarizing neuromuscular blocking agent that acts by competing with acetylcholine for receptors at the motor endplate. Causes histamine release in a small number of clients. Use must be accompanied by adequate anesthesia or sedation, as the drug has no effect on consciousness, pain threshold, or cerebration. Depending on the dose, it has a rapid to intermediate onset and an intermediate duration of action. $t^{1/2}$, **rapid distribution phase:** 1–2 min; $t^{1/2}$, **slower distribution phase:** 14–18 min. Metabolized by the liver.

**Uses:** As an adjunct to general anesthesia to facilitate rapid sequence and routine tracheal intubation; also, to cause relaxation of skeletal muscle during surgery or mechanical ventilation.

**Special Concerns:** Use with caution in clients with pulmonary hypertension, valvular heart disease, or significant hepatic disease. Burn clients may develop resistance to nondepolarizing neuromuscular blocking agents. Elderly clients may exhibit a slightly prolonged medical clinical duration of action. Use in children less than 3 months of age has not been studied.

**Side Effects:** *CV:* Arrhythmias, abnormal ECG, transient hypotension and hypertension, tachycardia. *GI:* N&V. *Respiratory:* Symptoms of asthma, including **bronchospasm,** wheezing, rhonchi; hiccup. *Dermatologic:* Rash, edema at injection site, pruritus.

**OD** **Overdose Management:** *Symptoms:* Neuromuscular blockade longer than needed for anesthesia and surgery. *Treatment:* Careful monitoring of client. Artificial respiration may be required.

**Dosage** —————————————
• **IV Only**
  *Rapid sequence intubation.*
0.6–1.2 mg/kg in appropriately premedicated and adequately anesthetized clients will result in good intubating conditions in less than 2 min.
  *Tracheal intubation.*
**Initial, regardless of anesthetic technique:** 0.6 mg/kg. Maximum blockade is noted in less than 3 min with a mean duration of 31 min. However, a dose of 0.45 mg/kg may also be used with maximum blockade in less than 4 min with a mean duration of 22 min. Initial doses of 0.6 mg/kg in children under halothane anesthesia produce good intubating conditions within 1 min with a mean duration of 41 min in children 3 months to 1 year and 27 min in children 1–2 years of age. Maintenance doses in children of 0.075–0.125 mg/kg, given upon return of $T_1$ of

25% of control provide muscle relaxation for 7–10 min.
  *Maintenance doses.*
0.1, 0.15, and 0.2 mg/kg, given at 25% recovery of control $T_1$ (defined as three twitches of train-of-four), provide a median of 12, 17, and 24 min of duration under opioid/nitrous oxide/oxygen anesthesia. The dose should not be administered until recovery of neuromuscular function is evident.
  *Continuous infusion.*
**Initial:** 0.01–0.02 mg/kg/min only after early evidence of spontaneous recovery from an intubating dose. Upon reaching the desired level of neuromuscular blockade, the infusion must be individualized for each client; the rate should be adjusted based on the twitch response (monitored with the use of a peripheral nerve stimulator) of the client. **Maintenance, usual:** 0.004–0.016 mg/kg/min.

---

## NURSING CONSIDERATIONS

See also *Nursing Considerations* for *Neuromuscular Blocking Agents.*
**Administration/Storage**
**IV** 1. Inhalation anesthetics (especially enflurane or isoflurane) may enhance the effects of rocuronium. When inhalation anesthetics are used, it may be necessary to reduce the rate of infusion by 30%–50% 45–60 min after the intubating dose.
2. Prepare solutions for infusion by mixing with D5W or RL solution. Drug is also compatible with 0.9% NaCl solution, sterile water for injection, and D5/NSS. Use solution within 24 hr after mixing; discard any unused solutions.
3. Spontaneous recovery occurs at about the same rate in children 3 months–1 year as in adults, but is more rapid in children 1–12 years old.
4. Do not mix rocuronium, which has an acid pH, with alkaline solutions (e.g., barbiturates) in the same syringe or give at the same time during

**R**

---

IV infusion through the same needle.

5. Store at 2°C–8°C (36°F–46°F); do not freeze.

**Assessment**

1. Obtain ECG, liver and renal function studies.

2. In the critically ill, intubate prior to rocuronium administration.

3. Use a peripheral nerve stimulator to assess neuromuscular function and to confirm recovery from neuromuscular blockade.

**Outcomes/Evaluate**

• Desired level of skeletal muscle relaxation

• Control of breathing during mechanical ventilation

# Ropinirole hydrochloride
(roh-**PIN**-ih-roll)
**Pregnancy Category:** C
Requip **(Rx)**
**Classification:** Antiparkinson agent

See also *Antiparkinson Agents.*

**Action/Kinetics:** Mechanism is not known but believed to involve stimulation of postsynaptic $D_2$ dopamine receptors in caudate-putamen in brain. Causes decreases in both systolic and diastolic BP at doses above 0.25 mg. Rapidly absorbed. **Peak plasma levels:** 1–2 hr. Food reduces maximum concentration. **t½, elimination:** 6 hr. First pass effect; extensively metabolized in liver.

**Uses:** Treat signs and symptoms of idiopathic Parkinson's disease.

**Contraindications:** Lactation.

**Special Concerns:** Safety and efficacy have not been determined in children.

**Side Effects:** *CNS:* Hallucinations, cause and/or exacerbate pre-existing dyskinesia. *CV:* Syncope (sometimes with bradycardia), postural hypotension.

**OD** **Overdose Management:** *Symptoms:* Agitation, increased dyskinesia, grogginess, sedation, orthostatic hypotension, chest pain, confusion, N&V. *Treatment:* General suppportive measures. Maintain vital signs. Gastric lavage.

**Drug Interactions**
*Ciprofloxacin* / Significant ↑ in ropinirole plasma levels
*Estrogens* / ↓ Oral clearance of ropinirole

**Dosage**

• **Tablets**
*Parkinson's disease.*

**Week 1:** 0.25 mg t.i.d. **Week 2:** 0.5 mg t.i.d. **Week 3:** 0.75 mg t.i.d. **Week 4:** 1 mg t.i.d. After week 4, daily dose, if necessary, may be increased by 1.5 mg/day on weekly basis up to dose of 9 mg/day. This may be followed by increase of up to 3 mg/day weekly to total dose of 24 mg/day.

## NURSING CONSIDERATIONS

See also *Nursing Considerations* for *Antiparkinson Agents.*

**Administration/Storage**

1. May be taken with or without food.

2. If taken with l-dopa, dose of l-dopa may be decreased gradually, as tolerated.

3. When discontinued, do so gradually over 7-day period. Reduce frequency of administration to twice daily for 4 days. For remaining 3 days, reduce frequency to once daily prior to complete withdrawal.

**Assessment**

1. Document disease onset, extent of motor function, reflexes, gait, strength of grip, and amount of tremor.

2. With tremor, note extent, muscle weakness, muscle rigidity, difficulty walking or changing direction.

3. Monitor VS, ECG.

**Client/Family Teaching**

1. May cause dizziness and syncope, use caution and report if persistent.

2. Report any loss of effect or evidence of dyskinesia.

3. Do not stop abruptly. Drug must be gradually withdrawn over seven day period.

**Outcomes/Evaluate:** Control of tremor

# S

# Salmeterol xinafoate

(sal-MET-er-ole)

**Pregnancy Category:** C

Serevent **(Rx)**

**Classification:** Beta-2 adrenergic agonist

See also *Sympathomimetic Drugs.*

**Action/Kinetics:** Selective for beta-2 adrenergic receptors which are located in the bronchi and heart. Acts by stimulating intracellular adenyl cyclase, the enzyme that converts ATP to cyclic AMP. Increased AMP levels cause relaxation of bronchial smooth muscle and inhibition of release of mediators of immediate hypersensitivity, especially from mast cells. Significantly bound to plasma proteins. Cleared by hepatic metabolism.

**Uses:** Long-term maintenance treatment of asthma. Prevention of bronchospasms in clients over 12 years of age with reversible obstructive airway disease, including nocturnal asthma. Prevention of exercise-induced bronchospasms. Inhalation powder for long-term maintenance treatment of asthma in clients aged 12 years or older.

**Contraindications:** Use in clients who can be controlled by short-acting, inhaled beta-2 agonists. Use to treat acute symptoms of asthma or in those who have worsening or deteriorating asthma. Lactation.

**Special Concerns:** The drug is not a substitute for PO or inhaled corticosteroids. The safety and efficacy of using salmeterol with a spacer or other devices has not been studied adequately. Use with caution in impaired hepatic function; with cardiovascular disorders, including coronary insufficiency, cardiac arrhythmias, and hypertension; with convulsive disorders or thyrotoxicosis; and in clients who respond unusually to sympathomimetic amines. Be-

cause of the potential of the drug interfering with uterine contractility, use of salmeterol during labor should be restricted to those in whom benefits clearly outweigh risks. Safety and efficacy have not been determined in children less than 12 years of age.

**Side Effects:** *Respiratory:* Paradoxical bronchospasms, upper or lower respiratory tract infection, nasopharyngitis, disease of nasal cavity/sinus, cough, pharyngitis, allergic rhinitis, laryngitis, tracheitis, bronchitis. *Allergic:* **Immediate hypersensitivity reactions,** including urticaria, rash, and **bronchospasm.** *CV:* Palpitations, chest pain, increased BP, tachycardia. *CNS:* Headache, sinus headache, tremors, nervousness, malaise, fatigue, dizziness, giddiness. *GI:* Stomachache. *Musculoskeletal:* Joint pain, back pain, muscle cramps, muscle contractions, myalgia, myositis, muscle soreness. *Miscellaneous:* Flu, dental pain, rash, skin eruption, dysmenorrhea.

**Laboratory Test Alterations:** ↓ Serum potassium.

**OD** **Overdose Management:** *Symptoms:* Tachycardia, arrhythmia, tremors, headache, muscle cramps, hypokalemia, hyperglycemia. *Treatment:* Supportive therapy. Consider judicious use of a beta-adrenergic blocking agent, although these drugs can cause bronchospasms. Cardiac monitoring is necessary. Dialysis is not an appropriate treatment of overdosage.

**Drug Interactions**

*MAO Inhibitors* / Potentiation of the effect of salmeterol

*Tricyclic antidepressants* / Potentiation of the effect of salmeterol

**Dosage**

• **Metered Dose Inhaler**

*Maintenance of bronchodilation, prevention of symptoms of asthma, including nocturnal asthma.*

---

★ = Available in Canada        **bold italic** = life threatening side effect

**Adults and children over 12 years of age:** Two inhalations (42 mcg) b.i.d. (morning and evening, approximately 12 hr apart)

*Prevention of exercise-induced bronchospasms.*

**Adults and children over 12 years of age:** Two inhalations (42 mcg) at least 30–60 min before exercise. Additional doses should not be used for 12 hr.

- **Inhalation Powder (Diskus)**
*Maintenance treatment of asthma.*

**Adults and children over 12 years of age:** 50 mcg (one inhalation) b.i.d. in the morning and evening.

*NOTE:* Even though the metered dose inhaler and the inhalation powder are used for the same conditions, they are not interchangeable.

## NURSING CONSIDERATIONS

See also *Nursing Considerations* for *Sympathomimetic Drugs.*

**Administration/Storage**

1. Ensure that doses are spaced q 12 hr.

2. The safety of more than 8 inhalations per day of short-acting beta-2 agonists with salmeterol has not been established.

3. If a previously effective dose fails to provide the usual response, contact provider immediately.

4. If using salmeterol twice daily, do not use additional doses to prevent exercise-induced bronchospasms.

5. Use only with the actuator provided. Do not use the actuator with other aerosol medications.

6. Store between 2°C and 30°C (36°F and 86°F). Store the canister nozzle end down and protect from freezing temperatures and direct sunlight.

7. Exercise caution so the drug is not sprayed in the eyes.

8. Shake canister well before using at room temperature; therapeutic effect may diminish if cold.

9. For the inhalation powder (Diskus), a built-in dose counter shows the number of doses remaining.

**Assessment**

1. Document onset, duration, and characteristics of symptoms; note other agents tried and the outcome.

2. Determine any history of cardiac or liver dysfunction, thyrotoxicosis, hypertension, or convulsive disorders.

3. Document pulmonary function status and lung sounds.

4. Monitor VS, liver enzymes, PFTs (ABGs, PEFR, and FEV at 1 sec).

**Client/Family Teaching**

1. Review proper use (with actuator) and obtain instruction. Record peak flows and identify critical zones.

2. Use only as prescribed and do not exceed prescribed dosage and administration frequency (drug effects last 12 hr).

3. Do not use this drug during an acute asthma attack.

4. Review procedure for use of the short-acting beta-2 agonist prescribed to treat symptoms of asthma that occur between the salmeterol dosing schedule. Increased utilization warrants medical evaluation (e.g., when used more than 4 times/day or more than one canister of 200 inhalations/8 weeks).

5. May experience palpitations, chest pain, headaches, tremors, and nervousness as side effects.

6. Report immediately if chest pain, fast pounding irregular heart beat, hives, increased wheezing, or difficulty breathing occurs.

7. Take 30–60 min before activity to prevent acute bronchospasms.

8. Salmeterol does not replace inhaled or systemic steroids; do not stop prescribed steroid therapy abruptly without approval.

9. Identify appropriate support groups that may assist to cope and live a normal life with asthma.

10. Stop smoking; avoid smokey environments and any other triggers that may aggravate condition.

**Outcomes/Evaluate**

- Prevention and control of asthmatic symptoms (e.g., decreased

wheezing, dyspnea, orthopnea, and cough)
• Prevention of exercise-induced bronchospasms

# Saquinavir mesylate
((sah-**KWIN**-ah-veer))
**Pregnancy Category:** B
Fortovase, Invirase **(Rx)**
**Classification:** Antiviral drug, protease inhibitor

See also *Antiviral Drugs.*
**Action/Kinetics:** HIV protease cleaves viral polyprotein precursors to form functional proteins in HIV-infected cells. Cleavage of viral polyprotein precursors is required for maturation of the infectious virus. Saquinavir inhibits the activity of HIV protease and prevents the cleavage of viral polyproteins. Has a low bioavailability after PO use, probably due to incomplete absorption and first-pass metabolism. A high-fat meal or high-calorie meal increases the amount of drug absorbed. Over 98% bound to plasma protein. About 87% metabolized in the liver by the cytochrome P450 system. Both metabolites and unchanged drug are excreted mainly through the feces. It is believed the bioavailability of Fortovase is greater than Invirase.
**Uses:** Combined with AZT or zalcitabine (ddC) for treatment of advanced HIV infection in selected clients. No data are available regarding the benefit of combination therapy of saquinavir with AZT or ddC on HIV disease progression or survival.
**Contraindications:** Lactation.
**Special Concerns:** Photoallergy or phototoxicity may occur; thus, clients should take protective measures against exposure to ultraviolet or sunlight until tolerance is assessed. Use with caution in those with hepatic insufficiency. Hemophiliacs treated with protease inhibitors for HIV infections may manifest spontaneous bleeding episodes. Safety and efficacy have not been determined in HIV-infected children or adolescents less than 16 years of age.
**Side Effects:** Side effects listed are for saquinavir combined with either AZT or ddC. *GI:* Diarrhea, abdominal discomfort, nausea, dyspepsia, abdominal pain, ulceration of buccal mucosa, cheilitis, constipation, dysphagia, eructation, blood-stained or discolored feces, gastralgia, gastritis, GI inflammation, gingivitis, glossitis, *rectal hemorrhage,* hemorrhoids, hepatomegaly, hepatosplenomegaly, melena, pain, painful defecation, pancreatitis, parotid disorder, pelvic salivary glands disorder, stomatitis, tooth disorder, vomiting, frequent bowel movements, dry mouth, alteration in taste. *CNS:* Headache, paresthesia, numbness of extremity, dizziness, peripheral neuropathy, ataxia, confusion, *convulsions,* dysarthria, dysesthesia, hyperesthesia, hyperreflexia, hyporeflexia, face numbness, facial pain, paresis, poliomyelitis, progressive multifocal leukoencephalopathy, spasms, tremor, agitation, amnesia, anxiety, depression, excessive dreaming, euphoria, hallucinations, insomnia, reduced intellectual ability, irritability, lethargy, libido disorder, overdose effect, psychic disorder, somnolence, speech disorder. *Musculoskeletal:* Musculoskeletal pain, myalgia, arthralgia, arthritis, back pain, muscle cramps, musculoskeletal disorder, stiffness, tissue changes, trauma. *Body as a whole:* Allergic reaction, chest pain, edema, fever, intoxication, external parasites, retrosternal pain, shivering, wasting syndrome, weight decrease, abscess, angina tonsillaris, candidiasis, hepatitis, herpes simplex, herpes zoster, infections (bacterial, mycotic, staphylococcal), influenza, lymphadenopathy, tumor. *CV:* Cyanosis, heart murmur, heart valve disorder, hypertension, hypotension, syncope, distended vein, HR disorder. *Metabolic:* Dehydration, hyperglycemia, weight decrease. *Hematologic:* Anemia, microhemorrhages, pancytopenia, splenomegaly, thrombocy-

**S**

---
✦ = Available in Canada    *bold italic* = life threatening side effect

topenia. *Respiratory:* Bronchitis, cough, dyspnea, epistaxis, hemoptysis, laryngitis, pharyngitis, pneumonia, respiratory disorder rhinitis, sinusitis, URTI. *GU:* Enlarged prostate, vaginal discharge, micturition disorder, UTI. *Dermatologic:* Acne, dermatitis, seborrheic dermatitis, eczema, erythema, folliculitis, furunculosis, hair changes, hot flushes, photosensitivity reaction, changes in skin pigment, maculopapular rash, skin disorder, skin nodules, skin ulceration, increased sweating, urticaria, verruca, xeroderma. *Ophthalmic:* Dry eye syndrome, xerophthalmia, blepharitis, eye irritation, visual disturbance. *Otic:* Earache, ear pressure, decreased hearing, otitis, tinnitus.

**Laboratory Test Alterations:** ↑ CPK, serum amylase, AST, ALT, total bilirubin. ↓ Neutrophils. Abnormal phosphorus.

**Drug Interactions**
*Astemizole* / Possibility of prolongation of QT intervals → serious CV adverse effects
*Carbamazepine* / ↓ Blood levels of saquinavir
*Dexamethasone* / ↓ Blood levels of saquinavir
*Phenobarbital* / ↓ Blood levels of saquinavir
*Phenytoin* / ↓ Blood levels of saquinavir
*Rifampin* / ↓ Blood levels of saquinavir
*Terfenadine* / Possibility of prolongation of QT intervals → serious CV adverse effects

**Dosage** ——————
• **Fortovase Capsules**
*HIV infections in combination with AZT or ddC.*
Six 200-mg capsules (i.e., 1,200 mg) taken t.i.d. with meals or up to 2 hr after meals.
• **Invirase Capsules**
*HIV infections in combination with AZT or ddC.*
Three 200-mg capsules of saquinavir t.i.d. taken within 2 hr of a full meal. The recommended doses of AZT or ddC as part of combination therapy are: AZT, 200 mg t.i.d., or ddC, 0.75

mg t.i.d. However, base dosage adjustments of AZT or ddC on the known toxicity profile of the individual drug. This form of the drug will be phased out.

## NURSING CONSIDERATIONS

See also *Nursing Considerations* for *Antiviral Drugs.*

**Administration/Storage**
1. Take within 2 hr of a full meal. If taken without food, blood levels may not be sufficiently high to exert an antiviral effect.
2. Doses less than 200 mg t.i.d. of Invirase are not recommended; lower doses have not shown antiviral activity.
3. Fortovase Capsules must be refrigerated.

**Assessment**
1. Document onset, duration, and type of symptoms manifested.
2. Monitor CBC, T-lymphocytes/viral load, liver and renal function tests.
3. List drugs currently prescribed; drug is metabolized hepatically via cytochrome P450 system.
4. If serious or severe toxicity occurs, interrupt therapy until cause is determined or toxicity resolves.

**Client/Family Teaching**
1. Take only as prescribed and within 2 hr of a full meal, as blood levels are markedly reduced when taken without food.
2. Drug is not a cure for HIV infections. It does not prevent the occurrence or decrease the frequency of opportunistic infections associated with HIV.
3. Avoid sun exposure; take protective measures against exposure to UV or sunlight until tolerance assessed.
4. Continue to use barrier contraception and practice safe sex; drug does not inhibit disease transmission.
5. Long-term drug effects are still unknown; report any unusual or adverse effects.

**Outcomes/Evaluate:** Control of progression of advanced HIV infections

# Sargramostim
(sar-**GRAM**-oh-stim)
**Pregnancy Category:** C
Leukine **(Rx)**
**Classification:** Colony-stimulating factor

**Action/Kinetics:** A granulocyte-macrophage colony-stimulating factor (rhu GM-CSF) produced by recombinant DNA technology in a yeast expression system. GM-CSF stimulates the proliferation and differentiation of hematopoietic progenitor cells. It stimulates partially committed progenitor cells to divide and differentiate in the granulocyte-macrophage pathways. Division, maturation, and activation are induced through GM-CSF binding to specific receptors located on the surface of target cells. Also activates mature granulocytes and macrophages. Increases the cytotoxicity of monocytes toward certain neoplastic cell lines as well as activates polymorphonuclear neutrophils, thus inhibiting the growth of tumor cells. Sargramostim differs from the naturally occurring GM-CSF by one amino acid and by a different carbohydrate moiety. **Peak levels:** 2–3 hr, depending on the dose. **t½, initial:** 12–17 min; **t½, terminal:** 1.6–2.6 hr, depending on the dose. Neutralizing antibodies have been detected in a small number of clients.

**Uses:** Increased myeloid recovery in clients with non-Hodgkin's lymphoma, acute lymphoblastic leukemia, and Hodgkin's disease undergoing autologous bone marrow transplantation. Bone marrow transplantation failure or engraftment delay. To shorten recovery time to neutrophil recovery and to decrease the incidence of severe and life-threatening infections in older adult clients with acute myelogenous leukemia. To mobilize hematopoietic progenitor cells into peripheral blood collection by leukapheresis. For acceleration of myeloid recovery in allogenic bone marrow transplantation from human lymphocyte antigen-matched related donors. *Investigational:* To increase WBC counts in clients with myelodysplastic syndrome and in AIDS clients taking AZT; to correct neutropenia in clients with aplastic anemia; to decrease the nadir of leukopenia secondary to myelosuppressive chemotherapy and to decrease myelosuppression in preleukemic clients; and to decrease organ system damage following transplantation, especially in the liver and kidney.

**Contraindications:** More than 10% leukemic myeloid blasts in the bone marrow or peripheral blood. Known hypersensitivity to GM-CSF, yeast-derived products, or any component of the product. Simultaneous use with cytotoxic chemotherapy or radiotherapy or use within 24 hr preceding or following chemotherapy or radiotherapy.

**Special Concerns:** Use with caution in clients with preexisting cardiac disease and hypoxia and during lactation. Safety and effectiveness have not been determined in children although it appears the drug is no more toxic in children than in adults. The drug may aggravate fluid retention in clients with preexisting peripheral edema, or pleural or pericardial effusion. Insufficient data are available to support the effectiveness of sargramostim in increasing myeloid recovery after peripheral blood stem cell transplantation. It is possible that sargramostim can act as a growth factor for any tumor type, especially myeloid malignancies; thus, use with caution in any malignancy with myeloid characteristics.

**Side Effects:** *First-dose effects (rare):* Respiratory distress, hypoxia, flushing, hypotension, syncope, tachycardia. *CV:* Hypertension, **hemorrhage,** edema, hypotension, peripheral edema, cardiac event, tachycardia, pericardial effusion, pleural effusion, capillary leak syndrome. *GI:* N&V, diarrhea, abdominal pain, GI disorder, stomatitis, dyspepsia, anorexia, hematemesis, dysphagia, **GI hemorrhage,** constipation, abdominal distension, liver damage. *CNS:* Neuroclinical, neuromotor, neuropsychiatric, and neurosensory side effects. Paresthesia, headache, CNS disorder, insomnia, anxiety. *Respiratory:* Pulmonary event, pharyngitis, lung disorder, epistaxis, dyspnea, rhinitis. *Hematologic:* Blood dyscrasias, thrombocytopenia, leukopenia, petechia, agranulocytosis, coagulation disorders. *Musculoskeletal:* Bone pain, arthralgia, asthenia. *Dermatologic:* Rash, alopecia, pruritus. *GU:* Urinary tract disorder, hematuria, abnormal kidney function. *Miscellaneous:* Fever, infection, malaise, weight loss, chills, pain, chest pain, allergy, **sepsis,** eye hemorrhage, back pain, weight gain, sweating.

**Laboratory Test Alterations:** ↑ Glucose, BUN, cholesterol, bilirubin, serum creatinine, ALT, alkaline phosphatase. ↓ Albumin, calcium.

**OD Overdose Management:** *Symptoms:* Dyspnea, malaise, nausea, fever, rash, sinus tachycardia, chills, headache. *Treatment:* Discontinue therapy. Monitor for increases in WBCs and for respiratory symptoms.

**Drug Interactions:** Drugs such as corticosteroids and lithium may ↑ the myeloproliferative effects of sargramostim. The effect of sargramostim may be limited in those who have received alkylating agents, anthracycline antibiotics, or antimetabolites.

## Dosage

• **IV Infusion, SC**

*Myeloid reconstitution after autologous or allogenic bone marrow transplantation.*

250 mcg/m²/day for 21 days as a 2-hr infusion beginning 2–4 hr after the autologous bone marrow infusion and greater than 24 hr after the last dose of chemotherapy and 12 hr after the last dose of radiotherapy. Clients should not receive the drug until the postmarrow infusion absolute neutrophil count is less than 500 cells/mm³.

*Bone marrow transplantation failure or engraftment delay.*

250 mcg/m²/day for 14 days as a 2-hr IV infusion. If engraftment has not occurred, therapy may be repeated after 7 days off therapy. A third course of 250 mcg/m²/day may be undertaken after another 7 days off therapy. However, if no response occurs after three courses, it is unlikely the drug will be beneficial.

*Neutrophil recovery following chemotherapy in acute myelogenous leukemia.*

250 mcg/m²/day given over a 4-hr period staring at about day 11 or 4 days following completion of induction chemotherapy. Use if the day 10 bone marrow is hypoplastic with less than 5% blasts. If a second cycle of therapy is needed, give about 4 days after the completion of chemotherapy if the bone marrow is hypoplastic with less than 5% blasts. Therapy should be continued until an absolute neutrophil count greater than 1,500/mm³ is noted for 3 consecutive days or a maximum of 42 days. If a severe adverse reaction occurs, the dose should be decreased by 50% or the drug temporarily discontinued until the drug reaction is reduced.

*Mobilization of peripheral blood progenitor cells (PBPCs).*

250 mcg/m²/day IV over 24 hr or SC once daily. This dose should be used throughout the PBPC collection period. If the WBC count is greater than 50,000 cells/mm³, the dose should be reduced by 50%. If sufficient numbers of progenitor cells are not collected, other mobilization therapy should be used.

*Postperipheral blood progenitor cell transplantation.*

250 mcg/m²/day IV over 24 hr or SC once daily beginning immediately after infusion of progenitor cells and continuing until an absolute neutrophil count greater than 1,500 is reached for 3 consecutive days.

## NURSING CONSIDERATIONS
### Administration/Storage

**IV** 1. Give daily dosage as a 2-hr IV infusion beginning 2–4 hr after the autologous bone marrow infusion making sure at least 24 hr have elapsed after the last dose of chemotherapy and 12 hr have elapsed since the last dose of radiotherapy.

2. Reduce the dose or temporarily discontinue if severe adverse reactions occur; resume therapy once the reactions abate.

3. Reconstitute the lyophilized powder with 1 mL of sterile water for injection without preservatives. Direct the sterile water at the side of the vial, followed by a gentle swirling of the contents to avoid foaming. Avoid excessive or vigorous agitation.

4. Reconstituted solutions are clear, colorless, and isotonic with a pH of 7.4.

5. Do not reenter or reuse the vial; discard unused portion.

6. Dilute with 0.9% NaCl injection for IV infusion. If the final concentration is less than 10 mcg/mL, add human albumin at a final concentration of 0.1% to the saline before adding sargramostim, to prevent adsorption to components of the drug delivery system.

7. Contains no preservatives; thus, give as soon as possible, but within 6 hr, following reconstitution or dilution for IV infusion. Store the sterile powder, reconstituted solution, and dilution solution in the refrigerator at 2°C–8°C (36°F–46°F). Do not freeze or shake solutions or use beyond the expiration date on the vial.

8. Do not add other drugs to infusion solutions containing sargramostim.

9. Use an in-line membrane filter for IV infusion.

### Assessment

1. Determine any sensitivity to yeast-derived products. Note any cardiac disease, hypoxia, peripheral edema, pleural or pericardial effusion, or myeloid-type malignancy.

2. Monitor CBC (ANC and platelets), liver and renal function studies.

3. Document any therapy with drugs or radiation. Drug should *not* be administered 24 hr before or after chemotherapy or within 12 hr preceding or following radiation therapy.

### Interventions

1. Monitor I&O, VS, and weight; assess for fluid retention or edema.

2. Monitor for respiratory symptoms during or immediately following infusion, especially with preexisting lung disease. Reduce rate of infusion by one-half if dyspnea occurs.

3. Monitor hematologic response with a CBC twice weekly. If the ANC exceeds 20,000/mm$^3$ or the platelet count exceeds 500,000/mm$^3$ or a severe reaction occurs, stop therapy and reduce the dose by one-half. Excessive blood counts have returned to normal levels within 3–7 days following termination of therapy.

4. Renal and hepatic function should be monitored every 2 weeks with hepatic or renal dysfunction.

5. Drug effectiveness may be limited in clients who, before autologous bone marrow transplantation, received extensive radiotherapy in the chest or abdomen to treat the primary disease; effectiveness is also limited in clients who have received multiple myelotoxic agents such as antimetabolites, alkylating agents, or anthracycline antibiotics.

### Outcomes/Evaluate

• Inhibition of tumor cell growth
• Improved hematologic parameters
• Mobilization of peripheral blood progenitor cells
• Neutrophil recovery following chemotherapy with AML

# Scopolamine hydrobromide

(scoh-**POLL**-ah-meen)
**Pregnancy Category:** C
Hyoscine Hydrobromide, Isopto Hyoscine Ophthalmic, Scopace **(Rx)**

---

# Scopolamine transdermal therapeutic system

(scoh-**POLL**-ah-meen)

**Pregnancy Category:** C
Transderm-Scop, Transderm-V ✤ **(Rx)**
**Classification:** Anticholinergic, antiemetic

See also *Cholinergic Blocking Agents.*
**Action/Kinetics:** Anticholinergic with CNS depressant effects which produces amnesia when given with morphine or meperidine. In the presence of pain, delirium may be produced. Causes pupillary dilation and paralyzes the muscle required to accommodate for close vision (cycloplegia). This enables the physician to examine the inner structure of the eye, including the retina, as well as to examine refractive errors of the lens without automatic accommodation by the client. Tolerance may develop if scopolamine is used alone. When used for refraction: **peak for mydriasis,** 20–30 min; **peak for cycloplegia,** 30–60 min; **duration:** 24 hr (residual cycloplegia and mydriasis may last for 3–7 days). Recovery time can be reduced by using 1–2 gtt pilocarpine (1% or 2%). To reduce absorption, pressure should be applied over the nasolacrimal sac for 2–3 min.

The transdermal therapeutic system contains 1.5 mg scopolamine, which is slowly released from a mineral oil–polyisobutylene matrix. Approximately 0.5 mg is released from the system per day.

**Uses: Ophthalmic:** For cycloplegia and mydriasis in diagnostic procedures. Preoperatively and postoperatively in the treatment of iridocyclitis. Dilate the pupil in treatment of uveitis or posterior synechiae. *Investigational:* Prophylaxis of synechaie, treatment of iridocyclitis. **Parenteral:** Antiemetic, antivertigo. Preanesthetic sedation and obstetric amnesia. Antiarrhythmic during anesthesia and surgery. **Oral:** Prevention of motion sickness. **Transdermal:** Antiemetic, antivertigo. Prevention of motion sickness.

**Additional Contraindications:** For transdermal therapeutic system: Children, lactating women. Ophthalmic use contraindicated in glaucoma, infants less than 3 months of age.

**Special Concerns:** Use with caution in children, infants, geriatric clients, diabetes, hypo- or hyperthyroidism, narrow anterior chamber angle. Use for prophylaxis of excess secretions is not recommended for children less than 4 months of age. The transdermal system is not recommended for children.

**Additional Side Effects:** Disorientation, delirium, increased HR, decreased respiratory rate. *Ophthalmologic:* Blurred vision, stinging, increased intraocular pressure. Long-term use may cause irritation, photophobia, conjunctivitis, hyperemia, or edema.

## Dosage

- **Ophthalmic Solution**
  *Cycloplegia/mydriasis.*
  **Adults:** 1–2 gtt of the 0.25% solution in the conjunctiva 1 hr prior to refraction; **children:** 1 gtt of the 0.25% solution b.i.d. for 2 days prior to refraction.
  *Uveitis.*
  **Adults and children:** 1 gtt of the 0.25% solution in the conjunctiva 1–4 times/day, depending on the severity of the condition.
  *Treatment of posterior synechiae.*
  **Adults and children:** 1 gtt of the 0.25% solution q min for 5 min. (1 gtt of either a 2.5% or 10% solution of phenylephrine instilled q min for 3 min will enhance the effect of scopolamine.)
  *Postoperative mydriasis.*
  **Adults:** 1 gtt of the 0.25% solution once daily. For dark brown irides, administration 2 or 3 times/day may be required.
  *Pre- or Postoperative iridocyclitis.*
  **Adults and children:** 1 gtt of the 0.25% solution 1–4 times/day as required. The pediatric dose should be individualized based on age, weight, and severity of the inflammation.
- **Injection (IM, IV, SC)**

*Anticholinergic, antiemetic.*
**Adults:** 0.3–0.6 mg (single dose).
**Pediatric:** 0.006 mg/kg (0.2 mg/m²) as a single dose.

*Prophylaxis of excessive salivation and respiratory tract secretions in anesthesia.*
**Adults:** 0.2–0.6 mg 30–60 min before induction of anesthesia. **Pediatric (given IM): 8–12 years:** 0.3 mg; **3–8 years:** 0.2 mg; **7 months–3 years:** 0.15 mg; **4–7 months:** 0.1 mg. Not recommended for children less than 4 months of age.

*Adjunct to anesthesia, sedative-hypnotic.*
**Adults:** 0.6 mg t.i.d–q.i.d.

*Adjunct to anesthesia, amnesia.*
**Adults:** 0.32–0.65 mg.
• **Tablets**
*Prevent motion sickness.*
0.4–0.8 mg taken 1 hr before travel.
• **Transdermal System**
*Antiemetic, antivertigo.*
**Adults:** 1 transdermal system placed on the postauricular skin to deliver 0.5 mg over 3 days (apply at least 4 hr before antiemetic effect is required). The Canadian product delivers 1 mg over a 3-day period; it should be applied about 12 hr before the antiemetic effect is desired.

## NURSING CONSIDERATIONS

See also *Nursing Considerations* for *Cholinergic Blocking Agents.*
**Administration/Storage**
1. Give drops into the conjunctival sac followed by digital pressure for 2–3 min after instillation.
2. Do not give alone for pain because it may cause delirium; use an analgesic or sedative as needed.
3. Protect solution from light.
**Assessment**
1. Document indications for therapy, type and onset of symptoms.
2. With eyedrops, check for angle-closure glaucoma; may precipitate an acute glaucoma crisis.
3. Some clients may experience toxic delirium with therapeutic doses. Observe closely and have physostigmine available to reverse effects.

**Client/Family Teaching**
1. Do not drive a car or operate dangerous machinery until drug effects realized; may cause drowsiness, confusion, disorientation, and, when used ophthalmologically, blurred vision and dilated pupils.
2. Wear dark glasses if photosensitivity occurs and report if eye pain occurs. May temporarily impair vision.
3. Wait 5 min before instilling other eye drops.
4. With the transdermal system:
• Wash hands before and after application
• Apply at least 4 hr before desired effect
• Apply to a clean, nonhairy site, behind the ear
• Use pressure to apply the patch to ensure contact with the skin
• Replace with a new system if patch becomes dislodged
• System is water-proof so bathing and swimming are permitted
• System effects last for 3 days
5. Report any extrapyramidal symptoms, urinary retention, and constipation. Increase fluids and bulk to prevent constipation.
6. Use gum, sugarless candies, and frequent mouth rinses to alleviate symptoms of dry mouth.
7. Avoid alcohol and any other CNS depressants.
**Outcomes/Evaluate**
• Control of vomiting
• Preoperative sedation; postoperative amnesia
• Desired mydriasis
• Prevention of motion sickness

# Secobarbital sodium
(see-koh-**BAR**-bih-tal)
**Pregnancy Category:** D
Novo-Secobarb ✦, Seconal Sodium
**(C-II) (Rx)**
**Classification:** Barbiturate sedative-hypnotic

See also *Barbiturates.*
**Action/Kinetics:** Short-acting. Distributed quickly due to high lipid solubility. **Onset:** 10–15 min. **t½:**

S

15–40 hr. **Duration:** 3–4 hr. Is 46%–70% protein bound.

**Uses: Parenteral:** Intermittent use as a sedative, hypnotic, or preanesthetic.

**Special Concerns:** Elderly or debilitated clients may be more sensitive to the drug and require reduced dosage.

**Dosage**

* **IM, IV**
  *Hypnotic.*
  **Adults:** 100–200 mg IM or 50–250 mg IV.
  *Preoperative sedative.*
  **Adults:** 1 mg/kg IM 10–15 min before procedure. **Children:** 4–5 mg/kg IM.
  *Dentistry in clients who will receive nerve block.*
  100–150 mg IV.
  *Status epilepticus.*
  **Children:** 15–20 mg/kg IV over 10–15 min.

**NURSING CONSIDERATIONS**

See also *Nursing Considerations* for *Barbiturates*.

**Administration/Storage**

1. Reduce dosage in impaired hepatic or renal function.

2. Following prolonged use, taper dosage and withdraw drug slowly to prevent precipitating withdrawal symptoms.

3. Refrigerate the parenteral solution and protect from light. Do not use if solution contains a precipitate.

**IV** 4. For adults, the aqueous parenteral solution is preferred to polyethylene glycol, which may be irritating to the kidneys, especially with signs of renal insufficiency.

5. Freshly prepare aqueous solutions for injection from dry-packed ampules.

6. Rapid IV administration may precipitate hypotension, respiratory depression, laryngospasm or apnea; do not exceed recommended rate (50 mg/15 sec).

7. Parenteral form may damage or necrose tissue if infiltrated due to high solution alkalinity.

**Client/Family Teaching**

1. Do not perform activities that require mental alertness until drug effects realized.

2. Avoid alcohol and any other CNS depressants.

3. Take analgesics as prescribed; does not control pain.

4. Carefully supervise for 6 to 8 hr after procedure as client may be irrational.

5. Drug may cause dependency. Review alternative methods that assist with sleeping, such as relaxation techniques, daily exercise, no napping, stress reduction, no caffeine, and/or white noise simulator.

**Outcomes/Evaluate**

* Improved sleeping patterns with less frequent awakenings
* Effective sedation

# Selegiline hydrochloride (Deprenyl)

(seh-**LEH**-jih-leen)

**Pregnancy Category:** C

Carbex, Eldepryl, Novo-Selegiline ✿ **(Rx)**

**Classification:** Antiparkinson agent

See also *Antiparkinson Agents*.

**Action/Kinetics:** Precise mechanism of action is not known; does inhibit MAO, type B. May act through other mechanisms to increase dopaminergic activity, including interference with dopamine uptake at the synapse. Metabolites include amphetamine and methamphetamine, which may contribute to the effects of the drug. Rapidly absorbed and metabolized. **Maximum plasma levels:** 0.5–2 hr.

**Uses:** Adjunct in the treatment of Parkinson's disease in clients being treated with levodopa/carbidopa who have manifested a decreased response to this therapy. *NOTE:* No evidence that selegiline is effective in clients not taking levodopa.

**Contraindications:** Hypersensitivity to the drug. Doses greater than 10 mg/day. Use with meperidine (and usually other opiates).

**Special Concerns:** Use with caution during lactation. Safety and efficacy in children have not been established.

**Side Effects:** *CNS:* Dizziness, light-headedness, fainting, confusion, hallucinations, vivid dreams/nightmares, headache, anxiety, drowsiness, depression, mood changes, delusions, fatigue, disorientation, apathy, malaise, vertigo, overstimulation, sleep disturbance, transient irritability, weakness, lethary, personality change. *Skeletal Muscle:* Tremor, chorea, loss of balance, blepharospasm, restlessness, increased bradykinesia, facial grimace, dystonic symptoms, tardive dyskinesia, dyskinesia, involuntary movements, muscle cramps, heavy leg, falling down, stiff neck, freezing, festination, increased apraxia. *Altered Sensations/pain:* Headache, tinnitus, migraine, back or leg pain, supraorbital pain, burning throat, chills, numbness of fingers/toes, taste disturbance, generalized aches. *CV:* Orthostatic hypotension, hypertension, arrhythmia, angina pectoris, palpitations, hypotension, tachycardia, syncope, peripheral edema, sinus bradycardia. *GI:* N&V, constipation, anorexia, weight loss, dry mouth, poor appetite, dysphagia, diarrhea, rectal bleeding, *GI bleeding (worsening of pre-existing ulcer disease),* heartburn. *GU:* Nocturia, slow urination, urinary hesitancy or retention, prostatic hypertrophy, urinary frequency, sexual dysfunction. *Miscellaneous:* Blurred vision, increased sweating, diaphoresis, facial hair, hair loss, rash, photosensitivity, hematoma, asthma, diplopia, SOB, speech affected.

**OD** **Overdose Management:** *Symptoms:* Hypotension, psychomotor agitation. Also, symptoms from overdose of nonselective MAO inhibitors (e.g., isocarboxazid, phenelzine, tranylcypromine). *Treatment:* IV fluids and a dilute pressor agent to treat hypotension and vascular collapse. Treat symptoms.

**Drug Interactions**
*Fluoxetine (Prozac)* / Possibility of death—five weeks should elapse

between discontinuing fluoxetine and beginning selegiline and 14 days between discontinuing selegiline and initiation of fluoxetine
*Meperidine* / Symptoms include stupor, muscle rigidity, severe agitation, hyperthermia, hallucinations, death.

**Dosage**
• **Capsules, Tablets**
*Parkinsonism in those receiving levodopa/carbidopa.*
**Adults:** 5 mg taken at breakfast and lunch, not to exceed 10 mg/day.

## NURSING CONSIDERATIONS

See also *Nursing Considerations* for *Antiparkinson Agents.*
**Administration/Storage**
1. No evidence exists that doses higher than 10 mg/day will result in additional beneficial effects.
2. Following 2 or 3 days of selegiline therapy, attempts may be made to decrease the dose of levodopa/carbidopa (10%–30%).
3. The tablet formulation of Eldepryl has been replaced by capsules; however, no dosage adjustment is necessary, as the capsules contain the same 5-mg dose.
**Assessment**
1. Document the level of tremor, rigidity, ROM, and ability to ambulate.
2. List agents currently prescribed or used within the last 2 weeks to ensure that none interact unfavorably.
**Client/Family Teaching**
1. Do not exceed prescribed daily dose. Take with breakfast and lunch.
2. Selegiline is to be taken concurrently with prescribed dose of levodopa/carbidopa. Drug enhances and prolongs the antiparkinsonism effects of levodopa, permitting a dosage reduction.
3. Report any bothersome and/or persistent side effects.
4. Rise slowly from a sitting or lying position to minimize drug's hypotensive effects.
5. Do not drive or operate hazardous

✽ = Available in Canada     ***bold italic*** = life threatening side effect

machinery until drug effects are realized.

6. Avoid tyramine-containing foods; may precipitate a hypertensive crisis.

7. Do not stop abruptly without provider approval.

**Outcomes/Evaluate:** Improved response to levodopa/carbidopa as evidenced by ↓ muscle weakness, ↓ rigidity, ↓ salivation, and improved mobility

# Sertraline hydrochloride

(**SIR**-trah-leen)
**Pregnancy Category:** B
Zoloft **(Rx)**
**Classification:** Antidepressant

**Action/Kinetics:** Believed to act by inhibiting CNS neuronal uptake of serotonin. No significant affinity for adrenergic, cholinergic, dopaminergic, histaminergic, serotonergic, GABA, or benzodiazepine receptors. Steady-state plasma levels are usually reached after 1 week of once daily dosing but is increased to 2–3 weeks in older clients. **Time to peak plasma levels:** 4.5–8.4 hr. **Peak plasma levels:** 20–55 ng/mL. **Time to reach steady state:** 7 days. **Terminal elimination t½:** 1–4 days (including active metabolite). Washout period is 7 days. Food decreases the time to reach peak plasma levels. Undergoes significant first-pass metabolism, significant (98%) binding to serum proteins. Excreted through the urine (40%–45%) and feces (40%–45%). Metabolized to N-desmethyl-sertraline, which has minimal antidepressant activity.

**Uses:** Treatment of depression with reduced psychomotor agitation, anxiety, and insomnia. Obsessive-compulsive disorders in adults and children as defined in DSM-III-R. Treatment of panic disorder, with or without agoraphobia.

**Contraindications:** Use in combination with a MAO inhibitor or within 14 days of discontinuing treatment with a MAO inhibitor.

**Special Concerns:** Use with caution in hepatic or renal dysfunction, with seizure disorders, during lactation, and in diseases or conditions that may affect hemodynamic responses or metabolism. Safety and efficacy have not been determined in children. The plasma clearance may be lower in elderly clients. The possibility of a suicide attempt is possible in depression and may persist until significant remission occurs.

**Side Effects:** A large number of side effects is possible; listed are those side effects with a frequency of 0.1% or greater. *GI:* Nausea and diarrhea (common), dry mouth, constipation, dyspepsia, vomiting, flatulence, anorexia, abdominal pain, thirst, increased salivation, increased appetite, gastroenteritis, teeth-grinding, dysphagia, eructation, taste perversion or change. *CV:* Palpitations, hot flushes, edema, hypertension, hypotension, peripheral ischemia, postural hypotension or dizziness, syncope, tachycardia. *CNS:* Headache (common), insomnia (common), somnolence, agitation, nervousness, anxiety, dizziness, tremor, fatigue, impaired concentration, yawning, paresthesia, hypoesthesia, twitching, hypertonia, confusion, ataxia or abnormal coordination, abnormal gait, hyperesthesia, hyperkinesia, abnormal dreams, aggressive reaction, amnesia, apathy, delusion, depersonalization, depression, aggravated depression, emotional lability, euphoria, hallucinations, neurosis, paranoid reaction, *suicide ideation or attempt,* abnormal thinking, hypokinesia, migraine, nystagmus, vertigo. *Dermatologic:* Rash, acne, excessive sweating, alopecia, pruritus, cold and clammy skin, facial edema, erythematous rash, maculopapular rash, dry skin. *Musculoskeletal:* Myalgia, arthralgia, arthrosis, dystonia, muscle cramps or weakness. *GU:* Urinary frequency, micturition disorders, menstrual disorders, dysmenorrhea, dysuria, painful menstruation, intermenstrual bleeding, sexual dysfunction and decreased libido, nocturia, polyuria, dysuria, urinary incontinence. *Respiratory:* Rhinitis, pharyngitis, yawning, bronchospasm, coughing, dyspnea, epistaxis. *Ophthalmologic:* Blurred vision, abnormal vision, abnormal accommodation, conjunctivitis, diplopia, eye pain, xerophthalmia. *Otic:* Tinnitus, earache. *Body as a whole:* Asthenia, fever, chest pain, chills, back pain, weight loss or weight gain, generalized edema, malaise, flushing, hot flashes, rigors, lymphadenopathy, purpura.

**Laboratory Test Alterations:** ↑ AST or ALT, total cholesterol, triglycerides. ↓ Serum uric acid.

**OD Overdose Management:** *Symptoms:* Intensification of side effects. *Treatment:*
• Establish and maintain an airway, ensuring adequate oxygenation and ventilation.
• Activated charcoal, with or without sorbitol, may be as or more effective than emesis or lavage.
• Cardiac and VS should be monitored.
• Provide general supportive measures and symptomatic treatment.
• Since sertraline has a large volume of distribution, it is unlikely that dialysis, forced diuresis, hemoperfusion, or exchange transfusion will be beneficial.

**Drug Interactions:** Because sertraline is highly bound to plasma proteins, its use with other drugs that are also highly protein bound may lead to displacement, resulting in higher plasma levels of the drug and possibly increased side effects.
*Alcohol* / Concurrent use is not recommended in depressed clients
*Benzodiazepines* / ↓ Clearance of benzodiazepines metabolized by hepatic oxidation
*Cimetidine* / ↑ Half-life and blood levels of sertraline
*Diazepam* / ↑ Plasma levels of desmethyldiazepam (significance not known)
*MAO inhibitors* / Serious and possibly fatal reactions including hyperthermia, rigidity, autonomic instability with possible rapid fluctuation of VS, myoclonus, changes in mental status (e.g., extreme agitation, delirium, coma)
*Warfarin* / ↑ PT and delayed normalization of PT

**Dosage** ————————
• **Tablets**
  *Depression.*
**Adults, initial:** 50 mg once daily either in the morning or evening. Clients not responding to a 50-mg dose may benefit from doses up to a maximum of 200 mg/day.
  *Obsessive-compulsive disorder.*
**Adults:** 50–200 mg/day. **Children, 6 to 12 years:** 25 mg once a day; **adolescents, 13 to 17 years:** 50 mg once a day.
  *Panic attacks.*
**Adults, initial:** 25 mg/day for the first week; **then,** dosage ranges from 50–200 mg/day, based on response and tolerance.

## NURSING CONSIDERATIONS
### Administration/Storage
1. Clients responding during an initial 8-week treatment period will likely benefit during an additional 8-week treatment period. The effectiveness of sertraline has not been evaluated for more than 16 weeks, although it is generally recognized that acute periods of depression require several months or longer of sustained drug therapy. Shown to be effective up to 52 weeks for depression.
2. Do not increase dosage at intervals of less than 1 week.
3. Beneficial effects may not be observed for 2–4 weeks after treatment is started.
4. Use for more than 12 weeks for panic attacks has not been studied.
### Assessment
1. Document indications for therapy, type, onset, and symptom characteristics.
2. List other drugs trialed and the outcome.
3. Note any seizure disorder.
4. Assess life-style, i.e., recent loss (death of loved one), stress, job change/loss, alcohol/drug use, or

**S**

---

other factors that may contribute to depression.

5. Monitor ECG, liver and renal function studies.

**Client/Family Teaching**

1. Take only as directed and remain under close medical supervision.

2. Do not perform activities that require mental and physical alertness until drug effects are realized.

3. Review side effects, noting those that require immediate medical attention.

4. Loss of appetite, persistent nausea, and diarrhea with excessive weight loss should be reported.

5. Report any suicidal thoughts or aggression. Attend counseling and maintain contact with provider so drug utilization can be assessed, as the risk of suicide is tantamount in a depressive phase.

6. Avoid OTC agents, alcohol, and any other CNS depressants.

7. Use reliable contraception; report if pregnancy suspected.

**Outcomes/Evaluate**

• Improved eating and sleeping patterns

• ↓ Levels of agitation and anxiety

• Relief of symptoms of depression

---

# Simvastatin
(**sim**-vah-**STAH**-tin)
**Pregnancy Category:** X
Zocor **(Rx)**
**Classification:** Antihyperlipidemic

See also *Antihyperlipidemic Agents HMG–CoA Reductase Inhibitors.*

**Action/Kinetics:** Inhibits HMG-CoA reductase, an enzyme that is necessary to convert HMG-CoA to mevalonate (an early step in the biosynthesis of cholesterol). Levels of VLDL and LDL cholesterol and plasma triglycerides are reduced while the plasma concentration of HDL cholesterol is increased. Does not reduce basal plasma cortisol or testosterone levels or impair renal reserve.
**Peak therapeutic response:** 4–6 weeks. Approximately 85% absorbed; significant first-pass effect with less than 5% of a PO dose

reaching the general circulation. Metabolites excreted in the feces (60%) and urine (13%).

**Uses:** Adjunct to diet for the reduction of elevated total and LDL cholesterol levels in types IIa and IIb hypercholesterolemia when the response to diet and other approaches have been inadequate. Prophylaxis of heart attack and decrease in incidence of cardiac death in those with CHD and elevated cholesterol levels. *Investigational:* Heterozygous familial hypercholesterolemia, familial combined hyperlipidemia, diabetic dyslipidemia in non-insulin-dependent diabetes, hyperlipidemia secondary to the nephrotic syndrome, and homozygous familial hypercholesterolemia in clients with defective LDL receptors.

**Contraindications:** Active liver disease or unexplained persistent increases in liver function tests. Use in pregnancy, during lactation, or in children.

**Special Concerns:** Use with caution in clients who have a history of liver disease/consume large quantities of alcohol or with drugs that affect steroid levels or activity. Higher plasma levels may be observed in clients with severe renal insufficiency. Safety and efficacy have not been determined in children less than 18 years of age.

**Side Effects:** *Musculoskeletal:* Rhabdomyolysis with renal dysfunction secondary to myoglobinuria, myopathy, arthralgias. *GI:* N&V, diarrhea, abdominal pain, constipation, flatulence, dyspepsia, pancreatitis, anorexia, stomatitis. *Hepatic:* Hepatitis (including chronic active hepatitis), cholestatic jaundice, cirrhosis, fatty change in liver, *fulminant hepatic necrosis, hepatoma. Neurologic:* Dysfunction of certain cranial nerves resulting in alteration of taste, impairment of extraocular movement, and facial paresis. Paresthesia, peripheral neuropathy, peripheral nerve palsy. *CNS:* Headache, tremor, vertigo, memory loss, anxiety, insomnia, depression. *Hypersensitivity Reactions:* Although rare, the following symptoms have been noted. ***Angioedema, anaphylaxis,*** lupus erythematous–like syndrome, vasculitis, purpura, thrombocytopenia, leukopenia, ***hemolytic anemia,*** polymyalgia rheumatica, positive ANA, ESR increase, arthritis, arthralgia, asthenia, urticaria, photosensitivity, chills, fever, flushing, malaise, dyspnea, ***toxic epidermal necrolysis, erythema multiforme (including Stevens-Johnson syndrome).*** *GU:* Gynecomastia, loss of libido, erectile dysfunction. *Ophthalmologic:* Lens opacities, ophthalmoplegia. *Hematologic:* Transient asymptomatic eosinophilia, anemia, thrombocytopenia, leukopenia. *Miscellaneous:* Upper respiratory infection, asthenia, alopecia, edema.

**Laboratory Test Alterations:** ↑ CPK, AST, ALT.

**Drug Interactions**
*Gemfibrozil* / Possible severe myopathy or rhabdomyolysis
*Warfarin* / ↑ Anticoagulant effect of warfarin

**Dosage**
• **Tablets**
**Adults, initially:** 5–10 mg once daily in the evening; **maintenance:** 5–40 mg/day as a single dose in the evening. Consider a starting dose of 5 mg/day for clients with LDL less than 190 mg/dL and 10 mg/day for clients with LDL greater than 190 mg/dL. For geriatric clients, the starting dose should be 5 mg/day with maximum LDL reductions seen with 20 mg or less daily.

## NURSING CONSIDERATIONS

See also *Nursing Considerations* for *Antihyperlipidemic Agents HMG–CoA Reductase Inhibitors.*
**Administration/Storage**
1. Place client on a standard cholesterol-lowering diet for 3–6 months before starting simvastatin. Continue the diet during drug therapy.
2. May be given without regard to meals.
3. Dosage may be adjusted at intervals of at least 4 weeks.

**Assessment**
1. Monitor CBC, cholesterol profile, liver and renal function studies. Schedule LFTs at the beginning of therapy and semiannually for the first year of therapy. Special attention should be paid to elevated serum transaminase levels.
2. List all medications prescribed to ensure none interact unfavorably.
3. Assess level of compliance with weight reduction, exercise, and cholesterol-lowering diet.
4. Note any alcohol abuse.

**Client/Family Teaching**
1. A low-cholesterol diet must continue to be followed during drug therapy. Consult dietitian for assistance in meal planning and food preparation.
2. Report any S&S of infections, unexplained muscle pain, tenderness or weakness (especially if accompanied by fever or malaise), surgery, trauma, or metabolic disorders.
3. Review importance of following a low-cholesterol diet, obtaining regular exercise, low alcohol consumption, and not smoking in the overall plan to reduce serum cholesterol levels.

**Outcomes/Evaluate:** ↓ Serum triglycerides and LDL cholesterol levels; ↑ HDL cholesterol

# Sodium bicarbonate
(**SO**-dee-um bye-**KAR**-bon-ayt)
**Pregnancy Category:** C
Arm and Hammer Pure Baking Soda, Bell/ans, Citrocarbonate, Neut, Soda Mint (Rx and OTC)
**Classification:** Alkalinizing agent, antacid, electrolyte

**Action/Kinetics:** The antacid action is due to neutralization of hydrochloric acid by forming sodium chloride and carbon dioxide (1 g of sodium bicarbonate neutralizes 12 mEq of acid). Provides temporary relief of peptic ulcer pain and of discomfort associated with indigestion. Although widely used by the public, sodium bicarbonate is rarely prescribed as an antacid because of its high sodium content, short duration of action, and ability to cause alkalosis (sometimes desired). Is also a systemic and urinary alkalinizer by increasing plasma and urinary bicarbonate, respectively.

**Uses:** Treatment of hyperacidity, severe diarrhea (where there is loss of bicarbonate). Alkalization of the urine to treat drug toxicity (e.g., due to barbiturates, salicylates, methanol). Treatment of acute mild to moderate metabolic acidosis due to shock, severe dehydration, anoxia, uncontrolled diabetes, renal disease, cardiac arrest, extracorporeal circulation of blood, severe primary lactic acidosis. Prophylaxis of renal calculi in gout. During sulfonamide therapy to prevent renal calculi and nephrotoxicity. Neutralizing additive solution to decrease chemical phlebitis and client discomfort due to vein irritation at or near the site of infusion of IV acid solutions. *Investigational:* Sickle cell anemia.

**Contraindications:** Chloride loss due to vomiting or from continuous GI suction. With diuretics known to produce a hypochloremic alkalosis. Metabolic and respiratory alkalosis. Hypocalcemia in which alkalosis may cause tetany. Hypertension, convulsions, CHF, and other situations where administration of sodium can be dangerous. As a systemic alkalinizer when used as a neutralizing additive solution. As an antidote for strong mineral acids because carbon dioxide is formed, which may cause discomfort and even perforation.

**Special Concerns:** Use with caution in impaired renal function, toxemia of pregnancy, with oliguria or anuria, during lactation, in edema, CHF, liver cirrhosis, with low-salt diets, and in geriatric or postoperative clients with renal or CV insufficiency with or without CHF.

**Side Effects:** *GI:* Acid rebound, gastric distention. *Milk-alkali syndrome:* Hypercalcemia, metabolic alkalosis (dizziness, cramps, thirst, anorexia,

N&V, hyperexcitability, tetany, diminished breathing, *seizures*), renal dysfunction. *Miscellaneous:* Systemic alkalosis after prolonged use. *Following rapid infusion:* Hypernatremia, alkalosis, hyperirritability, tetany, fluid or solute overload. Extravasation following IV use may manifest ulceration, sloughing, cellulitis, or tissue necrosis at the site of injection.

**OD** **Overdose Management:** *Symptoms:* Severe alkalosis that may be accompanied by tetany or hyperirritability. *Treatment:* Discontinue sodium bicarbonate. Reverse symptoms of alkalosis by rebreathing expired air from a paper bag or using a rebreathing mask. Use an IV infusion of ammonium chloride solution, 2.14%, to control severe cases. Treat hypokalemia by IV sodium chloride or potassium chloride. Calcium gluconate will control tetany.

**Drug Interactions**

*Amphetamines* / ↑ Effect of amphetamines by ↑ renal tubular reabsorption

*Antidepressants, tricyclic* / ↑ Effect of tricyclics by ↑ renal tubular reabsorption

*Benzodiazepines* / ↓ Effect due to ↑ alkalinity of urine

*Chlorpropamide* / ↑ Rate of excretion due to alkalinization of the urine

*Ephedrine* / ↑ Effect of ephedrine by ↑ renal tubular reabsorption

*Erythromycin* / ↑ Effect of erythromycin in urine due to ↑ alkalinity of urine

*Flecainide* / ↑ Effect due to ↑ alkalinity of urine

*Iron products* / ↓ Effect due to ↑ alkalinity of urine

*Ketoconazole* / ↓ Effect due to ↑ alkalinity of urine

*Lithium carbonate* / Excretion of lithium is proportional to amount of sodium ingested. If client on sodium-free diet, may develop lithium toxicity because less lithium is excreted

*Mecamylamine* / ↓ Excretion due to alkalinization of the urine

*Methenamine compounds* / ↓ Effect of methenamine due to ↑ alkalinity of urine

*Methotrexate* / ↑ Renal excretion due to alkalinization of the urine

*Nitrofurantoin* / ↓ Effect of nitrofurantoin due to ↑ alkalinity of urine

*Procainamide* / ↑ Effect of procainamide due to ↓ excretion by kidney

*Pseudoephedrine* / ↑ Effect of pseudoephedrine due to ↑ tubular reabsorption

*Quinidine* / ↑ Effect of quinidine by ↑ renal tubular reabsorption

*Salicylates* / ↑ Rate of excretion due to alkalinization of the urine

*Sulfonylureas* / ↓ Effect due to ↑ alkalinity of urine

*Sympathomimetics* / ↓ Renal excretion due to alkalinization of the urine

*Tetracyclines* / ↓ Effect of tetracyclines due to ↑ excretion by kidney

**Dosage** ————————————

• **Effervescent Powder**
  *Antacid.*
**Adults:** 3.9–10 g in a glass of cold water after meals. **Geriatric and pediatric, 6–12 years:** 1.9–3.9 g after meals.

• **Oral Powder**
  *Antacid.*
**Adults:** ½ teaspoon in a glass of water q 2 hr; adjust dosage as required.
  *Urinary alkalinizer.*
**Adults:** 1 teaspoon in a glass of water q 4 hr; adjust dosage as required. Dosage not established for this form for children.

• **Tablets**
  *Antacid.*
**Adults:** 0.325–2 g 1–4 times/day; pediatric, 6–12 years: 520 mg; may be repeated once after 30 min.
  *Urinary alkalinizer.*
**Adults, initial:** 4 g; **then,** 1–2 g q 4 hr. **Pediatric:** 23–230 mg/kg/day; adjust dosage as needed.

• **IV**
  *Cardiac arrest.*
**Adults:** 200–300 mEq given rapidly as a 7.5% or 8.4% solution. In emergencies, 300–500 mL of a 5% solution given as rapidly as possible without overalkalinizing the client. **Infants, less than 2 years of age, initial:** 1–2 mEq/kg/min given over 1–2 min; **then,** 1 mEq/kg q 10 min of arrest. Do not exceed 8 mEq/kg/day.
  *Severe metabolic acidosis.*
90–180 mEq/L (about 7.5–15 g) at a rate of 1–1.5 L during the first hour. Adjust to needs of client.
  *Less severe metabolic acidosis.*
Add to other IV fluids. **Adults and older children:** 2–5 mEq/kg given over a 4- to 8-hr period.
  *Neutralizing additive solution.*
One vial of neutralizing additive solution added to 1 L of commonly used parenteral solutions, including dextrose, NaCl, and Ringer's.

## NURSING CONSIDERATIONS
### Administration/Storage
**IV** 1. Hypertonic solutions must be administered by trained personnel. Avoid extravasation as tissue irritation or cellulitis may result.

2. Determine IV dose by arterial blood pH, $pCO_2$, and base deficit; may be given IV push in an arrest situation or may be diluted in dextrose or saline solution and administered over 4–8 hr.

3. Administer isotonic solutions slowly; too-rapid administration may result in death due to cellular acidity. Check rate of flow frequently.

4. If only the 7.5% or 8.4% solution is available, dilute 1:1 with D5W when used in infants for cardiac arrest.

5. Do not exceed a rate of administration of 8 mEq/kg/day in infants with cardiac arrest to guard against hypernatremia, induction of intracranial hemorrhage, and decreasing CSF pressure.

6. Have available a parenteral solution of calcium gluconate and 2.14% solution of ammonium chloride in the event of severe alkalosis or tetany.

7. Do not add to calcium-containing solutions, except where compatibility has been established.

---

✦ = Available in Canada      ***bold italic*** = life threatening side effect

8. Norepinephrine and dobutamine are incompatible with sodium bicarbonate.

**Assessment**

1. Note any history of renal impairment, CHF, or if prescribed a low-sodium diet.

2. Assess for edema, which may indicate inability to utilize sodium bicarbonate. May try potassium bicarbonate (sodium content is 27%).

3. If on low continuous or intermittent NG suctioning or vomiting, assess for evidence of excessive chloride loss.

4. Record I&O. Observe for dry skin and mucous membranes, polydipsia, polyuria, and air hunger; may indicate a reversal of symptoms of metabolic acidosis.

5. With acidosis, assess for the relief of dyspnea and hyperpnea.

6. If prescribed to counteract metabolic acidosis, monitor electrolytes and ABGs (pH, $pCO_2$, and $HCO_3$). Test urine periodically with nitrazine paper to determine if becoming alkaline.

**Client/Family Teaching**

1. If routinely taking excessive PO preparations of sodium bicarbonate to relieve gastric distress, a rebound reaction may occur, resulting either in an increased acid secretion or systemic alkalosis. Persistent symptoms of gastric distress require medical intervention.

2. Continuous, routine ingestion of sodium bicarbonate may cause formation of phosphate crystals in the kidney and fluid retention.

3. Consuming sodium bicarbonate with milk or calcium may result in a milk-alkali syndrome. Report immediately if anorexia, N&V, or mental confusion occurs.

4. Avoid OTC preparations that contain sodium bicarbonate, such as Alka-Seltzer or Fizrin.

**Outcomes/Evaluate**

- Reversal of metabolic acidosis
- ↑ Urinary and serum pH
- ↓ Gastric discomfort

# Sodium chloride

(**SO**-dee-um **KLOR**-eyed)

**Pregnancy Category:** C

**Topical:** Ayr Saline, HuMIST Saline Nasal, NaSal Saline Nasal, Ocean Mist, Saline From Otrivin ✦, Salinex Nasal Mist., Thalaris ✦, **Ophthalmic:** Adsorbonac Ophthalmic, AK-NaCl, Cordema ✦, Hypersal 5%, Muro-128 Ophthalmic, Muroptic-5, **Parenteral:** Sodium Chloride IV Infusions (0.45%, 0.9%, 3%, 5%), Sodium Chloride Injection for Admixtures (50, 100, 625 mEq/vial), Sodium Chloride Diluent (0.9%), Concentrated Sodium Chloride Injection (14.6%, 23.4%) (parenteral is Rx; topical and ophthalmic are OTC)

**Classification:** Electrolyte

**Action/Kinetics:** Sodium is the major cation of the body's extracellular fluid. It plays a crucial role in maintaining the fluid and electrolyte balance. Excess retention of sodium results in overhydration (edema, hypervolemia), which is often treated with diuretics. Abnormally low levels of sodium result in dehydration. Normally, the plasma contains 136–145 mEq sodium/L and 98–106 mEq chloride/L. The average daily requirement of salt is approximately 5 g.

**Uses: PO:** Prophylaxis of heat prostration or muscle cramps, chloride deficiency due to diuresis or salt restriction, prevention or treatment of extracellular volume depletion.

**Parenteral:**

*0.9% (Isotonic) NaCl.* To restore sodium and chloride losses; to dilute or dissolve drugs for IV, IM, or SC use; flushing of IV catheters; extracellular fluid replacement; priming solution for hemodialysis; initiate and terminate blood transfusions so RBCs will not hemolyze; metabolic alkalosis when there is fluid loss and mild sodium depletion.

*0.45% (Hypotonic) NaCl.* Fluid replacement when fluid loss exceeds depletion of electrolytes; hyperosmolar diabetes when dextrose should not be used (need for large volume of fluid but without excess sodium ions).

*3% or 5% (Hypertonic) NaCl.* Hyponatremia and hypochloremia due to electrolyte losses; to dilute body water significantly following excessive fluid intake; emergency treatment of severe salt depletion.

*Concentrated NaCl.* Additive in parenteral therapy for clients with special needs for sodium intake.

*Bacteriostatic NaCl.* Used only to dilute or dissolve drugs for IM, IV, or SC injection.

**Topical:** Relief of inflamed, dry, or crusted nasal membranes; irrigating solution. **Ophthalmic:** Use hypertonic solutions to decrease corneal edema due to bullous keratitis; as an aid to facilitate ophthalmoscopic examination in gonioscopy, biomicroscopy, and funduscopy.

**Contraindications:** Congestive heart failure, severely impaired renal function, hypernatremia, fluid retention. Use of the 3% or 5% solutions in elevated, normal, or only slightly depressed levels of plasma sodium and chloride. Use of bacteriostatic NaCl injection in newborns.

**Special Concerns:** Use with caution in CV, cirrhotic, or renal disease; in presence of hyperproteinemia, hypervolemia, urinary tract obstruction, and CHF; in those with concurrent edema and sodium retention and in clients receiving corticosteroids or corticotropin; and during lactation. Use with caution in geriatric or postoperative clients with renal or CV insufficiency with or without CHF.

**Side Effects:** Hypernatremia. Excessive NaCl may lead to hypopotassemia and acidosis. Fluid and solute overload leading to dilution of serum electrolyte levels, CHF, overhydration, *acute pulmonary edema* (especially in clients with CV disease or in those receiving corticosteroids or other drugs that cause sodium retention). Too rapid administration may cause local pain and venous irritation.

*Postoperative intolerance of NaCl:* Cellular dehydration, weakness, asthenia, disorientation, anorexia, nausea, oliguria, increased BUN levels, distention, deep respiration.

*Symptoms due to solution or administration technique:* Fever, abscess, tissue necrosis, infection at injection site, venous thrombosis or phlebitis extending from injection site, local tenderness, extravasation, hypervolemia.

***Inadvertent administration of concentrated NaCl (i.e., without dilution) will cause sudden hypernatremia with the possibility of CV shock, extensive hemolysis, CNS problems, necrosis of the cortex of the kidneys, local tissue necrosis (if given extravascularly).***

**OD** **Overdose Management:** *Symptoms:* Irritation of GI mucosa, N&V, abdominal cramps, diarrhea, edema. Hypernatremia symptoms include: irritability, restlessness, weakness, *seizures, coma,* tachycardia, hypertension, fluid accumulation, *pulmonary edema, respiratory arrest. Treatment:* Supportive measures, including gastric lavage, induction of vomiting, provide adequate airway and ventilation, maintain vascular volume and tissue perfusion. Magnesium sulfate given as a cathartic.

**Dosage** _____
• **Tablets (Including Extended-Release and Enteric-Coated)**
*Heat cramps/dehydration.*
0.5–1 g with 8 oz water up to 10 times/day; total daily dose should not exceed 4.8 g.
• **IV**
**Individualized.** Daily requirements of sodium and chloride can be met by administering 1 L of 0.9% NaCl.
*To calculate sodium deficit.* Amount of sodium to be given to raise serum sodium to the desired level:
Total body water (TBW): sodium deficit (mEq) = TBW × (desired plasma Na − observed plasma Na).
• **Ophthalmic Solution 2% or 5%**
1–2 gtt in eye q 3–4 hr.

**S**

---

• **Ophthalmic Ointment 5%**
A small amount (approximately ¼ in.) to the inside of the affected eye(s) (i.e., by pulling down the lower eyelid) q 3–4 hr.

## NURSING CONSIDERATIONS
### Administration/Storage
**IV** 1. Give hypertonic injections of NaCl slowly through a small-bore needle placed well within the lumen of a large vein (to minimize irritation). Avoid infiltration.
2. Concentrated NaCl injection must be diluted before use.
3. Flush IV catheters before and after the medications are given using 0.9% NaCl for injection.
4. Incompatibilities may occur when mixing NaCl injection with other additives; inspect the final product for cloudiness or a precipitate immediately after mixing, before administration, and periodically during administration. Do not store these mixtures.

### Assessment
1. Note indications for therapy; monitor electrolytes, ECG, liver and renal function studies.
2. Observe for S&S of hypernatremia: flushed skin, elevated temperature, rough dry tongue, and edema. Symptoms of hyponatremia may include N&V, muscle cramps, dry mucous membranes, increased HR, and headaches.
3. Monitor VS and I&O. Assess urine specific gravity and serum sodium levels. Report if urine specific gravity is above 1.020 and serum sodium level is above 146 mEq/L.
4. Note level of consciousness and periodically assess heart and lung sounds.
5. When administering IV the 0.45% NaCl is hypotonic, the 0.9% NaCl is isotonic, and the 3% and 5% NaCl solutions are hypertonic.

### Outcomes/Evaluate
• Prophylaxis of heat prostration during exposure to high temperatures or during increased activity
• Prevention of chloride deficiency R/T excessive diuresis or salt restriction or excessive sweating

# Sodium hyaluronate/ Hylan G-F 20
(**SO**-dee-um **high**-ah-**LUR**-ah-nayt)
Hyalgan, Synvisc **(Rx)**
**Classification:** Hyaluronic acid derivative

**Action/Kinetics:** Hyaluronic acid occurs naturally in body tissues and fluids. It is secreted by cells in synovial membranes and, in healthy synovial joints, maintains viscosity of synovial fluid and supports lubricating and shock-absorbing properties of the cartilage. In osteoarthritis, synovial fluid is decreased in viscosity and elasticity. Sodium hyaluronate and hylan G-F 20 replace diseased synovial fluid. Following intra-articular use, hylan G-F 20 permeates cartilage and slowly moves through joint tissues; it then passes through the lymph system into systemic circulation. Hyaluronic acid is metabolized by hyaluronidase in synovium.

**Uses:** Treatment of pain in osteoarthritis of knee in those who have not responded adequately to conservative non-drug therapy and to acetaminophen.

**Contraindications:** Hypersensitivity to hyaluronan. Use in infections or skin diseases in area of injection site or with skin disinfectants containing quaternary ammonium salts (drug may precipitate). Concomitant use with other intra-articular injectables.

**Special Concerns:** Safety and efficacy on intra-articular use in areas other than knee or use for conditions other than osteoarthritis have not been determined. Use with caution in severely inflamed knee joints, when lymphatic or venous stasis exists in treatment leg, during lactation, and in those allergic to avian proteins, feathers and egg products. Safety and efficacy may be altered by dilutional effects. Safety and efficacy have not been determined during pregnancy or in children.

**Side Effects:** *Sodium hyaluronate (Hyalgan):* Injection site pain, skin reaction (ecchymosis, rash), pruritus.

*Hylan G-F 20 (Synvisc):* Knee pain, swelling, thorax and back rash, pruritus, calf cramps, hemorrhoid problems, ankle edema, muscle pain, tonsillitis with nausea, tachyarrhythmia, phlebitis with varicosities, low back sprain.

**Dosage**
• **Intra-articular injection**
*Osteoarthritis of knee.*
*Hyalgan:* 2 mL once weekly for total of 5 injections using 20 gauge needle. *Synvisc:* 2 mL once weekly for total of 3 injections using 18-20 gauge needle. For both drugs, inject local anesthetic (e.g., lidocaine) SC prior to administration. Pain relief may not be noted until after last injection.

**NURSING CONSIDERATIONS**
**Administration/Storage**
1. If treatment is bilateral, use separate 2 mL vial/syringe for each knee.
2. Do not prepare injection site with skin disinfectants containing quaternary ammonium salts.
3. Remove joint effusion before giving drug. Do not use same syringe for removing fluid and injecting hyaluronic acid derivatives. However, use the same needle for injecting hylan G-F 20.
4. Drug products are intended for single use. Use immediately once opened and discard unused portion.
5. Safety and efficacy of repeat cycles have not been determined.
6. Store in original package at 25°C–30°C (77°F–86°F). Protect from light; do not freeze.
**Assessment**
1. Document other therapy utilized (nonpharmacologic and analgesic) and outcome.
2. Assess for effusion and remove prior to administering therapy.
3. Drug is derived from chicken/rooster coombs; assess for allergy to egg products, feathers, or avian proteins.

**Client/Family Teaching**
1. Review drug information sheet enclosed.
2. Drug is administered by provider into knee joint once weekly for 3-5 weeks, depending on agent used.
3. May experience swelling and pain in treated joints.
4. Do not perform strenuous or prolonged (>1 hr) weight bearing activities such as tennis or jogging within 48 hr of injection.
5. Pain relief usually lasts for up to 6 mo and may not be evident until after last injection.
**Outcomes/Evaluate:** Control of osteoarthritis knee pain; ↑ mobility

# Sodium polystyrene sulfonate
(SO-dee-um pol-ee-STY-reen SUL-fon-ayt)
**Pregnancy Category:** C
Kayexalate, K-Exit ✶, PMS Sodium Polystyrene Sulfonate ✶, SPS **(Rx)**
**Classification:** Potassium ion exchange resin

**Action/Kinetics:** Resin that exchanges sodium ions for potassium ions primarily in the large intestine. Thus, excess amounts of potassium (as well as calcium and magnesium) may be removed. Therapy is governed by daily monitoring of serum potassium levels. Discontinue therapy when serum potassium levels have reached 4–5 mEq/L. Monitor for serum calcium and magnesium levels. **Onset, PO:** 2–12 hr.
**Uses:** Hyperkalemia.
**Special Concerns:** Use with caution in geriatric clients because they are more likely to develop fecal impaction. Use with caution in clients sensitive to sodium overload (e.g., in CV disease) or for those receiving digitalis preparations because the action of these agents is potentiated by hypokalemia. Effective decreases in potassium may take several hours to accomplish; other treatment (e.g., IV calcium or

**S**

sodium bicarbonate or glucose and insulin) may be considered in states of severe hyperkalemia (e.g., burns, renal failure).

**Side Effects:** *GI:* N&V, constipation, anorexia, gastric irritation, diarrhea (rarely). Fecal impaction in geriatric clients. *Electrolyte:* Sodium retention, hypokalemia, hypocalcemia, hypomagnesemia. *Other:* Overhydration, *pulmonary edema.*

**Drug Interactions**
*Aluminum hydroxide* / ↑ Risk of intestinal obstruction
*Calcium- or magnesium-containing antacids or laxatives* / ↑ Risk of metabolic alkalosis

**Dosage** ———————
• **Powder for Suspension, Suspension**
    *Hyperkalemia.*
**Adults:** 15 g resin suspended in 20–100 mL water or syrup (to increase palatability) 1–4 times/day. Up to 40 g/day has been used. **Pediatric:** To calculate dose, use an exchange ratio of 1 mEq potassium/g resin (usually, 1 g/kg dose).
• **Enema**
    *Hyperkalemia.*
**Adults:** 30–50 g suspended in 100 mL sorbitol or 20% dextrose in water q 6 hr.

## NURSING CONSIDERATIONS
**Administration/Storage**
1. To treat or to prevent constipation, 10–20 mL of 70% sorbitol may be given PO q 2 hr (or as necessary) to produce 1–2 watery stools each day.
2. For PO administration, give the resin suspended in water or sorbitol syrup (3–4 mL/g resin). If necessary, the resin can be administered through a NGT, either as an aqueous suspension, mixed with dextrose, or as a peanut or olive oil emulsion.
3. Rectal administration:
• First, administer a cleansing enema.
• To administer medication, insert a large-size rubber tube (e.g., French 28) into the rectum for a distance of 20 cm until it is well into the sigmoid colon and tape in place.

• Suspend resin in appropriate vehicle (see *Dosage*) at body temperature. Administer by gravity while stirring suspension.
• Flush suspension that remains in the container with 50–100 mL fluid, clamp the tube, and leave in place.
• Elevate hips or ask client to assume a knee-chest position for a short time if there is back leakage.
• The enema should be kept in the colon as long as possible (3–4 hr).
• Resin is removed by colonic irrigation with 2 quarts of a *non-sodium*-containing solution warmed to body temperature. Returns are drained constantly through a Y tube.
4. Retention enemas are less effective than PO administration.
5. Use freshly prepared solutions within 24 hr. Do not heat resin.
6. Oral suspension products contain sorbitol and sodium.
7. Designate on orders the grams of powder and the percent sorbitol and volume to be used or the amount of premixed suspension. Specify the frequency and route of administration.
8. Avoid inhaling the powder for suspension when admixing.

**Assessment**
1. Document serum potassium levels. Attempt to identify cause for increased levels. Also monitor renal function studies and levels of sodium, magnesium, and calcium.
2. Determine any history of CV disease and/or if taking any digitalis preparations.
3. Assess clients on sodium restrictions closely; drug contains 100 mg Na/g.

**Client/Family Teaching**
1. The use of calcium- or magnesium-containing antacids during PO administration of sodium polystyrene may predispose one to metabolic alkalosis; use cautiously.
2. Report any increase in urinary output or constipation.
3. With enemas, retain the solution for several hours to ensure drug effectiveness.

**Outcomes/Evaluate:**    ↓    Serum

potassium levels to within desired range (4.0–5.5 mEq/L)

———COMBINATION DRUG———

# Soma Compound
(**SO**-mah)
**Pregnancy Category:** C
**(Rx)**

# Soma Compound with Codeine
(**SO**-mah, **KOH**-deen)
**Pregnancy Category:** C
**(Rx) (C-III)**
**Classification:** Analgesic/skeletal muscle relaxant

**Content:** Soma Compound contains: *Nonnarcotic analgesic:* Aspirin, 325 mg. *Centrally acting skeletal muscle relaxant:* Carisoprodol, 200 mg. In addition to the above, Soma Compound with Codeine contains: *Narcotic analgesic:* Codeine phosphate, 16 mg. See also information on individual components.

**Uses:** As an adjunct to rest and physical therapy for the relief of acute, painful musculoskeletal conditions including muscle spasm, pain, and conditions leading to limited mobility.

**Contraindications:** Acute intermittent porphyria, bleeding disorders, lactation. Use in children less than 12 years of age.

**Special Concerns:** Use with caution in clients with impaired hepatic or renal function, in elderly or debilitated clients, in clients with a history of gastritis or peptic ulcer, in those on anticoagulant therapy, and in individuals prone to addiction.

**Dosage** ————————
• **Tablets: Soma Compound and Soma Compound with Codeine**
    *Analgesia.*
**Adults:** 1–2 tablets q.i.d.

## NURSING CONSIDERATIONS

See *Nursing Considerations* for *Acetylsalicylic Acid* and *Narcotic Analgesics.*

**Assessment**
1. Document indications for therapy; note location, onset, duration, and frequency of symptoms. Rate pain using a pain-rating scale.
2. Document ROM, swelling, inflammation, and instability with acute injury. Assess for point tenderness and muscle spasm location.
3. List other agents/therapies trialed and the outcome.

**Outcomes/Evaluate:** Relief of musculoskeletal pain

# Somatrem
(**SO**-mah-trem)
**Pregnancy Category:** C
Protropin **(Rx)**

# Somatropin
(so-mah-**TROH**-pin)
**Pregnancy Category:** C, Serostim is B
Genotropin, Humatrope, Norditropin, Nutropin, Nutropin AQ, Saizen, Serostim **(Rx)**
**Classification:** Growth hormone

**Action/Kinetics:** Both somatrem and somatropin are derived from recombinant DNA technology. Somatrem contains the same sequence of amino acids (191) as human growth hormone derived from the pituitary gland plus one additional amino acid (methionine). Somatropin, on the other hand, has the identical sequence of amino acids as does human growth hormone of pituitary origin. These agents stimulate linear growth by increasing somatomedin-C serum levels, which, in turn, increases the incorporation of sulfate into proteoglycans, thereby stimulating skeletal growth. They also increase the number and size of muscle cells, increase synthesis of collagen, increase protein synthesis, and increase internal organ size. Serum insulin levels increase (indicative of insulin resistance), and there is acute mobilization of lipid. **Peak plasma levels, somatotropin:** 7.5 hr after SC. **t½, somatotropin:** 3.8 hr after SC and 4.9 hr after IM.

**S**

**Uses:** Treat growth failure associated with chronic renal insufficiency up to the time of renal transplantation. Except for Serostim to stimulate linear growth of children who suffer from lack of adequate levels of endogenous growth hormone. Humatrope and Genotropin have been approved for the treatment of somatropin deficiency syndrome in adults. In adults, Humatrope produces increased lean muscle mass and exercise capacity, decreased body fat, and normalized high-density lipoprotein cholesterol levels. Humatrope, Nutropin, and Nutropin AQ for long-term treatment of short stature associated with Turner's syndrome. Serostim is approved for the treatment of AIDS wasting (i.e., cachexia). *Investigational:* Short children due to intrauterine growth retardation.

**Contraindications:** In clients in whom epiphyses have closed. Active intracranial lesions, sensitivity to benzyl alcohol (somatrem); sensitivity to m-cresol or glycerin (diluent in Humatrope). Use of Gonotropin to treat acute catabolism in critically ill clients. *NOTE:* Hypothyroidism (which may be induced by the drug) decreases the response to somatrem.

**Special Concerns:** Use with caution during lactation. Concomitant use of glucocorticoids may decrease the response to growth hormone.

**Side Effects:** Development of persistent antibodies to growth hormone (30%–40% of clients taking somatrem and 2% of clients taking somatropin). Development of insulin resistance. Development of hypothyroidism. Sodium retention and mild edema (especially in adults). Slipped capital femoral epiphysis or avascular necrosis of the femoral head in children with advanced renal osteodystrophy. Intracranial hypertension manifested by papilledema, visual changes, headache, N&V. *In adults:* Hyperglycemia, glucosuria; mild, transient edema; headache, weakness, muscle pain. *In children:* Injection site pain, leukemia.

*Nutropin AQ:* Carpal tunnel syndrome, increased growth of preexisting nevi, gynecomastia, peripheral edema (rare), pancreatitis (rare). *Somatropin:* In adults, headache, localized muscle pain, weakness, mild hyperglycemia, glucosuria, mild transient edema during early treatment.

**OD** **Overdose Management:** *Symptons:* Acute overdose can cause hypoglycemia followed by hyperglycemia. Long-term overdose can result in S&S of acromegaly or gigantism.

**Drug Interactions:** Glucocorticoids inhibit the effect of somatrem on growth.

**Dosage**
SOMATREM (PROTROPIN)
• **IM, SC**
**Individualized. Usual:** Up to 0.1 mg/kg (0.26 IU/kg) 3 times/week, not to exceed a weekly dosage of 0.30 mg/kg (about 0.90 IU/kg). The incidence of side effects increases if the dose is greater than 0.1 mg/kg.
SOMATROPIN (GENOTROPIN)
• **SC**
0.16–0.24 mg/kg/week divided into 6 or 7 SC injections.
SOMATROPIN (HUMATROPE)
• **IM, SC**
**Adults: Individualized. Initial:** 0.006 mg/kg/day (0.018 IU/kg/day) or less SC. May be increased, depending on need, to a maximum of 0.0125 mg/kg/day (0.0375 IU/kg/day). **Pediatric:** 0.18 mg/kg/week (0.54 IU/kg/week) SC or IM divided into equal doses given either on 3 alternate days or 6 times a week. Maximum weekly dose is 0.3 mg/kg (0.9 IU/kg) divided into equal doses and given on 3 alternate days.
SOMATRIPIN (NORDITROPIN)
• **SC**
0.024–0.034 mg/kg 6 to 7 times a week.
SOMATROPIN (NUTROPIN, NUTROPIN AQ)
• **SC**
*Growth hormone deficiency.*
**Individualized. Usual:** Give a weekly dose of 0.3 mg/kg (about 0.9 IU/kg).

*Chronic renal insufficiency.*
**Individualized. Usual:** Give a weekly dose of 0.35 mg/kg (about 1.05 IU/kg). This dose can be given up to the time of renal transplantation.
*Turner Syndrome.*
Give a weekly dose of 0.375 (or less) mg/kg (about 1.125 IU/kg) divided into equal doses 3 to 7 times/week.
SOMATROPIN (SAIZEN)
• **IM, SC**
0.06 mg/kg (about 0.18 IU/kg) 3 times weekly. Discontinue when epiphyses fuse.
SOMATROPIN (SEROSTIM)
• **SC**
**Weight > 55 kg:** 6 mg daily; **45–55 kg:** 5 mg daily; **35–45 kg:** 4 mg daily; **less than 35 kg:** 0.1 mg/kg. Give daily dose at bedtime.

## NURSING CONSIDERATIONS
### Administration/Storage
1. Somatrem should be prescribed only by a physician experienced in the diagnosis and treatment of pituitary disorders.
2. Due to the development of insulin resistance, evaluate for possible glucose intolerance.
3. Reconstitue the powder for injection for somatrem *only* with bacteriostatic water for injection (benzyl alcohol preserved).
4. If used in newborns, it should be reconstituted with water for injection because benzyl alcohol can be toxic to newborns.
5. Inject only reconstituted somatrem solution that is clear and without particulate matter.
6. Be sure the needle used for injection is at least 1 in. or greater in length so that the injection reaches the muscle layer.
7. Use reconstituted somatrem within 7 days; do not freeze.
8. Genotropin is supplied in a two-chamber cartridge with the drug in the front chamber and the diluent in the rear chamber. Use a reconstitution device to co-mix the drug and diluent following the directions on the package. Gently tip the cartridge up-

side down a few times until complete dissolution occurs. Do not shake.
9. For Genotropin, the 1.5-mg cartridge may be refrigerated for 24 hr or less because it contains no preservative. Use once and discard any remaining solution. The 5.8- and 13.8-mg cartridges contain a preservative and may be stored under refrigeration for up to 14 days.
10. Give Genotropin in the thigh, buttocks, or abdomen; rotate the site daily to help prevent liopatrophy.
11. Humatrope is reconstituted by adding 1.5–5 mL of the diluent supplied for each 5-mg vial. Do not shake the vial. Do not give the reconstituted solution if it is cloudy or contains particulate material. Use a small enough syringe to ensure accuracy when the solution is withdrawn from the vial.
12. If sensitivity to the diluent for Humatrope occurs, reconstitute with sterile water for injection. The following guidelines must be followed.
• Use only one dose per reconstituted vial.
• Refrigerate solutions if not used immediately after reconstitution.
• Use the reconstituted dose within 24 hr.
• After the dose is administered, discard any unused portion.
13. Reconstitute either the 4- or 8-mg vial of Norditropin, with 2 mL diluent. Avoid direct sunlight. Refrigerate and use reconstituted vials within 14 days after dissolution.
14. Give Norditropin in the thighs and vary the injection site on the thigh on a rotating basis.
15. Reconstitute Nutropin by adding bacteriostatic water for injection, 1–5 mL for each 5-mg vial and 1–10 mL for each 10-mg vial. For use in newborns, use water for injection as the benzyl alcohol (preservative) used in the bacteriostatic water may cause toxicity.
16. Use the following guidelines when giving Nutropin for clients who require dialysis:

S

• Give hemodialysis clients Nutropin at night just prior to going to sleep or at least 3–4 hr after dialysis in order to prevent hematoma formation due to heparin.

• Give chronic cycling peritoneal dialysis clients Nutropin in the morning after they have completed dialysis.

• Give chronic ambulatory peritoneal dialysis clients Nutropin in the evening at the time of the overnight exchange.

17. Reconstitute Saizen with 1 to 3 mL bacteriostatic water for injection. Reconstituted solutions are stable, under refrigeration, for 14 days. Avoid freezing.

18. Reconstitute Serostim with 1 mL sterile water for injection. Use within 24 hr of reconstitution and refrigerate reconstituted solution.

19. Except for Genotropin, when reconstituting somatrem or somatropin, do not shake the vial. Rather, swirl with a gentle rotary motion. The solution should be clear immediately after reconstitution.

20. Before reconstitution, vials should be stored at 2°C–8°C (36°F–46°F).

**Assessment**

1. Note indications for therapy, age of client, and any other therapy trialed.

2. Determine that X-ray evidence of bone growth (wrists, hands) has been conducted. Record height and weight monthly. Generally a growth increase of 2 cm/year should be attained in order for treatment to be continued.

3. If growth is slow in the absence of rising antibody titers, hypopituitarism should be ruled out; untreated hypothyroidism or excessive glucocorticoid replacement can impair growth.

4. Monitor blood sugar and thyroid function studies; assess for diabetes or hypothyroidism. With diabetes, assess for hyperglycemia and acidosis.

5. Note any limps or knee/hip pain because a slipped capital epiphysis may occur.

**Client/Family Teaching**

1. Keep and review drug literature with guidelines for the appropriate method of administration, drug preparation, and storage, after instructed by provider.

2. Report as scheduled for F/U.

3. Report any adverse effects or any limps or knee or hip pain.

4. The cost per year is based on client's weight and typically runs $10,000–$30,000.

**Outcomes/Evaluate:** Evidence of desired skeletal growth; (growth hormone replacement with deficiency)

# Sotalol hydrochloride
(**SOH**-tah-lol)
**Pregnancy Category:** B
Alti-Sotalol ✦, Apo-Sotalol ✦, Betapace, Linsotalol ✦, Sotacor ✦ **(Rx)**
**Classification:** Beta-adrenergic blocking agent

See also *Beta-Adrenergic Blocking Agents.*

**Action/Kinetics:** Blocks both beta-1- and beta-2-adrenergic receptors; has no membrane-stabilizing activity or intrinsic sympathomimetic activity. Has both Group II and Group III antiarrhythmic properties (dose dependent). Significantly increases the refractory period of the atria, His-Purkinje fibers, and ventricles. Also prolongs the QTc and JT intervals. **t½:** 12 hr. Not metabolized; excreted unchanged in the urine.

**Uses:** Treatment of documented ventricular arrhythmias such as life-threatening sustained ventricular tachycardia.

**Contraindications:** Use in asymptomatic PVCs or supraventricular arrhythmias due to the proarrhythmic effects of sotalol. Congenital or acquired long QT syndromes. Use in clients with hypokalemia or hypomagnesemia until the imbalance is corrected, as these conditions aggravate the degree of QT prolongation and increase the risk for torsades de pointes.

**Special Concerns:** Clients with sustained ventricular tachycardia and a history of CHF appear to be at the

highest risk for serious proarrhythmia. Dose, presence of sustained
ventricular tachycardia, females,
excessive prolongation of the QTc
interval, and history of cardiomegaly
or CHF are risk factors for torsades de
pointes. Use with caution in clients
with chronic bronchitis or emphysema and in asthma if an IV agent is required. Use with extreme caution in
clients with sick sinus syndrome
associated    with    symptomatic
arrhythmias due to the increased
risk of sinus bradycardia, sinus paus-
es, or sinus arrest. Reduce dosage in
impaired renal function. Safety and
efficacy in children have not been
established.

**Additional Side Effects:** *CV: New
or worsened ventricular arrhythmias,
including sustained ventricular tachycardia or ventricular fibrillation that
might be fatal. Torsades de pointes.*

## Dosage
* **Tablets**
  *Ventricular arrhythmias.*

**Adults, initial:** 80 mg b.i.d. The
dose may be increased to 240 or 320
mg/day after appropriate evaluation.
**Usual:** 160–320 mg/day given in
two or three divided doses. Clients
with life-threatening refractory ventricular arrhythmias may require doses
ranging from 480 to 640 mg/day
(due to potential proarrhythmias,
these doses should only be used if the
potential benefit outweighs the increased risk of side effects).

## NURSING CONSIDERATIONS

See also *Nursing Considerations* for
*Beta-Adrenergic Blocking Agents.*
### Administration/Storage
1. Adjust dosage gradually, allowing
2–3 days between increments in
dosage. This allows steady-state
plasma levels to be reached and QT
intervals to be monitored.
2. Undertake initiation of and
increases in dosage in a hospital
with facilities for cardiac rhythm
monitoring and assessment. The
dose for each client must be individ-

ualized only after appropriate clinical
assessment.
3. Proarrhythmias can occur during
initiation of therapy and with each
increment in dosage.
4. In clients with impaired renal
function, alter the dosing interval as
follows: if $C_{CR}$ is 30–60 mL/min, the
dosing interval is 24 hr; if $C_{CR}$ is
10–30 mL/min, the dosing interval
should be 36–48 hr. If $C_{CR}$ is less
than 10 mL/min, dose must be individualized.    Undertake    dosage
adjustments in clients with impaired
renal function only after five to six
doses at the intervals described.
5. Before initiating sotalol, withdraw
previous   antiarrhythmic   therapy
with careful monitoring for a minimum of 2–3 plasma half-lives if condition permits.
6. After amiodarone is discontinued,
do not initiate sotalol until the QT
interval is normalized.
### Assessment
1. Perform a thorough nursing history; note any cardiomegaly or CHF.
2. Obtain ECG and document QT
interval; note symptoms associated
with arrhythmia.
3. Client should be in a closely
monitored environment with VS and
ECG monitored during initiation and
adjustment of sotalol.
4. Monitor VS, I&O, electrolytes,
magnesium level, liver and renal
function studies.
### Client/Family Teaching
1. Take on an empty stomach as
food decreases absorption.
2. Take exactly as directed and do not
stop abruptly; drug controls symptoms but does not cure condition.
3. Avoid activites that require mental
alertness until drug effects realized;
may cause dizziness and drowsiness.
4. Immediately report increased
chest pain, increased SOB, night
cough, swelling of feet and ankles, increased fatigue, low heart rate, or
unsteady gait.
5. Avoid alcohol and all OTC agents
without approval.

6. Continue dietary and exercise guidelines as prescribed and lifestyle changes compatible with healthy living.

**Outcomes/Evaluate:** Control/conversion of life-threatening arrhythmias to stable cardiac rhythm

# Sparfloxacin
(spar-**FLOX**-ah-sin)
**Pregnancy Category:** C
Zagam **(Rx)**
**Classification:** Fluoroquinolone antibiotic

See also *Fluoroquinolones*.
**Action/Kinetics:** Well absorbed. **Peak serum levels:** 4–5 hr. 50% excreted in the urine.
**Uses:** Community acquired pneumonia due to *Chlamydia pneumoniae, Haemophilus influenzae, Haemophilus parainfluenzae, Moraxella catarrhalis, Mycoplasma pneu-moniae,* or *Streptococcus pneu-moniae.* Acute bacterial exacerbations of chronic bronchitis caused by *C. pneumoniae, Enterobacter cloacae, H. influenzae, H. parainfluenzae, Klebsiella pneumoniae, M. catarrhalis, Staphylococcus aureus,* or S. pneumoniae.
**Special Concerns:** Safety and efficacy have not been determined in children less than 18 years of age.

**Dosage**
• **Tablets**
*Community-acquired pneumonia, acute bacterial exacerbations of chronic bronchitis.*
**Adults over 18 years of age:** Two - 200 mg tablets taken on the first day as a loading dose. Then, one - 200 mg tablet q 24 hr for a total of 10 days of therapy (i.e., a total of 11 tablets). For clients with a $C_{CR}$ less than 50 mL/min, the loading dose is two - 200 mg tablets taken on the first day. Then, one - 200 mg tablet q 48 hr for a total of 9 days (i.e., a total of 6 tablets).

## NURSING CONSIDERATIONS
See also *Nursing Considerations* for *Antiviral Drugs*.
**Assessment**
1. Document onset, location, duration, and characteristics of symptoms.
2. Monitor CBC, cultures, and renal function studies; reduce dose with impaired renal function.
**Client/Family Teaching**
1. Take exactly as directed; may be taken with or without food.
2. Complete entire prescription and do not skip or double up on doses other than the loading dose if directed.
3. Report any unusual side effects or lack of response after 72 hr of therapy.
**Outcomes/Evaluate**
• Symptomatic improvement
• Resolution of infection

# Spectinomycin hydrochloride
(speck-tin-oh-**MY**-sin)
Trobicin **(Rx)**
**Classification:** Antibiotic, miscellaneous

See also *Anti-Infectives*.
**Action/Kinetics:** Produced by *Streptomyces spectabilis.* It inhibits bacterial protein synthesis by binding to ribosomes (30S subunit), thereby interfering with transmission of genetic information crucial to life of microorganism. Mainly bacteriostatic. Only given IM. **Peak plasma concentration:** 100 mcg/mL (2-g dose) after 1 hr and 160 mcg/mL (4-g dose) after 2 hr. **t½:** 1.2–2.8 hr. Not significantly bound to protein. Excreted in urine.
**Uses:** Acute gonorrheal proctitis and urethritis in males and acute gonorrheal cervicitis and proctitis in females due to susceptible strains of *Neisseria gonorrhoeae.* It is ineffective against pharyngeal infections and against syphilis; is a poor drug to choose when mixed infections are present.

**Contraindications:** Sensitivity to drug.

**Special Concerns:** Safe use during pregnancy, in infants, and in children has not been established.

**Side Effects:** A single dose of spectinomycin has caused soreness at the site of injection, urticaria, dizziness, nausea, chills, fever, and insomnia. Multiple doses have caused a decrease in H&H and $C_{CR}$ and an increase in alkaline phosphatase, BUN, and ALT.

**Dosage**

• **IM Only**

*Gonorrheal urethritis in males, proctitis, and cervicitis.*

2 g. In geographic areas where antibiotic resistance is known to be prevalent, give 4 g divided between two gluteal injection sites.

*Alternative regimen for urethral, endocervical, or rectal gonococcal infections in clients who cannot take ceftriaxone.*

**Adults and children weighing more than 45 kg:** Spectinomycin, 2 g, as a single dose followed by doxycycline. **Children weighing less than 45 kg:** 40 mg/kg given IM once.

*Gonococcal infections in pregnancy where client is allergic to beta-lactams.*

2 g followed by erythromycin.

*Disseminated gonococcal infection where client is allergic to beta-lactams.*

2 g q 12 hr.

## NURSING CONSIDERATIONS

See also *General Nursing Considerations for All Anti-Infectives.*

**Administration/Storage**

1. Powder is stable for 3 years.
2. Use reconstituted solution within 24 hr.
3. Inject deeply into the upper, outer quadrant of the gluteus muscle.
4. Injections may be divided between two sites for clients requiring 4 g. Rotate and document injection sites.

**Client/Family Teaching**

1. Return for serologic tests monthly for at least 3 months if syphilis suspected; with gonorrhea, report for a repeat serologic test 3 months after treatment.
2. Obtain counseling and encourage treatment of sexual partners.
3. Abstain from intercourse until infection is resolved; follow safe sex practices to prevent reinfections.

**Outcomes/Evaluate**

• Negative serology/cultures for gonorrhea
• Symptomatic improvement with gonorrheal urethritis, cervicitis, and/or proctitis

# Spironolactone
(speer-oh-no-**LAK**-tohn)
Aldactone, Novo-Spiroton ✤ (Rx)
**Classification:** Diuretic, potassium-sparing

See also *Diuretics, Thiazides.*

**Action/Kinetics:** Mild diuretic that acts on the distal tubule to inhibit sodium exchange for potassium, resulting in increased secretion of sodium and water and conservation of potassium. It is also an aldosterone antagonist. Manifests a slight antihypertensive effect. It also interferes with synthesis of testosterone and may increase formation of estradiol from testosterone, thus leading to endocrine abnormalities. **Onset:** Urine output increases over 1–2 days. **Peak:** 2–3 days. **Duration:** 2–3 days, and declines thereafter. Metabolized to an active metabolite (canrenone). $t^{1/2}$: 13–24 hr for canrenone. Canrenone is excreted through the urine (primary) and the bile. Almost completely bound to plasma protein.

**Uses:** Primary hyperaldosteronism, including diagnosis, short-term preoperative treatment, long-term maintenance therapy for those who are poor surgical risks and those with bilateral micronodular or macronodular adrenal hyperplasia. To treat edema when other approaches are

**S**

inadequate or ineffective (e.g., CHF, cirrhosis of the liver, nephrotic syndrome). Essential hypertension (usually in combination with other drugs). Prophylaxis of hypokalemia in clients taking digitalis. *Investigational:* Hirsutism, treat symptoms of PMS, with testolactone to treat familial male precocious puberty (short-term treatment), acne vulgaris.

**Contraindications:** Acute renal insufficiency, progressive renal failure, hyperkalemia, and anuria. Clients receiving potassium supplements, amiloride, or triamterene.

**Special Concerns:** Use during pregnancy only if benefits clearly outweigh risks. Use with caution in impaired renal function. Geriatric clients may be more sensitive to the usual adult dose.

**Side Effects:** *Electrolyte:* Hyperkalemia, hyponatremia (characterized by lethargy, dry mouth, thirst, tiredness). *GI:* Diarrhea, cramps, ulcers, gastritis, gastric bleeding, vomiting. *CNS:* Drowsiness, ataxia, lethargy, mental confusion, headache. *Endocrine:* Gynecomastia, menstrual irregularities, impotence, bleeding in postmenopausal women, deepening of voice, hirsutism. *Dermatologic:* Maculopapular or erythematous cutaneous eruptions, urticaria. *Miscellaneous:* Drug fever, breast carcinoma, gynecomastia, hyperchloremic metabolic acidosis in hepatic cirrhosis (decompensated), **agranulocytosis.** *NOTE:* Spironolactone has been shown to be tumorigenic in chronic rodent studies.

**Laboratory Test Alterations:** Interference with radioimmunoassay for digoxin. False + plasma cortisol (as determined by fluorometric assay of Mattingly).

**Drug Interactions**
*Anesthetics, general* / Additive hypotension
*ACE inhibitors* / Significant hyperkalemia
*Anticoagulants, oral* / Inhibited by spironolactone
*Antihypertensives* / Potentiation of hypotensive effect of both agents.

Reduce dosage, especially of ganglionic blockers, by one-half
*Captopril* / ↑ Risk of significant hyperkalemia
*Digitalis* / ↑ Half-life of digoxin → ↓ clearance. Spironolactone may ↓ inotropic effect of digoxin. Spironolactone both ↑ and ↓ elimination t½ of digitoxin
*Diuretics, others* / Often administered concurrently because of potassium-sparing effect of spironolactone. Severe hyponatremia may occur. Monitor closely
*Lithium* / ↑ Chance of lithium toxicity due to ↓ renal clearance
*Norepinephrine* / ↓ Responsiveness to norepinephrine
*Potassium salts* / Since spironolactone conserves potassium excessively, hyperkalemia may result. Rarely used together
*Salicylates* / Large doses may ↓ effects of spironolactone
*Triamterene* / Hazardous hyperkalemia may result from combination

**Dosage** —————————
• **Tablets**
  *Treat edema.*
**Adults, initial:** 100 mg/day (range: 25–200 mg/day) in two to four divided doses for at least 5 days; **maintenance:** 75–400 mg/day in two to four divided doses. **Pediatric:** 3.3 mg/kg/day as a single dose or as two to four divided doses.
  *Antihypertensive.*
**Adults, initial:** 50–100 mg/day as a single dose or as two to four divided doses—give for at least 2 weeks; **maintenance:** adjust to individual response. **Pediatric:** 1–2 mg/kg in a single dose or in two to four divided doses.
  *Treat hypokalemia.*
**Adults:** 25–100 mg/day as a single dose or two to four divided doses.
  *Diagnosis of primary hyperaldosteronism.*
**Adults:** 400 mg/day for either 4 days (short-test) or 3–4 weeks (long-test).
  *Hyperaldosteronism, prior to surgery.*
**Adults:** 100–400 mg/day in two to four doses prior to surgery.

*Hyperaldosteronism, chronic-therapy.*
Use lowest possible dose.
*Hirsutim.*
50–200 mg/day.
*Symptoms of PMS.*
25 mg q.i.d. beginning on day 14 of the menstrual cycle.
*Familial male precocious puberty, short-term.*
Spironolactone, 2 mg/kg/day, and testolactone, 20–40 mg/kg/day, for at least 6 months.
*Acne vulgaris.*
100 mg/day.

## NURSING CONSIDERATIONS

See also *Nursing Considerations* for *Diuretics, Thiazides.*

### Administration/Storage

1. When used as the sole drug to treat edema, maintain the initial dose for at least 5 days. After that, adjustments may be made. If the dosage is not effective, a second diuretic may be added, especially one that acts in the proximal tubules.
2. When administered to small children, tablets may be crushed and given as suspension in cherry syrup.
3. Food may increase the absorption of spironolactone.
4. Protect the drug from light.

### Assessment

1. Document indications for therapy, other agents prescribed, and the outcome.
2. If history of cardiac disease, be alert for cardiac irregularities R/T hypokalemia.
3. Monitor ABGs, ECG, CBC, blood sugar, uric acid, serum electrolytes, and liver and renal function studies. Record VS, I&O, and weights.
4. If client develops dysuria, urinary frequency, or renal spasm, obtain a urinalysis and urine culture.
5. Assess for drug tolerance characterized by edema and reduced urine output.

### Client/Family Teaching

1. Take with a snack or meals to minimize GI upset. Report if nausea,

bloating, anorexia, vomiting, or diarrhea persist. discontinued.
2. Record BP for provider review.
3. Avoid foods or salt substitutes high in potassium; drug is potassium-sparing.
4. Record weight twice a week. Report any evidence of edema or weight gain/loss of more than 5 lb (2.2 kg) weekly.
5. Do not drive or operate dangerous machinery until drug effects realized; may cause drowsiness or ataxia.
6. Drug may cause gynecomastia and diminished libido by reducing testosterone levels.
7. Report if deep, rapid respirations, headaches, or mental slowing occurs; may indicate hyperchloremic metabolic acidosis.
8. Drug is metabolized in the liver. Report if jaundice, tremors, or mental confusion occurs; may develop hepatic encephalopathy with hepatic disease .

### Outcomes/Evaluate

• Enhanced diuresis with ↓ edema
• ↓ BP
• Antagonism of high levels of aldosterone
• Prevention of hypokalemia in those taking digitalis and/or other diuretics

———COMBINATION DRUG———

# Spironolactone and Hydrochlorothiazide

(speer-oh-no-**LAK**-tohn)
(hy-droh-**klor**-oh-**THIGH**-ah-zyd)
Aldactazide, Aldactazide 25 and 50 ✮, Apo-Spirozide ✮, Novo-Spirozine ✮ **(Rx)**
**Classification:** Antihypertensive, diuretic

See also *Spironolactone* and *Hydrochlorothiazide.*
**Content:** This drug is a combination of a thiazide and potassium-sparing diuretic. *Diuretic:* Spironolactone, 25 or 50 mg. *Diuretic/antihypertensive:* Hydrochlorothiazide, 25 or 50

mg. Also see information on individual components.

**Uses:** Congestive heart failure, essential hypertension, nephrotic syndrome. Edema and/or ascites in cirrhosis of the liver.

**Contraindications:** Use in pregnancy only if benefits outweigh risks.

**Dosage**
- **Tablets**
  *Edema.*
**Adults, usual:** 100 mg of each drug daily (range: 25–200 mg), given as single or divided doses. **Pediatric, usual:** equivalent to 1.65–3.3 mg/kg spironolactone.
  *Essential hypertension.*
**Adults, usual:** 50–100 mg of each drug daily in single or divided doses.

## NURSING CONSIDERATIONS

See *Nursing Considerations* for *Diuretics, Thiazides; Antihypertensive Agents;* and *Spironolactone.*

**Outcomes/Evaluate**
- Enhanced diuresis; ↓ edema
- ↓ BP

# Stavudine
(**STAH**-vyou-deen)
**Pregnancy Category:** C
Zerit
**Classification:** Antiviral agent

See also *Antiviral Agents.*

**Action/Kinetics:** Inhibits replication of HIV due to phosphorylation by cellular kinases to stavudine triphosphate, which has antiviral activity. The mechanism for the antiviral activity includes inhibition of HIV reverse transcriptase by competing with the natural substrate deoxythymidine triphosphate and by causing DNA chain termination, thereby inhibiting viral DNA synthesis. Rapidly absorbed. **Peak plasma levels:** 1 hr or less. **t½, terminal:** Approximately 1.2 hr. About 40% of the drug is eliminated through the kidney.

**Uses:** Treatment of adults with advanced HIV infection who cannot tolerate approved therapies or who have experienced significant clinical or immunologic deterioration while receiving such therapies (or for whom such therapies are contraindicated).

**Contraindications:** Lactation.

**Special Concerns:** The effect of stavudine on the clinical progression of HIV infection, such as incidence of opportunistic infections or survival, has not been determined.

**Side Effects:** *Neurologic:* Peripheral neuropathy (common), including numbness, tingling, or pain in feet or hands. *CNS:* Insomnia, anxiety, depression, nervousness, dizziness, confusion, migraine, somnolence, tremor, neuralgia, dementia. *GI:* Diarrhea, N&V, anorexia, dyspepsia, constipation, ulcerative stomatitis, aphthous stomatitis, pancreatitis. *Body as a whole:* Headache, chills, fever, asthenia, abdominal pain, back pain, malaise, weight loss, allergic reactions, flu syndrome, lymphadenopathy, pelvic pain, neoplasms, death. *CV:* Chest pain, vasodilation, hypertension, peripheral vascular disorder, syncope. *GU:* Dysuria, genital pain, dysmenorrhea, vaginitis, urinary frequency, hematuria, impotence, urogenital neoplasm. *Respiratory:* Dyspnea, pneumonia, asthma. *Dermatologic:* Rash, sweating, pruritus, maculopapular rash, benign skin neoplasm, urticaria, exfoliative dermatitis. *Ophthalmic:* Conjunctivitis, abnormal vision.

**Laboratory Test Alterations:** ↑ AST, ALT.

**Dosage**
- **Capsules**
  *Advanced HIV infections.*
**Adults, initial:** 40 mg b.i.d. for clients weighing 60 or more kg and 30 mg b.i.d. for clients weighing less than 60 kg. In clients developing peripheral neuropathy, the following dosage schedule may be used if symptoms of neuropathy resolve completely: 20 mg b.i.d. for clients weighing 60 or more kg and 15 mg b.i.d. for clients weighing less than 60 kg.

The following dosage schedule is recommended for clients with impaired renal function: (a) $C_{CR}$ greater than 50 mL/min: 40 mg q 12 hr for clients weighing 60 or more kg and 30 mg q 12 hr for clients weighing less than 60 kg; (b) $C_{CR}$ 26–50 mL/min: 20 mg q 12 hr for clients weighing 60 or more kg and 15 mg q 12 hr for clients weighing less than 60 kg; (c) $C_{CR}$ 10–25 mL/min: 20 mg q 24 hr for clients weighing 60 or more kg and 15 mg q 24 hr for clients weighing less than 60 kg. Insufficient data are available to recommend doses for a $C_{CR}$ less than 10 mL/min or for clients undergoing dialysis.

## NURSING CONSIDERATIONS

See *Nursing Considerations* for *Antiviral Agents*.

**Administration/Storage:** The interval between PO doses should be 12 hr.

**Assessment**

1. Document onset of symptoms, other agents prescribed, and date confirmed; note date of intolerance.
2. Obtain baseline CBC, $CD_4$ counts/viral load, PT/PTT, liver and renal function studies. Reduce dose with impaired renal function.

**Client/Family Teaching**

1. May be taken without regard to meals.
2. Take exactly as prescribed, do not exceed prescribed dose, and do not share medications.
3. Drug is not a cure, but alleviates/manages the symptoms of HIV infections. May continue to acquire illnesses associated with AIDS or ARC, including opportunistic infections; must remain under close medical supervision.
4. The risk of transmission of HIV to others through blood or sexual contact is not reduced with drug therapy. Review the criteria and precautions for safe sex and do not share needles.
5. Insomnia and GI upset usually resolve after 3–4 weeks of therapy.
6. Report any S&S of infection (i.e., sore throat, swollen glands, fever).

7. Report symptoms of peripheral neuropathy characterized by numbness and tingling or pain in the hands and/or feet. Discontinue drug if these symptoms are evident. Symptoms may temporarily worsen following cessation of drug therapy but, once completely resolved, drug may be reintroduced at a lower dose.
8. Report for all scheduled lab studies and follow-up visits to assess response to therapy and to identify any adverse drug effects.
9. Identify local support groups that may assist client/family to understand and cope with this disease.

**Outcomes/Evaluate:** Clinical/immunologic improvement with AIDS and ARC

# Streptokinase
(strep-toe-**KYE**-nayz)
**Pregnancy Category:** C
Kabikinase, Streptase **(Rx)**
**Classification:** Thrombolytic agent

**Action/Kinetics:** Most clients have a natural resistance to streptokinase that must be overcome with the loading dose before the drug becomes effective. Streptokinase acts with plasminogen to produce an "activator complex," which enhances the conversion of plasminogen to plasmin. Plasmin then breaks down fibrinogen, fibrin clots, and other plasma proteins, promoting the dissolution (lysis) of the insoluble fibrin trapped in intravascular emboli and thrombi. Also, inhibitors of streptokinase, such as alpha-2-macroglobulin, are rapidly inactivated by streptokinase. **Onset:** rapid; **duration:** 12 hr. **t½, activator complex:** 23 min.
**Uses:** DVT; arterial thrombosis and embolism; acute evolving transmural MI; pulmonary embolism. Also, clearing of occluded arteriovenous and IV cannulae.
**Contraindications:** Any condition presenting a risk of hemorrhage, such as recent surgery or biopsies, delivery within 10 days, ulcerative

disease. Arterial emboli originating from the left side of the heart. Also, hepatic or renal insufficiency, tuberculosis, recent cerebral embolism, thrombosis, hemorrhage, SBE, rheumatic valvular disease, thrombocytopenia. Streptokinase resistance in excess of 1 million IU.

**Special Concerns:** The use of streptokinase in septic thrombophlebitis may be hazardous. History of significant allergic response. Safety in children has not been established. Geriatric clients have an increased risk of bleeding during therapy.

**Side Effects:** *CV:* Superficial bleeding, *severe internal bleeding.* *Allergic:* Nausea, headache, breathing difficulties, *bronchospasm, angioneurotic edema,* urticaria, flushing, musculoskeletal pain, vasculitis, interstitial nephritis, periorbital swelling. *Other:* Fever, possible development of Guillain-Barre syndrome, development of antistreptokinase antibody (i.e., streptokinase may be ineffective if administered between 5 days and 6 months following prior use of streptokinase or following streptococcal infections.

**Laboratory Test Alterations:** ↓ Fibrinogen, plasminogen. ↑ Thrombin time, PT, and activated PTT.

**Drug Interactions:** The following drugs increase the chance of bleeding when given concomitantly with streptokinase: anticoagulants, aspirin, heparin, indomethacin, and phenylbutazone.

**Dosage** ————————
• **IV Infusion**
*DVT, pulmonary embolism, arterial thrombosis or embolism.*
**Loading dose:** 250,000 IU over 30 min (use the 1,500,000 IU vial diluted to 90 mL); **maintenance:** 100,000 IU/hr for 24–72 hr for arterial thrombosis or embolism, 72 hr for deep vein thrombosis, and 24 hr (72 hr if deep vein thrombosis is suspected) for pulmonary embolism.
*Acute evolving transmural MI.*
1,500,000 IU within 60 min (use the 1,500,000 IU vial diluted to a total of 45 mL).

*Arteriovenous cannula occlusion.* 250,000 IU in 2-mL IV solution into each occluded limb of cannula and clamp off; **then,** after 2 hr aspirate cannula limbs, flush with saline, and reconnect cannula.
• **Intracoronary Infusion**
*Acute evolving transmural MI.*
20,000 IU by bolus; **then,** 2,000 IU/min for 60 min (total dose of 140,000 IU). Use the 250,000 IU vial diluted to 125 mL.

——————————————

## NURSING CONSIDERATIONS

See also *Nursing Considerations* for *Alteplase, Recombinant.*

### Administration/Storage
**IV** 1. NaCl injection USP or 5% dextrose injection is the preferred diluent for IV use.
2. For AV cannulae, dilute 250,000 units with 2 mL of NaCl injection or 5% dextrose injection.
3. Reconstitute gently, as directed by manufacturer, without shaking vial.
4. Use within 24 hr after reconstitution.
5. Use an electronic infusion device to administer streptokinase and do not add any other medications to the line. Note any redness and/or pain at the site of infusion; may need to further dilute solution to prevent phlebitis.
6. Have emergency drugs and equipment available. Have corticosteroids and aminocaproic acid available in the event bleeding is excessive.

### Assessment
1. Document indications for therapy, type, onset, and duration of symptoms.
2. Note any history of tuberculosis, SBE, ulcerative disease, recent surgery, or streptococcal infection.
3. Assess for bleeding tendencies, heart disease, and/or allergic reaction to any drugs.
4. Identify other drugs taking such as aspirin or NSAIDs that could increase bleeding times.
5. Clients with high allergy potential or high streptokinase antibody titer

S

may benefit by skin testing prior to administering therapy. Drug may not be effective if administered within 5 days to 6 months of a strep infection.

6. Obtain baseline lab studies; ensure that bleeding studies, type and crossmatch, thrombin time, and streptokinase resistance have been completed before initiation of therapy.

**Interventions**

1. Observe in a closely monitored environment; document rhythm strips and VS q 15–30 min initially.

2. Check access sites for evidence of bleeding. Test stools, urine, and emesis for occult blood.

3. During IV therapy, arterial sticks require 30 min of manual pressure followed by application of a pressure dressing. To prevent bruising, avoid unnecessary handling of client.

4. If IM injections necessary, apply pressure after withdrawing the needle to prevent hematoma and bleeding from the puncture site. Observe injection sites and postoperative wounds for bleeding during therapy

5. If excessive bleeding develops from an invasive procedure, discontinue therapy and call for packed RBCs and plasma expanders *other than dextran.*

6. To prevent new thrombus formation, or rethrombosis, IV heparin and oral anticoagulants are used when therapy is concluded.

7. Note allergic reactions, ranging from anaphylaxis to moderate and mild reactions. These usually can be controlled with antihistamines and corticosteroids.

8. Fever reaction may be treated with acetaminophen.

9. Following recanalization of an occluded coronary artery, clients may develop reperfusion reactions; these may include:

• Reperfusion arrhythmias (accelerated idioventricular rhythm, sinus bradycardia) usually of short duration.

• Reduction of chest pain

• Return of elevated ST segment to near baseline levels

**Client/Family Teaching**

1. Review inherent benefits and risks of drug therapy.

2. To be effective, the therapy should be instituted within 4–6 hr of onset of symptoms of acute MI.

3. Report any symptoms or side effects immediately.

4. With CAD, encourage family members or significant other to learn CPR.

**Outcomes/Evaluate**

• Lysis of emboli/thrombi with restoration of normal blood flow

• ↓ Myocardial infarct size; improved ventricular function

• Catheter patency in previously occluded AV or IV cannulae

---

# Streptozocin

(strep-toe-**ZOH**-sin)
**Pregnancy Category:** C
Zanosar **(Rx)**
**Classification:** Antineoplastic, alkylating agent

---

See also *Antineoplastic Agents* and *Alkylating Agents.*

**Action/Kinetics:** Cell-cycle nonspecific although it does inhibit progression out of the $G_2$ phase of cell division. The drug forms methylcarbonium ions that alkylate or bind with intracellular substances such as nucleic acids. It is also cytotoxic by virtue of cross-linking of DNA strands resulting in inhibition of DNA synthesis. It may also cause hyperglycemia. Does not penetrate the blood-brain barrier well, although within 2 hr after administration, metabolites do and produce levels similar to those in plasma. **t½, unchanged drug, initial:** 35 min. **t½, metabolites, initial:** 6 min; **intermediate:** 3.5 hr; **terminal:** 40 hr. Unchanged drug and metabolites excreted in urine.

**Uses:** Metastatic islet cell pancreatic carcinomas (functional and nonfunctional) in clients with symptomatic or progressive metastases. *In-*

*vestigational:* Malignant carcinoid tumors.

**Contraindications:** Use during lactation.

**Special Concerns:** Dosage has not been determined for children.

**Additional Side Effects:** Renal toxicity (up to two-thirds of clients) manifested by anuria, azotemia, glycosuria, hypophosphatemia, and renal tubular acidosis. *Toxicity is dose-related and cumulative and may be fatal.* Glucose intolerance (reversible) or insulin shock with hypoglycemia, depression.

**Dosage** ⸺⸺⸺⸺⸺⸺⸺
• **IV**
*Daily schedule:* 500 mg/m² for 5 consecutive days q 6 weeks (until maximum benefit is achieved or toxicity occurs). Dose should not be increased. *Weekly schedule:* **Initial:** 1,000 mg/m²/week for 2 weeks; **then,** if no response or no toxicity, dose can be increased, not to exceed a single dose of 1,500 mg/m². Response should be seen in 17–35 days.

## NURSING CONSIDERATIONS

See also *Nursing Considerations* for *Antineoplastic Agents.*

**Administration/Storage**

**IV** 1. Reconstitute with 9.5 mL dextrose injection or 0.9% NaCl injection. Reconstituted solution is pale gold in color and contains 100 mg/mL streptozocin. This may be further diluted. Administer slowly over 1–2 hr.

2. Total storage time for reconstituted drug is 12 hr, as there are no preservatives present. The ampule is not considered to be multiple dose.

3. Caution should be observed (wear gloves) in handling the drug.

4. Drug is a vesicant. Infiltration may result in tissue ulceration and necrosis.

**Assessment**

1. Document indications for therapy, type and onset of symptoms, and other agents trialed.

2. Premedicate with antiemetic; may cause severe N&V.

3. Monitor I&O, lab studies, and weight. Consume 3 L/day of fluids to reduce the risk of renal damage; if urine output decreases streptozocin can cause anuria.

4. Monitor blood sugar, CBC, uric acid, liver and renal function studies. Drug may cause lymphocyte and platelet suppression. Nadir: 10 days; recovery: 14–17 days.

**Outcomes/Evaluate:** ↓ Tumor size and spread; suppression of malignant cell proliferation

# Strontium-89 Chloride

(**STRON**-shee-um)

**Pregnancy Category:** D
Metastron **(Rx)**
**Classification:** Antineoplastic, radiopharmaceutical

See also *Antineoplastic Agents.*

**Action/Kinetics:** Taken up preferentially in sites of active osteogenesis leading to significant accumulation in primary bone tumors and areas of metastatic involvement. As a beta emitter, it selectively irradiates primary metastatic bone involvement with minimal irradiation of soft tissues distant from bone lesions. Retained in metastatic areas significantly longer than in normal bone. **Physical t½:** 50.5 days. Two-thirds is excreted through the urine and one-third through the feces. Urinary excretion is greater in clients with no bone lesions.

**Uses:** Relief of bone pain in clients with painful skeletal metastases.

**Contraindications:** Use in clients with seriously compromised bone marrow from previous therapy or disease without an assessment of benefit vs. risk. Lactation.

**Special Concerns:** The drug is a potential carcinogen. Use with caution in clients with platelet counts below 60,000 and WBC counts less than 2,400. Safety and efficacy in children less than 18 years of age have not been determined.

**Side Effects:** Calcium-like flushing following rapid (< 30 sec) administration. Increase in bone pain between

36 and 72 hr following injection. Bone marrow depression.

## Dosage

- **Slow IV Injection**
  *Pain from bone metastases.*
148 MBq, 4 mCi, given by slow IV injection over 1–2 min. An alternative dose is 1.5–2.2 MBq/kg, 40–60 mcCi/kg.

## NURSING CONSIDERATIONS

See also *Nursing Considerations* for *Antineoplastic Agents.*

### Administration/Storage

**IV** 1. Administer only by those trained/experienced in safe use and handling of radiopharmaceuticals.
2. Pain relief is usually noted within 7–10 days after a dose and should last for several months.
3. Repeat doses are usually not recommended at intervals of less than 90 days.
4. The injection is preservative free.
5. The vial is shipped in a transportation shield of about 3 mm lead wall thickness. The vial and its contents are stored inside the transportation container at room temperature (15°C–25°C; 59°F–77°F) until used.

### Assessment

1. Confirm presence of bone metastases.
2. Note other procedures/agents utilized and the outcome. Include last dosage and type of chemotherapy/radiation therapy received.
3. Document dose and frequency of pain medications, if any relief attained, and for how long.
4. Drug is bone marrow toxic; monitor hematologic profile. Platelet nadir: 12–16 weeks.
5. Strontium-89 delivers a high dose of radioactivity. Ensure consent and carefully verify client and dose prior to administration.
6. Administration is not recommended in clients with a very short life expectancy, as it takes from 7 to 20 days to gain pain relief.

### Client/Family Teaching

1. Drug is an injectable radioisotope that accumulates in and irradiates metastatic bone lesions.
2. An increase in bone pain 36–72 hr after administration is usually mild and self-limiting and can be managed with analgesics. Continue analgesics until the strontium-89 becomes effective and then gradually reduce the analgesic dose.
3. Review the special precautions that must be taken when incontinent to minimize the risk of radioactive contamination of clothing, bed linen, and the environment. Strontium-89 will be present in urine and blood for the first week after an injection; take proper precautions to avoid contamination. Guidelines include:

- Wear gloves if available.
- Use toilet if able, and flush twice after use.
- Thoroughly wash and rinse bed pan or urinal after each use.
- If incontinence is a problem, a catheter may be considered to minimize the risk of radioactive contamination.
- When urine is dripped or spilled, wipe up immediately with a tissue and flush it away.
- Always wash hands thoroughly after toileting.
- Clothes or linens that become stained with urine or blood should be washed immediately; separate from other clothes and rinse thoroughly
- Cuts, scratches, or spilled blood should be washed and wiped with a tissue, which is properly discarded

4. May eat and drink normally; there is no need to avoid alcohol or caffeine.
5. Practice reliable contraception, as drug will cause fetal damage.
6. Repeat administrations will be based on client response, current symptoms, and hematologic status; generally not repeated for 90 days.

**Outcomes/Evaluate:** Relief of bone pain with skeletal metastases

# Succinylcholine chloride
(suck-sin-ill-**KOH**-leen)
**Pregnancy Category:** C
Anectine, Anectine Flo-Pack,
Quelicin, Succinylcholine Chloride
Min-I-Mix **(Rx)**
**Classification:** Depolarizing neuro-
muscular blocking agent

See also *Neuromuscular Blocking
Agents.*

**Action/Kinetics:** Initially excites
skeletal muscle by combining with
cholinergic receptors preferentially
to acetylcholine. Subsequently, it
prevents the muscle from contracting by prolonging the time during
which the receptors at the neuromuscular junction cannot respond to
acetylcholine. The order of paralysis
is levator muscles of the eyelid, mastication muscles, limb muscles,
abdominal muscles, glottis muscles,
the intercostals, the diaphragm, and all
other skeletal muscles. Prolonged
use may change from a depolarizing
neuromuscular block (phase I
block) to a block that resembles a
nondepolarizing block (phase II
block). This may be associated with
prolonged respiratory depression
and apnea. No effect on pain threshold, cerebration, or consciousness;
use with sufficient anesthesia. Effects are not blocked by anticholinesterase drugs and may even be
enhanced by them. May cause a
change in myocardial rhythm due to
vagal stimulation due to surgical
procedures (especially in children)
and from potassium-mediated alterations in electrical conductivity (enhanced by cyclopropane and halogenated anesthetics). **IV: onset,**
30–60 sec; **duration:** 4–6 min;
**recovery:** 8–10 min. **IM: Onset,** 2–3
min; **duration:** 10–30 min. Metabolized by plasma pseudocholinesterase to succinylmonocholine, which is
a nondepolarizing muscle relaxant,
and then to succinic acid and choline.
About 10% excreted unchanged in
the urine.

**Uses:** Adjunct to general anesthesia to
facilitate ET intubation and to induce relaxation of skeletal muscle
during surgery or mechanical ventilation. *Investigational:* Reduce intensity of electrically induced seizures
or seizures due to drugs.

**Contraindications:** Use in those
with genetically determined disorders of plasma pseudocholinesterase. Personal or family history of
malignant hyperthermia. Myopathies
associated with elevated CPK values.
Acute narrow-angle glaucoma or
penetrating eye injuries.

**Special Concerns:** Use with caution during lactation. Pediatric clients may be especially prone to
myoglobinemia, myoglobinuria, and
cardiac effects. Use of IV infusion is
not recommended in children due to
the risk of malignant hyperpyrexia.
Use with caution in clients with severe
liver disease, severe anemia, malnutrition, impaired cholinesterase
activity, fractures. Also, use with
caution in CV, pulmonary, renal, or
metabolic diseases. Use with great
caution in those with severe burns,
electrolyte imbalance, hyperkalemia,
those receiving quinidine, and those
who are digitalized or recovering
from severe trauma, as serious cardiac
arrhythmias or cardiac arrest may result. Clients with myasthenia gravis
may show resistance to succinylcholine. Those with fractures or muscle
spasms may manifest additional
trauma due to succinylcholine-in-
duced muscle fasciculations.

**Side Effects:** *Skeletal muscle:* May
cause **severe, persistent respiratory
depression or apnea.** Muscle fasciculations, postoperative muscle pain.
*CV:* Bradycardia or tachycardia,
hypertension, hypotension, **arrhythmias, cardiac arrest.** *Respiratory:* **Apnea,
respiratory depression.** *Other:* Fever,
salivation, hyperkalemia, postoperative muscle pain, **anaphylaxis,** myoglobinemia, myoglobinuria, skin
rashes, increased intraocular pressure, muscle fasciculation, myalgia,
jaw rigidity, perioperative dreams in
children, rhabdomyolysis with possible myoglobinuric acute renal failure. Repeated doses may cause
tachyphylaxis.

*Malignant hyperthermia:* Muscle rigidity (especially of the jaw), tachycardia, tachypnea unresponsive to increased depth of anesthesia, increased oxygen requirement and carbon dioxide production, increased body temperature, metabolic acidosis.

**OD** **Overdose Management:** *Symptoms:* Skeletal muscle weakness, decreased respiratory reserve, low tidal volume, apnea. *Treatment:* Maintain a patent airway and respiratory support until normal respiration is ensured.

**Drug Interactions**

*Aminoglycoside antibiotics* / Additive skeletal muscle blockade

*Amphotericin B* / ↑ Effect of succinylcholine due to induced electrolyte imbalance

*Antibiotics, nonpenicillin* / Additive skeletal muscle blockade

*Beta-adrenergic blocking agents* / Additive skeletal muscle blockade

*Chloroquine* / Additive skeletal muscle blockade

*Cimetidine* / Cimetidine inhibits pseudocholinesterase

*Clindamycin* / Additive skeletal muscle blockade

*Cyclophosphamide* / ↑ Effect of succinylcholine by ↓ breakdown of drug in plasma by pseudocholinesterase

*Cyclopropane* / ↑ Risk of bradycardia, arrhythmias, sinus arrest, apnea, and malignant hyperthermia

*Diazepam* / ↓ Effect of succinylcholine

*Digitalis glycosides* / ↑ Chance of cardiac arrhythmias, including ventricular fibrillation

*Echothiophate iodide* / ↑ Effect of succinylcholine by ↓ breakdown of drug in plasma by pseudocholinesterase

*Furosemide* / ↑ Skeletal muscle blockade

*Halothane* / ↑ Risk of bradycardia, arrhythmias, sinus arrest, apnea, and malignant hyperthermia

*Isoflurane* / Additive skeletal muscle blockade

*Lidocaine* / Additive skeletal muscle blockade

*Lincomycin* / Additive skeletal muscle blockade

*Lithium carbonate* / ↑ Skeletal muscle blockade

*Magnesium salts* / Additive skeletal muscle blockade

*Narcotics* / ↑ Risk of bradycardia and sinus arrest

*Nitrous oxide* / ↑ Risk of bradycardia, arrhythmias, sinus arrest, apnea, and malignant hyperthermia

*Oxytocin* / ↑ Effect of succinylcholine

*Phenelzine* / ↑ Effect of succinylcholine

*Phenothiazines* / ↑ Effect of succinylcholine

*Polymyxin* / Additive skeletal muscle blockade

*Procainamide* / ↑ Effect of succinylcholine

*Procaine* / ↑ Effect of succinylcholine by inhibiting plasma pseudocholinesterase activity

*Promazine* / ↑ Effect of succinylcholine

*Quinidine* / Additive skeletal muscle blockade

*Quinine* / Additive skeletal muscle blockade

*Tacrine* / ↑ Effect of succinylcholine

*Thiazide diuretics* / ↑ Effect of succinylcholine due to induced electrolyte imbalance

*Thiotepa* / ↑ Effect of succinylcholine by ↓ breakdown of drug in plasma by pseudocholinesterase

*Trimethaphan* / ↑ Effect of succinylcholine by inhibiting plasma pseudocholinesterase activity

**Dosage**
- **IM, IV**

  *Short or prolonged surgical procedures.*

  **Adults, IV, initial:** 0.3–1.1 mg/kg (average: 0.6 mg/kg); **then,** repeated doses can be given based on client response. **Adults, IM:** 3–4 mg/kg, not to exceed a total dose of 150 mg.
- **IV Infusion (Preferred)**

*Prolonged surgical procedures.*
**Adults:** Average rate ranges from 2.5 to 4.3 mg/min. Most commonly used are 0.1%–0.2% solutions in 5% dextrose, sodium chloride injection, or other diluent given at a rate of 0.5–10 mg/min depending on client response and degree of relaxation desired, for up to 1 hr.
• **Intermittent IV**
*Prolonged muscle relaxation.*
**Initial:** 0.3–1.1 mg/kg; **then,** 0.04–0.07 mg/kg at appropriate intervals to maintain required level of relaxation.
• **IM, IV**
*Electroshock therapy.*
**Adults, IV:** 10–30 mg given 1 min prior to the shock (individualize dosage). **IM:** Up to 2.5 mg/kg, not to exceed a total dose of 150 mg.
*ET intubation.*
**Pediatric, IV:** 1–2 mg/kg; if necessary, dose can be repeated. **IM:** 3–4 mg/kg, not to exceed a total dose of 150 mg.

## NURSING CONSIDERATIONS

See also *Nursing Considerations* for *Neuromuscular Blocking Agents.*
**Administration/Storage**
**IV** 1. Give an initial test dose of 0.1 mg/kg to assess sensitivity and recovery time.
2. Do not mix with anesthetic.
3. For IV infusion, use 1 or 2 mg/mL solution of drug in 5% dextrose injection, 0.9% NaCl, or other suitable IV solution; drug is not compatible with alkaline solutions.
4. To reduce salivation, premedicate with atropine or scopolamine.
5. Have neostigmine or pyridostigmine available to reverse neuromuscular blockade.
6. Store drug in the refrigerator at 2°C–8°C (36°F–46°F). Multidose vials are stable for 14 days or less at room temperature without significant loss of potency.
**Assessment**
1. List agents currently prescribed to ensure that none interact unfavorably. Note if the client is taking digitalis products or quinidine. These clients are sensitive to the release of intracellular potassium.
2. Obtain baseline lab studies and VS. Assess clients with low plasma pseudocholinesterase levels. They are sensitive to the effects of succinylcholine and require lower doses.
3. Document any evidence of a history of MS, malignant hyperthermia, CPK myopathy, acute glaucoma, or eye injury, as drug is generally contraindicated.
**Interventions**
1. A peripheral nerve stimulator should be used to assess neuromuscular response and recovery. The order of paralysis is levator muscles of the eyelid, mastication muscles, limb muscles, abdominal muscles, glottis muscles, the intercostals, the diaphragm, and all other skeletal muscles. This is reversed with recovery.
2. Monitor VS and ECG; can cause vagal stimulation resulting in bradycardia, hypotension, and cardiac arrhythmias, especially in children.
3. Observe for excessive, transient increase in intraocular pressure.
4. Muscle fasciculations may cause the client to be sore and injured after recovery. Administer prescribed nondepolarizing agent (i.e., tubocurarine) and reassure that the soreness is likely caused by the unsynchronized contractions of adjacent muscle fibers just before the onset of paralysis.
5. Monitor for evidence of malignant hyperthermia, unresponsive tachycardia, jaw spasm, or lack of laryngeal relaxation.
6. Drug should be used only on a short-term basis and in a continuously monitored environment. Prolonged use may change from a depolarizing neuromuscular block (phase I block) to a block that resembles a nondepolarizing block (phase II block) which may be associated with prolonged respiratory depression and apnea.
7. Client is fully conscious and aware of surroundings and conversations.
8. Drug does not affect pain or anx-

iety; administer analgesics and anti-anxiety agents as indicated.

9. When used for seizures, ensure that serum level of anticonvulsant agent is therapeutic. Succinylcholine does not cross the blood-brain barrier and will only suppress peripheral manifestations of seizures, not the central process.

**Outcomes/Evaluate**
• Muscle relaxation/paralysis
• Suppression of the twitch response
• Facilitation of ET intubation; control of breathing during mechanical ventilation

# Sucralfate
(sue-**KRAL**-fayt)
**Pregnancy Category:** B
Apo-Sucralfate ✹, Carafate, Novo-Sucralate ✹, Nu-Sucralfate ✹, Sulcrate ✹, Sulcrate Suspension Plus ✹
**(Rx)**
**Classification:** Antiulcer drug

**Action/Kinetics:** Thought to form an ulcer-adherent complex with albumin and fibrinogen at the site of the ulcer, protecting it from further damage by gastric acid. May also form a viscous, adhesive barrier on the surface of the gastric mucosa and duodenum. It adsorbs pepsin, thus inhibiting its activity. May be used in conjunction with antacids. Approximately 90% excreted in the feces. **Duration:** 5 hr.

**Uses:** Short-term treatment (up to 8 weeks) of active duodenal ulcers. Maintenance for duodenal ulcer at decreased dosage after healing of acute ulcers. *Investigational:* Hasten healing of gastric ulcers, chronic treatment of gastric ulcers. Treatment of reflux and peptic esophagitis. Treatment of aspirin- and NSAID-induced GI symptoms; prevention of stress ulcers and GI bleeding in critically ill clients. The suspension has been used to treat oral and esophageal ulcers due to chemotherapy, radiation, or sclerotherapy.

*Note:* Even though healing of ulcers may result, the frequency or severity of subsequent attacks is not altered.
**Special Concerns:** Safety for use in children and during lactation has not been fully established. A successful course resulting in healing of ulcers will not alter posthealing frequency or severity of duodenal ulceration.
**Side Effects:** *GI:* Constipation (most common); also, N&V, diarrhea, indigestion, flatulence, dry mouth, gastric discomfort. *Hypersensitivity:* Urticaria, *angioedema, respiratory difficulty,* rhinitis. *Miscellaneous:* Back pain, dizziness, sleepiness, vertigo, rash, pruritus, facial swelling, *laryngospasm.*

**Drug Interactions**
*Antacids containing aluminum* / ↑ Total body burden of aluminum
*Anticoagulants* / ↓ Hypoprothrombinemic effect of warfarin
*Cimetidine* / ↓ Absorption of cimetidine due to binding to sucralfate
*Ciprofloxacin* / ↓ Absorption of ciprofloxacin due to binding to sucralfate
*Digoxin* / ↓ Absorption of digoxin due to binding to sucralfate
*Ketoconazole* / ↓ Bioavailability of ketoconazole
*Norfloxacin* / ↓ Absorption of norfloxacin due to binding to sucralfate
*Phenytoin* / ↓ Absorption of phenytoin due to binding to sucralfate
*Quinidine* / ↓ Quinidine levels → ↓ effect
*Ranitidine* / ↓ Absorption of ranitidine due to binding to sucralfate
*Tetracycline* / ↓ Absorption of tetracycline due to binding to sucralfate
*Theophylline* / ↓ Absorption of theophylline due to binding to sucralfate

**Dosage**
• **Suspension, Tablets**
**Adults: usual:** 1 g q.i.d. (10 mL of the suspension) 1 hr before meals and at bedtime (it may also be taken 2 hr after meals). The drug should be taken for 4–8 weeks unless X-ray films or endoscopy have indicated signifi-

cant healing. **Maintenance (tablets only):** 1 g b.i.d.

## NURSING CONSIDERATIONS
### Assessment
1. Document indications for therapy, noting location, type, onset, and symptom characteristics.
2. List other agents prescribed and the outcome.
3. Ensure that tablets are reconstituted prior to administering through the NGT. Generally when placed in a medicine cup with a small amount of water and left for 10–15 min, the tablets will dissolve completely.
4. Assess and monitor gastric pH; maintain pH above 5.
5. Monitor CBC and serum phosphate levels. Drug binds phosphate and may lead to hypophosphatemia.
### Client/Family Teaching
1. Take on an empty stomach 1 hr before or 2 hr after meals. If antacids are used, take 30 min before or after sucralfate.
2. Do not crush or chew tablets.
3. Take medication exactly as prescribed. It binds to proteins at the site of the lesions to create a protective barrier that prevents diffusion of hydrogen ions at a normal gastric pH.
4. May cause constipation; increase fluids and bulk and exercise regularly.
5. Avoid smoking, alcohol, and caffeine to prevent a recurrence of duodenal ulcers. Even though healing of ulcers may result, the frequency or severity of subsequent attacks is not altered.
6. Report as scheduled for follow-up, upper GI, endoscopy, and labs.
### Outcomes/Evaluate
* ↓ Abdominal pain/discomfort
* Prophylaxis of GI bleeding
* Healing of duodenal ulcers

# Sufentanil
(soo-**FEN**-tah-nil)
**Pregnancy Category:** C
Sufenta **(Rx)**
**Classification:** Narcotic analgesic

See also *Narcotic Analgesics.*
**Action/Kinetics: Onset, IV:** 1.3–3 min. **Anesthetic blood concentration:** 8–30 mcg/kg. **t½:** 2.5 hr. Allows appropriate oxygenation of the heart and brain during prolonged surgical procedures. May be used in children.
**Uses:** Narcotic analgesic used as an adjunct to maintain balanced general anesthesia. To induce and maintain general anesthesia (with 100% oxygen), especially in neurosurgery or CV surgery.
**Additional     Contraindications:** Use during labor.
**Special Concerns:** Dosage must be decreased in the obese, elderly, or debilitated client.
**Additional Side Effects:** Erythema, chills, intraoperative muscle movement. *Extended postoperative respiratory depression.*

### Dosage
* **IV**
    *Analgesia.*
**Adults, individualized, usual initial:** 1–2 mcg/kg with oxygen and nitrous oxide; **maintenance:** 10–25 mcg as required.
    *For complicated surgery.*
**Adults:** 2–8 mcg/kg with oxygen and nitrous oxide; **maintenance:** 10–50 mcg.
    *To induce and maintain general anesthesia.*
**Adults:** 8–30 mcg/kg with 100% oxygen and a muscle relaxant; **maintenance:** 25–50 mcg. **Pediatric, less than 12 years:** 10–25 mcg/kg with 100% oxygen; **maintenance:** 25–50 mcg.
    *Induction and maintenance of general anesthesia in children less than 12 years of age undergoing CV surgery.*
**Initial:** 10–25 mcg/kg with 100% oxygen; **maintenance:** 25–50 mcg.

## NURSING CONSIDERATIONS

See also *Nursing Considerations* for *Narcotic Analgesics.*
### Administration/Storage
**IV** 1. Reduce the dose in the debilitated or elderly client.

2. Calculate the dose based on lean body weight.

**Client/Family Teaching**

1. Avoid activities that require mental alertness for at least 24 hr following procedure; dizziness and drowsiness may occur.

2. Call for assistance with ambulation and transfers.

3. Avoid alcohol and any other CNS depressants for 24 hr following procedure.

**Outcomes/Evaluate:** Desired level of analgesia

# Sulfacetamide sodium

(sul-fah-**SEAT**-ah-myd)

AK-Sulf, Balsulph ✿, Bleph-10, Bleph-10 Liquifilm ✿, Cetamide, Diosulf ✿, Isopto-Cetamide, I-Sulfacet, Ocu-Sul-10, Ocu-Sul-15, Ocu-Sul-30, Ocusulf-10, Ophthacet, Ophtho-Sulf ✿, PMS-Sulfacetamide Sodium ✿, Sebizon, Sodium Sulamyd, Spectro-Sulf, Steri-Units Sulfacetamide, Sulf-10, Sulfair, Sulfair 10, Sulfair 15, Sulfair Forte, Sulfamide, Sulfex 10% ✿, Sulten-10

**(Rx)**

**Classification:** Sulfonamide, topical

See also *Sulfonamides*.

**Uses:** Topically for conjunctivitis, corneal ulcer, and other superficial ocular infections. As an adjunct to systemic sulfonamides to treat trachoma.

**Contraindications:** In infants less than 2 months of age. Use in the presence of epithelial herpes simplex keratitis, vaccinia, varicella, and other viral diseases of the cornea and conjunctiva. Mycobacterial or fungal infections of the ocular structures. After uncomplicated removal of a corneal foreign body.

**Special Concerns:** Safe use during pregnancy and lactation or in children less than 12 years of age has not been established. Use with caution in clients with dry eye syndrome. Ophthalmic ointments may retard corneal wound healing.

**Side Effects:** *When used topically:* Itching, local irritation, periorbital edema, burning and transient stinging,

headache, bacterial or fungal corneal ulcers. *NOTE:* Sulfonamides may cause serious systemic side effects, including severe hypersensitivity reactions. Symptoms include fever, skin rash, GI disturbances, bone marrow depression, **Stevens-Johnson syndrome, toxic epidermal necrolysis,** exfoliative dermatitis, photosensitivity. Fatalities have occurred.

**Drug Interactions:** Preparations containing silver are incompatible with sulfacetamide sodium.

**Dosage**

• **Ophthalmic Solution, 10%, 15%, 20%**

*Conjunctivitis or other superficial ocular infections.*

1–2 gtt in the conjunctival sac q 1–4 hr. Doses may be tapered by increasing the time interval between doses as the condition improves.

*Trachoma.*

2 gtt q 2 hr with concomitant systemic sulfonamide therapy.

• **Ophthalmic Ointment (10%)**

Apply approximately ¼ in. into the lower conjunctival sac 3–4 times/day and at bedtime. Alternatively, 0.5–1 in. is placed in the conjunctival sac at bedtime along with use of drops during the day.

*For cutaneous infections.*

Apply locally (10%) to affected area b.i.d.–q.i.d.

• **Lotion**

*Seborrheic dermatitis.*

Apply 1–2 times/day (for mild cases, apply overnight).

*Cutaneous bacterial infections.*

Apply b.i.d.–q.i.d. until infection clears.

## NURSING CONSIDERATIONS

See also *General Nursing Considerations for All Anti-Infectives* and for *Sulfonamides*.

**Administration/Storage:** Solutions will darken in color if left standing for long periods; discard these products.

**Assessment**

1. Document indications for thera-

S

py, onset, duration, and characteristics of symptoms.

2. List other agents prescribed and the outcome.

3. Note any allergy to sulfa drugs.

**Client/Family Teaching**

1. Medication is for topical use only.

2. When used for seborrheic dermatitis of the scalp, apply at bedtime and allow to remain overnight. The hair and scalp may be washed the following morning or at least once a week. Apply lotion for 8–10 consecutive nights.

3. If hair and scalp are oily or if there is debris, shampoo scalp before application.

4. Ophthalmic products may cause sensitivity to bright light; wear sunglasses to minimize.

5. Report any purulent eye drainage as this inactivates sulfacetamide.

6. If prescribed additional eye drops, wait 5 min after sulfacetamide instillation.

7. Do not wear contact lenses until infection is resolved.

**Outcomes/Evaluate:** Resolution of inflammation/infection; symptomatic improvement

# Sulfadiazine
(sul-fah-**DYE**-ah-zeen)
**Pregnancy Category:** C
Microsulfon **(Rx)**

# Sulfadiazine sodium
(sul-fah-**DYE**-ah-zeen)
**Pregnancy Category:** C
**(Rx)**
**Classification:** Sulfonamide

See also *Sulfonamides.*

**Action/Kinetics:** Short-acting, and often combined with other anti-infectives.

**Uses:** Urinary tract infections caused by *Escherichia coli, Klebsiella, Enterobacter, Staphylococcus aureus, Proteus mirabilis,* and *Proteus vulgaris.* Chancroid, inclusion conjunctivitis, adjunct in treating chloroquine-resistant strains of *Plasmodium falciparum,* meningitis caused by *Haemophilus influenzae,* meningococcal

meningitis for sulfonamide-sensitive group A strains, nocardiosis, with penicillin to treat acute otitis media caused by *H. influenzae,* rheumatic fever prophylaxis, adjunct with pyrimethamine for toxoplasmosis in selected immunocompromised clients (e.g., those with AIDS, neoplastic disease, or congenital immune compromise), trachoma.

**Special Concerns:** Safe use during pregnancy has not been established. Should not be used in infants less than 2 months of age unless combined with pyrimethamine to treat congenital toxoplasmosis.

**Dosage** ———————————
• **Tablets**
*General use.*
**Adults, loading dose:** 2–4 g; **maintenance:** 2–4 g/day in 3 to 6 divided doses; **infants over 2 months, loading dose:** 75 mg/kg/day (2 g/m²); **maintenance:** 150 mg/kg/day (4 g/m²/day) in 4 to 6 divided doses, not to exceed 6 g/day.

*Rheumatic fever prophylaxis.*
**Under 30 kg:** 0.5 g/day; **over 30 kg:** 1 g/day.

*As adjunct with pyrimethamine in congenital toxoplasmosis.*
**Infants less than 2 months:** 25 mg/kg q.i.d. for 3 to 4 weeks. **Children greater than 2 months:** 25–50 mg/kg q.i.d. for 3 to 4 weeks.

## NURSING CONSIDERATIONS

See also *General Nursing Considerations for All Anti-Infectives* and for *Sulfonamides.*

**Assessment:** Document indications for therapy, onset, duration, and characteristics of symptoms. Obtain appropriate cultures.

**Outcomes/Evaluate**
• Negative culture reports
• Rheumatic fever prophylaxis during invasive procedures

# Sulfamethoxazole
(sul-fah-meth-**OX**-ah-zohl)
**Pregnancy Category:** C
Apo-Sulfamethoxazole ✤, Gantanol
**(Rx)**

**Classification:** Sulfonamide, intermediate-acting

See also *Sulfonamides*.
**Action/Kinetics:** t½: 8.6 hr.
**Uses:** Urinary tract infections caused
by *Escherichia coli, Klebsiella, Enterobacter, Staphylococcus aureus, Proteus mirabilis, and Proteus vulgaris*.
Chancroid, inclusion conjunctivitis,
adjunct in treating chloroquine-resistant strains of *Plasmodium falciparum*, meningococcal meningitis for
sulfonamide-sensitive group A
strains, nocardiosis, with penicillin
to treat acute otitis media caused by
*H. influenzae*, adjunct with pyrimethamine for toxoplasmosis in
selected immunocompromised clients (e.g., those with AIDS, neoplastic disease, or congenital immune
compromise), trachoma.
**Special Concerns:** May be an increased risk of severe side effects in
elderly clients.

**Dosage**
• **Tablets**
*Mild to moderate infections.*
**Adults, initially:** 2 g; **then,** 1 g in
morning and evening.
*Severe infections.*
**Adults, initially:** 2 g; **then,** 1 g t.i.d.
**Infants over 2 months, initial:**
50–60 mg/kg; **then,** 25–30 mg/kg in
morning and evening, not to exceed
75 mg/kg/day. Alternative dosing:
50–60 mg/kg/day divided q 12 hr,
not to exceed 3 g/24 hr.

**NURSING CONSIDERATIONS**

See also *General Nursing Considerations for All Anti-Infectives* and for
*Sulfonamides*.
**Client/Family Teaching**
1. Take only as directed and complete entire prescription.
2. May cause dizziness; assess response prior to any activity requiring
mental alertness.
3. Use sunglasses, sunscreens, and
protective clothing during sun exposure as a photosensitivity reaction
may occur.

**Outcomes/Evaluate:** Resolution of
infection; symptomatic improvement

# Sulfasalazine
(sul-fah-**SAL**-ah-zeen)
**Pregnancy Category:** B
Alti-Sulfasalazine ✦, Apo-
Sulfasalazine ✦, Azulfidine, Azulfidine
EN-Tabs, PMS Sulfasalazine ✦, Sala-
zopyrin ✦, Salazopyrin-EN Tabs ✦,
SAS-500 ✦ **(Rx)**
**Classification:** Sulfonamide

See also *Sulfonamides*.
**Action/Kinetics:** About one-third
of the dose of sulfasalazine is absorbed from the small intestine
while two-thirds passes to the colon,
where it is split to 5-aminosalicylic
acid and sulfapyridine. The drug
does not affect the microflora.
**Uses:** Ulcerative colitis. Azulfidine
EN-tabs are also used to treat rheumatoid arthritis in clients who do not
respond well to NSAIDs. *Investigational:* Ankylosing spondylitis, collagenous colitis, Crohn's disease,
psoriasis, juvenile chronic arthritis,
psoriatic arthritis.
**Additional      Contraindications:**
Children below 2 years, persons
with marked sulfonamide, salicylate,
or related drug hypersensitivity. Intestinal or urinary obstruction.
**Special Concerns:** Use with caution during lactation.
**Side Effects:** Most common include
anorexia, headache, N&V, gastric
distress, reversible oligospermia.
Less frequently, pruritus, urticaria,
fever, Heinz body anemia, hemolytic
anemia, cyanosis.
**Drug Interactions**
*Digoxin* / ↓ Absorption of digoxin
*Folic acid* / ↓ Absorption of folic
acid

**Dosage**
• **Enteric-Coated Tablets, Tablets**
*Ulcerative colitis.*
**Adults, initial:** 3–4 g/day in divided
doses (1–2 g/day may decrease side
effects); **maintenance:** 500 mg
q.i.d. **Pediatric, over 2 years of**

**S**

---

**age, initial:** 40–60 mg/kg/day in 3 to 6 equally divided doses; **maintenance:** 30 mg/kg/day in 4 divided doses.

*For desensitization to sulfasalazine.*
Reinstitute at level of 50–250 mg/day; **then,** give double dose q 4–7 days until desired therapeutic level reached. Do not attempt in those with a history of agranulocytosis or who have experienced anaphylaxis previously with sulfasalazine.

*Collagenous colitis.*
2–3 g/day.
*Psoriasis.*
3–4 g/day.
*Juvenile chronic arthritis.*
50 mg/kg.
*Psoriatic arthritis.*
2 g/day.

## NURSING CONSIDERATIONS

See also *General Nursing Considerations for All Anti-Infectives* and for *Sulfonamides.*

**Assessment**
1. Note indications for therapy, including onset, location, duration, and characteristics of symptoms.
2. Document frequency, quantity, and consistency of stool production as well as characteristics of abdominal pain.
3. Note joint deformity, pain, ROM, inflammation, and swelling with rheumatoid arthritis.
4. Monitor CBC, renal function studies, and urinalysis; with colitis, send stool for analysis.

**Client/Family Teaching**
1. Take with food to reduce GI upset.
2. Take exactly as ordered; intermittent therapy (2 weeks on, 2 weeks off) is generally recommended.
3. Drug may discolor urine or skin a yellow-orange color.
4. Take at least 2–3 L/day of water to decrease incidence of crystalluria and stone formation.
5. Avoid prolonged exposure to sunlight; may increase sensitivity. Wear protective clothing, sunglasses, and sunscreen.

**Outcomes/Evaluate**
• ↓ Frequency of loose stools; ↓ abdominal pain; ↓ colon inflammation
• Relief of pain from joint deformity, swelling, and inflammation

# Sulfinpyrazone
(sul-fin-**PEER**-ah-zohn)
Antazone ✤, Anturane, Apo-Sulfinpyrazone ✤, Novo–Pyrazone ✤, Nu-Sulfinpyrazone ✤ **(Rx)**
**Classification:** Antigout agent, uricosuric

**Action/Kinetics:** Inhibits tubular reabsorption of uric acid, thereby increasing its excretion. Also exhibits antithrombotic and platelet inhibitory actions. **Peak plasma levels:** 1–2 hr. **Therapeutic plasma levels:** Up to 160 mcg/mL following 800 mg/day for uricosuria. **Duration:** 4–6 hr (up to 10 hr in some). **t½:** 3–8 hr. Sulfinpyrazone is metabolized by the liver. Approximately 45% of the drug is excreted unchanged by the kidney, and a small amount is excreted in the feces.

**Uses:** Chronic and intermittent gouty arthritis. Sulfinpyrazone is not effective during acute attacks of gout and may even increase the frequency of acute episodes during the initiation of therapy. However, the drug should not be discontinued during acute attacks. Concomitant administration of colchicine during initiation of therapy is recommended. *Investigational:* To decrease sudden death during first year after MI.

**Contraindications:** Active peptic ulcer or symptoms of GI inflammation or ulceration. Blood dyscrasias. Sensitivity to phenylbutazone or other pyrazoles. Use to control hyperuricemia secondary to treatment of malignancies.

**Special Concerns:** Use with caution in pregnant women. Dosage has not been established in children. Use with extreme caution in clients with impaired renal function and in those with a history of peptic ulcers.

**Side Effects:** *GI:* N&V, abdominal discomfort. May reactivate peptic ulcer. *Hematologic:* Leukopenia, *agran-*

*ulocytosis,* anemia, thrombocytopenia, **aplastic anemia.** *Miscellaneous:* Skin rash (which usually disappears with usage), **bronchoconstriction in aspirin-induced asthma.** Acute attacks of gout may become more frequent during initial therapy. Give concomitantly with colchicine at this time.

**OD** **Overdose Management:** *Symptoms:* N&V, diarrhea, epigastric pain, labored respiration, ataxia, seizures, coma. *Treatment:* Supportive measures.

**Drug Interactions**
*Acetaminophen* / ↑ Risk of acetaminophen hepatotoxicity; ↓ effect of acetaminophen
*Anticoagulants* / ↑ Effect of anticoagulants due to ↓ plasma protein binding
*Niacin* / ↓ Uricosuric effect of sulfinpyrazone
*Salicylates* / Inhibit uricosuric effect of sulfinpyrazone
*Theophylline* / ↓ Effect of theophylline due to ↑ plasma clearance
*Tolbutamide* / ↑ Risk of hypoglycemia
*Verapamil* / ↓ Effect of verapamil due to ↑ plasma clearance

**Dosage** ———————
• **Capsules, Tablets**
*Gout.*
**Adults, initial:** 200–400 mg/day in two divided doses with meals or milk. Clients who are transferred from other uricosuric agents can receive full dose at once. **Maintenance:** 100–400 mg b.i.d. Maintain full dosage without interruption even during acute attacks of gout.
*Following MI.*
**Adults:** 300 mg q.i.d. or 400 mg b.i.d.

**NURSING CONSIDERATIONS**
**Assessment**
1. Assess joint(s) for pain, deformity, ROM, and inflammation.
2. Monitor CBC and uric acid levels.
**Client/Family Teaching**
1. If GI upset occurs, take with food, milk, or antacids. May still reactivate peptic ulcer.
2. Consume at least ten to twelve 8-oz glasses of fluid daily to prevent the formation of uric acid stones. Avoid cranberry juice or vitamin C preparations, as these acidify urine; acidification may cause formation of uric acid stones.
3. Sodium bicarbonate may be ordered to alkalinize the urine to prevent urates from crystallizing in acid urine and forming kidney stones.
4. Avoid alcohol and aspirin; may interfere with drug effectiveness.
5. During *acute* attacks of gout, concomitant administration of colchicine is indicated.
**Outcomes/Evaluate**
• ↓ Frequency and intensity of gout attacks
• ↓ Serum uric acid levels

# Sulfisoxazole
(sul-fih-**SOX**-ah-zohl)
**Pregnancy Category:** C
Apo-Sulfisoxazole ✦, Novo-Soxazole ✦, Sulfizole ✦ **(Rx)**

# Sulfisoxazole diolamine
(sul-fih-**SOX**-ah-zohl)
**Pregnancy Category:** C
**(Rx)**
**Classification:** Sulfonamide, short-acting

See also *Sulfonamides.*
**Action/Kinetics: t½:** 5.9 hr.
**Uses:** Urinary tract infections caused by *Escherichia coli, Klebsiella, Enterobacter, Staphylococcus aureus, Proteus mirabilis, and Proteus vulgaris.* Chancroid, inclusion conjunctivitis, adjunct in treating chloroquine-resistant strains of *Plasmodium falciparum,* meningitis caused by *Haemophilus influenzae,* meningococcal meningitis for sulfonamide-sensitive group A strains, nocardiosis, with penicillin to treat acute otitis media caused by *H. influenzae,* adjunct with pyrimethamine for toxoplasmosis in selected immunocompromised clients (e.g., those with AIDS, neoplas-

tic disease, or congenital immune compromise). Ophthalmically as an adjunct with systemic sulfonamides to treat trachoma.

**Additional Contraindications:** Use in infants less than 2 months of age except as adjunct with pyrimethamine to treat congenital toxoplasmosis. Use in the presence of epithelial herpes simplex keratitis, vaccinia, varicella, and other viral diseases of the cornea and conjunctiva. Mycobacterial or fungal infections of the ocular structures. After uncomplicated removal of a corneal foreign body.

**Special Concerns:** Safety and efficacy of the ophthalmic products have not been established in children. Use with caution in clients with severe dry eye.

**Additional Side Effects:** *Following ophthalmic use:* Blurred vision, itching, local irritation, epithelial keratitis, reactive hyperemia, conjunctival edema, burning, headache or browache, transient stinging.

**Additional Drug Interactions:** Sulfisoxazole may ↑ effects of thiopental due to ↓ plasma protein binding.

**Dosage** _____
• **Tablets**

**Adults, loading dose:** 2–4 g; **maintenance:** 4–8 g/day in 4 to 6 divided doses, depending on severity of the infection. **Infants over 2 months, initial:** 75 mg/kg/day; **maintenance:** 150 mg/kg/day (4 g/m²/day) in 4 to 6 divided doses, not to exceed 6 g/day.

• **Ophthalmic Solution (4%)**
*Conjunctivitis or corneal ulcer.*
1–2 gtt into conjunctival sac q 1–4 hr, depending on the severity of the infection. Dose may be tapered by increasing the time interval between doses as the condition improves.
*Trachoma.*
2 gtt q 2 hr with concomitant systemic therapy.

## NURSING CONSIDERATIONS

See also *General Nursing Considerations for All Anti-Infectives* and *Sulfonamides.*

**Administration/Storage:** Solutions will darken in color if left standing for long periods; discard these products.

**Assessment**
1. Document type, onset, and characteristics of symptoms. List other agents trialed and the outcome.
2. Monitor CBC and cultures.

**Client/Family Teaching**
1. Ophthalmic use may cause sensitivity to bright light; wear sunglasses to minimize.
2. With ophthalmic use, report if no improvement after 7–8 days, if the condition worsens, or if pain, increased redness, itching, or swelling of the eye occurs.

**Outcomes/Evaluate:** Negative cultures; symptomatic improvement

# Sulindac
(sul-**IN**-dak)
Apo-Sulin ✷, Clinoril, Novo–Sundac ✷, Nu-Sulindac ✷ **(Rx)**
**Classification:** Nonsteroidal anti-inflammatory drug

See also *Nonsteroidal Anti-Inflammatory Drugs.*

**Action/Kinetics:** Biotransformed in the liver to a sulfide, the active metabolite. **Peak plasma levels of sulfide:** after fasting, 2 hr; after food, 3–4 hr. **Onset, anti-inflammatory effect:** within 1 week; **duration, anti-inflammatory effect:** 1–2 weeks. t½, of sulindac: 7.8 hr; of metabolite: 16.4 hr. Excreted in both urine and feces.

**Uses:** Acute and chronic treatment of rheumatoid arthritis, osteoarthritis, ankylosing spondylitis, acute gouty arthritis; acute, painful shoulder; tendinitis, bursitis. *Investigational:* Juvenile rheumatoid arthritis, sunburn.

**Contraindications:** Use with active GI lesions or a history of recurrent GI lesions.

**Special Concerns:** Safety and efficacy have not been established for children. Safe use during pregnancy has not been established. Use with caution during lactation.

**Additional Side Effects:** Hypersensitivity, pancreatitis, GI pain (common), maculopapular rash. Stupor, *coma,* hypotension, and diminished urine output.

**Additional Drug Interactions:** Sulindac ↑ effect of warfarin due to ↓ plasma protein binding.

## Dosage
• **Tablets**

*Osteoarthritis, rheumatoid arthritis, ankylosing spondylitis.*
**Adults:** 150 mg b.i.d.

*Acute painful shoulder, acute gouty arthritis.*
**Adults:** 200 mg b.i.d. for 7–14 days.

*Antigout.*
**Adults:** 200 mg b.i.d. for 7 days.

## NURSING CONSIDERATIONS

See also *Nursing Considerations* for *Nonsteroidal Anti-Inflammatory Drugs.*

**Administration/Storage:** For acute conditions, reduce dosage when satisfactory response is attained.

**Assessment**
1. Document type, onset, and duration of symptoms.
2. Determine baseline ROM; describe location of pain, inflammation, and swelling; note functional class of arthritis.
3. If renal dysfunction evident, reduce dosage.
4. Monitor CBC, liver and renal function studies.

**Client/Family Teaching**
1. Take with food to decrease GI upset and consume plenty of water. A stomach protectant (i.e., misoprostol) may be prescribed with a history of ulcer disease.
2. Do not take aspirin because plasma levels of sulindac will be reduced. Avoid alcohol.
3. Report any incidence of unexplained bleeding such as oozing of blood from the gums, nosebleeds, or excessive bruising.
4. Drug may cause dizziness; assess response prior to any activity requiring mental alertness.

5. When used for arthritis, a favorable response usually occurs within 1 week.

**Outcomes/Evaluate:** ↓ Joint pain and inflammation with ↑ mobility

# Sumatriptan succinate
(**soo**-mah-**TRIP**-tan)
**Pregnancy Category:** C
Imitrex
**Classification:** Antimigraine drug

**Action/Kinetics:** Selective agonist for a vascular 5-HT$_1$ receptor subtype (probably 5-HT$_{1D}$) located on cranial arteries, on the basilar artery, and the vasculature of the dura mater. Sumatriptan activates the 5-HT$_1$ receptor, causing vasoconstriction and therefore relief of migraine. Transient increases in BP may be observed. No significant activity at 5-HT$_2$ or 5-HT$_3$ receptor subtypes; alpha-1-, alpha-2-, or beta-adrenergic receptors; dopamine-1 or dopamine-2 receptors; muscarinic receptors; or benzodiazepine receptors. **Time to peak effect after SC:** 12 min after a 6-mg SC dose. **t½ distribution, after SC:** 15 min; **terminal t½:** 115 min. Approximately 22% of a SC dose is excreted in the urine as unchanged drug and 38% as metabolites. Rapidly absorbed after PO administration, although bioavailability is low due to incomplete absorption and a first-pass effect (bioavailability may be significantly increased in those with impaired liver function). **PO, elimination t½:** About 2.5 hr. About 60% of a PO dose is excreted through the urine and 40% in the feces.

**Uses:** Treatment of acute migraine attacks with or without aura. Photophobia, phonophobia, nausea, and vomiting associated with migraine attacks are also relieved. Intended to relieve migraine, but not to prevent or reduce the number of attacks experienced. Treatment of cluster headaches.

**Contraindications:** Hypersensitivity to sumatriptan. IV use due to the possibility of coronary vasospasm.

S

SC use in clients with ischemic heart disease, history of MI, documented silent ischemia, Prinzmetal's angina, or uncontrolled hypertension. Concomitant use with ergotamine-containing products or MAO inhibitor therapy (or within 2 weeks of discontinuing an MAO inhibitor). Use in clients with hemiplegic or basilar migraine. Use in women who are pregnant, think they may be pregnant, or are trying to get pregnant.

**Special Concerns:** Use with caution during lactation, in clients with impaired hepatic or renal function, and in clients with heart conditions. Clients with risk factors for CAD (e.g., men over 40, smokers, postmenopausal women, hypertension, obesity, diabetes, hypercholesterolemia, family history of heart disease) should be screened before initiating treatment. Safety and efficacy have not been determined for use in children.

**Side Effects:** Side effects listed are for either SC or PO use of the drug. *CV:* Coronary vasospasm in clients with a history of CAD. ***Serious and/or life-threatening arrhythmias, including atrial fibrillation, ventricular fibrillation, ventricular tachycardia, MI, marked ischemic ST elevations,*** chest and arm discomfort representing angina pectoris. Flushing, hypertension, hypotension, bradycardia, tachycardia, palpitations, pulsating sensations, ECG changes (including nonspecific ST- or T-wave changes, prolongation of PR or QTc intervals, sinus arrhythmia, nonsustained ventricular premature beats, isolated junctional ectopic beats, atrial ectopic beats, and delayed activation of the right ventricle), syncope, pallor, abnormal pulse, vasodilatation, atherosclerosis, bradycardia, cerebral ischemia, CV lesion, heart block, peripheral cyanosis, thrombosis, transient myocardial ischemia, vasodilation, Raynaud's syndrome. *At injection site:* Pain, redness. *Atypical sensations:* Sensation of warmth, cold, tingling, or paresthesia. Localized or generalized feeling of pressure, burning, numbness, and tightness.

Feeling of heaviness, feeling strange, tight feeling in head. *CNS:* Fatigue, dizziness, drowsiness, vertigo, sedation, headache, anxiety, malaise, confusion, euphoria, agitation, relaxation, chills, tremor, shivering, prickling or stinging sensations, phonophobia, depression, euphoria, facial pain, heat sensitivity, incoordination, monoplegia, sleep disturbances, shivering. *EENT:* Throat discomfort, discomfort in nasal cavity or sinuses. Vision alterations, eye irritation, photophobia, lacrimation, otalgia, feeling of fullness in ear, disorders of sclera, mydriasis. *GI:* Abdominal discomfort, dysphagia, discomfort of mouth and tongue, gastroesophageal reflux, diarrhea, peptic ulcer, retching, flatulence, eructation, gallstones, taste disturbances, GI bleeding, hematemesis, melena. *Respiratory:* Dyspnea, diseases of the lower respiratory tract, hiccoughs, influenza, asthma. *Dermatologic:* Erythema, pruritus, skin rashes, skin eruptions, skin tenderness, dry or scaly skin, tightness or wrinkling of skin. *GU:* Dysuria, dysmenorrhea, urinary frequency, renal calculus, breast tenderness, increased urination, intermenstrual bleeding, nipple discharge, abortion, hematuria. *Musculoskeletal:* Weakness, neck pain or stiffness, myalgia, muscle cramps, joint disturbances (pain, stiffness, swelling, ache), muscle stiffness, need to flex calf muscles, backache, muscle tiredness, swelling of the extremities, tetany. *Endocrine:* Elevated TSH levels, galactorrhea, hyperglycemia, hypoglycemia, hypothyroidism, weight gain or loss. *Miscellaneous:* Chest, jaw, or neck tightness. Sweating, thirst, polydipsia, chills, fever, dehydration.

**Laboratory Test Alterations:** Disturbance of LFTs.

**OD** **Overdose Management:** *Symptoms:* Tremor, ***convulsions,*** inactivity erythema of extremities, reduced respiratory rate, cyanosis, ataxia, mydriasis, injection site reactions (desquamation, hair loss, scab formation), paralysis. *Treatment:* Continuous monitoring of client for at least 10 hr and especially when signs and symptoms persist.

**Drug Interactions**

*Ergot drugs* / Prolonged vasospastic reactions

*Monoamine oxidase A inhibitors* / ↑ t½ of sumatriptan

**Dosage**

- **SC**

    *Migraine headaches.*

    **Adults:** 6 mg. A second injection may be given if symptoms of migraine come back but no more than two injections (6 mg each) should be taken in a 24-hr period and at least 1 hr should elapse between doses.

- **Tablets**

    **Adults:** 25 mg with fluids as soon as symptoms of migraine appear. A second dose may be taken if symptoms return but not sooner than 2 hr following the first dose. **Maximum recommended dose:** 100 mg, with no more than 300 mg taken in a 24-hr period.

- **Nasal Spray**

    A single dose of 5, 10, or 20 mg given in one nostril. The 20 mg dose increases the risk of side effects. The 10 mg dose may be given as a single 5-mg dose in each nostril. If the headache returns, repeat the dose once after 2 hr; not to exceed a total daily dose of 40 mg. The safety of treating an average of more than 4 headaches in a 30-day period has not been studied.

---

## NURSING CONSIDERATIONS

**Administration/Storage**

1. No increased beneficial effect has been found with the administration of a second 6-mg dose in clients not responding to the first injection.

2. If side effects are dose limiting, a dose lower than 6 mg may be given; in such cases, only the single-dose vial dosage form should be used, as the autoinjection form delivers 6 mg.

3. Consideration should be given to administering the first dose of sumatriptan in the provider's office due to

the possibility (although rare) of coronary events.

4. Is equally effective at whatever stage of the attack given; advisable to take as soon as possible after the onset of a migraine attack.

5. Store away from heat (no higher than 30°C; 86°F) and light.

**Assessment**

1. Document headache characteristics, including onset, frequency, type, and duration of symptoms.

2. Determine any cardiac problems or ischemic CV disease.

3. Review neurologic exam and CT/MRI results. A clear diagnosis of migraine should be made; the drug should not be given for headaches due to other neurologic events.

4. Assess ECG, liver, and renal function studies. Monitor VS; expect transient increases in BP

5. Parenteral form is for SC use only. IV use may cause coronary vasospasm.

**Client/Family Teaching**

1. Review the appropriate method for administration. With SC form, administer (or have client self-administer) first dose in office to assess response.

2. Printed instructions concerning how to load the autoinjector, administer the medication, and remove the syringe, are enclosed and provided by the manufacturer.

3. The injection is given just below the skin as soon as migraine symptoms appear or any time during the attack. A second injection may be administered 1 hr later if migraine symptoms return; do *not* exceed two injections in 24 hr.

4. Practice safe handling, storage, and disposal of syringes.

5. Pain and tenderness may be evident at injection site for up to an hour after administration.

6. Check expiration date before use and discard all outdated drugs.

7. Report if chest, jaw, throat, and neck pain occur after injection; this should be medically evaluated before using more Imitrex.

**S**

---

8. Severe chest pain or tightness, wheezing, palpitations, facial swelling, or rashes/hives should be immediately reported.

9. Symptoms of flushing, tingling, heat and heaviness, as well as dizziness or drowsiness may occur and should be reported before taking more sumatriptan.

10. Practice barrier contraception and do not use Imitrex if pregnancy is suspected.

**Outcomes/Evaluate:** Reversal of acute migraine attack; relief of symptoms

# Suprofen
(sue-**PROH**-fen)
**Pregnancy Category:** C
Profenal **(Rx)**
**Classification:** Nonsteroidal anti-inflammatory drug, ophthalmic use

See also *Nonsteroidal Anti-Inflammatory Drugs.*

**Action/Kinetics:** By inhibiting prostaglandin synthesis, suprofen reverses prostaglandin-induced vasodilation, leukocytosis, increased vascular permeability, and increased intraocular pressure. Also inhibits miosis, which occurs during cataract surgery.

**Uses:** Inhibition of intraoperative miosis.

**Contraindications:** Dendritic keratitis.

**Special Concerns:** Use with caution during lactation, in clients sensitive to aspirin and other NSAIDs, and in surgical clients with a history of bleeding tendencies or who are on drugs that prolong bleeding time. Safety and efficacy have not been established in children.

**Side Effects:** *Ophthalmic:* Ocular irritation, transient burning, and stinging on installation. Redness, itching, discomfort, pain, iritis, allergy, chemosis, photophobia, punctate epithelial staining.

**Drug Interactions:** Acetylcholine and carbachol may be ineffective if used in combination with suprofen.

## Dosage
• **Ophthalmic Solution**
  *Day before surgery.*
2 gtt into the conjunctival sac q 4 hr during waking hours.
  *Day of surgery.*
2 gtt into the conjunctival sac 3, 2, and 1 hr prior to surgery.

## NURSING CONSIDERATIONS

See also *Nursing Considerations* for *Nonsteroidal Anti-Inflammatory Drugs.*

**Outcomes/Evaluate:** Control of inflammation; inhibition of abnormal pupillary contractions

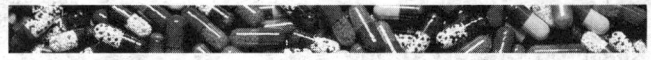

# T

# Tacrine hydrochloride (THA, Tetrahydro-aminoacridine)
(**TAH**-krin)
**Pregnancy Category:** C
Cognex **(Rx)**
**Classification:** Psychotherapeutic drug for Alzheimer's disease

**Action/Kinetics:** During early stages of Alzheimer's disease, cholinergic neuronal pathways that project from the basal forebrain to the cerebral cortex and hippocampus may be affected. Symptoms of dementia may be due to a deficiency of acetylcholine. As a reversible CNS cholinesterase inhibitor, tacrine elevates acetylcholine levels in the cerebral cortex. There is no evidence tacrine alters progression of dementia. Rapidly absorbed after PO administration. **Maximal plasma levels:** 1–2 hr. Food will affect the bioavailability of tacrine. Extensively metabolized in the liver. Undergoes first-pass metabolism; can be overcome by increasing the dose. **Elimination $t\frac{1}{2}$:** 2–4 hr. The average plasma levels are about 50% higher in females. Also, the mean tacrine levels in smokers are about one-third the levels of nonsmokers.

**Uses:** Treatment of mild to moderate dementia of the Alzheimer's type.

**Contraindications:** Hypersensitivity to tacrine or acridine derivatives. Use in clients previously treated with tacrine who developed jaundice (elevated total bilirubin > 3 mg/dL).

**Special Concerns:** May cause bradycardia—important in sick sinus syndrome. Use with caution in clients at risk for developing ulcers as the drug increases gastric acid secretion. Use with caution in clients with a history of abnormal liver function as indicated by abnormalities in serum ALT, AST, bilirubin, and GGT levels. Use with caution in clients with a history of asthma. There may be worsening of cognitive function following abrupt discontinuation of the drug. Safety and efficacy have not been determined in children with dementing illness.

**Side Effects:** *Hepatic:* Increased transaminase levels (most common reason for stopping the drug during treatment). *GI:* N&V, diarrhea, dyspepsia, anorexia, abdominal pain, flatulence, constipation, glossitis, gingivitis, dry mouth or throat, stomatitis, increased salivation, dysphagia, esophagitis, gastritis, gastroenteritis, *GI hemorrhage,* stomach ulcer, hiatal hernia, hemorrhoids, bloody stools, diverticulitis, fecal impaction, fecal incontinence, *rectal hemorrhage,* cholelithiasis, cholecystitis, increased appetite. *Musculoskeletal:* Myalgia, fracture, arthralgia, arthritis, hypertonia, osteoporosis, tendinitis, bursitis, gout, myopathy. *CNS:* **Precipitation of seizures** (may also be due to Alzheimer's), dizziness, confusion, ataxia, insomnia, somnolence, tremor, agitation, depression, abnormal thinking, anxiety, hallucinations, hostility, migraine, *convulsions,* vertigo, syncope, hyperkinesia, paresthesia, abnormal dreams, dysarthria,

aphasia, amnesia, twitching, hypesthesia, delirium, paralysis, bradykinesia, movement disorders, cogwheel rigidity, paresis, neuritis, hemiplegia, Parkinson's disease, neuropathy, extrapyramidal syndrome, decreased or absent reflexes, tardive dyskinesia, dysesthesia, dystonia, encephalitis, *coma,* apraxia, oculogyric crisis, akathisia, oral facial dyskinesia, Bell's palsy, nervousness, apathy, increased libido, paranoia, neurosis, *suicidal episodes,* psychosis, hysteria. *Respiratory:* Rhinitis, URI, coughing, pharyngitis, sinusitis, bronchitis, pneumonia, dyspnea, epistaxis, chest congestion, asthma, hyperventilation, lower respiratory infection, hemoptysis, lung edema, *lung cancer, acute epiglottitis. CV:* Hypotension, hypertension, *heart failure, MI, CVA,* angina pectoris, TIA, phlebitis, venous insufficiency, abdominal aortic aneurysm, atrial fibrillation or flutter, palpitation, tachycardia, bradycardia, *pulmonary embolus, heart arrest,* premature atrial contractions, *AV block,* bundle branch block. *Dermatologic:* Rash, facial and skin flushing, increased sweating, acne, alopecia, dermatitis, eczema, dry skin, herpes zoster, psoriasis, cellulitis, cyst, furunculosis, herpes simplex, hyperkeratosis, basal cell carcinoma, skin cancer, desquamation, seborrhea, squamous cell carcinoma, skin ulcer, skin necrosis, *melanoma. GU:* Bladder outflow obstruction, urinary frequency, urinary incontinence, UTI, hematuria, renal stone, kidney infection, glycosuria, dysuria, polyuria, nocturia, pyuria, cystitis, urinary retention, urinary urgency, *vaginal hemorrhage,* genital pruritus, breast pain, urinary obstruction, impotence, *prostate cancer, bladder tumor, renal tumor, renal failure, breast cancer, ovarian carcinoma,* epididymitis. *Body as a whole:* Headache, fatigue, chest pain, weight decrease, back pain, asthenia, chill, fever, malaise, peripheral edema, facial edema, dehydration, weight increase, cachexia, lipoma, heat

**T**

---

exhaustion, sepsis, **cholinergic crisis, death.** *Hematologic:* Anemia, lymphadenopathy, leukopenia, thrombocytopenia, hemolysis, pancytopenia. *Ophthalmologic:* Conjunctivitis, cataract, dry eyes, eye pain, visual field defect, diplopia, amblyopia, glaucoma, hordeolum, vision loss, ptosis, blepharitis. *Otic:* Deafness, earache, tinnitus, inner ear infection, otitis media, labyrinthitis, inner ear disturbance. *Miscellaneous:* Purpura, hypercholesterolemia, diabetes mellitus, hypothyroid, hyperthyroid, unusual taste.

**OD** **Overdose Management:** *Symptoms:* Cholinergic crisis characterized by severe N&V, sweating, bradycardia, salivation, hypotension, *collapse, seizures, and increased muscle weakness (may paralyze respiratory muscles leading to death).* *Treatment:* General supportive measures. IV atropine sulfate, titrated to effect, may be given in an initial dose of 1–2 mg IV with subsequent doses based on the response.

**Drug Interactions**

*Anticholinergic drugs* / Tacrine interferes with the action of these drugs

*Bethanechol* / Tacrine → synergistic effect with bethanechol

*Cholinesterase inhibitors* / Tacrine → synergistic effect with cholinesterase inhibitors

*Cimetidine* / Cimetidine ↑ maximum levels of tacrine

*Succinylcholine* / Tacrine ↑ muscle relaxation due to succinylcholine

*Theophylline* / Tacrine ↑ plasma levels of theophylline; ↓ theophylline dose recommended.

**Dosage** ⸻

• **Capsules**

*Alzheimer's disease.*

**Initial:** 10 mg q.i.d. for at least 6 weeks; **then,** after 6 weeks, increase the dose to 20 mg q.i.d., providing there are no significant transaminase elevations and the client tolerates the treatment. Based on the degree of tolerance, the dose may be titrated, at 6-week intervals, to 30 or 40 mg q.i.d.

If transaminase elevations occur, modify the dose as follows: If transaminase levels are 2 × ULN or less, discontinue the drug and monitor. If transaminse levels are greater than 2 but equal to or less than 3 × ULN, treatment is continued according to recommended titraiton but transaminase levels are monitored weekly until they return to normal levels. If transaminase levels are more than 3 but equal to or less than 5 × ULN, the daily dose is reduced by 40 mg/day. Dose titration is resumed and every other week monitoring is undertaken when transaminase levels return to within normal limits. If transaminase levels are greater than 5 × ULN, treatment is stopped and transaminase levels monitored until they are within normal limits.

Clients who are required to stop treatment due to elevated transaminase levels may be rechallenged once levels return to within normal range. Weekly monitoring of serum ALT levels should be undertaken after rechallenging occurs. If rechallenged, the initial dose is 10 mg t.i.d. with transaminase levels monitored weekly. After 6 weeks on this dose, the client may begin dose titration if transaminase levels are acceptable.

## NURSING CONSIDERATIONS
### Administration/Storage

1. Take drug between meals, if possible. If GI upset occurs, may take with meals; however, the plasma level will be decreased by 30%–40%.
2. The initial dose should not be increased for 6 weeks as there is the potential for delayed onset of transaminase elevations.

### Assessment

1. Assess mental status. Document onset and duration of symptoms and if this is a first drug trial or a rechallenge. If a rechallenge, document serum bilirubin and SGPT from previous treatment.
2. Note any ECG evidence of sick sinus syndrome or any ulcer disease, asthma, or liver disease.
3. List drugs currently prescribed to ensure none interact unfavorably.

Drug is a cholinesterase inhibitor; notify anesthesia before procedures.

4. Monitor ECG, hematologic, liver, and renal profiles. Serum transaminase levels (ALT/SGPT) should be monitored weekly for the first 18 weeks and then every 3 months unless dose is increased or the transaminase levels are mildly elevated; follow guidelines under *Dosage*.

5. Monitor VS; may cause bradycardia.

6. Observe and record response carefully; drug is titrated according to client tolerance.

**Client/Family Teaching**

1. Take between meals unless GI upset is experienced. With meals, the plasma drug level will be decreased by 30%–40%

2. Drug must be administered at regularly spaced intervals.Do not increase dose for the first 6 weeks until response and tolerance assessed.

3. Clinical manifestations of mild to moderate dementia in Alzheimer's disease are thought to be related to a deficiency of acetylcholine. Tacrine is thought to act to elevate acetylcholine concentrations in the cerebral cortex. As the disease progresses, tacrine's effect may lessen.

4. Report any new symptoms or any increase in existing symptoms.

5. Smoking may interfere with serum drug levels.

6. During initiation of therapy, N&V and diarrhea may be evident; report if persistent or bothersome. Delayed-onset side effects that should be reported include rashes, yellow skin discoloration, and changes in stool color.

7. Do not stop abruptly. Abrupt withdrawal may cause a decline in cognitive function and also contribute to behavioral disturbances.

8. Identify appropriate resources and support groups that may assist the family and caregivers in understanding and coping with this disorder.

**Outcomes/Evaluate:** Improved level of cognitive functioning with Alzheimer's disease

# Tacrolimus (FK506)
(tah-**KROH**-lih-mus)
**Pregnancy Category:** C
Prograf **(Rx)**
**Classification:** Immunosuppressive drug

**Action/Kinetics:** Produced by *Streptomyces tsukubaensis.* Mechanism of action is not known but it inhibits T-lymphocyte formation leading to immunosuppression. Absorption from the GI tract is variable. **t½, terminal elimination:** 11.7 hr in liver transplant clients and 21.2 hr in healthy volunteers. Food decreases both the absorption and bioavailability of tacrolimus. Significantly bound to proteins and erythrocytes; extensively metabolized by the liver and excreted through the urine.

**Uses:** Prophylaxis of organ rejection in allogeneic liver transplants and kidney transplants; usually used with corticosteroids. *Investigational:* Transplants of bone marrow, heart, pancreas, pancreatic island cells, and small bowel. Treatment of autoimmune disease and severe recalcitrant psoriasis.

**Contraindications:** Hypersensitivity to tacrolimus or HCO-60 polyoxyl 60 hydrogenated castor oil (vehicle used for the injection). Lactation. Concomitant use with cyclosporine.

**Special Concerns:** Increased risk of developing lymphomas and other malignancies (especially of the skin).

**Side Effects:** *CNS:* Headache, tremor, insomnia, paresthesia, ***seizures, coma,*** delirium, abnormal dreams, anxiety, agitation, confusion, depression, dizziness, emotional lability, hallucinations, hypertonia, incoordination, myoclonus nervousness, psychosis, somnolence, abnormal thinking. *Neurotoxicity:* Changes in motor function, mental status, and sensory function; tremor, headache. *GI:* Diarrhea, nausea, constipation, liver function test abnormal, anorexia, vomiting, dyspepsia, dysphasia, flatulence, ***GI hemorrhage, GI perfora-***

T

---

*tion,* ileus, increased appetite, oral moniliasis. *Hepatic:* Hepatitis, cholangitis, cholestatic jaundice, jaundice, liver damage. *CV:* Hypertension, chest pain, abnormal ECG, **hemorrhage,** hypotension, tachycardia. *Hematologic:* Anemia, thrombocytopenia, leukocytosis, coagulation disorder, ecchymosis, hypochromic anemia, leukopenia, decreased prothrombin. *GU:* Abnormal kidney function, nephrotoxicity, UTI, oliguria, hematuria, **kidney failure.** *Metabolic:* Hyperkalemia, hypokalemia, hyperglycemia, hypomagnesemia, acidosis, alkalosis, hyperlipemia, hyperphosphatemia, hyperuricemia, hypocalcemia, hypophosphatemia, hyponatremia, hypoproteinemia, bilirubinemia. *Respiratory:* Pleural effusion, atelectasis, dyspnea, asthma, bronchitis, increased cough, pulmonary edema, pharyngitis, pneumonia, lung disorder, respiratory disorder, rhinitis, sinusitis, alteration in voice. *Musculoskeletal:* Arthralgia, leg cramps, myalgia, myasthenia, osteoporosis, generalized spasm. *Dermatologic:* Pruritus, rash, alopecia, herpes simplex, sweating, skin disorder, herpes simplex. *Miscellaneous:* Hypersensitivity reactions (including **anaphylaxis**), increased incidence of malignancies, lymphoma, diabetes mellitus, pain, fever, asthenia, back pain, ascites, peripheral edema, abdominal pain, enlarged abdomen, abscess, chills, hernia, photosensitivity, peritonitis, abnormal healing.

**Laboratory Test Alterations:** ↑ Alkaline phosphatase, AST, ALT.

**Drug Interactions**

*Aminoglycosides* / Additive or synergistic impairment of renal function

*Amphotericin B* / Additive or synergistic impairment of renal function

*Antifungal drugs* / ↑ Tacrolimus blood levels

*Bromocriptine* / ↑ Tacrolimus blood levels

*Calcium channel blocking drugs* / ↑ Tacrolimus blood levels

*Carbamazepine* / ↓ Tacrolimus blood levels

*Cimetidine* / ↑ Tacrolimus blood levels

*Cisplatin* / Additive or synergistic impairment of renal function

*Clarithromycin* / ↑ Tacrolimus blood levels

*Cyclosporine* / Additive or synergistic nephrotoxicity; also, ↑ tacrolimus blood levels

*Danazol* / ↑ Tacrolimus blood levels

*Diltiazem* / ↑ Tacrolimus blood levels

*Erythromycin* / ↑ Tacrolimus blood levels

*Methylprednisolone* / ↑ Tacrolimus blood levels

*Metoclopramide* / ↑ Tacrolimus blood levels

*Phenobarbital* / ↓ Tacrolimus blood levels

*Phenytoin* / ↓ Tacrolimus blood levels

*Rifamycin* / ↓ Tacrolimus blood levels

*Vaccines* / ↓ Effectiveness of vaccines

**Dosage** ————————
- **IV Infusion Only**
  *Immunosuppression.*
**Initial:** 0.05–0.1 mg/kg/day as a continuous IV infusion. Early in the period following transplantation, concomitant adrenal corticosteroid use is recommended.
- **Capsules**
  *Immunosuppression.*
**Initial:** 0.15–0.3 mg/kg/day administered in two divided doses q 12 hr.
**Maintenance:** Titrate dose based on clinical assessment of rejection and tolerability. Lower doses may suffice for maintenance therapy.

**NURSING CONSIDERATIONS**
**Administration/Storage**

**IV** 1.   IV therapy may be started if unable to take capsules.

2. For both IV and PO administration, give doses for adult clients at the lower end of the dosage range and initiate doses for pediatric clients at the higher end of the dosage range (i.e., 0.1 mg/kg/day for IV use and 0.3 mg/kg/day for PO use).

3. Give the initial dose no sooner than 6 hr after implantation.

4. Prior to use dilute with either 0.9% NaCl injection or 5% dextrose injection to a concentration between 0.004 and 0.02 mg/mL.

5. Continue IV therapy only until client can be switched to PO therapy (usually within 2–3 days). Give the first PO dose 8–12 hr after discontinuing the IV infusion.

6. With renal or hepatic impairment administer at the lowest level of the dosage range.

7. Do not use tacrolimus and cyclosporine simultaneously; discontinue either agent at least 24 hr before initiating the other.

8. Store the diluted solution for infusion in glass or polyethylene containers and discard after 24 hr. Do not use PVC containers for storage due to decreased stability and the possiblity of extraction of phthalates.

**Assessment**

1. Injection contains castor oil derivatives; note any sensitivity.

2. Monitor serum electrolytes, CBC, uric acid, blood sugar, liver and renal function studies.

3. Determine time of transplantation; monitor in facilities equipped and staffed with adequate lab and supportive medical resources.

4. Monitor VS, labs, and I&O. Anticipate higher dosages in children to maintain trough levels and reduced dosage with impaired renal function.

5. During IV administration, observe continuously for the first 30 min and at frequent intervals until infusion completed; interrupt infusion if S&S of anaphylaxis occur.

6. Monitoring tacrolimus blood levels is helpful in the clinical evaluation of rejection and toxicity.

**Client/Family Teaching**

1. Review the risk of therapy associated with neoplasia (lymphomas and other malignancies).

2. Must follow the written guidelines for medication therapy explicitly. Call with questions or if problems arise. The drug must be taken throughout one's lifetime to prevent transplant rejection.

3. Because this drug is so important to transplant clients in preventing rejection, a written list of all possible side effects and how to identify which side effects need to be reported will be provided.

4. Perform daily weights and I&O. Take BP and keep a log of these values for provider review. Report any persistent diarrhea and N&V.

5. Report as scheduled and for labs to evaluate drug effectiveness, since dosage is based on clinical assessments of rejection and tolerability.

**Outcomes/Evaluate**

• Prophylaxis of organ rejection
• Immune suppression
• Median trough blood concentrations of 9.8–19.4 ng/mL

---

# Tamoxifen

(tah-**MOX**-ih-fen)
**Pregnancy Category:** D
Apo-Tamox ✿, Gen-Tamoxifen, Nolvadex, Nolvadex-D ✿, Novo-Tamoxifen ✿, Tamofen ✿, Tamone ✿, Tamoplex ✿ **(Rx)**
**Classification:** Antiestrogen

See also *Antineoplastic Agents.*

**Action/Kinetics:** Antiestrogen believed to compete with estrogen for estrogen-binding sites in target tissue (breast); also blocks uptake of estradiol. **Steady-state plasma levels (after 10 mg b.i.d. for 3 months):** 120 ng/mL for tamoxifen and 336 ng/mL for N-desmethyl tamoxifen. **Steady-state levels, tamoxifen:** About 4 weeks; **for N-desmethyl-tamoxifen:** About 8 weeks ($t\frac{1}{2}$ **for metabolite:** about 14 days). Metabolized to the equally active N-desmethyltamoxifen. Tamoxifen and metabolites are excreted mainly through the feces. Objective response may be delayed 4–10 weeks with bone metastases.

**Uses:** Adjuvant treatment of axillary node-negative or node-positive breast cancer in women following total or segmental mastectomy, axil-

T

lary dissection, and breast irradiation. Metastatic breast cancer in premenopausal women as an alternative to oophorectomy or ovarian irradiation (especially in wowen with estrogen-positive tumors). Advanced metastatic breast cancer in men. *Investigational:* Mastalgia, gynecomastia (to treat pain and size), prophylaxis of breast cancer in high-risk women, pancreatic carcinoma, advanced or recurrent endometrial and hepatocellular carcinoma.

**Contraindications:** Lactation.

**Special Concerns:** Use with caution in clients with leukopenia or thrombocytopenia. Women should not become pregnant while taking tamoxifen.

**Side Effects:** *GI:* N&V, distaste for food, anorexia, diarrhea, abdominal cramps. *CV:* Peripheral edema, superficial phlebitis, deep vein thrombosis, **pulmonary embolism, thromboembolic disorders (especially when tamoxifen is combined with other cytotoxic agents).** *CNS:* Depression, dizziness, lightheadedness, headache, fatigue. *Hepatic:* Rarely, fatty liver, cholestasis, hepatitis, **hepatic necrosis.** *GU:* Hot flashes, vaginal bleeding and discharge, menstrual irregularities, pruritus vulvae, ovarian cysts, hyperplasia of the uterus, polyps, uterine carcinoma. *Other:* Skin rash, skin changes, hypercalcemia, musculoskeletal pain, hyperlipidemias, weight gain or loss, increased bone and tumor pain, mild to moderate thrombocytopenia and leukopenia, retinopathy, hair thinning or partial loss, fluid retention, coughing. In men, may be loss of libido and impotency. Impotence and loss of libido in males after discontinuing therapy.

**Laboratory Test Alterations:** ↑ Serum calcium (transient), thyroid-binding globulin in postmenopausal women, BUN, AST, alkaline phosphatase, bilirubin, creatinine.

**Drug Interactions**
*Anticoagulants* / ↑ Hypoprothrombinemic effect

*Bromocriptine* / ↑ Serum levels of tamoxifen and N-desmethyl tamoxifen

**Dosage** ————————————
- **Tablets**
  *Breast cancer.*
  10–20 mg b.i.d. (morning and evening) or 20 mg daily. Doses of 10 mg b.i.d.–t.i.d. for 2 years and 10 mg b.i.d. for 5 years have been used. There is no evidence that doses greater than 20 mg daily are more effective.
  *Mastalgia.*
  10 mg/day for 4 months.

## NURSING CONSIDERATIONS

See also *Nursing Considerations* for *Antineoplastic Agents.*

**Assessment**
1. Document onset, duration, and characteristics of symptoms.
2. Assess hematologic profile and monitor. Drug may cause granulocyte suppression. Nadir: 14 days; recovery: 21 days.
3. The effect of the steroid and osteolytic metastases may result in hypercalcemia. Report symptoms of hypercalcemia (insomnia, lethargy, anorexia, N&V, coma, and vascular collapse).
4. With increased pain, administer adequate analgesics.

**Client/Family Teaching**
1. Review side effects that should be reported; a reduction in dosage or discontinuation may be indicated.
2. Increased bone and lumbar pain or local disease flares should subside and may be associated with a good (tumor) response to medication. Take analgesics as needed.
3. Consume 2–3 L/day of fluids to minimize hypercalcemia.
4. Exercise to reduce calcium levels, improve circulation, and prevent thrombophlebitis. (Perform ROM exercises if bedridden.)
5. Record weights weekly; report excessive weight gain or evidence of peripheral edema.
6. May cause "hot flashes" dress accordingly.
7. Wear protective clothing, sun-

screens, and sunglasses to prevent photosensitivity reactions.

8. Practice safe, nonhormonal methods of contraception during and for 1 mo following therapy.

9. Report decreased visual acuity. Have regular eye exams, especially if doses are higher than those generally used.

10. Obtain regular gynecologic exams; report any menstrual irregularities, abnormal vaginal bleeding, change in vaginal discharge, or pelvic pain or pressure.

**Outcomes/Evaluate**
• Suppression of tumor growth and malignant cell proliferation
• Relief of breast pain

# Tazarotene

(taz-**AR**-oh-teen)
**Pregnancy Category:** X
Tazorac **(Rx)**
**Classification:** Antipsoriasis topical drug

**Action/Kinetics:** A retinoid prodrug converted by deesterification to active cognate carboxylic acid of tazarotene. Mechanism not known. Little systemic absorption. **t½, after topical use:** About 18 hr. Parent drug and metabolite are further metabolized and excreted through urine and feces.

**Uses:** Stable plaque psoriasis. Mild to moderate facial acne vulgaris.

**Contraindications:** Pregnancy. Use on eczematous skin. Use of cosmetics or skin medications that have strong drying effect.

**Special Concerns:** Use with caution during lactation. Safety and efficacy have not been determined in children less than 12 years of age. Psoriasis may worsen from month 4 to 12 compared with first 3 months of therapy. Use with caution with drugs that cause photosensitivity.

**Side Effects:** *Dermatologic:* Pruritus, photosensitivity, burning/stinging, erythema, worsening of psoriasis, skin pain, irritation, rash, desquamation, contact dermatitis, skin inflamma-

tion, fissuring, bleeding, dry skin, localized edema, skin discoloration.

**OD** **Overdose Management:** *Symptoms:* Marked redness, peeling, discomfort. *Treatment:* Decrease or discontinue dose.

**Drug Interactions:** ↑ Risk of photosensitivity when used with fluoroquinolones, phenothiazines, sulfonamides, tetracyclines, thiazides.

**Dosage**
• **Gel**
  *Acne vulgaris, Psoriasis.*

After skin is dry following cleaning, apply thin film (2 mg/cm²) on lesions once daily in evening. Cover entire affected area. For psoriasis, do not apply to more than 20% of body surface area.

## NURSING CONSIDERATIONS

**Administration/Storage:**    Avoid application to unaffected skin due to increased susceptibility to irritation.

**Assessment**

1. Document condition requiring treatment; may photograph to assess response.

2. Determine if pregnant and begin therapy during menstrual cycle.

**Client/Family Teaching**

1. Cleanse face gently, pat dry, apply a thin film in evening only where lesions are present.

2. Apply once daily as directed. Avoid contact with eyes and mouth; rinse thoroughly if contact occurs.

3. Report excessive itching, redness, burning, or peeling of skin. Stop therapy until skin integrity restored.

4. Avoid weather extremes such as wind or cold; may increase irritation.

5. Practice reliable contraception; drug causes fetal damage.

6. May experience photosensitivity reaction; use sunscreens and protective clothing if exposed.

**Outcomes/Evaluate:** Clearing of psoriasis placques/acne lesions

# Temazepam

(teh-**MAZ**-eh-pam)
**Pregnancy Category:** X

T

Restoril **(C-IV) (Rx)**
**Classification:** Benzodiazepine hypnotic

See also *Tranquilizers, Antimanic Drugs, and Hypnotics.*

**Action/Kinetics:** Benzodiazepine derivative. Disturbed nocturnal sleep may occur the first one or two nights following discontinuance of the drug. Prolonged administration is not recommended because physical dependence and tolerance may develop. See also *Flurazepam.* **Peak blood levels:** 2–4 hr. **t½, initial:** 0.4–0.6 hr; **final:** 10 hr. **Steady-state plasma levels:** 382 ng/mL (2.5 hr after 30-mg dose). Accumulation of the drug is minimal following multiple dosage. Significantly bound (98%) to plasma protein. Metabolized in the liver to inactive metabolites.

**Uses:** Insomnia in clients unable to fall asleep, with frequent awakenings during the night and/or early morning awakenings.

**Contraindications:** Pregnancy.

**Special Concerns:** Use with caution in severely depressed clients. Use during lactation may cause sedation and feeding problems in the infant. Geriatric clients may be more sensitive to the effects of temazepam.

**Side Effects:** *CNS:* Drowsiness (after daytime use) and dizziness are common. Lethargy, confusion, euphoria, weakness, ataxia, lack of concentration, hallucinations. In some clients, paradoxical excitement (less than 0.5%), including stimulation and hyperactivity, occurs. *GI:* Anorexia, diarrhea. *Other:* Tremors, horizontal nystagmus, falling, palpitations. Rarely, blood dyscrasias.

**Dosage** —————————
• **Capsules**
**Adults, usual:** 15–30 mg at bedtime. **In elderly or debilitated clients, initial:** 15 mg; **then,** adjust dosage to response.

## NURSING CONSIDERATIONS

See also *Nursing Considerations* for *Tranquilizers, Antimanic Drugs, and Hypnotics.*
**Assessment**
1. Note indications for therapy, onset and duration of symptoms.
2. Assess sleep patterns; identify factors that may contribute to insomnia.
**Client/Family Teaching**
1. Take only as directed and do not increase dose.
2. May cause daytime drowsiness. Avoid activities that require mental alertness until drug effects realized.
3. Avoid alcohol and CNS depressants; may increase CNS depression.
4. Avoid tobacco; decreases drug's effect.
5. Review nonpharmacologic methods of sleep induction.
6. For short-term use only. Long-term use can cause dependence and withdrawal symptoms. After more than 3 weeks of continuous use may experience rebound insomnia.
**Outcomes/Evaluate:** Improved sleeping patterns with less frequent awakenings

# Teniposide (VM-26)
(teh-**NIP**-ah-side)
**Pregnancy Category:** D
Vumon **(Rx)**
**Classification:** Antineoplastic

See also *Antineoplastic Agents.*
**Action/Kinetics:** Derivative of podophyllotoxin that acts in the late S or early $G_2$ phase of the cell cycle, preventing cells from entering mitosis. Inhibits type II topoisomerase activity resulting in both single- and double-stranded breaks in DNA and DNA:protein cross-links. Active against sublines of certain murine leukemias that have developed resistance to amsacrine, cisplatin, daunorubicin, doxorubicin, mitoxantrone, or vincristine. **Terminal t½:** 5 hr. Significantly bound to plasma proteins (over 99%). Metabolized

in the liver and excreted mainly through the urine (4%–12% unchanged) with small amounts excreted in the feces.

**Uses:** In combination with other antineoplastic agents for induction therapy in clients with refractory childhood acute lymphoblastic leukemia (ALL). Has also been used for relapsed ALL.

**Contraindications:** Hypersensitivity to teniposide, etoposide, or the polyoxylethylated castor oil present in teniposide products. Lactation.

**Special Concerns:** Clients with both Down syndrome and leukemia may be especially sensitive to myelosuppressive chemotherapy; thus, reduce initial dosing. A life-threatening anaphylactic reaction may occur with the first dose (incidence appears to be greater in clients with brain tumors and neuroblastoma). Use with caution in clients with impaired hepatic function. Contains benzyl alcohol associated with a fatal "gasping" syndrome in premature infants.

**Side Effects:** *Hematologic:* **Severe myelosuppression,** leukopenia, neutropenia, thrombocytopenia, anemia. *Hypersensitivity reactions:* **Anaphylaxis** manifested by chills, fever, **bronchospasm,** dyspnea, facial flushing, hypertension or hypotension, tachycardia. *CV:* Hypotension. *GI:* Mucositis, N&V, diarrhea. *Dermatologic:* Alopecia (reversible), rash, hepatic dysfunction or toxicity, peripheral neurotoxicity, infection, bleeding, renal dysfunction, metabolic abnormalities.

**OD** **Overdose Management:** *Symptoms:* Myelosuppression, hypotension, anaphylaxis. *Treatment (Anaphylaxis or Overdose).*
• Treat anaphylaxis promptly with antihistamines, corticosteroids, epinephrine, IV fluids, and other supportive measures. If a client who manifested a hypersensitivity reaction must be retreated, undertake pretreatment with corticosteroids and

antihistamines; carefully observe client during and after the infusion.
• If hypotension occurs, stop the infusion and give fluids. Undertake other supportive therapy as needed.
• Myelosuppression may be treated with supportive care including blood products and antibiotics.

**Drug Interactions**
*Antiemetic drugs* / Acute CNS depression and hypotension in clients receiving high doses of teniposide and who were pretreated with antiemetics
*Methotrexate* / ↑ Plasma clearance of methotrexate
*Sodium salicylate* / ↑ Effect of teniposide due to displacement from plasma protein binding sites
*Sulfamethizole* / ↑ Effect of teniposide due to displacement from plasma protein binding sites
*Tolbutamide* / ↑ Effect of teniposide due to displacement from plasma protein binding sites

**Dosage**
• **IV Infusion**
*Regimen 1 for childhood ALL clients failing induction therapy with cytarabine.*
Teniposide, 165 mg/m², and cytarabine, 300 mg/m² IV twice weekly for eight to nine doses.
*Regimen 2 for childhood ALL refractory to vincristine/prednisone-containing regimens.*
Teniposide, 250 mg/m², and vincristine, 1.5 mg/m², IV weekly for 4–8 weeks, and prednisone, 40 mg/m² orally for 28 days.

## NURSING CONSIDERATIONS

See also *Nursing Considerations* for *Antineoplastic Agents* and *Etoposide*.

**Administration/Storage**
**IV** 1. Give over 30–60 min or longer; do not give by rapid IV infusion, as hypotension may occur.
2. The IV catheter or needle must be in the proper position and functional prior to infusion. Improper administration may cause extravasation resulting in local tissue necrosis

or thrombophlebitis. Also, occlusion of central venous access devices has occurred during 24-hr infusion at concentrations of 0.1–0.2 mg/mL.

3. Dilute with either 5% dextrose injection or 0.9% NaCl injection to give a final concentration of 0.1, 0.2, 0.4, or 1 mg/mL.

4. Contact of undiluted teniposide with plastic equipment or devices used to prepare IV infusions may result in softening, cracking, and possible drug leakage. To prevent extraction of plasticizer DEHP, prepare and give solutions in non-DEHP-containing LVP containers such as glass or polyolefin plastic bags or containers. Do not use PVC containers.

5. Lipid administration sets or low DEHP-containing nitroglycerin sets will keep exposure to DEHP at low levels and can be used. Diluted solutions are chemically and physically compatible with the recommended IV administration sets and LVP containers for up to 24 hr at ambient room temperature and lighting conditions.

6. Use caution in handling and preparing the solution as skin reactions may occur with accidental exposure and drug is cytotoxic. Use of gloves is recommended; if the solution comes in contact with the skin, wash immediately with soap and water. If the drug comes in contact with mucous membranes, flush thoroughly with water.

7. Heparin solution can cause precipitation of teniposide, flush administration apparatus thoroughly with 5% dextrose injection or 0.9% NaCl injection before and after administration.

8. Unopened ampules are stable until the date indicated if stored at 2°C–8°C (36°F–46°F) in the original package (protected from light).

9. Give solutions containing 1 mg/mL within 4 hr of preparation to reduce the potential for precipitation. Refrigeration of solutions is not recommended.

10. Precipitation of teniposide may occur at the recommended concentra-

tions, especially if the diluted solution is agitated more than recommended during preparation. Also, minimize storage time prior to administration; take care to avoid contact of the diluted solution with other drugs or fluids.

11. Not for use in premature infants; contains benzyl alcohol.

**Assessment**

1. Note any sensitivity to product derivatives, especially polyoxylethylated castor oil. Product also contains benzyl alcohol.

2. Premedicate with antiemetics. Observe for enhanced CNS effects when premedicated with antiemetics.

3. Reduce dose with liver or renal dysfunction or with Down syndrome.

4. If symptoms of anaphylaxis occur (chills, fever, tachycardia, chest pain, dyspnea, or altered BP), interrupt infusion and report.

5. Monitor hematologic profile, uric acid, liver and renal function studies. Drug may cause granulocyte and platelet suppression. Withhold if platelet count < 50,000/mm³ or ANC < 500/mm³ and do not resume treatment until hematologic recovery is evident. Nadir: 14 days; recovery: 21 days.

**Client/Family Teaching**

1. Drug is a "possible carcinogen"; review risk of developing secondary acute nonlymphocytic leukemia with intensive therapy schedules (1–2 times/week during remission).

2. Report promptly if fever, chills, rapid heartbeat, or difficulty in breathing occurs.

3. N&V and hair loss are frequent drug side effects.

4. Drug will cause fetal harm; use reliable contraceptive measures during treatment.

**Outcomes/Evaluate:** Remission of acute ALL with relapsed or refractory ALL

# Terazosin
(ter-**AY**-zoh-sin)
**Pregnancy Category:** C

Hytrin **(Rx)**
**Classification:** Antihypertensive, alpha-1-adrenergic receptor blocking agent

**Action/Kinetics:** Blocks postsynaptic alpha-1-adrenergic receptors, leading to a dilation of both arterioles and veins, and ultimately, a reduction in BP. Both standing and supine BPs are lowered with no reflex tachycardia. Also relaxes smooth muscle of the prostate and bladder neck. Usefulness in BPH is due to alpha-1 receptor blockade, which relaxes the smooth muscle of the prostate and bladder neck and relieves pressure on the urethra. Bioavailability is not affected by food. **Onset:** 15 min. **Peak plasma levels:** 1–2 hr. **t½:** 9–12 hr. **Duration:** 24 hr. Excreted unchanged and as inactive metabolites in both the urine and feces.

**Uses:** Alone or in combination with diuretics or beta-adrenergic blocking agents to treat hypertension. Treat symptoms of benign prostatic hyperplasia.

**Special Concerns:** Use with caution during lactation. Safety and efficacy have not been determined in children. Geriatric clients may be more sensitive to the hypotensive and hypothermic effects of terazosin.

**Side Effects:** *First-dose effect:* Marked postural hypotension and syncope. *CV:* Palpitations, tachycardia, postural hypotension, syncope, **arrhythmias,** chest pain, vasodilation. *CNS:* Dizziness, headache, somnolence, drowsiness, nervousness, paresthesia, depression, anxiety, insomnia, vertigo. *Respiratory:* Nasal congestion, dyspnea, sinusitis, epistaxis, bronchitis, **bronchospasm,** cold or flu symptoms, increased cough, pharyngitis, rhinitis. *GI:* Nausea, constipation, diarrhea, dyspepsia, dry mouth, vomiting, flatulence, abdominal discomfort or pain. *Musculoskeletal:* Asthenia, arthritis, arthralgia, myalgia, joint disorders, back pain, pain in extremities, neck and shoulder pain, muscle cramps.

*Miscellaneous:* Peripheral edema, weight gain, blurred vision, impotence, chest pain, fever, gout, pruritus, rash, sweating, urinary frequency, UTI, tinnitus, conjunctivitis, abnormal vision, edema, facial edema.

**Laboratory Test Alterations:** ↓ H&H, WBCs, albumin.

**OD Overdose Management:** *Symptoms:* Hypotension, drowsiness, shock. *Treatment:* Restore BP and HR. Client should be kept supine; vasopressors may be indicated. Volume expanders can be used to treat shock.

**Dosage**
• **Capsules**
*Hypertension.*
**Individualized, initial:** 1 mg at bedtime (this dose is not to be exceeded); **then,** increase dose slowly to obtain desired response. **Range:** 1–5 mg/day; doses as high as 20 mg may be required in some clients. Doses greater than 20 mg daily do not provide further BP control.
*Benign prostatic hyperplasia.*
**Initial:** 1 mg/day; dose should be increased to 2 mg, 5 mg, and then 10 mg once daily to improve symptoms and/or urinary flow rates. Doses greater than 20 mg daily have not been studied.

## NURSING CONSIDERATIONS

See also *Nursing Considerations* for *Antihypertensive Agents.*
**Administration/Storage**
1. The initial dosing regimen must be carefully observed to minimize severe hypotension.
2. Monitor BP 2–3 hr after dosing and at the end of the dosing interval to ensure BP control has been maintained.
3. Consider an increase in dose or b.i.d. dosing if BP control is not maintained at 24-hr interval.
4. To prevent dizziness or fainting due to a drop in BP, take the initial dose at bedtime; the daily dose can be given in the morning.
5. If terazosin must be discontinued

**T**

---

for more than a few days, reinstitute the initial dosing regimen if restarted.

6. Due to additive effects, caution must be exercised when combined with other antihypertensive agents.

7. When treating BPH, a minimum of 4–6 weeks of 10 mg/day may be needed to determine if a beneficial effect has occurred.

**Assessment**

1. Document onset, duration, and characteristics of symptoms.

2. Assess prostate gland, PSA level, and BPH score.

3. A gradual increase in dose, i.e., 1 mg/day for 7 days, then 2 mg/day for 7 days, then 3 mg/day for 7 days, then 4 mg/day for 7 days, and then 5 mg /day, may assist to diminish adverse effects and enhance compliance, especially in the elderly.

**Client/Family Teaching**

1. Take initial dose at bedtime to minimize side effects. Do not stop abruptly. Use caution when performing activities that require mental alertness until drug effects realized.

2. Do not drive or undertake hazardous tasks for 12 hr after the first dose and after increasing dose or reinstituting therapy.

3. Avoid symptoms of orthostatic hypotension by rising slowly from a sitting or lying position and waiting until symptoms subside.

4. Record weight 2 times/week; report persistent side effects or excessive weight gain or ankle edema.

**Outcomes/Evaluate**

• Control of BP

• Improvement in symptoms R/T prostate enlargement

# Terbinafine hydrochloride

(ter-**BIN**-ah-feen)
**Pregnancy Category:** B
Lamisil **(Rx)**
**Classification:** Antifungal agent

**Action/Kinetics:** Inhibits squalene epoxidase, a key enzyme in the sterol biosynthesis in fungi. Results in ergosterol deficiency and a corresponding accumulation of squalene leading to fungal cell death. Approximately 75% of cutaneously ab-

sorbed drug is excreted in the urine, mostly as metabolites. Well absorbed following PO administration, with first-pass metabolism being about 40%. **Peak plasma levels:** 1 mcg/mL within 2 hr. Food enhances absorption. Over 99% bound to plasma proteins. Slowly excreted from adipose tissue and skin. Extensively metabolized, with about 70% of the dose eliminated in the urine. Renal or hepatic disease decreases clearance from the body.

**Uses: Topical use:** Interdigital tinea pedis (athletes' foot), tinea cruris (jock itch), or tinea corporis (ringworm) due to *Epidermophyton floccosum, Trichophyton mentagrophytes,* or *T. rubrum*. Plantar tinea pedis. Tinea versicolor due to *Malassezia furfur. Investigational:* Cutaneous candidiasis and tinea versicolor. **Oral use:** Onychomycosis of the toenail or fingernail due to dermatophytes.

**Contraindications:** Ophthalmic or intravaginal use. PO use in preexisting liver disease or renal impairment ($C_{CR}$ less than 50 mL/min). Lactation.

**Special Concerns:** Safety and efficacy have not been determined in children less than 12 years of age.

**Side Effects:** *Following topical use. Dermatologic:* Irritation, burning, itching, dryness.

*Following oral use. GI:* Diarrhea, dyspepsia, abdominal pain, nausea, flatulence. *Dermatologic:* Rash, pruritus, urticaria. *Other:* Headache, taste or visual disturbances. Rarely, symptomatic idiosyncratic hepatobiliary dysfunction (including cholestatic hepatitis), serious skin reactions, severe neutropenia, allergic reactions (including *anaphylaxis*).

**Drug Interactions**

*Cimetidine* / Terbinafine clearance is ↓ by one-third

*Cyclosporine* / ↑ Clearance of cyclosporine

*Rifampin* / ↑ Clearance (100%) of terbinafine

*Terfenadine* / ↓ Clearance of terbinafine

**Laboratory Test Interferences:** Liver enzyme abnormalities that are two or more times the upper limit of the normal range. ↓ Absolute neutrophil counts.

## Dosage
### • Cream
*Interdigital tinea pedis.*

Apply to cover the affected and immediately surrounding areas b.i.d. until symptoms are significantly improved. Drug therapy should be maintained for a minimum of 1 week and should not exceed 4 weeks.

*Tinea cruris or tinea corporis.*

Apply to cover the affected and immediately surrounding areas 1–2 times/day until symptoms are significantly improved. Drug therapy should be maintained for a minimum of 1 week and should not exceed 4 weeks.

### • Spray
*Tinea pedis, Tinea versicolor.*

Spray b.i.d. for one week.

*Tinea corporis, Tinea cruris.*

Spray once daily for one week.

### • Tablets
*Onychomycosis.*

250 mg/day for 6 weeks if fingernails are affected and 250 mg/day for 12 weeks if toenails are affected. Alternatively, intermittent dosing may be used: 500 mg daily for one week each month (use 2 months for fingernails and 4 months for toenails). The optimal clinical effect is observed several months after mycologic cure and cessation of treatment due to slow period for outgrowth of healthy nails.

## NURSING CONSIDERATIONS
### Administration/Storage
1. Avoid contact of the cream with eyes, nose, mouth, or other mucous membranes.
2. Avoid occlusive dressings.
3. For topical use, many clients treated for 1–2 weeks continue to improve during the 2–4 weeks after drug therapy has been completed. Do not consider clients therapeutic failures until they have been observed for a period of 2–4 weeks off therapy.
4. Store the cream between 5°C and 30°C (41°F and 86°F). Protect tablets from light and store below 25°C (77°F).

### Assessment
1. Describe clinical presentation and note location, onset, duration, and characteristics of symptoms.
2. If presentation unclear, document infected tissue scrapings to confirm diagnosis.
3. Note any liver or renal dysfunction.

### Client/Family Teaching
1. Cream is for topical dermatologic use only; review appropriate method for application.
2. Wash hands before and after topical application. Use a clean towel and washcloth; avoid sharing with anyone.
3. Avoid contact of cream with mouth, nose, eyes, and other mucous membranes; do not cover treated areas with occlusive dressing.
4. Take tablets with food to ensure maximal absorption.
5. Report symptoms of increased irritation or possible sensitization such as redness, itching, burning, blistering, swelling, or oozing.
6. Use for the prescribed time frame; do not skip or double up on doses.
7. Continued improvement in skin condition and/or mycotic nails may be noted for 2–4 weeks following therapy.

### Outcomes/Evaluate
- Improvement in dermatologic condition
- Clearing/healing of mycotic nail beds

---

# Terbutaline sulfate
(ter-**BYOU**-tah-leen)
**Pregnancy Category:** B
Brethaire, Brethine, Bricanyl **(Rx)**
**Classification:** Sympathomimetic, direct-acting; bronchodilator

See also *Sympathomimetic Drugs.*

*bold italic* = life threatening side effect

**Action/Kinetics:** Specific beta-2 receptor stimulant, resulting in bronchodilation and relaxation of peripheral vasculature. Minimum beta-1 activity. Action resembles that of isoproterenol. **PO: Onset:** 30 min; **maximum effect:** 2–3 hr; **duration:** 4–8 hr. **SC: Onset,** 5–15 min; **maximum effect:** 30 min–1 hr; **duration:** 1.5–4 hr. **Inhalation: Onset,** 5–30 min; **time to peak effect:** 1–2 hr; **duration:** 3–6 hr.

**Uses:** Bronchodilator in asthma, bronchitis, emphysema, bronchiectasis, pulmonary obstructive disease, and other conditions associated with reversible bronchospasms. Relief of reversible bronchospasms in clients age six and up who suffer from obstructive airway diseases. *Investigational:* Inhibit premature labor.

**Contraindications:** Lactation.

**Special Concerns:** Safe use in children less than 12 years of age not established.

**Laboratory Test Alterations:** ↑ Liver enzymes.

**Additional Side Effects:** *CV:* PVCs, ECG changes (e.g., atrial premature beats, AV block, sinus pause, ST-T wave depression, T-wave inversion, sinus bradycardia, atrial escape beat with aberrant conduction), tachycardia. *Respiratory:* Wheezing. *Miscellaneous:* Hypersensitivity reactions (including vasculitis), flushing, sweating, bad taste or taste change, muscle cramps, CNS stimulation, pain at injection site.

**Dosage**

• **Tablets**
*Bronchodilation.*
**Adults and children over 15 years:** 5 mg t.i.d. q 6 hr during waking hours, not to exceed 15 mg q 24 hr. If disturbing side effects are observed, dose can be reduced to 2.5 mg t.i.d. without loss of beneficial effects. Anticipate use of other therapeutic measures if client fails to respond after second dose. **Children 12–15 years:** 2.5 mg t.i.d., not to exceed 7.5 mg q 24 hr.
*Premature labor.*
2.5 mg q 4–6 hr until term.

• **SC**
*Bronchodilation.*
**Adults:** 0.25 mg. May be repeated 1 time after 15–30 min if no significant clinical improvement is noted. If client does not respond to the second dose, undertake other measures. Do not exceed a dose of 0.5 mg over 4 hr.

• **IV Infusion**
*Premature labor.*
10 mcg/min initially; **then,** increase rate by 0.005 mg/min q 10 min until contractions cease or a maximum dose of 80 mcg/min is reached. Continue the minimum effective dose for 4–8 hr after contractions cease. Terbutaline may also be given SC for preterm labor.

• **Metered Dose Inhaler**
*Bronchodilation.*
**Adults and children over 12 years:** 0.2–0.5 mg (1–2 inhalations) q 4–6 hr. Inhalations should be separated by 60-sec intervals. Dosage may be repeated q 4–6 hr.

## NURSING CONSIDERATIONS

See also *Nursing Considerations* for *Sympathomimetic Drugs.*

**Assessment**

1. Document type, onset, duration, and characteristics of symptoms.
2. Auscultate and document lung assessments and PFTs. Observe respiratory client for evidence of drug tolerance and rebound bronchospasm.
3. Determine onset, frequency, and duration of contractions and fetal HR with preterm labor.
4. Observe mother for headache, tremor, anxiety, palpitations, symptoms of pulmonary edema, and tachycardia. Assess fetus for distress; report increased contractions. Monitor both for symptoms of hypoglycemia and mother for hypokalemia.

**Client/Family Teaching**

1. Take oral medication with meals to minimize GI upset.
2. Report any persistent or bothersome side effects. Do not increase dose or frequency if symptoms are not relieved. Report so dose can be reevaluated.

3. Increase fluid intake to help lique-fy secretions.

4. With preterm labor, notify provider immediately if labor resumes or unusual side effects are noted.

**Outcomes/Evaluate**
- Improved airway exchange
- Inhibition of premature labor

# Terconazole nitrate
(ter-**KON**-ah-zohl)
**Pregnancy Category:** C
Terazol ✤, Terazol 3, Terazol 7 **(Rx)**
**Classification:** Antifungal, vaginal

**Action/Kinetics:** May exert its antifungal activity by disrupting cell membrane permeability leading to loss of essential intracellular materials. Also inhibits synthesis of triglycerides and phospholipids as well as inhibiting oxidative and peroxidative enzyme activity. When used for *Candida,* terconazole inhibits transformation of blastospores into the invasive mycelial form.

**Uses:** Vulvovaginitis caused by *Candida.* Ineffective in infections due to *Trichomonas* or *Haemophilus vaginalis.*

**Special Concerns:** During lactation, consider discontinuing nursing or the drug. Safety and efficacy have not been established in children.

**Side Effects:** *GU:* Vulvovaginal burning, irritation, or itching; dysmenorrhea, pain of the female genitalia. *Miscellaneous:* Headache (most common), body pain, photosensitivity, abdominal pain, chills, fever.

**Dosage**
- **Vaginal Cream (0.4%, 0.8%)**
One applicator full (5 g) intravaginally, once daily at bedtime for 7 consecutive days for the 0.4% cream and for 3 consecutive days for the 0.8% cream.
- **Vaginal Suppository**
One 80-mg suppository once daily at bedtime for 3 consecutive days.

## NURSING CONSIDERATIONS
**Assessment**
1. Obtain a thorough nursing history

because recurrent candidiasis may be caused by oral contraceptives, antibiotics, or diabetes whereas intractable candidiasis may be the result of undetected diabetes mellitus or reinfection.

2. Prior to a second course of therapy, the diagnosis should be confirmed to rule out other pathogens associated with vulvovaginitis.

**Client/Family Teaching**
1. Review the appropriate method for administration and cleansing (the cream should be inserted high into the vagina). Sitz baths and vaginal douches may also be used.

2. Discontinue use and report if any burning, irritation, or pain occurs.

3. May stain clothes; use sanitary napkins during therapy and change frequently because damp sanitary napkins may harbor infecting organisms.

4. To avoid reinfection, refrain from sexual intercourse. Advise partner to use a condom as med may also irritate partner.

5. Use for prescribed time frame even if symptoms subside.

6. Continue to use during menses to ensure a full course of therapy.

**Outcomes/Evaluate:** Resolution of fungal infections; symptomatic improvement

# Terfenadine
(ter-**FEN**-ah-deen)
**Pregnancy Category:** C
Apo-Terfenadine ✤, Novo-Terfenadine ✤, Seldane **(Rx)**
**Classification:** Antihistamine, piperidine type

See also *Antihistamines.*

**Action/Kinetics:** Manifests significantly less drowsiness and anticholinergic effects than other antihistamines. **Onset:** 1–2 hr; **peak effect:** 3–4 hr; **peak plasma levels:** 2 hr. **t½:** About 20 hr. **Duration:** Over 12 hr. Metabolized in the liver and excreted in the urine and feces. *NOTE:* With the marketing of fexofenadine, it is likely terfenadine will be withdrawn from the market.

**Uses:** Seasonal allergic rhinitis. *Investigational:* Histamine-induced bronchoconstriction in asthmatics; exercise and hyperventilation-induced bronchospasm.

**Contraindications:** Significant hepatic dysfunction. Use with drugs that prolong the QT interval, such as disopyramide, procainamide, quinidine, most antidepressants, and most neuroleptics. Consumption of grapefruit juice.

**Special Concerns:** Safety and efficacy in children less than 12 years of age have not been established. Hepatic insufficiency and any drug or food (e.g., grapefruit juice) that blocks the metabolism of terfenadine may cause serious CV effects (see *Side Effects* that follow).

**Additional Side Effects:** *Doses of 360 mg or more may cause serious CV effects, including death, cardiac arrest, torsades de pointes, and other ventricular arrhythmias (including QT interval prolongation).* Syncope may precede severe arrhythmias.

**Drug Interactions**

*Azole antifungal drugs* / ↑ Risk of serious CV effects, including death, cardiac arrest, torsades de pointes, and other ventricular arrhythmias

*Clarithromycin* / ↑ Risk of serious CV effects, including death, cardiac arrest, torsades de pointes, and other ventricular arrhythmias

*Diltiazem* / Potential for ↑ risk of serious CV effects, including death, cardiac arrest, torsades de pointes, and other ventricular arrhythmias

*Erythromycins* / ↑ Risk of serious CV effects, including death, cardiac arrest, torsades de pointes, and other ventricular arrhythmias

*Itraconazole* / ↑ Risk of serious CV effects, including death, cardiac arrest, torsades de pointes, and other ventricular arrhythmias

*Ketoconazole* / ↑ Risk of serious CV effects, including death, cardiac arrest, torsades de pointes, and other ventricular arrhythmias

*Macrolide antibiotics* / ↑ Risk of serious CV effects, including death, cardiac arrest, torsades de pointes, and other ventricular arrhythmias

*Mibifradil* / ↑ Effect of terfenadine due to ↓ breakdown by the liver

*Sparfloxacin* / ↑ Effect of terfenadine due to ↓ breakdown by the liver

*Troleandomycin* / ↑ Risk of serious CV effects, including death, cardiac arrest, torsades de pointes, and other ventricular arrhythmias

**Dosage** —————
- **Tablets**

**Adults and children over 12 years:** 60 mg q 12 hr. Do not exceed this dose.

## NURSING CONSIDERATIONS

See also *Nursing Considerations* for *Antihistamines.*

**Administration/Storage:** Advise not to consume grapefruit juice when taking terfenadine.

**Assessment**

1. Document onset, duration, and characteristics of symptoms.

2. List other agents trialed and the outcome. Note agents that should be avoided during this therapy.

3. Describe pulmonary and ENT assessment findings; note any sinus pressure.

**Client/Family Teaching**

1. Take with food or milk to minimize GI upset, *not* with grapefruit juice.

2. *Do not* exceed prescribed dose or take with clarithomycin, macrolide antibiotics, azole antifungals, diltiazem, or troleandomycin because of the increased the risk of side effects, especially lethal arrhythmias. Review drug information or check with pharmacist and provider for any newly added adverse effects or contraindications.

3. With the $H_1$ antagonists, clinical effectiveness of one group may diminish with continuous use. Changing to another group may restore drug effectiveness.

**Outcomes/Evaluate:** Improved airway exchange; relief of allergic manifestations

————COMBINATION DRUG————

# Terfenadine and Pseudoephedrine hydrochloride

(ter-**FEN**-ah-deen **soo**-doh-eh-**FED**-rin)

**Pregnancy Category:** C

Seldane-D **(Rx)**

**Classification:** Antihistamine, decongestant

See also *Terfenadine* and *Pseudoephedrine hydrochloride*.

**Content:** Each extended-release tablet contains: *Antihistamine:* Terfenadine, 60 mg, and *Decongestant:* Pseudoephedrine hydrochloride, 120 mg. Ten milligrams of the pseudoephedrine is in an outer coat for immediate release while 110 mg is in an extended-release core. See also individual components.

**Action/Kinetics: Onset of terfenadine:** 1–2 hr. **Maximum effect of terfenadine:** 3–4 hr. **t½, terfenadine:** 8.5 hr. **Duration of terfenadine:** 12 hr. *Note:* With the marketing of fexofenadine, it is likely terfenadine will be withdrawn from the market.

**Uses:** Relief of symptoms associated with seasonal allergic rhinitis including sneezing, pruritus, rhinorrhea, lacrimation, and nasal congestion.

**Contraindications:** Lactation, severe hypertension, CAD, individuals taking MAO inhibitors.

**Special Concerns:** Use with caution in diabetes, CV disease, hypertension, hyperreactivity to ephedrine. Clients with impaired hepatic function, or who are taking ketoconazole or troleandomycin, or who have conditions leading to QT prolongation may experience QT prolongation and/or ventricular tachycardia. Safety and effectiveness in children less than 12 years of age have not been determined.

**Side Effects:** See individual components.

**Drug Interactions**

*Azole antifungal drugs* / ↑ Risk of serious CV effects, including death, cardiac arrest, torsades de pointes, and other ventricular arrhythmias

*Beta-adrenergic blocking agents* / ↑ Effect of pseudoephedrine

*Erythromycins* / ↑ Risk of serious CV effects, including death, cardiac arrest, torsades de pointes, and other ventricular arrhythmias

*Clarithromycin* / ↑ Risk of serious CV effects, including death, cardiac arrest, torsades de pointes, and other ventricular arrhythmias

*Itraconazole* / ↑ Risk of serious CV effects, including death, cardiac arrest, torsades de pointes, and other ventricular arrhythmias

*Ketoconazole* / ↑ Risk of serious CV effects, including death, cardiac arrest, torsades de pointes, and other ventricular arrhythmias

*MAO inhibitors* / ↑ Effect of pseudoephedrine

*Macrolide antibiotics* / ↑ Risk of serious CV effects, including death, cardiac arrest, torsades de pointes, and other ventricular arrhythmias

*Mecamylamine* / Pseudoephedrine ↓ antihypertensive effect of mecamylamine

*Methyldopa* / Pseudoephedrine ↓ antihypertensive effect of methyldopa

*Reserpine* / Pseudoephedrine ↓ antihypertensive effect of reserpine

**Dosage** ————————————

• **Extended-Release Tablets**

**Adults and children over 12 years:** 1 tablet morning and night.

## NURSING CONSIDERATIONS

See also *Nursing Considerations* for *Terfenadine* and *Pseudoephedrine hydrochloride*.

**Administration/Storage**

1. Swallow tablets whole; do not crush or chew.

2. Store in a tightly closed container in a cool, dry location away from heat, moisture, or direct sunlight.

**Assessment**

1. Note any history of hypertension, diabetes, or CAD.

2. List drugs currently prescribed to

ensure none interact unfavorably. Review client/family teaching guidelines from previous entry *(Terfenadine)* and list of drug interactions and contraindications; drug may cause lethal arrhythmias.

3. If insomnia occurs, advise not to take a dose within 8 hr of bedtime.

**Outcomes/Evaluate:** Relief of congestion and allergic manifestations

# Testolactone

(tes-toe-**LACK**-tohn)
**Pregnancy Category:** C
Teslac **(C-III) (Rx)**
**Classification:** Antineoplastic, androgen

See also *Antineoplastic Agents.*

**Action/Kinetics:** Synthetic steroid related to testosterone. May act to reduce synthesis of estrone from adrenal androstenedione by inhibiting steroid aromatase activity. Well absorbed from the GI tract. Metabolized in the liver and unchanged drug and metabolites are excreted through the urine. Does not cause virilization.

**Uses:** Palliative treatment of advanced disseminated mammary cancer in postmenopausal women or in premenopausal ovariectomized clients. Is effective in only 15% of clients.

**Contraindications:** Breast cancer in men. Lactation. Premenopausal women with intact ovaries.

**Special Concerns:** Safety and efficacy have not been determined in children.

**Laboratory Test Alterations:** ↑ Plasma calcium, urinary excretion of creatine (24 hr) and 17-ketosteroids. ↓ Estradiol levels using radioimmunoassays.

**Additional Side Effects:** *GI:* N&V, glossitis, anorexia. *CNS:* Numbness or tingling of fingers, toes, face. *Miscellaneous:* Inflammation and irritation at injection site; increased BP. Hypercalcemia. Maculopapular erythema, alopecia, aches and edema of the extremities, nail growth disturbances. See also *Testosterone.*

**Drug Interactions:** Testolactone may ↑ effect of oral anticoagulants.

**Dosage**
• **Tablets**
250 mg q.i.d. Therapy usually should be continued for 3 months unless there is active progression of the disease.

## NURSING CONSIDERATIONS

See also *Nursing Considerations* for *Antineoplastic Agents* and *Testosterone.*

**Assessment:** Document indications for therapy, noting onset, location, and duration of symptoms and other agents or therapies trialed.

**Interventions**
1. Reduce dose of anticoagulants with concomitant therapy and monitor INR.
2. The effect of the steroid and osteolytic metastases may result in hypercalcemia. Assess for symptoms of hypercalcemia (insomnia, lethargy, anorexia, N&V). Encourage high fluid intake (2–3 L/day) to minimize hypercalcemia.
3. Monitor BP and report any significant increases >20 mm Hg DBP.
4. Perform ROM exercises on bedridden clients and encourage others to exercise to reduce calcium levels, improve circulation, and prevent thrombophlebitis.

**Outcomes/Evaluate:** ↓ Tumor size and spread

# Testosterone aqueous suspension

(tess-**TOSS**-ter-ohn)
**Pregnancy Category:** X
Histerone 100, Malogen Aqueous ✤, Tesamone 100, Testandro **(Rx) (C-III)**

# Testosterone cypionate (in oil)

(tess-**TOSS**-ter-ohn)
**Pregnancy Category:** X
depAndro 100 and 200, Depotest 100 and 200, Depo-Testosterone, Depo-Testosterone Cypionate ✤,

Duratest-100 and -200, Scheinpharm
Testone-Cyp ✦ **(Rx) (C-III)**

# Testosterone enanthate (in oil)

(tess-**TOSS**-ter-ohn)
**Pregnancy Category:** X
Andro L.A. 200, Andropository-200,
Delatestryl, Depo-Testosterone
Enanthate ✦, Durathate-200,
Everone 200, Malogex LA ✦, PMS-
Testosterone Enanthate ✦ **(Rx) (C-III)**

# Testosterone propionate (in oil)

(tess-**TOSS**-ter-ohn)
**Pregnancy Category:** X
Malogen ✦ **(Rx) (C-III)**

# Testosterone transdermal system

(tess-**TOSS**-ter-ohn)
**Pregnancy Category:** X
Androderm, Testoderm, Testoderm
with Adhesive **(Rx) (C-III)**
**Classification:** Androgen, natural
hormone and salts of natural hormone

**Action/Kinetics:** Treatment with
testosterone and its congeners is
complicated by the fact that the
exogenous supply of the hormone
may depress secretion of the natural
hormone through inhibitory effects
on the pituitary. Too large a dose
may cause permanent damage.
Treatment is usually associated with a
feeling of well-being. Following PO
use, 44% of testosterone is cleared
by the liver in the first pass. Thus, the
parenteral forms are used. **t½, testosterone cypionate after IM:** 8 days.
Ninety percent is excreted through
the urine as metabolites and 6% is
excreted through the feces. Testosterone and testosterone propionate
are considered short-acting; testosterone enanthate and testosterone
cypionate are long-acting.

Following use of Testoderm on
the scrotal skin: **Maximum serum
levels:** 2–4 hr with return to baseline
in about 2 hr after system is re-

moved. Serum levels reach a plateau
in 3–4 weeks. Will not produce sufficient serum levels if applied to non-
genital skin. Following use of Androderm to nonscrotal skin, there is
continual absorption over 24 hr. Application of two systems at 10:00
p.m. results in serum testosterone
levels similar to normal circadian
variation with maximum levels
occurring in the early morning hours
and minimum levels in the evening.
**Uses: Parenteral products:** Replacement therapy in males for congenital or acquired primary hypogonadism or for congenital or acquired
hypogonadotropic hypogonadism.
Delayed puberty. In postmenopausal women to treat inoperable metastatic breast carcinoma or in premenopausal women following oophorectomy. Postpartum breast engorgement
(evidence for effectiveness is lacking). *Investigational:* Male contraceptive (testosterone enanthate).

**Transdermal products:** Replacement therapy for acquired or congenital primary hypogonadism or for
acquired or congenital secondary
hypogonadotropic hypogonadism.
**Contraindications:** Serious renal,
hepatic, or cardiac disease due to
edema formation. Prostatic or breast
(males) carcinoma. Pregnancy (masculinization of female fetus) and lactation. Discontinue if hypercalcemia
occurs.
**Special Concerns:** Use with caution in young males and females
who have not completed their
growth (because of premature epiphyseal closure). Androgens may
also cause virilization in females or
precocious sexual development in
males. Geriatric clients may manifest
an increased risk of prostatic hypertrophy or prostatic carcinoma. Androgen therapy occasionally seems
to accelerate metastatic breast carcinoma in women.
**Side Effects:** *Hepatic:* Liver toxicity is
the most serious side effect. Jaundice, cholestasis, alterations in BSP
retention, AST, and ALT. Rarely,

**T**

---

✦ = Available in Canada                    *bold italic* = life threatening side effect

*hepatic necrosis, hepatocellular neo-plasms,* peliosis hepatis, acute intermittent porphyria in clients with this disease. *GI:* N&V, diarrhea, anorexia, symptoms of peptic ulcer. *CNS:* Headache, anxiety, increased or decreased libido, insomnia, excitation, paresthesias, sleep apnea syndrome, *CNS hemorrhage,* chills, choreiform movements, habituation, confusion (toxic doses). *GU:* Testicular atrophy with inhibition of testicular function (e.g., oligospermia), impotence, epididymitis, irritable bladder, prepubertal phallic enlargement, gynecomastia. *Electrolyte:* Retention of sodium, chloride, calcium, potassium, phosphates. Edema. *Miscellaneous:* Acne, flushing, suppression of clotting factors (II, V, VII, X), polycythemia, leukopenia, rashes, dermatitis, *anaphylaxis (rare),* muscle cramps, hypercholesterolemia, male-pattern baldness, acne, seborrhea, hirsutism. Hypercalcemia, especially in immobilized clients or those with metastatic breast carcinoma. Virilization in women.

**In females,** menstrual irregularities (including amenorrhea), virilization, clitoral enlargement, hirsutism, increased libido, baldness (male pattern), virilization of external genitalia of female fetus.

**In males,** decreased ejaculatory volume, oligospermia (high doses), gynecomastia, increased frequency and duration of penile erections.

**In children,** disturbances of growth, premature closure of epiphyses, precocious sexual development.

Buccal preparations may cause stomatitis. Inflammation and pain at site of IM or SC injection.

*NOTE:* Side effects of the cypionate and enanthate products are not readily reversible due to the long duration of action of these dosage forms.

The patch may cause itching, irritation, erythema, or discomfort of the scrotum (Testoderm) or on skin areas where applied (Androderm). Potentially, small amounts of testosterone may be transferred to a sex partner.

**Laboratory Test Alterations:** Altered thyroid function tests. False + or ↑ BSP, alkaline phosphatase, bilirubin, cholesterol, and acid phosphatase (in women). Alteration of glucose tolerance tests.

**Drug Interactions**
*Anticoagulants, oral* / Anabolic steroids ↑ effect of anticoagulants
*Antidiabetic agents* / Additive hypoglycemia
*Barbiturates* / ↓ Effect of androgens due to ↑ breakdown by liver
*Corticosteroids* / ↑ Chance of edema
*Phenylbutazone* / Certain androgens ↑ effect of phenylbutazone

**Dosage**
• **Testosterone aqueous suspension and Testosterone propionate in oil**
• **IM Only**
*Replacement therapy.*
25–50 mg 2–3 times/week.
*Breast cancer.*
50–100 mg 3 times/week.
*Growth stimulation in Turner's syndrome or constitutional delay of puberty.*
40–50 mg/m²/dose given monthly for 6 months.
*Male hypogonadism, initiation of pubertal growth.*
40–50 mg/m²/month until growth rate falls to prepubertal levels (about 5 cm/year).
*Male hypogonadism, during terminal growth phase.*
100 mg/m²/month until growth ceases.
*Male hypogonadism, maintain virilization.*
100 mg/m² twice monthly or 50–400 mg/dose q 2–4 weeks.
*Postpartum breast engorgement.*
25–50 mg of testosterone propionate for 3–4 days.
• **Testosterone enanthate and cypionate**
• **IM Only**
*Hypogonadism, replacement therapy.*
50–400 mg q 2–4 weeks.
*Delayed puberty.*

50–200 mg q 2–4 weeks for no more than 4–6 months.

*Palliation of inoperable breast cancer in women.*
200–400 mg q 2–4 weeks.

• **Transdermal System**
*Replacement therapy (congenital or acquired primary hypogonadism, congenital or acquired hypogonado-tropic hypogonadism).*
*Testoderm:* One 6-mg patch applied daily on clean, dry scrotal skin that has been dry-shaved to remove hair. Clients with a smaller scrotum can use a 4-mg patch. The patch should be worn for 22–24 hr/day for 6–8 weeks.

*Androderm:* **Initial dose, usual:** Two systems applied nightly for 24 hr providing a total dose of 5 mg/day. The systems are applied to a clean, dry area of the skin on the back, abdomen, upper arms, or thighs.

## NURSING CONSIDERATIONS
### Administration/Storage
1. Redissolve crystals of testosterone enanthate or cipionate by warming and shaking the vial.
2. If needle or syringe is wet, the product may become cloudy; this does not affect potency.
3. For IM oil-based suspensions, warm the unopened vial in warm water to decrease the viscosity of the oil. Vigorously rotate the vial to resuspend the medication in the oil. A film may appear on the sides of the vial. When no more suspended particles are observed on the bottom or sides of the vial, the drug has been suspended appropriately. Administer the needle deep into the muscle; give slowly.
4. When parenteral injection is to be used, testosterone propionate is more effective than testosterone because it is released more slowly.
5. Continue therapy for at least 2 months for a satisfactory response and for 5 months for an objective response.
6. When used for delayed puberty, consider the chronological and skel-

etal ages when determining initial and subsequent doses. Use is for a limited time (e.g., 4–6 mo).
7. The patch is made of a cloth and co-polymer that sticks to the skin without a sticky adhesive. Warm the patch in the hands before applica-tion. Wear loose clothing to keep the patch in place.
8. Prior to sexual activity, remove the Testoderm patch from the scrotum and wash the scrotal area to remove residue.
9. Do not apply the Androderm patch to bony areas such as the shoulders or hips; it is *not* to be ap-plied to the scrotum. Sites of applica-tion should be rotated, with an inter-val of 7 days between applications to the same site. Areas should not be oily, damaged, or irritated.
10. Apply Androderm immediately after opening the pouch and remov-ing the protective liner. Press the system firmly in place, making sure there is good contact with the skin, especially around the edges of the patch. Excessive heat or pressure can cause the drug reservoir to burst.
11. Do not use damaged patches. Discard systems safely to prevent accidental application or ingestion by children, pets, or others.
### Assessment
1. Document indications for thera-py, type, onset, and characteristics of symptoms.
2. Assess for any cardiac, renal, or hepatic dysfunction. Document neu-rologic status, BP, respirations, heart sounds, and GU function.
3. Note hair distribution and skin texture.
4. Check prescribed medications for any drugs that may interact unfavor-ably (i.e., anticoagulants, hypoglyce-mic agents, and mineralocorticoids).
5. Determine if pregnant.
6. Monitor CBC, serum glucose, cal-cium, electrolytes, cholesterol, liver and renal function studies. Treat-ment with aplastic anemia has

T

resulted in several cases of hepatocellular carcinoma.

**Interventions**

1. Monitor for signs of mental depression such as insomnia, lack of interest in personal appearance, and a general withdrawal from social contacts.

2. Monitor weight, BP, pulse, and serum electrolytes. Auscultate lung sounds and note any distention of the jugular veins. Report edema, as sodium retention and edema can be easily treated with diuretics.

3. Assess for relaxation of the skeletal muscles and pain deep in the bones. The discomfort in the bones is caused by a honeycombing; often caused by increased calcium levels.

4. Flank pain may be caused by kidney stones from excessively high serum calcium levels. Administer large amounts of fluids to prevent renal calculi. If hypercalcemia is the result of metastases, initiate other appropriate therapy.

5. Observe for jaundice, malaise, complaints of right upper quadrant pain, pruritus, or a change in the color or consistency of the stools. Document LFTs.

6. Observe for easy bruising, bleeding, complaints of sore throat or the development of a fever. Obtain CBC to rule out polycythemia and leukopenia.

7. With a child, monitor closely for growth retardation and development of precocious puberty. Use with caution as the effect on the CNS in developing children is still being explored.

• Review therapy with parents; often intermittent to allow for periods of normal bone growth.

• Regular X rays to monitor bone maturation and effects on epiphyseal centers should be obtained every 6 mo.

• Record height and weight regularly.

8. If female, report the signs of virilization, such as deepening of the voice, hirsuitism, acne, menstrual irregularity, and clitoral enlarge-ment. Usually only evident with doses exceeding 200–300 mg/month.

9. Increased libido in females may be an early sign of serious drug toxicity.

10. Report if acne is severe; may be necessary to change dose.

11. May alter serum lipid levels enhancing susceptibility to arteriosclerotic heart disease in women; monitor cholesterol profiles periodically.

**Client/Family Teaching**

1. Review method for administration/application, dosage, frequency of administration, site preparation, and time of application for the transdermal patch.

2. Report any unusual incidents of bleeding or bruising. Androgens suppress clotting factors (II, V, VII, and X); polycythemia and leukopenia may occur.

3. If drug received via pellets, sloughing can occur; report if evident.

4. In older males, urinary obstruction may occur as a result of prostate hyperplasia.

5. Parents of children receiving testosterone should record weight twice a week and height every 2–3 mo. X rays will be performed periodically on prepubertal children to assess effect on bone growth.

6. Women with metastatic breast cancer need lab tests of serum and urine calcium levels, alkaline phosphatase, and serum cholesterol. If the serum cholesterol level is high, the dosage of drug may need to be changed. Follow a low-cholesterol diet and see dietitian for further assistance in meal planning and preparation.

7. Facial hair and acne in females are reversible once drug is withdrawn.

8. Drug may cause irregularities in the menstrual cycle; in postmenopausal women may cause withdrawal bleeding.

9. Use reliable birth control during and for several weeks after therapy withdrawn. Report if pregnancy sus-

pected; increased risk of fetal abnormalities with this drug.

10. Males should report gynecomastia or priapism; may necessitate drug withdrawal (at least temporarily).

11. Report any complaints of tingling of the fingers and toes or loss of appetite.

12. Follow a diet high in calories, proteins, vitamins, minerals, and other nutrients. Restrict sodium to reduce edema.

13. With diabetes, hypoglycemia may occur. Report extreme variations as diet and/or dose of antidiabetic agents may require modification.

14. Review potential for drug abuse. High doses of androgens for enhancement of athletic performance can result in serious irreversible side effects and permanent physical damage.

**Outcomes/Evaluate**

• Replacement therapy with control of S&S of androgen deficiency

• Male contraceptive agent

• Suppression of breast tumor size and spread

---

# Tetracycline
(teh-trah-**SYE**-kleen)
**Pregnancy Category:** D
Achromycin Ophthalmic Ointment, Achromycin Ophthalmic Suspension, Actisite Periodontal Fiber **(Rx)**

# Tetracycline hydrochloride
(teh-trah-**SYE**-kleen)
**Pregnancy Category:** D (topical solution is B)
Achromycin Topical Ointment, Achromycin V, Apo-Tetra ✤, Jaa Tetra ✤, Medicycline ✤, Nor-Tet, Novo-Tetra ✤, Nu-Tetra ✤, Panmycin, Robicaps, Sumycin 250 and 500, Sumycin Syrup, Tetracap, Tetracyn ✤, Topicycline Topical Solution **(Rx)**
**Classification:** Antibiotic, tetracycline

See also *General Information* on *Tetracyclines*.

**Action/Kinetics:** t½: 7–11 hr. From 40% to 70% excreted unchanged in urine; 65% bound to serum proteins. Always express dose as the hydrochloride salt.

**Additional Uses: Ophthalmic:** Superficial ophthalmic infections due to *Staphylococcus aureus, Streptococcus, Streptococcus pneumoniae, Escherichia coli, Neisseria,* and *Bacteroides.* Prophylaxis of *Neisseria gonorrhoeae* in newborns. With oral therapy for treatment of *Chlamydia trachomatis.* **Topical:** Acne vulgaris, prophylaxis or treatment of infection following skin abrasions, minor cuts, wounds, or burns. **Tetracycline fiber:** Adult periodontitis. *Investigational:* Pleural sclerosing agent in malignant pleural effusions (administered by chest tube); in combination with gentamicin for *Vibrio vulnificus* infections due to wound infection after trauma or by eating contaminated seafood. Mouthwash (use suspension) to treat nonspecific mouth ulcerations, canker sores, aphthous ulcers. Possible drug of choice for stage I Lyme disease.

**Contraindications:** Use of the topical ointment in or around the eyes. Ophthalmic products to treat fungal diseases of the eye, dendritic keratitis, vaccinia, varicella, mycobacterial eye infections, or following removal of a corneal foreign body.

**Special Concerns:** Use tetracycline fiber with caution in clients with a history of oral candidiasis. Use of the fiber in chronic abscesses has not been evaluated. Safety and efficacy of the fiber have not been determined in children.

**Additional Side Effects:** Temporary blurring of vision or stinging following administration. Dermatitis and photosensitivity following ophthalmic use. *Use of the tetracycline fiber:* Oral candidiasis, glossitis, staining of the tongue, severe gingival hyperplasia, minor throat irritation, pain following placement in an abscessed area, throbbing pain, hypersensitivity reactions.

T

---

✤ = Available in Canada          ***bold italic*** = life threatening side effect

## Dosage

• **Capsules, Syrup, Tablets**
*Mild to moderate infections.*
**Adults, usual:** 500 mg b.i.d. or 250 mg q.i.d.
*Severe infections.*
**Adult:** 500 mg q.i.d. **Children over 8 years:** 25–50 mg/kg/day in four equal doses.
*Brucellosis.*
500 mg q.i.d. for 3 weeks with 1 g streptomycin IM b.i.d. for first week and once daily the second week.
*Syphilis.*
Total of 30–40 g over 10–15 days.
*Gonorrhea.*
**Initially,** 1.5 g; **then,** 500 mg q 6 hr until 9 g has been given.
*Gonorrhea sensitive to penicillin.*
**Initially,** 1.5 g; **then,** 500 mg q 6 hr for 4 days (total: 9 g).
*GU or rectal Chlamydia trachomatis infections.*
500 mg q.i.d. for minimum of 7 days.
*Severe acne.*
**Initially,** 1 g/day; **then,** 125500 mg/day (long-term).
*NOTE:* The CDC have established treatment schedules for STDs.
**Initially,** 1 g/day; **then,** 125–500 mg/day (long-term).

• **Topical**
*Acne.*
Apply topical solution to affected areas in the morning and at night, making sure that skin is completely wet after each application.
*Infections.*
Apply OTC ointment (3%) to affected areas 1–4 times/day. A sterile bandage may be used.

• **Tetracycline Fiber**
*Adult periodontitis.*
Place the fiber into the periodontal pocket until the pocket is filled (amount of fiber will vary with pocket depth and contour) ensuring that the fiber is in contact with the base of the pocket. Retain the fiber in place for 10 days, after which it is to be removed. The effectiveness of subsequent therapy with the fiber has not been assessed.

## NURSING CONSIDERATIONS

See also *Nursing Considerations* for *Tetracyclines* and *General Nursing Considerations for All Anti-Infectives.*

### Administration/Storage

1. For IM administration, inject into a large muscle mass.
2. The tetracycline fiber product consists of a monofilament of ethylene/vinyl acetate copolymer evenly dispersed with tetracycline. The fiber provides for continuous release of tetracycline for 10 days. The fiber releases about 2 mcg/cm/hr of tetracycline.
3. Avoid actions that may dislodge the fiber; i.e., chewing hard, crusty, or sticky foods; brushing or flossing near any treated areas; engaging in hygienic practices that might dislodge the fiber; probing the treated area with tongue or fingers.
4. Contact the dentist if the fiber is dislodged or falls out before the next scheduled visit or if pain or swelling occurs.
**IV** 5. To reconstitute solutions for IV use, dilute vials containing 250 or 500 mg with 5 or 10 mL, respectively, of sterile water for injection. Further dilution (100–1,000 mL) can be done with NaCl injection, 5% dextrose injection, D5/NSS, Ringer's injection, and RL injection.
6. Except for Ringer's and RL injections, do not use calcium-containing solutions to dilute tetracycline HCl.

### Assessment

1. Document indications for therapy, type, onset, duration, and characteristics of symptoms.
2. Monitor cultures, CBC, liver and renal function studies.

### Client/Family Teaching

1. Take PO form 1 hr before or 2 hr after meals with a full glass of water. Avoid dairy products, antacids, or iron preparations for 2 hr of ingestion of drug.
2. May cause photosensitivity reaction; avoid exposure to sunlight and wear protective clothing and sunscreen when exposed.
3. Transient blurring of vision or

stinging may occur when instilled into the eye.

4. Topical ointment may stain clothing.

5. Drug may cause increased yellow-brown discoloration and softening of teeth and bones. *Not* advised for children under 8 years of age.

6. With oral application for gum disease, review proper care of site(s), foods to avoid, and proper cleaning while avoiding floss or pics for the entire length of therapy. Symptoms that require immediate reporting include pain, abnormal discharge, fever, swelling, expulsion of fiber; return as scheduled for removal and follow-up.

**Outcomes/Evaluate**
• Resolution of infection; symptomatic improvement
• ↓ Acne lesions
• Resolution of effusion with desired pleural sclerosing

# Theophylline
(thee-**OFF**-ih-lin)
**Pregnancy Category:** C
Immediate-release Capsules, Tablets, **Liquid Products:** Accurbron, Aquaphyllin, Asmalix, Bronkodyl, Elixomin, Elixophyllin, Lanophyllin, Lixolin, Pulmophylline ✦, Quibron-T/SR ✦, Quibron-T Dividose, Slo-Phyllin, Solu-Phyllin, Somnophyllin-T, Theo, Theoclear-80, Theolair, Theolixir ✦, Theomar, Theostat-80, Truxophyllin.
**Timed-release Capsules and Tablets:** Aerolate III, Aerolate Jr., Aerolate Sr., Apo-Theo LA ✦, Quibron-T/SR Dividose, Respid, Slo-Bid Gyrocaps, Slo-Phyllin Gyrocaps, Somophyllin-CRT, Sustaire, Theo-24, Theo 250, Theobid Duracaps, Theoclear L.A.-130 Cenules, Theoclear L.A.-260 Cenules, Theocot, Theochron, Theochron-SR ✦, Theo-Dur, Theo-SR ✦, Theolair ✦, Theolair-SR, Theospan-SR, Theo-Time, Theophylline SR, Theovent Long-Acting, Uni-Dur, Uniphyl **(Rx)**
**Classification:** Antiasthmatic, bronchodilator

See also *Theophylline Derivatives.*
**Action/Kinetics: Time to peak serum levels, oral solution:** 1 hr;

**uncoated tablets:** 2 hr; **chewable tablets:** 1–1.5 hr; **enteric-coated tablets:** 5 hr; **extended-release capsules and tablets:** 4–7 hr. In healthy adults, about 60% is bound to plasma protein whereas in neonates 36% is bound to plasma protein.
**Additional Uses: Oral liquid:** Neonatal apnea as a respiratory stimulant. Theophylline and dextrose injection: Respiratory stimulant in neonatal apnea and Cheyne-Stokes respiration.

**Dosage**
• **Capsules, Tablets, Elixir, Oral Solution, Syrup**
See *Dosage* for *Oral Solution, Tablets,* under *Aminophylline.*
• **Extended-Release Capsules, Extended-Release Tablets**
See *Dosage* for *Extended-Release Tablets,* under *Aminophylline.*
• **Elixir, Oral Solution, Oral Suspension, Syrup**
*Bronchodilator, chronic therapy.*
**9–12 years:** 20 mg/kg/day; **6–9 years:** 24 mg/kg/day.
*Neonatal apnea.*
**Loading dose:** Using the equivalent of anhydrous theophylline administered by NGT, 5 mg/kg; **maintenance:** 2 mg/kg/day in two to three divided doses given by NGT.

# NURSING CONSIDERATIONS

See also *Nursing Considerations* for *Theophylline Derivatives.*
**Administration/Storage**
1. Dosage is individualized to maintain serum levels of 10–20 mcg/mL.
2. Calculate dosage based on lean body weight (theophylline does not distribute to body fat).
3. Monitor serum theophylline levels in chronic therapy, especially if the maximum maintenance doses are used or exceeded.
4. The extended-release tablets or capsules are not recommended for children less than 6 years of age. Dosage for once-a-day products has not been established in children less than 12 years of age.

**Assessment**

1. Document onset, duration, and characteristics of symptoms, other agents prescribed, and the outcome.

2. Describe pulmonary assessment findings and note PFTs and ABGs.

3. If switching from IV therapy, wait 4 hr before administering intermediate-release forms; may administer extended-release when IV discontinued.

**Client/Family Teaching**

1. Take with food or milk to minimize GI upset.

2. Take only as prescribed; more is not better.

3. Do not crush or break slow-release forms of the drug.

4. Avoid cigarette smoking; decreases drug's effectiveness.

5. Caffeine- and xanthine-containing beverages and foods (chocolate, coffee, colas) and daily intake of charbroiled foods should be avoided; tend to increase drug side effects.

6. Fluid intake should be at least 2 L/day in order to decrease viscosity of secretions.

7. Do not take any OTC cough, cold, or breathing preparations without provider approval.

8. Report if symptoms do not improve or worsen with therapy.

9. Report any adverse side effects; report as scheduled for serum drug levels.

**Outcomes/Evaluate**

• Improved airway exchange; ease in secretion removal and breathing

• Stimulation of respirations in the neonate

• Therapeutic serum drug levels (10–20 mcg/mL)

# Thiabendazole

(thigh-ah-**BEN**-dah-zohl)
**Pregnancy Category:** C
Mintezol **(Rx)**
**Classification:** Anthelmintic

See also *Anthelmintics*.

**Action/Kinetics:** Interferes with the enzyme fumarate reductase, which is specific to several helminths. Readily absorbed from the GI tract.

**Peak plasma levels:** 1–2 hr. **t½:** 0.9–2 hr. Most excreted within 24 hr, mainly through the urine.

**Uses:** Primarily for threadworm infections, cutaneous larva migrans, visceral larva migrans when these infections occur alone or if pinworm is also present. Use in the following infections only if specific therapy is not available or cannot be used or if a second drug is desirable: hookworm, whipworm, large roundworm. To reduce symptoms of trichinosis during the invasive phase.

**Contraindications:** Lactation. Use in mixed infections with ascaris as it may cause worms to migrate.

**Special Concerns:** Safety and efficacy not established in children less than 13.6 kg. Use with caution in clients with hepatic disease or impaired hepatic function.

**Side Effects:** *GI:* N&V, anorexia, diarrhea, epigastric distress. *CNS:* Dizziness, drowsiness, headache, irritability, weariness, giddiness, numbness, psychic disturbances, collapse, *seizures. Allergic:* Pruritus, *angioedema,* flushing of face, chills, fever, skin rashes, *Stevens-Johnson syndrome, anaphylaxis,* lymphadenopathy, conjunctival injection, erythema multiforme. *Hepatic:* Jaundice, cholestasis, parenchymal liver damage. *GU:* Crystalluria, hematuria, enuresis, foul odor of urine. *Ophthalmic:* Blurred vision, abnormal sensation in the eyes, yellow appearance of objects, drying of mucous membranes. *Miscellaneous:* Tinnitus, hypotension, hyperglycemia, transient leukopenia, perianal rash, appearance of live *Ascaris* in nose and mouth.

**Laboratory Test Alterations:** Rarely, ↑ AST and cephalin flocculation.

**OD** **Overdose Management:** *Symptoms:* Psychic changes, transient vision changes. *Treatment:* Induce vomiting or perform gastric lavage. Treat symptoms.

**Drug Interactions:** ↑ Serum levels of xanthines to potentially toxic levels due to ↓ breakdown by liver.

## Dosage
- **Oral Suspension, Chewable Tablets**

**Over 68 kg:** 1.5 g/dose; **less than 68 kg:** 22 mg/kg/dose.

## NURSING CONSIDERATIONS

See also *Nursing Considerations* for *Anthelmintics*.

### Administration/Storage
1. Take with food to reduce stomach upset.
2. Chewable tablets should be chewed thoroughly before swallowing.
3. Cleansing enemas are not required after drug therapy.
4. For strongyloidiasis, cutaneous larva migrans, hookworm, whipworm, or roundworm; two doses daily are given for 2 days. For trichinelliasis, give two doses daily for 2–4 days. For visceral larva migrans, give two doses/day for 7 successive days.

### Assessment
1. Document indications for therapy, onset and duration of symptoms, and how and when acquired.
2. List agents currently prescribed to ensure none interact.

### Client/Family Teaching
1. Administer with food or after meals to decrease stomach upset; chew tablets thoroughly.
2. Report any CNS disturbances, including muscular weakness and loss of mental alertness.
3. Do not operate hazardous machinery; drug may cause dizziness and drowsiness.
4. May notice an odor to the urine 24 hr following ingestion; this is normal.
5. Report any evidence of rash, fever, or itching immediately.

### Outcomes/Evaluate
- Negative consecutive stool cultures
- Eradication of infestation

# Thiamine hydrochloride (Vitamin B₁)

(THIGH-ah-min)

**Pregnancy Category:** A (parenteral use)

Betaxin ✸, Bewon ✸, Thiamilate (Rx: Injection; OTC: Tablets)

**Action/Kinetics:** Water-soluble vitamin, stable in acid solution. Decomposed in neutral or acid solutions. Required for the synthesis of thiamine pyrophosphate, a coenzyme required in carbohydrate metabolism. The maximum amount absorbed PO is 8–15 mg/day although absorption may be increased by giving in divided doses with food.

**Uses:** Prophylaxis and treatment of thiamine deficiency states and associated neurologic and CV symptoms. Prophylaxis and treatment of beriberi. Alcoholic neuritis, neuritis of pellagra, and neuritis of pregnancy. To correct anorexia due to thiamine insufficiency. *Investigational:* Treatment of subacute necrotizing encephalomyelopathy, maple syrup urine disease, pyruvate carboxylase deficiency, hyperalaninemia.

**Special Concerns:** Use with caution during lactation.

**Side Effects:** *Serious hypersensitivity reactions;* thus, intradermal testing is recommended if sensitivity is suspected. *Dermatologic:* Pruritus, urticaria, sweating, feeling of warmth. *CNS:* Weakness, restlessness. *Other:* Nausea, tightness in throat, *angioneurotic edema,* cyanosis, *hemorrhage into the GI tract, pulmonary edema, CV collapse. Death has been reported.* Following IM use: Induration, tenderness.

**Drug Interactions:** Because vitamin B₁ is unstable in neutral or alkaline solutions, the vitamin should not be used with substances that yield alkaline solutions, such as citrates, barbiturates, carbonates, or erythromycin lactobionate IV.

## Dosage
- **Tablets, Enteric-Coated Tablets**

---

✸ = Available in Canada    ***bold italic*** = life threatening side effect

*Mild beriberi or maintenance following severe beriberi.*
**Adults:** 5–10 mg/day (as part of a multivitamin product); **infants:** 10 mg/day.

*Treatment of deficiency.*
**Adults:** 5–10 mg/day; **pediatric:** 10–50 mg/day.

*Alcohol-induced deficiency.*
**Adults:** 40 mg/day.

*Dietary supplement.*
**Adults:** 1–2 mg/day; **pediatric:** 0.3–0.5 mg/day for infants and 0.5 mg/day for children.

*Genetic enzyme deficiency disease.*
10–20 mg/day (up to 4 g/day has been used in some clients).
• **Slow IV**
*Wet beriberi with myocardial failure.*
**Adults:** 10–30 mg t.i.d.
• **IM**
*Beriberi.*
10–20 mg t.i.d. for 2 weeks. A PO multivitamin product containing 5–10 mg/day thiamine should be given for 1 month to cause body saturation.

*Recommended dietary allowance.*
**Adult males:** 1.2–1.5 mg; **adult females:** 1.1 mg.

## NURSING CONSIDERATIONS
### Administration/Storage
**IV** 1. May administer direct IV undiluted over at least 5 min or may be reconstituted in dextrose or saline solution and administered with daily solution therapy.
2. Drug may enhance the effects of neuromuscular blocking agents. Have epinephrine available to treat for anaphylactic shock if large dose of thiamine ordered.
### Assessment
1. Document type, onset, and characteristics of symptoms.
2. List other agents prescribed to ensure none interact.
3. Note neurologic assessment and clinical presentation.
### Client/Family Teaching: Review dietary sources high in thiamine (enriched and whole grain cereals, meats, especially pork, and fresh vegetables); consult dietitian for assistance in meal planning and preparation.
### Outcomes/Evaluate
• Prophylaxis/relief of thiamine deficiency
• Prevention/reduction of neuritis symptoms

# Thioguanine
(thigh-oh-**GWON**-een)
**Pregnancy Category:** D
Lanvis ✦, TG, 6-Thioguanine (Abbreviation: 6-TG) **(Rx)**
**Classification:** Antimetabolite, purine analog

See also *Antineoplastic Agents.*
**Action/Kinetics:** Purine antagonist that is cell-cycle specific for the S phase of cell division. Converted to 6-thioguanylic acid, which in turn interferes with the synthesis of guanine nucleotides by competing with hypoxanthine and xanthine for the enzyme phosphoribosyltransferase (HGPRTase). Ultimately the synthesis of RNA and DNA is inhibited. Resistance to the drug may result from increased breakdown of 6-thioguanylic acid or loss of HGPRTase activity. Partially absorbed (30%) from GI tract. **t½:** 80 min. Detoxified by liver and excreted in the urine. More effective in children than in adults. Cross-resistance with mercaptopurine. Perform platelet counts weekly; discontinue drug if abnormally large fall in blood count is noted, indicating severe bone marrow depression.
**Uses:** Acute and nonlymphocytic leukemias (usually in combination with other drugs such as cyclophosphamide, cytarabine, prednisone, vincristine). Chronic myelogenous leukemia (not first-line therapy).
**Contraindications:** Resistance to mercaptopurine or thioguanine. Lactation.
**Laboratory Test Alterations:** ↑ Uric acid in blood and urine.
**Additional Side Effects:** Loss of vibration sense, unsteadiness of gait. *Hepatotoxicity,* myelosuppression

(common), hyperuricemia. Adults tend to show a more rapid fall in WBC count than children.

**OD** **Overdose Management:** *Symptoms:* N&V, hypertension, malaise, and diaphoresis may be seen immediately, which may be followed by myelosuppression and azotemia. *Severe hematologic toxicity.* *Treatment:* Induce vomiting if client is seen immediately after an acute overdosage. Treat symptoms. Hematologic toxicity may be treated by platelet transfusions (for bleeding) and granulocyte transfusions. Antibiotics are indicated for sepsis.

**Dosage**
• **Tablets**
*Individualized and determined by hematopoietic response.* **Adults and pediatric, initial:** 2 mg/kg/day (or 75–100 mg/m²) given at one time. From 2 to 4 weeks may elapse before beneficial results become apparent. Compute dose to nearest multiple of 20 mg. If no response, dosage may be increased to 3 mg/kg/day. **Usual maintenance dose (even during remissions):** 2–3 mg/kg/day (or 100 mg/m²). Dosage of thioguanine does not have to be decreased during administration of allopurinol (to inhibit uric acid production).

## NURSING CONSIDERATIONS

See also *Nursing Considerations* for *Antineoplastic Agents.*
**Assessment**
1. Note indications for therapy, onset, duration, and characteristics of symptoms; list other agents trialed and the outcome.
2. Monitor CBC, uric acid, liver and renal function studies. Obtain CBC weekly and LFTs monthly during course of therapy; may cause granulocyte and platelet suppression. Nadir: 10 days; recovery: 21 days.
**Interventions**
1. Provide assistance to those who may experience loss of vibration sense and have unsteady gait (may be unable to rely on canes).

2. Expect hyperuricemia after tumor lysis, which may be reduced with administration of allopurinol, by preventing purine breakdown and excessive uric acid formation.
**Client/Family Teaching**
1. Take on an empty stomach for best results.
2. Increase fluid intake (2–3 L/day) to minimize hyperuricemia and hyperuricosuria.
3. Withhold drug and report if jaundice, decreased urine output, diarrhea, S&S of anemia (fatigue, dyspnea), or extremity swelling occurs.
4. Any sore throat, fever, or flu-like symptoms as well as increased bruising and bleeding tendencies require immediate reporting.
5. Avoid crowds, vaccinia, and persons with infectious diseases.
6. Practice reliable contraception.
**Outcomes/Evaluate**
• Suppression of malignant cell proliferation
• Hematologic evidence of leukemia remission

# Thioridazine hydrochloride
(thigh-oh-**RID**-ah-zeen)
Apo-Thioridazine ✦, Mellaril, Mellaril-S, Novo-Ridazine ✦, PMS-Thioridazine ✦, Thioridazine HCl Intensol Oral **(Rx)**
**Classification:** Antipsychotic, piperidine-type phenothiazine

See also *Antipsychotic Agents, Phenothiazines.*
**Action/Kinetics:** High incidence of hypotension; moderate incidence of sedative and anticholinergic effects and weak antiemetic and extrapyramidal effects. Can often be used in clients intolerant of other phenothiazines. **Peak plasma levels** (after PO administration): 1–4 hr. May impair its own absorption at higher doses due to the strong anticholinergic effects. **t½:** 10 hr. Metabolized in the liver to both active and inactive metabolites. **Uses:** Acute and chronic schizophrenia; moderate to marked depression

with anxiety; sleep disturbances. **In children:** Treatment of hyperactivity in clients and those with retarded and behavior problems. Geriatric clients with organic brain syndrome. Alcohol withdrawal. Intractable pain.

**Special Concerns:** Safe use during pregnancy has not been established. Dosage has not been established in children less than 2 years of age. Geriatric, emaciated, or debilitated clients usually require a lower initial dose.

**Additional Side Effects:** More likely to cause pigmentary retinopathy than other phenothiazines.

**Dosage**

- **Oral Suspension, Oral Solution, Tablets**

Highly individualized.

*Neurosis, anxiety states, sleep disturbances, tension, alcohol withdrawal, senility.*

**Adults, range:** 20–200 mg/day; **initial:** 25 mg t.i.d. **Maintenance,** mild cases: 10 mg b.i.d.–q.i.d.; severe cases: 50 mg t.i.d.–q.i.d.

*Psychotic, severely disturbed hospitalized clients.*

**Adults, initial,** 50–100 mg t.i.d. If necessary, increase to maximum of 200 mg q.i.d. When control is achieved, reduce gradually to minimum effective dosage. **Pediatric above 2 years:** 0.25–3.0 mg/kg/day.

*Hospitalized psychotic children.*

**Initial:** 25 mg b.i.d.–t.i.d. *Moderate problems:* **initial,** 10 mg b.i.d.–t.i.d. Increase gradually if necessary. **Not recommended for children under 2 years of age.**

## NURSING CONSIDERATIONS

See also *Nursing Considerations* for *Antipsychotic Agents, Phenothiazines.*

**Administration/Storage:** Dilute each dose just before administration with distilled water, acidified tap water, or suitable juices. Preparation and storage of bulk dilutions are not recommended.

**Assessment**

1. Document mental status; assess

behavioral manifestations. Note presence and type of hallucinations.

2. Monitor ECG, CBC, liver and renal function studies.

**Client/Family Teaching**

1. Take only as directed; do not stop abruptly, as withdrawal may activate N&V, gastritis, dizziness, tachycardia, headache, and insomnia.

2. Drug may cause drowsiness.

3. Wear protective clothing and sunscreens to prevent a photosensitivity reaction.

4. May cause retinal deposits viewed as a "browning of vision."

5. May impair temperature regulation; avoid temperature extremes and dress appropriately.

6. Doses exceeding 300 mg/day may cause reversible T-wave abnormalities on ECG. Doses above 800 mg/day have been associated with retinal deposits and cardiac toxicity.

**Outcomes/Evaluate**

- Improved behavioral patterns; ↓ agitation and improved coping mechanisms
- ↓ Anxiety levels; ↓ depression; ↓ sleep disturbances

# Thiotepa

(thigh-oh-**TEP**-ah)

**Pregnancy Category:** D

(Abbreviation: Thio), Thioplex **(Rx)**

**Classification:** Antineoplastic, alkylating agent

See also *Antineoplastic Agents* and *Alkylating Agents.*

**Action/Kinetics:** Cell-cycle non-specific; thought to act by causing the release of ethylenimmonium ions that bind or alkylate various intracellular substances such as nucleic acids. Is cytotoxic by virtue of cross-linking of DNA and RNA strands as well as by inhibition of protein synthesis. Rapidly cleared from the plasma following IV use. **t½, elimination:** About 2.3 hr. May be significantly absorbed through the bladder mucosa. Approximately 85% excreted through the urine, mainly as metabolites.

**Uses:** Adenocarcinoma of the breast or ovary. To control intracavitary effusions secondary to diffuse or localized neoplastic disease of various serosal cavities. Superficial papillary carcinoma of the urinary bladder. Lymphosarcoma and Hodgkin's disease, although other treatments are used more often.

**Contraindications:** Lactation. Pregnancy. Renal, hepatic, or bone marrow damage. Acute leukemia. Use with other alkylating agents due to increased toxicity.

**Special Concerns:** Is both carcinogenic and mutagenic. Use with caution in renal and hepatic dysfunction. Safety and efficacy have not been determined in children.

**Side Effects:** *GI:* N&V, abdominal pain, anorexia. *CNS:* Dizziness, headache, blurred vision, fatigue, weakness, febrile reaction. *Dermatologic:* Contact dermatitis, alopecia, pain at injection site, dermatitis, skin depigmentation following topical use. *GU:* Dysuria, urinary retention, chemical or hemorrhagic cystitis following intravesical use, amenorrhea, interference with spermatogenesis. *Hypersensitivity:* Rash, urticaria, wheezing, ***laryngeal edema, asthma, anaphylactic shock.*** *Miscellaneous:* Conjunctivitis, discharge from a SC lesion due to tumor tissue breakdown. Significant toxicity to the hematopoietic system.

**OD** **Overdose Management:** *Symptoms:* ***Hematopoietic toxicity.*** *Treatment:* Transfusions of whole blood, platelets, or leukocytes have been used.

**Drug Interactions**
*Alkylating agents* / Combination with other alkylating agents ↑ toxicity
*Pancuronium* / Prolonged muscle paralysis and respiratory depression
*Succinylcholine* / Risk of ↑ apnea

**Dosage**
• **IV (may be rapid)**
0.3–0.4 mg/kg at 1- to 4-week intervals by rapid administration or 0.2 mg/kg for 4–5 days q 2–4 weeks.
• **Intratumor or Intracavitary Administration**
0.6–0.8 mg/kg q 1–4 weeks; through the same tubing used to remove fluid from the cavity.
• **Intravesical Administration (Bladder Cancer)**
After dehydrating client with papillary carcinoma of the bladder for 8–12 hr, instill 60 mg thiotepa in 30–60 mL of sterile water for injection in the bladder using a catheter. Retain, if possible, for 2 hr. If it is not possible to retain 60 mL, give the dose in a volume of 30 mL. Reposition client q 15 min for maximum contact area. This dose is given once a week for 4 weeks.

## NURSING CONSIDERATIONS

See also *Nursing Considerations* for *Antineoplastic Agents.*
**Administration/Storage**
**IV** 1. Reconstitute with sterile water for injection (usually 1.5 mL to give a concentration of 5 mg/0.5 mL). The reconstituted solution can then be mixed with NaCl injection, dextrose injection, dextrose and NaCl injection, Ringer's injection, or RL injection (i.e., if a large volume is needed for intracavitary use, IV drip, or perfusion).
2. Minimize pain on injection and retard rate of absorption by simultaneous administration of local anesthetics. Drug may be mixed with procaine HCl 2% or epinephrine HCl 1:1,000, or both, as ordered.
3. Store vials in the refrigerator. Reconstituted solutions may be stored for 5 days in the refrigerator without substantial loss of potency.
4. Since thiotepa is not a vesicant, it may be injected quickly and directly into the vein with the desired volume of sterile water. Usual amount of diluent is 1.5 mL.
5. Do not use NSS as a diluent.
6. Discard solutions grossly opaque or with precipitate.

**T**

---

7. When used for bladder carcinoma, a second or third course of treatment may be undertaken, although bone marrow depression may be increased.

**Assessment**

1. Document indications for therapy, onset of symptoms, and any other agents trialed.

2. Monitor CBC, uric acid, liver and renal function studies. Drug causes platelet and granulocyte suppression. Nadir: 21 days; recovery: 40–50 days.

**Interventions**

1. Encourage clients who receive drug as bladder instillations to retain fluid for 2 hr. They should be NPO for 6 hr to ensure drug retention. Observe for hematuria and dysuria.

2. With bladder instillation, reposition q 15 min to ensure maximum bladder area contact.

3. Advise to practice contraception; drug is carcinogenic and mutagenic.

**Outcomes/Evaluate:** Control of tumor size and malignant cell proliferation

---

# Thiothixene

(thigh-oh-**THICKS**-een)

Navane **(Rx)**

**Classification:** Antipsychotic, miscellaneous

---

**Action/Kinetics:** Mechanism of action may be due to blockade of postsynaptic dopamine receptors in the brain, especially at subcortical levels in the reticular formation, hypothalamus, and limbic system. Also causes cholinergic and alpha-adrenergic blocking effects, adrenergic potentiating effects, antiserotonin effects, and prevention of uptake of biogenic amines. This results in significant extrapyramidal symptoms and antiemetic effects and minimal sedation, orthostatic hypotension, and anticholinergic symptoms. The margin between a therapeutically effective dose and one that causes extrapyramidal symptoms is narrow. Well absorbed from the GI tract. **Peak plasma levels, PO:** 1–3 hr. **t½:** 34 hr. A therapeutic response

may occur within 1 to 6 hr following IM use and within a few days to several weeks following PO use. Metabolized in the liver and excreted in the feces as both unchanged drug and metabolites.

**Uses:** Symptomatic treatment of psychotic disorders, including withdrawn, apathetic schizophrenia, delusions, and hallucinations.

**Contraindications:** Use in clients with circulatory collapse, comatose states, CNS depression due to any cause, and blood dyscrasias. Hypersensitivity to thiothixene and possibly phenothiazine derivatives. Use in children less than 12 years of age.

**Special Concerns:** Use with caution in CV disease, glaucoma, and prostatic hypertrophy, and in those exposed to extreme heat. Use with extreme caution in those with a history of seizure disorders, alcohol withdrawal, and in clients who develop akathisia and restlessness. Use during pregnancy only when potential benefits outweigh possible risks to the mother and/or fetus.

**Side Effects:** Since thiothixene has pharmacologic properties similar to phenothiazines, the side effects associated with phenothiazines should also be consulted. *CNS:* Drowsiness, extrapyramidal symptoms (especially akathisia and dystonia), persistent tardive dyskinesia (especially in female geriatric clients), lethargy, dizziness, restlessness, lightheadedness, agitation, insomnia, hyperpyrexia, weakness, fatigue. Rarely, seizures and paradoxical exacerbation of psychoses. *GI:* Dry mouth, constipation, increased salivation, adynamic ileus, anorexia, N&V, diarrhea, increase in appetite and weight, cholestatic jaundice. *CV:* Orthostatic hypotension, tachycardia, syncope, ECG changes. *Ophthlamic:* Blurred vision, miosis, mydriasis. *Hypersensitivity:* Rash, pruritus, urticaria, photosensitivity, **anaphylaxis (rare).** *GU:* Impotence, lactation, moderate breast enlargement in women, amenorrhea. *Hematologic:* Leukopenia, leukocytosis. *Miscellaneous:* **Neu-**

*roleptic malignant syndrome.* Increased sweating, nasal congestion, impotence, leg cramps, polydypsia, peripheral edema, fine lenticular pigmentation.

**Laboratory Test Alterations:** ↑ Serum transaminase, alkaline phosphatase, uric acid excretion. ↓ Prothrombin time.

**OD** **Overdose Management:** *Symptoms:* Muscle twitching, drowsiness, dizziness. In severe cases, symptoms include rigidity, weakness, torticollis, tremor, salivation, dysphagia, disturbance of gait, CNS depression, coma. *Treatment:* General supportive measures, including maintaining an adequate airway and oxygenation. Gastric lavage, if overdose found early. Hypotension and circulatory collapse may be treated with IV fluids and/or vasopressor agents (epinephrine is not to be used). Antiparkinson drugs may be used to treat extrapyramidal symptoms.Do *not* use analeptic drugs.

**Drug Interactions**
*Anticholinergic drugs* / Additive or potentiation of anticholinergic effect
*CNS depressants* / Additive or potentiation of depressant effect
*Hypotensive drugs* / Additive or potentiation of hypotensive effect

**Dosage** ————————————
• **Capsules, Concentrate**
*Mild to moderate psychoses.*
**Adults, initial:** 2 mg t.i.d., increased to 15 mg/day if necessary.
*Severe psychoses.*
**Adults, initial:** 5 mg b.i.d., increased to 60 mg/day if necessary. The usual optimum dose is 20–30 mg/day. Doses greater than 60 mg/day rarely increase the therapeutic effect.
• **IM**
*Acutely agitated clients or those unwilling or unable to take PO medication.*
**Adults, initial:** 4 mg b.i.d.–q.i.d. The dose may then be increased or decreased, depending on the response. **Usual dose:** 16–20 mg/day.

IM doses should not exceed 30 mg/day.

## NURSING CONSIDERATIONS

See also *Nursing Considerations* for *Antipsychotics.*
**Administration/Storage**
1. For maintenance therapy, a single daily dose may be adequate.
2. The preferred IM site is the upper outer quadrant of the gluteal muscle or the midlateral thigh.
3. The powder for injection is reconstituted by adding 2.2 mL of sterile water for injection to the 10 mg vial of drug. The reconstituted solution contains 5 mg of thiothixene/mL.
4. Replace IM therapy with PO therapy as soon as possible. An adjustment in dose may be required when switching from IM to PO and vice versa.
**Assessment**
1. Document onset, duration, and characteristics of symptoms. List other agents trialed and the outcome.
2. Assess baseline mental status, noting mood, behavior, and any evidence of depression.
3. List drugs currently prescribed to ensure none interact.
4. Avoid drug with CNS depression, circulatory collapse, coma, blood dyscrasias, or uncontrolled seizure disorder.
5. Monitor CBC, LFTs, and ECG.
**Client/Family Teaching**
1. Take exactly as prescribed; do not stop abruptly.
2. Drug may cause sedation, orthostatic hypotension, and visual disturbances. Do not engage in activities that require mental alertness.
3. Drug may cause tardive dyskinesias (slow, automatic movements) and extrapyramidal symptoms (tremor, twisting repetitive jerks); report if evident so dosage can be adjusted or other meds prescribed to combat symptoms.
4. Consume plenty of fluids to prevent dehydration and constipation.
5. Report any elevation in body

**T**

———————————————

temperature, feeling of weakness, or sore throat; S&S of blood dyscrasias.

6. May cause a photosensitivity reaction; use suncsreen and protective clothing when exposed.

7. Avoid alcohol and any other OTC agents or CNS depressants without approval.

8. Drug may cause menstrual irregularity, false positive pregnancy test, breast enlargement, decreased libido, and a pink brown discoloration of urine.

9. Report any evidence of yellow skin discoloration or RUQ abdominal pain as drug may cause cholestatic jaundice.

10. Report as scheduled for F/U ECG, lab work, psychotherapy, prescription renewal, and evaluation of mental status.

**Outcomes/Evaluate:** ↓ Excitable, withdrawn, agitated, or paranoid behaviors.

# Tiagabine hydrochloride
(tye-**AG**-ah-been)
**Pregnancy Category:** C
Gabatril **(Rx)**
**Classification:** Anticonvulsant, miscellaneous

See also *Anticonvulsants.*

**Action/Kinetics:** Mechanism not known but activity of GABA, an inhibitory neurotransmitter, may be enhanced. Drug may block uptake of GABA into presynaptic neurons allowing more GABA to bind to post-synaptic cells. This prevents propagation of neural impulses that contribute to seizures due to GABA-ergic action. **Peak plasma levels:** About 45 min when fasting. High fat meals decrease rate but not extent of absorption. Metabolized in liver; excreted in urine and feces. **t½, elimination:** 7–9 hr. Diurnal effect occurs with levels being lower in evening compared with morning.

**Uses:** Adjunctive therapy for partial seizures.

**Contraindications:** Lactation.

**Special Concerns:** Safety and efficacy have not been determined in children less than 12 years old.

**Side Effects:** *CNS:* Dizziness, asthenia, somnolence, nervousness, tremor, insomnia, difficulty with concentration or attention, ataxia, confusion, speech disorder, difficulty with memory, paresthesia, depression, emotional lability, abnormal gait, hostility, nystagmus, problems with language, agitation. *GI:* N&V, diarrhea, increased appetite, mouth ulceration. *Respiratory:* Pharyngitis, increased cough. *Dermatologic:* Rash, pruritus. *Miscellaneous:* Abdominal pain, unspecified pain, vasodilation, myasthenia.

**OD** **Overdose Management:** *Symptoms:* Somnolence, impaired consciousness, agitation, confusion, speech difficulties, depression, weakness, myoclonus. *Treatment:* Emesis or gastric lavage, maintain an airway. General supportive treatment.

**Drug Interactions**
*Carbamazepine* / ↑ Clearance due to ↑ metabolism
*Phenobarbital* / ↑ Clearance due to ↑ metabolism
*Phenytoin* / ↑ Clearance due to ↑ metabolism
*Valproate* / ↑ Clearance due to ↑ metabolism

**Dosage**
• **Tablets**
*Partial seizures.*
**Adults and children over 18 years, initial:** 4 mg once daily. Total daily dose may be increased by 4 to 8 mg at weekly intervals until clinical effect is observed or daily dose is 56 mg/day. **Children, 12 to 18 years, initial:** 4 mg once daily. Total daily dose may be increased by 4 mg at beginning of week 2. Thereafter, dose may be increased by 4 to 8 mg at weekly intervals until clinical effect is seen or dose is 32 mg/day. For all ages, give total daily dose in 2 to 4 divided doses.

## NURSING CONSIDERATIONS

See also *Nursing Considerations* for *Anticonvulsants.*

**Administration/Storage**
1. Take with food.
2. It is not necessary to modify dose of concomitant anticonvulsant drugs, unless clinically indicated.
3. Dose must be titrated in those taking enzyme-inducing anticonvulsant drugs. Package insert must be consulted.
**Assessment:**
1. Document indications for therapy, characteristics of seizures, other agents trialed and outcome.
2. Monitor LFTs; decrease dosage or dosing intervals with dysfunction.
**Client/Family Teaching**
1. Take with food as directed.
2. Do not perform activities requiring mental alertness until drug effects realized; may cause dizziness, sleepiness, or confusion.
3. Report any increased frequency or loss of seizure control, rash, weakness, or visual disturbances.
4. Do not stop abruptly; may trigger seizures.
5. Practice reliable contraception; do not breast feed.
**Outcomes/Evaluate:** Control of seizures

# Ticarcillin disodium
(tie-kar-**SILL**-in)
**Pregnancy Category:** B
Ticar **(Rx)**
**Classification:** Antibiotic, penicillin

See also *Anti-Infectives* and *Penicillins.*
**Action/Kinetics:** A parenteral, semisynthetic antibiotic with an antibacterial spectrum of activity resembling that of carbenicillin. **Peak plasma levels: IM,** 25–35 mcg/mL after 1 hr; **IV,** 15 min. **t½:** 70 min. Elimination complete after 6 hr.
**Uses:** Primarily suitable for treatment of gram-negative organisms but also effective for mixed infections. Bacterial septicemia, skin and soft tissue infections, acute and chronic respiratory tract infections caused by susceptible strains of *Pseudomonas aeruginosa, Proteus, Escherichia coli,* and other gram-negative organisms. Combined therapy with gentamicin or tobramycin is sometimes indicated for treatment of *Pseudomonas* infections. GU tract infections caused by the above organisms and by *Enterobacter* and *Streptococcus faecalis.* Anaerobic bacteria causing empyema, anaerobic pneumonitis, lung abscess, bacterial septicemia, peritonitis, intra-abdominal abscess, skin and soft tissue infections, salpingitis, endometritis, pelvic inflammatory disease, pelvic abscess. Ticarcillin may be used in infections in which protective mechanisms are impaired such as during use of oncolytic or immunosuppressive drugs or in clients with acute leukemia.
**Additional    Contraindications:** Pregnancy.
**Special Concerns:** Use with caution in presence of impaired renal function and for clients on restricted salt diets.
**Laboratory Test Alterations:** ↑ Alkaline phosphatase, AST, ALT.
**Additional Side Effects:** Neurotoxicity and neuromuscular excitability, especially in clients with impaired renal function.
**Additional Drug Interactions:** Effect of carbenicillin may be enhanced when used in combination with gentamicin or tobramycin for *Pseudomonas* infections.

**Dosage**
• **IV Infusion, Direct IV, IM**
   *Bacterial septicemia, intra-abdominal infections, skin and soft tissue infections, infections of the female genital system and pelvis, respiratory tract infections.*
**Adults:** 200–300 mg/kg/day by IV infusion in divided doses q 3, 4, or 6 hr, depending on the severity of the infection; **pediatric, less than 40 kg:** 200–300 mg/kg/day by IV infusion q 4 or 6 hr (daily dose should not exceed the adult dose).
   *UTIs, uncomplicated.*

**T**

**Adults:** 1 g IM or direct IV q 6 hr; **pediatric, less than 40 kg:** 50–100 mg/kg/day IM or direct IV in divided doses q 6 or 8 hr.

*UTIs, complicated.*

**Adults:** 150–200 mg/kg/day by IV infusion in divided doses q 4 or 6 hr (usual dose is 3 g q.i.d. for a 70-kg client).

*Neonates with sepsis due to* Pseudomonas, Proteus, *or* E. coli.

**Less than 7 days of age and less than 2 kg,** 75 mg/kg q 12 hr; **more than 7 days of age and less than 2 kg,** 75 mg/kg q 8 hr; **less than 7 days of age and more than 2 kg,** 75 mg/kg q 8 hr; **more than 7 days of age and more than 2 kg,** 100 mg/kg q 8 hr. Can be given IM or by IV infusion over 10–20 min.

Clients with renal insufficiency should receive a loading dose of 3 g **IV,** and subsequent doses, as indicated by creatinine clearance.

## NURSING CONSIDERATIONS

See also *Nursing Considerations* for *Penicillins.*

### Administration/Storage

1. Clients seriously ill should receive higher doses such as in serious urinary tract and systemic infections.

2. For IM use, reconstitute each gram with 2 mL sterile water for injection, NaCl injection, or 1% lidocaine HCl (without epinephrine) to prevent pain and induration. Use the reconstituted solution quickly; inject well into a large muscle.

3. Do not administer more than 2 g of the drug in each IM site.

4. Give the adult dose to children weighing over 40 kg.

5. Do not mix ticarcillin together with amikacin, gentamicin, or tobramycin due to the gradual inactivation of these aminoglycosides.

6. Discard unused reconstituted solutions after 24 hr when stored at room temperature and after 72 hr when refrigerated.

**IV** 7. For IV use, reconstitute each gram with 4 mL of the desired solution. Administer slowly to prevent vein irritation and phlebitis. A dilution of 1 g/20 mL (or more) will decrease the chance of vein irritation.

8. For an IV infusion, use 50 or 100 mL *ADD-Vantage* container of either D5W or NaCl injection and give by intermittent infusion over 30–120 min in equally divided doses.

### Assessment

1. Document type, onset, and characteristics of symptoms.

2. Monitor bleeding times, cultures, liver and renal function studies. Reduce dosage with liver or renal dysfunction.

3. With high doses, monitor for signs of electrolyte imbalance (especially Na and K levels).

4. Note sodium content of drug (usually 4.75 mEq Na/g) and calculate accordingly if Na restricted.

### Client/Family Teaching

1. Report any symptoms of bleeding abnormalities, such as petechiae, ecchymosis, or frank bleeding.

2. Edema, weight gain, or respiratory distress may be precipitated by drug's large sodium content.

3. Review drug side effects that should be reported if evident.

### Outcomes/Evaluate

- Negative cultures
- Symptomatic improvement

———*COMBINATION DRUG*———

# Ticarcillin disodium and Clavulanate potassium

(tie-kar-**SILL**-in, klav-you-**LAN**-ate poe-**TASS**-ee-um)

**Pregnancy Category:** B

Timentin **(Rx)**

**Classification:** Antibiotic, penicillin

See also *Ticarcillin disodium* and *Penicillins.*

**Content:** Each vial of the Powder for Injection and the Solution contains: ticarcillin disodium, 3.1 g, and clavulanate potassium, 0.1 g.

**Action/Kinetics:** Contains clavulanic acid, which protects the breakdown of ticarcillin by beta-lactamase enzymes, thus ensuring appropriate blood levels of ticarcillin.

**Uses:** Complicated and uncomplicated UTIs; infections of the bones and joints, lower respiratory tract, skin and skin structures; gynecologic infections, bacterial septicemia. In combination with an aminoglycoside for certain *Pseudomonas aeruginosa* infections.

**Dosage**
- **IV Infusion**
  *Systemic and UTIs.*
  **Adults more than 60 kg:** 3.1 g (containing 0.1 g clavulanic acid) q 4–6 hr for 10–14 days. **Adults less than 60 kg:** 200–300 mg ticarcillin/kg/day in divided doses q 4–6 hr for 10–14 days.
  *Gynecologic infections.*
  **Adults more than 60 kg, moderate infections:** 200 mg/kg/day in divided doses q 6 hr; **severe infections:** 300 mg/kg/day in divided doses q 4 hr.
  *In renal insufficiency.*
  **Initially,** loading dose of 3.1 g ticarcillin and 0.1 g clavulanic acid; **then,** dose based on $C_{CR}$ (see package insert).

## NURSING CONSIDERATIONS

See also *Nursing Considerations* for *Penicillins* and *Ticarcillin disodium.*
**Administration/Storage**
1. To attain the appropriate dilution for 3.1 g ticarcillin and 0.1 g clavulanic acid, dilute with 13 mL of either NaCl injection or sterile water for injection. Further dilutions can be undertaken with 5% dextrose injection, RL injection, or NaCl.
2. Administer over a 30-min period, either through a Y-type IV infusion or by direct infusion.
3. This product is incompatible with sodium bicarbonate.
4. Dilutions with NaCl injection or RL injection may be stored at room temperature for 24 hr or refrigerated for 7 days. Dilutions with 5% dextrose injection are stable at room temperature for 12 hr or for 3 days if refrigerated.
5. If used with another anti-infective agent (e.g., an aminoglycoside), give each drug separately.

**Outcomes/Evaluate:** Resolution of infection; symptomatic improvement

# Ticlopidine hydrochloride
(tie-**KLOH**-pih-deen)
**Pregnancy Category:** B
Ticlid **(Rx)**
**Classification:** Platelet aggregation inhibitor

**Action/Kinetics:** Irreversibly inhibits ADP-induced platelet-fibrinogen binding and subsequent platelet-platelet interactions. This results in inhibition of both platelet aggregation and release of platelet granule constituents as well as prolongation of bleeding time. **Peak plasma levels:** 2 hr. **Maximum platelet inhibition:** 8–11 days after 250 mg b.i.d. **Steady-state plasma levels:** 14–21 days. **t½, elimination:** 4–5 days. After discontinuing therapy, bleeding time and other platelet function tests return to normal within 14 days. Rapidly absorbed; bioavailability is increased by food. Highly bound (98%) to plasma proteins. Extensively metabolized by the liver with approximately 60% excreted through the kidneys; 23% is excreted in the feces (with one-third excreted unchanged). Clearance of the drug decreases with age.
**Uses:** To reduce the risk of fatal or nonfatal thrombotic stroke in clients who have manifested precursors of stroke or who have had a completed thrombotic stroke. Due to the risk of neutropenia or agranulocytosis, use should be reserved for clients who are intolerant to aspirin therapy. *Investigational:* Chronic arterial occlusion, coronary artery bypass grafts, intermittent claudication, open heart surgery, primary glomerulonephritis, subarachnoid hemorrhage, sickle cell disease, uremic clients with AV shunts or fistulas.
**Contraindications:** In the presence of neutropenia and thrombocytopenia, hemostatic disorder, or active pathologic bleeding such as bleeding peptic ulcer or intracranial

T

bleeding. Severe liver impairment. Lactation.

**Special Concerns:** Use with caution in clients with ulcers (i.e., where there is a propensity for bleeding). Consider reduced dosage in impaired renal function. Geriatric clients may be more sensitive to the effects of the drug. Safety and effectiveness have not been established in children less than 18 years of age.

**Side Effects:** *Hematologic:* Neutropenia, *agranulocytosis,* thrombocytopenia, pancytopenia, thrombotic thrombocytopenia purpura, immune thrombocytopenia, *hemolytic anemia with reticulocytosis. GI:* Diarrhea, N&V, GI pain, dyspepsia, flatulence, anorexia, GI fullness. *Bleeding complications:* Ecchymosis, hematuria, epistaxis, conjunctival hemorrhage, *GI bleeding,* perioperative bleeding, *intracerebral bleeding (rare). Dermatologic:* Maculopapular or urticarial rash, pruritus, urticaria. *CNS:* Dizziness, headache. *Neuromuscular:* Asthenia, SLE, peripheral neuropathy, arthropathy, myositis. *Miscellaneous:* Tinnitus, pain, allergic pneumonitis, vasculitis, hepatitis, cholestatic jaundice, nephrotic syndrome, hyponatremia, serum sickness.

**Laboratory Test Alterations:** ↑ Alkaline phosphatase, ALT, AST, serum cholesterol, and triglycerides.

**Drug Interactions**

*Antacids /* ↓ Plasma levels of ticlopidine

*Aspirin /* Ticlopidine ↑ effect of aspirin on collagen-induced platelet aggregation

*Cimetidine /* ↓ Clearance of ticlopidine probably due to ↓ breakdown by liver

*Digoxin /* Slight ↓ in digoxin plasma levels

*Theophylline /* ↑ Plasma levels of theophylline due to ↓ clearance

**Dosage**
- **Tablets**
  *Reduce risk of thrombotic stroke.*
  250 mg b.i.d.

**NURSING CONSIDERATIONS**
**Administration/Storage**
1. To increase bioavailability and decrease GI discomfort, take with food or just after eating.
2. If switched from an anticoagulant or fibrinolytic drug to ticlopidine, discontinue the former drug before initiation of ticlopidine therapy.
3. IV methylprednisolone (20 mg) may normalize prolonged bleeding times, usually within 2 hr.

**Assessment**
1. Note any liver disease, bleeding disorders, or ulcer disease.
2. Ascertain aspirin intolerance.
3. Determine baseline hematologic profile (e.g., CBC, PT, PTT, INR), liver and renal function studies.

**Client/Family Teaching**
1. Take with food or after meals to minimize GI upset.
2. It may take longer than usual to stop bleeding; unusual bleeding should be reported.
3. Brush teeth with a soft-bristle tooth brush, use an electric razor for shaving, wear shoes when ambulating, use caution and avoid injury, as bleeding times may be prolonged.
4. During the first 3 months of therapy, neutropenia can occur, resulting in an increased risk of infection. Come for scheduled blood tests and report any symptoms of infection (e.g., fever, chills, sore throat).
5. Any severe or persistent diarrhea, SC bleeding, skin rashes, or evidence of cholestasis (e.g., yellow skin or sclera, dark urine, light-colored stools) should be reported.

**Outcomes/Evaluate:** Prevention of a complete or recurrent cerebral thrombotic event

# Tiludronate disodium
(tye-**LOO**-droh-nayt)
**Pregnancy Category:** C
Skelid **(Rx)**
**Classification:** Bone growth regulator

**Action/Kinetics:** Inhibits activity of osteoclasts and decreases bone turnover. Does not interfere with bone mineralization. Poorly absorbed from GI tract when fasting and in presence of food. **Peak serum levels:** 2 hr. Not metabolized; excreted in urine. **t½:** About 150 hr.

**Uses:** Treatment of Paget's disease where level of serum alkaline phosphatase is at least twice upper limit of normal, in those who are symptomatic, or who are at risk for future complications of disease.

**Contraindications:** Not recommended for those with $C_{CR}$ less than 30 mL/min.

**Special Concerns:** Use with caution during lactation and in those with dysphagia, symptomatic esophageal disease, gastritis, duodenitis, or ulcers. Safety and efficacy have not been determined in children.

**Side Effects:** *GI:* Diarrhea, N&V, dyspepsia, flatulence, tooth disorder, abdominal pain, constipation, dry mouth, gastritis. *Body as whole:* Pain, back pain, accidental injury, flu-like symptoms, chest pain, asthenia, syncope, fatigue, flushing. *CNS:* Headache, dizziness, paresthesia, vertigo, anorexia, somnolence, anxiety, nervousness, insomnia. *CV:* Dependent edema, peripheral edema, hypertension. *Musculoskeletal:* Arthralgia, arthrosis, pathological fracture, involuntary muscle contractions. *Respiratory:* Rhinitis, sinusitis, URTI, coughing, pharyngitis, bronchitis. *Dermatologic:* Rash, skin disorder, pruritus, increased sweating. *Ophthalmic:* Cataract, conjunctivitis, glaucoma. *Miscellaneous:* Hyperparathyroidism, vitamin D deficiency, UTI.

**OD** **Overdose Management:** *Symptoms:* Hypocalcemia. *Treatment:* Supportive.

**Drug Interactions**

*Antacids, aluminum- or magnesium-containing* / ↓ Bioavailability of tiludronate when taken 1 hr before tiludronate

*Aspirin* / ↓ Bioavailability of tiludronate by 50% when taken 2 hr after tiludronate

*Calcium* / ↓ Bioavailability of tiludronate when taken at same time

*Indomethacin* / ↑ Bioavailability of tiludronate by two- to four-fold

**Dosage**

• **Tablets**

*Paget's disease.*

**Adults:** Single 400 mg dose/day taken with 6 to 8 oz of plain water for period of only 3 months.

## NURSING CONSIDERATIONS

### Administration/Storage

1. Take calcium or mineral supplements at least 2 hr before or after tiludronate. Take aluminum- or magnesium-containing antacids at least 2 hr after tiludronate.

2. Allow an interval of 3 months to assess response.

### Client/Family Teaching

1. Take with 6 to 8 oz of plain water. Do not take within 2 hr of food. Beverages other than water, food, and some medications reduce absorption of tiludronate.

2. Do not take aspirin, indomethacin, or calcium or mineral supplements within 2 hr before or after taking drug.

3. Do not remove tablets from foil strips until they are to be used.

4. May experience nausea, diarrhea, and GI upset; report if severe.

5. Report any rashes, itching, hives, severe stomach pains, bloody or black tarry stools.

6. Consume diet high in calcium and vitamin D.

**Outcomes/Evaluate:** Inhibition of Paget's disease progression

# Timolol maleate

(**TIE**-moh-lohl)

**Pregnancy Category:** C

Apo-Timol ♣, Apo-Timop ♣, Beta-Tim ♣, Blocadren, Gen-Timolol ♣, Med-Timolol ♣, Novo-Timol ♣, Nu-Timolol ♣, Tim-Ak ♣, Timoptic, Timoptic in Acudose, Timoptic-XE **(Rx)**

**Classification:** Ophthalmic agent, beta-adrenergic blocking agent

See also *Beta-Adrenergic Blocking Agents.*

**Action/Kinetics:** Exerts both beta-1- and beta-2-adrenergic blocking activity. Has minimal sympathomimetic effects, direct myocardial depressant effects, or local anesthetic action. Does not cause pupillary constriction or night blindness. The mechanism of the protective effect in MI is not known. **Peak plasma levels:** 1–2 hr. **t½:** 4 hr. Metabolized in the liver. Metabolites and unchanged drug excreted through the kidney.

Also reduces both elevated and normal IOP, whether or not glaucoma is present; thought to act by reducing aqueous humor formation and/or by slightly increasing outflow of aqueous humor. Does not affect pupil size or visual acuity. For use in eye: **Onset:** 30 min. **Maximum effect:** 1–2 hr. **Duration:** 24 hr.

**Uses: Tablets:** Hypertension (alone or in combination with other antihypertensives such as thiazide diuretics). Within 1–4 weeks of MI to reduce risk of reinfarction. Prophylaxis of migraine. *Investigational:* Ventricular arrhythmias and tachycardias, essential tremors.

**Ophthalmic solution (Timoptic):** Lower IOP in chronic open-angle glaucoma, selected cases of secondary glaucoma, ocular hypertension, aphakic (no lens) clients with glaucoma. *Ophthalmic gel forming solution (Timoptic-XE):* Reduce elevated IOP in glaucoma.

**Contraindications:** Hypersensitivity to drug. Bronchial asthma or bronchospasm including severe COPD.

**Special Concerns:** Use ophthalmic preparation with caution in clients for whom systemic beta-adrenergic blocking agents are contraindicated. Safe use in children not established.

**Side Effects:** *Systemic following use of tablets:* See *Beta-Adrenergic Blocking Agents.*

*Following use of ophthalmic product:* Few. Occasionally, ocular irritation, local hypersensitivity reactions, slight decrease in resting HR.

**Laboratory Test Alterations:** ↑ BUN, serum potassium, and uric acid. ↓ H&H.

**Drug Interactions:** When used ophthalmically, possible potentiation with systemically administered beta-adrenergic blocking agents.

## Dosage

- **Tablets**
  *Hypertension.*
  **Initial:** 10 mg b.i.d. alone or with a diuretic; **maintenance:** 20–40 mg/day (up to 80 mg/day in two doses may be required), depending on BP and HR. If dosage increase is necessary, wait 7 days.
  *MI prophylaxis in clients who have survived the acute phase.*
  10 mg b.i.d.
  *Migraine prophylaxis.*
  **Initially:** 10 mg b.i.d. **Maintenance:** 20 mg/day given as a single dose; total daily dose may be increased to 30 mg in divided doses or decreased to 10 mg, depending on the response and client tolerance. If a satisfactory response for migraine prophylaxis is not obtained within 6–8 weeks using the maximum daily dose, discontinue the drug.
  *Essential tremor.*
  10 mg/day.
- **Ophthalmic Solution (Timoptic 0.25% or 0.5%)**
  *Glaucoma.*
  1 gtt of 0.25%–0.50% solution in each eye b.i.d. If the decrease in intraocular pressure is maintained, reduce dose to 1 gtt once a day.
- **Ophthalmic Gel-Forming Solution (Timoptic-XE 0.25% or 0.5%)**
  *Glaucoma.*
  1 gtt once daily.

## NURSING CONSIDERATIONS

See also *Nursing Considerations* for *Beta-Adrenergic Blocking Agents* and *Antihypertensive Agents.*

**Administration/Storage**

**Ophthalmic Solution**

1. When client is transferred from another antiglaucoma agent, continue old medication on day 1 of timolol therapy (1 gtt of 0.25% solution). Then, discontinue former therapy. Initiate with 0.25% solution. Increase to 0.50% solution if response is

insufficient. Further increases in dosage are ineffective.

2. When transferred from several antiglaucoma agents, individualize the dose. If one of the agents is a beta-adrenergic blocking agent, discontinue it before starting timolol. Dosage adjustments should involve one drug at a time at 1-week intervals. Continue the antiglaucoma drugs with the addition of timolol, 1 gtt of 0.25% solution b.i.d. (if response is inadequate, 1 gtt of 0.5% solution may be used b.i.d.). The following day, discontinue one of the other antiglaucoma agents while continuing the remaining agents or discontinue based on client response.

3. Before using the gel, invert the closed container and shake once before each use.

4. Administer other ophthalmics at least 10 min before the gel.

5. The ocular hypotensive effect has been maintained when switching clients from timolol solution given b.i.d. to the gel once daily.

**Assessment**

1. Document indications for therapy; onset, duration, and characteristics of symptoms.

2. Monitor liver and renal function studies.

**Client/Family Teaching**

1. Review procedure for ophthalmic administration.

• Apply finger lightly to lacrimal sac for 1 min following administration.

• Regular intraocular measurements by an ophthalmologist are required because ocular hypertension may recur without any overt signs or symptoms.

2. When tablets used for long-term prophylaxis against MI, do not interrupt therapy; abrupt withdrawal may precipitate reinfarction.

3. Report any evidence of rash, dizziness, heart palpitations, SOB, edema, or depression.

4. Do not perform tasks such as driving or operating machinery until drug effects are realized; may cause dizziness.

5. May cause increased sensitivity to cold; dress appropriately.

6. With diabetes, monitor FS as drug may mask some symptoms of hypoglycemia.

7. Continue life-style modifications (i.e., weight reduction, regular exercise, reduced intake of sodium and alcohol, and no smoking) in the overall goal of BP control.

**Outcomes/Evaluate**

• ↓ BP

• Prevention of myocardial reinfarction

• Migraine prophylaxis

• ↓ Intraocular pressures

# Tioconazole
(tie-oh-**KON**-ah-zohl)
**Pregnancy Category:** C
Gynecure ✤, Trosyd AF ✤, Trosyd J ✤, Vagistat-1 **(Rx) (OTC)**
**Classification:** Antifungal, vaginal

**Action/Kinetics:** Antifungal activity thought to be due to alteration of the permeability of the cell membrane of the fungus, causing leakage of essential intracellular compounds. The systemic absorption of the drug in nonpregnant clients is negligible.

**Uses:** *Candida albicans* infections of the vulva and vagina. Also effective against *Torulopsis glabrata*. OTC for recurrent vaginal yeast infections in those who have previously been diagnosed and have the same symptoms again.

**Contraindications:** Use of a vaginal applicator during pregnancy may be contraindicated.

**Special Concerns:** Safety and effectiveness have not been determined during lactation or in children.

**Side Effects:** *GU:* Burning, itching, irritation, vulvar edema and swelling, discharge, vaginal pain, dysuria, dyspareunia, nocturia, desquamation, dryness of vaginal secretions.

**Dosage**
• **Vaginal Ointment, 6.5%**
One applicator full (about 4.6 g) should be inserted intravaginally at bedtime for 3 days. If needed, the

T

treatment period can be extended to 6 days.

## NURSING CONSIDERATIONS

**Administration/Storage:** The ointment base may interact with rubber and latex; thus, avoid use of condoms or diaphragms for 3 days following treatment.

**Assessment:** Obtain a thorough nursing history and carefully evaluate sources of infection.

**Client/Family Teaching**

1. Review appropriate method for administration (the cream should be inserted high into the vagina). Use just prior to bedtime.

2. Continue to take for prescribed time frame even if symptoms subside. Report if any burning, irritation, or pain occurs.

3. May stain clothes; use sanitary napkins during therapy and change frequently because damp sanitary napkins may harbor infecting organisms.

4. To avoid reinfection, refrain from sexual intercourse. The ointment base may interact with rubber and latex; thus, avoid use of condoms or diaphragms for 3 days following treatment.

5. Use during menses to ensure a full course of therapy. Effectiveness is not altered by menstruation.

**Outcomes/Evaluate:** Resolution of fungal infection; symptomatic improvement

## Tizanidine hydrochloride

(tye-ZAN-ih-deen)
**Pregnancy Category:** C
Zanaflex **(Rx)**
**Classification:** Skeletal muscle relaxant, centrally-acting

See also *Skeletal Muscle Relaxants, Centrally Acting.*

**Action/Kinetics:** Acts on central α-2 adrenergic receptors; reduces spasticity by increasing presynaptic inhibition of motor neurons. Greatest effects are on polysynaptic pathways. **Peak effect:** 1–2 hr. **Duration:** 3–6 hr. Extensive first pass metabolism. **t½:** About 2.5 hr. Excreted in urine and feces. Elderly clear drug more slowly.

**Uses:** Acute and intermittent management of muscle spasticity.

**Contraindications:** Use with α-2-adrenergic agonists.

**Special Concerns:** Use with caution in renal impairment, in elderly and during laction. Use with extreme caution in hepatic insufficiency. Safety and efficacy have not been determined in children.

**Side Effects:** *Note:* Side effects listed are those with a frequency of 0.1% or greater. *CV:* Hypotension, vasodilation, postural hypotension, syncope, migraine, arrhythmia. *GI:* Hepatotoxicity, dry mouth, constipation, pharyngitis, vomiting, abdominal pain, diarrhea, dyspepsia, dysphagia, cholelithiasis, fecal impaction, flatulence, *GI hemorrhage* hepatitis, melena. *CNS:* Dizziness, dyskinesia, nervousness, somnolence, sedation, hallucinations, psychotic-like symptoms, depression, anxiety, paresthesia, tremor, emotional lability, seizures, paralysis, abnormal thinking, vertigo, abnormal dreams, agitation, depersonalization, euphoria, stupor, dysautonomia, neuralgia. *GU:* Urinary frequency, UTI, urinary urgency, cystitis, menorrhagia, pyelonephritis, urinary retention, kidney calculus, enlarged uterine fibroids, vaginal moniliasis, vaginitis. *Hematologic:* Ecchymosis, anemia, leukopenia, leukocytosis. *Musculoskeletal:* Myasthenia, back pain, pathological fracture, arthralgia, arthritis, bursitis. *Respiratory:* Sinusitis, pneumonia, bronchitis, rhinitis. *Dermatologic:* Rash, sweating, skin ulcer, pruritus, dry skin, acne, alopecia, urticaria. *Body as a whole:* Flu syndrome, weight loss, infection, *sepsis, cellulitis, death,* allergic reaction, moniliasis, malaise, asthenia, fever, abscess, edema. *Ophthalmic:* Glaucoma, amblyopia, conjunctivitis, eye pain, optic neuritis, retinal hemorrhage, visual field defect. *Otic:* Ear pain, tinnitus, deafness, otitis media. *Miscellaneous:* Speech disorder.

**Laboratory Test Alterations:** ↑ ALT. Abnormal LFTs. Hypercholesterolemia, hyperlipemia, hypothyroidism, adrenal cortical insufficiency, hyperglycemia, hypokalemia, hyponatremia, hypoproteinemia.

**Drug Interactions**

*Alcohol /* ↑ Side effects of tizanidine; additive CNS depressant effects

*Alpha-2-Adrenergic agonists /* Additive hypotensive effects

*Oral contraceptives /* ↓ Clearance of tizanidine

**Dosage** ────────────
• **Tablets**
*Muscle spasticity.*
**Initial:** 4 mg; **then,** increase dose gradually in 2 to 4 mg steps to optimum effect. Dose can be repeated at 6–8-hr intervals, to maximum of 3 doses/24 hr, not to exceed 36 mg/day. There is no experience with repeated, single, daytime doses greater than 12 mg or total daily doses of 36 mg or more.

## NURSING CONSIDERATIONS

See also *Nursing Considerations* for *Skeletal Muscle Relaxants, Centrally Acting.*
**Assessment:** Monitor VS, liver, and renal function studies.
**Client/Family Teaching**
1. Do not perform activities that require mental alertness; drug causes sedation.
2. Report if hallucinations or delusions experienced.
3. May cause orthostatic hypotension; avoid sudden changes in position.
4. Avoid alcohol and any other CNS depressants.
**Outcomes/Evaluate:** ↓ Spasticity; ↑ muscle relaxation

# Tobramycin sulfate
(toe-brah-**MY**-sin)
**Pregnancy Category:** D (B for ophthalmic use)
**Inhalation:**Tobi, **Parenteral:** Nebcin, **Ophthalmic:** AKTob Ophthalmic

Solution, Tobrex Ophthalmic Ointment, Tobrex Ophthalmic Solution
**(Rx)**
**Classification:** Antibiotic, aminoglycoside

────────────

See also *Aminoglycosides.*
**Action/Kinetics:** Similar to gentamicin and can be used concurrently with carbenicillin. **Therapeutic serum levels: IM,** 4–8 mcg/mL. **t½:** 2–2.5 hr. **Toxic serum levels:** > 12 mcg/mL (peak) and > 2 mcg/mL (trough).
**Uses: Systemic:** Complicated and recurrent UTIs due to *Pseudomonas aeruginosa, Proteus, Escherichia coli, Klebsiella, Enterobacter, Serratia, Staphylococcus aureus, Citrobacter,* and *Providencia.* Lower respiratory tract infections due to *P. aeruginosa, Klebsiella, Enterobacter, E. coli, Serratia,* and *S. aureus.* Intra-abdominal infections (including peritonitis) due to *E. coli, Klebsiella,* and *Enterobacter.* Septicemia in neonates, children, and adults due to *P. aeruginosa, E. coli,* and *Klebsiella.* Skin, bone, and skin structure infections due to *P. aeruginosa, Proteus, E. coli, Klebsiella, Enterobacter,* and *S. aureus.* Serious CNS infections, including meningitis. Can be used with penicillins or cephalosporins in serious infections when results of susceptibility testing are not yet known.
**Ophthalmic:** Treat superficial ocular infections due to *Staphylococcus, S. aureus, Streptococcus, S. pneumoniae,* beta-hemolytic streptococci, *Corynebacterium, E. coli, Haemophilus aegyptius, H. ducreyi, H. influenzae, H. parainfluenzae, Klebsiella pneumoniae, Neisseria, N. gonorrhoeae, Proteus, Acinetobacter calcoaceticus, Enterobacter, Enterobacter aerogenes, Serratia marcescens, Moraxella, Pseudomonas aeruginosa,* and *Vibrio.*
**Inhalation:** Management of cystic fibrosis in clients with *P. aeruginosa.*
**Contraindications:** Ophthalmically to treat dendritic keratitis, vaccinia,

varicella, fungal or mycobacterial eye infections, after removal of a corneal foreign body. Lactation.

**Special Concerns:** Use with caution in premature infants and neonates. Ophthalmic ointment may retard corneal epithelial healing.

**Additional Side Effects:** *Ophthalmic use:* Transient irritation, burning, stinging, itching, inflammation, angioneurotic edema, urticaria, vesicular and maculopapular dermatitis.

**OD** **Overdose Management:** *Symptoms (Ophthalmic Use):* Edema, lid itching, punctate keratitis, erythema, lacrimation.

**Additional Drug Interactions:** With carbenicillin or ticarcillin, tobramycin may have an increased effect when used for *Pseudomonas* infections.

**Dosage** ————————

• **IM, IV**
*Non-life-threatening serious infections.*
**Adults:** 3 mg/kg/day in three equally divided doses q 8 hr.
*Life-threatening infections.*
Up to 5 mg/kg/day in three or four equal doses. **Pediatric:** Either 2–2.5 mg/kg q 8 hr or 1.5–1.9 mg/kg q 6 hr; **neonates 1 week of age or less:** up to 4 mg/kg/day in two equal doses q 12 hr.
*Impaired renal function.*
**Initially:** 1 mg/kg; **then,** maintenance dose calculated according to information supplied by manufacturer.

• **Ophthalmic Ointment (0.3%)**
*Acute infections.*
0.5-in. ribbon q 3–4 hr until improvement is noted.
*Mild to moderate infections.*
0.5-in. ribbon b.i.d.–t.i.d.

• **Ophthalmic Solution (0.3%)**
*Acute infections.*
**Initial:** 1–2 gtt q 15–30 min until improvement noted; **then,** reduce dosage gradually.
*Moderate infections.*
1–2 gtt 2–6 times/day.

• **Inhalation Solution**

*Pseudomonas aeruginosa in cystic fibrosis.*
Dose using a nebulizer b.i.d. for 10–15 min in cycles of 28 days on and then 28 days off.

## NURSING CONSIDERATIONS

See also *Nursing Considerations* for *Aminoglycosides.*
**Administration/Storage**
**IV** 1. Prepare IV solution by diluting calculated dose of tobramycin with 50–100 mL of dextrose or saline solution and infuse over 30–60 min.
2. Use proportionately less diluent for children than for adults.
3. Do not mix with other drugs for parenteral administration.
4. Discard solution of drug containing up to 1 mg/mL after 24 hr at room temperature.
5. Store drug at room temperature no longer than 2 years.
**Client/Family Teaching**
1. Drink plenty of fluids (2–3 L/day) during parenteral drug therapy.
2. With eye infections, avoid wearing contact lenses until infection is cleared and provider approves.
3. Report if symptoms do not improve or if they worsen after 3 days of therapy.
**Outcomes/Evaluate**
• Negative cultures; resolution of infection
• Therapeutic drug levels (peak: 4–10 mcg/mL; trough: 1–2 mcg/mL)

# Tocainide hydrochloride
(toe-**KAY**-nyd)
**Pregnancy Category:** C
Tonocard **(Rx)**
**Classification:** Antiarrhythmic, class IB

See also *Antiarrhythmic Agents.*
**Action/Kinetics:** Similar to lidocaine. Decreases the excitability of cells in the myocardium by decreasing sodium and potassium conductance. Increases pulmonary and aortic arterial pressure and slightly increases peripheral resistance. Effective in both digitalized and nondigitalized clients. **Peak plasma levels:** 0.5–2 hr. **t½:** 11–15 hr. **Therapeutic**

**serum levels:** 4–10 mcg/mL. **Duration:** 8 hr. Approximately 10% is bound to plasma protein. From 28% to 55% is excreted unchanged in the urine. Alkalinization decreases the excretion of the drug although acidification does not produce any changes in excretion.

**Uses:** Life-threatening ventricular arrhythmias, including ventricular tachycardia. Has not been shown to improve survival in clients with ventricular arrhythmias. *Investigational:* Myotonic dystrophy, trigeminal neuralgia.

**Contraindications:** Allergy to amide-type local anesthetics, second- or third-degree AV block in the absence of artificial ventricular pacemaker. Lactation.

**Special Concerns:** Increased risk of death when used in those with non-life-threatening cardiac arrhythmias. Safety and efficacy have not been established in children. Use with caution in clients with impaired renal or hepatic function (dose may have to be decreased). Geriatric clients may have an increased risk of dizziness and hypotension; the dose may have to be reduced in these clients due to age-related impaired renal function.

**Side Effects:** *CV: Increased arrhythmias,* increased ventricular rate (when given for atrial flutter or fibrillation), CHF, tachycardia, hypotension, *conduction disturbances,* bradycardia, chest pain, LV failure, palpitations. *CNS:* Dizziness, vertigo, headache, tremors, confusion, disorientation, hallucinations, ataxia, paresthesias, numbness, nervousness, altered mood, anxiety, incoordination, walking disturbances. *GI:* N&V, anorexia, diarrhea. *Respiratory: Pulmonary fibrosis, fibrosing alveolitis,* interstitial pneumonitis, *pulmonary edema,* pneumonia. *Hematologic:* Leukopenia, *agranulocytosis,* hypoplastic anemia, *aplastic anemia,* bone marrow depression, neutropenia, *thrombocytopenia and sequelae as septicemia and septic shock. Musculoskeletal:* Arthritis, arthralgia, myalgia.

*Dermatologic:* Rash, skin lesion, diaphoresis. *Other:* Blurred vision, visual disturbances, nystagmus, tinnitus, hearing loss, lupus-like syndrome.

**Laboratory Test Alterations:** Abnormal LFTs (esp. in early therapy). ↑ ANA.

**OD** **Overdose Management:** *Symptoms:* Initially are CNS symptoms including tremor (see above). GI symptoms may follow (see above). *Treatment:* Gastric lavage and activated charcoal may be useful. In the event of respiratory depression or arrest or seizures, maintain airway and provide artificial ventilation. An IV anticonvulsant (e.g., diazepam, thiopental, thiamylal, pentobarbital, secobarbital) may be required if seizures are persistent.

**Drug Interactions**
*Cimetidine* / ↓ Bioavailability of tocainide
*Metoprolol* / Additive effects on wedge pressure and cardiac index
*Rifampin* / ↓ Bioavailability of tocainide

**Dosage** ———————————
• **Tablets**
  *Antiarrhythmic.*
**Adults, individualized, initial:** 400 mg q 8 hr, up to a maximum of 2,400 mg/day; **maintenance:** 1,200–1,800 mg/day in divided doses. Total daily dose of 1,200 mg may be adequate in clients with liver or kidney disease.
  *Myotonic dystrophy.*
800–1,200 mg/day.
  *Trigeminal neuralgia.*
20 mg/kg/day in three divided doses.

## NURSING CONSIDERATIONS

See also *Nursing Considerations* for *Antiarrhythmic Agents.*
**Assessment**
1. Document indications for therapy, type, onset, and characteristics of symptoms.
2. Monitor ECG, CBC, electrolytes, liver and renal function studies; correct potassium deficits.

---

3. Document cardiac and pulmonary assessment findings.

**Client/Family Teaching**

1. Take with food to minimize GI upset.

2. Do not drive or operate machinery until drug effects are realized; may cause drowsiness or dizziness.

3. Report any abnormal bruising, bleeding, fever, sore throat, or chills (S&S of blood dyscrasia).

4. Pulmonary symptoms such as wheezing, coughing, or dyspnea should be reported immediately; may indicate pulmonary fibrosis.

**Outcomes/Evaluate**

• Control of lethal ventricular arrhythmias

• ↓ Muscle spasm and pain

• Therapeutic drug levels (4–10 mcg/mL)

# Tolazamide

(toll-**AZ**-ah-myd)
**Pregnancy Category:** C
Tolinase **(Rx)**
**Classification:** Sulfonylurea, first-generation

See also *Antidiabetic Agents, Hypoglycemic Agents.*

**Action/Kinetics:** Effective in some with a history of coma or ketoacidosis; may be effective in clients who do not respond well to other oral antidiabetics. Use with insulin is not recommended for maintenance. **Onset:** 4–6 hr. **t½:** 7 hr. **Time to peak levels:** 3–4 hr. **Duration:** 12–24 hr. Metabolized in liver to metabolites with minor hypoglycemic activity. Excreted through the kidneys (85%) and feces (7%).

**Additional Contraindications:** Renal glycosuria.

**Additional Drug Interactions:** Concomitant use of alcohol and tolazamide may → photosensitivity.

**Dosage**

• **Tablets**

*Diabetes.*

**Adults, initial:** 100 mg/day if fasting blood sugar is less than 200 mg/100 mL, or 250 mg/day if fasting blood sugar is greater than 200

mg/100 mL. Adjust dose to response, not to exceed 1 g/day. If more than 500 mg/day is required, it should be given in two divided doses, usually before the morning and evening meals. **Elderly, malnourished, underweight clients or those not eating properly:** 100 mg once daily with breakfast, adjusting dose by increments of 50 mg/day each week. Doses greater than 1 g/day will probably not improve control.

## NURSING CONSIDERATIONS

See also *Nursing Considerations* for *Antidiabetic Agents, Hypoglycemic Agents.*

**Client/Family Teaching**

1. Take 30 min before meals for best results; do not take if vomiting or unable to eat.

2. Monitor fingersticks and maintain a record (different times on different days) for provider review.

3. Avoid alcohol as a disulfiram-like reaction may occur.

4. Use caution; may cause dizziness.

5. Use a nonhormonal form of contraception.

6. Wear protective clothing and a sunscreen to prevent a photosensitivity reaction.

**Outcomes/Evaluate:** Normalization of serum glucose levels

# Tolbutamide

(toll-**BYOU**-tah-myd)
**Pregnancy Category:** C
APO-Tolbutamide ✹, Novo-Butamide ✹, Orinase **(Rx)**

# Tolbutamide sodium

(toll-**BYOU**-tah-myd)
**Pregnancy Category:** C
Orinase Diagnostic **(Rx)**
**Classification:** Sulfonylurea, first-generation

See also *Antidiabetic Agents, Hypoglycemic Agents.*

**Action/Kinetics: Onset:** 1 hr. **t½:** 4.5–6.5 hr. **Time to peak levels:** 3–4 hr. **Duration:** 6–12 hr. Changed in liver to inactive metabolites. Excreted through the kidney (75%) and feces (9%).

**Additional Uses:** Most useful for clients with poor general physical status who should receive a short-acting compound.

Tolbutamide sodium is used to diagnose pancreatic islet cell tumors. It causes blood glucose, in the presence of a tumor, to drop quickly after IV administration and remain low for 3 hr.

**Additional Side Effects:** Melena (dark, bloody stools) in some clients with a history of peptic ulcer. Relapse or secondary failure may occur a few months after therapy has been started. May cause hyponatremia and a mild goiter.

**Additional Drug Interactions**
*Alcohol* / Photosensitivity reactions
*Sulfinpyrazone* / ↑ Effect of tolbutamide due to ↓ breakdown by liver

**Dosage** ――――――――――
• **Tablets**
  *Diabetes mellitus.*
**Adults, initial:** 0.25–3 g/day (usually 1–2 g). Adjust dosage depending on response. **Usual maintenance:** 0.25–2 g/day). A daily dose greater than 2 g is rarely needed; maximum daily dose should not exceed 3 g.

## NURSING CONSIDERATIONS

See also *Nursing Considerations* for *Antidiabetic Agents, Oral.*
**Client/Family Teaching**
1. Take 30 min before meals for best results. May take as a single dose before breakfast or as divided doses before the morning and evening meals. Divided doses may improve GI tolerance.
2. Maintain log of blood sugar levels for provider review.
3. Drug may cause dizziness.
4. Avoid alcohol and any OTC meds without approval.
5. May cause a photosensitivity reaction; wear protective clothing and sunscreen when exposed.
6. Use a nonhormonal form of birth control.

**Outcomes/Evaluate**
• Serum glucose/HbA1C levels with-in desired range
• Pancreatic islet cell tumor presence

# Tolmetin sodium

(**TOLL**-met-in)
**Pregnancy Category:** C
Novo-Tolmetin ✦, Tolectin ✦, Tolectin 200, Tolectin 600, Tolectin DS **(Rx)**
**Classification:** Nonsteroidal, anti-inflammatory, analgesic

See also *Nonsteroidal Anti-Inflammatory Drugs.*

**Action/Kinetics: Peak plasma levels:** 30–60 min. **t½:** 1 hr. **Therapeutic plasma levels:** 40 mcg/mL. **Onset, anti-inflammatory effect:** within 1 week; **duration, anti-inflammatory effect:** 1–2 weeks. Inactivated in liver and excreted in urine.

**Uses:** Acute and chronic treatment of rheumatoid arthritis and osteoarthritis. Juvenile rheumatoid arthritis. *Investigational:* Sunburn.

**Special Concerns:** Use with caution during lactation. Dosage has not been determined in children less than 2 years of age.

**Laboratory Test Alterations:** Tolmetin metabolites give a false + test for proteinuria using sulfosalicylic acid.

**Dosage** ――――――――――
• **Capsules, Tablets**
  *Rheumatoid arthritis, osteoarthritis.*
**Adults:** 400 mg t.i.d. (one dose on arising and one at bedtime); adjust dosage according to client response. **Maintenance:** *rheumatoid arthritis,* 600–1,800 mg/day in three to four divided doses; *osteoarthritis,* 600–1,600 mg/day in three to four divided doses. Doses larger than 1,800 mg/day for rheumatoid arthritis and osteoarthritis are not recommended.
  *Juvenile rheumatoid arthritis.*
**2 years and older, initial:** 20 mg/kg/day in three to four divided doses to start; **then,** 15–30 mg/kg/day. Doses higher than 30 mg/kg/day

**T**

――――――――――――――――――――――――

are not recommended. Beneficial effects may not be observed for several days to a week.

## NURSING CONSIDERATIONS

See also *Nursing Considerations* for *Nonsteroidal Anti-Inflammatory Drugs*.

**Assessment**
1. Document indications for therapy; note joint pain, deformity, swelling, inflammation, and ROM.
2. Monitor CBC and renal function studies.

**Client/Family Teaching**
1. Doses should be spaced so that one dose is taken in the morning on arising, one during the day, and one at bedtime.
2. May administer with meals, milk, a full glass of water, or antacids if gastric irritation occurs. Never administer with sodium bicarbonate. Elderly clients are particularly susceptible to gastric irritation and should take with milk, meals, or an antacid.
3. Assess response; drug may cause drowsiness or dizziness.
4. Report any unusual bruising or bleeding or evidence of edema.
5. It may take several weeks before effects are evident.
6. Avoid alcohol and any OTC meds without approval.
7. Report for labs to evaluate renal function and hematologic parameters.

**Outcomes/Evaluate:** ↓ Joint pain and inflammation; ↑ mobility

---

# Tolnaftate
(toll-**NAF**-tayt)
Aftate for Athlete's Foot, Aftate for Jock Itch, Genaspor, NP-27, Pitrex ✿, Quinsana Plus, Tinactin, Tinactin for Jock Itch, Ting, Zeasorb-AF **(OTC)**
**Classification:** Topical antifungal

See also *Anti-Infectives*.
**Action/Kinetics:** Exact mechanism not known; is thought to stunt mycelial growth causing a fungicidal effect.
**Uses:** Tinea pedis, tinea cruris, tinea corporis, and tinea versicolor. Fungal infections of moist skin areas.

**Contraindications:** Scalp and nail infections. Avoid getting into eyes. Use in children less than 2 years of age.
**Side Effects:** Mild skin irritation.

**Dosage**
• **Topical: Aerosol Powder, Aerosol Solution, Cream, Ointment, Powder, Solution, Spray Solution**
Apply b.i.d. for 2–3 weeks although treatment for 4–6 weeks may be necessary in some instances.

## NURSING CONSIDERATIONS

See also *General Nursing Considerations for All Anti-Infectives*.
**Assessment**
1. Inspect source of infection; document presentation because the choice of vehicle is important for effective therapy.
• Powders are used in mild conditions as adjunctive therapy.
• For primary therapy and prophylaxis, creams, liquids, or ointments are used, especially if the area is moist.
• Liquids and solutions are used if the area is hairy.
2. Assess cultures; use concomitant therapy if bacterial or *Candida* infections are also present.
**Client/Family Teaching**
1. Skin should be thoroughly cleaned and dried before the medication is applied.
2. Use care; do not rub medication into or near the eye.
3. Report any bothersome side effects; local relief of symptoms should be evident within the first 24–48 hr. Report if no improvement noted within 10 days.
4. Continue to use as directed, despite improvement of symptoms. Takes 2–6 weeks to clear infection.
**Outcomes/Evaluate**
• Symptomatic relief; skin healing
• Eradication of fungal infection

---

# Topiramate
(toh-**PYRE**-ah-mayt)
**Pregnancy Category:** C
Topamax **(Rx)**

**Classification:** Anticonvulsant, miscellaneous

See also *Anticonvulsants.*

**Action/Kinetics:** Precise mechanism not known. The following effects may contribute to the anticonvulsant activity. (1) Action potentials seen repetitively by sustained depolarization of neurons are blocked in a time-dependent manner, suggesting an effect to block sodium channels. (2) Increases the frequency at which GABA activates GABA$_A$ receptors, thus enhancing the ability of GABA to cause a flux of chloride ions into neurons (i.e., enhanced effect of the inhibitory transmitter, GABA$_A$). (3) Antagonizes the ability of kainate to activate the kainate/AMPA subtype of excitatory amino acid aspartate, thus reducing the excitatory effect. Rapidly absorbed; **peak plasma levels:** About 2 hr. **t½, elimination:** 21 hr. Steady state is reached in about 4 days in those with normal renal function. Excreted mostly unchanged in the urine.

**Uses:** Adjunct to treat partial onset seizures in adults.

**Contraindications:** Lactation.

**Special Concerns:** Use with caution in impaired hepatic and renal function. Safety and efficacy have not been determined in children.

**Side Effects:** *Note:* Side effects with an incidence of 0.1% or greater are listed. *CNS:* Psychomotor slowing, including difficulty with concentration and speech or language problems. Somnolence, fatigue, dizziness, ataxia, nystagmus, paresthesia, nervousness, difficulty with memory, tremor, confusion, depression, abnormal coordination, agitation, mood problems, aggressive reaction, hypoesthesia, apathy, emotional lability, depersonalization, hypokinesia, vertigo, stupor, *clonic/tonic seizures,* hyperkinesia, hypertonia, insomnia, personality disorder, impotence, hallucinations, euphoria, psychosis, decreased libido, *suicide attempt,* hyporeflexia, neuropathy, migraine, apraxia, hyperesthesia, dyskinesia, hyperreflexia, dysphonia, scotoma, dystonia, coma, encephalopathy, upper motor neuron lesion, paranoid reaction, delusion, paranoia, delirium, abnormal dreaming, neuroses. *GI:* Nausea, dyspepsia, anorexia, abdominal pain, constipation, dry mouth, gingivitis, halitosis, diarrhea, vomiting, fecal incontinence, flatulence, gastroenteritis, gum hyperplasia, hemorrhoids, increased appetite, tooth caries, stomatitis, dysphagia, melena, gastritis, increased saliva, hiccough, gastroesophageal reflux, tongue edema, esophagitis, gall bladder disorder, gingival bleeding. *CV:* Palpitation, hypertension, hypotension, postural hypotension, AV block, bradycardia, bundle branch block, angina pectoris, vasodilation. *Body as a whole:* Asthenia, back pain, chest pain, flu-like symptoms, leg pain, hot flashes, body odor, edema, rigors, fever, malaise, syncope, enlarged abdomen. *Respiratory:* URI, pharyngitis, sinusitis, dyspnea, coughing, bronchitis, asthma, ***bronchospasm, pulmonary embolism.*** *Dermatologic:* Acne, alopecia, dermatitis, nail disorder, folliculitis, dry skin, urticaria, skin discoloration, eczema, photosensitivity reaction, erythematous rash, seborrhea, decreased sweating, abnormal hair texture, facial edema. *GU:* Breast pain, renal stone formation, dysmenorrhea, menstrual disorder, hematuria, intermenstrual bleeding, leukorrhea, menorrhagia, vaginitis, amenorrhea, UTI, micturition frequency, urinary incontinence, dysuria, renal calculus, ejaculation disorder, breast discharge, urinary retention, renal pain, nocturia, albuminuria, polyuria, oliguria. *Musculoskeletal:* Arthralgia, muscle weakness, arthrosis, osteoporosis, myalgia, leg cramps. *Metabolic:* Increased weight, decreased weight, dehydration, xeropthalmia. *Hematologic:* Anemia, leukopenia, lymphadenopathy, eosinophilia, lymphopenia, granulocytopenia, lymphocytosis, thrombocytothemia, purpura, thrombocytopenia. *Dermatologic:* Rash, pruritus, increased sweating, flushing. *Ophthalmic:* Diplopia, abnormal vision, eye pain, conjunctivitis, abnormal accommodation, photophobia, abnormal lacrimation, strabismus, color blindness, myopia, mydriasis, ptosis, visual field defect. *Miscellaneous:* Decreased hearing, epistaxis, taste perversion, tinnitus, taste loss, parosmia, goiter, basal cell carcinoma.

**Laboratory Test Alterations:** ↑ AST, ALT, alkaline phosphatase, creatinine. Hypokalemia, hypocalcemia, hyperlipemia, acidosis, hyperglycemia, hyperchloremia.

**OD** **Overdose Management:** *Symptoms:* See side effects. *Treatment:* Gastric lavage or induction of emesis if ingestion is recent. Supportive treatment. Hemodialysis.

**Drug Interactions**
*Alcohol* / CNS depression and cognitive and neuropsychiatric side effects
*Carbamazepine* / ↓ Plasma levels of topiramate
*Carbonic anhydrase inhibitors* / ↑ Risk of renal stone formation
*CNS depressants* / CNS depression and cognitive and neuropsychiatric side effects
*Oral contraceptives* / ↓ Effect of oral contraceptives
*Phenytoin* / ↓ Plasma levels of topiramate and ↑ plasma levels of phenytoin
*Valproic acid* / ↓ Plasma levels of both topiramate and valproic acid

**Dosage**
• **Tablets**
*Adjunctive therapy for treatment of partial onset seizures.*
**Initial:** 50 mg/day; **then,** titrate to an effective dose of 400 mg/day in 2 divided doses. Titrate by adding 50 mg each week for eight weeks, until the dose is 400 mg/day. Doses greater than 400 mg/day have not been shown to improve the response. If $C_{CR}$ < 70 mL/1.73 m², use one half of the usual adult dose.

**NURSING CONSIDERATIONS**

See also *Nursing Considerations* for Anticonvulsant Drugs.

**Assessment**
1. Document age at onset, cause, type, frequency, and characteristics of seizures.
2. Monitor CBC, liver and renal function studies; reduce dose with renal dysfunction.
3. List drugs currently prescribed to ensure none interact or lose effectiveness; MAO inhibitors may promote kidney stones.
4. Document baseline psychomotor and mental status; assess for psychomotor slowing, speech or expression problems, difficulty concentrating, fatigue, or sleepiness.

**Client/Family Teaching**
1. Take exactly as prescribed. Due to the bitter taste of the drug, do not break tablets. Can be taken without regard for meals.
2. Distinguish if drug affects motor or mental capacity before driving or performing activities that require mental alertness; may cause dizziness, confusion, drowsiness, and altered concentration.
3. Increase fluid intake to decrease substance concentration as drug may precipitate renal stone formation by increasing urinary pH and reducing urinary citrate excretion.
4. Use reliable, nonhormonal form of birth control; drug may compromise efficacy of PO contraceptives.
5. Do not stop drug abruptly due to risk of increased seizure frequency.
6. Review list of side effects, noting those that require immediate medical attention.

**Outcomes/Evaluate:**    Adjunctive therapy in the control of partial onset seizures.

# Topotecan hydrochloride
(toh-poh-**TEE**-kan)
**Pregnancy Category:** D
Hycamtin **(Rx)**
**Classification:** Antineoplastic, hormone

See also *Antineoplastic Agents.*

**Action/Kinetics:** An inhibitor of topoisomerase I. Topoisomerase I relieves torsional strain in DNA by causing reversible single-strand breaks. Topotecan binds to the topoisomerase I-DNA complex and prevents religation of single-strand breaks. Cytotoxicity thought to be caused by double-strand DNA damage produced during DNA synthesis when replication enzymes interact with the ternary complex formed by topotecan, topoisomerase I, and DNA. Hydrolyzed to the active lactone form of the drug. About 30% of the drug is excreted in the urine. **t½, terminal:** 2 to 3 hr.

**Uses:** Metastatic cancer of the ovary after failure of initial or subsequent chemotherapy.

**Contraindications:** Pregnancy, lactation. Severe bone marrow depression, including those with baseline neutrophil counts less than 1,500 cells/mm³.

**Special Concerns:** Safety and efficacy have not been determined in children.

**Side Effects:** *Hematologic:* Bone marrow suppression, including neutropenia, thrombocytopenia, anemia, sepsis or fever/infection with grade 4 neutropenia, platelet or RBC infusions. *GI:* N&V, abdominal pain, constipation, diarrhea, intestinal obstruction, stomatitis. *CNS:* Asthenia, headache, pain, paresthesias. *Musculoskeletal:* Arthralgia, myalgia. *Body as a whole:* Anorexia, fatigue, malaise. *Respiratory:* Dyspnea. *Dermatologic:* Total alopecia.

**Laboratory Test Alterations:** ↑ AST, ALT, bilirubin.

**Drug Interactions**
*Cisplatin* / More severe myelosuppression
*G-CSF* / Prolonged duration of neutropenia

**Dosage**
- **IV Infusion**
  *Metastatic ovarian cancer.*
  **Adults:** 1.5 mg/m² by IV infusion over 30 min daily for 5 consecutive days, starting on day 1 of a 21-day course of therapy. A minimum of four courses is recommended. If severe neutropenia occurs, reduce the dose by 0.25 mg/m² for subsequent courses. Also, for severe neutropenia, G-CSF may be given following the subsequent course and before dosage reduction starting from day 6 of the course (i.e., 24 hr after completion of topotecan administration).

  Reduce the dose to 0.75 mg/m² for clients with a C$_{CR}$ of 20–39 mL/min. No dosage reduction is required if the C$_{CR}$ is 40–60 mL/min.

## NURSING CONSIDERATIONS

See also *Nursing Considerations* for *Antineoplastic Agents.*

**Administration/Storage**

**IV** 1. To begin therapy, clients must have a baseline neutrophil count greater than 1,500 cells/mm³, a platelet count greater than 100,000 cells/mm³, and a hemoglobin level of 9 mg/dL or higher. Do not retreat until neutrophils are greater than 1,000 cells/mm³, platelets are greater than 100,000 cells/mm³, and hemoglobin levels are 9 mg/dL or greater.

2. Reconstitute the 4-mg topotecan vial with 4 mL of sterile water for injection. This may then be further diluted either with 0.9% NaCl or 5% dextrose IV infusion and administered over 30 min.

3. Reconstituted vials diluted for infusion are stable at controlled room temperature and ambient lighting conditions for 24 hr.

4. Store vials in their original carton, protected from light, at controlled room temperature of 20°C–25°C (68°F–77°F).

**Assessment**

1. Document indications for therapy, other agents/therapies trialed, and when administered.

2. Monitor CBC and renal function studies; reduce dose with C$_{CR}$ of 20–39 mL/m² . Ensure baseline neutrophil count above 1,500 cells/mm³ and platelet count at 100,000/mm³. Do not readminister until neutrophils

are above 1,000, platelets are 100,000 cells/mm³, and hemoglobin levels are at least 9 mg/dL. Drug causes neutropenia and anemia. Nadir: 15 days.

**Outcomes/Evaluate:** Control of malignant cell proliferation in metastatic ovarian cancer

---

# Toremifene citrate

(**TOR**-em-ih-feen)
**Pregnancy Category:** D
Fareston **(Rx)**
**Classification:** Antineoplastic, hormone

See also *Antineoplastic Agents*.

**Action/Kinetics:** Antiestrogen that binds to estrogen receptors and may cause estrogenic, antiestrogenic, or both effects, depending on duration of treatment, genders, and endpoint/target organ selected. Antitumor effect is likely due to antiestrogenic effect, i.e., competes for estrogen at receptor and blocks growth-stimulating effects of estrogen in tumor. Well absorbed from GI tract. **Peak plasma levels:** 3 hr. t½, **distribution:** About 4 hr. t½, **elimination:** About 5 days. Extensively metabolized in liver and mainly excreted in feces.

**Uses:** Metastatic breast cancer in postmenopausal women with positive estrogen-receptor (ER) or ER unknown tumors.

**Contraindications:** Use with history of thromboembolic disease.

**Special Concerns:** Hypercalcemia and tumor flare in some breast cancer clients with bone metastases during first weeks of treatment. Use with caution during lactation. No indication for use in pediatric clients.

**Side Effects:** *CV: **Cardiac failure, MI, pulmonary embolism, CVA,*** TIA. *GI:* Constipation, nausea. *Hematologic:* Leukopenia, thrombocytopenia. *Dermatologic:* Skin discoloration, dermatitis, alopecia, pruritus. *Ophthalmic:* Cataracts, dry eyes, abnormal visual fields, corneal keratopathy, glaucoma, reversible corneal opacity. *CNS:* Tremor, vertigo, depression. *Miscellaneous:* Dyspnea, paresis, anorexia, asthenia, jaundice, rigors, vaginal bleeding.

**Laboratory Test Alterations:** ↑ AST, alkaline phosphatase, bilirubin. Hypercalcemia.

**Drug Interactions**

*Carbamazepine* / ↓ Blood levels of toremifene due to ↑ breakdown in liver

*Clonazepam* / ↓ Blood levels of toremifene due to ↑ breakdown in liver

*Erythromycin* / Inhibition of breakdown of toremifene

*Ketoconazole* / Inhibition of breakdown of toremifene

*Macrolide antibiotics* / Inhibition of breakdown of toremifene

*Phenobarbital* / ↓ Blood levels of toremifene due to ↑ breakdown in liver

*Phenytoin* / ↓ Blood levels of toremifene due to ↑ breakdown in liver

*Warfarin* / ↑ PT

**Dosage** ⸺⸺⸺⸺⸺

• **Tablets**

*Metastatic breast cancer.*

**Adults:** 60 mg once daily. Continue until disease progression is observed.

## NURSING CONSIDERATIONS

See also *Nursing Considerations* for *Antineoplastic Agents*.

**Assessment**

1. Document indications for therapy, characteristics of symptoms, other agents trialed and outcome.

2. Note any history or evidence of thromboembolic disorders.

3. Monitor CBC, calcium, and LFTs.

**Client/Family Teaching**

1. Take once daily as directed.

2. Report any unusual vaginal bleeding.

3. May experience "tumor flare," syndrome of diffuse musculoskeletal pain and erythema with increased size of tumor lesions that regress later; usually accompanied by hypercalcemia. Must stop drug if hypercalcemia occurs.

**Outcomes/Evaluate:** Control of malignant cell proliferation

# Torsemide

(**TOR**-seh-myd)
**Pregnancy Category:** B
Demadex **(Rx)**
**Classification:** Loop diuretic

See also *Diuretics, Loop.*
**Action/Kinetics: Onset, IV:** Within 10 min; **PO:** within 60 min. **Peak effect, IV:** Within 60 min; **PO:** 60–120 min. **Duration:** 6–8 hr. **t½:** 210 min. Metabolized by the liver and excreted through the urine. Food delays the time to peak effect by about 30 min, but the overall bioavailability and the diuretic activity are not affected.
**Uses:** Congestive heart failure, acute or chronic renal failure, hepatic cirrhosis, hypertension.
**Contraindications:** Lactation.
**Special Concerns:** Clients sensitive to sulfonamides may show allergic reactions to torsemide. Safety and efficacy in children have not been determined.
**Side Effects:** *CNS:* Headache, dizziness, asthenia, insomnia, nervousness, syncope. *GI:* Diarrhea, constipation, nausea, dyspepsia, edema, *GI hemorrhage,* rectal bleeding. *CV:* ECG abnormality, chest pain, atrial fibrillation, hypotension, *ventricular tachycardia,* shunt thrombosis. *Respiratory:* Rhinitis, increase in cough. *Musculoskeletal:* Arthralgia, myalgia. *Miscellaneous:* Sore throat, excessive urination, rash.
**Laboratory Test Alterations:** Hyperglycemia, hyperuricemia, hypokalemia, hypovolemia.

## Dosage
• **Tablets, IV**
*Congestive heart failure.*
**Adults, initial:** 10 or 20 mg once daily.
*Chronic renal failure.*
**Adults, initial:** 20 mg once daily.
*Hepatic cirrhosis.*
**Adults, initial:** 5 or 10 mg once daily given with an aldosterone antagonist or a potassium-sparing diuretic.
*Hypertension.*

**Adults, initial:** 5 mg once daily. If this dose does not lead to an adequate decrease in BP within 4–6 weeks, the dose may be increased to 10 mg once daily. If the 10-mg dose is not adequate, an additional antihypertensive agent is added to the treatment regimen.

## NURSING CONSIDERATIONS

See also *Nursing Considerations* for *Diuretics, Loop.*
**Administration/Storage**
1. If the response is inadequate for the initial dose used for CHF, chronic renal failure, or hepatic cirrhosis, the dose can be doubled until the desired diuretic response is obtained. Doses greater than 200 mg for CHF or chronic renal failure and greater than 40 mg for hepatic cirrhosis have not been adequately studied.
2. May be given without regard for meals.
3. It is not necessary to adjust the dose for geriatric clients.
**IV** 4. Give the IV dose slowly over a period of 2 min.
5. Oral and IV doses are therapeutically equivalent; may switch to and from the IV form with no change in dose.
**Assessment**
1. Document indications for therapy, type and onset of symptoms. List other agents trialed and the outcome.
2. Note any sensitivity to sulfonamides.
3. Monitor VS, weight, I&O, blood sugar, uric acid, and potassium; drug may increase blood sugar and uric acid levels.
4. Document pulmonary, renal, and CV assessments.
**Client/Family Teaching**
1. Take only as directed. May take with food to decrease GI upset.
2. With hypertension, keep a BP log for provider review.
3. Report immediately any chest pain, increased SOB, or sudden weight gain with evidence of extremity edema.

**T**

---

4. Drug may cause dizziness, light-headedness, and fatigue.

5. Rise slowly from a sitting or lying position to minimize orthostatic drug effects.

6. May experience blurred vision, yellowing of vision, or sensitivity to sunlight. Report any unusual or persistent symptoms.

**Outcomes/Evaluate**

- ↓ Edema; ↑ diuresis
- ↓ BP
- Reduction of interdialysis weight gain and promotion of Na, Cl, and water excretion

---

# Tramadol hydrochloride
(**TRAM**-ah-dol)
**Pregnancy Category:** C
Ultram **(Rx)**
**Classification:** Analgesic, centrally acting

---

**Action/Kinetics:** A centrally acting analgesic not related chemically to opiates. Precise mechanism is not known. It may bind to mu-opioid receptors and inhibit reuptake of norepinephrine and serotonin. The analgesic effect is only partially antagonized by the antagonist naloxone. Causes significantly less respiratory depression than morphine. In contrast to morphine, tramadol does not cause release of histamine. Produces dependence of the mu-opioid type (i.e., like codeine or dextropropoxyphene); however, there is little evidence of abuse. Tolerance occurs but is relatively mild; the withdrawal syndrome is not as severe with other opiates. Rapidly absorbed after PO administration. Food does not affect the rate or extent of absorption. **Onset:** 1 hr. **Peak effect:** 2–3 hr. **Peak plasma levels:** 2 hr. **t½, plasma:** Approximately 7 hr after multiple doses. Extensively metabolized by one of the P-450 isoenzymes. Excreted in the urine, with about 30% excreted unchanged and 60% as metabolites. The M-metabolite is active.

**Uses:** Management of moderate to moderately severe pain.

**Contraindications:** Hypersensitivity to tramadol. In acute intoxication with alcohol, hypnotics, centrally acting analgesics, opiates, or psychotropic drugs. Use in clients with past or present addiction or opiate dependence or in those with a prior history of allergy to codeine or opiates. Use for obstetric preoperative medication or for postdelivery analgesia in nursing mothers. Use in children less than 16 years of age, as safety and efficacy have not been determined.

**Special Concerns:** Use with great caution in those taking MAO inhibitors, as tramadol inhibits norepinephrine and serotonin uptake. Dosage reduction is recommended with impaired hepatic or renal function and in clients over 75 years of age. Use with caution in increased intracranial pressure or head injury, in epilepsy, or in clients with an increased risk for seizures, including head trauma, metabolic disorders, alcohol or drug withdrawal, and CNS infections. Tramadol may complicate the assessment of acute abdominal conditions.

**Side Effects:** *CNS:* Dizziness, vertigo, headache, somnolence, CNS stimulation, anxiety, confusion, incoordination, euphoria, nervousness, sleep disorders, *seizures,* paresthesia, cognitive dysfunction, hallucinations, tremor, amnesia, concentration difficulty, abnormal gait, migraine, development of drug dependence. *GI:* Nausea, constipation, vomiting, dyspepsia, dry mouth, diarrhea, abdominal pain, anorexia, flatulence, GI bleeding, hepatitis, stomatitis, dysgeusia. *CV:* Vasodilation, syncope, orthostatic hypotension, tachycardia, abnormal ECG, hypertension, myocardial ischemia, palpitations. *Dermatologic:* Pruritus, sweating, rash, urticaria, vesicles. *Body as a whole:* Asthenia, malaise, allergic reaction, accidental injury, weight loss, *suicidal tendency. GU:* Urinary retention, urinary frequency, menopausal symptoms, dysuria, menstrual disorder. *Miscellaneous:* **Anaphylaxis,** visual disturbances, cataracts, deafness, tinnitus, hypertonia, dyspnea.

**Laboratory Test Alterations:** ↑ Creatinine, liver enzymes. ↓ Hemoglobin. Proteinuria.

**OD Overdose Management:** *Symptoms:* Extension of side effects, especially ***respiratory depression and seizures.*** *Treatment:* Naloxone will reverse some, but not all, of the symptoms of overdose. General supportive treatment, with special attention to maintenance of adequate respiration. Diazepam or barbiturates may help if seizures occur. Hemodialysis is not helpful.

**Drug Interactions**
*Alcohol* / Enhanced respiratory depression
*Anesthetics, general* / Enhanced respiratory depression
*Carbamazepine* / ↓ Effect of tramadol due to ↑ metabolism induced by carbamazepine
*CNS depressants* / Additive CNS depression
*MAO Inhibitors* / Tramadol may ↑ the risk of seizures in those taking MAO inhibitors
*Naloxone* / Use of naloxone for tramadol overdose may ↑ risk of seizures.
*Quinidine* / Quinidine inhibits the isoenzyme that metabolizes tramadol → ↑ levels of tramadol and ↓ levels of M1

**Dosage**
- **Tablets**
  *Management of pain.*

**Adults:** 50–100 mg q 4–6 hr, as needed, but not to exceed 400 mg/day. For moderate pain, 50 mg, initially, may be adequate, and for severe pain, 100 mg, initially, is often more effective. For clients over 75 years of age, the recommended dose is no more than 300 mg/day in divided doses. In impaired renal function with a $C_{CR}$ less than 30 mL/min, the dosing interval should be increased to 12 hr, with a maximum daily dose of 200 mg. The recommended dose for clients with cirrhosis is 50 mg q 12 hr.

## NURSING CONSIDERATIONS

See also *Nursing Considerations* for *Narcotic Analgesics.*

**Assessment**
1. Document indications for therapy, location, onset, and characteristics of symptoms. Use a pain-rating scale to rate pain; note any associated factors.
2. Assess for history of drug addiction, allergy to opiates or codeine, or seizures; drug may increase the risk of convulsions.
3. Monitor liver and renal function studies; reduce dose with dysfunction and if over 75 years old.

**Client/Family Teaching**
1. Take only as directed. May be taken without regard to meals. Do not exceed single or daily doses of tramadol in order to enhance pain relief.
2. Do not perform activities that require mental alertness; drug may impair mental or physical performance.
3. Review list of side effects (nausea, dizziness, constipation, somnolence, pruritus, and constipation) that one may experience; report if persistent or intolerable.
4. May mask abdominal pathology and obscure intracranial pathology due to miosis. Always alert provider and carry ID of drugs currently prescribed.

**Outcomes/Evaluate:** Pain control

# Trandolapril
(tran-**DOHL**-ah-pril)
**Pregnancy Category:** C (first trimester); D (second and third trimesters)
Mavik **(Rx)**
**Classification:** Antihypertensive

See also *Angiotensin Converting Enzyme (ACE) Inhibitors.*
**Action/Kinetics:** Rapidly absorbed; food slows rate, but not amount absorbed. **Peak plasma levels, trandolapril:** 30–60 min; **trandolaprilat:**

4–10 hr. **t½, trandoprilat:** 15–24 hr.
Metabolized in liver to active trandolaprilat. About ⅓ trandolaprilat is
excreted in urine and ⅔ in feces.

**Uses:** Hypertension, alone or in
combination with other antihypertensives such as hydrochlorothiazide.

**Contraindications:** In those with
history of angioedema with ACE
inhibitors.

**Special Concerns:** Safety and efficacy have not been determined in children.

**Side Effects:** See also *ACE Inhibitors. Hypersensitivity: **Angioedema**. CNS:* Dizziness, headache, fatigue. *GI:* Diarrhea, dyspepsia, gastritis. *CV:* Hypotension, bradycardia,
***cardiogenic shock*** , intermittent claudication, stroke. *Pulmonary:* Cough,
*Hepatic:* **Hepatic failure,** including
cholestatic jaundice, ***fulminant hepatic necrosis, death.*** *Miscellaneous:* Neutropenia, syncope, myalgia, asthenia.

**Laboratory Test Alterations:** Hyperkalemia, hypocalcemia. ↑ Serum
uric acid, BUN, creatinine.

**Drug Interactions**
*Diuretics* / Excessive hypotensive
effects
*Diuretics, Potassium-sparing:* / ↑
Risk of hyperkalemia
*Lithium* / ↑ Risk of lithium toxicity

**Dosage** ─────────────
- **Tablets**
  *Hypertension.*
**Initial:** 1 mg once daily in nonblack
clients and 2 mg once daily in black
clients. Adjust dosage according to
response; usually, adjustments are
made at intervals of 1 week. **Maintenance, usual:** 2–4 mg once daily.
Those inadequately treated with
once-daily dosing can be treated
with twice-daily dosing. If BP is still
not adequately controlled, diuretic
may be added. If $C_{CR}$ is less than 30
mL/min or if there is hepatic cirrhosis, initial dose is 0.5 mg daily.

## NURSING CONSIDERATIONS

See also *Nursing Considerations* for
*Angiotensin Converting Enzyme
(ACE) Inhibitors.*

**Administration/Storage:** If client
is on diuretic, discontinue 2 to 3
days prior to beginning therapy with
trandolapril to reduce likelihood of
hypotension. If diuretic can not be discontinued, use initial dose of trandolapril of 0.5 mg. Titrate subsequent dosage.

**Assessment**
1. Note indications for therapy, disease onset, other agents trialed and
outcome.
2. Monitor liver and renal function
studies; reduce dosage with impairment.

**Client/Family Teaching**
1. Take only as directed.
2. May experience cough, dizziness,
and diarrhea; report if persistent.
3. Practice reliable contraception,
stop drug and report if pregnancy
suspected.
4. Continue lifestyle changes i.e.,
regular exercise, smoking/alcohol
cessation, low fat, low salt diet in
overall goal of BP control.

**Outcomes/Evaluate:** ↓ BP

# Tranylcypromine sulfate
(**tran**-ill-**SIP**-roh-meen)
Parnate **(Rx)**
**Classification:** Antidepressant, mono-
amine oxidase inhibitor

**Action/Kinetics:** A MAO inhibitor
with a rapid onset of activity. Due to
inhibition of MAO, the concentration
of epinephrine, norepinephrine, and
serotonin increases in storage sites
throughout the nervous system. This
increase has been alleged to be the
basis for the antidepressant effects.
MAO activity recovers in 3–5 days
after drug withdrawal.

**Uses:** Treatment of major depressive
episode without melancholia. Not a
first line of therapy; is used when
clients have failed to respond to other drug therapy. *Investigational:*
Alone or as an adjunct to treat bulimia,
obsessive compulsive disorder, and
manifestations of psychotic disorders. Also, treatment of social phobia,
seasonal affective disorders, adjunct to
treat multiple sclerosis, and to treat
idiopathic orthostatic hypotension

(e.g., Shy-Drager syndrome), refractory to conventional therapy.

**Contraindications:** Use in those with a confirmed or suspected CV defect or in anyone with CV disease, hypertension, or history of headache. In the presence of pheochromocytoma. History of liver disease or in those with abnormal liver function. Use in combination with a large number of other drugs, especially other MAO inhibitors, tricyclic antidepressants, serotonin-reuptake inhibitors, buspirone, sympathomimetics, meperidine, CNS depressants (e.g., alcohol and narcotics), hypotensive drugs, excessive caffeine, and dextromethorphan (see *Drug Interactions*). Use with tyramine-containing foods (see Drug Interactions).

**Special Concerns:** Assess benefits versus risks before using during pregnancy and lactation. Use with caution in clients taking antiparkinson drugs, in impaired renal function, in those with seizure disorders, in diabetics, in hyperthyroid clients, and in those taking disulfiram. Geriatric clients may be more sensitive to the drug.

**Side Effects:** *CNS:* Anxiety, agitation, headaches (without elevation of BP), manic symptoms, restlessness, insomnia, weakness, drowsiness, dizziness, significant anorexia. *GI:* Dry mouth, nausea, diarrhea, abdominal pain, constipation. *CV:* Tachycardia, edema, palpitation. *GU:* Impotence, urinary retention, impaired ejaculation. *Musculoskeletal:* Muscle spasm, tremors, myoclonic jerks, numbness, paresthesia. *Hematologic:* Anemia, leukopenia, agranulocytosis, thrombocytopenia. *Miscellaneous:* Blurred vision, chills, impotence, hepatitis, skin rash, impaired water excretion, tinnitus.

**OD** **Overdose Management:** *Symptoms:* Insomnia, restlessness, anxiety, agitation, mental confusion, incoherence, hypotension, dizziness, weakness, drowsiness, shock, hypertension with severe headache. Rarely, hypertension accompanied by twitching or myoclonic fibrillation of skeletal muscles with *hyperprexia, generalized rigidity, and coma.* The toxic effects may be delayed or prolonged following the last dose of the drug; thus, the client should be closely observed for at least a week. *Treatment:* Gastric lavage, if performed early. General supportive measures. Treat hypertensive crisis using phentolamine 5 mg IV. External cooling to treat hyperprexia. Standard measures to treat circulatory shock. Myoclonic effects may be relieved by using barbiturates; however, tranylcypromine may prolong the effects of barbiturates.

**Drug Interactions**

*Alcohol* / Possibility of excitation, seizures, delirium, hyperpyrexia, circulatory collapse, coma, death

*Anesthetics, general* / Hypotensive effect; use together with caution. Phenelzine should be discontinued at least 10 days before elective surgery

*Anticholinergic drugs, atropine* / MAO inhibitors effect of anticholinergic drugs

*Antidepressants, tricyclic* / Concomitant use may result in excitation, sweating, tachycardia, tachypnea, hyperpyrexia, disseminated intravascular coagulation, delirium, tremors, convulsions, death. At least 7-10 days should elapse between discontinuing a MAO inhibitor and initiating a new drug. However, such combinations have been used together successfully

*Antihypertensive drugs* / Exaggerated hypotensive effects

*Beta-adrenergic blocking drugs* / Exaggerated hypotensive effects

*Buspirone* / Elevated BP

*Dextromethorphan* / Brief episodes of psychosis or bizarre behavior

*Fluoxetine* / Possibility of hyperthermia, rigidity, myoclonic movements, death. At least 10 days should elapse between discontinuation of phenelzine and initiation of fluoxetine; and, at least 5 weeks should elapse between discontinu-

T

ing fluoxetine and beginning phenelzine

*MAO Inhibitors* / Concomitant use of tranylcypromine with other MAO inhibitors may cause a hypertensive crisis or severe seizures

*Meperidine* / See *Narcotics*

*Narcotics* / Possibility of excitation, seizures, delirium, hyperpyrexia, circulatory collapse, coma, death

*Selective serotonin reuptake inhibitors* /See *Fluoxetine*

*Sympathomimetic drugs—amphetamine, cocaine, dopa, ephedrine, epinephrine, metaraminol, methyldopa, methylphenidate, norepinephrine, phenylephrine, phenylpropanolamine. Many OTC cold products, hay fever medications, and nasal decongestants contan one or more of these drugs* / All peripheral, metabolic, cardiac, and central effects are potentiated for up to 2 weeks after termination of MAO inhibitor therapy. Symptoms include acute hypertensive crisis with possible intracranial hemorrhage, hyperthermia, coma, and possibly death

*Thiazide diuretics* / Exaggerated hypotensive effects

*Tryptophan* / Possibility of behavioral and neurologic effects, including disorientation, confusion, amnesia, delirium, agitation, hypomania, ataxia, myoclonus, hyperreflexia, shivering, ocular oscillation,and Babinski signs

*Tyramine-rich foods—beer, broad beans, certain cheeses (Brie, cheddar, Camembert, Stilton), Chianti wine, chicken livers, caffeine, cola beverages, figs, licorice, liver, pickled or kippered herring, dry sausage (Genoa salami, hard salami, pepperoni, Lebanon bologna), tea, cream, yogurt, yeast extract, and chocolate* / Possible precipitation of hypertensive crisis, including severe headache, hyperension, intracranial hemorrhage, death

## Dosage

- **Tablets**

   *Major depressive syndrome without melancholia.*

Individualize the dose. **Usual effective dose:** 30 mg/day given in divided doses. If there are no signs of improvement in 2 weeks, the dose can be increased by 10 mg/day at intervals of 1 to 3 weeks, up to a maximum of 60 mg/day.

## NURSING CONSIDERATIONS

**Administration/Storage:** Improvement should be observed within 2 days to three weeks after beginning treatment.

**Assessment**

1. Document indications for therapy, onset and duration of symptoms, previous agents trialed and the outcome. Note clinical presentation and failure with other classes of antidepressants. These drugs have a narrow safety margin and require close supervision and restriction of foods and drugs and use with other medical conditions.

2. List all drugs currently prescribed and those used within the past two weeks (especially sympathomimetic drugs) to ensure none interact unfavorably.

3. Determine if pregnant; drugs cross placenal barrier and may be teratogenic.

4. Monitor VS, ECG, electrolytes, liver and renal function studies.

5. Determine if on any special diet and if foods on the diet affect MAO inhibitors (especially tyramine-rich foods).

**Interventions**

1. Monitor VS q 4 to 8 hr when initiating therapy and at regular intervals thereafter to detect any hypertension or arrhythmias.

2. Observe for symptoms of CHF, such as rales, SOB, or the presence of peripheral edema.

3. Monitor closely for indications of suicidal ideations. Suicide attempts are more frequent during this period when the client emerges from the deepest phases of depression.

**Client/Family Teaching**

1. Take as directed and with meals to decrease GI irritation. Do not take in the evening; may cause insomnia.

2. Avoid taking other drugs while

on this therapy and for two week after therapy has been discontinued unless specifically ordered. This includes OTC preparations for coughs, colds, congestion, or allergic reactions.

3. Review list of tyramine-containing foods to avoid (i.e. beer, Chianti wine, chicken livers, caffeine, cola beverages, certain cheeses such as Brie, cheddar, Camembert, and Stilton; figs, licorice, liver, pickled or kippered herring, dried fish, bananas, raisins, tenderizers, game meats, avocados, dry sausage such as Genoa salami, hard salami, pepperoni, and Lebanon bologna; tea, sour cream, yogurt, yeast extract, and chocolate.

4. Several weeks of therapy are required before significant changes in condition may be evident. Report increased agitation, anxiety, mania, suicidal ideations, or any marked changes in behavior. Must continue taking even if there appears to be improvement; continued therapy is necessary to maintain proper blood levels of the drug.

5. Report any visual changes, stiff neck, photophobia, unusual soreness or sweating, or changes in pupil size immediately; may signal a hypertensive crisis.

6. Practice reliable birth control during and for several weeks before and after therapy.

7. Frequent mouth rinses, sugarless gum or hard candy, and increased fluid intake may diminish dry mouth side effects.

8. If feeling faint lie down immediately. Rise slowly from a supine position and dangle legs before standing to minimize orthostatic hypotension.

9. Maintain activity in moderation. MAO inhibitors suppress anginal pain which may indicate myocardial ischemia.

10. May experience weight loss, nausea, anorexia, and/or diarrhea. If weight gain becomes significant, i.e., more than 5 lb/week for more than 2 weeks, may need reducing diet or a change in drug therapy or dosage may be warranted.

11. Report any urinary retention or bladder distension. Retention is more common among the elderly, males and those who are immobilized.

12. Increase fluids to 3 L/day and the intake of fuits, fruit juices, and fiber to avoid constipation.

13. Reports of red-green vision warrant further evaluation as this may indicate ophthalmic damage.

14. If taking elevated doses of MAO inhibitors over a long period of time, any drug withdrawal should be accomplished by gradually reducing the dosage of drug to a maintenance level before discontinuing the drug entirely.

15. Need regular F/U care since the dose will be gradually increased until the desired response is obtained. (Generally if there is no response observed by the third week of therapy, it is not likely client will respond to increased dosages.)

**Outcomes/Evaluate**

• Improvement in mood, energy, and interest levels; ↓ somatic complaints
• Normal sleep patterns
• Improved sense of self and abilty to problem solve

# Trazodone hydrochloride
(**TRAYZ**-oh-dohn)
**Pregnancy Category:** C
Alti-Trazodone ✤, Alti-Trazodone Dividose ✤, Apo-Trazodone ✤, Apo-Trazodone D ✤, Desyrel, Desyrel Dividose, Dom-Trazodone ✤, Novo-Trazodone ✤, Nu-Trazodone ✤, Nu-Trazodone-D ✤, PMS-Trazodone ✤, Trazon, Trialodine **(Rx)**
**Classification:** Antidepressant, miscellaneous

**Action/Kinetics:** A novel antidepressant that does not inhibit MAO and is also devoid of amphetamine-like effects. Response usually occurs after 2 weeks (75% of clients), with the remainder responding after 2–4 weeks. May inhibit serotonin uptake by brain cells, therefore increasing serotonin concentrations in the synapse. May also cause changes in binding of serotonin to receptors. Causes moderate sedative and orthostatic hypotensive effects and slight anticholinergic effects. **Peak plasma levels:** 1 hr (empty stomach) or 2 hr (when taken with food). **t½, initial:** 3–6 hr; **final:** 5–9 hr. **Effective plasma levels:** 800–1,600 ng/mL. **Time to reach steady state:** 3–7 days. Three-fourths of those with a therapeutic effect respond by the end of the second week of therapy. Metabolized in liver and excreted through both the urine and feces. **Uses:** Depression with or without accompanying anxiety. *Investigational:* In combination with tryptophan for treating aggressive behavior. Panic disorder or agoraphobia with panic attacks. Treatment of cocaine withdrawal. Chronic pain including diabetic neuropathy. **Contraindications:** During the initial recovery period following MI. Concurrently with electroshock therapy. **Special Concerns:** Use with caution during lactation. Safety and efficacy in children less than 18 years of age have not been established. Geriatric clients are more prone to the sedative and hypotensive effects. **Side Effects:** *General:* Dermatitis, edema, blurred vision, constipation, dry mouth, nasal congestion, skeletal muscle aches and pains. *CV:* Hypertension or hypotension, syncope, palpitations, tachycardia, SOB, chest pain. *GI:* Diarrhea, N&V, bad taste in mouth, flatulence. *GU:* Delayed urine flow, priapism, hematuria, increased urinary frequency. *CNS:* Nightmares, confusion, anger, excitement, decreased ability to concentrate, dizziness, disorientation, drowsiness, lightheadedness, fatigue, insomnia, nervousness, impaired memory. Rarely, hallucinations, impaired speech, hypomania. *Other:* Incoordination, tremors, paresthesias, decreased libido, appetite disturbances, red eyes, sweating or clamminess, tinnitus, weight gain or loss, anemia, hypersalivation. Rarely, akathisia, muscle twitching, increased libido, impotence, retrograde ejaculation, early menses, missed periods.

**OD** **Overdose Management:** *Symptoms:* **Respiratory arrest, seizures,** ECG changes, hypotension, priapism as well as an increase in the incidence and severity of side effects noted above (vomiting and drowsiness are the most common). *Treatment:* Treat symptoms (especially hypotension and sedation). Gastric lavage and forced diuresis to remove the drug from the body.

**Drug Interactions**
*Alcohol* / ↑ Depressant effects of alcohol
*Antihypertensives* / Additive hypotension
*Barbiturates* / ↑ Depressant effects of barbiturates
*Clonidine* / Trazodone ↓ effect of clonidine
*CNS depressants* / ↑ CNS depression
*Digoxin* / Trazodone may ↑ serum digoxin levels
*MAO inhibitors* / Initiate therapy cautiously if trazodone is to be used together with MAO inhibitors
*Phenytoin* / Trazodone may ↑ serum phenytoin levels

**Dosage**
• **Tablets**
  *Antidepressant.*
**Adults and adolescents, initial:** 150 mg/day; **then,** increase by 50 mg/day every 3–4 days to maximum of 400 mg/day in divided doses (outpatients). Inpatients may require up to, but not exceeding, 600 mg/day in divided doses. **Maintenance:** Use lowest effective dose. **Geriatric clients:** 75 mg/day in divided doses; dose can then be increased, as needed and tolerated, at 3- to 4-day intervals.
  *Treat aggressive behavior.*
Trazodone, 50 mg b.i.d., with tryptophan, 500 mg b.i.d. Dosage adjustments may be required to reach a therapeutic response or if side effects develop.

*Panic disorder or agoraphobia with panic attacks.* 300 mg/day.

## NURSING CONSIDERATIONS
### Administration/Storage
1. Initiate dose at the lowest possible level; increase gradually.
2. Beneficial effects may be observed within 1 week with optimal effects seen within 2 weeks.
### Assessment
1. Document indications for therapy, onset of symptoms, and any associated causative factors.
2. Note any history of recent MI.
3. Monitor ECG, CBC, liver and renal function studies.
### Client/Family Teaching
1. Take with food to enhance absorption and minimize dizziness and/or lightheadedness. Take major portion of dose at bedtime to reduce daytime side effects.
2. Use caution when driving or when performing other hazardous tasks; may cause drowsiness or dizziness.
3. Avoid alcohol and CNS depressants.
4. Report any persistent/bothersome side effects.
5. Use sugarless gum or candies and frequent mouth rinses to diminish dry mouth effects.
6. Inform surgeon if elective surgery is planned to minimize interaction with anesthetic agent.
7. Encourage family to to share responsibility for drug therapy to optimize treatment, prevent overdosage, and observe for any suicidal cues. Clients taking antidepressants and emerging from the deepest phases of depression are more prone to suicide.
8. May take 2–4 weeks for full drug effects to be realized.
### Outcomes/Evaluate:
• ↓ Depression (e.g., improved sleeping/eating patterns, ↓ fatigue, and ↑ social interactions)
• Control of overwhelming anxiety/panic symptoms

• ↓ Aggressive behavior

# Tretinoin (Retinoic acid, Vitamin A acid)
(TRET-ih-noyn)
**Pregnancy Category:** C (Topical products), D (Oral products)
Avita, Renova, Retin-A, Retin-A Micro, Retisol-A ✦, StieVA-A ✦, StieVA-A Forte ✦, Vesanoid, Vitinoin ✦ (Rx)
**Classification:** Antiacne drug

**Action/Kinetics:** Topical tretinoin is believed to decrease microcomedone formation by decreasing the cohesiveness of follicular epithelial cells. Also believed to increase mitotic activity and increase turnover of follicular epithelial cells as well as decrease keratin synthesis. Some systemic absorption occurs (approximately 5% is recovered in the urine).

The mechanism of action for PO use in acute promyelocytic leukemia (APL) is not known. Absorption is enhanced when the drug is taken with food. **Time to peak levels:** 1–2 hr. Is over 95% bound to plasma proteins (mainly to albumin). **Terminal elimination t½:** 0.5–2 hr in APL clients. Metabolized by the liver, with about two-thirds excreted in the urine and one-third in the feces.
**Uses: Dermatologic:** *Retin-A:* Acne vulgaris. *Retin-A* and *Renova:* As an adjunct to comprehensive skin care and sun avoidance to treat fine wrinkles, mottled hyperpigmentation, and roughness of facial skin caused by age and the sun. For those individuals who do not achieve palliation using comprehensive skin care and sun avoidance programs alone. *Investigational (Retin-A):* Treat various forms of skin cancer. Dermatologic conditions including lamellar ichthyosis, mollusca contagiosa, verrucae plantaris, verrucae planae juveniles, ichthyosis vulgaris, bullous congenital ichthyosiform, and pityriasis rubra pilar-

is. To enhance the percutaneous absorption of topical minoxidil.

**Oral:** To induce remission in APL. After induction therapy with tretinoin, clients should be given a standard consolidation or maintenance chemotherapy regimen for APL, unless contraindicated.

**Contraindications:** Eczema, sunburn. Use if inherently sensitive to sunlight or if taking other drugs that increase sensitivity to sunlight. Use of Renova if client is also taking drugs known to be photosensitizers (e.g., fluoroquinolones, phenothiazines, sulfonamides, tetracyclines, thiazides). Those allergic to parabens (preservative in the gelatin capsules). Use of PO form during lactation. Use around the eyes, mouth, angles of the nose, and mucous membranes.

**Special Concerns:** Use with caution during lactation. Safety and effectiveness have not been determined in children. Excessive sunlight and weather extremes (e.g., wind and cold) may be irritating. Use Renova with caution with concomitant topical medications, medicated or abrasive soaps, shampoos, cleansers, cosmetics with a strong drying effect, permanent wave solutions, electrolysis, hair depilatories or waxes, and products with high concentrations of alcohol, astringents, spices, or lime. Safety and efficacy of Renova have not been determined in children less than 18 years of age, in individuals over the age of 50 years, or in individuals with moderately or heavily pigmented skin. Use of the PO form has resulted in retonic acid-APL syndrome, especially during the first month of treatment. The safety and efficacy of oral tretinoin at doses less than 45 mg/m²/day have not been evaluated in children.

**Side Effects: Following topical use.** Dermatologic: Red, edematous, crusted, or blistered skin; hyperpigmentation or hypopigmentation, increased susceptibility to sunlight, erythema, pruritus, burning, dryness. Excessive application will cause redness, peeling, or discomfort with no increase in results.

**Following oral use.** Retinoic acid-APL syndrome: Fever, dyspnea, weight gain, radiographic pulmonary infiltrate, pleural or pericardial effusions. Occasional impaired myocardial contractility and episodic hypotension; possibility of concomitant leukocytosis. *Progressive hypoxemia with possible fatal outcome.* Respiratory symptoms, including upper respiratory tract disorders, respiratory insufficiency, pneumonia, rales, expiratory wheezing, lower respiratory tract disorders, bronchial asthma, *pulmonary or larynx edema,* unspecified pulmonary disease. *Pseudotumor cerebri (especially in children):* Papilledema, headache, N&V, visual disturbances. *Typical retinoid toxicity (similar to ingestion of high doses of vitamin A):* Headache, fever, dryness of skin and mucous membranes, bone pain, N&V, rash, mucositis, pruritus, increased sweating, visual disturbances, ocular disorders, alopecia, skin changes, changed visual acuity, bone inflammation, visual field defects. *Body as a whole:* Malaise, shivering, *hemorrhage, disseminated intravascular coagulation,* infections, peripheral edema, pain, chest discomfort, edema, weight increase, anorexia, weight decrease, myalgia, flank pain, cellulitis, facial edema, fluid imbalance, pallor, lymph disorders, acidosis, hypothermia, ascites. GI: **GI hemorrhage,** abdominal pain, various GI disorders, diarrhea, constipation, dyspepsia, abdominal distension, hepatosplenomegaly, hepatitis, ulcer, unspecified liver disorders. *CV:* Arrhythmias, flushing, hypotension, hypertension, phlebitis, *cardiac failure, cardiac arrest, stroke,* MI, enlarged heart, heart murmur, ischemia, myocarditis, pericarditis, pulmonary hypertension, secondary cardiomyopathy. *CNS:* Dizziness, paresthesias, anxiety, insomnia, depression, confusion, *cerebral hemorrhage, intracranial hypertension* , agitation, hallucinations, abnormal gait, agnosia, aphasia, asterixis, cerebellar edema, cerebellar disorders, **convulsions, coma** , CNS depression, dysarthria, encephalopathy, facial paralysis, hemiplegia, hyporeflexia, hypotaxia, no light reflex, neurologic reaction, spinal cord disorder, tremor, leg weakness, unconsciousness, dementia, forgetfulness, somnolence, slow speech. *GU:* Renal insufficiency, dysuria, acute renal failure, micturition frequency, renal tubular necrosis, enlarged prostate. *Otic:* Earache, feeling of fullness in the ears, hearing loss, unspecified auricular disorders, irreversible hearing loss. *Other:* Erythema nodosum, basophilia, hyperhistaminemia, Sweet's syndrome, organomegaly, hypercalcemia, pancreatitis, myositis.

**Laboratory Test Alterations:** Elevated LFTs following use of PO product.

**Drug Interactions:** Concomitant use with sulfur, resorcinol, benzoyl peroxide, or salicylic acid may cause significant skin irritation.

## Dosage

• **Cream, Gel, or Liquid**
*Acne vulgaris.*
Apply lightly over the affected areas once daily at bedtime. Beneficial effects many not be seen for 2–6 weeks.

• **Cream, 0.025%, 0.05%, 0.1%**
*Palliation for skin conditions.*
Apply a pea-sized amount once daily at bedtime, using only enough to lightly cover the entire affected area. Up to 6 months of therapy may be needed before effects are seen.

• **Capsules**
*APL.*
**Adults:** 45 mg/m²/day given as two evenly divided doses. Given until complete remission is obtained. Therapy should be discontinued 30 days after achieving complete remission or after 90 days of treatment, whichever comes first.

## NURSING CONSIDERATIONS

### Administration/Storage

1. Apply the liquid carefully with the fingertip, cotton swab, or gauze pad only to affected areas.

2. Excessive amounts of the gel will cause a "pilling" effect which minimizes the likelihood of overapplication.

3. Wash hands thoroughly immediately after applying tretinoin.

4. Before applying Renova, wash the face gently with a mild soap and pat the skin dry, waiting 20–30 min before applying. When applied, take care to avoid contact with eyes, ears, nostrils, and mouth.

5. Do not freeze Renova cream.

6. Treatment with Renova for more than 24 weeks does not appear to increase improvement. The results of continued irritation of the skin for more than 48 weeks are not known.

### Assessment

1. Note indications for therapy, type, onset, and characteristics of symptoms.

2. With acne, thoroughly describe pretreatment skin condition; obtain photographs to compare with results of therapy.

3. Determine if pregnant.

4. Monitor hematologic, liver, and renal function studies.

**Client/Family Teaching:** Topical:

1. Keep away from normal skin, mucous membranes, eyes, ears, mouth, nostrils, and the angles of the nose.

2. Wash with mild soap and warm water and pat skin dry. Wait 20–30 min before applying tretinoin.

3. On application there will be a transitory feeling of warmth and stinging.

4. Wash hands thoroughly before and immediately after applying tretinoin.

5. Expect dryness and peeling of skin from the affected areas.

6. May be more sensitive to wind and cold. Do not apply to wind or sunburned skin or to open wounds.

7. Avoid alcohol-containing preparations such as shaving lotions and creams, perfumes, cosmetics with drying effects, skin cleansers, and medicated soaps.

---

8. Initially, the lesions may worsen. This is caused by the effect of the drug on deep lesions that had been previously undetected. Report if lesions become severe; drug should be discontinued until skin integrity restored.

9. Improvement should be evident in 6 weeks but therapy should be continued for at least 3 months.

10. Practice reliable form of birth control.

11. Avoid excessive exposure to sunlamps and to the sun. If in sunlight while using medication, use a sunscreen and protective clothing over affected areas.

**Oral:**

1. Drug will be administered until complete remission is obtained. It will be stopped 30 days after remission or after 90 days of therapy, whichever comes first. This does not replace standard maintenance chemotherapy for APL.

2. Take with food to enhance absorption.

3. Take exactly as prescribed; do not exceed or skip doses.

4. Review list of potential drug side effects, noting those that require immediate reporting.

**Outcomes/Evaluate**
- ↓ Size/number of acne eruptions
- Clearing of skin condition; symptomatic improvement
- Remission with APL

# Triamcinolone
(try-am-**SIN**-oh-lohn)
**Pregnancy Category:** C
**Dental Paste:** Kenalog in Orabase, Oracort, Oralone **(Rx)**. **Tablets:** Aristocort, Atolone, Kenacort **(Rx)**

# Triamcinolone acetonide
(try-am-**SIN**-oh-lohn)
**Pregnancy Category:** C
**Dental Paste:** Oracort ✹. **Inhalation Aerosol:** Azmacort, Nasacort, Nasacort AQ **(Rx)**. **Parenteral:** Kenaject-40, Kenalog-10 and -40, Scheinpharm Triamcine-A ✹, Tac-3 and -40, Triam-A, Triamonide 40, Tri-Kort, Trilog **(Rx)**. **Topical Aerosol:** Kenalog **(Rx)**. **Topical Cream:** Aristocort, Aristocort

A, Delta-Tritex, Flutex, Kenac, Kenalog, Kenalog-H, Kenonel, Triacet, Triaderm ✹, Trianide Mild, Trianide Regular, Triderm, Trymex **(Rx)**. **Topical Lotion:** Kenalog, Kenonel **(Rx)**. **Topical Ointment:** Aristocort, Aristocort A, Kenac, Kenalog, Kenonel, Triaderm ✹, Trymex **Topical Spray:** Nasacort AQ **(Rx)**

# Triamcinolone diacetate
(try-am-**SIN**-oh-lohn)
**Pregnancy Category:** C
**Parenteral:** Amcort, Aristocort Forte, Aristocort Intralesional, Aristocort Parenteral ✹, Articulose L.A., Kenacort Diacetate, Triam-Forte, Triamolone 40, Trilone, Tristoject.
**Syrup:** Aristocort Syrup ✹ **(Rx)**

# Triamcinolone hexacetonide
(try-am-**SIN**-oh-lohn)
**Pregnancy Category:** C
Aristospan Intra-Articular, Aristospan Intralesional **(Rx)**
**Classification:** Corticosteroid, synthetic

See also *Corticosteroids*.

**Action/Kinetics:** More potent than prednisone. Intermediate-acting. Has no mineralocorticoid activity. **Onset:** Several hours. **Duration:** One or more weeks. **t½:** Over 200 min.

**Additional Uses:** Pulmonary emphysema accompanied by bronchospasm or bronchial edema. Diffuse interstitial pulmonary fibrosis. With diuretics to treat refractory CHF or cirrhosis of the liver with ascites. Multiple sclerosis. Inflammation following dental procedures. Triamcinolone acetonide for PO inhalation is used for maintenance treatment of asthma. Triamcinolone hexacetonide is restricted to intra-articular or intralesional treatment of rheumatoid arthritis and osteoarthritis.

**Special Concerns:** Use during pregnancy only if benefits clearly outweigh risks. Use with special caution with decreased renal function or renal disease. Dose must be highly individualized.

**Additional Side Effects:** Intra-articular, intrasynovial, or intrabursal administration may cause transient flushing, dizziness, local depigmentation, and rarely, local irritation. Exacerbation of symptoms has also been reported. A marked increase in swelling and pain and further restricted joint movement may indicate septic arthritis. Intradermal injection may cause local vesicular ulceration and persistent scarring. *Syncope and anaphylactoid reactions* have been reported with triamcinolone regardless of route of administration.

## Dosage

TRIAMCINOLONE

• **Tablets**

*Adrenocortical insufficiency (with mineralocorticoid therapy).*
4–12 mg/day.
*Acute leukemias (children).*
1–2 mg/kg.
*Acute leukemia or lymphoma (adults).*
16–40 mg/day (up to 100 mg/day may be necessary for leukemia).
*Edema.*
16–20 mg (up to 48 mg may be required until diuresis occurs).
*Tuberculosis meningitis.*
32–48 mg/day.
*Rheumatic disease, dermatologic disorders, bronchial asthma.*
8–16 mg/day.
*SLE.*
20–32 mg/day.
*Allergies.*
8–12 mg/day.
*Hematologic disorders.*
16–60 mg/day.
*Ophthalmologic diseases.*
12–40 mg daily.
*Respiratory diseases.*
16–48 mg/day.

TRIAMCINOLONE ACETONIDE

• **IM Only (Not for IV Use)**
2.5–60 mg/day, depending on the disease and its severity.

• **Intra-articular,    Intrabursal, Tendon Sheaths**
2.5–5 mg for smaller joints and 5–15 mg for larger joints, although up to 40 mg has been used.

• **Intradermal**
1 mg/injection site (use 3 mg/mL or 10 mg/mL suspension only).

• **Topical: 0.025%, 0.1%, 0.5% Ointment or Cream; 0.025%, 0.1% Lotion; Paste: 0.1%; Aerosol—to deliver 0.2 mg)**
Apply sparingly to affected area b.i.d.–q.i.d. and rub in lightly.

• **Metered Dose Inhaler (Azmacort)**
**Adults, usual:** 2 inhalations (200 mcg) t.i.d.–q.i.d. or 4 inhalations (400 mcg) b.i.d., not to exceed 1,600 mcg/day. **High initial doses** (1,200–1,600 mcg/day) may be needed in some clients with severe asthma. **Pediatric, 6–12 years:** 1–2 inhalations (100–200 mcg) t.i.d.–q.i.d. or 2–4 inhalations b.i.d., not to exceed 1,200 mcg/day. Use in children less than 6 years of age has not been determined.

• **Intranasal Spray (Nasacort)**
*Seasonal and perennial allergic rhinitis.*
**Adults and children over 12 years of age:** 2 sprays (110 mcg) into each nostril once a day (i.e., for a total dose of 220 mcg/day). The dose may be increased to 440 mcg/day given either once daily or q.i.d. (1 spray/nostril).

TRIAMCINOLONE DIACETATE

• **IM Only**
40 mg/week.

• **Intra-articular, Intrasynovial**
5–40 mg.

• **Intralesional, Sublesional**
5–48 mg (no more than 12.5 mg/injection site and 25 mg/lesion).

TRIAMCINOLONE HEXACETONIDE

**NOT FOR IV USE.**

• **Intra-articular**
2–6 mg for small joints and 10–20 mg for large joints.

• **Intralesional/Sublesional**
Up to 0.5 mg/sq. in. of affected area.

## NURSING CONSIDERATIONS

See also *Nursing Considerations* for *Corticosteroids.*
**Administration/Storage**
1. Initially, use the aerosol concomi-

**T**

tantly with a systemic steroid. After 1 week, initiate a gradual withdrawal of systemic steroid. Make the next reduction after 1–2 weeks, depending on the response. If symptoms of insufficiency occur, the dose of systemic steroid can be increased temporarily. Also, the dose of systemic steroid may need to be increased in times of stress or a severe asthmatic attack.

2. Do not use the acetonide products if they clump due to exposure to freezing temperatures.

3. A single IM dose of the diacetate provides control from 4–7 days up to 3–4 weeks.

4. Triamcinolone acetonide nasal spray for allergic rhinitis may be effective as soon as 12 hr after initiation of therapy. Reevaluate if improvement is not seen within 2–3 weeks.

5. For best results, store the canister at room temperature and shake well before use.

6. Nasacort AQ is viscous at rest but a liquid when shaken. This allows the drug to stay in the nasal airways at the site of inflammation for up to 2 hr.

**Assessment**

1. Document indications for therapy; note type, onset, and characteristics of symptoms.

2. Assess area/condition requiring treatment and describe findings.

3. Monitor blood sugar, CBC, electrolytes, and renal function.

**Client/Family Teaching**

1. Take at the same time each morning.

2. Ingest a liberal amount of protein; with regular use may experience gradual weight loss, associated with anorexia, muscle wasting, and weakness. See dietitian for assistance in meal planning and preparation.

3. Lie down if feeling faint; report if syncopal episodes persist and interfere with daily activities.

4. Report any evidence of abnormal bruising, bleeding, weight gain, edema, or dyspnea.

5. Drug may suppress reactions to skin allergy testing.

6. With topical therapy, apply to clean, slightly moist skin. Report if area does not improve with therapy or if symptoms worsen.

7. With nasal spray or inhaler, review appropriate method of administration and proper care and storage of equipment. Always rinse mouth and equipment after use.

8. Report immediately any new onset of depression as well as aggravation of existing depressive symptoms.

**Outcomes/Evaluate**

• ↓ Immune and inflammatory responses in autoimmune disorders and allergic reactions

• Improved airway exchange

• Restoration of skin integrity

• Relief of pain/inflammation; improved joint mobility

# Triamterene

(fry-**AM**-ter-een)

**Pregnancy Category:** B

Dyrenium **(Rx)**

**Classification:** Diuretic, potassium-sparing

See also *Diuretics*.

**Action/Kinetics:** A mild diuretic that acts directly on the distal tubule. It promotes the excretion of sodium—which is exchanged for potassium or hydrogen ions—bicarbonate, chloride, and fluid. It increases urinary pH and is a weak folic acid antagonist. **Onset:** 2–4 hr. **Peak effect:** 6–8 hr. **Duration:** 7–9 hr. **t½:** 3 hr. From one-half to two-thirds of the drug is bound to plasma protein. Metabolized to hydroxytriamterene sulfate, which is also active. About 20% is excreted unchanged through the urine.

**Uses:** Edema due to CHF, hepatic cirrhosis, nephrotic syndrome, steroid therapy, secondary hyperaldosteronism, and idiopathic edema. May be used alone or with other diuretics. *Investigational:* Prophylaxis and treatment of hypokalemia, adjunct in the treatment of hypertension.

**Contraindications:** Hypersensitivity to drug, severe or progressive renal insufficiency, severe hepatic disease, anuria, hyperkalemia, hyperuricemia, gout, history of nephrolithiasis. Lactation.

**Special Concerns:** Safety and efficacy have not been determined in children.

**Side Effects:** *Electrolyte:* Hyperkalemia, electrolyte imbalance. *GI:* Nausea, vomiting (may also be indicative of electrolyte imbalance), diarrhea, dry mouth. *CNS:* Dizziness, drowsiness, fatigue, weakness, headache. *Hematologic:* Megaloblastic anemia, thrombocytopenia. *Renal:* Azotemia, interstitial nephritis. *Miscellaneous:* **Anaphylaxis,** photosensitivity, hypokalemia, jaundice, muscle cramps, rash.

**Laboratory Test Alterations:** Triamterene may impart blue fluorescence to urine, interfering with fluorometric assays (e.g., lactic dehydrogenase, quinidine). ↑ BUN, creatinine. ↑ Serum uric acid in clients predisposed to gouty arthritis.

**OD** **Overdose Management:** *Symptoms:* Electrolyte imbalance, especially hyperkalemia. Also, nausea, vomiting, other GI disturbances, weakness, hypotension, reversible acute renal failure. *Treatment:* Immediately induce vomiting or perform gastric lavage. Evaluate electrolyte levels and fluid balance and treat if necessary. Dialysis may be beneficial.

**Drug Interactions**
*Amantadine* / ↑ Toxic effects of amantadine due to ↓ renal excretion
*Angiotensin-converting enzyme inhibitors* / Significant hyperkalemia
*Antihypertensives* / Potentiated by triamterene
*Captopril* / ↑ Risk of significant hyperkalemia
*Cimetidine* / ↑ Bioavailability and ↓ clearance of triamterene
*Digitalis* / Inhibited by triamterene
*Indomethacin* / ↑ Risk of nephrotoxicity and acute renal failure

*Lithium* / ↑ Chance of lithium toxicity due to ↓ renal clearance
*Potassium salts* / Additive hyperkalemia
*Spironolactone* / Additive hyperkalemia

**Dosage**
- **Capsules.**
  *Diuretic.*
  **Adults, initial:** 100 mg b.i.d. after meals; **maximum daily dose:** 300 mg.

## NURSING CONSIDERATIONS

See also *Nursing Considerations* for *Diuretics.*

**Administration/Storage**
1. Minimize nausea by giving the drug after meals.
2. Dosage is usually reduced by one-half when another diuretic is added to the regimen.

**Assessment**
1. Document indications for therapy; list agents prescribed to ensure none interact.
2. Assess for alcoholism; megaloblastic anemia may occur because triamterene is a weak antagonist of folic acid.
3. Monitor ECG, CBC, uric acid, electrolytes, and renal function studies.

**Client/Family Teaching**
1. Take with food to minimize GI upset/nausea.
2. Report any sore throat, rash, or fever (S&S of blood dyscrasia).
3. Persistent headaches, drowsiness, vomiting, restlessness, mental wandering, lethargy, and foul breath may be signs of uremia; report if evident.
4. Drug may cause dizziness.
5. Avoid alcohol and any OTC agents. Also avoid potassium supplements, salt substitutes that contain potassium, and foods high in potassium; drug is potassium-sparing.
6. Urine may appear pale fluorescent blue.
7. Avoid direct sunlight for pro-

longed periods; may cause a photosensitivity reaction. Use sunscreens, sunglasses, hat, and long sleeves and pants when exposed.

**Outcomes/Evaluate**
- ↓ Edema; ↑ diuresis
- ↓ BP

————COMBINATION DRUG————

# Triamterene and Hydrochlorothiazide Capsules

(try-**AM**-ter-een, hy-droh-**klor**-oh-**THIGH**-ah-zyd)
**Pregnancy Category:** C
Dyazide **(Rx)**

# Triamterene and Hydrochlorothiazide Tablets

(try-**AM**-teh-reen, hy-droh-**kloh**-roh-**THIGH**-ah-zyd)
**Pregnancy Category:** C
Apo-Triazide ✤, Dyazide, Maxide, Maxide-25 MG, Novo-Triamzide ✤, Nu-Triazide ✤, Pro-Triazide ✤ **(Rx)**
**Classification:** Diuretic, antihypertensive

See also *Hydrochlorothiazide* and *Triamterene*.

**Content: Capsules.** D*iuretic:* Hydrochlorothiazide, 25 or 50 mg. D*iuretic:* Triamterene, 50 or 100 mg.
**Tablets.** D*iuretic:* Hydrochlorothiazide, 25 or 50 mg. D*iuretic:* Triamterene, 37.5 or 75 mg. (In Canada the tablets contain 25 mg of hydrochlorothiazide and 50 mg triamterene.)
**Uses:** To treat hypertension or edema in clients who manifest hypokalemia on hydrochlorothiazide alone. In clients requiring a diuretic and in whom hypokalemia cannot be risked (i.e., clients with cardiac arrhythmias or those taking digitalis). Usually not the first line of therapy, except for clients in whom hypokalemia should be avoided.
**Contraindications:** Clients receiving other potassium-sparing drugs such as amiloride and spironolactone. Use in anuria, acute or chronic renal insufficiency, significant renal impairment, preexisting elevated serum potassium.
**Special Concerns:** Use with caution during lactation. Geriatric clients may be more sensitive to the hypotensive and electrolyte effects of this combination; also, age-related decreases in renal function may require a decrease in dosage.

**Dosage** ————
- **Capsules**
  *Hypertension or edema.*
**Adults:** Triamterene/hydrochlorothiazide: 37.5 mg/25 mg—1–2 capsules given once daily with monitoring of serum potassium and clinical effect. Triamterene/hydrochlorothiazide: 50 mg/25 mg—1–2 capsules b.i.d. after meals. Some clients may be controlled using 1 capsule every day or every other day. No more than 4 capsules should be taken daily.
- **Tablets**
  *Hypertension or edema.*
**Adults:** Triamterene/hydrochlorothiazide: 37.5 mg/25 mg—1–2 tablets/day (determined by individual titration with the components). Or, triamterene/hydrochlorothiazide: 75 mg/50 mg—1 tablet daily.

## NURSING CONSIDERATIONS

See also *Nursing Considerations* for *Antihypertensive Agents, Triamterene,* and *Hydrochlorothiazide*.
**Administration/Storage:** Monitor clients who are transferred from less bioavailable formulations of triamterene and hydrochlorothiazide for serum potassium levels following the transfer.
**Outcomes/Evaluate**
- Control of hypertension
- Resolution of edema

# Triazolam

(try-**AYZ**-oh-lam)
**Pregnancy Category:** X
Alti-Triazolam ✤, Apo-Triazo ✤, Gen-Triazolam ✤, Halcion, Novo-Triolam ✤ **(C-IV) (Rx)**
**Classification:** Benzodiazepine sedative-hypnotic

See also *Tranquilizers, Antimanic Drugs, and Hypnotics.*

**Action/Kinetics:** Decreases sleep latency, increases the duration of sleep, and decreases the number of awakenings. **Time to peak plasma levels:** 0.5–2 hr. **t½:** 1.5–5.5 hr. Metabolized in liver; inactive metabolites excreted in the urine.

**Uses:** Insomnia (short-term management, not to exceed 1 month). May be beneficial in preventing or treating transient insomnia from a sudden change in sleep schedule.

**Contraindications:** Use concomitantly with itraconazole, ketoconazole, nefaxodone. Lactation (may cause sedation and feeding problems in infants).

**Special Concerns:** Safety and efficacy in children under 18 years of age not established. Geriatric clients may be more sensitive to the effects of triazolam.

**Side Effects:** *CNS:* Rebound insomnia, anterograde amnesia, headache, ataxia, decreased coordination, "traveler's" amnesia. Psychologic and physical dependence. *GI:* N&V.

**Dosage** ————————————
• **Tablets**
**Adults, initial:** 0.25–0.5 mg before bedtime. **Geriatric or debilitated clients, initial:** 0.125 mg; **then,** depending on response, 0.125–0.25 mg before bedtime.

## NURSING CONSIDERATIONS

See also *Nursing Considerations* for *Tranquilizers, Antimanic Drugs, and Hypnotics.*
**Assessment**
1. Document indications for therapy, onset, duration, and characteristics of symptoms.
2. Assess mental status and note behavioral manifestations.
3. Monitor CBC and LFTs.
4. Evaluate sleep patterns; determine underlying cause of insomnia so that source may be removed. With simple insomnia, try nonpharmacologic interventions to induce sleep,

such as soft music, guided imagery, or progressive muscle relaxation.
5. Initiate safety precautions (i.e., side rails up, supervised ambulation, frequent observations) at bedtime, especially with elderly clients and confused clients.
6. Assess for tolerance and for psychologic and physical dependence. Monitor closely for CNS toxic effects especially during prolonged therapy (longer than 2 weeks).
**Client/Family Teaching**
1. Take only as directed. Store away from bedside.
2. Avoid alcoholic and other CNS depressants.
3. Use caution when driving or operating machinery until daytime sedative effects have been evaluated.
4. Drug is for short-term use only; may cause physical and psychologic dependence. Try warm baths, warm milk, and other methods to induce sleep, such as white noise simulator, soft music, guided imagery, or progressive muscle relaxation, rather than become dependent on drugs for insomnia.
5. Report immediately any unusual side effects including hallucinations, nightmares, depression, or periods of confusion.
**Outcomes/Evaluate:** Improved sleeping patterns; relief from insomnia

# Trientine hydrochloride
(**TRY**-en-teen)
**Pregnancy Category:** C
Syprine **(Rx)**
**Classification:** Chelating agent

**Action/Kinetics:** A chelating agent that binds copper, thus facilitating its excretion from the body.
**Uses:** Wilson's disease (a metabolic defect resulting in excess copper accumulation) who are intolerant of penicillamine.
**Contraindications:** Use in cystinuria, rheumatoid arthritis, biliary cirrhosis.

T

**Special Concerns:** Use with caution during lactation. Safety and effectiveness in children have not been determined although the drug has been used in children as young as 6 years of age.

**Side Effects:** Iron deficiency anemia, SLE.

## Dosage
• **Capsules**
   *Wilson's disease.*
**Adults, initial:** 750 mg/day–1.25 g/day in divided doses b.i.d., t.i.d., or q.i.d.; **then,** may increase to a maximum of 2 g/day. **Children less than 12 years of age, initial:** 500–750 mg/day in divided doses b.i.d., t.i.d., or q.i.d.; **then,** may increase to a maximum of 1.5 g/day.

### NURSING CONSIDERATIONS
**Administration/Storage**
1. Increase the daily dose only if the response is not adequate or the serum copper level is consistently greater than 20 mcg/dL.
2. At 6- to 12-month intervals, determine the optimal long-term maintenance dosage.
3. If the contents of the capsule come in contact with any site on the body, promptly wash with water to avoid contact dermatitis.
4. Store capsules at 2°C–8°C (36°F–46°F).

**Assessment:** Monitor CBC and serum copper levels. Note previous treatment regimens and results.

**Client/Family Teaching**
1. Take on an empty stomach at least 1 hr before meals or 2 hr after meals and at least 1 hr apart from any other drug, food, or milk.
2. Swallow capsules whole with water; do not chew or open capsules.
3. Iron deficiency anemia may develop in children, in menstruating or pregnant women, or as a result of the low-copper diet necessary to treat Wilson's disease. Iron may be given in such cases but allow 2 hr between administration of iron and trientine.
4. Record temperature nightly for the first month of treatment; report any fever or skin eruptions.
5. Report for labs; serum copper levels will be followed, and periodically a 24-hr urinary copper analysis will be requested. Free serum copper is the most reliable way to monitor the effectiveness of therapy. Clients responsive to therapy will have less than 10 mcg/dL of free copper in the serum.

**Outcomes/Evaluate:** ↓ Serum copper levels; relief of symptoms of copper toxicity

# Trifluoperazine
(try-**flew**-oh-**PER**-ah-zeen)
Apo-Trifluoperazine ✹, Novo-Flurazine ✹, Novo-Trifluzine ✹, PMS-Trifluoperazine ✹, Stelazine, Terfluzine ✹ **(Rx)**

**Classification:** Antipsychotic, antiemetic, piperazine-type phenothiazine

See also *Antipsychotic Agents, Phenothiazines.*

**Action/Kinetics:** Causes a high incidence of extrapyramidal symptoms and antiemetic effects and a low incidence of sedation, orthostatic hypotension, and anticholinergic side effects. **Maximum therapeutic effect:** Usually 2–3 weeks after initiation of therapy.

**Uses:** Schizophrenia. Suitable for clients with apathy or withdrawal. Anxiety, tension, agitation in neuroses. Recommended only for hospitalized or well-supervised clients.

**Special Concerns:** Use during pregnancy only when benefits clearly outweigh risks. Dosage has not been established in children less than 6 years of age. Geriatric, emaciated, or debilitated clients usually require a lower initial dose.

## Dosage
• **Oral Solution, Tablets**
   *Psychoses.*
**Adults and adolescents, initial:** 2–5 mg (base) b.i.d.; **maintenance:** 15–20 mg/day in two or three divided doses. **Pediatric, 6–12 years:** 1 mg

(base) 1–2 times/day; adjust dose as required and tolerated.

*Anxiety/tension.*

**Adults and adolescents:** 1–2 mg/day up to 6 mg/day. Not to be given for this purpose longer than 12 weeks.

• **IM**

*Pyschoses.*

**Adults:** 1–2 mg q 4–6 hr, not to exceed 10 mg/day. Switch to PO therapy as soon as possible. **Pediatric:** *Severe symptoms only:* 1 mg 1–2 times/day.

## NURSING CONSIDERATIONS

See also *Nursing Considerations* for *Antipsychotic Agents, Phenothiazines.*

**Administration/Storage**

1. Dilute concentrate just before administration with 60 mL of juice (tomato or fruit), carbonated drinks, water, milk, orange or simple syrup, coffee, tea, or semisolid foods (e.g., applesauce, pudding, soup).

2. Protect liquid forms from light.

3. Discard strongly colored solutions.

4. Avoid skin contact with liquid form to prevent contact dermatitis.

5. To prevent cumulative effects, at least 4 hr should elapse between IM injections.

**Assessment**

1. Document indications for therapy, onset of symptoms, and behavioral manifestations.

2. Note other agents prescribed and the outcome.

3. Assess mental status and note findings.

4. Monitor CBC, ECG, and LFTs.

**Outcomes/Evaluate**

• Reduction in paranoid, excitable, or withdrawn behaviors

• ↓ Levels of anxiety, agitation, and tension

# Triflupromazine hydrochloride

(try-flew-**PROH**-mah-zeen)

Vesprin **(Rx)**

**Classification:** Antipsychotic, dimethylaminopropyl-type phenothiazine

See also *Antipsychotic Agents, Phenothiazines.*

**Action/Kinetics:** Produces significant anticholinergic and antiemetic effects; moderate to strong extrapyramidal and sedative effects; and moderate hypotensive effects.

**Uses:** Severe N&V. Psychotic disorders (do not use for psychotic disorders with depression).

**Special Concerns:** Use during pregnancy only if benefits clearly outweigh risks. Dosage has not been established for children less than 30 months of age. IV use not recommended for children because of hypotension and rapid onset of extrapyramidal side effects. Geriatric, emaciated, or debilitated clients may require a lower initial dose.

**Dosage**

• **IM**

*Psychoses.*

**Adults and adolescents:** 60 mg up to maximum of 150 mg/day. **Pediatric:** 0.2–0.25 mg/kg to maximum of 10 mg/day.

*N&V.*

**Adults and adolescents:** 5–15 mg as single dose repeated q 4 hr up to maximum of 60 mg/day (for elderly or debilitated clients: 2.5 mg up to maximum of 15 mg/day). **Pediatric, over 2½ years:** 0.2–0.25 mg/kg up to maximum of 10 mg/day.

• **IV**

*Psychoses.*

**Adults and adolescents:** 1 mg as required, up to a maximum of 3 mg/day.

## NURSING CONSIDERATIONS

See also *Nursing Considerations* for *Antipsychotic Agents, Phenothiazines.*

**Administration/Storage**

1. Avoid excessive heat and freezing.

2. Store in amber-colored containers.

3. Do not use discolored (darker than light amber) solutions.

**Assessment:** Document indications for therapy; note source, onset, and duration of symptoms. List other agents trialed.

**Client/Family Teaching**
1. Avoid skin contact with liquid form to prevent contact dermatitis.
2. May discolor urine reddish brown.
3. When used in children for N&V, the duration may be 12 hr.

**Outcomes/Evaluate**
• Control of N&V
• ↓ Agitated and hyperactive behaviors

# Trifluridine
(try-**FLUR**-ih-deen)
**Pregnancy Category:** C
Viroptic **(Rx)**
**Classification:** Antiviral, ophthalmic

See also *Anti-Infectives.*

**Action/Kinetics:** Closely resembles thymidine; inhibits thymidylic phosphorylase and specific DNA polymerases necessary for incorporation of thymidine into viral DNA. Trifluridine, instead of thymidine, is incorporated into viral DNA, resulting in faulty DNA and the ability to infect or reproduce in tissue. Also incorporated into mammalian DNA. **t½:** 12–18 min.

**Uses:** Primary keratoconjunctivitis and recurrent epithelial keratitis caused by HSV types 1 and 2. Epithelial keratitis resistant to idoxuridine or if ocular toxicity or hypersensitivity to idoxuridine has occurred. Is also indicated for infections resistant to vidarabine.

**Contraindications:** Hypersensitivity or chemical intolerance to drug.

**Special Concerns:** Safe use during pregnancy not established. Use with caution during lactation.

**Side Effects:** *Ophthalmic:* Mild, transient burning or stinging when instilled. Palpebral edema, superficial punctate keratopathy, epithelial keratopathy, hypersensitivity reaction, stomal edema, irritation, eratitis sicca, hyperemia, increased intraocular pressure.

**Dosage**
• **Solution, 1%**
1 gtt solution q 2 hr onto cornea, up to maximum of 9 gtt/day in each eye during acute stage (presence of corneal ulcer). Following reepithelialization, decrease dosage to 1 gtt/4 hr (or minimum of 5 gtt/day in each eye) for 7 days. Do not use for more than 21 days.

## NURSING CONSIDERATIONS

See also *General Nursing Considerations for All Anti-Infectives.*

**Administration/Storage**
1. May be used concomitantly in the eye with antibiotics (chloramphenicol, bacitracin, polymyxin B sulfate, erythromycin, neomycin, gentamicin, tetracycline, sulfacetamide sodium), corticosteroids, anticholinergics, epinephrine HCl, and sodium chloride.
2. Drug is heat-sensitive. Store in refrigerator at 2°C–8°C (35.6°F–46.4°F).

**Client/Family Teaching**
1. Instill drop onto cornea. Apply finger pressure lightly to lacrimal sac for 1 min after instillation.
2. A mild, transient burning sensation may occur on instillation.
3. Report any new or bothersome side effects but do not stop medication without specific instructions as herpetic keratitis may recur. Have regular exams by an ophthalmologist.
4. Improvement usually occurs within 7 days and healing takes place within 14 days. Thereafter, 7 more days of therapy are necessary to prevent recurrence. Report if no improvement noted within 7 days.
5. Do not administer for more than 21 days because toxicity may occur (discard remaining drug after 21 days).
6. Store drug in refrigerator.

**Outcomes/Evaluate**
• Resolution of infection
• Reepithelialization of herpetic eye lesions

# Trihexyphenidyl hydrochloride

(try-hex-ee-**FEN**-ih-dill)
**Pregnancy Category:** C
Aparkane ✿, Apo-Trihex ✿, Artane, Artane Sequels, Novo-Hexidyl ✿, PMS-Trihexyphenidyl ✿, Trihexy-2 and -5, Trihexyphen ✿ **(Rx)**
**Classification:** Antiparkinson agent, anticholinergic

See also *Cholinergic Blocking Agents* and *Antiparkinson Drugs*.
**Action/Kinetics:** Synthetic anticholinergic, which relieves rigidity but has little effect on tremors. Causes a direct antispasmodic effect on smooth muscle. High incidence of side effects. Small doses cause CNS depression, whereas larger doses may result in CNS excitation. **Onset, PO:** 60 min. **Duration, PO:** 6–12 hr.
**Uses:** Adjunct in the treatment of all types of parkinsonism (often used as adjunct with levodopa). Drug-induced extrapyramidal symptoms. Sustained-release medication is for maintenance dosage only.
**Additional Contraindications:** Arteriosclerosis and hypersensitivity to drug.
**Additional Side Effects:** Serious CNS stimulation (restlessness, insomnia, delirium, agitation) and psychotic manifestations.
**Additional Drug Interactions:** ↑ Effectiveness of levodopa if used together; such combined use not recommended in clients with psychoses.

**Dosage** —————
• **Elixir, Tablets**
  *Parkinsonism.*
**Initial (day 1):** 1–2 mg; **then,** increase by 2 mg q 3–5 days until daily dose is 6–10 mg given in divided doses. Some clients may require 12–15 mg/day (especially those with postencephalitic parkinsonism).
  *Adjunct with levodopa.*
**Adults:** 3–6 mg/day in divided doses.
  *Drug-induced extrapyramidal reactions.*

**Initial:** 1 mg/day; **then,** increase as needed to total daily dose of 5–15 mg.

## NURSING CONSIDERATIONS

See also *Nursing Considerations* for *Cholinergic Blocking Agents* and *Antiparkinson Drugs*.
**Assessment:** Assess for and note extent of involuntary movements, drooling, pill rolling, and muscle spasms/rigidity. Note mental status.
**Client/Family Teaching**
1. Take with or after meals to minimize GI upset.
2. May cause dizziness or drowsiness and othostatic effects.
3. Increase fluids and bulk in diet to prevent constipation.
4. May impair perspiration; avoid overheating and hot weather exposures. Report urinary retention.
5. This drug has a high incidence of side effects; report as early detection and intervention are imperative.
6. Report any evidence of extrapyramidal symptoms or an increase in restlessness, insomnia, agitation, or psychotic manifestations as dosage may need adjusting.
**Outcomes/Evaluate**
• Control of symptoms of parkinsonism
• Prevention of drug-induced extrapyramidal symptoms

# Trimethobenzamide hydrochloride

(try-meth-oh-**BENZ**-ah-myd)
Arrestin, Hymetic, Tebamide, T-Gen, Ticon, Tigan **(Rx)**
**Classification:** Antiemetic

See also *Antiemetics*.
**Action/Kinetics:** Related to the antihistamines but with weak antihistaminic properties. Less effective than the phenothiazines but has fewer side effects. Not suitable as sole agent for severe emesis. Can be used PR. Appears to control vomiting by depressing the CTZ in the medulla. **Onset: PO and IM,** 10–40 min.

**T**

**Duration:** 3–4 hr after PO and 2–3 hr after IM. 30%–50% of drug excreted unchanged in urine in 48–72 hr.

**Uses:** Nausea and vomiting.

**Contraindications:** Hypersensitivity to drug, benzocaine, or similar local anesthetics. Do not use suppositories for neonates; do not use IM in children.

**Special Concerns:** Use during pregnancy only if benefits outweigh risks. Use with caution during lactation.

**Side Effects:** *CNS:* Depression of mood, disorientation, headache, drowsiness, dizziness, *seizures, coma,* Parkinson-like symptoms. *Other:* Hypersensitivity reactions, hypotension, blood dyscrasias, jaundice, muscle cramps, opisthotonos, blurred vision, diarrhea, allergic skin reactions. *After IM injection:* Pain, burning, stinging, redness at injection site.

**Drug Interactions:** Concomitant use with atropine-like drugs and CNS depressants including alcohol should be avoided.

**Dosage** ────────────

• **Capsules**

**Adults:** 250 mg t.i.d.–q.i.d.; **pediatric, 13.6–40.9 kg:** 100–200 mg t.i.d.–q.i.d.

• **Suppositories**

**Adults:** 200 mg t.i.d.–q.i.d.; **pediatric, under 13.6 kg:** 100 mg t.i.d.–q.i.d.; **13.6–40.9 kg:** 100–200 mg t.i.d.–q.i.d.

• **IM**

**Adults only:** 200 mg t.i.d.–q.i.d. *IM route not to be used in children.*

## NURSING CONSIDERATIONS

See also *Nursing Considerations* for *Antiemetics.*

**Administration/Storage**

1. Inject drug IM deeply into the upper, outer quadrant of the gluteus muscle. Be careful to avoid escape of fluid from the needle so as to minimize local reaction.

2. Do not administer suppositories to clients allergic to benzocaine or similar anesthetics.

**Assessment**

1. Identify cause for N&V.

2. Document any sensitivity to benzocaine. Assess for any skin reaction (first sign of hypersensitivity to the drug).

3. Note any local reaction to the suppositories.

**Client/Family Teaching**

1. Use only as directed; report any adverse drug effects.

2. Do not drive or operate machinery until drug effects are realized; may cause drowsiness and dizziness.

3. Avoid alcohol and any other CNS depressants.

**Outcomes/Evaluate:** Prevention/control of N&V

────────*COMBINATION DRUG*────────

# Trimethoprim and Sulfamethoxazole

(try-**METH**-oh-prim, sul-fah-meh-**THOX**-ah-zohl)

**Pregnancy Category:** C

Apo-Sulfatrim ✹, Bactrim, Bactrim DS, Bactrim IV, Bactrim Pediatric, Bactrim Roche ✹, Cotrim, Cotrim D.S., Cotrim Pediatric, Novo-Trimel ✹, Novo-Trimel D.S. ✹, Nu-Cotrimix ✹, Pro-Trin ✹, Roubac ✹, Septra, Septra DS, Septra Injection ✹, Septra IV, Sulfatrim, Trisulfa ✹, Trisulfa DS ✹ **(Rx)**

**Classification:** Antibacterial

See also *Sulfonamides.*

**Content:** These products contain the antibacterial agents sulfamethoxazole and trimethoprim. See also *Sulfamethoxazole.*

  **Oral Suspension:** Sulfamethoxazole, 200 mg and trimethoprim, 40 mg/5 mL.

  **Tablets:** Sulfamethoxazole, 400 mg and trimethoprim, 80 mg/tablet.

  **Double Strength (DS) Tablets:** Sulfamethoxazole, 800 mg and trimethoprim, 160 mg/tablet.

  **Concentrate for injection:** Sulfamethoxazole, 80 mg and trimethoprim, 16 mg/mL.

**Uses: PO, Parenteral:** UTIs due to *Escherichia coli, Klebsiella, Enterobacter, Pseudomonas mirabilis* and *vulgaris,* and *Morganella morganii.* Enteritis due to *Shigella flexneri* or *S. sonnei.*

*Pneumocystis carinii* pneumonitis in children and adults. **PO:** Acute otitis media in children due to *Haemophilus influenzae* or *Streptococcus pneumoniae*. Traveler's diarrhea in adults due to *E. coli*. Prophylaxis of *P. carinii* pneumonia in immunocompromised clients (including those with AIDS). Acute exacerbations of chronic bronchitis in adults due to *H. influenzae* or *S. pneumoniae*. *Investigational:* Cholera, salmonella, nocardiosis, prophylaxis of recurrent UTIs in women, prophylaxis of neutropenic clients with *P. carinii* infections or leukemia clients to decrease incidence of gram-negative rod bacteremia. Treatment of acute and chronic prostatitis. Decrease chance of urinary and blood bacterial infections in renal transplant clients.

**Additional Contraindications:** Infants under 2 months of age. During pregnancy at term. Megaloblastic anemia due to folate deficiency. Lactation.

**Special Concerns:** Use with caution in impaired liver or kidney function and in clients with possible folate deficiency. AIDS clients may not tolerate or respond to this product.

**Laboratory Test Alterations:** Jaffe alkaline picrate reaction overestimation of creatinine by 10%.

**Additional Drug Interactions**

*Cyclosporine* / ↓ Effect of cyclosporine; ↑ risk of nephrotoxicity

*Dapsone* / ↑ Effect of both dapsone and trimethoprim

*Methotrexate* / ↑ Risk of methotrexate toxicity due to displacement from plasma protein binding sites

*Phenytoin* / ↑ Effect of phenytoin due to ↓ hepatic clearance

*Sulfonylureas* / ↑ Hypoglycemic effect of sulfonylureas

*Thiazide diuretics* / ↑ Risk of thrombocytopenia with purpura in geriatric clients

*Warfarin* / ↑ PT

*Zidovudine* / ↑ Serum levels of AZT due to ↓ renal clearance

**Dosage** —————
• **Oral Suspension, Double-Strength Tablets, Tablets**

*UTIs, shigellosis, bronchitis, acute otitis media.*

**Adults:** 1 DS tablet, 2 tablets, or 4 teaspoonfuls of suspension q 12 hr for 10–14 days. **Pediatric:** Total daily dose of 8 mg/kg trimethoprim and 40 mg/kg sulfamethoxazole divided equally and given q 12 hr for 10–14 days. (*NOTE:* For shigellosis, give adult or pediatric dose for 5 days.) For clients with impaired renal function the following dosage is recommended: $C_{CR}$ of 15–30 mL/min: one-half the usual regimen and for $C_{CR}$ less than 15 mL/min: use is not recommended.

*Chancroid.*

1 DS tablet b.i.d. for at least 7 days (alternate therapy: 4 DS tablets in a single dose).

*Pharyngeal gonococcal infection due to penicillinase-producing* Neisseria gonorrhoeae.

720 mg trimethoprim and 3,600 mg sulfamethoxazole once daily for 5 days.

*Prophylaxis of* P. carinii *pneumonia.*

**Adults:** 160 mg trimethoprim and 800 mg sulfamethoxazole q 24 hr. **Children:** 150 mg/m² of trimethoprim and 750 mg/m² sulfamethoxazole daily in equally divided doses b.i.d. on three consecutive days per week. Do not exceed a total daily dose of 320 mg trimethoprim and 1,600 mg sulamethoxazole.

*Treatment of* P. carinii *pneumonia.*

**Adults and children:** Total daily dose of 15–20 mg/kg trimethoprim and 100 mg/kg sulfamethoxazole divided equally and given q 6 hr for 14–21 days.

*Prophylaxis of* P. carinii *pneumonia in immunocompromised clients.*

1 DS tablet daily.

*Traveler's diarrhea.*

**Adults,** 1 DS tablet q 12 hr for 5 days.

*Prostatitis, acute bacterial.*

T

---

✦ = Available in Canada | ***bold italic*** = life threatening side effect

1 DS tablet b.i.d. until client is afebrile for 48 hr; treatment may be required for up to 30 days.

*Prostatitis, chronic bacterial.*

1 DS tablet b.i.d. for 4–6 weeks.

• **IV**

*UTIs, shigellosis, acute otitis media.*

**Adults and children:** 8–10 mg/kg/day (based on trimethoprim) in two to four divided doses q 6, 8, or 12 hr for up to 14 days for severe UTIs or 5 days for shigellosis.

*Treatment of* P. carinii *pneumonia*

**Adults and children:** 15–20 mg/kg/day (based on trimethoprim) in 3–4 divided doses q 6–8 hr for up to 14 days.

## NURSING CONSIDERATIONS

See also *General Nursing Considerations for All Anti-Infectives* and for *Sulfonamides.*

**Administration/Storage**

**IV** 1. The IV infusion must be administered over a period of 60–90 min.

2. Each 5-mL vial must be diluted to 125 mL with D5W and used within 6 hr. If the amount of fluid should be restricted, each 5 mL can be diluted up to 75 mL with D5W and used within 2 hr. Do not refrigerate the diluted solution.

3. Do not mix the IV infusion with any other drugs or solutions.

4. If the diluted IV infusion is cloudy or precipitates after mixing, discard and prepare a new solution.

**Assessment**

1. Document indications for therapy, onset, duration, and characteristics of symptoms.

2. Monitor cultures, CBC, liver and renal function studies; reduce dose with renal dysfunction.

3. Assess for megaloblastic anemia; drug inhibits ability to produce folinic acid. Simultaneous administration of folinic acid (6–8 mg/day) may prevent antifolate drug effects.

4. Document if clients infected with AIDS virus; may be intolerant to this product.

**Client/Family Teaching**

1. Take only as directed. Complete entire prescription and do not share meds.

2. Report any symptoms of drug fever, vasculitis, N&V, or CNS disturbances immediately.

3. Consume 2.5–3 L of fluids/day.

**Outcomes/Evaluate**

• Resolution of infection; negative cultures

• Prophylaxis of *P. carinii* pneumonia.

# Trimetrexate glucuronate
(**try**-meh-**TREX**-ayt gloo-**KYOU**-roh-nayt)

**Pregnancy Category:** D
NeuTrexin **(Rx)**
**Classification:** Miscellaneous anti-infective

See also *Anti-Infectives.*

**Action/Kinetics:** Inhibits the enzyme dihydrofolate reductase resulting in interference with thymidylate biosynthesis and inhibition of folate-dependent formyltransferases. This leads to inhibition of purine synthesis and disruption of DNA, RNA, and protein synthesis and ultimately cell death. Must be given with leucovorin to prevent serious or life-threatening complications, including bone marrow suppression, oral and GI mucosal ulceration, and renal and hepatic dysfunction. **t½:** 11 hr. Highly bound to plasma protein and metabolized by the liver. Metabolites also appear to have an inhibitory effect on dihydrofolate reductase.

**Uses:** As alternative therapy with concurrent leucovorin for the treatment of moderate to severe *Pneumocystis carinii* pneumonia in immunocompromised clients. Treatment is indicated in clients with AIDS who are intolerant of or refractory to trimethoprim-sulfamethoxazole (TMP/SMZ) therapy or in whom this combination is contraindicated. *Investigational:* Treatment of non-small-cell lung, prostate, or colorectal cancer.

**Contraindications:** Hypersensitivity to trimetrexate, leucovorin, or methotrexate. Lactation.

**Special Concerns:** Use with caution in clients with impaired hematologic, renal, or hepatic function. Safety and efficacy have not been determined for clients less than 18 years of age for use in treating histologically confirmed PCP.

**Side Effects:** *GI:* N&V. *Hematologic:* Neutropenia, thrombocytopenia, anemia. *Hepatic:* Hepatic toxicity manifested by increased ALT, AST, alkaline phosphatase, and bilirubin. *Renal:* Increased serum creatinine. *Electrolytes:* Hyponatremia, hypocalcemia.

**OD** **Overdose Management:** *Symptoms:* Primarily hematologic. *Treatment:* Discontinue trimetrexate and administer leucovorin at a dose of 40 mg/m² q 6 hr for 3 days.

**Drug Interactions:** Since trimetrexate is metabolized by the P-450 enzyme system in the liver, drugs that stimulate or inhibit this enzyme system may cause drug interactions that may alter plasma levels of trimetrexate (e.g., erythromycin, rifabutin, rifampin).

*Acetaminophen* / May alter the levels of trimetrexate metabolites
*Cimetidine* / May ↓ metabolism of trimetrexate
*Clotrimazole* / ↓ Metabolism of trimetrexate
*Ketoconazole* / ↓ Metabolism of trimetrexate
*Miconazole* / ↓ Metabolism of trimetrexate

**Dosage** —————
• **IV Infusion**
Pneumocystis carinii *pneumonia*.
**Adults:** 45 mg/m² once daily by IV infusion over 60–90 min. Leucovorin is given IV at a dose of 20 mg/m² over 5–10 min q 6 hr for a total daily dose of 80 mg/m². Leucovorin may also be given orally in four doses of 20 mg/m² spaced equally throughout the day (the oral dose should be rounded up to the next higher 25-mg

increment). Doses of trimetrexate and leucovorin are modified depending on hematologic toxicity. If neutrophils are between 750 and 1,000/mm³ and platelets between 50,000 and 75,000/mm³, the dose of trimetrexate remains at 45 mg/m² once daily but the dose of leucovorin is increased to 40 mg/m² q 6 hr. If neutrophils are between 500 and 749/mm³ and platelets between 25,000 and 49,999, the dose of trimetrexate is reduced to 22 mg/m² once daily and the dose of leucovorin is 40 mg/m² q 6 hr. If neutrophils are less than 500/mm³ and platelets are less than 25,000/mm³, trimetrexate is discontinued for 9 days with leucovorin still given at a dose of 40 mg/m² q 6 hr; from days 10 to 21, trimetrexate should be interrupted up to 96 hr.

# NURSING CONSIDERATIONS

See also *General Nursing Considerations for All Anti-Infectives.*
**Administration/Storage**
**IV** 1. Leucovorin therapy must be given for 72 hr after the last dose of trimetrexate.
2. The recommended course of therapy is 21 days for trimetrexate and 24 days for leucovorin.
3. Reconstitute the lyophilized powder with 2 mL of 5% dextrose injection or sterile water for injection to yield a concentration of 12.5 mg/mL. The reconstituted product appears as a pale greenish-yellow solution. Do not use the solution if it is cloudy or a precipitate is observed. Filter the solution before dilution.
4. Do not reconstitute the powder with solutions containing either chloride ion or leucovorin as precipitation occurs immediately.
5. The reconstituted solution may be further diluted with 5% dextrose injection to yield a final concentration of from 0.25 to 2 mg/mL.
6. Before and after administering trimetrexate, the IV line must be flushed thoroughly with at least 10 mL of 5% dextrose injection.

**T**

---

7. Trimetrexate and leucovorin solutions must be given separately.

8. If trimetrexate comes in contact with the skin or mucosa, immediately and thoroughly wash areas with soap and water.

9. After reconstitution, the solution is stable under refrigeration or at room temperature for at least 24 hr. Do not freeze the reconstituted solution. Discard any unused portion after 24 hr.

**Assessment**

1. Document indications for therapy, any other agents prescribed, and the outcome. Note if client intolerant or refractory to trimethoprim-sulfamethoxazole.

2. Determine any hypersensitivity to leucovorin, methotrexate, or trimetrexate.

3. Monitor CBC, liver and renal function studies twice a week during therapy.

**Interventions**

1. Drug is to be administered concurrently with leucovorin to avoid its hematologic, hepatic, renal, and GI toxicities.

2. If also receiving myelosuppressive, nephrotoxic, or hepatotoxic drugs, monitor carefully.

3. To allow for use of full therapeutic doses of trimetrexate, AZT should be discontinued during therapy.

4. Observe client carefully and report any changes. It may be difficult to distinguish side effects caused by trimetrexate from symptoms due to underlying medical conditions.

5. Trimetrexate should be discontinued for the following:

• Serum transaminase or alkaline phosphatase increases to > 5x the ULN.

• Serum creatinine increases to 2.5 mg/dL.

• Mucosal toxicity becomes so severe it interferes with oral intake.

• Body temperature increases to more than 40.5°C (105°F) when taken PO.

**Client/Family Teaching:** Identify local support groups that may assist client to understand and cope with this disease.

**Outcomes/Evaluate:** Resolution of PCP in immunocompromised clients

# Trimipramine maleate
(try-**MIP**-rah-meen)
**Pregnancy Category:** C
Apo-Trimip ✤, Novo-Tripramine ✤,
Nu-Trimipramine ✤, Rhotrimine ✤,
Surmontil **(Rx)**
**Classification:** Antidepressant, tricyclic

See also *Antidepressants, Tricyclic.*
**Action/Kinetics:** Causes moderate anticholinergic and orthostatic hypotensive effects and significant sedative effects. **Effective plasma levels:** 180 ng/mL. **Time to reach steady state:** 2–6 days. t½: 7–30 hr.
**Uses:** Treatment of symptoms of depression. PUD. Seems more effective in endogenous depression than in other types of depression.
**Contraindications:** Use in children less than 12 years of age.

**Dosage** ⎯⎯⎯⎯⎯⎯⎯⎯
• **Capsules**
  *Antidepressant.*
**Adults, outpatients, initial:** 75 mg/day in divided doses up to 150 mg/day. Daily dosage should not exceed 200 mg; **maintenance:** 50–150 mg/day. Total dose can be given at bedtime. **Adults, hospitalized, initial:** 100 mg/day in divided doses up to 200 mg/day. If no improvement in 2–3 weeks, increase to 250–300 mg/day. **Adolescent/geriatric clients, initial:** 50 mg/day up to 100 mg/day. Not recommended for children.

## NURSING CONSIDERATIONS

See also *Nursing Considerations* for *Antidepressants, Tricyclic.*
**Administration/Storage:** To minimize relapse, continue maintenance therapy for about 3 months.
**Assessment:** Document indications for therapy, onset, duration, and characteristics of symptoms. Note any predisposing factors/events.

**Outcomes/Evaluate**
- ↓ Depression symptoms
- Control of symptoms of PUD

————COMBINATION DRUG————

# Trinalin
**(TRIN**-al-in)
**Pregnancy Category:** D
**(Rx)**
**Classification:** Antihistamine, decongestant

**Content:** *Antihistamine:* Azatadine maleate, 1 mg. *Decongestant:* Pseudoephedrine sulfate, 120 mg in a long-acting formulation. See also information on individual components.

**Action/Kinetics:** The tablet is formulated so that the azatadine and one-half of the pseudoephedrine are released immediately; the remaining one-half of the pseudoephedrine is released after several hours.

**Uses:** Symptoms of allergic rhinitis and perennial rhinitis, nasal and eustachian tube congestion.

**Contraindications:** Lactation. Children under 12 years of age. Use to treat lower respiratory tract symptoms, including asthma. Narrow-angle glaucoma, urinary retention, clients taking MAO inhibitors, severe hypertension, severe CAD, hyperthyroidism, clients hypersensitive to adrenergic agents.

**Special Concerns:** Use with caution in clients with stenosing peptic ulcer, pyloroduodenal obstruction, urinary bladder obstruction due to prostatic hypertrophy or narrowing of the bladder neck, hypertension, ischemic heart disease, increased intraocular pressure, and diabetes mellitus and in clients taking digitalis or oral anticoagulants.

**Dosage**
- **Tablets**
**Adults:** 1 tablet b.i.d.

## NURSING CONSIDERATIONS

See also *Nursing Considerations* for *Antihistamines* and *Sympathomimetic Drugs*.

**Administration/Storage:** May be used in conjunction with other analgesics and/or antibiotics.
**Outcomes/Evaluate:** Relief of congestion; ↓ allergic manifestations

# Tripelennamine hydrochloride
(try-pell-**EN**-ah-meen)
PBZ, PBZ-SR, Pyribenzamine ✽ **(Rx)**
**Classification:** Antihistamine, ethylenediamine derivative

See also *Antihistamines.*
**Action/Kinetics:** GI effects more pronounced than other antihistamines. Moderate sedative effects and low to no anticholinergic activity.
**Duration:** 4–6 hr.
**Contraindications:** Use in neonates.
**Special Concerns:** Safe use during pregnancy has not been established. Geriatric clients may be more sensitive to the usual adult dose.
**Side Effects:** Low incidence. Moderate sedation, mild GI distress, paradoxical excitation, hyperirritability.

**Dosage**
- **Tablets**
**Adults, usual:** 25–50 mg q 4–6 hr; as little as 25 mg or as high as 600 mg may be given to control symptoms.
**Pediatric:** 5 mg/kg/day or 150 mg/m²/day divided into 4–6 doses, not to exceed 300 mg/day.
- **Extended-Release Tablets**
**Adults:** 100 mg q 8–12 hr as needed, up to a maximum of 600 mg/day. Do not use sustained-release form in children.

## NURSING CONSIDERATIONS

See also *Nursing Considerations* for *Antihistamines.*
**Administration/Storage:** Swallow extended-release tablets whole; never crush or chew.
**Outcomes/Evaluate:** ↓ Allergic manifestations

# Troglitazone
(troh-**GLIH**-tah-zohn)
**Pregnancy Category:** B
Rezulin **(Rx)**
**Classification:** Oral hypoglycemic

See also *Hypoglycemic Agents.*

**Action/Kinetics:** Lowers blood glucose by improving the target cell response to insulin without increasing pancreatic insulin secretion. Decreases hepatic glucose output and increases insulin-dependent glucose disposal in skeletal muscle and perhaps liver and adipose tissue. This effect may be due to a binding of the drug to nuclear receptors that regulate the transcription of a number of insulin responsive genes required for the control of glucose and lipid metabolism. Troglitazone is not an insulin secretagogue. Rapidly absorbed; **maximum plasma levels:** 2–3 hr. Steady-state plasma levels are reached in 3–5 days. Food increases the rate of absorption. **t½, elimination:** 16–34 hr. Metabolized in the liver and excreted mainly in the feces.

**Uses:** Alone or in combination with a sulfonylurea for treatment of type II diabetes with poor glucose control despite insulin therapy. *Investigational:* Use in the productive and metabolic consequences of polycystic ovary syndrome.

**Contraindications:** Lactation. Use for type I diabetes or for the treatment of diabetic ketoacidosis.

**Special Concerns:** Use with caution in those with liver disease. Ovulation may resume in premenopausal anovulatory clients, leading to an increased risk of pregnancy. Safety and efficacy have not been determined in children.

**Side Effects:** *GI:* Nausea, diarrhea. *CNS:* Headache, dizziness. *Metabolic:* Hypoglycemia. *Hematologic:* Decreased hemoglobin, hematocrit, and white blood cell counts. *Nose/throat:* Rhinitis, pharyngitis. *Miscelleaneous:* Infection, pain, accidental injury, asthenia, back pain, UTI, peripheral edema.

**Laboratory Test Alterations:** ↑ AST, ALT, both of which are reversible. Small changes in serum lipids.

**Drug Interactions**
*Cholestyramine* / ↓ Absorption of troglitazone → ↓ effect
*Cyclosporine* / ↓ Effect of cyclosporine due to ↑ breakdown by the liver
*HMG-CoA reductase inhibitors (antihyperlipidemics)* / Effect of antihyperlipidemic due to breakdown by the liver
*Oral contraceptives containing ethinyl estradiol/norethindrone* / ↓ Plasma levels of the hormones → ↓ contraceptive effect
*Tacrolimus* / Effect of tacrolimus due to breakdown by the liver
*Terfenadine* / ↓ Plasma levels of terfenadine → ↓ effect

**Dosage**
• **Tablets**
   *With insulin in type II diabetes mellitus.*
**Adults:** 200 mg daily while continuing the insulin dosage. If the response is inadequate, the dose may be increased after 2 to 4 weeks. **Usual daily dose:** 400 mg/day. **Maximum daily dose:** 600 mg/day. The insulin dose should be decreased by 10% to 25% when fasting plasma glucose levels decrease to less than 120 mg/dL in clients receiving both insulin and troglitazone.
   *Polycystic ovary syndrome.*
**Adults:** 400 mg/day.

## NURSING CONSIDERATIONS

See also *Nursing Considerations* for *Hypoglycemic Agents.*
**Assessment**
1. Document indications for therapy, onset, duration, and characteristics of disease. Note other agents trialed and the outcome.
2. Assess finger stick values at different times throughout the day; review exercise and dietary habits.
3. Monitor ECG, CBC, urinalysis, HbA1-C, liver and renal function studies.

4. Avoid with CHF or liver dysfunction.

5. New FDA warnings to monitor for signs of liver damage. Liver enzyme studies are to be undertaken at the start of therapy, every month for the first 6 months of treatment, every other month for the next 6 months, and periodically thereafter. Also, obtain LFTs in clients who develop symptoms of liver dysfunction.

**Client/Family Teaching**

1. Take with meals to increase absorption. If a dose is missed, it should be taken at the next meal. If the dose is missed on one day, the dose is not to be doubled the next day.

2. Continue diet, weight loss, regular exercise, and alcohol and tobacco cessation, in the overall management of diabetes.

3. Drug is only active in the presence of insulin; do not use with type I diabetes or with diabetic ketoacidosis.

4. Monitor fingersticks regularly; report persistent hypoglycemia, as a reduction in insulin dosage may needed.

5. Practice reliable birth control.

6. Report any evidence of CHF (i.e., increased cough, SOB, or edema) or hepatotoxicity (i.e., abdominal pain or yellow discoloration of skin) immediately.

7. Report as scheduled for F/U evaluation: frequent lab studies for liver function (q mo for the first six mo of treatment, every other mo for the next six mo, and periodically thereafter) and ECG to assess drug effectiveness.

**Outcomes/Evaluate**

• HbA1-C less than 8.5%
• Control of BS with reduced insulin requirements with Type II diabetes

# Tromethamine
(troh-**METH**-ah-meen)
**Pregnancy Category:** C
Tham, Tham-E **(Rx)**
**Classification:** Systemic alkalizing and buffering agent

**Action/Kinetics:** Actively binds hydrogen ions, thereby decreasing and correcting acidosis. It promotes the excretion of acids, carbon dioxide, and electrolytes and is thought to be able to neutralize some intracellular acid. It acts as an osmotic diuretic, increasing urine flow. Seventy-five percent of the drug is eliminated within 8 hr, the remainder within 3 days.

**Uses:** Prevention and correction of systemic acidosis, especially that accompanying cardiac bypass surgery, correction of acidity of acid citrate dextrose (ACD) blood in cardiac bypass surgery, and cardiac arrest.

**Contraindications:** Uremia and anuria.

**Special Concerns:** Use with caution in newborns and infants and in clients with renal disorders.

**Side Effects:** *Respiratory:* Respiratory depression, especially in those with chronic hypoventilation or getting drugs that depress respiration. *Other:* Fever, hypervolemia, transient decrease of blood glucose. *At injection site:* Extravasation may cause inflammation, vascular spasms, and tissue damage (e.g., chemical phlebitis, thrombosis, necrosis, sloughing). *In newborn: **Hemorrhagic liver necrosis when given by umbilical vein.***

**OD** **Overdose Management:** *Symptoms:* Alkalosis, overhydration, hypoglycemia (severe and prolonged), solute overload. *Treatment:* Discontinue the infusion and treat symptoms.

**Dosage** ——————————

Minimum amount to correct acid-base imbalance. The amount of tromethamine can be estimated using the buffer base deficit of the extracellular fluid: mL of 0.3 M tromethamine solution required = body weight (kg) × base deficit (mEq/L) × 1.1

• **Slow IV Infusion**
*Acidosis in cardiac bypass surgery.*

**Adults:** 500 mL (150 mEq or 18 g) as a single dose. Severe cases may require 1,000 mL. The dose should not exceed 500 mg/kg over a period of not less than 1 hr.

- **Injection into Ventricular Cavity or Large Peripheral Vein**
  *Acidosis in cardiac arrest (given at the same time as other standard procedures are being applied).*

**If chest is open. Adults:** 62–185 mL (2–6 g) into the ventricular cavity (not into the cardiac muscle). **If chest closed. Adults:** 111–333 mL (3.6–10.8 g) into a large peripheral vein.

- **Addition to Pump Oxygenator Acid Citrate Dextrose Blood**
  *For acidity in ACD blood.*
  15–77 mL (0.5–2.5 g) added to each 500 mL of ACD blood. Usually 62 mL (2 g) added to 500 mL of ACD blood is adequate.

---

## NURSING CONSIDERATIONS
### Administration/Storage
**IV** 1. Undertake tests on blood pH, $pCO_2$, bicarbonate, glucose, and electrolytes before, during, and after administration of tromethamine.
2. Concentration of solution administered *must not* exceed 0.3 M.
3. Prepare a 0.3-M solution of tromethamine by adding 1,000 mL of sterile water for injection to 36 g of lyophilized tromethamine.
4. Infuse slowly.
5. Administer into the largest antecubital vein through a large needle or indwelling catheter and elevate limb.
6. For treatment of cardiac arrest, the drug may be injected into the ventricular cavity if the chest is open. If the chest is not open, the drug may be injected into a large peripheral vein.
7. Do not administer longer than 1 day unless acute life-threatening situation exists.
8. Discontinue administration *immediately,* if extravasation occurs:
- Administer 1% procaine hydrochloride with hyaluronidase to reduce venospasm and to dilute the drug in the tissues.

- Phentolamine mesylate (Regitine) has been used for local infiltration for its adrenergic blocking properties.
- If necessary, a nerve block of the autonomic fibers may be done.

### Assessment
1. Note any history of urinary or bladder problems.
2. Determine if pregnant.
3. Obtain and analyze baseline pH, $pCO_2$, bicarbonate, glucose, electrolytes, liver and renal function studies.

### Interventions
1. Observe for respiratory depression; have mechanical ventilatory equipment available.
2. Document and report any complaints of weakness, presence of moist pale skin, tremors, and a full bounding pulse (symptoms of hypoglycemia, which can occur after rapid- or high-dose administration).
3. Record I&O. Assess for nausea, diarrhea, tachycardia, oliguria, weakness, numbness, or tingling sensations (symptoms of hyperkalemia).
4. Observe closely for extravasation; drug is extremely irritating to veins.

### Outcomes/Evaluate
- Neutralization of ACD blood in pump oxygenator
- Correction of systemic acidosis; serum pH within desired range

---

# Tubocurarine chloride
(too-boh-kyour-**AR**-een)
**Pregnancy Category:** C
**(Rx)**
**Classification:** Nondepolarizing neuromuscular blocking agent

See also *Neuromuscular Blocking Agents.*

**Action/Kinetics:** Cumulative effects may occur. Most likely of the nondepolarizing drugs to cause histamine release. Narrow margin between therapeutic dose and toxic dose. **Onset, IV:** 1 min; **IM:** 15–25 min. **Time to peak effect, IV:** 2–5 min. **Duration, IV:** 20–90 min. **t½:** 1–3 hr. About 43% excreted unchanged in urine.

**Uses:** Muscle relaxant during surgery or setting of fractures and dislocations; spasticity caused by injury to or disease of CNS. Treat seizures electrically induced or induced by drugs. Diagnosis of myasthenia gravis.
**Additional Contraindications:** Clients in whom release of histamine is hazardous.

**Special Concerns:** Use with caution during pregnancy and lactation and in children. If repeated doses are used before delivery, the newborn may manifest decreased skeletal muscle activity. Children up to 1 month of age may be more sensitive to the effects of tubocurarine. Use with extreme caution in clients with renal dysfunction, liver disease, or obstructive states.

**Additional Side Effects:** *Allergic reactions.* Excessive secretion and circulatory collapse.

**OD**  **Overdose Management:** *Treatment:* Overdosage chiefly treated by artificial respiration, although neostigmine, atropine, and edrophonium chloride should also be on hand.

**Additional Drug Interactions**
*Acetylcholine* / Acetylcholine antagonizes effect of tubocurarine
*Anticholinesterases* / Anticholinesterases antagonize effect of tubocurarine
*Calcium salts* / ↑ Effect of tubocurarine
*Diazepam* / Diazepam may cause malignant hyperthermia with tubocurarine
*Potassium* / Antagonizes effect of tubocurarine
*Propranolol* / ↑ Effect of tubocurarine
*Quinine* / ↑ Effect of tubocurarine
*Succinylcholine chloride* / ↑ Relaxant effect of both drugs

**Dosage** ⎯⎯⎯⎯⎯⎯⎯⎯⎯
• **IV, IM**
   *Adjunct to surgical anesthesia.*
**Adults, IM, IV, initial:** 6–9 mg (40–60 units); **then,** 3–4.5 mg (20–30 units) in 3–5 min if needed. Supplemental doses of 3 mg (20 units) can be given for prolonged procedures. Dosage can be calculated on the basis of 1.1 units/kg. **Pediatric, up to 4 weeks of age, IV, initial:** 0.3 mg/kg; **then,** give subsequent doses in increments of ⅕–⅙ the initial dose. **Infants and children, IV:** 0.6 mg/kg.
   *Electroshock therapy.*
**Adults, IV:** 0.165 mg/kg (1.1 units/kg) given over 30–90 sec. It is recommended that the initial dose be 3 mg less than the calculated total dose.
   *Diagnosis of myasthenia gravis.*
**Adults, IV:** 0.004–0.033 mg/kg. A test dose should be given within 2–3 min with IV neostigmine, 1.5 mg, to minimize prolonged respiratory paralysis.

## NURSING CONSIDERATIONS

See also *Nursing Considerations* for *Neuromuscular Blocking Agents.*
**Administration/Storage**
**IV** 1. Give IV as a sustained injection over 1–1.5 min. May also be given IM.
2. Give in incremental doses until relaxation is reached.
3. Decrease the initial dose if the inhalation anesthetic used enhances the action of curariform drugs or if the client has compromised renal function.
4. Review the drugs with which tubocurarine interacts.
5. Tubocurarine is incompatible with alkaline solutions and may form a precipitate when mixed with them (e.g., methohexital sodium or thiopental sodium).
6. Have neostigmine methylsulfate available as an antidote.
**Assessment**
1. Document indications for therapy, onset, duration, and characteristics of symptoms.
2. Utilize a peripheral nerve stimulator to assess neuromuscular response and recovery.
3. Document length of time receiving the drug. It should be used only on a short-term basis and in a continuously monitored environment.

T

---

4. Remember that client may be fully conscious and aware of surroundings and conversations.

5. Drug does not affect pain or anxiety; administer analgesics and anti-anxiety agents as needed.

6. Monitor VS, ECG, and lab studies. Drug can cause vagal stimulation resulting in bradycardia, hypotension, and cardiac arrhythmias.

**Outcomes/Evaluate**

- Skeletal muscle relaxation
- Control of drug or electrically induced seizures
- Diagnosis of myasthenia gravis

————COMBINATION DRUG————

# Tylenol with Codeine Elixir or Tablets

(**TIE**-leh-noll, **KOH**-deen)
**Pregnancy Category:** C
(Tablets are C-III and Elixir is C-V) **(Rx)**
**Classification:** Analgesic

See also *Acetaminophen* and *Narcotic Analgesics.*

**Content:** *Nonnarcotic analgesic:* Acetaminophen, 300 mg in each tablet, and 120 mg/5 mL elixir. *Narcotic analgesic:* Codeine phosphate, 15 mg (No. 2 Tablets), 30 mg (No. 3 Tablets), 60 mg (No. 4 Tablets), and 12 mg/5 mL (Elixir).

**Uses: Tablets:** Mild to moderately severe pain. **Elixir:** Mild to moderate pain.

**Special Concerns:** Use with caution during lactation. Safety has not been determined in children less than 3 years of age. May be habit-forming due to the codeine component.

**Dosage**

- **Tablets, Capsules**
  *Analgesia.*

**Adults, individualized, usual:** 1–2 No. 2 or No. 3 Tablets or No. 3 Capsules q 2–4 hr as needed for pain. Or, 1 No. 4 Tablet or Capsule q 4 hr as required. Maximum 24-hr dose is 360 mg codeine phosphate and 4,000 mg acetaminophen. **Pediatric:** Dosage equivalent to 0.5 mg/kg codeine.

- **Elixir**
  *Analgesia.*

**Adults, individualized, usual:** 15 mL q 4 hr as needed; **pediatric, 7–12 years:** 10 mL t.i.d.–q.i.d.; **3–6 years:** 5 mL t.i.d.–q.i.d.

## NURSING CONSIDERATIONS

See also *Nursing Considerations* for *Narcotic Analgesics* and *Acetaminophen.*

**Administration/Storage**

1. Adjust dosage depending on the response of the client and the severity of the pain.

2. Doses of codeine greater than 60 mg do not provide additional analgesia but may lead to an increased incidence of side effects.

**Assessment:** Note location, onset, duration, and characteristics of symptoms. Use a pain-rating scale to rate pain.

**Client/Family Teaching**

1. Take only as directed.

2. Report any loss of pain control because drug and/or dosage may require adjustment.

**Outcomes/Evaluate:** Relief of pain

**U**

# Urofollitropin for injection

(**YOUR**-oh-foll-ee-**troh**-pin)
**Pregnancy Category:** X
Metrodin **(Rx)**

# Urofollitropin for injection, purified

(**YOUR**-oh-foll-ee-**troh**-pin)

**Pregnancy Category:** X
Fertinex, Fertinorm HP ✸ **(Rx)**
**Classification:** Ovarian stimulant

**Action/Kinetics:** Prepared from the urine of postmenopausal women. Is a gonadotropin that stimulates follicular growth in the ovaries of women without primary ovarian failure. Because treatment with urofollitropin only causes growth and maturation of a follicle, HCG must also be given to effect ovulation. **Time to peak effect:** 32–36 hr after HCG.

**Uses:** To cause ovulation in women with polycystic ovarian disease; such clients should have an elevated LH/FSH ratio and should have failed to respond to therapy with clomiphene. In conjunction with HCG to stimulate development and maturation of ovarian follicles and subsequent ovulation in clients with polycystic ovary syndrome and infertility. Use of the purified urofollitropin is said to cause less discomfort than use of the less purified urofollitropin product.

**Contraindications:** Primary ovarian failure (as indicated by high levels of both LH and FSH), adrenal dysfunction, thyroid dysfunction, pituitary tumor, abnormal uterine bleeding of unknown cause, ovarian cysts, enlarged ovaries (not as a result of polycystic disease), infertility due to causes other than failure to ovulate. Pregnancy.

**Special Concerns:** Use with caution in lactation. There is the potential for multiple births.

**Side Effects:** *Ovarian hyperstimulation syndrome:* Severe ovarian enlargement, abdominal pain or distention, N&V, diarrhea, dyspnea, oliguria, ascites, pleural effusion, hypovolemia, electrolyte imbalance, **hemoperitoneum, thromboembolic events.** *Ovarian:* Hyperstimulation resulting in ovarian enlargement with abdominal distention or pain. *GI:* N&V, diarrhea, bloating, abdominal cramps. *CV:* Thromboembolic events resulting in venous thrombophlebitis, arterial occlusion, **pulmonary embolism, pulmonary infarction, CVA.** *Respiratory:* Atelectasis, **acute respiratory distress syndrome.** *Pyrogenic or allergic reaction:* Chills, fever, muscle aches or pains, joint pain, headache, fatigue, malaise. *Dermatologic:* Hives, dry skin, loss of hair, rash. *Other:* Headache, **ectopic pregnancy,** breast tenderness.

**OD   Overdose Management:** *Symptoms:* Hyperstimulation of the ovary, multiple gestations.

**Dosage**
• **IM (Metrodin)**
*Polycystic ovary syndrome.*
**Adults, initial:** 75 IU urofollitropin daily for 7–12 days followed by 5,000–10,000 IU HCG 24 hr after the last dose of urofollitropin. If ovulation has occurred but pregnancy has not resulted, this dosage regimen may be repeated for two more courses of therapy. If pregnancy still has not resulted, the dose of urofollitropin may be increased to 150 IU/day for 7–12 days followed by 5,000–10,000 IU HCG 24 hr after the last dose of urofollitropin. This regimen may be repeated for two additional courses if pregnancy has not occurred.
*In vitro fertilization.*
**Adults:** 150 IU/day beginning on day 2 or 3 of the cycle followed by 5,000–10,000 IU of HCG 1 day after the last dose of urofollitropin. Treatment is usually limited to 10 days.
• **SC (Fertinex)**
*Induction of ovulation in polycystic ovary syndrome and infertility.*
**Adults:** 75–300 IU urofollitropin daily with HCG, as above.

**NURSING CONSIDERATIONS**
**Administration/Storage**
1. Reconstitute the powder for injection by dissolving in 1–2 mL of sterile saline immediately before use.
2. Discard any unused drug.
3. Protect from light and store at 3°C–25°C (37°F–77°F).
**Assessment**
1. A thorough gynecologic and endocrinologic evaluation and examination should be completed before initiating urofollitropin therapy.
2. Note any renal or thyroid dysfunction or abnormal uterine bleeding from an unknown cause.
3. Monitor CBC, electrolytes, liver and renal function studies.

**Client/Family Teaching**

1. Treatment usually consists of daily injections for 7–12 days.

2. Engage in daily intercourse, beginning 1 day prior to the administration of HCG until ovulation occurs.

3. During the treatment and for 2 weeks thereafter, client should be examined at least every other day for hyperstimulation of the ovaries; if evident, the drug will be stopped immediately.

4. Avoid having intercourse if symptoms of hyperstimulation occur (sudden abdominal pain or tenderness). A ruptured ovarian cyst could occur resulting in hemoperitoneum.

5. This drug enhances the risk of multiple births.

6. Report all side effects to the provider and report for all scheduled exams.

**Outcomes/Evaluate:** Stimulation of ovulation to enhance fertility

# Urokinase

(your-oh-**KYE**-nayz)
**Pregnancy Category:** B
Abbokinase, Abbokinase Open-Cath
**(Rx)**
**Classification:** Thrombolytic agent

**Action/Kinetics:** Urokinase converts plasminogen to plasmin; plasmin then breaks down fibrin clots and fibrinogen. **Onset:** rapid; **duration:** 12 hr. **t½:** <20 min, although effect on coagulation disappears after a few hours.

**Uses:** Acute pulmonary thromboembolism. To clear IV catheters that are blocked by fibrin or clotted blood. Coronary artery thrombosis. *Investigational:* Acute arterial thromboembolism, acute arterial thrombosis, to clear arteriovenous cannula.

**Contraindications:** Active internal bleeding, history of CVA, within 2 months of intracranial or intraspinal surgery or trauma, recent cardiopulmonary resuscitation, intracranial neoplasm, arteriovenous malformation or aneurysm, known bleeding diathesis, severe uncontrolled arterial hypertension. Any condition pre-

senting a risk of hemorrhage, such as recent surgery or biopsies, delivery within 10 days, pregnancy, ulcerative disease. Also hepatic or renal insufficiency, tuberculosis, recent cerebral embolism, thrombosis, hemorrhage, SBE, rheumatic valvular disease, thrombocytopenia.

**Special Concerns:** The use of the drugs in septic thrombophlebitis may be hazardous. Use with caution during lactation. Safe use in children has not been established.

**Side Effects:** *CV:* Superficial bleeding, *severe internal bleeding,* transient hypotension or hypertension, tachycardia. *Allergic:* Rarely, skin rashes, *bronchospasm. Other:* Fever, chills, rigors, N&V, dyspnea, cyanosis, back pain, hypoxemia, acidosis.

**Drug Interactions:** The following drugs increase the chance of bleeding when given concomitantly with urokinase: Anticoagulants, aspirin, heparin, indomethacin, and phenylbutazone.

**Dosage**

• **IV Infusion Only**

*Acute pulmonary embolism.*

**Loading dose:** 4,400 IU/kg administered over 10 min at a rate of 90 mL/hr; **maintenance:** 4,400 IU/kg administered continuously at a rate of 15 mL/hr for 12 hr. May be followed by continuous IV heparin infusion to prevent recurrent thrombosis (start only after thrombin time has decreased to less than twice the normal control value).

*Coronary artery thrombi.*

**Initial bolus:** Heparin, as a bolus of 2,500–10,000 units **IV; then,** begin infusion of urokinase at a rate of 6,000 IU/min (4 mL/min) for up to 2 hr (average total dose of urokinase may be 500,000 IU). Urokinase should be administered until the artery is opened maximally (15–30 min after initial opening although it has been given for up to 2 hr).

*Clear IV catheter.*

Instill into the catheter 1–1.8 mL of a solution containing 5,000 IU/mL.

## NURSING CONSIDERATIONS

See also *Nursing Considerations* for *Streptokinase* and *Alteplase, Recombinant.*

**Administration/Storage**

**IV** 1. Reconstitute only with sterile water for injection without preservatives. Do not use bacteriostatic water.

2. The vial should be rolled and tilted, but not shaken, during reconstitution.

3. Reconstitute immediately before using.

4. Discard any unused portion.

5. Dilute reconstituted urokinase before IV administration in 0.9% NSS or 5% dextrose injection.

6. Type and cross and have blood for transfusion available. Aminocaproic acid may be employed with severe bleeding or hemorrhage.

7. Store the powder for injection at 2°C–8°C (35°F–47°F). Store the powder for catheter clearance below 25°C (77°F) and avoid freezing.

**Assessment**

1. Note indications for therapy, type, onset, and characteristics of symptoms.

2. Monitor ECG, CBC, PT, PTT, liver and renal function studies.

3. Assess for conditions that may preclude drug therapy (recent surgery, cerebral embolism, thrombosis, hemorrhage, SBE, thrombocytopenia, pregnancy, TB).

**Outcomes/Evaluate**

• Lysis of thrombi with restoration of blood flow and prevention of tissue infarction

• Restoration of catheter/cannula patency

# Ursodiol
(ur-so-**DYE**-ohl)
**Pregnancy Category:** B
Actigall, Ursofalk ✽ **(Rx)**
**Classification:** Gall stone solubilizer

**Action/Kinetics:** Naturally occurring bile acid that inhibits the hepatic synthesis and secretion of cholesterol; it also inhibits intestinal absorption of cholesterol. Acts to solubilize cholesterol in micelles and to cause dispersion of cholesterol as liquid crystals in aqueous media. Undergoes a significant first-pass effect where it is conjugated with either glycine or taurine and then secreted into hepatic bile ducts.

**Uses:** Dissolution of gallstones in clients with radiolucent, noncalcified gallstones (<20 mm) in whom elective surgery would be risky (i.e., systemic disease, advanced age, idiosyncratic reactions to general anesthesia) or in those who refuse surgery. Prevent gallstones in obese clients undergoing rapid weight loss.

**Contraindications:** Clients with calcified cholesterol stones, radiopaque stones, or radiolucent bile pigment stones. Acute cholecystitis, cholangitis, biliary obstruction, gallstone pancreatitis, biliary-gastrointestinal fistula, allergy to bile acids, chronic liver disease.

**Special Concerns:** Use with caution during lactation. Safety and efficacy have not been determined in children. Safety for use beyond 24 months is not known.

**Side Effects:** *GI:* N&V, dyspepsia, metallic taste, abdominal pain, biliary pain, cholecystitis, constipation, stomatitis, flatulence, diarrhea (rare). *Skin:* Pruritus, rash, dry skin, urticaria. *CNS:* Headache, fatigue, anxiety, depression, sleep disorders. *Other:* Sweating, thinning of hair, back pain, arthralgia, myalgia, rhinitis, cough.

**OD** **Overdose Management:** *Symptoms:* Diarrhea. *Treatment:* Treat with supportive measures.

**Drug Interactions**

*Antacids, aluminum-containing* / ↓ Effect of ursodiol due to ↓ absorption from GI tract

*Cholestyramine* / ↓ Effect of ursodiol due to ↓ absorption from GI tract

*Clofibrate* / ↓ Effect of ursodiol by ↑ hepatic cholesterol secretion

*Colestipol* / ↓ Effect of ursodiol due to ↓ absorption from GI tract

**U**

---

***bold italic*** = life threatening side effect

*Contraceptives, oral* / ↓ Effect of ursodiol by ↑ hepatic cholesterol secretion

*Estrogens* / ↓ Effect of ursodiol by ↑ hepatic cholesterol secretion

## Dosage
• **Capsules**

*Gallstones.*

**Adults:** 8–10 mg/kg/day in two or three divided doses, usually with meals.

*Prevent gallstones in rapid weight loss in obesity.*

**Adults:** 300 mg b.i.d. during period of weight loss.

## NURSING CONSIDERATIONS
### Administration/Storage
1. If partial stone dissolution is not observed within 12 months, the drug will probably not be effective.
2. For the first year of therapy, perform ultrasound of the gallbladder every 6 months to determine the response.

### Assessment
1. Document indications for therapy, expected duration of therapy, and any conditions that may preclude drug therapy.
2. The drug is not indicated for calcified cholesterol stones, radiopaque stones, or radiolucent bile pigment stones.
3. Obtain ultrasound of gallbladder and LFTs; monitor q 6 mo.
4. Determine if pregnant.

### Client/Family Teaching
1. Avoid taking antacids unless prescribed. Many antacids have an aluminum base, which adsorbs the drug.
2. Ursodiol therapy may take up to 24 months; drug will need to be taken 2–3 times/day.
3. Stones may recur after the dissolution of the current stones.
4. Report any persistent N&V, abdominal pain, diarrhea, presence of a metallic taste in the mouth, headaches, itching, rash, or altered bowel function.
5. Any new-onset headache, anxiety, depression, and sleep disorders should also be reported.
6. Practice reliable birth control to avoid pregnancy. The use of estrogens and oral contraceptives may decrease the effectiveness of the drug; use alternative forms of birth control.
7. Report for follow-up medical visits and routine lab studies and ultrasonography to evaluate the effectiveness of therapy.
8. Ursodiol therapy will be continued for 1–3 months following stone dissolution and then status of stones is reconfirmed with another ultrasound.

### Outcomes/Evaluate
• Radiographic evidence of a reduction or complete dissolution of radiolucent, noncalcified gallstones.
• Reversal of intracellular accumulation of toxic bile acids

---

**V**

# Valacyclovir hydrochloride
(**val**-ah-**SIGH**-kloh-veer)
**Pregnancy Category:** B
Valtrex (**Rx**)
**Classification:** Antiviral drug

See also *Antiviral Drugs.*
**Action/Kinetics:** Rapidly converted to acyclovir, which has inhibitory activity against herpes simplex virus types 1 (HSV-1) and 2 (HSV-2) and varicella-zoster virus. Acts by inhibiting replication of viral DNA by competitive inhibition of viral DNA polymerase, incorporation and termination of the growing viral DNA chain, and inactivation of the viral DNA polymerase. Rapidly absorbed after PO administration and is rapidly and nearly completely converted to acyclovir and l-valine by first-pass intes-

tinal or hepatic metabolism. **Time to peak levels:** Approximately 1.5 hr. **Peak plasma levels:** Less than 0.5 mcg/mL of valacyclovir at all doses. **t½, acyclovir:** 2.5–3.3 hr. Approximately 50% is excreted through the urine.

**Uses:** Treatment of recurrent episodes of genital herpes in immunocompetent adults. Treatment of herpes zoster in immunocompetent adults. Suppression of genital herpes in adults who have experienced previous outbreaks.

**Contraindications:** Hypersensitivity or intolerance to acyclovir or valacyclovir. Use in immunocompromised individuals. Lactation.

**Special Concerns:** Use with caution in renal impairment or in those taking potentially nephrotoxic drugs. Dosage reduction may be necessary in geriatric clients depending on the renal status. Safety and efficacy have not been determined in children.

**Side Effects:** *GI:* N&V, diarrhea, constipation, abdominal pain, anorexia. *CNS:* Headache, dizziness. *Miscellaneous:* Asthenia, precipitation of acyclovir in renal tubules resulting in acute renal failure and anuria.

**OD** **Overdose Management:** *Symptoms:* Precipitation of acyclovir in renal tubules if the solubility (2.5 mg/mL) is exceeded in the intratubular fluid. *Treatment:* Hemodialysis until renal function is restored. About 33% of acyclovir in the body is removed during a 4-hr hemodialysis session.

**Drug Interactions:** Administration of cimetidine and/or probenecid decreased the rate, but not the extent, of conversion of valacyclovir to acyclovir. Also, the renal clearance of acyclovir was decreased.

**Dosage** ————————
• **Tablets**
  *Herpes zoster (shingles).*
**Adults:** 1 g t.i.d. for 7 days. Dosage adjustment is necessary in renal

impairment. If $C_{CR}$ is between 30 and 49 mL/min, the dose of valacyclovir is 1 g q 12 hr; if $C_{CR}$ is between 10 and 29 mL/min, the dose is 1 g q 24 hr; and if $C_{CR}$ is less than 10 mL/min, the dose is 500 mg q 24 hr.
  *Recurrent genital herpes.*
**Adults:** 500 mg b.i.d. for 5 days. Dosage adjustment is necessary in renal impairment. If $C_{CR}$ is between 30 and 49 mL/min, the dose of valacyclovir is 500 mg q 12 hr; if $C_{CR}$ is between 10 and 29 mL/min, the dose of valacyclovir is 500 mg q 24 hr; and if $C_{CR}$ is less than 10 mL/min, the dose is 500 mg q 24 hr.
  *Suppression of genital herpes.*
**Adults:** 1,000 mg once daily (500 mg once daily for those who have 9 or fewer recurrences per year).

## NURSING CONSIDERATIONS

See also *Nursing Considerations* for *Antiviral Drugs.*
**Administration/Storage**
1. Begin therapy as soon as possible after herpes zoster has been diagnosed. The drug is most effective when started within 48 hr after the onset of rash. For recurrent genital herpes, initiate therapy at the first S&S of a flare.
2. May be given without regard to meals.
**Assessment**
1. Document indications for therapy and onset. With herpes zoster, note dermatone(s) location and characteristics of lesions. Drug is most effective if initiated within 48 hr of rash or within 72 hr of any symptoms.
2. With recurrent genital herpes, note extent of lesions; initiate at first S&S of outbreak.
3. Monitor CBC and renal function studies; reduce dose if $C_{CR}$ below 50 mL/min.
**Client/Family Teaching**
1. Take exactly as prescribed; do not share meds or skip or double up on doses.
2. Vesicles usually become red or pustular after 4 or 5 days and by the

**V**

7th to 10th day dry up and crust over. The acute phase is completed by approximately 3 weeks, when the scabs slough from the skin.

3. Immunocompromised clients usually experience a more severe case and the disease course usually doubles.

4. During the acute stage, cover the area and avoid contact with immuno-compromised individuals, pregnant women, or anyone else that has not had the chicken pox virus.

5. Report any persistent pain once lesions have healed (postherpetic neuralgia) or if there is ocular involvement or any other unusual symptoms or behaviors.

6. Report any recurrence since these tend to be rare and may signal an underlying malignancy or immune system dysfunction.

7. With genital herpes, abstain from sexual contact during acute out-breaks to prevent infecting partner; use condoms during all other times.

**Outcomes/Evaluate**

• ↓ Duration/progression of herpes zoster outbreak with reduced healing time; symptomatic relief

• ↓ Pain, ↓ duration, and ↓ intensity with genital herpes outbreak

# Valproic acid

(val-**PROH**-ick)
**Pregnancy Category:** D
Alti-Valproic ✹, Depakene, Gen-Valproic ✹, Novo-Valproic ✹ **(Rx)**
**Classification:** Anticonvulsant, miscellaneous

See also *Anticonvulsants*.

**Action/Kinetics:** The following information also applies to dival-proex sodium (Depakote, Epival ✹). The precise anticonvulsant action is unknown, but activity is believed to be caused by increased brain levels of the neurotransmitter GABA. Other possibilities include acting on postsyn-aptic receptor sites to mimic or en-hance the inhibitory effect of GABA, inhibiting an enzyme that catabolizes GABA, affecting the potassium chan-nel, or directly affecting membrane

stability. Absorption from the GI tract is more rapid following admin-istration of the syrup (sodium salt) than capsules, with peak levels follow-ing administration of the syrup in 15 min–2 hr. Equivalent PO doses of divalproex sodium and valproic acid deliver equivalent amounts of val-proate ion to the system. **Peak serum levels, capsules and syrup:** 1–4 hr (delayed if the drug is taken with food); **peak serum levels, en-teric-coated tablet (divalproex sodium):** 3–4 hr. t½: 9–16 hr, with the lower time usually seen in clients taking other anticonvulsant drugs (e.g., primidone, phenytoin, pheno-barbital, carbamazepine). Half-lives in children less than 10 days range 10–67 hr, compared to 7–13 hr in children over 2 months of age. The half-life may be up to 18 hr in those with cirrhosis or acute hepatitis. **Therapeutic serum levels:** 50–100 mcg/mL. Approximately 90% bound to plasma protein. Metabolized in the liver and inactive metabolites are excreted in the urine; small amounts of valproic acid are excreted in the fe-ces.

**Uses:** Alone or in combination with other anticonvulsants for treatment of simple and complex absence sei-zures (petit mal). As an adjunct in multiple seizure patterns that in-clude absence seizures. Alone or as adjunct to treat complex partial sei-zures that occur either in isolation or in association with other types of seizures. Divalproex sodium de-layed release used for the acute treatment of manic episodes in bipo-lar disorder and for prophylaxis of migraine headaches. *Investigational:* Alone or in combination to treat atypical absence, myoclonic, and grand mal seizures; also, atonic, complex partial, elementary partial, and infantile spasm seizures. Pro-phylaxis of febrile seizures in chil-dren, to treat anxiety disor-ders/panic attacks, and subchroni-cally to treat minor incontinence after ileoanal anastomosis. Manage-ment of anxiety disorders or panic attacks.

**Contraindications:** Liver disease or dysfunction.

**Special Concerns:** Use with caution during lactation. Use with caution in children 2 years of age or less as they are at greater risk for developing fatal hepatotoxicity. Geriatric clients should receive a lower daily dose because they may have increased free, unbound valproic acid levels in the serum. Safety and efficacy of divalproex sodium have not been determined for treating acute mania in children less than 18 years of age or for treating migraine in children less than 16 years of age.

**Side Effects:** *GI:* (most frequent): N&V, indigestion. Also, abdominal cramps, abdominal pain, dyspepsia, diarrhea, constipation, anorexia with weight loss or increased appetite with weight gain. *CNS:* Sedation, psychosis, depression, emotional upset, aggression, hyperactivity, deterioration of behavior, tremor, headache, dizziness, somnolence, dysarthria, incoordination, coma (rare). *Ophthalmologic:* Nystagmus, diplopia, "spots before eyes." *Hematologic:* Thrombocytopenia, leukopenia, eosinophilia, anemia, bone marrow suppression, relative lymphocytosis, hypofibrinogenemia, myelodysplastic-type syndrome. *Dermatologic:* Transient alopecia, petechiae, erythema multiforme, skin rashes. photosensitivity, pruritus, ***Stevens-Johnson syndrome***. *Hepatic:* Hepatotoxicity. Also, minor increases in AST, ALT, LDH, serum bilirubin, and serum alkaline phosphatase values. *Endocrine:* Menstrual irregularities, secondary amenorrhea, breast enlargement, galactorrhea, swelling of parotid gland, abnormal thyroid function tests. *Miscellaneous:* Also asterixis, weakness, asthenia, bruising, hematoma formation, frank hemorrhage, acute pancreatitis, hyperammonemia, hyperglycinemia, hypocarnitinemia, edema of arms and legs, weakness, inappropriate ADH secretion, Fanconi's syndrome (rare and seen mostly in children), lupus erythematosus, fever, enuresis, hearing loss .

**Laboratory Test Alterations:** False + for ketonuria. Altered thyroid function tests.

**OD** **Overdose Management:** *Symptoms:* Motor restlessness, asterixis, visual hallucinations, somnolence, heart block, ***deep coma.*** *Treatment:* Perform gastric lavage if client is seen early enough (valproic acid is absorbed rapidly). Undertake general supportive measures making sure urinary output is maintained. Naloxone has been used to reverse the CNS depression (however, it could also reverse the anticonvulsant effect). Hemodialysis and hemoperfusion have been used with success.

**Drug Interactions**

*Alcohol* / ↑ Incidence of CNS depression

*Carbamazepine* / Variable changes in levels of carbamazepine with possible loss of seizure control

*Charcoal* / ↓ Absorption of valproic acid from the GI tract

*Chlorpromazine* / ↓ Clearance and ↑ t½ of valproic acid → ↑ pharmacologic effects

*Cimetidine* / ↓ Clearance and ↑ t½ of valproic acid → ↑ pharmacologic effects

*Clonazepam* / ↑ Chance of absence seizures (petit mal) and ↑ toxicity due to clonazepam

*CNS depressants* / ↑ Incidence of CNS depression

*Diazepam* / ↑ Effect of diazepam due to ↓ plasma binding and ↓ metabolism

*Erythromycin* / ↑ Serum valproic acid levels → valproic acid toxicitiy

*Ethosuximide* / ↑ Effect of ethosuximide due to ↓ metabolism

*Felbamate* / ↑ Mean peak valproic acid levels

*Lamotrigine* / ↓ Valproic acid serum levels and ↑ lamotrigine serum levels (reduce dose of lamotrigine)

*Phenobarbital* / ↑ Effect of phenobarbital due to ↓ breakdown by liver

**V**

---

✦ = Available in Canada          ***bold italic*** = life threatening side effect

*Phenytoin* / ↑ Effect of phenytoin due to ↓ breakdown by liver or ↓ effect of valproic acid due to ↑ metabolism

*Salicylates (aspirin)* / ↑ Effect of valproic acid due to ↓ plasma protein binding and ↓ metabolism

*Warfarin sodium* / ↑ Effect of valproic acid due to ↓ plasma protein binding. Also, additive anticoagulant effect

*AZT* / ↓ Clearance of AZT in HIV-seropositive clients

**Dosage**

• **Capsules, Syrup, Enteric-Coated Capsules and Tablets (Divalproex)**

*Complex partial seizures.*

**Adults and children 10 years and older:** 10–15 mg/kg/day. Increase by 5–10 mg/kg/week until seizures are controlled or side effects occur, up to a maximum of 60 mg/kg/day. If the total daily dose exceeds 250 mg, the dosage should be divided. Dosage of concomitant anticonvulsant drugs can usually be reduced by about 25% every 2 weeks. Divalproex sodium may be added to the regimen at a dose of 10–15 mg/kg/day; the dose may be increased by 5–10 mg/kg/week to achieve the optimal response (usually less than 60 mg/kg/day).

*Simple and complex absence seizures.*

**Initial:** 15 mg/kg/day, increasing at 1-week intervals by 5–10 mg/kg/day until seizures are controlled or side effects occur.

*Acute manic episodes in bipolar disorder (use divalproex).*

**Initial:** 250 mg t.i.d.; **then,** increase dose q 2–3 days until a trough serum level of 50 mcg/mL is reached. The maximum dose is 60 mg/kg/day.

*Prophylaxis of migraine (divalproex sodium).*

250 mg/day b.i.d., although some may require up to 1,000 mg daily.

• **Rectal**

*Intractable status epilepticus that has not responded to other treatment.*

**Adults:** 200–1,200 mg q 6 hr rectally with phenytoin and phenobarbital.
**Children:** 15–20 mg/kg.

## NURSING CONSIDERATIONS

See also *Nursing Considerations* for *Anticonvulsants.*

**Administration/Storage**

1. Divide daily dosage if it exceeds 250 mg/day.

2. Initiate at lower dosage level, give with food, or use the delayed-release form (Depakote) to minimize GI irritation.

3. Giving the drug at bedtime may minimize CNS depression.

4. Valproic acid capsules should be swallowed whole to avoid local irritation. However, divalproex sodium capsules can either be swallowed whole or the contents sprinkled on a teaspoonful of a soft food (e.g., applesauce, pudding) and swallowed immediately without chewing.

5. Do not administer valproic acid syrup to clients whose *sodium* intake must be restricted. Consult provider if a sodium-restricted client is unable to swallow capsules.

6. In clients taking valproic acid, conversion to divalproex sodium can be undertaken at the same total daily dose and dosing schedule.

7. Reduce the starting dose in geriatric clients, depending on the response. Younger children will require larger maintenance doses, especially if they are receiving enzyme-inducing drugs.

**Assessment**

1. Note indications for therapy, type, onset, and duration of symptoms.

2. Document characteristics of seizure activity, including onset and prodrome if evident.

3. Identify type, frequency, and duration of behaviors that warrant therapy; list other agents prescribed and the outcome.

4. Monitor LFTs due to increased potential for hepatoxicity.

**Client/Family Teaching**

1. Take with or after meals to mini-

mize GI upset and at bedtime to minimize sedative effects.

2. Take only as directed and do not stop suddenly because seizures may occur.

3. Do not drive or perform activities that require mental alertness until drug effects realized and seizure control verified.

4. Any unexplained fever, sore throat, skin rash, yellow skin discoloration, or unusual bruising or bleeding should be reported immediately.

5. With diabetes, drug may cause a false positive urine test for ketones. Report symptoms of ketoacidosis (dry mouth, thirst, and dry flushed skin).

6. Report any loss of seizure control.

7. Avoid alcohol and any other CNS depressants or OTC products without approval.

8. Report as scheduled for periodic CBC, serum glucose/acetone, and LFTs.

**Outcomes/Evaluate**

• Control of seizures

• Migraine headache prophylaxis

• Control of manic episodes in bipolar disorder

• Therapeutic drug levels (50–100 mcg/mL)

# Vancomycin hydrochloride

(van-koh-**MY**-sin)

**Pregnancy Category:** C

Lyphocine, Vancocin, Vancoled **(Rx)**

**Classification:** Antibiotic, miscellaneous

See also *Anti-Infectives.*

**Action/Kinetics:** Appears to bind to bacterial cell wall, arresting its synthesis and lysing the cytoplasmic membrane by a mechanism that is different from that of penicillins and cephalosporins. May also change the permeability of the cytoplasmic membranes of bacteria, thus inhibiting RNA synthesis. The drug is bactericidal for most organisms and bacteriostatic for enterococci. It is poorly absorbed from the GI tract. Diffuses in pleural, pericardial, ascitic, and synovial fluids after parenteral administration. **Peak plasma levels, IV:** 33 mcg/mL 5 min after 0.5-g dosage. **t½, after PO:** 4–8 hr for adults and 2–3 hr for children; **t½, after IV:** 4–11 hr for adults and ranging from 2–3 hr in children to 6–10 hr for newborns. The half-life is increased markedly in the presence of renal impairment (240 hr has been noted). Primarily excreted in urine unchanged. Auditory and renal function tests are indicated before and during therapy.

**Uses: PO:** Antibiotic-induced pseudomembranous colitis due to *Clostridium difficile*. Staphylococcal enterocolitis. Severe or progressive antibiotic-induced diarrhea caused by *C. difficile* that is not responsive to the causative antibiotic being discontinued; also for debilitated clients.

**IV:** Severe staphylococcal infections in clients who have not responded to penicillins or cephalosporins, who cannot receive these drugs, or who have resistant infections. Infections include lower respiratory tract infections, bone infections, endocarditis, septicemia, and skin and skin structure infections. Alone or in combination with aminoglycosides to treat endocarditis caused by *Streptococcus viridans* or *S. bovis*. Must combine with an aminoglycoside to treat endocarditis due to *Streptococcus faecalis*. Used with rifampin, an aminoglycoside (or both) to treat early onset prosthetic valve endocarditis caused by *Staphylococcus epidermidis* or other diphtheroids. Prophylaxis of bacterial endocarditis in penicillin-allergic clients who have congenital heart disease or rheumatic or other acquired or valvular heart disease if such clients are undergoing dental or surgical procedures of the upper respiratory tract. The parenteral dosage form

**V**

---

may be given PO to treat pseudo-membranous colitis or staphylococcal enterocolitis due to *C. difficile.*

**Contraindications:** Hypersensitivity. Minor infections. Lactation.

**Special Concerns:** Use with extreme caution in the presence of impaired renal function or previous hearing loss. Geriatric clients are at a greater risk of developing ototoxicity.

**Side Effects:** Ototoxicity (may lead to deafness), nephrotoxicity (may lead to uremia). *Red-neck syndrome:* Chills, erythema of neck and back, fever, paresthesias. *Dermatologic:* Urticaria, macular rashes. *Allergic:* Drug fever, hypersensitivity, **anaphylaxis.** *Miscellaneous:* Nausea, tinnitus, eosinophilia, neutropenia (reversible), hypotension (due to rapid administration). Thrombophlebitis at site of injection. Deafness may progress after drug is discontinued.

**Drug Interactions**

*Aminoglycosides* / ↑ Risk of nephrotoxicity

*Anesthetics* / Risk of erythema and histamine-like flushing in children

*Muscle relaxants, nondepolarizing* / ↑ Neuromuscular blockade

**Dosage** ——————————

• **Capsules, Oral Solution**

**Adults:** 0.5–2 g/day in three to four divided doses for 7–10 days. Alternatively, 125 mg t.i.d.–q.i.d. for *C. difficile* may be as effective as the 500-mg dosage. **Children:** 40 mg/kg/day in three to four divided doses for 7–10 days, not to exceed 2 g/day. **Neonates:** 10 mg/kg/day in divided doses.

• **IV**

*Severe staphylococcal infections.*

**Adults:** 500 mg q 6 hr or 1 g q 12 hr. **Children:** 10 mg/kg/6 hr. **Infants and neonates, initial:** 15 mg/kg for one dose; **then,** 10 mg/kg q 12 hr for neonates in the first week of life and q 8 hr thereafter up to 1 month of age.

*Prophylaxis of bacterial endocarditis in dental, oral, or upper respiratory tract procedures in penicillin-allergic clients.*

**Adults:** 1 g vancomycin over 1 hr plus 1.5 mg/kg gentamicin (IV or IM), not to exceed 80 mg, 1 hr before the procedure. May repeat once, 8 hr after the initial dose. **Children:** 20 mg/kg vancomycin plus 2 mg/kg gentamicin (IV or IM), not to exceed 80 mg, 1 hr before the procedure. May repeat once, 8 hr after the initial dose.

## NURSING CONSIDERATIONS

See also *General Nursing Considerations for All Anti-Infectives.*

**Administration/Storage**

1. Dosage must be reduced in clients with renal disease; see package insert for procedure.

2. The PO solution is prepared by adding 115 mL distilled water to the 10-g container. The appropriate dose of PO solution may be mixed with 1 oz of water or flavored syrup to improve the taste. The diluted drug may also be given by NGT.

3. The parenteral form may be administered PO by diluting the 1-g vial with 20 mL distilled or deionized water (each 5 mL contains about 250 mg vancomycin).

**IV** 4. For IV use, dilute each 500-mg vial with 10 mL of sterile water. This may be further diluted in 200 mL of dextrose or saline solution and infused over 60 min.

5. Intermittent infusion is the preferred route, but continuous IV drip may be used.

6. Avoid rapid IV administration because this may result in hypotension, nausea, warmth, and generalized tingling. Administer over 1 hr in at least 200 mL of NSS or D5W.

7. Avoid extravasation during injections as this may cause tissue necrosis.

8. Reduce risk of thrombophlebitis by rotating injection sites or adding additional diluent.

9. Aqueous solution is stable for 2 weeks.

10. Once rubber stopper is punctured, ampule should be refrigerated to maintain stability.

**Assessment**

1. Document indications for thera-

**V**

py, type, onset, and characteristics of symptoms.

2. Assess renal and auditory functions (including 8th cranial nerve function).

3. Monitor CBC, cultures, and renal function studies; reduce dose with renal dysfunction.

**Interventions**

1. Record weight, VS, and I&O; ensure adequate hydration.

2. Report any adverse drug effects, such as:

• Ototoxicity, demonstrated by tinnitus, progressive hearing loss, dizziness, and/or nystagmus

• Nephrotoxicity, demonstrated by albuminuria, hematuria, anuria, casts, edema, and uremia

3. During IV administration ensure that peak and trough drug levels are performed at the prescribed dosing interval, usually 30 min prior to scheduled IV dose (trough) and 1 hr following IV dose (peak) to accurately assess serum levels.

**Outcomes/Evaluate**

• Negative cultures

• Relief of S&S R/T infection

• Serum levels within therapeutic range (trough 1–5 mcg/mL; peak 20–50 mcg/mL)

# Vasopressin
(vay-so-**PRESS**-in)
**Pregnancy Category:** C
Pitressin Synthetic, Pressyn ✿ **(Rx)**
**Classification:** Pituitary (antidiuretic) hormone

**Action/Kinetics:** Vasopressin (ADH) is released from the anterior pituitary gland. The hormone regulates water conservation by promoting reabsorption of water by increasing the permeability of the collecting ducts in the kidney. Depending on the concentration, the hormone acts on both $V_1$ and $V_2$ receptors. Also causes vasoconstriction (pressor effect) of the splanchnic and portal vessels (and to a lesser extent of peripheral, cerebral, pulmonary, and coronary vessels). Also increases the smooth

muscular activity of the bladder, GI tract, and uterus. **IM, SC: Onset,** variable; **duration,** 2–8 hr. **t½:** 10–20 min. **Effective plasma levels:** 4.5–6 microunits.

**Uses:** Neurogenic (central) diabetes insipidus (ineffective when diabetes insipidus is of renal origin—nephrogenic diabetes insipidus). Relief of postoperative intestinal gaseous distention, to dispel gas shadows in abdominal roentgenography. *Investigational:* Bleeding esophageal varices.

**Contraindications:** Vascular disease, especially when involving coronary arteries; angina pectoris. Chronic nephritis until reasonable blood nitrogen levels are attained. Never give the tannate IV.

**Special Concerns:** Pediatric and geriatric clients have an increased risk of hyponatremia and water intoxication. Use caution in the presence of asthma, epilepsy, migraine, CAD, and CHF. Use with caution during lactation.

**Side Effects:** *GI:* N&V, increased intestinal activity (e.g., belching, cramps, urge to defecate), abdominal cramps, flatus. *Miscellaneous:* Facial pallor, tremor, sweating, ***allergic reactions,*** vertigo, skin blanching, ***bronchoconstriction,*** ***anaphylaxis,*** "pounding" in head, water intoxication (drowsiness, headache, ***coma,*** ***convulsions***).

IV use of vasopressin may result in severe vasoconstriction; local tissue necrosis if extravasation occurs. IM use of tannate may cause pain and sterile abscesses at site of injection.

**OD** **Overdose Management:** *Symptoms:* Water intoxication. *Treatment:* Withdraw vasopressin until polyuria occurs. If water intoxication is serious, administration of mannitol (i.e., an osmotic diuretic), hypertonic dextrose, or urea alone (or with furosemide) is indicated.

**Drug Interactions:** Carbamazepine, chlorpropamide, or clofibrate may ↑ antidiuretic effects of vasopressin.

**V**

---

## Dosage

• **IM, SC**

*Diabetes insipidus.*

**Adults:** 5–10 units b.i.d.–t.i.d.; **pediatric:** 2.5–10 units t.i.d.–q.i.d.

*Abdominal distention.*

**Adults, initial:** 5 units IM; **then,** 10 units IM q 3–4 hr; **pediatric:** dose should be individualized (usual: 2.5–5 units).

*Abdominal roentgenography.*

**IM, SC:** 2 injections of 10 units each 2 hr and ½ hr before X rays are taken.

*Esophageal varices.*

**Initial:** 0.2 units/min IV or selective IA; **then,** 0.4 units/min if bleeding continues. The maximum recommended dose is 0.9 units/min.

• **Intrannasal (Using Injection Solution)**

*Diabetes insipidus.*

The dose is individualized using the injection solution on cotton pledgets, by nasal spray, or by dropper.

## NURSING CONSIDERATIONS

### Administration/Storage

1. Administration of 1–2 glasses of water prior to use for diabetes insipidus will reduce side effects such as nausea, cramps, and blanching of the skin.

2. Warm the vial (of vasopressin tannate in oil) in the hands and mix until the hormone is distributed throughout the solution before withdrawing the dose.

### Assessment

1. Document indications for therapy, type, onset, and characteristics of symptoms.

2. Note any history of vascular disease, especially involving the coronary arteries (e.g., hypertension, CHF, CAD).

3. Document any asthma, seizures, or migraine headaches.

### Interventions

1. Monitor weights and I&O to assess response to therapy.

2. Check skin turgor, mucous membranes, and presence of thirst to determine presence of dehydration.

3. Monitor BP and report any excessive elevation or lack of response characterized by a lowering of BP.

4. Record weight daily and assess for edema; report any rapid weight gain.

5. Perform urine specific gravity and report if < 1.005 or > 1.030. Determine urine osmolarity.

6. With abdominal distention, assess and document presence and characteristics of bowel sounds and the passage of flatus and/or stool. A rectal tube may assist with the expulsion of gas.

### Client/Family Teaching

1. Review appropriate method for administration or instillation.

2. Avoid alcohol and OTC agents without approval.

### Outcomes/Evaluate

• Prevention of dehydration: ↓ urinary frequency, ↑ urine osmolarity

• Control of intra-arterial bleeding

• ↓ Abdominal distention/discomfort; elimination of intestinal gas

# Vecuronium bromide

(vh-kyour-**OH**-nee-um)

**Pregnancy Category:** C

Norcuron **(Rx)**

**Classification:** Nondepolarizing neuromuscular blocking agent

See also *Neuromuscular Blocking Agents.*

**Action/Kinetics:** Less likely than other agents to cause histamine release. Effects can be antagonized by anticholinesterase drugs. **Onset:** 2.5–3 min; **peak effect:** 3–5 min; **duration:** 25–40 min using balanced anesthesia. About one-third more potent than pancuronium, but its duration of action is shorter at initial equipotent doses. No cumulative effects noted after repeated administration. **t½, elimination:** 65–75 min; a shortened half-life (35–40 min) has been noted in late pregnancy. Metabolized in liver and excreted through the kidney and bile. Is bound to plasma protein. Recovery may be doubled in clients with cirrhosis or cholestasis; renal failure does not affect recovery time.

**Uses:** To induce skeletal muscle relaxation during surgery or mechanical ventilation. To facilitate ET intubation. As an adjunct to general anesthesia. *Investigational:* To treat electrically induced seizures or seizures induced by drugs.

**Additional Contraindications:** Use in neonates, obesity. Sensitivity to bromides.

**Special Concerns:** Pediatric clients from 7 weeks to 1 year of age are more sensitive to the effects of vecuronium leading to a recovery time up to 1½ times that for adults. The dose for children aged 1–10 years of age must be individualized and may, in fact, require a somewhat higher initial dose and a slightly more frequent supplemental dosing schedule than adults. Clients with myasthenia gravis or Eaton-Lambert syndrome may experience profound effects with small doses of vecuronium. Cardiovascular disease, old age, and edematous states result in increased volume of distribution and thus a delay in onset time—the dose should *not* be increased.

**Additional Side Effects:** Moderate to severe skeletal muscle weakness, which may require artificial respiration. *Malignant hyperthermia.*

**Additional Drug Interactions**
*Bacitracin* / ↑ Muscle relaxation following high IV or IP doses of bacitracin
*Sodium colistimethate* / ↑ Muscle relaxation following high IV or IP doses of sodium colistimethate
*Tetracyclines* / ↑ Muscle relaxation following high IV or IP doses of tetracyclines
*Succinylcholine* ↑ Effect of vecuronium.

**Dosage** —————
• **IV Only**
  *Intubation.*
**Adults and children over 10 years of age.** 0.08–0.1 mg/kg.
  *For use after succinylcholine-assisted ET intubation.*
0.04–0.06 mg/kg for inhalation anes-

thesia and 0.05–0.06 mg/kg using balanced anesthesia. (*NOTE:* For halothane anesthesia, doses of 0.15–0.28 mg/kg may be given without adverse effects.)

  *For use during anesthesia with enflurane or isoflurane after steady state established.*
0.06–0.085 mg/kg (about 15% less than the usual initial dose).

  *Supplemental use.*
**IV only:** 0.01–0.015 mg/kg given 25–40 min following the initial dose; **then,** given q 12–15 min as needed.
**IV infusion:** Initiated after recovery from effects of initial IV dose of 0.08–0.1 mg/kg has started. **Initial:** 0.001 mcg (1 mg)/kg; **then** adjust according to client response and requirements. Average infusion rate: 0.0008–0.0012 mg/kg/min (0.8–1.2 mcg/kg/min). After steady-state enflurane, isoflurane, and possibly halothane anesthesia has been established: IV infusion should be reduced by 25%–60%.

---

## NURSING CONSIDERATIONS

See also *Nursing Considerations* for *Neuromuscular Blocking Agents.*
**Administration/Storage**
**IV** 1. Dosage must be individualized and depends on prior or concomitant use of anesthetics or succinylcholine.
2. Vecuronium may be mixed with saline, 5% dextrose alone or with saline, RL solution, and sterile water for injection.
3. Refrigerate after reconstitution. Use within 8 hr of reconstitution.
4. Have neostigmine, pyridostigmine, or edrophonium available to reverse vecuronium; atropine helps counteract muscarinic effects.
**Assessment**
1. Document indications for therapy and anticipated time frame for utilization.
2. Monitor ECG, VS, CBC, electrolytes, liver and renal function studies.
**Interventions**
1. Use a peripheral nerve stimulator

**V**

---

to assess neuromuscular response and recovery.

2. Monitor VS and ECG. Drug can cause vagal stimulation resulting in bradycardia, hypotension, and cardiac arrhythmias.

3. Muscle fasciculations may cause soreness or injury after recovery. Administer prescribed nondepolarizing agent and reassure that the soreness is likely caused by the unsynchronized contractions of adjacent muscle fibers just before the onset of paralysis.

4. Monitor closely for any evidence of malignant hyperthermia, unresponsive tachycardia, jaw spasm, or lack of laryngeal relaxation. Stop infusion and report; temperature elevations are a late sign of this condition.

5. Drug should only be used on a short-term basis and in a continuously monitored environment.

6. Client is fully conscious and aware of surroundings and conversations. Drug does not affect pain or anxiety; give analgesics and antianxiety agents as needed.

7. Prolonged use, as in an ICU setting, may lead to skeletal muscle weakness and symptoms consistent with muscle disuse atrophy. This may complicate ventilator weaning; some clients may require extensive physical therapy.

**Outcomes/Evaluate**
- Skeletal muscle relaxation
- Facilitation of intubation; tolerance of mechanical ventilation
- Suppression of the twitch response when tested with a peripheral nerve stimulator

# Venlafaxine hydrochloride
(ven-lah-**FAX**-een)
**Pregnancy Category:** C
Effexor, Effexor XR **(Rx)**
**Classification:** Antidepressant, miscellaneous

**Action/Kinetics:** Not related chemically to any of the currently available antidepressants. A potent inhibitor of the uptake of neuronal serotonin and norepinephrine in the CNS and a weak inhibitor of the uptake of dop-amine. Has no anticholinergic, sedative, or orthostatic hypotensive effects. The major metabolite—O-desmethylvenlafaxine (ODV)—is active. The drug and metabolite are eliminated through the kidneys. **t½, venlafaxine:** 5 hr; **t½, ODV:** 11 hr. **Time to reach steady state:** 3–4 days. The half-life of the drug and metabolite are increased in clients with impaired liver or renal function. Food has no effect on the absorption of venlafaxine.

**Uses:** Treatment of depression.

**Contraindications:** Use with a MAO inhibitor or within 14 days of discontinuation of a MAO inhibitor. Use of alcohol.

**Special Concerns:** Use with caution with impaired hepatic or renal function, during lactation, in clients with a history of mania, and in those with diseases or conditions that could affect the hemodynamic responses or metabolism. Although it is possible for a geriatric client to be more sensitive, dosage adjustment is not necessary. Use for more than 4–6 weeks has not been evaluated.

**Side Effects:** Side effects with an incidence of 0.1% or greater are listed.

*CNS:* Anxiety, nervousness, insomnia, mania, hypomania, *seizures, suicide attempts,* dizziness, somnolence, tremors, abnormal dreams, hypertonia, paresthesia, decreased libido, agitation, confusion, abnormal thinking, depersonalization, depression, twitching, migraine, emotional lability, trismus, vertigo, apathy, ataxia, circumoral paresthesia, CNS stimulation, euphoria, hallucinations, hostility, hyperesthesia, hyperkinesia, hypertonia, hypotonia, incoordination, increased libido, myoclonus, neuralgia, neuropathy, paranoid reaction, psychosis, psychotic depression, sleep disturbance, abnormal speech, stupor, torticollis. *CV:* Sustained increase in BP (hypertension), vasodilation, tachycardia, postural hypotension, angina pectoris, extrasystoles, hypotension, peripheral vascular disorder, syncope, thrombophlebitis, peripheral edema.

*GI:* Anorexia, N&V, dry mouth, constipation, diarrhea, dyspepsia, flatulence, dysphagia, eructation, colitis, edema of tongue, esophagitis, gastroenteritis, gastritis, glossitis, gingivitis, hemorrhoids, **rectal hemorrhage,** melena, stomatitis, stomach ulcer, mouth ulceration. *Body as a whole:* Headache, asthenia, infection, chills, chest pain, trauma, yawn, weight loss, accidental injury, malaise, neck pain, enlarged abdomen, allergic reaction, cyst, facial edema, generalized edema, hangover effect, hernia, intentional injury, neck rigidity, moniliasis, substernal chest pain, pelvic pain, photosensitivity reaction. *Respiratory:* Bronchitis, dyspnea, asthma, chest congestion, epistaxis, hyperventilation, laryngismus, laryngitis, pneumonia, voice alteration. *Dermatologic:* Acne, alopecia, brittle nails, contact dermatitis, dry skin, herpes simplex, herpes zoster, maculopapular rash, urticaria. *Hematologic:* Ecchymosis, anemia, leukocytosis, leukopenia, lymphadenopathy, lymphocytosis, thrombocytopenia, thrombocythemia, abnormal WBCs. *Endocrine:* Hypothyroidism, hyperthyroidism, goiter. *Musculoskeletal:* Arthritis, arthrosis, bone pain, bone spurs, bursitis, joint disorder, myasthenia, tenosynovitis. *Ophthalmic:* Blurred vision, mydriasis, abnormal accommodation, abnormal vision, cataract, conjunctivitis, corneal lesion, diplopia, dry eyes, exophthalmos, eye pain, photophobia, subconjunctival hemorrhage, visual field defect. *GU:* Urinary retention, abnormal ejaculation, impotence, urinary frequency, impaired urination, disturbed orgasm, menstrual disorder, anorgasmia, dysuria, hematuria, metrorrhagia, vaginitis, amenorrhea, kidney calculus, cystitis, leukorrhea, menorrhagia, nocturia, bladder pain, breast pain, kidney pain, polyuria, prostatitis, pyelonephritis, pyuria, urinary incontinence, urinary urgency, enlarged uterine fibroids, **uterine hemorrhage, vaginal hemorrhage,** vaginal moniliasis. *Miscellaneous:* Sweating, tinnitus, taste perversion, thirst, diabetes mellitus, alcohol intolerance, gout, hypoglycemic reaction, hemochromatosis, ear pain, otitis media.

**Laboratory Test Alterations:** ↑ Alkaline phosphatase, creatinine, AST, ALT. Glycosuria, hyperglycemia, hyperlipemia, bilirubinemia, hyperuricemia, hypercholesterolemia, hypoglycemia, hypokalemia, hyperkalemia, hyperphosphatemia, hyponatremia, hypophosphatemia, hypoproteinemia, uremia, albuminuria.

**OD** **Overdose Management:** *Symptoms:* Extensions of side effects, especially somnolence. Other symptoms include prolongation of QTc, mild sinus tachycardia, and *seizures.* *Treatment:* General supportive measures; treat symptoms. Ensure an adequate airway, oxygenation, and ventilation. Monitor cardiac rhythm and VS. Activated charcoal, induction of emesis, or gastric lavage may be helpful.

**Drug Interactions**
*Cimetidine* / ↓ First-pass metabolism of venlafaxine
*MAO inhibitors* / Serious and possibly fatal reaction, including hyperthermia, rigidity, myoclonus, autonomic instability with rapid changes in VS, extreme agitation, coma

**Dosage** ─────────
• **Tablets**
*Depression.*
**Adults, initial:** 75 mg/day given in two or three divided doses. Depending on the response, the dose can be increased to 150–225 mg/day in divided doses. Dosage increments should be made up to 75 mg/day at intervals of 4 or more days. Severely depressed clients may require 375 mg/day in divided doses. **Maintenance:** Sufficient studies have not been undertaken to determine how long a client should continue to take venlafaxine.
• **Tablets, Extended-Release**
*Depression.*

**V**

**Adults, initial:** 75 mg once daily. Dose can be increased by up to 75 mg no more often than every 4 days, to a maximum of 225 mg/day.

## NURSING CONSIDERATIONS
### Administration/Storage
1. Take with food.
2. Reduce the dose by 50% with moderate hepatic impairment and by 25% with mild to moderate renal impairment.
3. When discontinuing venlafaxine after more than 1 week of therapy, taper the dose to minimize the risk of symptoms of discontinuation. If receiving for 6 or more weeks, taper doses over a 2-week period.
4. At least 14 days should elapse between discontinuation of a MAO inhibitor and initiation of venlafaxine therapy; at least 7 days should elapse after stopping venlafaxine before starting a MAO inhibitor.
5. Take the extended-release form in the morning.
### Assessment
1. Document indications for therapy, type, onset, and duration of symptoms.
2. List other agents prescribed to ensure none interact unfavorably.
3. Monitor CBC, serum lipid levels, liver and renal function studies; reduce dose with hepatic or renal impairment.
4. Due to possible sustained hypertension, HR and BP should be monitored regularly.
### Client/Family Teaching
1. Take only as directed; *do not* stop abruptly.
2. Do not perform activities that require mental alertness until drug effects realized; may cause dizziness or drowsiness.
3. Any rash, hives, or other allergic manifestations should be reported immediately.
4. Drug may impair appetite and induce weight loss; report if excessive.
5. May experience anxiety, palpitations, headaches, and constipation; report if persistent or intolerable.
6. Avoid alcohol and any unprescribed or OTC preparations without approval.
7. Use birth control. Notify provider if pregnant or intends to become pregnant while taking drug.
8. Any suicide ideations or abnormal behaviors should be reported. Due to the possibility of suicide, high-risk clients should be observed closely during initial therapy. Prescriptions should be written for the smallest quantity to reduce the risk of overdose. Have family supervise medication administration with severely depressed clients.
**Outcomes/Evaluate:** Improvement in symptoms of depression

# Verapamil
(ver-**AP**-ah-mil)
**Pregnancy Category:** C
Alti-Verapamil HCl ✸, Apo-Verap ✸, Calan, Calan SR, Covera HS, Gen-Verapamil SR ✸, Isoptin, Isoptin I.V. ✸, Isoptin SR, Novo-Veramil ✸, Novo-Veramil SR ✸, Nu-Verap ✸, Taro-Verapamil ✸, Verelan **(Rx)**
**Classification:** Calcium channel blocking agent

See also *Calcium Channel Blocking Agents*.
**Action/Kinetics:** Slows AV conduction and prolongs effective refractory period. IV doses may slightly increase LV filling pressure. Moderately decreases myocardial contractility and peripheral vascular resistance. Worsening of heart failure may result if verapamil is given to clients with moderate to severe cardiac dysfunction. **Onset: PO,** 30 min; **IV,** 3–5 min. **Time to peak plasma levels (PO):** 1–2 hr (5–7 hr for extended-release). **t½, PO:** 4.5–12 hr with repetitive dosing; **IV, initial:** 4 min; **final:** 2–5 hr. **Therapeutic serum levels:** 0.08–0.3 mcg/mL. **Duration, PO:** 8–10 hr (24 hr for extended-release); **IV:** 10–20 min for hemodynamic effect and 2 hr for antiarrhythmic effect. Verapamil is metabolized to norverapamil, which possesses 20% of the activity of verapamil.

*NOTE:* Covera HS is designed to

deliver verapamil in concert with the 24-hr circadian variations in BP.

**Uses: PO:** Angina pectoris due to coronary artery spasm (Prinzmetal's variant), chronic stable angina including angina due to increased effort, unstable angina (preinfarction, crescendo). With digitalis to control rapid ventricular rate at rest and during stress in chronic atrial flutter or atrial fibrillation. Prophylaxis of repetitive paroxysmal supraventricular tachycardia. Essential hypertension. Sustained-release tablets are used to treat essential hypertension (Step I therapy). **IV:** Supraventricular tachyarrhythmias. Atrial flutter or fibrillation *Investigational:* PO for prophylaxis of migraine, manic depression (alternate therapy), exercise-induced asthma, recumbent nocturnal leg cramps, hypertrophic cardiomyopathy, cluster headaches.

**Contraindications:** Severe hypotension, second- or third-degree AV block, cardiogenic shock, severe CHF, sick sinus syndrome (unless client has artificial pacemaker), severe LV dysfunction. Cardiogenic shock and severe CHF unless secondary to SVT that can be treated with verapamil. Lactation. Use of verapamil, IV, with beta-adrenergic blocking agents (as both depress myocardial contractility and AV conduction). Ventricular tachycardia.

**Special Concerns:** Infants less than 6 months of age may not respond to verapamil. Use with caution in hypertrophic cardiomyopathy, impaired hepatic and renal function, and in the elderly.

**Side Effects:** *CV:* CHF, bradycardia, *AV block, asystole,* premature ventricular contractions and tachycardia (after IV use), peripheral and pulmonary edema, hypotension, syncope, palpitations, AV dissociation, *MI, CVA. GI:* Nausea, constipation, abdominal discomfort or cramps, dyspepsia, diarrhea, dry mouth. *CNS:* Dizziness, headache, sleep disturbances, depression, amnesia, paranoia, psychoses, hallucinations, jitteri-

ness, confusion, drowsiness, vertigo. IV verapamil may increase intracranial pressure in clients with supratentorial tumors at the time of induction of anesthesia. *Dermatologic:* Rash, dermatitis, alopecia, urticaria, pruritus, erythema multiforme, *Stevens-Johnson syndrome. Respiratory:* Nasal or chest congestion, dyspnea, SOB, wheezing. *Musculoskeletal:* Paresthesia, asthenia, muscle cramps or inflammation, decreased neuromuscular transmission in Duchenne's muscular dystrophy. *Other:* Blurred vision, equilibrium disturbances, sexual difficulties, spotty menstruation, sweating, rotary nystagmus, flushing, gingival hyperplasia, polyuria, nocturia, gynecomastia, claudication, hyperkeratosis, purpura, petechiae, bruising, hematomas, tachyphylaxis.

**Laboratory Test Alterations:** ↑ Alkaline phosphatase, transaminase.

**OD** **Overdose Management:** *Symptoms:* Extension of side effects. *Treatment:* Beta-adrenergics, IV calcium, vasopressors, pacing, and resuscitation.

**Additional Drug Interactions**

*Antihypertensive agents* / Additive hypotensive effects

*Barbiturates* / ↓ Bioavailability of verapamil

*Calcium salts* / ↓ Effect of verapamil

*Carbamazepine* / ↑ Effect of carbamazepine due to ↓ breakdown by liver

*Cimetidine* / ↑ Bioavailability of verapamil

*Cyclosporine* / ↑ Plasma levels of cyclosporine possibly leading to renal toxicity

*Digoxin* / ↑ Risk of digoxin toxicity due to ↑ plasma levels

*Disopyramide* / Additive depressant effects on myocardial contractility and AV conduction

*Etomidate* / Anesthetic effect of etomidate may be ↑ with prolonged respiratory depression and apnea

*Lithium* / ↓ Lithium plasma levels; lithium toxicity also observed

**V**

---

*Muscle relaxants, nondepolarizing /* ↑ Neuromuscular blockade due to effect of verapamil on calcium channels
*Prazosin /* Acute hypotensive effect
*Quinidine /* Possibility of bradycardia, hypotension, AV block, ventricular tachycardia, and pulmonary edema
*Ranitidine /* ↑ Bioavailability of verapamil
*Rifampin /* ↓ Effect of verapamil
*Sulfinpyrazone /* ↑ Clearance of verapamil
*Theophyllines /* ↑ Effect of theophyllines
*Vitamin D /* ↓ Effect of verapamil
*Warfarin /* Possible ↑ effect of either drug due to ↓ plasma protein binding
*NOTE:* Since verapamil is significantly bound to plasma proteins, interaction with other drugs bound to plasma proteins may occur.

**Dosage**
• **Tablets**
*Angina at rest and chronic stable angina.*
**Individualized. Adults, initial:** 80–120 mg t.i.d. (40 mg t.i.d. if client is sensitive to verapamil); **then,** increase dose to total of 240–480 mg/day. Covera HS is given once daily at bedtime in doses of either 180 or 240 mg.
*Arrhythmias.*
Dosage range in digitalized clients with chronic atrial fibrillation: 240–320 mg/day in divided doses t.i.d.–q.i.d. For prophylaxis of nondigitalized clients: 240–480 mg/day in divided doses t.i.d.–q.i.d. Maximum effects are seen within 48 hr.
*Essential hypertension.*
**Initial, when used alone:** 80 mg t.i.d. Doses up to 360 mg daily may be used. Effects are seen in the first week of therapy. In the elderly or in people of small stature, initial dose should be 40 mg t.i.d.
• **Extended-Release Capsules and Tablets**
*Essential hypertension.*
**Initial:** 240 mg/day in the a.m (120 mg/day in the elderly or people of

small stature). If response is inadequate, increase dose to 240 mg in the a.m. and 120 mg in the evening and then 240 mg q 12 hr. Covera HS is given once daily at bedtime in doses of either 180 or 240 mg.
• **IV, Slow**
*Supraventricular tachyarrhythmias.*
**Adults, initial:** 5–10 mg (0.075–0.15 mg/kg) given over 2 min (over 3 min in older clients); **then,** 10 mg (0.15 mg/kg) 30 min later if response is not adequate. **Infants, up to 1 year:** 0.1–0.2 mg/kg (0.75–2 mg) given as an IV bolus over 2 min; **1–15 years:** 0.1–0.3 mg/kg (2–5 mg, not to exceed 5 mg total dose) over 2 min. If response to initial dose is inadequate, it may be repeated after 30 min, but not more than a total of 10 mg should be given to clients from 1 to 15 years of age.

## NURSING CONSIDERATIONS

See also *Nursing Considerations* for *Calcium Channel Blocking Agents.*
**Administration/Storage**
1. The SR tablets (120 mg) may be useful for small stature and elderly clients who require less medication.
2. Take the SR tablets with food.
3. Verelan pellet filled capsules may be carefully opened and the contents sprinkled on a spoonful of applesauce. Swallow the applesauce immediately without chewing and follow with a glass of cool water to ensure complete swallowing of the pellets. Subdividing the contents of a capsule is not recommended.
**IV** 4. Before administration, inspect ampules for particulate matter or discoloration.
5. Administer IV dosage under continuous ECG monitoring with resuscitation equipment readily available.
6. Give as a slow IV bolus (5–10 mg) over 2 min (3 min to elderly clients) to minimize toxic effects.
7. Store ampules at 15°C–30°C (59°F–86°F) and protect from light.
8. Do not give verapamil in an infusion line containing 0.45% NaCl with

sodium bicarbonate because a crystalline precipitate will form.

9. Do not give verapamil by IV push in the same line used for nafcillin infusion because a milky white precipitate will form.

10. Do not mix with albumin, amphotericin B, hydralazine, trimethoprim/sulfamethoxazole, or diluted with sodium lactate in PVC bags.

11. Verapamil will precipitate in any solution with a pH greater than 6.

12. Always individualize dose in the elderly because the pharmacologic effects are more pronounced and more prolonged.

**Assessment**

1. Document indications for therapy, onset and duration of symptoms. List other agents trialed and the outcome.

2. Review list of prescribed medications to ensure none interact unfavorably.

3. Monitor ECG, CBC, liver and renal function studies; reduce dose with hepatic or renal impairment.

**Interventions**

1. Monitor VS; assess for bradycardia and hypotension, symptoms that may indicate overdosage. Verapamil may lower BP to dangerously low levels if BP already low.

2. *Do not* administer concurrently with IV beta-adrenergic blocking agents.

3. Unless treating verapamil overdosage, withhold any med that elevates serum calcium levels without approval.

4. Clients receiving concurrent digoxin therapy should be assessed for symptoms of toxicity and have digoxin levels checked periodically.

5. If disopyramide is to be used, do not administer for at least 48 hr before verapamil to 24 hr after verapamil administration.

6. Administer extended-release tablets with food to minimize fluctuations in serum levels.

**Client/Family Teaching**

1. Drug may cause dizziness and orthostatic effects; use caution.

2. Keep a log of BP and pulse for provider review.

3. Avoid alcohol, CNS depressants, and any OTC preparations without approval.

4. Continue life-style modifications (low-fat and low-salt diet, decreased alcohol consumption, no smoking, and regular exercise) in the overall goal of BP control.

5. Increase bulk and fiber in diet to prevent constipation. With higher doses constipation occurs more frequently. Report if bothersome or pronounced, as psyllium may be prescribed or, if severe, drug therapy may be changed.

**Outcomes/Evaluate**

• ↓ Frequency/severity of anginal attacks

• Control of BP

• Restoration of stable rhythm

• Therapeutic drug levels (0.08–0.3 mcg/mL)

# Vidarabine
(vye-**DAIR**-ah-been)
**Pregnancy Category:** C
Vira-A **(Rx)**
**Classification:** Antiviral

See also *Antiviral Agents* and *Anti-Infectives*.

**Action/Kinetics:** Phosphorylated in the cell to arabinosyl adenosine monophosphate (ara-AMP) or the triphosphate (ara-ATP). These compounds cause inhibition of viral DNA polymerase, inhibition of virus-induced ribonucleotide reductase. The drug may also incorporate into the viral DNA molecule leading to chain termination. Rapidly metabolized to ara-HX, which has decreased antiviral activity. **Peak plasma levels:** Vidarabine, 0.2–0.4 mcg/mL; ara-HX, 3–6 mcg/mL. **t½: IV,** vidarabine, 1 hr; ara-HX, 3.3. hr. Drug and metabolites excreted by kidneys. Due to low solubility, very little vidarabine penetrates following ophthalmic use.

**Uses: Systemic:** Herpes simplex virus encephalitis. Neonatal herpes simplex viral infections including disseminated infection with encephalitis, visceral involvement, and infections of the eyes, mouth, and skin. Herpes zoster in immunocompromised clients.

**Ophthalmic:** Acute keratoconjunctivitis and recurrent epithelial keratitis caused by HSV types 1 and 2. Superficial keratitis caused by HSV that is resistant to idoxuridine or when toxic or hypersensitivity reactions have resulted from idoxuridine. It is more effective than idoxuridine for deep recurrent infections.

**Contraindications:** Hypersensitivity to drug. Concomitant use of corticosteroids usually contraindicated. Lactation. IM, SC, or IV use by rapid or bolus injection. Ophthalmic use in presence of sterile trophic ulcers.

**Special Concerns: Systemic:** Use with caution in clients susceptible to fluid overload, cerebral edema, or with impaired renal or hepatic function. May be carcinogenic and mutagenic. Early diagnosis and treatment of viral infections are essential. Ineffective against infections due to adenovirus or RNA viruses, bacteria, fungi, or chlamydial infections of the cornea.

**Side Effects: Systemic.** *GI:* N&V, diarrhea, anorexia, hematemesis. *CNS:* Tremor, dizziness, ataxia, confusion, malaise, headache, hallucinations, psychoses, metabolic encephalopathy (may be fatal). *Hematologic:* Decrease in reticulocytes, H&H, WBC count, and platelet count. *Miscellaneous:* Weight loss, rash, pruritus, pain at injection site, neurologic abnormalities in infants. **Ophthalmic.** Photophobia, lacrimation, conjunctival injection, foreign body sensation, temporal visual haze, burning, irritation, superficial punctate keratitis, pain, punctal occlusion, sensitivity to bright light.

**Laboratory Test Alterations:** ↑ Bilirubin, AST.

**OD** **Overdose Management:** *Symptoms:* Bone marrow depression with thrombocytopenia and leukopenia. Acute fluid overloading may pose a greater risk than vidarabine itself. *Treatment:* Monitor hematologic as well as liver and kidney function.

**Drug Interactions:** Allopurinol may interfere with the metabolism of vidarabine.

**Dosage** ─────────────

• **Slow IV Infusion**
*Herpes simplex viral encephalitis, neonatal herpes simplex viral infections.*
15 mg/kg/day for 10 days.
*Herpes zoster.*
10 mg/kg/day for 5 days.

• **Ophthalmic Ointment**
½ in. of 3% ointment applied to lower conjunctival sac 5 times/day at 3-hr intervals. Continue therapy for 7 days after complete reepithelialization but at reduced dosage (e.g., b.i.d.). If there are no signs of improvement after 7 days or if complete reepithelialization has not occurred within 21 days, consider other therapy.

## NURSING CONSIDERATIONS

See also *General Nursing Considerations for All Anti-Infectives.*

**Administration/Storage**

1. To be effective, initiate therapy as soon as possible, but no later than 72 hr after the appearance of vesicular lesions.

2. Topical corticosteroids or antibiotics may be used concomitantly with vidarabine, but benefits and risks must be assessed.

3. Wait 10 min before use of an additional topical ointment.

4. Ophthalmic use may result in sensitivity to bright light that can be minimized by wearing sunglasses.

**IV** 5. Systemic: slowly infuse total daily dose at constant rate over 12–24 hr.

6. A total of 2.2 mL of IV solution is required to dissolve 1 mg of medication. A maximum of 450 mg may be dissolved in 1 L and administered over 12–24 hr. Should be used with-

in 48 hr after dilution. Do not refrigerate solution.

7. Since such a small amount is needed for newborns, 1 mL of the injection should be added to 9 mL of sterile NSS or sterile water for injection to provide a suspension of 20 mg/mL.

8. Any carbohydrate or electrolyte solution is suitable as diluent. Do not use biologic or colloidal fluids.

9. Shake vidarabine vial well before withdrawing dosage. Add to prewarmed (35°C–40°C; 95°F–104°F) infusion solution. Shake mixture until completely clear.

10. For final filtration use an in-line filter (0.45 µm).

11. Dilute just before administration and use within 48 hr.

12. Due to insolubility, the drug may have to be given in a large fluid volume. Care should be exercised in administering such a volume to clients susceptible to fluid overloading or with cerebral edema (e.g., with CNS infections or renal impairment).

**Assessment**

1. Document indications for therapy, type, onset, and duration of symptoms. Describe clinical presentation. Drug must be initiated within 72 hr of lesion appearance to be effective.

2. Monitor CBC, liver and renal function studies; assess for any dysfunction precipitated by drug therapy.

**Client/Family Teaching**

1. Take only as directed and do not share medications. Drug must be initiated within 72 hr of appearance of vesicular lesions to be effective.

2. Wash hands before and after applying ointment. If other agents prescribed, wait 10 min before application.

3. Ophthalmic ointment will cause a temporary haze after instillation. Avoid hazardous activities until vision clears.

4. Report any new, persistent, or bothersome side effects.

5. Wear sunglasses outside and avoid bright lights; may cause photophobic reactions.

6. Do not wear contact lenses until eye infection clears.

7. Remain under close ophthalmic supervision while receiving therapy for eye problem.

**Outcomes/Evaluate**

• Resolution of infection; negative cultures

• Healing of skin lesions

• Reepithelialization of herpetic eye lesions with complete healing in 1–3 weeks

# Vinblastine sulfate

(vin-**BLAS**-teen)

**Pregnancy Category:** D

Velban, Velbe ✦(Abbreviation: VLB)

**(Rx)**

**Classification:** Antineoplastic, plant alkaloid

See also *Antineoplastic Agents.*

**Action/Kinetics:** Alkaloid believed to interfere with metabolic pathways of amino acids leading from glutamic acid to the citric acid cycle and urea. It also affects cell energy production needed for mitosis (affects growing cells in metaphase) and interferes with nucleic acid synthesis. Rapidly cleared from plasma but poor penetration to the brain. About 75% bound to serum proteins. Almost completely metabolized in the liver after IV administration. **t½, triphasic:** initial, 3.7 min; intermediate, 1.6 hr; final, 24.8 hr. Metabolites are excreted in the bile with smaller amounts in the urine. No cross-resistance with vincristine.

**Uses:** Palliative treatment of generalized Hodgkin's disease (stages III and IV, Ann Arbor modification of Rye staging system); lymphocytic lymphoma (nodular and diffuse, poorly and well differentiated); histiocytic lymphoma; advanced stages of mycosis fungoides; advanced testicular carcinoma; Kaposi's sarcoma; Letterer-Siwe disease (histiocytosis X).

Less effective for palliative treat-

V

ment of coriocarcinoma resistant to other chemotherapy; breast cancer unresponsive to endocrine surgery and hormonal therapy.

Usually given in combination therapy. However, it has been used as a single agent to treat Hodgkin's disease and advanced testicular germinal-cell cancers (although combination therapy is more effective).

**Contraindications:** Leukopenia, granulocytopenia. Bacterial infections. Lactation.

**Additional Side Effects:** Toxicity is dose-related and more pronounced in clients over age 65 or in those suffering from cachexia (profound general ill health) or skin ulceration. *GI:* Ileus, rectal bleeding, *hemorrhagic enterocolitis,* vesiculation of the mouth, *bleeding from a former ulcer. Dermatologic:* Total epilation, skin vesiculation. *Respiratory:* Acute SOB, *severe bronchospasm. Neurologic:* Paresthesias, neuritis, mental depression, loss of deep tendon reflexes, *seizures.* Extravasation may result in phlebitis and cellulitis with sloughing.

**OD Overdose Management:** *Symptoms:* Exaggeration of side effects (see the above). Neurotoxicity. *Treatment:*
• If ingestion is discovered early enough, oral activated charcoal slurry should be given followed by a cathartic.
• Treat side effects due to inappropriate secretion of ADH.
• Prevent ileus (e.g., enemas, cathartic).
• Administer an anticonvulsant (e.g., phenobarbital), if necessary.
• Monitor the CV system.
• Monitor blood counts daily to determine risk of infection and whether blood transfusions are necessary.

**Drug Interactions**
*Bleomycin sulfate and cisplatin /* Combination of bleomycin, cisplatin, and vinblastine may produce signs of Raynaud's disease in clients with testicular cancer
*Erythromycin /* Severe myalgia, neutropenia, and constipation

*Glutamic acid /* Inhibits effect of vinblastine
*Mitomycin C /* Severe bronchospasm with SOB
*Phenytoin /* ↓ Effect of phenytoin due to ↓ plasma levels
*Tryptophan /* Inhibits effect of vinblastine

**Dosage** ————————
• **IV**
**Individualized, using WBC count as guide.** Vinblastine is administered once every 7 days. **Adults, initial:** 3.7 mg/m²; **then,** after 7 days, graded doses of 5.5, 7.4, 9.25, and 11.1 mg/m² at intervals of 7 days (maximum dose should not exceed 18.5 mg/m²). **Children, initial:** 2.5 mg/m²; **then,** after 7 days, graded doses of 3.75, 5.0, 6.25, and 7.5 mg/m² at intervals of 7 days (maximum dose should not exceed 12.5 mg/m²). **Maintenance** doses are calculated based on WBC count—at least 4,000/mm³.

## NURSING CONSIDERATIONS

See also *Nursing Considerations* for *Antineoplastic Agents.*
**Administration/Storage**
**IV** 1. Dilute vinblastine with 10 mL of bacteriostatic NaCl injection.
2. Inject into tubing of flowing IV infusion or directly into vein and administer over 1 min. May be further diluted in 50–100 mL of NSS and infused over 15–30 min.
3. Assess peripheral IV site for patency to prevent extravasation and local irritation and pain. If extravasation occurs, move infusion to another vein. Treat affected area with injection of hyaluronidase and application of moderate heat to decrease local reaction.
4. After reconstitution and removal of a portion from the vial, the remainder may be stored in the refrigerator for 30 days. Unopened vials should be refrigerated at temperatures of 2°C–8°C (36° F–46°F).
5. If drug gets into the eye, immediately wash eye thoroughly with water to prevent irritation and ulceration.
6. To reconstitute, under a laminar

V

flow hood, add 10 mL NaCl injection, which is preserved with either benzyl alcohol or phenol for a final concentration of 1 mg/mL.

7. Do not reconstitute with solutions that raise or lower the pH from between 3.5 and 5.5.

**Assessment**

1. Take a thorough drug history; note indications for therapy.

2. Document any evidence of neuropathies.

3. Monitor uric acid, renal function, and hematologic profiles. Drug may cause granulocyte and platelet suppression. Nadir: 10 days; recovery: 21 days.

**Interventions**

1. Administer antiemetic to control N&V.

2. Monitor I&O. Encourage fluid intake of 2–3 L/day.

3. Observe for cyanosis and pallor of extremities and signs of Raynaud's disease if also receiving bleomycin.

4. Check for manifestations of neurotoxicity and report if evident; dosage may need to be adjusted. Monitor neurologic toxicity by checking reflexes and strength of hand grip.

5. Observe for symptoms of gout. May empirically add allopurinol to decrease uric acid levels.

**Client/Family Teaching**

1. Report any signs of infection, fever, sore throat, unusual bruising, or bleeding.

2. Practice barrier contraception.

3. Avoid vaccinations and exposure to persons with infectious diseases.

4. To prevent constipation, eat a high-fiber diet, increase intake of fluids, remain active, and take stool softeners as prescribed.

5. Wear protective clothing, sunglasses, and a sunscreen if exposure to sunlight is necessary.

6. Partial hair loss may occur; plan for cosmetic replacement.

7. Report any evidence of jaw pain, numbness, tingling, and deep tendon loss as well as diminished reflexes (S&S of neurotoxicity) in the lower extremities; indication to discontinue drug therapy.

**Outcomes/Evaluate:** Control/regression of malignant process

# Vincristine sulfate

(vin-**KRIS**-teen)

**Pregnancy Category:** D

Oncovin, Vincasar PFS, Vincrex (Abbreviation: VCR or LCR) **(Rx)**

**Classification:** Antineoplastic, plant alkaloid

See also *Antineoplastic Agents.*

**Action/Kinetics:** Vincristine inhibits mitosis at metaphase. The antineoplastic effect is due to interference with intracellular tubulin function by binding to microtubule and spindle proteins in the S phase. After IV use, drug is distributed within 15–30 min to tissues. Poorly penetrates blood-brain barrier. **t½, triphasic:** initial, 5 min; intermediate, 2.3 hr; final, 85 hr. Approximately 80% is excreted in the feces and up to 20% in the urine. No cross-resistance with vinblastine.

**Uses:** Frequently used in combination therapy. Acute lymphocytic leukemia in children. Hodgkin's and non-Hodgkin's lymphomas (lymphocytic, mixed-cell, histiocytic, undifferentiated, nodular, and diffuse). Wilms' tumor, neuroblastoma, lymphosarcoma, rhabdomyosarcoma, reticulum cell sarcoma. *Investigational:* Idiopathic thrombocytopenic purpura; cancer of the breast, ovary, cervix, lung, colorectal area; malignant melanoma, osteosarcoma, multiple myeloma, ovarian germ cell tumors, mycosis fungoides, chronic lymphocytic leukemia, chronic myelocytic leukemia. Kaposi's sarcoma.

**Contraindications:** Clients with demyelinating Charcot-Marie-Tooth syndrome. Lactation. Use during radiation therapy.

**Special Concerns:** Geriatric clients are more susceptible to the neurotoxic effects. Intrathecal use may cause death.

V

---

**Additional Side Effects:** *Neurologic:* Paresthesias, depression of deep tendon reflexes, foot drop, *seizures,* difficulties in gait. *GI: Intestinal necrosis or perforation.* Constipation, paralytic ileus. *Renal:* Inappropriate ADH secretion (polyuria or dysuria). Acute uric acid nephropathy. *Ophthalmic:* Blindness, ptosis, diplopia, photophobia. *Miscellaneous:* CNS leukemia, leukopenia or complicating infection, *bronchospasm,* SOB. Less bone marrow depression than vinblastine. Significant tissue irritation if leakage occurs during IV use.

**OD** **Overdose Management:** *Symptoms:* Exaggeration of side effects. *Treatment:*
• Treat side effects due to inappropriate secretion of ADH.
• Use an anticonvulsant (e.g., phenobarbital), if necessary.
• Prevent ileus by use of enemas, cathartics, or decompression of the GI tract.
• Monitor the CV system.
• Monitor blood counts daily to determine risk of infection and whether blood transfusions are necessary.
• Folinic acid, 100 mg IV q 3 hr for 24 hr and then q 6 hr for a minimum of 48 hr, may help with treating the symptoms of overdose.

**Drug Interactions**
*L-Asparaginase* / Asparaginase ↓ liver clearance of vincristine
*Calcium channel blocking drugs* / ↑ Accumulation of vincristine in cells
*Digoxin* / Vincristine ↓ effect of digoxin
*Glutamic acid* / Inhibits effect of vincristine
*Methotrexate* / Combination may cause hypotension
*Mitomycin C* / Severe bronchospasm and acute SOB
*Phenytoin* / ↓ Effect of phenytoin due to ↓ plasma levels

**Dosage**
• **IV Only (Direct, Infusion)**
*Individualized with extreme care as overdose can be fatal.* **Adults, usual, initial:** 0.4–1.4 mg/m² (or 0.01–0.03

mg/kg) 1 time/week; **children:** 1.5–2 mg/m² 1 time/week. **Children less than 10 kg or with body surface area less than 1 m²:** 0.05 mg/kg 1 time/week.
   *For hepatic insufficiency.* If serum bilirubin is 1.5–3, administer 50% of the dose; if serum bilirubin is more than 3.1 or AST is more than 180, omit the dose.

## NURSING CONSIDERATIONS

See also *Nursing Considerations* for *Antineoplastic Agents* and *Vinblastine.*

**Administration/Storage**
**IV** 1. Dissolve powder in sterile water or isotonic saline injection to a concentration ranging from 0.01 to 1 mg/mL.
2. Medication is injected either directly into a vein or into the tubing of a flowing IV infusion over a period of 1 min.
3. If extravasation occurs, move infusion to another vein. Treat affected area with injection of hyaluronidase (150 U/mL in 1 mL NaCl) and application of moderate heat to decrease local reaction.
4. Store in refrigerator. Dry powder is stable for 6 mo. Solutions are stable for 2 weeks under refrigeration.
5. Protect drug from exposure to light.
6. Do not mix with any solution that alters the pH outside the range of 3.5–5.5.
7. Do not mix with anything other than NSS or glucose in water.

**Assessment**
1. Note indications for therapy. Document neurologic assessment; monitor for early S&S of neurologic and neuromuscular side effects (e.g., sensory impairment and paresthesias) before neuritic pain and motor difficulties are apparent because neuromuscular manifestations are irreversible.
2. Monitor CBC, uric acid, liver and renal function studies. May cause granulocyte suppression. Nadir: 10 days; recovery: 21 days.

V

## Interventions

1. Premedicate and regularly administer antiemetic to control N&V.

2. Record I&O, weights, and assess nutritional status.

3. Observe for symptoms of gout. Add allopurinol empirically to decrease uric acid levels.

4. Use laxatives and enemas to treat high colon impaction caused by vincristine.

5. Assess for absence of bowel sounds indicative of paralytic ileus; requires temporary discontinuation of drug therapy.

### Client/Family Teaching

1. Prevent constipation by increased intake of fluids (2–3 L/day), regular exercise, a high-fiber diet, and stool softeners as needed.

2. Report any S&S of neurotoxicity: paresthesias, difficulty walking, and diminished reflexes.

3. Avoid vaccinations and persons with infectious diseases.

4. Practice reliable birth control during and for 2 mo following therapy.

5. Report any increased dyspnea, cough, or fatigue.

6. Avoid alcohol and all OTC agents without approval.

**Outcomes/Evaluate:** Inhibition of malignant cell proliferation

---

# Vinorelbine tartrate

(vin-OR-el-been)

**Pregnancy Category:** D

Navelbine **(Rx)**

**Classification:** Antineoplastic agent

---

**Action/Kinetics:** Semisynthetic vinca alkaloid thought to act by inhibiting mitosis at metaphase through the drug's interaction with tubulin. Other possible actions may include interference with (a) amino acid, cyclic AMP, and glutathione metabolism, (b) calmodulin-dependent calcium transport ATPase activity, (c) cellular respiration, and (d) nucleic acid and lipid biosynthesis. Following IV administration, the concentration of vinorelbine in plasma decays in a triphasic manner. The initial rapid decline is due to distribution of the drug to peripheral compartments. The prolonged terminal phase is due to a slow efflux of the drug from peripheral compartments. **Terminal phase t½:** Averages 27.7–43.6 hr. Metabolized by the liver and excreted through the urine and feces.

**Uses:** Alone or in combination with cisplatin for first-line treatment of ambulatory clients with unresectable, advanced non-small-cell lung cancer. *Investigational:* Breast cancer, cisplatin-resistant ovarian carcinoma, and Hodgkin's disease.

**Contraindications:** Clients with pretreatment granulocyte counts less than 1,000 cells/mm³. Use during lactation.

**Special Concerns:** Use with caution in clients with severe hepatic injury or impairment. Use with extreme caution in clients whose bone marrow reserve may have been compromised by chemotherapy or prior to irradiation; also, in those whose bone marrow function is recovering from the effects of previous chemotherapy. Older clients may be more sensitive to the effects of the drug. Safety and efficacy have not been determined in children.

**Side Effects:** *Hematologic:* Granulocytopenia (may require hospitalization), leukopenia, thrombocytopenia, anemia. *GI:* N&V, constipation, diarrhea, paralytic ileus, anorexia, stomatitis. *CNS:* Mild to severe peripheral neuropathy including paresthesia and hypesthesia, loss of deep tendon reflexes. *CV:* Chest pain, especially in those with a history of CV disease or tumor within the chest; phlebitis. *Respiratory:* SOB (may be severe), dyspnea, interstitial pulmonary changes. *Dermatologic:* Erythema, pain at injection site and vein discoloration, chemical phlebitis along the vein proximal to the site of injection. *Miscellaneous:* Alopecia, asthenia, fatigue, jaw pain, myalgia, arthralgia, rash, hemorrhag-

V

---

ic cystitis, syndrome of inappropriate ADH secretion.

**Laboratory Test Alterations:** ↑ Total bilirubin, AST. Transient elevations of liver enzymes.

**OD** **Overdose Management:**
*Symptoms:* Bone marrow suppression, peripheral neurotoxicity. *Treatment:* There is no known antidote
for vinorelbine. For overdosage, begin general supportive measures
together with appropriate blood
transfusions and antibiotics, as necessary.

**Drug Interactions**
*Cisplatin* / ↑ Incidence of granulocytopenia
*Mitomycin* / Acute pulmonary reactions

**Dosage**
• **IV Only**
*Non-small-cell lung cancer.*
**Granulocytes (1,500 or more
cells/mm³) on the day of treatment:** 30 mg/m² weekly given over
6–10 min into the side port of a free-
flowing IV closest to the IV bag followed by flushing with at least
75–125 mL of the solution used to
dilute the product. May also be given,
at the same dose level, with cisplatin,
120 mg/m² on days 1 and 29 and
then q 6 weeks. **Granulocytes
(1,000–1,499 cells/mm³) on the
day of treatment:** 15 mg/m² weekly given over 6–10 min as described
previously.
*Breast cancer, Hodgkin's disease.*
30 mg/m²/week.

## NURSING CONSIDERATIONS

See also *Nursing Considerations* for
*Antineoplastic Agents.*
**Administration/Storage**
**IV** 1. During therapy, if clients
have manifested fever or sepsis
while granulocytopenic or had two
consecutive weekly doses held due to
granulocytopenia, give subsequent
doses of vinorelbine as follows: 22.5
mg/m² for granulocytes equal to or
greater than 1,500 cells/mm³ or
11.25 mg/m² for granulocytes from
1,000 to 1,499 cells/mm³.
2. Ensure granulocyte counts are

equal to or greater than 1,000
cells/mm³ prior to giving vinorelbine. Base dosage on granulocyte
counts on the day of drug treatment.
3. If hyperbilirubinemia develops
during treatment, adjust the dose of
vinorelbine as follows: 30 mg/m² for
a total bilirubin of 2 or less mg/dL, 15
mg/m² for a total bilirubin of 2.1–3
mg/dL, and 7.5 mg/m² for a total
bilirubin greater than 3 mg/dL.
4. The drug must be given IV with the
IV needle or catheter properly positioned before any drug is given.
Leakage into surrounding tissue may
cause considerable irritation, local
tissue necrosis, or thrombophlebitis. If
extravasation occurs, stop the injection
immediately and give the remaining
dose in another vein. Use institutional guidelines to treat extravasation
injuries.
5. Due to the toxicity of vinorelbine,
use caution in handling and preparing the solution. The use of gloves is
recommended. If the solution comes
in contact with skin or mucosa,
wash the area immediately with
soap and water. If the eye is affected,
flush with water immediately and
thoroughly.
6. Vinorelbine must be diluted in either a syringe or IV bag. If an IV bag
is used, dilute the dose to a concentration between 0.5 and 2 mg/mL using one of the following solutions:
5% dextrose injection, 0.45% or 0.9%
NaCl injection, D5/0.45% NaCl injection, Ringer's injection, or RL injection.
When dilution in a syringe is used, dilute the dose to a concentration between 1.5 and 3 mg/mL with 5%
dextrose injection or 0.9% NaCl
injection.
7. Diluted vinorelbine solutions may
be used for up to 24 hr under normal
room light when stored in polypropylene syringes or PVC bags at
5°C–30°C (41°F–96°F). Unopened
vials are stable until the expiration
date indicated if stored under refrigeration at 2°C–8°C (36°F–46°F). Protect unopened vials from light and
do not freeze. Do not use if particulate matter is seen.

## Assessment

1. Document indications for therapy, other agents and therapies prescribed and when administered.
2. Monitor CBC, uric acid, and renal function studies. Do not administer if granulocyte counts are not at least 1,000 cells/mm³. Granulocyte nadir 7–10 days; recovery 7–14 days thereafter.

## Client/Family Teaching

1. Report any fever or chills immediately because drug-induced granulocytopenia makes one much more susceptible to infections.
2. Avoid crowds, persons with infectious diseases, and vaccinations during therapy.
3. Practice reliable contraception during and for several months after therapy.
4. Rinse mouth frequently and brush teeth often to prevent stomatitis; use unwaxed floss.

**Outcomes/Evaluate:** Control of malignant cell proliferation.

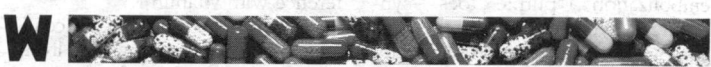

# Warfarin sodium

(**WAR**-far-in)
**Pregnancy Category:** X
Coumadin, Warfilone ✹ **(Rx)**
**Classification:** Anticoagulant

See also *Anticoagulants*.

**Action/Kinetics:** Interferes with synthesis of vitamin K–dependent clotting factors resulting in depletion of clotting factors VII, IX, X, and II. Has no direct effect on an established thrombus although therapy may prevent further extension of a formed clot as well as secondary thromboembolic problems. Well absorbed from the GI tract although food affects the rate (but not the extent) of absorption. Suitable for parenteral administration. **Peak activity:** 1.5–3 days; **duration:** 2–5 days. **t½:** 1–2.5 days. Highly bound to plasma proteins. Metabolized in the liver and inactive metabolites are excreted through the urine and feces.

**Uses:** Prophylaxis and treatment of venous thrombosis and its extension. Prophylaxis and treatment of atrial fibrillation with embolization. Prophylaxis and treatment of pulmonary embolism. Prophylaxis and treatment of thromboembolic complications associated with atrial fibrillation. *Investigational:* Adjunct to treat small cell carcinoma of the lung with chemotherapy and radiation. Prophylaxis of recurrent transient ischemic attacks and to reduce the risk of recurrent MI.

**Additional Contraindications:** Lactation. IM use. Use of a large loading dose (30 mg) is not recommended due to increased risk of hemorrhage and lack of more rapid protection.

**Special Concerns:** Geriatric clients may be more sensitive. Anticoagulant use in the following clients leads to increased risk: trauma, infection, renal insufficiency, sprue, vitamin K deficiency, severe to moderate hypertension, polycythemia vera, severe allergic disorders, vasculitis, indwelling catheters, severe diabetes, anaphylactic disorders, surgery or trauma resulting in large exposed raw surfaces. Use with caution in impaired hepatic and renal function. Safety and efficacy have not been determined in children less than 18 years of age. Careful monitoring and dosage regulation are required during dentistry and surgery.

**Side Effects:** *CV: **Hemorrhage*** is the main side effect and may occur from any tissue or organ. Symptoms of hemorrhage include headache, paralysis; pain in the joints, abdomen, or chest; difficulty in breathing or swal-

---

lowing; SOB, unexplained swelling or shock. *GI:* N&V, diarrhea, sore mouth, mouth ulcers, anorexia, abdominal cramping, paralytic ileus, intestinal obstruction (due to intramural or submucosal hemorrhage). *Hepatic:* Hepatotoxicity, cholestatic jaundice. *Dermatologic:* Dermatitis, exfoliative dermatitis, urticaria, alopecia, necrosis or gangrene of the skin and other tissues (due to protein C deficiency). *Miscellaneous:* Pyrexia, red-orange urine, priapism, leukopenia, systemic cholesterol microembolization ("purple toes" syndrome), hypersensitivity reactions, compressive neuropathy secondary to hemorrhage adjacent to a nerve (rare).

**Laboratory Test Alterations:** False ↓ levels of serum theophylline determined by Schack and Waxler UV method (warfarin and dicumarol). Metabolites of indanedione derivatives may color alkaline urine red; color disappears upon acidification.

**OD** **Overdose Management:** *Symptoms:* Early symptoms include melena, petechiae, microscopic hematuria, oozing from superficial injuries (e.g., nicks from shaving, excessive bruising, bleeding from gums after teeth brushing), excessive menstrual bleeding. *Treatment:* Discontinue therapy. Administer oral or parenteral phytonadione (e.g., 2.5–10 mg PO or 5–25 mg parenterally). In emergency situations, 200–250 mL fresh frozen plasma or commercial factor IX complex. Fresh whole blood may be needed in clients unresponsive to phytonadione.

**Drug Interactions:** Warfarin is responsible for more adverse drug interactions than any other group. Clients on anticoagulant therapy must be monitored carefully each time a drug is added or withdrawn. Monitoring usually involves determination of PT. In general, a lengthened PT means potentiation of the anticoagulant. Since potentiation may mean hemorrhages, a lengthened PT warrants **reduction of the dosage of the anticoagulant.** However, the anticoagulant dosage must again be increased when the second drug is discontinued. A shortened PT means inhibition of the anticoagulant and may require an increase in dosage.

*Acetaminophen* / ↑ Anticoagulant effect

*Alcohol, ethyl* / Chronic alcohol use ↓ effect of oral anticoagulants

*Aminoglutethimide* / ↓ Effect of anticoagulants due to ↑ breakdown by liver

*Aminoglycoside antibiotics* / ↑ Effect of anticoagulants due to interference with vitamin K

*Amiodarone* / ↑ Effect of anticoagulants due to ↓ breakdown by liver

*Androgens* / ↑ Effect of anticoagulants

*Ascorbic acid* / ↓ Effect of anticoagulants by unknown mechanism

*Barbiturates* / ↓ Effect of anticoagulants due to ↑ breakdown by liver

*Beta-adrenergic blockers* / ↑ Effect of anticoagulants

*Carbamazepine* / ↓ Effect of anticoagulants due to ↑ breakdown by liver

*Cephalosporins* / ↑ Effect of anticoagulants due to effects on platelet function

*Chloral hydrate* / ↑ Effect of anticoagulant due to ↓ binding to plasma proteins

*Chloramphenicol* / ↑ Effect of anticoagulant due to ↓ breakdown by liver

*Cholestyramine* / ↓ Anticoagulant effect due to binding in and ↓ absorption from GI tract

*Cimetidine* / ↑ Anticoagulant effect due to ↓ breakdown by liver

*Clofibrate* / ↑ Anticoagulant effect

*Contraceptives, oral* / ↓ Anticoagulant effect by ↑ activity of certain clotting factors (VII and X); rarely, the opposite effect of ↑ risk of thromboembolism

*Contrast media containing iodine* / ↑ Effect of anticoagulants by ↑ PT

*Corticosteroids* / ↑ Effect of anticoagulants; also ↑ risk of GI bleeding due to ulcerogenic effect of steroids

*Cyclophosphamide* / ↑ Anticoagulant effect

*Dextrothyroxine* / ↑ Effect of anticoagulants

*Dicloxacillin* / ↓ Effect of anticoagulants

*Diflunisal* / ↑ Anticoagulant effect and ↑ risk of bleeding due to effect on platelet function and GI irritation

*Disulfiram* / ↑ Effect of anticoagulants

*Erythromycin* / ↑ Effect of anticoagulants

*Estrogens* / ↓ Anticoagulant response by ↑ activity of certain clotting factors; rarely, the opposite effect of ↑ risk of thromboembolism

*Ethchlorvynol* / ↓ Effect of anticoagulants

*Etretinate* / ↓ Effect of anticoagulants due to ↑ breakdown by liver

*Fluconazole* / ↑ Effect of anticoagulants

*Gemfibrozil* / ↑ Effect of anticoagulants

*Glucagon* / ↑ Effect of anticoagulants

*Glutethimide* / ↓ Effect of anticoagulants due to ↑ breakdown by liver

*Griseofulvin* / ↓ Effect of anticoagulants

*Hydantoins* / ↑ Effect of anticoagulants; also, ↑ hydantoin serum levels

*Hypoglycemics, oral* / ↑ Effect of anticoagulants due to ↓ plasma protein binding; also, ↑ effect of sulfonylureas

*Ifosfamide* / ↑ Effect of anticoagulants due to ↓ breakdown by liver and displacement from protein binding sites

*Indomethacin* / ↑ Effect of anticoagulants by an effect on platelet function; also, indomethacin is ulcerogenic cause GI hemorrhage

*Isoniazid* / ↑ Effect of anticoagulants

*Ketoconazole* / ↑ Effect of anticoagulants

*Loop diuretics* / ↑ Effect of anticoagulants by displacement from protein binding sites

*Lovastatin* / ↑ Effect of anticoagulants due to ↓ breakdown by liver

*Metronidazole* / ↑ Effect of anticoagulants due to ↓ breakdown by liver

*Miconazole* / ↑ Effect of anticoagulants

*Mineral oil* / ↑ Hypoprothrombinemia by ↓ absorption of vitamin K from GI tract; also mineral oil may ↓ absorption of anticoagulants from GI tract

*Moricizine* / ↑ Effect of anticoagulants

*Nafcillin* / ↓ Effect of anticoagulants

*Nalidixic acid* / ↑ Effect of anticoagulants due to displacement from protein binding sites

*Nonsteroidal anti-inflammatory agents* / ↑ Effect of anticoagulants and ↑ risk of bleeding due to effects on platelet function and GI irritation

*Omeprazole* / ↑ Effect of anticoagulant due to ↓ breakdown by liver

*Penicillins* / ↑ Effect of anticoagulants and ↑ risk of bleeding due to effects on platelet function

*Phenylbutazone* / ↑ Effect of anticoagulants due to ↓ breakdown by liver and ↑ displacement from protein binding sites

*Propafenone* / ↑ Effect of anticoagulant due to ↓ breakdown by liver

*Propoxyphene* / ↑ Effect of anticoagulants

*Quinidine, quinine* / ↑ Effect of anticoagulants due to ↓ breakdown by liver

*Quinolones* / ↑ Effect of anticoagulants

*Rifampin* / ↓ Anticoagulant effect due to ↑ breakdown by liver

*Salicylates* / ↑ Effect of anticoagulants and ↑ risk of bleeding due to effect on platelet function and GI irritation

*Spironolactone* / ↓ Effect of anticoagulants due to hemoconcentration of clotting factors due to diuresis

*Streptokinase* / ↑ Effect of anticoagulants

*Sucralfate* / ↓ Effect of anticoagulants

**W**

*Sulfamethoxazole and Trimethoprim* / ↑ Effect of anticoagulants due to ↓ breakdown by liver

*Sulfinpyrazone* / ↑ Anticoagulant effect due to ↓ breakdown by liver and inhibition of platelet aggregation

*Sulfonamides* / ↑ Effect of sulfonamides

*Sulindac* / ↑ Effect of anticoagulants

*Tamoxifen* / ↑ Effect of anticoagulants

*Tetracyclines* / ↑ Effect of anticoagulants due to interference with vitamin K

*Thiazide diuretics* / ↓ Effect of anticoagulants due to hemoconcentration of clotting factors

*Thioamines* / ↑ Effect of anticoagulants

*Thiopurines* / ↓ Effect of anticoagulants due to ↑ synthesis or activation of prothrombin

*Thyroid hormones* / ↑ Anticoagulant effect

*Trazodone* / ↓ Effect of anticoagulants

*Thiazide diuretics* / ↓ Effect of anticoagulants due to hemoconcentration of clotting factors due to diuresis

*Urokinase* / ↑ Effect of anticoagulants

*Vitamin E* / ↑ Effect of anticoagulants due to interference with vitamin K

*Vitamin K* / ↓ Effect of anticoagulants

**Dosage** ——————
• **Tablets, IV**
*Induction.*
**Adults, initial:** 5–10 mg/day for 2–4 days; **then,** adjust dose based on prothrombin or INR determinations. A lower dose should be used in geriatric or debilitated clients or clients with increased sensitivity. Dosage has not been established for children.
*Maintenance.*
**Adults:** 2–10 mg/day, based on prothrombin or INR.
*Prevent blood clots with prosthetic heart valve replacement.*
2–5 mg daily.

## NURSING CONSIDERATIONS

See also *Nursing Considerations* for *Anticoagulants*.

**Administration/Storage**

1. Daily monitoring of PT is recommended during the first week of therapy, or during adjustment periods, and weekly thereafter.

2. Do not change brands of warfarin sodium. There may be differences in bioavailability.

3. To transfer from heparin therapy, give heparin and warfarin together from the first day (as there is a delayed onset of oral anticoagulant effects). Alternatively, warfarin may be started on the third to sixth day of heparin therapy.

4. Levels of anticoagulation that are recommended for specific indications by the American College of Chest Physicians and the National Heart, Lung, and Blood Institute should be followed.

5. Protect from light; store at controlled room temperature. Dispense in a tight, light-resistant container.

**IV** 6. Give IV as a slow bolus injection over 1–2 min into a peripheral vein.

7. Reconstitute for IV use by adding 2.7 mL sterile water for injection. Inspect for particulate matter and discoloration.

8. After reconstitution, the injection is stable for 4 hr at room temperature. There is no preservative; take care to assure sterility of the prepared solution.

9. Do not use the vial for multiple use; discard unused solution.

**Assessment**

1. Document indications for therapy, type and onset of symptoms.

2. List drugs currently prescribed to ensure that none interacts unfavorably by increasing or decreasing PT as a result of competition for protein binding at receptor sites.

3. Note any bleeding tendencies.

4. Determine if pregnant. May cause fetal malformations and neonatal hemorrhage.

5. Monitor ECG, CBC, PT/PTT, INR, liver and renal function studies.

**Interventions**

1. Request written parameters noting the desired range for PT or INR, once anticoagulated (orally). It usually takes 36–48 hr for drug to reach steady state; therefore allow time to equilibrate. The INR is the PT ratio (test/control) obtained from human brain thromboplastin and is universally considered most accurate to calculate dosage.

2. Drug inhibits production of factors II, VII, IX, and X; onset in response is delayed because of degradation of clotting factors that have already been synthesized.

3. Observe for "purple toes" syndrome related to inhibition of protein C and S.

**Client/Family Teaching**

1. Take oral warfarin as prescribed and at the same time each day.

2. This drug does not dissolve clots but decreases the clotting ability of the blood and helps to prevent the formation of harmful blood clots in the blood vessels and heart valves.

3. Avoid activities and contact sports that may cause injury or cuts and bruises. Use a soft toothbrush, electric razor to shave, wear shoes and use a night light to avoid falls at night.

4. Report immediately any unusual bruising or bleeding, dark brown or blood-tinged body secretions, injury or trauma, dizziness, abdominal pain or swelling, back pain, severe headaches, and joint swelling and pain.

5. May carry vitamin K for emergency use. (The usual dosage is 5–20 mg, to be used in the event of excessive bleeding.)

6. Avoid foods high in vitamin K: asparagus, broccoli, cabbage, brussels sprouts, spinach, turnips, milk, and cheese.

7. Use reliable birth control measures.

8. Menstruation may be prolonged and flow slightly increased. Report if excessive and unusual.

9. Skin eruptions may develop as an allergic reaction and should be reported.

10. Do not change brands of drug unless approved because response may be altered.

11. Wear identification and alert all providers of anticoagulant therapy.

12. Report as scheduled for labs to evaluate effectiveness of therapy and need for dosage changes.

**Outcomes/Evaluate**

• Prevention of thrombus formation
• PT within desired range (1.5–2 times the control)
• INR within desired range (2.0–3.0 with standard therapy; 2.5–3.5 with high-dose therapy)

---

# Z

# Zafirlukast
(zah-**FIR**-loo-kast)
**Pregnancy Category:** B
Accolate **(Rx)**
**Classification:** Antiasthmatic

**Action/Kinetics:** A selective and competitive antagonist of leukotriene receptors $D_4$ and $E_4$, which are components of slow-reacting substance of anaphylaxis. It is believed that cysteinyl leukotriene occupation of receptors causes asthma, including airway edema, smooth muscle constriction, and altered cellular activity associated with the inflammatory process. Zafirlukast inhibits bronchoconstriction caused by sulfur dioxide and cold air in clients with asthma. It also attenuates the early- and late-phase reaction in asthmatics caused by inhalation of antigens such as grass, cat dander, ragweed, and mixed antigens. Rapidly absorbed after PO use; bioavailabilty may be decreased when taken with food. **Peak plasma levels:** 3 hr. **t½, terminal:** About 10 hr. Over 99% bound to plasma proteins. Extensively metabolized in the liver, with about 90% excreted in the feces and 10% in the urine. Inhibits certain cytochrome P450 isoenzymes.

**Uses:** Prophylaxis and chronic treatment of asthma in adults and children 12 years of age and older.

**Contraindications:** Use to terminate an acute asthma attack, including status asthmaticus. Lactation.

**Special Concerns:** The clearance is reduced in clients 65 years of age and older. Safety and efficacy have not been determined in children less than 12 years of age.

**Side Effects:** *GI:* N&V, diarrhea, abdominal pain, dyspepsia. *CNS:* Headache, dizziness. *Miscellaneous:* Infection, generalized pain, asthenia, accidental injury, myalgia, fever, back pain.

**Laboratory Test Alterations:** ↑ ALT.

**Drug Interactions**
*Aspirin* / ↑ Plasma levels of zafirlukast
*Erythromycin* / ↓ Plasma levels of zafirlukast
*Terfenadine* / ↓ Plasma levels of zafirlukast
*Theophylline* / ↓ Plasma levels of zafirlukast
*Warfarin* / Significant ↑ PT

**Dosage** ————————
• **Tablets**
  *Asthma.*
**Adults and children aged 12 and older:** 20 mg b.i.d.

## NURSING CONSIDERATIONS
**Administration/Storage:** Protect from light and moisture and store at controlled room temperatures of 20°C–25°C (68°F–77°F).

**Assessment**
1. Document indications for therapy, onset, duration, and characteristics of symptoms. List other agents trialed with the outcome.
2. Note cardiopulmonary assessment findings.
3. Monitor labs and pulmonary function studies.

**Client/Family Teaching**
1. Take 1 hr before or 2 hr after meals to prevent loss of bioavailability.
2. Take drug regularly during symptom-free periods. Do not increase or decrease dose without approval.
3. Drug is not appropriate for acute episodes of asthma. Continue all other antiasthma medications as prescribed.
4. Review peak flow meter use and set targets for intervention or additional therapy.
5. Avoid triggers, i.e., dust, chemicals, cigarette smoke, pollutants, pets, and perfumes.
6. Practice reliable birth control; do not breast feed during therapy.

**Outcomes/Evaluate:** Inhibition of bronchoconstriction; improved breathing patterns

# Zalcitabine (Dideoxycytidine, ddC)
(zal-**SIGH**-tah-been)
**Pregnancy Category:** C
Hivid **(Rx)**
**Classification:** Antiviral

See also *Antiviral Drugs,* and *Anti-Infectives.*

**Action/Kinetics:** Converted in cells to the active metabolite, dideoxycytidine 5'-triphosphate (ddCTP), by cellular enzymes. ddCTP serves as an alternative substrate to deoxycytidine triphosphate for HIV-reverse transcriptase, thereby inhibiting the in vitro replication of HIV-1 and inhibiting viral DNA synthesis. The incorporation of ddCTP into the growing DNA chain leads to premature chain termination. ddCTP serves as a competitive inhibitor of the natural substrate for deoxycytidine triphosphate for the active site of the viral reverse transcriptase, which further inhibits viral DNA synthesis. Food reduces the rate of absorption. Does not appear to undergo significant metabolism by the liver. **Elimination t½:** 1–3 hr. Approximately 70% of a PO dose is excreted through the kidneys and 10% in the feces. Prolonged elimination (t½ up to 8.5 hr) is observed in clients with impaired renal function.

**Uses:** In combination with AZT in advanced HIV infections (CD$_4$ cell count of 300/mm³ or less and who have shown significant clinical or immunologic deterioration). Alone for HIV-infected adults with advanced disease who are intolerant to AZT or where the disease has progressed while taking AZT.

**Contraindications:** Hypersensitivity to zalcitabine or any components of the product. Use in clients with moderate or severe peripheral neuropathy or with drugs that have the potential to cause peripheral neuropathy (see *Drug Interactions*). Concomitant use with didanosine. Lactation.

**Special Concerns:** Use with extreme caution in clients with low CD$_4$ cell counts (< 50/mm³). Use with caution in clients with a history of pancreatitis or known risk factors for the development of pancreatitis. Clients with a creatinine clearance less than 55 mL/min may be at a greater risk for toxicity due to decreased clearance. Clients may continue to develop opportunistic infections and other complications of HIV infection. Safety and efficacy have not been determined in HIV-infected children less than 13 years of age.

**Side Effects:** The incidence of certain side effects is dependent on the duration of use and the dose of the drug. *Neurologic:* Peripheral neuropathy (may be severe) characterized by numbness and burning dysesthesia involving the distal extremities; this may be followed by sharp shooting pains or severe continuous burning pain if the drug is not withdrawn. The neuropathy may progress to severe pain requiring narcotic analgesics and may be irreversible. *GI:* **Fatal pancreatitis** when given alone or with AZT. Esophageal ulcers, oral ulcers, nausea, dysphagia, anorexia, abdominal pain, vomiting, constipation, ulcerative stomatitis, aphthous stomatitis, diarrhea, dry mouth, dyspepsia, glossitis, **rectal hemorrhage,** hemorrhoids, enlarged abdomen, gum disorders, flatulence, anorexia, tongue ulceration, dysphagia, eructation, gastritis, **GI hemorrhage,** left quadrant pain, salivary gland enlargement, esophageal pain, esophagitis, rectal ulcers, melena, painful swallowing, mouth lesion, acute pharyngitis, abdominal bloating or cramps, anal/rectal pain, colitis, dental abscess, epigastric pain, gagging with pills, gingivitis, heartburn, **hemorrhagic pancreatitis,** increased salivation, odynophagia, painful sore gums, rectal mass, sore tongue, sore throat, tongue disorder, toothache, unformed/loose stools. *Dermatologic:* Rash (including erythematous, maculopapular, follicular), pruritus, night sweats, dermatitis, skin lesions, acne, alopecia, bullous eruptions, increased sweating, urticaria, hot flashes, lip blister or lesions, carbuncle/furuncle, cellulitis, dry skin, dry rash desquamation, exfoliative dermatitis, finger inflammation, impetigo, infection, itchy rash, moniliasis, mucocutaneous/skin disorder, nail disorder, photosensitivity, skin fissure, skin ulcer. *CNS:* Headache, dizziness, seizures, ataxia, abnormal coordination, Bell's palsy, dysphonia, hyperkinesia, hypokinesia, migraine, neuralgia, neuritis, stupor, aphasia, decreased neurologic function, disequilibrium, facial nerve palsy, focal motor seizures, memory loss, paralysis, speech disorder, **status epilepticus,** tremor, vertigo, hypertonia, hand tremor, twitching, confusion, impaired concentration, insomnia, agitation, depersonalization, hallucinations, emotional lability, nervousness, anxiety, depression, euphoria, manic reaction, dementia, amnesia, somnolence, abnormal thinking, crying, loss of memory, decreased concentration, acute psychotic disorder, acute stress reaction, decreased motivation, decreased sexual desire,

---

mood swings, paranoid states, *suicide attempt*. *Respiratory:* Coughing, dyspnea, respiratory distress, rales/rhonchi, nasal discharge, flu-like symptoms, cyanosis, acute nasopharyngitis, chest congestion, dry nasal mucosa, hemoptysis, sinus congestion, sinus pain, sinusitis, wheezing. *Musculoskeletal:* Myalgia, arthralgia, arthritis, arthropathy, cold extremities, leg cramps, myositis, joint pain or inflammation, weakness in leg muscle, generalized muscle weakness, back pain, backache, bone aches and pains, bursitis, pain in extremities, joint swelling, muscle disorder, muscle stiffness, muscle cramps, arthrosis, myopathy, neck pain, rib pain, stiff neck. *Hepatic:* Exacerbation of hepatic dysfunction, especially in those with preexisting liver disease or with a history of alcohol abuse. Abnormal hepatic function, hepatitis, jaundice, hepatocellular damage, hepatomegaly with steatosis, cholecystitis. *CV:* **Cardiomyopathy,** CHF, abnormal cardiac movement arrhythmia, atrial fibrillation, **cardiac failure,** cardiac dysrhythmias, heart racing, hypertension, palpitations, **subarachnoid hemorrhage,** syncope, tachycardia, ventricular ectopy, epistaxis. *Hematologic:* Anemia, leukopenia, thrombocytopenia, alteration of absolute neutrophil count, granulocytosis, eosinophilia, neutropenia, hemoglobinemia, neutrophilia, platelet alteration, purpura, thrombus, unspecified hematologic toxicity, alteration of WBCs. *Hypersensitivity:* Urticaria, **anaphylaxis** (rare). *Endocrine:* Diabetes mellitus, gout, hot flushes, hypoglycemia, hyperglycemia, hypocalcemia, hypophosphatemia, hypernatremia, hyponatremia, hypomagnesemia, hyperkalemia, hypokalemia, hyperlipidemia, polydipsia. *GU:* Dysuria, toxic nephropathy, polyuria, renal calculi, **acute renal failure,** hyperuricemia, increased frequency of micturition, abnormal renal function, renal cyst, albuminuria, bladder pain, genital lesion/ulcer, nocturia, painful/sore penis, penile edema, testicular swelling, urinary retention, vaginal itch/ulcer/pain,

vaginal/cervix disorder. *Ophthalmologic:* Abnormal vision, burning or itching eyes, xerophthalmia, eye pain or abnormality, blurred or decreased vision, eye inflammation/irritation, eye redness/hemorrhage, increased tears, mucopurulent conjunctivitis, photophobia, dry eyes, unequal sized pupils, yellow sclera. *Otic:* Ear pain/blockage, fluid in ears, hearing loss, tinnitus. *Body as a whole:* Fatigue, fever, rigors, chest pain or tightness, weight decrease, pain, malaise, asthenia, generalized edema, general debilitation, chills, difficulty moving, facial pain or swelling, flank pain, flushing, pelvic/groin pain. *Miscellaneous:* Lymphadenopathy, taste perversion, decreased taste, parosmia, lactic acidosis.

**Laboratory Test Alterations:** ↑ ALT, AST, alkaline phosphatase, CPK, amylase, nonprotein nitrogen. Abnormal gamma-glutamyl transferase, GGT, LDH, lactate dehydrogenase, triglycerides, lipase. Bilirubinemia. ↓ Hematocrit.

**Drug Interactions:** The following drugs have the potential to cause peripheral neuropathy and should probably not be used concomitantly with zalcitabine: chloramphenicol, cisplatin, dapsone, disulfiram, ethionamide, glutethimide, gold, hydralazine, iodoquinol, isoniazid, metronidazole, nitrofurantoin, phenytoin, ribavirin, vincristine. Drugs such as amphotericin, foscarnet, and aminoglycosides may increase the risk of peripheral neuropathy by interfering with the renal clearance of zalcitabine, thus increasing plasma levels.
*Antacids (Mg/Al-containing)* / ↓ Absorption of zalcitabine
*Cimetidine* / ↓ Elimination of zalcitabine by ↓ renal tubular secretion
*Pentamidine* / ↑ Risk of fulminant pancreatitis
*Probenecid* / ↓ Elimination of zalcitabine by ↓ renal tubular secretion

**Dosage**
• **Tablets**
*In combination with AZT in advanced HIV infection.*

**Adults:** 0.75 mg given at the same time with 200 mg AZT q 8 hr for a total daily dose of 2.25 mg zalcitabine and 600 mg AZT.

*Alone in advanced HIV infection.* 0.75 mg q 8 hr (2.25 mg/day).

## NURSING CONSIDERATIONS
### Administration/Storage

1. If $C_{CR}$ is 10–40 mL/min, reduce the dose to 0.75 mg/12 hr; if $C_{CR}$ is less than 10 mL/min, reduce the dose to 0.75 mg/24 hr.

2. Reduction of dosage is not required for client weights down to 30 kg.

### Assessment

1. Clients with a history of pancreatitis or elevated serum amylase should be followed closely while on zalcitabine therapy.

2. Baseline serum amylase and triglyceride levels should be performed in clients with a history of pancreatitis, increased amylase, those on parenteral nutrition, or those with a history of drug abuse.

3. Frequent monitoring of hematologic indices is recommended to detect serious anemia or granulocytopenia. In clients manifesting hematologic toxicity, decreases in hemoglobin may occur as early as 2–4 weeks after beginning therapy, whereas granulocytopenia may be seen after 6–8 weeks of therapy.

4. Monitor CBC, $CD_4$ counts/viral loads, liver and renal function studies.

5. Assess for symptoms of peripheral neuropathy: pain, numbness, and tingling. If symptoms evident, the drug may be reintroduced at 50% of the initial dose (i.e., 0.375 mg/8 hr) once all symptoms related to the peripheral neuropathy have improved to mild symptoms. The drug should be permanently discontinued if severe discomfort due to peripheral neuropathy progresses for 1 week or longer.

### Client/Family Teaching

1. Take only as directed on an empty stomach (with concurrently pre-scribed AZT) q 8 hr around the clock.

2. May continue to develop opportunistic infections and other complications of HIV infection; remain under close medical supervision.

3. Use reliable contraceptive and practice safe sex.

4. Drug is not a cure, but helps to alleviate and manage the symptoms of HIV infections.

5. Discontinue and report if symptoms of peripheral neuropathy occur, especially if the symptoms are bilateral and progress for more than 72 hr. Peripheral neuropathy may continue to worsen despite interruption of therapy. If the symptoms improve, then drug may be reintroduced.

6. Schedule retinal exams every 6 mo to assess for retinal depigmentation.

7. Identify local support groups that may assist client/family to understand and cope with this disease.

**Outcomes/Evaluate:** Improved $CD_4$ cell counts, ↓ viral load, ↓ incidence of opportunistic infection, and improved survival rates in clients with advanced HIV infections

# Zidovudine (Azidothymidine, AZT)

(zye-**DOH**-vyou-deen, ah-**zee**-doh-**THIGH**-mih-deen)
**Pregnancy Category:** C
Apo-Zidovudine ✹, Novo-AZT ✹, Retrovir **(Rx)**
**Classification:** Antiviral

See also *Antiviral Drugs* and *Anti-Infectives.*

**Action/Kinetics:** The active form of the drug is AZT triphosphate, which is derived from AZT by cellular enzymes. AZT triphosphate competes with thymidine triphosphate (the natural substrate) for incorporation into growing chains of viral DNA by retroviral reverse transcriptase. Once incorporated, AZT triphosphate causes premature termination of the growth of the DNA chain. Low concentrations of AZT also inhibit the activity of *Shigella, Klebsiella, Salmonella, Enterobacter, Escherichia coli,* and *Citrobacter,* although resistance develops rapidly. Rapidly absorbed from the GI tract and is distributed to both plasma and CSF. **Peak serum levels:** 0.1–1.5 hr. **t½:** approximately 1 hr. Metabolized rapidly by the liver and excreted through the urine.

**Uses: PO:** Initial treatment of HIV-infected adults who have a CD₄ cell count of 500/mm³ or less. Has been found superior to either didanosine or zalcitabine monotherapy for initial treatment of HIV-infected clients who have not had previous antiretroviral therapy. To prevent HIV transmission from pregnant women to their fetuses. For HIV-infected children over 3 months of age who have HIV-related symptoms or are asymptomatic with abnormal laboratory values indicating significant immunosuppression. In combination with zalcitabine in selected clients with advanced HIV disease (CD₄ cell count of 300 cells/mm³ or less).

**IV:** Selected adults with symptomatic HIV infections who have a history of confirmed *Pneumocystis carinii* pneumonia or an absolute CD₄ (T₄ helper/inducer) lymphocyte count of less than 200 cells/mm³ in the peripheral blood prior to therapy.

**Contraindications:** Allergy to AZT or its components. Lactation.

**Special Concerns:** Use with caution in clients who have a hemoglobin level of less than 9.5 g/dL or a granulocyte count less than 1,000/mm³. AZT is not a cure for HIV; thus, clients may continue to acquire opportunistic infections and other illnesses associated with ARC or HIV. AZT has not been shown to reduce the risk of HIV transmission to others through sexual contact or blood contamination.

**Side Effects: Adults.** *Hematologic:* Anemia (severe), granulocytopenia. *Body as a whole:* Headache, asthenia, fever, diaphoresis, malaise,

body odor, chills, edema of the lip, flu-like syndrome, hyperalgesia, abdominal/chest/back pain, lymphadenopathy. *GI:* Nausea, GI pain, diarrhea, anorexia, vomiting, dyspepsia, constipation, dysphagia, edema of the tongue, eructation, flatulence, bleeding gums, mouth ulcers, *rectal hemorrhage. CNS:* Somnolence, dizziness, paresthesia, insomnia, anxiety, confusion, emotional lability, depression, nervousness, vertigo, loss of mental acuity. *CV:* Vasodilation, syncope, vasculitis (rare). *Musculoskeletal:* Myalgia, myopathy, myositis, arthralgia, tremor, twitch, muscle spasm. *Respiratory:* Dyspnea, cough, epistaxis, rhinitis, pharyngitis, sinusitis, hoarseness. *Dermatologic:* Rash, pruritus, urticaria, acne, pigmentation changes of the skin and nails. *GU:* Dysuria, polyuria, urinary hesitancy or frequency. *Other:* Amblyopia, hearing loss, photophobia, *severe hepatomegaly with steatosis,* lactic acidosis, change in taste perception, hepatitis, pancreatitis, hypersensitivity reactions, including *anaphylaxis,* hyperbilirubinemia (rare), *seizures.*

**Children.** The following side effects have been observed in children, although any of the side effects reported for adults can also occur in children. *Body as a whole:* Granulocytopenia, anemia, fever, headache, phlebitis, bacteremia. *GI:* N&V, abdominal pain, diarrhea, weight loss. *CNS:* Decreased reflexes, nervousness, irritability, insomnia, *seizures. CV:* Abnormalities in ECG, left ventricular dilation, CHF, generalized edema, *cardiomyopathy,* S₃ gallop. *GU:* Hematuria, viral cystitis

**OD** **Overdose Management:** *Symptoms:* N&V. Transient hematologic changes. Headache, dizziness, drowsiness, confusion, lethargy. *Treatment:* Treat symptoms. Hemodialysis will enhance the excretion of the primary metabolite of AZT.

**Drug Interactions**
*Acetaminophen* / ↑ Risk of granulocytopenia

*Adriamycin* / ↑ Risk of cytotoxicity, nephrotoxicity, or hematologic toxicity

*Dapsone* / ↑ Risk of cytotoxicity, nephrotoxicity, or hematologic toxicity

*Flucytosine* / ↑ Risk of cytotoxicity, nephrotoxicity, or hematologic toxicity

*Fluconazole* / ↑ Levels of AZT

*Ganciclovir* / ↑ Risk of hematologic toxicity

*Interferon alfa* / ↑ Risk of hematologic toxicity

*Interferon beta-1b* / ↑ Serum levels of AZT

*Phenytoin* / Levels of phenytoin may ↑ , ↓ , or remain unchanged; also, ↓ excretion of AZT

*Probenecid* / ↓ Biotransformation or renal excretion of AZT → flu-like symptoms, including myalgia, malaise or fever, and maculopapular rash

*Rifampin* / ↓ Levels of AZT

*Trimethoprim* / ↑ Serum levels of AZT

*Vinblastine* / ↑ Risk of cytotoxicity, nephrotoxicity, or hematologic toxicity

*Vincristine* / ↑ Risk of cytotoxicity, nephrotoxicity, or hematologic toxicity

## Dosage

• **Capsules, Syrup**

*Symptomatic HIV infections.*

**Adults:** 100 mg (one 100-mg capsule or 10 mL syrup) q 4 hr around the clock (i.e., total of 600 mg daily).

*Asymptomatic HIV infections.*

**Adults:** 100 mg q 4 hr while awake (500 mg/day); **Pediatric, 3 months–12 years, initial:** 180 mg/ $m^2$ q 6 hr (720 mg/$m^2$/day, not to exceed 200 mg q 6 hr).

*Prevent transmission of HIV from mothers to their fetuses (after week 14 of pregnancy).*

**Maternal dosing:** 100 mg 5 times a day until the start of labor. During labor and delivery, AZT IV at 2 mg/kg over 1 hr followed by continuous IV infusion of 1 mg/kg/hr until clamping

of the umbilical cord. **Infant dosing:** 2 mg/kg PO q 6 hr beginning within 12 hr after birth and continuing through 6 weeks of age. Infants unable to take the drug PO may be given AZT IV at 1.5 mg/kg, infused over 30 min q 6 hr.

*In combination with zalcitabine.* Zidovudine, 200 mg, with zalcitabine, 0.75 mg, q 8 hr.

• **IV**

1–2 mg/kg infused over 1 hr. The IV dose is given q 4 hr around the clock only until PO therapy can be instituted. Dosage adjustment may be necessary due to hematologic toxicity.

## NURSING CONSIDERATIONS

See also *General Nursing Considerations for All Anti-Infectives.*

### Administration/Storage

1. Protect capsules and syrup from light.

**IV** 2. Do not mix with blood products or protein solutions.

3. Remove dose from 20-mL vial and dilute in 5% dextrose injection to a concentration not to exceed 4 mg/mL. Administer calculated dose IV at a constant rate over 1 hr .

4. After dilution, the solution is stable at room temperature for 24 hr and if refrigerated (2°C–8°C, 35.6°F– 46.4°F) for 48 hr. However, to ensure safety from microbial contamination, give within 8 hr if stored at room temperature and 24 hr if refrigerated.

### Assessment

1. Document indications for therapy, onset, other therapies trialed and baseline $CD_4$ counts and viral load.

2. Initially monitor CBC at least q 2 weeks. If anemia or granulocytopenia severe, the dose must be adjusted or discontinued. Epoetin alfa recombinant may be administered with iron to stimulate RBC production. A blood transfusion may also be required.

3. Safety and effectiveness of chronic AZT therapy in adults are not known, especially in clients who

have a less advanced form of disease.

4. When used to prevent maternal-fetal transmission of HIV, AZT should be initiated in pregnant women between 14 and 24 weeks of gestation; also, IV AZT should be given during labor up until the cord is clamped, and newborn infants should receive AZT syrup. Mothers may not breast feed.

**Client/Family Teaching**

1. Take on an empty stomach q 4 hr ATC as ordered; sleep must be interrupted to take medication.

2. Report for all labs, especially CBC, because drug causes anemia, and additional medications or blood transfusions may be necessary.

3. Report early S&S of anemia, such as SOB, weakness, lightheadedness, or palpitations, and increased tiredness.

4. Consume 2–3 L/day fluids to ensure adequate hydration. Maintain a record of weights and I&O.

5. Report any symptoms of superinfections (e.g., furry tongue, mouth lesions, vaginal or rectal itching, thrush).

6. Avoid acetaminophen and any other unprescribed drugs that may exacerbate the toxicity of AZT.

7. Drug is not a cure but helps to alleviate and manage symptoms of HIV infections. May continue to develop opportunistic infections and other complications due to AIDS or ARC.

8. Do not share meds and do not exceed the recommended dose of AZT.

9. The risk of transmission of HIV to others through blood or sexual contact is not reduced in individuals on AZT therapy. Practice safe sex and do not share needles.

10. With pregnancy, AZT therapy should start after the 14-week gestation period to help prevent the transmission from mother to infant. Once delivered, do not nurse infant.

11. Identify local support groups that may assist client/family to understand and cope with this disease.

**Outcomes/Evaluate**

• Control of symptoms of HIV, AIDS, or ARC

• ↑ $CD_4$ counts; ↓ viral load (HIV RNA)

• ↓ Maternal fetal HIV transmission

# Zileuton
(zye-**LOO**-ton)
**Pregnancy Category:** C
Zyflo **(Rx)**
**Classification:** Antiasthmatic, leukotriene receptor inhibitor

**Action/Kinetics:** As a specific inhibitor of 5-lipoxygenase, zileuton inhibits the formation of leukotrienes. Leukotrienes are substances that induce various biological effects including aggregation of neutrophils and monocytes, leukocyte adhesion, increase of neutrophil and eosinophil migration, increased capillary permeability, and contraction of smooth muscle. These effects of leukotrienes contribute to edema, secretion of mucus, inflammation, and bronchoconstriction in asthmatic clients. By inhibiting leukotriene formation, zileuton reduces bronchoconstriction due to cold air challenge in asthmatics. Rapidly absorbed from the GI tract; **peak plasma levels:** 1.7 hr. Metabolized in liver and mainly excreted through the urine. t½: 2.5 hr.

**Uses:** Prophylaxis and chronic treatment of asthma in adults and children over 12 years of age.

**Contraindications:** Active liver disease or transaminase elevations greater than or equal to three times the upper limit of normal. Hypersenstivity to zileuton. Treatment of bronchoconstriction in acute asthma attacks, including status asthmaticus. Lactation.

**Special Concerns:** Use with caution in clients who ingest large quantities of alcohol or who have a past history of liver disease. Safety and efficacy have not been determined in children less than 12 years of age.

**Side Effects:** *GI:* Dyspepsia, nausea, constipation, flatulence, vomiting.

Z

*CNS:* Headache, dizziness, insomnia, malaise, nervousness, somnolence. *Body as a whole:* Unspecified pain, abdominal pain, chest pain, asthenia, accidental injury, fever. *Musculoskeletal:* Myalgia, arthralgia, neck pain/rigidity. *GU:* Urinary tract infection, vaginitis. *Miscellaneous:* Conjunctivitis, hypertonia, lymphadenopathy, pruritus.

**Laboratory Test Alterations:** ↑ Liver enzyme tests. Low WBC count.

**Drug Interactions**
*Propranolol* / ↑ Effect of propranolol
*Terfenadine* / ↑ Effect of terfenadine due to ↓ clearance
*Theophylline* / Doubling of serum theophylline levels → ↑ effect
*Warfarin* / ↑ Prothrombin time

**Dosage** —————————————
• **Tablets**
*Symptomatic treatment of asthma.*
**Adults and children over 12 years of age:** 600 mg q.i.d.

## NURSING CONSIDERATIONS
**Administration/Storage**
1. May be taken with meals and at bedtime.
2. Do not decrease the dose or stop taking any other antiasthmatics when taking zileuton.
**Assessment**
1. Document onset, characteristics, and severity of disease. Note triggers and list currently prescribed medications.
2. Monitor CBC, PFTs, and LFTs.
3. Screen for excessive alcohol use and any evidence of liver disease.
**Client/Family Teaching**
1. Take regularly as directed (may take with meals and at bedtime) and continue other antiasthmatic medications as prescribed.
2. Drug will not reverse bronchospasm during acute asthma attack; use bronchodilators and seek medical attention if symptoms are severe or peak flow readings indicate need.
3. Drug inhibits formation of those

substances that cause bronchoconstrictive symptoms in asthmatics.
4. Use peak flow meter readings to monitor airway effectiveness, to increase medications, and to seek immediate medical attention.
5. Report immediately if experiencing RUQ pain, lethargy pruritus, jaundice, fatigue, or flu-like symptoms (S&S of liver toxicity).
6. Report for CBC, regularly scheduled LFTs and evaluation of pulmonary status. Bring record of peak flow readings.
7. Review triggers (i.e., smoke, cold air, and exercise) that may cause increased hyperresponsiveness which can last up to a week. If more than the usual or maximum number of inhalations of short-acting bronchodilator treatment in a 24-hr period are required, notify the provider.

**Outcomes/Evaluate:** Asthma prophylaxis; improved airway exchange.

# Zolpidem tartrate
(**ZOL**-pih-dem)
**Pregnancy Category:** B
Ambien **(Rx) (C-IV)**
**Classification:** Nonbarbiturate, nonbenzodiazepine sedative-hypnotic

**Action/Kinetics:** May act by subunit modulation of the GABA receptor chloride channel macromolecular complex resulting in sedative, anticonvulsant, anxiolytic, and myorelaxant properties. Although unrelated chemically to the benzodiazepines or barbiturates, it interacts with a GABA-benzodiazepine receptor complex and shares some of the pharmacologic effects of the benzodiazepines. Specifically, it binds the omega-1 receptor preferentially. No evidence of residual next-day effects or rebound insomnia at usual doses; little evidence for memory impairment. Sleep time spent in stage 3 to 4 (deep sleep) was comparable to placebo with only inconsistent, minor changes in REM sleep at recommended doses. Rapidly absorbed

---

from the GI tract. **t½:** About 2.5 hr (increased in geriatric clients and those with impaired hepatic function). Bound significantly (92.5%) to plasma proteins. Food decreases the bioavailability of zolpidem. Metabolized in the liver; inactive metabolites are excreted primarily through the urine.

**Uses:** Short-term treatment of insomnia.

**Contraindications:** Lactation.

**Special Concerns:** Use with caution and at reduced dosage in clients with impaired hepatic function, in compromised respiratory function, in those with impaired renal function, and in clients with S&S of depression. Impaired motor or cognitive performance after repeated use or unusual sensitivity to hypnotic drugs may be noted in geriatric or debilitated clients. Closely observe individuals with a history of dependence on or abuse of drugs or alcohol. Safety and efficacy have not been determined in children less than 18 years of age.

**Side Effects:** *Symptoms of withdrawal:* Although there is no clear evidence of a withdrawal syndrome, the following symptoms were noted with zolpidem following placebo substitution: fatigue, nausea, flushing, lightheadedness, uncontrolled crying, emesis, stomach cramps, panic attack, nervousness, abdominal discomfort.

The most common side effects following use for up to 10 nights included drowsiness, dizziness, and diarrhea. The side effects listed in the following are for an incidence of 1% or greater. *CNS:* Headache, drowsiness, dizziness, lethargy, drugged feeling, lightheadedness, depression, abnormal dreams, amnesia, anxiety, nervousness, sleep disorder, ataxia, confusion, euphoria, insomnia, vertigo. *GI:* Nausea, diarrhea, dyspepsia, abdominal pain, constipation, anorexia, vomiting. *Musculoskeletal:* Myalgia, arthralgia. *Respiratory:* Upper respiratory infection, sinusitis, pharyngitis, rhinitis. *Body as a whole:* Allergy, back pain,

flu-like symptoms, chest pain, fatigue. *Ophthalmologic:* Diplopia, abnormal vision. *Miscellaneous:* Rash, UTI, palpitations, dry mouth, infection.

**Laboratory Test Alterations:** ↑ ALT, AST, BUN. Hyperglycemia, hypercholesterolemia, hyperlipidemia, abnormal hepatic function.

**OD** **Overdose Management:** *Symptoms:* Symptoms ranging from somnolence to light coma. Rarely, CV and respiratory compromise. *Treatment:* Gastric lavage if appropriate. General symptomatic and supportive measures. IV fluids as needed. Flumazenil may be effective in reversing CNS depression. Monitor hypotension and CNS depression and treat appropriately. Sedative drugs should not be used, even if excitation occurs. Zolpidem is not dialyzable.

**Drug Interactions:** Additive CNS depressant effects are possible when combined with alcohol and other drugs with CNS depressant effects.

**Dosage** ——————
• **Tablets**
  *Hypnotic.*
**Adults, individualized, usual:** 10 mg just before bedtime. An initial dose of 5 mg is recommended in clients with hepatic insufficiency.

---

## NURSING CONSIDERATIONS
### Administration/Storage
1. Limit therapy to 7–10 days. Reevaluate if the drug is required for more than 2–3 weeks.
2. Do not prescribe in quantities exceeding a 1-month supply.
3. Do not exceed 10 mg daily.

### Assessment
1. Document indications for therapy, onset, duration, and characteristics of symptoms.
2. Note any respiratory dysfunction (sleep apnea).
3. Note any drug or alcohol dependence; assess for symptoms of depression.
4. Monitor LFTs.
5. Review sleep patterns and lifestyle. Identify underlying cause(s) of

insomnia (i.e., napping during the daytime, lack of exercise, ↑ stress, depression).

**Client/Family Teaching**

1. Take only as directed, on an empty stomach at bedtime.

2. Do not perform any activities that require mental or physical alertness after ingesting medication. Evaluate response the following day to ensure that no residual depressant effects are evident.

3. Avoid alcohol and any unprescribed or OTC drugs.

4. Drug is only for short-term use; keep a log and identify factors that may be contributing to insomnia.

5. Review alternative methods for inducing sleep such as relaxation techniques, daily exercise, soft music, no daytime napping, guided imagery, white noise or special effects simulator.

6. Those with depression are at a higher risk for suicide or intentional overdose. Advise family that these clients warrant closer observation and limited prescriptions and to report any evidence of suicidal thoughts or aggressive behavior.

7. Keep out of reach of children and store in a safe place; drug has a high potential for abuse.

**Outcomes/Evaluate:** Relief of insomnia

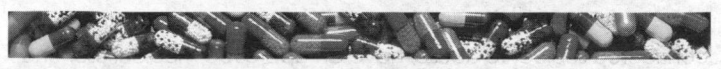

# APPENDIX 1
# Controlled Substances in the United States and Canada

### Controlled Substances Act—United States

The U.S. Federal Controlled Substances Act of 1970 placed drugs controlled by the Act into five categories or schedules based on their potential to cause psychologic and/or physical dependence as well as on their potential for abuse. The schedules are defined as follows:

**Schedule (C-I):** Includes substances for which there is a high abuse potential and no current approved medical use (e.g., heroin, marijuana, LSD, other hallucinogens, certain opiates and opium derivatives).

**Schedule (C-II):** Includes drugs that have a high abuse potential and a high ability to produce physical and/or psychologic dependence and for which there is a current approved or acceptable medical use.

**Schedule (C-III):** Includes drugs for which there is less potential for abuse than drugs in Schedule II and for which there is a current approved medical use. Certain drugs in this category are preparations containing limited quantities of codeine. Also, anabolic steroids are classified in Schedule III.

**Schedule (C-IV):** Includes drugs for which there is a relatively low abuse potential and for which there is a current approved medical use.

**Schedule (C-V):** Drugs in this category consist mainly of preparations containing limited amounts of certain narcotic drugs for use as antitussives and antidiarrheals. Federal law provides that limited quantities of these drugs (e.g., codeine) may be bought without a prescription by an individual at least 18 years of age. The product must be purchased from a pharmacist who must keep appropriate records. However, state laws vary, and in many states such products require a prescription.

### Controlled Substances—Canada

In Canada, narcotics are governed by the Narcotics Control regulations and are designated by the letter N. Drugs that are considered subject to abuse, have an approved medical use, and are not narcotics are designated by the letter C.

Generally prescriptions for Schedule II (high-abuse-potential) drugs cannot be transmitted over the phone and they cannot be refilled. Prescriptions for Schedule III, IV, and V drugs may be refilled up to five times within 6 months. Schedule II drugs are not necessarily "stronger" than drugs in Schedules III, IV, or V; Schedule II drugs are classified as such due to their high abuse potential.

| | Drug Schedule | |
|---|---|---|
| Drug | United States | Canada |
| Alfentanil | II | N |
| Alprazolam | IV | * |
| Amobarbital | II | C |
| Amphetamine | II | Not available |
| Aprobarbital | III | * |
| Benzphetamine | III | Not available |
| Buprenorphine | V | * |
| Butabarbital | III | C |
| Butorphanol | * | C |
| Chloral hydrate | IV | * |
| Chlordiazepoxide | IV | * |
| Clonazepam | IV | * |
| Clorazepate | IV | * |
| Codeine | II | N |
| Dextroamphetamine | II | C |
| Diazepam | IV | * |
| Diethylpropion | IV | C |
| Estazolam | IV | * |
| Ethchlorvynol | IV | * |
| Fenfluramine | IV | * |
| Fentanyl | II | N |
| Fluoxymesterone | III | * |
| Flurazepam | IV | * |
| Glutethimide | III | * |
| Halazepam | IV | Not available |
| Hydrocodone | Not available | N |
| Hydromorphone | II | N |
| Levomethadyl acetate HCl | II | Not available |
| Levorphanol | II | N |
| Lorazepam | IV | * |
| Mazindol | IV | * |
| Meperidine | II | N |
| Mephobarbital | IV | C |
| Meprobamate | IV | * |
| Methadone | II | N |
| Methamphetamine | II | Not available |
| Metharbital | III | C |
| Methylphenidate | II | C |
| Methyltestosteone | III | * |
| Methyprylon | III | * |
| Midazolam | IV | * |
| Morphine | II | N |
| Nalbuphine | * | C |

| | | |
|---|---|---|
| Nandrolone decanote | III | * |
| Nandrolone phenpropionate | III | * |
| Opium | II | N |
| Oxandrolone | III | * |
| Oxazepam | IV | * |
| Oxycodone | II | N |
| Oxymetholone | III | * |
| Oxymorphone | II | N |
| Paraldehyde | IV | * |
| Paregoric | III | N |
| Pemoline | IV | * |
| Pentazocine | IV | N |
| Pentobarbital | | |
|   PO, parenteral | II | C |
|   Rectal | III | C |
| Phendimetrazine | III | Not available |
| Phenmetrazine | II | Not available |
| Phenobarbital | IV | C |
| Phentermine | IV | C |
| Prazepam | IV | Not available |
| Propoxyphene | IV | N |
| Quazepam | IV | Not available |
| Secobarbital | | |
|   PO | II | C |
|   Parenteral | II | * |
|   Rectal | III | * |
| Stanozolol | III | * |
| Sulfentanil | II | N |
| Talbutal | III | * |
| Temazepam | IV | * |
| Testosterone cypionate in oil | III | * |
| Testosterone enanthante in oil | III | * |
| Testosterone in aqueous suspension | III | * |
| Testosterone propionate in oil | III | * |
| Testosterone transdermal system | III | * |
| Triazolam | IV | * |
| Zolpidem tartrate | IV | * |

*Not controlled

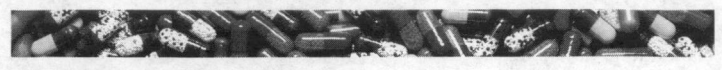

# APPENDIX 2
# Elements of a Prescription

In order to safely communicate the exact elements desired on a prescription, the following items should be addressed:

**A.** The prescriber: Name, address, and phone number and associated practice/speciality

**B.** The client: Name, age, address and social security number

**C.** The prescription itself: Name of the medication (generic or trade); quantity to be dispensed (e.g., tablets or capsules, 1 vial, 1 tube, volume of liquid); the strength of the medication (e.g., 125-mg tablets, 250 mg/5 mL, 80 mg/1 mL, 10%); and directions for use (e.g., 1 tablet po t.i.d.; 2 gtt to each eye q.i.d.; 1 teaspoonful po q 8 hr for 10 days; apply a thin film to lesions b.i.d. for 14 days)

**D.** Other elements: Date prescription is written, signature of the provider, number of refills; provider number: state license number and Drug Enforcement Agency (DEA) number (when applicable); and brand-product-only indication (when applicable)

A typical prescription is depicted as follows:

---

**A.**　　　　**Julia Bryan, MSN, RN, CPNP**
**Pediatric Associates**
**1611 Kirkwood Highway**
**Wilmington, DE 19805**
**302-645-8261**

　　　　　　　　　　　　　　　　**Date: July 10, 1999**

**B.**　**For: Kathryn Woods, Age 8**
　　　**27 East Parkway**
　　　**Lewes, DE 19958**
　　　**123-555-1234**

**C.**　**Rx**　　　**Amoxicillin susp. 250 mg/5 mL**
　　　　　　　**Disp. 150 mL**
　　　　　　　**Sig: 1 teaspoon PO q 8 hr x 10 days**

**D.**　**Refills: 0**

　　　　　　　　　　　　　　　**Provider signature**
　　　　　　　　　　　　**Provider/State license number**

---

*Interpretation of prescription:* The above prescription is written by Pediatric Nurse Practitioner Julia Bryan for Kathryn Woods and is for amoxicillin suspension. The concentration desired is 250 mg/5 mL. The directions for taking the medication are 1 teaspoon (i.e., 5 mL) by mouth every 8 hr for 10 days. The prescriber wants 150 mL dispensed and there are no refills allowed.

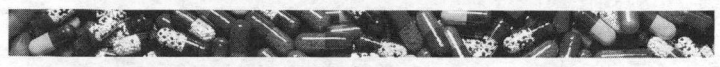

# APPENDIX 3
# Pregnancy Categories: FDA Assigned

The U.S. Food and Drug Administration's use-in-pregnancy rating system weighs the degree to which available information has ruled out risk to the fetus against the drug's potential benefit to the patient. The ratings, and their interpretation, are as follows:

| Category | Interpetation |
| --- | --- |
| A | **CONTROLLED STUDIES SHOW NO RISK.** Adequate, well-controlled studies in pregnant women have failed to demonstrate a risk to the fetus in any trimester of pregnancy. |
| B | **NO EVIDENCE OF RISK IN HUMANS.** Adequate, well-controlled studies in pregnant women have not shown increased risk of fetal abnormalities despite adverse findings in animals, or, in the absence of adequate human studies, animal studies show no fetal risk. The chance of fetal harm is remote, but remains a possibility. |
| C | **RISK CANNOT BE RULED OUT.** Adequate, well-controlled human studies are lacking, and animal studies have shown a risk to the fetus or are lacking as well. There is a chance of fetal harm if the drug is administered during pregnancy; but the potential benefits may outweigh the potential risk. |
| D | **POSITIVE EVIDENCE OF RISK.** Studies in humans, or investigational or post-marketing data, have demonstrated fetal risk. Nevertheless, potential benefits from the use of the drug may outweigh the potential risk. For example, the drug may be acceptable if needed in a life-threatening situation or serious disease for which safer drugs cannot be used or are ineffective. |
| X | **CONTRAINDICATED IN PREGNANCY.** Studies in animals or humans, or investigational or post-marketing reports, have demonstrated positive evidence of fetal abnormalities or risk which clearly outweighs any possible benefit to the patient. |

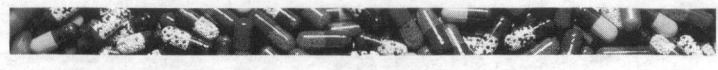

# APPENDIX 4

# Nomogram for Estimating Body Surface Area

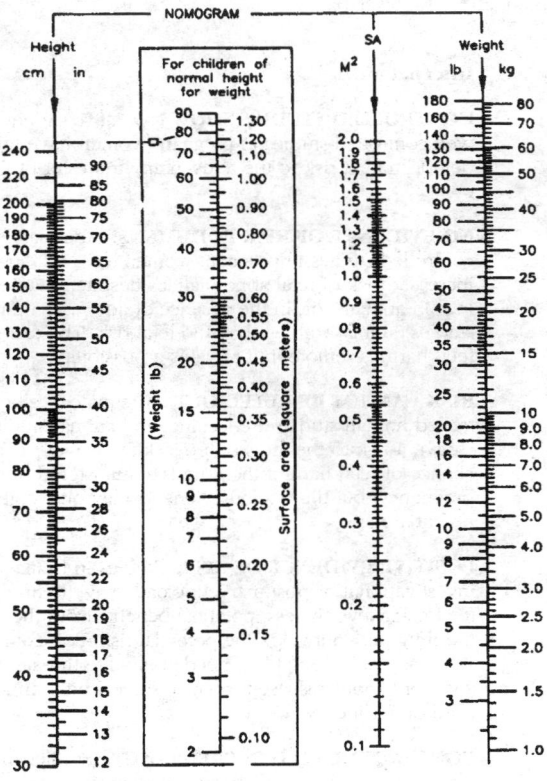

Directions for use: (1) Determine client height. (2) Determine client weight. (3) Draw a straight line to connect the height and weight. Where the line intersects on the surface area line is the derived body surface area (M²).

Reprinted with permission from Behrman, R. E., Kliegman, R., and Arvin, A. M., eds. *Nelson Textbook of Pediatrics,* 15th ed. (Philadelphia: W. B. Saunders Company, 1996).

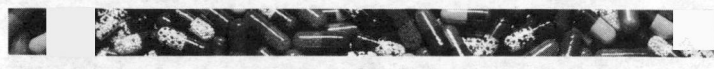

# APPENDIX 5
# Easy Formulas for IV Rate Calculation

In order to calculate the continuous drip rate for an IV infusion, the following information is necessary:

    a. amount of solution to be infused
    b. time for infusion to be administered
    c. *drop factor (found in the tubing package)

$$\frac{\text{Total volume to be infused}}{\text{Total hours for infusion}} \times \frac{\text{*drop factor}}{60 \text{ min/hr}} = \text{gtt/min or cc/hr or mL/hr}$$

    *If drop factor is:    60 gtt/min, then use 1 in the formula
                                 10 gtt/min, then use ⅙ in the formula
                                 15 gtt/min, then use ¼ in the formula
                                 20 gtt/min, then use ⅓ in the formula

*Example:*    Infuse 1,000 cc over 8 hr using tubing with a drop factor of 10 gtt/min.

$$\frac{1,000 \text{ cc}}{8 \text{ hr}} \times \frac{1}{6} = 20.8 \text{ or } 21 \text{ cc/hr}$$

When administering intermittent infusions, as with antibiotic therapy, use the following formula:

$$\text{Total volume to be infused} \div \frac{\text{minutes to administer}}{60 \text{ min/hr}} = \frac{\text{mL}}{\text{hr}}$$

*Example:*    Administer 3 g Zosyn in 100 cc of D5W over 45 min

$$100 \div \frac{45}{60} \text{ (invert to multiply)}$$

or

$$100 \times \frac{60}{45} = 133.3 \text{ or } 134 \ \frac{\text{mL}}{\text{hr}}$$

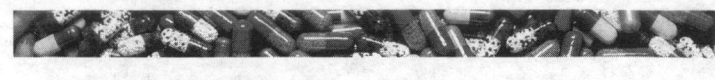

# APPENDIX 6
# Adult IVPB Medication Administration Guidelines and Riders

**Adult IVPB Medication Guidelines**

| Medication | Solutions(s) | Amount | Infuse Over |
|---|---|---|---|
| Amikin (Amikacin) | D5W; NSS | 250–500 mg/ 100 mL | 30–60 min |
| Amphotericin B (Fungizone) | D5W | 50 mg/500 mL | 6 hr |
| Ampicillin (Polycillin-N) | NSS | 1 g/50 mL | 15–30 min |
| Ancef (Cefazolin Na) | D5W; NSS | 1 g/50 mL | 40 min |
| Azactam (Aztreonam) | D5W; NSS | 1 g/50 mL | 20–30 min |
| Bactrim (Septra/ Co-Trimoxazole) | D5W | Premixed, usually 5 mL/125 mL | 60–90 min |
| Cefotan (Cefotetan disodium) | D5W; NSS | 1–2 g/75 mL | 30 min |
| Cipro (Ciprofloxacin) | D5W; NSS | 400 mg/200 mL | 60 min |
| Claforan (Cefotaxime) | D5W; NSS | 1 g/50 mL | 30 min |
| Cleocin (Clindamycin) | D5W; NSS | 300–900 mg/ 100 mL | 20–40 min |
| Decadron (Dexamethasone) | D5W; NSS | 40 mg/50 mL | 15–30 min |
| Doxycycline (Vibramycin) | D5W; NSS | 100 mg/100 mL | 1–2 hr |
| Erythromycin (Erythrocin) | NSS, RL | 500 mg/100 mL | 30–60 min |
| Famotidine (Pepcid) | D5W; NSS | 20 mg/50–100 mL | 15–30 min |
| Flagyl (Metronidazole) | Prepackaged | — | 60 min |
| Foscavir (Foscarnet) | D5W | 60–90 mg/kg q 8 hr | 2 hr |
| Fortaz (Ceftazidime) | D5W; NSS | 1–2 g/100 mL | 30 min |
| Gentamycin (Garamycin) | D5W; NSS | 80 mg/50 mL | 30–60 min |
| Nafcillin (Nafcin) | D5W; NSS | 1 g/50–100 mL | 30–60 min |
| Penicillin G | D5W; NSS | 5,000,000 U/ 100 mL | 40 min |
| Primaxin (Imipenem-Cilastatin Na) | D5W; NSS | 500 mg/100 mL | 20–30 min |
| Rocephin (Ceftri-axone Na) | D5W; NSS | 1–2 g/100 mL | 30 min |
| Solumedrol (Methyl-prednisolone) | D5W; NSS | 10–250 mg/50 mL | 20 min |

| Tagamet (Cimetidine) | D5W; NSS | 300 mg/50 mL | 15–20 min |
| Tetracycline (Achromycin IV) | D5W; NSS | 250–500 mg/100 mL | 60 min |
| Tobramycin (Nebcin) | D5W; NSS | 80 mg/100 mL | 30 min |
| Vancomycin (Vancocin) | D5W; NSS | 1 g/200 mL | 60 min |
| Zantac (Ranitidine HCl) | D5W; NSS | 50 mg/100 mL | 15–20 min |

## Riders

When ordered for nonemergent IV infusion, the following guidelines may be used for administration:

- Calcium gluconate: 1 ampule Ca gluconate in 100 mL D5W given over 1 hr (each ampule contains approximately 940 mg Ca)

- Magnesium sulfate: 1 g in 100 mL D5W given over 1 hr

- Potassium chloride: 40 mEq in 150 mL D5W given over 4 hr or 60 mEq in 250 mL D5W given over 6 hr. With KCl, a good rule of thumb is not to infuse more than 10 mEq/hr.

- Potassium phosphate: 15 mM phosphate (contains 22 mEq K) in 100 mL D5W given over 2–3 hr

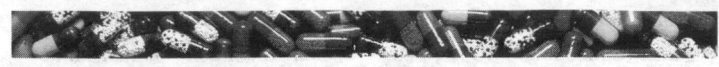

# APPENDIX 7
# Therapeutic Classification of Wounds and Dressings

The nineties have brought a proliferation of products to enhance wound care management. Wounds heal best in a moist environment; thus moisture-retentive or occlusive dressings should be utilized. With a moist wound environment, granulation tissue formation and collagen synthesis are improved, cell migration and epithelial resurfacing occur faster, and crusts, scabs, and eschars do not form. Dressing categories will be listed with some sample product names, indications for therapy, action/kinetics, contraindications, adverse reactions, and evaluation/outcome criteria.

A careful wound assessment should be performed to determine the ulcer stage and any other factors contributing to the skin breakdown, such as infection or necrotic tissues. Wounds are staged by determining which tissue layers are involved:

## WOUND STAGING

**Stage I:** Erythema of intact skin; nonblanchable

**Stage II:** Partial-thickness skin loss involving epidermis and/or dermis; appears as a shallow crater, blister, or abrasion. Includes partial or complete skin tear.

**Stage III:** Full-thickness skin loss of subcutaneous tissue involving damage or necrosis that may extend down to the fascia; appears as a deep crater.

**Stage IV:** Full-thickness skin loss with extensive necrosis, destruction, or damage to muscle, bone, or supporting structures; may also see sinus tracts or undermining with this stage.

Once the wound has been staged, an appropriate dressing choice may be made.

## DRESSING CHOICE
by Wound Stage

**Stage I:** Wounds; management options:

Nonadherent dressing or
Barrier product
Moisture product or

Extra thin hydrocolloid or
Transparent dressing

**Stage II** Wounds with

**A:** Scant or minimal drainage; management options:
Non-adherent gauze or
Transparent dressing or
Hydrogel or
Extra thin or Foam dressing

**B:** Moderate drainage; protect surrounding tissue and consider:
Hydrocolloid or
Continually moist saline soaked dressings or
Foam dressing

**C:** Extensive drainage, consider:
Absorption dressing or
Alginate (especially if drainage is sanguinous) or
Fibergel

**Stage III:** Wounds; protect surrounding tissue; check for undermining
wound margins, as debridement of edges may be necessary

**A.** Scant or minimal drainage, consider:
Hydrogel or
Hydrocolloid paste with wafer or
Continually moist saline soaked dressing or
Foam dressing
**B.** Moderate drainage, consider:
Hydrocolloid paste with wafer or
Continually moist saline soaked packing or
Hypertonic saline gauze or
Fibergel or foam dressing
Alginate if drainage sanguinous
**C.** Excessive drainage, consider:
Absorption packing (hydrophillic) or
Continually moist saline soaked packing with hydrophillic
sponge or
Fibergel or
Alginate (especially if sanguinous drainage)

**Stage IV:** Wounds, evaluate for surgical debridement and repair; with

**A.** Scant or minimal drainage, consider:
Hydrogel-soaked packing
**B.** Moderate drainage, consider:
Hypertonic saline gauze or
Fibergel or
Continually moist saline-soaked dressings
**C.** Excessive drainage, consider adding a:
Hydrophillic topper or packing or
Alginate dressing or
Fibergel

*Dressing Category of*
## WOUND CARE PRODUCTS

I. <u>Nonadherent Dressings</u>—use on stage I and stage IIA with minimal drainage;

> *Nonimpregnated:* Telfa, Release, Metalline, EXU-DRY, ETE-sterile Protective dressing
>
> *Impregnated:* Adaptic, Scarlet Red, Vaseline Gauze, Xeroflo, xeroform

**USE/ACTION:** useful for skin tears, skin grafts, and donor sites; occlusive, nontraumatic, nonadhesive. May require secondary dressing, such as gauze, to wrap area. Use an ATX ointment to keep wound bed moist and to prevent dressing adherence.

II. <u>Transparent Films</u>—use on stage I and stage IIA with minimal drainage

> OpSite, Tegaderm, Transite, Bioclusive, Blister Film, Ensure-It, Omiderm, OpraFlex, Bioclusive, UniFlex, Varilmoist, Polyderm

**USE/ACTION:** adhesive elastomeric copolymer dressing; use with superficial wounds such as superficial burns, abrasions, wounds, donor sites; water resistant, permits easy wound visualization, nonbulky, comfortable, semipermeable, moisture retentive. Useful for autolytic debridement and does not require secondary dressing; minimally absorbent.

III. <u>Hydrocolloids</u>—use extra thin or transparent hydrocolloid on stage I and IIA; all others on Stage II and III wounds

> DuoDERM, Restore, Hydrapad, Intact, IntraSite, 3M Tegasorb, ULTEC

**USE/ACTION:** adhesive wafers containing colloids and elastomers; may see wafer, powder or paste forms; water resistant, nonbulky, comfortable, occlusive or semipermeable, moisture retentive, excellent bacterial barrier, high tack (adhesive), useful for autolytic debridement and does not require secondary dressing.

IV. <u>Gels/Hydrogels</u>—use on stage IIA, IIIA, IVA wounds

> Biolex, Carrington Dermal Wound Gel, Clear Site, Elasto-Gel, Gelicerm Wet/Granulate, Hydron Wound Dressing, IntraSite Gel, Nu-Gel, Second Skin, Spand-Gel, Vigilon.

**USE/ACTION:** single-polymer formulations; adhesive or nonadhesive; sheet or gel form; moisture retentive, lowers wound temperature resulting in decreased inflammation and pain, with cooling, soothing effects; autolysis of necrotic tissue; can be useful when infection is present; permits easy wound visualization, may use a transparent film or gauze dressing over gel forms to contain.

V. <u>Exudate Absorbers</u>—use on stage IIB, IIC, and IIIC wounds

> Allevyn Cavity Wound Dressing, Bard Absorption dressing, Debrisan, Envisan Hydragran, Kaltostat, Mesalt hypertonic saline gauze, Sorosan, Algosteril, Aquacel

**USE/ACTION:** only for highly exudating wounds; can absorb several times their weight in exudate; materials such as starch, paste, beads, hypertonic saline gauze; moisture retentive, requires secondary dressing to contain. Nonadhesive, useful for autolytic debridement.

VI. <u>Foams</u>—nonadhesive, nonadhering polymeric dressings

> Mitraflex, EPIGARD, Epi-Lock, LYOfoam, Allevyn

**USE/ACTION:** moisture retentive, comfortable, moderately absorptive, insulates the wound, nonadherent, compressible; very useful on leg ulcers.

VII: <u>Cotton Mesh Gauzes</u>—use cotton mesh gauze with large interstices, such as, Kerlix for debridement; use nonwoven gauze, such as Sof-Kling for secondary dressings, wrapping, or absorption

> For heavy exudating wounds use absorbent toppers: Topper, ABD, Surgipad Combine dressing; or Hypertonic saline gauze (Mesalt) or wound pouches.
>
> Use Montgomery straps to secure dressings or protect wound margins with a skin sealant.

**USE/ACTION:** wet to dry for debridement, packing of tunneling or undermining wounds, moderately absorptive, may be combined with NSS for granulation or antibiotic solutions for infections; dressings tend to be bulky and uncomfortable.

Moisture-Retentive Dressings
**Side Effects:**
> Increased number of bacteria
> Silent infections
> Accumulation of exudates
> Maceration of wound margins
> Hypergranulation

**Contraindications/Precautions:**
> Active cellulitis/vasculitis
> Wound infection
> Some are not appropriate for stage IV full-thickness wounds

**Outcome/Evaluation:**
> Prevent further skin breakdown
> Decreased infection
> Promote healing of wound
> Decreased pain
> Enhancement of wound-healing process

Finally, dressing choice should change as the wound changes during the healing process. A good rule of thumb is to use wet-dry for debridement, and moisture-retentive for granulation, and always have someone experienced/trained in wound assessment and management evaluate your client.

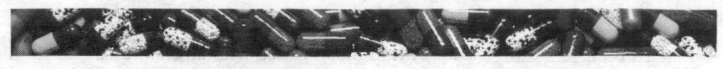

# APPENDIX 8
# Drug Preview

Information of the following drugs was received subsequent to the submission of the manuscript for PDR-99. This appendix contains limited information for these drugs; a more complete profile will be included in next year's edition of this book.

## Becaplermin
(beh-**KAP**-ler-min)
**Pregnancy Category:** C
Regranex **(Rx)**
**Classification:** Topical wound healing drug

**Action/Kinetics:** Topical recombinant human platelet-derived growth factor. Promotes chemotactic recruitment and proliferation of cells involved in wound repair and enhances formation of granulation tissue.

**Uses:** As adjunct to good ulcer care practices to treat lower extremity diabetic neuropathic ulcers that extend into SC tissue or beyond and have adequate blood supply. Use for diabetic neuropathic ulcers that do not extend through dermis into SC tissue or ischemic ulcers has not been studied.

**Contraindications:** Known neoplasms at application site. Use in wounds that close by primary intention.

**Special Concerns:** Effect on exposed joints, tendons, ligaments, and bone has not been established. Use with other topical drugs has not been studied. Use with caution during lactation. Safety and efficacy have not been determined in children less than 16 years of age.

**Side Effects:** *General:* Infection, cellulitis, osteomyelitis, erythematous rashes.

**Dosage** ————————————
• **Gel, 0.01%**
 *Lower extremity diabetic neuropathic ulcers.*

Dose depends on size of ulcer area. To determine length of gel to be applied, measure greatest length of ulcer by greatest width of ulcer in either inches or centimeters. To calculate length of gel in inches:
7.5 g or 15 g tube: length x width x 0.6
2 g tube: length x width x 1.3
Generally, each square inch of ulcer surface will require about ⅔ inch from 7.5 g or 15 g tube and about 1¼ inches from 2 g tube.
To calculate length of gel in centimeters:
7.5 g or 15 g tube: length x width divided by 4
2 g tube: length x width divided by 2
Generally, each square centimeter of ulcer surface will require about 0.25 cm of gel from 7.5 or 15 g tube or about 0.5 cm of gel from 2 g tube. Calculate amount to be applied at weekly or biweekly intervals depending on rate of change in ulcer area.

## NURSING CONSIDERATIONS
### Administration/Storage
1. Squeeze calculated length of gel onto a clean measuring surface (e.g., wax paper). Gel is transferred from clean measuring surface using an application aid and then spread over entire ulcer area. This should yield thin continuous layer of about ¹⁄₁₆ inch thickness.
2. Cover site with saline moistened dressing and leave in place about 12 hr.

3. Remove dressing after 12 hr and rinse ulcer with saline or water to remove residual gel. Cover again with second moist dressing without gel for remainder of day.

4. Apply once daily until complete ulcer healing has occurred.

5. If ulcer does not decrease in size by about 30% after 10 weeks of therapy or complete healing has not occurred in 20 weeks, reassess treatment.

6. Refrigerate gel but do not freeze. Do not use gel after expiration date at bottom of tube.

**Assessment**

1. Document onset, duration, size, and characteristics of area requiring treatment. May record initial wound assessment with photographs.

2. Assess area to ensure it is free from infection, cellulitis, rash, and osteomyelitis.

3. Ensure client is enrolled in active wound management program with ongoing debridement, relief of pressure (e.g., wheel chair, wedge shoe), systemic management of infections, and moist dressings changed bid.

**Client/Family Teaching**

1. Wash hands before application.

2. Apply gel with cotton swab or tongue depressor; do not let tube tip come in contact with wound or skin surfaces and cap tightly.

3. Squeeze calculated length of gel on firm, dry, surface. Spread gel over area requiring treatment and cover with saline moistened gauze dressing.

4. Gently rinse wound after 12 hr with saline or water to remove gel; cover wound with saline moistened dressing.

5. Report any changes in wound that resemble infection, such as purulent drainage, odor, swelling, redness, or increased pain.

**Outcomes/Evaluate:** Healing of diabetic neuropathic foot ulcers.

# Cerivastatin sodium
(seh-**RIHV**-ah-stat-in)
**Pregnancy Category:** X
Baycol **(Rx)**
**Classification:** HMG-CoA reductase inhibitor

See also *HMG-CoA Reductase Inhibitors.*

**Action/Kinetics:** Competitive inhibitor of HMG-CoA reductase leading to inhibition of cholesterol synthesis and decrease in plasma cholesterol levels. **Peak plasma levels:** 2.5 hr. **t½, terminal:** 2–3 hr. Food does not affect blood levels. Metabolized in liver and excreted through urine and feces.

**Uses:** Adjunct to diet to reduce elevated total and LDL cholesterol in clients with primary hypercholesterolemia and mixed dyslipidemia when response to diet or other nonpharmacologic approaches have not been adequate.

**Contraindications:** Use in active liver disease or unexplained elevation of serum transaminases. Pregnancy, lactation.

**Special Concerns:** Use in women of child-bearing age only when pregnancy is unlikely and they have been informed of potential risks. Drug has not been evaluated in rare homozygous familial hypercholesterolemia. Due to interference with cholesterol synthesis and lower cholesterol levels, may be blunting of adrenal or gonadal steroid hormone production. Use with caution in renal or hepatic insufficiency. Safety and efficacy have not been determined in children.

**Side Effects:** See also *HMG-CoA Reductase Inhibitors. Musculoskeletal:* Rarely, rhabdomyolysis with acute renal failure secondary to myoglobinemia.

**Laboratory Test Alterations:** ↑ ALT, AST.

**Drug Interactions:** ↑ Risk of myopathy when used with azole antifungals, cyclosporine, erythromycin, fibric acid derivatives, and lipid-lowering doses of niacin.

## Dosage

- **Tablets**

*Hypercholesterolemia.*

**Adults:** 0.3 mg once daily in evening. Recommended starting dose in those with significant renal impairment ($C_{CR}$ less than 60 mL/min/1.73 m²) is 0.2 mg once daily in evening.

## NURSING CONSIDERATIONS

See also *Nursing Considerations* for *HMG-CoA Reductase Inhibitors.*

### Administration/Storage

1. Place client on standard cholesterol-lowering diet before giving cerivastatin. Diet should continue during therapy.
2. When given with bile-acid-binding resin (e.g., cholestyramine), give cerivastatin at least 2 hr after resin.

### Assessment

1. Document indications for therapy, previous agents/therapies trialed, and outcome.
2. Assess liver and renal function; reduce dose with dysfunction. Monitor LFTs at 6 and 12 weeks initially and with dose increases, then biannually.

### Client/Family Teaching

1. Take as directed. May be taken with or without food.
2. Continue regular exercise and low fat, low cholesterol diet during therapy.
3. Report any unexplained muscle pain, weakness, or tenderness, especially if malaise or fever present.
4. Report for F/U labs as scheduled.

**Outcomes/Evaluate:** ↓ Total and LDL cholesterol

# Daclizumab

(dah-**KLIZ**-you-mab)
**Pregnancy Category:** C
Zenapax **(Rx)**
**Classification:** Immunosuppressive drug

**Action/Kinetics:** Daclizumab is a humanized IgG1 monoclonal antibody produced by recombinant DNA technology. As an antagonist, it binds to the alpha subunit (Tac subunit) of the human high affinity interleukin-2 (IL-2) receptor found on the surface of activated lymphocytes. This results in inhibition of IL-2 mediated activation of lymphocytes, a critical pathway in the cellular immune response involved in allograft rejection. **t½, terminal:** Estimated to be 20 days.

**Uses:** Prophylaxis of acute organ rejection in renal transplants. Used with cyclosporine and corticosteroids.

**Contraindications:** Lactation.

**Special Concerns:** Increased risk for developing lymphoproliferative disorders and opportunistic infections. Use with caution in geriatric clients. Adequate studies have not been performed in children.

**Side Effects:** Incidence of 2% or more is reported. *GI:* Constipation, N&V, abdominal pain, pyrosis, dyspepsia, abdominal distention, epigastric pain, flatulence, gastritis, hemorrhoids. *CNS:* Tremor, headache, dizziness, prickly sensation, depression, anxiety. *CV:* Hypertension, hypotension, aggravated hypertension, tachycardia, thrombosis, bleeding. *Respiratory:* Dyspnea, pulmonary edema, coughing atelectasis, congestion, pharyngitis, rhinitis, hypoxia, rales, abnormal breathing sounds, pleural effusion. *GU:* Oliguria, dysuria, renal tubular necrosis, renal damage, hydronephrosis, urinary tract bleeding, urinary tract disorder, renal insufficiency, urinary retention. *Dermatologic:* Impaired wound healing without infection, acne, pruritus, hirsutism, rash, night sweats, increased sweating. *Musculoskeletal:* Musculoskeletal pain, back pain, arthralgia, leg cramps, myalgia. *Body as a whole:* Post-traumatic pain, chest pain, fever, pain, fatigue, insomnia, lymphocele, shivering, general weakness, injection site reaction, infections. *Metabolic:* Peripheral edema, edema, fluid overload, diabetes mellitus, hyperglycemia. *Miscellaneous:* Blurred vision.

## Dosage

• **IV**

*Prevent kidney transplant rejection.*

1 mg/kg q 14 days for total of five doses. Regimen also includes cyclosporine and corticosteroids.

## NURSING CONSIDERATIONS

### Administration/Storage

**IV** 1. Give the first dose 24 hr or less before transplantation.

2. The calculated volume of daclizumab is mixed with 50 mL of sterile 0.9% NaCl solution. Give via a peripheral or central vein over 15-min period.

3. When mixing, gently invert bag to avoid foaming; do not shake.

4. Product contains no preservatives or bacteriostatic agents. Once infusion is prepared, give within 4 hr. If solution must be held longer, refrigerate between 2°C–8°C (36°F–46°F); discard after 24 hr. Discard any unused portion of solution.

5. Do not add or infuse other drugs simultaneously through same IV line.

### Assessment

1. Document date/time of kidney transplant.

2. Therapy includes cyclosporine and corticosteroids. Initiate therapy within 24 hr pretransplant and subsequent doses every 14 days for total of 5 doses.

3. Monitor VS, I&O, suture line, CBC, lytes, liver and renal function studies.

**Outcomes/Evaluate:** Prophylaxis of acute organ rejection

# Ipratropium bromide and Albuterol sulfate

(eye-prah-**TROH**-pee-um/ al-**BYOU**-ter-ohl)

**Pregnancy Category:** C

Combivent **(Rx)**

**Classification:** Drug for chronic obstructive pulmonary disease

See also *Ipratropium bromide* and *Albuterol sulfate.*

**Content:** Each actuation of metered dose inhaler delivers: *Cholinergic blocking drug:* Iptratropium bromide, 18 mcg; and *Sympathomimetic:* Albuterol sulfate, 103 mcg.

**Uses:** Treatment of chronic obstructive pulmonary disease in those who are on regular aerosol bronchodilator therapy and who require a second bronchodilator.

**Contraindications:** History of hypersensitivity to soya lecithin or related food products, such as soybean and peanuts. Lactation.

**Special Concerns:** Use with caution in CV disorders, especially coronary insufficiency, cardiac arrhythmias, and hypertension. Use with caution in narrow-angle glaucoma, prostatic hypertrophy, bladder-neck obstruction, convulsive disorders, hyperthyroidism, diabetes mellitus, in those unusually responsive to sympathomimetic amines, and renal or hepatic disease. Safety and efficacy have not been determined in children.

**Side Effects:** *Respiratory: **Paradoxical bronchospasm,*** bronchitis, dyspnea, coughing, respiratory disorders, pneumonia, URTI, pharyngitis, sinusitis, rhinitis. *CV:* ECG changes including flattening of T wave, prolongation of QTc interval, and ST segment depression. Also, arrhythmias, palpitation, tachycardia, angina, hypertension. *Hypersensitivity, immediate:* Urticaria, **angioedema, bronchospasm, anaphylaxis, oropharyngeal edema.** *Body as a whole:* Headache, pain, flu, chest pain, edema, fatigue. *GI:* N&V, dry mouth, diarrhea, dyspepsia. *CNS:* Dizziness, nervousness, paresthesia, tremor, dysphonia, insomnia. *Miscellaneous:* Arthralgia, increased sputum, taste perversion, UTI, dysuria.

**Drug Interactions:** See individual drugs.

**Dosage**
- **Inhalation**
  *COPD.*
  2 inhalations q 6 hr not to exceed 12 inhalations/24-hr.

## NURSING CONSIDERATIONS

See also *Nursing Considerations* for *Ipratropium bromide* and *Albuterol sulfate.*

**Administration/Storage**

1. Canister provides sufficient medication for 200 inhalations.
2. Discard canister after labeled number of inhalations have been used.
3. Store between 15°C–30°C (59°F–86°F).
4. Avoid excessive humidity. For best results, canister should be at room temperature before use.
5. Shake canister well before using.
6. Test spray 3 times before first use and again if the canister has not been used for 24 hr.

**Assessment**

1. Assess for any soybean or peanut allergy.
2. Note indications for therapy, characteristics and frequency of symptoms, other agents trialed, and outcome.
3. Assess breath sounds and PFTs.

**Client/Family Teaching**

1. Use as directed; do not increase dose or frequency of administration unless specifically directed.
2. Report any loss of effectiveness.
3. Avoid eye contact; report any visual disturbances or eye irritation.

**Outcomes/Evaluate:** Improved airway exchange

---

# Montelukast sodium
(mon-teh-**LOO**-kast)
**Pregnancy Category:** B
Singulair **(Rx)**
**Classification:** Antiasthmatic

**Action/Kinetics:** Cysteinyl leukotrienes and leukotriene receptor occupation are associated with symptoms of asthma, including airway edema, smooth muscle contraction, and inflammation. Montelukast binds with cysteinyl leukotriene receptors thus preventing the action of cysteinyl leukotrienes. Rapidly absorbed after PO use. **Time to peak levels:** 3–4 hr for 10 mg tablet and 2–2.5 hr for 5 mg tablet. Metabolized in liver and mainly excreted in feces. **t½:** 2.7–5.5 hr.

**Uses:** Prophylaxis and chronic treatment of asthma in adults and children aged 6 years of age and older.

**Contraindications:** Use to reverse bronchospasm in acute asthma attacks, including status asthmaticus. Use to abruptly substitute for inhaled or oral corticosteroids. Use as monotherapy to treat and manage exercise-induced bronchospasm. Use with known aspirin or NSAID sensitivity.

**Special Concerns:** Use with caution during lactation. Safety and efficacy have not been determined for children less than 6 years of age.

**Side Effects:** *Adolescents and adults aged 15 and older. GI:* Dyspepsia, infectious gastroenteritis, abdominal pain, dental pain. *CNS:* Headache, dizziness. *Body as a whole:* Asthenia, fatigue, trauma. *Respiratory:* Influenza, cough, nasal congestion. *Dermatologic:* Rash. *Miscellaneous:* Pyuria.

*Children, aged 6 to 14 years. GI:* Nausea, diarrhea. *Respiratory:* Pharyngitis, laryngitis, otitis, sinusitus. *Miscellaneous:* Viral infection.

**Laboratory Test Alterations:** ↑ ALT, AST.

**Dosage**
- **Tablets**
  *Asthma.*
  **Adolescents and adults age 15 years and older:** 10 mg daily taken in evening.
- **Chewable tablets**
  *Asthma.*
  **Pediatric clients aged 6 to 14 years:** 5 mg chewable tablet daily taken in evening.

## NURSING CONSIDERATIONS

**Administration/Storage:** Drug is to be taken daily as prescribed, even when client is asymptomatic.

Provider is to be contacted if asthma is not well controlled.

**Assessment**

1. Document indications for therapy, onset, triggers, and characteristics of disease. List other agents trialed and outcome.

2. Note other agents prescribed for asthma and reinforce which should be continued.

3. Document pulmonary assessments, PFTs, and xrays when indicated.

4. Chewable 5 mg tablet contains 0.842 mg of phenylalanine and should not be used with phenylketonurics.

5. Assist to identify and eliminate/minimize triggers.

**Client/Family Teaching**

1. Take once daily in evening as directed.

2. Drug should be continued during acute attacks as well as during symptom free periods.

3. Use short-acting prescribed β-agonist inhalers to treat acute asthma attacks. Report if increased use and frequency of inhalers is needed for symptom control.

4. Continue other prescribed antiasthma meds during this therapy.

5. With exercise-induced asthma, must continue to use prescribed inhaler for prophylaxis unless otherwise instructed.

6. Report any unusual side effects, changes in disease, or significant drop in peak flow readings.

7. Notify provider if pregnancy suspected or planned.

8. Ensure that environment is assessed for triggers and that appropriate steps are taken to minimize or avoid exposures.

**Outcomes/Evaluate:** Prophylaxis of asthma attack; asthma control; ↑ FEV$_1$

# Naratriptan hydrochloride

(**NAR**-ah-trip-tan)
**Pregnancy Category:** C

**Amerge (Rx)**
**Classification:** Antimigraine drug

**Action/Kinetics:** Binds to serotonin 5-HT$_{1D}$ and 5-HT$_{1B}$ receptors. Activation of these receptors located on intracranial blood vessels, including those on arteriovenous anastomoses, leads to vasoconstriction and thus relief of migraine. Another possibility is that activation of these receptors on sensory nerve endings in trigeminal system causes inhibition of pro-inflammatory neuropeptide release. Well absorbed from GI tract. **Peak levels:** 2–3 hr. Unchanged drug and metabolites are primarily eliminated in urine. **t½, elimination:** 6 hr.

**Uses:** Acute treatment of migraine attacks in adults with or without aura.

**Contraindications:** Use for prophylaxis of migraine or for management of hemiplegic or basilar migraine. Use in clients with ischemic cardiac, cerebrovascular, or peripheral vascular syndromes; use in uncontrolled hypertension; severe renal impairment (C$_{CR}$ less than 15 mL/min); severe hepatic impairment; within 24 hr of treatment with another 5-HT$_1$ agonist, dihydroergotamine, or methysergide.

**Special Concerns:** Safety and efficacy have not been determined for use in cluster headaches. Use with caution with diseases that may alter the absorption, metabolism, or excretion of drugs, such as impaired renal or hepatic function.

**Side Effects:** Most common side effects follow. *CNS:* Paresthesia, dizziness, drowsiness, malaise, fatigue. *GI:* Nausea. *Miscellaneous:* Throat and neck symptoms, pain and pressure sensation.

Side effects that occurred in 0.1% to 1% of clients follow. *GI:* Hyposalivation, vomiting, dyspeptic symptoms, diarrhea, GI discomfort and pain, gastroenteritis, constipation. *CNS:* Vertigo, tremors, cognitive function disorders, sleep disorders,

disorders of equilibrium, anxiety, depression, detachment. *CV:* Palpitations, increased BP, tachyarrhythmias, syncope, abnormal ECG (PR prolongation, QTc prolongation, ST/T wave abnormalities, premature ventricular contractions, atrial flutter, or atrial fibrillation). *Musculoskeletal:* Muscle pain, arthralgia, articular rheumatism, muscle cramps and spasms, joint and muscle stiffness, tightness, and rigidity. *Dermatologic:* Sweating, skin rashes, pruritus, urticaria. *GU:* Bladder inflammation, polyuria, diuresis. *Body as a whole:* Chills, fever, descriptions of odor or taste, edema and swelling, allergies, allergic reactions, warm/cold temperature sensations, feeling strange, burning/stinging sensation. *Respiratory:* Bronchitis, cough, pneumonia. *Ophthalmic:* Photophobia, blurred vision. *ENT:* Ear, nose, and throat infections; phonophobia, sinusitis, upper respiratory inflammation, tinnitus. *Endocrine/Metabolic:* Thirst, polydipsia, dehydration, fluid retention. *Hematologic:* Increased WBCs.

**OD** **Overdose Management:** *Symptoms:* Increased BP, chest pain. *Treatment:* Standard supportive treatment. Possible use of antihypertensive therapy. Monitor ECG if chest pain presents.

**Drug Interactions**
*Dihydroergotamine* / Additive effects
*Methysergide* / Additive effects
*Selective serotonin reuptake inhibitors* / Possible weakness, hyperreflexia, and incoordination
*Serotonin 5-HT₁ agonists* / Additive effects

**Dosage**
• **Tablets**
  *Migraine headaches.*
**Adults:** Either 1 mg or 2.5 mg taken with fluid. If headache returns or client has had only partial response, dose may be repeated once after 4 hr, for maximum of 5 mg in a 24-hr period.

## NURSING CONSIDERATIONS
**Administration/Storage**
1. Dose of 2.5 mg is usually more effective but causes more side effects. Choice of dose is made on individual basis, weighing possible benefit of 2.5-mg dose with greater risk for side effects.
2. Safety of treating, on average, more than 4 headaches in 30-day period has not been established.
3. Store medication at controlled room temperature away from light.
**Assessment**
1. Document onset, frequency, duration, and characteristics of migraines.
2. List all drugs consumed to ensure none interact.
3. Monitor ECG, liver, and renal function studies; assess for dysfunction.
**Client/Family Teaching**
1. Take exactly as directed to relieve headache. Will not reduce or prevent number of attacks experienced.
2. Review patient information brochure.
3. May repeat once every 4 hr if headache returns or if only partial response attained. Do not exceed 5 mg/24 hr.
4. Report any unusual side effects including chest pain, SOB, or palpitations.
5. Practice reliable contraception.
6. Attempt to identify migraine triggers.
**Outcomes/Evaluate:** Relief of migraine headache

---

# Sibutramine hydrochloride monohydrate
(sih-**BYOU**-trah-meen)
**Pregnancy Category:** C
Meridia **(Rx) (C-IV)**
**Classification:** Anti-obesity drug

---

**Action/Kinetics:** Main effect is likely due to primary and secondary amine metabolites of sibutramine.

Inhibits reuptake of norepinephrine (NE) and serotonin (5HT), resulting in enhanced NE and 5HT activity and reduced food intake. Significant improvement in serum uric acid. Rapidly absorbed from GI tract. Extensive first-pass metabolism in liver. **Peak plasma levels of active metabolites:** 3–4 hr. **t½, sibutramine:** 1.1 hr; **t½, active metabolites:** 14–16 hr. Excreted in urine and feces.

**Uses:** Management of obesity, including weight loss and maintenance of weight loss. Recommended for obese clients with initial body mass index of 30 kg/m² or more or 27 kg/m² in presence of hypertension, diabetes, or dyslipidemia. Use in conjunction with reduced calorie diet. Safety and efficacy have not been determined for more than 1 year.

**Contraindications:** Lactation. Use in clients receiving MAO inhibitors, who have anorexia nervosa, those taking centrally-acting appetite suppressant drugs, those with history of coronary artery disease, CHF, arrhythmias, or stroke. Use in severe renal impairment or hepatic dysfunction. Use with serotonergic drugs, such as fluoxetine, fluvoxamine, paroxetine, sertraline, venlafaxine, sumatriptan, and dihydroergotamine; also, use with dextromethorphan, meperidine, pentazocine, fentanyl, lithium, or tryptophan.

**Special Concerns:** Use with caution in geriatric clients. Safety and efficacy have not been determined in children less than 16 years of age. Use with caution in narrow angle glaucoma, history of seizures, or with drugs that may raise BP (e.g., phenylpropanolamine, ephedrine, pseudoephedrine). Exclude organic causes (e.g., untreated hypothyroidism) before use.

**Side Effects:** *Body as a whole:* Headache, back pain, flu syndrome, injury/accident, asthenia, chest pain, neck pain, allergic reaction. *GI:* Dry mouth, anorexia, abdominal pain, constipation, N&V, rectal disorder, increased appetite, dyspepsia, gastritis. *CNS:* Insomnia, dizziness, paresthesia, nervousness, anxiety, depression, somnolence, CNS stimulation, emotional lability. *CV:* Increased blood pressure, tachycardia, vasodilation, migraine, palpitation. *Dermatologic:* Sweating, rash, herpes simplex, acne. *Musculoskeletal:* Arthralgia, myalgia, tenosynovitis, joint disorder. *Respiratory:* Rhinitis, pharyngitis, sinusitis, increase cough, laryngitis. *GU:* Dysmenorrhea, UTI, vaginal monilia, metrorrhagia. *Otic:* Ear disorder, ear pain. *Miscellaneous:* Thirst, generalized edema, taste perversion.

**Dosage** ─────────────
- **Capsules**
  *Obesity.*
**Adults, initial:** 10 mg once daily (usually in morning) with or without food. If there is adequate weight loss, dose may be titrated after 4 weeks to total of 15 mg once daily. Daily dose should not exceed 15 mg.

## NURSING CONSIDERATIONS
### Administration/Storage
1. May be taken with or without food.
2. Re-evaluate therapy if client has not lost at least 4 pounds in first 4 weeks of treatment.
3. At least 2 weeks should clapse between discontinuation of MAO inhibitor and initiation of sibutramine. Also, at least 2 weeks should elapse between discontinuation of sibutramine and initiation of MAO inhibitor.
4. Store at controlled room temperature. Protect from heat and moisture and dispense in tight, light-resistant container.
### Assessment
1. Document indications for therapy, length of weight problem, other agents/therapies trialed and outcome.

---

2. Assess for anorexia nervosa and MAO use.

3. Obtain weight and calculate BMI.

4. Monitor ECG, VS and labs; assess for increased BP or increased HR.

**Client/Family Teaching**

1. Take only as directed with or without food.

2. Continue regular exercise, weight counselling, and low calorie diet during therapy.

3. Review package insert before starting therapy and review with each refill.

4. Report any signs of allergic reaction including rash or hives.

5. Avoid all OTC agents and report all prescribed meds to prevent interactions.

6. Report as scheduled for F/U visits; record BP and pulse for review.

**Outcomes/Evaluate:** Desired weight loss

---

# Sildenafil citrate

(sill-**DEN**-ah-fill)

**Pregnancy Category:** B

Viagra **(Rx)**

**Classification:** Drug for erectile dysfunction

---

**Action/Kinetics:** Nitric oxide activates the enzyme guanylate cyclase, which causes increased levels of guanosine monophosphate (cGMP) and subsequently smooth muscle relaxation in the corpus cavernosum and allowing inflow of blood. Sildenafil enhances effect of nitric oxide by inhibiting phosphodiesterase type 5 which is responsible for degradation of cGMP in the corpus cavernosum. When sexual stimulation causes local release of nitric oxide, inhibition of phosphodiesterse type 5 by sildenafil causes increased levels of cGMP in the corpus cavernosum and thus smooth muscle relaxation and inflow of blood resulting in an erection. Drug has no effect in absence of sexual stimulation. Rapidly absorbed after PO use. Absorption is decreased when taken with high fat meal. Metabolized in liver where it is converted to active metabolite (N-desmethyl sildenafil). **t½, sildenafil and metabolite:** 4 hr. Excreted mainly in feces (80%) with about 13% excreted in urine. Reduced clearance is seen in geriatric clients.

**Uses:** Treatment of erectile dysfunction.

**Contraindications:** Concomitant use with organic nitrates in any form or with other treatments for erectile dysfunction. Use in newborns, children, or women.

**Special Concerns:** Use with caution in clients with anatomical deformation of penis, in those with predisposition to priapism (e.g., sickle cell anemia, multiple myeloma, leukemia), in bleeding disorders or active peptic ulceration, and in those with genetic disorders of retinal phosphodiesterases.

**Side Effects:** Listed are side effects with incidence of 2% or greater. *CNS:* Headache, dizziness. *GI:* Dyspepsia, diarrhea. *Dermatologic:* Flushing, rash. *Ophthalmic:* Mild and transient predominantly color tinge to vision, increased sensitivity to light, blurred vision. *Respiratory:* Nasal congestion, respiratory tract infection. *Miscellaneous:* UTI, back pain, flu syndrome, arthralgia.

**OD** **Overdose Management:** *Symptoms:* Extension of side effects. *Treatment:* Standard supportive measures.

**Drug Interactions**

*Cimetadine* / ↑ Plasma levels of sildenafil

*Erythromycin* / ↑ Plasma levels of sildenafil

*Itraconazole* / ↑ Plasma levels of sildenafil

*Ketoconazole* / ↑ Plasma levels of sildenafil

*Mibefradil* / ↑ Plasma levels of sildenafil

*Rifampin* / ↓ Plasma levels of sildenafil

---

**Dosage**

• **Tablets**

*Treat erectile dysfunction.*

For most clients, 50 mg no more than once daily, as needed, about 1 hr before sexual activity. May be taken anywhere from 0.5 hr to 4 hr before sexual activity. Depending on tolerance and effectiveness, dose may be increased to maximum of 100 mg or decreased to 25 mg. Starting dose of 25 mg should be considered in those with hepatic or renal impairment or if taken with erythromycin, itraconzole, or ketoconazole.

## NURSING CONSIDERATIONS
### Assessment
1. Note onset and cause of erectile dysfunction, i.e., organic, psychogenic, or combined.
2. Assess cardiovascular status and obtain ECG. Clients using nitrates should not use this drug or should be nitrate free for 24 hr prior to use.
3. List drugs prescribed as some may potentiate drug effects.
4. Assess for any retinal or bleeding disorders or active ulcers.
5. Note any conditions that may predispose client to priapism, i.e., multiple myelomas, sickle cell anemia, or leukemia.
6. Assess for any anatomical deformation of penis (Peyronie's disease, angulation, or cavernosal fibrosis).
### Client/Family Teaching
1. Take only as directed; high fat meal may slow absorption.
2. May experience headache, flushing, upset stomach, stuffy nose, or abnormal vision; report any unusual, persistant or bothersome effects.
3. Do not use any other agent for erections with this therapy.
4. Report all meds currently prescribed to ensure none alter effects.
5. Practice safe sex; drug does not prevent disease transmission.
6. Plan some form of stimulation after ingestion to ensure desired erection obtained.
### Outcomes/Evaluate: Acquisition and maintenance of penile erection

# Tamsulosin hydrochloride
(tam-**SOO**-loh-sin)
**Pregnancy Category:** B

Flomax **(Rx)**
**Classification:** Alpha-1 adrenergic blocking agent

**Action/Kinetics:** Blockade of alpha-1 receptors (probably alpha$_{1A}$) in prostate results in relaxation of smooth muscles in bladder neck and prostate; thus, urine flow rate is improved and there is a decrease in symptoms of BPH. Food interferes with the rate of absorption. **t½, elimination:** 5–7 hr. Significantly bound to plasma proteins. Extensively metabolized in liver; excreted through urine and feces.
**Uses:** Treatment of signs and symptoms of BPH. Rule out prostatic carcinoma before using tamsulosin.
**Contraindications:** Use to treat hypertension, with other alpha-adrenergic blocking agents, or in women or children.
**Special Concerns:** Use with caution with concurrent administration of warfarin.
**Side Effects:** *Body as a whole:* Headache, infection, asthenia, back pain, chest pain. *CV:* Postural hypotension, syncope. *GI:* Diarrhea, nausea, tooth disorder. *CNS:* Dizziness, vertigo, somnolence, insomnia, decreased libido. *Respiratory:* Rhinitis, pharyngitis, increased cough, sinusitis. *GU:* Abnormal ejaculation. *Miscellaneous:* Amblyopia.
**OD** **Overdose Management:** *Symptoms:* Hypotension. *Treatment:* Keep client in supine position to restore BP and normalize HR. If this is inadequate, consider IV fluids. Vasopressors may also be used; monitor renal function.
**Drug Interactions:** Cimetidine causes significant ↓ in clearance of tamsulosin.

### Dosage
• **Capsules**
   *Benign prostatic hypertrophy.*
**Adult males:** 0.4 mg daily given about 30 min after same meal each day. If, after 2 to 4 weeks, clients have not responded, dose can be increased to 0.8 mg daily.

---

## NURSING CONSIDERATIONS
### Administration/Storage
1. If dose is discontinued or interrupted for several days after either 0.4 mg or 0.8 mg dose, start therapy again with 0.4 mg dose.
2. Store at 20°C–25°C (68°F–77°F).
### Assessment
1. Document indications for therapy, onset, and characteristics of symptoms. Note BPH score.
2. List drugs prescribed to ensure none interact; especially cimetidine and coumadin.
3. Note PSA levels and digital rectal exam findings.
### Client/Family Teaching
1. Take as directed, do not chew, crush, or open capsule.
2. Do not perform activities that require mental/physical alertness until drug effects realized; may cause dizziness and syncope.
**Outcomes/Evaluate:** Improvement in BPH symptoms; decreased nocturia

# Trovafloxacin mesylate
(**TROH**-vah-**FLOX**-ah-sin)
**Pregnancy Category:** C
Trovan **(Rx)**

# Alatrofloxacin mesylate injection
(al-**AY**-troh-**flox**-ah-sin)
**Pregnancy Category:** C
Trovan I.V. **(Rx)**
**Classification:** Broad-spectrum antibiotic related to fluoroquinolines

See also *Fluoroquinolines.*
**Action/Kinetics:** After IV use, alatrofloxacin is rapidly converted to trovafloxacin. Trovafloxacin is rapidly absorbed from GI tract. **t½, trovafloxacin:** 10.5–12.2 hr, depending on dose and after multiple doses. **t½, alatrofloxacin:** 11.7–12.7 hr, depending on dose and after multiple doses. About 50% excreted unchanged in urine and feces; remainder is metabolized by liver.

**Uses: IV, PO:** Nosocomial pneumonia caused by *Escherichia coli, Pseudomonas aeruginosa, Haemophilus influenzae,* or *Staphylococcus aureus.* Community acquired pneumonia caused by *Streptococcus pneumoniae, H. influenzae, Klebsiella pneumoniae, S. aureus, Mycoplasma pneumoniae, Moraxella catarrhalis, Legionella pneumophila,* or *Chlamydia pneumoniae.* Acute bacterial exacerbation of chronic bronchitis caused by *H. influenzae, M. catarrhalis, S. pneumoniae, S. aureus,* or *Haemophilus parainfluenzae.* Acute sinusitis caused by *H. influenzae, M. catarrhalis,* or *S. pneumoniae.* Complicated intra-abdominal infections, including post-surgical infections caused by *E. coli, Bacteroides fragilis,* viridans group streptococci, *P. aeruginosa, K. pneumoniae, Peptostreptococcus* species, or *Prevotella* species. Gynecologic or pelvic infections, including endomyometritis, parametritis, septic abortion, and post-partum infections caused by *E. coli, B. fragilis,* viridans group streptococci, *Enterococcus faecalis, Streptococcus agalactiae, Peptostreptococcus* species, *Prevotella* species, or *Gardnerella vaginalis.*

Prophylaxis of infection associated with elective colorectal surgery, vaginal, and abdominal hysterectomy. Uncomplicated skin and skin structure infections due to *S. aureus, S. pyogenes,* or *S. agalactiae.* Complicated skin and skin structure infections, including diabetic foot infections due to *S. aureus, S. agalactiae, P. aeruginosa, E. faecalis, E.coli,* or *Proteus mirabilis.* Uncomplicated urinary tract infections (cystitis) due to *E. coli.* Chronic bacterial prostatitis due to *E. coli, E. faecalis,* or *Staphylococcus epidermidis.* Uncomplicated urethral gonorrhea in males and endocervical and rectal gonorrhea in females due to *Neisseria gonorrhoeae.* Cervicitis due to *Chlamydia trachomatis.* Pelvic inflammatory disease due to *N. gonorrhoeae* or *C. trachomatis.*

**Contraindications:** Use in those with history of hypersensitivity to trovafloxacin, alatrofloxacin, or quinolone antimicrobial agents.

**Special Concerns:** Safety and efficacy in children less than 18 years of age, in pregnant women, and during lactation have not been studied.

**Side Effects:** Side effects listed occur at rate of 1% or greater. *GI:* N&V, diarrhea, abdominal pain. *CNS:* Dizziness, headache, lightheadedness. *Dermatologic:* Pruritus, rash. *Miscellaneous:* Vaginitis, reaction at injection site, eosinophila.

**Laboratory Test Alterations:** ↑ Platelets, ALT, AST, alkaline phosphatase, BUN, creatinine. ↓ Hemoglobin, hematocrit, protein, albumin, sodium, bicarbonate. ↑ or ↓ WBCs.

**Drug Interactions**

*Aluminum hydroxide* / ↓ Plasma levels of trovafloxacin

*Ferrous sulfate* / ↓ Plasma levels of trovafloxacin

*Magnesium hydroxide* / ↓ Plasma levels of trovafloxacin

*Morphine* / ↓ Plasma levels of trovafloxacin

*Omeprazole* / ↓ Plasma levels of trovafloxacin

*Sucralfate* / ↓ Plasma levels of trovafloxacin

**Dosage** —————————
- **IV, Tablets**

  *Nosocomial pneumonia.*

300 mg IV followed by 200 mg PO for 10–14 days. If due to *P. aeruginosa,* combination therapy with either aminoglycoside or aztreonam may be indicated.

  *Community acquired pneumonia.*

200 mg PO or 200 mg IV followed by 200 mg PO for 7–14 days.

  *Acute bacterial exacerbation of chronic bronchitis.*

100 mg PO for 7–10 days.

  *Acute sinusitis.*

200 mg PO for 10 days.

  *Complicated intra-abdominal infections, including post-surgical infections.*

300 mg IV followed by 200 mg PO for 7–14 days.

  *Gynecologic and pelvic infections.*

300 mg IV followed by 200 mg PO for 7–14 days.

  *Surgical prophylaxis for elective colorectal surgery or abdominal or vaginal hysterectomy.*

200 mg as a single IV or PO dose within 30 min to 4 hr before surgery.

  *Skin and skin structure infections, uncomplicated.*

100 mg PO for 7–10 days.

  *Skin and skin structure infections, complicated, including diabetic foot infections.*

200 mg PO or 200 mg IV, followed by 200 mg PO for 10–14 days.

  *UTIs, uncomplicated (cystitis).*

100 mg PO for 3 days.

  *Chronic bacterial prostatitis.*

200 mg PO for 28 days.

  *Uncomplicated urethral gonorrhea in males; endocervical and rectal gonorrhea in females.*

100 mg PO as single dose.

  *Cervicitis due to* C. trachomatis.

200 mg PO for 5 days.

  *Pelvic inflammatory disease, mild to moderate.*

200 mg PO for 14 days.

## NURSING CONSIDERATIONS

See also *Nursing Considerations* for *Fluoroquinolines.*

**Administration/Storage**

1. Doses are given once q 24 hr.

2. Tablets can be given without regard to food.

3. Give PO doses at least 2 hr before or 2 hr after antacids containing magnesium or aluminum, sucralfate, citric acid buffered with sodium citrate, or ferrous sulfate.

4. Give IV morphine at least 2 hr after PO trovafloxacin in fasting state and at least 4 hr after PO trovafloxacin is taken with food.

5. No dosage adjustment is necessary when switching from IV or PO dosing. Switching is at discretion of provider.

6. Reduce dose in mild to moderate cirrhosis. If indicated dose in normal hepatic function is 300 mg IV, give 200 mg IV in chronic hepatic disease. If indicated dose in normal hepatic function is 200 mg IV or PO, give 100 mg IV or PO in chronic hepatic disease. If indicated dose is 100 mg in normal hepatic function, do not decrease dose in chronic hepatic disease.

**IV** 7. Alatrofloxacin mesylate injection is given only by IV infusion. It is not for IM, SC, intrathecal, or intraperitoneal use.

8. Give IV by direct infusion or through Y-type IV infusion set over period of 60 min.

9. Trovan I.V. single use vials, containing 5 mg/mL must be further diluted with appropriate solution before IV administration.

10. Compatible IV solutions include 5% dextrose solution, 0.45% NaCl injection, D5%/0.45% NaCl injection, D5%/0.2% NaCl injection, and lactated Ringer's (RL) and 5% dextrose injection.

11. There is no preservative or bacteriostatic in Trovan I.V. Thus, discard any unused portion.

12. Do not add any additives or other medications to single use vials or through same IV line.

13. If the same IV line is used for sequential infusion of different drugs, flush the line before and after infusion of Trovan I.V. with an infusion solution compatible with Trovan I.V. and any other drugs to be given in same line.

14. Diluted Trovan I.V. concentrations of 0.5 to 2 mg/mL (as trovafloxacin) are stable for up to 7 days when refrigerated or up to 3 days at room temperature if stored in glass bottles or plastic (PVC type) IV containers.

15. Store Trovan I.V. vials, prior to dilution, at 15°C–30°C (59°F–86°F). Protect from light and do not freeze.

**Assessment:** Document indications for therapy noting onset, duration, culture results, and characteristics of symptoms.

**Client/Family Teaching**
1. May take without regard to meal. Avoid antacids, vitamins, or minerals with iron, or sucralfate 2 hr before or 2 hr after dose.
2. May cause dizziness and lightheadedness; avoid activities requiring mental/physical alertness until response evaluated.
3. Stop drug and report any pain, inflammation, rash, or tendon rupture.
4. If skin rash, hives, or other skin reactions occur, or difficulty swallowing or breathing occurs, report immediately; may indicate hypersensitivity reaction.
5. Avoid excessive sunlight or UV exposure; stop drug and report if phototoxicity reaction occurs.
6. Report if symptoms do not improve or worsen after 3-4 days of therapy.

**Outcomes/Evaluate:** Resolution of infection

# Valsartan
(val-**SAR**-tan)
**Pregnancy Category:** C (1st trimester), D (2nd and 3rd trimesters)
Diovan **(Rx)**
**Classification:** Antihypertensive, angiotensin II receptor blocker

**Action/Kinetics:** Angiotensin II receptor blocker specific for $AT_1$ receptors, which are responsible for cardiovascular effects of angiotensin II. Drug blocks vasoconstrictor and aldosterone-secreting effects of angiotensin II. **Peak plasma levels:** 2–4 hr. Highly bound to plasma proteins. Eliminated mostly unchanged in feces (83%) and urine (13%).

**Uses:** Treat hypertension alone or in combination with other antihypertensive drugs.

**Contraindications:** Lactation.

**Special Concerns:** Use with caution in impaired hepatic and renal function. Safety and efficacy have not been determined in children.

**Side Effects:** *CNS:* Headache, dizziness, fatigue, anxiety, insomnia, paresthesia, somnolence. *GI:* Abdominal pain, diarrhea, nausea, constipation, dry mouth, dyspepsia, flatulence. *Respiratory:* URI, cough, rhinitis, sinusitis, pharyngitis, dyspnea. *Body as a whole:* Viral infection, edema, asthenia, allergic reaction. *Musculoskeletal:* Arthralgia, back pain, muscle cramps, myalgia. *Dermatologic:* Pruritus, rash. *Miscellaneous:* Palpitations, vertigo, neutropenia, impotence.

**Laboratory Test Alterations:** ↓ Hemoglobin and hematocrit. ↑ Serum potassium, liver chemistries.

**Dosage** ⎯⎯⎯⎯⎯⎯⎯⎯⎯⎯⎯
• **Capsules**
  *Hypertension.*
**Adults, initial:** 80 mg once daily as monotherapy. **Dose range:** 80–320 mg once daily. If additional antihypertensive effect is needed, dose may be increased to 160 mg or 320 mg once daily or diuretic may be added.

⎯⎯⎯⎯⎯⎯⎯⎯⎯⎯⎯⎯⎯⎯⎯⎯⎯

## NURSING CONSIDERATIONS

**Administration/Storage**
1. May be given with or without food.
2. Antihypertensive effect is usually seen within 2 weeks with maximum reduction after 4 weeks.

**Client/Family Teaching**
1. May take with or without food and with other prescribed antihypertensive agents.
2. Change positions slowly and avoid dehydration to prevent postural effects and dizziness.
3. Practice reliable contraception; report if pregnancy suspected as drug may cause fetal death.
4. Continue low fat, low sodium diet, regular exercise, weight loss, smoking and alcohol cessation, and stress reduction in overall goal of BP control.
5. May experience headaches, coughing, diarrhea, nausea, and joint aches; report if persistent.

**Outcomes/Evaluate:** ↓ BP

⎯⎯⎯⎯⎯⎯⎯⎯⎯⎯⎯⎯⎯⎯⎯⎯⎯

# Zolmitriptan
(zohl-mih-**TRIP**-tin)

**Pregnancy Category:** C
Zomig **(Rx)**
**Classification:** Antimigraine drug
⎯⎯⎯⎯⎯⎯⎯⎯⎯⎯⎯⎯⎯⎯⎯⎯⎯

**Action/Kinetics:** Binds to serotonin 5-HT$_{1B/1D}$ receptors on intracranial blood vessels and in sensory nerves of trigeminal system. This results in cranial vessel constriction and inhibition of pro-inflammatory neuropeptide release. Well absorbed after PO use. **Peak plasma levels:** 2 hr. **t½, elimination:** 3 hr (for zolmitriptan and active metabolite). Excreted in feces and urine.

**Uses:** Treatment of acute migraine in adults with or without aura. Use only when there is clear diagnosis of migraine.

**Contraindications:** Prophylaxis of migraine or management of hemiplegic or basilar migraine. Use in angina pectoris, history of MI, documented or silent ischemia, ischemic heart disease, coronary artery vasospasm (including Prinzmetal's variant angina), other significant underlying CV disease. Also use in uncontrolled hypertension, within 24 hr of treatment with another serotonin HT$_1$ agonist or an ergotamine-containing or ergot-type drug (e.g., dihydroergotamine, methysergide). Concurrent use with MAO A inhibitor or within 2 weeks of discontinuing MAO A inhibitor.

**Special Concerns:** Use with caution in liver disease. Safety and efficacy have not been determined for cluster headache.

**Side Effects:** *GI:* Dry mouth, dyspepsia, dysphagia, nausea, increased appetite, tongue edema, esophagitis, gastroenteritis, abnormal liver function, thirst. *CV:* Palpitations, arrhythmias, hypertension, syncope. *Atypical sensations:* Hypesthesia, paresthesia, warm/cold sensation. *CNS:* Dizziness, somnolence, vertigo, agitation, anxiety, depression, emotional lability, insomnia. *Pain pressure sensations:* Chest pain, tightness, pressure and/or heaviness. Pain, tightness, or heaviness in the neck, throat, or jaw. Heaviness,

⎯⎯⎯⎯⎯⎯⎯⎯⎯⎯⎯⎯⎯⎯⎯⎯⎯

pressure, tightness other than in the chest or neck. *Musculoskeletal:* Myalgia, myasthenia, back pain, leg cramps, tenosynovitis. *Respiratory:* Bronchitis, **bronchospasm,** epistaxis, hiccup, laryngitis, yawn. *Dermatologic:* Sweating, pruritus, rash, urticaria, ecchymosis, photosensitivity. *GU:* Hematuria, cystitis, polyuria, urinary frequency or urgency. *Body as a whole:* Asthenia, allergic reaction, chills, facial edema, edema, fever, malaise. *Miscellaneous:* Dry eye, eye pain, hyperacusis, ear pain, parosmia, tinnitus.

**Drug Interactions**
*Cimetidine* / Half life of zolmitriptan is doubled

**Dosage**
• **Tablets**
  *Migraine headaches.*
**Adults, initial:** 2.5 mg or lower. Dose of 5 mg may be required. If headache returns, repeat dose after 2 hr, not to exceed 10 mg in 24-hr period.

# NURSING CONSIDERATIONS
## Administration/Storage
1. Doses less than 2.5 mg may be obtained by manually breaking 2.5 mg tablet in half.

2. Safety of treating more than 3 headaches in 30 day period has not been established.
**Assessment**
1. Document frequency, duration, and characteristics of migraines. Note neurologist headache evaluation/diagnosis.
2. Note any evidence or history or cardiovascular disease as this precludes therapy.
3. List all drugs prescribed to ensure none interact unfavorably.
4. Determine if pregnant.
5. Monitor VS, ECG, liver, and renal function studies; reduce dose with dysfunction.
**Client/Family Teaching**
1. Take exactly as directed. Do not exceed dosage or dosing intervals of 2 hr apart and total of 10 mg/24 hr. Drug is strictly for migraine headaches.
2. Report if chest pain, SOB, chest tightness, or wheezing persists.
3. Do not perform activities that require mental alertness until drug effects realized.
4. Practice reliable contraception; report if pregnancy suspected.
5. Report any loss of effect, unusual, or adverse side effects.
6. Attempt to identify triggers.
**Outcomes/Evaluate:** Relief of migraine headache

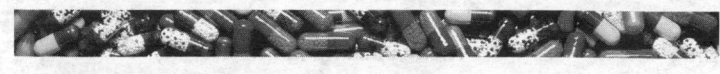

# APPENDIX 9

# Commonly Accepted Therapeutic Drug Levels

| Drug | Peak | Trough |
|------|------|--------|
| Amikacin | 20–30 mcg/mL | 1–5 mcg/mL |
| Gentamicin | 5–10 mcg/mL | 1–2 mcg/mL |
| Netilmicin | 4–10 mcg/mL | 1–2 mcg/mL |
| Streptomycin | 25 mcg/mL | – |
| Tobramycin | 4–10 mcg/mL | 1–2 mcg/mL |
| Vancomycin | 20–50 mcg/mL | 1–5 mcg/mL |

| Drug | Therapeutic Range |
|------|-------------------|
| Amiodarone | 0.5–2.5 mcg/mL |
| Amitriptyline | 50–200 ng/mL |
| Bepridil HCl | 1–2 ng/mL |
| Carbamazepine | 4–10 mcg/mL |
| Desipramine | 50–200 ng/mL |
| Digoxin | 0.5–2.2 ng/mL |
| Disopyramide | 2–8 mcg/mL |
| Doxepin | 50–200 ng/mL |
| Flecainide acetate | 0.2–1.0 mcg/mL |
| Haloperidol | 3–10 ng/mL |
| Heparin | 1.5–3 times normal clotting time |
| Lidocaine | 1.5–5 mcg/mL |
| Lithium | 0.4–1.0 mEq/mL (maintenance) |
| Mezlocillin sodium | 35–45 mcg/mL |
| Mexiletine HCl | 0.5 mcg/mL |
| Milrinone | 150–250 ng/mL |
| Nicardipine | 0.028–0.05 mcg/mL |
| Nifedipine | 0.025–0.1 mcg/mL |
| Phenobarbital | 15–40 mcg/mL (as anticonvulsant) |
| Phenytoin | 10–20 mcg/mL |
| Primidone | 5–12 mcg/mL |
| Procainamide | 4–8 mcg/mL |
| Propafenone | 0.5–3 mcg/mL |
| Propranolol | 50–200 ng/mL |

| Drug | Therapeutic Range |
|------|-------------------|
| Quinidine | 2–6 mcg/mL |
| Salicylic acid | 150–300 mcg/mL (as anti-inflammatory) |
| Theophylline | 10–20 mcg/mL |
| Tocainide HCl | 4–10 mcg/mL |
| Valproic acid | 50–100 mcg/mL |
| Verapamil | 0.08–0.3 mcg/mL |

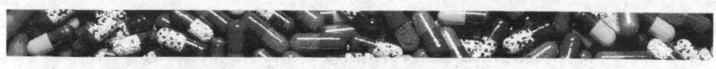

# APPENDIX 10
# Tables of Weights and Measures

| Weights | Exact Equivalents | Approximate Equivalents |
|---|---|---|
| 1 ounce (oz) | 28.35 g | 30 g |
| 1 pound (lb) | 453.6 g | 454 g |
| 1 gram (g) | 0.0353 oz | 0.035 oz |
| 1 kilogram (kg) | 2.205 lb | 2.2 lb |

| Fluid Measures | | |
|---|---|---|
| 1 teaspoon (t) | | 5 mL |
| 1 tablespoon (T) | 3 tsp | 15 mL (½ fl oz) |
| 1 fluid ounce (fl oz) | 29.57 mL | 30 mL |
| 1 pint (16 fl oz) | 473.0 mL | 473 mL |
| 1 quart (32 fl oz) | 946 mL | 945 mL |
| 1 gallon (128 fl oz) | 3.785 L | 3.8 L |
| 1 milliliter (mL) | 0.0352 fl oz (Imperial) | 0.0345 fl oz |
| 1 liter (L) | 2.11 pt | 2 pt |

| Lengths | | |
|---|---|---|
| 1 inch (in) | 2.54 cm | 2.5 cm |
| 1 foot (ft) | 30.48 cm | 30.0 cm |
| 1 yard (yd) | 0.914 m | 0.9 m |
| 1 centimeter (cm) | 0.3937 in | |
| 1 meter (m) | 39.4 in | |

### Approximate Conversions to Metric Measures

| To Convert | To | Multiply By |
|---|---|---|
| Inches | Centimeters | 2.54 |
| Feet | Centimeters | 30.48 |
| Grains | Grams | 0.065 |
| Ounces | Grams | 28.35 |
| Pounds | Kilograms | 0.45 |
| Teaspoons, Medical | Milliliters | 5.0 |
| Tablespoons | Milliliters | 15.0 |
| Fluid ounces | Milliliters | 29.57 |
| Cups | Liters | 0.24 |
| Pints | Liters | 0.47 |
| Quarts | Liters | 0.95 |
| Gallons | Liters | 3.8 |

## Approximate Conversions to Metric Measures

| To Convert | To | Multiply By |
|---|---|---|
| Millimeters | Inches | 0.039 |
| Centimeters | Inches | 0.39 |
| Grams | Grains | 15.432 |
| Kilograms | Pounds | 2.2 |
| Milliliters | Fluid ounces | 0.034 |
| Liters | Pints | 2.1 |
| Liters | Quarts | 1.06 |
| Liters | Gallons | 0.26 |
| Deg. Fahrenheit | Deg. Celsius | 5/9 (after subtracting 32) |
| Deg. Celsius | Deg. Fahrenheit | 9/5 (then add 32) |

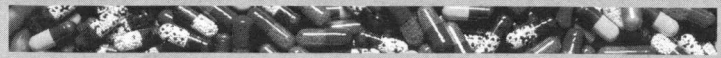

# Index

---

**Boldface** = generic drug name
*italics* = therapeutic drug class

Regular type = trade names
CAPITALS = combination drugs

---

**Boldface** = generic drug name    Regular type = trade names
*italics* = therapeutic drug class    CAPITALS = combination drugs

---

Boldface = generic drug name
*italics* = therapeutic drug class
Regular type = trade names
CAPITALS = combination drugs

---

**Boldface** = generic drug name
*italics* = therapeutic drug class

Regular type = trade names
CAPITALS = combination drugs

Becloforte Inhaler ✹ **(Beclomethasone dipropionate)**, 301

**Beclomethasone dipropionate** (Beclovent, Vanceril), **301**

Beclovent **(Beclomethasone dipropionate)**, 301

Beclovent Rotacaps or Rotahaler ✹ **(Beclomethasone dipropionate)**, 301

Beconase AQ Nasal **(Beclomethasone dipropionate)**, 301

Beconase Inhalation **(Beclomethasone dipropionate)**, 301

Beepen-VK **(Penicillin V potassium)**, 1015

Bell/ans **(Sodium bicarbonate)**, 1165

Benadryl **(Diphenhydramine hydrochloride)**, 529

Benadryl Allergy **(Diphenhydramine hydrochloride)**, 529

Benadryl Allergy Ultratabs **(Diphenhydramine hydrochloride)**, 529

Benadryl Dye-Free Allergy **(Diphenhydramine hydrochloride)**, 529

Benadryl Dye-Free Allergy Liqui Gels **(Diphenhydramine hydrochloride)**, 529

**Benazepril hydrochloride** (Lotensin), **303**

Benefix **(Factor IX Complex (Human))**, 597

Benemid **(Probenecid)**, 1083

Bentyl **(Dicyclomine hydrochloride)**, 511

Bentylol ✹ **(Dicyclomine hydrochloride)**, 511

Benuryl ✹ **(Probenecid)**, 1083

Benylin DM **(Dextromethorphan hydrobromide)**, 501

Benylin DM for Children **(Dextromethorphan hydrobromide)**, 501

Benylin-E ✹ **(Guaifenesin)**, 678

**Benzonatate** (Tessalon Perles), **304**

**Benztropine mesylate** (Cogentin), **305**

**Bepridil hydrochloride** (Vascor), **306**

**Beractant** (Survanta), **308**

Berubigen **(Cyanocobalamin 12)**, 459

*Beta-Adrenergic Blocking Agents*, 92

Betacort ✹ **(Betamethasone valerate)**, 310

Betaderm ✹ **(Betamethasone valerate)**, 310

Betagan ✹ **(Levobunolol hydrochloride)**, 785

Betagan Liquifilm **(Levobunolol hydrochloride)**, 785

Betaloc ✹ **(Metoprolol tartrate)**, 878

Betaloc Durules ✹ **(Metoprolol tartrate)**, 878

**Betamethasone** (Celestone), **310**

**Betamethasone dipropionate** (Diprosone), **310**

**Betamethasone sodium phosphate** (Celestone Phosphate), **310**

**Betamethasone sodium phosphate and Betamethasone acetate** (Celestone Soluspan), **310**

**Betamethasone valerate** (Valisone), **310**

Betapace **(Sotalol hydrochloride)**, 1176

Betapen-VK **(Penicillin V potassium)**, 1015

Betaprolene ✹ **(Betamethasone dipropionate)**, 310

Betaprone ✹ **(Betamethasone dipropionate)**, 310

Betaseron **(Interferon beta-1b)**, 739

Beta-Tim ✹ **(Timolol maleate)**, 1241

Betatrex **(Betamethasone valerate)**, 310

Betaxin ✹ **(Thiamine hydrochloride$_1$)**, 1229

**Betaxolol hydrochloride** (Betoptic, Betoptic S, Kerlone), **311**

Beta-2 **(Isoetharine hydrochloride)**, 748

**Bethanechol chloride** (Urecholine), **312**

Betnesol ✹ **(Betamethasone sodium phosphate)**, 310

Betnovate ✹ **(Betamethasone valerate)**, 310

Betnovate-1/2 ✹ **(Betamethasone valerate)**, 310

Betoptic **(Betaxolol hydrochloride)**, 311

Betoptic S **(Betaxolol hydrochloride)**, 311

Bewon ✹ **(Thiamine hydrochloride$_1$)**, 1229

Biaxin **(Clarithromycin)**, 425

**Bicalutamide** (Casodex), **314**

Bicillin C-R (PENICILLIN G BENZATHINE AND PROCAINE COMBINED), 1011

Bicillin C-R 900/300 (PENICILLIN G BENZATHINE AND PROCAINE COMBINED), 1011

Bicillin L-A **(Penicillin G benzathine, parenteral)**, 1011

Bicillin 1200 L-A ✹ **(Penicillin G benzathine, parenteral)**, 1011

BiCNU **(Carmustine)**, 361

---

**Boldface** = generic drug name
*italics* = therapeutic drug class

Regular type = trade names
CAPITALS = combination drugs

---

**Boldface** = generic drug name
*italics* = therapeutic drug class

Regular type = trade names
CAPITALS = combination drugs

---

**Boldface** = generic drug name
*italics* = therapeutic drug class

Regular type = trade names
CAPITALS = combination drugs

---

**Boldface** = generic drug name
*italics* = therapeutic drug class

Regular type = trade names
CAPITALS = combination drugs

**Boldface** = generic drug name
*italics* = therapeutic drug class

Regular type = trade names
CAPITALS = combination drugs

---

**Boldface** = generic drug name
*italics* = therapeutic drug class

Regular type = trade names
CAPITALS = combination drugs

---

**Boldface** = generic drug name
*italics* = therapeutic drug class

Regular type = trade names
CAPITALS = combination drugs

---

**Boldface** = generic drug name
*italics* = therapeutic drug class
Regular type = trade names
CAPITALS = combination drugs

---

**Boldface** = generic drug name   Regular type = trade names
*italics* = therapeutic drug class   CAPITALS = combination drugs

---

**Boldface** = generic drug name        Regular type = trade names
*italics* = therapeutic drug class        CAPITALS = combination drugs

---

**Boldface** = generic drug name  
*italics* = therapeutic drug class  

Regular type = trade names  
CAPITALS = combination drugs

---

**Boldface** = generic drug name          Regular type = trade names
*italics* = therapeutic drug class          CAPITALS = combination drugs

---

Boldface = generic drug name
*italics* = therapeutic drug class

Regular type = trade names
CAPITALS = combination drugs

---

**Boldface** = generic drug name
*italics* = therapeutic drug class

Regular type = trade names
CAPITALS = combination drugs

---

**Boldface** = generic drug name
*italics* = therapeutic drug class

Regular type = trade names
CAPITALS = combination drugs

---

**Boldface** = generic drug name
*italics* = therapeutic drug class

Regular type = trade names
CAPITALS = combination drugs

---

**Boldface** = generic drug name
*italics* = therapeutic drug class

Regular type = trade names
CAPITALS = combination drugs

---

**Boldface** = generic drug name
*italics* = therapeutic drug class

Regular type = trade names
CAPITALS = combination drugs

---

**Boldface** = generic drug name
*italics* = therapeutic drug class

Regular type = trade names
CAPITALS = combination drugs

---

**Boldface** = generic drug name
*italics* = therapeutic drug class

Regular type = trade names
CAPITALS = combination drugs

---

**Boldface** = generic drug name          Regular type = trade names
*italics* = therapeutic drug class          CAPITALS = combination drugs

---

**Boldface** = generic drug name
*italics* = therapeutic drug class

Regular type = trade names
CAPITALS = combination drugs

Tiazac **(Diltiazem hydrochloride)**, 523

Ticar **(Ticarcillin disodium)**,    1237

**Ticarcillin disodium** (Ticar),    **1237**

TICARCILLIN DISODIUM AND CLAVULANATE POTASSIUM (Timentin),    1238

Ticlid **(Ticlopidine hydrochloride)**, 1239

**Ticlopidine hydrochloride** (Ticlid), **1239**

Ticon **(Trimethobenzamide hydrochloride)**,    1275

Tigan **(Trimethobenzamide hydrochloride)**,    1275

Tilade **(Nedocromil sodium)**,    931

**Tiludronate disodium** (Skelid),    **1240**

Tim-Ak ✿ **(Timolol maleate)**,    1241

Timentin (TICARCILLIN DISODIUM AND CLAVULANATE POTASSIUM),    1238

**Timolol maleate** (Blocadren, Timoptic), **1241**

Timoptic **(Timolol maleate)**,    1241

Timoptic in Acudose **(Timolol maleate)**, 1241

Timoptic-XE **(Timolol maleate)**,    1241

Tinactin **(Tolnaftate)**,    1250

Tinactin for Jock Itch **(Tolnaftate)**, 1250

Ting **(Tolnaftate)**,    1250

**Tioconazole** (Gyno-Trosyd, Trosyd, Vagistat-1),    **1243**

**Tizanidine hydrochloride** (Zanaflex), **1244**

Tobi **(Tobramycin sulfate)**,    1245

**Tobramycin sulfate** (Nebcin),    **1245**

Tobrex Ophthalmic Ointment **(Tobramycin sulfate)**,    1245

Tobrex Ophthalmic Solution **(Tobramycin sulfate)**,    1245

**Tocainide hydrochloride** (Tonocard), **1246**

Toesen ✿ **(Oxytocin, parenteral)**,    986

Tofranil **(Imipramine hydrochloride)**, 717

Tofranil-PM **(Imipramine pamoate)**, 717

**Tolazamide** (Tolinase),    **1248**

**Tolbutamide** (Orinase),    **1248**

**Tolbutamide sodium** (Orinase Diagnostic),    **1248**

Tolectin ✿ **(Tolmetin sodium)**,    1249

Tolectin DS **(Tolmetin sodium)**,    1249

Tolectin 200 **(Tolmetin sodium)**,    1249

Tolectin 600 **(Tolmetin sodium)**,    1249

Tolinase **(Tolazamide)**,    1248

**Tolmetin sodium** (Tolectin),    **1249**

**Tolnaftate** (Tinactin),    **1250**

Tonocard **(Tocainide hydrochloride)**, 1246

Topamax **(Topiramate)**,    1250

Topicycline Topical Solution **(Tetracycline hydrochloride)**, 1225

Topilene ✿ **(Betamethasone dipropionate)**,    310

**Topiramate** (Topamax),    **1250**

Topisone ✿ **(Betamethasone dipropionate)**,    310

**Topotecan hydrochloride** (Hycamtin), **1252**

Toprol XL **(Metoprolol succinate)**, 878

Toradol **(Ketorolac tromethamine)**, 767

Toradol IM **(Ketorolac tromethamine)**, 767

**Toremifene citrate** (Fareston),    **1254**

Tornalate Aerosol **(Bitolterol mesylate)**, 319

**Torsemide** (Demadex),    **1255**

Totacillin **(Ampicillin oral)**,    260

Totacillin-N **(Ampicillin sodium, parenteral)**,    260

Tracrium Injection **(Atracurium besylate)**,    281

**Tramadol hydrochloride** (Ultram), **1256**

Trandate **(Labetalol hydrochloride)**, 769

**Trandolapril** (Mavik),    **1257**

*Tranquilizers/Antimanic Drugs/Hypnotics*,    *178*

Transderm-Nitro 0.1 mg/hr, 0.2 mg/hr, 0.4 mg/hr, and 0.6 mg/hr **(Nitroglycerin transdermal system)**,    959

Transderm-Scop **(Scopolamine transdermal therapeutic system)**, 1158

Transderm-V ✿ **(Scopolamine transdermal therapeutic system)**, 1158

Tranxene-SD **(Clorazepate dipotassium)**,    441

Tranxene-T **(Clorazepate dipotassium)**, 441

**Tranylcypromine sulfate** (Parnate), **1258**

Trasylol **(Aprotinin)**;    271

Travamine **(Dimenhydrinate)**,    525

Travel Tabs ✿ **(Dimenhydrinate)**,    525

Traveltabs ✿ **(Dimenhydrinate)**,    525

**Trazodone hydrochloride** (Desyrel), **1261**

Trazon **(Trazodone hydrochloride)**, 1261

---

**Boldface** = generic drug name
*italics* = therapeutic drug class

Regular type = trade names
CAPITALS = combination drugs

---

**Boldface** = generic drug name
*italics* = therapeutic drug class

Regular type = trade names
CAPITALS = combination drugs

---

**Boldface** = generic drug name      Regular type = trade names
*italics* = therapeutic drug class      CAPITALS = combination drugs

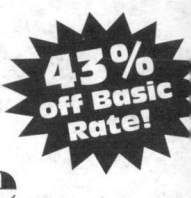
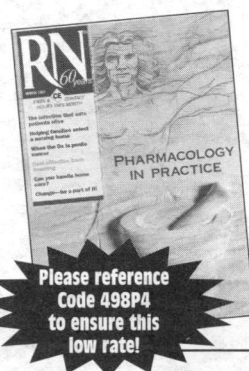

# A GUIDE TO DRUG COMPATIBILITY

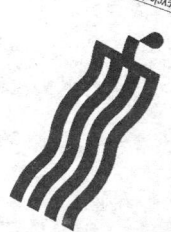

| | Acyclovir Sodium | Amiodarone HCl | Amikacin Sulfate | Aminophylline | Amphotericin B | Ampicillin Sodium | Ampicillin Sodium-Sulbactam Sodium | Amrinone Lactate | Atracurium Besylate | Atropine Sulfate | Aztreonam | Bretylium Tosylate | Calcium Chloride | Calcium Gluconate | Cefazolin Sodium | Cefoperazone Sodium | Cefotaxime Sodium | Cefotetan Disodium | Cefoxitin Sodium | Ceftazidime | Ceftizoxime Sodium | Ceftriaxone Sodium |
|---|---|---|---|---|---|---|---|---|---|---|---|---|---|---|---|---|---|---|---|---|---|---|
| Acyclovir Sodium | | | C | | | C | | | | | I | | | | C | C | C | | C | C | C | C |
| Amiodarone HCl | | | C | I | | | | | | | | C | | | | | | | | | | |
| Amikacin Sulfate | C | C | | | I | I | | | | | C | | C | C | I | | | | | | | |
| Aminophylline | | I | | | | | | C | I | | C | C | | C | | | I | C | | | | I |
| Amphotericin B | | | I | | | | | | | | I | | I | I | | | | | | | | |
| Ampicillin Sodium | C | | I | | | | | | | | | | | | | | | C | | | | |
| Ampicillin Sodium-Sulbactam Sodium | | | | | | | | | | | C | | | | | | | | | | | |
| Amrinone Lactate | | | | C | | | | | | C | | C | C | | | | | | | | | |
| Atracurium Besylate | | | | I | | | | | | | | C | | | | | | | | | | |
| Atropine Sulfate | | | | | | | | C | | | | | | | | | | C | | | | |
| Aztreonam | I | | C | C | I | | C | | | | | | | C | C | C | C | C | | C | C | C |
| Bretylium Tosylate | | C | | C | | | | C | C | | | | C | C | | | | | | | | |
| Calcium Chloride | | | C | | I | | | C | | | | C | | | | | | | | | | |
| Calcium Gluconate | | | C | C | I | | | | | | C | C | | | | | | | | | | |
| Cefazolin Sodium | C | | I | | | | | | | | C | | | | | | | | | | | |
| Cefoperazone Sodium | C | | | | | | | | | | C | | | | | | | | | | | |
| Cefotaxime Sodium | C | | | I | | | | | | | C | | | | | | | | | | | |
| Cefotetan Disodium | | | | C | | C | | | | C | C | | | | | | | | | | | |
| Cefoxitin Sodium | C | | | | | | | | | | | | | | | | | | | | | |
| Ceftazidime | C | | | | | | | | | | C | | | | | | | | | | | |
| Ceftizoxime Sodium | C | | | | | | | | | | C | | | | | | | | | | | |
| Ceftriaxone Sodium | C | | | I | | | | | | | C | | | | | | | | | | | |
| Cefuroxime Sodium | C | | | | | | | | C | | C | | | | | | | | | | | |
| Cimetidine HCl | C | | C | C | I | | | C | C | C | C | | | | | C | | C | C | | | |
| Ciprofloxacin | | | C | I | | | I | | | | C | | | C | | | | | | C | | |
| Clindamycin Phosphate | C | C | C | I | | | | | | | C | | | I | C | C | C | | C | C | C | I |
| Dexamethasone Sodium Phosphate | C | | | C | | | | | | | C | | | | | | | | | | | |
| Digoxin | | | | | | | | C | | | | C | | | | | | C | | | | |
| Diltiazem HCl | | | C | | C | | | | | | C | C | | | C | | C | C | C | C | | C |
| Diphenhydramine HCl | C | | C | C | I | | | | | C | C | | | | | | | | | | | |
| Dobutamine HCl | I | C | | I | | | | C | C | C | C | | | | | | | | | | | |
| Dopamine HCl | I | C | | C | I | I | | C | C | | C | C | C | | | | | C | | | | |
| Droperidol | | | | | | | | | | C | C | | | | | | | | | | | |
| Enalaprilat | | | C | C | I | C | C | | | | C | | | C | C | C | | | | C | C | |
| Epinephrine HCl | | | C | I | | I | | C | C | | | | C | C | | | | C | | | | |
| Erythromycin Lactobionate | C | C | | C | | | | | | | | | | | | | | C | | | | |
| Esmolol HCl | | C | C | C | | C | | | C | | | C | C | | C | C | | | | C | C | |
| Famotidine | | | | C | | C | C | C | | C | C | C | | C | C | C | C | C | C | C | C | |
| Fentanyl Citrate | | | | | | C | | | C | C | | | | C | C | | C | | | | | |
| Filgrastim | C | | C | C | I | C | C | | | | C | | | C | C | I | I | C | I | C | I | I |
| Fluconazole | C | | C | C | | I | C | | | | C | | | I | C | | I | C | C | | | I |
| Foscarnet Sodium | I | | C | C | I | C | | | | | C | | | | C | C | | | C | C | C | C |
| Furosemide | | | C | C | | C | | I | | C | C | | | C | | C | | C | | | | |

| | Cefuroxime Sodium | Cimetidine HCl | Ciprofloxacin | Clindamycin Phosphate | Dexamethasone Sodium Phosphate | Digoxin | Diltiazem HCl | Diphenhydramine HCl | Dobutamine HCl | Dopamine HCl | Droperidol | Enalaprilat | Epinephrine HCl | Erythromycin Lactobionate | Esmolol HCl | Famotidine | Fentanyl Citrate | Filgrastim | Fluconazole | Foscarnet Sodium | Furosemide | Gentamicin Sulfate |
|---|---|---|---|---|---|---|---|---|---|---|---|---|---|---|---|---|---|---|---|---|---|---|
| Acyclovir Sodium | C | C | | C | C | | | C | I | I | | | | C | | | | C | C | I | | C |
| Amiodarone HCl | | | | C | | | | | C | C | | | | C | C | | | | | | | C |
| Amikacin Sulfate | | C | C | C | | | C | C | | | | C | C | | C | | | C | C | C | C | |
| Aminophylline | C | C | I | I | C | | | C | I | C | | C | I | C | C | C | | C | C | C | C | |
| Amphotericin B | | I | | | | | C | I | | I | | I | | | | | | I | | I | | I |
| Ampicillin Sodium | | | | | | | | | | I | | C | I | | C | C | C | C | I | C | C | I |
| Ampicillin Sodium-Sulbactam Sodium | | | I | | | | | | | | | C | | | | C | | C | C | | | |
| Amrinone Lactate | | C | | | | C | | | C | C | | | C | | | C | | | | | I | |
| Atracurium Besylate | C | C | | | | | | | C | C | | | C | | C | | C | | | | | C |
| Atropine Sulfate | | C | | | | | | C | C | | C | | | | | C | C | | | | C | |
| Aztreonam | C | C | C | C | C | | C | C | C | C | C | C | | | | C | | C | C | C | C | C |
| Bretylium Tosylate | | | | | | C | C | | | C | | | | | C | C | | | | | | |
| Calcium Chloride | | | | | | | | | | C | | | C | | C | | | | | | | |
| Calcium Gluconate | | | C | I | | | | | | | | C | C | | | C | C | C | I | | C | |
| Cefazolin Sodium | | | | C | | | C | | | | | C | | | C | C | C | C | C | C | | |
| Cefoperazone Sodium | | C | | C | | | | | | | | C | | | C | C | | I | | C | C | |
| Cefotaxime Sodium | | | | C | | | C | | | | | | | | | C | C | I | I | | | |
| Cefotetan Disodium | | C | | | | C | C | | | C | | | C | C | | C | | C | C | | C | |
| Cefoxitin Sodium | | C | | C | | | C | | | | | | | | | C | | I | C | C | | |
| Ceftazidime | | | C | C | | | C | | | | | C | | | C | C | | C | I | C | | |
| Ceftizoxime Sodium | | | | C | | | | | | | | C | | | C | C | | I | | C | | |
| Ceftriaxone Sodium | | | | I | | | C | | | | | | | | | | | I | I | C | | |
| Cefuroxime Sodium | | | | C | | | C | | | | | | | | | C | C | I | I | C | C | |
| Cimetidine HCl | | | | C | C | C | C | C | | | C | C | C | C | C | | C | C | C | C | C | C |
| Ciprofloxacin | | | | I | I | C | C | C | C | C | | | | | | | | | | | I | C |
| Clindamycin Phosphate | C | C | I | | | | C | | | | | C | | | C | | C | I | | C | | |
| Dexamethasone Sodium Phosphate | | C | I | | | | | | | | | | | | | C | C | C | C | C | C | |
| Digoxin | | C | C | | | | C | | I | | | | | | | C | C | | I | I | C | |
| Diltiazem HCl | C | C | C | C | | C | | | C | C | | | C | C | C | | | | C | | I | C |
| Diphenhydramine HCl | | C | C | | | | | | | | C | | | C | | | C | C | C | I | | |
| Dobutamine HCl | | | C | | | I | C | | | C | | C | C | | | C | C | | C | I | | |
| Dopamine HCl | | | C | | | | C | | C | | | C | | | C | C | C | | C | C | | |
| Droperidol | | C | | | | | | C | | | | | | | | | C | C | C | I | I | |
| Enalaprilat | | C | | C | | | | | C | C | | | | C | C | C | C | C | | | | C |
| Epinephrine HCl | | C | | | | | C | | C | | | | | | | C | | | | | C | |
| Erythromycin Lactobionate | | C | | | | | C | C | | | | C | | | C | C | | | I | C | I | |
| Esmolol HCl | | C | | C | | | C | | | C | | C | | C | | C | C | | | | I | C |
| Famotidine | C | | | | C | C | | | C | C | | C | C | C | C | | | C | C | | C | C |
| Fentanyl Citrate | C | C | | C | C | C | | C | C | C | C | C | | | C | | | | | | C | C |
| Filgrastim | I | C | | I | C | | | C | | | C | C | | | | C | | | C | | I | C |
| Fluconazole | I | C | | | C | I | C | C | C | C | C | | | I | | C | | C | | C | I | C |
| Foscarnet Sodium | C | C | | C | C | I | | I | I | C | I | | | C | | | | | C | | C | C |
| Furosemide | C | C | I | | C | C | I | | | | I | | C | I | I | C | C | I | I | C | | |

| | Heparin Sodium | Hydrocortisone Sodium Succinate | Hydromorphone HCl | Imipenem-Cilastatin Sodium | Isoproterenol HCl | Labetalol HCl | Lidocaine HCl | Magnesium Sulfate | Meperidine HCl | Methylprednisolone Sodium Succinate | Metoclopramide HCl | Metronidazole | Mezlocillin Sodium | Midazolam HCl | Milrinone Lactate | Morphine Sulfate | Nafcillin Sodium | Nitroglycerin | Nitroprusside Sodium | Norepinephrine Bitartrate | Ondansetron HCl | Oxacillin Sodium |
|---|---|---|---|---|---|---|---|---|---|---|---|---|---|---|---|---|---|---|---|---|---|---|
| Acyclovir Sodium | C | C | C | C | | | | C | | C | C | C | | | | | C | | | | I | C |
| Amiodarone HCl | I | | | | C | C | C | | | | | C | I | C | | C | | C | | C | | |
| Amikacin Sulfate | I | C | C | | | C | | C | C | | | C | | C | | C | | | | C | C | |
| Aminophylline | C | C | | | I | C | C | | I | | C | | | | | | | C | | I | I | |
| Amphotericin B | | C | | | | | | I | | | | | | | | | | | | | I | |
| Ampicillin Sodium | C | | | | | C | | C | C | | I | | | I | | C | | | | | I | |
| Ampicillin Sodium-Sulbactam Sodium | C | | | | | | | | C | | | | | | | C | | | | | I | |
| Amrinone Lactate | | C | | | C | | C | | | C | | | | | | | | C | C | C | | |
| Atracurium Besylate | | C | | | C | | C | | | | | | | C | | C | | C | | | | |
| Atropine Sulfate | C | C | C | | | | | | C | | C | | | C | C | C | C | | | | | |
| Aztreonam | C | C | C | C | | | | C | C | C | C | I | C | | | C | I | | | | C | |
| Bretylium Tosylate | | | | | C | | C | | | | | | | | | | | | | | | |
| Calcium Chloride | | C | | | C | | C | | | | | | | | C | C | | | | C | | |
| Calcium Gluconate | C | C | | | | C | C | C | | I | I | | | C | | | | | | C | | |
| Cefazolin Sodium | C | | | | | C | | C | C | | | C | | C | | C | | | | | C | |
| Cefoperazone Sodium | C | | C | | | I | | C | I | | | | | | | C | | | | | I | |
| Cefotaxime Sodium | C | | C | | | | | C | C | | | C | | | | C | | | | | C | |
| Cefotetan Disodium | | | | | | | | | C | | | | C | | | C | | | | | | |
| Cefoxitin Sodium | C | | C | | | | | C | C | | | | | | | C | | | | | C | |
| Ceftazidime | C | | C | | | C | | | C | | | C | | I | | C | | | | | C | |
| Ceftizoxime Sodium | | | C | | | C | | | C | | | C | | | | C | | | | | C | |
| Ceftriaxone Sodium | C | | | | | | | | C | | | C | | | | C | | | | | | |
| Cefuroxime Sodium | | | C | | | | | | C | | | C | | I | | C | | | | | C | |
| Cimetidine HCl | C | | C | | C | C | C | | C | C | | | | C | | C | C | | C | C | C | |
| Ciprofloxacin | I | I | | | | | C | | | I | C | C | I | C | | | | | | | | |
| Clindamycin Phosphate | C | C | C | | | C | | | C | C | C | C | | C | | C | | | | | C | |
| Dexamethasone Sodium Phosphate | C | C | | | | | C | | C | | C | | | I | | C | C | | | | C | |
| Digoxin | C | C | | | | | C | | C | | | | | C | C | C | | | | | | |
| Diltiazem HCl | | | | C | | | C | | C | | C | C | | | | C | I | C | C | C | | C |
| Diphenhydramine HCl | C | C | C | | | | C | | C | | | C | | C | | C | C | | | | C | |
| Dobutamine HCl | | | | | C | C | C | | C | | | | | I | | C | | C | C | C | | |
| Dopamine HCl | C | C | | | | C | C | | C | C | | | | C | | C | | C | C | | | C |
| Droperidol | | C | | | | | | | C | | C | | | C | | C | I | | | | C | |
| Enalaprilat | C | C | | | | C | C | C | | C | | C | | | | C | C | C | C | | | |
| Epinephrine HCl | C | C | | | | | | | | | | | | | C | | | | | | | |
| Erythromycin Lactobionate | | C | C | | | C | C | C | C | | I | | | C | | C | | | | | | |
| Esmolol HCl | C | C | | | | | | C | | | | C | | | | C | C | | | | | |
| Famotidine | C | C | | C | C | C | C | C | C | C | C | | C | C | | C | C | C | C | C | C | C |
| Fentanyl Citrate | C | C | C | | | C | | | C | | C | C | | C | | C | C | C | | | | |
| Filgrastim | I | C | C | C | | | | | C | I | C | I | I | | | C | | | | | C | |
| Fluconazole | C | | | I | | | | | C | | C | C | | C | | C | C | C | | | C | C |
| Foscarnet Sodium | C | C | C | C | | | | | | | C | C | | I | | C | C | | | | | C |
| Furosemide | C | | | | I | I | C | | | | I | | | I | I | I | | C | | | I | |

| | Pancuronium Bromide | Penicillin G Potassium | Phenylephrine HCl | Phenytoin Sodium | Piperacillin Sodium | Piperacillin Sodium-Tazobactam Sodium | Potassium Chloride | Procainamide HCl | Ranitidine HCl | Sargramostim | Sodium Bicarbonate | Tacrolimus | Theophylline | Ticarcillin Disodium | Ticarcillin Disodium-Clavulanate Potassium | Tobramycin Sulfate | Trimethoprim-Sulfamethoxazole | Vancomycin HCl | Vecuronium Bromide | Verapamil HCl | Zidovudine |
|---|---|---|---|---|---|---|---|---|---|---|---|---|---|---|---|---|---|---|---|---|---|
| Acyclovir Sodium | | C | | | C | I | C | | C | I | C | C | C | C | | C | C | C | | | C |
| Amiodarone HCl | | C | C | | | | C | C | | | I | | | | | C | | C | | C | |
| Amikacin Sulfate | | | | I | | | | | C | C | C | | | | | | | C | | C | C |
| Aminophylline | C | I | | | C | C | C | | C | C | C | C | | | | | | | C | | |
| Amphotericin B | | I | | | | I | I | | I | | C | C | | | | | | | | I | C |
| Ampicillin Sodium | | | | | | | C | | | I | | C | C | | | | | | | | |
| Ampicillin Sodium-Sulbactam Sodium | | | | | | | | | | I | | C | C | | | | | | | | |
| Amrinone Lactate | | | C | | | | C | | | | I | | | | | | | | | C | |
| Atracurium Besylate | | | | | | | C | C | | | | | | | | | C | C | | | |
| Atropine Sulfate | | | | | | | C | | C | | C | | | | | | | | | C | |
| Aztreonam | | | | | C | C | C | | C | C | C | | C | C | C | C | C | | | | C |
| Bretylium Tosylate | | | | I | | | C | | C | | C | | | | | | | | | C | |
| Calcium Chloride | | C | | | | | | | | | | | | | | | | | | C | |
| Calcium Gluconate | | C | | | | C | C | | | C | | C | | | | C | | C | | C | |
| Cefazolin Sodium | C | | | | | | | | | C | | C | C | | | | | | C | C | |
| Cefoperazone Sodium | | | | | | | | | | I | | | | | | I | | | | | |
| Cefotaxime Sodium | | | | | | | | | | C | I | | | | | | | | | C | |
| Cefotetan Disodium | | C | | | C | | | | | C | | C | C | C | | | | | | | |
| Cefoxitin Sodium | | | | | | | | | | | C | | | | | | | | | C | |
| Ceftazidime | | | | | | | C | | C | | | C | C | | | | | | | | C |
| Ceftizoxime Sodium | | | | | | | | | | C | | | | | | | | | | | |
| Ceftriaxone Sodium | | | | | | | | | | C | C | C | | | | | | I | | | C |
| Cefuroxime Sodium | C | | | | | | C | | | C | | C | | | | | | | C | | |
| Cimetidine HCl | C | | | | | C | C | | | C | C | C | C | | | | | C | C | C | C |
| Ciprofloxacin | | | | I | C | | C | | C | | | C | | | | C | | | | C | |
| Clindamycin Phosphate | | C | | I | C | C | C | | | C | C | C | C | | | | | | | C | C |
| Dexamethasone Sodium Phosphate | | | | | | C | C | | C | C | C | C | C | | | | | I | | C | C |
| Digoxin | | | | | | | C | | C | | | C | | | | | | | | C | |
| Diltiazem HCl | | C | | I | C | | C | | C | | | | C | C | C | C | C | C | | | |
| Diphenhydramine HCl | | C | | I | | C | C | | C | C | | C | | | | | | | | | |
| Dobutamine HCl | C | | C | I | | I | | C | C | | I | C | C | | | | | | C | | C |
| Dopamine HCl | C | I | | | | C | C | | C | C | I | C | C | | | | | | C | C | C |
| Droperidol | | | | | | I | C | | | C | | | | | | | | | | | |
| Enalaprilat | | C | | I | C | C | C | | C | | | | | | | C | C | C | | | |
| Epinephrine HCl | C | | | | | | C | | C | | I | | | | | | | | C | C | |
| Erythromycin Lactobionate | | C | | | | | C | | C | | C | C | C | | | | | | | C | C |
| Esmolol HCl | C | C | | C | C | | C | I | C | | C | C | | | | C | C | C | C | | |
| Famotidine | | | C | C | C | I | C | C | | C | C | | C | C | C | | | | | C | |
| Fentanyl Citrate | C | | | | | | C | | C | C | C | | C | | | C | | C | C | | |
| Filgrastim | | | | | I | | C | | C | | C | | | C | C | C | C | C | | | C |
| Fluconazole | C | C | | C | C | C | C | | C | C | | C | C | I | C | C | I | C | C | | C |
| Foscarnet Sodium | | C | | C | C | | | | C | | | | | | C | C | | | | | |
| Furosemide | | C | | | | C | C | | C | C | C | C | | | | C | | | | | |

## Drug compatibility chart (row labels)

- Labetalol HCl
- Lidocaine HCl
- Magnesium Sulfate
- Meperidine HCl
- Methylprednisolone Sodium Succinate
- Metoclopramide HCl
- Metronidazole
- Mezlocillin Sodium
- Midazolam HCl
- Milrinone Lactate
- Morphine Sulfate
- Nafcillin Sodium
- Nitroglycerin
- Nitroprusside Sodium
- Norepinephrine Bitartrate
- Ondansetron HCl
- Oxacillin Sodium
- Pancuronium Bromide
- Penicillin G Potassium
- Phenylephrine HCl
- Phenytoin Sodium
- Piperacillin Sodium
- Piperacillin Sodium-Tazobactam Sodium
- Potassium Chloride
- Procainamide HCl
- Ranitidine HCl
- Sargramostim
- Sodium Bicarbonate
- Theophylline
- Ticarcillin Disodium
- Ticarcillin Disodium-Clavulanate Potassium
- Tobramycin Sulfate
- Trimethoprim-Sulfamethoxazole
- Vancomycin HCl
- Vecuronium Bromide
- Verapamil HCl
- Zidovudine

## LEGEND

**i** Incompatible

**c** Compatible

**blank** No information available or conflicting information. The primary literature should be consulted.
*Compatibility should not be assumed.*

## REFERENCES

1. Trissel, LA: Handbook on Injectable Drugs, ninth edition, American Society of Health-System Pharmacists, Bethesda, MD, 1996.
2. King, JC: Guide to Parenteral Admixtures, Pacemarq, Inc., St. Louis, 1996.

## REVIEWERS

1. David DiPersio, Pharm D., Critical Care Pharmacist, Vanderbilt University Medical Center, Nashville, TN
2. Jim Pierce, Pharm D, Clinical Specialist, Trauma Critical Care, University of Tennessee, Knoxville, TN.

*Compatibility may be affected by numerous factors including temperature, drug concentration, other medications present, diluent and contact time.*
This chart is not intended to be an exhaustive review. The clinician is encouraged to compare conditions in their institutions with conditions tested in the literature.
All clinicians involved in the prescribing, compounding and administration of medications have the responsibility of ensuring that medications delivered are compatible.
Abbott Laboratories cannot be responsible for events arising from use of this chart

Abbott Laboratories
Hospital Products Division
Abbott Park, IL 60064

1-800-ABBOTT 3
1-800-222-6883
Abbott HPD Internet Address: http://www.abbotthosp.com

96-4457-20-Feb. 97

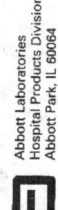

# Incredible

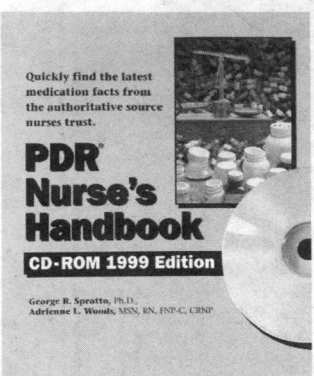

# SEARCHING

# Accuracy
# and
# Precision

## PDR® NURSE'S HANDBOOK
## CD-ROM 1999 EDITION

*George R. Spratto, Ph.D.*
*Adrienne L. Woods, MSN, CRNP, FNP-C*

SYSTEM REQUIREMENTS: *Minimum:* 386 IBM-compatible PC,
4 MB memory, Microsoft Windows 3.1 or higher, 14 MB hard disk space,
CD-ROM drive. *Recommended:* 486 IBM-compatible PC,
8 MB memory, VGA monitor
ISBN: 0-7668-0639-1, List Price: $39.95

Now the information nurses need to know about medications is instantly available.

- Instant access to vital information—the database is searchable by trade and generic name or disorder.
- Customize the information you give to clients—each monograph can be printed in its entirety or just print the patient education portion for each client.
- Free, easy access to 1999 PDR Nurse's Handbook Online Service, where users can get monographs on newly approved drugs over the Internet.

Delmar products are available wherever quality nursing products are sold. For more information contact your book retailer or computer store.

To order Delmar products, call 1-800-347-7707. You can also reach us at www.DelmarNursing.com.

Prices and availability are subject to change.

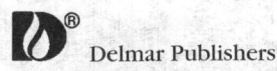

**Delmar Publishers**
*an International Thomson Publishing Company* I(T)P

**Medical Economics Company**